Hypertension

Pathophysiology, Diagnosis, and Management

Volume 2

Hypertension

Pathophysiology, Diagnosis, and Management

Volume 2

Editors

John H. Laragh, M.D.
Director, Cardiovascular Center and
Hypertension Center
Chief, Cardiology Division
Hilda Altschul
Master Professor of Medicine
The New York Hospital–
Cornell Medical Center
New York, New York

Barry M. Brenner, M.D.
Director, Renal Division
Department of Medicine
Brigham and Women's Hospital, and
Director, Harvard Center for the Study of Kidney Disease, and
Samuel A. Levine Professor of Medicine
Harvard Medical School
Boston, Massachusetts

RAVEN PRESS NEW YORK

Raven Press, Ltd., 1185 Avenue of the Americas, New York, New York 10036

Made in the United States of America

Library of Congress Cataloging-in-Publication Data

Hypertension: pathophysiology, diagnosis, and
management.

Includes bibliographies and index.
1. Hypertension. I. Laragh, John H., 1924–
II. Brenner, Barry M., 1937–
RC685.H8H9144 1990 616.1'32 87-45367
ISBN 0-88167-493-1

---

9 8 7 6 5 4 3 2

To my teachers and colleagues who taught me physiology, clinical medicine, and the disciplines of research. In particular my physiology professor, Robert Pitts, a man of penetrating logic, showed me how to design, perform, and analyze an experiment. Harry Goldblatt taught me about experimental hypertension. Homer Smith introduced me to free water clearance and taught me how to tell a good experiment from a bad one. Marcel Goldenberg, who found norepinephrine in adrenal tissue and differentiated its action in humans from that of epinephrine, showed me the excitement of clinical discovery and convinced me anew that cardiology had to involve hormonal signals, chemical transmitters, and cellular mechanisms. This warm, gentle, volatile man died prematurely of malignant hypertension. He asked me to care for him but, sadly, there was little to do. I am especially fortunate to work with my wife, Dr. Jean Sealey, a creative scientist with unique skills that I lack who always gives more than she expects in return.

These scientists, a number of others like them, and my trainees with whom I have worked side by side make every working day a joy. Asking questions and discovering new things to be true has its own rewards.

J.H.L.

To my students and trainees—for they shared heavily in the toil that created and continues to create the richness of new knowledge that has been my lodestar.

B.M.B.

Preface

This textbook is the most ambitious yet attempted in the field of hypertension, which has seen a swiftly accelerating interest and knowledge base over the past 25 years. In these two volumes we have assembled 150 generously referenced and indexed chapters written by over 250 internationally recognized authorities and their colleagues. Even so, inevitably, there will be gaps—nobody can fully contain such a fast moving knowledge base. We have given great thought to the choice of authors and subjects, and we hope that our vertical cut into a growing mass, selective as it must be, will provide a valuable source of information for a respectable number of years.

Our aim is that this work will be a useful reference for clinicians, scientists, and related health care professionals who practice their many disciplines in this large, expanding field. These volumes should also appeal to scientists and health planners from academia, industry, and government.

Hypertension is unique as a biomedical discipline. Unlike the fields of cardiology, nephrology, or neurology, it is not organ-oriented. Neither is it identified with a discrete disease process such as cancer or arthritis. Rather, hypertension is a physical sign common to a large group of pathophysiologic disorders that appear to express basic disturbances in integrative physiology. Whatever the origin of the sign, the whole body becomes involved and the involvement is mediated by, or reflected in, demonstrably abnormal endocrine, paracrine, and neural signals. Sooner or later, the heart, brain, and kidney are involved.

That is why there is something in it for everybody. The field of hypertension brings together basic biomedical scientists and clinicians, epidemiologists, and health planners. It is not surprising that this melting pot of disciplines has spawned a rich store of knowledge and created innovative drugs with broad applications in cardiology, nephrology, endocrinology, and general medicine, all with enormous economic and social impact on the health care system.

We felt it appropriate to begin this book with a historical section that reprints a classic treatise by the late Sir George Pickering on the nature of essential hypertension. This is accompanied by an afterword by his son, Dr. Thomas Pickering, a hypertension scholar in his own right. Two following chapters by distinguished contemporary scientists recount other landmark contributions: Dr. Peter Goldblatt reviews and interprets his father's research and Dr. John Ledingham considers anew Byrom's classic work on the vascular fault in hypertension. The historical section concludes with viewpoints from two senior contemporary scientists that provide a historical orientation on the roles of adrenal cortical function and of dietary sodium and potassium as factors in hypertension. This leads naturally into the chapters that review the epidemiologic dimensions of human hypertension.

The remainder of these volumes is organized into sections that address overall circulatory physiology and blood pressure regulation by cardiovascular, neural, and hormonal mechanisms, including what we have lately come to know about the atrial hormone and such local transmitters as endothelin and EDRF. We then consider the role of genetic and metabolic factors in the expression or mediation of these mechanisms in experimental models or humans. This is followed by two renal sections, one on intrarenal hemodynamic mechanisms and the other on renal-endocrine mechanisms as they regulate blood pressure over the long term and contribute to the causation or maintenance of hypertensive states. In these discussions, the reader will find considerable overlap, but this is by design, reflecting an intent to present different lines of evidence and perception in order to provide a diversity of perspectives and interpretations of data on unresolved issues.

In this setting, these volumes then deal comprehensively with the latest concepts of clinical and laboratory diagnosis and the treatment, with and without drugs, of the entire spectrum of human hypertensive disorders. This includes full discussions of presently available classes of drugs as well as agents not yet available for human use but which are of theoretical interest and promise in pre-clinical testing. These volumes conclude with a provocative discussion of changing strategies for drug design, development, and clinical evaluation.

Overall, this was a larger undertaking than we anticipated when we first conceived it during an intermission at a scientific meeting—such breaks often provide more valuable opportunities to exchange information than the formal sessions. We were in solid agreement that the currently enormous hypertension knowledge base needed a new attempt at organization and synthesis. Traditional academic societies and their meetings seem neither inclined nor able to bring together, in one place, all the relevant scientific activity on this topic.

There was a kind of inevitability in this collaboration, for we have known each other a long time. Many years ago we shared an interest in natriuretic hormone research but our concentrations later diverged into different aspects of renal phenomena. However, our research approaches and our dialogue have always been complementary—and this book is a happy outcome of that. But then, we are only the taskmasters. Whatever this book accomplishes, of course, is owed to the authors who toiled only for love of their subject, tolerating our prodding with grace and enthusiasm. To each of them we express our gratitude for their fine contributions and splendid cooperation.

Last, but most of all, we sincerely hope that from these pages readers will conceive novel ideas for great new experiments. Advancement in understanding of hypertension will only come from creative research.

John H. Laragh, M.D.
Barry M. Brenner, M.D.
September, 1989

Acknowledgments

We express our appreciation to many dedicated professionals at Raven Press for their guidance and assistance in matters pertaining to the publication of this work. In particular, we acknowledge the enormous efforts of Dr. Alan Edelson, Rita Scheman, John Molyneux, Denise Watov, Bob Golden, and Louise Fecher. It is with pleasure that we also acknowledge several extremely able editorial assistants in our respective offices who not only provided invaluable help in the preparation of this book but also enabled us to delegate many other responsibilities in order to devote extensive time and effort to this project: Virginia Otis Locke, Deena Spaulding, and Michelle Hardiman.

Contents

Volume 1

Section I. Background and Historical Aspects

1 Hypertension: Definitions, Natural Histories, and Consequences 3
Sir George Pickering
Afterword by Thomas G. Pickering 17

2 The Goldblatt Experiment: A Conceptual Paradigm 21
Peter J. Goldblatt

3 The Vascular Fault in Hypertension: Byrom's Work Revisited 33
John M. Ledingham

4 The Protective Effects of High-Potassium Diets in Hypertension, and the Mechanisms by Which High-NaCl Diets Produce Hypertension—A Personal View 49
Louis Tobian

5 The Adrenal Cortex in Hypertension: DOCA/Salt Hypertension and Beyond 63
Alexander C. Brownie

Section II. Epidemiological Dimensions of Hypertension

6 Familial Aggregation and Genetic Epidemiology of Blood Pressure 81
Ryk Ward

7 Hypertension and the Risk of Cardiovascular Disease 101
William B. Kannel

8 Does Hypertension Predispose to Coronary Disease? Conflicting Epidemiological and Experimental Evidence 119
Austin E. Doyle

9 Genes, Hypertension, and Early Familial Coronary Heart Disease 127
Roger R. Williams, Steven C. Hunt, Paul N. Hopkins, Lily L. Wu, Sandra J. Hasstedt, Barry M. Stults, and Hiroshi Kuida

10 Human Population Biology and Hypertension: Evolutionary and Ecological Aspects of Blood Pressure 137
Gary D. James and Paul T. Baker

11 Societal and Community Effects on Blood Pressure 147
Felix Gutzwiller, Ulrich Keil, and Jaakko Tuomilehto

12 Socioeconomic Status, Age, and Sex in the Prevalence and Prognosis of Hypertension in Blacks and Whites 159
Herman A. Tyroler

13 Hypertension and Longevity 175
Edward A. Lew

14 Epidemiology of Hypertension in the Elderly 191
C. M. Viscoli and Adrian Ostfeld

Section III. Diet and Hypertension

15 Blood Pressure and Sodium Intake 205
F. Olaf Simpson

16 Blood Pressure and Potassium Intake 217
Laura P. Svetkey and Paul E. Klotman

17 Blood Pressure and Calcium and Magnesium Intake 229
William R. Harlan and Linda C. Harlan

18 Vegetarian and Other Complex Diets, Fiber Intake, and Blood Pressure 241
Ian L. Rouse and Lawrence J. Beilin

19 Blood Pressure and Fat Intake 257
James M. Iacono and Rita M. Dougherty

20 Blood Pressure and Alcohol Intake 277
Arthur L. Klatsky

21 The Role of Dietary Protein in Hypertensive Disease 295
Walter Lovenberg and Yukio Yamori

Section IV. Circulatory and Target Organ Pathophysiology of Hypertensive Disease

22 Hemodynamic Patterns of Untreated Hypertensive Disease 305
Per Lund-Johansen and Per Omvik

23 Blood Viscosity as a Factor in Human Hypertension 329
Anne Chabanel and Shu Chien

24 Blood Volume Measurements in Hypertensive Disease 339
Joseph Feldschuh

25 The Cardiopulmonary Reflex in Hypertension 349
Alberto U. Ferrari, Guido Grassi, and Giuseppe Mancia

26 Hypertensive Cardiac Hypertrophy: Pathophysiologic and Clinical Characteristics 359
Richard B. Devereux

27 Frequency of Systemic Hypertension in Various Cardiovascular Diseases 379
William C. Roberts

28 Hypertensive Disease and Kidney Structure 389
Michael Kashgarian

29 Hypertensive Disease and the Cerebral Circulation 399
Svend Strandgaard and Olaf B. Paulson

30 Hypertension and Stroke 417
Stephen J. Phillips and Jack P. Whisnant

31 Hypertensive Retinopathy, Choroidopathy, and Optic Neuropathy of Hypertensive Ocular Disease: A Clinical and Pathophysiologic Approach to Classification 433
Mark O. M. Tso and Lee M. Jampol

Section V. Blood Pressure Regulation in Normal and Hypertensive States

Part A. Arteriolar Physiology and Pathophysiology

32 Calcium, a Neglected Key Factor in Hypertension and Arteriosclerosis: Experimental Vasoprotection with Calcium Antagonists or ACE Inhibitors 471
A. Fleckenstein, M. Frey, J. Zorn, and G. Fleckenstein-Grün

33 Protective Effects of Calcium Channel Antagonists in Experimental Models of Atherogenesis and Vascular Disease 511
David B. Weinstein

34 Vascular Remodeling in Hypertension and Atherosclerosis 521
Stephen M. Schwartz, Mark W. Majesky, and Rodney J. Dilley

35 Similarities in Cellular Proliferative Mechanisms in Hypertension and Neoplasia 541
Philippe Meyer

36 Calcium Mobilization in Vascular Smooth Muscle and Its Relevance to the Etiology of Hypertension 547
R. A. Khalil, N. J. Lodge, K. Saida, C. H. Gelband, and Cornelis van Breemen

37 The "Structural Factor" in Hypertension: With Special Emphasis on the Hypertrophic Adaptation of the Systemic Resistance Vessels 565
Björn Folkow

38 Angiotensin, Other Pressors, and the Transduction of Vascular Smooth Muscle Contraction 583
Kathy K. Griendling and R. Wayne Alexander

39 The Phosphoinositide Signaling System and the Pathogenesis of Hypertension 601
Anthony M. Heagerty and J. D. Ollerenshaw

40 Cyclic Nucleotides in the Pathogenesis of Hypertension 617
Pavel Hamet and Johanne Tremblay

41 Interactions Between Platelets and the Vessel Wall: Role of Endothelium-Derived Vasoactive Substances 637
Thomas F. Lüscher, Dennis Diederich, Fritz R. Bühler, and Paul M. Vanhoutte

42 Endothelin: A Potent Vasoactive Peptide of Endothelial Origin 649
Andrew J. King, Philip A. Marsden, and Barry M. Brenner

43 Vascular Muscle Electrophysiology and Platelet Calcium in Hypertension .. 661
Kent Hermsmeyer and Paul Erne

44 Role of Products of Univalent Reduction of Oxygen in Hypertensive Vascular Injury 667
Hermes A. Kontos

Part B. Neural and Other Humoral Factors in the Control of Arterial Pressure

45 The Role of the Central Nervous System in Hypertension 679
J. Michael Wyss, Suzanne Oparil, and Yiu-Fai Chen

46 Intracranial Disorders and Hypertension 703
Gordon M. Bell

47 The Autonomic Nervous System and Catecholamines in Normal Blood Pressure Control and in Hypertension 711
David S. Goldstein and Irwin J. Kopin

48 Dopamine-β-Hydroxylase Deficiency and Cardiovascular Control 749
David Robertson, Alan S. Hollister, and Italo Biaggioni

49 Serotonin and Hypertension 761
J. P. Chalmers, J. A. Angus, G. L. Jennings, and J. B. Minson

50 Role of Vasopressin in Hypertensive Disorders 779
Irene Gavras and Haralambos Gavras

51 Neuropeptides in Blood Pressure Control 791
Sami I. Said

52 Kinins as Regulators of Blood Flow and Blood Pressure 805
Oscar A. Carretero and A. Guillermo Scicli

53 Renal Kallikrein 819
Carlos P. Vio

54 Eicosanoids and Hypertension 829
J. Quilley, C. P. Quilley, and J. C. McGiff

55 Role of Medullipin: The Renomedullary Vasodepressor Lipid 841
E. Eric Muirhead, James A. Pitcock, Lawrence W. Byers, Bennie Brooks, and Peggy S. Brown

56 Atrial Natriuretic Factor and Its Involvement in Hypertensive Disorders . . . 861
Steven A. Atlas and John H. Laragh

57 Calcium-Regulatory Hormones in Hypertension 885
Michael B. Zemel and James R. Sowers

Part C. Genetic and Metabolic Factors in Hypertension

58 Lessons from Experimental Genetic Hypertension 901
Giuseppe Bianchi, Patrizia Ferrari, and Barry R. Barber

59 Proposed Defects in Membrane Transport and Intracellular Ions as Pathogenic Factors in Essential Hypertension 923
Abraham Aviv and Norman Lasker

60 Circulating Natriuretic Factors in Hypertension 939
Vardaman M. Buckalew, Jr. and Francis J. Haddy

61 Genetic Hypertension: Classical and Molecular Genetic Concepts as Applied to the Renin Gene 955
John P. Rapp and Sue-May Wang

62 The Membrane Carriers Related to Intracellular Calcium Regulation 965
Ernesto Carafoli, Michele Chiesi, and Paolo Gazzotti

63 Calcium Metabolism in Experimental Genetic Hypertension 977
Eric W. Young, Richard D. Bukoski, and David A. McCarron

64 Hemodynamic Effects of Potassium in Experimental Hypertension 989
Michael E. Ullian and Stuart L. Linas

65 Role of Magnesium in the Pathogenesis of Hypertension: Relationship to Its Actions on Cardiac and Vascular Smooth Muscle 1003
Burton M. Altura and Bella T. Altura

Part D. The Kidneys: Role in Volume Homeostasis and Pathogenesis of Hypertension

66 The Dominant Role of the Kidneys in the Long-Term Regulation of Arterial Pressure in Normal and Hypertensive States 1029
Arthur C. Guyton, John E. Hall, Thomas G. Coleman, and R. Davis Manning, Jr.

67 The Juxtaglomerular Apparatus: A Morphologic Perspective 1053
Luciano Barajas, Eduardo C. Salido, and Kenneth V. Powers

68 The Tubuloglomerular Feedback Mechanism 1067
Josephine P. Briggs and Jurgen Schnermann

69 On the Renal Basis for Essential Hypertension: Nephron Heterogeneity with Discordant Renin Secretion and Sodium Excretion Causing a Hypertensive Vasoconstriction–Volume Relationship 1089
Jean E. Sealey, Jon D. Blumenfeld, Gordon M. Bell, Mark S. Pecker, Sheldon C. Sommers, and John H. Laragh

70 Control of Sodium Excretion and Arterial Pressure by Intrarenal Mechanisms and the Renin–Angiotensin System 1105
John E. Hall and Arthur C. Guyton

71 Potassium Homeostasis and Blood-Pressure and Sodium-Volume Regulation 1131
David B. Young

72 The Renal Abnormality in Hypertension: A Proposed Defect in Glomerular Filtration Surface Area 1151
Barry M. Brenner, Diego L. Garcia, and Sharon Anderson

73 The Critical Role of Nephron Mass and of Intraglomerular Pressure for Initiation and Progression of Experimental Hypertensive-Renal Disorders . . 1163
Sharon Anderson and Barry M. Brenner

Part E. The Renin–Angiotensin–Aldosterone System: Biochemistry and Pathophysiology

74 The Biochemistry and Molecular Biology of Recombinant Human Renin and Prorenin 1179
Robert L. Heinrikson and Roger A. Poorman

75 Angiotensinogen: Biochemistry and Molecular Biology 1197
Duane A. Tewksbury

76 Angiotensin-Converting Enzyme: Biochemistry and Molecular Biology 1217
Mario R. W. Ehlers and James F. Riordan

77 First and Second Messengers in Renin Secretion 1233
Paul C. Churchill

78 Mechanisms of Angiotensin Action on Vascular Smooth Muscle, the Adrenal, and the Kidney 1247
Philip A. Marsden, Barry M. Brenner, and Barbara J. Ballermann

79 Physiologic Actions of Aldosterone on the Kidney 1273
Michael J. Field and Gerhard H. Giebisch

80 The Renin–Angiotensin–Aldosterone System for Normal Regulation of Blood Pressure and Sodium and Potassium Homeostasis 1287
Jean E. Sealey and John H. Laragh

81 Tissue Renin Systems as a Possible Factor in Hypertension 1319
Tomas Lenz and Jean E. Sealey

82 The Renin–Angiotensin–Aldosterone System in Hypertensive Disorders: A Key to Two Forms of Arteriolar Vasoconstriction and a Possible Clue to Risk of Vascular Injury (Heart Attack and Stroke) and Prognosis 1329
John H. Laragh and Jean E. Sealey

83 Abnormal Renal Function, Sodium-Volume Homeostasis, and Renin System Behavior in Normal-Renin Essential Hypertension 1349
Norman K. Hollenberg and Gordon H. Williams

84 Renal Hemodynamic Patterns and the Autonomic Control of Renal Renin Secretion in Essential Hypertension 1371
P. W. de Leeuw and W. H. Birkenhäger

Subject and Author Indexes follow page 1382

Volume 2

Section VI. Clinical and Laboratory Evaluation of Hypertensive Disorders

85 Clinical Evaluation and Differential Diagnosis of the Individual Hypertensive Patient 1385
Franco B. Müller and John H. Laragh

86 Diurnal Rhythms and Other Sources of Blood Pressure Variability in Normal and Hypertensive Subjects 1397
Thomas G. Pickering

87 Pseudohypertension 1407
J. David Spence

88 Labile Hypertension, Vasomotor Instability, and Postural Syndromes 1415
Joseph L. Izzo, Jr.

89 Blood Pressure Measurement and Ambulatory Blood Pressure Monitoring: Evaluation of Available Equipment 1429
Thomas G. Pickering and Seymour G. Blank

90 Hormone Assays: Renin, Aldosterone, Peripheral Vein, Renal Vein, and Urinary Assays. Guidelines to Methodology and Interpretation 1443
Jean E. Sealey, Gordon A. Campbell, and Jacek J. Preibisz

91 Laboratory Evaluation of Autonomic Nervous System Function 1461
Addison A. Taylor and Jerry R. Mitchell

92 Evaluation of Cardiac Structure and Function by Echocardiography and Other Noninvasive Techniques 1479
Richard B. Devereux

93 The Evaluation of Kidney Function in Hypertensive Patients 1493
Susanne Ljungman and Göran Granerus

94 Role of Nuclear Medicine Techniques for Evaluating Hypertensive Disease 1509
M. Donald Blaufox and Eugene J. Fine

Section VII. Pathophysiology, Diagnosis, and Treatment of Specific Forms of Hypertension

Part A. Secondary Forms of Hypertension

95 Renovascular Hypertension: Medical Evaluation and Non-Surgical Treatment 1539
Thomas G. Pickering

96 Renovascular Hypertension: Surgical Treatment 1561
Andrew C. Novick

97 Primary Reninism 1573
P. Corvol, F. Pinet, F. X. Galen, P. F. Plouin, G. Chatellier, J. Y. Pagny, P. Bruneval, J. P. Camilleri, and J. Ménard

98 Hypertension in Renal Parenchymal Disease 1583
Michael C. Smith and Michael J. Dunn

99 Hypertension and Hydronephrosis 1601
E. Darracott Vaughan, Jr. and R. Ernest Sosa

100 Adrenocortical Forms of Human Hypertension 1609
Edward G. Biglieri, Ilan Irony, and Claudio E. Kater

101 The Syndrome of Hypertension with Hyperkalemia and Normal Glomerular Filtration Rate: A Rare Form of Hypertension 1625
Richard D. Gordon, Terence J. Tunny, Shelley A. Klemm, and Stephen M. Hamlet

102 Pheochromocytoma 1639
William M. Manger and Ray W. Gifford, Jr.

103 Thyroid Hormone and Blood Pressure Regulation 1661
Irwin Klein

Part B. Diabetes and Obesity

104 Experimental Diabetes and Hypertensive Vascular Disease 1677
Sharon Anderson and Barry M. Brenner

105 Mechanisms of Hypertension in Diabetes Mellitus 1689
Naftali Stern and Michael L. Tuck

106 Hypertension and Vascular Disease as Complications of Diabetes 1703
Eberhard Ritz, Christoph Hasslacher, Johannes Mann, and Ji-Zhen Guo

107 Management of the Diabetic Patient with Hypertension: Early Screening and Treatment Programs 1717
C. E. Mogensen

108 Obesity and Hypertension 1741
Diane R. Krieger and Lewis Landsberg

Part C. Hypertension in Special Situations

109 The Renin–Angiotensin System in Normal and Hypertensive Pregnancy and in Ovarian Function 1761
Phyllis August and Jean E. Sealey

110 Abnormal Placentation in Hypertensive Disorders of Pregnancy 1779
Frederick P. Zuspan

111 Eicosanoids in the Pathogenesis of Preeclampsia 1789
Desmond J. Fitzgerald and Garret A. FitzGerald

112 Management of Hypertension During Pregnancy 1809
William M. Barron, Michael B. Murphy, and Marshall D. Lindheimer

113 Cyclosporine-Induced Hypertension 1829
John J. Curtis

114 Hypertension in Black Populations 1837
Daniel D. Savage, Laurence O. Watkins, Clarence E. Grim, and Shiriki K. Kumanyika

115 Childhood Hypertension 1853
Alan R. Sinaiko and Thomas G. Wells

116 Hypertension in the Elderly 1869
Richard L. Byyny

117 Anesthesia in the Hypertensive Patient 1889
Leroy D. Vandam

Part D. Iatrogenic Forms of Hypertension

118 Cyclo-oxygenase Inhibitors and Blood Pressure: Interaction with Antihypertensive Drugs 1905
John A. Oates

119 Phenylpropanolamine 1911
Emmanuel L. Bravo

120 Smoking and Cardiovascular Disease 1917
Henry R. Black

Section VIII. Management of the Hypertensive Patient

Part A. Application and Value of Nonpharmacologic Therapies

121 Clinical Trials as a Guide to Intervention 1941
Michael H. Alderman and Paul R. Marantz

122 The Meaning of Clinical Trials: Controversies in the Treatment of Hypertension ... 1955
Göran Berglund

123 What Blood Pressure Level Should Be Treated? ... 1967
Alberto Zanchetti

124 Physical Exercise in Hypertension ... 1985
R. Fagard, E. Bielen, P. Hespel, P. Lijnen, J. Staessen, L. Vanhees, R. Van Hoof, and A. Amery

125 Clinical Studies of the Role of Dietary Sodium in Blood Pressure ... 1999
Myron H. Weinberger

126 Dietary Sodium Restriction in Hypertension ... 2011
John D. Swales

127 Role of Dietary Chloride in Hypertension ... 2021
R. Curtis Morris, Jr., Hamoudi Al-Bander, and Theodore Kurtz

128 Weight Reduction as a Therapeutic Modality in Hypertension: The Influence of Concurrent Sodium Deprivation ... 2025
Efrain Reisin

129 The Role of Dietary Calcium and Magnesium in the Therapy of Hypertension ... 2037
Lawrence M. Resnick

130 Nursing Management of the Hypertensive Patient ... 2061
RoseMerie Marion and Carolyn Ryan

131 Physician–Patient Interaction in the Treatment of Hypertension ... 2073
Jay I. Meltzer

132 Autonomic Nervous and Behavioral Factors in Hypertension: A Rationale for Treatment ... 2083
Stevo Julius and Jurij Petrin

Part B. Drug Therapy

133 Origins and Development of Antihypertensive Treatment ... 2093
Edward D. Freis

134 Issues, Goals, and Guidelines for Choosing First-Line and Combination Antihypertensive Drug Therapy ... 2107
Franco B. Müller and John H. Laragh

135 Effects of Antihypertensive Drugs on Cardiovascular Hemodynamics ... 2117
Arie J. Man in't Veld and Anton H. van den Meiracker

136 What Are We Really Achieving with Long-Term Antihypertensive Drug Therapy? ... 2131
Lennart Hansson and Björn Dahlöf

137 Pathophysiologic Effects and Strategies for Long-Term Diuretic Treatment of Hypertension ... 2143
Mark S. Pecker

138 Calcium Antagonists ... 2169
Fritz R. Bühler

139 Beta-Blockers in the Treatment of Hypertension 2181
Peter Bolli, Peter G. Fernandez, and Fritz R. Bühler

140 Angiotensin-Converting-Enzyme Inhibitors in Hypertension 2209
Bernard Waeber, Jürg Nussberger, and Hans R. Brunner

141 Alpha-Adrenoceptor-Blocking Agents in the Treatment of Hypertension 2233
Peter A. van Zwieten

142 Centrally Acting Sympathetic Inhibitors 2251
Michael A. Weber, William F. Graettinger, and Deanna G. Cheung

143 Vasodilators 2263
Brian F. Robinson and N. Benjamin

144 Hypertensive Emergencies 2275
Samuel J. Mann and Steven A. Atlas

145 The Pharmacology of Antihypertensive Drugs and Drug–Drug Interactions 2291
K. R. Lees and J. L. Reid

146 Withdrawal of Drug Therapy: A Component of the Proper Management of the Hypertensive Patient 2301
Michael H. Alderman and Bernard Lamport

147 Medication-Taking in Hypertension 2309
Peter Rudd and Gary Marshall

Part C. Future Horizons in Therapy

148 Clinical Development of Antihypertensive Drugs: Can We Perform Better? 2331
Joël Ménard, Marc Bellet, and Hans R. Brunner

149 Specific Renin Inhibitors: The Concept and the Prospects 2343
Edgar Haber and Kwan Y. Hui

150 The Discovery and Physiological Effects of a New Class of Highly Specific Angiotensin II-Receptor Antagonists 2351
Pieter B. M. W. M. Timmermans, David J. Carini, Andrew T. Chiu, John V. Duncia, William A. Price, Jr., Gregory J. Wells, Pancras C. Wong, Ruth R. Wexler, and Alexander L. Johnson

Subject and Author Indexes follow page 2360

Contributors

Hamoudi Al-Bander, M.D.
General Clinical Research Center
The Moffit Hospital
University of California at San Francisco
San Francisco, California 94143

Michael H. Alderman, M.D.
Department of Epidemiology and Social Medicine
Albert Einstein College of Medicine
1300 Morris Park Avenue
Bronx, New York 10461

R. Wayne Alexander, M.D.
Division of Cardiology
Department of Medicine
Emory University
Atlanta, Georgia 30322

Bella T. Altura, Ph.D.
Department of Physiology
State University of New York
Health Science Center at Brooklyn
450 Clarkson Avenue
Brooklyn, NY 11203

Burton M. Altura, Ph.D.
Department of Physiology
State University of New York
Health Science Center at Brooklyn
450 Clarkson Avenue
Brooklyn, New York 11203

A. Amery, M.D.
Hypertension and Cardiovascular Rehabilitation Unit
Department of Pathophysiology
Faculty of Medicine
University of Leuven
Leuven, Belgium

Sharon Anderson, M.D.
Renal Division
Department of Medicine
Brigham and Women's Hospital, and
The Harvard Center for the Study of Kidney Disease
Harvard Medical School
75 Francis Street
Boston, Massachusetts 02115

J. A. Angus, M.D.
Baker Medical Research Institute
Commercial Road
Prahran, Victoria, Australia

Steven A. Atlas, M.D.
Cardiovascular Center
The New York Hospital–Cornell Medical Center
525 East 68th Street
New York, New York 10021

Phyllis August, M.D.
Cardiovascular Center
The New York Hospital–Cornell Medical Center
525 East 68th Street
New York, New York 10021

Abraham Aviv, M.D.
Hypertension Research Center
University of Medicine and Dentistry of New Jersey
185 South Orange Avenue
Newark, New Jersey 07103

Paul T. Baker, Ph.D.
Department of Anthropology
The Pennsylvania State University
University Park, PA 16802
Current Address
47-450 Lulani Street
Kaneohe, Hawaii 96744

Barbara J. Ballermann, M.D.
Renal Division
Department of Medicine
Brigham and Women's Hospital, and
The Harvard Center for the Study of Kidney Disease
Harvard Medical School
75 Francis Street
Boston, Massachusetts 02115

Luciano Barajas, M.D.
Department of Pathology
Harbor-UCLA Medical Center
1000 West Carson Street
Torrance, California 90509

Barry R. Barber, A.I.A.T.
Centro Ricerche Farmitalia-C. Erba
Via Giovanni XXIII
20014 Nerviano (Milano), Italy

William M. Barron, M.D.
Department of Medicine and Obstetrics and Gynecology
University of Chicago
5841 South Maryland Avenue
Chicago, Illinois 60637

Lawrence J. Beilin, M.D.
Department of Medicine
University of Western Australia
35 Victoria Square
Perth 6000, Western Australia

Gordon M. Bell, M.D.
Cardiovascular Center
The New York Hospital–Cornell Medical Center
525 East 68th Street
New York, New York 10021; and
Department of Medicine
Royal Liverpool Hospital
Prescott Street
Liverpool L7 8XP, England

Marc Bellet, M.D.
International Clinical Research and Development
Ciba-Geigy, Ltd.
4002 Basel, Switzerland

N. Benjamin, M.D.
Department of Pharmacology
St. George's Hospital Medical School
Jenner Wing, Cranmer Terrace
Tooting, London SW17 ORE, England

Göran Berglund, M.D.
Department of Medicine
University of Lund
Lund, Sweden; and
Department of Medicine
Malmö General Hospital
S-214 01 Malmö, Sweden

Italo Biaggioni, M.D.
Departments of Medicine and Pharmacology
Autonomic Dysfunction Center
Vanderbilt University
Nashville, Tennessee 37232

Giuseppe Bianchi, M.D.
Instituto di Scienze Mediche
Universita di Milano
Via Francesco Sforza, 35
20122 Milano, Italy

E. Bielen, M.D.
Hypertension and Cardiovascular Rehabilitation Unit
Department of Pathophysiology
Faculty of Medicine
University of Leuven
Leuven, Belgium

Edward G. Biglieri, M.D.
Department of Medicine
Clinical Study Center
San Francisco General Hospital
1001 Petrero
San Francisco, California 94110

W. H. Birkenhäger, M.D.
Department of Medicine
Zuiderziekenhuis
Groene Hilledijk 315
3075 EA Rotterdam, The Netherlands

Henry R. Black, M.D.
Department of Internal Medicine
Yale University School of Medicine
333 Cedar Street
New Haven, Connecticut 06510

Seymour G. Blank, Ph.D.
Cardiovascular Center
The New York Hospital–Cornell Medical Center
525 East 68th Street
New York, New York 10021

M. Donald Blaufox, M.D., Ph.D.
Department of Nuclear Medicine
Albert Einstein College of Medicine/ Montefiore Medical Center
1300 Morris Park Avenue
Bronx, New York 10461

Jon D. Blumenfeld, M.D.
Cardiovascular Center
The New York Hospital–Cornell Medical Center
525 East 68th Street
New York, New York 10021

Peter Bolli, M.D.
Division of Clinical Pharmacology
Department of Medicine
Health Science Centre
Memorial Medical School
St. John's, Newfoundland, Canada A1B 3V6

Emmanuel L. Bravo, M.D.
Department of Heart and Hypertension Research Institute
The Cleveland Clinic Foundation
9500 Euclid Avenue
Cleveland, Ohio 44106

Barry M. Brenner, M.D.
Renal Division
Department of Medicine
Brigham and Women's Hospital, and
The Harvard Center for the Study of Kidney Disease
Harvard Medical School
75 Francis Street
Boston, Massachusetts 02115

Josephine P. Briggs, M.D.
Departments of Internal Medicine and Physiology
Division of Nephrology
University of Michigan Medical School
3916 Taubman Center
Ann Arbor, Michigan 48109

Bennie Brooks
Department of Pathology
University of Tennessee
858 Madison Avenue
Memphis, Tennessee 38163; and
Department of Pathology
Baptist Memorial Hospital
899 Madison Avenue
Memphis, Tennessee 38146

Peggy S. Brown, B.A.
Department of Pathology
University of Tennessee
858 Madison Avenue
Memphis, Tennessee 38163; and
Department of Pathology
Baptist Memorial Hospital
899 Madison Avenue
Memphis, Tennessee 38146

Alexander C. Brownie, Ph.D.
Department of Biochemistry
State University of New York at Buffalo School of Medicine
102 Cary Hall
Buffalo, New York 14214

P. Bruneval, M.D.
Service d'Anatomopathologie
Hôpital Broussais
96, rue Didot
75674 Paris, France

Hans R. Brunner, M.D.
Division of Nephrology and Hypertension
Centre Hospitalier Universitaire Vaudois
1011 Lausanne, Switzerland

Vardaman M. Buckalew, Jr., M.D.
Department of Medicine/Nephrology
Bowman Gray School of Medicine
Wake Forest University
300 South Hawthorne Road
Winston-Salem, North Carolina 27103

Fritz R. Bühler, M.D.
Department of Research and Division of Cardiology, Department of Internal Medicine
University Hospital
CH-4031 Basel, Switzerland

Richard D. Bukoski, Ph.D.
Departments of Medicine (Division of Nephrology and Hypertension) and Physiology
Oregon Health Sciences University
3181 S.W. Sam Jackson Park Road
Portland, Oregon 97201

Lawrence W. Byers, Ph.D.
Department of Pathology
University of Tennessee
858 Madison Avenue
Memphis, Tennessee 38163; and
Department of Pathology
Baptist Memorial Hospital
899 Madison Avenue
Memphis, Tennessee 38146

Richard L. Byyny, M.D.
Division of Internal Medicine
University of Colorado Health Science Center
4200 East Ninth Avenue
Denver, Colorado 80262

J. P. Camilleri, M.D.
Service d'Anatomopathologie
Hôpital Broussais
96, rue Didot
75674 Paris, France

Gordon A. Campbell, Ph.D.
Cardiovascular Center
The New York Hospital–Cornell Medical Center
525 East 68th Street
New York, New York 10021

Ernesto Carafoli, M.D.
Laboratory of Biochemistry
Swiss Federal Institute of Technology (ETH)
8092 Zurich, Switzerland

David J. Carini, M.D.
Experimental Station
Medical Products Department
E.I. du Pont de Nemours & Company
P.O. Box 80400
Wilmington, Delaware 19880

Oscar A. Carretero, M.D.
Hypertension Research Division
Department of Medicine and Heart and Vascular Institute
2799 West Grand Boulevard
Detroit, Michigan 48202

Anne Chabanel, M.D.
Department of Physiology and Cellular Biophysics
Columbia University College of Physicians and Surgeons
630 West 168th Street
New York, New York 10032

J. P. Chalmers, M.D.
Department of Medicine
Flinders Medical Centre
Bedford Park SA 5042, Australia

G. Chatellier, M.D.
Service d'Hypertension Artérielle et Médecine Interne
Hôpital Broussais
96, rue Didot
75674 Paris, France

Yiu-Fai Chen, Ph.D.
The Hypertension Program of the Division of Cardiovascular Disease
Department of Medicine
University of Alabama at Birmingham
Birmingham, Alabama 35294

Deanna G. Cheung, M.D.
Veterans Administration Medical Center
5901 East 7th Street
Long Beach, California 90822

Shu Chien, M.D., Ph.D.
Department of Physiology and Cellular Biophysics
Columbia University College of Physicians and Surgeons
630 West 168th Street
New York, New York 10032

Michele Chiesi, Ph.D.
Department of Research
Pharmaceutical Division
Ciba-Geigy, Ltd.
4002 Basel, Switzerland

Andrew T. Chiu, M.D.
Experimental Station
Medical Products Department
E.I. du Pont de Nemours & Company
P.O. Box 80400
Wilmington, Delaware 19880

Paul C. Churchill, M.D.
Department of Physiology
Wayne State University
School of Medicine
5263 Scott Hall
540 East Canfield
Detroit, Michigan 48201

Thomas G. Coleman, Ph.D.
Department of Physiology and Biophysics
University of Mississippi Medical Center
2500 North State Street
Jackson, Mississippi 39216

P. Corvol, M.D.
Vascular Pathology and Renal Endocrinology Division
Institut National de la Santé et de la Recherche Médicale
U36
17, rue du Fer-à-Moulin
75005 Paris, France; and
Service d'Hypertension Artérielle et Médecine Interne
Hôpital Broussais
96, rue Didot
75674 Paris, France

John J. Curtis, M.D.
Department of Medicine and Surgery
Nephrology Research and Training Center
University of Alabama Medical Center
Birmingham, Alabama 35294

Björn Dahlöf, M.D.
Hypertension Section
Department of Medicine
Östra Hospital
S-416 85 Göteborg, Sweden

P. W. de Leeuw, M.D.
Department of Medicine
Zuiderziekenhuis
Groene Hilledijk 315
3075 EA Rotterdam, The Netherlands

Richard B. Devereux, M.D.
Division of Cardiology
The New York Hospital–Cornell Medical Center
525 East 68th Street
New York, New York 10021

Dennis Diederich, M.D.
Departments of Internal Medicine (Division of Cardiology) and Research
University Hospital
Petersgraben 4
CH-4031 Basel, Switzerland

Rodney J. Dilley, M.D.
Department of Pathology
Health Science Center
University of Washington
Seattle, Washington 98195

Rita M. Dougherty, B.A.
U.S. Department of Agriculture, ARS
Western Nutrition Research Center
P.O. Box 29997
Presidio of San Francisco, California 94129

Austin E. Doyle, M.D.
Department of Physiology
University of Melbourne
Grattan Street
Parkville, Victoria 3052, Australia

John V. Duncia, Ph.D.
Experimental Station
Medical Products Department
E.I. du Pont de Nemours & Company
P.O. Box 80400
Wilmington, Delaware 19880

Michael J. Dunn, M.D.
Department of Medicine
Case Western Reserve University
University Hospitals of Cleveland
Cleveland, Ohio 44106; and
Division of Nephrology
University Hospitals of Cleveland
2074 Abington Road
Cleveland, Ohio 44106

Mario R. W. Ehlers, M.D., Ph.D.
Center for Biochemical and Biophysical Sciences and Medicine
Harvard Medical School
Seeley G. Mudd Building
250 Longwood Avenue
Boston, Massachusetts 02115; and
M.R.C. Liver Research Centre
Department of Medicine
University of Cape Town Medical School
Cape Town, South Africa

Paul Erne, M.D.
Chiles Research Institute
Providence Medical Center and Oregon Health Sciences University
4805 NE Glisan Street
Portland, Oregon 97213

R. Fagard, M.D.
Hypertension and Cardiovascular Rehabilitation Unit
Department of Pathophysiology
Faculty of Medicine
University of Leuven
Leuven, Belgium

Joseph Feldschuh, M.D.
The New York Hospital–Cornell Medical Center
525 East 68th Street
New York, New York 10021
Private Office
645 Madison Avenue
New York, NY 10022

Peter G. Fernandez, M.D.
Division of Clinical Pharmacology
Department of Medicine
Health Sciences Centre
Memorial Medical School
St. John's Newfoundland, Canada A1B 3V6

Alberto U. Ferrari, M.D.
Cattedra di Semeiotica Medica
Clinica Medica Generale e Terapia Medica
CNR e Università di Milano
Centro di Fisiologia Clinica e Ipertensione
Via Francesco Sforza, 35
Ospedale Maggiore
20122 Milano, Italy

Patrizia Ferrari, M.D.
Centro Ricerche Farmitalia-C. Erba
Via Giovanni XXIII
20014 Nerviano (Milano), Italy

Michael J. Field, M.D.
Department of Medicine
University of Sydney
Concord Hospital
New South Wales 2139, Australia

Eugene J. Fine, M.D.
Department of Nuclear Medicine
Albert Einstein College of Medicine/ Montefiore Medical Center
1300 Morris Park Avenue
Bronx, New York 10461

Desmond J. Fitzgerald, M.D.
Department of Clinical Pharmacology
Vanderbilt University School of Medicine
Nashville, Tennessee 37232

Garret A. FitzGerald, M.D.
Department of Clinical Pharmacology
Vanderbilt University School of Medicine
Nashville, Tennessee 37232

A. Fleckenstein, Dr. Med. h.c. mult.
Study Group for Calcium Antagonism
Physiological Institute
University of Freiburg
Hermann-Herder-Strasse 7
D-7800 Freiburg, Federal Republic of Germany

G. Fleckenstein-Grün, M.D.
Study Group for Calcium Antagonism
Physiological Institute
University of Freiburg
Hermann-Herder-Strasse 7
D-7800 Freiburg, Federal Republic of Germany

Björn Folkow, M.D.
Department of Physiology
University of Göteborg
400 33 Göteborg, Sweden

Edward D. Freis, M.D.
Hypertension Research Unit
Veterans Administration Medical Center
50 Irving Street, N.W.
Washington, D.C. 20422

M. Frey, M.D.
Study Group for Calcium Antagonism
Physiological Institute
University of Freiburg
Hermann-Herder-Strasse 7
D-7800 Freiburg, Federal Republic of Germany

F. X. Galen, D.Sc.
Department of Physiology
Faculté de Pharmacie
Université de Limoges
Limoges, France

Diego L. Garcia, M.D.
Renal Division
Department of Medicine
Brigham and Women's Hospital, and
The Harvard Center for the Study of Kidney Disease
Harvard Medical School
75 Francis Street
Boston, Massachusetts, 02115

Haralambos Gavras, M.D.
Hypertension Section
Department of Medicine
Boston City Hospital and Boston University School of Medicine
80 East Concord Street
Boston, Massachusetts 02118

Irene Gavras, M.D.
Department of Medicine
Boston City Hospital and Boston University School of Medicine
80 East Concord Street
Boston, Massachusetts 02118

Paolo Gazzotti, Ph.D.
Laboratory of Biochemistry
Swiss Federal Institute of Technology (ETH)
8092 Zurich, Switzerland

C. H. Gelband, M.D.
Department of Pharmacology
University of Miami School of Medicine
P.O. Box 016189
Miami, Florida 33101

Gerhard H. Giebisch, M.D.
Department of Physiology
Yale University School of Medicine
333 Cedar Street
New Haven, Connecticut 06510

Ray W. Gifford, Jr., M.D.
The Cleveland Clinic Foundation
9500 Euclid Avenue
Cleveland, Ohio 44106

Peter J. Goldblatt, M.D.
Department of Pathology
Dean, Graduate School
Medical College of Ohio
C.S. 10008
Toledo, Ohio 43699

David S. Goldstein, M.D.
Hypertension-Endocrine Branch
National Heart, Lung, and Blood Institute
National Institutes of Health
Building 10 8C103
Bethesda, Maryland 20892

Richard D. Gordon, M.D., Ph.D., F.R.A.C.P.
Endocrine-Hypertension Research Unit
Department of Medicine
University of Queensland
Greenslopes Hospital
Brisbane, Australia 4120

William F. Graettinger, M.D.
Veterans Administration Medical Center
5901 7th Street
Long Beach, California 90822

Göran Granerus, M.D.
Department of Clinical Physiology
Sahlgrenska Hospital
University of Göteborg
S-413 45 Göteborg, Sweden

Guido Grassi, M.D.
Cattedra di Semeiotica Medica
Clinica Medica Generale e Terapia Medica
CNR e Università di Milano
Centro di Fisiologia Clinica e Ipertensione
Ospedale Maggiore
Via Francesco Sforza, 35
20122 Milano, Italy

Kathy K. Griendling, M.D.
Division of Cardiology
Department of Medicine
Emory University
Atlanta, Georgia 30322

Clarence E. Grim, M.D., M.S.
Department of Medicine
Charles R. Drew University of Medicine and Science
University of California at Los Angeles
Los Angeles, California 90059

Ji-Zhen Guo, M.D.
Department of Internal Medicine
University of Heidelberg
Bergheimer Strasse 56a
D-6900 Heidelberg, Federal Republic of Germany

Felix Gutzwiller, M.D., Dr. P.H.
Institute of Social and Preventive Medicine
University of Zurich
Sumatrastrasse 30
CH-8006 Zurich, Switzerland

Arthur C. Guyton, M.D.
Department of Physiology and Biophysics
University of Mississippi Medical Center
2500 North State Street
Jackson, Mississippi 39216

Edgar Haber, M.D.
Cardiac Unit
Massachusetts General Hospital
Boston, Massachusetts 02114

Francis J. Haddy, M.D.
Department of Physiology
Uniformed Services University of the Health Sciences
4301 Jones Bridge Road
Bethesda, Maryland 20814

John E. Hall, Ph.D.
Department of Physiology and Biophysics
University of Mississippi Medical Center
2500 North State Street
Jackson, Mississippi 39216

Pavel Hamet, M.D., Ph.D.
Laboratory of Molecular Pathophysiology
Clinical Research Institute of Montreal
110 Pine Avenue West
Montreal, Quebec H2W 1R7, Canada

Stephen M. Hamlet, M.Sc.
Endocrine-Hypertension Research Unit
Department of Medicine
University of Queensland
Greenslopes Hospital
Brisbane, Australia 4120

Lennart Hansson, M.D., Ph.D.
Hypertension Section
Department of Medicine
Östra Hospital
S-416 85 Göteborg, Sweden

Linda C. Harlan, Ph.D.
Department of Biostatistics
The University of Michigan School of Public Health
Ann Arbor, Michigan 48109
Current Address
Division of Cancer Prevention and Control
National Cancer Institute
Bethesda, Maryland 20892

William R. Harlan, M.D.
Department of Medicine
The University of Michigan School of Medicine
Ann Arbor, Michigan 48109
Current Address
Division of Epidemiology and Clinical Applications
National Heart, Lung, and Blood Institute
National Institutes of Health
Bethesda, Maryland 20892

Christoph Hasslacher, M.D.
Department of Internal Medicine
University of Heidelberg
Bergheimer Strasse 56a
D-6900 Heidelberg, Federal Republic of Germany

Sandra J. Hasstedt, Ph.D.
Cardiovascular Genetics Research Clinic
University of Utah School of Medicine
410 Chipeta Way, Room 161
Salt Lake City, Utah 84108

Anthony M. Heagerty, M.D., M.R.C.P.
Department of Medicine
Clinical Sciences Building
Leicester Royal Infirmary
Leicester LE2 7LX, England

Robert L. Heinrikson, Ph.D.
Department of Biopolymer Chemistry
The Upjohn Company
Kalamazoo, Michigan 49001

Kent Hermsmeyer, Ph.D.
Chiles Research Institute
Providence Medical Center and Oregon Health Sciences University
4805 NE Glisan Street
Portland, Oregon 97213

P. Hespel, M.D.
Hypertension and Cardiovascular Rehabilitation Unit
Department of Pathophysiology
Faculty of Medicine
University of Leuven
Leuven, Belgium

Norman K. Hollenberg, M.D., Ph.D.
Department of Medicine and Radiology
Harvard Medical School and Brigham and Women's Hospital
75 Francis Street
Boston, Massachusetts 02115

Alan S. Hollister, M.D., Ph.D.
Department of Medicine and Pharmacology
Autonomic Dysfunction Center
Vanderbilt University
Nashville, Tennessee 37232

Paul N. Hopkins, M.D., M.S.P.H.
Cardiovascular Genetics Research Clinic
University of Utah School of Medicine
410 Chipeta Way, Room 161
Salt Lake City, Utah 84108

Kwan Y. Hui, Ph.D.
Eli Lilly and Company
Lilly Corporate Center
Indianapolis, Indiana 46285

Steven C. Hunt, Ph.D.
Cardiovascular Genetics Research Clinic
University of Utah School of Medicine
410 Chipeta Way, Room 161
Salt Lake City, Utah 84108

James M. Iacono, Ph.D.
U.S. Department of Agriculture, ARS
Western Nutrition Research Center
P.O. Box 29997
Presidio of San Francisco, California 94129

Ilan Irony, M.D.
Department of Medicine
Clinical Study Center
San Francisco General Hospital
1001 Petrero
San Francisco, California 94110

Joseph L. Izzo, Jr., M.D.
Medicine Nephrology Unit
Hypertension Service
University of Rochester
601 Elmwood Avenue
Rochester, New York 14642

Gary D. James, Ph.D.
Cardiovascular Center
The New York Hospital–Cornell Medical Center
525 East 68th Street
New York, New York 10021

Lee M. Jampol, M.D.
Department of Ophthalmology
Northwestern University Medical School
303 East Chicago Avenue
Chicago, Illinois 60611

G. L. Jennings, M.D.
Baker Medical Research Institute
Commercial Road
Prahran, Victoria, Australia

Alexander L. Johnson, Ph.D.
Experimental Station
Medical Products Department
E.I. du Pont de Nemours & Company
P.O. Box 80400
Wilmington, Delaware 19880

Stevo Julius, M.D., Sc.D.
Division of Hypertension
Department of Internal Medicine
University of Michigan
3918 Taubman Center
Ann Arbor, Michigan 48109

William B. Kannel, M.D., M.P.H.
Section of Preventive Medicine and Epidemiology
Evans Department of Clinical Research
University Hospital
Boston University Medical Center
Boston, Massachusetts 02118

Michael Kashgarian, M.D.
Department of Pathology
Yale University School of Medicine
333 Cedar Street
New Haven, Connecticut 06510

Claudio E. Kater, M.D.
Department of Medicine
Section of Endocrinology
Escola Paulista de Medecine
Sao Paulo, Brazil

Ulrich Keil, M.D., M.Sc.
Department of Social Medicine and Epidemiology
Ruhr-Universität Bochum
Stiepelerstrasse 129
D-4630 Bochum, Federal Republic of Germany

R. A. Khalil, M.D.
Department of Medicine
University of Miami School of Medicine
P.O. Box 016189
Miami, Florida 33101

Andrew J. King, M.D.
Renal Division
Department of Medicine
Brigham and Women's Hospital, and
The Harvard Center for the Study of Kidney Disease
Harvard Medical School
75 Francis Street
Boston, Massachusetts 02115

Arthur L. Klatsky, M.D.
Division of Cardiology
Department of Medicine
Kaiser Permanente Medical Center
280 West MacArthur Boulevard
Oakland, California 94611

Irwin Klein, M.D.
Division of Endocrinology and Metabolism
Department of Medicine
North Shore University Hospital
300 Community Drive
Manhasset, New York 11030; and
Department of Medicine
Cornell University Medical College
New York, New York 10021

Shelley A. Klemm, Ph.D.
Endocrine-Hypertension Research Unit
Department of Medicine
University of Queensland
Greenslopes Hospital
Brisbane, Australia 4120

Paul E. Klotman, M.D.
Department of Medicine
Duke University Medical Center
Box 3014
Durham, North Carolina 27710

Hermes A. Kontos, M.D., Ph.D.
Department of Medicine
Medical College of Virginia
11th and Marshall Streets
Richmond, Virginia 23298

Irwin J. Kopin, M.D.
Intramural Research Program
National Institute of Neurological and Communicative Disorders and Stroke
National Institutes of Health
Bethesda, Maryland 20892

Diane R. Krieger, M.D.
Division of Endocrinology and Metabolism
Beth Israel Hospital
339 Brookline Avenue
Boston, Massachusetts 02115

Hiroshi Kuida, M.D.
Cardiovascular Genetics Research Clinic
University of Utah School of Medicine
410 Chipeta Way, Room 161
Salt Lake City, Utah 84108

Shiriki K. Kumanyika, Ph.D., M.P.H.
Department of Epidemiology
Johns Hopkins School of Public Health and Hygiene
Baltimore, Maryland 21205

Theodore Kurtz, M.D.
General Clinical Research Center
The Moffit Hospital
University of California at San Francisco
San Francisco, California 94143

Bernard Lamport, M.D.
Department of Epidemiology and Social Medicine
Albert Einstein College of Medicine
1300 Morris Park Avenue
Bronx, New York 10461

Lewis Landsberg, M.D.
Division of Endocrinology and Metabolism
Beth Israel Hospital
339 Brookline Avenue
Boston, Massachusetts 02116

John H. Laragh, M.D.
Cardiovascular Center
The New York Hospital–Cornell Medical Center
525 East 68th Street
New York, New York 10021

Norman Lasker, M.D.
Division of Nephrology
Department of Medicine
University of Medicine and Dentistry of New Jersey
185 South Orange Avenue
Newark, New Jersey 07103

John M. Ledingham, M.D.
University of London
11 Montpelier Walk
London SW7 1JL, England

K. R. Lees, M.D., M.R.C.P.
Department of Materia Medica
Stobhill General Hospital
University of Glasgow
Glasgow G21 3UW, Scotland

Tomas Lenz, M.D.
Cardiovascular Center
The New York Hospital–Cornell Medical Center
525 East 68th Street
New York, New York 10021

Edward A. Lew, A.M., F.S.A.
Retired Vice-President of Metropolitan Life Insurance Company
Past President of the American Society of Actuaries
Honorary Member Association of Life Insurance Medical Directors
Punta Gorda, Florida
Current Address
1750 Jamaica Way, Unit 213
Punta Gorda, Florida 33950

P. Lijnen, M.D.
Hypertension and Cardiovascular Rehabilitation Unit
Department of Pathophysiology
Faculty of Medicine
University of Leuven
Leuven, Belgium

Stuart L. Linas, M.D.
Department of Medicine
Denver General Hospital
777 Bannock Street
Denver, Colorado 80204

Marshall D. Lindheimer, M.D.
Departments of Medicine and Obstetrics and Gynecology
University of Chicago
5841 South Maryland Avenue
Chicago, Illinois 60637

Susanne Ljungman, M.D.
Department of Nephrology
Sahlgrenska Hospital
University of Göteborg
S-413 45 Göteborg, Sweden

N. J. Lodge, M.D.
Department of Pharmacology
University of Miami School of Medicine
P.O. Box 016189
Miami, Florida 33101

Walter Lovenberg, M.D.
Merrell Dow Research Institute
Strasbourg Center
16 Rue D'Ankara
Strasbourg 67084, France

Per Lund-Johansen, M.D.
Section of Cardiology
Haukeland Hospital
University of Bergen School of Medicine
Bergen 5016, Norway

Thomas F. Lüscher, M.D.
Departments of Internal Medicine (Division of Cardiology) and Research
University Hospital
Petersgraben 4
CH-4031 Basel, Switzerland

Mark W. Majesky, M.D.
Department of Pathology
Health Science Center
University of Washington
Seattle, Washington 98195

Giuseppe Mancia, M.D.
Cattedra di Semeiotica Medica
Clinica Medica Generale e Terapia Medica
CNR e Università di Milano
Clinica e Ipertensione
Via Francesco Sforza, 35
Ospedale Maggiore
20122 Milano, Italy

William M. Manger, M.D., Ph.D.
Department of Clinical Medicine
New York University Medical Center
400 East 34th Street
New York, New York 10016
Private Practice
324 East 30th Street
New York, New York 10016

Arie J. Man in't Veld, M.D.
Department of Internal Medicine
University Hospital Dijksigt
Erasmus University Rotterdam
Dr. Molewaterplein 40
3015 GD Rotterdam, The Netherlands

Johannes Mann, M.D.
Department of Internal Medicine
University of Heidelberg
Bergheimer Strasse 56a
D-6900 Heidelberg, Federal Republic of Germany

Samuel J. Mann, M.D.
Cardiovascular Center
The New York Hospital–Cornell Medical Center
525 East 68th Street
New York, New York 10021

R. Davis Manning, Jr., Ph.D
Department of Physiology and Biophysics
University of Mississippi Medical Center
2500 North State Street
Jackson, Mississippi 39216

Paul R. Marantz, M.D., M.P.H.
Department of Epidemiology and Social Medicine
Albert Einstein College of Medicine
1300 Morris Park Avenue
Bronx, New York 10461

RoseMerie Marion, R.N.
Cardiovascular Center
The New York Hospital–Cornell Medical Center
525 East 68th Street
New York, New York 10021

Philip A. Marsden, M.D.
Renal Division and Department of Medicine
Brigham and Women's Hospital, and
The Harvard Center for the Study of Kidney Disease
Harvard Medical School
75 Francis Street
Boston, Massachusetts 02115

Gary Marshall, Ph.D.
Research Associate
693 Wildwood Lane
Palo Alto, California 94303

David A. McCarron, M.D.
Departments of Medicine (Division of Nephrology and Hypertension) and Physiology
Oregon Health Sciences University
3181 S.W. Sam Jackson Park Road
Portland, Oregon 97201

J. C. McGiff, M.D.
Department of Pharmacology
New York Medical College
Valhalla, New York 10595

Jay I. Meltzer, M.D.
Department of Medicine
Columbia Presbyterian Medical Center
New York, New York 10032
Private Practice
903 Park Avenue
New York, New York 10021

Joël Ménard, M.D.
Vascular Pathology and Renal Endocrinology Division
Institute Nationale de la Sante et de la Recherche Medicale
U36
17, rue du Fer-à-Moulin

Joël Ménard, M.D. (cont'd)
75005 Paris, France; and
Service d'Hypertension Artérielle
Hôpital Broussais
96, rue Didot
75014 Paris, France; and
International Clinical Research and Development
Ciba-Geigy, Ltd.
4002 Basel, Switzerland

Philippe Meyer, M.D.
Départment de Pharmacologie
Hôpital Necker
161, rue de Sévres
75015 Paris, France

J. B. Minson, M.D.
Department of Medicine
Flinders Medical Centre
Beford Park SA 5042, Australia

Jerry R. Mitchell, M.D., Ph.D.
Department of Medicine
Section of Hypertension and Clinical Pharmacology
Center for Experimental Therapeutics
Baylor College of Medicine
1 Baylor Plaza
Houston, Texas 77030

C. E. Mogensen, M.D.
Second University Clinic of Internal Medicine
Kommunehospitalet
University of Aarhus
DK-8000 Aarhus C, Denmark

R. Curtis Morris, Jr., M.D.
General Clinical Research Center
The Moffit Hospital
University of California at San Francisco
San Francisco, California 94143

E. Eric Muirhead, M.D.
Department of Pathology
University of Tennessee
858 Madison Avenue
Memphis, Tennessee 38163; and
Department of Pathology
Baptist Memorial Hospital
899 Madison Avenue
Memphis, Tennessee 38146

Franco B. Müller, M.D.
Cardiovascular Center
The New York Hospital–Cornell Medical Center
525 East 68th Street
New York, New York 10021

Michael B. Murphy, M.D.
Department of Medicine
University of Chicago
5841 South Maryland Avenue
Chicago, Illinois 60637

Andrew C. Novick, M.D.
Department of Urology
The Cleveland Clinic Foundation
9500 Euclid Avenue
Cleveland, Ohio 44106

Jürg Nussberger, M.D.
Division of Nephrology and Hypertension
Centre Hospitalier Universitaire Vaudois
1011 Lausanne, Switzerland

John A. Oates, M.D.
Department of Medicine
Vanderbilt University School of Medicine
B-3218 Medical Center North
Nashville, Tennessee 37232

J. D. Ollerenshaw, H.N.D.
Department of Medicine
Clinical Sciences Building
Leicester Royal Infirmary
Leicester LE2 7LX, England

Per Omvik, M.D.
Section of Cardiology
Haukeland Hospital
University of Bergen School of Medicine
Bergen 5016, Norway

Suzanne Oparil, Ph.D.
The Hypertension Program of the Division of Cardiovascular Disease
Department of Medicine
University of Alabama at Birmingham
Birmingham, Alabama 35294

Adrian Ostfeld, M.D.
Department of Epidemiology and Public Health
Yale University School of Medicine
60 College Street
P.O. Box 3333
New Haven, Connecticut 06510

J. Y. Pagny, M.D.
Service d'Hypertension Artérielle et Médecine Interne
Hôpital Broussais
96, rue Didot
75674 Paris, France

Olaf B. Paulson, M.D.
Department of Neurology
Rigshospitalet
DK-2100 Copenhagen, Denmark

Mark S. Pecker, M.D.
Cardiovascular Center
The New York Hospital–Cornell Medical Center
525 East 68th Street
New York, New York 10021

Jurij Petrin, M.D.
Division of Hypertension
Department of Internal Medicine
University of Michigan
3918 Taubman Center
Ann Arbor, Michigan 48109

Stephen J. Phillips, M.D.
Department of Health Sciences Research
Department of Neurology, and the Cerebrovascular Research Center
Mayo Clinic
200 1st Street, SW
Rochester, Minnesota 55905
Current Address
Department of Medicine
Camp Hill Hospital
1763 Robie Street
Halifax, Nova Scotia B3H 3G2, Canada

Sir George Pickering, M.D.
(Deceased)

Thomas G. Pickering, M.D.
Cardiovascular Center
The New York Hospital–Cornell Medical Center
525 East 68th Street
New York, New York 10021

F. Pinet, Ph.D.
Vascular Pathology and Renal Endocrinology Division
Institut Nationale de la Santé et de la Recherche Medicale
U36
17, rue du Fer-à-Moulin
75005 Paris, France

James A. Pitcock, M.D.
Department of Pathology
University of Tennessee
858 Madison Avenue
Memphis, Tennessee 38163; and
Department of Pathology
Baptist Memorial Hospital
899 Madison Avenue
Memphis, Tennessee 38146

P. F. Plouin, M.D.
Service d'Hypertension Artérielle et Médecine Interne
Hôpital Broussais
96, rue Didot
75674 Paris, France

Roger A. Poorman, Ph.D.
Department of Biopolymer Chemistry
The Upjohn Company
Kalamazoo, Michigan 49001

Kenneth V. Powers, M.S.
Department of Pathology
Harbor-UCLA Medical Center
1000 West Carson Street
Torrance, California 90509

Jacek J. Preibisz, M.D.
Cardiovascular Center
The New York Hospital–Cornell Medical Center
525 East 68th Street
New York, New York 10021

William A. Price, Jr., Ph.D.
Experimental Station
Medical Products Department
E.I. du Pont de Nemours & Company
P.O. Box 80400
Wilmington, Delaware 19880

C. P. Quilley, M.D.
Department of Pharmacology
New York Medical College
Valhalla, New York 10595

J. Quilley, M.D.
Department of Pharmacology
New York Medical College
Valhalla, New York 10595

John P. Rapp, M.D.
Department of Medicine
Medical College of Ohio
Toledo, Ohio 43699

J. L. Reid, M.D., F.R.C.P.
Department of Materia Medica
Stobhill General Hospital
University of Glasgow
Glasgow G21 3UW, Scotland

Efrain Reisin, M.D.
Department of Medicine
Nephrology Section
Louisiana State University Medical Center
1542 Tulane Avenue
New Orleans, Louisiana 70112

Lawrence M. Resnick, M.D.
Cardiovascular Center
The New York Hospital–Cornell Medical Center
525 East 68th Street
New York, New York 10021

James F. Riordan, Ph.D.
Center for Biochemical and Biophysical Sciences and Medicine
Harvard Medical School
Seeley G. Mudd Building
250 Longwood Avenue
Boston, Massachusetts 02115

Eberhard Ritz, M.D.
Department of Internal Medicine
University of Heidelberg
Bergheimer Strasse 56a
D-6900 Heidelberg, Federal Republic of Germany

William C. Roberts, M.D.
Pathology Branch
National Heart, Lung, and Blood Institute
National Institutes of Health
Bethesda, Maryland 20892

David Robertson, M.D.
Departments of Medicine and Pharmacology
Vanderbilt University
Nashville, Tennessee 37232

Brian F. Robinson, M.D.
Department of Pharmacology
St. George's Hospital Medical School
Jenner Wing, Cranmer Terrace
Tooting, London SW 17 ORE, England

Ian L. Rouse, M.D.
Department of Medicine
University of Western Australia
35 Victoria Square
Perth 6000, Western Australia

Peter Rudd, M.D.
Internal Medicine and Hypertension Clinics
Stanford University Medical Center
Stanford, California 94305

Carolyn Ryan, M.S., R.N.
Cardiovascular Center
The New York Hospital–Cornell Medical Center
525 East 68th Street
New York, New York 10021

Sami I. Said, M.D.
Department of Medicine
University of Illinois
College of Medicine
P.O. Box 6998
Chicago, Illinois 60680; and
Department of Medicine
West Side VAMC
Chicago, Illinois 60612

K. Saida, M.D.
Department of Pharmacology
University of Miami School of Medicine
P.O. Box 016189
Miami, Florida 33101

Eduardo C. Salido, M.D.
Department of Pathology
Harbor-UCLA Medical Center
1000 West Carson Street
Torrance, California 90509

Daniel D. Savage, M.D., Ph.D.
Department of Medicine
Uniformed Services University of the Health Sciences
4301 Jones Bridge Road
Bethesda, Maryland 20814; and
Department of Medicine
Morehouse School of Medicine
Atlanta, Georgia 30310

Jurgen Schnermann, M.D.
Department of Internal Medicine and Physiology
Division of Nephrology
University of Michigan Medical School
3916 Taubman Center
Ann Arbor, Michigan 48109

Stephen M. Schwartz, M.D.
Department of Pathology
Health Science Center
University of Washington
Seattle, Washington 98195

A. Guillermo Scicli, Ph.D.
Hypertension Research Division
Department of Medicine and Heart Vascular Institute
Henry Ford Hospital
2799 West Grand Boulevard
Detroit, Michigan 48202

Jean E. Sealey, D.Sc.
Cardiovascular Center
The New York Hospital–Cornell Medical Center
525 East 68th Street
New York, New York 10021

F. Olaf Simpson, M.D.
Wellcome Medical Research Institute
University of Otago Medical School
P.O. Box 913
Dunedin, New Zealand 9001

Alan R. Sinaiko, M.D.
Division of Clinical Pharmacology
Departments of Pediatrics and Pharmacology
University of Minnesota Health Sciences Center
Mayo Building
420 Delaware Street S.E.
Minneapolis, Minnesota 55455

Michael C. Smith, M.D.
Department of Medicine
Case Western Reserve University
Cleveland, Ohio 44106; and
Division of Nephrology
University Hospitals of Cleveland
2074 Abington Road
Cleveland, Ohio 44106

Sheldon C. Sommers, M.D.
Cardiovascular Center
The New York Hospital–Cornell Medical Center
525 East 68th Street
New York, New York 10021

R. Ernest Sosa, M.D.
Department of Surgery
Division of Urology
The New York Hospital–Cornell Medical Center
525 East 68th Street
New York, New York 10021

James R. Sowers, M.D.
Division of Endocrinology, Nutrition, and Hypertension
Wayne State University School of Medicine
University Health Center
4201 St. Antoine Avenue
Detroit, Michigan 48201

J. David Spence, M.D.
Department of Internal Medicine
Clinical Neurological Sciences and Pharmacology and Toxicology
University of Western Ontario, and
Hypertension Clinics
Victoria Hospital
London, Ontario N6A 4G5, Canada

J. Staessen, M.D.
Hypertension and Cardiovascular Rehabilitation Unit
Department of Pathophysiology
Faculty of Medicine
University of Leuven
Leuven, Belgium

Naftali Stern, Ph.D.
Department of Medicine
UCLA School of Medicine, and
Endocrine Hypertension Research
VA Medical Center
16111 Plummer Street
Sepulveda, California 91343

Svend Strandgaard, M.D.
Department of Medicine and Nephrology B
Herlev Hospital
DK-2730 Herlev, Denmark

Barry M. Stults, M.D.
Cardiovascular Genetics Research Clinic
University of Utah School of Medicine
410 Chipeta Way, Room 161
Salt Lake City, Utah 84108

Laura P. Svetkey, M.D.
Department of Medicine
Duke University Medical Center
Box 3075
Durham, North Carolina 27710

John D. Swales, M.D.
Department of Medicine
Clinical Sciences Building
Leicester Royal Infirmary
P.O. Box 65
Leicester L32 6LX, England

Addison A. Taylor, M.D., Ph.D.
Section of Hypertension and Clinical Pharmacology (Department of Medicine)
Center for Experimental Therapeutics
Baylor College of Medicine
1 Baylor Plaza
Houston, Texas 77030

Duane A. Tewksbury, Ph.D.
Marshfield Medical Foundation, Inc.
510 North St. Joseph Avenue
Marshfield, Wisconsin 54449

Pieter B. M. W. M. Timmermans, Ph.D.
Experimental Station
Medical Products Department
E.I. du Pont de Nemours & Company
P.O. Box 80400
Wilmington, Delaware 19880

Louis Tobian, M.D.
Mayo Building, Box 285
University of Minnesota Hospital
420 Delaware Street
Minneapolis, Minnesota 55455

Johanne Tremblay, M.D.
Laboratory of Molecular Pathophysiology
Clinical Research Institute of Montreal
110 Pine Avenue West
Montreal, Quebec, H2W 1R7, Canada

Mark O. M. Tso, M.D.
Georgiana Theobald Ophthalmic Pathology Laboratory
Department of Ophthalmology
University of Illinois College of Medicine at Chicago
1855 West Taylor Street
Chicago, Illinois 60612

Michael L. Tuck, M.D.
Department of Medicine
UCLA School of Medicine, and
Endocrinology Division
VA Medical Center
16111 Plummer Street
Sepulveda, California 91343

Terence J. Tunny, M.Appl.Sc.
Endocrine-Hypertension Research Unit
Department of Medicine
University of Queensland
Greenslopes Hospital
Brisbane, Australia 4120

Although bruits are premonitory of subsequent cardiovascular disease, they do not predict the location of the lesion. Our experience has been that patients with carotid bruits are more apt to have heart attacks than cerebrovascular accidents.

A systolic bruit over the femoral artery suggests atherosclerotic disease but does not necessarily imply that it is occlusive. When pulses in the lower extremities are absent or dampened in a young person, coarctation of the aorta should be suspected; in an older patient, occlusive aortic femoral disease is possible.

Examination of the Abdomen

The aorta should be carefully palpated in all patients, since aortic dilation or aneurysm is a highly treatable condition often identifiable on the physical examination. A systolic and diastolic bruit in the upper epigastrium or in one or both upper quadrants of the abdomen suggests renal artery stenosis, a diagnosis that should be pursued if other criteria are compatible. A palpable enlargement of one or both kidneys can suggest polycystic renal disease, hydronephrosis, or a renal tumor. Very rarely is a pheochromocytoma large enough to be palpable.

Neurologic Examination

Gross deficits in sensory or motor function, mentation, or mood are not likely to be missed, but more subtle deficits indicating transient cerebral ischemia or autonomic dysfunction should be sought for clinically, especially if the history is suggestive.

Laboratory and Instrumented Evaluation

Together with the history and the physical examination, the purpose of the laboratory and instrumented evaluation is to:

1. Identify specifically all curable causes of hypertension (Table 1);
2. Stratify pathophysiologically the remaining heterogeneous group with essential hypertension; and
3. Assess and characterize the risk profile of the individual patient by identifying target organ damage, the presence of coexisting disease, and the presence of attendant biochemical risk factors.

The initial laboratory work-up should include a complete blood count and hematocrit together with a complete urinalysis, blood urea nitrogen, serum creatinine, serum uric acid, fasting blood sugar, lipid profile, and serum electrolytes. If the serum potassium level is borderline or low (i.e., equal to or below 3.6 mEq/liter), it should be repeated on two or three separate occasions. A low potassium level often provides the first laboratory clue to the presence of aldosterone excess.

Since plasma renin is part of a cybernetic control system that responds to changes in sodium balance, an evaluation of the renin system in hypertensive patients (carried out under standardized conditions) should be part of the initial laboratory work-up (see Chapters 80 and 82). This enables the clinician to rule out or go on to diagnose curable disorders (i.e., renovascular disease and primary aldosteronism). Also, it stratifies all patients pathophysiologically according to the degree of their renin and sodium involvement.

The renin–sodium profile, plasma potassium, serum urea and creatinine, and 4-hr urinary microalbumin excretion rate, together with the 24-hr urinary sodium and potassium values, comprise an especially valuable primary biochemical package to screen for and then identify secondary causes of hypertension and characterize all patients pathophysiologically. Plasma renin levels in curable renovascular disease or coarctation are often increased and are never low, whereas they are markedly suppressed in primary aldosteronism. The assay is no more expensive or complicated than the cholesterol assays so common nowadays, and it is potentially far more relevant, not only because it can enable the absolute diagnosis of curable forms but also because it can be used for evaluating the pathophysiology of essential hypertension and for planning its treatment. The test involves the collection of a 24-hr urine for measurement of sodium excretion and a venous blood sample for renin measurement, the latter being collected while the patient is seated quietly in the office (see Chapters 80, 82, 90). The plasma renin activity value is plotted against the 24-hr urinary sodium level, thereby correcting for the fact that renin, a regulatory hormone, rises normally in response to a low-salt diet and declines in response to a high-salt diet (see Chapter 90). Where the test is done while the patient is on his or her own diet, it provides basic information about salt appetite. If the kidneys are healthy and there is no edema, it can be presumed that the daily sodium output reliably reflects the sodium intake.

Since all antihypertensive medications can affect plasma renin values, accurate interpretation of a renin–sodium profile requires that the test be carried out with the patient off drugs for at least 3 weeks in the case of diuretics, 6 weeks for spironolactone, and 2 weeks for all other antihypertensive treatments. The renin–sodium profile as a diagnostic test, like most other laboratory tests, is most powerful when the deviations are extreme. Patients exhibiting very high or very low plasma renin levels can be immediately selected for special work-ups.

The simultaneous measurement of the 24-hr urinary potassium helps evaluate the normalcy of aldosterone secretion. If urinary potassium excretion exceeds 40 mEq/day when plasma levels are less than 3.6 mEq/liter, the pattern suggests oversecretion of aldosterone (perhaps due to an adenoma) and thus suggests the need for more diagnostic testing. (See Chapters 90, 100.)

Furthermore, the determination of albumin in the 24-hr urine helps to identify renal hypertension or microalbuminuria reflecting a degree of renal damage in essential hypertension or in diabetic nephropathy (42–44). In our own laboratory, normal values are less than 10 mg/day (42–44). This test is a valuable guide to occult renal damage in hypertensive patients and can be used to follow effects of drug therapy (44). (See Chapter 93.)

With the current widespread use of automated laboratory testing, a variety of other relevant tests may be added at little or no extra cost. Serum calcium and circulating thyroid hormone levels may point to parathyroid or thyroid disease, which can sometimes exist without clear-cut clinical evidence.

Tests of lipid, cholesterol, and triglyceride metabolism are usually offered as part of these automated testing profiles. However, even the advocates of this group of tests (45) agree that over the age of 60 and perhaps over the age of 50, blood lipids have less prognostic value except when markedly abnormal (see Chapter 7). Recent national guidelines, while probably overly enthusiastic (45), provide one basis for antilipid therapy. A more cautious viewpoint has recently been offered (46,47).

When pheochromocytoma is suspected, measurements of plasma and/or urinary catecholamines or of their urinary metabolites can be extremely helpful (48,49). Also, measurement of urinary free cortisol or urinary 17-hydroxycorticosteroids can be suggestive, but sometimes the dexamethasone suppression test may be necessary to define the nature of Cushing's syndrome (37).

Determination of urinary aldosterone levels is most valuable for revealing the rate of adrenal aldosterone secretion. This test is essential for establishing the diagnosis of primary or pseudoprimary aldosteronism (see Chapters 90 and 100) and is very helpful in evaluating other hypertensive situations associated with high renin level and/or potassium wasting, but it is not necessary to perform it routinely. However, it is very useful to store a urine sample for later determination of urinary aldosterone if plasma renin is low.

The *chest x-ray* is highly desirable as part of every initial workup, particularly in patients over age 40. It can reveal coarctation of the aorta and can be useful in assessing cardiac hypertrophy.

A routine *electrocardiogram* should be part of the evaluation of every new patient with established high blood pressure. Manifestations of hypertensive heart disease include T-wave abnormalities, expressed either by notching or a biphasic form, particularly in the precordial leads. As left ventricular hypertrophy progresses, there is increased voltage of the R-waves and then a characteristic strain pattern involving ST segment depressions and T-wave inversion (50).

Studies show that patients with electrocardiographic or radiographic abnormalities have twofold or greater increases in premature mortality rates (51–53). Yet, electrocardiography and chest radiography detect left ventricular hypertrophy in only about 5% (or fewer) of unselected hypertensive patients (52,54). Significantly greater sensitivity has been demonstrated by *echocardiography* (54–56). In recent years it has become apparent that a routine M-mode echocardiogram can provide more sensitive information than an electrocardiogram or a chest x-ray with regard to the presence and degree of left ventricular hypertrophy and enlargement of chamber size (see Chapter 26). Moreover, recent studies from two groups (55,56) indicate that the finding of increased left ventricular mass by echocardiographic studies has prognostic reference and may be even more prognostic than the blood pressure level itself for anticipating subsequent morbidity (i.e., stroke, heart attack, sudden death). Nevertheless, it should be remembered that left ventricular hypertrophy may occasionally be identified by electrocardiographic criteria when echocardiographic results are normal. This may occur when cardiac enlargement is still minimal, in the presence of myocardial ischemia sufficient to produce the inverted T-waves of the so-called *strain pattern* (57).

The *intravenous pyelogram* (IVP) should not be routinely used to screen for surgically curable renovascular disease. It has now been shown to be inefficient for that purpose. False-negative results occur in 10–30% of patients subsequently treated surgically (58,59). False-positive results of a similar degree also occur (58,60). At best, a positive IVP merely indicates more specific testing, and a negative IVP should not deter the physician from more specific tests when he strongly suspects renovascular disease.

In patients diagnosed as having renal disease, the IVP remains useful for defining renal architecture, size, and capacity for concentrating dye. However, as a screening procedure, it is relatively expensive, invasive, and carries some hazard. Simpler, more practical, and more specific screening tests are now available.

Identifying Curable Forms of Hypertension

The importance of identifying curable hypertension has been magnified nowadays by recent technologic advances —in particular, the advent of balloon angioplasty as a treatment for renovascular disease. With the development of the simple and inexpensive *captopril test* (61–64), to be discussed below, increasing numbers of candidates for balloon angioplasty are being found. In the last 3 years at The New York Hospital–Cornell Medical Center, more than 400 successful balloon dilatations have been carried out. Similar experiences are being reported from other large centers. It is safe to say that if not for the availability of the new diagnostic technology, a very large proportion (perhaps the majority) of these patients might have been assigned erroneously to the category of "essential hypertension" and placed on a regimen of antihypertensive drugs for the rest of their lives.

In view of this experience, it is now particularly unreasonable for the physician to apply long-term drug therapy before employing this technology to identify curable forms of hypertension. Rather, after a significant and sustained hypertension has been demonstrated, the first step is the establishment of normokalemia or hypokalemia and the determination of a normal renal function by serum urea and creatinine assays and a 24-hr urine for albumin. These are simple, but highly relevant, primary screening procedures, because they make it unnecessary to pursue identification of mineralocorticiod causes in the normokalemic group.

The *renin–sodium profile* is also included in the initial evaluation (9) (see Chapters 80, 82, 90). As indicated in the flow diagram (Fig. 1), low-renin patients who have hypokalemia are evaluated for curable adrenocortical disease. Curable primary aldosteronism is characterized typically by the diagnostic triad of: (i) serum potassium below 3.5

Hypertension: Pathophysiology, Diagnosis, and Management, edited by J. H. Laragh and B. M. Brenner. Raven Press, Ltd., New York © 1990.

CHAPTER 86

Diurnal Rhythms and Other Sources of Blood Pressure Variability in Normal and Hypertensive Subjects

Thomas G. Pickering

Changes of Blood Pressure During Sleep and Wakefulness, 1397
Hemodynamic and Neurohormonal Changes During Sleep, 1398
Is There a Circadian Rhythm of Blood Pressure?, 1398
Ultradian Rhythms, 1399
Effects of Physical and Mental Activity on Blood Pressure Patterns, 1399
Physical Activity, 1399
Ingestion, 1400
Mental Activity, 1400
Can the Effects of Factors Influencing Diurnal Variations of Blood Pressure be Quantified?, 1400
Comparison of Diurnal Patterns in Normal and Hypertensive Subjects, 1400
Sleep Apnea Syndrome, 1401
Other Conditions in Which the Normal Diurnal Pattern of Blood Pressure Is Altered, 1401
Seasonal Variations of Blood Pressure, 1401
Physiologic Regulation of Blood Pressure Variability, 1402
Effects of Antihypertensive Treatment on Blood Pressure Variability, 1402
Does Blood Pressure Variability Contribute to Cardiovascular Damage?, 1403
References, 1403

Blood pressure is not a fixed entity but, instead, fluctuates continuously throughout the day and night. Such fluctuations may be of very short duration (e.g., the changes associated with respiration) or of longer duration (e.g., diurnal or seasonal variations). This chapter will review what is known about the sources of such variability, how it is altered in disease, and its pathologic significance.

CHANGES OF BLOOD PRESSURE DURING SLEEP AND WAKEFULNESS

Sleep is an active process regulated by centers in the brain stem and composed of distinct cycles that recur regularly throughout the course of the night (1). Two basic varieties are recognized: nondreaming, or slow-wave sleep [so called because of low-frequency, high-amplitude waves on the electroencephalogram (EEG)], and dreaming, or REM (rapid eye movement) sleep, which occurs when the EEG shows low-voltage high-frequency activity similar to the pattern of wakefulness. The deepest stages of slow-wave sleep (Stages 3 and 4) occur in the first two hours of sleep; periods of REM sleep occur in 90-min cycles, with episodes lasting longer during the latter part of the night.

Blood pressure changes are closely linked to the level of arousal. During the first hour of sleep there is normally a progressive fall of blood pressure, which usually shows its maximal decrease of 15–20% two hours after sleep onset (2–9). This coincides with the deepest stages of slow-wave sleep (Stages 3 and 4). During REM sleep the blood pressure is at about the same level as in Stage 2 (approximately 10% less than during wakefulness) but is much more variable, with fluctuations of as much as 30 mmHg over a few minutes (2). Similar surges of pressure mediated by sympathetic vasoconstriction are also seen during K complexes, which are brief periods of arousal during Stages 1 and 2 sleep and which occur in response to external stimuli (5). Blood pressure rises immediately on waking. The close association between blood pressure and the level of arousal is further shown by the fact that in a drowsy subject the appearance of episodes of alpha rhythm is accompanied by surges of arterial pressure (5). The contrasting effects of sleep and wakefulness on blood pressure were well demonstrated in a study by Athanassiadis et al. (8); in patients in an accident ward, whose physical activity was limited by plaster casts, blood pressure remained relatively constant during the day and fell consistently by about 25% during sleep.

HEMODYNAMIC AND NEUROHORMONAL CHANGES DURING SLEEP

The fall of blood pressure during sleep is accompanied by a decreased heart rate (see Fig. 1). Cardiac output decreases by a modest amount (10), but there may also be vasodilation (9). Cerebral blood flow has been reported to be increased during sleep (11). Renal blood flow falls slightly (12), but there is a much more pronounced decrease in urine flow, which has been attributed to increased tubular reabsorption (12,13). This nocturnal oliguria is not a direct consequence of sleep, since it can persist independently of the sleep–wakefulness cycle (14), and is also not dependent on changes of posture (12). The composition of the urine also changes: There are large decreases in the excretion of sodium and chloride, but there are relatively small decreases in potassium and bicarbonate (13).

Plasma catecholamine levels fall during sleep, which would be consistent with a diminished sympathetic activity (15,16).

Plasma renin and aldosterone levels have usually been found to begin to rise steadily at the onset of sleep and reach their highest levels during the second half of the night (17,18). However, the nocturnal rise of renin is not directly related to sleep, since it persists in subjects who remain awake during the night (18,19). In such subjects the blood pressure does not change, so that the increase of renin release cannot be due to hypotension. It also does not appear to be due to a decreased sodium delivery to the macula densa, since it is not abolished by a saline infusion (18). It can be abolished by beta blockade, and so it is presumably mediated (at least in part) by the sympathetic nervous system (19). This subject remains confused, however, because the only study to use electroencephalographic monitoring of sleep failed to show any significant diurnal rhythm of renin secretion in normal subjects (20). This same study reported that renin secretion was shut off during episodes of REM sleep, which occur mainly during the second half of the night. It might be assumed that the rise of aldosterone is a consequence of increased renin and angiotensin formation, but it has been reported that while beta blockade prevents the nocturnal rise of renin, that of aldosterone persists (19).

Antidiuretic hormone (ADH) levels rise during the night, which could contribute to the nocturnal oliguria (21). Plasma atrial natriuretic peptide (ANP) was reported in one study to be elevated at night (21), but this does not occur if subjects remain recumbent throughout the entire 24-hr period (22).

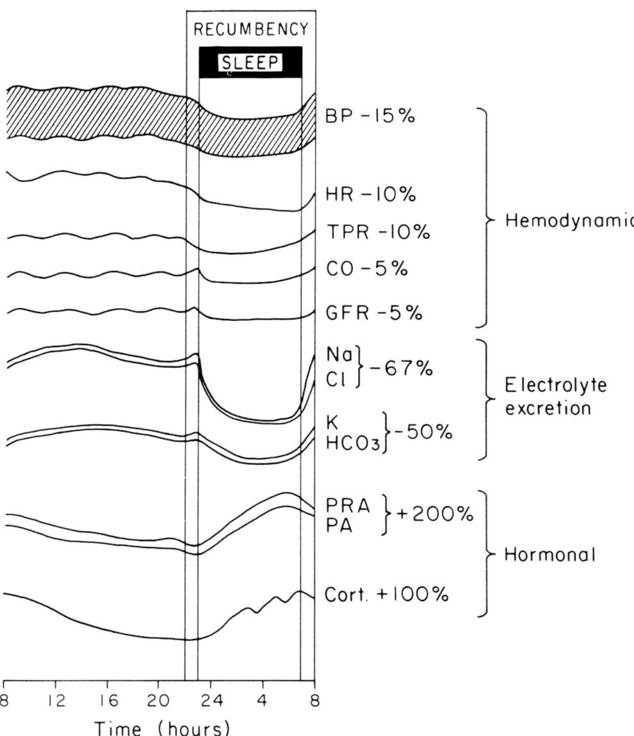

FIG. 1. Normal physiologic changes during sleep and wakefulness. From top to bottom: blood pressure (BP), heart rate (HR), total peripheral resistance (TPR), cardiac output (CO), glomerular filtration rate (GFR), electrolyte excretion (Na, Cl, K, HCO_3), plasma renin activity (PRA), plasma aldosterone (PA), and cortisol (Cort).

IS THERE A CIRCADIAN RHYTHM OF BLOOD PRESSURE?

Recordings made over 24 hours in ambulatory subjects, using either invasive (23) or noninvasive recorders (24), have typically shown that blood pressure tends to be highest in the morning, with a gradual decrease over the course of the day, and lowest during the night. This observation led to the suggestion that there might be an intrinsic circadian rhythm of blood pressure analogous to the circadian pattern of cortisol or body temperature. This led to the further suggestion that there might be a gradual increase of blood pressure during the early morning hours (3 a.m. to 6 a.m.) before the time of wakening and that this increase could contribute to the high incidence of cerebral hemorrhage and myocardial infarction in the early morning (23). Other workers, however, presented data which indicate that the apparently sinusoidal pattern of blood pressure was most probably an artifact attributable to the averaging of records from individuals who woke at different times: When the recordings are synchronized to the time of waking rather than the time of day, the early morning rise of pressure is no longer seen (25,26). Instead, blood pressure remains relatively stable during the hour before waking but rises abruptly at the moment of waking. This pattern is consistent with the changes described earlier (9), in studies where EEG was recorded as well as blood pressure.

The case for an intrinsic sinusoidal pattern of blood pressure variation has been argued most forcefully by Halberg et al. (27), who found that such curves fitted the blood pressure pattern of subjects kept in a confined environment for a period of several days.

The question as to whether there is an endogenous circadian rhythm of blood pressure, or whether the change can be accounted for by changes of activity, is an important one. It can best be answered by removing the influence of external stimuli, so that if the rhythm persists, it can be attributed to endogenous factors. This was done in the study by Athanassiadis et al. (8), in which blood pressure was monitored noninvasively for 24 hours in patients in an orthopedic ward who were immobilized by plaster casts. In this situation the blood pressure showed no evidence of any sinusoidal change, being relatively constant during the day but decreasing during sleep. Similar observations were made by Mann et al. (28) in hospitalized patients kept on bed rest. In the latter study, diurnal variations of pressure became more pronounced when subjects were studied a second time, but while being physically active during the day. Similar changes based on our own observations are shown in Fig. 2.

ULTRADIAN RHYTHMS

Circadian rhythms normally have a periodicity of approximately 24 hours, but there may also exist ultradian rhythms, which have a periodicity of approximately 90 min. These were first described for REM sleep (29) but may also be apparent during the day. Thus, a study using continuous monitoring of heart rate, blood pressure, and cardiac output in conscious dogs showed a 90-min periodicity of all three (30). It was concluded that the rhythm was due to phasic variations in the level of sympathetic drive to the heart, because this periodicity of both pressure and heart rate can be suppressed by clonidine (31). The amplitude of this ultradian rhythm of blood pressure may actually exceed the amplitude of the circadian rhythm in dogs.

It is not known to what extent ultradian rhythms of heart rate and blood pressure exist in humans. It seems reasonable to suppose that they do, but they might not be readily detectable in studies of free-ranging individuals, because they would be obscured by extraneous stimuli.

EFFECTS OF PHYSICAL AND MENTAL ACTIVITY ON BLOOD PRESSURE PATTERNS

A large number of activities have been identified which are likely to exert a significant influence on cardiovascular variables that are studied by ambulatory monitoring. Most of the published studies have dealt with blood pressure, but their findings are in many cases likely to apply to heart rate as well.

If the effects of environmental stimuli and changes in physical activity are minimized, the profile of blood pressure during the day becomes relatively flat, with a fall of about 20% occurring during sleep (8,28). It has also been shown that diurnal blood pressure changes are less pronounced in hospitalized patients than in patients studied in their natural environment (32). Both the average level of blood pressure and its variability are reduced during periods of bed rest as compared to periods of physical activity (33). Some of the more relevant activities influencing the changes of blood pressure and other variables that might be detected by ambulatory monitoring are briefly reviewed below; they are divided into physical and mental activities, although obviously there is considerable overlap.

Physical Activity

Blood pressure, heart rate, and plasma norepinephrine are usually at their maximum during intense physical exercise and are at their lowest level during sleep (34). The percentage changes of pressure are generally similar in normal and hypertensive subjects. A mildly hypertensive patient with a resting systolic pressure of 140 mmHg might be expected to reach a level of 240 mmHg during exercise and 120 mmHg during sleep (34). The position of the subject is also important. Large increases of pressure and heart rate are also seen during another form of exercise, sexual intercourse, ranging from 25 to 120 mmHg in systolic pressure and from 24 to 48 mmHg in diastolic pressure. These changes are reversed within a few minutes after orgasm

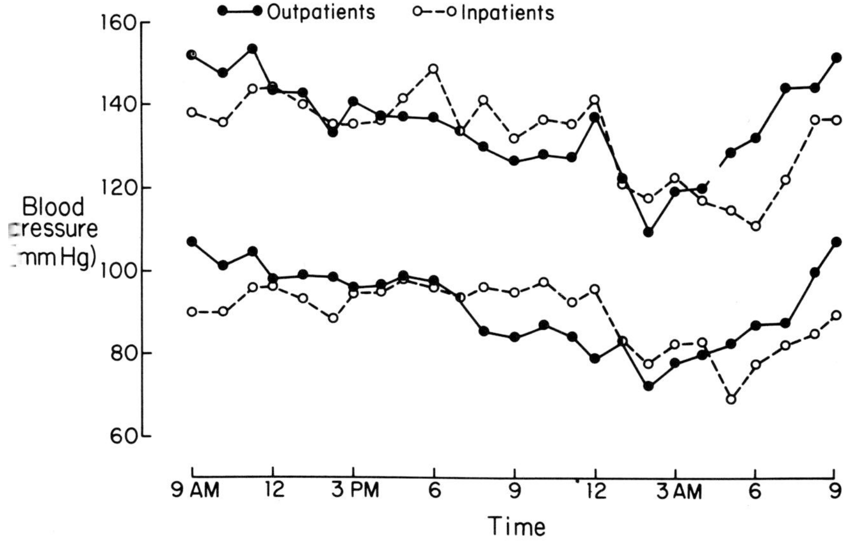

FIG. 2. Comparison of diurnal blood pressure patterns in two groups of subjects: inpatients, studied in hospital with restricted activities, and outpatients, studied during normal activities. Note the greater diurnal variation in the latter. The apparent early morning rise of pressure in the outpatients may be attributed to different times of waking.

(35). Transient changes occur during micturition and defecation (36). Laboratory studies by Lynch's group have shown that talking is also a potent pressor stimulus; the cardiovascular changes depend both on physical factors such as the rate of talking (37) and on psychological factors such as the size of the audience (38). Both systolic and diastolic pressure increase, and the absolute changes are somewhat bigger in hypertensive than in normotensive subjects (39).

Ingestion

Most of the studies investigating the effects of ingested substances have been carried out in the laboratory, but their results may in most cases be extrapolated to the field. For three hours after a meal there is an increase of heart rate, a decrease of diastolic pressure, and little change of systolic pressure (40). In older subjects there may be a pronounced fall of both systolic and diastolic pressure after food (41). Smoking a cigarette raises both heart rate and blood pressure for about 15 min (42,43). Alcohol may increase heart rate, with small but variable effects on blood pressure in normal subjects (44–46). Caffeine can increase blood pressure, plasma catecholamines, and renin, but not heart rate (47), although these changes are diminished in people who take it regularly (48). Older subjects show a bigger increase of blood pressure (48). Caffeine may also augment the blood pressure response to acute psychologic stress (49). Coffee and cigarettes are often taken together, and a study by Freestone and Ramsey showed that they may have an additive effect, causing blood pressure to remain elevated for two hours or longer (50).

It is likely that other factors such as dietary sodium intake may influence blood pressure variations during ambulatory monitoring (51), although little direct information is available concerning it.

Mental Activity

At least two studies have reported some correlation between self-rated mental "stress" or "arousal" and blood pressure during noninvasive ambulatory monitoring (52,53). We have reported higher levels of blood pressure when people are at work than when they are at home (as shown in Fig. 2), which we have attributed to mental factors rather than physical factors, because most of our subjects had sedentary jobs (54,55).

Mood has also been reported to be a potent determinant of blood pressure during ambulatory monitoring. We have found that self-reported levels of anger, anxiety, and happiness are correlated with pressure: systolic pressure decreased as the intensity of happiness increased, and diastolic pressure increased with the intensity of anxiety (56). A number of other factors may be expected to influence blood pressure changes during ambulatory monitoring, although they have not yet been studied in this context. They include both genetic factors (family history of hypertension) and environmental factors (e.g., seasonal variations, noise, and crowding).

CAN THE EFFECTS OF FACTORS INFLUENCING DIURNAL VARIATIONS OF BLOOD PRESSURE BE QUANTIFIED?

In the past, analyses of ambulatory recordings of heart rate and blood pressure have typically expressed the data in terms of the mean level plus an overall measure of variability. While this approach provides much useful information, students of behavior are going to want to quantify the effects of specific activities or moods on such variables. In the case of blood pressure, we were interested to see how much of the overall variance could be accounted for by changes of activity (24). We found that the average effect of 15 commonly occurring activities (including sleep) on blood pressure (using the patient's clinic pressure as a covariate) accounted for 41% of systolic variance and 36% of diastolic variance. Time of day was a less important determinant of blood pressure.

Although these modeling techniques can account for a sizable portion of the overall variation of blood pressure or other variables, it is only a first approximation. Thus, the idea that the effects of each activity can be represented by a single coefficient is an oversimplification, because the intensity of any activity may vary, and individual subjects will have different pressure responses to the same activity, e.g., from differences in baroreflex sensitivity. Furthermore, it is not clear to what extent the effects of one activity "carry over" to another. We are currently exploring the hypothesis that blood pressures measured at home in the evening are higher if the subject has been to work earlier in the day as compared to being at home all day.

COMPARISON OF DIURNAL PATTERNS IN NORMAL AND HYPERTENSIVE SUBJECTS

In patients with hypertension the diurnal pattern of blood pressure change is generally similar to the changes occurring in normotensive subjects, except that the entire blood pressure profile is shifted upward (Fig. 3). Thus, the differences between work and home pressures and between home and sleep pressures are approximately the same in normotensive and hypertensive subjects (about a 20% decrease during sleep in both cases) when expressed on a percentage basis, although in absolute terms they may be greater in hypertensives (6,55,57). Similar changes have been reported for subjects with essential and renovascular hypertension (58). There are some situations in which the fall of blood pressure during sleep in hypertensive patients may be absent or reversed. It has been reported that blood pressure does not fall during sleep in patients with malignant hypertension (59) or with pheochromocytoma (60). During normal pregnancy there is a normal fall of blood pressure during sleep (61), but in patients with preeclamptic toxemia this fall may be absent or reversed, with an increase of pressure during sleep (62).

The diurnal hormonal patterns are also altered in hypertension. The nocturnal rise of renin is still seen in patients with borderline hypertension but is absent in those with more severe hypertension (19). Aldosterone, however, rises in both situations. In hypertensive subjects the decrease of

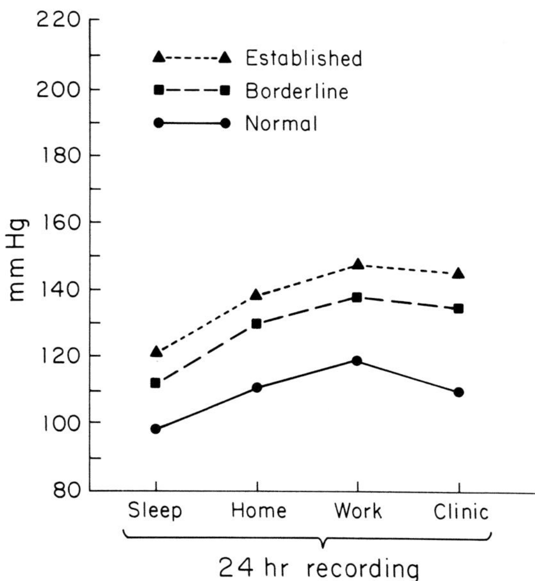

FIG. 3. Diurnal blood pressure profile in normotensive subjects and in patients with mild (borderline) or moderate (established) hypertension.

plasma norepinephrine that is normally seen during sleep still occurs but is somewhat less pronounced (63). When hypertensive subjects are studied in the recumbent position for 24 hours, with the influence of extraneous stimuli removed, there is a good correlation between plasma norepinephrine and arterial pressure (63). Diurnal changes of blood pressure have also been reported to correlate with changes of plasma renin activity and of norepinephrine (64) in patients with renovascular hypertension. In hypertensive subjects the normal diurnal pattern of sodium excretion, with a pronounced decrease during the night, may be absent or even reversed (65). This is of potential practical importance because overnight urine collections are sometimes used in lieu of 24-hr collections and, hence, may give misleading results.

In preeclampsia the normal hormonal patterns may be altered: Although both renin and angiotensin II are generally lower than in normal pregnancies, angiotensin II levels show a smaller decrease during the night. Plasma norepinephrine shows a normal pattern, but plasma epinephrine may rise. Thus, it has been suggested that the nocturnal rise of blood pressure in these patients might be caused by the relative elevation of either epinephrine or angiotensin II (66).

Conditions in which the diurnal rhythm of pressure is absent or reversed are listed in Table 1.

SLEEP APNEA SYNDROME

Sleep apnea syndrome is a condition that is probably underdiagnosed. It mainly effects middle-aged men, and its hallmark is episodic and repetitive apneic episodes occurring throughout the night, probably as a result of mechanical obstruction of the airways. The patient's spouse may complain that he snores; snoring is associated with an increased risk of cerebral infarction, independently of blood pressure (67). During the end of each apneic period, blood pressure may rise, so that such patients may have significant hypertension during the night (68). There is also evidence that a sizable proportion of such patients may be hypertensive during the day (69). Characteristic symptoms include daytime sleepiness, snoring, disturbed sleep, morning headaches, and fatigue. One recent survey of patients with essential hypertension found that 22% had sleep apnea syndrome (70). That the apneic episodes may be responsible for the daytime hypertension is suggested by a report of two hypertensive adolescents whose sleep apnea was relieved by tracheostomy and whose hypertension was also cured (71).

OTHER CONDITIONS IN WHICH THE NORMAL DIURNAL PATTERN OF BLOOD PRESSURE IS ALTERED

Patients suffering from idiopathic orthostatic hypotension have been found to exhibit (a) a paradoxical elevation of pressure during the first part of the night and (b) the lowest pressures of the day during the morning, when they are typically most symptomatic (72). These pressure changes are associated with less consistent changes of heart rate, which may either decrease during the night or show little change. The nocturnal rise of pressure cannot be explained purely on the basis of recumbency, because it is still seen in patients who are recumbent for the full 24 hours. This increase of pressure is associated with a nocturnal polyuria, which has been attributed to a pressure natriuresis.

Cardiac denervation is another situation where pressure increases at night. This has been observed in patients with cardiac transplants (73) and has also been observed in diabetics, where autonomic neuropathy may also cause partial denervation of the heart (73). The mechanism is unexplained but could, in part, be due to increased venous filling of the heart associated with recumbency.

SEASONAL VARIATIONS OF BLOOD PRESSURE

At any rate in temperate climates, blood pressure is about 5 mmHg higher in winter than in summer. The effect appears to be a direct consequence of changes of environmental temperature and is more marked in older subjects than in younger ones (74,75). It has also been observed in children, however (76).

TABLE 1. *Conditions in which the normal diurnal rhythm of blood pressure is altered*

Sleep apnea syndrome
Preeclamptic toxemia
Pheochromocytoma
Malignant hypertension
Cardiac transplantation
Idiopathic orthostatic hypotension
Diabetes mellitus (with autonomic neuropathy)

PHYSIOLOGIC REGULATION OF BLOOD PRESSURE VARIABILITY

Blood pressure variability is a term that is often used rather loosely, and it can be used to describe a variety of sources of variation having a time course ranging from a few seconds (respiratory variations) to 1 year (seasonal variations), as shown in Fig. 4. Thus it may include situations as diverse as (a) variations in clinic pressure from one visit to another or (b) variability over 24 hours.

Short-term blood pressure variability, of which respiratory fluctuation is the dominant cause, can only be assessed by beat-to-beat monitoring, e.g., using intra-arterial recording. Blood pressure normally falls during inspiration as stroke volume falls, and the heart slows. This variability seems to be largely under vagal control (presumably via the effect on heart rate), since it persists despite blockade of either the alpha- or beta-adrenergic system, but is attenuated by vagal blockade with atropine (77,78). Thus, such blood pressure variations are significantly correlated with variations of cardiac output and heart rate, but not of stroke volume or peripheral resistance (79). Such variability is more pronounced in patients with higher pressures (80).

Variability of blood pressure during the course of the day has been the subject of several studies using intra-arterial ambulatory monitoring. When the distribution of blood pressure values over a full 24-hr period is plotted, the result is a bimodal plot: One mode corresponds to daytime values, and the other one corresponds to sleep (81). A consistent finding from these studies has been that subjects with diminished baroreflex sensitivity show increased blood pressure variability, with an inverse correlation between the two (82,83). In this situation the heart rate changes are buffering rather than causing the variations of blood pressure. Conway et al. (84) found that subjects with high baroreflex sensitivity showed greater heart rate variability during ambulatory monitoring, and a smaller fall of blood pressure during the night, than subjects with lower reflex sensitivity.

The autonomic nervous system is thought to play the dominant role in regulating blood pressure changes during normal activities, including the diurnal or circadian changes. Thus, blood pressure varies over 24 hours in parallel with changes in plasma catecholamines (63). In the rat, much of the apparently spontaneous variability of blood pressure can be attributed to activities such as eating, drinking, grooming, and exploring (85). The effects of these activities on pressure are greatly attenuated by chemosympathectomy. Individual differences in plasma catecholamine levels are not correlated with differences in blood pressure variability (86). Variability also increases as a function of age (86); this can only be partly attributed to the diminished baroreflex sensitivity associated with aging (87). Blood pressure variability may also be increased when plasma renin activity is high (86).

These changes of variability depend to some extent on which measure is used. Thus, the increased variability in hypertensive individuals is much less pronounced if expressed as the coefficient of variation (which allows for differences in baseline levels) rather than as the standard deviation (which does not).

EFFECTS OF ANTIHYPERTENSIVE TREATMENT ON BLOOD PRESSURE VARIABILITY

Since there is abundant evidence to indicate that the autonomic nervous system, and perhaps also the renin–angiotensin system, modulates short-term blood pressure variability, it would be expected that antihypertensive medications, particularly those which specifically block the actions of one of these mechanisms, would reduce blood pressure variability. Surprisingly, this is not the case.

In ambulatory monitoring studies of hypertensive pa-

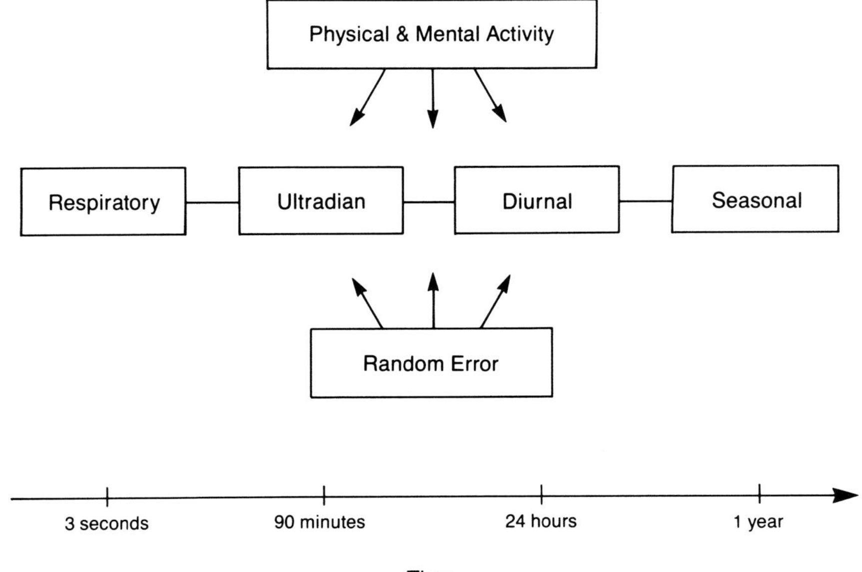

FIG. 4. Sources of blood pressure variability. There are basic rhythms of varying periodicity (respiratory, ultradian, diurnal, and seasonal) upon which are superimposed effects of physical and mental activity and random error.

tients, it has often been observed that the changes of blood pressure during sleep are similar on and off treatment. This has been observed for diuretics, beta-blockers (6,58), and nifedipine (88). In other studies (e.g., with verapamil or enalapril), treatment resulted in a slightly smaller decrease during sleep (88).

Daytime variability of blood pressure has been studied in two ways: first, by measuring the blood pressure response to specific tests, which may be physical (e.g., exercise) or behavioral (e.g., mental arithmetic); and second, by computing blood pressure variability on and off treatment during normal activities. Several studies have reported that the increase of pressure occurring in response to specific challenges is little affected by treatment, even though the basal level of pressure is lowered. This has been reported for calcium antagonists (88), diuretics (89), reserpine (90), and beta blockers (91,92). Some attenuation may occur with (a) peripheral adrenergic antagonists such as bethanidine (92) and (b) prazosin (93).

Spontaneous blood pressure variability measured by intra-arterial blood pressure monitoring is affected little, if at all, by treatment. This has been reported for a number of agents, including (a) those which act directly on the sympathetic nervous system, such as clonidine (94), and (b) beta blockers (95,96).

DOES BLOOD PRESSURE VARIABILITY CONTRIBUTE TO CARDIOVASCULAR DAMAGE?

It is not known what component of the arterial pressure leads to vascular damage. Hypertension leads to morbid events by two main processes: first, by causing blood vessels to burst (as in cerebral hemorrhage); and second, by accelerating the formation of atheromatous plaques. In both cases it is likely that mechanical factors play a major role, although hormonal factors may contribute independently of blood pressure (97). As O'Rourke (98) has observed, physical materials are relatively resistant to continuous levels of stress and are more susceptible to intermittent stress. If this also applies to the effects of blood pressure on the arterial wall, the mean arterial pressure may be much less important than the rate of change of pressure. Hence, it might be expected, on theoretical grounds, that individuals with increased lability of blood pressure would suffer more vascular damage.

Unfortunately, no definitive answer can be given to this question at the present time. In experimental animals, blood pressure variability can be increased by sectioning the carotid sinus and aortic baroreceptor nerves (99,100). This does not necessarily lead to sustained hypertension, however, and so far as is known, it does not lead to accelerated vascular damage, although this latter question has received relatively little attention.

In humans there is even less information, although there have been case reports of individuals who appear to have increased blood pressure lability secondary to a greatly impaired baroreflex sensitivity and who also do not have sustained hypertension (101). A small number of cross-sectional studies have attempted to get at this problem, but their findings must be interpreted with great caution, because it is difficult to draw causal inferences from them. Kobrin et al. (102) classified elderly hypertensive patients in two groups according to whether or not blood pressure fell during the night. Patients whose pressure did not fall had a higher prevalence of atherosclerotic complications and left ventricular hypertrophy than those whose pressure showed the normal decline. In another study using intra-arterial monitoring, Parati et al. (103) found that subjects whose 24-hr variability was higher than the group average were more likely to have target organ damage. In this study, variability was measured over 30-min epochs, so that this would not be influenced by circadian variations of pressure to a great extent. However, it is not clear from these studies which is cause and which is effect, because subjects with more advanced hypertension and more target organ damage are likely to have a diminished baroreflex sensitivity and, hence, more labile blood pressure.

REFERENCES

1. Kleitman N. *Sleep and wakefulness.* Chicago: University of Chicago Press, 1963.
2. Snyder F, Hobson JA, Morrison DF, et al. Changes in respirations, heart rate, and systolic blood pressure in human sleep. *J Appl Physiol* 1964;19:417–422.
3. Coccagna G, Mantovani M, Brignani F, et al. Arterial pressure changes during spontaneous sleep in man. *Electroencephalogr Clin Neurophysicl* 1971;31:277–281.
4. Khatri IM, Fries ED. Hemodynamic changes during sleep. *J Appl Physiol* 1967;22:867–873.
5. Richardson DW, Honour AJ, Goodman AC. Changes in arterial pressure during sleep in man. *Hypertension* 1968;16:62–78.
6. Littler WA, Honour AJ, Carter RD, Sleight P. Sleep and blood pressure. *Br Med J* 1975;3:346–348.
7. Pickering TG. Sleep, circadian rhythms and cardiovascular disease. *Cardiovasc Rev Rep* 1980;1:37–47.
8. Athanassiadis D, Draper GJ, Honour AJ, Cranston WI. Variability of automatic blood pressure measurements over 24 hour periods. *Clin Sci* 1969;36:147–156.
9. Bristow JD, Honour AJ, Pickering TG, Sleight P. Cardiovascular and respiratory changes during sleep in normal and hypertensive subjects. *Cardiovasc Med* 1969;3:476–486.
10. Khatri IM, Fries ED. Hemodynamic changes during sleep. *J Appl Physiol* 1967;22:867–873.
11. Townsend RE, Prinz PN, Abrist WD. Human cerebral blood flow during sleep and waking. *J Appl Physiol* 1973;35:620–625.
12. Stanbury SW, Thompson AE. Diurnal variations in electrolyte excretion. *Clin Sci* 1951;10:267–293.
13. Sirota JH, Baldwin DW, Villareal H. Diurnal variations of renal function in man. *J Clin Invest* 1950;29:187–192.
14. Mills JN. Diurnal rhythm in urine flow. *J Physiol* 1950;113:528–536.
15. Dollery CT, Hamilton CA, Maling TJB. Changes in sleep pattern, blood pressure, heart rate, and plasma noradrenaline after night-time administration of slow release clonidine. *Clin Sci* 1979;57:509–514.
16. Watson RDS, Reid JL, Hamilton CA, Littler WA. Plasma noradrenaline, physical activity and systolic blood pressure in hypertension. *Clin Sci Mol Med* 1978;54:26P.
17. Brever H, Kaulhausen H, Mühlbauer W. Circadian rhythm of the renin–angiotensin–aldosterone system. In: *Chronobiological aspects of endocrinology.* Symposia Medica Hoechst. 9. Stuttgart: Schattauer Verlag, 1974;101–109.
18. Modlinger RS, Scharif-Zadeh K, Ertel NH, et al. The circadian rhythm of renin. *J Clin Endocrinol Metab* 1976;43:1276–1282.
19. Stumpe KO, Kolloch R, Vetter H, et al. Acute and long-term studies of the mechanisms of action of beta-blocking drugs in lowering blood pressure. *Am J Med* 1976;60:853–865.

20. Mullen PE, James VHT, Lightman SL, Linsell C, Peart WS. A relationship between plasma renin activity and the rapid eye movement phase of sleep in man. *J Clin Endocrinol Metab* 1980;50:466–469.
21. Donckier J, Anderson JV, Yeo T, Bloom SR. Diurnal rhythm in the plasma concentration of atrial natriuretic peptide. *N Engl J Med* 1986;315:710–711.
22. Richards AM, Tonolo G, Fraser R, Morton JJ, Leckie BJ, Ball SG, Robertson JIS. Diurnal changes in plasma atrial natriuretic peptide concentrations. *Clin Sci* 1987;73:489–495.
23. Millar-Craig MW, Bishop CN, Raftery EB. Circadian variation of blood-pressure. *Lancet* 1978;1:795–797.
24. Clark LA, Denby L, Pregibon D, Harshfield GA, Pickering TG, Blank S, Laragh JH. The effects of activity and time of day on the diurnal variations of blood pressure. *J Chronic Dis* 1987;40:671–681.
25. Littler WA, Watson RDS. Circadian variation in blood pressure. *Lancet* 1978;1:995–996.
26. Floras JS, Jones JV, Johnston JA, Brooks DE, Hussan MO, Sleight P. Arousal and the circadian rhythm of blood pressure. *Clin Sci Mol Med* 1978;55:395S–397S.
27. Halberg F, Halberg E, Halberg J, Halberg F. Chronobiologic assessment of human blood pressure variation in health and disease. In: Weber MA, Drayer JIM, eds. *Ambulatory blood pressure monitoring.* Darmstadt: Steinkopff, 1984;137–156.
28. Mann S, Millar-Craig MW, Melville DI, Balasubramanian V, Raftery EB. Physical activity and the circadian rhythm of blood pressure. *Clin Sci* 1979;57:291S–294S.
29. Aserinsky E, Kleitman N. Regularly occurring periods of eye motility, and concomitant phenomena, during sleep. *Science* 1953;118:273–274.
30. Shimada SG, Marsh DJ. Oscillations in mean arterial pressure in conscious dogs. *Circ Res* 1979;44:692–700.
31. Livnat A, Zehr JE, Broten TP. Ultradian oscillations in blood pressure and heart rate in free-running dogs. *Am J Physiol* 1984;246:R817–R824.
32. Young MA, Rowlands DB, Stallard TH, Watson RDS, Littler WA. Effect of environment on blood pressure: home versus hospital. *Br Med J* 1983;286:1235–1236.
33. Rowlands DB, Stallard TJ, Watson RDS, Littler WA. The influence of physical activity on arterial pressure during ambulatory recordings in man. *Clin Sci* 1980;58:115–117.
34. Watson RDS, Hamilton CA, Reid JL, Littler WA. Changes in plasma norepinephrine, blood pressure and heart rate during physical activity in hypertensive man. *Hypertension* 1979; 1:341–346.
35. Littler WA, Honour AJ, Sleight P. Direct arterial pressure, heart rate, and electrocardiogram during human coitus. *J Reprod Fertil* 1974;40:321–331.
36. Littler WA, Honour AJ, Sleight P. Direct arterial pressure, pulse rate, and electrocardiogram during micturition and defecation in unrestricted man. *Am Heart J* 1974;88:205–210.
37. Friedman E, Thomas SA, Kulick-Ciuffo D, Lynch JJ, Suginahara M. The effects of normal and rapid speech on blood pressure. *Psychosom Med* 1982;44:545–553.
38. Thomas SA, Friedman E, Lottes LS, Gresty S, Miller C, Lynch JJ. Changes in nurses' blood pressure and heart rate while communicating. *Res Nurs Health* 1984;7:119–126.
39. Lynch JJ, Long JM, Thomas SA, Malinow KL, Katcher AH. The effects of talking on the blood pressure of hypertensive and normotensive individuals. *Psychosom Med* 1981;43:25–33.
40. Fagan TC, Conrad KA, Mar HJ, Nelson L. Effects of meals on hemodynamics: implications for antihypertensive drug studies. *Clin Pharmacol Ther* 1986;39:255–260.
41. Lipsitz LA, Nyquist RP, Wei JY, Rowe JW. Postprandial reduction in blood pressure in the elderly. *N Engl J Med* 1983;309:81–83.
42. Cellina GU, Honour AJ, Littler WA. Direct arterial pressure, heart rate, and electrocardiogram during cigarette smoking in unrestricted patients. *Am Heart J* 1975;89:18–25.
43. Roth GM, McDonald JB, Sheard C. The effect of smoking cigarettes, and of intravenous administration of nicotine on the electrocardiogram, basal metabolic rate, cutaneous temperature, blood pressure, and pulse rate of normal persons. *JAMA* 1944;125:751–767.
44. Larbi EB, Cooper RS, Stamler J. Alcohol and hypertension. *Arch Intern Med* 1983;143:28–29.
45. Orlando J, Aronow WS, Cassidy J, Prakash R. Effect of ethanol on angina pectoris. *Ann Intern Med* 1976;84:652–655.
46. Gould L, Zahir M, DeMartino A, Gomprecht RF. The cardiac effects of a cocktail. *JAMA* 1971;218:1799–1802.
47. Robertson D, Frolich JC, Carr RK, Watson JT, Hollifield JW, Shand DG, Oates JA. Effects of caffeine on plasma renin activity, catecholamines and blood pressure. *N Engl J Med* 1978; 298:181–186.
48. Izzo JL, Ghosal A, Kwong T, Freeman RB, Jaenike JR. Age and prior caffeine use alter the cardiovascular and adrenomedullary responses to oral caffeine. *Am J Cardiol* 1983;52:769–773.
49. Lane JD. Caffeine and cardiovascular response to stress. *Psychosom Med* 1983;45:447–451.
50. Freestone S, Ramsey LE. Effect of coffee and cigarette smoking on the blood pressure of untreated and diuretic-treated hypertensive patients. *Am J Med* 1982;73:348–353.
51. Richards AM, Nicholls MG, Espiner EA, Ikram H, Maslowski AH, Hamilton EJ, Wells JE. Blood-pressure response to moderate sodium restriction and to potassium supplementation in mild essential hypertension. *Lancet* 1984;1:757–761.
52. Dembroski TM, MacDougall JM. Validation of the Vita-Stat automated noninvasive ambulatory blood pressure recording device. In: Herd JA, Gotto AM, Kaufmann PG, Weiss SM, ed. *Cardiovascular instrumentation.* Bethesda, MD: NIH publication no. 84-1654, 1984;55–77.
53. Schmieder R, Rüddel H, Langewitz W, Neus J, Wagner O, von Eiff AW. The influence of monotherapy with oxprenolol and nitrendipine on ambulatory blood pressure in hypertensives. *Clin Exp Hypertens* 1985;A7:445–454.
54. Harshfield GA, Pickering TG, Kleinert HD, Blank S, Laragh JH. Situational variation of blood pressure in ambulatory hypertensive patients. *Psychosom Med* 1982;44:237–245.
55. Pickering TG, Harshfield GA, Kleinert HD, Blank S, Laragh JH. Blood pressure during normal daily activities, sleep, and exercise. Comparison of values in normal and hypertensive subjects. *JAMA* 1982;247:992–996.
56. James GD, Yee LS, Harshfield GA, Blank SG, Pickering TG. The influence of happiness, anger, and anxiety on the blood pressure of borderline hypertensives. *Psychosom Med* 1986;48:502–508.
57. Messerli FH, Glade LB, Ventura HO, Dreslinski GR, Suarez DH, MacPhee AA, Aristimuno GG, Cole FE, Frohlich ED. Diurnal variations of cardiac rhythm, arterial pressure, and urinary catecholamines in borderline and established essential hypertension. *Am Heart J* 1982;104:109–113.
58. Reeves RA, Johnson AM, Shapiro AP, Traub YM, Jacob R. Ambulatory blood pressure monitoring: methods to assess severity of hypertension, variability and sleep changes. In: Weber MA, Drayer JIM, eds. *Ambulatory blood pressure monitoring.* Darmstadt: Steinkopff, 1984;27–34.
59. Shaw DB, Knapp MS, Davies DH. Variations in blood pressure in hypertensives during sleep. *Lancet* 1963;1:797–798.
60. Littler WA, Honour AJ. Direct arterial pressure, heart rate, and electrocardiogram in unrestricted patients before and after removal of a phaeochromocytoma. *Am J Med* 1979;53:441–449.
61. Seligman SA. Diurnal blood pressure variation in pregnancy. *Obstet Gynecol* 1971;79:417–422.
62. Redman CWG, Beilin LJ, Bonnar J. Reversed diurnal blood pressure rhythm in hypertensive pregnancies. *Clin Sci Mol Med* 1976;51:687s–689s.
63. Sowers JR. Dopaminergic control of circadian norepinephrine levels in patients with essential hypertension. *J Clin Endocrinol Metab* 1981;53:1133–1137.
64. Maslowski AH, Nicholls MG, Espiuner EA, Ikram H, Bones PJ. Mechanisms in human renovascular hypertension. *Hypertension* 1983;5:597–602.
65. Dyer AR, Stamler R, Grimm R, Stamler J, Berman R, Gosch FC, Emidy LA, Elmer P, Fishman J, Van Heel N, Civinelli G. Do

hypertensive patients have a different diurnal pattern of electrolyte excretion? *Hypertension* 1987;10:417–424.

66. Beilin LJ, Deacon J, Michael CA, Vandougen R, Labor CM, Barden AE, Davidson L, Rouse I. Diurnal rhythms of blood pressure, plasma renin activity, angiotensin II and catcholamines in normotensive and hypertensive pregnancies. *Clin Exp Hypertens—Hypertens Pregnancy* 1983;B2(2):271–293.
67. Partinen M, Palomaki H. Snoring and cerebral infarction. *Lancet* 1985;2:1325–1326.
68. Tilkian AG, Guilleminault C, Schroeder JS, et al. Hemodynamics in sleep-induced apnea studies during wakefulness and sleep. *Ann Intern Med* 1976;85:714.
69. Guilleminault C, Tilkian A, Dement W. The sleep apnea syndromes. *Annu Rev Med* 1976;27:465–484.
70. Lavie P, Ben-Yosef R, Rubin A-H. Prevalence of sleep apnea syndrome among patients with essential hypertension. *Am Heart J* 1984;108:373–376.
71. Guilleminault C, Eldridge FL, Simmons FB, Dement WC. Sleep apnea in eight children. *Pediatrics* 1976;58:23–30.
72. Mann S, Altman DG, Raftery EB, Bannister R. Circadian variation of blood pressure in autonomic failure. *Circulation* 1983;68:477–483.
73. Reeves RA, Shapiro AP, Thompson ME, Johnsen AM. Loss of nocturnal decline in blood pressure after cardiac transplantation. *Circulation* 1986;73:401–408.
74. Brennan PJ, Greenberg G, Miall WE, Thompson SG. Seasonal variations in arterial blood pressure. *Br Med J* 1982;285:919–923.
75. Khaw K-T, Barrett-Connor E, Suarez L. Seasonal and secular variation in blood pressure in man. *J Cardiac Rehabil* 1984;4:440–444.
76. Jenner DA, English DR, Vandongen R, Beilin LJ, Armstrong BK, Dunbar D. Environmental temperature and blood pressure in 9-year old Australian children. *J Hypertens* 1987;5:683–686.
77. Clement DL, DePue N, Jordaens LJ, Packet L. Adrenergic and vagal influences on blood pressure variability. *Clin Exp Hypertens* 1985;A7(2&3):159–166.
78. Clement DL, Jordaens LJ, Heyndrickx GR. Influence of vagal nervous activity on blood pressure variability. *J Hypertens* 1984;2(Suppl 3):391–393.
79. Anderson DE, Yaighing JE, Sagawa K. Minute-to-minute covariations in cardiovascular activity of conscious dogs. *Am J Physiol* 1979;236:H434–H439.
80. Clement DL, Mussche MM, Vanhoutte G, Pannier R. Is blood pressure variability related to the activity of the sympathetic system? *Clin Sci* 1979;57:217S–219S.
81. Littler WA, West MJ, Honour AJ, Sleight P. The variability of arterial pressure. *Am Heart J* 1978;95:180–186.
82. Mancia G, Ferrari A, Gregorini L, Parati G, Pomidossi G, Bertinieri G, Grassi G, Zanchetti A. Blood pressure variability in man: Its relation to high blood pressure, age, and baroreflex sensitivity. *Clin Sci* 1980;59:401S–410S.
83. Mancia G, Parati G, Pomidossi G, Casadei R, Di Rienzo M, Zanchetti A. Arterial baroreflexes and blood pressure and heart rate variabilities in humans. *Hypertension* 1985;8:147–153.
84. Conway J, Boon N, Vann Jones J, Sleight P. Mechanisms concerned with blood pressure variability throughout the day. *Clin Exp Hypertens* 1985;A7(2&3):153–157.
85. Le Doux JR, Del Bo A, Tucker LW, Harshfield G, Talman WT, Reis DJ. Hierarchic organization of blood pressure responses during the expression of natural behaviors in rat: medication by sympathetic nerves. *Exp Neurol* 1982;78:121–133.
86. Watson RDS, Stallard TJS, Flinn RM, Littler WA. Factors determining direct arterial pressure and its variability in hypertensive man. *Hypertension* 1980;2:333–341.
87. Mancia G, Ferrari A, Gregorini L, Parati G, Pomidossi G, Bertinieri G, Grassi G, Zanchetti A. Blood pressure variability in man: its relation to high blood pressure, age, and baroreflex sensitivity. *Clin Sci* 1980;59:401s–404s.
88. Jones RI, Gould RA, Hornung RS, Mann S, Raftery EB. Intra-arterial ambulatory blood pressure monitoring in the assessment of antihypertensive drugs. In: Weber MA, Drayer JIM, eds. *Ambulatory blood pressure monitoring.* Darmstadt: Steinkopff, 1984;233–241.
89. Falkner B, Onesti G, Affrime MB, Lowenthal DT. Effects of clonidine and hydrochlorothiazide in the cardiovascular response to mental stress in adolescent hypertension. *Clin Sci* 1982;63:455s–458s.
90. Shapiro AP. Pressor response to noxious stimuli in hypertensive patients. Effects of reserpine and chlorothiazide. *Circulation* 1962;26:242–250.
91. Bonelli J, Hörtnagl DH, Brücke T, Magometschnigg D, Locks H, Kaik G. Effects of calculation stress on hemodynamics and plasma catecholamines before and after β-blockade with propranolol (Inderal) and mepindolol sulfate (Corindolam). *Eur J Clin Pharmacol* 1979;15:1–8.
92. Watt SH, Thomas RD, Belfield PW, Goldstraw PW, Taylor SH. Influence of sympatholytic drugs on the cardiovascular response to isometric exercise. *Clin Sci* 1981;60:139–143.
93. Harmada M, Kazatani Y, Shigematsu Y, Ito T, Kokubu T, Ishise S. Enhanced blood pressure response to isometric handgrip exercise in patients with essential hypertension: effects of propranolol and prazosin. *J Hypertens* 1987;5:305–309.
94. Mancia G, Ferrari A, Gregorini L, Parati G, Pomidossi G, Grassi G, Bertinieri G, Zanchetti A. Evaluation of a slow-release clonidine preparation by direct continuous blood pressure recording in essential hypertensive patients. *J Cardiovasc Pharmacol* 1981;3:1193–1202.
95. West MJ, Sleight P, Honour AJ. Clinical trial of the β-adrenoreceptor-blocking agent tolamolol with the use of 24 hour blood pressure recordings. *Clin Sci* 1976;51:545s–547s.
96. Mancia G, Ferrari A, Pomidossi G, Parati G, Bertinieri G, Grassi G, Gregovini L, Zanchetti A. Twenty-four-hour hemodynamic profile during treatment of essential hypertension by once-a-day nadolol. *Hypertension* 1983;5:573–578.
97. Giese J. Renin, angiotensin and hypertensive vascular damage: a review. In: Laragh JH, ed. *Hypertension manual.* New York: Yorke Medical. 1973;371–403.
98. O'Rourke MF. Basic concepts for the understanding of large arteries in hypertension. *J Cardiovasc Pharmacol* 1985;7:S14–S21.
99. Cowley AW, Liard JF, Guyton AC. Role of the baroreceptor reflex in daily control of arterial pressure and other variables in the dog. *Circ Res* 1973;32:564–576.
100. Ferrario CM, McCubbin JW, Page IH. Hemodynamic changes of chronic experimental neurogenic hypertension in unanesthetized dogs. *Circ Res* 1969;24:911–922.
101. Kuchel O, Cusson JR, Larochelle P, Boo NT, Genest J. Case report. Posture- and emotion-induced severe hypertensive paroxysms with baroreceptor dysfunction. *J Hypertens* 1987;5:277–283.
102. Kobrin I, Oigman W, Kuman A, et al. Diurnal variation of blood pressure in elderly patients with essential hypertension. *J Ann Geriatr Soc* 1984;312:896–899.
103. Parati G, Pomidossi G, Albini F, Malaspina D, Mancia G. Relationship of 24-hour blood pressure mean and variability to severity of target-organ damage in hypertension. *J Hypertens* 1987;5:93–98.

Hypertension: Pathophysiology, Diagnosis, and Management, edited by J. H. Laragh and B. M. Brenner. Raven Press, Ltd., New York © 1990.

CHAPTER 87

Pseudohypertension

J. David Spence

Blood Pressure Lability, 1408
The White Coat Syndrome, 1408
Iatrophobia, 1408
An Approach to the Problem of Suspected White Coat Syndrome, 1408
Cuff Artifact Due to Obesity, 1408
Cuff Artifact Due to Arterial Stiffness, 1409
Pseudohypertension in the Elderly, 1409
The Osler Maneuver, 1409
Clinical Presentation of Patients with Pseudohypertension, 1410
Pseudonormotension, 1411
The Effects of Antihypertensive Drugs on Arterial Compliance, 1413
Conclusions, 1413
References, 1413

Since hypertension often requires treatment for life, the appropriate identification of those patients who require treatment is of great importance. The negative situation caused by labeling patients as hypertensive, which involves the increased requirement for attendance at medical facilities, laboratory testing, and the requirement for medication, with the attendant costs and adverse effects, is a significant burden. Those patients identified as hypertensive often experience reduced well-being, impaired sexual function, and other manifestations of impaired well-being, including increased absenteeism from work (1).

Adverse effects of medications may include (a) symptoms due to the pharmacology of the drugs, (b) symptoms due to the psychology of drug-taking, which also occur on placebos (e.g., impotence), (c) asymptomatic adverse effects such as changes in lipoprotein metabolism, and (d) adverse effects on arterial flow patterns which may offset the benefits of lowering blood pressure (35). Thus, if at all possible, the unnecessary treatment of patients who appear to be hypertensive but are not should be avoided.

One question raised by the Framingham data on vascular risk factors has recently come into focus as a result of the increased availability of noninvasive ambulatory blood-pressure-recording devices. For some time, it has been a puzzle why left ventricular hypertrophy as identified by electrocardiogram would be a risk factor for vascular disease, independent of blood pressure. The reverse side of the coin had been highlighted by Perloff et al. (3) using cuff ambulatory monitoring, and by Floras et al. (4) using intra-arterial ambulatory monitoring; they showed that high ambulatory pressures identify more accurately than clinic pressures the patients who have end-organ disease such as left ventricular hypertrophy. In addition to the differences between clinic readings and ambulatory pressures, the findings of Floras et al. (4) may in part be explained by cuff artifact, since these investigators used intra-arterial ambulatory monitoring (see discussion below of cuff artifact).

Recently, Deming (5) pointed out that the thickness of the left ventricle gives, in a sense, an integral of the ambulatory pressure and is probably a more accurate reflection of the blood pressure throughout the day than is a single reading taken in a doctor's office. Thus, patients with true hypertension might be expected to develop thickening of the left ventricle, whereas patients with pseudohypertension might well have high blood pressure readings in the doctor's office, without developing ventricular hypertrophy. Thus, the presence of left ventricular hypertrophy (LVH) would identify true hypertension more accurately than would blood pressure readings, explaining why LVH could be an independent risk factor. On the other hand, we have pointed out that the presence of stiff arteries due to atherosclerosis would identify patients at risk of vascular disease and would cause false elevation of the diastolic pressure (6,7), so that high blood pressure readings might be an independent risk factor for vascular disease, but in a way not intended by those taking the blood pressure. Falsely high blood pressure measured with a cuff would identify patients with arterial disease and normal true blood pressures, misidentified as hypertensive because of the cuff artifact but correctly identified as being at increased risk! This rather unusual viewpoint is supported by the observations of Kannel et al. (8) on the contribution of arterial rigidity to risk; it is also supported by the observations of Farrar et al. (9), who showed that regression of atherosclerosis in a monkey model decreased arterial stiffness.

BLOOD PRESSURE LABILITY

In recent large-scale studies of the treatment of mild hypertension, it has become apparent why it is so difficult to demonstrate the benefit of treating mild hypertension: It is very difficult to show that a treatment is beneficial if a significant proportion of those receiving the treatment do not need it in the first place. In the Australian Mild Hypertension Study (10) and in the British MRC study of mild hypertension (11), up to 40% of those patients receiving placebo became normotensive within a few months of the beginning of the study. The normalization of the blood pressure with repeated measurement while on treatment with placebo most likely represents misidentification of normotensives at the beginning of the study, even though the studies required several readings above the entry criteria before the patients could be entered into the study.

The White Coat Syndrome

Mancia et al. (12) has provided evidence to explain this phenomenon. He showed, using intra-arterial continuous ambulatory blood pressure recording equipment, that the act of taking a person's blood pressure with a cuff elevates blood pressure. He also showed that the presence of a physician elevates blood pressure to a greater extent than does the presence of a nurse. Amazingly, the average rise in blood pressure when a physician was present in the room was 27 mmHg systolic and 15 mmHg diastolic. This syndrome, which he called the *white coat syndrome,* makes it extremely difficult to know the meaning of blood pressure readings taken in the setting of a clinic. Blood pressure readings obtained in the clinical setting are only a small sample of the blood pressure readings throughout the day, and the presence of a physician in the clinic can be expected to elevate the blood pressure; the extent to which this elevation will occur will differ between individual patients.

Recently, Pickering et al. (13) showed in a hypertension clinic population that, on the basis of their clinical readings, 21% of patients thought to have borderline hypertension, as well as 5% of patients thought to have sustained hypertension, were actually normotensive (i.e., had ambulatory readings below the 90th percentile of readings seen in normotensives); these patients were therefore diagnosed as having "white coat syndrome." In that study it was also shown that young women experienced a more exaggerated elevation of their clinic readings when the blood pressure was measured by a male physician.

Iatrophobia

In our hypertension clinic, we have observed three extreme examples (among a referral clinic population of over 2000 patients) that we believe represent cases of "iatrophobia." These patients all have normal home blood pressures ranging from 110/60 to 130/80 mmHg but exhibit pressures in clinic ranging from 180/100 to 190/130 mmHg. The most striking of these cases is a young man whose father died when the patient was 3 years old. His mother became extremely protective of him, to the point of imagining illness in the child. This resulted in a series of hospital admissions from age 3 to age 5, during which he was subjected to a number of laboratory tests and became phobic with regard to needles used for blood sampling, white coats, and, eventually, hospitals. This man, whenever he attended clinic, was tremulous and sweaty, with a heart rate ranging from 100 to 120 beats per minute, accompanied by marked elevations of blood pressure, commonly to 190/130. He had (a) normal optic fundi, (b) a normal electrocardiogram with no LVH, (c) normal renal function, and (d) absolutely normal blood pressure while at home, typically ranging from 110/70 to 130/80. His management has been with self-recording of home blood pressure, combined with avoidance of clinics and hospitals.

An Approach to the Problem of Suspected White Coat Syndrome

When faced with patients in whom the white coat syndrome is suspected, the physician is in a dilemma, highlighted recently by Kaplan (14), which has no definitive solution. At present, the following approach is suggested:

1. Hypertension should be diagnosed on the basis of a series of blood pressure readings over a significant interval of time. The Canadian Hypertension Society, in its consensus conference on mild hypertension (15), recommended that before a decision is made to treat hypertension with drugs, diastolic pressures above 100 mmHg should be present on at least three occasions over a period of 6 months.
2. Home blood pressure recordings should be evaluated by comparing the device used with a mercury manometer, recording pressures simultaneously. To validate its performance, and if home blood pressures differ significantly from office readings, the patient should probably be evaluated by using an ambulatory blood pressure device (see Chapter 89 by Pickering for discussion of these devices).

Additionally, it may be reasonable, in trying to evaluate patients with major discrepancies between clinic and home blood pressures, to obtain an echocardiogram at baseline and repeat it at intervals of 6 months or a year. Patients who exhibit thickening of their left ventricle should be regarded as true hypertensives and treated accordingly.

CUFF ARTIFACT DUE TO OBESITY

The problem of blood pressure evaluation in obese subjects is a difficult one. Obesity appears to contribute to true hypertension as well as to cuff artifact in the measurement of blood pressure (16,17). Weight reduction also has a tendency to reduce cuff artifact and the severity of the hypertension. It is now clear from a number of earlier studies (16,18), as well as from the recent studies of Porter and Rangno (19) in Vancouver, Canada, that weight loss will reduce blood pressure; the studies of Porter and Rangno also show a reduction in the extent of cuff artifact by weight loss (19).

They showed that in obese hypertensive subjects, a regular adult cuff underestimated systolic pressure by a mean of 4 mmHg, while diastolic pressure was overestimated by a mean of 11 mmHg, with a maximum overestimate of diastolic pressure by 23 mmHg. A large cuff underestimated systolic pressure by a mean of 8 mmHg and overestimated diastolic pressure by a mean of 7 and a maximum of 13 mmHg. Interestingly, large-cuff diastolic pressures were accurate in normotensive obese subjects and weight loss eliminated the cuff artifact in the obese hypertensive subjects, suggesting the possibility that the cuff artifact may not always be attributable to arm size but that there may, instead, be other factors, such as arterial compliance, involved in the degree of inaccuracy of the cuff measurements. A similar problem of cuff artifact has been observed in elderly patients with stiff arteries, as described below.

CUFF ARTIFACT DUE TO ARTERIAL STIFFNESS

Pseudohypertension in the Elderly

Although blood pressure was probably first measured in 1733 by Stephen Hales, hypertension was possibly first described by Chinese physicians, who spoke of the "hard pulse" 2000 years ago. As pointed out by Messerli et al. (20), Osler wrote in his 1892 text that he mistrusted the blood pressure cuff in patients in whom the brachial artery was still palpable after the cuff was inflated above the systolic pressure. Among the first systematic studies to evaluate the relationship between cuff pressure and intra-arterial pressure were studies done by Steele in 1941 (21) and by Roberts et al. in 1953 (22). The latter study, along with a subsequent study by Van Bergen et al. (23), was the basis of the recommendation (24) that diastolic pressure be taken as the fourth Korotkoff sound (muffling), because they found that the fourth phase corresponded more closely to the intra-arterial diastolic pressure than did the fifth phase. This conclusion was subsequently challenged by London and London (25), among others; it is interesting that their work showed that the cuff method was subject to great error, depending on interobserver variability and the decision to choose muffling versus disappearance of Korotkoff sounds, and that commonly the error in measurement was 30 mmHg.

The first descriptions of pseudohypertension due to arterial stiffness were three single case reports of pseudohypertension attributed to "pipe stem brachial arteries" in patients who had intra-arterial pressure recording, usually as a part of anesthetic monitoring for general surgery (26–28). Subsequently, we studied the problem of cuff artifact in patients whose blood pressure readings by cuff were at odds with the clinical findings (6,7). We studied patients who had a diastolic pressure greater than 100 mmHg but who exhibited no evidence of end-organ disease. Thus, the patients had apparent hypertension but exhibited normal optic fundi, normal renal function, and no evidence of LVH on a chest x-ray or electrocardiogram. In these patients we found a significant discrepancy (Table 1) between the intra-arterial pressure and the cuff pressure, particularly in patients above age 60. In the older age group, half the patients had a significant (30 mmHg or more) elevation of the cuff diastolic pressure as compared to the intra-arterial diastolic pressure. Somewhat surprisingly, the systolic pressure was falsely reduced by the cuff; this has also been observed by others (19,20,25). These findings had in fact been predicted by Sacks et al. (29), whose studies in simulated arteries showed that a doubling of arterial thickness would cause a false elevation of the diastolic pressure by 30 mmHg.

Subsequently, a number of studies were done in which elderly individuals had intra-arterial pressures which did not appear to differ significantly from cuff pressure (30). However, in those studies, the patients were not selected because of any discrepancy between the cuff pressure and the clinical findings; they were simply elderly individuals who had intra-arterial pressures compared with cuff pressures.

This issue was addressed further in a study by Finnigan et al. (31), who studied the difference between intra-arterial pressure and cuff pressure in 55 healthy elderly volunteers. In that study, the average cuff artifact was (a) an 8-mm false reduction of systolic pressure by the cuff and (b) a 5-mm false elevation of the diastolic pressure by the cuff. In those healthy ambulatory elderly volunteers, therefore, there was much less discrepancy between intra-arterial and cuff pressures than had been observed in patients selected because of a suspected discrepancy. In that study, we also examined the relationship between (a) arterial stiffness as reflected in pulse wave velocity and (b) extent of cuff artifact: A significant, though not very strong, correlation was observed.

The Osler Maneuver

These findings were validated by Messerli et al. (20), who cited Osler's misgivings about cuff readings. Messerli et al. described a maneuver derived from Osler's observation, which they called the *Osler maneuver.* In their study, they divided elderly subjects into (a) Osler-positive patients, in whom a palpable brachial artery was observed after inflation of the cuff above the systolic pressure, and (b) Osler-negative patients, in whom the brachial artery was not palpable after inflation of the cuff above the systolic pressure. In the Osler-positive patients, they observed false elevation of the diastolic blood pressure by the cuff method, which exactly paralleled our observations in patients with pseudohypertension: They found that diastolic pressures were falsely elevated by 10–54 mmHg in the Osler-positive patients, whereas the Osler-negative patients had much smaller discrepancies between the cuff and the intra-arte-

TABLE 1. *Intra-arterial pressures compared with cuff pressures using an adult cuff and large thigh cuff, in patients with clinic diastolic pressures above 100 mmHg but no end-organ disease*[a]

		Method of measurement			
		Indirect			
Sex	Age	Adult cuff	Thigh cuff	Direct	Mean (electronic)
		Patients under 60			
M	29	122/90	118/80	118/73	88[b]
M	35	156/106 . . . 88	130/86 . . . 78	142/95	115[b]
M	38	158/100 . . . 96	146/96	141/84	100[b]
M	43	162/110	162/110	145/67	97
F	49	210/110	200/100	233/108	152[b]
M	50	242/140 . . . 134	190/108 . . . 100	207/91	132
F	51	144/80	100/64	154/84	108
M	52	228/116	190/104	135/68	89
M	53	138/98	126/85	136/84	102[c]
F	54	168/110 . . . 100	154/100 . . . 96	153/107	120[b]
F	55	220/110	224/120 . . . 90	272/98	149[b]
F	55	210/118 . . . 110	200/102	186/92	130
F	56	150/90		134/94	113
F	56	162/108	140/88 . . . 80	135/68	97[b]
M	57	188/102	176/98	186/81	78
M	59	228/118	180/108 . . . 98	208/98	140
		Patients over 60			
M	62	260/118	220/100	244/106	157[b]
M	62	190/95	165/100	145/74	102
M	62	170/110	150/105	166/85	114
F	63	>300/168	>300/188	292/131	195
F	64	190/120	180/110	180/80	123
F	64	220/90	235/90	260/82	154
F	65	198/100	190/90	193/82	128[b]
F	65	238/140	230/120 . . . 100	175/98	138
F	65	150/88	150/88	156/76	105
F	67	245/120	230/110	184/86	122
M	71	210/158	200/160	227/115	158
M	72	178/130 . . . 112	180/110	162/112	140
F	72	224/118	252/112	235/87	144
F	73	220/108	200/90	197/77	112[b]
F	73	250/135	250/130	219/88	142
M	74	170/94		203/60	100
F	74	160/120		184/109	139
F	75	188/118 . . . 110	140/90	165/77	110
M	77	158/96	140/84 . . . 70	155/64	106
F	79	190/100	190/90	209/81	124
M	79	226/130	220/120	230/106	153
F	80	240/110	250/100	220/66	115
M	83	180/100	170/110	160/90	128
F	84	186/88	198/94	236/83	130[c]

[a] From ref. 28.
[b] Fat arms.
[c] Thin arms.

rial pressures. Messerli et al. (20) also found a correlation between pulse wave velocity and the magnitude of cuff artifact.

Clinical Presentation of Patients with Pseudohypertension

Misidentification of normotensive patients as hypertensive can lead to excessive lowering of blood pressure, which may account for (a) the observations of Jackson et al. (32) and (b) their suggestion that treatment of hypertension in the elderly may be dangerous. The following cases (reprinted by permission of *Clinical and Investigative Medicine*) illustrate some of the problems associated with pseudohypertension (27).

Case 1. A 74-year-old man was referred for assessment of episodes of cerebral ischemia, several of which had occurred while standing. Five years prior to referral, he had an episode of postural syncope; 1 year prior to admission, he experienced impairment of vision in the left eye for several hours; 6 months prior to admission he experienced, while walking, two episodes of ataxia and dysarthria, the latter persisting for several days; 3 months prior to admission, he woke up one morning with numbness and weakness of the left leg, which partially improved over months. He had been treated for hypertension for 15 years and had been taking debrisoquin (20 mg) daily and hydrochlorothiazide (50 mg) daily for 2 years. Physical findings included subtle long-tract weakness and hyperreflexia of the left arm and leg, with an equivocal plantar response. There were no cardiovascular abnormalities; the optic fundi revealed some atherosclerosis but no hemorrhages, exudates, or microaneurysms. His cuff pressure during debrisoquin therapy was striking: 200/120 recumbent and 70/60 after standing 3 min. Despite the drop in pressure, he was asymptomatic at the time.

The blood urea nitrogen (BUN) concentration was 25 mg/dl, the serum creatinine value was 1.4 mg/dl, and the hemoglobin value was 14.6 g/dl; urinalysis was normal. An electrocardiogram showed no evidence of LVH, and a chest radiograph gave no indication of cardiomegaly.

Because of the apparent discrepancy, in a man with a 15-year history of hypertension, between the rather high diastolic blood pressure of 120 mmHg and the paucity of evidence of hypertensive change in the heart or fundi, the blood pressure was measured by direct means. By that time, with the combination of propranolol (40 mg q.i.d.), hydralazine (25 mg q.i.d.), and hydrochlorothiazide (50 mg daily), pressure had been maintained at about 170/100 mmHg after lying and standing for several days.

In the intensive care unit, his indirect (cuff) blood pressure, using an adult-size cuff and mercury manometer, was 170/94 mmHg in the left arm, recumbent (mean of six readings; three before and three after the intra-arterial recording). His direct intra-arterial blood pressure (mean of three readings) was 203/60 mmHg (mean arterial pressure 100 mmHg).

It was concluded that indirect blood pressure measurement was misleading in his case and that it may have contributed to his overtreatment with antihypertensive drugs. It was suggested to the family doctor that about 30 mmHg could be subtracted from his diastolic readings obtained by indirect measurement.

Case 2. A 56-year-old woman was referred for evaluation of hypertension. Treatment with hydrochlorothiazide had been started 1 month earlier by her referring physician, because of a high blood pressure reading during an episode of vertigo. She was obese, with fat arms, but had no cardiomegaly or hypertensive changes in the fundi. An electrocardiogram was normal, with no evidence of cardiomegaly; routine urinalysis was normal; the hemoglobin concentration was 16.0 g/dl; the BUN value was 14 mg/dl; and the creatinine value was 0.85 mg/dl. Indirect blood pressures were as follows: adult cuff, 162/108 mmHg; thigh cuff applied to the arm, 140/88–80 mmHg. The direct intra-arterial pressure was 135/68 mmHg [mean arterial pressure (MAP) was 97 mmHg]. Her referring physician was advised that because her arms were fat there was a significant error in indirect measurement of her blood pressure and that she did not require treatment for arterial hypertension.

Case 3. A 57-year-old male biophysics technician was referred for assessment of "hypertension." Though unusually intelligent, he was referred as a problem in difficult management because he was said to be obstinate, refusing to take his antihypertensive drugs. He was said to have had hypertension for 12 years, by four physicians consulted in that period, including nephrologists and cardiologists. His chief complaint was that antihypertensive drugs made him feel sick. A combination of methyldopa and hydrochlorothiazide caused lethargy and postural hypotension, propranolol made him feel generally weak, and thiazides alone made him nauseated. He had been taking no medications for 1 year.

He looked fit and was not overweight. There were old stasis changes on the left leg, along with a pansystolic aortic murmur; there were no hypertensive changes in the fundi. Echocardiography revealed evidence of a bicuspid aortic valve, with aortic regurgitation. An electrocardiogram showed left axis deviation but no LVH; a chest radiograph indicated some left ventricular predominance. The hemoglobin concentration was 16.9 g/dl, the BUN value was 17 mg/dl, and the serum creatinine value was 1.0 mg/dl. Indirect blood pressures were as follows: adult cuff, 188/102 mmHg; thigh cuff, 176/98 mmHg. Direct intra-arterial pressure was 186/81 mmHg (MAP 78 mmHg).

The patient was referred for further cardiologic assessment, since his problem was not arterial hypertension.

Case 4. A 73-year-old woman was referred for assessment of hypertension, since she had a family history of hypertension and stroke. Her gynecologist had found that her blood pressure was 200/100 mmHg. She had been treated for hypertension 10 years before but had stopped taking medications because of symptoms of postural hypotension. Physical examination revealed some copper-wiring and arteriovenous nicking, but no hemorrhages or exudates. Both brachial arteries were palpably hardened. The hemoglobin value was 14.7 g/dl; the BUN value was 11 mg/dl; and the serum creatinine value was 0.5 mg/dl; results of urinalysis, chest radiography, and electrocardiography were normal; and there was no evidence of cardiomegaly. In this woman, whose arms were thin, indirect blood pressure readings were as follows: adult cuff, 250/135 mmHg; thigh cuff; 250/130 mmHg. At the same time, her direct intra-arterial pressure was 219/88 mmHg (MAP 142 mmHg).

Because of the high systolic and mean blood pressures, propranolol (10 mg q.i.d.) was started. Her family doctor was advised that she did not have diastolic hypertension and that there was an error of 40 mmHg in indirect blood pressure estimation.

PSEUDONORMOTENSION

Occasionally, there may be patients who appear to have normal blood pressures but who have true hypertension. These patients are at grave risk if their falsely normal cuff pressures are used to withhold treatment. The following cases illustrate two such instances.

Case 1. The first patient was a lady of 76, referred to our stroke prevention clinic in March 1986 because retinal hemorrhages, discovered when she complained of episodic impairment of vision, had raised the question of whether the patient was suffering from carotid stenosis, with the ocular ischemic syndrome. Her blood pressure had repeatedly been checked in her doctor's office, and she had been thought to be normotensive. In the clinic, the pressures measured by the nurse were 174/66 in the left arm recumbent, 177/72 in the right arm recumbent, and 170/76 in the right arm standing. Because of suspicion raised by examination of the optic fundi, I took particular pains to avoid an auscultatory gap and found a recumbent pressure in the right arm of 260/90, repeated several times. (The white coat syndrome may have been responsible for some of the discrepancy between pressures measured by the nurse and the physician.)

A Doppler ultrasound scan of her cervical vessels revealed bilateral subclavian stenosis. She was brought in for treatment of her presumed hypertension and for further evaluation of her cuff artifact. She was treated initially with hydrochlorothiazide (25 mg) spironolactone (25 mg) twice daily, combined with hydralazine (25 mg) every 6 hours, by mouth. After 2 days, when her blood pressures on the ward were 130/70 to 150/70, measured by the nurse with a mercury cuff on either arm, she was taken to the intensive care unit for intra-arterial blood pressure recording.

Table 2 gives the pressures obtained by intra-arterial recording in the right femoral artery and right radial artery, as well as in the right and left arm, by an appropriate size cuff and mercury manometer (the physician taking the arm cuff pressures was blinded as to the intra-arterial readings); the last two readings also give the intra-arterial MAP.

It is presumed that the pressures after 2 days of treatment were lower than they had been before treatment and, thus, that this lady had significant hypertension but, because of bilateral subclavian artery stenosis, had falsely normal blood pressure cuff readings in the arms. The pressures in the left arm, which showed more severe stenosis on the Doppler study, were more discrepant. One feature of these readings is that she had a significant cuff artifact, comparing the intra-arterial pressures in the right arm with the cuff pressures in the right arm, and showed the usual pattern of damping, with (a) the systolic pressures falsely lowered by the cuff and (b) the diastolic pressures falsely elevated by the cuff. The discrepancy between the two arms illustrates why, in our earlier studies, we chose to measure the pressure in the same arm when using both the cuff method and the intra-arterial method. [We had been criticized by O'Callaghan et al. (30) for not measuring the pressure simultaneously in the two arms, i.e., by the cuff method in one and by the intra-arterial method in the other. However, my background is that of a vascular neurologist, with a rather large referral practice of patients with atherosclerosis of the cervical vessels, including more than 20 patients with subclavian steal syndrome; this background led to our preference for measurement of the pressures in the same arm by the two methods, and for using the mean of several cuff recordings before and after the three meaned intra-arterial recordings, to take account of the variability of pressure over time.]

TABLE 2. *Intra-arterial pressures in the right radial and right femoral artery, compared with cuff pressures in the arms, in an elderly woman with hypertensive retinal hemorrhages and pseudonormotension due to bilateral subclavian stenosis*

Time	Right radial	Right femoral	Right arm cuff	Left arm cuff
13:00	196/50	204/66	—	—
13:30	190/58	226/60	158/72	148/80
13:50	190/55	210/53	160/80	178/60
14:05	195/55 (92)	211/52 (92)	158/90	130/52
14:16	186/46 (97)	196/44 (98)	190/90	152/80

TABLE 3. *Ambulatory automated cuff pressures in a young pregnant woman with normal clinic pressures but hypertensive retinopathy*

Time	Systolic	Diastolic	MAP	Heart rate
10:44	130	91	104	73
11:55	125	84	98	68
12:54	118	65	83	72
13:53	124	76	91	82
14:53	153	101	118	104
15:53	128	88	100	89
16:51	148	89	108	86
17:50	163	96	118	115
18:56	158	96	116	109
19:55	181	109	133	111
21:07	160	135	150	104
22:06	185	114	145	87
23:07	155	110	135	89

The case points out the need for interpretation of blood pressure readings in light of clinical findings.

Case 2. The second case was a pregnant 20-year-old woman who was referred to the hypertension clinic because of a single high blood pressure reading in her obstetrician's office. She had first been told that her pressure was slightly elevated about 2 years previously, at a time when she was taking birth control pills. Her pressure in the obstetrician's office was 138/80 early in the pregnancy, but at 26 weeks her pressure was up to 130/100, and she was referred.

When she visited the hypertension clinic, her cuff blood pressures, obtained by the nurse with a mercury manometer and cuff of appropriate size, were 130/90 recumbent and 124/88 standing. Her physical examination was unremarkable except for slight obesity, the signs of pregnancy, and abnormal optic fundi. She had arteriolar narrowing, some irregularity of arteriolar caliber, retinal microaneurysms, and loss of retinal sheen, suggesting retinal edema. These findings suggested that her blood pressure may have been significantly elevated at times, requiring further investigation.

A 24-hr ambulatory blood pressure recording was done, using a Spacelabs 5200 recorder, the results of which are shown in Table 3. The patient had falsely normal clinical readings, with clearly abnormal ambulatory blood pressure readings, the only clue to which was a careful ophthalmoscopic examination. She was treated with oral hydralazine and atenolol, and she successfully completed the pregnancy. This case again illustrates the importance of interpreting cuff blood pressure readings in light of all the clinical evidence available.

THE EFFECTS OF ANTIHYPERTENSIVE DRUGS ON ARTERIAL COMPLIANCE

As observed in the studies by Finnigan et al. (31) and Messerli et al. (20), cuff artifact is influenced by arterial stiffness. Arterial stiffness is related to blood pressure, and it can be expected therefore that the cuff artifact will be greater in magnitude (i.e., cuff readings will be more inaccurate) at higher pressures.

Additionally, it may be expected that antihypertensive drugs may influence the extent to which cuff readings are inaccurate and that the magnitude of this influence may differ between drugs, according to their effects on arterial stiffness.

Recently, Safar and his colleagues in Paris have been using ultrasound methods to measure arterial compliance. They have developed a device which uses two Doppler probes, aimed so that the angle of insonation between the two probes is exactly 90°. This arrangement cancels out the effect of the angle of incidence in the Doppler equation, and it permits them to use their device to accurately assess changes in blood velocity simultaneously with changes in arterial diameter. Together with a pressure recording, this permits measurement of arterial compliance (2). They have studied the effects of various antihypertensive drugs on arterial compliance and have shown that there are significant differences: Angiotensin converting enzyme (ACE) inhibitors, some calcium-channel antagonists, and nitrates increase arterial compliance (33), whereas beta-adrenergic blockers (given acutely as an intravenous dose) decrease arterial compliance (34); thus, it may be expected that in patients with stiff arteries, ACE inhibitors, nitrates, and calcium-channel antagonists may make blood pressure readings more accurate, whereas beta blockers may increase the extent to which diastolic pressure is falsely elevated by the cuff method. Conversely, in patients with accurate readings, it might be expected that nitrates, calcium-channel antagonists, and ACE inhibitors might lead to falsely low diastolic cuff readings. To my knowledge, this possibility has not yet been tested.

CONCLUSIONS

The accurate identification of true hypertensives is of paramount importance in the decision to initiate and maintain lifelong therapy. In the measurement of blood pressure by the standard cuff methods, in addition to the problems of cuff size and inaccurate measurement technique, three major problems require awareness by physicians: Firstly, blood pressures in the clinic may be falsely elevated because of the White Coat Syndrome, leading to misidentification of normotensives as hypertensives. Secondly, significant false elevation of the diastolic pressure because of cuff artifact may be a major problem in obese patients. Thirdly, false elevation of the diastolic pressure by the cuff method is an important source of error in blood pressure measurement in elderly patients with stiff arteries. In elderly patients with high cuff readings but no end-organ disease, cuff readings commonly overestimate the diastolic pressure by 20 mmHg and occasionally overestimate it by 40–50 mmHg. Occasionally, patients with true hypertension will have falsely normal pressures. These problems demand intelligent interpretation of blood pressure readings in light of all the clinical findings. Blind acceptance of blood pressure readings must be resisted.

REFERENCES

1. Haynes RB, Sackett DL, Taylor DW, Gibson ES, Johnson AL. Increased absenteeism from work after detection and labelling of hypertensive patients. *N Engl J Med* 1978;299:741–744.
2. Simon AC, Laurent S, Levenson JA, Bouthier JE, Safar ME. Estimation of forearm arterial compliance in normal and hypertensive men from simultaneous pressure and flow measurements in the brachial artery, using a pulsed Doppler device and a first-order arterial model during diastole. *Cardiovasc Res* 1983;17:331–338.
3. Perloff D, Sokolow M, Cowan R. The prognostic value of ambulatory blood pressures. *JAMA* 1983;249:2792–2798.
4. Floras JS, Jones JV, Hassan MO, Osikowska B, Sever PS, Sleight P. Cuff and ambulatory blood pressure in subjects with essential hypertension. *Lancet* 1981;ii:107–109.
5. Deming Q. How important is ambulatory BP monitoring in blood pressure monitoring? Presented at: Symposium on controversies in the management of hypertension. American Society of Hypertension, May 16, 1987, New York.
6. Spence JD, Sibbald WJ, Cape RD. Pseudohypertension in the elderly. *Clin Sci Mol Med* 1978;55(Suppl 4):399s–402s.
7. Spence JD, Sibbald WJ, Cape RD. Direct, indirect and mean blood pressures in hypertensive patients: the problem of cuff artefact due to arterial wall stiffness and a partial solution. *Clin Invest Med* 1980;2:165–173.
8. Kannel WB, Wolf PA, McGee DL, Dawber TR, McNamara P, Castelli WP. Systolic blood pressure, arterial rigidity, and risk of stroke. The Framingham study. *JAMA* 1981;245:1225–1229.
9. Farrar DJ, Green HD, Wagner WD, Bond MG. Reduction in pulse wave velocity and improvement of aortic distensibility accompanying regression of atherosclerosis in the rhesus monkey. *Circ Res* 1980;47:425–432.
10. Australian National Blood Pressure Study Management Committee. The Australian Therapeutic Trial in Mild Hypertension. *Lancet* 1980;i:1261–1267.
11. Medical Research Council Working Party. MRC Trial of Treatment of Mild Hypertension: principal results. *Br Med J* 1985;291:97–104.
12. Mancia G, Bertinieri G, Grassi G, Parati G, Pomidossi G, Ferrari A, Gregorini L, Zanchetti A. Effects of blood pressure measurement by the doctor on patient's blood pressure and heart rate. *Lancet* 1983;ii:695–697.
13. Pickering TG, James GD, Boddie C, Harshfield GA, Laragh JH. How common is the white coat syndrome? *JAMA* 1987;259:225–228.
14. Kaplan NM. Misdiagnosis of systemic hypertension and recommendations for improvement. *Am J Cardiol* 1987;60:1383–1386.
15. Logan AG. Report of the Canadian Hypertension Society's Consensus Conference on Mild Hypertension. *Can Med Assoc J* 1984;131:1053–55.
16. Staessen J, Fagard R, Amery A. Blood pressure, calorie intake and obesity. In: Bulpitt CJ, ed. *Handbook of hypertension.* New York: Elsevier, 1985;131–158.

17. Trout KW, Bertrand CA, Williams MH. Measurement of blood pressure in obese persons. *JAMA* 1956;162:970–971.
18. MacMahon SW, MacDonald GJ, Bernstein L, Andrews G, Blacket RB. Comparison of weight reduction with metoprolol in treatment of hypertension in young overweight patients. *Lancet* 1985;1233–1236.
19. Porter R, Rangno R. Hypertension in obesity: measurement error and effect of weight loss [Abstract]. *Clin Invest Med* 1987;10(Suppl):B88.
20. Messerli FH, Ventura HO, Amodeo C. Osler's maneuver and pseudohypertension. *N Engl J Med* 1985;312:1548–1551.
21. Steele JM. Comparison of simultaneous indirect (auscultatory) and direct (intra-arterial) measurements of blood pressure in man. *J Mt Sinai Hosp* 1941;8:1042–1050.
22. Roberts LN, Smiley JR, Manning GW. Comparison of direct and indirect blood pressure determinations. *Circulation* 1953;8:232–242.
23. Van Bergen FH, Weatherhead DH, Treloar AE, Doblan AB, Buckley JJ. A comparison of indirect and direct methods of measuring blood pressure. *Circulation* 1954;10:481–490.
24. Report of the Joint National Committee on detection, evaluation and treatment of high blood pressure. *JAMA* 1977;237:255–261.
25. London SB, London RE. Comparison of indirect pressure measurements (Korotkoff) with simultaneous direct brachial artery pressure distal to the cuff. *Adv Intern Med* 1967;13:127–142.
26. Sprague DH, Kim DI. Pseudohypertension due to Monkeberg's arteriosclerosis. *Anesth Analg* 1978;57:588–589.
27. Taguchi JT, Suwangoal P. Pipe-stem brachial arteries. A cause of pseudohypertension. *JAMA* 1974;288:733.
28. Wallace CT, Carpenter FA, Evins CS, Mahaffey JE. Acute pseudohypertensive crisis. *Anaesthesiology* 1975;43:588–589.
29. Sacks AH, Raman KR, Burnell JA. A study of auscultatory blood pressure in simulated arteries. *Symposium on Biorheology* 1963;215–230.
30. O'Callaghan W, Fitzgerald DJ, O'Malley K, O'Brien E. Accuracy of indirect blood pressure measurement in the elderly. *Br Med J* 1983;286:1545–1546.
31. Finnegan TP, Spence JD, Wong DG, Wells GA. Blood pressure measurement in the elderly: correlation of arterial stiffness with difference between intra-arterial and cuff pressures. *J Hypertens* 1985;3:231–235.
32. Jackson G, Pierscianowski TA, Mahon W, Condon J. Inappropriate antihypertensive therapy in the elderly. *Lancet* 1976;ii:1317–1318.
33. Safar ME, Bouthier JA, Levenson JA, Simon AC. Peripheral large arteries and the response to antihypertensive treatment. *Hypertension* 1983;5:(Suppl III):III-63–III-68.
34. Levenson JA, Simon AC, Fiessinger JN, Safar ME, London GM, Housset EM. Systemic arterial compliance in patients with arteriosclerosis obliterans of the lower limbs. Observations on the effect of intravenous propranolol. *Arteriosclerosis* 1982;2:266–271.
35. Spence JD. Antihypertensive therapy and atherosclerosis. In: Rapaport E, ed. *Cardiology update.* New York: Elsevier, 1986; 137–155.

Hypertension: Pathophysiology, Diagnosis, and Management, edited by J. H. Laragh and B. M. Brenner. Raven Press, Ltd., New York © 1990.

CHAPTER 88

Labile Hypertension, Vasomotor Instability, and Postural Syndromes

Joseph L. Izzo, Jr.

Pathophysiology of Blood Pressure Variation, 1416
Vascular Compliance and Physical Factors in Blood Pressure Regulation, 1416
Integrative Role of the Sympathoadrenal System (SAS) in the Control of Systemic Hemodynamics and Blood Volume, 1416
The Carotid Baroreflex and the Buffering of Systolic Pressure and Heart Rate, 1417
Central Blood Volume, Cardiopulmonary Baroreflex Interactions, and Postural Adaptation, 1417
Central Blood Volume and the Control of Renal Sympathetic Nervous Activity and Renal Sodium Excretion, 1417
A Simplified Model of Blood Pressure Counterregulation, 1418
Common Causes of Variation, 1418
Sleep/Arousal, 1418
Respiratory Variation, 1418
Postural Adaptation, 1419
Physical Exercise, 1419
Pain, 1419
White Coat Hypertension, 1419
Postprandial Hemodynamic Changes, 1419
Hypoglycemic Recovery, 1420
Temperature Change, 1420
Cigarette Smoking, 1420
Dehydration/Volume Depletion, 1420
Diurnal Variation, 1420
Menstrual Cycle, 1420
Seasonal Variation, 1420
Psychological Stress Responses, 1420
Syndromes of Abnormal Sympathoadrenal Discharge, 1421
Neurologic Abnormalities and Sleep Apnea, 1421
Postanesthesia and Postsurgical Hypertension, 1421
Alcoholism and Withdrawal Syndromes, 1421
Panic Attacks, 1421
Autonomic Dysfunction and Orthostatic Hypotension, 1422
Syndromes of Apparent Central-Volume–Sympathoadrenal Dysregulation, 1422
Transient Left Ventricular Dysfunction (Silent Ischemia), 1422
Pulmonary Hypertension, 1423
Mitral Valve Prolapse (MVP), 1423
Orthostatic Hypertension and Postdialysis Hypertension, 1423
Idiopathic Hypovolemia, 1423
Episodic Dopamine Discharge, 1424
Neurocirculatory Asthenia (Soldier's Heart), 1424
Other Neurohumoral Syndromes, 1424
Histamine and Systemic Mastocytosis, 1424
Hyperbradykininism, 1424
Serotonin and Carcinoid Syndrome, 1424
Porphyria, 1424
Drugs and Drug Dosing Effects, 1424
Dosing Effects, 1424
Pressor Substances, 1425
References, 1425

Arterial pressure normally exhibits extremely wide variability, with the range of blood pressures within a given individual being far greater than the range of average blood pressures between individuals. Common physiologic stresses such as exercise significantly increase blood pressure. However, these increases range from a few mmHg in certain individuals to over 100 mmHg in others. If these excursions were predictable or consistent, then resting blood pressure would accurately reflect all values in that individual. However, basal blood pressures are not always proportional to stress-related increases, and different stressors elicit different responses within and between individuals.

Even "normal" arterial pressure variability confounds the diagnosis of hypertension. About 25% of all patients labeled as hypertensive by blood pressure elevations observed in their physicians' offices are actually normotensive at home ("white coat hypertension"). The simple act of having the physician measure the blood pressure has a highly variable effect between individuals. New emphasis on home blood pressures and ambulatory monitoring techniques provides the practitioner with a better appreciation of the true lability of blood pressure. Yet this new understanding of blood pressure variation carries with it many vexing problems that remain to be solved. Most importantly, the definition and therapeutic goals of the syndrome of essential hypertension are now substantially less clear. The possibility also exists that many patients are misclassified or inappropriately treated by using a narrow definition of hypertension based on office blood pressures.

The clinical situation is further confounded by excessive blood pressure lability, postural differences in blood pressure, and the existence of several syndromes of vasomotor instability that are commonly mistaken for pheochromocytoma. Such vasomotor instability is usually exacerbated by volume depletion or may be caused by an imbalance between central blood volume and peripheral vasoconstriction. Treatment for many of these conditions commonly includes volume repletion.

The intent of this chapter is to provide a framework that will aid the clinician in the differentiation of pathologic conditions from common variations in arterial pressure. Repeated reference will be made to central blood volume, the sympathoadrenal system, and other opposing physiologic mechanisms that counterregulate blood pressure. Although distinctions will be drawn between "normal" and "abnormal" variation, it should be emphasized that such a division is often arbitrary and that a continuum of physiologic and pathologic states exists. Appropriate diagnosis and therapy of hypertensive patients depends heavily on an understanding of these graded phenomena.

PATHOPHYSIOLOGY OF BLOOD PRESSURE VARIATION

Vascular Compliance and Physical Factors in Blood Pressure Regulation

Systolic blood pressure varies more than diastolic pressure because it is dependent on several highly variable factors, including the volume and force of cardiac contraction, compliance of large blood vessels, and total systemic vascular resistance. In general, the systolic hypertension in elderly individuals is related to the relative degree of arteriosclerosis (1). In contrast, diastolic pressure relates most closely to systemic vascular resistance and is less affected by cardiac function or vascular compliance. In part, these phenomena led to early emphasis on diastolic blood pressure as the most important marker of essential hypertension. Yet, systolic hypertension is the more potent predictor of true cardiovascular risk (2).

The development of noninvasive ambulatory monitoring techniques (see chapter entitled "Blood Pressure Measurement and Ambulatory Blood Pressure Monitoring: Evaluation of Available Equipment") has broadened the experience gained from direct intra-arterial techniques, but much pathophysiologic research in the area still relies on the latter. The complex mathematical formulae employed in harmonic or spectral analysis (3,4) are useful for pathophysiologic research. A more straightforward but cumbersome approach is the use of diaries of activities combined with multivariate analysis (5). Despite a necessary reliance on esoteric methods, the problem of blood pressure variability has many practical implications that will subsequently be discussed.

In general, the degree of variability of both systolic and diastolic blood pressure is proportional to the mean or arithmetic average of all blood pressures for that individual (6). Although there is greater absolute variability in a patient whose average blood pressure is 180/120 than in a patient whose average blood pressure is 130/85, the coefficient of variation (standard deviation/mean) of blood pressure tends to be equal in both cases. Thus, it has been argued by some that "labile hypertension" does not really exist.

Nevertheless, it is the experience of many clinicians that certain individuals have far greater variability of blood pressure than others at the same level of "average" pressure. These are usually older patients who have marked decreases in vascular compliance (2,7,8) and diminished baroreflex function. The contribution of each of these two components to arterial pressure variation will be discussed in the following sections.

Treatment of these individuals with advanced arteriosclerosis is difficult because therapy often results in side effects such as hypotensive episodes, particularly with orthostasis (9). Therapeutic goals must therefore be tailored to the individual patient (10). In practice, home blood pressures and office readings can be used in parallel, trying on the one hand to optimize office readings, while minimizing symptomatology. Simply noting the time of day of each reading gives close enough approximation to dosing, meals, and activity to be interpretable later. Alternatively, patients may keep a diary of events for later analysis.

Integrative Role of the Sympathoadrenal System (SAS) in the Control of Systemic Hemodynamics and Blood Volume

Any short-term fluctuation in arterial pressure affects, and is affected by, the SAS. This complex regulatory network serves several purposes simultaneously. In its simplest form, the "fight or flight" response of the SAS causes selective vasoconstriction, redistribution of blood flow to the central nervous system and skeletal muscle, and increased oxygen and substrate delivery to these tissues in times of stress. Concomitant cardiac excitation is mediated through beta-1 adrenergic receptor activation and sympathetic neurons that are parallel to, but anatomically different from, the peripheral vasomotor fibers that trigger alpha-adrenergic receptor-mediated vasoconstriction (11). Rapid blood pressure adaptations to posture, exercise, mental stress, pain, and other stimuli may be modulated by hormonal influences but are predominantly the result of changes in SAS activity. The SAS also modulates certain longer-term basal regulatory functions, including thermoregulation, metabolic counterregulation, cardiovascular adaptation, extracellular fluid volume regulation, and arousal state (12).

The Carotid Baroreflex and the Buffering of Systolic Pressure and Heart Rate

Acute increases in systolic and mean arterial pressure distend the carotid sinus, stimulate local stretch receptors to increase afferent nerve traffic to the nucleus tractus solitarius (NTS) in the brain stem, and subsequently *inhibit* further efferent sympathetic outflow to the heart and blood vessels (13,14). This instantaneous baroreflex response acts to limit increases in systolic blood pressure, providing a rapid buffering function that protects the cerebral and peripheral microcirculations.

Despite this acute buffering function, the arterial baroreflex is not thought by most experts to be a major force in the long-term regulation of arterial pressure. This statement is based on the repeatedly observed phenomenon of baroreflex "resetting." Studies by Cowley et al. in dogs elegantly demonstrate that baroreflex deafferentation results in increased blood pressure lability, yet the 24-hr average blood pressures of these "debuffered" dogs are similar to those of the control animals (15). In humans, it is common to encounter labile systolic hypertension in elderly individuals, who have reduced baroreflex sensitivity due to arteriosclerosis, with decreased arterial compliance of the carotid sinus and peripheral arteries, as already discussed.

During earlier stages of hypertension, baroreflex control of SAS activity is already blunted (13,16). However, cause and effect in this resetting cannot be readily separated, and a few investigators still envision a role of defective arterial baroreflexes in the genesis of chronic hypertension.

Central Blood Volume, Cardiopulmonary Baroreflex Interactions, and Postural Adaptation

It is well accepted that central and peripheral blood volume, stroke volume, and cardiac output are directly and proportionally related. However, when central blood volume is reduced acutely, activation of the SAS acts to restore central blood volume through peripheral venoconstriction, which centralizes blood volume and increases cardiac output. Thus, the SAS affects, and is affected by, central blood *volume* changed in similar fashion to its interrelationship with arterial pressure.

The role of the SAS as a determinant of venous return and cardiac output is often inapparent, largely because most cardiac diagnostic procedures are performed in the supine position, when (a) the SAS is not activated and (b) venous return is passive and not rate-limiting. Respiratory patterns, postural adaptation, hydration state, and a variety of other stimuli alter central blood volume and critically affect cardiopulmonary baroreflexes (atrial stretch).

Examination of available information suggests that atrial stretch receptors may be more important than arterial baroreflexes in the chronic activation of the SAS that, in turn, allows blood pressure to be maintained in the upright position. This statement is made on the basis of several observations. First, lower body suction activates the SAS without affecting the carotid sinus (17). Secondly, postural change also activates the SAS independent of effects on the carotid sinus. Julius and co-workers have used passive tilt to reproducibly decrease central blood volume and cause SAS activation. Subsequently, while subjects remained tilted, external compression of the lower extremities with a water-filled suit restored central blood volume to values identical to those observed during the supine baseline period. Despite the fact that this last maneuver did not significantly affect carotid sinus pressure, plasma norepinephrine (NE) was suppressed back to baseline levels (18). Finally, our laboratory has found that the increases in plasma NE that occur with postural stimulation are much more closely related to changes in stroke volume than to changes in carotid sinus pressure (J. L. Izzo, Jr., *unpublished observations*). These findings underscore the importance of the cardiopulmonary baroreflex in the "volume-vasoconstrictor" continuum. Its control of sympathetic outflow and systemic vascular resistance suggests a possible, though controversial, role of the cardiopulmonary baroreflex in the pathogenesis of hypertension (19,20).

Central Blood Volume and the Control of Renal Sympathetic Nervous Activity and Renal Sodium Excretion

Cardiac output remains a critical determinant of renal blood flow, which, in turn, is a major determinant of glomerular filtration rate and salt excretion. Salt depletion reduces blood volume and cardiac output, causing renal vasoconstriction, increased urinary concentration, and "prerenal azotemia."

However, more subtle relationships between blood volume and natriuresis also exist. For example, both cardiac denervation (21) and supraventricular arrhythmias (22) can be associated with exaggerated diuresis and natriuresis, even when cardiac output is constant. Clinical clues relating the SAS to volume control and salt and water homeostasis include the observations that sympatholytic drugs (23) and autonomic insufficiency (24) are associated with renal sodium wasting.

Atrial stretch receptors are connected, via vagal afferent fibers, to hypothalamic nuclei that control vasopressin release. They are also connected to brain-stem vasomotor control centers, which, in turn, control renal nerves. In elegant dog studies, Thames et al. (25) and Morita and Vatner (26) have demonstrated that renal sympathetic nervous activity is tightly and predominantly controlled by cardiac atrial pressure and stretch when renal nerve activity increases, renal vasoconstriction occurs and renal blood flow decreases. The functional significance of these neural connections has also been documented by DiBona and other investigators, who have shown that renal nerves are critical controllers of renal sodium excretion (27,28).

Demonstration of cardiopulmonary baroreflex control of renal sympathetic nerve activity and sodium excretion remains difficult in humans. Stimuli that affect cardiopulmonary receptors usually cause parallel stimulation of the carotid sinus baroreflex, making separation of the two afferent reflex arcs difficult. In addition, we do not have any way to measure human renal sympathetic nervous traffic.

The redundancy of the control mechanisms modifying renal vasoconstriction causes further confounding in the interpretation of data obtained from intact humans. Using head-out water immersion, Epstein (29) and other investigators have shown that natriuresis and diuresis occur. However, the reason for the natriuresis in this model may be more complicated than simple central blood volume increases and may be due to altered renal perfusion pressure, atrial peptides, or other mechanisms.

Parenthetically, the control of atrial peptide release by atrial distension, along with the subsequent effects on renal hemodynamics and natriuresis, has received much fanfare. Yet there is no convincing evidence that atrial peptides play any greater role in natriuretic control than the "volume-vasoconstrictor" effects mediated via cardiopulmonary baroreflex control of renal nerve activity. Both mechanisms appear to operate in parallel, with decreased central blood volume simultaneously stimulating renal sympathetic nerve traffic and suppressing atrial peptide release, thereby limiting natriuresis. The opposite effects occur when central blood volume is increased.

A Simplified Model of Blood Pressure Counterregulation

In both physiologic experiments and clinical medicine, it is useful to employ a model of blood pressure counterregulation. Arterial pressure is stabilized by a series of redundant mechanisms similar to those defending blood glucose. Two-way mutually reinforcing interactions between the two major blood pressure defense mechanisms—the SAS and the renin–angiotensin system—are responsible for maintaining systemic vascular resistance. We now know that a functional "volume-vasoconstrictor" continuum is largely controlled by central blood volume and cardiac atrial stretch balanced against systemic and renal hemodynamics (and natriuresis) (17,18,22–27). Figure 1 demonstrates a model of these interactions. During periods of volume depletion, the vasoconstrictors are activated; when volume is repleted, the vasoconstrictor systems are suppressed. The concept of central blood volume thus replaces the incorrect notion of "effective arterial volume" and helps explain physiologic phenomena such as postural adaptation as well as various pathologic syndromes.

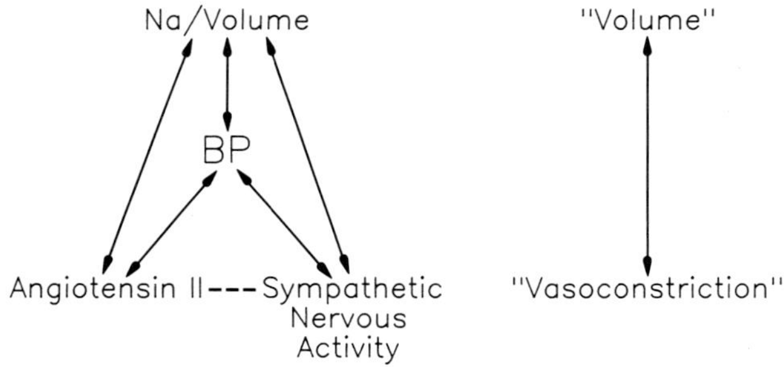

FIG. 1. A highly simplified model of blood pressure counterregulation. Multiple physiologic interactions act to keep blood pressure constant over wide ranges of extracellular fluid volume. Mutually reinforcing interactions of the SAS and angiotensin II (dashed line) counterbalance (double-headed arrows) any decreases in central blood volume through cardiopulmonary baroreflexes or any decreases in blood pressure through arterial baroreflexes. Volume loading or hypertension reverses these processes. Other compensations also exist. For example, increases in pressure directly and indirectly cause diuresis, whereas volume depletion directly and indirectly favors renal sodium retention.

COMMON CAUSES OF VARIATION

Most blood pressure fluctuations can be traced to altered SAS activity. For convenience, they can be divided into categories based on the speed of the response (Table 1).

Sleep/Arousal

Blood pressure normally declines 10–30 mmHg during deep sleep (30). There are small variations of blood pressure during sleep, probably related to sleep cycles or dream periods. Sleep blood pressures are markedly elevated in a number of conditions in which there are abnormalities of autonomic function and in which chronic steroid levels are pathologically or therapeutically elevated. These include cardiac transplantation (31) and Cushing's syndrome (32).

Respiratory Variation

With inspiration, increased venous return to the right heart improves right ventricular stroke volume, while simultaneous decreases in left atrial filling decrease left ventricular stroke volume. After a lag of two to four cardiac cycles, the transiently increased right ventricular stroke volume is transferred to the left ventricle. This tends to occur at about the time of exhalation, reversing the phenomena observed during inspiration and further augmenting the transient increase in left ventricular stroke volume. Respiratory-cycle-related changes in blood flow are partially

TABLE 1. *Cyclic or episodic changes related to sympathoadrenal activation*

Instantaneous (seconds)	*Intermediate (hours)*
Sleep/arousal	Volume depletion
Respiration	Diurnal variation
Posture	Withdrawal syndromes
Pain	
Exercise	*Slow (days to weeks)*
"White coat" hypertension	Menstrual cycle
	Seasonal change
Rapid (minutes)	
Postprandial alterations	*Chronic (months to years)*
Hypoglycemia	Life crises and chronic stress
Temperature change	
Cigarette smoking	

buffered by neural reflexes that control vascular resistance reciprocally through inputs of arterial and venous baroreflexes (4).

The net effect of the respiratory cycle on cardiac output and vascular resistance is (a) a decrease in systolic pressure during inspiration and (b) a proportional increase in systolic pressure during expiration. Diastolic pressure usually follows the same pattern as systolic pressure but varies less. Under normal circumstances, respiratory variation of blood pressure is less than 5 mmHg. However, variations can exceed 10 mmHg during periods of low cardiac output, such as pericardial tamponade or severe congestive heart failure, or in syndromes of marked changes of intrapleural pressure, such as severe asthma. At this point they are considered pathologic and are called "pulsus paradoxus."

Postural Adaptation

An understanding of postural adaptation requires a knowledge of "cardiopulmonary baroreflex interactions," already discussed. Successful maintenance of blood pressure during positional change requires an instantaneous set of responses that depends on the two major afferent stimuli that activate the SAS (Fig. 2). First, the venous pooling caused by gravitational pull reduces central blood volume, disinhibiting the cardiopulmonary baroreflex. Simultaneous decreases in carotid sinus pressure act in concert via the brain-stem control centers to increase SAS activity, causing both arterial and venous constriction. The syndromes of abnormal orthostasis discussed in the following sections reflect alterations in at least one of these interactions.

Physical Exercise

Under conditions of dynamic exercise, increased cardiac output is manifested by a decrease in diastolic pressure and an increase in systolic pressure and heart rate. The use of exercise may be an overlooked modality in the assessment of hypertension in that it defines a certain form of cardiovascular "reactivity." It has been found that if blood pressure exceeds 230/90 during moderate activity, cardiovascular risk increases over twofold, even when basal blood pressures are normal (33). Such blood pressure increases

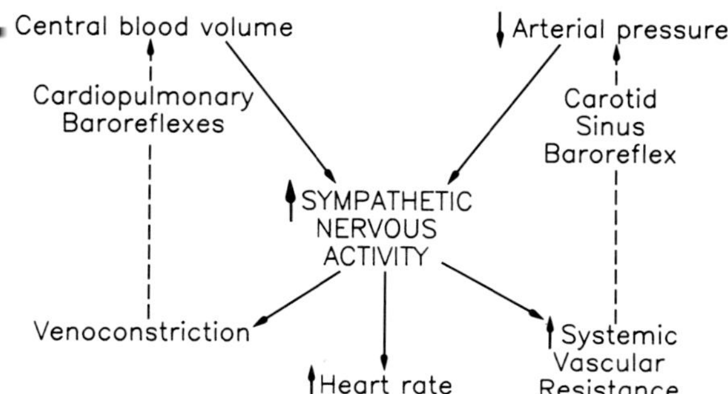

FIG. 2. A simplified schema for postural adaptation. Both carotid sinus and cardiopulmonary stimulation are required for optimal postural adaptation. When pressure and central volume are restored, the baroreflexes are again quiescent (dashed arrows).

during exercise are not predicted by resting parameters. Physical conditioning markedly attenuates the SAS and blood pressure increases caused by exercise (34,35) and also lowers resting heart rate and blood pressure (35).

Pain

Headache and other forms of chronic pain may actually contribute to elevated blood pressure. A systematic study has not been conducted in this area, however.

White Coat Hypertension

The etiology of this condition is not really known, but most experts consider it to be a classic stress response mediated by the SAS. This form of "reactive" blood pressure change differs from sustained hypertension in that target organ damage is reduced (36) and serious cardiovascular complications are less (37). Some current estimates based on ambulatory monitoring data suggest that about 25% of "office" hypertensives are normotensive at home (see Afterword to Chapter 1). Mancia et al. have found extreme variability in the "reactivity" of various hypertensive subjects simultaneously studied with cuff and intra-arterial monitoring. After simple cuff blood pressure measurement, some patients had no changes in intra-arterial pressure, while others had as much as a 75/40 mmHg increase (38).

The white coat syndrome presents one of the most vexing practical problems in the definition of hypertension. This syndrome also confounds data submitted by pharmaceutical firms claiming drug efficacy and makes therapeutic assessment in patients difficult. Frequently these individuals experience numerous drug side effects and present the practitioner with difficult therapeutic choices. On the one hand, many patients now demand treatment for syndromes that may not actually require drug therapy. On the other hand, drug therapy is not totally benign. At present, it seems fair to recommend that all patients be counseled in nonpharmacologic modalities such as exercise and weight reduction. If target organ damage is present or if there are other significant cardiovascular risks (such as hypercholesterolemia), treatment with drugs is probably warranted. In individuals who elect not to take medications, careful follow-up is indicated. It is also prudent to teach many of these individuals to perform home blood pressure monitoring and to assess trends in both office and home blood pressures. Despite the general tendency for repeated office measurements to eventually become similar to those taken by the patient at home (39), the white coat syndrome persists indefinitely in many patients.

Postprandial Hemodynamic Changes

A large meal can increase cardiac output by 20–25%, which is often reflected in an increased heart rate and pulse pressure (40). It has also been described that blood pressure in elderly individuals can fall dramatically after a meal (41,42). This may result from splanchnic vasodilatation in individuals who exhibit some degree of abnormal baroreflex function, vascular volume depletion, and diminished cardiac function.

Hypoglycemic Recovery

A rapid decrease in blood sugar is a marked stimulus to the sympathoadrenal system to liberate catecholamines (43). The predominant release of epinephrine stimulates cardiac output, but the concomitant sympathetic excitation also increases systemic vascular resistance and tends to increase blood pressure (44), particularly in patients taking beta blockers. We have observed patients with hypoglycemia whose blood pressures have transiently reached the range of 250/150. Restoration of blood sugar or a central sympatholytic agent will rapidly lower blood pressure in this condition.

Temperature Change

SAS-mediated systemic vasoconstriction is a reflex response to cold exposure (45). The processes that regulate basal metabolism appear to be influenced by the SAS, but the area remains strongly controversial. The cold pressor test (46) may separate one form of blood pressure "reactivity" from basal hypertension, but it depends on different pain thresholds and other variables.

Cigarette Smoking

Despite the transient increase in blood pressure caused by each cigarette smoked (47), epidemiologists have consistently failed to find a causal relationship between smoking and sustained hypertension. Nevertheless, the increased incidence of peripheral vascular disease and cardiovascular fatalities in cigarette smokers is unquestioned.

As with alcoholism and other addictive syndromes, therapy to induce cessation can be difficult. Combined approaches are best, and clonidine is showing some promise as adjunctive therapy in early studies, presumably by helping to diminish the SAS-mediated symptoms of withdrawal (see section entitled "Alcoholism and Withdrawal Syndromes," below).

Dehydration/Volume Depletion

As already discussed in the description of cardiopulmonary baroreflexes in the control of extracellular fluid volume, severe volume depletion or dehydration can elicit a sympathetic response (48,49). In those individuals with a high degree of vascular reactivity and a marked SAS response, mild volume depletion can increase, rather than decrease, blood pressure (see section entitled "Orthostatic Hypertension and Postdialysis Hypertension," below). When any individual is markedly volume depleted, hypotension inevitably ensues.

Diurnal Variation

This phenomenon has been discussed in detail (see chapter entitled "Diurnal Rhythms and Other Sources of Blood Pressure Variability in Normal and Hypertensive Subjects"). In addition to sleep–waking differences, it is more common to have higher blood pressure in the morning than in the afternoon. The reasons for this variation probably include morning diurnal peaks in total blood volume, central blood volume, sympathoadrenal activity, and plasma renin activity.

Menstrual Cycle

In addition to extracellular fluid volume changes, SAS activity is related to the menstrual cycle (50).

Seasonal Variation

New data indicate that there are predictable increases in blood pressure in the winter in Northern latitudes (51,52), averaging 9 mmHg systolic pressure (52). Data from our laboratory indicate that this phenomenon relates to an activation of the sympathetic nervous system with attendant increases in systemic vascular resistance (20%) during the colder months. During these times when blood pressures are the highest, there are marked decreases in blood volume and cardiac output (15%), underscoring the importance of systemic vascular resistance in the overall determination of arterial pressure. Seasonal variation may also confound the diagnosis of hypertension.

Psychological Stress Responses

The "fight or flight" mechanism has already been mentioned as the hallmark response of the SAS. However, there are different patterns of stress responses within the same individual. These patterns also vary between individuals, making stress research very difficult. For example, blood pressure increases during mental arithmetic may be larger than those with video game stress in one individual, yet the pattern may be reversed in the next (53).

A pragmatic way to approach this problem might be to initially separate patients who are "reactors" to various stressors from those who have unstressed (basal) hypertension. This classification generates four basic groups: one group with hypertension and reactive blood pressure, a second with reactive blood pressure without basal hypertension, a third with basal hypertension only, and a fourth with true normotension. Such distinctions are important for both definition of hypertension and assessment of therapeutic efficacy. Yet one can predict major disagreements among experts about which stressors to use and what cutoffs are important. A consensus has not yet emerged regarding the proper way to address these differences.

There may also be more chronic forms of stress in patients who experience "life crises" or "passages." During such times, blood pressure may be difficult to control.

However, when the conflicts are resolved, blood pressure may spontaneously decline or drug responsiveness may be restored. Such individuals may have significant "suppressed hostility" or high "anger-in" (54).

SYNDROMES OF ABNORMAL SYMPATHOADRENAL DISCHARGE

Neurologic Abnormalities and Sleep Apnea

Strokes, subarachnoid hemorrhage, and other forms of increased intracranial pressure (55) are often associated with marked increases in blood pressure. In these conditions of massive SAS discharge, beta-adrenergic blocking drugs may be useful in lowering pressure and restoring more normal hemodynamics (56).

Patients with spinal cord injuries also manifest an interesting form of episodic hypertension (57). With bladder or bowel distention and rapid decompression, autonomic discharge can cause paroxysmal hypertension, diaphoresis, and other symptoms of autonomic hyperreflexia. As with other syndromes of vascular instability, blood volume depletion exacerbates these problems. Care must be taken in bladder catheterization, and adequate hydration must be maintained in these patients.

Another syndrome recently recognized to have a high degree of association with hypertension is sleep apnea (58). Although obesity confounds existing studies of pathogenesis, abnormal SAS discharge has been postulated to result from hypoxia. Further studies are needed with regard to this condition.

Postanesthesia and Postsurgical Hypertension

Stresses of anesthesia and surgery often result in postoperative hypertension. The most severe cases seem to occur after cardiopulmonary bypass (59), carotid endarterectomy (60), and other vascular and neurosurgical procedures. In a few of these cases, the hypertension is extremely severe and is resistant to nitroprusside. In such cases, the addition of intravenous methyldopa or labetalol often attenuates the blood pressure elevations, presumably by diminishing the component of hypertension related to SAS activation.

Alcoholism and Withdrawal Syndromes

The relationship of alcoholism and alcohol withdrawal to blood pressure is complex and is described in detail (see chapter entitled "Blood Pressure and Alcohol Intake"). Some alcoholics experience (a) a marked increase in blood pressure during periods of consumption (61,62) and (b) normalized blood pressures when abstinent (62). These changes are commonly attributed to "volume overload"; however, that mechanism alone is an unlikely cause of the hypertension, which must involve vascular smooth muscle metabolic effects and possibly neurohumoral cardiovascular regulatory changes as well (63). Alcoholic hypertension may be refractory not only to diuretic therapy but also to potent antihypertensive combinations.

Withdrawal hypertension is quite clearly related to a marked SAS discharge and can be blocked by clonidine (64). The similarity to other withdrawal syndromes probably reflects the role of other modulators in central vasomotor control mechanisms. Therapy is beyond the scope of this chapter and is best carried out by experienced personnel using a multidisciplinary approach.

Panic Attacks

It is generally recognized that the classic symptoms of severe anxiety are similar to those achieved by the infusion of catecholamines (65,66). In true panic attacks, patients often have severe cardiac awareness, tachycardia and palpitations, sensations of impending doom, peripheral vasoconstriction, paroxysmal hypertension (67,68), and other vasomotor symptoms. However, as described in the preceding and following sections, these same symptoms can result from central blood volume dysregulation or other forms of SAS discharge. The question arises whether many physicians are missing these more esoteric diagnoses, writing them off as simple anxiety neuroses. Much more work must be done in these areas to understand and treat these patients.

When the diagnosis of a panic disorder is firm, there are several therapeutic modalities. First, it is common experience that beta-blockers are helpful to many patients in controlling symptoms of catecholamine excess (such as tachycardia and tremor) and even exert a mild anxiolytic effect (69). In our experience, *intermittent* therapy can be preferable to chronic therapy.

More recently, alprazolam and other benzodiazepines have been employed in anxiety syndromes to control symptoms such as tremor, tachycardia, and cardiac awareness (70). However, alprazolam only partially blunts anxiety-dependent blood pressure "reactivity," and is largely ineffective in controlling blood pressure in those patients with both essential hypertension and panic attacks.

This selective ability of benzodiazepines to blunt cardiac (but not vascular) events gives rise to a highly simplified model for approaching the clinical physiology and pharmacology of anxiety syndromes (Fig. 3). Because alprazolam is specific for GABA-binding proteins (particularly in the locus ceruleus region of the basal ganglia), responses to alprazolam have physiologic as well as therapeutic significance. Stratton and Halter have shown that exercise-induced epinephrine, but not norepinephrine, release is blocked by alprazolam (71). This fits well with the ability of the drug to diminish beta-adrenoceptor–mediated signs and symptoms such as tachycardia and tremor through selective action on the locus ceruleus. In contrast, the vasomotor center controls both sympathetic ("noradrenergic") and adrenal medullary ("adrenergic") functions. Thus, actions of benzodiazepines further suggest the separability of "reactive" and "basal" forms of hypertension.

Alprazolam must be used cautiously and tapered very slowly over many weeks because of its propensity to cause a severe withdrawal syndrome, even at low doses. In many patients, high-dose (2–4 mg daily) maintenance therapy is required. In some hypertensives with panic syndromes, we

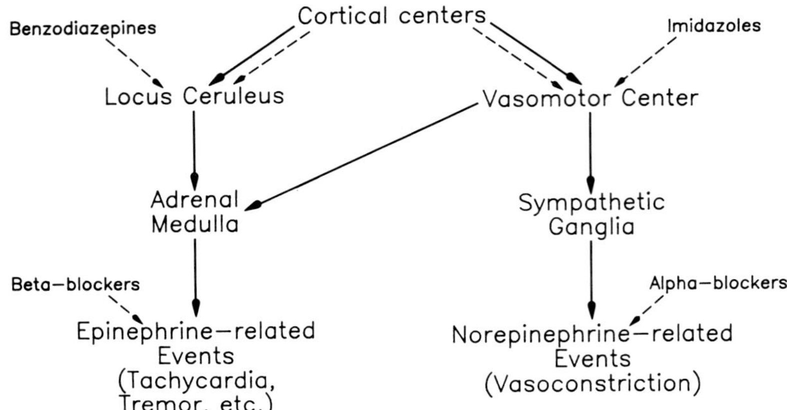

FIG. 3. A highly simplified model of dual efferent sympathoadrenal control. The vasomotor center (C1 neurons) of the brain stem controls both the adrenal medulla and peripheral sympathetic neurons. A separate input from other brain centers (locus ceruleus) affects the adrenal medulla without significantly affecting sympathetic neurons. Inhibitory effects of cortical centers, as well as sites of action of various blocking drugs, are shown by interrupted lines.

have combined angiotensin-converting-enzyme (ACE) inhibitors or calcium-channel blockers with benzodiazepines. In this way we have avoided the use of beta blockers in patients with easily triggered depressive episodes.

Autonomic Dysfunction and Orthostatic Hypotension

Failure to stimulate the SAS after a decrease in arterial pressure or central blood volume constitutes autonomic insufficiency. In practice, Valsalva maneuvers and plasma norepinephrine values are used to help establish the diagnosis of "central" versus "peripheral" autonomic failure (69), although plasma catecholamines do not always clearly differentiate these groups. A high degree of blood pressure variability occurs in both forms of the disease. Generalized lesions can be found in "central" control centers including basal ganglia (Shy–Drager syndrome), in brain-stem control centers, or in the peripheral sympathetic nervous system (72,73). Various subtypes of autonomic dysfunction have been described, including congenital deficiencies of dopamine beta-hydroxylase (74), or "preganglionic" versus "postganglionic" disease (75). Some diabetics appear to have hyperresponsiveness of the SAS, while others demonstrate hyporesponsiveness (76). In all of these cases, there is an inability to maintain blood pressure in the upright position. Because these patients have renal sodium wasting (23), small degrees of blood volume depletion can precipitate hypotensive crises. Clinically, a volume challenge helps to separate simple dehydration from autonomic insufficiency. Patients with intact autonomic function do not immediately excrete a saline load, whereas patients with autonomic insufficiency cannot retain a saliva load.

Therapy of autonomic insufficiency is difficult. Elastic stockings can be employed to compress the lower extremities and improve venous return. However, many patients object to wearing these uncomfortable garments. Pharmacotherapy is also problematic. Fludrocortisone causes symptomatic improvement in the upright position but exacerbates supine hypertension and increases sequelae such as strokes and ventricular hypertrophy (77). Sympathomimetic amines (78), monoamine oxidase inhibitors (79), and vasodilators (80) are occasionally useful. Reports of beneficial effects of nonsteroidal anti-inflammatory drugs (81), nonspecific vasoconstrictors (82), beta-blockers (83), and yohimbine (84) also exist.

SYNDROMES OF APPARENT CENTRAL-VOLUME–SYMPATHOADRENAL DYSREGULATION

Transient Left Ventricular Dysfunction (Silent Ischemia)

When there is a sudden decrease in the forward flow of blood, brain-stem centers stimulate the SAS. The release of catecholamines, which is well documented in angina pectoris (85), myocardial infarction (86), and ventricular failure (87), probably occurs via (a) hypoxic stimulation of chemoreceptors and (b) transient drops in arterial pressure. The role of the atrial stretch receptors is unclear; at first blush, it would appear that atrial distension should inhibit SAS outflow. However, the rate of change in atrial stretch may be crucial. Rapid central volume expansion may result in SAS-mediated vasoconstriction, whereas slow volume loading suppresses peripheral SAS activity (25,26).

Clinically milder forms of ventricular dysfunction can also affect the SAS. "Silent ischemia" may be accompanied by large blood pressure surges and symptoms of catecholamine release similar to those observed in patients with panic attacks (arrhythmias, tachycardia, diaphoresis, pallor, and cold extremities). In a recent study, emotional stimuli proved to be more effective than exercise in induction of ventricular wall motion abnormalities in these patients (88). It is the opinion of this author that transitory episodes of ventricular ischemia/dysfunction are among the most common pathophysiologic reasons for paroxysmal elevations of blood pressure in elderly individuals. Systematic studies are just now being undertaken to determine the severity and prevalence of this condition using a combination of ambulatory electrocardiogram (ECG) and blood pressure monitoring.

Anecdotally, ACE inhibitors may be effective in reducing the number and severity of these paroxysmal episodes, but no controlled-trial data are available. Alprazolam may also be effective in the reduction of tachycardia, arrhythmias, ECG changes, and other SAS-related symptoms in patients with silent ischemia (89), similar to its effects in panic syndromes (see above).

Pulmonary Hypertension

Paroxysmal hypertension in this syndrome has been mistaken for anxiety (90). The etiology of the lability of blood pressure in pulmonary hypertension is unknown, but it may relate to abnormally disparate right and left heart pressures.

Mitral Valve Prolapse (MVP)

There is no direct association between this condition and sustained hypertension, and one report suggests that patients with MVP have a reduced prevalence rate of hypertension (91). However, there can be marked lability of blood pressure in many of these patients. The clinical similarities of MVP patients and individuals with hyperdynamic circulatory states or panic syndromes (92,93) also deserves mention.

In theory, many of the clinical features of MVP may be related to alterations in atrial stretch and central blood volume and, in turn, to secondary effects on the SAS. These patients often have long symptom-free periods and shorter periods of apparent decompensation. It is the experience of this author that the winter and early spring are the peak periods for symptomatic episodes (see section entitled "Seasonal Variation"). During these times of relative central blood volume decrease and increased SAS activity, smaller ventricular volume may cause the mitral leaflets to prolapse farther back into the atrium, worsening the mitral regurgitation. Concomitant increases in stroke volume variability would be expected to cause greater variability of atrial pressures and SAS activity, predisposing to the well-known arrhythmias and catecholamine-related somatic symptoms that accompany MVP.

Therapeutically it is important to maximize blood volume in MVP patients by rehydrating or withdrawing diuretics. Beta-blockade also has been helpful in managing tachycardia, arrhythmias, and somatic symptoms (94). Anecdotally, vasodilator therapy, particularly with such agents as low-dose ACE inhibitors, may also help, although controlled trials are not available. ACE inhibitors may work because they expand blood volume while blunting SAS activity (95).

Orthostatic Hypertension and Postdialysis Hypertension

Streeten et al. have described a group of patients with normal supine blood pressures and markedly abnormal increases in blood pressure on standing (96). These patients have (a) abnormally low blood volumes, (b) excessive (proportional) venous pooling with upright posture or tilt, (c) marked stimulation of the cardiopulmonary baroreceptors, and (d) an exaggerated sympathoadrenal response to orthostatic stress. This orthostatic SAS discharge causes a marked increase in upright systemic vascular resistance, which results in orthostatic hypertension.

Postdialysis hypertension appears to have the same etiology as orthostatic hypertension. Although the cardiopulmonary baroreflexes in these groups have not been formally tested, it appears that patients with postdialysis hypertension have an exaggerated vasoconstrictor response to mild central volume depletion. This group also tends to have a higher plasma renin activity than those patients whose blood pressures fall after dialysis (97). Recalling the facilitating effects of angiotensin II on the sympathetic nervous system, these syndromes fit neatly into the blood pressure counterregulation model, but exhibit increased SAS-dependent vasoconstriction.

Therapy in these conditions is initially directed toward restoration of the depleted blood volume. In those patients not on dialysis, diuretic therapy should be withdrawn. In dialysis patients, less vigorous ultrafiltration should be employed. Whether or not drug therapy is necessary in uncomplicated orthostatic hypertension is a matter for considerable debate. In either group, appropriate vasodilator therapy can be effective. ACE inhibitors or calcium-channel blockers are good choices, and many patients also respond well to alpha-blockers, as might be predicted.

Idiopathic Hypovolemia

Frohlich, Cohn and coworkers originally described a subgroup of individuals initially thought to have a hyperdynamic circulation (98), who instead proved to have low cardiac output and high systemic vascular resistance (99). More recently, Fouad et al. reported more extensive studies in this same group. Included in the presenting symptomatology were orthostatic tachycardia (despite a normal response of blood pressure to tilt), frequent flushing attacks, syncope, and extreme blood pressure lability. These individuals had high-normal plasma catecholamines and normal autonomic reflexes. The most salient finding was that blood volume averaged 73% of predicted normal values (100).

As already described in patients with orthostatic hypertension, such a syndrome fits well within the framework of blood pressure counterregulation and the "volume-vasoconstrictor" concept. The differences between individuals with hypovolemia and those with orthostatic hypertension is not clear, but the former group seems to have a more "vascular reactivity," whereas the latter manifests more "cardiac reactivity" to catecholamines. Adrenergic receptors have not been studied in these populations, and the reasons for inappropriate volume depletion are unknown (see section entitled "Episodic Dopamine Discharge," below). It is unclear from the reports whether some or all of these individuals may have had mitral valve prolapse, but it is the experience of this author that some do. Therapy is similar to that described for orthostatic hypertension. Fludrocortisone has been employed, but this therapy is poorly tolerated by many patients as a result of peripheral edema, supine headaches (due to supine hypertension), and bloating.

Episodic Dopamine Discharge

In attempting to further characterize the ailments of those patients without pheochromocytoma who had paroxysmal elevations of blood pressure, Kuchel et al. discovered that some were polyuric and had exceptionally high plasma levels of free and sulfoconjugated dopamine (101,102). These authors likened their patients to those females described by Page, who had flushing and other vasomotor symptoms, diaphoresis, palpitations, and extreme paroxysms of hypertension (103). Page coined the term "diencephalic hypertension," though this diagnosis has never been substantiated. Whatever its true etiology, this fairly common syndrome is interesting to compare with "idiopathic hypovolemia." When one remembers that dopamine is both natriuretic and diuretic (104), the possibility is raised that the two syndromes are the same. Kuchel claims therapeutic success with beta-blockers, but the experience is still rather small.

Neurocirculatory Asthenia (Soldier's Heart)

This diagnostic category includes many eponyms, synonyms, and phrases too numerous to mention (105). The diagnosis exists more commonly in the European literature than in the United States. In brief, this syndrome was recognized in foot soldiers who were said to experience "battle fatigue." Included in the symptom complex were syncopal and hypotensive attacks, autonomic symptomatology, and asthenia. Whether or not these individuals may have had variants of hypovolemic syndromes or mitral valve prolapse is reasonable speculation.

OTHER NEUROHUMORAL SYNDROMES

Other hormones and autacoids may influence arterial pressure through alterations in vasomotor tone, vascular permeability, extracellular fluid compartmentation, natriuresis, or autonomic control mechanisms. A variety of amines, peptides, prostaglandins, cyclic nucleotides, and other substances may affect blood pressure at physiologic or pathologic extremes but may have only a minor role in more typical circumstances. In many cases, the role of these factors is still theoretical.

Histamine and Systemic Mastocytosis

Patients with urticaria pigmentosa or systemic mastocytosis are known to have vasomotor instability. The mechanism of their blood pressure lability is probably complex, including effects on catecholamine release, stimulation of various autacoids, and permeability and volume alterations. Recently, Roberts and coworkers described a cohort of patients with dermographism, increased cutaneous mast cell numbers on skin biopsy, and cardiovascular instability (106). These patients commonly had flushing attacks, and some had bouts of severe hypotension with cardiac arrhythmias that simulated an epinephrine-secreting pheochromocytoma. Not only did they have increased levels of circulating histamine, but they were also found to have large excesses of the vasodilatory prostaglandins of the D2 series.

This condition may require intensive drug therapy. In the Vanderbilt experience, both H1 and H2 blockade are combined with high-dose prostaglandin synthetase inhibition. It is not uncommon for some of these individuals to require chlorphenirimine (12–24 mg/day), cimetidine (600–1200 mg/day), and aspirin (12–24 g/day) to prevent episodes of cardiovascular collapse. In our experience, smaller doses of these drugs can be effective in milder cases, and intermittent therapy is sometimes possible. In general, both H1 and H2 receptors must be blocked to achieve efficacy.

Hyperbradykininism

The existence of this syndrome is still debated by experts in the field. It was originally described by Streeten et al. in a group of individuals with cutaneous flushing and orthostatic hypotension (107). Two major problems have plagued investigation of the kallikrein–kinin system: the lack of sensitive, reliable assays for bradykinin and the lack of specific inhibitors of this peptide. More recently, specific bradykinin inhibition has been reported, but application to specific syndromes remains to be accomplished. Diagnosis and treatment of any possible bradykinin-related syndrome is not currently possible.

Serotonin and Carcinoid Syndrome

Although flushing can occur in carcinoid syndrome, it is generally limited to those with hepatic metastases. Hypertension has been also reported as a sequela of this syndrome (108). The diagnosis is suggested by the presence of elevated urinary 5-hydroxyindoleacetate excretion in a patient with strong clinical history, but the cost-effectiveness of screening for this condition is highly questionable. Therapy is directed at surgical removal of the tumor, with the possibility of adjunctive chemotherapy.

Porphyria

Paroxysms of blood pressure in the syndrome have been ascribed to abnormal catecholamine metabolism (109). Its diagnosis should be entertained in patients with cardiovascular instability and hepatic or cutaneous abnormalities. Various tests for bilirubin metabolites are available, but therapy is largely symptomatic.

DRUGS AND DRUG DOSING EFFECTS

Dosing Effects

Early formulations of many antihypertensive drugs were actually quite short-acting and therefore had to be given too frequently for patients to be able to readily comply with

TABLE 2. *Common drugs that can raise blood pressure*

Prescription drugs
Amphetamines
MAO inhibitors (+tyramine in food)
Oral contraceptives
Nonsteroidal anti-inflammatory drugs (NSAIDs)
Cyclosporine
Imidazole withdrawal (clonidine, guanabenz)
Beta-blockers (elderly patients)
Over-the-counter drugs
Phenylpropanolamine (diet pills)
Pseudoephedrine (cold pills)
Phenylephrine (nasal drops)
NSAIDs
Antacids (sodium content)
"Street drugs"
Cocaine
Amphetamines and congeners
Nicotine
Caffeine

the regimen. At best, the result was equivalent to converting sustained to labile hypertension. Short-acting drugs are still a problem today, though long-acting formulations are available in almost all classes of antihypertensive drugs. The shortest-acting drugs still in widespread clinical use are hydralazine, nifedipine capsules, and diltiazem. Each of these drugs usually must be given at least three (and preferably four) times daily. Clonidine and guanabenz are also relatively short-acting, but they can usually be given twice daily. Short-acting drugs not only fail to keep the blood pressure under tight control, but they often cost more and are more likely to be associated with side effects related to marked differences in peak and trough effects.

Pressor Substances

Many commonly ingested substances can raise blood pressure. A partial list of these compounds is presented in Table 2; this list was formulated from a similar list modified by Dr. Norman Kaplan from an article by Messerli and Frohlich (110). A careful history of ingestion of these substances can be extremely valuable to the clinician and the patient, who may be unaware of such effects.

REFERENCES

1. Koch-Weser J. Correlation of pathophysiology and pharmacology in primary hypertension. *Am J Cardiol* 1973;32:499.
2. Kannel WB. Role of blood pressure in cardiovascular morbidity and mortality. *Prog Cardiovasc Dis* 1974;17:5.
3. Clark LA, Denby L, Pregibon D, et al. A quantitative analysis of the effects of activity and time of day on the diurnal variations of blood pressure. *J Chronic Dis* 1987;40:671–681.
4. deBoer RW, Karemaker JM, Strackee J. Hemodynamic fluctuations and baroreflex sensitivity in humans: a beat-to-beat model. *Am J Physiol* 1987;253(2):H680–H689.
5. Pickering TG, Harshfield GA, Blank S, et al. Behavioral determinants of 24-hour blood pressure patterns in borderline hypertension. *J Cardiovasc Pharmacol* 1986;8:89–92.
6. Mancia G. Blood pressure variability at normal and high blood pressure. *Chest* 1983;83:317–320.
7. Rowe JW. Clinical consequences of age-related impairments in vascular compliance. *Am J Cardiol* 1987;60:68G–71G.
8. Safar ME, London GM. Arterial and venous compliance in sustained essential hypertension. *Hypertension* 1987;10:133–139.
9. Lipsitz LA, Storch HA, Minaker KL, Rowe JW. Intra-individual variability in postural blood pressure in the elderly. *Clin Sci* 1985;69:337–341.
10. Izzo JL Jr. Hypertension in the elderly: a pathophysiologic approach to therapy. *J Am Geriatr Soc* 1982;30:352–359.
11. Abboud FM. Sympathetic nervous system in hypertension. *Hypertension* 1982;4(Suppl II):208–225.
12. Izzo JL Jr. The sympathoadrenal system in the maintenance of elevated arterial pressure. *J Cardiovasc Pharmacol* 1984;6:s514–s521.
13. Gribbin B, Pickering TG, Sleight P, Peto R. Effect of age and high blood pressure on baroreflex sensitivity in man. *Circ Res* 1971;29:424–430.
14. Eckberg DL, Harkins SW, Fritsch JM, Musgrave GE, Gardner DF. Baroreflex control of plasma norepinephrine and heart period in healthy subjects and diabetic patients. *J Clin Invest* 1986;78:366–374.
15. Cowley AW, Monos E, Guyton AC. Interaction of vasopressin and the baroreceptor reflex system in the regulation of arterial pressure in the dog. *Circ Res* 1974;34:505.
16. Mancia G, Parati G, Pomidossi G, Casadei R, Di Rienzo M, Zanchetti A. Arterial baroreflexes and blood pressure and heart rate variabilities in humans. *Hypertension* 1986;8:147–153.
17. Mark AL, Kerber RE. Augmentation of cardiopulmonary baroreflex control of forearm vascular resistance in borderline hypertension. *Hypertension* 1982;4:39–46.
18. Egan BM, Julius S, Cottier C, Osterziel KJ, Ibsen H. Role of cardiovascular receptors on the neuroregulation of renin release in normal men. *Hypertension* 1983;5:779–786.
19. Sowers JR, Mohanty PK. Effect of advancing age on cardiopulmonary baroreceptor function in hypertensive men. *Hypertension* 1987;10:274–279.
20. Mancia G, Grassi G, Parati G, et al. Control of circulation by arterial baroreceptors and cardiopulmonary receptors in hypertension. *J Cardiovasc Pharmacol* 1988;8(Suppl 5):s82–s88.
21. Mohanty PK, Thames MD, Arrowood JA, Sowers JR, McNamara C, Szentpetery S. Impairment of cardiopulmonary baroreflex after cardiac transplantation in humans. *Circulation* 1987;75:914–921.
22. Wood P. Polyuria in paroxysmal tachycardia and paroxysmal atrial flutter and fibrillation. *Br Heart J* 1963;25:273.
23. Gill JR Jr, Bartter FC. Adrenergic nervous system in sodium metabolism. II. Effects of guanethidine on the renal response to sodium deprivation in normal man. *N Engl J Med* 1966;275:1466–1471.
24. Wagner HN Jr. The influence of autonomic vasoregulatory reflexes on the rate of sodium and water excretion in man. *J Clin Invest* 1957;36:1319–1327.
25. Thames MD, Miller BD, Abboud FM. Baroreflex regulation of renal nerve activity during volume expansion. *Am J Physiol* 1982;243:810–814.
26. Morita H, Vatner SF. Effects of volume expansion on renal nerve activity, renal blood flow, and sodium and water excretion in conscious dogs. *Am J Physiol* 1985;249(5):F680–F687.
27. DiBona GF. Neural control of renal tubular sodium reabsorption in the dog. *Fed Proc* 1978;37:1214–1217.
28. Winternitz SR, Oparil S. Importance of the renal nerves in the pathogenesis of experimental hypertension. *Hypertension* 1982;5:108–114.
29. Epstein M. Renal effects of head out water immersion in men: implications for an understanding of volume homeostasis. *Physiol Rev* 1978;58:529–581.
30. Littler WA, West MJ, Honour AJ, Sleight P. The variability of arterial pressure. *Am Heart J* 1978;95:180–186.
31. Reeves RA, Shapiro AP, Thompson ME, Johnsen AM. Loss of

nocturnal decline in blood pressure after cardiac transplantation. *Circulation* 1986;73(3):401–408.
32. Imai Y, Abe K, Sasaki S, et al. Daily variation of blood pressure in patients with Cushing's syndrome. *Tohoku J Exp Med* 1987;153:67–74.
33. Wilson NV, Meyer BM. Early prediction of hypertension using exercise blood pressure. *Prev Med* 1981;10:62–68.
34. Urata H, Tanabe Y, Kiyonaga A, et al. Antihypertensive and volume-depleting effects of mild exercise on essential hypertension. *Hypertension* 1987;9:245–252.
35. Kaplan NM. Therapy for mild hypertension: toward a more balanced view. *JAMA* 1983;249:365–367.
36. Floras JS, Jones JV, Hassan MD. Cuff and ambulatory blood pressure in subjects with essential hypertension. *Lancet* 1981;2:107–109.
37. Sokolow M, Werdegar D, Kain HK, Hinman AT. Relationship between level of blood pressure measured casually and by portable recorders and severity of complications in essential hypertension. *Circulation* 1966;34:279.
38. Mancia G, Ferrari A, Gregorini L. Blood pressure and heart rate variabilities in normotensive and hypertensive human beings. *Circ Res* 1983;53:96.
39. Padfield PL, Lindsay BA, McLaren JA, Pirie A, Rademaker M. Changing relation between home and clinic blood-pressure measurements: do home measurements predict clinic hypertension? *Lancet* 1987;8554:322–324.
40. Cowley AJ, Stainer K, Murphy DT, Murphy J, Hampton JR. A non-invasive method for measuring cardiac output: the effect of Christmas lunch. *Lancet* 1986;2:1422–1424.
41. Lipsitz LA, Pluchino FC, Wei JY, Minaker KL, Rowe JW. Cardiovascular and norepinephrine responses after meal consumption in elderly (older than 75 years) persons with postprandial hypotension and syncope. *Am J Cardiol* 1986;58:810–815.
42. Lipsitz LA, Nyquist RP Jr, Wei JY, Rowe JW. Postprandial reduction in blood pressure in the elderly. *N Engl J Med* 1983;309:81–83.
43. Garber AJ, Cryer PE, Santiago JV, et al. The role of adrenergic mechanisms in the substrate and hormonal response to insulin-induced hypoglycemia in man. *J Clin Invest* 1976;58:7–15.
44. Farr MJ. Diazoxide, glipizide, hypertension, and hypoglycemia. *Lancet* 1976;2:1138.
45. Landsberg L, Young JB. Catecholamines and the adrenal medulla. In: Wilson JD, Foster DW, eds. *Textbook of endocrinology.* Philadelphia: WB Saunders, 1985:891–965.
46. Thomas CB, Duszynski KR. Blood pressure levels in young adulthood as predictors of hypertension and the fate of the cold pressor test. *Johns Hopkins Med J* 1982;151:93.
47. Cryer PE, Haymond MW, Shah SD, Santiago JV. Norepinephrine and epinephrine release and adrenergic medication of smoking-associated hemodynamic and metabolic effects. *N Engl J Med* 1976;295:573–577.
48. Romoff MS, Kreusch G, Campese VM, et al. Effect of sodium intake on plasma catecholamines in normal subjects. *J Clin Endocrinol Metab* 1979;48:26–31.
49. Luft FC, Rankin LI, Henry DP, et al. Plasma and urinary norepinephrine at extremes of sodium intake in normal man. *Hypertension* 1979;1:261–266.
50. Goldstein DS, Levinson P, Keiser HR. Plasma and urinary catecholamines during the human ovulatory cycle. *Am J Obstet Gynecol* 1983;146:824–829.
51. Hata T, Ogihara T, Maruyama A, et al. The seasonal variation of blood pressure in patients with essential hypertension. *Clin Exp Hypertens* 1982;3:341–354.
52. Brennan PJ, Greenberg G, Miall WE, Thompson SG. Seasonal variation in arterial blood pressure. *Br Med J* 1982;285:919–923.
53. Ewart CK, Harris WL, Zeger S, Russell GA. Diminished pulse pressure under mental stress characterizes normotensive adolescents with parental high blood pressure. *Psychosom Med* 1986;48:489–501.
54. Schneider RH, Egan BM, Johnson EH, Drobny H, Julius S. Anger and anxiety in borderline hypertension. *Psychosom Med* 1986;48:242–248.
55. Clifton GI, Robertson CS, Kyper K. Cardiovascular response to severe head injury. *J Neurosurg* 1983;59:447.
56. Colgan JJ, Sawa T, Ten Eyck LG, Izzo JL Jr. Protective effects of beta blockade on pulmonary function when intracranial pressure is elevated. *Crit Care Med* 1983;11:368–372.
57. Naftchi NE, Demeny M, Lowman EW, Tuckman J. Hypertensive crises in quadriplegic patients. Changes in cardiac output, blood volume, serum dopamine-beta-hydroxylase activity, and arterial prostaglandin PGE2. *Circulation* 1978;57:336–341.
58. Kales A, Bixler EO, Cadieux RJ. Sleep apnea in a hypertensive population. *Lancet* 1984;2:1005–1008.
59. Estanfous FG, Tarazi RC, et al. Systemic arterial hypertension associated with cardiac surgery. *Am J Cardiol* 1980;46:685–694.
60. Caplan LR, Skillman J, Ojemann R, Fields WS. Intracerebral hemorrhage following carotid endarterectomy: a hypertensive complication? *Stroke* 1978;9:457–460.
61. Criqui MH, Wallace RB, MM. Alcohol consumption and blood pressure: the lipid clinics prevalence study. *Hypertension* 1981;3:557–565.
62. Saunders JB, Beevers DG, Paton A. Factors influencing blood pressure in chronic alcoholics. *Clin Sci* 1979;57:295s.
63. Arkwright P, Beilin LJ, Vandongen R, Armstrong BK, Masarei JR. Alcohol and hypertension. *Aust NZ J Med* 1984;14(4):463–469.
64. Abrams WB. In summary: satellite symposium on central alpha-adrenergic blood pressure regulating mechanisms. *Hypertension* 1984;6(Suppl II):II87–II93.
65. Pyke RE, Greenberg HS. Norepinephrine challenges in panic patients. *J Clin Psychopharmacol* 1986;6:279–285.
66. Frohlich ED, Tarazi RC, Dustan HP. Hyperdynamic beta-adrenergic circulatory state. *Arch Intern Med* 1969;123:1.
67. White WB, Baker LH. Episodic hypertension secondary to panic disorder. *Arch Intern Med* 1986;146:1129–1130.
68. White WB, Baker LH. Ambulatory blood pressure monitoring in patients with panic disorder. *Arch Intern Med* 1987;147:1973–1975.
69. Granvill-Grossman KL, Turner P. The effect of propranolol on anxiety. *Lancet* 1966;1:788.
70. Ballenger JC, Burrows GD, Dupont RL Jr, et al. Alprazolam in panic disorder and agoraphobia: results from a multicenter trial. *Arch Gen Psychiatry* 1988;45:413–443.
71. Stratton JR, Halter JB. Effect of a benzodiazepine (alprazolam) on plasma epinephrine and norepinephrine levels during exercise stress. *Am J Cardiol* 1985;56:136–139.
72. Ziegler MG, Lake CR, Kopin IJ. The sympathetic-nervous-system defect in primary orthostatic hypotension. *N Engl J Med* 1977;296:293–297.
73. Shy GM, Drager GA. A neurological syndrome associated with orthostatic hypotension: a clinical-pathologic study. *Arch Neurol* 1960;2:511–527.
74. Man In't Veld AJ, Boomsma F, Moleman P, Schalekamp MA. Congenital dopamine-beta-hydroxylase deficiency. *Lancet* 1987;1:183–188.
75. Cryer PE. Physiology and pathophysiology of the human sympathoadrenal neuroendocrine system. *N Engl J Med* 1980;303:436–444.
76. Cryer PE, Silverberg AB, Santiago JV, Shah SD. Plasma catecholamines in diabetes: the syndromes of hypoadrenergic and hyperadrenergic postural hypotension. *Am J Med* 1978;64:407–416.
77. Chobanian AV, Volicer L, Tifft CP, Gavras H, Liang C, Faxon D. Mineralocorticoid-induced hypertension in patients with orthostatic hypotension. *N Engl J Med* 1979;301:68–73.
78. Biaggioni I, Onrot J, Stewart CK, Robertson D. The potent pressor effet of phenylpropanolamine in patients with autonomic impairment. *JAMA* 1987;258:236–239.
79. Nanda RN, Johnson RH, Keogh HJ. Treatment of neurogenic orthostatic hypotension with a monoamine oxidase inhibitor and tyramine. *Lancet* 1976;2:1164–1167.
80. Jones DH, Reid JL. Volume expansion and vasodilators in the treatment of idiopathic postural hypotension. *Postgrad Med J* 1980;56:234–235.
81. Kochar MS, Itskovitz HD. Treatment of idiopathic orthostatic hypotension (Shy–Drager syndrome) with indomethacin. *Lancet* 1978;1(8072):1011–1014.
82. Jennings G, Esler M, Holmes R. Treatment of orthostatic hypotension with dihydroergotamine. *Br Med J* 1979;2:307.
83. Man In't Veld AJ, Boomsma F, Schalekamp MADH. Effects of

beta-adrenoceptor agonists and antagonists in patients with peripheral autonomic neuropathy. *Br J Clin Pharmacol* 1982;13:367s–374s.
84. Onrot J, Goldberg MR, Biaggioni I, Wiley RG, Hollister AS, Robertson D. Oral yohimbine in human autonomic failure. *Neurology* 1987;37:215–220.
85. Schwartz L, Sole MJ, Vaughan-Neil EF, Hussain NM. Catecholamines in coronary sinus and peripheral plasma during pacing-induced angina in man. *Circulation* 1979;59:37–43.
86. Nadeau RA, de Champlain J. Plasma catecholamines in acute myocardial infarction. *Am Heart J* 1979;98:548–554.
87. Cohn JN, Levine TB, Olivari MT, et al. Plasma norepinephrine as a guide to prognosis in patients with chronic congestive heart failure. *N Engl J Med* 1984;311:819–823.
88. Rozanski A, Bairey CN, Krantz DS, et al. Mental stress and the induction of silent myocardial ischemia in patients with coronary artery disease. *N Engl J Med* 1988;318:1005–1012.
89. Shell WE, Swan HJC. Treatment of silent myocardial ischemic with transdermal nitroglycerine aded to beta-blockers and alprazolam. *Cardiol Clin* 1986;4:697–703.
90. Sietsema KE, Simon JI, Wasserman K. Pulmonary hypertension presenting as a panic disorder. *Chest* 1987;91:910–912.
91. Holgado GM, Prakash R. Prevalence of mitral valve prolapse in hypertension. *J Nat Med Assoc* 1987;79:966–968.
92. Weissman NJ, Shear MK, Kramer Fox R, Devereux RB. Contrasting patterns of autonomic dysfunction in patients with mitral valve prolapse and panic attacks. *Am J Med* 1987;82:880–888.
93. Davies AO, Mares A, Pool JL, Taylor AA. Mitral valve prolapse with symptoms of beta-adrenergic hypersensitivity. *Am J Med* 1987;82:193–201.
94. Winkle RA, Lopes MG, Goodman DS. Propranolol for patients with mitral valve prolapse. *Am Heart J* 1970;93:422.
95. Izzo JL Jr, Licht MR, Smith RJ, Larrabee PS, Radke KJ, Kallay MC. Chronic effecs of direct vasodilation (pinacidil), alpha-adrenergic blockade (prazosin) and angiotensin-converting enzyme inhibition (captopril). *Am J Cardiol* 1987;60:303–308.
96. Streeten DH, Auchincloss JH Jr, Anderson GH Jr, Richardson RL, Thomas FD, Miller JW. Orthostatic hypertension: pathogenetic studies. *Hypertension* 1985;7:196–203.
97. Textor SC, Gavras H, Tifft CP, Bernard DB, Idelson B, Brunner HR. Norepinephrine and renin activity in chronic renal failure. Evidence for interacting roles in hemodialysis hypertension. *Hypertension* 1981;3:294–299.
98. Frohlich ED, Kozul VN, Tarazi RC, Dustan HP. Physiological comparison of labile and essential hypertension. *Circ Res* 1970;27:55–69.
99. Cohn JN. Blood pressure measurement in shock: mechanism of inaccuracy in ausculatory and palpatory methods. *JAMA* 1967;199:118–122.
100. Fouad FM, Tadena-Thome L, Bravo EL, Tarazi RC. Idiopathic hypovolemia. *An Intern Med* 1986;104:298–303.
101. Kuchel O, Buu NT, Larochelle P, Hamet P, Genest J. Episodic dopamine discharge in paroxysmal hypertension. *Arch Intern Med* 1986;146:1315–1320.
102. Kuchel O, Buu NT, Hamet P. Orthostatic hypotension: a posture-induced hyperdopaminergic state. *Am J Med Sci* 1985;289:3–11.
103. Page IH. A syndrome simulating diencephalic stimulation occurring in patients with essential hypertension. *Am J Med Sci* 1935;190:9–14.
104. Weiner N. Norepinephrine, epinephrine, and the sympathomimetic amines. In: Gilman AG, Goodman LS, Rall TW, Murad F, eds. *The pharmacological basis of therapeutics.* New York: Macmillan, 1985:145–180.
105. Wheeler EO, White PD, Reed EW. Neurocirculatory asthenia (anxiety neurosis, effort syndrome, neurasthenia). *JAMA* 1950;142:878.
106. Kootte AM, Haak A, Roberts LJ. The flush syndrome: an expression of systemic mastocytosis with increased prostaglandin D2 production. *Neth J Med* 1983;26:18–20.
107. Streeten DH, Kerr CB, Kerr LP, Prior JC, Dalakos TG. Hyperbradykininism: a new orthostatic syndrome. *Lancet* 1972;2:1048–1053.
108. Rosenberg FB. The carcinoid syndrome and hypertension. *Arch Intern Med* 1968;121:95–96.
109. Beal MF, Atuk NO, Westfall TC, Turner SM. Catecholamine uptake, accumulation, and release in acute porphyria. *J Clin Invest* 1977;60:1141–1148.
110. Messerli FH, Frohlich ED. High blood pressure: a side effect of drugs, poisons, and food. *Arch Intern Med* 1979;139:682–687.

Hypertension: Pathophysiology, Diagnosis, and Management, edited by J. H. Laragh and B. M. Brenner. Raven Press, Ltd., New York © 1990.

CHAPTER 89

Blood Pressure Measurement and Ambulatory Blood Pressure Monitoring

Evaluation of Available Equipment

Thomas G. Pickering and Seymour G. Blank

Invasive Techniques for Measuring Blood Pressure, 1429
Noninvasive Techniques for Measuring Blood Pressure, 1430
Korotkoff Sound Technique, 1430
Random-Zero Sphygmomanometer, 1432
Oscillometric Technique, 1432
Ultrasound Techniques, 1432
Pulse Transit-Time Technique, 1432
Finger-Cuff Method of Penaz, 1432
Korotkoff Signal (K2) Technique, 1433
Recommendations for Evaluation of Noninvasive Blood Pressure Monitors and Observers, 1433
Automatic and Semiautomatic Home Blood Pressure Monitors, 1434
Telephonic Transmission of Home Blood Pressures, 1435
Ambulatory Blood Pressure Monitors, 1435
Invasive Recorders, 1435
Noninvasive Recorders, 1436
Accuracy of Noninvasive Ambulatory Recorders, 1437
Reproducibility of Ambulatory Recordings, 1437
Evaluation of Ambulatory Recordings, 1437
Clinical Relevance of Ambulatory Blood Pressure Recordings, 1437
Measurement of Blood Pressure in Special Populations and Circumstances, 1438
Infants and Children, 1438
Elderly Subjects, 1438
Obese Subjects, 1439
Exercise, 1439
References, 1439

For most hypertensive patients, a mildly elevated level of blood pressure is the only abnormality that can be detected on routine examination. Since it is beyond dispute that blood pressure is not a fixed entity, its measurement is often the single most important component in the evaluation of the hypertensive patient. The problem is compounded by the fact that management decisions may be based on differences of blood pressure of 5 mmHg or less. When a blood pressure reading is taken, it has traditionally been assumed that the reading will give a reliable measure of that particular individual's "true" level of pressure, which is conceived as being the average level over time, and that it is this level of pressure which is responsible for the development of morbid events.

There are two reasons for wishing to extend the measurement of blood pressure beyond single clinic readings: First, the inherent variability of blood pressure means that multiple measurements may be expected to give a closer approximation to the "true" level of pressure than single ones; and second, clinic readings may give a spuriously high level of blood pressure that is not representative of the pressure outside the clinic. At the same time it must be remembered that such clinic readings form the basis of the epidemiological data relating blood pressure, risk, and the benefits of treatment.

INVASIVE TECHNIQUES FOR MEASURING BLOOD PRESSURE

Although measurement of intra-arterial pressure is generally accepted as being the most accurate method of blood pressure recording, its clinical use is limited by virtue of its invasiveness. It is still often used for the evaluation of noninvasive blood pressure recorders, however. The shape of the arterial pressure wave varies according to a number of

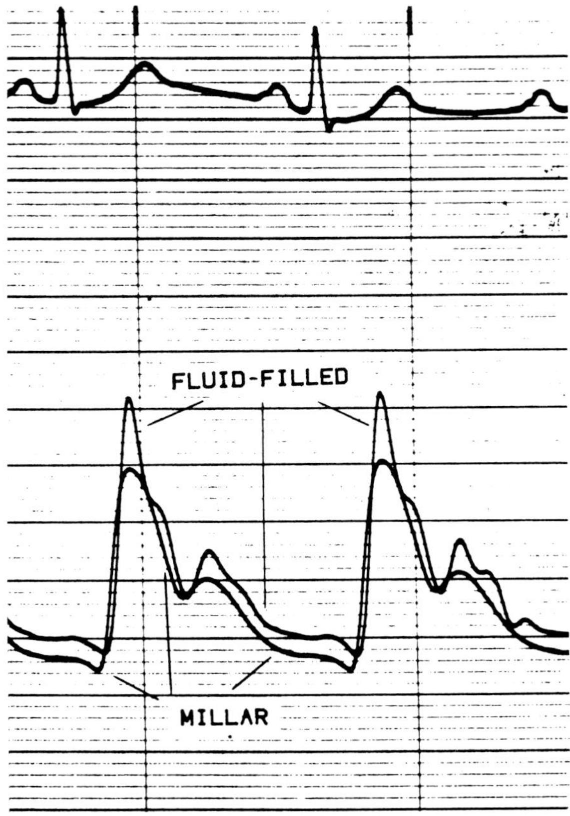

FIG. 1. Intra-arterial measurements from brachial artery using both a fluid-filled catheter and a Millar solid-state catheter-tip transducer. Note the overshoot from the fluid-filled system due to underdamping.

factors. It can be considered as being the summation of an incident and reflected wave, and it is generally agreed that wave reflection and the physical properties of the arterial wall are significant factors responsible for the propagating arterial pressure pulse changes (1). Progressive changes occur as the wave proceeds to the peripheral circulation, with an increase of pulse pressure and the maximal rate of rise (*dp*/*dt*). Thus, since mean pressure decreases slightly at more peripheral sites, there is an increase of systolic pressure and a decrease of diastolic pressure (2). For a person with an aortic pressure of 122/81 mmHg the corresponding pressure might be 131/79 in the brachial artery and 136/77 in the radial.

The sites most commonly used for intra-arterial pressure recording are the brachial and radial arteries. While intra-arterial recording is potentially the most accurate method, its accuracy may be limited by the frequency response of the recording system. Such recordings are commonly made with a long, thin, fluid-filled line connecting the artery and the transducer. This low-compliance coupling may adversely affect the fidelity of the intra-arterial pressure being recorded, often taking the form of an overshoot of systolic pressure. In addition, such lines may contain small air bubbles, and these factors may interact to cause substantial damping and distortion of the signal (3). It is now possible to obtain catheter-tip transducers of sufficiently small size to be inserted in the brachial artery, which avoid these problems and which also give recordings that are free of artifact. Figure 1 compares measurement of intra-arterial pressure made with a conventional fluid-filled system and a Millar solid-state catheter-tip transducer.

NONINVASIVE TECHNIQUES FOR MEASURING BLOOD PRESSURE

Korotkoff Sound Technique

Despite continued efforts to find a superior method, the technique first described by Korotkoff in 1905 is still the most widely used, both for clinical measurement of blood pressure and for automatic recorders. The mechanism of the origin of the Korotkoff sounds has been a subject of debate for many years. The two most popular theories are that they are caused by pressure-induced movement of the arterial wall, or by turbulent flow through the compressed arterial lumen. Most of the evidence favors the former; thus, McCutcheon and Rushmer (4) showed that the sounds occur before there is any real increase of flow, and Dock (5), using a model with isolated segments of artery, concluded that they are due to a sudden tautening of the arterial wall.

Several studies have compared measurements taken by the auscultatory Korotkoff sound method and intra-arterial recordings and have generally reported correlations better than 0.9. Systolic pressure is more reliably detected than diastolic pressure, since, as conventionally recorded, there is a gradual diminution in the intensity of the sounds at around diastolic pressure.

The human ear can only detect vibrations above a frequency of around 20 Hz. In fact, as shown in Fig. 2, most of the energy that is generated under a sphygmomanometer cuff during blood pressure measurement is below the audible range and shows no sudden change at systolic or diastolic pressure, in contrast to the more abrupt changes in energy above 20 Hz.

There is still no universal agreement as to which phase of the Korotkoff sounds should be used for recording diastolic pressure. Phase four (muffling) is about 8 mmHg higher than the intra-arterial diastolic pressure and is more subject to interobserver error; phase five (disappearance) is about 2 mmHg lower than the true diastolic pressure (6).

Formerly, the official recommendation of the American Heart Association (AHA) was to report both the fourth and fifth phases (7); more recently, however, the AHA recommended using only the fifth phase, except in children (8). Most of the large-scale clinical trials which have evaluated the benefits of treating hypertension have used the fifth phase, although the Framingham study, which has given us much of our knowledge about the risks associated with hypertension, used the fourth phase. Most people today use the fifth phase.

A number of factors may lead to inaccuracies with the Korotkoff sound technique. The size of the cuff relative to the diameter of the arm is critical. Maxwell et al. (9) compared readings in obese subjects taken with the three gener-

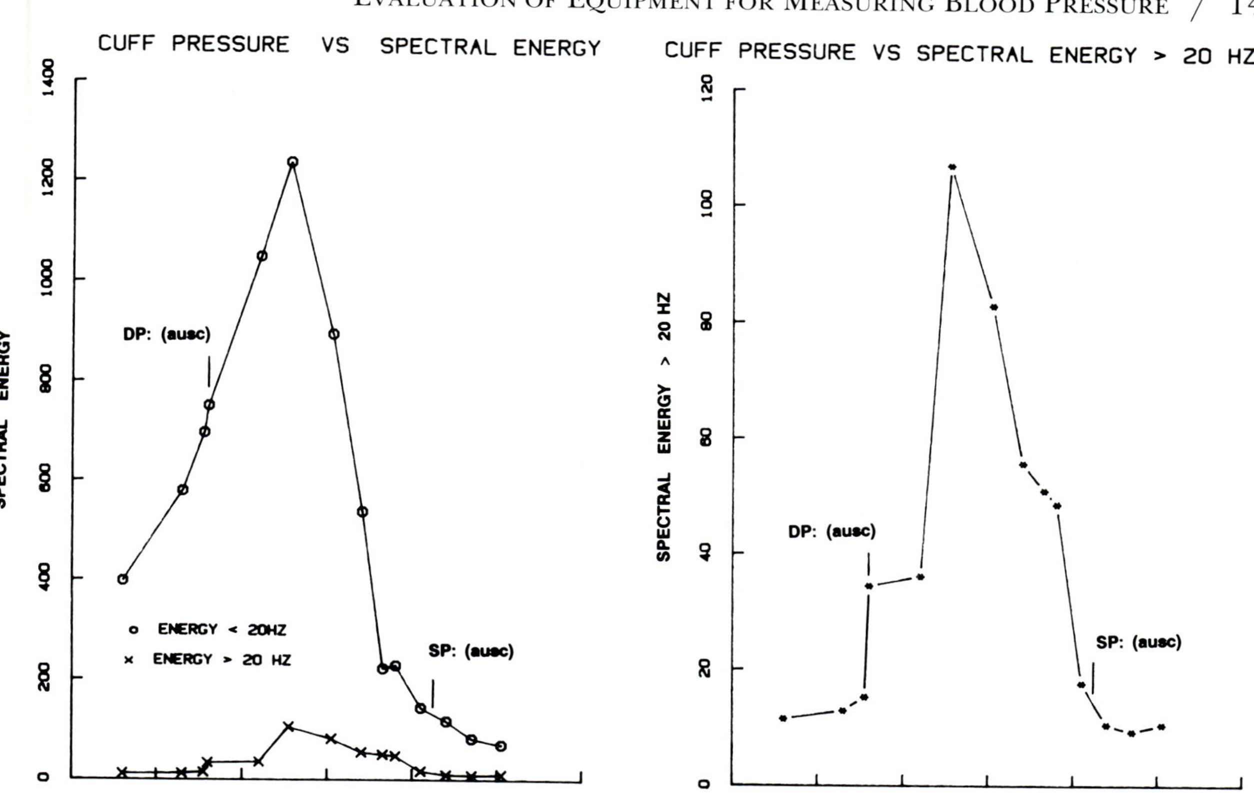

FIG. 2. Recordings obtained with a high-fidelity transducer placed under a sphygmomanometer cuff during deflation. (**a**) The spectral energy of the signal has been separated into components above and below 20 Hz. Note that most of the energy is below this level. (**b**) An amplified plot of the energy above 20 Hz, corresponding to the audible Korotkoff sounds. With the oscillometric technique, low-frequency vibrations in the cuff are detected.

ally available cuff sizes for adults and recommended that the appropriate cuff size be selected according to the arm diameter, as shown in Table 1. In general, the error can be reduced by using a large adult sized cuff for all except the skinniest arms (10). Blood pressure measurements are also influenced by the position of the arm. Both systolic and diastolic readings may change by as much as 20 mmHg by moving the arm through 90° (11).

Observer error and observer bias are important sources of error when conventional sphygmomanometers are used. Differences of auditory acuity between observers may lead to consistent errors, and digit preference is very common, with most observers recording a disproportionate number of readings ending in 5 or 0 (12). The level of pressure that is recorded may also be profoundly influenced by behavioral factors related to the effects of the observer on the subject, the best known of which is the presence of a physician. It has been known for more than 40 years that blood pressures recorded by a physician can be as much as 30 mmHg higher than pressures taken by the patient at home, using the same technique and in the same posture (13). Physicians also record higher pressures than nurses or technicians (14,15). In our own population of patients with mild hypertension (diastolic pressures between 90 and 104 mmHg), we have estimated that approximately 20% have "white coat" hypertension, that is, pressures that are persistently high when in the presence of a physician but normal at other times (15). Other factors that influence the pressure that is recorded may include both the race and sex of the observer: Comstock (16) found that men tended to have higher pressures when taken by a woman than by a man, whereas the opposite was true for women. Whether or not the person taking the blood pressure is of the same race as the subject is also important (17).

There are also technical sources of error with the auscul-

TABLE 1. *Recommended cuff sizes for auscultatory measurement of blood pressure*

Arm circumference (cm)	Cuff type	Cuff size (cm) Frohlich (1988)	Maxwell (1982)
<7.5	Newborn	3 × 5	—
7.5–13	Infant	5 × 8	—
13–20	Child	8 × 13	—
17–26	Small adult	11 × 17	—
24–32	Adult	13 × 24	12 × 23
32–42	Large adult	17 × 32	15 × 33
>42	Thigh	20 × 42	18 × 36

tatory method, although these are usually much fewer when a mercury column is used than with many of the semiautomatic methods (see below). These include the position of the column, which should be at approximately the level of the heart. The mercury should read zero when no pressure is applied, and it should fall freely when the pressure is reduced (this may not occur if the mercury is not clear or if the pinhole connecting the mercury column to the atmosphere is blocked). With aneroid meters, it is essential that they be checked against a mercury column both at zero pressure and when pressure is applied to the cuff. Surveys of such devices used in clinical practice have shown them to be frequently inaccurate (18).

Random-Zero Sphygmomanometer

Some of the sources of observer error (e.g., digit preference) may be reduced by the use of a random-zero (Hawksley) sphygmomanometer (19). This device is a mercury sphygmomanometer whose zero point may be varied randomly; after a reading is taken, the zero value is subtracted from it to give the true reading. The elimination of digit preference is more apparent than real, however, because although it may not appear in the final value, it may still occur when the pressures are read off the mercury column. It does not, of course, eliminate the more subtle psychosocial effects due to the interaction of the observer and the subject.

Oscillometric Technique

This was first demonstrated by Marey in 1876 (20), and it was subsequently shown that when the oscillations of pressure in a sphygmomanometer cuff are recorded during gradual deflation, the point of maximal oscillation corresponds to the mean intra-arterial pressure (21). The oscillations begin above systolic pressure and continue below diastolic (see Fig. 2), so that systolic and diastolic pressure can only be estimated indirectly according to some empirically derived algorithm. One advantage of the method is that no transducer need be placed over the brachial artery, so that placement of the cuff is not critical. The method works reasonably well in general, but it may be seriously in error in some patients (22,23). It has recently been used successfully in ambulatory blood pressure monitors (such as the Spacelabs 90202).

It is customary to validate noninvasive blood pressure recorders against simultaneously determined auscultatory readings. This presents somewhat of a problem, because the pressure is computed in a manner different from that in Korotkoff sound recorders. With the oscillometric technique, all the data are gathered and then smoothed to allow for respiratory fluctuations of blood pressure. When blood pressure is continually changing in this way, the first Korotkoff sound is likely to be heard at the peak of systolic pressure, whereas the last one is likely to be heard at the trough of diastolic pressure, so it might be expected that an oscillometric recorder, which computes the average level of both, would give lower systolic and higher diastolic readings than those obtained by the Korotkoff sound method. In practice, however, this does not appear to be a problem.

Other potential advantages of the oscillometric method for ambulatory monitoring are that it is less susceptible to external noise (but not to low-frequency mechanical vibration) and that the cuff can be removed and replaced by the patient (e.g., when taking a shower).

Ultrasound Techniques

Devices incorporating this technique use an ultrasound transmitter and receiver placed over the brachial artery under a sphygmomanometer cuff. As the cuff is deflated, the movement of the arterial wall at systolic pressure causes a Doppler phase shift in the reflected ultrasound, and diastolic pressure is recorded as the point at which diminution of arterial motion occurs (24). Another variation of this method detects the onset of blood flow at systolic pressure and has been found to be of particular value for measuring pressure in infants and children (25,26). Such devices compare favorably with ones using other techniques (27), although their accuracy for measuring diastolic pressure in infants and children has been questioned (28).

Pulse Transit-Time Technique

The velocity of the pulse wave along an artery is proportional to the arterial pressure, and this principle has been used to evaluate changes of blood pressure by measuring changes of pulse wave velocity, by recording either (a) the interval between the R wave of the electrocardiogram and the radial pulse or (b) the interval between brachial and radial pulses. Although the method has the advantages of not requiring a cuff and being theoretically suitable for beat-to-beat measurement of blood pressure, its accuracy has been found to be unacceptably low (29,30).

Finger-Cuff Method of Penaz

This interesting method, developed by Penaz (31), works on the principle of the "unloaded arterial wall." Arterial pulsation in a finger is detected by a photoplethysmograph under a pressure cuff. The output of the plethysmograph is used to drive a servo-loop which rapidly changes the cuff pressure to keep the output constant, so that the artery is held in a partially opened state. The oscillations of pressure in the cuff are measured, and they have been found to resemble the intra-arterial pressure wave in most subjects (see Fig. 3). This method gives an accurate estimate of systolic and diastolic pressure, although both may be underestimated when compared to brachial artery pressures (32); the cuff can be kept inflated for up to 2 hours. It is now commercially available as the FINAPRESS recorder, and it has been validated in several studies against intra-arterial pressures, mostly during anesthesia for surgical operations (32–34). These studies have shown that while there may be a sizable systematic error in the recorded pressure (particularly in hypertensive patients), the device can accu-

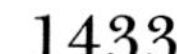

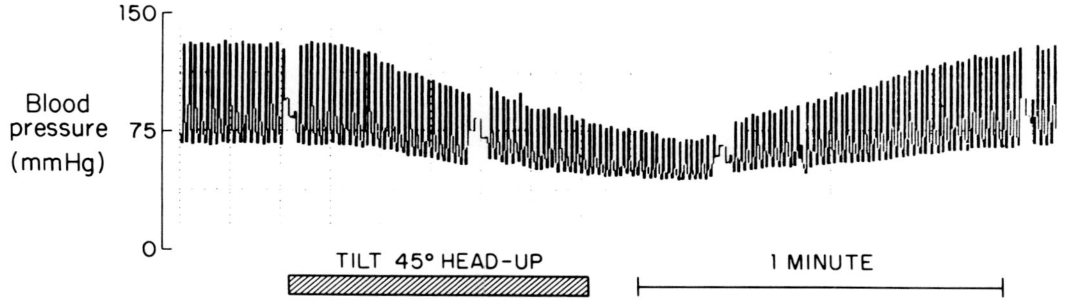

FIG. 3. Recording from FINAPRESS blood pressure monitor during head-up tilt in a patient with orthostatic hypotension.

rately monitor changes of pressure. However, when there is intense peripheral vasoconstriction, the pressure recorded in the finger may be considerably lower than that recorded in the systemic circulation (35). Its application is likely to be greatest in situations where short-term blood pressure changes are being monitored (e.g., in tests of blood pressure reactivity or baroreflex sensitivity). Figure 3 shows a recording obtained during tilting in a patient with orthostatic hypotension.

A variant of this method has been described by Aaslid and Brubakk (36), who measured flow with an ultrasound transducer placed over the brachial artery distal to a cuff. A servo-loop system operated to keep the artery partly compressed with a constant flow. This method also correlated well with intra-arterial pressures.

Korotkoff Signal (K2) Technique

We have recently described a technique of indirect blood pressure measurement which is based on waveform analysis of the Korotkoff signal (37,38) and uses a specially designed transducer called a *foil electret sensor,* which gives an accurate rendition of both the low-frequency and high-frequency components of the signal. With this technique, we have identified three components, which we have termed K1, K2, and K3 (see Fig. 4). K1 is a low-frequency–low-amplitude signal that can be detected at cuff pressures above systolic (Fig. 4a). As cuff pressure is reduced, a high-frequency component (K2) develops (Fig. 4b and 4c), and we have found that its appearance corresponds precisely to systolic pressure. With further reduction of cuff pressure, a third component (K3) appears, which resembles the arterial pressure waveform (Fig. 4d and 4e). K2 disappears at diastolic pressure and therefore corresponds roughly to the audible Korotkoff sound. The potential advantage of blood pressure measurement by the "K2 algorithm" is that it can be done on the basis of pattern recognition rather than by an absolute level of sound, which varies greatly from one individual to another. We suspect that K2 originates from sudden movement of the arterial wall. We have shown that the K2 method gives readings that are closer to true intra-arterial pressure than those given by the auscultatory method. Although this technique is not yet generally available, it can be replicated using any sensor–amplifier system that has an appropriately wide frequency response (including low frequencies).

RECOMMENDATIONS FOR EVALUATION OF NONINVASIVE BLOOD PRESSURE MONITORS AND OBSERVERS

There are no standardized criteria for evaluating such devices, but the most widely used technique has been to compare the readings obtained by the automatic recorder with simultaneously determined auscultatory readings, using either one or two observers. The Association for the Advancement of Medical Instrumentation (AAMI) has published recommendations (39), one of which is that three sets of measurements should be made simultaneously by two observers using the device being tested, on at least 85 subjects. This number is needed to cover (a) an age range from 15 to 80 years and (b) a pressure range of 100/60 to 200/110 mmHg. The automatic device should give readings that are within ±5 mmHg of the auscultatory readings, with a standard deviation of ±8 mmHg.

Any automatic or semiautomatic blood pressure device that is used in behavioral studies needs to be calibrated against standard methods. Ideally, intra-arterial pressures should be used as a reference, but this is often not feasible in practice. Most of the noninvasive methods cannot be expected to give readings that are any more accurate than the auscultatory method, which remains the usual method for comparison. At the present time, there is no automatic or semiautomatic recoder that is universally reliable, so we would strongly recommend that every time such a device is used it should be calibrated against a standard method, which, for practical reasons, means a mercury sphygmomanometer. It is possible that, in the future, the K2 method may be used rather than the auscultatory method.

Calibration against a mercury column is best performed using readings taken simultaneously from the same arm by the device being tested and by an observer with a stethoscope placed just distal to the cuff, reading a mercury column connected to the cuff. With this technique, a satisfactory device should give readings that are within 5 mmHg of the observer's. If this technique is not practical, the observer can take auscultatory readings from the opposite arm. This is less satisfactory for two reasons: There may be differences between the two arms, and it may be difficult to

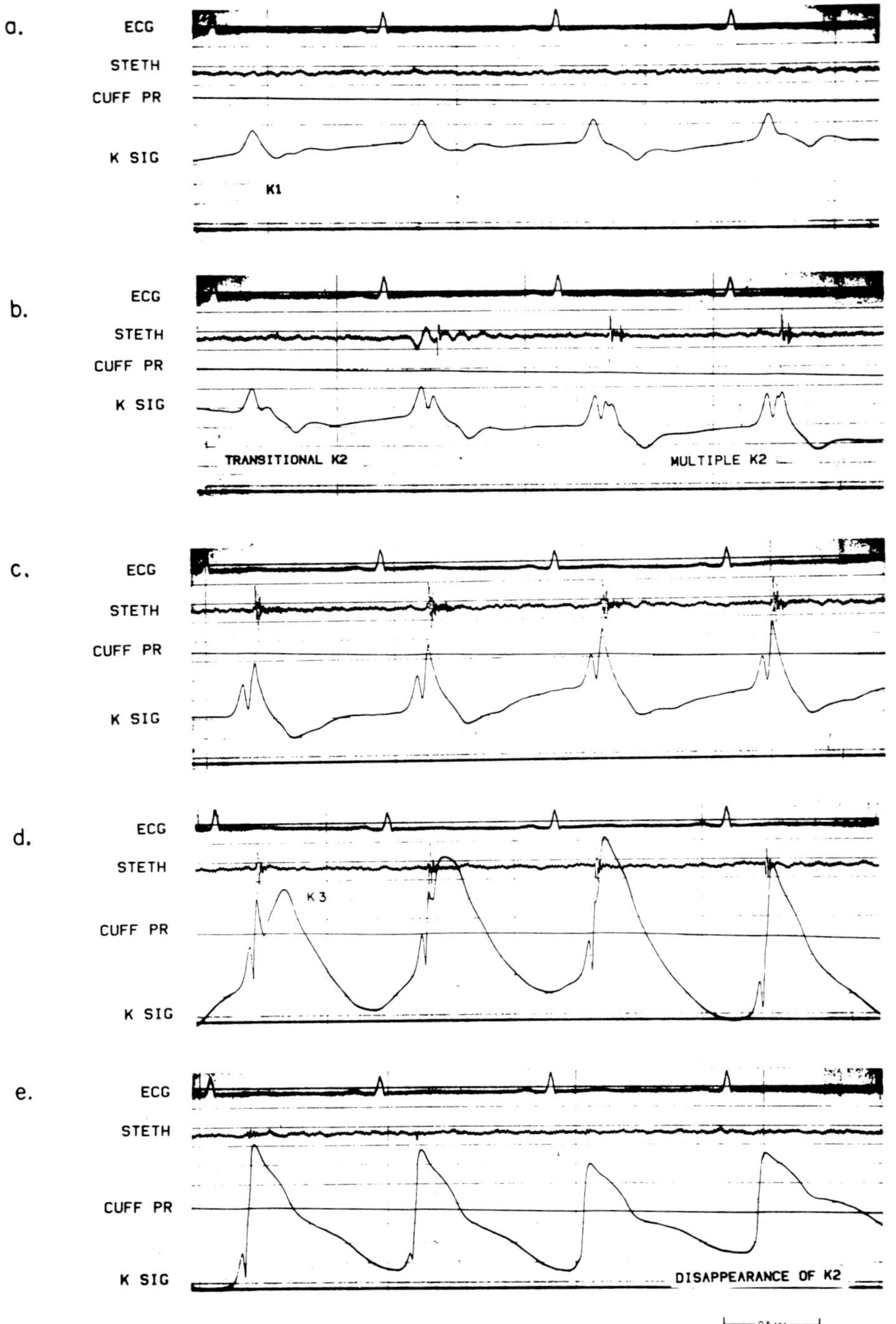

FIG. 4. Five consecutive panels recorded during gradual deflation of sphygmomanometer cuff from above systolic pressure to below diastolic pressure. Four channels were recorded: ECG; steth (recording from microphone placed in stethoscope earpiece, corresponding to audible Korotkoff sound); cuff Pr (cuff pressure); and K sig (recording from high-fidelity transducer placed over brachial artery). K sig trace shows low-frequency component (K1) when cuff pressure is above systolic (**a**); at lower pressures (**b** and **c**) a high-frequency component (K2) appears, audible in stethoscope (steth). At lower pressures (**d** and **e**) a low frequency component (K3) appears.

obtain the two sets of readings simultaneously. We have found that with the latter technique, two observers with mercury sphygmomanometers can get correlation coefficients between the two arms of 0.98 for systolic pressure and 0.94 for diastolic pressure; 70% of readings should be within 5 mmHg of each other (40).

Validation of each observer's technique is also necessary; for this purpose, training videotapes are available, and a double-headed stethoscope is advisable, so that two observers may listen to the same Korotkoff sounds. With this technique, differences in auditory acuity can be evaluated; under ideal circumstances, more than 90% of readings taken by the two observers should be within 5 mmHg of each other.

AUTOMATIC AND SEMIAUTOMATIC HOME BLOOD PRESSURE MONITORS

A large number of devices which monitor blood pressure automatically are now available. Virtually all use a sphygmomanometer cuff, and they operate either by Korotkoff sound detection, oscillometry, or ultrasound. Some are suitable for home monitoring of blood pressure, whereas

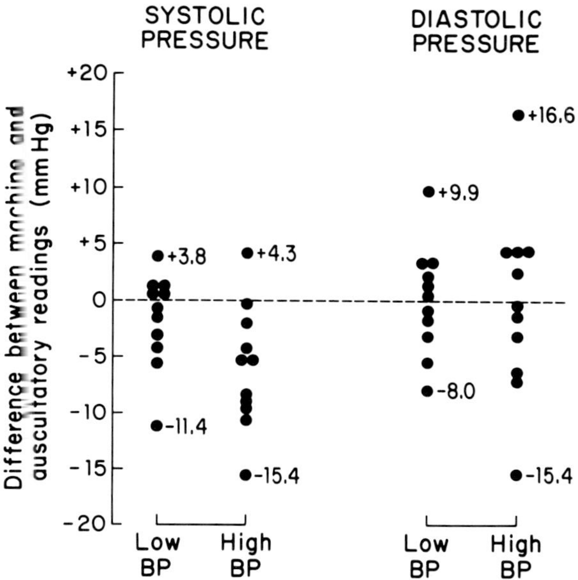

FIG. 5. Comparisons of blood pressure readings obtained with 11 different home monitors and auscultatory readings, in normotensive and hypertensive subjects. Each point represents average differences between a recorder and an observer.

others are better for laboratory studies. They have several obvious advantages: One is that they eliminate observer error and observer bias; another is that they may print out the readings as well as displaying them. We have evaluated a number of such devices and have come to the following conclusions (40): First, many of the recorders are inaccurate, giving readings that are consistently more than 5 mmHg in error when compared with simultaneously determined auscultatory values (see Fig. 5); second, no single method of recording (e.g., oscillometric or Korotkoff sound) is consistently superior; and third, there is no correlation between the price and the accuracy of the recorders. It is essential that any automatic recorder be calibrated against auscultatory readings in each subject.

Telephonic Transmission of Home Blood Pressures

Recently, a home blood pressure monitor (the Telelabs Barograf) has been developed which has the ability not only of storing the readings in a memory chip but also of transmitting them over a telephone via a modem to a personal computer, on which the data can be stored and analyzed (Fig. 6). This promising development is analogous to the technique of transmitting pacemaker signals over the telephone. It has great potential both for research purposes and for monitoring patients' response to treatment, but in its present form it is prohibitively expensive.

AMBULATORY BLOOD PRESSURE MONITORS

The development of devices which can automatically monitor blood pressure over periods of 24 hours or more in subjects who are going about their normal daily activities has added a new dimension to the evaluation of hypertensive patients. Two types of recorders have been developed —invasive and noninvasive. The former have the advantages of the greater accuracy of intra-arterial recording and of giving continuous beat-to-beat measurements, but they are unsuited for widespread clinical or epidemiological use. The noninvasive recorders are less accurate and give intermittent readings, but they can be used for routine clinical evaluation. Both types are described below.

Invasive Recorders

The most widely used invasive ambulatory recorder has been the Oxford Medilog device, which records blood pressure continuously from a catheter in the brachial artery (41). The central unit containing the transducer and tape recording system is worn in a harness on the chest so that the transducer is always at the level of the heart. Since every pressure wave is recorded, it is theoretically possible to obtain a complete picture of blood pressure and heart rate

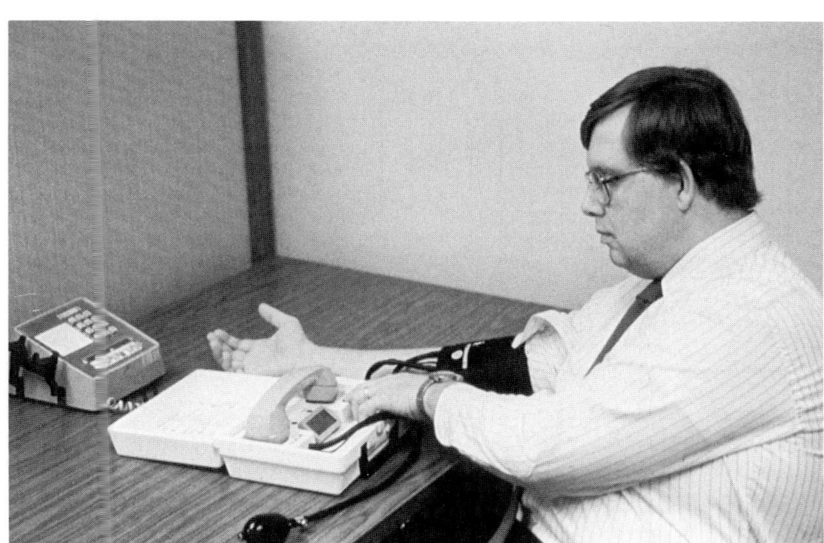

FIG. 6. Telephonic transmission of blood pressure readings by the Telelabs Baro-Graf recorder.

TABLE 2. *Noninvasive ambulatory blood pressure monitors*

Type	Mode of operation	Weight	Cuff inflation	Accuracy[a]	Author	Reference
Spacelabs 5200	Oscillometric/K sound	1.9 kg	Pump	+7/+3	Light et al.	61
				−2/−4	Pagny et al.	57
Suntech Accutracker	K sound	1 kg	Pump	+13/+3	Light et al.	61
Remler M2000	K sound	0.7 kg	Patient	0/−4	Pagny et al.	57
Spacelabs 90202	Oscillometric	0.7 kg	Pump	+1/−2.5	Santucci et al.	63
Del Mar Avionics P IV	K sound	0.8 kg	Pump	+1/−2	Harshfield et al.	62
Oxford Medilog	K sound	0.5 kg	Pump	+2/−1	Hope et al.	64
Colin	Oscillometric + K sound	0.8 kg	CO_2 cylinder			

[a] Accuracy: Mean difference between monitor and observer for systolic and diastolic pressure.

changes over 24 hours. In practice there is some loss of data due to movement artifact and damping of the catheter, but at the present time this technique provides the only method for obtaining a true measure of the range of blood pressure and its variability in ambulatory patients.

The technique has been used mainly in studies of blood pressure variability (42–44), as well as for documenting the effects of antihypertensive medications (45–48).

Noninvasive Recorders

Several noninvasive ambulatory recorders have been developed, and more are likely to follow. Most of these have a conventional blood pressure cuff, and they operate either by the Korotkoff sound technique or by oscillometry (see Table 2). One (the Colin device) takes readings by both techniques and gives simultaneous printouts of both sets. This procedure has the theoretical advantage of enabling a check on the internal consistency of the readings. Ambulatory recorders using finger cuffs have also been developed (49) but may be susceptible to artifacts from movement and changes of environmental temperature. All except the Remler M2000 are fully automatic, and most use a pump to inflate and deflate the cuff at preset intervals. The subject can also inflate the cuff on demand. The pumps tend to be noisy, which may prove embarrassing to the subject. The Colin recorder uses a CO_2 cylinder, which inflates the cuff noiselessly.

Such recorders typically give 50–100 readings over a 24-hr period (see Fig. 7). The blood pressure readings and/or the Korotkoff sounds are stored in the memory of the recorder, and at the end of the 24-hr period they can be unloaded into a personal computer. None of the currently available devices works in every patient, and problems are most pronounced in the elderly and the obese. It is important to calibrate the recorder against simultaneously determined auscultatory readings, which can be done using a mercury column. Some of the devices can be manually deflated during calibration (e.g., the Del Mar Pressurometer IV). Ideally, it should be possible to obtain paired readings that are within 5 mmHg of each other; furthermore, it is desirable to have the patient fill out a diary describing his or her activity, posture, and location at the time of each reading, since these variables may have a substantial influence on blood pressure.

None of the recorders so far evaluated gives good readings during physical exercise, nor in environments where there is a lot of vibration, although the oscillometric technique may be less adversely affected than the Korotkoff

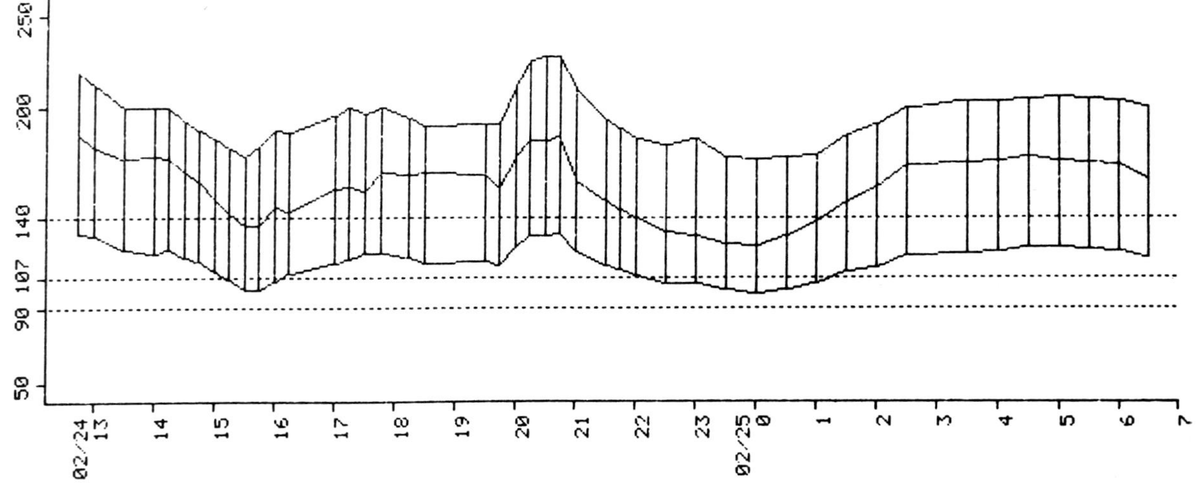

FIG. 7. Variability of blood pressure during a 24-hr recording. Blood pressure is shown on vertical axis; each vertical line represents one reading (systolic and diastolic). Horizontal axis shows time of day. Recording made with Colin ABPM.

sound technique. It is our policy to tell patients that they should keep their arm motionless by their side while a reading is being taken. Even with such precautions, there is still a proportion of readings that are artifactual; these readings must be edited out for the final analysis.

Accuracy of Noninvasive Ambulatory Recorders

The accuracy of such recorders is limited by the inherent limitations of the noninvasive techniques used. Thus they are less accurate than direct intra-arterial recording. A number of validation studies have been published in which readings taken by the noninvasive recorders have been compared with either (a) simultaneously determined auscultatory readings taken with a mercury column or (b) intra-arterial readings. On the whole, these reports have shown reasonably satisfactory correlations for the devices that have been used most extensively—the Del Mar Avionics recorder (50–54), the Spacelabs recorder (55–57), the Remler (58,59), and the Accutracker (60,61). There is now a second generation of ambulatory recorders (such as the Del Mar Avionics PIV and the Spacelabs 90202) which have also been validated (62,63). The new Oxford Medilog (64) also looks very promising. As with all noninvasive methods, systolic pressure is more reliably recorded than diastolic. There does not appear to be any systematic difference between (a) the accuracy of recorders which use the Korotkoff sound technique and (b) the accuracy of the oscillometric technique.

Reproducibility of Ambulatory Recordings

One of the problems associated with clinic readings, which was particularly pronounced in the clinical trials of the treatment of mild hypertension (65,66), is that the blood pressure tends to fall with repeated visits. An important question is whether this change is a genuine one, or merely a consequence of habituation to the clinic setting. We compared the reproducibility of three measures of blood pressure: clinic readings, ambulatory readings, and home readings, taken on two occasions 2 weeks apart. Where possible, subjects went to work on both days during which they wore the ambulatory recorders (67). The average levels of clinic systolic pressure decreased from the first to the second occasion in the hypertensives but not in the normotensives. This change, however, was not associated with any change of either ambulatory or home pressures, both of which were highly reproducible. These findings indicate that the apparent fall of clinic pressures, which can be regarded as an artifact, is presumably an instance of regression to the mean. For all three measures of pressure, the correlation coefficients between the levels on the first and second occasion were high, ranging from 0.87 to 0.96.

A number of other studies have evaluated the reproducibility of ambulatory blood pressure recordings, over periods as short as 48 hours (68–70) and as long as 4 months (71). Most of these studies have found that the reproducibility is high and that there is little tendency for the level of pressure to be lower on the second occasion. These other studies did not compare the ambulatory pressures to home and clinic pressures, however.

In contrast to the highly reproducible average levels of pressure, measures of blood pressure variability (e.g., the variance) are unreliable, unless steps are taken to reduce the random error (e.g., by matching for equal numbers of readings on the two occasions, and by the use of robust statistical techniques) (72).

Evaluation of Ambulatory Recordings

One of the problems with 24-hr recorders is that large numbers of readings whose interpretation is not necessarily straightforward, are produced. As shown in Fig. 7, the blood pressure may show substantial variations over 24 hours, depending on the activity of the patient. The valid interpretation of such recordings can only be made in the context of the circumstances in which they were made. Relatively little information is currently available as to ambulatory blood pressures in normotensive subjects, although some norms have been proposed (73). For the clinical evaluation of hypertensive patients, most authors take the 24-hr or daytime average. The potential importance of including sleep readings is illustrated by Fig. 8, which shows a 24-hr blood pressure profile in a patient with diabetic autonomic neuropathy, who was hypertensive only during the night.

Although the 24-hr average pressure is probably the most appropriate measure for establishing the diagnosis of hypertension, a number of caveats should be stated. First, the quality of the sleep readings varies considerably. In our experience, sleep may be interrupted by the inflation of the cuff, so that the variability of the blood pressure readings may be spuriously high. Many subjects disconnect the recorders at night as a consequence of this. Second, the daytime level of blood pressure varies considerably according to the activity of the patient during the recording period. Most important is whether or not the patient went to work or stayed at home: We have found that this variable alone may influence the average daytime pressure by 5–10 mmHg. Thus we normally analyze the recordings in terms of (a) the average 24-hr pressure, (b) the average daytime pressure, and (c) the pressures at work, at home, and during sleep (74,75). It is also possible to analyze the effects of specific activities on blood pressure (76).

Clinical Relevance of Ambulatory Blood Pressure Recordings

The correlations between blood pressure measured in the clinic and by ambulatory monitoring are typically around 0.6. This means that there are many individuals for whom the clinic pressures are not in good agreement with the pressures at other times, thus raising the question as to which measure of pressure gives the best prediction of prognosis.

This question can be resolved in two ways: (i) indirectly, by cross-sectional studies relating blood pressure to target organ damage, and (ii) directly, by studies relating blood

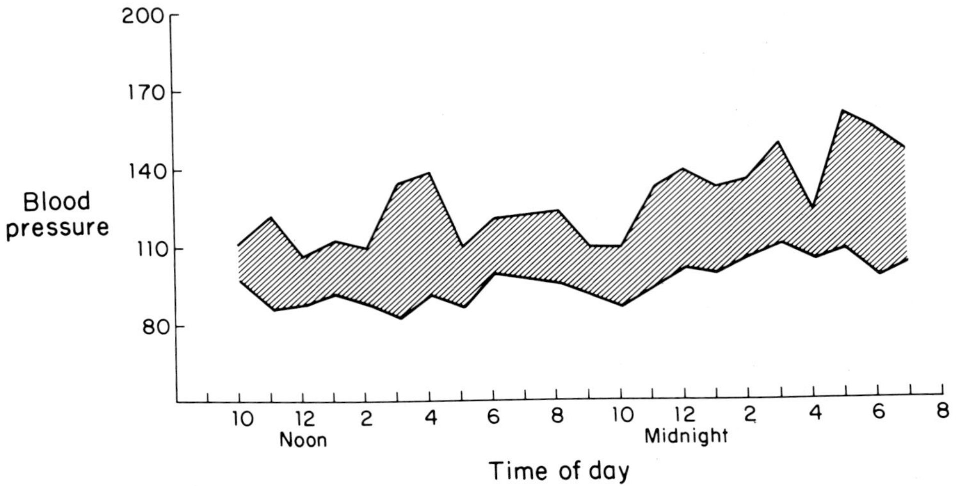

FIG. 8. Nocturnal hypertension in a patient with diabetic autonomic neuropathy.

pressure and morbidity. The first cross-sectional study was reported by Sokolow et al. (77), who classified target organ damage as the aggregate of changes seen on the electroencephalogram (ECG), the chest x-ray, and funduscopic examination. The overall severity of these hypertensive complications was more closely related to ambulatory pressures than to casual pressures. More recent studies have used echocardiography for evaluating left ventricular hypertrophy, since this is much more sensitive than either the ECG or the chest x-ray. So far, four published studies have all reported that ambulatory blood pressures give a better correlation with echocardiographically determined left ventricular hypertrophy than do clinic pressures (78). In another study, Littler et al. compared the differences between clinic and ambulatory blood pressures in (a) eight untreated hypertensive patients and (b) eight other patients who had persistently high levels of clinic pressure but no detectable target organ damage (79). In the former group, clinic and ambulatory pressures were similar; in the latter group, however, the clinic readings were 30 mmHg higher. Similar findings were obtained by Floras et al. (80), who classified 59 patients with mild hypertension according to whether clinic pressure was higher than or similar to ambulatory pressure. Clinic pressures were the same in the two groups; however, in the group in which both clinic and ambulatory pressures were elevated, target organ damage was present in 64%, whereas in the group who had a high clinic pressure and lower ambulatory pressure, it was present in only 19%. Thus, there is a general consensus that target organ damage is more closely related to ambulatory pressure than to clinic pressure.

Only one published study has related outcome to ambulatory pressures. Perloff et al. followed 1076 patients for 5 years and classified them according to the differences between their clinic and ambulatory pressures at the start of the study (81). Those patients whose ambulatory pressures were higher than their clinic pressures had a higher mortality and incidence of first morbid events than those in whom the clinic pressures were higher. Of particular interest was their finding that the predictive power of ambulatory readings was greatest in mildly hypertensive patients who had experienced no prior cardiovascular morbid event.

At the present time, ambulatory monitoring is in a transitional phase between being a research procedure and a clinically relevant tool. Although its use has not yet been officially endorsed by government bodies or organizations such as the American College of Physicians (82), other independent review panels have been more enthusiastic (83). It is our belief that clinicians are increasingly using it for the evaluation of patients with borderline hypertension.

MEASUREMENT OF BLOOD PRESSURE IN SPECIAL POPULATIONS AND CIRCUMSTANCES

Infants and Children

Conventional techniques such as the auscultatory method may give systematic errors in infants, where the true systolic pressure may be underestimated (25). For indirect measurements the best technique is using an ultrasonic flow detector (e.g., a Parks Doppler unit) coupled with an appropriately designed (e.g., Pedisphyg) cuff (25,26,28). In children over the age of 12 the auscultatory method may be used, provided that the appropriate-sized cuff be used (Table 1).

Elderly Subjects

In older people there is often an increase of systolic pressure without a corresponding increase of diastolic. This has been attributed to a diminished distensibility of the arteries with increasing age. In extreme cases this may result in a diminished compressibility of the artery by the sphygmomanometer cuff, so that falsely high readings may be recorded, often referred to as *pseudohypertension of the elderly* (84). In such individuals the only accurate method of measuring the arterial pressure is with direct intra-arterial recordings, which may reveal pressures 30 mmHg lower than those revealed by noninvasive techniques.

Obese Subjects

It is well known that the accurate estimate of blood pressure using the auscultatory method requires an appropriate match between cuff size and arm diameter. In obese subjects the regular adult cuff (12 × 23 cm) may seriously overestimate blood pressure (85). Maxwell et al. (9) compared readings in obese subjects taken with the three available cuff sizes for adults, and recommended that the appropriate cuff size be selected according to the arm diameter, as shown in Table 1. These recommendations are somewhat different than the recommendations of the American Heart Association, which are also shown in Table 1.

Exercise

During dynamic exercise the auscultatory method may underestimate systolic pressure by up to 15 mmHg, while during recovery it may be overestimated by 30 mmHg (86 87). Errors in diastolic pressure are unlikely to be as large, except during the recovery period, when falsely low readings may be recorded (87). This is the reason why the American Heart Association recommends taking the fourth phase of the Korotkoff sound after exercise.

REFERENCES

1. O'Rourke M. Wave reflection and the arterial pulse. *Arch Intern Med* 1984;144:366–371.
2. Kroeker EJ, Wood EH. Beat-to-beat alterations in relationship to simultaneously recorded central and peripheral arterial pressure pulses during Valsalva maneuver and prolonged expiration in man. *J Appl Physiol* 1956;8:483–494.
3. Geddes LA. *Cardiovascular devices and their applications.* New York: Wiley, 1984.
4. McCutcheon EP, Rushmer RF. Korotkoff sounds. An experimental critique. *Circ Res* 1967;20:149–161.
5. Dock W. Occasional notes—Korotkoff sounds. *N Engl J Med* 1980;302:1264–1267.
6. Short D. The diastolic dilemma. *Br Med J* 1976;2:685–686.
7. Kirkendall WM, Burton AC, Epstein FH, Fries ED. American Heart Association Recommendations for human blood pressure determinations by sphygmomanometers. *Circulation* 1967; 36:980–987.
8. Frohlich ED, Grim C, Labarthe DR, Maxwell MH, Perloff D, Weidman WH. Recommendations for human blood pressure determination by sphygmomanometers. *Hypertension* 1988; 11:210A–222A.
9. Maxwell MH, Waks AV, Schroth PC, Karam M, Dornfeld L. Error in blood pressure measurement due to incorrect cuff size in obese patients. *Lancet* 1982;2:33–35.
10. Van Montfrans GA, Van Der Hoeven GMA, Karemaker JM, Wieling W, Dunning AJ. Accuracy of auscultatory blood pressure measurement with a long cuff. *Br Med J* 1987;295:354–355.
11. Webster J, Newnham D, Petrie JC, Lovell HG. Influence of arm position on measurement of blood pressure. *Br Med J* 1984;228:1574–1575.
12. Pickering GW. *High blood pressure.* London: Churchill, 1968.
13. Ayman P, Goldshine AD. Blood pressure determinations by patients with essential hypertension. I. The difference between clinic and home readings before treatment. *Am J Med Sci* 1940;200:465–474.
14. Mancia G, Bertini G, Grassi G, Pomidossi G, Gregorini L, Bertinieri G, Parati G, Ferrari A, Zanchetti A. Effects of blood pressure measurement by the doctor on patients' blood pressure and heart rate. *Lancet* 1983;2:695–697.
15. Pickering TG, James GD, Boddie C, Harshfield GA, Blank S, Laragh JH. How common is white coat hypertension? *JAMA* 1988;259:225–228.
16. Comstock GW. An epidemiologic study of blood pressure levels in a biracial community in the southern United States. *Am J Hygiene* 1957;65:271–315.
17. Murphy JK, Alpert BS, Moes DM, Somes GW. Race and cardiovascular reactivity. A neglected relationship. *Hypertension* 1986;3:1075–1083.
18. Burke MJ, Towers HM, O'Malley K, Fitzgerald DJ, O'Brien ET. Sphygmomanometers in hospital and family practice: problems and recommendations. *Br Med J* 1982;285:469–471.
19. Wright BM, Dore CF. A random-zero sphygmomanometer. *Lancet* 1970;1:337–338.
20. Marey EJ. Pression et vitesse du sang. Physiologie Experimentale, Paris. Pratique des hautes etudes lab de M. Marey, 1876.
21. Mauck GB, Smith CR, Geddes LR, Bourland JD. The meaning of the point of maximum oscillations in cuff pressure in the indirect measurement of blood pressure II. *J Biomech Eng* 1980;102:28–33.
22. Ramsey M. Noninvasive automatic determination of mean arterial pressure. *Med Biol Eng Comput* 1979;17:11–18.
23. Yelderman M, Ream AK. Indirect measurement of mean blood pressure in the anesthetized patient. *Anesthesiology* 1979;50:253–256.
24. Ware RW, Laenger CJ. Indirect blood pressure measurement by Doppler ultrasonic kinetoarteriography. *Proc 20th Ann Conf Eng Med Biol* 1967;9:27–30.
25. Elseed AM, Shinebourne EA, Joseph MC. Assessment of techniques for measurement of blood pressure in infants and children. *Arch Dis Child* 1973;48:932–936.
26. Steinfeld L, Dimich I, Reder R, Cohen M, Alexander H. Sphygmomanometry in the pediatric patients. *J Pediatr* 1978;92:934–938.
27. Hochberg HM, Solomon H. Accuracy of an automated ultrasound blood pressure monitor. *Curr Ther Res* 1971;13:129–138.
28. Reder RF, Dimich I, Cohen ML, Steinfeld L. Evaluating indirect blood pressure measurement techniques: a comparison of three systems in infants and children. *Pediatrics* 1978;62:326–330.
29. Pollack MH, Obrist PA. Aortic–radial pulse transit time and ECG Q-wave to radial pulse wave interval as indices of beat-to-beat blood pressure change. *Psychophysiology* 1983;20:21–28.
30. Steptoe A, Smulyan H, Gribbin B. Pulse wave velocity and blood pressure change: calibration and applications. *Psychophysiology* 1976;13:488–493.
31. Penaz J. Photo-electric measurement of blood pressure, volume and flow in the finger. *Digest Tenth Int Conf Med Biol Eng (Dresden)* 1973:104.
32. Wesseling KH, deWit B, Settels JJ, Klawer WH. On the indirect registration of finger blood pressure after Penaz. *Funkt Biol Med J* 1982;245:245–250.
33. Ty Smith N, Wesseling KH, de Wit B. Evaluation of two prototype devices producing noninvasive, pulsatile, calibrated blood pressure measurement from a finger. *J Clin Monitoring* 1985;1:17–29.
34. Van Egmond J, Hasenbos M, Crul JF. Invasive v. noninvasive measurement of arterial pressure. Comparison of two automatic methods and simultaneously measured direct intra-arterial pressure. *Br J Anesth* 1985;57:434–444.
35. Kurki T, Ty Smith N, Head N, Dec-Silver H, Quinn A. Noninvasive continuous blood pressure measurement from the finger: optional measurement conditions and factors affecting reliability. *J Clin Monitoring* 1987;3:6–13.
36. Aaslid R, Brubakk AO. Accuracy of an ultrasound Doppler servo method for noninvasive determination of instantaneous and mean arterial blood pressure. *Circulation* 1981;64:753–759.

37. Blank S, West JE, Muller FB, Cody R, Harshfield GA, Pecker MS, Laragh JH, Pickering TG. Wideband external pulse recording during cuff deflation: a new technique for evaluation of the arterial pressure pulse and measurement of blood pressure. *Circulation* 1988.
38. West JE, Busch-Vishniac IJ, Harshfield GA, Pickering TG. Foil electret transducer for blood pressure monitoring. *J Acoust Soc Am* 1983;74:680–686.
39. Association for the Advancement of Medical Instrumentation. Proposed Standard for Electronic or Automated Sphygmomanometers. Arlington, VA: AAMI, 1985.
40. Pickering TG, Cvetkovski B, James GD. An evaluation of electronic recorders for self monitoring of blood pressure. *J Hypertens* 1986;4(Suppl 5):S328–S330.
41. Bevan AT, Honour AJ, Scott FG. Direct arterial pressure recording in unrestricted man. *Clin Sci* 1969;36:329–344.
42. Conway J. Blood pressure and heart rate variability. *J Hypertens* 1986;4:261–263.
43. Watson RD, Stallard TJ, Flinn RM, Littler WA. Factors determining direct arterial pressure and its variability in hypertensive man. *Hypertension* 1986;2:333–341.
44. Mancia G, Ferrari A, Gregorini L, Parati G, Pomidossi G, Bertinlen G, Grassi G, Zandetti A. Blood pressure variability in man: its relation to high blood pressure, age, and baroreflex sensitivity. *Clin Sci* 1980;59:401s–404s.
45. Mann S, Millar-Craig MW, Balasubramanian V, Cashman PMM, Raftery EB. Ambulant blood pressure: reproducibility and the assessment of interventions. *Clin Sci* 1980;59:497–500.
46. Gould BA, Mann S, Davies AB, Altman DG, Raftery EB. Does placebo lower blood-pressure? *Lancet* 1981;2:1377–1381.
47. Goldberg AD, Raftery EB. Patterns of blood-pressure during chronic administration of postganglionic sympathetic blocking drugs for hypertension. *Lancet* 1976;2:1052–1054.
48. Floras JS, Jones JV, Hassan MO, Sleight P. Ambulatory blood pressure during once-daily randomized double-blind administration of atenolol, metoprolol, pindolol, and slow-release propranolol. *Br Med J* 1982;285:1387–1392.
49. Yamakoshi K, Kawarada A, Kamiya A, Shimazu H, Ito H. Long-term ambulatory monitoring of indirect arterial blood pressure using a volume-oscillometric method. *Med Biol Eng Comput* 1985;23:459–465.
50. Harshfield GA, Pickering TG, Laragh JH. A validation study of the Del Mar Avionics ambulatory blood pressure system. *Ambul Electrocardiogr* 1979;1:7–12.
51. Sheps SG, Elvebach LR, Close EL, Kleven MK, Bissen C. Evaluation of the Del Mar Avionics ambulatory blood pressure recording device. *Mayo Clin Proc* 1981;56:740–743.
52. Messerli FH, Glade LB, Ventura HO, et al. Diurnal variations of cardiac rhythm, arterial pressure and urinary catecholamines in borderline and established essential hypertension. *Am Heart J* 1982;104:109–114.
53. Ward A, Hanson P. Accuracy and reproducibility of ambulatory blood pressure recorder measurements during rest and exercise. In: Weber MA, Dreyer JIM, eds. *Ambulatory blood pressure monitoring.* Darmstadt: Steinkopff, 1984;51–56.
54. Gould BA, Horning RS, Cashman PMM, Raftery EB. Ambulatory blood pressure: direct and indirect. In: Weber MA, Drayer JIM, eds. *Ambulatory blood pressure monitoring.* Darmstadt: Steinkopff, 1984;9–20.
55. Harshfield GA, Pickering TG, Blank S, Lindahl C, Stroud L, Laragh JH. Ambulatory blood pressure monitoring: recorders, applications, and analysis. In: Weber MA, Drayer JIM, eds. *Ambulatory blood pressure monitoring.* Darmstadt: Steinkopff, 1984;1–8.
56. Dembroski TM, MacDougall TM. Validation of the Vita-Stat automated noninvasive blood pressure recording device. In: Herd JA, Gotto AM, Kaufman PC, Weiss SM, eds. *Cardiovascular instrumentation: applicability of new technology to biobehavioral research.* Bethesda, MD: National Institutes of Health, 1984;53–77.
57. Pagny J-Y, Chatellier G, Devries C, Janod J-P, Corvol P, Menard J. Evaluation of the Spacelabs ambulatory blood pressure recorder: comparison with the Remler M2000. *Cardiovasc Rev Rep* 1987;8:31–36.
58. Hinman AT, Engel BT, Bickford AF. Portable blood pressure records: accuracy and preliminary use in evaluating intradaily variations in pressure. *Am Heart J* 1962;64:663–668.
59. Waeber B, Jacot des Gombes B, Porchet M, Brunner HR. Accuracy, reproducibility and usefulness of ambulatory blood pressure recordings obtained with the Remler system. In: Weber MA, Drayer JIM, eds. *Ambulatory blood pressure monitoring.* Darmstadt: Steinkopff, 1984;65–70.
60. White WB, Schulman P, McCabe EJ, Nardone M. Clinical validation of the Accutracker ambulatory blood pressure monitor. *Clin Pharm Ther* 1987;41:191 (Abstr).
61. Light KC, Obrist PA, Cubeddu LX. Evaluation of a new ambulatory blood pressure monitor (Accutracker 102): laboratory comparisons with direct arterial pressure, stethoscopic auscultatory pressure, and readings from a similar monitor (Spacelabs Model 5200). *Psychophysiology* 1988;25:107–116.
62. Harshfield GA, Hwang C, Grim CE. A validation study of the Del Mar Avionics Pressurometer IV according to AAMI guidelines. Submitted for publication.
63. Santucci S, Steiner D, Zimbler M, James GD, Pickering TG. A validation study of the Spacelabs 90202 and 5200 ambulatory blood pressure monitors. Submitted for publication.
64. Hope SL, Alun-Jones E, Sleight P. Validation of the accuracy of the Medilog ABP noninvasive blood pressure monitor. *J Ambulatory Monitoring* 1988;1:39–51.
65. A report by the Management Committee of the Australian Therapeutic Trial in Mild Hypertension: untreated mild hypertension. *Lancet* 1982;1:185–191.
66. Medical Research Council Working Party. MRC Trial of treatment of mild hypertension: principal results. *Br Med J* 1985;291:97–104.
67. James GD, Pickering TG, Yee LS, Harshfield GA, Riva S, Laragh JH. The reproducibility of average ambulatory, home, and clinic pressures. *Hypertension* 1989;in press.
68. Weber MA, Drayer JIM, Wyle GA, Young JL. Reproducibility of the whole-day blood pressure pattern in essential hypertension. *Clin Exp Hypertens* 1982;A4(8):1377–1390.
69. Mann S, Miller-Craig WM, Balasubramanian V, Cashman PMM, Raftery EB. Ambulant blood pressure: reproducibility and the assessment of interventions. *Clin Sci* 1980;59:497–500.
70. Fitzgerald DJ, O'Malley K, O'Brien ET. Reproducibility of ambulatory blood pressure recordings. In: Weber MA, Drayer JIM, eds. *Ambulatory blood pressure monitoring.* Darmstadt: Steinkopff, 1984;71–74.
71. Jacot des Combes B, Porchet M, Waeber G, Brunner HR. Ambulatory blood pressure recordings. Reproducibility and unpredictability. *Hypertension* 1984;6:C110–C115.
72. Clark L, Denby L, Pregibon D, James GD, Pickering TG. Methods for analyzing the reproducibility of noninvasive ambulatory blood pressure recordings. Submitted for publication.
73. Pickering TG, Harshfield GA, Devereux RB, Laragh JH. What is the role of ambulatory blood pressure monitoring in the management of hypertensive patients? *Hypertension* 1985;7:171–177.
74. Pickering TG, Harshfield GA, Kleinert HD, Blank S, Laragh JH. Comparisons of blood pressure during normal daily activities, sleep, and exercise in normal and hypertensive subjects. *JAMA* 1982;247:992–996.
75. Harshfield GA, Pickering TG, Kleinert HD, Blank S, Laragh JH. Situational variations of blood pressure in ambulatory hypertensive patients. *Psychsom Med* 1982;44:237–245.
76. Clark LA, Denby L, Pregibon D, Harshfield GA, Pickering TG, Blank S, Laragh JH. A quantitative analysis of the effects of activity and time of day on the diurnal variations of blood pressure. *J Chronic Dis* 1987;40:671–681.
77. Sokolow M, Werdegar D, Keim HK, Hinman AT. Relationship between level of blood pressure measured casually and by portable records and severity of complications in essential hypertension. *Circulation* 1966;34:279–298.
78. Pickering TG, Devereux R. Ambulatory monitoring of blood pressure as a predictor of cardiovascular risk. *Am Heart J* 1987;114:925–928.

79 Littler WA, Honour AJ, Pugsley DJ, Sleight P. Continuous recording of direct arterial pressure in unrestricted patients: its role in the diagnosis and management of high blood pressure. *Circulation* 1975;51:1101–1106.

80. Floras JS, Hassan MO, Sever PS, Sleight P. Cuff and ambulatory blood pressure in subjects with essential hypertension. *Lancet* 1981;2:107–109.

81. Perloff D, Sokolow M, Cowan R. The prognostic value of ambulatory blood pressure. *JAMA* 1983;249:2792–2798.

82. Health and Public Policy Committee, American College of Physicians. Automated ambulatory blood pressure monitoring. *Ann Intern Med* 1986;104:275–278.

83. National Health Services and Practice Patterns Survey. Report on Fully Automated Blood Pressure Monitoring. Current and Future Applications. Institute for Health Policy Analysis. Georgetown University Medical Center, 1986.

84. Spence JD, Sibbald WJ, Cape RD. Direct, indirect and mean blood pressures in hypertensive patients: the problem of cuff artifact due to arterial wall stiffness, and a partial solution. *Clin Invest Med* 1980;2:165–173.

85. Nielsen PE, Janniche H. The accuracy of auscultatory measurement of arm blood pressure in very obese subjects. *Acta Med Scand* 1974;195:403–409.

86. Henschel A, DeLaVega F, Taylor HL. Simultaneous direct and indirect blood pressure measurements in man at rest and work. *J Appl Physiol* 1954;5:506–508.

87. Gould BA, Hornung RS, Altman DG, Cashman PMM, Raftery EB. Indirect measurement of blood pressure during exercise testing can be misleading. *Br Heart J* 1985;53:611–615.

TABLE 4. *Complete list of foods to eat or avoid on a moderate low-sodium diet*

Food	Not allowed	Allowed
Milk	Buttermilk	Regular homogenized milk, skimmed milk, cream, yogurt
Meat	All dried, salted, smoked, or canned meat such as bacon, ham, bologna, salami, sausage, and kosher meats	Beef, veal, chicken, pork, lamb, turkey, duck, rabbit
Fish	Fish with salt added	Fresh fish, shrimp, lobster; unsalted tuna and salmon
Cheese	None except those listed	Unsalted cottage cheese or pot cheese; low-salt dietetic cheese
Eggs		Use as a substitute, 1 egg for 1 oz meat
Butter and fats	Mayonnaise, regular salad dressing (you can make your own)	Use sweet butter or margarine; unsalted oils and fats for frying
Potato and pastas	Potato chips, instant potatoes	White and sweet potatoes, rice, spaghetti, noodles, macaroni
Breads and cereals	Baking powder biscuits and other hot breads unless low salt; pretzels; self-rising flour mixes; regular crackers	White and whole wheat flour, unsalted matzos, cornmeal, low-salt cereals: cream of wheat, puffed wheat, puffed rice, shredded wheat, Maltex, oatmeal, Ralston, Wheatena
Fruits	Dried fruits or fruits with sodium added in preparation; read label	Fresh, frozen, and canned
Vegetables	Artichokes, beets, beet greens, celery, dandelion greens, kale, hominy, mustard greens, spinach, sauerkraut, swiss chard, white turnip. The following frozen vegetables (usually frozen with salt): lima beans, mixed vegetables, peas, peas and carrots, succotash	Fresh, frozen, or low-salt canned: asparagus, beans (green, lima, soy, navy, wax), broccoli, brussels sprouts, cabbage, carrots, corn, cauliflower, cow peas, cucumber, eggplant, endive, escarole, lettuce, mushroom, okra, onions, parsnips, parsley, peas, peppers (green), pumpkin, radishes, rutabaga, squash, tomato, yellow turnip, turnip greens
Dessert	Cakes, cookies, ice cream, sherbet, pastry, prepared mixes, Jell-O	Fruit; fruit ices; special low-salt dessert pudding and custard made with allowed milk and eggs; pie made without salt
Sweets	Molasses, corn syrup, brown sugar, chocolate	Sugar; honey; maple syrup; jelly and jam without added sodium; chewing gum; candies: gumdrops, marshmallows, sour balls, Lifesavers
Beverages	Beverages containing milk; mineral water; sodas not listed in next column	Coffee, Sanka, tea (regular and instant), milk in allowed amounts, Coke, ginger ale, 7-Up, low-calorie soda, orange Crush, root beer
Miscellaneous	Baking powder and soda; bouillon cubes and broth; catsup, chili sauce, pickles, relishes; canned, frozen, or powdered soup; Worcestershire sauce, soy sauce, other meat sauces	Low-salt baking powder, bakers' compressed dry yeast, unflavored gelatin, unsalted nuts, coconut; seasonings: allspice, bay leaf, cinnamon, cloves, garlic, lemon juice, dry mustard, nutmeg, basil, paprika, oregano, parsley, vinegar, pepper, vanilla extract

It should be appreciated that various drugs can modify plasma renin and aldosterone activity. As might be expected from the previous discussion, these include agents that affect (a) sodium or potassium balance, (b) blood pressure, or (c) the β-adrenergic nervous system. Diuretics, antihypertensive drugs, oral contraceptives, and excessive laxative usage are examples. Ideally, patients should be studied after these agents have been withdrawn for at least 3 weeks.

TABLE 5. *Proper collection of a 24-hr urine sample*

To start, empty the bladder and discard this first specimen.
From then on, *all* specimens must be saved *complete.*
At the end of 24 hrs, empty the bladder and *save* this last specimen.
Samples should be pooled together and refrigerated throughout.
No preservative is added to the collection vessels.

Very recently, highly specific renin inhibitors have been developed. These are currently being investigated as antihypertensive agents. For unknown reasons the measurement of renin activity in plasma during administration of these inhibitors seems to be falsely low. A likely explanation is that the inhibitors bind to albumin and that the equilibrium *in vitro* shifts from albumin to renin, so that as the enzymatic incubation progresses, less and less angiotensin I is formed. Renin assays that employ a short incubation time—e.g., the antibody trapping method of Poulsen et al. (16), as performed by Nussberger and Brunner—give higher values for PRA in the presence of renin inhibitors than do other types of assays.

Renal-Vein Renin Measurements and the Diagnosis of Renovascular Hypertension

Renal-vein renin measurements can provide the clinician with useful information about renal pathology and

TABLE 6. *Abnormal renal renin secretion in human disorders*

A. Subnormal plasma renin activity (low plasma angiotensin II)
  I. Hypertensive disorders
    a. Consequent to aldosterone excess:
      1. Primary aldosteronism (discrete adrenal cortical adenoma)
      2. Pseudoprimary aldosteronism (idiopathic aldosteronism, bilateral hyperplasia)
    b. Consequent to other mineralocorticoid excess:
      1. 11-beta-hydroxylase deficiency
      2. 17-alpha-hydroxylase deficiency
      3. Other adrenal enzyme defects with overproduction of precursor mineralocorticoid (e.g., Liddle's syndrome)
      4. Glucocorticoid suppressible hyperaldosteronism
      5. Mineralocorticoid excess from adrenal carcinoma
      6. (Ectopic) ACTH-secreting tumors
      7. Iatrogenic: mineralocorticoid, licorice, or butisolidine abuse
    c. Without demonstrable mineralocorticoid excess:
      1. Low-renin essential hypertension
      2. Parenchymal renal disease with sodium–volume retention
      3. Uninephrectomized or other renoprival states
      4. Gordon's hyperkalemic hypertensive syndrome
  II. Normotensive or hypotensive disorders with low plasma renin activity (low plasma angiotensin II and aldosterone)
    a. Renal parenchymal insufficiency with failure of renin secretion (e.g., "hyporeninemic hypoaldosteronism")
    b. Autonomic dysfunction with attendant postural hypotension
    c. Drug induced: beta blockers (low plasma renin), converting-enzyme inhibitors (high plasma renin but low angiotensin II and low aldosterone)
B. Increased plasma renin activity (high plasma angiotensin II)
  I. Hypertensive disorders
    a. With consequent secondary aldosteronism:
      1. Malignant hypertension (i.e., malignant nephrosclerosis)
      2. Unilateral renovascular disease
      3. High-renin essential hypertension
      4. Bilateral renovascular or renal parenchymal disease (e.g., collagen disease) with renin oversecretion
      5. Renin-secreting tumors
      6. Pheochromocytoma
      7. Iatrogenic: oral contraceptive, estrogen or corticosteroid use, renin incompletely suppressed, angiotensin and aldosterone increased due to high plasma renin substrate levels
    b. Without consequent secondary aldosteronism:
      1. Potassium-depleted patients with all of the above (i.e., listed under heading "a") disorders.
  II. Normotensive or hypotensive high-renin disorders
    a. With consequent hyperaldosteronism:
      1. Edematous states (reduced effective blood volume)
        i. Congestive heart failure
        ii. Nephrotic syndrome
        iii. Cirrhosis with ascites
      2. Hypokalemic states (often stimulated by aldosterone consequent to renal sodium wasting)
        i. Renal tubular acidosis
        ii. Bartter's syndrome
        iii. Other nephropathies
      3. Physiologic or iatrogenic induced hyperreninemia and hyperaldosteronism
        i. Dietary sodium depletion
        ii. Diuretic usage
        iii. Laxative abuse
        iv. Alimentary disorders, gastroenteritis, vomiting
        v. Other causes of reduced effective blood volume (hemorrhage, dehydration, sweat loss, posture)
    b. Without expected secondary aldosteronism:
      1. Adrenal cortical failure (i.e., Addison's disease)
      2. Converting-enzyme inhibitor drugs (renin and angiotensin I high but angiotensin II and aldosterone low)
      3. Potassium-depleted hypokalemic states (or when potassium depletion accompanies sodium depletion, e.g., alimentary disorders or thiazide diuretics)
C. Disorders producing variable renin secretory responses
  I. Bilateral renovascular stenosis or coarctation of aorta: The initially high renin secretion becomes dampened as impaired renal sodium excretion volume expansion and hypertension finally restores renal perfusion pressure beyond the arterial occlusion.
  II. Bilateral renal parenchymal disease: Renin secretion is usually suppressed by sodium retention from impaired renal excretory capacity. Less commonly, renin secretion may be increased if there is ischemia in a subpopulation of nephrons or impaired if the disease process damages the juxtaglomerular apparatus (hyporeninemic hypoaldosteronism).

renal blood flow. A key fact to remember is that renal-vein renin levels do not give information about the secretion rate of renin. The peripheral plasma renin reflects the secretion rate of renin. Under steady-state conditions the secretion rate of renin per minute is 144 times the peripheral renin level (2). Several facts can help the clinician to understand the meaning of peripheral and renal-vein renin measurements. The kidneys do not clear appreciable amounts of renin from the circulation. If a kidney completely shuts off its secretion of renin, the renal-vein renin concentration (V) will be exactly the same as the renal-artery renin concentration (A). If the two kidneys contribute equally to the circulating renin, under steady-state conditions each V will be 25% higher than A (2); if one kidney secretes all of the renin, this increment $[(V - A)/A]$ will be 50%. These relationships are constant because the liver always clears the same *fraction* of renin from blood per minute, regardless of the circulating renin level. Only a change in hepatic blood flow can cause a change in these relationships in the patient with normal renal blood flow. Of significance, however, is the fact that renal blood flow can have a marked effect on the relationship between V and A. This can be best understood if one first examines the relationship between V and A in a patient who fails to secrete renin from one kidney and who secretes all of the renin from the other. (This occurs frequently in patients with renovascular hypertension.) As just described, the V values of the ischemic kidney will be at least 50% higher than the A values, but this increment will be higher if renal blood flow is subnormal because, *ceteris paribus,* the renin will be secreted into a smaller volume of blood per minute. As described by Fick's principle, the lower the renal blood flow, the higher the concentration of renin. This means that the renal venous–arterial renin relationship $[(V - A)/A]$ is inversely related to renal blood flow (Fig. 3). Thus, a renal-vein renin concentration that is more than 50% higher than the simultaneously collected peripheral renin concentration, in a patient whose opposite kidney secretes no renin ($V = A$), tells the clinician that the renal blood flow to that kidney is subnormal. Because of the errors in sampling and in assays, etc., an increment of 75% or more may be needed to be sure that renal blood flow is indeed reduced. This increment is almost always exceeded in patients with functional unilateral renal artery stenosis.

The demonstration of suppression of renin secretion from the contralateral kidney of the patient with unilateral renovascular hypertension is an additional piece of diagnostically useful information. It is most easily documented 30 min after administration of a rapidly acting CEI, since this induces massive reactive renin secretion from the ischemic kidney while the contralateral kidney remains suppressed. Under baseline conditions (i.e., before CEI), one cannot always be sure that the contralateral kidney is completely suppressed because the normal 25% renal venous increment falls close to the combined potential errors of the procedures. Suppression of renin secretion (and no response to CEI) means that the kidney in question is exposed to abnormally high pressure (baroreceptor renin suppression) and is also excreting most of the dietary sodium chloride (macula densa renin suppression). Unfortunately, this does not necessarily mean that the kidney is normal; rather, it just means that it is not as ischemic as the other one. If the blood urea nitrogen (BUN) and serum creatinine values are elevated, bilateral renal pathology is present, but the renal-vein renin measurement can still help the clinician to decide which kidney is more ischemic. When renal function tests (BUN and serum creatinine) are normal, a completely suppressed renin secretion from the contralateral kidney is a good sign that the contralateral kidney may be normal.

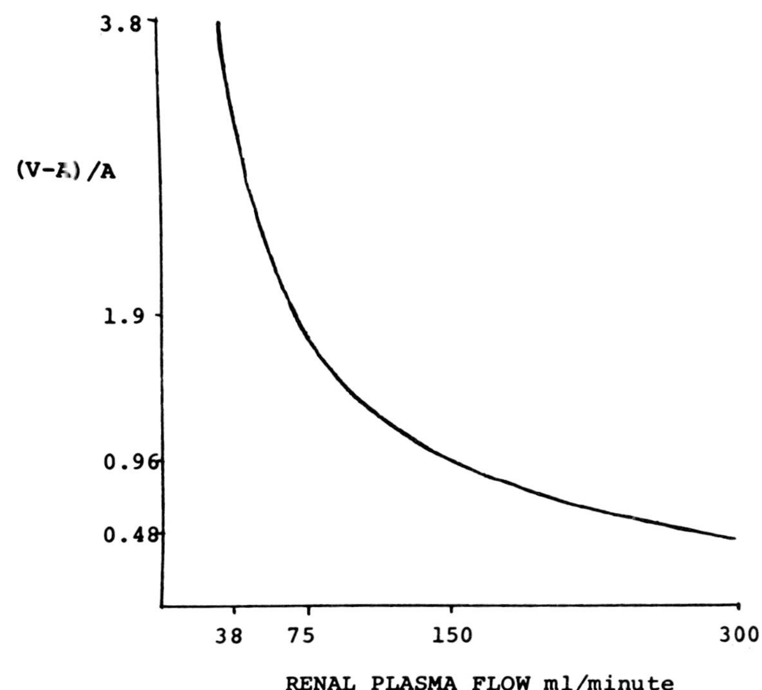

FIG. 3. Nomogram for estimating renal plasma flow in the suspect kidney using only renal-vein and peripheral renin measurements. The plot describes the relationship of renal plasma flow to $(V - A)/A$ in patients with unilateral renal renin secretion. (From ref. 49.)

When renal-vein renin levels are equal and more than 25% higher than the arterial renin, renal blood flow is most likely reduced to both kidneys and bilateral renal disease should be suspected. Bilateral renin secretion and unequal renal-vein renin levels are difficult to interpret. In this situation it is important to remember that renal-vein renin levels do not indicate the level of renin secretion from either kidney. The peripheral plasma level of renin reflects the combined rate of secretion of renin from both kidneys, but it is difficult to distinguish which kidney is secreting the most renin. A renal-vein renin increment of more than 50% over the peripheral level indicates reduction in renal blood flow. However, if one kidney is secreting most of the renin and is causing a high peripheral renin level, a renal-vein renin increment much less than 50% in the contralateral kidney may also be associated with marked reduction in flow, because the peripheral renin is much higher than it would be if that kidney were contributing all of the renin to the circulation; this leads to underestimation of $(V-A)/A$. In this situation, increased BUN and serum creatinine levels will indicate whether bilateral renal disease is present or not, which can help in the decision of whether or not to perform arteriography. Notwithstanding all these factors, in the presence of bilateral disease, the renal vein with the highest $(V-A)/A$ value is more likely to be the kidney with the lowest flow and secreting the most renin.

Table 7 indicates how to collect samples for renal-vein renin measurements and how to interpret these measurements.

Urine and Plasma Aldosterone

Aldosterone is a mineralocorticoid that is synthesized and secreted from the zona glomerulosa of the adrenal cortex. Table 8 summarizes the disorders of aldosterone secretion. Aldosterone has relevance to the work-up of the hypertensive patient because excessive secretion of aldosterone can cause hypertension. In addition, angiotensin II stimulates aldosterone biosynthesis and secretion, and the consequent sodium-retaining effect of aldosterone helps to maintain blood pressure in the presence of angiotensin-II-induced arteriolar vasoconstriction. During excessive aldosterone secretion, derangements in potassium and hydrogen ion homeostasis can occur; a low serum potassium and high serum bicarbonate often provide the first clues that the circulating level of aldosterone is high.

Aldosterone's principal target tissue is the kidney where it acts in the connecting and collecting tubules of the distal nephron to enhance sodium reabsorption and potassium secretion. Aldosterone also promotes hydrogen ion secretion at the same site. The coordination of aldosterone's effect with intrarenal physical factors to maintain both sodium and potassium homeostasis is discussed in another chapter by Sealey and Laragh, entitled "The Renin–Angiotensin–Aldosterone System for Normal Regulation of Blood Pressure and Sodium and Potassium Homeostasis" (17).

Factors Affecting Urine and Plasma Aldosterone Levels

Changes in PRA, via angiotensin II, play a leading role in determining the rate of aldosterone secretion (Fig. 1). As illustrated in Fig. 2, during changes in sodium intake, parallel changes occur in PRA and urinary aldosterone excretion. During sodium depletion, aldosterone secretion increases; however, during sodium loading, it falls.

In addition, potassium has a marked effect on aldosterone secretion (18). Figure 4 illustrates the influence of potassium intake on the aldosterone–sodium relationship in normal subjects. The lower the rate of urine potassium excretion, the lower the excretion rate of aldosterone for a given level of sodium excretion. The opposite is also true. In normal subjects, differences in potassium intake are not accompanied by any change in serum potassium, most likely because the response of aldosterone and concurrent changes in intrarenal physical factors perfectly compensate.

Adrenocorticotropic hormone (ACTH) plays a second-

TABLE 7. *Renovascular hypertension: renal-vein renin samples for diagnosis*

1. Samples to collect
   A. Simultaneous collection, from each kidney, of supine renal vein renin (V_1, V_2) and inferior vena caval renin (A_1, A_2)
   B. Oral administration of 25 mg captopril; then 30 min later, repeat collections as described in A.
2. Interpretation of results
   A. Pre-captopril
      1. $V_1/A_1 = 1.0$
         No renin secretion from that kidney. Indicator of contralateral suppression.
      2. $V_2/A_2 \geq 1.5$
         The degree to which this value exceeds 1.5 in the presence of contralateral suppression is a measure of the reduction in flow to that kidney (see Fig. 3).
      3. $V_1/A_1 > 0$ and $V_2/A_2 > 0$ and $(V_2/A_2 + V_2/A_2) \geq 2.5$
         An indicator of bilateral disease; the more ischemic kidney is likely to be the one with the higher V/A.
      4. $(V_1/A_1 + V_2/A_2) < 2.5$
         This occurs when the samples are not collected under steady-state conditions or when the renal vein blood is contaminated with blood from another source (e.g., ovarian vein or vena cava). The study may have to be repeated.
   B. Post-captopril
      1. $V_1/A_1 = 1.0$
         A more reliable indicator of contralateral suppression than the pre-captopril V_1/A_1.
      2. $V_2/A_2 > 2.0$
         An indicator of renal ischemia.

TABLE 8. *Disorders of aldosterone secretion*

A Oversecretion (aldosteronism)
- I. Primary aldosteronism (adrenal in origin)
  - a. Primary aldosteronism due to adenoma
  - b. Pseudoprimary aldosteronism (bilateral adrenal hyperplasia)
- II. Secondary aldosteronism (driven by an extra-adrenal signal that activates renin secretion)
  - a. Hypertensive states:
    1. Malignant hypertension
    2. Malignant or severe hypertension due to unilateral renovascular disease
    3. High-renin essential hypertension
    4. Renin-secreting tumors
  - b. Edematous states:
    1. Cirrhosis
    2. Nephrosis
    3. Heart failure
  - c. Hypokalemic normotensive states:
    1. Juxtaglomerular cell hyperplasia with sodium and potassium wastage and retarded growth
    2. Renal tubular acidosis
    3. Other sodium-wasting renal diseases
- II. Physiologic aldosteronism
  - a. Via activation of renin secretion: sodium–volume depletion (alimentary loss, diuretic usage trauma, hemorrhage, burns, antihypertensive vasodilator drugs which reflexly activate the renin system via a renal baroreceptor as pressure falls
  - b. Via a direct stimulation of the adrenal cortex: from potassium ingestion

B. Lack of aldosterone secretion
- I. Adrenal cortical insufficiency (Addison's disease)
  - a. Pure mineralocorticoid failure (e.g., hyporeninemic hypoaldosteronism)
  - b. Combined cortisol–aldosterone failure (Waterhouse–Friedrickson syndrome)

ary supportive role in the physiologic regulation of aldosterone secretion (19). ACTH appears to be responsible for acute stress-related changes in plasma aldosterone and for the diurnal pattern of secretion. Diurnal changes in plasma aldosterone are most apparent in patients with primary aldosteronism, in whom the renin–angiotensin system is completely suppressed. In such patients the counteracting effects of the postural induced rise in angiotensin II and aldosterone in the morning do not occur, so that the effect of falling ACTH levels is mirrored by a fall in aldosterone (see below for the interpretation of plasma aldosterone measurements).

As discussed in the next section, it is not possible to explain all of the changes in aldosterone in pathologic situations based on the known effects of these three stimuli to aldosterone secretion. Other undefined factors clearly participate, including atrial natriuretic peptide (ANP), which suppresses (a) basal aldosterone levels and (b) the aldosterone response to angiotensin II stimulation (20). However, even when ANP is taken into account, unexplained differences in aldosterone levels do occur.

How to Use Urine and Plasma Aldosterone Measurements in the Work-up of the Hypertensive Patient

The 24-hr rate of urinary excretion of the acid labile conjugate of aldosterone is a reliable index of the daily adrenal secretion rate of aldosterone (21). Since this conjugate is converted back to free aldosterone during the assay, results are reported as micrograms of aldosterone secreted per day. Measurement of this conjugate may not entirely parallel the secretion rate of aldosterone, and it may be less reliable in the presence of impaired liver or kidney function as discussed below. Such situations are usually readily apparent in the clinic. There is an important advantage in measuring the 24-hr urinary excretion of aldosterone rather than the blood levels, since the urinary measurement integrates the 24-hr secretion rate and eliminates the considerable effect of minute-to-minute changes in secretion. A 24-hr urine is usually collected anyway to assess the concurrent level of sodium and potassium excretion.

About 10% of secreted aldosterone is excreted into the urine as the acid-labile conjugate; the biologically active hormone can be liberated from this conjugate at pH 1. This metabolite is unusual because approximately 50% of it is formed by kidney tissue (22,23). Because of this, in the presence of liver disease as much as 50% of the aldosterone may be metabolized and excreted in the urine as this conjugate. Its rapid rate of excretion by the kidneys (6 hr) also makes the acid-labile conjugate especially suitable for the estimation of aldosterone (24). This is to be contrasted with the relatively slow rate of excretion (48 hr) of the major metabolite of aldosterone, tetrahydroaldosterone, which is formed by the liver (25).

The normal rates of excretion of the acid-labile conjugate are illustrated in Figs. 2 and 4. It is quite clear that the normalcy of an aldosterone measurement should be assessed in relation to the concurrent state of both sodium and potassium balance. In normal subjects the urinary potassium excretion provides a reliable index of net "balance," but this is not so in patients with hyperaldosteronism. They excrete large amounts of potassium per day even when intake and serum potassium are low. In fact, a urine potassium excretion greater than 40 mEq/day in the pres-

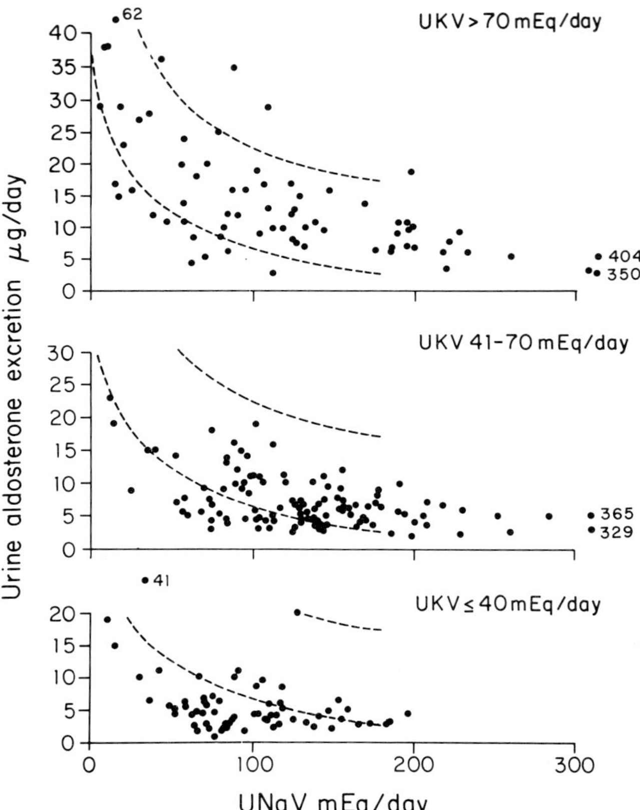

FIG. 4. Relationship of urinary aldosterone excretion to the daily rate of urinary sodium excretion in normal subjects eating a random diet divided according to the concurrent rate of urinary potassium excretion. The dashed lines are replotted from Fig. 2. Subjects excreting over 70 mEq K^+ per day fall within the previously defined normal range. Those excreting between 40 and 70 mEq/day have, on average, a lower aldosterone excretion for a given rate of sodium excretion. Those who excrete below 40 mEq K^+ per day have very low levels of aldosterone excretion, even when they receive a relatively low sodium diet.

ence of a serum K^+ of less than 3.5 mEq/liter is a good indicator of hyperaldosteronism. Because the serum potassium level has such a profound effect on aldosterone secretion, both urine and plasma aldosterone measurements in patients must be considered in relationship to the concurrent serum potassium level. An apparently "normal" level of aldosterone can actually be abnormally high in the patient with hypokalemia. Potassium repletion of the hypokalemic patient will often increase the aldosterone level out of the normal range.

Interpretation of plasma aldosterone measurements from a single sample or during a particular intervention (e.g., captopril test or ACTH test) should be made with caution. Several factors make it difficult to get a good baseline measurement. Firstly, a falling ACTH during the day (especially in the morning) results in a steadily falling baseline as the day progresses. Secondly, even when ACTH is unchanged it takes close to an hour for aldosterone to reach a new steady state. In addition, the stress caused by drawing blood can transiently increase aldosterone as can the earlier consumption of a potassium-rich meal. Ideally, the profile baseline plasma aldosterone should be established on a different day from the one on which any testing procedure is carried out. When this is done, useful information about the factors controlling aldosterone secretion can be derived from administration of CEIs (to block the effect of angiotensin II) or dexamethasone (to block the effects of ACTH).

The patient with hypokalemia, alkalosis, high plasma and urine aldosterone levels, completely suppressed renins, and no increase (or even a fall) in plasma aldosterone between 8 a.m. (supine) and noon (upright) and who exhibits no fall in plasma aldosterone in response to converting-enzyme inhibition almost certainly has primary aldosteronism due to an adrenal cortical tumor. About 50% of patients with primary aldosteronism fall into this group. The problem is that not all patients with primary aldosteronism have completely suppressed renins, and such patients are hard to distinguish from patients with adrenal hyperplasia (pseudo-primary aldosteronism) who do not have a discrete tumor and who do not respond to even total adrenalectomy with cure of their hypertension. It is not clear why some patients with discrete aldosterone-secreting tumors do not shut off their renin completely. Concurrent renal impairment may be an answer, since some of them develop essential hypertension in later years after "cure" of their primary aldosteronism. The reader is referred to several

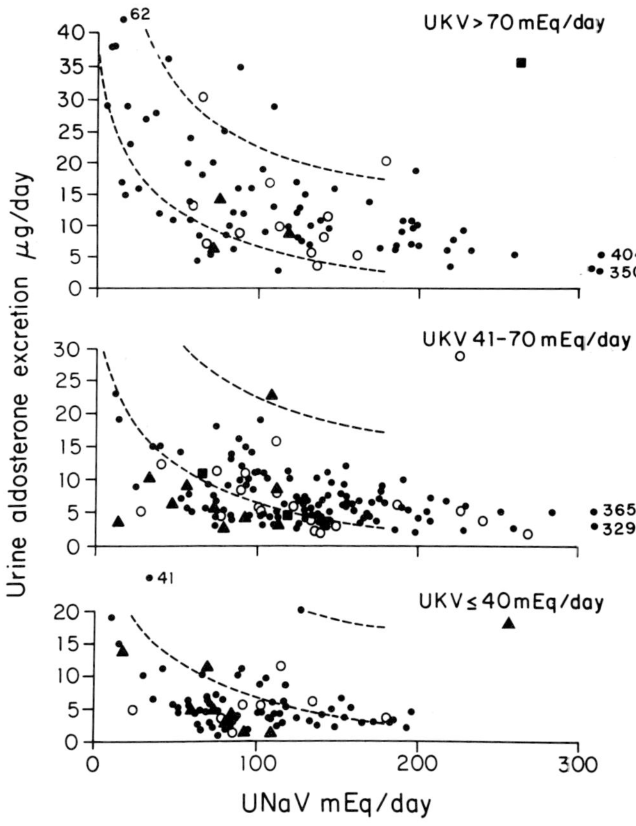

FIG. 5. Untreated hypertensive patients usually exhibit a normal rate of aldosterone excretion when their concurrent rate of potassium excretion is taken into account, whether or not they have low (▲), medium (○), or high (■) plasma renin levels.

reports by Biglieri describing in detail how to use aldosterone measurements and other adrenal steroid measurements to diagnose patients with primary aldosteronism and other adrenal disorders (see chapter by Biglieri et al., entitled "Adrenocortical Forms of Human Hypertension") (13).

Essential hypertensive patients have been thought to exhibit a wider range of urine aldosterone levels than do normal subjects. This may not be correct because when we took the concurrent urinary potassium excretion into account, these differences almost completely disappeared (Fig. 5). This means that patients with low-renin essential hypertension do not have commensurately low aldosterone levels (26). The cause of this abnormal relationship between renin and aldosterone is not clear, since there are no differences in potassium homeostasis or ACTH secretion. For unknown reasons, these patients appear to have increased adrenal sensitivity to angiotensin II (27). This phenomenon can also occur in normal subjects. Those with the lowest renins for a given rate of sodium excretion have high aldosterone/renin ratios. The reciprocal phenomenon also occurs. Patients with renovascular hypertension often have very high renin levels, but their aldosterone levels are not proportionally elevated and they rarely exhibit hypokalemia. A normal secretion rate of aldosterone appears to be physiologically appropriate for the essential hypertensive patient, regardless of the renin level, since normokalemia is almost uniformly maintained. However, it is possible that a consequence of this may be high blood pressure, since treatment with the aldosterone receptor antagonist spironolactone often lowers blood pressure, especially in low-renin patients.

Plasma Angiotensin II

Angiotensin II measurements have rarely been used clinically. This is because of the lack of availability of a sensitive and accurate assay (see below) and the concurrent availability of sensitive renin assays which provide very similar information and which, in addition, can be used for renal-vein renin measurements. Measurement of angiotensin II in renal vein bloods could not substitute for the renin measurement as a guide to renal function.

Two potential uses for plasma angiotensin II measurements can be envisioned. During converting-enzyme inhibition and during administration of renin inhibitors, angiotensin II measurements could be used to assess the effectiveness of blockade. This could be important clinically. Unfortunately, this requires a most sensitive and specific assay because angiotensin II levels are very low after CEI inhibition and angiotensin I levels are high. Interference by angiotensin I is a major problem in angiotensin II assays.

A second potential use of angiotensin II assays is for assessment of the contribution of extrarenal renin to the circulating angiotensin II level. There is evidence that there is uptake of renal renin by vascular tissues (28), and some investigators believe that it may contribute to the circulating angiotensin II level. In addition, although active renin disappears from the circulation after nephrectomy, a few investigators have suggested that locally active tissue renin systems exist in heart and vascular tissues and contribute to circulating angiotensin II levels. So far, the evidence for vascular and cardiac renin biosynthesis is very weak, but the possible contribution of vascular uptake of renal renin (or prorenin) to the circulating angiotensin II level needs to be assessed.

Plasma Angiotensinogen (Renin Substrate)

Unlike that of renin, angiotensin II, and aldosterone, secretion of angiotensinogen is not regulated on a minute-by-minute basis, and its blood level does not normally vary much. The stimuli that affect its blood level take several days to have significant effect. Nonetheless, the concentration of angiotensinogen in blood is rate-limiting, and a change in its concentration can effect the PRA measurement (29). The normal circulating level of angiotensinogen is close to K_m, which means that, *ceteris paribus,* a fall in plasma angiotensinogen can cause close-to-linear fall in the rate of angiotensin formation. On the other hand, the maximum increase in rate of angiotensin formation that can occur with an increase in plasma angiotensinogen is twofold, since K_m is that concentration at which half-maximum velocity occurs.

Under most circumstances, an increase in plasma angiotensinogen will not increase the rate of angiotensin production *in vivo,* since the secretion rate of renin normally has a feedback relationship with angiotensin II and with those parameters regulated by angiotensin II so as to maintain a physiologically appropriate rate of formation of angiotensin II. Exceptions do occur, however, as discussed below.

Factors Affecting Plasma Angiotensinogen Levels

We do not know what factors determine the normal blood level of angiotensinogen, but we do know what factors can change those levels. In humans, the most potent stimulus to circulating angiotensinogen is estrogen (30). High estrogen levels can increase plasma angiotensinogen more than fivefold. This occurs during pregnancy (14), in ovarian hyperstimulated women who develop many ovarian follicles (31), and in women taking oral contraceptives (29). The changes in plasma estrogen that occur during the normal menstrual cycle are either not great enough or not sustained enough to significantly affect plasma angiotensinogen levels (5).

Glucocorticoids also increase plasma angiotensinogen, but the effect is much less than that of estrogen and rarely causes more than a twofold increase (32).

Patients with liver disease (e.g., cirrhosis) (33) or reduced hepatic blood flow (e.g., congestive heart failure) often have low levels of renin substrate, most likely due to impaired production. For unknown reasons, binephrectomy leads to a rise in plasma angiotensinogen, but this is most apparent in animal models and does not markedly affect levels in humans (34).

The Meaning of Angiotensinogen Levels in Hypertensive Patients

It is rare that angiotensinogen affects the rate of angiotensin generation *in vivo,* since, as discussed above, renin concentration falls to compensate for a rise in circulating renin substrate. However, when renin secretion is unresponsive to feedback stimuli, a rise in angiotensinogen can be pathologic. For example, patients taking oral contraceptives sometimes develop hypertension which disappears when the pill is discontinued. In most of these subjects, PRA levels are in the normal range. But renin ought to be suppressed by the activation of the renal baroreceptor mechanism. It is possible that in such patients, ischemic nephrons cannot turn off their renin secretion appropriately. In the presence of high angiotensinogen, this would lead to a circulating angiotensin II level that was too high in relationship to the blood pressure and state of sodium balance. Similarly, renin secretion may fail to turn off in malignant and advanced hypertension. For unknown reasons, these patients often have elevated angiotensinogen levels which could contribute to pathogenesis of the disease if uncontrolled renin secretion is a factor.

Angiotensinogen levels may fall in patients taking ACE inhibitors. While angiotensin II may be able to directly stimulate angiotensinogen synthesis, concurrently high levels of renin may cause excessive utilization. This is rarely important clinically, but it could lead to underestimation of endogenous PRA *in vitro.* For example, if renin substrate were depleted during the assay, the estimation of PRA would be falsely low. This underestimation of renin might be important in renal-vein samples in which a difference in the relative renin concentrations from the two kidneys might be missed. The highest renal-vein renin value we have measured is close to 1000 ng/ml/hr. A normal level of plasma angiotensinogen is close to 1800 ng/ml (Table 9). Such a high renin would totally exhaust renin substrate before the end of a 3-hr incubation.

Plasma Prorenin

Close to 90% of total renin in human plasma is prorenin, the inactive biosynthetic precursor (35). Plasma prorenin has had impact clinically only because of its interference with renin assays. It has rarely been used as a tool for clinical diagnosis. The reason that the clinician needs to know about prorenin is that misconceptions about renin measurements (during antihypertensive therapy and after nephrectomy) in relation to hypertensive disease have occurred because two previously commonly used renin methods (36,37) actually measured total renin, i.e., prorenin plus active renin. Since renin and prorenin do not occur in plasma in a fixed ratio, and since certain factors that affect renin release may have the opposite effect on prorenin, the measurement of total plasma renin can lead to wrong conclusions about the functioning of the renin system. For example, groups that inadvertently measured total renin thought that patients with primary aldosteronism or who were bilaterally nephrectomized always had a small amount of circulating renin. In fact they do not, but they do have low but detectable levels of prorenin. They also thought that β-blockers did not suppress renin, since β-blockers lower active renin but do not suppress the total renin. In addition, whereas most patients with low-renin essential hypertension have suppressed prorenin, 20% or so have quite high levels, so that certain investigators who inadvertently divided patients with essential hypertension according to a total renin assay were studying different subgroups than those who divided the patients on the basis of active renin. This most likely contributed to some of the controversy about the characteristics of renin subgroups in essential hypertension.

Although these methodological flaws have now been corrected, there remains one other way that prorenin can interfere with renin assays. This is especially a problem in patients who have a high percentage of prorenin in their blood (35). Examples are pregnant women (about 98%

TABLE 9. *Renin, prorenin, and renin substrate values in normal subjects*[a]

	Age			*P* (old vs. young)	Females	Males	Whites	Blacks
	22–30	31–50	51–68					
Number of subjects:	12	50	55		56	66	70	52
PRA (ng/ml · hr):	4.5 ± 0.6[b]	2.3 ± 0.2	2.1 ± 0.2	<0.001	2.3 ± 0.2	2.4 ± 0.2	2.6 ± 0.2[c]	2.0 ± 0.2
Prorenin (*t*) (ng/ml · hr):	14.5 ± 2.0	16.0 ± 1.1	16.2 ± 1.9	<0.05	14.0 ± 1.3[d]	17.5 ± 1.4	15.4 ± 1.4	16.8 ± 1.4
Renin substrate (ng/ml):	1490 ± 115	1700 ± 65	1690 ± 40		1750 ± 60	1615 ± 40	1600 ± 45[c]	1775 ± 55
Age (years):	26.9 ± 0.7	39.8 ± 0.8	57.7 ± 0.7		46.3 ± 1.6	47.3 ± 1.5	47.3 ± 1.5	46.1 ± 1.6

[a] From ref. 35. Values are the mean ± SE. Statistical significance was determined by unpaired Wilcoxon test. Prorenin (*t*) measured following liquid-phase trypsin activation (47). Prorenin is about 60% higher when measured using solid-phase trypsin (5).

[b] $p < 0.01$, age 22–30 vs. age 31–50.

[c] $p < 0.05$, whites vs. blacks.

[d] $p < 0.05$, females vs. males.

prorenin), ovarian hyperstimulated women (about 98%), low-renin hypertensive patients with normal to high prorenin (98%), and patients with ectopic renin-secreting tumors (over 98%). When the plasma is chilled after collection, a small fraction of prorenin is irreversibly changed to active renin. Some methods, kits, and clinical labs still advocate chilling bloods for renin immediately upon collection or they may thaw frozen plasmas in a refrigerator. Even a short exposure to cold can activate a fraction of the prorenin reservoir. When the prorenin concentration is more than 10 times that of active renin, cryoactivation of as little as 2% can appreciably increase the PRA measurement. This has especially been a problem in determining normal values in pregnant women. The whole problem can be avoided by collecting samples at room temperature and then freezing the separated plasma.

Prorenin levels have proven to be diagnostically useful in identifying patients with ectopic renin-secreting tumors. Such patients usually have extremely high plasma prorenin levels. Such is not necessarily the case for renal renin-secreting tumors, with the exception of Wilms' tumors. Prorenin levels could theoretically be used to diagnose early pregnancy because a 10-fold rise in plasma prorenin occurs in the first 2 weeks after conception. This increased ovarian secretion of prorenin is maintained throughout gestation.

Prorenin is the only form of renin that is secreted from extrarenal sources. So far, no method is available to separately identify the organ sources of prorenin. We have demonstrated that the ovary secretes prorenin at mid-menstrual cycle and during pregnancy. The blood level of prorenin increases about twofold at mid-menstrual cycle and about 10-fold following conception. The testis and adrenal also secrete some prorenin, but only very low amounts that may not significantly affect the normal circulating level.

METHODOLOGY

Plasma Renin

Collection of Blood

Blood for renin measurement should be collected into a lavender-topped EDTA Vacutainer and centrifuged *at room temperature.* Serum or plasma collected into another anticoagulant can also be used as long as EDTA is added before the sample is assayed. It should be recognized, however, that prorenin is more likely to cryoactivate in serum than in plasma. Following centrifugation of the blood, plasma can be stored frozen until assay. It should be emphasized that the freezer should be able to maintain the sample *completely frozen.* Plasma can thaw transiently in an automatically defrosting freezer, especially one that is opened and closed frequently. The blood or plasma should not be placed on ice because inadvertent cryoactivation of prorenin can occur, which leads to falsely high estimates of plasma renin activity (see above). To evaluate the baseline renin–sodium profile, patients should be untreated, ideally for at least 3 weeks. A 24-hr urine should be collected on the day before the renin test for measurement of sodium excretion. The patient should have been ambulatory for at least 1 hr before blood collection, which makes the test ideal for outpatients who must travel to reach the doctor's office. Inpatients who are capable should ambulate for half an hour or more before blood is drawn. See the section entitled "How to Use the Renin Test in the Work-up of the Hypertensive Patient" for other factors that should be considered in relation to blood collection.

Description of the Assay

PRA is commonly measured by incubating plasma at 37°C for a fixed time in the presence of angiotensinase and CEIs, followed by radioimmunoassay to quantitate the amount of formed angiotensin I (9,10). The assay thus consists of two steps: (i) cleavage of angiotensin I from plasma angiotensinogen by renin and (ii) radioimmunoassay of angiotensin I. The measurement is expressed as an hourly rate of angiotensin I generation (ng/ml/hr). The method is described in detail in refs. 8 and 34. In this approach to the measurement of plasma renin, the rate of angiotensin generation is a function of the plasma concentration of both renin and renin substrate. For clinical purposes this is useful, since the measurement reflects the net capacity of the blood to generate angiotensin II (converting enzyme is not normally rate-limiting unless it is pharmacologically blocked). Investigators occasionally prefer to measure the concentration of renin in blood independently of differences in renin substrate. This can be achieved by adding excess substrate (usually heterologous) to the plasma prior to enzymatic incubation (37,38). Alternatively, the rate of angiotensin I generation can be compared to that of several concentrations of purified renin added to the same blood; the renin concentration is then derived by extrapolation (39).

Direct radioimmunoassays for the measurement of renin have recently been developed and may reach the market in the near future. So far they have had problems of sensitivity and/or specificity (one of them measures total renin, i.e., active renin plus prorenin). No doubt these deficiencies will be overcome, making the renin assay much simpler and avoiding some of the problems described below.

Factors to Consider in Selecting a Renin Assay for Clinical Use

Since the renin test is potentially very simple, and since radioimmunoassay of angiotensin I provides no unusual complications, one might wonder why the renin test has been performed inadequately in so many laboratories. There are several reasons (40):

1. *pH control.* Plasma that has been separated from blood in which EDTA was used as an anticoagulant may have a pH ranging from 7.6 to 8.2. If the sample is not buffered, the pH rises during the 37°C enzymatic incubation, and the rate of angiotensin generation falls because of

a gradual shift in the enzyme kinetics and because renin is destroyed at 37°C above pH 8. This can result in renin values that are falsely low and unreproducible. The problem of pH control during the enzymatic incubation of renin in plasma has now been resolved by most laboratories and commercial kits, but it should be noted that Haber's original method (41) did not advocate pH control.

2. *Prorenin.* Prorenin comprises a variable but large proportion (close to 90%) of renin in human blood (35). As just discussed, it can be activated by certain *in vitro* procedures. It is converted to active renin in human plasma during dialysis to pH 3.3 and then to pH 7.4, a technique that was used in certain early renin assays to destroy renin substrate and angiotensinases (36). In addition, when plasma is chilled but not frozen, some activation of prorenin occurs. Such cryoactivation occurs even more rapidly in serum. To avoid cryoactivation, plasma (or serum) should *not be chilled* before renin assay. It should be processed at room temperature or stored completely frozen (35).

3. *Blank subtraction and angiotensinase inhibition.* This becomes an issue when renin is low, e.g., less than 1 ng/ml/hr. The problem is that nonspecific substances in plasma cross-react with angiotensin I antibodies (called the *blank*) and contribute to the measured renin value. This blank partially disappears during incubation at 37°C, and it does not have the same characteristics as true angiotensin I in the radioimmunoassay (42). The correct result cannot be obtained by measuring and subtracting the blank. But by prolonging the enzymatic incubation of renin until the true angiotensin I is much higher than the nonspecific immunoreactive component, the blank can be ignored.

Prolonged incubations of renin (for 18 hr) can be accurate only if angiotensinases are completely inhibited, and this depends on the pH chosen for enzymatic reaction. (Converting enzyme is completely inhibited by EDTA.) To our knowledge, no one has reported any combination of angiotensinase inhibitors that is effective in plasma for more than 3 hr at pH 7.4. For that reason we incubate plasma renin at pH 5.7, where complete angiotensinase inhibition can be achieved for up to 18 hr with EDTA and PMSF. An additional advantage of pH 5.7 is that the pH of plasma is quite stable if it is adjusted with maleic acid. The one disadvantage of incubating for 18 hr is that low-renin samples require 2 days to assay. To avoid waiting overnight for all renin results, and to avoid excessive substrate utilization in samples with high PRA, we divide each plasma sample into two parts and incubate one part for 3 hr and the remainder for 18 hr. The latter sample is assayed only if the renin value falls below 1 ng/ml/hr.

In summary, we consider that the ideal human plasma renin assay (10,43) is one which is carried out in plasma that has not been exposed to temperatures between +6°C and freezing, and in which the enzymatic incubation is carried out at the pH optimum (pH 5.7–6.0) in the presence of EDTA and PMSF, long enough to eliminate the need for blank subtraction (i.e., 3 hr for most samples, 18 hr for low-renin samples).

TABLE 10. *What to look for in a renin assay*

Best assays
1. Samples not chilled during collection.
2. Three-hour incubation for generation of Ang I; 18-hr incubation for low renin samples.
3. pH 5.7–6 used for Ang I generation; EDTA and PMSF used as angiotensinase and ACE inhibitors.
Compromises
If pH 7.4 used for Ang I generation, 8-OH quinoline added in addition to EDTA and PMSF as angiotensinase inhibitors.
Techniques that could cause errors
1. Chilled tubes used for blood collection.
2. Plasma placed on ice during processing before pH adjusted to 6 or below.
3. Frozen plasma placed in refrigerator to thaw.
4. Dimercaprol as angiotensinase inhibitor; it can interfere with the radioimmunoassay.
5. No pH control during Ang I generation.
6. Less than 2-hr incubation for Ang I generation.

Commercial Kits and Clinical Laboratories

The renin test is available in kit form and from clinical laboratories. Table 10 lists the important criteria for a good assay. Unfortunately, the absolute values for renin often differ between kits and assays, making it necessary to make use of correction factors when comparing values. It is also necessary to change the criteria for the captopril test depending on the renin method used. The conversion factors and the criteria for the captopril test from different sources are listed in Table 11. They were derived by sending samples to each clinical laboratory or by running each kit (20 or more samples each) as described by the manufacturers. A conversion factor was then derived for each source. For simplicity, the sources with similar conversion factors were grouped together. Locations of the different sources and a more detailed description of the methods are listed in Table 12.

Urinary or Plasma Aldosterone

Collection of Urine and Blood

A complete 24-hr urine sample should be collected as described in Table 5. It should be kept in a refrigerator during collection and should remain there for no more than 48 hr before delivery to the laboratory. Boric acid can be added to the urine as a stabilizing agent during the collection, or can be added afterwards to a well-mixed aliquot, to a final concentration of 1 g/100 ml urine. Some laboratories suggest that the urine pH be adjusted to 4.0 with 30% acetic acid, but urine should not be acidified with hydrochloric acid during collection because this could lead to hydrolysis of the acid-labile conjugate and destruction of some of the liberated aldosterone.

TABLE 11. *Conversion factors and three renin criteria for positive captopril test result using renin values from kits or clinical laboratories*

Source	Conversion factor	Stimulated PRA (ng/ml/hr)	Absolute increase in PRA (ng/ml/hr)	Cutoff point for % increase in PRA[a]
Laragh	1.0	≥12	≥10	3.0
Biotecx kit	1.3	≥9.2	≥7.7	2.3
Travenol–Genentech kit[b] New England Nuclear kit Nichols Institute Roche Clinical Labs Metpath Labs Smith Kline Clinical Labs	1.6	≥7.3	≥6.1	1.8
Mayo Medical Labs	2.1	≥5.7	≥4.7	1.4

[a] Percent increase in plasma renin activity of 150% or more if baseline plasma renin activity is above or equal to this value; percent increase in plasma renin activity of 400% or more if baseline plasma renin activity is below this value (11).
[b] Previously known as Clinical Assays.

Heparinized, EDTA-treated, or citrated plasma or serum can be used for plasma aldosterone. Factors to consider in the collection of blood and urine samples are similar to those discussed for renin (see sections entitled "Factors Affecting Plasma Renin Levels" and "Collection of Blood") and in the section entitled "Urine and Plasma Aldosterone."

Description of the Assays

Both urinary and plasma aldosterone are measured by radioimmunoassay. A problem with both urinary and plasma aldosterone radioimmunoassay measurements is that other steroids are recognized by anti-aldosterone antibodies. Although the cross-reactivity is relatively low, the

TABLE 12. *Plasma renin: kits and clinical laboratories*

Source	Reference or catalog number	Blood collection: Room temperature	Blood collection: On ice	ACE and angiotensinase inhibitors: EDTA	ACE and angiotensinase inhibitors: PMSF	BAL and 8-OH Q[a]	Incubation at 37°C: pH	Incubation at 37°C: hours
Sealey–Laragh	Ref. 10	+		+	+		5.7	3/18[b]
Kits								
Biotecx[d]	BL-860		+	+	+		6.0	2/18[b]
New England Nuclear[e]	RIA NEN NEA-104		+	+		+	6.0[c]	1
Travenol–Genentech Clinical Assays[f]	CA-533		+	+	+		6.0	1.5/18[b]
Clinical laboratories								
Nichols Institute[g]	In house		+	+	+		5.5	1/3[b]
Mayo Medical Labs[h]	In house		+	+		+	6.0	1/18
Roche Clinical Labs[i]	CA-533		+	+	+		6.0	1.5/18[b]
Smith Kline Labs[j]	CA-533		+	+	+		6.0	1.5/18[b]
Metpath Labs[k]	RIA NEN NEA-104		+	+		+	6.0[c]	1

[a] Dimercaprol and 8-OH quinoline.
[b] Eighteen-hour incubation used for samples with PRA < 1.0.
[c] A threefold dilution is used to adjust pH to 6.0, thereby making the assay insensitive and highly dependent on differences in angiotensinogen.
[d] Biotecx Laboratories Inc., P.O. Box 1421, Friendswood, TX 77546.
[e] Dupont–New England Nuclear, 331 Treble Cove Road, Billerica, MA 01862.
[f] Travenol–Genentech Diagnostics, 600 Memorial Drive, Cambridge, MA 02139.
[g] Nichols Institute, 26441 Via deAnza, San Juan Capistrano, CA 92675.
[h] Mayo Medical Laboratories, 200 1st Street SW, Rochester, MN 55905.
[i] Roche Biomedical Laboratories, 69 First Avenue, Raritan, NJ 08869.
[j] Smith Kline Bioscience Laboratories, 1075 First Avenue, King of Prussia, PA 19406.
[k] Metpath Laboratories, 1 Malcolm Avenue, Teterboro, NJ 07608.

concentration of the other steroids is often very high, which means that aldosterone must often be separated from them prior to assay. The acid-labile conjugate of aldosterone can be easily separated from cross-reacting steroids by taking advantage of the fact that it is present in urine in a form that is insoluble in organic solvents (44). Cross-reacting steroids can be separated by extraction into an organic solvent such as methylene chloride or ethyl acetate, and then the conjugate can be converted to aldosterone by acidification to pH 1. The aldosterone thus formed is then extracted into the same organic solvent. The solvent is evaporated, and radioimmunoassay is performed on the dried extract.

Plasma aldosterone is routinely measured by radioimmunoassay. Many claims have been made of highly specific antibodies that do not require purification of aldosterone prior to assay. In our limited experience, few of these claims have been substantiated, and we have often found it necessary to perform a chromatographic separation procedure prior to radioimmunoassay (45). The clinician may have to decide how specific the aldosterone assay needs to be for the particular diagnostic problem. This will depend on the type of patient and the type of intervention. For example, specificity is less of a problem in normal adults and in hypertensive patients without adrenal disease. But greater specificity may be needed for children, adolescents, patients with adrenal disease, and pregnant women.

Commercial Kits and Clinical Laboratories

Many organizations such as New England Nuclear (now DuPont) and Serono no longer produce a commercial kit for the radioimmunoassay of urinary or plasma aldosterone. We recommend two kits still in production, namely, (i) the RSL (^{125}I) Aldosterone Kit (Radioassay Systems Laboratories, Inc./Immunochem Corp., Domingues Technology Center, 2015 East University Drive, P.O. Box 6227, Carson, CA 90746) for plasma aldosterone and (ii) the DPC Coat-a-Count Aldosterone Extraction Kit (Diagnostic Products Corp., 5700 West 96th Street, Los Angeles, CA 90045). Our laboratory and RSL have independently found that for plasma the RSL kit, used according to instructions, gives results that compare favorably with results obtained using celite column purification of extracted plasma, indicating that the antibody has good specificity for aldosterone. We did not obtain satisfactory comparison between the DPC kit and our procedures for plasma, but the comparison was not done with heparinized plasma, which the DPC kits call for. We did, however, find that urine aldosterone results using the DPC kit compared favorably with our reported method (44).

Table 13 presents a list of reference laboratories which offer blood and urine aldosterone determinations. Included are (a) methods for collecting samples, (b) some characteristics of these methods, and (c) kit usage.

Plasma Angiotensin II

This is the most difficult component of the renin cascade to measure accurately—and in many ways the most important. Angiotensin II is measured by radioimmunoassay. The problems are due to: (i) very low levels of angiotensin II in blood; (ii) cross-reactivity of antibodies with (a) angiotensin I which can be present in much higher concentrations than angiotensin II, (b) degraded fragments of angiotensin I and II, and (c) nonspecific substances in plasma; and (iii) the fact that the level of angiotensin II actually increases during storage of plasma in the frozen state. The reason for this is unclear, but it is not prevented by the presence of CEIs.

Nussberger et al. (46) developed a method for measurement of angiotensin II which involves (a) removal of proteins by passage through a C-18 cartridge, (b) separation of angiotensin II from angiotensin I by high-pressure liquid chromatography (HPLC), and (c) quantitation of angiotensin II by radioimmunoassay in several HPLC fractions. The method is accurate but extremely time-consuming and it strains the sensitivity of most radioimmunoassays because the angiotensin II is divided between several tubes. For this method to work, step (a) should be carried out on the day of blood collection to avoid further production of angiotensin II. In addition, very sensitive antibodies are needed for the radioimmunoassay step.

The HPLC step to remove angiotensin I may be avoidable in the near future, since the majority of the angiotensin I appears to be formed *in vitro.* By adding a renin inhibitor to the anticoagulant and by ensuring that complete mixing with this inhibitor occurs within seconds of blood collection, the angiotensin I in blood may be kept to a level that does not interfere with the angiotensin II radioimmunoassay, which usually has only a 1% cross-reactivity of angiotensin I. This assay is constantly under development, and hopefully it will soon be simple enough to be commercially available. However, an assay carried out by a clinical laboratory may not be practical as long as the plasma has to be passed through a C-18 cartridge on the day of collection.

Plasma Renin Substrate

Renin substrate is normally measured by incubating a small amount of plasma with excess renin in the presence of angiotensinase and CEIs, and then measuring by radioimmunoassay the amount of angiotensin I formed (9). Human angiotensinogen can only be cleaved by human renin. This has not been readily available. However, the recent production of recombinant human renin should make this reagent more accessible. The results are expressed in molar terms or as nanograms of angiotensin I per milliliter.

Plasma Prorenin

Prorenin is measured in human plasma after it is converted to active renin, usually by limited proteolysis with trypsin; total renin is then measured in the same way as active renin, and prorenin is calculated as the difference between the two measurements. There are several different procedures reported for activation with trypsin. We currently incubate plasma for 18 hr at 4°C at pH 7.8 with

TABLE 13. *Plasma and urine aldosterone assays*

Source	Plasma (P), serum (S), or urine (U)	Collection instructions	Chromatography	Radioimmunoassay method	Cross-reactivity of relevant steroids
Commercial kits					
RSL[a]	P	Heparin	None		DOC < .09%
#1003 or #1004	S				B < .04%
	U				Others < .01%
DPC[b]	P	Heparin only	None		<.01%
#TKAL[b]	S				
	U				
Biotecx[c]	P	Heparin or EDTA	None		<.001%
BL-270	S				
	U				
Clinical laboratories					
Sealey–Laragh	P	EDTA	None	RSL kit	
	U			DPC kit	
Endocrine sciences[d]	P	Heparin or EDTA	None	In house	DOC < .04%
	S				Prednisolone < .02%
	U				<.01%
Mayo Medical Labs[e]	P	Heparin or EDTA	None	In house	
	S (preferred)			DPC kit	
Metpath Labs[f]	P	Heparin	None	DPC kit	
	S				
	U			DPC kit	
Nichols Institute[g]	P	Heparin or EDTA	Celite gel[j]	In house	
	S		Celite gel[j]		
	U			In house	
Roche Clinical Labs[h]	P	Heparin or EDTA	None	DPC kit	
	S				
	U			DPC kit	
Smith Kline Labs[i]	P	Heparin	None	DPC kit	
	S				
	U			DPC kit	

[a] Radioassay Systems Laboratories/Immunochem Corp., Dominguez Technology Center, 2015 E. University Drive, P.O. Box 6227, Carson, CA 90746.
[b] Diagnostic Products Corp., 5700 W. 96 Street, Los Angeles, CA 90045.
[c] Biotecx Laboratories, Inc., P.O. Box 1384, Friendswood, TX 77546.
[d] Endocrine Sciences, 18418 Oxnard Street, Tarzana, CA 91356.
[e] Mayo Medical Laboratories, 200 1st Street S.W., Rochester, MN 55905.
[f] Metpath Laboratories, 1 Malcolm Avenue, Teterboro, NJ 07608.
[g] Nichols Institute, 26441 Via DeAnza, San Juan Capistrano, CA 92675.
[h] Roche Clinical Laboratories, 69 First Avenue, Raritan, NJ 08869.
[i] Smith Kline Laboratories, 1075 First Avenue, King of Prussia, PA 19406.
[j] Ref. 50.
B, corticosterone.

trypsin bound to sepharose and remove the trypsin by centrifugation before carrying out the renin assay (5).

ACKNOWLEDGMENT

This work was supported, in part, by National Heart, Lung and Blood Institute grant HL-18323SCR.

REFERENCES

1. Laragh JH, Sealey JE. The renin–angiotensin–aldosterone hormonal system and regulation of sodium, potassium, and blood pressure homeostasis. In: Orloff J, Berliner RW, eds. *Handbook of physiology: renal physiology.* Baltimore: American Physiological Society, 1973;831–908.
2. Sealey JE, Buhler FR, Laragh JH, Vaughan ED Jr. The physiology of renin secretion in essential hypertension: estimation of renin secretion rate and renal plasma flow from peripheral and renal vein renin levels. *Am J Med* 1973;55:391–401.
3. Laragh JH, Baer L, Brunner HR, Buhler FR, Sealey JE, Vaughan ED Jr. Renin, angiotensin and aldosterone system in pathogenesis and management of hypertensive vascular disease. *Am J Med* 1972;52:633–652.
4. Sealey JE, Blumenfeld JD, Bell GM, Pecker MS, Sommers SC, Laragh JH. Presidential address. On the renal basis for essential hypertension: nephron heterogeneity with discordant renin secretion and sodium excretion. *J Hypertens* 1988;6:763–777.
5. Sealey JE, Atlas SA, Glorioso N, Manapat H, Laragh JH. Cyclical secretion of prorenin during the menstrual cycle: synchronization with luteinizing hormone and progesterone. *Proc Natl Acad Sci USA* 1985;82:8705–8709.

6. James GD, Sealey JE, Mueller F, Alderman M, Madhavan S, Laragh JH. Renin relationship to sex, race and age in a normotensive population. *J Hypertens* 1986;4(Suppl 5):S387–S389.
7. Laragh JH, Sealey JE. The renin–angiotensin–aldosterone system and the renal regulation of sodium, potassium, and blood pressure homeostasis. In: Windhager EE, ed. *Handbook of physiology.* New York: Oxford University Press, 1988; in press.
8. Sealey JE, Clark I, Bull MB, Laragh JH. Potassium balance and the control of renin secretion. *J Clin Invest* 1970;49:2119–2127.
9. Sealey JE, Gerten-Banes J, Laragh JH. The renin system: variations in man measured by radioimmunoassay or bioassay. *Kidney Inte* 1972;1:240–253.
10. Preibisz JJ, Sealey JE, Aceto RM, Laragh JH. Plasma renin activity measurements: an update. *Cardiovasc Rev Rep* 1982;5:787–804.
11. Müller FB, Sealey JE, Case DB, et al. The captopril test for identifying renovascular disease in hypertensive patients. *Am J Med* 1986;80:633–644.
12. Müller FB. Clinical evaluation and differential diagnosis of the patient with hypertension. In: Laragh JH, Brenner BM, eds. *Hypertension: pathophysiology, diagnosis and management.* New York: Raven Press, 1990; in press.
13. Biglieri E, Kater CE, Irony I. Adrenocortical forms of human hypertension. In: Laragh JH, Brenner BM, eds. *Hypertension: pathophysiology, diagnosis and management.* New York: Raven Press, 1990; in press.
14. Wilson M, Morganti AA, Zervoudakis I, et al. Blood pressure, the renin–aldosterone system and sex steroids throughout normal pregnancy. *Am J Med* 1980;68:97–104.
15. August P, Sealey JE. The renin–angiotensin system in normal and hypertensive pregnancy. In: Laragh JH, Brenner BM, eds. *Hypertension: pathophysiology, diagnosis and management.* New York: Raven Press, 1990; in press.
16. Poulsen K, Jorgensen J. An easy radioimmunological microassay of renin activity, concentration and substrate in human and animal plasma and tissues based on angiotensin I trapping by antibody. *J Clin Endocrinol Metab* 1974;39:816–825.
17. Sealey JE, Laragh JH. The renin–angiotensin–aldosterone system for regulation of sodium and potassium balance and arterial blood pressure. In: Laragh JH, Brenner BM, eds. *Hypertension: pathophysiology, diagnosis and management.* New York: Raven Press, 1990; in press.
18. Cannon PJ, Ames RP, Laragh JH. Relation between potassium balance and aldosterone secretion in normal subjects and in patients with hypertensive or renal tubular disease. *J Clin Invest* 1966;45:865–879.
19. Newton MA, Laragh JH. Effect of corticotropin on aldosterone excretion and plasma renin in normal subjects, in essential hypertension and in primary aldosteronism. *J Clin Endocrinol Metab* 1968;28:1006–1013.
20. Laragh JH. Atrial natriuretic hormone, the renin–aldosterone axis, and blood pressure–electrolyte homeostasis. *N Engl J Med* 1985;313:1330–1340.
21. Laragh JH, Sealey JE, Sommers SC. Patterns of adrenal secretion and urinary excretion of aldosterone and plasma renin activity in normal and hypertensive subjects. *Circ Res* 1966;18&19(Suppl I):158–174.
22. Bledsoe T, Liddle GW, Riondel A, Island DP, Bloomfield D, Sinclair-Smith B. Comparative fates of intravenously and orally administered aldosterone: evidence for extrahepatic formation of acidlabile conjugate in man. *J Clin Invest* 1966;45:264–269.
23. Cheville RA, Luetscher JA, Hancock EW, Dowdy AJ, Nokes GW. Distribution, conjugation and excretion of labeled aldosterone in congestive heart failure and in controls with normal circulation: development and testing of a model with an analog computer. *J Clin Invest* 1966;45:1302–1316.
24. Pasqualini JR. Aldosterone and tetrahydroaldosterone conjugation in human urine and plasma. In: Baulieu EE, Robel P, eds. *Aldosterone.* Oxford: Blackwell, 1964;131–143.
25. Laragh JH, Ulick S, Januszewicz W, Kelly WG, Lieberman S. Electrolyte metabolism and aldosterone secretion in benign and malignant hypertension. *Ann Intern Med* 1960;53:259–272.
26. Laragh JH, Sealey JE, Brunner HR. The control of aldosterone secretion in normal and hypertensive man: abnormal renin–aldosterone patterns in low renin hypertension. *Am J Med* 1972;53:649–663.
27. Wisgerhof M, Brown RD. Increased adrenal sensitivity to angiotensin II in low renin essential hypertension. *J Clin Invest* 1978;61:1456–1462.
28. Swales JD, Abramovici A, Beck F, Bing RF, Loudon M, Thurston H. Arterial wall renin. *J Hypertens* 1983;13(Suppl 1):17–22.
29. Newton MA, Sealey JE, Ledingham JGG, Laragh JH. High blood pressure and oral contraceptives. *Am J Obstet Gynecol* 1968;101:1037–1045.
30. Helmer OM, Griffith RS. The effect of the administration of estrogens on the renin-substrate (hypertensinogen) content of rat plasma. *Endocrinology* 1952;51:421–426.
31. Glorioso N, Atlas SA, Laragh JH, Jewelewicz R, Sealey JE. Prorenin in high concentrations in human ovarian follicular fluid. *Science* 1986;233:1422–1424.
32. Krakoff LR. Measurement of plasma renin substrate by radioimmunoassay of angiotensin I: concentration in syndromes associated with steroid excess. *J Clin Endocrinol Metab* 1973;37:110–117.
33. Ayers CR. Plasma renin activity and renin-substrate concentration in patients with liver disease. *Circ Res* 1967;20:594–598.
34. Sealey JE, White RP, Laragh JH, Case DB, Rubin AL. Studies of plasma aldosterone in anephric people: evidence for fundamental role of the renin system in maintaining aldosterone secretion. *J Clin Endocrinol Metab* 1978;47:52–60.
35. Sealey JE, Atlas SA, Laragh JH. Prorenin and other large molecular weight forms of renin. *Endocr Rev* 1980;1:365–391.
36. Skinner SL. Improved assay methods for renin concentration and activity in human plasma. Methods using selective denaturation of renin substrate. *Circ Res* 1967;20:391–402.
37. Brown JJ, Davies DL, Lever AF, Robertson JIS, Tree M. Estimation of renin in human plasma. *Biochem J* 1964;93:594–600.
38. Stockigt JR, Colling RD, Biglieri EG. Determination of plasma renin concentration by angiotensin I immunoassay. *Circ Res* 1971;28/29(Suppl II):175–189.
39. Haas E, Goldblatt H. Indirect assay of plasma renin. *Lancet* 1972;i:1330–1332.
40. Sealey JE. Measurement of the hormones of the renin system in hypertensive patients. *Clin Biochem* 1981;14:273–281.
41. Haber E, Koerner T, Page LB, Kliman B. Application of a radioimmunoassay for angiotensin I to the physiologic measurements of plasma renin activity in normal human subjects. *J Clin Endocrinol* 1969;29:1349–1355.
42. Sealey JE, Laragh JH. Radioimmunoassay of plasma renin activity. *Semin Nucl Med* 1975;5:189–202.
43. Sealey JE, Laragh JH. How to measure plasma renin activity and its applications. In: Berman DS, Mason DT, eds. *Clinical nuclear cardiology.* New York: Grune & Stratton, 1981;440–461.
44. Sealey JE, Buhler FR, Laragh JH, Manning EL, Brunner HR. Aldosterone excretion: physiologic variations in man measured by radioimmunoassay or double isotope dilution. *Circ Res* 1972;31:367–378.
45. Buhler FR, Laragh JH, Sealey JE, Brunner HR. Plasma aldosterone–renin interrelationships in various forms of essential hypertension: studies using a rapid assay of plasma aldosterone. *Am J Cardiol* 1973;32:554–561.
46. Nussberger J, Brunner DB, Waeber B, Brunner HR. True versus immunoreactive angiotensin II in human plasma. *Hypertension* 1985;70:I-1–I-7.
47. Sealey JE, Atlas SA, Laragh JH, Oza NB, Ryan JW. Activation of prorenin-like substance in human plasma by trypsin and by urinary kallikrein. *Hypertension* 1979;1:179–189.
48. Sealey JE, Laragh JH. The renin system in its pathophysiology in disease. In: Seldin DW, Giebisch G, eds. *The regulation of sodium and chloride balance.* New York: Raven Press, 1989; in press.
49. Laragh JH, Sealey JE, Buhler FR, Vaughan ED Jr, Brunner HR, Gavras H, Baer L. The renin axis and vasoconstriction volume analysis for understanding and treating renovascular and renal hypertension. *Am J Med* 1975;58:4–11.
50. Abraham GE. The use of diatomite microcolumns for the chromatographic separation of steroids prior to radioimmunoassay. *Pathol Biol* 1975;23:889–893.

Hypertension: Pathophysiology, Diagnosis, and Management, edited by J. H. Laragh and B. M. Brenner. Raven Press, Ltd., New York © 1990.

CHAPTER 91

Laboratory Evaluation of Autonomic Nervous System Function

Addison A. Taylor and Jerry R. Mitchell

Physiologic and Pharmacologic Evaluation of Autonomic Control of Cardiovascular Function, 1461
Tests of Baroreflex Control of the Circulation, 1461
Evaluation of Arterial Baroreflex Sensitivity, 1462
Evaluation of Cardiopulmonary Baroreflexes, 1465
Evaluation of Adrenergic Receptors, 1466
Norepinephrine as an Index of Sympathetic Nervous System Activity in Hypertension, 1467
Use of Autonomic Nervous System Tests in Clinical Practice, 1469
Protocol for Formal ANS Testing, 1469
Carotid Sinus Hypersensitivity, 1470
Hyperadrenergic Dysautonomias, 1471
Hypoadrenergic Dysautonomias, 1474
Clinical Recommendations, 1475
References, 1475

The autonomic nervous system participates in the development of, or serves a permissive role in the maintenance of, almost all forms of hypertension. Abnormalities in either peripheral or central components of the sympathetic nervous system have been clearly documented in experimental animals. Involvement of the autonomic nervous system has been demonstrated in genetic models of hypertension, such as the spontaneously hypertensive and the Dahl salt-sensitive rat, and in animal models of hypertension initially thought to result exclusively from excess production of vasoactive hormones, such as the DOCA–salt and renovascular hypertensive rat models. The evidence for participation of the sympathetic nervous system in the development or maintenance of hypertension in these models has been provided by sophisticated neurophysiologic and neuropharmacologic techniques, including the alteration of putative brain-stem pathways or the iontophoretic application of small amounts of agonist or antagonist chemicals into specific areas of the brain or spinal cord. These techniques are obviously not applicable to investigations of autonomic involvement in the cardiovascular maladaptations that accompany human hypertension. Nevertheless, these elegant studies in experimental models of hypertension have made it possible to draw inferences about the role of the autonomic nervous system in human hypertension using more indirect and less invasive methods of evaluation.

A diverse group of laboratory tests have been used over the past half-century to evaluate autonomic nervous system regulation of cardiovascular function in hypertensive humans. These tests have included (a) traditional neurophysiologic and pharmacologic perturbations of neuronal–cardiovascular reflex arcs, (b) measurements of the synthesis and/or release of neurotransmitter and neurohumoral substances that modulate cardiovascular function, (c) direct biochemical measurements of adrenergic receptor number and function, and, most recently, (d) direct measurements of sympathetic nerve activity in nerves to muscle and skin in humans.

This chapter will focus on those laboratory approaches that have been used in both clinical and clinical research settings to evaluate various aspects of autonomic nervous system function in hypertensive patients and will summarize the results of some of those investigations.

PHYSIOLOGIC AND PHARMACOLOGIC EVALUATION OF AUTONOMIC CONTROL OF CARDIOVASCULAR FUNCTION

Tests of Baroreflex Control of the Circulation

The central nervous system regulates all aspects of cardiac and peripheral vascular function through a series of highly differentiated, but closely integrated, cardiovascular reflex arcs. The principal efferent components of these reflex arcs are the sympathetic and parasympathetic divisions of the autonomic nervous system that connect the central nervous system with all segments of the arterial and venous circulation. Autonomic neuronal regulation of cardiovascular function is modulated by input from sensory nerves located in cardiovascular and other tissues, from the hypothalamus and higher cortical centers, and by local tissue factors. Maintenance of blood pressure—and, more importantly, maintenance of blood flow to vital organs—under a wide variety of diverse physiologic conditions such as standing, sleeping, emotional arousal, and exercise depends upon the integrity of afferent, central, and autonomic efferent neurons that comprise several key baroreflex arcs. A comprehensive review of the detailed neuroanatomy and neurophysiology of these reflex arcs is beyond the scope of this chapter. The reader is referred to several excellent reviews of this topic for more information than can be provided here (1–4).

The two baroreflex arcs most often evaluated in humans are the arterial (carotid and aortic) and the cardiopulmonary baroreceptor reflexes, usually referred to as high- and low-pressure baroreflexes, respectively. Studies in experimental animals indicate that the afferent limb of both arterial and cardiopulmonary baroreflex arcs can be activated by stimulating either mechanoreceptors or chemoreceptors located in the great vessels, lungs, and heart (see ref. 2 for review). It is presumed, but not proven, that most of the stimuli used by investigators to assess autonomic function in humans activate or deactivate mechanoreceptors rather than chemoreceptors.

Other baro- and chemoreflexes well described in experimental animals are undoubtedly also present in humans but are much less amenable to evaluation than are arterial and cardiopulmonary reflexes. For example, there is growing indirect evidence to support the existence of a renorenal reflex in humans similar to that documented in the one-kidney–one-clip model of renovascular hypertension (5). Activation of renal afferent nerves in experimental animals activates a renorenal reflex arc that increases blood pressure and heart rate while producing variable and species-dependent effects on renal vascular resistance and renal handling of sodium (6–9). More indirect evidence suggests that the renal nerves may participate in the maintenance of elevated blood pressure in some patients with essential hypertension (5,10,11). Additional studies will be needed to clarify the role of renorenal reflexes in the pathogenesis of renovascular hypertension and of other forms of human hypertension.

TABLE 1. *Some factors affecting cardiovascular responses to baroreflex activation*

1. The specific baroreflex activated.
2. The activating stimulus.
3. The influence of brain-stem, hypothalamic, and cortical modulation of the neurons involved in the reflex at the time of activation.
4. The responsiveness of the cardiovascular end-organ(s) involved in completing the reflex, including the state of specific adrenergic receptors that mediate the response.
5. Modulatory effects of circulating neurohumoral or vasoactive substances (such as catecholamines, arginine vasopressin, atrial peptides, angiotensin II, and prostaglandins) on baroreflexes.
6. Interaction of individual baroreflex arcs (such as cardiopulmonary) with arterial baroreflexes.

TABLE 2. *Tests of arterial baroreflex function*

Stimulus[a]	Response	References
Valsalva, phase IV (+)	BP ↑, HR ↓	17, 22, 25, 29
Deep breath	HR ↑ and ↓	142
Neck suction (+)	BP ↑, HR ↓	17, 19, 26, 36
Neck pressure (+)	BP ↑, HR ↑	17, 19, 26, 35
Passive tilt (−)	BP ↓ HR, NE, PRA ↑	24, 61, 143
Phenylephrine (+)	BP ↑, HR ↓	14, 15, 17, 19, 26, 27
Nitroglycerine (−)	BP ↓, HR ↑	17, 19, 26
Amyl nitrite (−)	BP ↓, HR ↑	14, 15
Nitroprusside (−)	BP ↓, HR ↑	144

[a] +, activates reflex; −, deactivates reflex.

The cardiovascular responses to baroreflex activation depend on several factors, which are outlined in Table 1. It is not possible to control closely each of these variables during human experimentation as can be done in the animal laboratory. The unrecognized influence of changes in one or more of these diverse factors during experiments conducted in humans may account for some of the reported discrepancies in the voluminous literature addressing this area of investigation.

In the absence of methods for measuring nerve traffic directly in afferent, central, and most sympathetic efferent neurons, alternative techniques for evaluating arterial and cardiopulmonary baroreflex function in the clinical setting have been devised. The tests most commonly used to study alterations in the function of these two baroreflex arcs in patients with cardiovascular diseases, including hypertension, are summarized in Table 2. References included in the table are not intended to be comprehensive but, instead, are meant to provide representative examples of studies in which each of these techniques have been employed.

Evaluation of Arterial Baroreflex Sensitivity

Control of Heart Rate

Many investigations of arterial baroreflex function in hypertensive patients have focused on the measurement of a change in heart rate (usually expressed as the increase in R–R interval) following an acute perturbation in blood pressure by a physiologic or pharmacologic stimulus. A wide range of stimuli have been employed to raise blood pressure acutely, including Valsalva maneuver, exposure of an extremity to cold (cold pressor test), and injection of pressor agents such as phenylephrine. Alternatively, to lower blood pressure acutely, passive head-up tilt or administration of vasodilators such as amyl nitrite, nitroprusside, or nitroglycerin have been utilized. Regardless of the stimulus, the magnitude of the change in systolic blood pressure from baseline is plotted against the change in pulse interval between the subsequent two cardiac cycles. The slope of the line determined by this relationship is taken as an index of baroreceptor sensitivity (12–15). The method for determining baroreceptor sensitivity after neck suction or neck pressure is the only major exception to this general approach. Since graded application of subatmospheric (neck suction) or superatmospheric (neck pressure) pressure to the neck produces a stimulus-dependent reduction (carotid baroreceptor activation) or augmentation (carotid baroreceptor deactivation) of both heart rate and arterial pressure, baroreceptor sensitivity is usually expressed as the change in R–R interval per mmHg suction or pressure applied to the neck when this technique is employed (16–18).

Apparent baroreflex sensitivity is influenced by the direction in which the blood pressure is changed by the acute stimulus. Baroreflex sensitivity is less when measured after administration of a vasodilator (such as nitroglycerin), which lowers blood pressure, than when measured after injection of a vasopressor (such as phenylephrine), which increases blood pressure (14,17,19,20). The diminished heart rate response to acute increases in blood pressure is mediated primarily by the parasympathetic (rather than the sympathetic) component of the autonomic nervous system (15,21). In contrast, the reflex increase in heart rate caused by a reduction in arterial pressure is presumably due to predominant activation of sympathetic efferents, with less influence from withdrawal of parasympathetic tone.

Several variables have been reported to influence the calculated arterial baroreflex sensitivity in controlling heart rate. These include age (12,19,22), the absolute level of blood pressure (12,22), and the state of the subject at the time of measurement. Apparent baroreflex sensitivity is lowest during sleep (19,23) but is highest during emotional arousal (19), when blood pressure and heart rate variations are at their minimum and maximum, respectively.

Choice of the stimulus has important effects on the observed cardiovascular response. For example, some maneuvers such as neck pressure and suction affect arterial baroreceptors almost exclusively, whereas others, such as passive tilt, may unload cardiopulmonary and arterial baroreflexes simultaneously (24). Using these techniques, numerous investigators have demonstrated diminished arterial baroreflex control of heart rate in humans with moderate to severe hypertension as well as in those with milder or "borderline" elevations in blood pressure (12,13, 15,18,19,25–28).

In the majority of studies, baroreflex control of heart rate has been calculated from direct intra-arterial recordings of blood pressure. An alternative noninvasive technique in which R–R interval on the electrocardiogram is plotted against arterial pressure measured in the finger by a "vascular unloading" technique has recently been compared with baroreceptor sensitivity determinations made in the same patient by invasive intra-arterial monitoring as described above (29). The correlation coefficient for the two techniques was 0.81 when phenylephrine was used and 0.90 after nitroglycerin administration. Although such noninvasive techniques need further validation under a wider variety of conditions, they may be sufficiently sensitive and reproducible to allow repetitive long-term evaluation of changes in baroreflex sensitivity in large numbers of patients under a wide variety of clinical and experimental conditions.

Control of Blood Pressure and Vascular Resistance

In addition to control of blood pressure, arterial baroreflexes are also involved in the regulation of regional vascular resistance and cardiac output, both important determinants of blood pressure. These latter baroreflex functions are less well studied (especially in hypertensive humans) than the reflex control of heart rate. Mancia et al. have studied baroreflex control of arterial pressure using a neck chamber device (26,30). Graded increments or decrements in carotid transmural pressure produced by this device cause reciprocal changes in blood pressure. The magnitude of this change is dependent upon the baseline blood pressure and on the direction of the blood pressure change induced by the alteration in transmural carotid pressure (Fig. 1). A decrease in carotid transmural pressure causes a much greater increase in mean arterial pressure in normotensive than in hypertensive subjects, whereas an increase in carotid transmural pressure produces the reverse effect in these two groups. The blood pressure responses of patients with moderate hypertension to changes in carotid transmural pressure are intermediate between those in normotensive and severely hypertensive subjects. These results suggest that the sensitivity of the carotid (and presumably aortic) baroreceptor for control of blood pressure is not significantly altered in hypertensive patients, although the threshold for receptor activation is reset.

Pressor responses to norepinephrine or phenylephrine

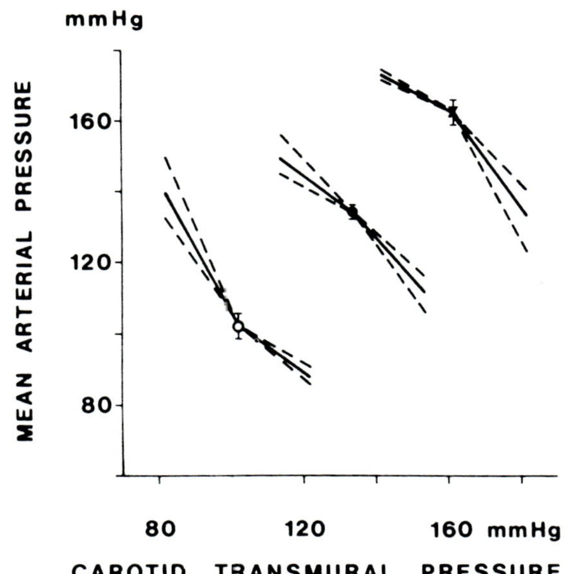

FIG. 1. Relation between absolute values of carotid transmural pressure and mean arterial pressure in normotensive, moderately hypertensive, and severely hypertensive subjects. In each group, the symbol represents the average mean arterial pressure prior to neck suction or pressure, the solid lines represent the average regression coefficients, and the dashed lines represent the standard errors of the regression coefficients. The absolute values of carotid transmural pressure were obtained by the difference between mean arterial pressure and neck tissue pressure during the steady-state part of the neck chamber stimulus. (From ref. 26, with permission.)

remain largely unchanged in humans (26,31) with established hypertension compared to normotensive controls, although other factors such as age, race, dietary sodium intake, and baroreceptor sensitivity can affect this response independent of blood pressure (31,32). Furthermore, the slope of the linear relationship between diastolic blood pressure and muscle sympathetic nerve traffic is similar in normotensive and hypertensive humans (33). However, during the development of hypertension, augmentation of the pressor responses to bilateral carotid occlusion in conscious dogs has been observed that is not maintained as the hypertension becomes established (34). Changes in pressor responses during the development of hypertension have not yet been examined in humans.

Control of Cardiac Output

During the development of perinephritic hypertension in the conscious dog (34), an increase in cardiac output associated with an increase in heart rate, arterial pressure, and total peripheral resistance in response to bilateral carotid occlusion has been observed that is not sustained after the hypertension becomes established for several weeks.

Baroreflex control of cardiac output has been evaluated to only a limited extent in hypertensive humans. Activation of carotid baroreceptors by application of neck suction to patients with established hypertension resulted in reflex hypotension which was accompanied by a reduction in both cardiac output and peripheral vascular resistance (30). The change in cardiac output was due primarily to a reduction in heart rate, since stroke volume did not change significantly. Conversely, increases in mean arterial pressure produced by deactivation of carotid baroreceptors was due almost exclusively to an increase in peripheral resistance, since neither heart rate nor cardiac output changed significantly. Unfortunately, the responses of normotensive subjects to these maneuvers were not investigated.

Interaction of Arterial and Cardiopulmonary Baroreceptors

Only a few studies have examined the interactions between cardiopulmonary and arterial baroreflex in humans. Victor and Mark (35) have demonstrated that nonhypotensive lower-body negative pressure to unload cardiopulmonary baroreceptors selectively augments carotid baroreflex control of forearm vascular resistance induced by neck pressure in normotensive subjects. Using a different experimental approach, Parati et al. (36) reported that immersion of normal subjects in water to increase right atrial pressure and stimulate cardiopulmonary baroreceptors reduced the degree of reflex bradycardia produced by carotid baroreceptor stimulation with neck suction. The results of this latter study are difficult to interpret, however, since immersion alone caused bradycardia and a reduction in mean arterial pressure, either of which could have modified the heart rate response to carotid baroreceptor stimulation.

These studies underscore the significant effect that stimulus strength can have on hemodynamic response to baroreflex activation in humans. In the studies described by Victor and Mark (35), application of +20 mmHg pressure to the neck of normotensive volunteers raised mean arterial pressure but had no significant effect on forearm vascular resistance. If the neck pressure was increased to +30 mmHg, a significant rise in arterial pressure, heart rate, and forearm vascular resistance occurred. Conversely, application of −10 mmHg negative pressure to the lower-body negative pressure decreased forearm blood flow but had no effect on heart rate or arterial pressure, whereas lower-body negative pressure (LBNP) at −40 mmHg or greater, a stimulus that affects high- as well as low-pressure baroreceptors, decreased arterial pressure and increased heart rate as it simultaneously increased forearm vascular resistance (37).

Modulation of Arterial Baroreflexes by Humoral Substances

Studies in animal models and in humans suggest that a variety of vasoactive humoral substances such as vasopressin, angiotensin, prostaglandins, and atrial natriuretic peptide (ANP) may modulate autonomic neural control of the circulation. The subsequent brief review is confined to a discussion of vasopressin and ANP, since these two vasoactive hormones have been shown to influence arterial baroreflex function under certain experimental circumstances.

The role of arginine vasopressin (AVP) in the genesis or maintenance of experimental and human hypertension is reviewed elsewhere (see ref. 38). It is important to recognize that AVP may influence autonomic nervous system evaluation in hypertensive patients if conditions that promote or suppress AVP secretion are not carefully controlled. Several lines of evidence are consistent with the view that AVP facilitates arterial and cardiopulmonary baroreflexes. AVP blunts its own direct pressor effect by reflex inhibition of sympathetic nerve activity, with a consequent reduction in heart rate, cardiac output, and peripheral resistance in both humans and other animals (38,39). Infusion of AVP in doses that produce maximal antidiuretic effect but little or no increase in arterial pressure when the sympathetic nervous system is intact causes an exaggerated pressor effect in animals with sinoaortic denervation and in patients with autonomic failure (38,40). In addition, blunted baroreceptor reflexes in rats with diabetes insipidus are restored by AVP infusion. Studies in experimental animals have suggested that several neuronal sites are affected by AVP, including aortic baroreceptor nerves (41,42) and the area postrema (43); other sites are also affected by AVP, including those in the brain that still need to be clearly defined (38,44). The results of a recent study suggest that part of this effect is mediated by a specific AVP vascular receptor. The exaggerated depressor effect of veratrum alkaloids that accompanied infusion of hypertonic saline to dogs with or without sinoaortic denervation was prevented by pretreatment with an AVP vascular receptor antagonist as well as by lesion of the area postrema (43). AVP has been shown to cause forearm vasodilation (41) and to inhibit muscle sympathetic nerve activity in normotensive humans by an action not due to ganglionic blockade (39). The contribution of mildly elevated plasma antidiuretic hormone (ADH) concentrations [reported in many patients with hypertension (38,45)] to abnormal autonomic control of the circulation in hypertensive patients requires further clarification.

The myriad actions of ANP, including its interactions with the autonomic nervous system, has recently been reviewed (see ref. 46). Certain specific investigations are germane to the issue of ANP modulation of arterial and cardiopulmonary baroreceptor function. The possibility that ANP may inhibit cardiac and renal sympathetic nerve activity by stimulation of cardiac chemoreceptors attached to vagal afferent nerves is suggested by the results of studies in both experimental animals (47) and humans (48). Infusion of α-human ANP in normotensive subjects at a dose that decreased central venous pressure but had no other hemodynamic or humoral effects blunted reflex tachycardia induced by neck pressure but did not blunt the reflex bradycardia produced by neck suction. Other neuronal sites of action of ANP have also been implicated; ANP has been reported to block vasopressin secretion in isolated perfused rat neurohypophyses (49) and to blunt the increase in plasma AVP concentrations produced by hemorrhage, dehydration, or hypotension (50,51). As a corollary, progressive declines in plasma concentrations of immunoreactive ANP accompanied sympathetic activation produced by graded application of neck pressure to deactivate carotid baroreflexes; both ANP and sympathetic responses were prevented by pretreatment with phentolamine and propranolol (52). These provocative results should stimulate further investigation of the interaction between ANP and the autonomic nervous system in patients with hypertension.

Evaluation of Cardiopulmonary Baroreflexes

Cardiopulmonary baroreflexes have been implicated in the control of (a) regional vascular resistance, renin secretion, and sodium excretion by the kidney and (b) vasopressin secretion by the posterior pituitary. Elucidation of the role of cardiac reflexes in regulating each of these processes is of interest because of their participation in one or more forms of experimental and human hypertension (2). Some of the diverse methods used to activate or deactivate cardiopulmonary baroreflexes are listed in Table 3.

The application of negative pressure to the lower extremities [lower-body negative pressure (LBNP)] has been used extensively to investigate the function of these receptors in both physiologic and pathologic states. Graded reductions in central venous and right atrial pressure with increasingly negative lower-body pressure, head-up tilt, or thigh-cuff inflation results in unloading of cardiopulmonary mechanoreceptors, with consequent reflex increases in sympathetic activity determined either directly by increased number and amplitude of sympathetic bursts in muscle branches of the median nerve (53) or indirectly by increases in forearm vascular resistance (FVR) using venous occlusion plethysmographic methods (30,35,54). This reflex forearm vasoconstriction is accompanied by an increase in plasma norepinephrine, the magnitude of which roughly parallels the change in FVR (54–57). The rise in plasma renin activity (PRA) and in plasma aldosterone that occurs following LBNP-induced reflex sympathetic activation is not only related to the stimulus magnitude but is also delayed for 20 min or longer following the initiation of lower-body suction (54,58–61); those studies that have not extended the LBNP or their measurements of plasma renin activity beyond 5–10 min have not consistently observed an increase in PRA with this stimulus (62).

The slopes of the regression line for changes in central venous pressure versus changes in forearm vascular resistance during application of graded LBNP were similar in individuals that were normotensive or hypertensive with cardiac left ventricular hypertrophy. The changes in FVR were inversely related to the changes in central venous pressure in both groups. Propranolol, which has been reported to selectively reduce the firing rate of left ventricular mechanoreceptors (63,64), blunted the LBNP-induced reflex forearm vasoconstriction in hypertensive, but not normotensive, subjects. In contrast, propranolol did not attenuate the vasoconstrictor response to hand-grip or to a cold pressor challenge (65,66).

The reflex vasoconstriction and neurohumoral changes that accompany the application of LBNP persist for at least 20 min; the magnitude of the response is related to the intensity of the LBNP stimulus. The increase in plasma norepinephrine following LBNP was maximal after 3 min but persisted for the entire 20 min over which the stimulus was applied. PRA and plasma aldosterone, however, were highest at the 20-min sampling time (54), indicating a time difference in these two responses to this low-pressure baroreceptor stimulus.

TABLE 3. *Tests of cardiopulmonary baroreflex function*

Stimulus[a]	Response	References
Lower-body negative pressure (−)	CVP, MAP ↓ FVR, HR, NE, PRA ↑	35, 37, 54, 55, 59, 62, 65, 145
Lower-body positive pressure (+)		143
Thigh-cuff inflation (−)	RAP ↓, PRA ↑	60, 143, 146
Passive leg raise (+)	CVP ↑ NE, FVR ↓	55, 59
Water immersion (+)	MAP, HR, FVR ↓	36
Volume expansion (+)	FVR ↓	147
Passive tilt (−)	FVR, HR, NE, PRA ↑	24, 58, 143

[a] +, activates reflex; −, deactivates reflex.

Evaluation of Adrenergic Receptors

Major advances have occurred in the molecular biology and biochemistry of receptor identification and purification and in the availability of receptor-specific agonist and antagonist radioligands in the past decade. Coupling these new techniques with classic pharmacologic methods for determining receptor affinity for agonists and antagonists has made it possible to study alterations in adrenergic receptor number and affinity in specific tissues of experimental animal models of hypertension. Based on these sophisticated methods, subtypes of both α- and β-adrenergic receptors have been identified in neural and vascular tissues (67,68). Activation of α_1-adrenergic receptors, located on the vascular side of the sympathetic nerve synaptic cleft, results in vasoconstriction. In contrast, α_2-adrenergic receptors are located on the prejunctional and postjunctional sides of the synaptic cleft. Postjunctional α_2-receptors are actually located extrasynaptically and are more responsive to circulating norepinephrine than are postjunctional α_1-receptors, although both mediate vascular constriction. Activation of prejunctional α_2-adrenergic receptors on sympathetic nerve terminals in the periphery or on noradrenergic neurons in the brain inhibits subsequent release of norepinephrine from the nerve. Receptors for other substances such as angiotensin II, dopamine, and prostaglandins also modulate release of norepinephrine from noradrenergic sympathetic neurons. Beta$_1$-adrenergic receptors are located primarily in the heart; their activation augments cardiac chronotropy and inotropy. Alpha$_2$-adrenergic receptors are found in many organs of the body, including the kidney, pancreas, and skeletal muscle. Those located on the walls of peripheral blood vessels mediate vasodilation.

Alpha-Adrenergic Receptors

Both pharmacologic and biochemical methods have been employed to evaluate the role of α-adrenergic receptors in hypertension. The state of α-adrenergic responsiveness in various types of human hypertension has been inferred from measurements of change in blood pressure or vascular resistance after intravenous or intra-arterial administration of α-adrenergic agonists or antagonists to hypertensive patients, as compared to the responses in normotensive subjects studied under similar conditions. Interpretation of the results from these studies is complicated by the possibility that structural changes in the vessel wall resulting from hypertension account for at least part of the observed response (69–71). Regardless of these potential pitfalls, most investigations have addressed the question of whether the abnormal autonomic neural control of the circulation in hypertension is mediated in part by α-adrenergic receptor supersensitivity or is due entirely to augmented sympathetic neural drive.

The results of sophisticated laboratory studies defining receptor type, distribution, and function have been applied to the study of hypertension in humans in two ways. The first involves classic pharmacologic methods for evaluating receptor–effector function; this approach provides much of the scientific rationale for the choice of a particular antihypertensive drug. For example, it was empirically noted many years ago that hypertensive patients became tolerant to nonselective α-adrenergic blockers such as phentolamine. The discovery that nonselective α-adrenergic antagonists increase release of norepinephrine from sympathetic nerve terminals by antagonizing the inhibitory α_2-adrenergic receptor on sympathetic nerve terminals provided a rational basis for this observation and for the development and therapeutic use of antagonists that are relatively selective for the α_1-adrenergic receptor. The development of relatively selective α_2-adrenergic (yohimbine) and α_1-adrenergic (prazosin, terazosin, and doxazosin) receptor antagonists and α_2-receptor partial agonists (clonidine) provided tools to study the contributions of specific α-adrenergic receptor subtypes to the control of blood pressure (72,73) and to renin secretion (74) and regional vascular sympathetic tone (74–77). Relatively selective β_1-adrenergic receptor antagonists have been available for many years (metoprolol, atenolol), but only recently has the development of agents relatively specific for β_2-adrenergic receptors become available for studies in humans. The studies with these agents have provided important practical therapeutic information that is useful in the treatment of hypertensive patients. However, conclusions about the role of α- or β-adrenergic receptors in the development or maintenance of hypertension based on hemodynamic responses to these agents should be interpreted with caution, since the actions of these drugs may extend beyond their effect on the adrenergic nervous system. A second approach to the study of adrenergic receptor function is the direct assessment of both the number and the affinity of these receptors on the tissues involved in the control of blood pressure. These types of studies in human hypertension have been limited by the inability to sample cardiovascular tissues directly, repetitively, and noninvasively. Alternatively, adrenergic receptors on the surface of the formed elements of blood have been studied with the assumption that changes in these receptors reflect changes in similar types of receptors located on sympathetic nerves or vascular tissues. Beta$_2$-receptors have been identified on human polymorphonuclear leukocytes and lymphocytes, and α_2-adrenergic receptors have been found on human platelets, but tissues containing β_1- and α_1-adrenergic receptors are not readily accessible (78). In fact, a recent report in which human right atrial β_1- and β_2-receptor number and function were compared with lymphocyte β_2-receptors suggests that lymphocyte β_2-adrenoceptors may not accurately reflect alterations in β_1-adrenoceptors in solid tissues (79).

Possible explanations for the exaggerated pressor responses of hypertensive patients to α-adrenergic agonists (17,80,81) have been sought by examination of platelet α_2-adrenergic receptors. Although it is assumed that the function of these platelet receptors reflects that of vascular and neuronal α_2-receptors, this has not been tested experimentally. Indirect evidence that these receptors may be abnormal in hypertensive patients arose from an early report (82) of exaggerated adhesiveness and catecholamine-induced aggregation of platelets in hypertensive, as compared to normotensive, persons. Such abnormalities could be due to a higher receptor density per platelet, to an increased affinity of each receptor for agonist, or to an exaggerated effector response to receptor activation. With few exceptions (83), no differences have been noted in the number of platelet α_2-adrenergic receptors among hypertensive and normotensive subjects (84–86), nor were differences found in the affinity of these receptors for agonists or antagonists (84,86). Platelet α_2-adrenergic receptors from hypertensive patients, however, were desensitized more slowly by physiologic concentrations of epinephrine than were those from normotensive subjects (84). Additional studies will be needed to determine whether these subtle abnormalities in platelet α_2-adrenergic receptor function have pathophysiologic significance in hypertensives and whether they reflect changes in α_2-receptors located on sympathetic nerve terminals.

Beta-Adrenergic Receptors

A decrease in beta-adrenergic receptor sensitivity (isoproterenol-induced cardiac chronotropic responses) with increasing age and blood pressure has been noted in some studies (87). Inferences about myocardial and vascular beta-adrenergic receptor function in human hypertension have been made based on evaluation of beta-adrenergic receptors on human leukocytes. Although no difference in [^{3}H]dihydroalprenolol binding to lymphocytes was noted in one study of hypertensive patients (88), the methods used may not have detected the leukocyte beta-adrenergic receptor abnormalities described by Feldman et al. (49). They reported diminished lymphocyte β_2-adrenergic receptor affinity for isoproterenol, with reduced binding sites in the high-affinity state associated with diminished adenyl cyclase activity. They have recently reported that reduced lymphocyte β_2-adrenoceptor responsiveness in hypertensive patients is corrected by severe reductions in dietary sodium intake (89). These provocative findings will require corroboration by others. Indeed, the role of altered adrenergic receptor function in the pathophysiology of human hypertension remains unclear at this time.

Norepinephrine as an Index of Sympathetic Nervous System Activity in Hypertension

Since von Euler's demonstration over 40 years ago that norepinephrine was the principal neurotransmitter of the sympathetic nervous system, the potential value of an accurate and sensitive biochemical index of sympathetic nerve activity for the study of cardiovascular disease has been apparent. Studies of catecholamines in animals *in vivo* and *in vitro* have provided invaluable basic information about the electrophysiologic and biochemical processes involved in norepinephrine synthesis and release from noradrenergic neurons and the adrenal medulla and about intraneuronal and extraneuronal metabolism of norepinephrine in tissues and organs throughout the body. The intricacies of using norepinephrine turnover to assess sympathetic nervous system activity in humans has been elegantly reviewed recently (90). Although the general concepts as they pertain to the evaluation of sympathetic involvement in hypertension will be highlighted here, this and other reviews (90–94) should be consulted for more specific details.

Measurements of Urinary Norepinephrine and Metabolites

Increased urinary excretion of norepinephrine has been reported in a relatively small number (10–15%) of patients with essential hypertension (95–97). The inclusion of the principal *O*-methylated and/or deaminated metabolites of norepinephrine, normetanephrine, dihydroxyphenylethylene glycol, dihydroxymandelic acid, 3-methoxy-4-hydroxyphenylglycol, and vanillylmandelic acid in these urinary measurements has not provided significantly greater sensitivity in detecting hypertensive patients (98) with increased sympathetic nervous system activity. These observations speak less to a lack of involvement of the sympathetic nervous system in the pathogenesis of hypertension than they do to the limitations of using urinary norepinephrine or metabolite determinations as a general integrated index of sympathetic neural firing rate as discussed below.

Measurements of Plasma Norepinephrine

Measurements of norepinephrine in peripheral venous plasma have provided a more dynamic, but still imprecise, index of sympathetic neuronal activity in humans than have urinary catecholamine measurements. Replacement of cumbersome and relatively insensitive fluorometric or double isotope dilution methods for measuring norepinephrine in plasma by either sensitive radioenzymatic methods or techniques that combine the specificity of high-pressure liquid chromatographic separation with the sensitivity of electrochemical detection has made it possible to compare changes in venous plasma norepinephrine with hemodynamic and electroneurographic indices of sympathetic nervous system activation in both normotensive and hypertensive subjects.

The popularity of using plasma norepinephrine to compare sympathetic nervous system activation in normotensive and hypertensive patients is reflected in the large number of studies available for review by Goldstein in 1981 (99). Plasma norepinephrine concentrations in hypertensive patients were higher than those in normotensive controls in 88% of the studies, although this difference achieved statistical significance in only 40% of the studies. Age was likely an important confounding but frequently uncontrolled variable in these studies since, in an additional study, the expected age-related increase in plasma norepinephrine was observed in normotensive subjects but not in hypertensive ones (100). The failure of plasma norepinephrine values to increase with age was due to significantly higher values in hypertensive patients less than 40 years old as compared to their age-related normotensive controls, a difference that was not present in these two groups of subjects over age 40. The results of a study using radiotracer methods for measuring the spillover of norepinephrine from specific organs into plasma suggests that this exaggerated release of norepinephrine into plasma of younger hypertensives is due, in part, to increased renal (42%) and cardiac (4%) norepinephrine spillover (92).

There are several theoretical and practical limitations to the use of urinary or plasma norepinephrine measurements as accurate indices of overall sympathetic nervous system activity. These limitations are best appreciated by identifying the multiple factors that influence the amount of norepinephrine that ultimately enters the circulation after release from the sympathetic neuron. A part of the norepinephrine released into the synaptic cleft is taken back into the nerve (reuptake 1), where it is subject to intraneuronal metabolism (primarily monoamine oxidase), and into non-neuronal cells (reuptake 2), where it is subject to metabolism by *O*-methylation. The quantity of norepinephrine that ultimately enters the circulation from an organ is also dependent, in part, on (a) the width of the synaptic cleft and (b) the capillary permeability to norepinephrine. Other factors influencing the contribution of each organ to the circulating pool of norepinephrine include the density of sympathetic innervation, the firing rates of these sympathetic nerves, the size of the organ, the organ's capacity for norepinephrine metabolism, and the organ's blood flow. The adrenal medulla also contributes a small quantity of norepinephrine, variably estimated as 2–7.5% (101,102), to the circulating pool by direct secretion rather than by organ spillover. Clearance of norepinephrine from the plasma is dependent primarily on direct excretion by the kidney and on metabolism by organs such as the liver to biologically inactive products.

Another limitation to the use of norepinephrine as an index of overall sympathetic activity is its inability to evaluate a highly differentiated neuronal system that may increase firing rates in some organs and decrease them in others in response to a particular stimulus. For example, mental stress is accompanied by an increase in both heart rate and blood pressure but a reduction in systemic vascular resistance and hence does not invariably produce changes in venous plasma norepinephrine (103,104). Thus, increased norepinephrine spillover due to exaggerated sympathetic stimulation of selected organs such as the brain, heart, or kidneys may be obscured by greater contributions to the circulating norepinephrine pool from organs in which sympathetic activity remains normal or is reduced (101,105,106). The site from which the plasma sample is drawn may also be a factor. Peripheral venous blood obtained from the antecubital fossa may, under certain circumstances, be more reflective of forearm release and metabolism of norepinephrine than it is of the average circulating concentration of norepinephrine throughout the body (104,107). Although urinary catecholamines provide a more integrated index of sympathetic activity over time than do single plasma norepinephrine determinations, their specificity is diminished by (a) a variable contribution to the total catecholamine pool of epinephrine metabolites, (b) variability in intraneuronal versus extraneuronal metabolism of norepinephrine by various organs, and (c) inability of norepinephrine formed in certain organs such as the brain to mix freely with the catecholamine pool available for excretion.

Despite these limitations, measurements of peripheral venous plasma norepinephrine provide a useful but indirect clinical index of overall sympathetic nervous system activity in many circumstances. Norepinephrine concentrations in peripheral venous plasma have been reported to change in parallel with increases in forearm vascular resistance after stimulation or deactivation of low-pressure baroreceptors (55,59) and in parallel with muscle sympathetic nerve activity both at rest and during isometric hand-grip exercise (108,109). Concentrations of this neurotransmitter in venous plasma increase with Valsalva maneuver, standing, passive tilt, and stimulation by cold, pain, mental stress, caffeine, cigarette smoking, vasodilators, and isometric exercise (107,110–114) and are reduced by drugs (clonidine) or diseases (autonomic failure) in which sympathetic efferent activity is decreased (115,116).

Measurement of Cerebrospinal Fluid Norepinephrine

A close correlation between cerebrospinal fluid (CSF) and plasma norepinephrine in the same individual (117–119), failure of norepinephrine from the periphery to enter the CSF in appreciable concentrations or of norepinephrine in the central nervous system to enter the periphery unmetabolized because of the blood–brain barrier (120), and reports of higher CSF norepinephrine concentrations in hypertensive than in normotensive subjects (117–119,121–124) all suggest that CSF norepinephrine concentrations might serve as a useful index of central noradrenergic neurotransmission. The recent demonstration of a parallel decrease in plasma and CSF norepinephrine after peripheral ganglionic blockade with trimethaphan (which does not cross the blood–brain barrier), along with the absence of a reflex increase in CSF norepinephrine in ganglion-blocked dogs made hypotensive with trimethaphan (125), is inconsistent with this view and suggests that a more precise localization of the source of norepinephrine in the CSF is needed.

Norepinephrine Turnover

Application of radiotracer methods to the study of sympathetic nervous system function in cardiovascular diseases has circumvented some, but not all, of the limitations imposed by plasma or urinary norepinephrine determinations. The primary advantage of these methods, based on isotope dilution principles, is that they allow separate estimates of (a) spillover of norepinephrine into plasma and (b) metabolic clearance of norepinephrine from plasma (90,126–128), under steady-state conditions. Total norepinephrine (NE) spillover rate is calculated from the ratio of the infusion rate of ^{3}H-NE divided by the specific radioactivity of ^{3}H-NE in plasma. NE plasma clearance is estimated by the ratio of ^{3}H-NE infusion rate and the plasma ^{3}H-NE concentration. Assumptions upon which these calculations are based include the following: (a) infusion of ^{3}H-NE to constant specific radioactivity; (b) steady-state concentrations of endogenous plasma NE; (c) all unlabeled endogenous and infused radioactive NE are well mixed in a central pool; (d) plasma samples obtained for determination of NE radioactivity and mass accurately reflect the central NE pool; and (e) any re-release of ^{3}H-NE from sympathetic nerves is negligible in comparison with the rate of infusion of ^{3}H-NE (94). The same methods can be applied to the estimation of organ-specific contributions to the plasma NE pool if the NE arteriovenous difference, the fractional extraction of NE, and the blood flow of the organ can be determined (129).

Findings in normal healthy subjects evaluated using these methods demonstrate the following: (a) The spillover rate from all organs into plasma is only about 22% of the total NE released based on measurements of radiolabeled NE metabolites in urine (127); (b) there is spillover of NE into plasma from all organs except the gut and liver; (c) whether there is net NE spillover from the lung (which, along with the liver, is one of the primary sites of NE removal from the circulation) is disputed; (d) the major sources of release of NE into the plasma are the kidneys (22%) and skeletal muscle (20%), with the heart and the skin each contributing 5% or less; (e) calculations of NE spillover rates tend to be influenced by the site from which the samples are obtained.

Studies of hypertensive patients using radiotracer methods have reported an exaggerated total spillover of NE into plasma in only a limited number of these patients, primarily those who are young (<40 years old) and have other evidence of hyperkinetic circulation (90,93,126). There have been no reported differences in the plasma clearance of NE in these hypertensive patients compared to normotensive subjects, but abnormalities in reuptake have been noted in a few. The kidneys and heart were identified as the source for 46% of the increased spillover of NE into plasma in these young hypertensives, whereas 54% of the increase was unaccounted for by NE spillover from any of the other organs studied (92). Defective neuronal NE reuptake does not appear to account for these observations (90). Although these findings are consistent with other, more indirect indices of increased renal and cardiac sympathetic activity in some young hypertensive patients (130,131), their precise contributions to the pathophysiology of the hypertension of these patients remains to be determined.

USE OF AUTONOMIC NERVOUS SYSTEM TESTS IN CLINICAL PRACTICE

The above investigations of autonomic nervous system (ANS) function in hypertensive patients have been conducted primarily in the research setting. Not only have they contributed to an understanding of the pathophysiology of human hypertension, but they also have provided direction and focus to the development of new drugs for the treatment of this disorder. In the clinical setting, therapeutic response to antihypertensive agents with defined actions usually takes precedent over formal laboratory evaluation of ANS function in most hypertensive patients. However, our laboratory has found that one hypertensive population in whom ANS testing has been clinically helpful is the group of patients with hypertension–hypotension syndromes who present with clear clinical evidence of dysautonomias (72,132,133) (Table 4). These patients not only have a history of orthostatic syncope (or near-syncope), palpitations, or sensation of rapid heart beat but also objectively demonstrate one or more of the following findings during routine examination: supine hypertension, orthostatic hypotension, orthostatic tachycardia, bradycardia or hypotension with carotid massage, or evidence of peripheral vasospasm.

Protocol for Formal ANS Testing

We have studied 354 patients with dysautonomias, including 32 patients with idiopathic orthostatic hypotension, 25 patients with evidence of multiple system atrophy (Shy–Drager syndrome), 26 patients with carotid sinus hypersensitivity of either the cardioinhibitory or vasodepressor type (or both), 102 patients with mitral valve prolapse and symptoms of hyperadrenergic dysautonomia, and 53 patients with symptoms of hyperadrenergic dysautonomia but no evidence of mitral valve prolapse. In 48 patients the pattern of cardiovascular responses was not sufficiently distinct to allow identification of the underlying autonomic abnormality. Normal volunteers (26) and asymptomatic patients with mitral valve prolapse by echocardiogram (12) also have been studied for comparison with symptomatic patients (132).

The majority of patients and control subjects have been evaluated by a standardized protocol that includes measurement of cardiovascular (heart rate and intra-arterial blood pressure) responses to the following maneuvers: (a) quantitative Valsalva maneuver; (b) slow, deep breathing; (c) bilateral sequential carotid sinus massage; (d) standing for 5–15 min; (e) incremental phenylephrine or tyramine injection until systolic blood pressure increases 25–30 mmHg above baseline values; and (f) incremental isoproterenol injections until heart rate increases 25–30 beats/min. In addition, plasma renin activity and plasma aldosterone have been measured after 45–60 min in the supine position, and plasma NE and epinephrine have been measured by high-performance liquid chromatography with electrochemical detection after 30 min of supine rest and

TABLE 4. *Recommendations for patient selection for ANS testing*

Clinical condition	Recommendation
Carotid sinus hypersensitivity	Test all patients
Hyperadrenergic dysautonomias (e.g., MVP syndrome)	Test only symptomatic patients without objective evidence of dysautonomia at bedside
Hypoadrenergic dysautonomias (multiple-systems atrophy, diabetes, etc.)	Test for research purposes only (see Table 5 for rationale)

again after 5 min of quiet standing. The details of these procedures have been described previously (133).

Carotid Sinus Hypersensitivity

Patients with carotid sinus hypersensitivity (CSH) provide a dramatic clinical example of the devastating hemodynamic consequences of pathologically supersensitive carotid baroreflexes (134,135). These patients present with recurrent episodes of syncope, frequently produced by sudden changes in head position. In approximately 20% of the 26 individuals we have studied, either a head or neck tumor had occurred or irradiation to the head and neck for such a tumor had been given. Two individuals had sustained traumatic injury to the neck many years before symptoms developed. No specific event could be identified in the other patients, although evidence of atherosclerotic cardiovascular disease was present in most. All patients met the prevailing criteria for diagnosis of carotid sinus hypersensitivity by demonstrating a fall in systolic blood pressure of (a) ≥50 mmHg but no symptoms or (b) ≥30 mmHg associated with symptoms of near-syncope or syncope after carotid sinus massage (135). A modest to very dramatic fall in heart rate accompanied the fall in blood pressure produced by carotid sinus massage in most of these patients (see Fig. 2A). It is important to identify the existence of a vasodepressor component in CSH, since effective therapeutic modalities in mixed cardioinhibitory–vasodepressor CSH or in pure vasodepressor CSH depend on surgical interruption of either the afferent or efferent components of the carotid baroreflex, whereas a pacemaker is adequate treatment if only the cardioinhibitory type of CSH is present. In our experience it is necessary to test for the presence of a vasodepressor component by repeating the carotid sinus massage during cardiac pacing (Fig. 2C), since atropine alone is frequently not sufficient to prevent the decrease in heart rate during carotid sinus massage (Fig. 2B) in patients with mixed cardioinhibitory–vasodepressor syndrome (134). Figure 2 illustrates the changes in heart rate and blood pressure in a patient with carotid sinus hypersensitivity produced by right neck massage for 10 sec before (Fig. 2A) and after (Fig. 2B) atropine and again during continuous cardiac pacing (Fig. 2C). The persistent effect of right glossopharyngeal nerve root section 12 months previously to block the hypotensive response to right carotid sinus massage (Fig. 2D), but not left carotid sinus massage (not shown), is also illustrated. Stripping of

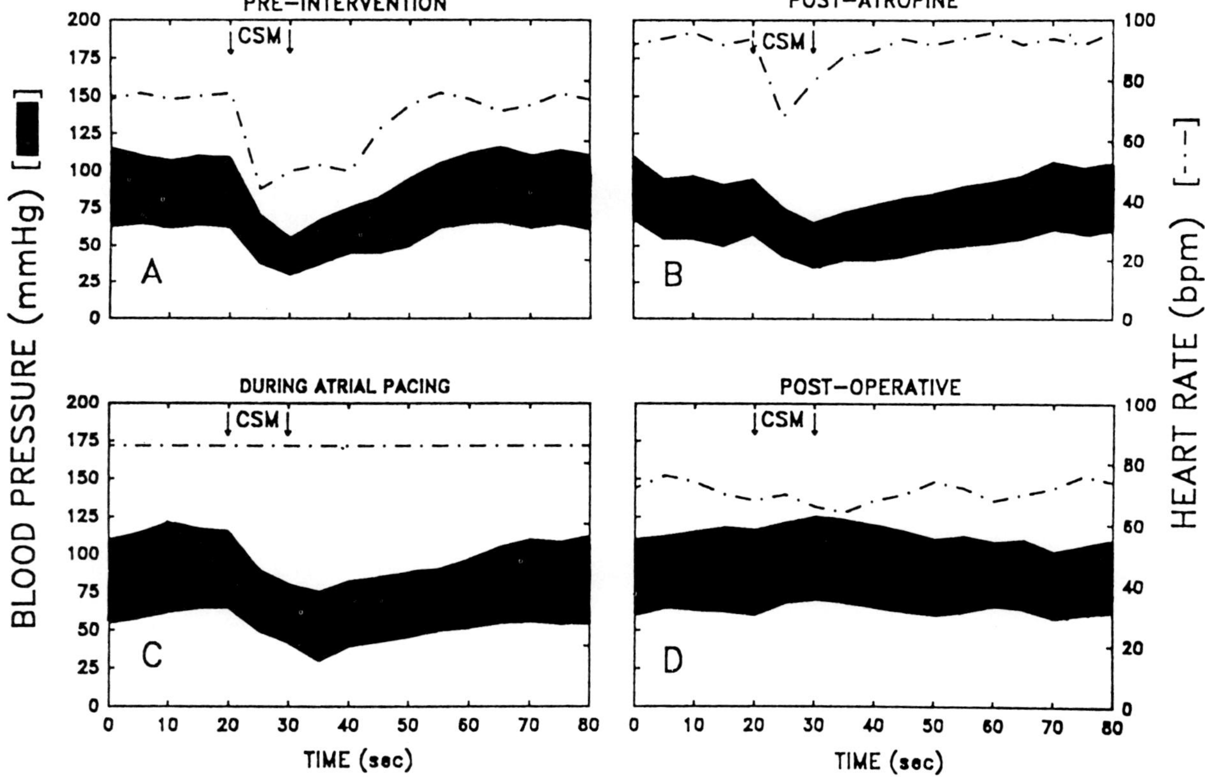

FIG. 2. Effect of right carotid sinus massage (CSM) on intra-arterial pressure (*solid line*) and heart rate (dashed line) in a patient with mixed cardioinhibitory–vasodepressor carotid sinus hypersensitivity. Note that 1 mg of intravenous atropine (**B**) only partly blunts the decrease in heart rate produced by CSM prior to any intervention (**A**). When heart rate is maintained at a constant rate by cardiac atrial pacing, the vasodepressor component produced by CSM is unmasked (**C**). Both the cardioinhibitory and vasodepressor components of the CSH are abolished 12 months after interruption of the carotid arterial baroreflex arc by extracranial right glossopharyngeal nerve root section (**D**); the unoperated left carotid remained supersensitive (data not shown).

the vascular adventitia in area of the carotid sinus also interrupts the baroreceptor reflex arc and represents an alternative form of therapy for CSH patients with a significant vasodepressor contribution to their symptoms, especially if the disease is bilateral, since both right and left glossopharyngeal nerve root section will likely produce vocal cord paralysis requiring permanent tracheostomy.

Hyperadrenergic Dsyautonomias

Another clinically challenging group of dysautonomic patients are those who present with (a) recurrent lightheadedness or syncope and (b) evidence of exaggerated hemodynamic responses to bedside maneuvers mediated by the ANS, such as standing or Valsalva maneuver. Of 118 patients with these symptoms referred to our laboratory for formal evaluation, we were unable to distinguish, by clinical characteristics alone, the 78 patients with mitral valve prolapse (MVP) from the 40 patients without it (132). The cardiovascular responses of these 118 patients to a series of maneuvers which affected the ANS were therefore compared with those of 12 asymptomatic patients with MVP and those of 23 normal volunteers to determine if unique patterns of responses to these maneuvers could distinguish patients in one subgroup from those in another. The most common pattern of abnormal responses in symptomatic patients was (a) an increased heart rate and plasma NE, both in the supine position and after standing quietly for 5 min (Figs. 3 and 4), (b) an exaggerated heart rate response during phase II of a quantitated Valsalva maneuver (Fig. 5), (c) a diminished bradycardic response during phase IV of the Valsalva maneuver (Fig. 5), and (d) an exaggerated heart rate response to administration of isoproterenol (Figs. 6 and 7). Noted in a minority of patients were (a) an exaggerated hypertensive overshoot during phase IV of the Valsalva maneuver, (b) an increased vascular response to α-adrenergic agonists, and (c) an excessive vasodilation after isoproterenol. There was no consistent pattern of abnormal cardiovascular responses to these maneuvers that uniquely identified a particular patient subgroup.

A subgroup of nine patients with MVP and symptoms of dysautonomia who demonstrated exaggerated heart rate and vasodilatory responses to isoproterenol was also

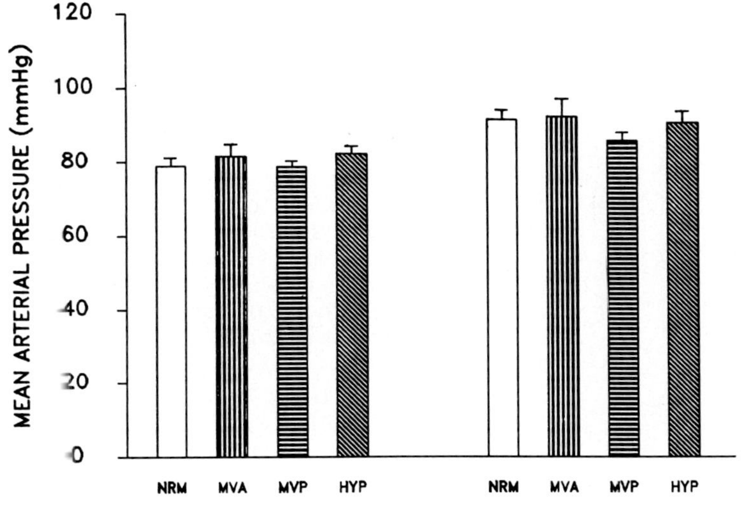

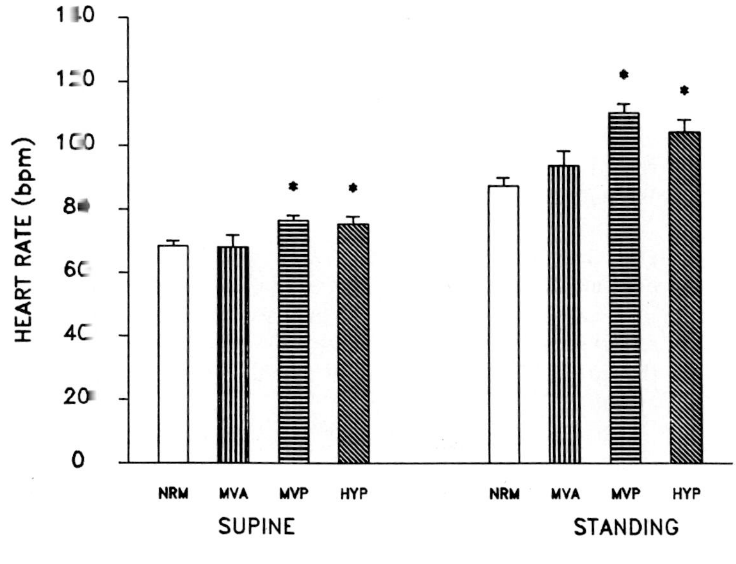

FIG. 3. Average (±) values for heart rate (**bottom**) and mean arterial pressure (**top**) after 30 min supine rest (*left*) and again after 5 min of quiet standing (*right*) in 23 normal volunteers (NRM), 12 asymptomatic (MVA) and 78 symptomatic mitral valve prolapse patients, and 40 symptomatic patients without mitral valve prolapse (HYP). *$p < 0.05$ compared to corresponding values in NRM. (From ref. 132, with permission.)

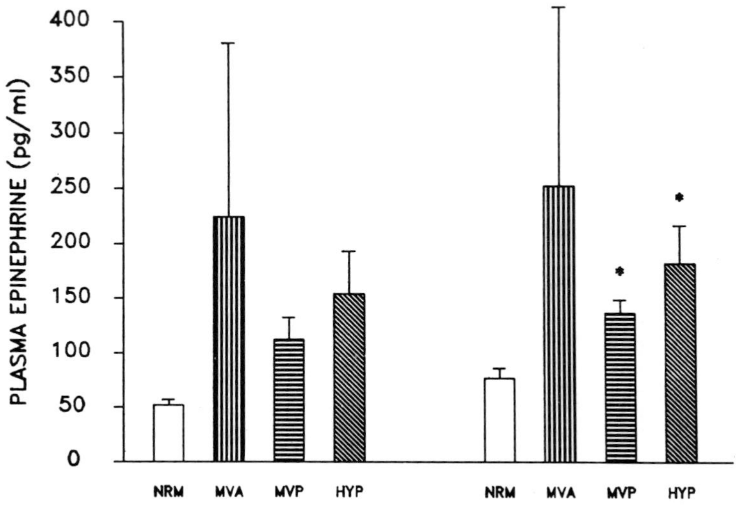

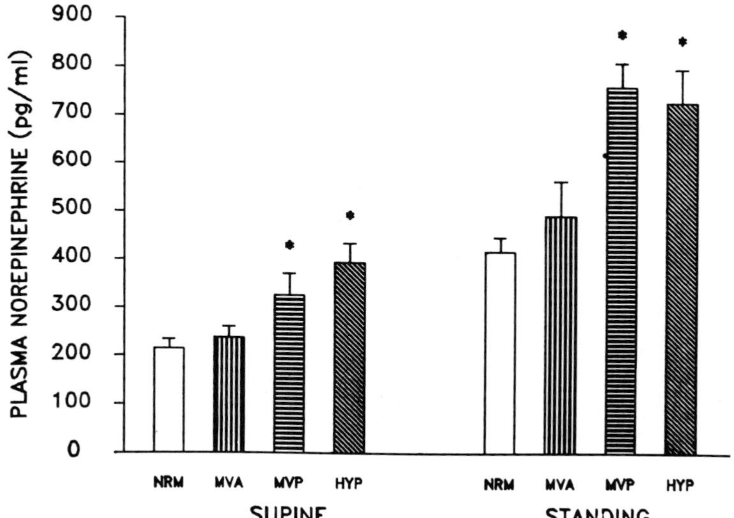

FIG. 4. Average (±) values for plasma norepinephrine (**bottom**) and epinephrine (**top**) after 30 min of supine rest (*left*) and again after 5 min of quiet standing (*right*) in 20 normal volunteers (NRM), 12 asymptomatic (MVA) and 75 symptomatic mitral valve prolapse patients, and 37 symptomatic patients without mitral valve prolapse (HYP). $^*p < 0.05$ compared to corresponding values in NRM. (From ref. 132, with permission.)

found to have biochemical evidence of supersensitive β_2-adrenoceptors on polymorphonuclear leukocytes (PMNs) (133). Although the density of β_2-receptors on PMNs was not different than that of normal volunteers, receptor affinity in MVP patients was augmented as determined by an increased ratio of receptors in the high-affinity state as compared to the low-affinity state and by more cAMP production by PMN membranes of MVP patients than by those of normal subjects upon exposure to isoproterenol. This functional alteration in β_2-adrenoceptors is a dynamic one, since infusion of isoproterenol for 4 hours at a rate that increased heart rate 10–15 beats/min normalized receptor affinity and the hemodynamic response to isoproterenol in MVP patients but in normal volunteers had no hemodynamic effect on cardiovascular β_2-adrenoceptors and no biochemical effect on PMN β_2-adrenoceptors.

Several diagnostic and therapeutic implications of these studies in patients with hyperadrenergic dysautonomias are worthy of mention. First, it is not possible to distinguish patients with MVP from those without it either by clinical criteria or by cardiovascular responses to autonomic stimuli. Thus, a decision to treat a patient's dysautonomic symptoms should be based on the severity of the symptoms rather than on the anatomic identification of a mitral valvular abnormality. Second, therapeutic agents (132,136) should be chosen with caution for the patient in whom there is no clear definition of site of abnormal autonomic control of cardiovascular function. Because of their marked orthostatic tachycardia, many of these patients have been empirically treated with β-adrenoceptor blockers without regard to other possible pathophysiologic derangements. We have seen several patients whose reflex tachycardia was compensating for their excessive peripheral vasodilation and whose symptoms therefore were greatly exacerbated by β-blocker therapy. In those patients, concomitant fluid volume expansion with high dietary sodium intake is often required to balance the undesirable aspects of β-blocker treatment; if necessary, a sodium-retaining hormone such as fludrocortisone is also used.

One rational approach to the treatment of patients with evidence of β-adrenergic receptor supersensitivity would be to desensitize the receptor with β-agonists. A pilot trial of

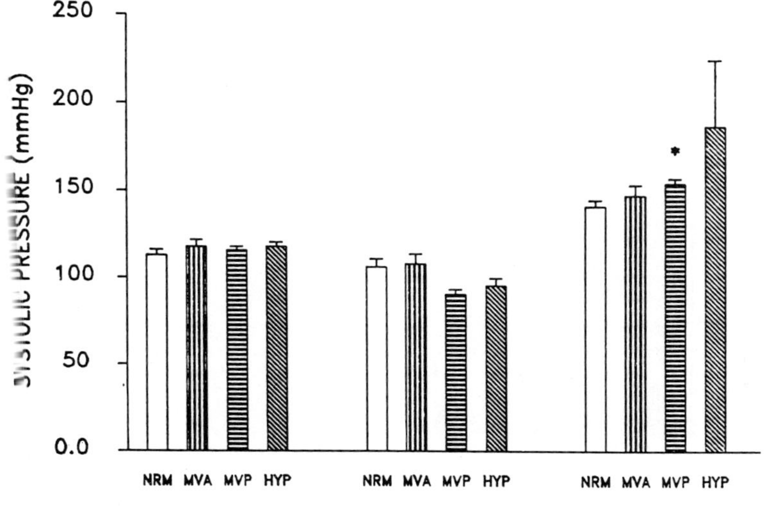

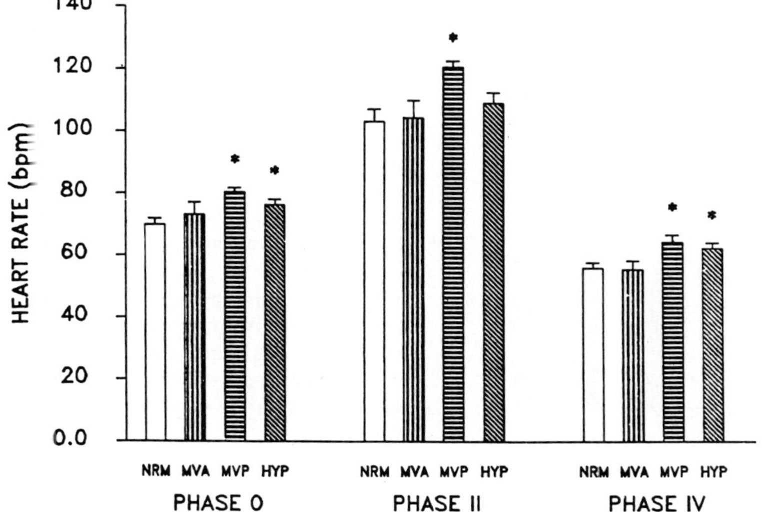

FIG. 5. Average (±) values for systolic blood pressure (**top**) and heart rate (**bottom**) prior to (phase 0), during (phase II), and after (phase IV) Valsalva maneuver (forced exhalation to 40 mmHg for 15 sec) in 23 normal volunteers (NRM), 12 asymptomatic (MVA) and 78 symptomatic mitral valve prolapse patients, and 40 symptomatic patients without mitral valve prolapse (HYP). $^*p < 0.05$ compared to corresponding values in NRM. (From ref. 132, with permission.)

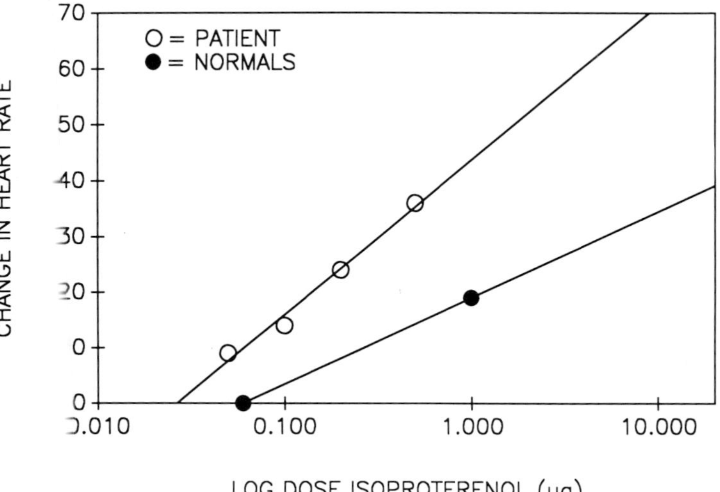

FIG. 6. Typical heart rate response of a single patient with mitral valve prolapse to graded intravenous injections of isoproterenol. The change in the heart rate from control in the patient (○) is exaggerated at each dose of isoproterenol compared to the average response in normal subjects (●). Thus, the dose of isoproterenol required to raise heart rate 25 beats/min, calculated from regression coefficient for the patient data, is less than that in normal subjects.

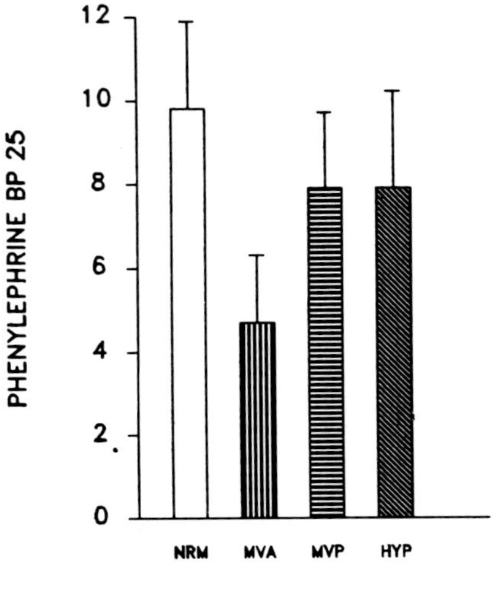

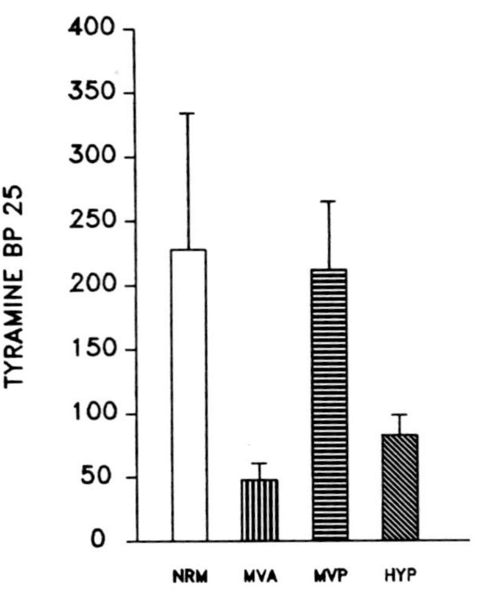

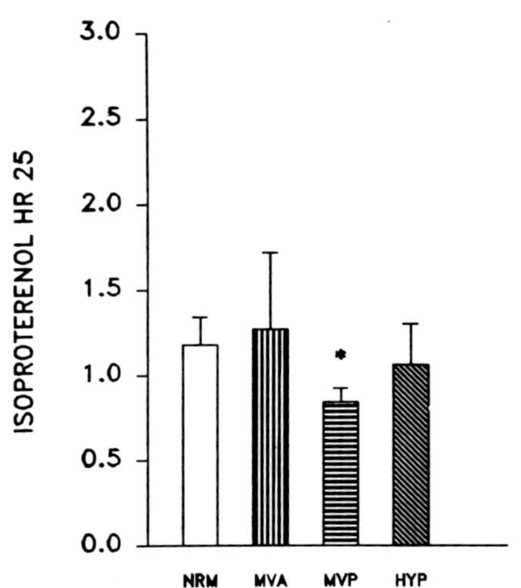

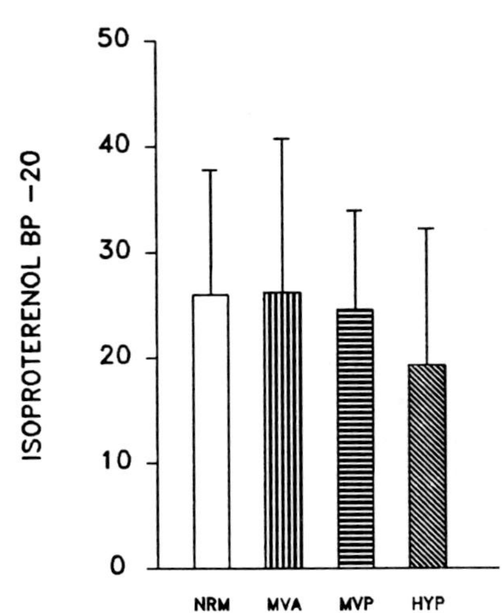

FIG. 7. Doses of pharmacologic agonists required to change mean arterial pressure (BP) or heart rate (HR) by specified amounts in 22 normal volunteers (NRM), 12 asymptomatic (MVA) and 77 symptomatic mitral valve prolapse patients, and 39 symptomatic patients without mitral valve prolapse (HYP). Isoproterenol BP20 is the dose of isoproterenol needed to lower BP 20 mmHg, whereas tyramine BP25 and phenylephrine BP25 are the doses of these agonists required to raise mean arterial pressure 25 mmHg. Isoproterenol HR25 is the dose of isoproterenol needed to raise heart rate 25 beats/min. *$p < 0.05$ compared to corresponding values in NRM. (From ref. 132, with permission.)

administering either terbutaline or metaproterenol to MVP patients with this abnormality has been performed (Davies, Mares, and Taylor, *unpublished observations*). Although patients demonstrated objective evidence of decreased β-receptor sensitivity as assessed by heart rate responses to graded injections of isoproterenol, the improvement in clinical symptoms was disappointing. A similar trial has not yet been carried out in patients with β-adrenergic supersensitivity who do not have MVP.

Hypoadrenergic Dysautonomias

Finally, specific identification of the site(s) of adrenergic abnormalities may guide rational therapy for patients with autonomic failure. Functionally, patients with autonomic insufficiency can be divided into those whose disease affects primarily the preganglionic sympathetic neuron versus those who have predominantly postganglionic sympathetic neuronal involvement (116,137,138). Formal autonomic evaluation in a research setting helps to identify into which of these two categories a patient with autonomic failure should be placed (72). Patients with preganglionic disease will have relatively normal supine values for plasma NE but will exhibit little increase in plasma NE with standing; these patients will also show normal blood pressure responses to graded injections of the direct-acting adrenergic agonist, phenylephrine, and to the indirect-acting agonist, tyramine. Patients with postganglionic disease, on the other hand, will have (a) subnormal plasma NE values at rest which also fail to rise with standing, (b) exaggerated blood pressure responses to phenylephrine, and (c) diminished or absent blood pressure increases after tyramine injection. Patients whose autonomic failure is due primarily to dysfunction of the postganglionic sympathetic neuron may respond best to (a) sympathomimetic drugs such as phenylpropanolamine (139), (b) the partial α_1-adrenergic agonist, clonidine (140), or (c) the α_2-adrenergic receptor antagonist, yohimbine (72). In contrast, patients with evidence of preganglionic sympathetic neuron dysfunction respond best to regimens like a high-tyramine diet combined with monoamine oxidase inhibitors; this combination promotes the release of NE from the intact postganglionic sympathetic neuron and also decreases the metabolic clearance of the NE that is released from these neurons (141).

TABLE 5. *Treatment recommendations for patients with dysautonomias*

Condition	Treatment (rationale)
Carotid sinus hypersensitivity	
Cardioinhibitory type	1. Cardiac pacemaker 2. Glossopharyngeal nerve root section
Mixed and vasodepressor types	1. Carotid adventitial stripping
Hyperadrenergic dysautonomia (e.g., MVP syndrome)	1. NaCl tablets, 3–24 g/day ± fludrocortisone, 0.1–0.5 mg/day (fluid volume expansion) 2. Cardioselective β-adrenergic blockers (tachycardia) 3. Calcium antagonists (chest pain, headache, and vasospasm) 4. Clonidine, 0.1–0.3 mg/day (vasospasm and tachycardia)
Hypoadrenergic dysautonomia Preganglionic (e.g., Shy–Drager) diseases[a] versus Postganglionic (e.g., diabetes) diseases[a]	1. NaCl tablets, 3–24 g/day 2. Jobst stockings—waist-high (mechanical venous compression) ± fludrocortisone, 0.1–0.5 mg/day 3. High-tyramine diet + monoamine oxidase inhibitors (MAOI) (raise blood pressure) 4. Phenylpropanolamine, 6.25–50 mg/day (sympathomimetic raises blood pressure) 5. Clonidine, 0.1–0.6 mg/day (α_1-agonist effect raises blood pressure) 6. Yohimbine, 2.5–15 mg/day (α_2-antagonist raises blood pressure) 7. Arginine vasopressin (DDAVP), 1 or 2 squirts in each nostril every 4–6 hours (exaggerated pressor effect) 8. Nonselective β-receptor antagonists, e.g., propranolol 30–60 mg/day (increase peripheral resistance by antagonizing vasodilatory β_2-receptors)

[a] When neuronal involvement is limited (early stages of disease), patients with either pre- or postganglionic disease may respond to a high-tyramine diet + MAOI regimen. Response can be predicted by blood pressure response to intravenous tyramine injections. When neuronal involvement is more extensive (later stages of disease), patients with both types of lesions respond better to sympathomimetic drugs or direct vasoconstrictors (DDAVP).

Clinical Recommendations (see Tables 4 and 5)

In summary, these studies in dysautonomic patients who represent the extremes of abnormal autonomic control of cardiovascular function demonstrate that laboratory tests of autonomic function can define the site of the patient's autonomic abnormality, thereby guiding the physician toward a more rational approach to therapy (Table 5).

REFERENCES

1. Mark AL. Sensitization of cardiac vagal afferent reflexes at the sensory receptor level: an overview. *Fed Proc* 1987;46:36–40.
2. Mark AL. The Bezold–Jarisch reflex revisited: clinical implications of inhibitory reflexes originating in the heart. *J Am Coll Cardiol* 1983;1:90–102.
3. Abboud FM. Integration of reflex responses in the control of blood pressure and vascular resistance. *Am J Cardiol* 1979;44:903–911.
4. Korner PI. Central nervous control of autonomic cardiovascular function. In: Berne RM, Sperelakis N, Geiger SR, eds. *Handbook of physiology. The cardiovascular system.* Bethesda, MD: American Physiological Society, 1979;691–739.
5. Oparil S. The sympathetic nervous system in clinical and experimental hypertension. *Kidney Int* 1986;30:437–452.
6. Stella A, Weaver L, Golin R, Genovesi S, Zanchetti A. Cardiovascular effects of afferent renal nerve stimulation. *Clin Exp Hypertens* [*A*] 1987;9:97–111.
7. Katholi RE, Woods WT. Afferent renal nerves and hypertension. *Clin Exp Hypertens* [*A*] 1987;9:211–226.
8. Stella A, Golin R, Genovesi S, Zanchetti A. Renal reflexes in the regulation of blood pressure and sodium excretion. *Can J Physiol Pharmacol* 1987;65:1536–1539.
9. Kopp UC, Smith LA. Renorenal reflex responses to renal sensory receptor stimulation in normotension and hypertension. *Clin Exp Hypertens* [*A*] 1987;9:113–125.
10. Mathias CJ, Kooner JS, Peart S. Neurogenic components of hypertension in human renal artery stenosis. *Clin Exp Hypertens* [*A*] 1987;9:293–306.
11. de Leeuw PW, Birkenhager WH. Efferent renal nerve activity in hypertensive man. *Clin Exp Hypertens* [*A*] 1987;9:281–292.
12. Gribbin B, Pickering TG, Sleight P, Peto R. Effect of age and high blood pressure on baroreflex sensitivity in man. *Circ Res* 1971;19:424–431.
13. Bristow JD, Honour AJ, Pickering GW, Sleight P, Smyth HS. Diminished baroreflex sensitivity in high blood pressure. *Circulation* 1969;39:48–54.
14. Pickering TG, Gribbin B, Sleight P. Comparison of the reflex heart rate response to falling and rising arterial pressure in man. *Cardiovasc Res* 1972;6:277–283.
15. Pickering TG, Gribbin B, Strange Peterson E, Cunningham DJC, Sleight P. Effects of autonomic blockade on the baroreflex in man at rest and during exercise. *Circ Res* 1972;30:177–185.
16. Bevegard BS, Shepherd JT. Circulatory effects of stimulating the carotid arterial stretch receptors in man at rest and during exercise. *J Clin Invest* 1966;45:132–142.
17. Goldstein DS. Arterial baroreflex sensitivity, plasma catecholamines, and pressor responsiveness in essential hypertension. *Circulation* 1983;68:234–240.
18. Eckberg DL. Carotid baroreflex function in young men with borderline blood pressure elevation. *Circulation* 1979;59:632–636.
19. Mancia G, Parati G, Pomidossi G, Casadei R, Di Rienzo M,

Zanchetti A. Arterial baroreflexes and blood pressure and heart rate variabilities in humans. *Hypertension* 1986;8:147–153.
20. Mancia G, Ferrari A, Gregorini L, Valentini R, Ludbrook J, Zanchetti A. Circulatory reflexes from carotid and extracarotid baroreceptor areas in man. *Circ Res* 1977;53:165–171.
21. Mancia G, Grassi G, Parati G, et al. Control of circulation by arterial baroreceptors and cardiopulmonary receptors in hypertension. *J Cardiovasc Pharmacol* 1986;8:82–88.
22. Shimada K, Kitazumi T, Ogura H, Sadakane N, Ozawa T. Effects of age and blood pressure on the cardiovascular responses to the Valsalva maneuver. *J Am Geriatr Soc* 1986;34:431–434.
23. Littler WA. Sleep and blood pressure: further observations. *Am Heart J* 1979;97:35–37.
24. London GM, Weiss YA, Pannier BP, Laurent SL, Safar ME. Tilt test in essential hypertension. Differential responses in heart rate and vascular resistance. *Hypertension* 1987;10:29–34.
25. Trimarco B, Volpe M, Ricciardelli B, et al. Valsalva maneuver in the assessment of baroreflex responsiveness in borderline hypertensives. *Cardiology* 1983;70:6–14.
26. Mancia G, Ludbrook J, Ferrari A, Gregorini L, Zanchetti A. Baroreceptor reflex in human hypertension. *Circ Res* 1978; 43:170–177.
27. Floras JS, Hassan MO, Jones JV, Osikowska BA, Sever PS, Sleight P. Factors influencing blood pressure and heart rate variability in hypertensive humans. *Hypertension* 1988;11:273–281.
28. Berdeaux A, Giudicelli JF. Antihypertensive drugs and baroreceptor reflex control of heart rate and blood pressure. *Fundam Clin Pharmacol* 1987;1:257–282.
29. Tochikubo O, Kaneko Y, Yukinari Y, Takeda I. Noninvasive measurement of baroreflex sensitivity index using an indirect and continuous blood-pressure recorder. *Jpn Heart J* 1986;27:849–857.
30. Mancia G, Ferrari A, Gregorini L, et al. Control of blood pressure by carotid sinus baroreceptors in human beings. *Am J Cardiol* 1979;44:895–902.
31. Dimsdale JE, Graham RM, Ziegler MG, Zusman RM, Berry CC. Age, race, diagnosis, and sodium effects on the pressor response to infused norepinephrine. *Hypertension* 1987;10:564–569.
32. Conway J, Boon N, Davies C, Jones JV, Sleight P. Neural and humoral mechanisms involved in blood pressure variability. *J Hypertens* 1984;2:203–208.
33. Wallin BG, Sundlof G. A quantitative study of muscle nerve sympathetic activity in resting normotensive and hypertensive subjects. *Hypertension* 1979;1:67–77.
34. Kirby DA, Vatner SF. Enhanced responsiveness to carotid baroreceptor unloading in conscious dogs during development of perinephritic hypertension. *Circ Res* 1987;61:678–686.
35. Victor RG, Mark AL. Interaction of cardiopulmonary and carotid baroreflex control of vascular resistance in humans. *J Clin Invest* 1985;76:1592–1598.
36. Parati G, Grassi G, Coruzzi P, et al. Influence of cardiopulmonary receptors on the bradycardic responses to carotid baroreceptor stimulation in man. *Clin Sci* 1987;72:639–645.
37. Zoller RP, Mark AL, Abboud FM, Schmid PG, Heistad DD. The role of low pressure baroreceptors in reflex vasoconstrictor responses in man. *J Clin Invest* 1972;51:2967–2972.
38. Cowley AW Jr, Liard JF. Vasopressin and arterial pressure regulation. *Hypertension* 1988;11(Suppl I):I25–I32.
39. Floras JS, Aylward PE, Abboud FM, Mark AL. Inhibition of muscle sympathetic nerve activity in humans by arginine vasopressin. *Hypertension* 1987;10:409–416.
40. Mohring J, Glanzer K, Maciel JA Jr, et al. Greatly enhanced pressor response to antidiuretic hormone in patients with impaired cardiovascular reflexes due to idiopathic orthostatic hypotension. *J Cardiovasc Pharmacol* 1980;2:367–376.
41. Floras JS, Aylward PE, Gupta BN, Mark AL, Abboud FM. Modulation of cardiovascular reflexes by arginine vasopressin. *Can J Physiol Pharmacol* 1987;65:1717–1723.
42. Abboud FM, Aylward PE, Floras JS, Gupta BN. Sensitization of aortic and cardiac baroreceptors by arginine vasopressin in mammals. *J Physiol (Lond)* 1986;377:251–265.
43. Hasser EM, DiCarlo SE, Applegate RJ, Bishop VS. Osmotically released vasopressin augments cardiopulmonary reflex inhibition of the circulation. *Am J Physiol* 1988;254:R815–R820.
44. Unger T, Rohmeiss P, Demmert G, Ganten D, Lang RE, Luft FC. Differential modulation of the baroreceptor reflex by brain and plasma vasopressin. *Hypertension* 1986;8(Suppl II):II157–II162.
45. Robertson GL, Ganguly A. Osmoregulation and baroregulation of plasma vasopressin in essential hypertension. *J Cardiovasc Pharmacol* 1986;8:87–91.
46. Lang RE, Unger T, Ganten D. Atrial natriuretic peptide: a new factor in blood pressure control. *J Hypertens* 1987;5:255–271.
47. Thoren P, Mark AL, Morgan DA, ONeill TP, Needleman P, Brody MJ. Activation of vagal depressor reflexes by atriopeptins inhibits renal sympathetic nerve activity. *Am J Physiol* 1986;251:H1252–H1259.
48. Ebert TJ, Cowley AW Jr. Atrial natriuretic factor attenuates carotid baroreflex-mediated cardioacceleration in humans. *Am J Physiol* 1988;254:R590–R594.
49. Feldman RD, Limbird LE, Nadeau J, Robertson D, Wood AJJ. Leukocyte beta-receptor alterations in hypertensive subjects. *J Clin Invest* 1984;73:648–653.
50. Madden DJ, Blumenthal JA, Ekelund LG. Effects of β-blockade and exercise on cardiovascular and cognitive functioning. *Hypertension* 1988;11:470–476.
51. Davidson WR Jr, Kawashima S, Banerjee SP, Liang CS. Preserved cardiac beta-adrenergic sensitivity in early renovascular hypertension. *Hypertension* 1987;9:467–472.
52. Volpe M, DeLuca N, Atlas SA, et al. Reduction of atrial natriuretic factor circulating levels by endogenous sympathetic activation in hypertensive patients. *Circulation* 1988;77:997–1002.
53. Sundlof G, Wallin BG. Effect of lower body negative pressure on human muscle nerve sympathetic activity. *J Physiol Lond* 1978;278:525–532.
54. Mohanty PK, Sowers JR, McNamara C, Thames MD. Reflex effects of prolonged cardiopulmonary baroreceptor unloading in humans. *Am J Physiol* 1988;254:R320–R324.
55. Grassi G, Gavazzi C, Capozi A, Galva MD, Picotti GB, Mancia G. Alterations in plasma noradrenaline in response to reflex modulation of sympathetic vasoconstrictor tone to skeletal muscles. *J Hypertens [Suppl]* 1984;2:131–133.
56. Mohanty PK, Sowers JR, Beck FW, et al. Catecholamine, renin, aldosterone, and arginine vasopressin responses to lower body negative pressure and tilt in normal humans: effects of bromocriptine. *J Cardiovasc Pharmacol* 1985;7:1040–1047.
57. Trimarco B, Vigorito C, Cuocolo A, et al. Reflex control of coronary vascular tone by cardiopulmonary receptors in humans. *J Am Coll Cardiol* 1988;11:944–952.
58. Grassi G, Gavazzi C, Ramirez A, Sabadini E, Turolo L, Mancia G. Role of cardiopulmonary receptors in reflex control of renin release in man. *J Hypertens [Suppl]* 1984;2:263–265.
59. Grassi G, Gravazzi C, Cesara AM, Picotti GB, Mancia G. Changes in plasma catecholamines in response to reflex modulation of sympathetic vasoconstrictor tone by cardiopulmonary receptors. *Clin Sci* 1985;68:503–510.
60. Kiowski W, Julius S. Renin response to stimulation of cardiopulmonary mechanoreceptors in man. *J Clin Invest* 1978;62:656–663.
61. Fasola AF, Martz BL. Peripheral venous renin activity during 70 degree tilt and lower body negative pressure. *Aerospace Med* 1972;43:713–715.
62. Mark AL, Abboud FM, Fitz AE. Influence of low- and high-pressure baroreceptors on plasma renin activity in humans. *Am J Physiol* 1978;235:H29–H33.
63. Thoren P. Characteristics of left ventricular receptors with nonmedullated vagal afferents in cats. *Circ Res* 1977;40:415–421.
64. Thames MD. Effects of *d*- and *l*-propranolol on the discharge of cardiac vagal C-fibers. *Am J Physiol* 1980;238:H465–H470.
65. Trimarco B, De Luca N, Ricciardelli B, et al. Effects of lower body negative pressure in hypertensive patients with left ventricular hypertrophy. *J Hypertens [Suppl]* 1986;4:306–309.
66. Ferguson DW, Thames MD, Mark AL. Effects of propranolol on reflex vascular responses to orthostatic stress in humans. Role of ventricular baroreceptors. *Circulation* 1983;67:802–807.
67. Stiles GL, Caron MG, Lefkowitz RJ. Beta-adrenergic receptors: biochemical mechanisms of physiological regulation. *Physiol Rev* 1984;64:661–743.

68. Starke K, Docherty JR. Recent developments in alpha-adrenoceptor research. *J Cardiovasc Pharmacol* 1980;2:S269–S286.
69. Mark AL. Structural changes in resistance and capacitance vessels in borderline hypertension. *Hypertension* 1984;6(Suppl III):III-69–III-73.
70. Schulte KL, Braun J, Meyer-Sabellek W, Wegscheider K, Gotzen R, Distler A. Functional versus structural changes of forearm vascular resistance in hypertension. *Hypertension* 1988;11:320–325.
71. Takeshita A, Mark AL. Decreased vasodilator capacity of forearm resistance vessels in borderline hypertension. *Hypertension* 1980;2:610–616.
72. Robertson D, Goldberg MR, Tung CS, Hollister AS, Robertson RM. Use of alpha-2-adrenoreceptor agonists and antagonists in the functional assessment of the sympathetic nervous system. *J Clin Invest* 1986;78:576–581.
73. Goldberg MR, Hollister AS, Robertson D. Influence of yohimbine on blood pressure, autonomic reflexes, and plasma catecholamines in humans. *Hypertension* 1983;5:772–778.
74. DeLeeuw PW, van Es PN, De Bos R, Birkenhager WH. Role of alpha-1- and alpha-2-adrenergic receptors in the human hypertensive kidney. *Hypertension* 1987;9(Suppl III):III-210–III-212.
75. Buhler FR, Bolli P, Amann WF, Erne P, Kiowski W. Sympathetic nervous system in essential hypertension and antihypertensive response to alpha-2-adrenoreceptor stimulation. *J Cardiovasc Pharmacol* 1984;6:S753–S756.
76. Bolli P, Erne P, Ji BH, Block LH, Kiowski W, Buhler FR. Adrenaline induces vasoconstriction through post-junctional alpha-2-adrenoreceptors and this response is enhanced in patients with essential hypertension. *J Hypertens [Suppl]* 1984;2:115–118.
77 Egan B, Panis R, Hinderliter A, Schork N, Julius S. Mechanism of increased alpha adrenergic vasoconstriction in human essential hypertension. *J Clin Invest* 1987;80:812–817.
78. Motulsky HJ, Insel PA. Adrenergic receptors in man. *N Engl J Med* 1982;307:18–29.
79. Michel MC, Beckeringh JJ, Ikezono K, Kretsch R, Brodde OE. Lymphocyte beta-2-adrenoceptors mirror precisely beta-2-adrenoceptor, but poorly beta-1-adrenoceptor changes in the human heart. *J Hypertens [Suppl]* 1986;4:S215–S218.
80. Doyle AE, Fraser JRE, Marshall RJ. Reactivity of forearm vessels to vasoconstrictor substances in hypertensive and normotensive subjects. *Clin Sci* 1959;18:441–454.
81. Weidmann P, Grimm M, Meier A, et al. Pathogenic and therapeutic significance of cardiovascular pressor reactivity as related to plasma catecholamines in borderline and established essential hypertension. *Clin Exp Hypertens [A]* 1980;2:427–449.
82. Coccheri S, Fiorentini P. Platelet adhesiveness and aggregation in hypertensive patients. *Acta Med Scand* 1971;525:273–275.
83. Continsouza-Blanc D, Elghozi JL, Dausse JP. Alteration of platelet alpha2-adrenoceptors in human hypertension. *J Hypertens [Suppl]* 1984;2:155–157.
84. Hollister AS, Onrot J, Lonce S, Nadeau JH, Robertson D. Plasma catecholamine modulation of alpha-2-adrenoreceptor agonist affinity and sensitivity in normotensive and hypertensive human platelets. *J Clin Invest* 1986;77:1416–1421.
85. Pfeifer MA, Ward K, Malpass T, et al. Variations in circulating catecholamines fail to alter human platelet alpha-2-adrenergic receptor number or affinity for [3H]yohimbine or [3H]-dihydroergocryptine. *J Clin Invest* 1984;74:1063–1072.
86. Motulsky H O'Connor, Insel P. Platelet alpha-2-adrenergic receptors in treated and untreated essential hypertension. *Clin Sci* 1983;64:265–272.
87. Bertel O, Buhler FR, Kiowski W, Lutold BE. Decreased beta-adrenergic responsiveness as related to age, blood pressure, and plasma catecholamines in patients with essential hypertension. *Hypertension* 1980;2:130–138.
88. Kafka MS, Lake CR, Gullner HG, Tallman JF, Bartter FC, Fujita T. Adrenergic receptor function is different in male and female patients with essential hypertension. *Clin Exp Hypertens [A]* 1979;1:613–627.
89. Feldman RD, Lawton WJ, McArdle WL. Low sodium diet corrects the defect in lymphocyte beta-adrenergic responsiveness in hypertensive subjects. *J Clin Invest* 1987;79:290–294.
90. Esler M, Jennings G, Korner P, et al. Assessment of human sympathetic nervous system activity from measurements of norepinephrine turnover. *Hypertension* 1988;11:3–20.
91. Esler M, Jackman G, Bobik A, et al. Norepinephrine kinetics in essential hypertension: defective neuronal uptake of norepinephrine in some patients. *Hypertension* 1981;3:149–156.
92. Esler M, Jennings G, Biviano B, Lambert G, Hasking G. Mechanism of elevated plasma noradrenaline in the course of essential hypertension. *J Cardiovasc Pharmacol* 1986;8(Suppl 5):S39–S43.
93. Esler M, Jennings G, Korner P, et al. Total, and organ-specific, noradrenaline plasma kinetics in essential hypertension. *Clin Exp Hypertens [A]* 1984;6:507–521.
94. Esler M, Jennings G, Korner P, Blombery P, Sacharias N, Leonard P. Measurement of total and organ-specific norepinephrine kinetics in humans. *Am J Physiol* 1984;247:E21–E28.
95. Henry DP, Luft FC, Weinberger MH, Fineberg NS, Grim CE. Norepinephrine in urine and plasma following provocative maneuvers in normal and hypertensive subjects. *Hypertension* 1980;2:20–28.
96. Von Euler US, Hellner S, Purkhold A. Excretion of noradrenaline in urine in hypertension. *Scand J Clin Lab Invest* 1954;6:54–59.
97. Weidmann P, Hirsch D, Beretta-Piccoli C, Reubi FC, Ziegler WH. Interrelations among blood pressure, blood volume, plasma renin activity and urinary catecholamines in benign essential hypertension. *Am J Med* 1977;62:209–218.
98. Eliasson K, Sjoquist B. Urinary catecholamine metabolites in borderline and established hypertension. *Acta Med Scand* 1984;216:369–375.
99. Goldstein DS. Plasma norepinephrine in essential hypertension: a study of the studies. *Hypertension* 1981;3:48–52.
100. Goldstein DS, Lake CR, Chernow B, et al. Age-dependence of hypertensive–normotensive differences in plasma norepinephrine. *Hypertension* 1983;5:100–104.
101. Brown MJ, Jenner DA, Allison DJ, Dollery CT. Variations in individual organ release of noradrenaline measured by an improved radioenzymatic technique; limitations of peripheral venous measurements in the assessment of sympathetic nervous activity. *Clin Sci* 1981;61:585–590.
102. Planz G, Planz R, Persigehl M, Bundschu HD, Heintz R. Adrenaline and noradrenaline concentration in blood of suprarenal and renal vein in man with normal blood pressure and with essential hypertension. *Klin Wochenschr* 1978;56:1109–1112.
103. Floras J, Vann Jones J, Hassan MO, Osikowska BA, Sever PS, Sleight P. Failure of plasma norepinephrine to consistently reflect sympathetic activity in humans. *Hypertension* 1986;8:641–649.
104. Hjemdahl P, Freyschuss U, Juhlin-Dannfelt A, Linde B. Differentiated sympathetic activation during mental stress evoked by the Stroop test. *Acta Physiol Scand [Suppl]* 1984;527:25–29.
105. Mancia G, Ferrari A, Gregorini L, et al. Plasma catecholamines do not invariably reflect sympathetically induced changes in blood pressure in man. *Clin Sci* 1983;65:227–235.
106. Folkow B, DiBona GF, Hjemdahl P, Toren PH, Wallin BG. Measurements of plasma norepinephrine concentrations in human primary hypertension: a word of caution on their applicability for assessing neurogenic contributions. *Hypertension* 1983;5:399–403.
107. Watson RDS, Page AJF, Littler WA, Jones DH, Reid JL. Plasma noradrenaline concentrations at different vascular sites during rest and isometric and dynamic exercise. *Clin Sci* 1979;57:545–547.
108. Wallin BG. Muscle sympathetic activity and plasma concentrations of noradrenaline. *Acta Physiol Scand [Suppl]* 1984;527:21–24.
109. Wallin BG, Morlin C, Hjemdahl P. Muscle sympathetic activity and venous plasma noradrenaline concentrations during static exercise in normotensive and hypertensive subjects. *Acta Physiol Scand* 1987;129:489–497.
110. Johnson DG, Hayward JS, Jacobs TP, Collis ML, Eckerson JD, Williams RH. Plasma norepinephrine responses of man in cold water. *J Appl Physiol* 1977;43:216–220.
111. LeBlanc J, Cote J, Jobin M, Labrie A. Plasma catecholamines and cardiovascular responses to cold and mental activity. *J Appl Physiol* 1979;47:1207–1211.

112. Watson RDS, Hamilton CA, Reid JL, Littler WA. Changes in plasma norepinephrine, blood pressure and heart rate during physical activity in hypertensive man. *Hypertension* 1979; 1:341–346.
113. Robertson D, Frolich JC, Carr RK, et al. Effects of caffeine on plasma renin activity, catecholamines and blood pressure. *N Engl J Med* 1978;298:181–186.
114. Cryer PE. Physiology and pathophysiology of the human sympathoadrenal neuroendocrine system. *N Engl J Med* 1980;303:436–444.
115. Goldstein DS, Levinson PD, Zimlichman R, Pitterman A, Stull R, Keiser HR. Clonidine suppression testing in essential hypertension. *Ann Intern Med* 1985;102:42–48.
116. Bannister R. *Autonomic failure: a textbook of clinical disorders of the autonomic nervous system.* New York: Oxford University Press, 1983.
117. Kawano Y, Fukiyama K, Takeya Y, Abe I, Omae T. Catecholamines, angiotensin II and sodium concentrations in cerebrospinal fluid in young men with borderline hypertension. *Clin Exp Hypertens* [*A*] 1984;A6:1131–1145.
118. Lake CR, Gullner HG, Polinsky RJ, Ebert MH, Ziegler MG, Bartter FC. Essential hypertension: central and peripheral norepinephrine. *Science* 1981;211:955–957.
119. Eide I, Kolloch R, DeQuattro V, Miano L, Dugger R, Van der Meulen J. Raised cerebrospinal fluid norepinephrine in some patients with primary hypertension. *Hypertension* 1979;1:255–260.
120. Ziegler MG, Lake CR, Wood JH, Brooks BR, Ebert MH. Relationship between norepinephrine in blood and cerebrospinal fluid in the presence of a blood–cerebrospinal fluid barrier for norepinephrine. *J Neurochem* 1977;28:677–679.
121. Vlachakis ND, Lampano C, Alexander N, Maronde RF. Catecholamines and their major metabolites in plasma and cerebrospinal fluid of man. *Brain Res* 1981;229:67–74.
122. Ziegler MG, Milano AJ, Lake CR. Increased cerebrospinal fluid norepinephrine in essential hypertension. *Clin Exp Hypertens* [*A*] 1982;4:663–674.
123. Cubeddu LX, Hoffman IS, Davila J, Barbells YR, Ordaz P. Clonidine reduces elevated cerebrospinal fluid catecholamine levels in patients with essential hypertension. *Life Sci* 1984;35:1365–1371.
124. DeQuattro V, Sullivan P, Minagawa R, et al. Central and peripheral noradrenergic tone in primary hypertension. *Fed Proc* 1984;43:47–51.
125. Goldstein DS, Zimlichman R, Kelly GD, Stull R, Bacher JD, Keiser HR. Effect of ganglion blockade on cerebrospinal fluid norepinephrine. *J Neurochem* 1987;49:1484–1490.
126. Goldstein DS, Horwitz D, Keiser HR, Polinsky RJ. Plasma *l*-[^{3}H]-norepinephrine, *d*-[^{14}C]norepinephrine, and *d,l*-[^{3}H]-isoproterenol kinetics in essential hypertension. *J Clin Invest* 1983;72:1748–1758.
127. Hoeldtke RD, Climi KM, Reichard GA, Boden G, Owen OE. Assessment of norepinephrine secretion and production. *J Lab Clin Med* 1983;101:772–782.
128. Christensen NJ, Galbo H, Gjerris A, et al. Whole body and regional clearances of noradrenaline and adrenaline in man. *Acta Physiol Scand* [*Suppl*] 1984;527:17–20.
129. Esler M, Jennings G, Leonard P, et al. Contribution of individual organs to total noradrenaline release in humans. *Acta Physiol Scand* [*Suppl*] 1984;527:11–16.
130. Julius S, Esler MD, Randall OS. Role of the autonomic nervous system in mild human hypertension. *Clin Sci Mol Med* 1975;48:243S–252S.
131. Esler M, Julius S, Zweifler A, et al. Mild high-renin essential hypertension. Neurogenic human hypertension? *N Engl J Med* 1977;296:405–411.
132. Taylor AA, Davies AO, Mares A, et al. The spectrum of dysautonomia in mitral valvular prolapse. *Am J Med* 1989;86:267–274.
133. Davies AO, Mares A, Pool JL, Taylor AA. Mitral valve prolapse with symptoms of beta-adrenergic hypersensitivity. Beta 2-adrenergic receptor supercoupling with desensitization on isoproterenol exposure. *Am J Med* 1987;82:193–201.
134. Davies AO, Taylor AA, Pool JL, Nelson EB, Mitchell JR. Carotid sinus syndrome: atropine alone does not distinguish cardioinhibitory from vasodepressor mechanisms [Abstract]. *Clin Res* 1986;34:397A.
135. Simpson RK, Pool JL, Grossman RG, Rose JE, Taylor AA. Neurosurgical management of carotid sinus hypersensitivity. *J Neurosurg* 1987;67:757–759.
136. Gaffney FA, Lane LB, Pettinger W, Blomqvist CG. Effects of long-term clonidine administration on the hemodynamic and neuroendocrine postural responses of patients with dysautonomia. *Chest* 1983;83:436–438.
137. Shy GM, Drager GA. A neurological syndrome associated with orthostatic hypotension: a clinical-pathologic study. *Arch Neurol* 1960;2:511–527.
138. Hines S, Houston M, Robertson D. The clinical spectrum of autonomic dysfunction. *Am J Med* 1981;70:1091–1096.
139. Biaggioni I, Onrot J, Stewart CK, Robertson D. The potent pressor effect of phenylpropanolamine in patients with autonomic impairment. *JAMA* 1986;258:236–239.
140. Robertson D, Goldberg MR, Hollister AS, Wade D, Robertson RM. Clonidine raises blood pressure in severe idiopathic orthostatic hypotension. *Am J Med* 1983;74:193–200.
141. Davies B, Bannister R, Sever P. Pressor amines and monoamine-oxidase inhibitors for treatment of postural hypotension in autonomic failure. Limitations and hazards. *Lancet* 1978;1:172–175.
142. Johnston LC. The abnormal heart rate response to a deep breath in borderline labile hypertension: a sign of autonomic nervous system dysfunction. *Am Heart J* 1980;99:487–493.
143. Julius S, Cottier C, Egan B, Ibsen H, Kiowski W. Cardiopulmonary mechanoreceptors and renin release in humans. *Fed Proc* 1983;42:2703–2708.
144. Shepherd AMM, Lin MS, McNay JL, Musgrave GE, Keeton TK. Baroreflex sensitivity modulates vasodepressor response to nitroprusside. *Hypertension* 1983;5:79–85.
145. Grassi G, Giannattasio C, Saino A, et al. Cardiopulmonary receptor modulation of plasma renin activity in normotensive and hypertensive subjects. *Hypertension* 1988;11:92–99.
146. Fitzpatrick MA, Hinderliter AL, Egan BM, Julius S. Decreased venous distensibility and reduced renin responsiveness in hypertension. *Hypertension* 1986;8(Suppl II):II-36–II-43.
147. London GM, Safar ME, Safar AL, Simon AC. Blood pressure in the 'low-pressure system' and cardiac performance in essential hypertension. *J Hypertens* 1985;3:337–342.

Hypertension: Pathophysiology, Diagnosis, and Management, edited by J. H. Laragh and B. M. Brenner. Raven Press, Ltd., New York © 1990.

CHAPTER 92

Evaluation of Cardiac Structure and Function by Echocardiography and Other Noninvasive Techniques

Richard B. Devereux

General Principles of Echocardiography, 1479
Physical Properties of Ultrasound, 1480
Fundamentals of the Echocardiographic Examination, 1480
Echocardiographic Evaluation of Left Ventricular Structure, Load, and Performance, 1482
M-Mode Echocardiographic Methods, 1482
Two-Dimensional Echocardiographic Methods, 1485
Doppler Echocardiographic Evaluation of Left Ventricular Diastolic Performance and Pump Function, 1488
Other Noninvasive Methods of Evaluating the Left Ventricle, 1488
Evaluation of Regional Circulations by Ultrasound Techniques, 1489
Technology and Cost-Effectiveness, 1489
References, 1490

The finding of electrocardiographic or roentgenographic evidence of left ventricular hypertrophy or enlargement has long been known to predict an adverse prognosis in patients with hypertension (1–3). Although evaluation of the heart by these methods has been incorporated in the World Health Organization system for classifying the severity of hypertension (4), it is well recognized that their sensitivity for detection of cardiac abnormalities is relatively low (5–7). Beginning in the late 1970s, methods have been developed that allow accurate noninvasive measurement of cardiac size and performance. Because of its simplicity, lack of radiation exposure, and lower cost than other techniques of promising accuracy, echocardiography has been most extensively applied for research and clinical evaluation of hypertensive patients. Of particular importance, several studies have shown that echocardiographically measured left ventricular mass is a strong predictor of cardiovascular morbidity in hypertensive patients and in the general population (8–11), possibly having greater predictive value than blood pressure itself. Accordingly, this chapter will focus primarily on imaging and Doppler echocardiographic methods of evaluating cardiac structure and function as well as systemic hemodynamics, with briefer consideration given to ultrasound evaluation of peripheral arteries and to other noninvasive methods of cardiac imaging. Aspects of echocardiography of specific relevance to evaluation of the heart in hypertension will be considered here, while uses of echocardiography for the broad spectrum of other heart diseases are well covered in standard textbooks (12–14).

GENERAL PRINCIPLES OF ECHOCARDIOGRAPHY

Echocardiography, like other applications of ultrasound, relies on the fact that ultrasound, generated by the vibration of piezoelectric crystals at frequencies from 2 to 10 MHz or higher, can be formed into a beam that (a) propagates at a uniform speed through most body tissues and (b) is reflected from structures in the body to return to strike the piezoelectric crystal from which it originated, which, in turn, generates an electrical signal. The time interval between transmission of a burst of ultrasound a few microseconds in duration and generation of an electrical signal by the returning "echo," taken together with the known velocity of ultrasound in the body, allows one to determine the distance along the ultrasound beam from the transducer to a reflecting structure, providing information used to image the heart. Increases or decreases of the frequency of the reflected ultrasound can be used, according to the Doppler principle, to determine the velocity of the reflecting structure's motion toward or away from the transducer. Use of the Doppler shift to determine the velocity along the ultrasound beam of red blood cells forms the basis of Doppler echocardiographic evaluation of blood flow.

Physical Properties of Ultrasound

An appreciation of physical properties of ultrasound that determine the information that can be obtained is valuable to understand the strengths and limitations of various echocardiographic modalities. One of these is that with an average speed of ultrasound of 1540 m/sec in body tissues, the cycle of ultrasound transmission and echo reception can be repeated 1000–1500 times per second in adults, in whom cardiac structures may be as far as 20 cm from body surface transducers. Nearly instantaneous tracking of rapidly moving structures is obtained when the echocardiographic beam interrogates the same portion of the heart throughout the cardiac cycle, as in M-mode echocardiography. Alternatively, the beam can be swept, mechanically or electronically, through an arc of up to 90° to create a tomographic slice. Because it is desirable to have at least 50 lines of primary information to produce a good quality "sector scan," these can be obtained no more frequently than 20–30 times per second. Thus, M-mode echocardiography has superior temporal resolution, whereas the better spatial orientation of two-dimensional echocardiography is obtained at a cost of a somewhat slow frame rate.

The spatial resolution of echocardiography is influenced by several additional factors. The ability to discriminate two nearby objects along the axis of the echocardiographic beam ("depth resolution") is directly related to the ultrasound wavelength and, hence, is inversely proportional to its frequency. The theoretical limit of depth resolution is about 1 mm at a frequency of 2.25 MHz and 0.5 mm at a frequency of 5 MHz. That these limits may be achieved *in vivo,* or even exceeded because of the effect of temporally (M-mode) or spatially (two-dimensional) adjacent lines of echoes to reduce ambiguity about the location of interfaces, is demonstrated by our ability to determine accurately, by echocardiography, left ventricular masses as low as 0.3 g in rabbits and rats (15; G. deSimone, D. C. Wallerson, M. Volpe, and R. B. Devereux, *unpublished data*). High ultrasound frequency thus enhances depth resolution; however, the inverse relation between ultrasound frequency and depth penetration into the body has so far limited transthoracic echocardiography to maximum frequencies between 3 and 5 MHz, whereas frequencies between 7 and 15 MHz may be used for other applications such as imaging superficial arteries transcutaneously, evaluating coronary arteries during open heart surgery (16), or measuring arterial lumen and wall dimensions and characteristics by catheter-tip ultrasound transducers (17).

The ability to discriminate two objects side-by-side perpendicular to the ultrasound beam (lateral resolution) is determined by beam width and the extent to which it is focused. Difficulties with lateral resolution, causing echoes from solid structures to extend laterally into what should have been echo-free spaces containing blood, appear to be the reason why two-dimensional echocardiograms obtained using early-generation echographs tended to overstate the cross-sectional area of the left ventricular myocardium and understate that of the ventricular cavity (18,19). This problem has been reduced by technologic advances that produce narrower ultrasound beams, including use of annular array transducers (20) and improved processing of signals from the multiple crystals of electronic sector scanners. Improved lateral resolution in both the x-axis and the unseen z-axis (perpendicular to the tomographic plane of two-dimensional echocardiography) has made possible some new applications of echocardiography such as imaging coronary arteries by transducers on the chest wall (21).

Evaluation of blood flow by Doppler echocardiography is also influenced by several properties of ultrasound. The most important of these is that the maximum frequency shift—and, hence, velocity of blood flow that can be accurately detected—is proportional to the frequency with which pulses of ultrasound are repeated (the so-called Nyquist limit). This is no problem in continuous-wave Doppler, where ultrasound is continuously emitted from one transducer and the returning signal is received by another, but this modality has the limitation that the recorded velocity may be due to blood flow at any depth along the ultrasound beam ("range ambiguity"). Range ambiguity is eliminated by pulsed-mode Doppler, in which bursts of ultrasound are emitted intermittently and the returning signal is interrogated at an interval thereafter determined to allow the ultrasound to travel from transducer to target and back. However, the slow pulse repetition frequency this entails may, at greater depths within the heart, limit the maximum velocity that can be resolved to 1 m/sec or less, well within the physiologic range.

Fundamentals of the Echocardiographic Examination

The most important primary measurements and derived variables for assessment of the heart in hypertension can be obtained from a relatively simple echocardiographic examination, provided that the ultrasound beam and imaging planes are correctly oriented to cardiac structures and blood flow. Because of the central importance in hypertension of left ventricular structure and performance, the following discussion will focus on this chamber.

The left ventricle may be thought of as a prolate ellipsoid, relatively circular in short-axis views, with a long-axis approximately twice its minor axis (22,23). To measure the left ventricular minor axis dimension accurately, it is necessary to orient the echocardiographic beam from the parasternal (or less commonly the subcostal) window to pass perpendicularly through the interventricular septum and posterolateral left ventricular wall at the level of the junction of the papillary muscle tips and mitral chordae, as may be performed under two-dimensional guidance (Fig. 1A) or by a careful M-mode long-axis sweep in which the ventricu-

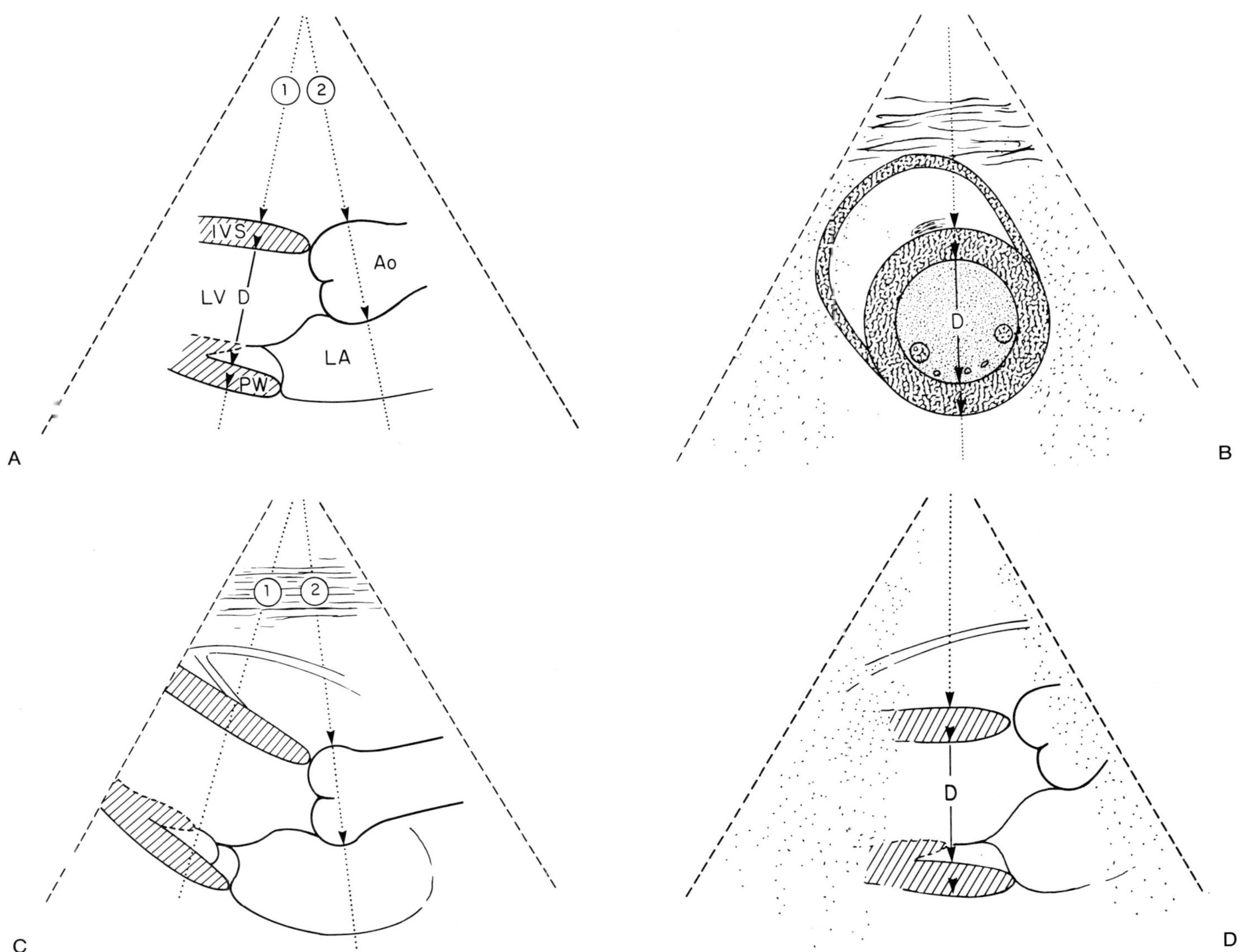

FIG. 1. Orientation of parasternal long- and short-axis two-dimensional echocardiographic imaging planes. **A:** Long-axis view in which the M-mode cursor would be correctly oriented to both the left ventricle and the aorta and left atrium. **B:** Rotation of the transducer approximately 90° results in an optimally oriented short-axis view. **C:** Long-axis view from a lower parasternal window in which the M-mode beam or short-axis tomographic plane is obliquely oriented to the left ventricle, as is common in older individuals. **D:** Movement of the transducer one interspace higher than used for part C permits correctly oriented views of the left ventricle, albeit with a narrower field of vision.

lar septum and aorta are shown to be equidistant from the transducer. Rotation of the two-dimensional sector approximately 90° to the short-axis projection allows one to measure the true, maximum left ventricular diameter (Fig. 1B) as does an M-mode T-scan (24). If, as commonly occurs in older subjects, the best parasternal window is in a low interspace, left ventricular M-mode dimension and short-axis two-dimensional cross-sectional areas should not be measured in the usual fashion, although it may be possible to measure correctly other structures such as the aortic root and left atrium (Fig. 1C). Instead, a higher interspace should be used even though this may image only a narrow sector that includes the left ventricular minor axis (Fig. 1D).

A major advantage of two-dimensional echocardiographic imaging is its ability to visualize the left ventricular long axis and ventricular wall segments near the apex. To use these measurements to calculate variables such as left ventricular mass and ejection fraction, one must obtain the true (longest) long-axis dimension and visualize the ventricular walls in approximately orthogonal planes (e.g., apical four- and two-chamber views). The left ventricular long axis is commonly foreshortened in the four-chamber view (Fig. 2C), as may be seen when the transducer is rotated to the two-chamber view; the ventricular apex is observed to be out of the field of view (25) (Fig. 2D). The transducer should then be moved inferolaterally until the left ventricular apex is as nearly centered at the top of the image "fan"

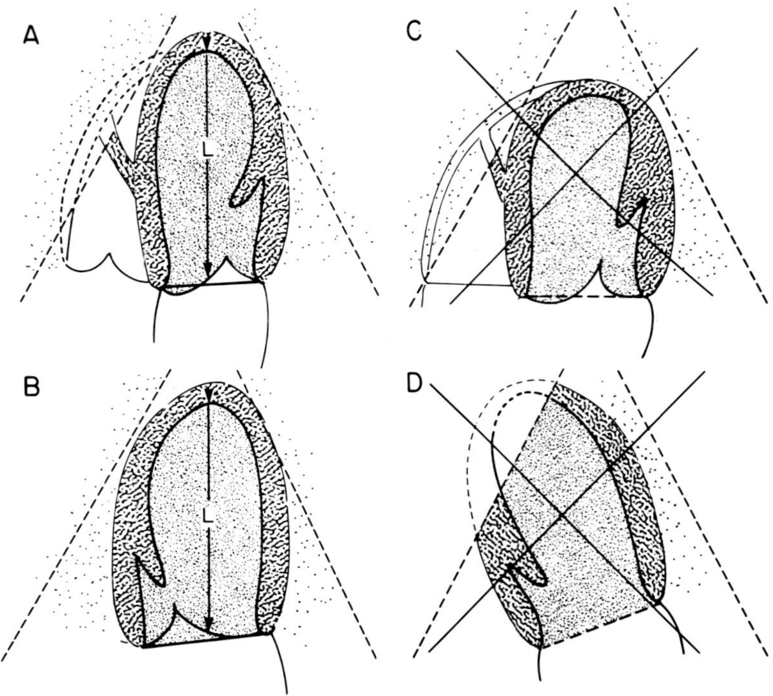

FIG. 2. Orientation of apical four- and two-chamber two-dimensional echocardiographic views. In optimally oriented views the left ventricular apex is centered at the top of the sector "fan" in both four-chamber (**A**) and two-chamber (**B**) projections. The left ventricular long-axis is commonly foreshortened in the four-chamber view (**C**), as is demonstrated by protrusion of the ventricular apex out of the field of vision in the two-chamber view (**D**).

in both views as possible (Fig. 2A and B). Additional rules for obtaining optimal two-dimensional images are given in Table 1.

The accuracy of Doppler recordings depends on interrogating the flow of interest with the ultrasound beam parallel to the axis of flow. Because the direction of blood flow is not always exactly what it would seem to be from the imaging echocardiogram, Doppler recordings of flow through a particular orifice should be performed from several potentially appropriate chest wall locations. Variants of the apical four-chamber view should be used to sample left ventricular inflow at the levels of the mitral annulus or valve orifice, whereas the apical long-axis view is best to measure systolic flow across the aortic annulus for calculation of stroke volume and systemic hemodynamic parameters (Fig. 3).

ECHOCARDIOGRAPHIC EVALUATION OF LEFT VENTRICULAR STRUCTURE, LOAD, AND PERFORMANCE

Extensive information about the structure and systolic function of a normally shaped left ventricle, such as occurs in patients with uncomplicated systemic hypertension, may be obtained by M-mode echocardiography. Because the relatively low cost of M-mode echocardiography appears to make it cost-effective compared to either older, less accurate methods of evaluating the heart in hypertension (7) or new, more expensive ones, this modality will be considered first.

M-Mode Echocardiographic Methods

Recordings with the M-mode beam oriented along the left ventricular minor axis by procedures described above permits visualization of the left ventricle's internal dimension (LVID) as well as interventricular septal and posterior wall thickness (IVS and PWT, respectively). For accurate and reproducible measurement of these structures, dominant lines representing the necessary interfaces should exhibit continuous motion in the correct pattern for the structure for at least 0.10 sec but should ideally do so throughout the entire cardiac cycle (26–28). Other recommendations concerning echocardiographic technique derived from a National Institutes of Health workshop devoted to the use of echocardiography in hypertension (29) are summarized in Table 2.

Evaluation of Left Ventricular Structure

Two methods of making M-mode echocardiographic left ventricular measurements are currently in widespread use.

TABLE 1. *Identification of most accurate two-dimensional echocardiographic left ventricular internal diameter*

	Parasternal		Apical	Subcostal	
	Long-axis	Short-axis	Four- and two-chamber views	Long-axis	Short-axis
Internal diameter	Largest	Smallest	Largest	Largest	Smallest
Wall thickness	Smallest	Smallest	Smallest	Smallest	Smallest

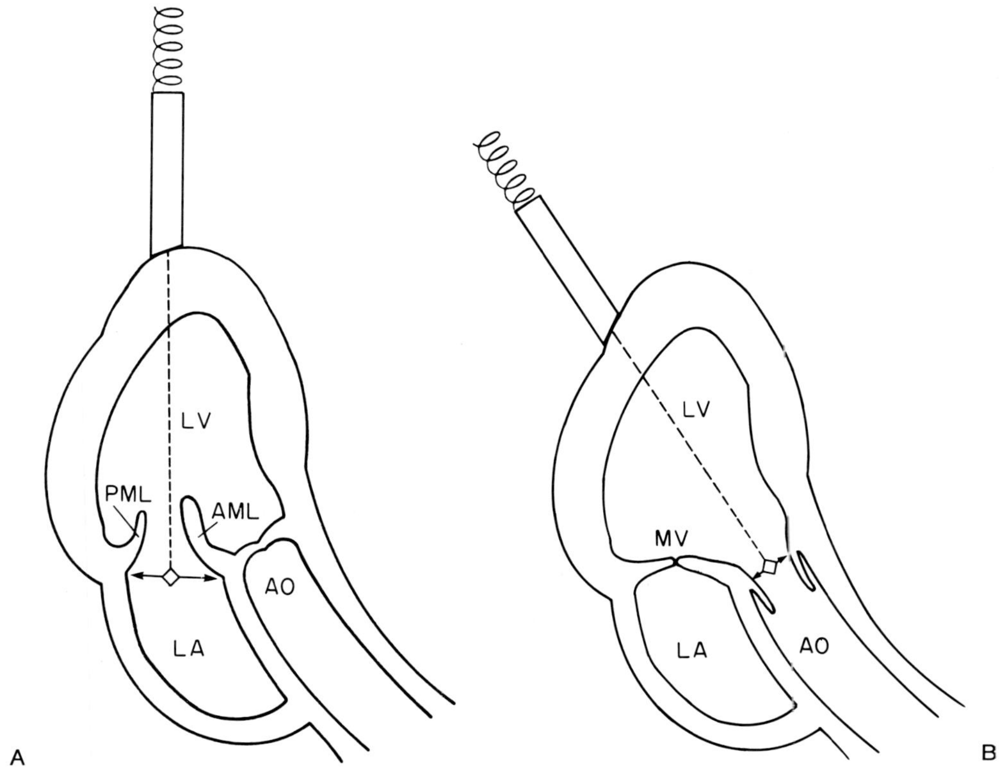

FIG. 3. A: Schematic diagram showing the location of pulsed Doppler sample volume for evaluation of left ventricular diastolic inflow at the level of the mitral valve orifice (◊) in an apical long-axis view oriented to maximize the diameter of the mitral annulus. **B:** Location of pulsed Doppler sample volume (◊) at the level of the aortic annulus in apical long-axis view. Abbreviations: AML, anterior mitral leaflet; Ao, aorta; LA, left atrium; LV, left ventricle; MV, mitral valve; PML, posterior mitral leaflet.

TABLE 2. *Recommendations concerning echocardiographic technique for left ventricular measurements* [a]

Instrument calibration: Calibrate against phantom at installation and at regular intervals thereafter.
Echocardiographic performance: Standardize and record decubitus position. Use mattress cutout for apical imaging. Record images in held expiration.
Location of imaging planes
Independent M-mode: Below mitral leaflet tips on long-axis sweep; maximum dimension on transverse scan.
Two-dimensionally guided M-mode: From short-axis view with correct angulation of short-axis plane defined in long-axis view.
Two-dimensional echo: Define correct orientation of short-axis and apical views by use of 90° orthogonal planes.
Recognition of measurable images
M-mode: Dominant lines with correct motion representing interfaces for at least 0.10 sec (5 mm at standard recording speed).
Two-dimensional echo: Visualization of complete interface in motion with persistence in stop-frame mode.
Enhancement of reproducibility: Use three or more cardiac cycles. Record imaging window location and patient position. For research, use independent readings by two or three investigators.

[a] Modified from ref. 29.

The first of these to be proposed, the Penn method, is commonly used to measure left ventricular mass. The thickness of the echocardiographic lines representing endocardial interfaces is excluded from wall thickness measurements and is included in chamber dimensions by the Penn Convention (Fig. 4, right panel). The more recent recommendations of the American Society of Echocardiography (30), in which all measurements are made from leading edge to leading edge (Fig. 4, left panel), have been widely adopted and may be used for measurement of left ventricular mass and other variables. End-diastolic measurements are made at the peak of the R wave of the simultaneous electrocardiogram by the Penn Convention and at the QRS onset according to the American Society of Echocardiography.

M-mode measurements made at end-diastole by either the Penn or American Society of Echocardiography conventions may be used to calculate left ventricular mass by anatomically validated formulae. For Penn measurements the formula to be used is (27,31)

$$\text{Left ventricular mass}_{(\text{Penn})} = 1.04[(\text{IVS} + \text{LVID} + \text{PWT})^3 - \text{LVID}^3] - 13.6\ \text{g}$$

Estimates of left ventricular mass by this method were closely correlated to actual ventricular weight measured at

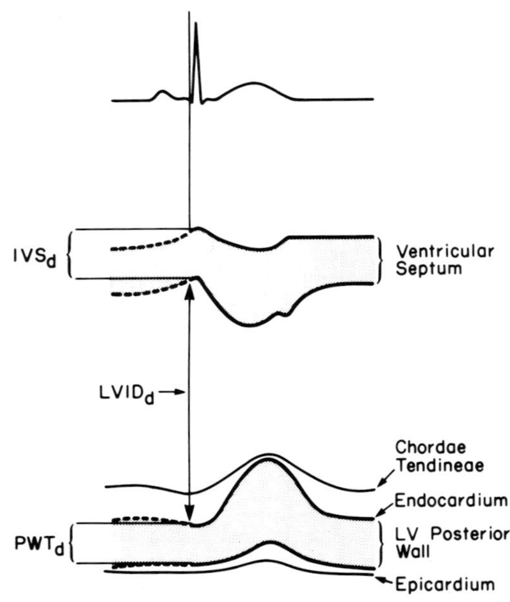

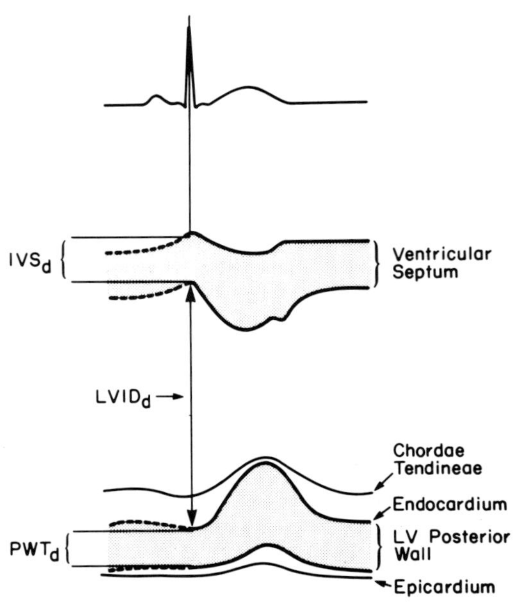

FIG. 4. Schematic depiction of M-mode echocardiographic left ventricular (LV) anatomic measurements. **Left:** The American Society of Echocardiography (30) recommended that end-diastolic measurements be made at the onset of the QRS complex using the leading edge of interfaces for all measurements. **Right:** Penn convention measurements are made at the peak of the electrocardiographic R wave with exclusion of endocardial interface thickness from measurements of ventricular septal and posterior LV wall thickness. IVS$_d$, interventricular septum and end-diastole; LVID$_d$, end-diastolic LV internal dimension; PWT$_d$, end-diastolic posterior wall thickness. (From ref. 29.)

necropsy ($r = 0.96$ and $r = 0.92$, both $p < 0.001$) in separate series of 34 and 52 necropsied patients. This formula used with postmortem ventricular dimensions also performed well ($r = 0.89$, $p < 0.001$) compared to autopsy ventricular weight in cardiovascularly normal children and adolescents (32).

Left ventricular mass may also be measured using American Society of Echocardiography measurements. However, similar to the findings of Woythaler et al. (33) in human patients and of Crawford et al. in baboons (34), we found that anatomic left ventricular mass was systematically overstated, by a mean of nearly 20%, when end-diastolic American Society of Echocardiography measurements were used in the cube-function formula (31,35). This error could be corrected to give values closely correlated to necropsy ventricular weight ($r = 0.90$, $p < 0.001$) by a simple regression equation (31):

$$\text{Left ventricular mass}_{(ASE)} = 0.8[1.04((\text{IVS} + \text{LVID} + \text{PWT})^3 - \text{LVID}^3)] + 0.6 \text{ g}$$

Other methods combining M-mode left ventricular measurements with the angiographically derived formulae of Troy et al. (22) and Teichholz et al. (36) were less accurate than the Penn or corrected-ASE methods when compared to anatomic ventricular weight (27,31).

Although left ventricular mass is, overall, the best measure of myocardial cell size (since the number of cardiac myocytes remains relatively constant after infancy in humans) and is more sensitive for detection of ventricular hypertrophy than other primary or derived echocardiographic measurements (37,38), valuable information about hypertensive cardiac hypertrophy can also be obtained from measures of ventricular wall thickness. Of these the most useful is the left ventricular wall thickness/chamber radius ratio, termed "relative wall thickness," which should increase in proportion to chronic elevations of ventricular systolic pressure if adaptive left ventricular hypertrophy develops (39–41). Relative wall thickness may be calculated simply from M-mode echocardiographic measurements as 2PWT/LVID (42).

In patients with systemic hypertension, wall thicknesses have been found to be most closely correlated with diastolic blood pressure (43–45), in keeping with the parallelism we have noted between concentric left ventricular hypertrophy and elevated peripheral resistance (43,46). Conversely, left ventricular mass is most closely related to systolic blood pressure in hypertensive patients (43,44,47–51), in accord with the concept that both systolic blood pressure and left ventricular mass reflect the summated effect of the combined hemodynamic pressure and volume load components of hypertension (52).

Evaluation of Ventricular Performance and Load

Systolic function of a symmetrically contracting ventricle, such as occurs in patients with uncomplicated systemic hypertension, can be easily assessed by measurement of the fractional shortening between end-diastole (d) and end-systole (s) of the left ventricular internal dimension (23,53):

$$\text{Fractional shortening (\%)} = [(\text{LVIDd} - \text{LVIDs})/\text{LVIDd}] \times 100$$

If ventricular wall motion is uniform, fractional shortening is closely correlated with global left ventricular ejection fraction and is a simple substitute for it.

Because ejection-phase indices of cardiac performance are highly dependent on afterload, measurement of myocardial afterload is helpful in determining whether or not observed ventricular function reflects normal myocardial contractile performance. The most direct measure of myocardial afterload is end-systolic stress, which can be measured noninvasively using (a) end-systolic echocardiographic left ventricular measurements by the American Society of Echocardiography convention and (b) simultaneous cuff blood pressure in a catheterization-validated formula (54):

$$\text{End-systolic stress} = \frac{0.334 \times \text{SBP} \times \text{LVIDs}}{\text{PWTs} \times \left(1 + \dfrac{\text{PWTs}}{\text{LVIDs}}\right)}$$

A close inverse relationship exists between fractional shortening or other ejection-phase indices and end-systolic stress in both normal and hypertensive subjects (43,55–57); this relationship becomes most linear when end-systolic stress is plotted on a logarithmic scale (ESS_{10}). When fractional shortening is afterload-corrected by expressing it as a percent of the mean value predicted for observed fractional shortening based on findings in 103 normal subjects (56,58), namely,

$$\text{Predicted fractional shortening (\%)} = 200.3 - 34.48\ (\text{ESS}_{10}),$$

deviations from normal in left ventricular contractile performance may be identified. This analytical approach reveals (a) reduced values in patients with congestive cardiomyopathy and (b) normal or elevated values in patients with uncomplicated essential hypertension (52) (Fig. 5).

Detection of Abnormal Left Ventricular Structure and Function

Although measurements of left ventricular structure and function are continuous variables that vary across the entire range of normal and abnormal values, it is often convenient—and, at times, necessary for clinical decision-making—to use partition values to separate abnormal from normal findings. This requires use of appropriate normal limits derived from study of reasonably large apparently normal populations, that take into account demographic and body habitus variables that influence normal findings. For left ventricular mass, gender and a measure of body size (such as body surface area or height) need to be taken into account; however, for relative wall thickness, no such adjustment is needed (37,38,51,59–62). Preliminary evidence suggests that left ventricular performance also differs between normal women and normal men (63). Available partition values for recognition of abnormal left ventricular structure and function by well-validated M-mode and two-dimensional echocardiographic methods (42,55,57–59,61–65) are given in Table 3.

Two-Dimensional Echocardiographic Methods

Despite the accuracy and practical advantages of M-mode echocardiographic methods, this technique has limitations that make two-dimensional echocardiography desirable, or even necessary, for evaluation of certain patients. Chief among these are patients in whom the shape of the left ventricle is distorted by ventricular aneurysms resulting from coronary artery disease or other severe geometric abnormalities, in whom M-mode echocardiographic measurements of left ventricular mass or other variables may be seriously erroneous (66).

Evaluation of Left Ventricular Structure

Two methods for determination of left ventricular mass by two-dimensional echocardiography have been anatomically validated. The first and simpler of these methods, proposed by Reichek et al. (66), employs an ellipsoidal model that requires measurement of the left ventricular long-axis and of the cross-sectional area (CSA) of left ventricular myocardium and cavity in short-axis projection (67). The measurements required are illustrated in Fig. 6. Left ventricular mass by the long-axis length–short-axis area method is calculated by the following anatomically validated formula (66,68):

$$\text{Left ventricular mass} = 1.055 \times 0.833 \times [(\text{CSA}_{\text{total}} \times \text{Long-axis}) - (\text{CSA}_{\text{cavity}} \times \text{Long-axis})]$$

Although echocardiographic measurements were originally adjusted for imaging errors produced by early-generation echocardiographs by regression equations (18,66), we have obtained data to indicate that technologic improvements have effectively eliminated the advantage of this procedure (20).

The other method for two-dimensional echocardiographic determination of left ventricular mass utilizes a truncated ellipsoid formula that corresponds more precisely to the shape of this chamber (69,70). The measurements needed for this method are given in Fig. 7, but computation by the relatively complex formula (69) requires use of a programmable calculator or computer. Anatomic validation of the truncated ellipsoid method of Schiller et al. has been obtained in both human patients and experimental animals (69,71,72). Preliminary evidence suggests that ventricular mass measurements by this method may be somewhat more reproducible than M-mode measurements (73), making its greater computational complexity (and hence cost) justifiable under certain circumstances, such as serial assessment of cardiac effects of antihypertensive treatment in small groups of patients. Upper normal

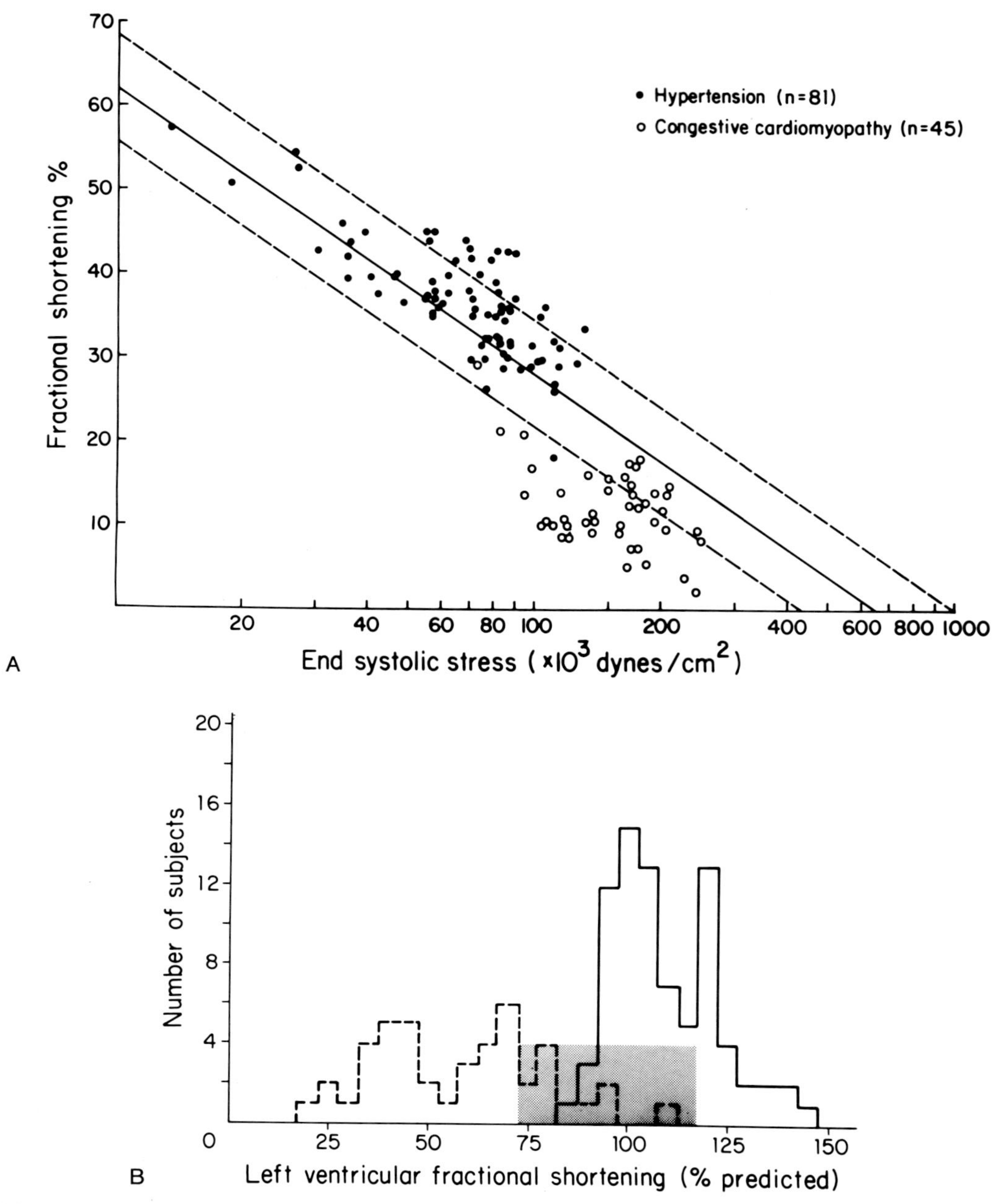

FIG. 5. Relation between echocardiographic fractional shortening and end-systolic meridional wall stress. **A:** Individual data points for 81 patients with mild essential hypertension and 45 patients with congestive cardiomyopathy are superimposed on the mean regression line and 95% confidence interval of this relationship in normal adults. **B:** Distribution of values of afterload-corrected fractional shortening reveals a bimodal distribution in hypertensive populations with one mode above the upper end of the normal range (*stippled area*), whereas downward displacement of a unimodal distribution is evident in patients with congestive cardiomyopathy. (From ref. 52.)

limits of left ventricular mass by this method are given in Table 3.

Evaluation of Left Ventricular Performance and Load

Two-dimensional echocardiography may be used to assess left ventricular volumes, ejection fraction, and load by a variety of methods. When left ventricular geometry is normal, as it usually is in patients with uncomplicated hypertension, left ventricular volumes may be most simply calculated by the long-axis length–short-axis cross-sectional area method (67). If ventricular shape or contraction pattern is abnormal, as is commonly the case when coronary artery disease coexists with hypertension, left ventricular volumes may be most accurately calculated by planimetry of the ventricular outline at end-diastole and end-systole in approximately orthogonal apical views (74). With either method of determining left ventricular volumes, the ejection fraction is calculated as follows:

TABLE 3. *Partition values for echocardiographic detection of abnormal left ventricular structure and function*

Left ventricular mass
M-mode echocardiography (Penn method):
Men: >134 g/m^2; Women: >110 g/m^2 (59)
Men: >131 g/m^2; Women: >100 g/m^2 (61)
Men: >143 g/m; Women: >102 g/m (62)
Two-dimensional truncated ellipsoid (64):
Men: >110 g/m^2; Women: >90 g/m^2
Relative wall thickness
M-mode echocardiography (ASE measurements) (42,61):
>0.45 (no gender differences)
M-mode echocardiographic measures of ventricular systolic performance and load
Fractional shortening (65):
≤26% [possible gender difference (63)]
Velocity of circumferential fiber shortening (57):
≤0.88 circumferences/second
End-systolic stress (56,58):
≤102 × 10^3 dynes/cm^2

Ejection fraction (%)

$$= \frac{\text{End-diastolic volume} - \text{End-systolic volume}}{\text{End-diastolic volume}} \times 100$$

Two-dimensional echocardiography makes it possible to assess myocardial afterload comprehensively by measuring meridional wall stress by methods analogous to those used for M-mode echocardiography and by measuring end-systolic circumferential wall stress. The best method for the latter purpose appears to utilize a formula adapted from that of Sandler and Dodge (75), which combines accuracy of absolute values with relatively low sensitivity to errors in measurement of the ventricular long-axis (72,76):

Circumferential wall stress

$$= \left(\frac{1333 \times \text{SBP} \times b^2}{h}\right) \times \left(1 - \left[\left(\frac{b}{a}\right)^{3/2} \times (2b + h)\right]\right)$$

in dynes/cm^2 where b, h, and a represent, respectively, the midwall radius and mean wall thickness in short-axis view, and the hemi-major axis.

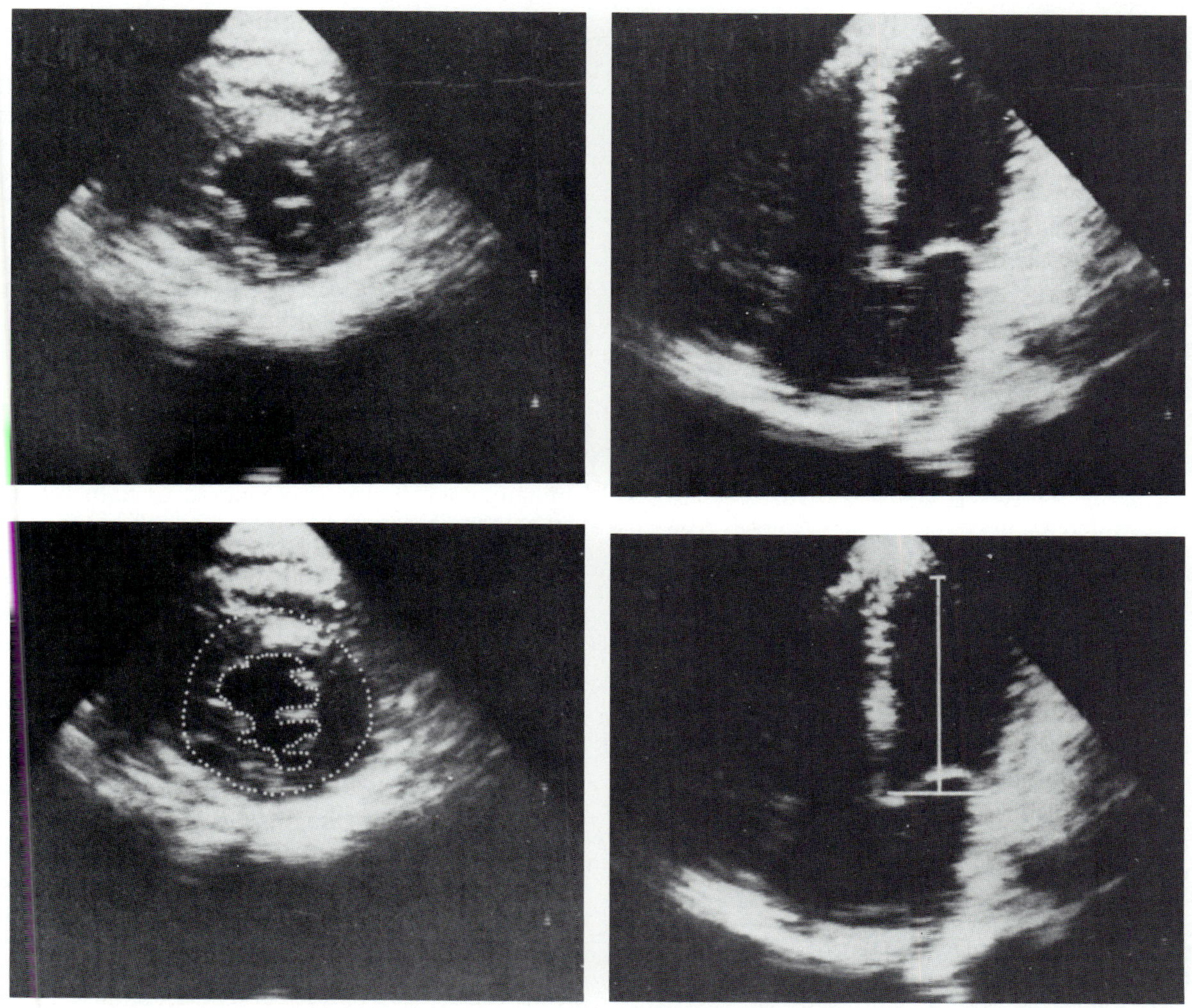

FIG. 6. Two-dimensional echocardiographic measurements needed to determine left ventricular mass by the short-axis area–long-axis length method. **A:** Planimetry of left ventricular cavity and myocardial area in short-axis views at the level of the papillary muscle tips. **B:** Measurement of long-axis length from apex to mid-mitral annular plane in apical four-chamber view. (From ref. 66.)

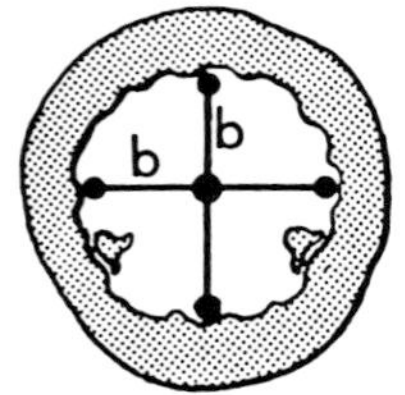

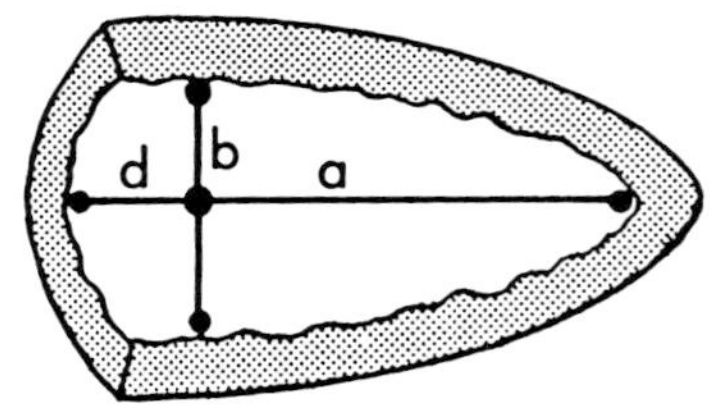

FIG. 7. Schematic depiction of measurements needed to measure left ventricular mass by the truncated ellipsoid method. a, hemi-long axis; b, hemi-short axis; d, truncated hemi-long axis at base of left ventricle. (From ref. 69.)

Doppler Echocardiographic Evaluation of Left Ventricular Diastolic Performance and Pump Function

Numerous studies have documented the frequent occurrence in patients with hypertension of abnormal left ventricular diastolic function (which may precede detectable left ventricular hypertrophy) and of deviations of cardiac output to sub- or supranormal levels. Doppler echocardiography may be used to evaluate both these facets of left ventricular performance.

For evaluation of ventricular diastolic function, reliance is placed on measurement of transmitral blood flow during the early and late phases of ventricular filling (77) (Fig. 8). The normality of early diastolic ventricular relaxation may be assessed, albeit indirectly, by measuring (a) the peak flow velocity in early diastole ("E" velocity) or (b) the integral of early diastolic flow (78,79). Similarly, the peak flow velocity in late systole ("A" velocity) and the integral of late diastolic flow will be increased by enhanced venous return or atrial Starling forces and diminished by impaired left ventricular compliance (78,79). Interpretation of Doppler findings as abnormal must be undertaken with caution because normal values are influenced by both subject age and echocardiographic technique (the E/A ratio declines with age in normal adults and is lower when measured at the mitral annular plane than at the level of the mitral orifice), whereas filling rates of diseased ventricles are affected by the level of atrial pressure (80).

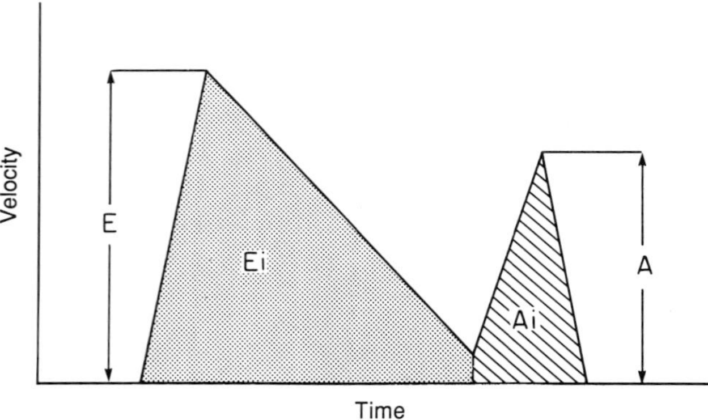

FIG. 8. Schematic depiction of transmitral blood flow in diastole as measured by Doppler echocardiography from an apical window. Early diastolic filling of the left ventricle, affected by ventricular relaxation and left atrial pressure, can be assessed by measurement of the peak early diastolic filling velocity (E) and the time–velocity integral of early diastolic filling (Ei) (*stippled area*). Late diastolic left ventricular filling, affected by ventricular stiffness, atrial pressure, and the forcefulness of atrial contraction, can be assessed by measurement of peak filling rate during atrial systole (A) and of the time–velocity integral of atrial filling (Ai) (*cross-hatched area*).

Doppler echocardiography can also be used to assess cardiac pump performance by measurement of left ventricular stroke volume. This is accomplished by measuring both the time–velocity integral of flow across a particular orifice (velocity × time = distance) and the cross-sectional area of that orifice, which yields volume as the product of cross-sectional area times the distance that blood flows per beat. In our experience and that of others (81,82), this may be most readily and accurately accomplished by using (a) Doppler recording from apical windows to record blood flow velocity across the aortic annulus and (b) two-dimensional echocardiography in the parasternal long-axis view to measure the aortic annular diameter and calculate its cross-sectional area. Normal values for this noninvasive method are not yet well established.

OTHER NONINVASIVE METHODS OF EVALUATING THE LEFT VENTRICLE

Information about the structure and function of the left ventricle can also be obtained by non-ultrasound methods that involve relatively simple or quite complex technology. Because of the desirability of obtaining prognostically important information about the heart in hypertension at the lowest possible cost, considerable effort has gone into developing improved methods for electrocardiographic detection of left ventricular hypertrophy. The most promising of these methods for routine clinical application are the Cornell voltage criteria, in which left ventricular hypertrophy is considered to be present if the sum of SV_3 and RaVL exceeds 20 mm (2.0 mV) in women or 28 mm (2.8 mV) in men (83,84). These criteria have been shown to enhance sensitivity for detection of hypertrophy with unimpaired specificity as compared to both echocardiographic and necropsy reference standards in patients with a variety of cardiovascular diseases, including hypertension (83–85). Further refinement has been achieved by use of multivariate equations that incorporate electrocardiographic voltage and other variables such as QRS duration to predict left ventricular mass (84,86). However, while Cornell voltage and multivariate methods represent improvements over traditional methods, the strength of correlation with left ventricular mass ($r^2 = 0.20–0.49$) remains considerably weaker than for echocardiographic methods ($r = 0.79–0.92$), thus limiting their usefulness in individual patients. The fact that statistically significant information about left ventricular hypertrophy continues to be detected by clinicians' qualitative electrocardiographic interpretations after application of the newer criteria (84,87) suggests that further improvement may be attained, possibly by systematic analysis of ventricular repolarization abnormalities (88,89).

At the other end of the technologic spectrum are new methods that produce highly accurate, electrocardiographically gated tomographic views of the heart. The most promising of these are cine-computed tomography and magnetic resonance imaging, both of which have been shown to yield highly accurate measurements of anatomic left ventricular mass (90,91) and of left ventricular volumes (92) in experimental animals. As yet there are no data available assessing the accuracy of these methods in determining the left ventricular mass under the difficult circumstances encountered in ill patients who come to necropsy, but it is likely that their accuracy will be at least slightly superior to that of echocardiography. Another appealing feature of cine-computed tomography of the heart is its capability of measuring coronary blood flow relatively noninvasively, with useful estimates being obtained after peripheral venous injection of radiographic contrast (93); however, precise measurements of myocardial blood flow require aortic injection of contrast (94).

EVALUATION OF REGIONAL CIRCULATIONS BY ULTRASOUND TECHNIQUES

The importance of hypertension as a cardiovascular disease depends, in large part, on its production of "target organ" damage due to coronary and cerebrovascular disease and on the compromise of organ perfusion that may ensue. Imaging and Doppler echocardiographic methods have been developed that allow measurement of the structure and blood flow characteristics of medium-sized arteries.

With use of transducers of relatively high frequency (5–10 MHz or higher), it is possible to obtain high-quality images of relatively superficial vessels such as the carotid and brachial arteries (95,96). Recent improvements in lateral and *z*-axis resolution make it possible to obtain echocardiographic images of long segments of the coronary arteries in as many as 85% of patients (21), suggesting that this technique may eventually play a role in screening for coronary artery disease. Determination of the blood flow profile across an artery and of its diameter allows measurement of regional blood flow and vascular resistance (96). Measurement of the step-up of blood flow velocity across an arterial stenosis, as in the carotid artery, allows calculation of the trans-stenosis pressure gradient as an index of its severity (14). Recent studies suggest that Doppler and imaging ultrasound techniques may permit reliable noninvasive screening for renal artery stenosis and at least qualitative assessment of its severity (97–100) (Table 4).

TECHNOLOGY AND COST-EFFECTIVENESS

Because of the high population prevalence and frequently benign long-term prognosis of essential hypertension, a screening method for accurate detection of patients at greatest risk is highly desirable. This would aid in detection of cardiovascularly normal subjects with "white coat hypertension" (101) and in assigning patients correctly to pharmacologic or nonpharmacologic treatment. M-mode echocardiographic measurement of left ventricular mass appears to be such a method based on its ability to predict prognosis in hypertensive and normotensive adults (8–11). However, because of the frequency and chronicity of essential hypertension, careful attention must be paid to the costs entailed by routine application of any laboratory test. Judged by the reference standards of cost per instance of left ventricular hypertrophy detected and of impact on several measures of research study design, echocardiography appears to be cost-effective compared to electrocardiography, when the cost of the latter is 40% that of echocardiography (7). The apparent cost-effectiveness of M-mode echocardiography as compared to electrocardiography needs to be verified by additional study using other patient populations and test costs and by assessing the relative usefulness of the techniques for prediction of prognosis.

Despite the desirable information that can be obtained by more refined methods, including two-dimensional and Doppler echocardiography as well as cine-computed tomography and nuclear magnetic resonance techniques, their higher costs (for equipment and skilled personnel to perform and interpret tests) necessitate careful scrutiny of indications for their use in patients with hypertension. Based on our experience with evaluation of large numbers of patients, it appears that the yield of information not detectable by M-mode echocardiography (e.g., regional wall motion abnormalities, unsuspected regurgitant valvular disease, etc.) is low among patients with clinically un-

TABLE 4. *Detection of renal artery stenosis by echo-Doppler methods*

			Diagnostic performance			
Number of vessels	Reference standard	Ultrasound measurement	Sensitivity (%)	Specificity (%)	Overall performance (%)	Reference
52	>50% diameter reduction of renal artery by conventional or digital subtraction angiography	Stenosis if: peak velocity > 1 m/sec; no diastolic flow; no blood flow; broad-band Doppler spectrum	89	73	81	97
44	>50% diameter reduction by contrast angiography	End systolic/peak systolic flow velocity ratio < 0.33	100	93	95	98
43	>60% diameter reduction by contrast angiography	Stenosis if renal artery/aortic peak velocity	91	95	93	100
149	>50% diameter reduction by contrast angiography	Acceleration time	100	83	87	99
		Acceleraton index	100	93	95	

complicated essential hypertension, making the cost of the incremental data quite high. Therefore, these methods should be reserved for selected clinical or research indications.

If current suggestions that M-mode echocardiographic measurements provide information of value for the routine management of patients with hypertension are verified, it would be desirable to refine methods to provide high-quality studies at the most affordable price. Because of the desirability of using two-dimensional echocardiography for M-mode beam guidance and to screen for segmental wall motion abnormalities, an echocardiograph designed for this purpose should have simple two-dimensional capabilities. However, image-enhancement algorithms and hard-copy recording and measurement systems could be optimized for M-mode measurements. Simplification of echocardiographic equipment and examination protocol might allow performance of a study suitable for hypertensive patients at as little as half the current cost of a comprehensive M-mode and two-dimensional imaging echocardiogram, although freedom should be retained to shift some patients to a complete study if findings suggestive of other heart disease are detected.

ACKNOWLEDGMENT

I would like to thank Drs. Thomas Giles, Philip R. Liebson, Riccardo Pini, and Donald C. Wallerson for their helpful suggestions on this topic, and I would also like to thank Virginia Burns for her assistance in preparation of the manuscript.

REFERENCES

1. Sokolow M, Perloff D. The prognosis of essential hypertension treated conservatively. *Circulation* 1961;23:697–713.
2. Breslin DJ, Gifford RW Jr, Fairbairn JF II. Essential hypertension: a twenty-year follow-up study. *Circulation* 1966;33:87–97.
3. Kannel WB, Abbott RD. A prognostic comparison of asymptomatic left ventricular hypertrophy and unrecognized myocardial infarction in the Framingham Study. *Am Heart J* 1986;111:391–397.
4. World Health Organization Expert Committee on Arterial Hypertension. *Arterial hypertension.* WHO Technical Report Series, No. 628. Geneva: World Health Organization, 1978.
5. Chikos PM, Figley MM, Fisher L. Correlation between chest film and angiographic assessment of left ventricular size. *AJR* 1977;128:367–373.
6. Reichek N, Devereux RB. Left ventricular hypertrophy: relationship of anatomic, echocardiographic and electrocardiographic findings. *Circulation* 1981;63:1391–1398.
7. Devereux RB, Casale PN, Wallerson DC, et al. Cost-effectiveness of echocardiography versus electrocardiography for detection of left ventricular hypertrophy in patients with systemic hypertension. *Hypertension* 1987;9(Suppl II):II-69–II-76.
8. Casale PN, Devereux RB, Milner M, et al. Value of echocardiographic measurement of left ventricular mass in predicting cardiovascular morbid events in hypertensive men. *Ann Intern Med* 1986;105:173–178.
9. Nestrova AZ, Navikov ID, Yurenev AP. Prognostic significance of blood pressure and left ventricular hypertrophy in systematic and non-systematic treatment of essential hypertension. *Kardiologia* 1986;8:89–91.
10. Levy D, Garrison RJ, Savage DD, Kannel WB, Castelli WP. Left ventricular mass and incidence of coronary heart disease in an elderly cohort: the Framingham Heart Study. *Ann Intern Med* 1989;110:101–107.
11. Koren MJ, Devereux RB, Pappas TW, et al. Echocardiographic left ventricular mass predicts complications of hypertension in both men and women [Abstract]. *Am J Hypertens* 1988;1:12A.
12. Feigenbaum H. *Echocardiography,* 4th edition. Philadelphia: Lea and Febiger, 1986.
13. Weyman AE. *Cross-sectional echocardiography.* Philadelphia: Lea and Febiger, 1982.
14. Hatle L, Angelson B. *Doppler ultrasound in cardiology: physical principles and clinical applications,* 2nd edition. Philadelphia: Lea and Febiger, 1985.
15. Young M, Goldweit R, Magid N, et al. Anatomic validation of echocardiographic left ventricular mass measurement in normal and aortic regurgitation rabbits [Abstract]. *Clin Res* 1987; 35:336A.
16. McPherson DD, Hiratka LF, Lamberth WC, et al. Delineation of the extent of coronary atherosclerosis by high-frequency epicardial echocardiography. *N Engl J Med* 1987;316:304–309.
17. Yock PG, Linker DT, Thapliyal HV, et al. Real-time two-dimensional catheter ultrasound: a new technique for high-resolution intravascular imaging [Abstract]. *J Am Coll Cardiol* 1988;11:130A.
18. Helak JW, Plappert T, Muhammed A, Reichek N. Two-dimensional echocardiographic imaging of the left ventricle: comparison of mechanical and phased-array systems *in vitro. Am J Cardiol* 1981;48:728–735.
19. Conetta DA, Geiser EA, Skorton DJ, Pandian NG, Kerber RE, Conti CR. *In vitro* analysis of boundary identification techniques used in quantification of two-dimensional echocardiograms. *Am J Cardiol* 1984;53:1374–1379.
20. Pini R, Ferruci L, DiBari M, et al. Two-dimensional echocardiographic imaging: *in vitro* comparison of conventional and dynamically focused annular array transducers. *Ultrasound Med Biol* 1987;13:643–650.
21. Douglas PS, Fiolkoski J, Berko B, Reichek N. Echocardiographic visualization of coronary artery anatomy in the adult. *J Am Coll Cardiol* 1988;11:565–571.
22. Troy BL, Pombo J, Rackley CE. Measurement of left ventricular wall thickness and mass by echocardiography. *Circulation* 1972;45:602–611.
23. Quinones MA, Pickering E, Alexander JK. Percentage of shortening of the echocardiographic left ventricular dimension: its use in determining ejection fraction and stroke volume. *Chest* 1978;74:59–65.
24. Henry WL, Clark CE, Epstein SE. Asymmetric septal hypertrophy: echocardiographic identification of the pathognomonic anatomic abnormality of IHSS. *Circulation* 1973;47:225–233.
25. Erbel R, Schweizer P, Lambertz H, et al. Echoventriculography —a simultaneous analysis of two-dimensional echocardiography and cineventriculography. *Circulation* 1983;67:205–213.
26. Schieken RM, Clarke WR, Mahoney LT, Lauer RM. Measurement criteria for group echocardiographic studies. *Am J Epidemiol* 1979;110:504–514.
27. Devereux RB, Reichek N. Echocardiographic determination of left ventricular mass in man: anatomic validation of the method. *Circulation* 1977;55:613–618.
28. Wallerson DC, Devereux RB. Reproducibility of echocardiographic left ventricular measurements. *Hypertension* 1987; 9(Suppl II):II-6–II-18.
29. Devereux RB, Liebson PR, Horan MJ. Recommendations concerning use of echocardiography in hypertension and general population research. *Hypertension* 1987;9(Suppl II):II-97–II-104.
30. Sahn DJ, DeMaria A, Kisslo J, Weyman A. The Committee on M-mode Standardization of the American Society of Echocardiography. Recommendations regarding quantitation in M-mode echocardiography: results of a survey of echocardiographic measurements. *Circulation* 1978;58:1072–1083.
31. Devereux RB, Alonso DR, Lutas EM, et al. Echocardiographic assessment of left ventricular hypertrophy: comparison to necropsy findings. *Am J Cardiol* 1986;57:450–458.
32. Daniels SR, Meyer RA, Liang Y, Bove KE. Echocardiographically determined left ventricular mass index in normal children,

adolescents and young adults. *J Am Coll Cardiol* 1988;12:703–708.

33. Woythaler JN, Singer SL, Kwan OLA. Accuracy of echocardiography versus electrocardiography in detecting left ventricular hypertrophy: comparison with post-mortem mass measurements. *J Am Coll Cardiol* 1983;2:305–311.
34. Crawford MH, Walsh RA, Cragg D, Freeman GL, Miller J. Echocardiographic left ventricular mass and function in the hypertensive baboon. *Hypertension* 1987;10:339–345.
35. Devereux RB. Detection of left ventricular hypertrophy by M-mode echocardiography. Anatomic validation, standardization, and comparison to other methods. *Hypertension* 1987;9(Suppl II):II-19–II-26.
36. Teichholz LE, Kreulen T, Herman MV, Gorlin R. Problems in echocardiographic volume determinations: echocardiographic–angiographic correlations in the presence or absence of asynergy. *Am J Cardiol* 1976;37:7–11
37. Devereux RB, Casale PN, Kligfield P, et al. Performance of primary and derived M-mode echocardiographic measurements for detection of left ventricular hypertrophy in necropsied subjects and in patients with systemic hypertension, mitral regurgitation and dilated cardiomyopathy. *Am J Cardiol* 1986;57:1388–1393.
38. Devereux RB, Casale PN, Hammond IW, Savage DD, Alonso DR, Laragh JH. Echocardiographic detection of pressure-overload left ventricular hypertrophy: effect of criteria and patient population. *J Clin Hypertension* 1987;3:66–78.
39. Grant C, Greene DG, Bunnell IL. Left ventricular enlargement and hypertrophy. A clinical and angiocardiographic study. *Am J Med* 1965;39:895–904.
40. Grossman W, Jones D, McLaurin LP. Wall stress and patterns of hypertrophy in the human left ventricle. *J Clin Invest* 1975;56:56–64.
41. Ford LE. Heart size. *Circ Res* 1976;39:297–303.
42. Reichek N, Devereux RB. Reliable estimation of peak left ventricular systolic pressure by M-mode echographic determined end-diastolic relative wall thickness: identification of severe valvular aortic stenosis in adult patients. *Am Heart J* 1982; 103:202–209.
43. Devereux RB, Savage DD, Sachs I, Laragh JH. Relation of hemodynamic load to ventricular hypertrophy and performance in hypertension. *Am J Cardiol* 1983;51:171–176.
44. Devereux RB, Pickering TG, Harshfield GA, et al. Left ventricular hypertrophy in patients with hypertension: importance of blood pressure response to regularly recurring stress. *Circulation* 1983;68:470–476.
45. Carr AA, Drexinger BR, Prisant LM. Left ventricular hypertrophy and ambulatory blood pressure [Abstract]. *Clin Res* 1986;34:476A.
46. Blake J, Devereux RB, Herrold EMcM, et al. Relation of concentric left ventricular hypertrophy and extracardiac target organ damage to supranormal left ventricular performance in established essential hypertension. *Am J Cardiol* 1988;62:246–252.
47. Rowlands DB, Glover DR, Ireland MA, et al. Assessment of left ventricular mass and its response to antihypertensive treatment. *Lancet* 1982;1:467–470.
48. Lattuada S, Rindi M, Antivalle M, Mutinelli MR, Corallo S, Libretti A. Ambulatory blood pressure monitoring (24 h), basal blood pressure and left ventricular echocardiographic findings in young adults. *J Hypertens* 1985;3(Suppl 3):s339–s341.
49. Palatini P, Mormino P, DiMarco A, et al. Ambulatory blood pressure versus casual blood pressure for the evaluation of target organ damage in hypertension: complications of hypertension. *J Hypertens* 1985;3(Suppl 3):s425–s427.
50. Gosse P, Campello G, Aouizerate E, Roudaut R, Broustet J-P, Dallochio M. Left ventricular hypertrophy in hypertension: correlation with rest, exercise and ambulatory systolic blood pressure *J Hypertens* 1986;4(Suppl 5):s297–s299.
51. Hammond IW, Devereux RB, Alderman MH, Laragh JH. Relation of blood pressure and body build to left ventricular mass in normotensive and hypertensive employed adults. *J Am Coll Cardiol* 1988;12:996–1004.
52. Devereux RB. Echocardiographic insights into the pathophysiology and prognostic significance of hypertensive cardiac hypertrophy. *Am J Hypertension* 1989;in press.
53. Gutgesell HP, Paquet M, Duff DF, McNamara DG. Evaluation of left ventricular size and function by echocardiography: results in normal children. *Circulation* 1977;56:457–462.
54. Reichek N, Wilson J, St. John Sutton M, Plappert TA, Goldberg S, Hirshfeld JW. Noninvasive determination of left ventricular end-systolic stress: validation of the method and initial application. *Circulation* 1982;65:99–108.
55. Borow KM, Green LH, Grossman W, Braunwald E. Left ventricular end-systolic stress-shortening and stress-length relations in humans: normal values and sensitivity to inotropic state. *Am J Cardiol* 1982;50:1301–1308.
56. Lutas EM, Devereux RB, Reis G, et al. Increased cardiac performance in mild essential hypertension: left ventricular mechanics. *Hypertension* 1985;7:979–988.
57. Colan SD, Borow KM, Neumann A. The left ventricular end-systolic wall stress-velocity of fiber shortening relation: a load-independent index of myocardial contractility. *J Am Coll Cardiol* 1984;4:715–724.
58. Narayan S, Devereux RB, Lutas EM, et al. Supernormal left ventricular function in essential hypertension: evidence for increased contractility [Abstract]. *J Am Coll Cardiol* 1984;3:515.
59. Devereux RB, Lutas EM, Casale PN, et al. Standardization of M-mode echocardiographic left ventricular anatomic measurements. *J Am Coll Cardiol* 1984;4:1222–1230.
60. Gardin JM, Savage DD, Ware JM, Henry WL. Effect of age, sex, and body surface area on echocardiographic left ventricular wall mass in normal subjects. *Hypertension* 1987;9(Suppl II):II-36–II-39.
61. Savage DD, Garrison RJ, Kannel WB, et al. The spectrum of left ventricular hypertrophy in a general population sample: the Framingham Study. *Circulation* 1987;75(Suppl I):I-26–I-33.
62. Levy D, Anderson KM, Savage DD, Kannel WB, Christiansen JC, Castelli WP. Echocardiographically detected left ventricular hypertrophy: prevalence and risk factors. *Ann Intern Med* 1988;108:7–13.
63. Pappas TW, Devereux RB, Blake J, Hammond IW, Alderman MH, Laragh JH. Systolic left ventricular performance is lower in normotensive and hypertensive men than women [Abstract]. *Am J Hypertens* 1988;1:12A.
64. Byrd BF III, Wahr D, Wang YS, Bouchard A, Schiller NB. Left ventricular mass and volume/mass ratio determined by two-dimensional echocardiography in normal adults. *J Am Coll Cardiol* 1985;6:1021–1025.
65. Devereux RB, Savage DD, Drayer JIM, Laragh JH. Left ventricular hypertrophy and function in patients with patients with high, normal and low-renin forms of essential hypertension. *Hypertension* 1982;4:524–531.
66. Reichek N, Helak J, Plappert T, St. John Sutton M, Weber KT. Anatomic validation of left ventricular mass estimates from clinical two-dimensional echocardiography: initial results. *Circulation* 1983;67:348–352.
67. Wyatt HL, Heng MK, Meerbaum S, et al. Cross-sectional echocardiography. I. Analysis of mathematic models for quantifying mass of the left ventricle in dogs. *Circulation* 1979;60:1104–1113.
68. Stack RS, Ramage JE, Bauman RP, Rembert JC, Phillips HR, Kisslo JA. Validation of *in vivo* two-dimensional echocardiographic dimension measurements using myocardial mass estimates in dogs. *Am Heart J* 1987;113:725–731.
69. Schiller NB, Skioldebrand CG, Schiller EJ, et al. Canine left ventricular mass estimation by two-dimensional echocardiography. *Circulation* 1983;68:210–216.
70. Geiser EA, Bove KE. Calculation of left ventricular mass and relative wall thickness. *Arch Pathol* 1974;97:13–21.
71. Byrd B III, Finkbeiner W, Bouchard A, Silverman N, Schiller NB. Factors influencing accuracy of two-dimensional echocardiographic left ventricular mass assessment [Abstract]. *J Am Coll Cardiol* 1984;3:515.
72. Florenzano F, Glanz SA. Left ventricular mechanical adaptation to chronic aortic regurgitation in intact dogs. *Am J Physiol* 1987;252:H969–H984.
73. Byrd BF III, Collins HW, Hartness WO, Kronenberg MW. Superior reproducibility of serial left ventricular mass measurements

by two-dimensional vs M-mode echocardiography [Abstract]. *J Am Coll Cardiol* 1988;11:146A.

74. Schiller NB, Acquatella H, Ports TA, et al. Left ventricular volume from paired biplane two-dimensional echocardiography. *Circulation* 1979;60:547–555.
75. Sandler H, Dodge HT. Left ventricular tension and stress in man. *Circ Res* 1963;13:91–104.
76. McHale PA, Greenfield JC Jr. Evaluation of several geometric models for estimation of left ventricular circumferential wall stress. *Circ Res* 1973;33:303–312.
77. Pearson AC, Labovitz AJ, Mrosek D, Williams GA, Kennedy HL. Assessment of diastolic function in hypertrophied hearts: comparison of Doppler echocardiography and M-mode echocardiography. *Am Heart J* 1987;113:1417–1425.
78. Stoddard MF, Pearson AC, Kern MJ, Ratcliff J, Mrosek DG, Labovitz AJ. Left ventricular diastolic function: comparison of pulsed Doppler echocardiographic and hemodynamic indexes in subjects with and without coronary artery disease. *J Am Coll Cardiol* 1989;in press.
79. Devereux RB. Left ventricular diastolic dysfunction: early diastolic relaxation and late diastolic compliance. *J Am Coll Cardiol* 1989;in press.
80. Ishida Y, Meisner JS, Tsujioka K, et al. Left ventricular filling dynamics: influence of left ventricular relaxation and left atrial pressure. *Circulation* 1986;74:187–196.
81. Wallerson DC, Dubin J, Devereux RB. Assessment of cardiac hemodynamics and valvular function by Doppler echocardiography. *Bull NY Acad Med* 1987;63:762–796.
82. Dittman H, Voelker W, Karsch K-R, Seipel L. Influence of sampling site and flow area on cardiac output measurements by Doppler echocardiography. *J Am Coll Cardiol* 1987;10:818–823.
83. Casale PN, Devereux RB, Kligfield P. Electrocardiographic detection of left ventricular hypertrophy: development and prospective validation of improved criteria. *J Am Coll Cardiol* 1985;6:572–580.
84. Casale PN, Devereux RB, Alonso DR, Campo E, Kligfield P. Improved sex-specific criteria of left ventricular hypertrophy for clinical and computer electrocardiogram interpretation: validation with autopsy findings. *Circulation* 1987;75:565–572.
85. Fiuza M, Turkman MA, Ferreira TC, Pereirinha A, dePadua F, Lopes MG. Left ventricular hypertrophy by ECG—how important is the underlying disease? [Abstract] *J Electrocardiol* 1987;20:70.
86. Rautaharju PM, LaCroix AZ, Savage DD, et al. Electrocardiographic estimate of left ventricular mass versus radiographic cardiac size and the risk of cardiovascular disease mortality in the epidemiologic follow-up study of the first National Health and Nutrition Examination Survey. *Am J Cardiol* 1988;62:59–66.
87. Devereux RB, Casale PN, Eisenberg RR, Miller DH, Kligfield P. Electrocardiographic detection of left ventricular hypertrophy using echocardiographic determination of left ventricular mass as the reference standard: comparison of standard criteria, computer diagnosis and physician interpretation. *J Am Coll Cardiol* 1984;3:82–87.
88. Devereux RB, Reichek N. Repolarization abnormalities of left ventricular hypertrophy. Clinical, echocardiographic and hemodynamic correlates. *J Electrocardiol* 1982;15:47–54.
89. Roman MJ, Kligfield P, Devereux RB, et al. Geometric and functional correlates of electrocardiographic repolarization and voltage in aortic regurgitation. *J Am Coll Cardiol* 1987;9:500–508.
90. Feiring AJ, Rumberger JA, Reiter SJ, et al. Determination of left ventricular mass in dogs with rapid-acquisition cardiac computed tomographic scanning. *Circulation* 1985;72:1355–1364.
91. Keller AM, Peshock RM, Malloy CR, et al. *In vivo* measurement of myocardial mass using nuclear magnetic resonance imaging. *J Am Coll Cardiol* 1986;8:113–117.
92. Reiter SJ, Rumberger JA, Feiring AJ, Stanford W, Marcus ML. Precision of measurements of right and left ventricular volume by cine computed tomography. *Circulation* 1986;74:890–900.
93. Rumberger JA, Feiring AJ, Lipton MJ, Higgins CB, Ell SR, Marcus ML. Use of ultrafast computed tomography to quantitate regional myocardial perfusion: a preliminary report. *J Am Coll Cardiol* 1987;9:59–69.
94. Wang T, Ritman EL. Regional myocardial perfusion—quantitation with high speed, volume scanning CT [Abstract]. *Circulation* 1987;76(Suppl IV):IV-5.
95. Langlois YE, Roederer GO, Strandness DE Jr. Ultrasonic evaluation of the carotid bifurcation. *Echocardiography* 1987;4:141–159.
96. Safar ME, Peronneau PA, Levenson JA, Toto-Moukouo JA, Simon AC. Pulsed Doppler: diameter, blood flow velocity and volumic flow of the brachial artery in sustained essential hypertension. *Circulation* 1981;63:393–400.
97. Avasthi PS, Voyles WG, Green ER. Noninvasive diagnosis of renal artery stenosis by echo-Doppler velocimetry. *Kidney Int* 1984;25:824–829.
98. Jenni R, Luscher TF, Schneider E, Vetter W, Auliker M. Combined two-dimensional ultrasound Doppler technique. *Nephron* 1986;44(Suppl 1):2–4.
99. Handa N, Fukuragu R, Etani H, Yaneda S, Kimura K, Kamada T. Efficacy of echo-Doppler examinations for the evaluation of renovascular disease. *Ultrasound Med Biol* 1988;14:1–5.
100. Kohler TR, Zierler RE, Martin RL, et al. Noninvasive diagnosis of renal artery stenosis by ultrasonic duplex scanning. *J Vasc Surg* 1986;4:450–456.
101. Pickering TG, James GD, Boddie C, Harshfield GA, Blank S, Laragh JH. How common is white coat hypertension? *JAMA* 1988;259:225–228.

Hypertension: Pathophysiology, Diagnosis, and Management, edited by J. H. Laragh and B. M. Brenner. Raven Press, Ltd., New York © 1990.

CHAPTER 93

The Evaluation of Kidney Function in Hypertensive Patients

Susanne Ljungman and Göran Granerus

Glomerular Filtration Rate, 1493
Indirect Methods for Determination of GFR, 1493
Direct Methods for Determination of GFR, 1495
Renal Circulation, 1498
Renal Plasma Flow, 1498
Renal Blood Flow, 1499
Filtration Fraction, 1499
Normal Values for RPF, RBF, and FF, 1500
Separate Kidney Function, 1500
Separate Clearance, 1500
Renography (Radioisotope Renography), 1501
Tubular Function, 1502
Proximal Tubular Function, 1502
Distal Tubular Function, 1502
Proteinuria, 1502
Albuminuria, 1502
β_2-Microglobulinuria, 1503
Kidney Function in Essential Hypertension, 1503
References, 1505

The kidney is a main target of organ damage in hypertension. Although renal hemodynamics become abnormal even in early stages of essential hypertension (1,2), the glomerular filtration rate (GFR) is usually not significantly reduced until late in the course of the disease (3,4). Elevated serum creatinine is therefore a late sign of renal damage in essential hypertension and indicates a poorer prognosis, as does the presence of proteinuria (5–9). The prevalence of renal involvement in hypertension varies with the population studied and is greater in selected patients referred to hypertension clinics than in unselected patients found by blood-pressure screening (10). The prevalence of renal involvement is also greater in studies that include patients with secondary hypertension (9,11) than in studies of patients with essential hypertension only (12), and it increases with the severity and duration of the hypertensive disease (6,11,13). This explains why the prevalence of proteinuria varies from 5% in unselected (12,14) to 18% in selected (9) hypertensive patients. The prevalence of elevated serum creatinine (>1.3 mg/100 ml or >115 μmol/liter) was 3.2% initially and 10% after 5 years of treatment in a random sample of middle-aged men with essential hypertension in the Primary Prevention Trial in Göteborg (12). In the Hypertension Detection and Follow-Up Program, which included patients with both essential and secondary hypertension, the baseline prevalence of increased serum creatinine (≥1.7 mg/100 ml or >150 μmol/liter) was 2.7% (14).

This chapter will mainly discuss the evaluation of GFR, renal circulation, tubular function, and proteinuria in the hypertensive patient.

GLOMERULAR FILTRATION RATE

GFR is often estimated by indirect methods such as the determination of serum creatinine and blood urea nitrogen (BUN) concentration. However, these methods are insensitive for the detection of early reductions in GFR and for monitoring changes in GFR. Direct methods for GFR determination are therefore used when more precise measurement of GFR is necessary.

Indirect Methods for Determination of GFR

Serum Creatinine

Creatinine is the end product of creatine metabolism in the muscles. The amount of creatinine formed is proportional to the muscle mass and is relatively constant, with a variation of about 10–15% from the mean value from day to day (15,16). Creatinine is excreted mainly by glomerular filtration and is therefore used as a marker of GFR. Since creatinine is also secreted by the tubules and may even be reabsorbed at low urine flow rates (17), it is not an ideal marker of GFR but serves as a practical index of GFR. The serum and urine concentration of creatinine varies throughout the day, with the highest values occurring in the afternoon and the lowest values occurring after midnight during sleep (16), and serum creatinine concentration may increase significantly for several hours after ingestion of well-cooked or boiled meat, which is rich in creatinine (18). Blood samples for serum creatinine should therefore be drawn in the morning under fasting conditions.

Analysis of creatinine is usually performed with the AutoAnalyzer method, which measures some noncreatinine chromogens in addition to creatinine chromogens and overestimates serum creatinine in the normal range by about 10% (19). Since these noncreatinine chromogens are not filtered, they do not appear in the urine. The analysis of creatinine with the AutoAnalyzer method therefore yields values which are closer to the true creatinine value for urine than for plasma.

Normal serum creatinine is in the range of 0.8–1.3 mg/100 ml (70–115 μmol/liter; conversion factor from mg/100 ml to μmol/liter = 88) in men and 0.6–1.2 mg/100 ml (55–105 μmol/liter) in women (16,20,21) and remains practically constant with age in adults (20–22). The serum creatinine level depends on both the muscle mass and the GFR. The greater muscle mass in relation to body size in men than in women (Table 1) explains why serum and urinary creatinine values are higher in men. The urinary creatinine excretion varies with age, from about 9 to 24 mg/kg/24 hr in males and from 8 to 20 mg/kg/24 hr in females (20) (Table 1). The relationship of serum creatinine to GFR at various amounts of muscle mass, reflected by the urinary creatinine excretion, is illustrated in Fig. 1. A subject with a serum creatinine value of 1.0 mg/100 ml may thus have a GFR of 30 ml/min to 130 ml/min, depending on the amount of muscle mass. In general, serum creatinine is unlikely to be elevated until GFR has fallen by at least 50% below normal values (23,24).

Plotting of reciprocal values of serum creatinine versus time may yield a linear relationship (16). The slope of the linear regression line for the relationship between the reciprocal of serum creatinine and time has therefore been used as a measure of the rate of change in a patient's kidney function. This procedure may, however, give misleading results if changes in the patient's muscle mass, tubular secretion of creatinine, or other factors (such as diet) that influence the serum creatinine level appear during the observation period.

To improve the estimation of GFR from serum creatinine, several formulas in which sex, age, and weight are taken into account have been developed (20,21,25). In the formula of Kampmann et al. (20) the expected urinary creatinine excretion for age and sex can be taken from a table (Table 1), and the C_{cr} can be calculated as follows:

$$C_{cr}\ (\text{ml/min}) = \frac{\text{Urinary creatinine (mg/kg/min)} \times \text{Weight (kg)} \times 100}{\text{Serum creatinine (mg/100 ml)}}$$

However, the estimated C_{cr} may also give erroneous values and may even provide a false sense of security, especially in chronically diseased patients (26,27).

TABLE 1. *Normal values for creatinine clearance, serum creatinine, and urinary creatinine excretion in males and females at different ages (mean ± SD)*[a]

Age (years)	Clearance ml/min	Clearance per 1.73 m²	Serum creatinine (mg/100 ml)	Urinary creatinine mg/24 hr	Urinary creatinine mg/kg/24 hr	Urinary creatinine mg/kg/min × 100
Males						
20–29	117 ± 23	110	0.99 ± 0.16	1625 ± 137	23.8 ± 2.3	1.65
30–39	98 ± 39	97	1.14 ± 0.22	1520 ± 130	21.9 ± 1.5	1.52
40–49	98 ± 22	88	1.10 ± 0.20	1544 ± 421	19.7 ± 3.2	1.37
50–59	88 ± 21	81	1.16 ± 0.17	1445 ± 252	19.3 ± 2.9	1.34
60–69	76 ± 22	72	1.15 ± 0.14	1252 ± 364	16.9 ± 2.9	1.17
70–79	64 ± 15	64	1.03 ± 0.22	919 ± 132	14.2 ± 3.0	0.99
80–89	45 ± 15	47	1.06 ± 0.25	651 ± 238	11.7 ± 4.0	0.81
90–99	35 ± 9	34	1.20 ± 0.16	612 ± 188	9.4 ± 3.2	0.65
Females						
20–29	91 ± 19	95	0.89 ± 0.17	1135 ± 224	19.7 ± 3.9	1.37
30–39	96 ± 25	103	0.91 ± 0.17	1218 ± 191	20.4 ± 3.9	1.42
40–49	76 ± 26	81	1.00 ± 0.24	1056 ± 256	17.6 ± 3.9	1.22
50–59	74 ± 24	74	0.99 ± 0.26	989 ± 246	14.9 ± 3.6	1.04
60–69	60 ± 15	63	0.97 ± 0.17	871 ± 283	12.9 ± 2.6	0.90
70–79	49 ± 12	54	1.02 ± 0.23	685 ± 184	11.8 ± 2.2	0.82
80–89	41 ± 14	46	1.05 ± 0.22	578 ± 154	10.7 ± 2.5	0.74
90–99	34 ± 8	39	0.91 ± 0.12	433 ± 113	8.4 ± 1.4	0.58

[a] From ref. 20.

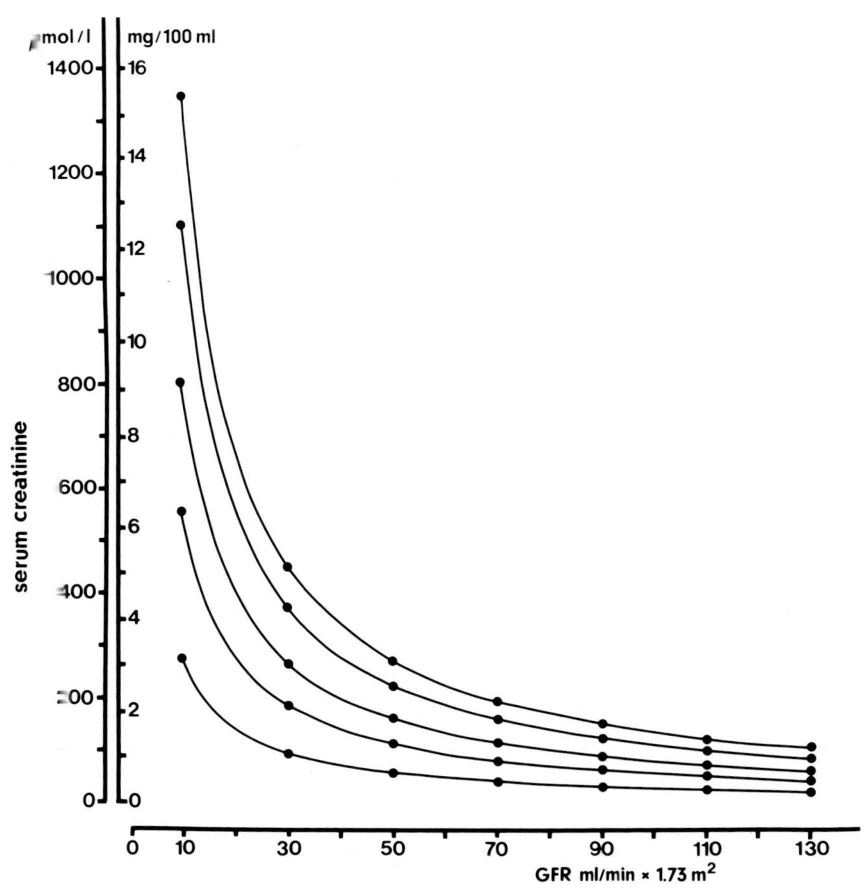

FIG. 1. The relationship between GFR and serum creatinine at different amounts of muscle mass expressed as the urinary creatinine excretion, constructed for urinary excretions of creatinine from 2.2 (*top curve*) to 1.8, 1.3, 0.9, and 0.45 (*bottom curve*) g/24 hr. (For conversion to mmol/24 hr, multiply by 88.)

BUN and Urea

Urea represents the primary end product of the hepatic protein metabolism and is measured in blood directly or as blood urea nitrogen (BUN). Urea is filtered in the kidney, and 30–70% of the filtered urea is reabsorbed by the tubules (17). The reabsorption varies with the diuresis and is highest at low urine flows (28). Urea clearance is therefore always lower than GFR, and in normal subjects it is about three-fifths of the GFR (28). Because of the variability in tubular reabsorption and in the production of urea, urea clearance does not give an accurate estimation of GFR, has a low precision, and is therefore seldom used for this purpose nowadays.

The plasma urea concentration is also influenced by the protein intake, the endogenous protein catabolism, and the state of hydration (28,29). The serum urea level can therefore vary markedly without changes in GFR and is a less reliable estimate of GFR than is serum creatinine. In patients with severely impaired renal function, urea is used as an indicator of the catabolic state and the dietary compliance with protein restriction and is better correlated with the symptoms of uremia than with the serum creatinine concentration (29). BUN gives a rough estimate of glomerular function and normally varies from 8 to 25 mg/100 ml. Plasma urea (= BUN × 2.14) is normally 15–40 mg/100 ml (3–10 mmol/liter; for conversion of mg/100 ml to mmol/liter, divide by 6).

Direct Methods for Determination of GFR

The Concept of Clearance

Clearance of a substance is defined as the volume of plasma which is completely cleared of the substance per unit time (30). The derivation of the clearance formula is based on the notion that the rate of removal of a substance "s" from plasma equals the urinary excretion of "s" at steady-state conditions. The product of the plasma concentration of "s" (P_s) and the renal plasma clearance of "s" (C_s) thus equals the product of the urinary concentration of "s" (U_s) and the urine flow (V):

$$P_s \times C_s = U_s \times V; \quad C_s = \frac{U_s \times V}{P_s}$$

For an ideal marker of GFR like inulin, which is freely filtered and neither reabsorbed nor secreted by the tubules (30), C_s equals GFR. Clearance values of substances that undergo tubular reabsorption (e.g., urea) or tubular secretion (e.g., creatinine) have also been used for estimation of GFR, but they give an underestimation and an overestimation, respectively, of GFR.

Clearance is usually expressed in ml/min and is corrected to 1.73 m² body surface area (BSA); BSA is calculated either according to the formula of Du Bois (31) or by the simpler formula of Isaksson (32), each of which gives equal values:

$$\text{BSA (m}^2) = 1 + \frac{\text{Height (cm)} - 160 + \text{Weight (kg)}}{100}$$

The corrected clearance is equal to the uncorrected clearance × 1.73 m^2, divided by the subject's BSA (m^2).

The choice of clearance method is influenced by the accuracy and precision needed, the renal function level, the laboratory equipment available, time, and cost aspects.

Clearance with Urine Collection (Standard Bladder Clearance, Renal Clearance)

Clearance with urine collection (renal clearance) is the original clearance method and necessitates a constant plasma concentration of the marker while timed complete urine collections at regular intervals are performed. This method is described in detail, for example, by Wesson (33) and Duarte (19) and will only be summarized here. After injection of the priming dose of the marker, a constant infusion is given. After an equilibrium period of about 45 min, the bladder is emptied; thereafter the first clearance period starts. The bladder must be emptied completely after each period, which is usually 30–40 min long when free voiding is practiced but may be shorter if a bladder catheter is used. The patient is hydrated before the clearance procedure, and water is then given to maintain a constant hydration. Blood samples are drawn at the midpoint of each period, and the plasma and urine concentration of the marker and the urine flow rate are determined for each period. At least three periods are needed, and the clearance values for the periods are averaged. This standard method can be used for all levels of renal function but has certain drawbacks. The procedure is time consuming, it necessitates a constant infusion, and it is not always possible to obtain complete emptying of the bladder without catheterization. If radiolabeled markers are used, the analysis of the samples is simplified. Other sources of error are (a) rapid changes in the plasma concentration of the marker, which makes it difficult to obtain a representative plasma sample, and (b) rapid increases and decreases in the urine flow rate, which cause erroneously high and low clearance values, respectively (17). The coefficient of variation (C.V.) between clearance periods is reported to be less than 10% (34).

Clearance without Urine Collection (Plasma Clearance)

The plasma clearance is determined from the plasma disappearance curve of a marker after a single injection. After equilibrium of the marker in its volume of distribution, the rate of decline in plasma concentration of the marker is assumed to be (a) constant and (b) related to the elimination of the marker by the kidney. In order for the plasma clearance to equal the renal clearance, the ideal marker for plasma clearance would be stable and would be eliminated only by the kidneys. Some radiolabeled tracers used for the determination of plasma clearance have a small extrarenal elimination, which is of practical importance only when very low renal function is measured (35) and can usually be corrected (36). It is also important that the tracer is stable and not protein bound.

Clearance Calculated from the Infusion Rate

When the continuous infusion technique is used, clearance may also be accurately calculated from only the infusion rate and the plasma levels of the marker during steady-state conditions without urine collection (37,38). The excretion rate is then assumed to equal the infusion rate. The product of the concentration of the marker in the infusion fluid and the velocity of the infusion is used instead of $U \times V$ in the clearance formula. Clearance of para-aminohippurate (PAH) is, however, overestimated by this method (37), presumably due to extrarenal elimination of PAH, even after an equilibration period as long as 4 hours.

Inulin Clearance (C_{in})

Inulin is a polymer of fructose (M.W. 5200) and fulfills all the requirements of an ideal marker of GFR (30). C_{in} has been used for more than 50 years and is a reference method for determination of GFR. The inulin analog polyfructosan (Inutest) has the same properties as inulin but is more water-soluble (39) and is therefore more widely used than inulin. It is determined by the same method and is equally as good a marker of GFR as inulin (39). Inulin is analyzed by a colorimetric technique (19,40).

Other Markers for GFR

A number of isotope-labeled indicators have been tested and found to correlate well with the results obtained with inulin (Table 2). Iothalamate labeled with ^{131}I (or ^{125}I) and ^{51}Cr-EDTA are widely used as markers of GFR. The latter is extensively used in Europe but is not approved for GFR measurements in the United States. ^{99m}Tc-DTPA is much used as an agent for gamma camera renography. Its usefulness for GFR measurement is well documented, but the accuracy of the results will depend on the extent of plasma protein binding, which varies with the source of preparation (41). A comprehensive survey of the characteristics of these tracers has been published by Dubovsky and Russel (42).

Because of the high reliability of the method (27) and lack of need for urine collection, the plasma clearance of ^{51}Cr-EDTA has become the routine method in many centers. The strictly standardized procedure makes the method particularly useful for research purposes as well as in all clinical conditions where serum creatinine is not reliable. The current status of assessment of GFR by different techniques has recently been summarized by Bröchner-Mortensen (27).

TABLE 2. *Indicators used for GFR and ERPF measurements*

Compound	Isotope	Measurement
Inulin	—	GFR
Iothalamate (Conray)	^{125}I, ^{131}I	GFR
Diatrizoate (Hypaque)	^{131}I	GFR
EDTA	^{51}Cr	GFR
DTPA	^{99m}Tc, ^{113}In, ^{140}La, ^{169}Yb	GFR
PAH	—	ERPF
Iodohippurate (Hippuran)	^{123}I, ^{125}I, ^{131}I	ERPF
Iodopyracet (Diodrast)	^{131}I	ERPF
MAG_3 (Mercaptoacetylglycylglycylglycine)	^{99m}Tc	ERPF

Creatinine Clearance (C_{cr})

The endogenous creatinine clearance is widely used as a measure of GFR. C_{cr} is calculated as the urinary concentration of creatinine (mg/100 ml) multiplied by the urine flow rate (ml/min), divided by the serum creatinine concentration (mg/100 ml); the value is corrected for 1.73 m^2 BSA. Urine is usually collected over a 24-hr period, but an accurate 24-hr urine collection is extremely difficult to achieve. This is one of the reasons why the day-to-day variation of C_{cr} is about 25% (C.V.) (27). Another explanation for the variation of C_{cr} is the day-to-day variation of the urinary creatinine excretion, which varies between 5% and 15% (C.V.) in outpatients (19) and is more than 10% among hospitalized patients (21,43). To increase the precision of the method, the mean of at least two or three consecutive C_{cr} determinations should be used.

The C_{cr} exceeds the inulin clearance by 10–40% (35,44–46) because creatinine is eliminated by tubular secretion as well as by glomerular filtration. With increasing impairment of renal function, the tubular excretion of creatinine is enhanced, and the creatinine/inulin clearance ratio increases with falling renal function to a GFR of about 20 ml/min; thereafter C_{cr} comes closer to GFR (47). This ratio normally varies and is found to increase after hydration and decrease after dehydration (48). When creatinine is

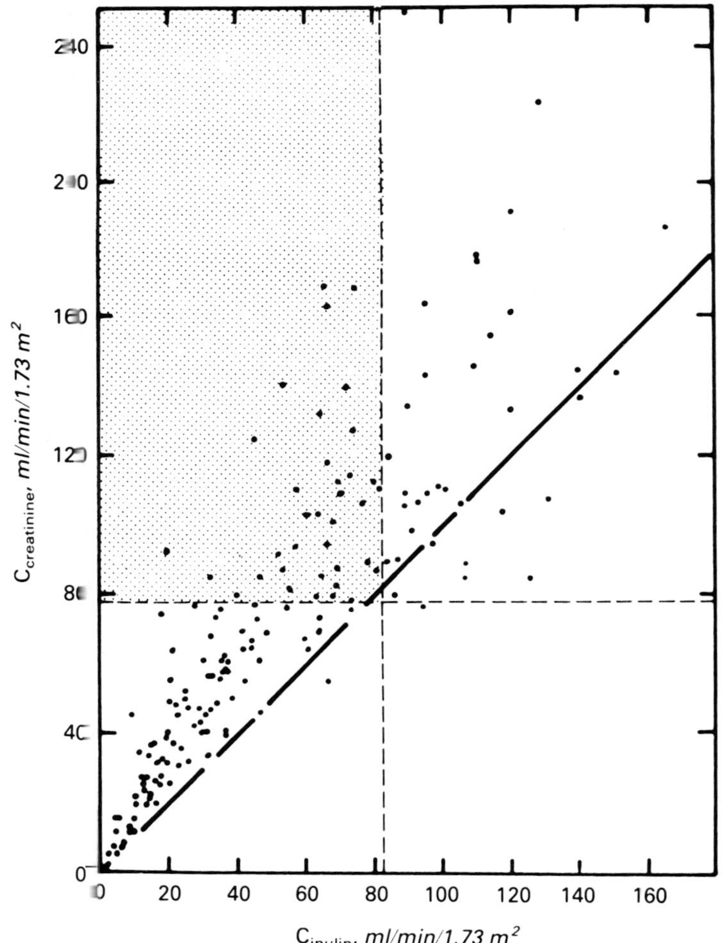

FIG. 2. The relationship between creatinine clearance (C_{cr}) and inulin clearance (C_{in}) in glomerulopathic patients. C_{cr} was generally higher than C_{cr}, and many patients having C_{cr} values within the normal range had a reduced C_{in} (*stippled zone*). (From ref. 24.)

determined by autoanalyzer or similar methods, the creatinine/inulin clearance ratio is normally 1.2–1.3 (2,44) and remains at this level in mild to moderate essential hypertension (2) but may be as high as 2.0–4.0 in some glomerular disorders (49).

For these reasons, C_{cr} gives only an approximation of the true GFR (29). For the detection of early impairment of GFR, C_{cr} is not a reliable method. For example, in a study of patients who were considered to have normal renal function ($C_{cr} \geq 90$ ml/min), 42% of the patients had GFRs of 61–70 ml/min while 23% had GFRs of 51–60 ml/min (44). The poor correlation of C_{cr} to C_{in} is illustrated in Fig. 2. Because of the low precision and the spontaneous variation of C_{cr}, the use of this method as the sole method for measurement of GFR is not recommendable in clinical trials of specific therapies or in studies of the progression of disease, especially not in glomerulopathic patients (24).

Normal Values for GFR

GFR starts to decline after the age of 30 according to Davies and Shock (50). They found that GFR dropped by 46% (from 123 to 65 ml/min) between 20 and 80 years of age. The decline of GFR is about 4 ml/min per decade below the age of 50 and about 10 ml/min per decade thereafter (51,52). Figure 3 shows the normal range for GFR in relation to age in terms of ^{51}Cr-EDTA plasma clearance, which is 105 ± 26 (mean ± 2 S.D.) ml/min/1.73 m^2 at 30 years, 98 ± 23 ml/min/1.73 m^2 at 50 years, and 78 ± 24 ml/min/1.73 m^2 at 70 years (52). Both GFR and renal blood flow decline during exercise and after emotional stress (33) and increase after high protein intake (33,53) and during pregnancy (33).

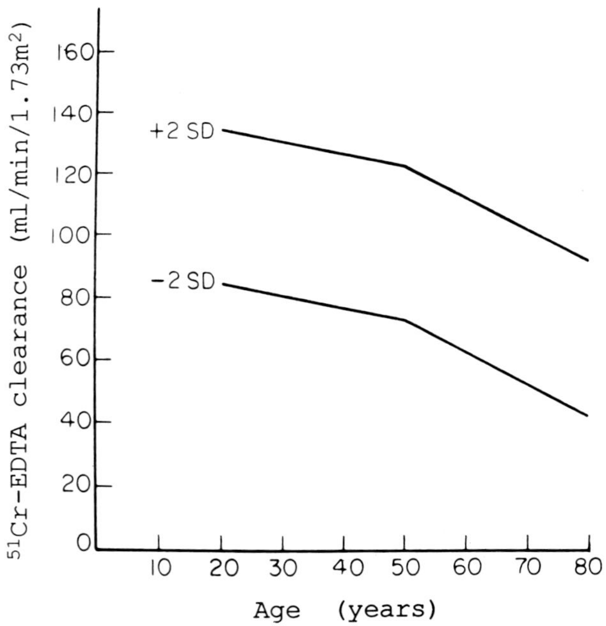

FIG. 3. Normal range of ^{51}Cr-EDTA-clearance in relation to age. Upper and lower normal limits are defined by mean ± 2 S.D. (n = 503). There is no sex difference after correction to 1.73 m^2 BSA. (From ref. 52.)

RENAL CIRCULATION

Renal Plasma Flow

Measurement of renal plasma flow (RPF) by the clearance technique is based on Fick's principle for the removal of an indicator substance (30). The ideal indicator for RPF measurement would be eliminated only through the kidneys, would be cleared unchanged, and would be cleared completely in one passage through the kidney by glomerular filtration and tubular secretion without being reabsorbed, and its arteriovenous difference would be so high that the renal venous concentration of the marker would be close to zero (30). According to Fick's principle the excreted amount of the indicator substance, "s", equals RPF multiplied by the arteriovenous difference of "s":

$$U_s \times V = \text{RPF}(A_s - V_s)$$

where U_s is the urinary concentration of "s", V is the urine flow rate, and A_s and V_s are the arterial and renal venous plasma concentrations of "s". This gives

$$\text{RPF} = \frac{U_s \times V}{A_s - V_s}$$

All clinically used indicators of RPF are not totally cleared from plasma after one passage through the kidney, and their clearances thus underestimate the renal plasma flow. The ability of the kidney to clear a substance is determined by the extraction ratio (E), which is calculated as

$$E_s = \frac{A_s - V_s}{A_s}$$

where E_s is the extraction ratio of "s". The extraction determination thus requires renal vein catheterization for the sampling of renal venous blood. Arterial blood can be substituted by a peripheral vein sample at steady state.

Given the extraction ratio of a substance, the true RPF can be calculated from its clearance (C_s) as

$$\text{True RPF} = \frac{C_s}{E_s}$$

In clinical studies, the true RPF flow is seldom determined because the error introduced by incomplete extraction is small and relatively constant. The renal plasma flow determined without correction for the extraction ratio is called the *effective renal plasma flow* (ERPF). One of the earliest markers of RPF was iodopyracet (Diodrast), but it was soon replaced by para-aminohippurate (PAH) because PAH has a higher extraction ratio (30,54).

PAH Clearance

PAH is an almost ideal marker of RPF, and PAH clearance (C_{PAH}) is the most widely used method clinically and experimentally for determination of ERPF. PAH is filtered

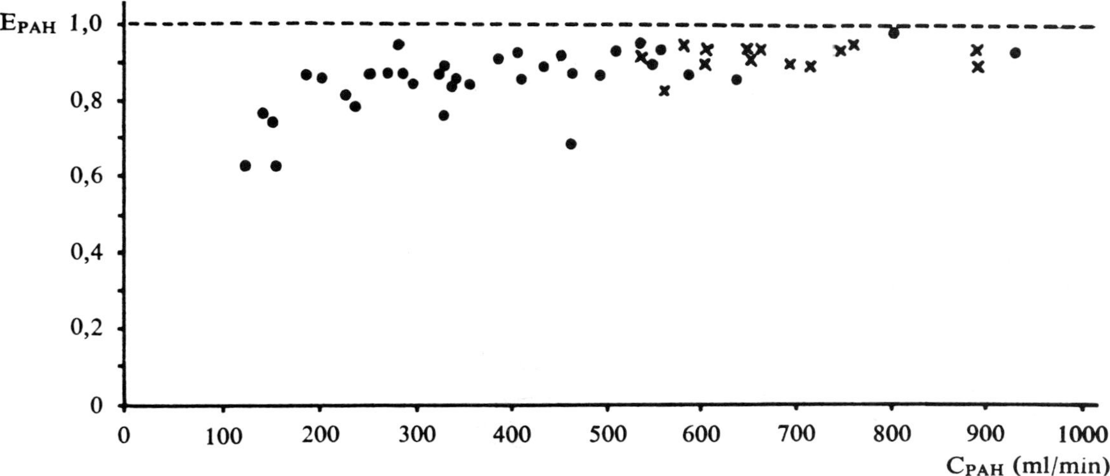

FIG. 4. Extraction of PAH (E_{PAH}) in relation to PAH clearance in patients with essential hypertension (●) and in healthy controls (×). (From ref. 57.)

at the glomerulus and excreted by the tubules and has an average extraction ratio (E_{PAH}) of 0.91 (range 0.81–1.0) in normal subjects (30). The variation of E_{PAH} is dependent on (a) the tubular load of PAH, (b) tubular function, and (c) plasma flow rate. Thus, E_{PAH} will fall if the plasma concentration of PAH exceeds a certain level (30,33). E_{PAH} may also fall if RPF is much increased in normal subjects —for example, by plasma volume expansion (55), which may be explained by reduced time available for complete PAH extraction.

C_{PAH} is determined in the same way as C_{in} (19,33) and often simultaneously with the determination of GFR. E_{PAH} is reduced in various renal diseases (30,56). In essential hypertension, however, E_{PAH} is found to be normal except in very advanced stages (57), as illustrated in Fig. 4, and is not considered to be substantially reduced until C_{PAH} is reduced below 300 ml/min (30).

^{131}I-Hippurate Clearance

The PAH analog ^{131}I-hippurate (Hippuran) is the radiolabeled marker most widely used for measurement of RPF. The error of estimation was found to be lower than with the more classic PAH clearance. The extraction of Hippuran is, however, lower than for PAH, and an average Hippuran extraction of 0.74 was found in a study of hypertensive patients (58). Hippuran clearance therefore underestimates PAH clearance by 10–20% (59).

ERPF can be estimated by means of a single plasma concentration determination after injection of ^{131}I-Hippuran (60). This test is based on a regression equation which relates (a) the plasma concentration of injected Hippuran at a specific sampling time to (b) ERPF derived by other means. A blood sample drawn at 44 min after the injection gives the most accurate estimate of ERPF compared to conventional PAH clearance. This method was recently compared with the two-sample method described by Blaufox and Merrill (61). The correlation between the methods was excellent although the two-sample method gave values of ERPF, which were 15% higher than those obtained with the one-sample method (62).

Renal Blood Flow

Renal blood flow (RBF) can be calculated from ERPF if the hematocrit (Hct; normal range 0.40–0.50) is known:

$$\text{RBF} = \frac{\text{ERPF}}{1 - \text{Hct}}$$

If E_{PAH} is known, the true RBF is obtained by dividing the achieved value of effective RBF (ERBF) by E_{PAH} (30).

RBF can also be measured by indicator dilution (e.g., with dye) as well as by washout of radioactive inert gas (krypton and xenon) injected into the renal artery (63). RBF can be measured separately in the two kidneys by thermodilution technique, but this method is invalidated by many sources of error (64,65). Noninvasive measurement of RBF by echo Doppler technique has lately been used (66).

Renal Vascular Resistance

The renal vascular resistance (RVR) is calculated as the ratio of mean arterial pressure (MAP) and RBF and is usually expressed in mmHg × min/liter or dynes × sec/cm^{-5}.

Filtration Fraction

The filtration fraction (FF) gives the fraction of renal plasma flow that is filtered at the glomerulus and is usually calculated as the inulin/PAH clearance ratio. The renal clearance of inulin provides the correct value of GFR,

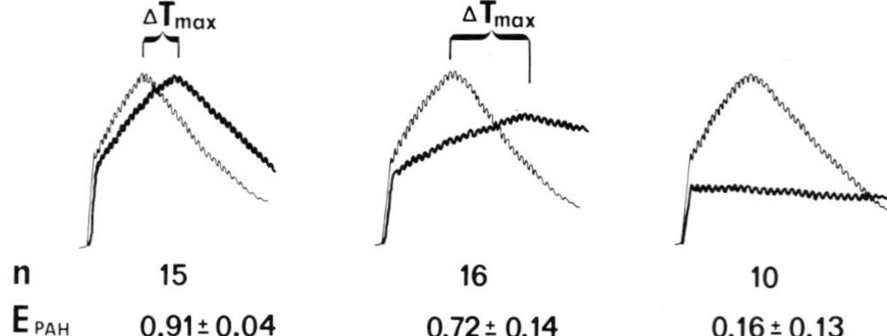

FIG. 5. ^{131}I-Hippuran renograms in three groups of patients with unilateral renal artery stenosis and mean PAH extraction (E_{PAH}) on the stenotic side ($n = 41$). Patients were divided into three groups, depending on the severity of the depression of the uptake phase on the stenotic side. ΔT is the interpeak interval between the renogram of the stenotic side (*thick lines*) and the renogram of the normal contralateral side (*thin lines*). The E_{PAH} values decreased with increasing severity of the renographic changes. The E_{PAH} values for the contralateral kidney were in the normal range in all three groups, 0.93 ± 0.03 (mean ± S.D.). (Granerus, Delin, and Aurell, *unpublished observations*).

whereas PAH clearance underestimates true RPF by a factor corresponding to E_{PAH}. Thus,

$$FF = \frac{GFR}{RPF} = \frac{C_{in}}{C_{PAH}/E_{PAH}} = \frac{E_{PAH} \times C_{in}}{C_{PAH}}$$

In normal kidneys, E_{PAH} is above 0.90 and the FF can be measured with reasonable accuracy by clearance measurements alone. Since E_{PAH} may be considerably reduced in diseased kidneys (30,56), the factor E_{PAH} should be measured together with the clearances. This is especially important in patients with renal vascular hypertension (RVH), because the renal extraction could be severely disturbed on the stenotic side (see Fig. 5), causing a falsely high calculated FF value on that side. In fact, such a reduction in extraction capacity can normalize a low true FF, and similar filtration fractions in the two kidneys in patients with unilateral renal artery stenosis have therefore been a common finding (67,68).

There are few published data regarding true FF values in patients with essential hypertension. The inulin/PAH clearance results are not misleading, however, because (a) the destruction of renal tissue is a late phenomenon in hypertension and (b) E_{PAH} declines slowly, attaining values of 0.6–0.7 only when GFR is 25–30% of normal (33,57). In hypertension, the FF is usually increased because of the proportionally greater impairment of RPF than of GFR. Although a pure increase in preglomerular arteriolar resistance in a circulatory model will lower FF while a pure increase in postglomerular resistance will raise FF (30,69), the pre- and postglomerular resistances may change in parallel in response to a vasoconstrictor or a vasodilator agent; changes in FF alone can therefore not be used as measures of alterations in segmental vascular resistances (69).

Another way of determining the FF is by measuring the renal extraction of a filtration marker, inulin (70) [or, more conveniently, ^{125}I-iothalamate (71), ^{51}Cr-EDTA (72), or ^{99m}Tc-DTPA], according to the formula

$$FF = \frac{GFR}{RPF} = \frac{E_{in} \times RPF}{RPF} = E_{in}$$

This approach is preferred when one is interested in the FF of the individual kidney, and it is easily applied to patients who are subjected to bilateral renal vein catheterization for renin analysis (71,73).

A third technique which might be useful in clinical practice is the simultaneous measurement of GFR and RPF by gamma camera renography (74). GFR is estimated from (a) the uptake slope of a filtration marker like ^{99m}Tc-DTPA and (b) the plasma flow from the initial flow peak of the same renographic curve. In the near future, noninvasive determination of split-kidney FF will probably be an important tool in the investigation of renal hemodynamics in patients with unilateral renal disease as well as during treatment with drugs affecting the GFR. The diagnostic value of separate FF determination in differentiating patients with renal artery stenosis (RAS) from patients with essential hypertension or pyelonephritis was demonstrated by Bianchi et al. (75) in 1978 by a somewhat different technique.

Normal Values for RPF, RBF, and FF

ERPF declines successively with age, from a mean value of 614–619 ml/min/1.73 m^2 at the age of 20, to 500–516 ml/min/1.73 m^2 at the age of 40, to 431–442 ml/min/1.73 m^2 at the age of 60, to less than 300 ml/min/1.73 m^2 at the age of 80 (50,51). The mean ERPF values are slightly lower in women than in men according to nomograms of C_{PAH} in relation to age presented by Wesson (33).

ERBF declines with age in men, from a mean of 1077 ml/min/1.73 m^2 at 20 years, to 1008 ml/min/1.73 m^2 at 40 years, to 775 ml/min/1.73 m^2 at 60 years, to 475 ml/min/1.73 m^2 at 80 years (50).

FF normally varies between 0.18 and 0.22 and increases slightly with age, from a mean of 0.19 at 20 years, to 0.21 at 40 years, to 0.22 at 60 years (51).

SEPARATE KIDNEY FUNCTION

Separate Clearance

The main purpose of performing a split function test in hypertensive patients is to exclude secondary forms of hypertension, primarily renal artery stenosis (RAS). There are three methods available for this purpose: (i) isotope renography, (ii) clearance measurements with bilateral ureteral catheters, and (iii) rapid sequence urography. Isotope renography has been the method of choice in many centers since its introduction in 1956 (76). It is cheap, rapid, and noninvasive and has completely replaced separate clearance measurements with bilateral ureteral catheterization. In fact, there is no routine method other than renography for correct evaluation of the side distribution of kidney function. It is also possible to obtain an estimation of the absolute value of GFR for each kidney without any blood sample or urine collection by utilizing modern gamma camera technique (77,78).

RAS may be detected by rapid sequence urography if the stenosis is severe, but this method has low sensitivity and specificity (79). Although all renal artery stenoses are discovered by renal angiography, many of them are not clinically significant, since the renin secretion from the affected kidney may not be increased. Renal vein renin measurements are therefore also needed.

Renography (Radioisotope Renography)

Renography performed with two separate detectors located over each kidney region is called *probe renography* or *two-detector renography*. The fundamentals of the method are elaborately described by Britton and Brown (80), and only a few aspects of the renographic technique in the screening of RVH will be discussed here.

In skilled hands, probe renography with ^{131}I-Hippuran may be quite useful for screening of RVH. Sensitivity and specificity around 90% have been reported for this type of study (81). Normal renograms without significant side differences effectively rule out RAS as the cause of hypertension. In patients with significant RAS, Hippuran renography shows the typical stenotic pattern on the affected side as demonstrated in Fig. 5. This pattern is caused by a reduced urine flow on the stenotic side, affecting the time to maximum curve (T_{max}) and the excretory phase, which are delayed. The uptake phase may not be affected at all, because Hippuran uptake is mainly the result of an active secretion by the tubular cells and because this process is often well preserved in patients with moderate stenosis and short duration of the disease.

The delay in T_{max}, or rather the difference in T_{max} between the two sides (ΔT_{max}), is highly dependent on the overall diuresis, i.e., the combined urine flow of the two kidneys that can be measured at the investigation. During low diuresis, ΔT_{max} increases substantially, whereas during high diuresis the side difference in T_{max} may not be detectable, as illustrated in Fig. 6. In our experience, the overall diuresis during the renographic examination should ideally be 2–3 ml/min (in the sitting position) in order to obtain the highest sensitivity and specificity; this is because with high diuresis the sensitivity decreases as a result of the less prominent stenotic pattern of the renogram, whereas with low diuresis the specificity decreases as a result of the appearance of side differences in the excretory phase produced by normally occurring small variations in pelvic volumes or by peristaltic activity of the urinary tracts. It should be noted that these normal variations are more often seen on the right side than on the left side, especially in women who have been pregnant (82). We strongly advocate measurement of the diuresis during the test and recommend repeating the renographic examination after hydration or dehydration of the patient if the diuresis was too low or too high, respectively.

The inherent problem with Hippuran renography in the screening of RVH is that it cannot differentiate between RAS and dilatation of the renal pelvis, since a reduced urine flow and an increased pelvic volume affect the renographic curve in the same way (83). Furthermore, the change in ΔT_{max} produced by these two mechanisms runs a parallel course at all levels of urinary flow rate, as shown in Fig. 6. Additional diagnostic problems arise when there are

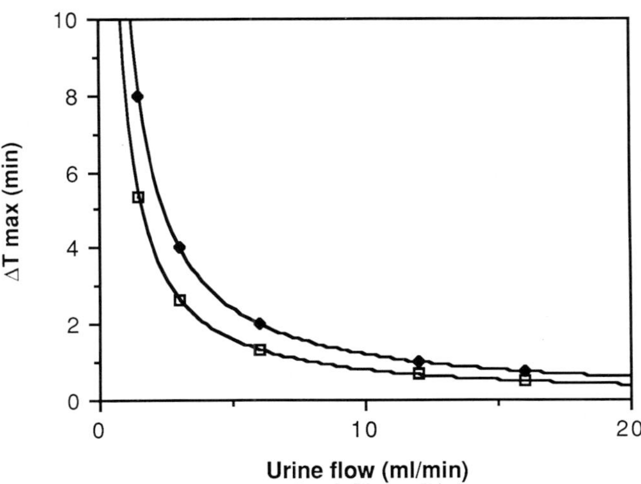

FIG. 6. Relationship between urine flow and difference in time to peak of the renogram on the affected side compared to the contralateral side (interpeak interval, ΔTmax). Filled symbols represent renal artery stenosis producing 50% lower urine flow on the stenotic side. Unfilled symbols represent pelvic dilatation with 50% larger pelvic volume on the affected side.

bilateral stenoses or when the kidneys have reduced function as a result of conditions other than RAS.

To increase the specificity of the renographic technique, one possibility is to make use of the hemodynamic influence of the artery stenosis on GFR and FF. The GFR and FF in a kidney with reduced perfusion pressure tend to be lower than in a normally perfused kidney, although compensatory mechanisms, including the renin–angiotensin system, strive to counteract the drop in filtration pressure by vasoconstriction of the efferent arteriole. Renography performed with an indicator excreted by glomerular filtration, like ^{99m}Tc-DTPA, before and after acute inhibition of the renin–angiotensin system by converting-enzyme inhibition (CEI), is therefore a logical step to achieve higher specificity of the test (71). The full diagnostic potential of renography during CEI is not yet settled, partly because the complex physiologic mechanisms regulating GFR are not fully clarified and partly because the renographic technique with ^{99m}Tc-DTPA requires sophisticated subtraction of background activity for the precise determination of changes in split-kidney GFR. A modern gamma camera with a computer provides these technical facilities, and the renographic examination is basically equivalent to probe renography. Because the location of the kidneys with a gamma camera is no longer a problem, side differences in GFR of each kidney and the excretory phases can be recorded with high reproducibility (78). When the uptake of the indicator in the parenchyma is of primary interest, it is not necessary to control the urine flow rate.

Theoretically, Hippuran or any other tubular-secreted indicator like MAG_3 (84) is less suitable for the captopril radionuclide test for two reasons. Firstly, the possibility of studying changes in GFR is lost; secondly, the renographic pattern will be diuresis-dependent. However, in patients with very tight RAS or poor renal function, Hippuran may provide a more sensitive alternative, since GFR on the stenotic side is close to zero and can change only marginally (85). It is important to stress that the renal uptake of Hippuran or MAG_3 (uptake = clearance = RPF × extracting capacity) does not represent the side distribution of RPF in patients with RAS, since the extraction capacity of the tubular cells is often impaired on the stenotic side (Fig. 5). In contrast, Hippuran renograms could be very useful for follow-up studies after reconstructive surgery or percutaneous transluminal angioplasty of the renal artery to record the gradual restitution of tubular cell function. In our experience, the stenotic pattern disappears immediately after successful intervention, whereas the recovery of Hippuran uptake can progress for months. This slow improvement of the active secretion of Hippuran may reflect a reversible tubular cell atrophy behind the stenosis.

TUBULAR FUNCTION

Disturbances in the tubular reabsorption or secretion capacity may influence the handling of substances used for determination of GFR and RPF. The maximal tubular function is dependent not only on the tubular mass but also on the renal circulation and may be inhibited by various drugs (33).

Proximal Tubular Function

PAH Extraction

PAH is secreted in the proximal tubules, and the E_{PAH} is maximal only when the plasma concentration of PAH is below 3–4 mg/100 ml (33). E_{PAH} remains normal until parenchymal loss is severe (33), and it is therefore reduced in chronic parenchymal renal disease (33,56). The secretion is depressed by probenecid, phenylbutazone, barbiturates, and diodrast, presumably competitively (33).

Lithium Clearance (C_{Li})

Lithium ions are reabsorbed in the proximal tubules only. Since these ions are reabsorbed in the same proportion as sodium and water, lithium clearance can be used as a measure of proximal sodium reabsorption (86). By the simultaneous determination of sodium clearance, C_{Li}, and GFR, the reabsorption of sodium and water in the proximal and distal tubule can be separated. C_{Li} is normal in patients with essential hypertension, but it increases in response to infusion of isotonic saline (87).

β_2-Microglobulin

β_2-Microglobulin (M.W. 11,600) is freely filtered at the glomerulus and is almost totally reabsorbed in the proximal tubules. It is mostly used as an indicator of proximal tubular damage (e.g., due to heavy metal poisoning) but has also been proposed as a better marker of GFR than endogenous creatinine clearance, especially for the detection of early impairment of GFR (27). However, the plasma concentration of β_2-microglobulin becomes elevated without relation to GFR in certain malignant disorders, immunological diseases, and septicemia (27). β_2-microglobulin is analyzed by radioimmunoassay.

Distal Tubular Function

Renal Concentrating Capacity

The concentration of urine in response to the antidiuretic hormone takes place in the distal tubule. The human kidney can maximally concentrate to 1300 mOsm/kg H_2O [specific gravity (S.G.) 1.040] (88). Deterioration of the urine concentrating capacity is characteristic of tubulo-interstitial diseases even before GFR is reduced, and it is seen in late stages of essential hypertension (89). The osmolality of urine is measured by determination of its freezing point depression (88).

The maximal concentrating capacity can be determined after fluid deprivation for 24 hours or more (the fluid deprivation test), after which the urine osmolality should be ≥800 mOsm/kg H_2O (S.G. 1.022) (88).

The vasopressin tannate-in-oil test (the Pitressin test) has been the standard concentration test for many years. It necessitates fluid deprivation for about 16 hours and may raise the blood pressure. Pitressin has been replaced by Desmopressin, a synthetic analog of vasopressin (desamino-*d*-arginine-vasopressin, DDAVP) which has no vasoactive effects in antidiuretic doses, has a shorter duration of action and can be administered after minimal or no fluid restriction (90). However, overnight fluid deprivation is recommended before desmopressin is administered. It is usually given intranasally (90,91) but can also be injected intramuscularly (90) or subcutaneously (92). The osmolality is determined in urine passed 1 and 3 hours after the administration of Desmopressin. The urine osmolality after Desmopressin correlates well with the values for the Pitressin test (91) and the 24-hr fluid deprivation test (93). The renal concentrating capacity declines with age, from 982 ± 214 mOsm/kg H_2O (mean ± 2 S.D.) at 20 years to 823 ± 278 mOsm/kg H_2O at 80 years (92). A nomogram is shown in Fig. 7. According to this, the lowest acceptable value for maximal urine osmolality (mean–2 S.D.) is 850 mOsm/kg H_2O at 20 years, 800 mOsm/kg H_2O at 40 years, 700 mOsm/kg H_2O at 60 years, and 600 mOsm/kg H_2O at 80 years.

PROTEINURIA

The mean normal urinary protein excretion is found to vary from 24 to 133 mg/24 hr in different studies, depending on the determination method used (94).

Albuminuria

Approximately 40% of the urinary protein consists of albumin (M.W. 69,000) (94), which is normally filtered to a

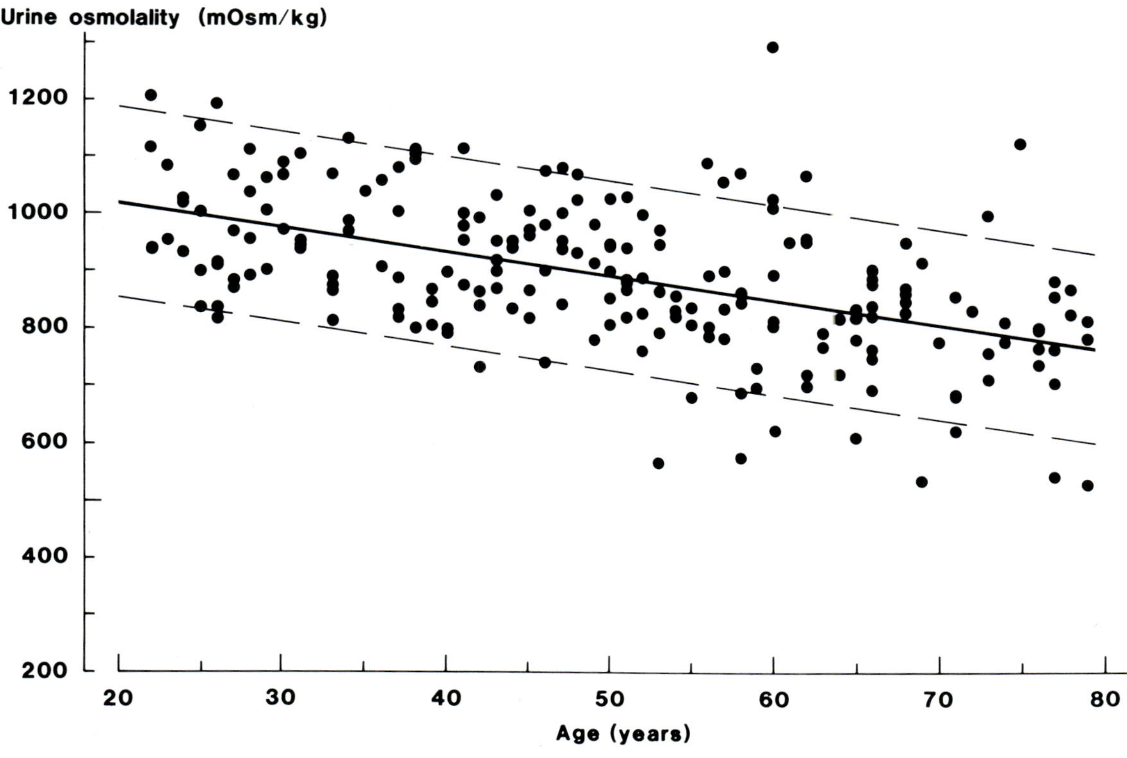

FIG. 7. Nomogram of renal concentrating capacity (Desmopressin test) in relation to age (mean ± S.D.). (From ref. 92.)

minimal extent. The urinary albumin excretion averages 7.1–8.5 mg/24 hr in normal humans (94–96). The commonly used qualitative dipstick test (Albustix) can only detect albumin concentrations of >200 mg/l (97), which explains why the urinary albumin excretion may be increased even if no proteinuria is detected by Albustix. The urinary albumin excretion within the range from the normal level to the detection limit for Albustix (approximately 30–300 mg/24 hr) is referred to as *microalbuminuria* (98). It can be detected by a new rapid qualitative latex agglutination test, which has a sensitivity of 25 mg/liter (99). The quantitation of the 24-hr urinary albumin excretion may give useful information for the treatment of hypertensive patients. The quantitative urinary albumin concentration is determined by radioimmunoassay, immunochemical techniques, and other methods, as reviewed by Mogensen (98).

Albuminuria and Hypertension

In hypertension, the urinary albumin excretion is increased and is correlated to the blood-pressure level (95,100,101). It has been suggested that the enhanced urinary albumin excretion in hypertension is a consequence of increased permeability of the glomerular filter due to increased glomerular transcapillary hydraulic pressure, but other factors may also be involved (102).

The average urinary albumin excretion in essential hypertension varies with the severity of the disease, from 16 to 90 mg/24 hr in mild or moderate hypertension (96,100) to 633 ± 645 mg/24 hr (mean ± S.D.) in severe essential hypertension (101); in primary malignant hypertension the proteinuria may be as heavy as in primary renal disease (range 0.4–12 g/24 hr) (103).

Albuminuria, detected by the dipstick test, is a significant and independent risk factor for cardiovascular disease in both untreated and treated hypertensive patients (8). Whether microalbuminuria is also a marker of increased risk in essential hypertension is still unclear. However, antihypertensive treatment does not appear to reduce the prevalence or incidence of dipstick-positive albuminuria (11,12). In contrast, the quantitated urinary albumin excretion has invariably been found to decrease after antihypertensive treatment (95,100,101,104), and the fall in albumin excretion parallels the blood-pressure reduction (95).

β_2-Microglobulinuria

β_2-Microglobulin excretion is usually normal in essential hypertension (95,96) but may be moderately increased in severe hypertension with dipstick-positive albuminuria (101).

KIDNEY FUNCTION IN ESSENTIAL HYPERTENSION

Most studies of mild and moderate essential hypertension have shown increased renal vascular resistance, reduced RBF, and normal or subnormal GFR accompanied by raised FF (1–4,58,105–108). These renal hemodynamic changes appear to develop successively with increasing

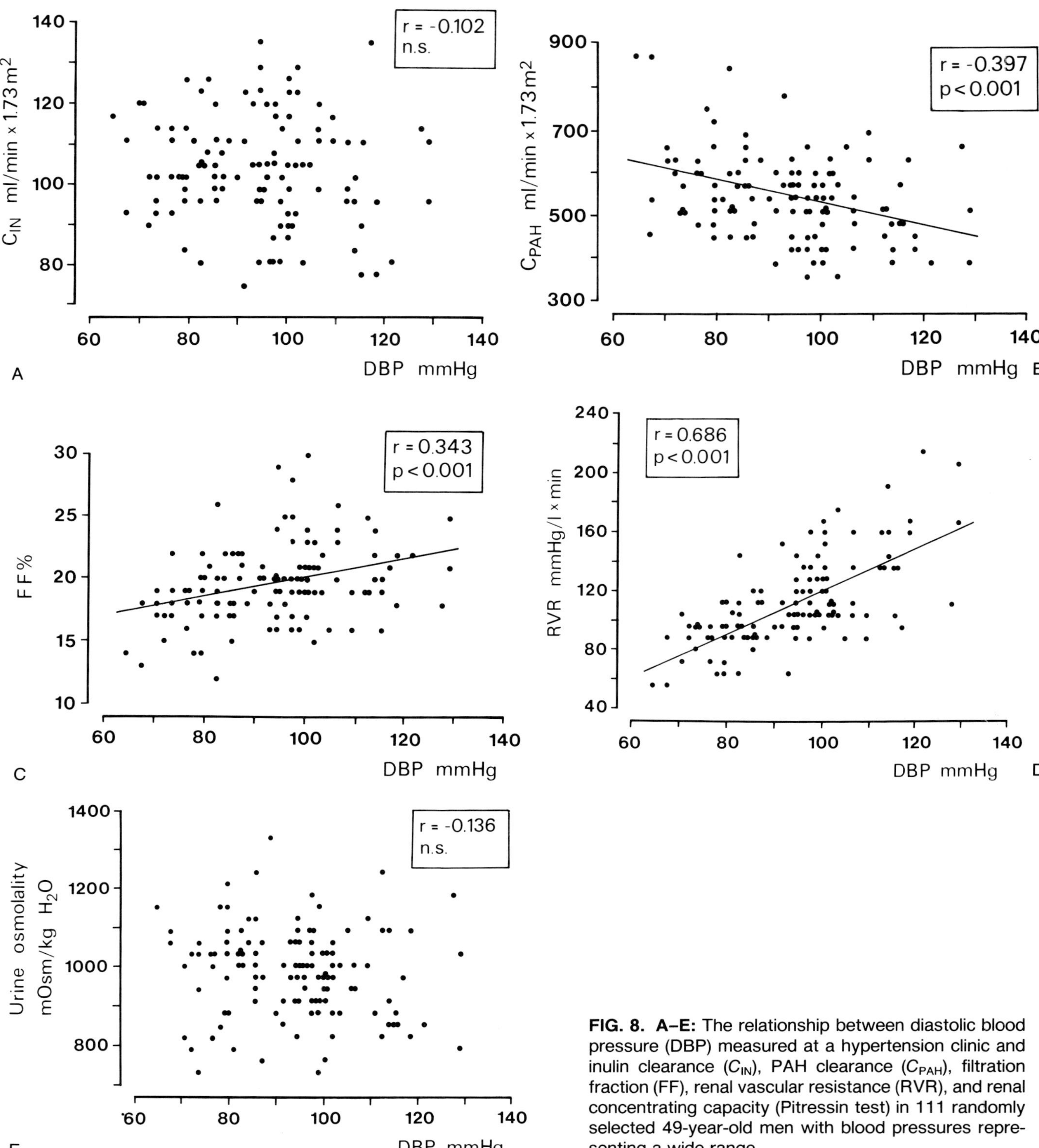

FIG. 8. A–E: The relationship between diastolic blood pressure (DBP) measured at a hypertension clinic and inulin clearance (C_{IN}), PAH clearance (C_{PAH}), filtration fraction (FF), renal vascular resistance (RVR), and renal concentrating capacity (Pitressin test) in 111 randomly selected 49-year-old men with blood pressures representing a wide range.

blood pressure and do not seem to start at any particular blood-pressure level, as illustrated in Fig. 8 by data from an investigation of a random sample of 49-year-old normotensive and hypertensive untreated men representing a wide range of blood pressures (109). The changes in renal vascular resistance, RBF, and FF become pronounced and GFR starts to decline only in more severe hypertension (1,3,4,110).

The renal concentrating capacity did not change significantly with increasing blood pressure in the study of 49-year-old men (Fig. 8E), and it is usually maintained until late stages of essential hypertension (89).

The changes in the different renal function parameters in patients with essential hypertension in relation to the severity of the disease are summarized in Fig. 9. The deviations from normal are partly a consequence of the pathophysiol-

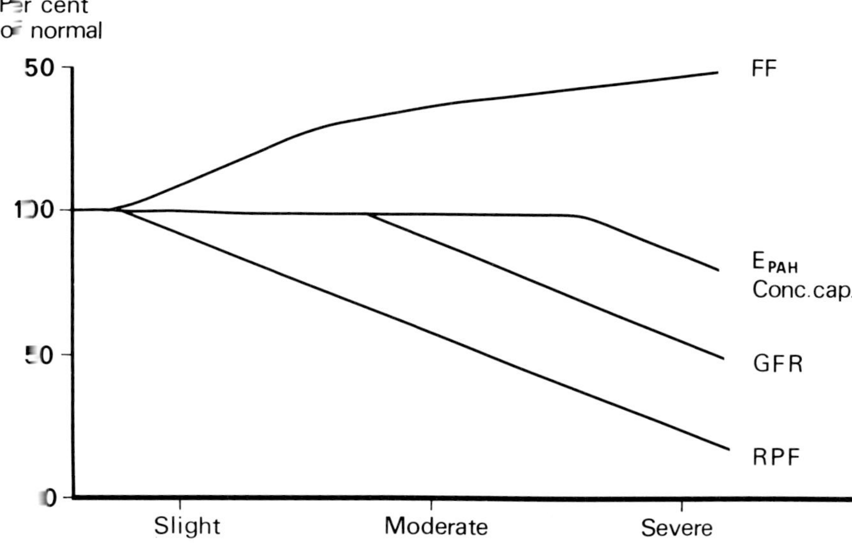

FIG. 9. A schematic presentation of the changes in some renal function parameters in patients with essential hypertension. FF, filtration fraction; E_{PAH}, renal extraction of PAH; Conc. cap., urine concentrating capacity; GFR, glomerular filtration rate; RPF, renal plasma flow, i.e., PAH clearance. "Slight," "moderate," and "severe" are arbitrarily chosen to indicate the severity of the disease.

ogy of hypertension and partly the result of developing structural damage. In the mild and moderate stages of hypertension, reduced RPF and increased FF are to be expected with our investigation techniques. The method of choice is simultaneous measurement of the renal clearance of a filtration marker and of PAH to obtain GFR and ERPF. The extraction of PAH is normal at this stage of the disease, and ERPF will be an acceptable approximation of RPF. However, it is desirable to measure the extraction level in all situations where it can be expected to be altered —for example, during therapeutic interventions with antihypertensive drugs.

The reduction in GFR in more advanced hypertension is probably due to loss of functioning nephrons and represents the onset of a state of irreversible morphological damage due to focal glomerulosclerosis. The very late appearance of abnormalities in E_{PAH} and urine concentration ability in relation to the other functional parameters indicates a well-preserved function of the proximal and distal tubular cells in residual nephrons and is in great contrast to pyelonephritic damage of the kidney (57).

It is evident from the above that evaluation of GFR only —for example, by creatinine clearance or measurement of serum creatinine—will not be an efficient diagnostic test for detection of slight or moderate kidney involvement in essential hypertension.

ACKNOWLEDGMENTS

The authors are greatly indebted to Prof. M. Aurell, Department of Nephrology, University of Göteborg, for his helpful suggestions and criticism.

REFERENCES

1. Reubi FC, Weidmann P, Hodler J, Cottier PT. Changes in renal function in essential hypertension. *Am J Med* 1978;64:556–563.
2. Ljungman S, Aurell M, Hartford M, Wikstrand J, Wilhelmsen L, Berglund G. Blood pressure and renal function. *Acta Med Scand* 1980;208:17–25.
3. Corcoran AC, Taylor RD, Page IH. Functional patterns in renal disease. *Ann Intern Med* 1948;28:560–582.
4. Birkenhäger WH, Schalekamp MADH. *Control mechanisms in essential hypertension.* Amsterdam: Elsevier, 1976.
5. Palmer RS, Muench H. Course and prognosis of essential hypertension: follow-up of 453 patients ten years after original series was closed. *JAMA* 1953;153:1–4.
6. Sokolow M, Perloff D. The prognosis of essential hypertension treated conservatively. *Circulation* 1961;23:697–713.
7. Bechgaard P. The natural history of benign hypertension—one thousand hypertensive patients followed for 26 to 32 years. In: Stamler J, Stamler R, Pullman TN, eds. *The epidemiology of hypertension. Proceedings of an international symposium.* New York: Grune and Stratton, 1967;357–363.
8. Samuelsson O, Wilhelmsen L, Elmfeldt D, Pennert K, Wedel H, Wikstrand J, Berglund G. Predictors of cardiovascular morbidity in treated hypertension: results from the Primary Prevention Trial in Göteborg, Sweden. *J Hypertens* 1985;3:167–176.
9. Bulpitt CJ, Beevers DG, Butler A, Coles EC, Hunt D, Munro-Faure AD, Newson RB, et al. The survival of treated hypertensive patients and their causes of death: a report from the DHSS hypertensive care computing project (DHCCP). *J Hypertens* 1986;4:93–99.
10. Hartford M, Ljungman S, Andersson O, Wikstrand J, Berglund G. Heart and kidney involvement in hypertension. *Acta Med Scand* 1979;205:563–568.
11. Kannel WB, Stampfer MJ, Castelli WP, Verter J. The prognostic significance of proteinuria: the Framingham study. *Am Heart J* 1984;108:1347–1352.
12. Samuelsson O, Wikstrand J, Wilhelmsen L, Berglund G. Heart and kidney involvement during antihypertensive treatment. *Acta Med Scand* 1984;215:305–311.
13. Moyer JH, Heider C, Pevey K, Ford R. The effect of treatment on the vascular deterioration associated with hypertension, with particular emphasis on renal function. *Am J Med* 1958;24:177–192.
14. Lewin A, Blaufox MD, Castle H, Entwisle G, Langford H. Apparent prevalence of curable hypertension in Hypertension Detection and Follow-up Program. *Arch Intern Med* 1985; 145:424–427.
15. Vestergaard P, Leverett R. Constancy of urine creatinine excretion. *J Lab Clin Med* 1958;51:211–218.
16. Doolan PD, Alpen EL, Theil GB. A clinical appraisal of the plasma concentration and endogenous clearance of creatinine. *Am J Med* 1962;32:65–79.
17. Levinsky NG, Levy M. Clearance techniques. In: Orloff J, Berliner RW, Geiger SR, eds. *Handbook of physiology. Section 8:*

renal physiology. Washington DC: American Physiological Society, 1973;103–117.
18. Jacobsen FK, Christensen CK, Mogensen CE, Heilskov NSC. Evaluation of kidney function after meals. *Lancet* 1980;i:319.
19. Duarte CG. *Renal function tests. Clinical laboratory procedures and diagnosis.* Boston: Little, Brown and Company, 1980.
20. Kampmann J, Siersbaek-Nielsen K, Kristensen M, Molholm Hansen J. Rapid evaluation of creatinine clearance. *Acta Med Scand* 1974;196:517–520.
21. Cockcroft DW, Gault MH. Prediction of creatinine clearance from serum creatinine. *Nephron* 1976;16:31–41.
22. Bröchner-Mortensen J, Jensen S, Rödbro P. Delimitation of plasma creatinine concentration values for assessment of relative renal function in adult patients. *Scand J Urol Nephrol* 1977;11:257–262.
23. Bauer JH, Brooks CS, Burch RN. Clinical appraisal of creatinine clearance as a measurement of glomerular filtration rate. *Am J Kidney Dis* 1982;2:337–346.
24. Shemesh O, Golbetz H, Kriss JP, Myers BD. Limitations of creatinine as a filtration marker in glomerulopathic patients. *Kidney Int* 1985;28:830–838.
25. Jeliffe RW. Creatinine clearance: bedside estimate. *Ann Intern Med,* 1973;79:604–605.
26. Rolin HA, Hall PM, Wei R. Inaccuracy of estimated creatinine clearance for prediction of iothalamate glomerular filtration rate. *Am J Kidney Dis* 1984;4:48–54.
27. Bröchner-Mortensen J. Current status on assessment and measurement of glomerular filtration rate. *Clin Physiol* 1985;5:1–17.
28. Chasis H, Smith HW. The excretion of urea in normal man and in subjects with glomerulonephritis. *J Clin Invest* 1938;17:347–358.
29. Kassirer JP. Clinical evaluation of kidney function—glomerular function. *N Engl J Med* 1971;285:385–389.
30. Smith HW. *The kidney: structure and function in health and disease.* New York: Oxford University Press, 1951.
31. Du Bois EF, Du Bois D. A formula to estimate the approximate surface area if height and weight be known. *Arch Intern Med* 1916;17:863–871.
32. Isaksson B. A simple formula for the mental arithmetic of the human body surface area. *Scand J Clin Lab Invest* 1958;10:283–289.
33. Wesson LG. *Physiology of the human kidney.* New York: Grune and Stratton, 1969.
34. Davies DF, Shock NW. The variability of measurement of inulin and diodrast tests of kidney function. *J Clin Invest* 1950;29:491–495.
35. Jagenburg R, Attman PO, Aurell M, Bucht H. Determination of glomerular filtration rate in advanced renal insufficiency. *Scand J Urol Nephrol* 1978;12:133–137.
36. Bröchner-Mortensen J, Rödbro P. Comparison between total and renal plasma clearance of (^{51}Cr) EDTA. *Scand J Clin Lab Invest* 1976;36:247–249.
37. Cole BR, Giangiacomo J, Ingelfinger JR, Robson AM. Measurement of renal function without urine collection. A critical evaluation of the constant-infusion technic for determination of inulin and para-aminohippurate. *N Engl J Med* 1972;287:1109–1114.
38. Schnurr E, Lahme W, Küppers H. Measurement of renal clearance of inulin and PAH in the steady state without urine collection. *Clin Nephrol* 1980;13:26–29.
39. Mertz DP, Sarre H. Polyfructosan-S. Eine neue inulinartige Substanz zur Bestimmung des Glomerulusfiltrates und des physiologisch aktiven extracellulären Flüssigkeitsvolumens beim Menschen. *Klin Wochenschr* 1963;41:868–872.
40. Hubbard RS, Loomis TA. The determination of inulin. *J Biol Chem* 1942;145:641–645.
41. Carlsen JE, Lehd Möller M, Lund JO, Trap-Jensen J. Comparison of four commercial Tc-99m (Sn) DTPA preparations used for the measurement of glomerular filtration rate: concise communication. *J Nucl Med* 1980;21:126–129.
42. Dubovsky EV, Russel CD. Quantitation of renal function with glomerular and tubular agents. *Semin Nucl Med* 1982;12:308–329.
43. Heymsfield SB, Arteaga C, McManus C, Smith J, Moffitt S. Measurement of muscle mass in humans: validity of the 24-hour urinary creatinine method. *Am J Clin Nutr* 1983;37:478–494.
44. Kim KE, Onesti G, Ramirez O, Brest AN, Swartz C. Creatinine clearance in renal disease. A reappraisal. *Br Med J* 1969;4:11–14.
45. Skov PE, Hansen HE. Glomerular filtration rate, renal plasma flow and filtration fraction in living donors before and after nephrectomy. *Acta Med Scand* 1974;195:97–103.
46. Hagstam KE, Nordenfelt I, Svensson L, Svensson SE. Comparison of different methods for determination of glomerular filtration rate in renal disease. *Scand J Clin Lab Invest* 1974;34:31–36.
47. Lubowitz H, Slatopolsky E, Shankel S, Rieselbach RE, Bricker NS. Glomerular filtration rate. Determination in patients with chronic renal disease. *JAMA* 1967;199:252–256.
48. Sjöström PA, Odlind BG, Wolgast M. Extensive tubular secretion and reabsorption of creatinine in humans. *Scand J Urol Nephrol* 1988;22:129–131.
49. Hood B, Attman P-O, Ahlmén J, Jagenburg R. Renal hemodynamics and limitations of creatinine clearance in determining filtration rate in glomerular disease. *Scand J Urol Nephrol* 1971;5:154–161.
50. Davies DF, Shock NW. Age changes in glomerular filtration rate, effective renal plasma flow, and tubular excretory capacity in adult males. *J Clin Invest* 1950;29:496–507.
51. Slack TK, Wilson DM. Normal renal function. C_{IN} and C_{PAH} in healthy donors before and after nephrectomy. *Mayo Clin Proc* 1976;51:296–300.
52. Granerus G, Aurell M. Reference values for ^{51}Cr-EDTA clearance as a measure of glomerular filtration rate. *Scand J Clin Lab Invest* 1981;41:611–616.
53. Bergström J, Ahlberg M, Alvestrand A. Influence of protein intake on renal hemodynamics and plasma hormone concentrations in normal subjects. *Acta Med Scand* 1985;217:189–196.
54. Bergström J, Bucht H, Josephson B. Determination of the renal blood flow in man by means of radioactive diodrast and renal vein catheterization. *Scand J Clin Lab Invest* 1959;11:71–81.
55. Aurell M, Fritjofsson Å, Granerus G, Grimby G. Renal extraction of *p*-aminohippurate: physiological and clinical observations. *Contrib Nephrol* 1978;11:14–18.
56. Bergström J, Bucht H, Ek J, Josephson B, Sundell H, Werkö L. The renal extraction of para-aminohippurate in normal persons and in patients with diseased kidneys. *Scand J Clin Lab Invest* 1959;11:361–375.
57. Reubi F. *Nierenkrankheiten,* 2nd edition. Bern: Verlag Hans Huber, 1970.
58. de Leeuw PW, Kho TL, Falke HE, Birkenhäger WH, Wester A. Haemodynamic and endocrinological profile of essential hypertension. *Acta Med Scand* 1978;(Suppl 622):9–86.
59. Smart R, Trew P, Burke J, Lyons N. Simplified estimation of glomerular filtration rate and effective renal plasma flow. *Eur J Nucl Med* 1981;6:249–253.
60. Tauxe WN, Dubovsky EV, Kidd T Jr, Diaz F, Smith LR. New formulas for the calculation of effective renal plasma flow. *Eur J Nucl Med* 1982;7:51–54.
61. Blaufox MD, Merrill JP. Simplified Hippuran clearance: measurement of renal function in man with simplified Hippuran clearances. *Nephron* 1966;3:274–281.
62. Fine EJ, Axelrod M, Gorkin J, Saleemi K, Blaufox MD. Measurement of effective renal plasma flow: a comparison of methods. *J Nucl Med* 1987;28:1393–1400.
63. Brenner BM, Zatz R, Ichikawa I. The renal circulations. In: Brenner BM, Rector FC, eds. *The kidney,* 3rd edition. Philadelphia: WB Saunders, 1986;93–123.
64. Hornych A, Brod J, Slechta V. The measurement of the renal venous outflow in man by the local thermodilution method. *Nephron* 1971;8:17–32.
65. Magrini F, Guo-Quing L. A critical improvement of the local thermodilution method for measuring renal blood flow in man. *Cardiovasc Res* 1982;16:350–354.
66. Greene ER, Venters MD, Avasthi PS, Conn RL, Jahnke RW. Noninvasive characterization of renal artery blood flow. *Kidney Int* 1981;20:523–529.
67. Britton KE, Brown NJG. *Clinical renography.* London: Lloyd-Luke (Medical Books) Ltd, 1971.
68. Stamey TA. Some observations on the filtration fraction, on the transport of sodium and water in the ischemic kidney, and on the prognostic importance of R.P.F. to the contralateral kidney in renovascular hypertension. In: Gross F, Naegeli SR, Kirkwood

paper chart recorders. Attempts were made to obtain qualitative (28–31) and quantitative (6,8,9,32–34) information about kidney function. Initial enthusiasm for the "cross-over" pattern (see Fig. 3A and B) as diagnostic for renovascular hypertension (7) soon waned because this pattern was seen in many other unrelated renal conditions. Patterns of renal parenchymal disease were also nonspecific. Unfortunately the failure of the nuclear medicine physician to recognize the lack of specificity of the test led to many diagnostic errors. This has created a distrust in the mind of the nephrologist which persists even today (35).

Tc-99m-labeled agents include DTPA (36), DMSA (37), and GHA (38); the first is commonly used for both qualitative imaging and quantitative functional assessment, whereas the latter two are used for morphological evaluation of the kidneys and, to a lesser degree, for functional assessment. Tc-99m bone-seeking agents such as methylene diphosphonate (MDP) often yield serendipitous information about the kidneys because of their high renal uptake. Sodium Tc-99m pertechnetate may be used in rapid sequence images to assess renal perfusion.

There are a number of Tc-99m-labeled tubular agents under investigation as potential alternatives to OIH. The advantages of such an agent are numerous. It is not possible at this time, however, to determine which, if any, of these agents will prove superior for clinical use, although Tc-99m-MAG$_3$ appears to be the most promising and may have FDA approval in 1989.

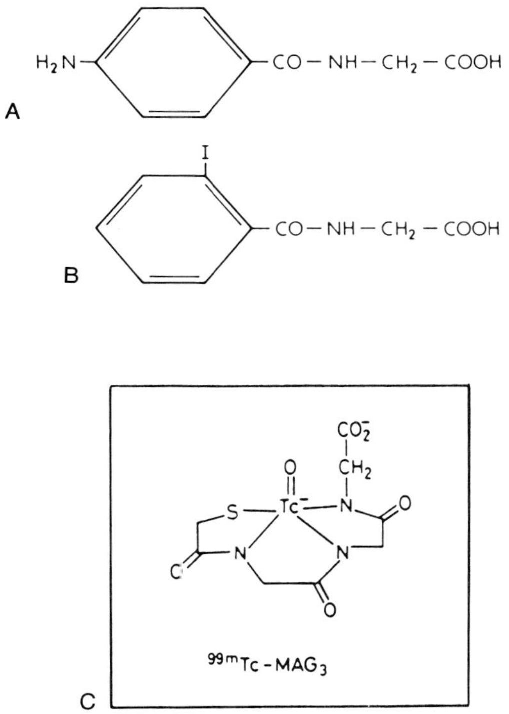

A: $H_2N-C_6H_4-CO-NH-CH_2-COOH$

B: (I)$C_6H_4-CO-NH-CH_2-COOH$

C: $^{99m}Tc-MAG_3$

FIG. 4. The structural formulas of (**A**) PAH, (**B**) OIH, and (**C**) MAG$_3$. Although MAG$_3$ has not achieved general clinical use, it is shown because it is the most promising 99m-Tc-labeled tubular agent available at this time and may replace OIH in some uses.

Orthoiodohippurate

This agent (24,25,27) is related structurally to para-aminohippurate (PAH) (see Fig. 4). The structural similarity of OIH to PAH is not a guarantee of identical physiologic behavior. In fact, OIH does behave qualitatively like PAH but differs quantitatively. Approximately 70% of OIH is extracted from renal arterial blood in one pass through the kidney; most of the clearance is due to proximal tubular secretion, but about 20% of its total excretion is from glomerular filtration (23,26). After blocking tubular secretion of OIH with probenicid, some investigators have used this compound to measure the glomerular filtration rate (39). In tracer quantities, after intravenous administration, approximately 70% of OIH is weakly protein-bound in the serum (40), in contrast to only a few percent of PAH (when administered in macroscopic quantities). However, the protein binding appears to be reversible *in vivo*. The binding of I-131 or I-123 to OIH is greater than 99% *in vitro* and is stable; a small amount of free radioiodine does appear in the circulation (23) when these agents are used. In commercial preparations, the maximum amount of free radioiodine is limited to 2%. This can expose a patient to significant thyroidal radiation, especially from I-131, although the risk can be reduced significantly by blocking thyroid uptake with Lugol's solution prior to tracer injec-

←

FIG. 3. A: I-131-OIH (300 μCi) was administered intravenously for a scintirenogram in this 33-year-old woman with difficult-to-control hypertension (BP 220/130 mmHg). The left kidney demonstrates normal function on the 0–3-min image, normal transit into the collecting system by the 3–6-min image, and normal excretion during the remainder of the study. The right kidney is small and demonstrates diminished function in proportion to its size on the 0–3-min image. Transit and excretion are both delayed on the right side. There is a normal renogram curve on the left, and there is diminished uptake with delayed transit (as measured by a delayed time to peak) and excretion on the right renogram curve. **B:** An angiogram obtained in the same patient as in part A, demonstrating fibromuscular dysplasia of the right renal artery. **C:** Percutaneous transluminal angioplasty (PCTA) was performed on the right renal artery in the same patient as in parts A and B. There is improvement in the transluminal diameter. **D:** Two weeks after the PCTA, a repeat scintirenogram was obtained. Perceptible changes in the scinti-images are subtle when compared to part A but are better appreciated on the renogram curve. The "time to peak" is now equal between the kidneys. This reflects a normalization of the transit time of the right kidney after PCTA. The height of the peaks has also been normalized, reflecting equalization of renal function. More important, this patient's blood pressure was controllable at 140/95 mmHg after the procedure.

tion. Various investigators have reported good correlations between (a) total effective renal plasma flow (ERPF) obtained from PAH measurements and (b) estimates from various measures of OIH clearance (23,26,41). Liver excretion is quite low (40), an advantage for quantitative renal functional evaluation and for imaging in advanced renal insufficiency.

OIH Scintigraphy/Scintirenography

Although only 25–50 μCi of I-131 OIH (6,23,32–34) need be administered for determination of renal function by nonimaging methods, reasonable images require 200–300 μCi. The major limitation on the administered dose is thyroid uptake of free I-131. A medium-energy parallel-hole collimator, interfaced to a standard scintillation camera with a 12-in. crystal, usually is sufficient to include both kidneys within the field of view. Detailed descriptions of the procedure can be found elsewhere (42). Briefly, a normally hydrated patient is given 3–5 drops of Lugol's iodine in orange juice before radiotracer administration, to block potential thyroidal uptake of unbound, free radioiodine. The patient is injected in the prone position with 150 μCi of I-131-OIH per kidney. Some institutions perform the test with the patient seated. Sequential images are obtained for 30 min, with each image taking 3 min. If a computer interface is available, sequential 32- × 32-byte matrix images are obtained at 15-sec intervals during the 30-min acquisition. A large-field-of-view camera sometimes enables bladder incorporation in the field of view, but standard field cameras generally do not permit this. A bladder (and/or urine collection bag) image is obtained at the end of the study to evaluate qualitatively for excretion, and a postvoiding image and/or count data is obtained for residual urine estimation (43).

The major uses of OIH scintirenography include evaluation of (a) total and individual renal function (either qualitatively or quantitatively), (b) parenchymal transit time, and (c) urinary excretion. The patient should be normally hydrated, since dehydration or overhydration may affect the appearance of the renal uptake (31). It should be noted that dealing with uncertainties of hydration remains an unsolved technical problem of renal scintigraphy. Delayed images of the kidneys are frequently helpful in the evaluation of ureteral obstruction, particularly after ambulating or voiding (44).

The normal appearance of the OIH scintirenogram appears in Fig. 5. There should be bilaterally symmetric uptake of tracer in the first 3-min image, with a high kidney-to-background ratio. The intensity of renal visualization on this first image in comparison to background activity is a qualitative index of renal function. More precise quantification of the kidney uptake using the computerized images allows one to measure total and individual effective renal plasma flow. This is described in greater detail below. Since the normal transit time of OIH through the kidney is 3–5 min (28), the renal pelves usually can be identified on the second-frame image (i.e., the image taken during minutes

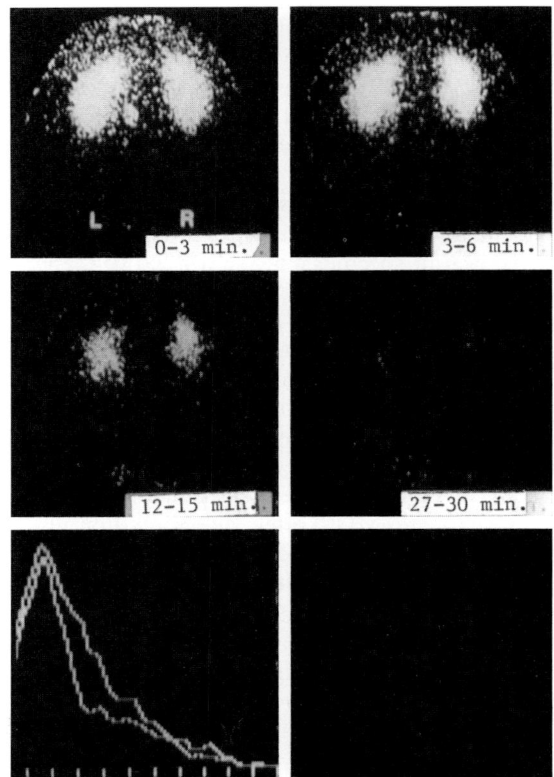

FIG. 5. Four weeks after passage of a right renal calculus, this 32-year-old woman was injected with 300 μCi I-131-OIH, and sequential posterior view scinti-images of the kidneys were obtained. This normal study demonstrates prompt symmetrical renal uptake of tracer on the 0–3-min image. There is normal bilateral transit, with both collecting systems visualized on the 3–6-min image. Finally, normal excretion is seen through the remainder of the study. The computer-generated renogram curves, below the images, demonstrate the normal renogram appearance. This is characterized by the following: a steep ascending portion, reflecting good uptake (and function); a sharp peak, indicating normal transit into the collecting system; and a subsequent rapid decline on renal activity, reflecting radioactive urine leaving the kidneys.

3–6). Progressive cortical and pelvic emptying occurs through the remainder of the normal exam. The computerized acquisition of these images enables us to identify regions of interest around the kidneys, and it also makes possible the generation of the time–activity histograms, known as *renograms.*

Abnormalities which may be detected by OIH scintirenography include ureteral obstruction, acute tubular necrosis, acute renal failure, renal artery stenosis, and chronic renal failure. Other purposes to which this exam is applicable include (a) detection of a kidney which is nonvisualized by intravenous urogram, (b) monitoring of qualitative or quantitative individual and/or total renal functional changes following interventional procedures such as nephrostomy, angioplasty, lithotripsy, and antibiotic therapy for pyelonephritis, and (c) determination of renal salvageability.

Clearance of OIH

Total ERPF

The classic measurement of ERPF utilizes a constant infusion of PAH (45) which is cumbersome for both patient and physician. The exam requires a constant intravenous infusion of PAH and multiple venipunctures for sampling of blood to ensure a constant serum PAH concentration. Once this state of equilibrium has been achieved, the rate of influx must equal the rate of efflux (excretion by the kidneys) and is measured by carefully timed urine collections.

Theoretically, the rate of disappearance of PAH from the plasma after bolus injection can provide the same information. In practice, however, a bolus of PAH in amounts sufficient for chemical analysis of delayed blood samples produces early plasma concentrations that may exceed the tubular maximum for PAH secretion by the kidneys (46). Alternatively, a small bolus of PAH initially would lead to serum concentrations of PAH in delayed blood samples which are too low for accurate chemical measurement. OIH may be used as a reasonable analog of PAH (23,26) and suffers none of the above problems. On the other hand, in the face of marked ERPF reductions, tracer doses of OIH may not be extracted as efficiently as macroscopic quantities of PAH. The typical disappearance of I-131-OIH from the plasma is shown in Fig. 6. Evaluation of a complete curve in a given subject requires multiple blood samples, but various compartmental analyses (47–49) of this type of disappearance curve have led to simplified methods requiring fewer blood specimens.

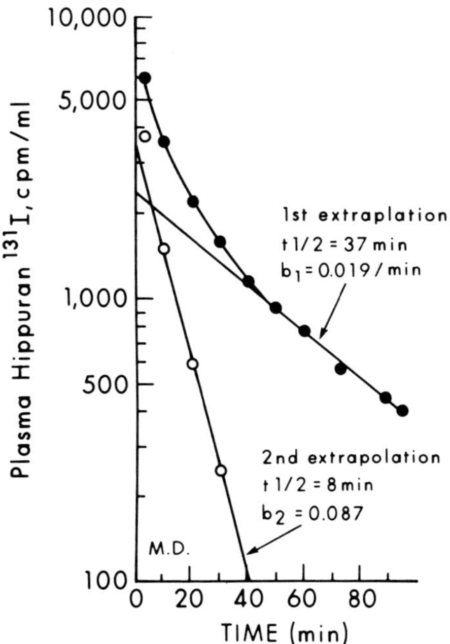

FIG. 6. A disappearance curve of I-131-OIH after a single injection. The log plasma concentration is plotted against time. The unfilled circles represent subtractive values obtained after extrapolating the line fitting the terminal portion of the curve to time 0. The use of this analytic approach to calculate renal clearance is described in the text. (From ref. 47, with permission.)

An open two-compartment model requires four to six blood specimens, minimally, for measurement of OIH activity. Two slopes and two intercepts may be obtained by curve stripping (48,49), and ERPF may be calculated as follows:

$$\text{ERPF} = \frac{\text{Dose} \times b_1 b_2}{Ab_2 - Bb_1}$$

where A and B are intercepts, and b_1 and b_2 are slopes of the slow and fast compartments, respectively (see Fig. 6).

Further simplification into a one compartment model requires only two blood specimens (41). Specimens obtained at 20 and 30 min after OIH injection are used to calculate ERPF:

$$\text{ERPF} = \text{Dose} \times \frac{\text{Slope}}{\text{Intercept}}$$

Only one slope and one intercept are derivable from two blood specimens. This introduces a potential loss of accuracy in exchange for the greater simplicity and convenience of a reduced number of blood samples. Nonetheless, good correlations with PAH clearances are obtained with this method as well. Although it has excellent precision, it tends to overestimate the true clearance by about 10%.

Even further simplifications have been attempted. A single sample technique attributable to Tauxe et al. (50,51) has surprising accuracy, nearly comparable to the two sample method (52). Another technique described by Schlegel and Hamway (53) requires no blood samples, since it utilizes the gamma-camera-derived renal uptake from computerized images. This, however, appears less accurate than the blood-sampling *in vitro* procedures (52).

Individual Renal Function

Divided renal function may be derived from computerized gamma-camera data. After the OIH injection, computer matrix images are obtained (usually at 15-sec intervals). After the first 3 min, the likelihood of pelvic accumulation and excretion becomes high (28,54). Therefore, only data obtained during the first 3 min may be used for evaluation of split renal function. For individual renal function measurements, the relative function is determined quite simply by the relative activity accumulated in one kidney compared with the other, usually during the interval between the first and second minute after injection (Fig. 7). The major problems are twofold: (i) selecting appropriate background regions to approximate nonrenal activity measured within the renal region of interest (ii) correcting for renal depth. To date, there is no consensus on how to choose renal background (6,53,55–57) (see Fig. 7). Renal depth correction also has been attempted by a variety of means, including (a) formulas based on height and weight (53,58), (b) the use of ultrasonography (58), and (c) single- (59,60) and double-isotope (61) depth-finding techniques. Formulas based on height and weight are not sufficiently reliable to recommend their general use (52,62).

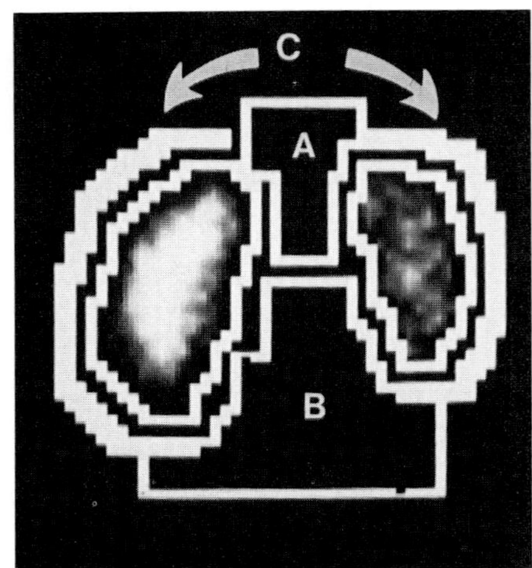

FIG. 7. In this patient with asymmetric renal function and size, a variety of radionuclide techniques could be used to evaluate individual renal function. This patient was injected with 300 μCi I-131-OIH. Relative renal function is proportional to the integrated radioactivity measured with each kidney, most reliably obtained during the interval 1–2 min after injection. The selection of an appropriate "background" region is controversial, and region A (between the upper poles), region B (between the lower poles), and region C (crescent-shaped regions adjacent and lateral to the kidneys) have all been proposed. Overlap of liver (on the right) and, to a lesser degree, spleen (on the left), although not seen in this high-contrast image, may influence the apparent background and therefore the calculated relative renal function. In this case the renal function was good enough that background contributed a small difference to the measured function. Using region A or B as background, the left kidney had 71%, the right 29%. Using region C as background, the left kidney was calculated as 76% of total function, the right 24%. A similar approach can be used for Tc-99m-DMSA, Tc-99m-GHA, and Tc-99m-DTPA. For DMSA and GHA, quantitation cannot begin before 1 hr after injection. (From ref. 52, with permission.)

Quantitative total and split renal-function measurements enable clinicians to follow the progress of a patient's renal function objectively and noninvasively. The utility of this method of studying renal pathophysiology is only beginning to show its promise. Other agents used to measure individual renal function include Tc-99m-DTPA, -DMSA, and -GHA (see below).

Transit Time Estimate

The transit time of OIH through the renal parenchyma varies according to the length of the nephron being traversed and the urine flow rate. Juxtaglomerular nephrons extend more deeply into the renal medulla than cortical nephrons and require a correspondingly longer time for OIH to transit to the collecting system. Since 90% of renal blood flow normally is directed toward the renal cortex, the normal transit of OIH reflects predominantly cortical transit. In normals, the mean transit time of OIH ranges from about 3 to 5 min (28,54). This reflects itself in the scintigram by the appearance of the renal collecting system on the 3- to 6-min image. The renogram curve correspondingly shows its peak at that time, after which OIH begins to leave the area of the kidney. The actual calculation of the mean transit time is performed from data obtained during a standard scintirenogram acquired on a computer matrix. Any alteration in intrarenal blood flow distribution will increase the mean transit time, since blood flow will be redirected toward the longer juxtaglomerular nephrons. This will reflect itself in the scintigram by a delay in the appearance of the collecting system, and in the renogram by a delayed peak. Unfortunately, these patterns of delayed or prolonged transit appear to be nonspecific. Britton and co-workers have attempted to examine the mean transit time as well as the distribution of transit times within the kidney by the technique of deconvolution analysis (63–65). Deconvolution analysis mathematically reconstructs the passage of activity through the kidney as if a single compact bolus of OIH entered the renal artery. The division of this bolus into many fragments with different transit times through the kidney allows determination of the distribution of transit times. Britton and co-workers have obtained interesting correlations in obstructive uropathies. They have observed prolonged parenchymal transit in patients with obstruction but have found no such prolongation in nonobstructed dilated systems.

Tc-99m-Labeled Agents

Sodium Tc-99m Pertechnetate (Na^+ $^{99m}TcO_4^-$)

Sodium Tc-99m pertechnetate is the chemical form in which Tc-99m is eluted from commercial molybdenum-99 generators. It is widely available and inexpensive. The chemical form of pertechnetate is similar to perchlorate and other iodide-like monovalent anions. Pertechnetate, too, concentrates in tissues with an affinity for such anions, such as the thyroid gland, salivary glands, gastric mucosa, and choroid plexus. Renal handling of $^{99m}TcO_4^-$ is complex, involving GFR and net tubular reabsorption. Its slow renal clearance and complex handling make this agent a poor choice in renal imaging. Pertechnetate may be administered as an intravenous bolus for a rapid sequence renal scintiangiogram. Choice of the appropriate form of Tc-99m usually depends on the clinical context. If perfusion information is all that is required, 10–15 mCi of $^{99m}TcO_4$ may be used. The major advantage of this agent is its low cost. If information about renal function, transit, and/or excretion is desired, Tc-99m-DTPA would be far more valuable. If morphologic information is needed, Tc-99m-GHA could be used.

Tc-99m-Diethylenetriaminepentaacetic Acid (DTPA) (36)

This chelate, available since 1970, is excreted by glomerular filtration and may be used to measure the glomerular filtration rate (39). Its clearance is usually a few percent lower than that of inulin (66), the physiologic standard for this measurement. The reason for this is not entirely clear, although the presence of a small amount of tin in the preparation appears to cause approximately 3–5% of the DTPA to be protein-bound in the serum. In addition, some renal parenchymal binding of Tc-99m-DTPA may occur, since it is not uncommon to be able to image the kidney at 24 hr, when all activity theoretically should be gone. The favorable imaging and dosimetric properties of Tc-99m compared with I-131 would appear to make the Tc-99m-DTPA superior to I-131-OIH for scintigraphic evaluation of qualitative renal function (see Table 4). In fact, significantly higher background activity is noted with Tc-99m-DTPA as a result of the much lower extraction efficiency for the glomerular agent compared with a tubular agent such as OIH (67). In recent years, scintillation cameras have become more sophisticated electronically. The modifications have included increasing the number of photomultiplier tubes to improve spatial resolution, decreasing crystal detector thickness for the same purpose, and decreasing electronic "dead time" between scintillations to improve detector sensitivity at high count rates. Collimators have been changed as well. The net result has been a dramatic improvement in the imaging of Tc-99m-labeled agents. Unfortunately the image quality for agents labeled with I-131 has deteriorated (68). Many institutions with modern scintillation cameras will find Tc-99m-DTPA to be their agent of choice for renal functional imaging. Although this may be justified for technical reasons, a tubular agent provides significant advantages. Reliable evaluation of tubular function with modern detectors requires the use of I-123-OIH (69). Such a tubular agent provides greater renal concentration than a glomerular agent such as DTPA, and this is an advantage in the evaluation of renal failure. Validation, approval, and commercial availability of a Tc-99m-labeled tubular agent is, therefore, anxiously awaited. Tc-99m-MAG_3 appears to be a promising possibility at this time (Fig. 4C). Tc-99m-DTPA may be used quite similarly to OIH, although Lugol's solution is not required. Modern gamma scintillation cameras produce high-quality images with Tc-99m-DTPA when fitted with a parallel-hole all-purpose low-energy collimator. Image quality is usually quite a bit better than with OIH (70). Technical factors aside, the amount of administered activity alone (10 mCi of Tc-99m-DTPA) usually provides improved images for scintirenography compared with only 300 μCi of I-131- or I-123-labeled OIH. The renal transit time of DTPA is approximately 3–5 min, just as for OIH, so that the renal pelvis is visualized during that time interval in the normal study. Higher tissue and liver background may make interpretation of renal images and renal function difficult in the face of renal insufficiency. As with OIH, an interface with a computer is a valuable adjunct for simultaneous computer matrix images and allows for generation of a renogram curve.

Measurement of Renal Function: Glomerular Filtration Rate (GFR)

Total GFR. The same general techniques for measuring the clearance of PAH apply to the use of inulin for the determination of total GFR. Like the PAH clearance, the inulin clearance procedure has inherited the distinction of standard use as well as the inconvenience of the constant infusion procedure. Unlike PAH, single-injection clearances can be performed accurately using inulin and chemical analysis (71) since GFR is independent of plasma concentration.

The radionuclide used clinically to measure GFR is Tc-99m-DTPA (39). The plasma disappearance rate after a single injection may be used to determine the GFR in ways completely analogous to ERPF determinations described above. Multicompartmental models of the disappearance curve require multiple blood samples for analysis (39,66). The equations for calculating GFR are similar to those for ERPF. The only significant difference is related to the time of blood-sample collection. Since the GFR is approximately 20% of the ERPF, the rate of Tc-99m-DTPA disappearance from plasma is correspondingly much slower than OIH. Sampling must be carried out for a longer period of time to derive the GFR accurately. A two-sample method analogous to that applied to OIH requires samples at approximately 1 and 3 hr after injection, instead of 20- and 30-min measurements for OIH (see above). One-sample methods (60) can be performed as well, analogous to the Tauxe method (50,51) for ERPF. An *in vivo* method requiring no samples has been suggested (72) which is analogous to the comparable method of Schlegel and Hamway (53) for ERPF (see above). Higher tissue background activity may produce greater problems quantifying renal function by the *in vivo* procedure for this glomerular agent when compared to OIH.

Individual Renal Function. Computer interfacing allows determination of relative renal uptake of DTPA and therefore allows the assessment of relative renal function. Again, this is analogous to the procedures described above for OIH, and this suffers from the same problems of proper background determination (73) and accurate depth correction (62). Other tracers used to determine relative renal function are Tc-99m-DMSA and GHA (see below).

Filtration Fraction. The ratio of GFR to ERPF is known as the *filtration fraction* (FF). Therefore it is a derived quantity and not an independent parameter of renal function. The radiotracer methods used to determine this parameter have been described above. The FF is not used widely in current clinical practice, but there is greater interest in it as a tool for physiologic research. Certain pathologic states appear to selectively affect GFR or ERPF disproportionately. Recently, this has been described as an effect of angiotensin-converting-enzyme inhibitors such as captopril, particularly in renal artery stenosis (74,75). Whether the FF will become a clinically useful marker of disease awaits further investigation.

Radionuclide Angiography and Transit Times. Rapid sequence imaging, in the posterior projection, after bolus Tc-99m-DTPA administration, in amounts exceeding 10 mCi, yields qualitative information about relative arterial flow to the kidney (76). Images obtained at intervals of 1 or 2 sec usually are used. The resultant radionuclide angiogram may be stored in a computer for generation of time–activity histograms derived from renal regions of interest.

Actually, any Tc-99m agent may be used, but DTPA is preferred because its rapid excretion causes lower absorbed radiation doses per millicurie administered. Tc-99m-DMSA should not be used for perfusion studies because of the high renal dose (see Table 4). It is also not acceptable to perform perfusion studies using OIH. I-131-OIH in millicurie amounts would provide too high a dose to the kidneys, bladder, and thyroid. I-123-OIH, although dosimetrically safe in millicurie amounts, is prohibitively expensive, although technically acceptable.

Figure 8A shows a normal "flow study" performed with Tc-99m-DTPA. This type of exam provides crude visual information about the symmetry and existence of renal flow. Asymmetry of flow is a rather nonspecific finding (Fig. 8B); consequently the imaging portion of a radionuclide angiogram has rather limited utility. Interest has been revived in the procedure, however, because the transit time of the bolus (derivable by deconvolution analysis from the computerized study only) may have interesting properties more specific to different disease states (77). This is currently under investigation.

Tc-99m-Glucoheptonate and Tc-99m-Dimercaptosuccinic Acid

The use of these compounds is mostly in the scintigraphic evaluation of renal morphology (78–81). There has been a fair amount of investigation, particularly with DMSA (2–5,42,82,83), evaluating split renal function with these agents. After intravenous administration they are extensively but reversibly protein-bound (84). They are handled by the kidney in a rather complex way. About 85% of GHA and 50% of DMSA are excreted by a combination of glomerular filtration and tubular secretion (79). The remainder binds to renal tubular cells (GHA) or to cortical cells (DMSA) by uncertain mechanisms. It should be noted that absorbed radiation dosages of DMSA are generally about three to five times those of equal millicurie doses of GHA (Tables 4 and 5). DMSA has greater renal absorbed dose as a result of its greater renal retention. The renal binding makes possible the scintigraphic evaluation of renal morphology once the collecting systems are clear of activity. This is usually $1\frac{1}{2}$–2 hr after injection of the tracer. In the presence of obstruction, morphology may be difficult to evaluate because of increased retained activity within the renal pelvis. Severe parenchymal renal dysfunction results in poor activity within the renal pelvis. Severe parenchymal renal dysfunction also is associated with poor background clearance and enhanced alternate routes of excretion. Images are therefore poor in this clinical situation. Biochemical disturbances may alter the body distribution of DMSA (84); furthermore, renal morphology may be difficult to evaluate under these circumstances, as a result of poor physiologic concentration of the radiotracer in the kidney compared to background at the usual imaging times.

Polycystic kidneys, which are usually associated with hypertension, may be identified readily using GHA or DMSA. In most cases, however, sonography, CT, or intravenous urography will be more helpful.

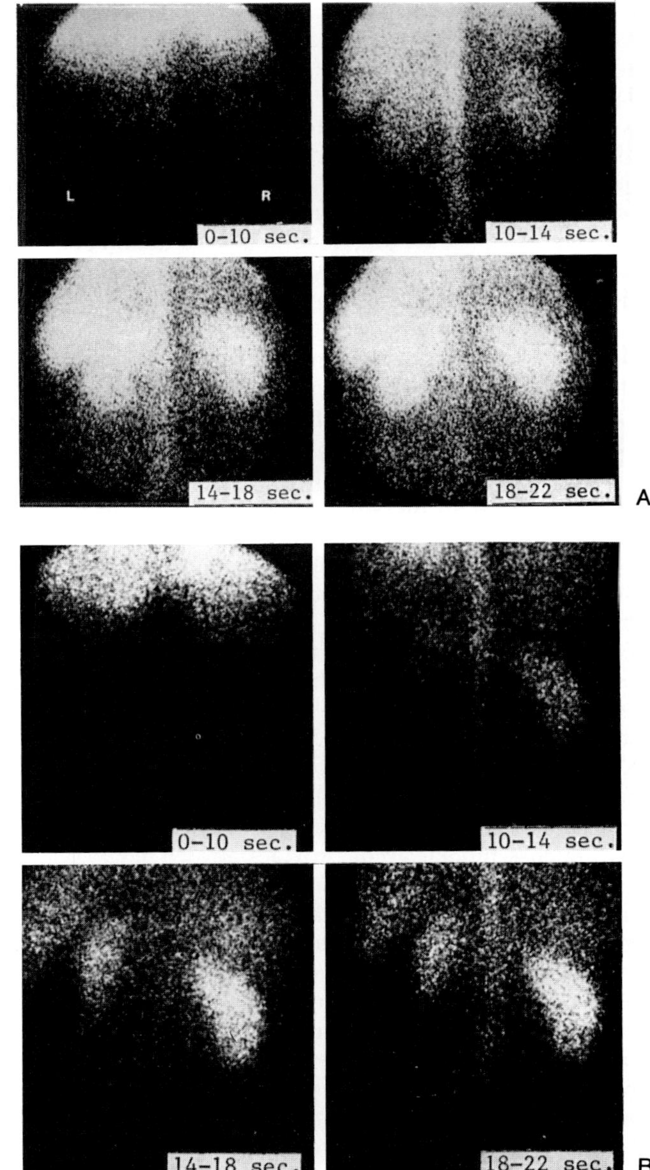

FIG. 8. A: Rapid sequential posterior images are obtained after intravenous injection of 10 mCi of Tc-99m-DTPA. Representative 2-sec scinti-images are displayed and demonstrate normal and symmetric appearance of radiotracer in the kidneys. This is a normal "flow study" or radionuclide angiogram. **B:** Rapid sequential images are obtained after bolus intravenous injection of 10 mCi Tc-99m-DTPA in a hypertensive female. The left kidney is smaller in size than the right and demonstrates decreased relative uptake of radiotracer. This abnormal flow study demonstrates the kind of asymmetry that may be seen in renal artery stenosis. It may also be seen in a wide variety of other processes that produce asymmetric renal size and function, and therefore it is not specific for renal artery stenosis. This patient was proven by angiography to have a left renal artery stenosis.

Quantification of Individual Renal Function Using 99m-Tc Agents

Subjective evaluation of the percentage of relative renal function estimated from scinti-images of GHA correlates well with quantitation by computer (82). This mirrors the comparable accuracy for detection of asymmetric flow by quantitative or qualitative means using $^{99m}TcO_4^-$ (76). Two hours after injection of radiotracer, the renal pelvices usually are free of activity. The relative counts within one kidney compared with the other gives the relative function. Although attempts to quantitate differential renal function have been made with GHA (85,86), DMSA has been used more extensively (2,5,87,88). Both agents have been used for the scintigraphic evaluation of renovascular hypertension (2–4,87,89). They may not be used to reproducibly quantitate total renal function, as a result of their complex handling by the kidney.

ROLE OF NUCLEAR MEDICINE PROCEDURES IN ESSENTIAL HYPERTENSION

Radionuclides may play a useful role in the evaluation of patients with end-organ damage whose primary disease is essential hypertension. These applications include evaluation of cardiac function (gated blood pool studies), evaluation of stroke, and evaluation of renal function. Numerous other complications arising in the patient with essential hypertension are also approachable by nuclear medicine techniques but are considered to be beyond the scope of this chapter, and the reader is referred to standard nuclear medicine texts for further information. Since the heart, kidney, and brain are the primary target organs of hypertension, they are briefly considered in this section.

Assessment of Renal Size and Function

Assessment of renal function has already been discussed. The assessment of renal size is of considerable importance to the nephrologist in many conditions, especially in renal insufficiency in the hypertensive patient. Normal size is usually compatible with recent onset and potential reversibility of the renal condition, whereas small kidneys suggest long-standing disease.

Plain radiographs of the abdomen or intravenous urography with nephrotomography will often demonstrate the size of each kidney. Unfortunately, poor preparation, overlying bowel contents, impaired concentration, or contraindications due to renal impairment limit their general value. Since ultrasound can provide information on renal size independently of renal function and without any radiation hazard to the patient, it usually is considered to be the procedure of choice. Where a simple estimate of renal length and calyceal pattern is required, this is entirely justified. Timmermans (90) found ultrasound estimates of renal size to differ from actual (nephrectomy) size by less than 15% in 9 of 10 cases examined.

In spite of its obvious value, however, the information provided by ultrasound is entirely structural, and it is often useful to combine an estimate of renal size with an evaluation of underlying function. Radionuclides can provide such information.

I-131-OIH, as a result of its prolonged transit time in renal failure (91), provides a useful image even by the obsolete rectilinear scanning technique. In 18 of 19 patients with advanced renal failure with a mean blood urea of 34 mmol/liter (BUN 96 mg/dl) and a creatinine level of 0.67 mmol/liter (7.6 mg/dl), successful visualization has been reported by Freeman et al. (92). Other reports confirm the value of I-131 Hippuran in assessing renal size in the presence of severe renal impairment (16). It has been suggested that renal concentration of OIH occurs with as little as 3% of normal renal function (93).

Tc-99m, as a chelate, has been used in renal failure. It has been estimated that renal size can be determined with Tc-99m-DTPA in 75% of patients with blood urea over 23 mmol/liter (BUN over 65 mg/dl) (94). Tc-99m glucoheptonate has also been reported to be imaged in all but "very extreme" renal failure (39,69), whereas DMSA was similarly successful in four of five patients with blood urea greater than 36 mmol/liter (BUN > 100 mg/dl) (95).

Routine radionuclide scanning techniques may underestimate renal size because of aberrant renal position. Lateral scanning of the kidneys has been recommended when this possibility exists (59,96). Virtually any agent is adequate for estimation of renal size in patients whose kidney function is good. Tc-99m glucoheptonate and DMSA are preferred because of better resolution and the potential for multiple views. In the presence of renal failure, I-131-OIH or I-123-OIH appears to be the single most reliable agent with good uptake and minimal interference from surrounding organs. The overriding usefulness of OIH lies in its important prognostic and functional information.

Assessment of Stroke

The presence of hypertension is well accepted as a contributing risk factor for the development of several common forms of stroke. In particular, hypertension is correlated with intracerebral hemorrhagic infarcts, as well as with ruptured saccular aneurysms. In addition, hypertension is a risk factor for cerebral atherosclerosis, a common setting for cerebrovascular thrombosis.

A more indirect relationship exists between hypertension and embolic stroke. Emboli usually originate in atherosclerotic plaques in the carotid arteries or the aorta, or they originate in mural thrombi within the left ventricle or atrium. Hypertension is a risk factor for development of atherosclerotic disease in the aorta, carotid arteries, and coronary arteries. Myocardial infarction of the left ventricle is, of course, an undesirable but common consequence of coronary artery disease; and mural thrombus is a not infrequent sequela of large transmural infarction, especially in infarctions with aneurysm formation.

Left atrial thrombus usually arises in the setting of atrial fibrillation, which may be a consequence of hypertensive cardiomyopathy, ischemic heart disease (again, increased in hypertensives), and thyrotoxicosis (a cause for systolic hypertension).

In any event, the control of hypertension is indicated to reduce the risk of stroke (71). Assessment of cerebral circulation in patients with suspected cerebrovascular disease may be performed in a variety of ways, including radionuclide techniques, computed tomography (CT), and magnetic resonance imaging (MRI), as well as direct contrast angiography and digital subtraction angiography (DSA) of the brain. CT and MRI do not become abnormal until the stroke has been completed and until edema, infarction, or some other gross anatomic change has taken place. Contrast angiography is invasive as is DSA, and both involve the use of potentially toxic contrast material.

Radionuclide techniques have the following advantages: (a) They demonstrate flow and/or metabolic abnormalities, even in vascular disease that has not led to completed stroke; (b) they are relatively noninvasive; and (c) they demonstrate the extent of metabolic and/or flow derangements in tissues surrounding completed stroke (i.e., tissues still at risk).

Older radionuclide techniques employed tracers which are either nondiffusible (with respect to the blood–brain barrier), such as Tc-99m-DTPA, or diffusible, such as ^{133}Xe (97). Tc-99m-DTPA, after bolus intravenous injection, can be used to provide gross flow information to the hemispheres. Multiple-probe detectors have been used to measure regional blood flow information after inhalation of Xe-133 gas by recording the rate of xenon washout. Unfortunately, these multiple-probe devices are rather cumbersome to use.

Recently, single-photon emission computer tomography (SPECT) of the brain has been performed with rotating gamma cameras, interfaced to a computer, analogous to radiographic CT. The utility of this procedure has begun to be demonstrated with the recently approved diffusible radiotracer I-123 iodoamphetamine (I-123-IMP), whose distribution after injection closely parallels cerebral blood flow (98,99). Three-dimensional information in multiple slices from several projections, analogous to CT displays, allow accurate assessment of regional blood flow information. A disadvantage of the procedure is the expense of I-123-IMP. Newer Tc-99m-labeled agents with properties somewhat similar to those of IMP are in the developmental stage (100,101) and are likely to be less costly.

The possibility of developing radiotracers for SPECT imaging that demonstrate regional metabolism will add additional power to this diagnostic modality (102).

There has already been substantial development of flow, metabolic, and brain-receptor tracers that require positron emitters as radiolabels (103). Positron emission tomography (PET) is an even more exciting application of nuclear medicine technology. This technique allows for radiolabeling of true metabolic substrates with isotopes of carbon, hydrogen, nitrogen, and oxygen. As such, glucose, fatty acids, and synaptic neurotransmitters may be labeled and imaged. The possibilities for exploring central-nervous-system regional biochemistry are extraordinarily rich, but they far exceed the scope of this chapter. The contribution of the central nervous system (and, in particular, the autonomic nervous system) to the pathophysiology of hypertension will undoubtedly be explored with PET, but at present it is purely at a speculative stage.

Assessment of the Heart

The mechanisms by which left ventricular hypertrophy and changes in cardiac contractility result from acute and chronic increases in afterload are just beginning to be understood at the cellular and molecular level. More poorly understood are the cellular changes that lead to an increase in atherosclerotic coronary artery disease among hypertensives compared to normotensive individuals. Nonetheless, the existence of hypertensive cardiomyopathy and the increased prevalence of ischemic cardiomyopathy among hypertensive individuals are accepted clinically (104,105). Evaluation of the heart for prognosis and management of ischemic heart disease is beyond the scope of this chapter. Further comments therefore are restricted to evaluation of hypertensive heart disease.

Nuclear medicine cardiac evaluation currently requires either Tl-201 for measurements of regional cardiac perfusion and cardiac mass (see below) or Tc-99m-labeled erythrocytes. Human erythrocytes may be labeled with Tc-99m by several variations of a rather simple technique (106). An intravenous injection, first of approximately 1 mg of nonradioactive stannous ion (usually given in the form of stannous pyrophosphate), prepares the patient's erythrocytes by "tinning" them intravascularly. A subsequent injection of $^{99m}TcO_4^-$ then chemically binds to the intracellular hemoglobin–tin complex. The value of this intravascular label has been demonstrated repeatedly in cardiac applications. In 1971 (107), using related equilibrium "blood pool" labeling techniques, separate scinti-images of the heart were obtained at end-diastole and end-systole. Subsequent refinements in the procedure, resulting from the use of computer technology, have allowed equilibrium "cine" images of the beating heart to be obtained in multiple projections (108). This noninvasive radionuclide ventriculogram (RNV) may be used to evaluate for regional wall motion abnormalities and to accurately calculate the left ventricular ejection fraction. Furthermore, the procedure has been adapted to a stationary bicycle and can, therefore, be performed during exercise. The response of the left ventricular ejection fraction and regional wall motion to maximum bicycle exercise has become an important adjunct to the stress-electrocardiogram in the assessment of patients for ischemic heart disease. In hypertensive heart disease, the left ventricular ejection fraction has become an important parameter when measured at rest and during stress. The simplicity, accuracy, and noninvasive character of the RNV have made this radionuclide exam of paramount importance in assessing end-organ damage to the heart in hypertensive heart disease.

Cardiac adaptation to hypertension of any etiology is complex. Several investigators using nuclear medicine techniques have shown a correlation between systolic hypertension and ejection fraction (109–111). One may hypothesize that this response of the heart to the increased "afterload" due to hypertension is analogous to the increased ejection fraction often seen due to increased afterload in early aortic stenosis. Ultimately, the heart will begin to fail, and a correlation between systolic pressure and ejection fraction may no longer apply.

On the other hand, a subset of hypertensives have isolated diastolic dysfunction only, presumably before the onset of systolic dysfunction (112). In these individuals, hypertensive changes in the left ventricle lead to hypertrophy and decreased compliance, requiring high pressures to fill the ventricle (113).

These ventricles maintain normal or even supranormal systolic function as measured by the ejection fraction; but the high diastolic pressures required to fill the stiff-walled ventricle imply high left atrial pressures and ultimately pulmonary alveolar edema. Early detection of cardiac end-organ responses to hypertension have important therapeutic and probably prognostic importance. Congestive heart failure accompanied by a dilated left ventricle with poor systolic function (as measured in the usual clinical setting by a low ejection fraction) has a much poorer prognosis than congestive heart failure accompanied by left ventricular hypertrophy with preserved systolic function but isolated diastolic dysfunction. Furthermore, therapy differs markedly in the two groups. The familiar dilated failing ventricle responds best to inotropes (e.g., digoxin), preload reducers (e.g., nitrates and diuretics), and afterload reducers (e.g., hydralazine and captopril). These drugs are of no value or are harmful in treating the ventricle afflicted with isolated diastolic dysfunction (113). Instead, selective diastolic dysfunction is treated with calcium channel blockers or with beta blockers, both of which have mild to moderate anionotropic effects. As such, these agents are likewise contraindicated in treating patients with low ejection fractions.

The radionuclide equilibrium blood pool ventriculogram (RNV) provides an accurate means of measuring the left ventricular ejection fraction (108). The ejection fraction (EF) is by no means a pure measure of left ventricular contractility, since it is influenced as well by preload and afterload. However, in the usual clinical setting, a normal or supranormal ejection fraction in the face of clinical and/or radiologic evidence for congestive heart failure strongly suggests diastolic dysfunction. Similarly, an ejection fraction less than 35% in the same clinical and radiological setting strongly suggests that the heart failure is due to a dilated cardiomyopathy with both systolic and diastolic dysfunction.

Some investigators have examined the diastolic portion of the ventricular time–activity curve that may be generated from the RNV. They have described differences in the diastolic portion of the curve in patients with ischemia (114), valve disease, and hypertensive heart disease (112). These changes of slowed diastolic filling, therefore, are not specific for hypertensive heart disease but, in the appropriate clinical setting, may be used to strengthen the diagnosis of diastolic dysfunction.

Measurement of the extent of end-organ damage to the heart from hypertension using the RNV is important not only for prognosis and management of congestive heart failure but also for management of the patient's hypertension. The choice of medication must first be those agents that would improve the patient's heart failure. Since dilated cardiomyopathies are treated with diuretics and afterload reducers, these medications assume "first-line" significance in the management of these patients' hypertension. Similarly, beta-adrenergic blockers and/or calcium channel blockers assume primacy in the management of hypertension for those hypertensives suffering from selective diastolic dysfunction. Selection of second- and third-line antihypertensives continues to differ in the two groups according to potential adverse effects on cardiac function.

Further studies of hypertensive heart disease with radionuclide techniques have led to additional physiologic information. Blaufox and co-workers (109,115) have demonstrated a reduced ability of certain subsets of hypertensive patients to increase their ejection fraction in response to stress. These early studies recently have been confirmed (110,111).

Ejection fraction responses to antihypertensive therapy also vary with the drug used (109,115,116). Studies of these kinds suggest further potential to provide a rational approach for selecting specific antihypertensive therapeutic programs in individual patients.

Thallium-201, when reduced to the +1 valence state, acts as a K^+ analog when administered in tracer quantities (117,118). Its relatively rapid accumulation in perfused cells following intravenous administration makes it an agent suitable for use for measurement of regional blood flow. As such, Tl-201 myocardial scintigraphy is employed primarily as a radiotracer for diagnosis of the extent of ischemic heart disease. However, it has been used as well for quantitation of left ventricular mass (119), particularly when imaged with single-photon emission computed tomography (SPECT). At present, echocardiography is more practical and is a more established tool for this purpose (120).

ROLE OF NUCLEAR MEDICINE IN DIFFERENTIAL DIAGNOSIS OF RENOVASCULAR HYPERTENSION

The role of nuclear medicine in the differential diagnosis of renovascular hypertension (RVH) has been controversial. The various tests to evaluate renal function which have been described in this chapter have a potential role in the evaluation of the patient with RVH.

To begin with, an effective screening test is needed. The intravenous urogram (IVU), widely used in the past as a screening test for RVH, has an estimated sensitivity of 78% and specificity of 89% for detection of RVH (121–126). Extensive costs–benefit analyses have clearly shown the IVU to not be a satisfactory screening test for RVH (124). Plasma renin assays, with or without captopril augmentation, performed even more poorly (127,128). The saralasin test has proven impractical (85,128,129).

There has been much interest in the use of intravenous digital subtraction angiography (IVDSA) in screening for RVH. IVDSA represents an improvement compared with the IVU. However, the improvement is insufficient to merit employment as a general screening test.

Renography in the Diagnosis of RVH and Renal Artery Stenosis (RAS)

I-131-OIH (13,23–27) (see earlier sections on OIH), a chemical and biological analog of PAH, was used in 1960 to demonstrate an abnormal renogram in RVH using dual detector probes (25). Decreased renal blood flow due to a stenotic vessel may produce a variety of findings on the renogram. (Decreased initial uptake reflecting decreased renal function is seen commonly on the affected side, but delayed transit and excretion due to increased water reabsorption may be seen also.) Enthusiasm for the test as pathognomonic for RVH faded as the sensitivity and specificity of the test were established, in the following 10 years, to be approximately 80–85% (10,12,17,25,124). These values are approximately the same as those reported for the rapid sequence IVU (121–126), despite the absence of imaging information in these early OIH renograms. Specificity suffers from false-positive (FP) exams resulting from virtually any unilateral renal disease with attendant compromised renal function, including chronic pyelonephritis, obstruction, perinephric abscess, perinephric hematoma, ptosis, renal vein thrombosis, or asymmetric parenchymal disease of any etiology, such as the nephrosclerosis of essential hypertension (130,131). Dehydration may increase detection of FPs by exaggerating what would normally be small differences in renal excretion. Sensitivity is affected by false negatives (FNs) in patients with mild RAS or symmetric bilateral disease. Overhydration may contribute to FN exams.

Scintirenography

Since the late 1960s, the gamma camera with computer interface has been employed, thereby allowing scinti-images, as well as renography, to be performed (Figs. 3 and 9). Visualization of the collecting system contributes to fewer FP exams from unilateral obstruction (Fig. 10). The time–activity histogram in obstruction may be just what one would see in classic RVH (Figs. 3A and 9A). This may be particularly confusing to the referring physician, since obstruction itself may be associated with hypertension (132). The scintigrams, however, demonstrate progressive accumulation of activity in a dilated collecting system with no apparent further emptying. This is the pattern of obstruction. Resolution following the passage of a renal stone is seen in Fig. 5. The relative percent of FP exams remains the critical determinant for any study that may be used to improve identification of renovascular hypertensives from a group of unselected hypertensives.

Although reliable data concerning the specificity and sensitivity of the dual-probe renogram are available, we do not have similar data for Tc-99m-DTPA or I-131-OIH renography with imaging. Data using Tc-99m flow studies with imaging yielded specificities and sensitivities similar to that observed with dual probes (11,85) (Table 6).

Importance of Decreasing False-Positive (FP) Rate

The prevalence of renovascular hypertension among unselected hypertensives is probably less than 1% (71,128,133). Assuming optimistic sensitivities and specificities of 90% by gamma-camera scintirenography, we would find the following: Among 1000 unselected hypertensives, 10 would have RVH, nine of whom would be detected; but among the 990 essential hypertensives in the group, the 10% FP rate would falsely identify 99 as having RVH. This would imply a post-test positive predictive value of only 10/109, or approximately 9%. Clearly, even such excellent sensitivities and specificities as 90% are inadequate to screen a disease with such a low prevalence, and substantial improvement must be made, particularly in the FP rate (134).

Improved accuracy of renography for the differential diagnosis of renovascular hypertension has been reported by Gruenewald and Collins (135). They studied 32 normal patients, 188 patients with essential hypertension, and 15 patients with RVH. They utilized a bolus slope ratio (BSR); this gives an index of renal perfusion and parenchymal transit time (PTT), which reflects tracer kinetics in the kidney. The BSR was 1.2 ± 0.2, 1.0 ± 0.25, and 0.5 ± 0.2 in normals, essential hypertensives, and RVH patients, respectively. The PTT was 1.35 ± 0.4, 1.35 ± 0.5, and 3.0 ± 1.4 in these groups, respectively. Four kidneys were omitted because of absent renal function, and 13 were omitted because of hold-up of activity in the collecting system. Detailed analyses of the results of this technique are limited, but the authors suggest that the finding of an abnormal BSR, PTT, and reduced renal function in a single kidney is highly specific for RVH (136). Careful inspection of their data suggests that their sensitivities and specificities are no better than those shown in Table 6.

The use of the Tc-99m-DTPA radionuclide angiogram also was greeted enthusiastically when first proposed as a diagnostic test for RVH. Unfortunately, it also may be influenced by asymmetric renal disease of multiple etiologies, and therefore it suffers from the same lack of specificity (see Fig. 8B and Table 6) (11) as its predecessor, the radiohippuran renogram.

The report of the Working Group on Renovascular Hypertension (1987) (136) summarizes its impression of radionuclide methods:

> *Nuclear Imaging Techniques.* Safe, noninvasive, and relatively inexpensive isotope renography has proved less accurate than hypertensive urography in screening for renovascular disease, largely because of an unacceptable frequency of abnormal results in patients with essential hypertension. Radionuclide imaging techniques can provide information regarding both renal blood flow and excretory function, and renal perfusion–excretion ratios may increase the predictive value of radionuclide screening for renovascular hypertension. Assessing of transit times by this method has proved to be an important advance in the use of renography for diagnosing renovascular hypertension. The most appropriate contemporary use of renography is for longitudinal assessment of total and individual renal blood flow, particularly for patients with impaired renal function who are at increased risk from contrast media. More sophisticated computer programs and the increased ability to assess individual kidney function may further improve the value of isotope renography in assessing renovascular hypertension. Renographic changes after captopril administration may prove useful in demonstrating functional renal artery stenosis before, or after, surgical or catheter intervention.

The authors do not agree that isotope renography is less accurate than the urogram. Table 7 shows data from a number of studies which suggest that the urogram is no better than the renogram in the diagnosis of RVH. Regardless of their relative merits, however, there is still a great need for improvement in sensitivity and specificity of these

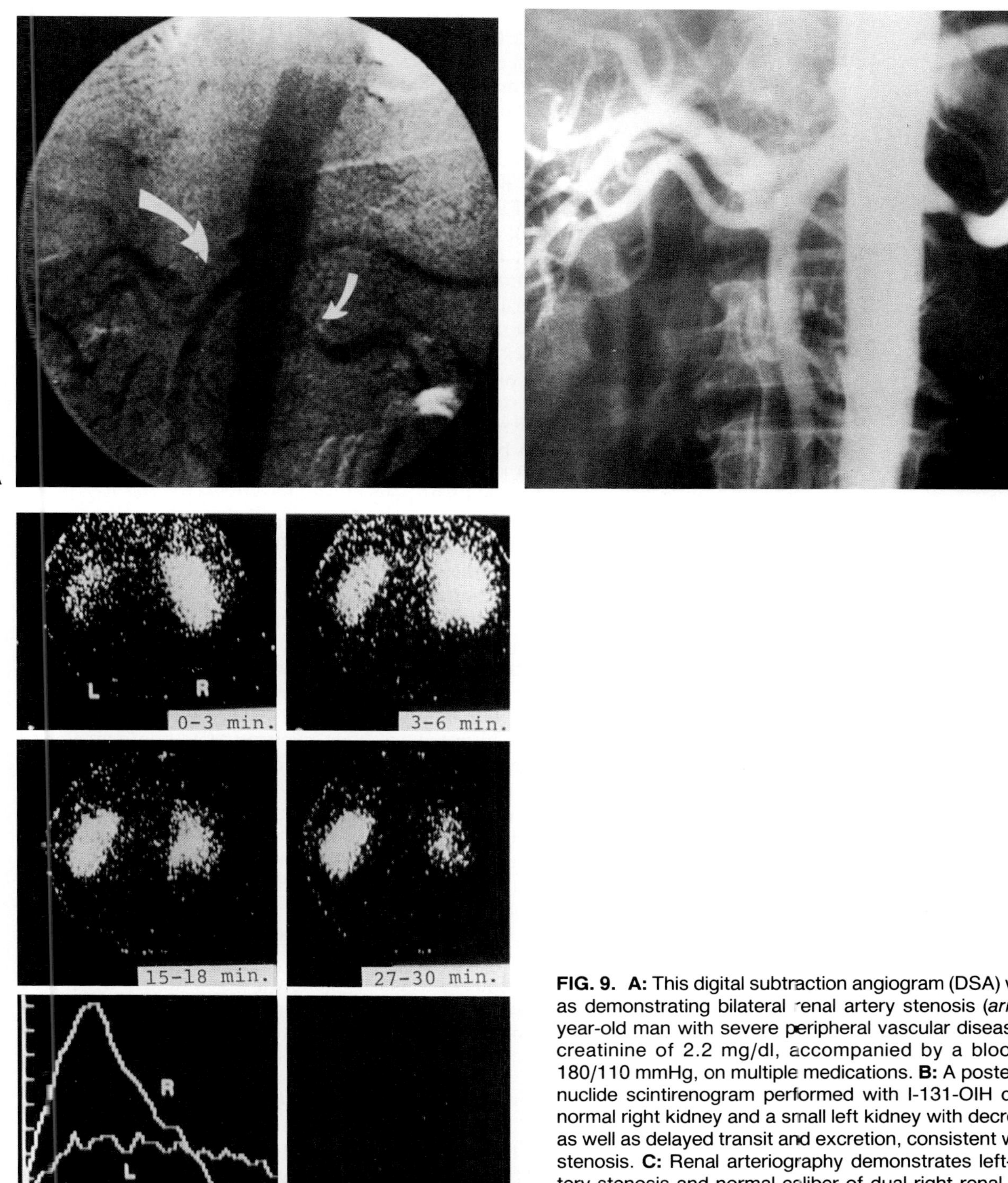

FIG. 9. **A:** This digital subtraction angiogram (DSA) was interpreted as demonstrating bilateral renal artery stenosis (*arrows*). This 55-year-old man with severe peripheral vascular disease had a serum creatinine of 2.2 mg/dl, accompanied by a blood pressure of 180/110 mmHg, on multiple medications. **B:** A posterior-view radionuclide scintirenogram performed with I-131-OIH demonstrates a normal right kidney and a small left kidney with decreased function, as well as delayed transit and excretion, consistent with renal artery stenosis. **C:** Renal arteriography demonstrates left-sided renal artery stenosis and normal caliber of dual right renal arteries. It was difficult to appreciate renal arteries on the right side on the DSA (part A), presumably because of oversubtraction near the origin of the dual right renal arteries.

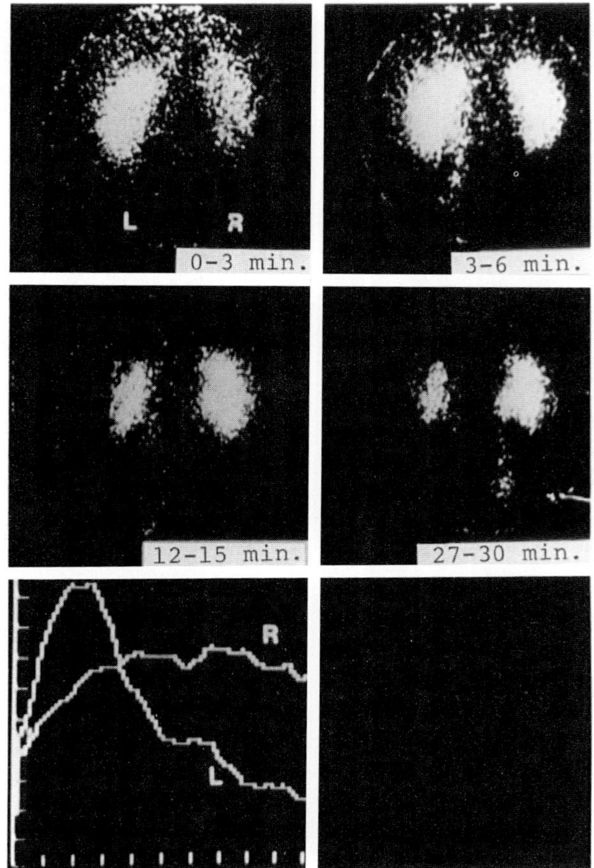

FIG. 10. This 34-year-old woman presented with acute right flank pain and evidence for a calculus on abdominal plain film. Her blood pressure was 160/100 mmHg. This scintirenogram, performed with I-131-OIH, demonstrates normal left-sided function, transit, and excretion. The right side, however, shows diminished initial uptake (representing decreased function) with delayed transit into a dilated collecting system (beginning to visualize by 12–15 min). The right collecting system is dilated down to the distal ureter and demonstrates minimal excretion by the 27–30-min image. The right renogram curve confirms and amplifies the scinti-images, showing slowed initial uptake and no identifiable peak of activity, with a plateau indicating no significant excretion. This patient passed a calculus, and the repeat scintirenogram was normal (see Fig. 5). Incidentally, the repeat blood pressure was 135/85 mmHg.

tests. Angiotensin-converting-enzyme inhibitors (ACEIs) may offer a chance to greatly improve the diagnostic accuracy of nuclear medicine procedures in RVH.

ACEI Scintirenography

There is growing interest in the use of ACEIs to enhance the specificity, and perhaps the sensitivity, of radionuclide studies in the diagnosis of renal artery stenosis (74,75,137).

Angiotensin II is thought to mediate RVH by potent arteriolar vasoconstriction as well as by stimulation of aldosterone-mediated renal salt and water retention (74,137,138). Blockade of angiotensin II formation by ACEIs lowers blood pressure effectively among patients with RVH (140). ACEIs were noted serendipitously to enhance the discrepancy in renal function between the abnormal and normal kidney in patients with unilateral RAS, by both Tc-99m-DTPA (75,140,141) and I-131-OIH scintirenography (142,143). Some investigators report a disproportionate decrease in GFR compared with ERPF on the affected side (75,141,144); others report an increase in ERPF but no change in GFR in the contralateral kidney (96). A hypothesis to explain the action of ACEIs suggests that angiotensin II enhances efferent arteriolar tone to maintain high perfusion and filtration pressure in the glomerular vessels despite lowered renal blood flow (138,145,146). Consequently, GFR is maintained. ACEIs block this effect and cause a disproportionate fall in GFR in the angiotensin-dependent kidney. Elevations in ERPF in the contralateral kidney probably result from decreased intrarenal resistance. The fall in GFR on the affected side can be detected by Tc-99m-DTPA scintirenography (75, 140,141,143,144), and the enhanced discrepancy due to elevated ERPF on the contralateral side may be detected by OIH (140,142,143). Alterations in OIH transit also have been reported (140,147).

Regardless of the precise mechanism, many investigators have reported both (a) enhanced detection of RVH using DTPA and OIH and, more importantly, (b) increased specificity, because ACEIs appear to produce no significant or worsened asymmetries of the renogram pattern in patients with essential hypertension or other conditions that might otherwise mimic RAS (Figs. 11 and 12).

Unanswered questions involving ACEI scintirenography include the following: the appropriate amount of oral medication (25 versus 50 mg of captopril) for optimum effect; the component of ACEI scintirenographic change due solely to the hypotensive effect of ACEI alone; the effects of hydration and patient medications on FP and FN rates; the relative merits of Tc-99m-DTPA versus I-131-OIH; the incidence of side-effects due to ACEI (111,148); the magnitude of changes in renal function induced by ACEI and their measurability by tracer techniques. The answers to these questions can be obtained only through meticulous evaluation of diagnostic technique accompanied by population-based studies.

Potential Advantages of ACEI Scintirenography

The potential ability of ACEI scintirenography to reduce FP exams cannot be overemphasized. Improvement in the FP rate is a critical component in developing a useful screening exam in the identification of patients with RAS. Other advantages of scintirenography are considerable: (a) The exam is relatively noninvasive, requiring a simple venipuncture to administer the tracer; (b) the tracer itself has no untoward side-effects; (c) the amount of whole-body radiation from the procedure is on the order of 16 mrad/mCi for Tc-99m-DTPA and 24 mrad/mCi for I-131-OIH (both substantially lower than absorbed in an IVU, IVDSA, or standard angiogram); (d) the technique is quite practical, since the equipment is standard in the vast majority of nuclear medicine departments throughout the country.

TABLE 6. *Nuclear medicine tests in renovascular hypertension*

	Tc-99m perfusion studies[a]			
	True negatives		Specificity	
Group	Visual	Quantitative	Visual	Quantitative
Essential hypertensives (n = 33)	27/33	29/33	42/54 = 85%	29/33 = 88%
Controls	19/21	—		
	True positives		Sensitivity	
Renovascular hypertensives (n = 8) (16 quantitated)	17/18	13/16	94%	81%

	I-131 Hippuran studies[b]	
Study	True positives	False positives
Renogram	85	10
Urogram	78	11
Both	91	18

[a] Adapted from ref. 11, with permission.
[b] From ref. 124, with permission.

Although ACEI scintirenography offers great promise to improve diagnostic screening for RVH (Fig. 13), it must still be considered unproven. OIH or DTPA scintigraphy, radionuclide angiography, transit time estimates, bolus–slope ratios, and other radionuclide techniques all offer noninvasive diagnostic means to evaluate for RVH. To date, none of these procedures recommends itself for mass screening of a general population of hypertensives.

On the other hand, in selected populations with an intermediate prevalence of RVH (i.e., approximately 20–30%), the authors recommend a radionuclide procedure as the first choice in the diagnostic work-up. It may be necessary to perform two tests (149) in certain instances. Two positive tests (e.g., scintirenogram and DSA in RVH) raise a pre-test likelihood of disease of 30%, for example, to over 93%, while two negative tests reduce the likelihood of disease to well under 5%. Two positive tests in RVH may then be followed by split-renal-vein renin determinations before arteriography (with or without angioplasty, as indicated). Two negative tests effectively rule out RVH, even with a relatively high (30%) pre-test probability. A positive and a negative test or equivocal results may mandate an arteriogram for diagnostic certainty, depending on the clinical urgency.

There are, of course, alternatives. One can choose to proceed directly to renal-vein renin determinations or angiography. IVUs and renograms play a role in helping to make this decision, which may be modified by a wide variety of clinical circumstances. Regardless of the work-up chosen, radionuclides are extremely valuable for follow-up. All patients who are submitted to surgery for RVH or who undergo angioplasty should have renal scintigrams, pre-op for baseline, and follow-up of the surgical result. This is especially important in patients undergoing balloon dilatation, where several procedures may be necessary before success is achieved (127).

Regardless of the individualized approach, there is a significant role for the use of nuclear medicine procedures in the evaluation of the hypertensive patient.

ADRENAL SCINTI-IMAGING IN THE EVALUATION OF HYPERTENSION

Several cholesterol congeners labeled with I-131 have been utilized in attempts to image the adrenal cortex (150) (see Fig. 14). These agents depend upon uptake and storage of cholesterol and its analogs by the adrenal cortex. Most bodily tissues contain cholesterol, but only the adrenal cortex, the ovary (corpora luteal cells), and the testes (Sertoli cells) normally store it, by esterification, to any degree. Historically, 19-iodocholesterol was first used in 1970 (151). However, the most successful adrenocortical agent to date has been I-131-6-beta iodomethyl-19-norcholest-5-

TABLE 7. *The IVU in the diagnosis of RAS*

Series	Sensitivity[a]	Specificity[a]
Bookstein et al. (121)	83% (138 RAS)	88.6% (771) (essential hypertensives)
Maxwell et al. (12)	93% (42 RAS)	83% (121) (61 normotensives)
Wilson et al. (125)	72% (128 RAS)	92% (125) (60 hypertensives)
Stewart et al. (126)	86% (22 RAS)	75% (105)
Thornbury et al. (123)	60.2% (197 RAS)	—

[a] Number of cases are in parentheses.

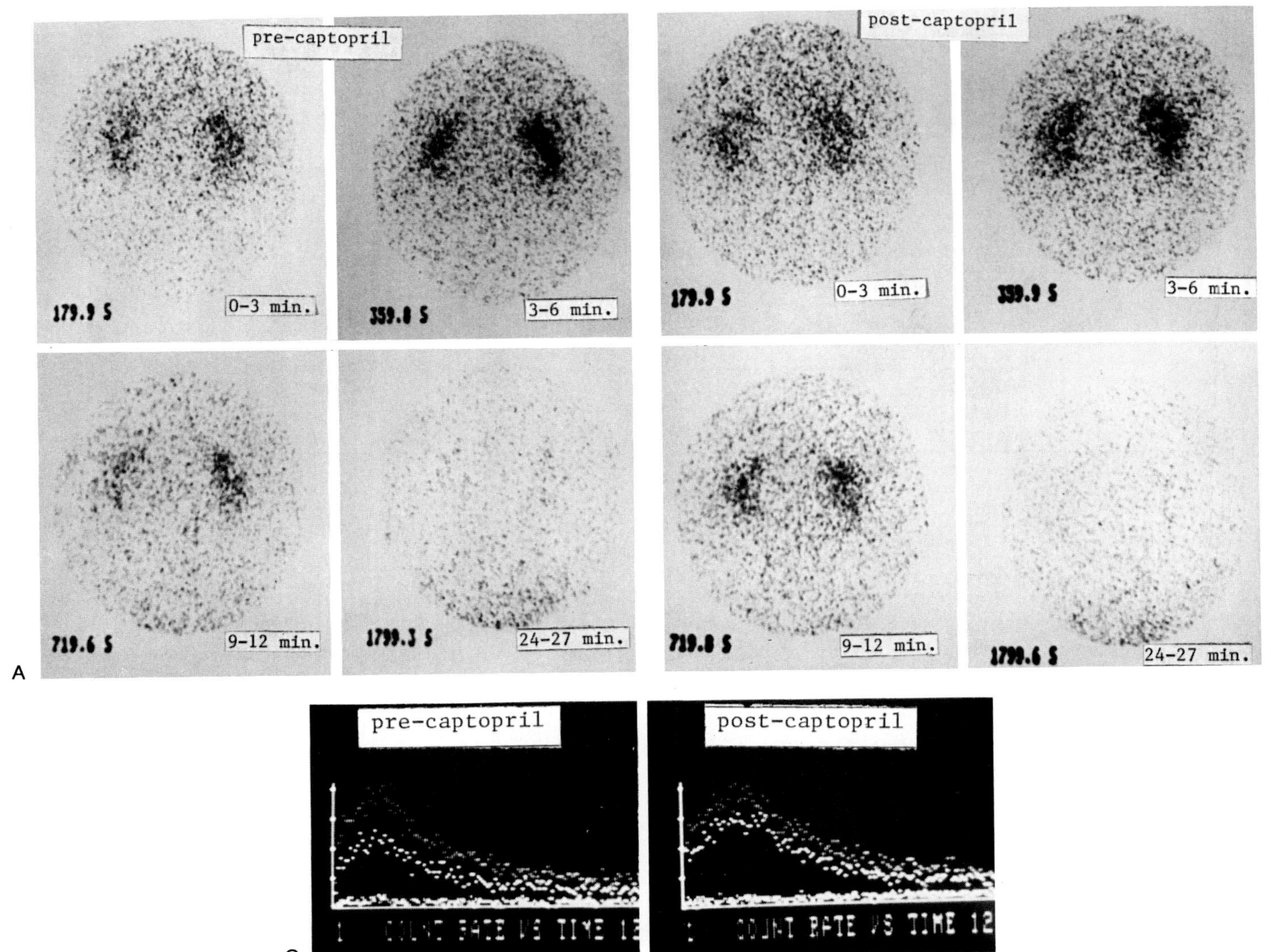

FIG. 11. This 49-year-old black male had hypertension (210/130 mmHg) before medication; diastolic blood pressure was still 110 mmHg after medication. **A:** A scintirenogram was obtained after injection of 150 μCi I-131-OIH. Sequential scinti-images in the posterior projection reveal slightly diminished left-sided uptake, as seen on the 0–3-min image. Subsequent images demonstrate normal excretion bilaterally. The above pattern is consistent with renal artery stenosis on the left side, although other asymmetric renal diseases may produce a similar pattern. **B:** The patient was administered 25 mg of oral captopril. After 1 hr a repeat scintirenogram was obtained with 300 μCi of I-131-OIH. There is no substantive change in the uptake or excretion pattern in comparison with the pre-captopril study represented in part A. **C:** Renogram curves before and after captopril are not substantially different. The absence of a change after captopril administration suggests asymmetric renal function for reasons other than renal artery stenosis. On the basis of this finding, the patient continues to be treated medically.

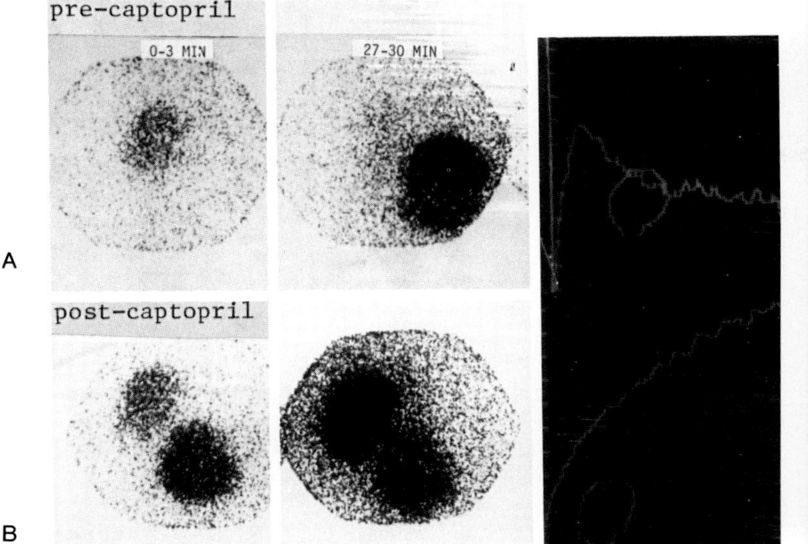

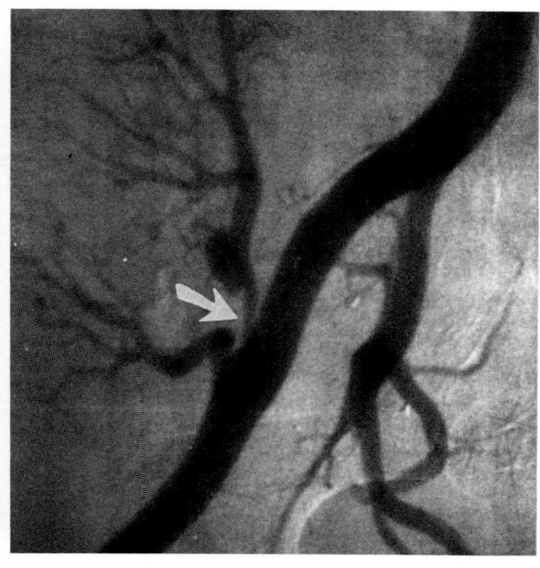

FIG. 12. This 31-year-old male transplant recipient had new onset of hypertension (170/110 mmHg sitting, 160/106 mmHg supine). **A:** After intravenous injection of 150 μCi I-131-OIH, sequential scintiphotos reveal normal initial uptake and good subsequent excretion. The renogram curve to the right parallels the scintigraphic findings and demonstrates a rapid upslope, early peak, and normal excretion. On its own merits, this study would not be suggestive of renal artery stenosis. **B:** The patient was given 25 mg of oral captopril, with a resultant fall in blood pressure to 130/90 mmHg in 30 min. A repeat scintirenogram after a second injection of I-131-OIH demonstrates satisfactory uptake, but progressive cortical accumulation without evidence for excretion, reflected in the scinti-images as well as in the renogram curve. This dramatic delay in renal transit with OIH has been reported (140). **C:** The angiogram demonstrates two renal arteries supplying the transplant. There is a stenosis of the upper renal artery (*arrow*). (From ref. 177, with permission.)

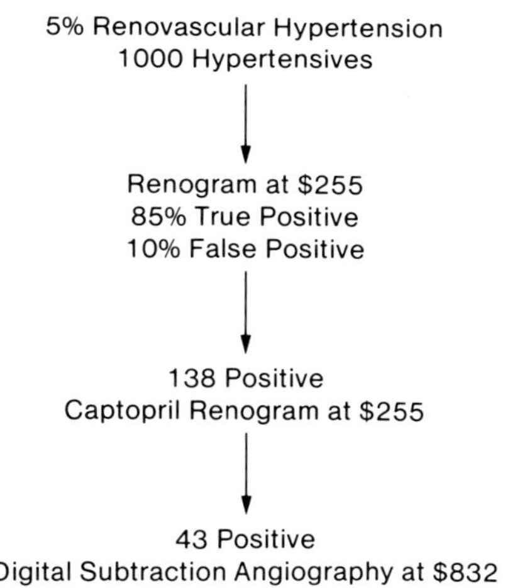

FIG. 13. Screening with captopril test. This flow scheme is based on the assumption that captopril renography may theoretically reduce the false positives in renography to nearly zero. This remains to be proven. A major benefit would be that 95 persons would be spared the discomfort and risk of digital subtraction angiography. (From ref. 175, with permission.)

(10)-ene-3 beta 1, known as NP-59 (152). None of these radiopharmaceuticals has been approved for routine use at this time.

The presence of free I-131, as well as expected further deiodination *in vivo,* mandates patient preparation including 1 day (preferably 2 days) of pretreatment with Lugol's iodine (3 drops, twice a day). This should be continued daily for 2 weeks after the exam. The patient is given 1–2 mCi per 1.7 m^2 of body surface area of high-specific activity NP-59 (1–5 mCi per milligram of cholesterol) by slow intravenous injection (over a period of 1–2 min) (153). Imaging is performed with a gamma camera which is combined with a medium-energy collimator and which is then interfaced with a computer. The imaging should begin 4–5 days following NP-59 injection, to allow background to clear (153). An additional 1 or 2 days may sometimes be helpful to improve image quality. The studies are limited by the fact that the absorbed radiation doses to the adrenal are higher than those associated with any other procedure or organ in current diagnostic nuclear studies (see Table 8).

Quantitation of adrenal uptake, analogous to that of thyroid uptake, may be performed; this is most readily done with a computer interface. Percent uptake of the initial dose then may be calculated after the correction for depth attenuation. Normal uptake ranges have been determined for NP-59 (154) as well as for I-131 19-iodocholesterol (155). Supranormal values have been reported to be associated with adrenocortical hypersecretion (154).

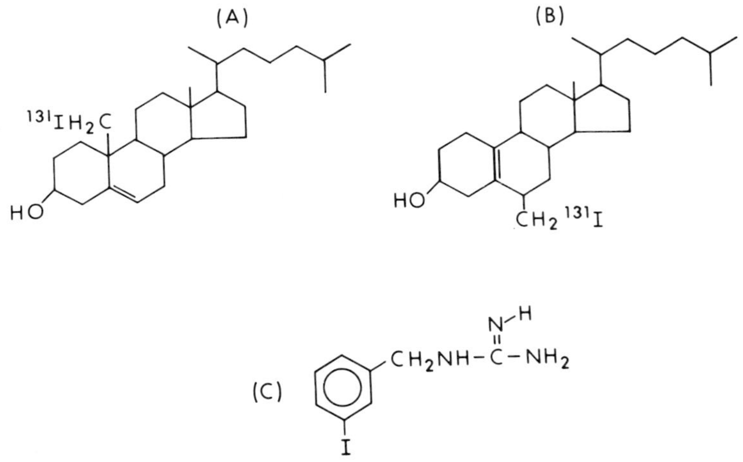

FIG. 14. The major adrenal cortical scanning agents. **A:** I-131 19-iodocholesterol. **B:** I-131 NP-59. **C:** The medullary agent I-131 meta-iodobenzylguanidine.

Hypercortisolism (Cushing's Syndrome)

The patient's clinical status, including serum cortisol levels and information about steroid medication, is essential for interpretation (Fig. 15) of these studies. The right adrenal normally is visualized slightly better than the left on the posterior view (vice versa on the anterior view) as a result of normal differences in depth of the adrenals. In the presence of documented cortisol excess, bilateral visualization (even if asymmetrical) represents adrenal hyperplasia (ACTH overproduction usually due to pituitary hyperfunction or ectopic ACTH overproduction). Rarely, bilateral hyperplasia plus unilateral adenoma may coexist; this situation is associated with greater than a 50% difference in uptake between the adrenals (153).

Unilateral visualization in the face of cortisol excess represents an adrenal adenoma suppressing ACTH production (thereby suppressing contralateral adrenal uptake) (155). Adenomas as small as 5 mm have been reported to be identified by this technique.

Bilateral nonvisualization in the face of cortisol excess may be due to corticosteroid administration or to adrenal cortical carcinoma. The carcinoma concentrates NP-59 less well than does normal tissue (155) (analogous to thyroid carcinoma) but still produces excess cortisol sufficient to suppress contralateral uptake, thereby resulting in bilateral nonvisualization.

TABLE 8. *Absorbed dose*

Tissue	I-131 NP-59[a] (rad/mCi)	I-123 NaI (rad/300 μCi)[b]
Total body	1.2	0.01
Adrenals	150.0[c]	—
Ovaries	8.0	—
Testes	2.3	—
Liver	2.4	—
Thyroid	—	4.5

[a] From refs. 150,151.

[b] Based on 27% uptake at 24 hr.

[c] Based on uptake data in experimental animals. In normal human adrenals, according to Beierwaltes et al. (151), the average dose is 27.5 rad.

Persistent cortisol excess due to adrenal remnants may be readily located using NP-59 or I-131 cholesterol (156).

The administration of dexamethasone aids in the distinction of hyperplasia from adenoma. Two milligrams of dexamethasone every 6 hours are administered by mouth, 2–3 days before NP-59, and continued until scanning is complete. Scanning should begin 1 day after NP-59 injection and should continue daily for 4 days (152). The normal response is bilateral nonvisualization. Persistent unilateral visualization is highly predictive for aldosterone adenoma (see section on hyperaldosteronism, below). Bilateral visualization by 4 days indicates macronodular hyperplasia. Bilateral visualization after 4 days has been associated with micronodular hyperplasia.

Hyperaldosteronism (Conn's Syndrome) (157)

The patient's clinical status, including medication, is essential for proper physiologic scan interpretation (Fig. 16).

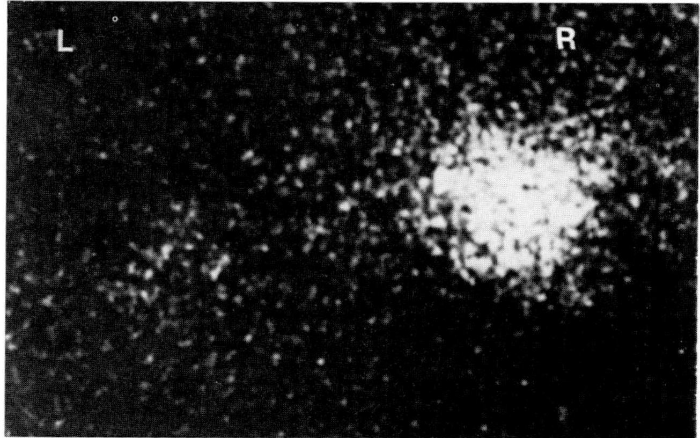

FIG. 15. In this patient with Cushing's syndrome and elevation of plasma cortisols, I-131-NP-59 (a cholesterol analog) was administered and posterior view scinti-images were obtained 72 hr after administration. These images reveal striking accumulation of I-131-NP-59 in the region of the right adrenal gland. There is no discernible activity in the region of the left adrenal gland. This pattern is that of an adrenal adenoma producing excessive cortisol. (From ref. 153, with permission.)

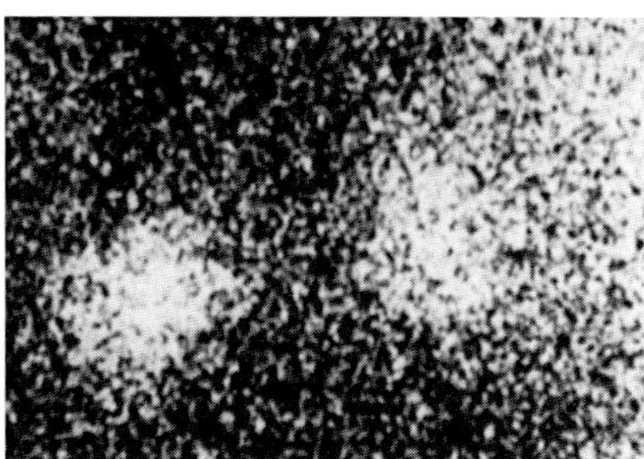

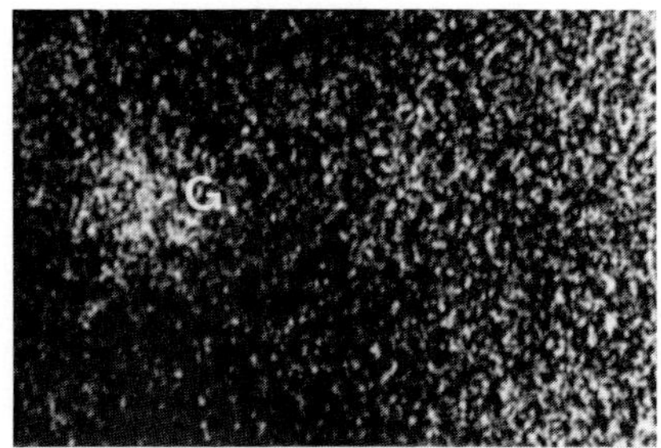

FIG. 16. A: I-131 NP-59 was administered to this patient with hyperaldosteronism. This scinti-image reflects concentration of NP-59 bilaterally in cells producing cortisol as well as in cells producing aldosterone. **B:** A repeat study was performed several weeks later in which the patient was pretreated with oral administration of dexamethasone. In principle, dexamethasone should suppress ACTH production by the pituitary gland. This, in turn, should suppress accumulation and metabolism of a cholesterol analog in cortisol-producing cells but not in aldosterone-producing cells (which are independent of ACTH). Accordingly, there is suppression of activity in both adrenals, but particularly there is suppression on the right side. There is persistent left-sided activity, indicating an aldosterone-producing adenoma on the left. (From ref. 153, with permission.)

Hyperaldosteronism, like hypercortisolism, may be due to unilateral or bilateral adenomas or to hyperplasia. Aldosterone hypersecretion, however, does not suppress pituitary ACTH production, and therefore an adenoma cannot suppress contralateral adrenal uptake. Asymmetry of uptake may be seen in normal subjects, particularly in the presence of macronodular hyperplasia, a nonpathologic variant.

Baseline scans performed in the same manner as above cannot distinguish hyperplasia from adenoma. If one gland fails to visualize, this may represent aldosterone-producing adrenal carcinoma of the nonvisualized side.

Pheochromocytoma

The development of I-131-labeled meta-iodobenzylguanidine (MIBG) has proven very exciting. This compound (Fig. 14) is concentrated in the adrenal medulla where its uptake is competitively inhibited by norepinephrine (159). The half-time for disappearance from the blood is approximately 15 min, and about 65% is excreted in the urine in the first 24 hr.

Pheochromocytomas are not common; however, when present, they are almost always accompanied by hypertension. Since up to 90% of pheochromocytomas are benign intra-abdominal tumors, they represent a surgically curable etiology of hypertension. The hypertension in such patients is due to excessive secretion of norepinephrine (usually) and epinephrine (less frequently) (149). Symptoms of palpatations, sweating, and headaches may be present in the afflicted individuals as a result of the effects of these hormones. The hypertension and symptoms are classically paroxysmal, but they may be sustained.

Diagnosis is suspected in the setting of severe hypertension, accompanied by the clinical symptoms described above. Urinary excretion of epinephrine and norepinephrine and of metabolites such as metanephrine, normetanephrine, and vanillylmandelic acid (VMA) may be quantitated to make the diagnosis. Plasma levels of norepinephrine and epinephrine may be more sensitive for diagnosis but are probably less specific than the urinary tests. Plasma levels are likely to be transiently influenced by emotions such as fear and pain, which commonly accompany the venipuncture needed to obtain the sample.

Until MIBG's very recent development (159), there had been no satisfactory radionuclide agents for physiologic visualization of the adrenal medulla. I-131-labeled cholesterol congeners such as NP-59 have not been satisfactory as medullary imaging agents.

The University of Michigan group has imaged the adrenal medulla successfully—first in dogs (159), then in primates (160), and most recently in humans (161). The affinity of this agent for pheochromatin tissue is such that MIBG has been used successfully to visualize many examples of adrenal disease. This may constitute an advantage over CT scanning or ultrasound, neither of which can specifically identify the tissue type of origin (162). Extra-adrenal chromatin tissue has been imaged in many patients (Fig. 17). In selected patients, I-131-labeled MIBG may even be used to treat metastatic pheochromocytoma.

EVALUATION OF MISCELLANEOUS DISEASES ASSOCIATED WITH HYPERTENSION

Hyperthyroidism

It should be recognized that an occasional patient with hyperthyroidism will present with hypertension. This diagnosis is easily excluded by *in vitro* measurements of serum thyroxine and of T3 uptake.

The 24-hr radioactive iodine uptake (RAIU) is a standard measure of thyroid function and is performed after oral administration of 100–300 μCi of I-123 sodium iodide (163). At 24 hr the thyroid uptake reflects both trapping and organification of iodine. In some cases, discharge of T4 labeled by I-123 has already begun. The normal range of uptake varies from lab to lab and is dependent on the patient population as well as on various technical factors (19). Labs report normal values anywhere from 5% to 50%, although 10% to 35–40% is quite common. The characteristically increased 24-hr RAIU of Graves' disease may not be seen in toxic nodular goiter.

In hyperthyroidism, nuclear procedures are useful in patient management, both diagnostically and therapeutically.

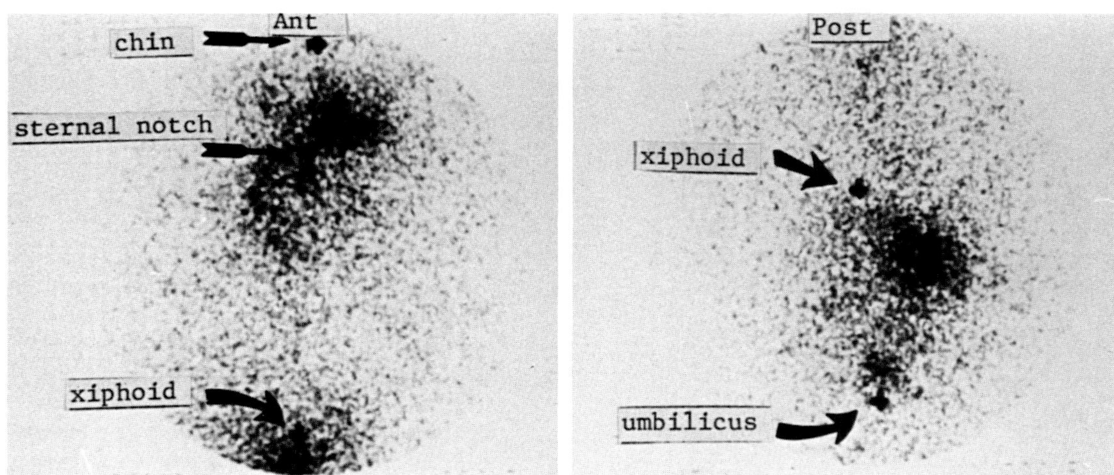

FIG. 17. In this patient with diastolic hypertension (125/100 mmHg on phenoxybenzamine and propranolol) and clinical evidence for pheochromocytoma, I-131-MIBG was administered; scans were obtained at 24 hr. There are multiple areas of focal accumulation of I-131-MIBG. These represent areas of metastatic pheochromocytoma.

The RAIU is necessary for radioiodine therapy and should always be preceded by *in vitro* serum testing.

Acute Interstitial Nephritis

Interstitial nephritis (noninfectious) is an occasional cause of hypertension which is susceptible to nuclear medicine diagnosis. Wood et al. (164) first noted the intense, diffuse, 48-hr uptake of gallium in three patients with biopsy evidence of this disorder. Linton et al. (165) described the same finding on gallium scanning in drug-induced interstitial nephritis. In addition, they studied patients with other renal disorders (e.g., acute tubular necrosis) in whom there was no uptake of the radionuclide.

Gallium scanning may help distinguish acute interstitial nephritis from acute tubular necrosis and other forms of renal disease.

Renal Artery Embolism

Renal artery embolism should be considered as a cause of acute hypertension, particularly in patients with atrial fibrillation or acute myocardial infarction. Radionuclide studies can play a major diagnostic role in this disorder and are especially helpful after angioplasty, when atherosclerotic plaques may be dislodged and cause infarction.

Early reports on patients with renal artery embolism noted the good correlation between Tc-99m-pertechnetate flow studies and renal arteriography (166–168). Tc-99m-pertechnetate perfusion scanning showed unilateral or bilateral absence of renal perfusion in 9 of 10 cases studied, and the remaining patient had bilateral perfusion defects. More recently, Tc-99m-DTPA (169), Tc-99m-glucoheptonate (170), and Tc-99m-DMSA (171) have been used and advocated for recognition of this problem.

Chronic Pyelonephritis

Chronic pyelonephritis, especially in the diabetic patient, is frequently associated with hypertension. Recognition of chronic nonobstructive pyelonephritis in the adult is not always simple, since a positive urine culture and pyuria are nonspecific. The "classical" changes on urography (calyceal blunting and deformity with depression of the overlying cortex) are seen most commonly in childhood as a result of vesicoureteric reflux (172). Adults with pyelonephritis may have advanced histological damage without an apparent abnormality on urography (173). The problem is further compounded by the continuing debate of the criteria for diagnosis of pyelonephritis and the fact that the end-stage kidney shares a common histological appearance with many other disease entities. The use of radionuclides is supported even by outdated Hg-197 chlormerodrin studies (174). In one such investigation, 50 patients with the clinical diagnosis of chronic pyelonephritis and normal urography were reviewed. Despite the poor image resolution of obsolete equipment and an imaging agent no longer in use, localized renal defects were seen in 10 patients.

McAfee (80) reported on 31 patients with chronic pyelonephritis (seven with renal insufficiency) who had urography and renal scans with Tc-99m-glucoheptonate and I-131 Hippuran and had abnormalities in at least one of these studies. Though the overall sensitivity to renal morphological abnormalities in this study was greater with urography than with scanning, focal parenchymal damage was seen better with nuclear imaging in eight patients; furthermore, glucoheptonate was reported to be more useful than Hippuran. Tc-99m-DMSA is also shown to be of great value in the assessment of cortical scarring in pyelonephritis (87,95).

An advantage over urography is that renal scans can demonstrate intraparenchymal abnormalities which do not deform the collecting system or renal outline. Nuclear imaging, therefore, may be a useful supplement to urography for detection of renal damage due to chronic pyelonephritis. The gallium scan is also of value in patients with renal infection.

Coarctation of the Aorta

Coarctation is usually diagnosed by physical examination. However, flow studies similar to the one shown in Fig. 8 demonstrate the abdominal aorta quite nicely and may be helpful in confirming the diagnosis and/or planning for angiography.

Polycystic Kidney

Polycystic kidney is commonly associated with hypertension. The role of nuclear medicine techniques in the diagnosis of polycystic kidney was discussed earlier, but this condition is evaluated best with ultrasonography.

Obstructive Uropathy

Obstructive uropathy may occasionally cause hypertension (Fig. 10). Renal imaging clarifies the diagnosis promptly.

Neuroblastoma

See discussion of pheochromocytoma.

Hyperparathyroidism

Hypertension may occur in hyperparathyroidism. The diagnosis is made by biochemical testing, but parathyroid scans may be helpful to the surgeon preoperatively.

REFERENCES

1. Patton DD. Introduction to clinical decisionmaking. *Semin Nucl Med* 1978;8(4):273.
2. Daly J, Jones W, Rudd TG, Tremann J. Differential renal function using technetium-99m,dimercapto succinic acid (DMSA): *in vitro* correlation. *J Nucl Med* 1979;20:63.
3. Kawamura J, Hosokawa S, Yoshida O, Fugita T, Ishii Y, Torizuka K. Validity of ^{99m}Tc dimercaptosuccinic acid renal uptake for an assessment of individual kidney function. *J Urol* 1978;119:305.
4. Kawamura J, Hosokara J, Yoshida O. Renal function studies using ^{99m}Tc-dimercaptosuccinic acid. *Clin Nucl Med* 1979;4:39.
5. Price RR, Born ML, Jones JP, Tonya J, Grove JB, Nadeau JH, Branch RA, Rhamy RH, Hallifield JW, Brill AB, Rollo FD. Comparison of differential renal function by Tc-99m DMSA, Tc-99m DTPA, I-131 hippuran and ureteral catheterization [Abstract]. *J Nucl Med* 1979;20:631.
6. Britton KE, Brown NJ. The clinical use of CABBS renography. Investigation of the "non-functioning kidney" and renal artery stenosis by the use of 131-hippuran renography by computer assisted blood background subtraction (CABBS). *Br J Radiol* 1968;41:570.
7. Doig A, Lawrence JR, Philip T, Tothill P, Donald KR. I-131 hippuran renography in detection of unilateral renal disease in patients with HTN. *Br Med J* 1963;1:500.
8. Fair WR. Renal perfusion/excretion determination renogram. *J Urol* 1975;113:535.
9. Gault MH, Sidhu JS, Fuks A. The ^{131}I-hippurate renogram as a quantitative test function in renal parenchymal disease. *Nephron* 1973;11:354.
10. Keane JM, Schlegel JU. The use of a scintillation camera system for scanning of hypertensive patients. *J Urol* 1972;108:12.
11. Keim HJ, Johnson PM, Vaughan DR Jr, Beg K, Follett DA, Freeman LM, Laragh JH. Computer-assisted static/dynamic renal imaging: a screening test for renovascular hypertension. *J Nucl Med* 1979;20(1):11.
12. Maxwell MH, Lupu AN, Taplin GV. Radioisotope renogram in renal arterial hypertension. *J Urol* 1968;100:376.
13. Nordyke RA, Gilbert FI Jr, Simmons EL. Screening for kidney disease with radioisotopes. *JAMA* 1969;208:493.
14. Rosenthall L. Ortho-iodohippurate ^{131}I kidney scanning in renal failure. *Radiology* 1966;87:298.
15. Schlegel JU, Ballule PT. A diagnostic approach in detecting renal and urinary tract disease. *J Urol* 1970;104:2.
16. Schoutens A, Dupuis F, Toussaint C. ^{131}I-Hippuran scanning in severe renal failure. *Nephron* 1972;9:275–290.
17. Wall CA, Hilario EM, Whalen JJ. An orderly search for a vascular lesion producing hypertension. *J Urol* 1972;108:511.
18. Wax SH, Frank IN, McDonald DF. Usefulness of the radioactive hippuran renogram in the differential diagnosis of azotemia. *J Urol* 1962;88:433.
19. Chervu S, Chervu LR, Goodwin PN, Blaufox MD. Thyroid uptake measurements with I-123. Problems and pitfalls: concise communication. *J Nucl Med* 1982;23:667.
20. Gillet R, Cogneaus M, Mathy R. The preparation of ^{123}I labelled sodium-ortho-iodohippurate for medical research. *Int J Appl Radiol Isot* 1976;27:61.
21. Heidenreich P, Lauer O, Fendel H, Oberdorfer M, Pabst HW. Total and individual renal function in children by means of ^{123}I-hippuran whole body clearance and scintillation camera. *Pediatr Radiol* 1981;11(1):17.
22. Stadalnik RL, Vogel JM, Jansholt A, Krohn KA, Matola NM, Lagunas-Solar MC, Zielinski FW. Renal clearance and extraction parameters of ortho-iodohippurate (I-123) compared with orthoiodohippurate (I-131) and para-aminohippurate. *J Nucl Med* 1980;21:168.
23. Burbank MK, Tauxe WN, Maher K, Hunt JC. Evaluation of radioiodohippuran for the estimation of renal plasma flow. *Proc Staff Meeting, Mayo Clin* 1961;36:372.
24. Mitta AEA, Fraga A, Veall N. A simplified method for preparing ^{131}I-labeled hippuran. *Int J Appl Radiol* 1961;12:146.
25. Nordyke RA, Tubis M, Blahd WH. Use of radioiodinated hippuran for individual kidney function tests. *J Lab Clin Med* 1960;56:438.
26. Schwartz FD, Madeloff MS. Simultaneous renal clearances of radiohippuran and para-aminohippurate in man. *Clin Res* 1961;9:208.
27. Tubis M, Posnick E, Nordyke RA. Preparation and use of ^{131}I labeled sodium iodohippurate in kidney function tests. *Proc Soc Exp Biol Med* 1960;109:497.
28. Dore EJ, Taplin GU, Johnson DE. Current interpretation of the sodium iodohippuran I-131 renocystogram. *JAMA* 1963; 185:925.
29. Magnusson G. Kidney function studies with I-131 tagged sodium orthoiodohippurate. *Acta Med Scand* 1962;171(Suppl 378):7.
30. Wax SH, McDonald DF. Analysis of the I-131 sodium *o*-iodohippurate renogram. *JAMA* 1962;179:140.
31. Wedeen RP, Goldstein MH, Levitt MF. The radioisotope renogram in normal subjects. *Am J Med* 1963;34:765.
32. Bianchi C, Coli A, Palla R, Rindi P. Divided renal plasma flow measurement. The improvement of a new technique. In: Timmermans L, Merchi G, eds. *Radioisotopes in the diagnosis of disease of the kidney and urinary tract.* Amsterdam: Excerpta Medica Fndn, 1967;273–280.
33. Koplowitz JM, Mitchel JF, Blahd WH. The radioisotope renogram. A comparison of qualitative and quantitative interpretation. *JAMA* 1963;192:12.

34. Taplin GU, Dore EJ, Johnson EE. The quantitative radiorenogram for total and differential renal blood flow measurement. *J Nucl Med* 1963;4:409.
35. Blaufox MD, Fine E, Lee HB. The role of nuclear medicine in clinical urology and nephrology. *J Nucl Med* 1984;25(5):619.
36. Hauser W, Atkins HL, Nelson KG. ^{99m}Tc-DTPA—a new radiopharmaceutical for brain and kidney imaging. *Radiology* 1970;94:679.
37. Lin TH, Khentigan A, Winchell HS. A ^{99m}Tc chelate substitute for organo-radiomercurial renal agents. *J Nucl Med* 1974;11:34.
38. Charamaza O, Budikova M. Method of preparation of a ^{99m}Tc-complex for renal scintigraphy. *Nucl Med (Stuttgart)* 1969;8:301.
39. Klopper JF, Hauser W, Atkins HL, Eckelman WC, Richards P. Evaluation of ^{99m}Tc-DTPA for the measurement of glomerular filtrate rate. *J Nucl Med* 1971;13:107.
40. Smith WW, Smith HW. Protein binding of phenol red, diodrast and other substances in plasma. *J Biol Chem* 1938;124:107.
41. Blaufox MD, Merrill JP. Simplified hippuran clearance: measurement of renal function in man with simplified hippuran clearances. *Nephron* 1966;3:274.
42. Freeman LM. The kidney. In: Freeman LM, Johnson PM, eds. *Clinical scintillation imaging.* New York: Grune and Stratton, 1975;332–333.
43. Rosenthall L. Residual urine determination by roentgenographic and isotopic means. *Radiology* 1963;80:454.
44. Rosenthall L, Tyler JL, Arzoumanian A. A crossover study comparing delayed radiohippurate images with furosemide renograms. *Diagn Imag* 1983;52:267–275.
45. Smith HW, Finkelstein N, Aluminosa L, Crawford B, Graber M. The renal clearance of substituted hippuric acid derivatives and other aromatic acids in dog and man. *J Clin Invest* 1945;24: 388–404.
46. Landowne M, Alving A. A method of determining the specific renal functions of glomerular filtration, maximum tubular excretion (or reabsorption) and "effective blood flow" using a single injection of a single substance. *J Lab Clin Med* 1947;32:931.
47. Blaufox MD. A compartmental analysis of the radiorenogram and uretics of ^{131}I-hippuran. In: Blaufox MD, ed. *Evaluation of renal function and disease with radionuclides.* Baltimore: Karger, 1972;107.
48. Blaufox MD, Orvis A, Owen CA Jr. Compartmental analysis of the radiorenogram and distribution of hippuran ^{131}I in dogs. *Am J Physiol* 1963;204:1059.
49. Blaufox MD, Merrill JP. Compartmental analysis of the hippuran I-131 renogram in man. *Fed Proc* 1965;24:405.
50. Tauxe WN, Dubovsky EV, Kidd T Jr, et al. New formulas for the calculation of effective renal plasma flow. *Eur J Nucl Med* 1982;7:51.
51. Tauxe WN, Maher FT, Taylor WF. Effective renal plasma flow: estimation from theoretical volumes of distribution of intravenously injected ^{131}I-ortho-iodohippurate. *Mayo Clin Proc* 1971;46:524.
52. Fine EJ, Axelrod M, Gorkin J, Saleemi K, Blaufox MD. Measurement of effective renal plasma flow: a comparison of methods. *J Nucl Med* 1987;28:1393–1400.
53. Schlegel JU, Hamway SA. Individual renal plasma flow determination in 2 minutes. *J Urol* 1976;116:282.
54. Kenny RW, Ackery DM, Fleming JS, Goddard BA, Grant RW. Deconvolution analysis of the scintillation camera renogram. *Br J Radiol* 1975;48:481.
55. Farmelant MH, Sachs CE, Burrows BA. The influence of tissue background activity on the apparent renal accumulation of radioactive compounds. *J Nucl Med* 1970;11:112.
56. Mlodkowska E, Liniecki B, Surma M. A method for subtraction of the extrarenal "background" in dynamic ^{131}I-hippurate renoscintigraphy. *Nucl Med (Stuttgart)* 1979;18:36.
57. Rosenthall L, Damtew B, Kloiber R. Selection of renal background for quantitative ^{131}I-hippurate relative renal function studies. *Diagn Imag* 1981;50:159.
58. Tonnesen KH, Munck O, Haid T, et al. Influence on the radiorenogram of variation in skin to kidney distance and the clinical importance thereof. In: zumWinkel K, Blaufox MD, Funck-Brentano JL, eds. *Radionuclides in nephrology.* Stuttgart: Georg Thieme, 1975;79.
59. Kohn HD, Mostbeck A. Value of additional lateral scans in renal scintigraphy. *Eur J Nucl Med* 1979;4:21–25.
60. Piepsz A, Denis R, Ham HR, Dobbeleir A, Schulman C, Erbsmann F. A simple method for measuring separate glomerular filtration rate using a single injection of ^{99m}Tc-DTPA and the scintillation camera. *J Pediatr* 1978;93:769.
61. Ostrowski ST, Tothill P. Kidney depth measurements using a double isotope technique. *Br J Radiol* 1975;48:291.
62. Gruenewald SM, Collins LT, Fawdry RM. Kidney depth measurement and its influence on quantitation of function from gamma camera renography. *Clin Nucl Med* 1984;10:338.
63. Britton KE, Whitfield HN, Nimmon CC, Hendry WF, Wickham JEA. Obstructive nephropathy: successful evaluation with radionuclides. *Lancet* 1979;1:905.
64. Gruenewald SM, Nimmon CC, Nawaz MK, Britton KE. A noninvasive gamma camera technique for the measurement of intrarenal flow distribution in man. *Clin Sci* 1981;61:385.
65. Whitfield HN, Britton KE, Nimmon CC, Hendry WF, Wallace DMA, Wickham JEA. Renal transit time measurements in the diagnosis of ureteric obstruction. *Br J Urol* 1981;53:500.
66. Braren V, Versage PN, Touya JJ, Brill AB, Goddard J, Rhamy RK. Radioisotopic determination of glomerular filtration rate. *J Urol* 1979;121:145.
67. Kempi V, Persson BRR. Evaluation of renal function parameters with simultaneously administered ^{99m}Tc-DTPA and ^{131}I-hippuran. *Eur J Nucl Med* 1983;8:65.
68. Zuckier LS, Axelrod MS, Wexler JP, Heller SL, Blaufox MD. The implications of decreased performance of new generation gamma-cameras on the interpretation of ^{131}I-hippuran renal images. *Nucl Med Commun* 1987;8:49.
69. Jewkes RF, Jayasingh K. Comparison of ^{123}I-hippuran and ^{99m}Tc-DTPA. *Nucl Med Commun* 1981;2:278.
70. Buck AC, Macleod MA, Blacklock NJ. The advantages of ^{99m}Tc-DTPA (Sn) in dynamic renal scintigraphy and measurement of renal function. *Br J Urol* 1980;52:174.
71. Hypertension Detection and Follow-up Program Cooperative Group. Five year findings of the Hypertension Detection and Follow-up Program. I. Reduction in mortality of persons with high blood pressure, including mild hypertension. *JAMA* 1979;242:2562.
72. Gates GF. Glomerular filtration rate: estimation from fractional renal accumulation of ^{99m}Tc-DTPA (stannous). *Am J Radiol* 1982;138:565–570.
73. Harris CC, Ford KK, Coleman RE, Dunnick NR. Effect of region assignment on relative renal blood flow estimates using radionuclides. *Radiology* 1984;151:791.
74. Blythe WB. Captopril and renal autoregulation. *N Engl J Med* 1983;308:390.
75. Nally JV, Clarke HS Jr, Grecos GP, Saunders M, Gross ML, Potvin WJ, Windham JP. Effect of captopril on ^{99m}Tc-diethylenetriaminepentaacetic acid renograms in two kidney, one clip hypertension. *Hypertension* 1986;8:685.
76. Koenigsberg M, Novich I, Lory M, Blaufox MD. Limits of sensitivity of radiopertechnetate flow studies in the detection of asymmetrical renal perfusion. In: Berlyne GM, et al, eds. *Contributions to nephrology.* Basel: S Karger, 1978;73.
77. Conrad GR, Wesolowski C, Kirchner PT. Intrarenal blood flow distributions from first transit recording of Tc-99m radiochelates [Abstract]. *J Nucl Med* 1985;26(5):132.
78. Bingham JB, Maisey MN. An evaluation of the use of ^{99m}Tc-dimercaptosuccinic acid (DMSA) as a static imaging agent. *Br J Radiol* 1978;51:599.
79. Enlander D, Weber PM, dos Remedios LV. Renal cortical imaging in 35 patients: superior quality with ^{99m}Tc-DMSA. *J Nucl Med* 1974;15:743–749.
80. McAfee JG. Radionuclide imaging in the assessment of primary chronic pyelonephritis. *Radiology* 1979;133:203–206.
81. Older RA, Korobkin M, Workman J, Cleeve DM, Cleeve LK, Sullivan D, Webster GD. Accuracy of radionuclide imaging in distinguishing renal masses from normal variants. *Radiology* 1980;136:443.
82. Kipper MF, Witztum KF, Taylor A. Visual determination of relative renal function: what to do until the computer comes [Abstract]. *J Nucl Med* 1982;23:P64.

83. Taylor A. Delayed scanning with DMSA. A simple index of relative renal plasma flow. *Radiology* 1980;136:449.
84. Yee CA, Lee HB, Blaufox MD. Tc-99m DMSA renal uptake influence of biochemical and physiologic factor. *J Nucl Med* 1981;22:1054.
85. McAfee JG, Thomas FD, Grossman Z, Streeten DHP, Dailey E, Gagne G. Diagnosis of angiotensinogenic hypertension: the complementary roles of renal scintigraphy and the saralasin infusion test. *J Nucl Med* 1977;18(7):669.
86. Pieretti R, Gilday D, Jeffs R. Differential kidney scan in pediatric urology. *Urology* 1974;4:665.
87. Ash JM, Antizo VF, Gilday DL, Houle S. Special considerations in the pediatric use of radionuclides for kidney studies. *Semin Nucl Med* 1982;12:345.
88. Atkins HL, Freeman LM. The investigation of renal disease using radionuclides. *Postgrad Med J* 1973;49:503–516.
89. Gordon I. A sensitive index of renal perfusion in hypertension. In: Joekes AM, et al, eds. *Radionuclides in nephrology.* London: Academic Press, 1982;205–209.
90. Timmermans L. A comparison of radioisotopic and ultrasonic scanning of the kidney. In: zumWinkel K, Blaufox MD, Funck-Brentano JL, eds. *Radionuclides in nephrology.* Stuttgart: Georg Thieme, 1975;101–106.
91 Blaufox MD, Conroy M. Measurement of renal mean transit time of hippuran ^{131}I with external counting. *J Nucl Biol Med* 1968;12:107–116.
92. Freeman LM, Goldman SM, Shaw RK, Blaufox MD. Kidney visualization with ^{131}I-ortho-iodohippurate in patients with renal insufficiency. *J Nucl Med* 1969;10:545–549.
93. O'Reilly PH, Shields RA, Testa HJ. Renovascular hypertension and renal failure. In: *Nuclear medicine in urology and nephrology.* London: Butterworths, 1979;81–85.
94. Reba RC, Poulouse KP, Kirchner PR. Radiolabeled chelates for visualization of kidney function and structure with emphasis on their use in renal insufficiency. *Semin Nucl Med* 1974;4:151.
95. Handmaker H, Young BW, Lowenstein JM. Clinical experience with ^{99m}Tc-DMSA (dimercaptosuccinic acid), a new renal imaging agent. *J Nucl Med* 1975;16:28–32.
96. Bradley-Moore PR, Nagel JS, Cano RA, Minker RG, Shapiro M, Jones AE, Johnstone GS. Kidney size measurement—mathematical solution to problems of angulation on two axes [Abstract]. *J Nucl Med* 1982;23:111.
97. Lassen NA, Henriksen L, Paulsen O. Regional cerebral blood flow in stroke by 133-xenon inhalation and emission tomography. *Stroke* 1981;12:284–288.
98. Kuhl DE, Wu JL, Lin TH, Senin C, Phelps M. Mapping local cerebral blood flow by use of emission computed tomography with *N*-isopropyl-*p* (123-I)-iodoamphetamine (IMP). *J Cereb Blood Flow Metab* 1981;1(Suppl 1):525–526.
99. Winchell HS, Horrt WD, Braun L, Hendorf WH, Hattner R, Parker H. *N*-Isopropyl-^{123}I-iodoamphetamine: single-pass brain uptake and washout; binding to brain synaptosomes; and localization in dog and monkey brain. *J Nucl Med* 1980;21:947–952.
100. Ell PJ, Cullum I, Costa DC. A new regional cerebral blood flow mapping with ^{99m}Tc-labeled compound. *Lancet* 1985;2:50–51.
101. Ell PJ, Jarritt PA, Costa DC, Cullum ID, Lui D. Functional imaging of the brain. *Semin Nucl Med* 1987;17:214–229.
102. Eckleman WC, Reba RC, Rzeszotarski WJ, et al. External imaging of cerebral muscarinic acetylcholine receptors. *Science* 1984; 223:291–292.
103. Blau M. Radiotracers for functional brain imaging. *Semin Nucl Med* 1985;15(4):329–334.
104. Borhani N, Blaufox MD, Oberman A, Polk F. Incidence of coronary heart disease and left ventricular hypertrophy in the Hypertension, Detection and Follow-up Program. *Prog Cardiovasc Dis* 1986;29(S-1):55–62.
105. Kannel WB, Schwartz MJ, McNamara PB. Blood pressure and risk of coronary heart disease. The Framingham Study. *Dis Chest* 1969;56:43–52.
106. Patel DG, Zimmer AM, Patterson VN. *In vivo* labeling of red blood cells with ^{99m}Tc: a new approach to blood pool visualization. *J Nucl Med* 1977;18:305.
107. Strauss HW, Zaret BL, Hurley PJ. A scintiphotographic method for measuring left ventricular ejection fraction in man without cardiac catheterization. *Am J Cardiol* 1971;28:575–580.
108. Borer JF, Bacharach SL, Green MV. Real time radionuclide cineangiography in the noninvasive evaluation of global and regional left ventricular function at rest and during exercise in patients with coronary artery disease. *N Engl J Med* 1977;296:839–844
109. Blaufox MD, Wexler JP, Sherman RA, Scharf SC, Sonnenblick EH, Strom JA, Lee HB. Left ventricular ejection fraction and its response to therapy in essential hypertension. *Nephron* 1981;28:112–117.
110. Borer JF, Jason M, Devereux R, Fisher J, Green MV, Bacharach S, Pickering T, Laragh JH. Function of the hypertrophied left ventricle at rest and exercise: Hypertension and aortic stenosis. *Am J Med* 1983;75(Suppl 3A):34–39.
111. Melin JA, Wijns W, Pouleur H, Robert A, Nannan M, DeCoster PM, Becker C, Detry JMR. Ejection fraction response to upright exercise in hypertension: relation to loading conditions and contractility. *Int J Cardiol* 1987;17:37–49.
112. Inouye I, Massie B, Lode D. Abnormal left ventricular filling on early finding in mild to moderate systemic hypertension. *Am J Cardiol* 1984;53:130.
113. Topol EJ, Traill TA, Fortuin NJ. Hypertensive hypertrophic cardiomyopathy of the elderly. *N Engl J Med* 1985;312:277.
114. Bonow RC, Bacharach SV, Green MV. Impaired left ventricular diastolic filling in patients with coronary artery disease assessment with radionuclide angiography. *Circulation* 1981;64:315.
115. Blaufox MD, Ross L, Koshy K, Lee HB. Physiologic effects of prazosin HCl: consequences of diuretic combination therapy. *Nephron* 1981;29:85–89.
116. Scharf SC, Lee HB, Wexler JP, Blaufox MD. Cardiovascular consequences of primary antihypertensive therapy with prazosin hydrochloride. *Am J Cardiol* 1984;53:32A–36A.
117. Gehring PJ, Hammond PB. The interrelationship between thallium and potassium in animals. *J Pharmacol Exp Ther* 1967;55:187.
118. Lebowitz E, Greene MW, Bradley-Moore P. Thallium-201 for medical use. *J Nucl Med* 1973;14:421.
119. Wolfe CL, Corbett JR, Levine SE. Determination of left ventricular mass by single photon emission computed tomography with thallium-201. *Am J Cardiol* 1984;53:1365–1368.
120. Liebson PR. Hypertension research: echocardiography in the measurement of left ventricular wass mass. *Hypertension* 1987;9(Suppl):11–12.
121. Bookstein JJ, Abrams HL, Buenger RE, Lecky J, Franklin SS, Reiss SS, Bleifer KH, Klatte EC, Varady PD, Maxwell MH. The role of urography in unilateral renovascular disease. *JAMA* 1972;220:1225.
122. Maxwell MH, Goonick HC, Witz R, Kaufman JJ. Use of the rapid sequence intravenous pyelogram in the diagnosis of renovascular hypertension. *N Engl J Med* 1964;270:213.
123. Thornbury JR, Stanley JC, Fryback DG. Hypertensive urogram: a nondiscriminatory test for renovascular hypertension. *Am J Radiol* 1982;138:43.
124. McNeil BJ, Varady PD, Burrows BA, Adelstein SJ. Measures of clinical efficacy. Cost-effectiveness calculations in the diagnosis and treatment of hypertensive renovascular disease. *N Engl J Med* 1975;293:216–221.
125. Wilson L, Dustan HP, Page IH, Foutasse EF. Diagnosis of renal arterial lesions. *Arch Intern Med* 1963;112:270.
126. Stewart PH, DeWeese MS, Conway J, Correa RJ. Renal hypertension: an appraisal of diagnostic studies and of direct operative treatment. *Arch Surg* 1962;85:617.
127. Pickering TG, et al. Predictive value and changes of renin secretion in hypertensive patients with unilateral renovascular disease. Successful renal angioplasty. *Am J Med* 1984;76:398–404.
128. Rudnick MR, Maxwell MH. Diagnosis of renovascular hypertension: limitations of renin assay. In: Narins RG, ed. *Controversies in nephrology.* New York: Churchill Livingstone, 1984;123.
129. Hollenberg NK. Response to saralasin and angiotensin's role in essential and renal hypertension. *Medicine* 1979;58(2):115–127.
130. Clorius JH, Schmidlin P. The exercise renogram. A new approach to current renal involvement in systemic hypertension. *J Nucl Med* 1983;24(2):104.

131. Mogensen P, Munck O, Giese J. ^{131}I-Hippuran renography in normal subjects and in patients with essential hypertension. *Scand J Clin Lab Invest* 1975;35:301.
132. Belman AB, Kropp KA, Simon NM. Renal pressor hypertension secondary to unilateral hydronephrosis. *N Engl J Med* 1968;278:1133.
133. Lewin A, Blaufox MD, Castle H, Entwisle G, Langford H, on behalf of the Hypertension Detection and Follow-up Program. Apparent prevalence of curable hypertension in the Hypertension Detection and Follow-up Program. *Arch Intern Med* 1985;145:424–427.
134. Fine EJ, Scharf SC, Blaufox MD. The role of nuclear medicine in evaluating the hypertensive patient. In: Freeman LM, Weismann HD, eds. *Nuclear medicine annual.* New York: Raven Press, 1984;23.
135. Gruenewald S, Collins L. Renovascular hypertension quantitative renography as a screening test. *Radiology* 1983;149:287–291.
136. Working Group on Renovascular Hypertension. Hypertension, detection, evaluation and treatment of renovascular hypertension. *Arch Intern Med* 1987;147:820–829.
137. Drew H, LaFrance N, Bender W, Walker G, Wagner H Jr. Renal function in patients with renovascular hypertension following inhibition of angiotensin converting enzyme [Abstract]. *J Nucl Med* 1984;25:P36.
138. Johnston CI, Jackson B. Overview: angiotensin converting enzyme inhibition in renovascular hypertension. *Kidney Int* 1987;31(Suppl 20):S154–S156.
139. Atkinson AB, Brown JJ, Cumming AMM, Fraser R, Lever AF, Leckie BJ, Morton JJ, Robertson JIS. Captopril in renovascular hypertension: long-term use in predicting surgical outcome. *Br Med J* 1982;284:689.
140. Geyskes CC, Oei Y, Puylaert AJ. Renography with captopril. Changes in patients with hypertension and unilateral renal artery stenosis. *Arch Intern Med* 1986;146:1705.
141. Jackson B, McGrath BP, Matthews G. Differential renal function during angiotensin converting enzyme inhibition in renovascular hypertension. *Hypertension* 1986;8(8):650.
142. Lee HB, Blaufox MD. Renal functional changes after converting enzyme inhibition or nitroprusside in hypertensive rats. *J Nucl Med* 1986;27(6):1053.
143. Wenting GJ, Tan-Tjiong HL, Derkx FH. Split renal function after captopril in unilateral renal artery stenosis. *Br Med J* 1984;288:886.
144. Miyamori I, Yasuhara S, Takeda Y. Effects of converting enzyme inhibition on split renal function in renovascular hypertension. *Hypertension* 1986;8(5):415.
145. Levenson DJ, Dzau VJ. Effects on angiotensin-converting enzyme inhibition on renal hemodynamics in renal artery stenosis. *Kidney Int* 1987;31(Suppl 20):S173–S179.
146. Tillman DM, Malatino LS, Lever AF, Robertson JIS. Transrenal changes in active and inactive renin and angiotensin II in renal artery stenosis: effects of converting enzyme inhibition. *Kidney Int* 1987;31(Suppl 20):S184–S190.
147. Sfakianikis G, Kyriakides G, Jaffe D. Single visit captopril renography for the diagnosis of curable renovascular hypertension. *J Nucl Med* 1985;26(5):P133.
148. Wenting GJ, Derkx FHM, Tan-Tjiong LH, van Seyen AJ, Man in't Veld AJ, Schalekamp MAD. Risks of angiotensin converting enzyme inhibition in renal artery stenosis. *Kidney Int* 1987;31(Suppl 20):S180–S183.
149. Aronoff SL, Passamani E, Borowski X. Norepinephrine and epinephrine secretion from a clinically epinephrine secretory pheochromocytoma. *Am J Med* 1980;69:321–324.
150. Beierwaltes WH, Wieland DM, Yu T, Swanson DP, Mosley ST. Adrenal imaging agents: rationale, synthesis, formulation and metabolism. *Semin Nucl Med* 1978;8(1):5.
151. Beierwaltes WH, Lieberman LM, Ansari AN, Nishiyama H. Visualization of human adrenal glands *in vivo* by scintillation scanning. *JAMA* 1971;216:275.
152. Sarkar SO, Cohen EL, Beierwaltes WH, et al. A new and superior adrenal imaging agent ^{131}I-6 iodomethyl-19-noncholesterol (NP-59): evaluation in humans. *J Clin Endocrinol Metab* 1977;45:333.
153. Thrall JH, Freitas JE, Beierwaltes WH. Adrenal scintigraphy. *Semin Nucl Med* 1978;8(1):23.
154. Freitas JE, Thrall JH, Swanson DP, Rifai AN, Beierwaltes WH. Normal adrenal imaging [Abstract]. *J Nucl Med* 1977;18:599.
155. Moses DC, Schteingart DE, Sturman MF, Beierwaltes WH, Ice RD. Efficacy of radiocholesterol imaging of the adrenal glands in Cushing's syndrome. *Surg Gynecol Obstet* 1974;139:201.
156. Schteingart DW, Conn JW, Lieberman LM, et al. Persistent or recurrent Cushing's syndrome after "total" adrenalectomy. *J Clin Endocrinol Metab* 1971;83:713.
157. Seabold JE, Cohen EL, Beierwaltes WH, Hinerman DL, Nishiyama RH. Adrenal imaging with ^{131}I-19 iodocholesterol in the diagnostic evaluation of patients with aldosteronism. *J Clin Endocrinol Metab* 1976;42:41.
158. Cryer PE. Physiology and pathophysiology of the human sympatho-adrenal neuroendocrine system. *N Engl J Med* 1980;303:436–444.
159. Wieland DM, Jiann-Long W, Brown LE, Mangner TJ, Swanson DP, Beierwaltes WH. Radiolabelled adrenergic neuron-blocking agents: adrenomedullary imaging with (^{131}I) iodobenzylguanidine. *J Nucl Med* 1980;21:349.
160. Wieland DM, Brown LE, Tobes MC, Rogers L, March DD, Mangner TJ, Swanson DP, Beierwalte WH. Imaging the primate adrenal medulla with ^{123}I and ^{131}I metaiodobenzylguanidine. *J Nucl Med* 1981;22:358.
161. Sisson JC, Fager MS, Valk TW, Gross MD, Swanson PP, Weiland DM, Tobes MC, Beierwaltes WH, Thompson NW. Scintigraphic localization of pheochromocytoma. *N Engl J Med* 1981;305:12.
162. Chatal JF, Charbonnel B. Comparison of iodo-benzylguanidine imaging with computed tomography in locating pheochromocytoma. *J Clin Endocrinol Metab* 1985;61(4):769–772.
163. Dorfman SG, Young RL, Nusynowitz ML. Thyroiditis and thyrotoxicosis. *JAMA* 1978;240:1520–1521.
164. Wood BC, Sharma JN, Germann DR, Wood WG, Crouch TT. Gallium citrate Ga-67 imaging in non-infectious interstitial nephritis. *Arch Intern Med* 1978;138:1665–1666.
165. Linton AL, Clark WF, Driedger AA, Turnbull DS, Lindsay RM. Acute interstitial nephritis due to drugs. *Ann Intern Med* 1980;93:735–741.
166. Hartenbower DL, Winston MA, Weiss ER, Coburn JW. The scintillation camera in embolic acute renal failure. *J Urol* 1970;104:799–802.
167. Freeman LM, Meng CH, Richter MW, et al. Patency of major renal vascular pathways demonstrated by rapid blood flow scintigraphy. *J Urol* 1971;105:473–481.
168. Lessman RK, Johnson SF, Coburn JW, Kaufman JJ. Renal artery embolism. *Ann Intern Med* 1978;89:477–482.
169. Sanders RC, Menon S, Sanders AD. The complementary uses of nuclear medicine and ultrasound in the kidney. *J Urol* 1978;120:521–527.
170. Kahn PC. Renal imaging with radionuclides, ultrasound and computed tomography. *Semin Nucl Med* 1979;9:43–57.
171. Arnold RW, Subramanian G, McAfee JG, Blair RJ, Thomas FD. Comparison of ^{99m}Tc complexes for renal imaging. *J Nucl Med* 1975;16:357–367.
172. Hodson CJ. The radiological contribution toward the diagnosis of chronic pyelonephritis. *Radiology* 1967;88:857–871.
173. Saunders CD, Corriere JN. The inability to diagnose chronic pyelonephritis on the excretory urogram in adults. *J Urol* 1974;111:560–562.
174. Davies ER, Roberts M, Roylance J, Penry JB, Stadden G. The renal scintigram in pyelonephritis. *Clin Radiol* 1972;23:370–376.
175. Blaufox MD, Freeman LM. Renewed role of nuclear medicine in renovascular hypertension. *Urol Radiol* 1988;10:35–38.

SECTION VII

Pathophysiology, Diagnosis, and Treatment of Specific Forms of Hypertension

PART A

Secondary Forms of Hypertension

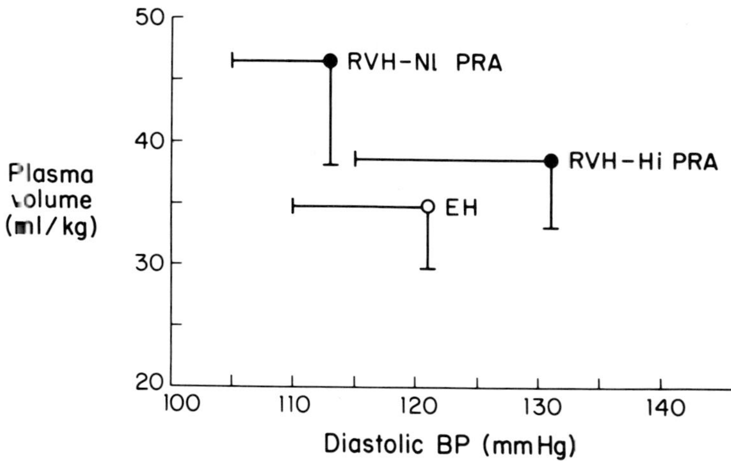

FIG. 2. Relationships between blood pressure, renin, and plasma volume in human renovascular and essential hypertension. (Data are from ref. 38.)

et al. (43), who reported nephroptosis in 70% of patients with fibromuscular dysplasia.

Despite this evidence for an apparent association between nephroptosis and hypertension, the physiologic mechanism remains obscure. It has been postulated that the renal mobility causes kinking of the renal artery, leading to fibrosis and obstruction, although this mechanism could be only contributory at best, since fibromuscular dysplasia also occurs in other less mobile arteries (e.g., celiac); other arteries subjected to much greater mobility (e.g., brachial) do not develop any similar lesions. Support for a functional significance of nephroptosis comes from a study by Bianchi et al. (44), who found that patients with nephroptosis show an exaggerated fall of glomerular filtration rate (GFR) on assuming the upright posture. It is equally possible that the nephroptosis is a consequence of the abnormal development of the renal arteries and plays no direct causal role.

Pathophysiologic Differences Between Unilateral and Bilateral Stenoses

In human renovascular hypertension the two most common patterns are unilateral and bilateral renal artery stenosis. Stenosis of the artery to a solitary kidney (equivalent to the one-clip one-kidney model in experimental animals) does of course occur, but only rarely. An important question, then, is whether the pathophysiology of the two common human patterns can be equated with the two animal models.

As discussed above, the resemblance between unilateral human renal artery stenosis and the one-clip two-kidney model is close (see Table 2). What is much less clear is what occurs with bilateral stenoses. Relatively little information is available concerning peripheral PRA levels, partly because it is often difficult to study patients with bilateral disease who are entirely free of antihypertensive medications. Two studies, however, have reported that PRA may be high in patients with both unilateral and bilateral disease (44,45). Consistent with this finding, it has been reported that patients with bilateral renal artery stenosis are just as likely to show a decrease of blood pressure when given converting-enzyme inhibitors (45). It is well recognized that in some patients with bilateral renal artery stenosis, converting-enzyme inhibitors may provoke azotemia, which would not occur if they did not also lower blood pressure. Not only are the levels of renin in the general circulation similar whether the stenoses are unilateral or bilateral, but the pattern of renal-vein renin is also indistinguishable. In patients with bilateral renal artery stenosis, we found that the renins tend to lateralize to the most ischemic kidney (46). Indeed, the most markedly asymmetrical patterns occur when one artery is totally occluded and the other stenosed. Figure 3 shows renal-vein renin patterns and peripheral (inferior vena cava) renin in patients with unilateral and bilateral renal artery stenosis. In both conditions, converting-enzyme inhibition with captopril, whether acute or chronic, has little effect on this asymmetrical pattern.

Despite these differences in renin between human bilateral disease and the one-kidney animal model, a number of circumstantial pieces of evidence suggest that there may be an increased effective blood volume in both cases. First, in our study of hemodynamic patterns comparing patients with unilateral and bilateral disease, using echocardiography, we found that in the patients with bilateral disease the cardiac output was higher than in patients with unilateral

TABLE 2. *Comparison of human and animal models of renovascular hypertension*[a]

	Animal	Human
	Two-kidney one-clip	Unilateral stenosis
Renin:	High	High
Volume:	Normal	Normal
Response to ACEI:	BP falls	BP falls
	One-kidney one-clip	Bilateral stenosis
Renin:	Normal	Normal/high
Volume:	Raised	? Raised
Response to ACEI:	Little change	BP falls

[a] ACEI, angiotensin-converting-enzyme inhibitor; BP, blood pressure.

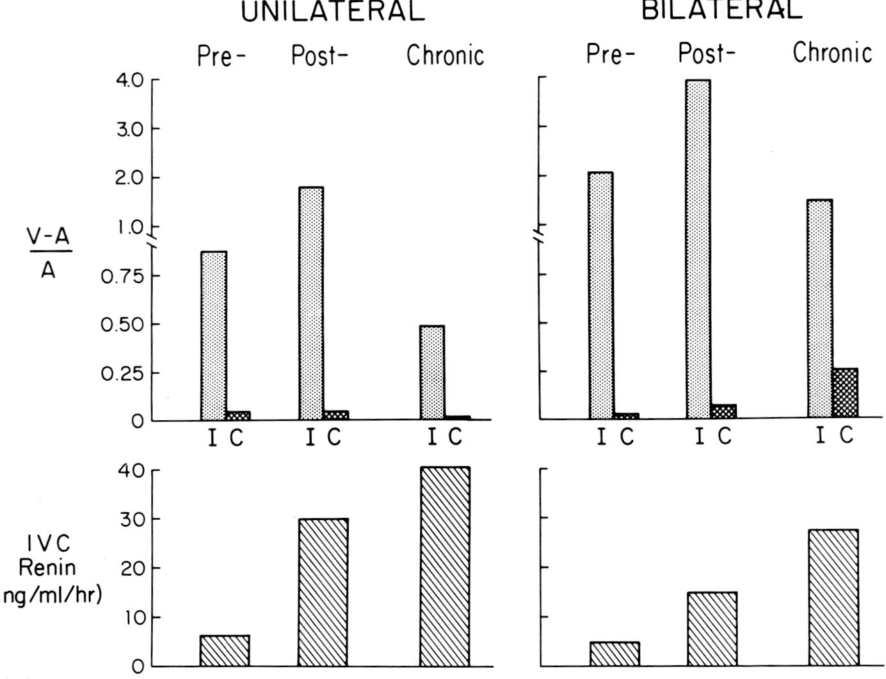

FIG. 3. Renal-vein renin patterns in patients with unilateral and bilateral renal-artery stenosis before (Pre-) and after (Post-) acute administration of captopril and during chronic treatment. I, most ischemic kidney; C, contralateral kidney; V, renin in renal vein; A, renin in inferior vena cava (equivalent to renal artery). Corresponding inferior vena cava (IVC) renins are shown in lower panels. (Data from ref. 47.)

disease (47). Second, as described in more detail below, we have found that recurrent pulmonary edema is more common in patients with bilateral disease than in those with unilateral disease (48). Third, we, as well as others (49), have observed that successful revascularization by angioplasty in a patient with bilateral renal artery stenosis or a solitary kidney is frequently followed by a diuresis, which is not seen in patients with unilateral disease (Fig. 4).

The overall picture in patients with bilateral renal artery stenosis is thus a mixed one, with both renin and volume factors typically being involved (Table 2). In this respect it differs from the one-kidney animal model. The most likely reason for this is that bilateral disease almost never develops symmetrically in the two kidneys, as witnessed by the common finding of (a) unequal kidney sizes and (b) asymmetrical renal-vein renin patterns. All bilateral cases presumably start out with unilateral disease. During the early stages of unilateral involvement there may well be parenchymal disease developing in the contralateral kidney, which would impair the pressure natriuresis by which the contralateral kidney normally maintains the classic high-renin normal-volume pattern of unilateral renal artery stenosis. This volume retention would be further exacerbated when the second stenosis develops in the contralateral renal artery.

The reason for the dissimilarity in renin levels between the one-kidney one-clip animal model and bilateral human renal artery stenosis deserves comment. The major influences affecting renin secretion are (a) delivery of sodium to the distal tubule (macula densa mechanism), (b) angiotensin II, (c) intrarenal arterial pressure acting via the renal baroreceptors, and (d) sympathetic nerve stimulation (50). In the one-clip two-kidney animal, sodium excretion occurs predominantly via the contralateral kidney, and renin secretion is suppressed by the increased sodium load at the macula densa. In the one-kidney model, all the sodium is excreted via the ischemic kidney, so that the renin secretion is suppressed, or at least normalized. In bilateral human renovascular disease the pattern of sodium excretion is often asymmetrical (51), with most of the excretion

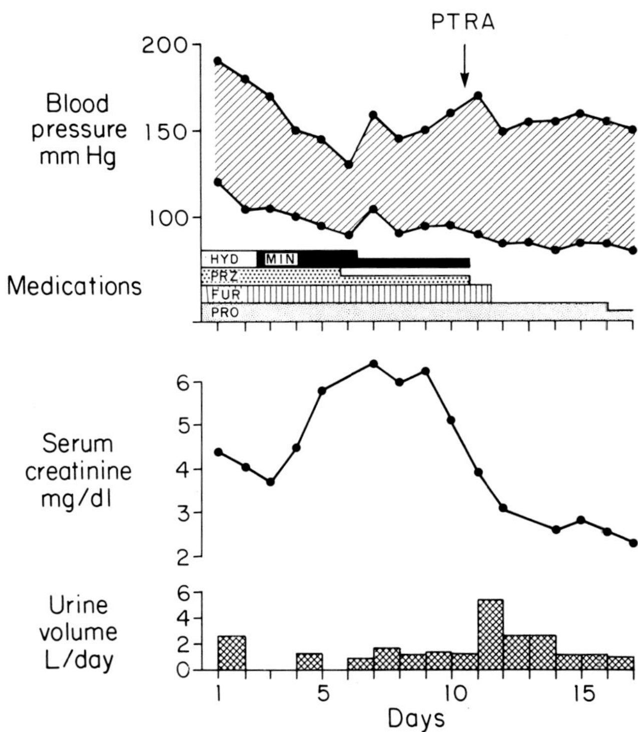

FIG. 4. Blood pressure, serum creatinine, and urine volume in a patient with bilateral renal-artery stenosis before and after renal angioplasty (PTRA). Note elevation of creatinine when minoxidil (MIN) was added to regimen, and also note improvement following PTRA, together with diuresis.

occurring via the less ischemic kidney. Thus, even though there may be net sodium and volume retention in such patients, there may be little or no increase of sodium delivery to the macula densa of the most ischemic kidney, which hence continues to secrete renin.

Role of Other Hormonal Factors

Many patients with renovascular hypertension have mild to moderate secondary hyperaldosteronism. However, in our experience, aldosterone excretion is generally less elevated for a given level of PRA than in other high-renin states (e.g., malignant hypertension). Two possible explanations for this observation are that there may be a dissociation between PRA and plasma levels of angiotensin II in some patients. The other, more likely hypothesis is that the state of sodium balance may alter the adrenal sensitivity to angiotensin II (AII), since it has been established that sodium depletion augments the aldosterone response to AII in isolated glomerulosa cells (52). Thus the degree of hyperaldosteronism may be a marker of volume status.

Plasma catecholamines are probably normal in human renovascular hypertension (53), unless there is azotemia (54). It has been suggested that the sympathetic nervous system contributes to short-term fluctuations of blood pressure, because a positive correlation has been observed (over a 24-hr period) between plasma norepinephrine and blood pressure and between plasma norepinephrine and renin (53).

ANATOMY AND PATHOLOGY OF RENAL ARTERIES

Normal Patterns

Although the most common pattern is a single renal artery and vein on each side, this actually only applies to a minority (38.5%) of people (55), since the majority of people have either multiple renal arteries or veins on one side, as shown in Table 3.

TABLE 3. *Anatomy of renal arteries (A) and veins (V)*

Percent of subjects	Right	Left
38.5	1A–1V	1A–1V
31.5	1A–1V	2A–1V
10	2A–1V	1A–1V
9.5	1A–2V	1A–1V
28.5	Complex patterns	

Atheromatous Lesions

Atheromatous plaques occur most commonly in the proximal third of the renal artery; in many cases, plaques in the wall of the aorta may encroach the ostium of the renal artery. If atheromatous lesions are left untreated, there is a high probability of progression to complete occlusion: In one series the average rate of progression of the percentage of transluminal diameter stenosed was estimated to be about 1.5% per month (56). Thus for patients with stenoses measuring 75–99% of luminal diameter at angiography, 40% had progressed to complete occlusion after 1 year.

Fibromuscular Dysplasia

Fibromuscular dysplasia of the renal arteries is the most common cause of renovascular hypertension in younger patients, and it has been classified into five types according to the pathologic differences in the lesions (Table 4). Medial fibroplasia is the most common variety in adults (accounting for at least 70% of cases) but is rare in children, and it produces the classical beaded appearance on angiography due to areas of thickening of the media, interspersed by areas of aneurysmal dilatation. This type of lesion is not confined to the renal arteries, since it may also occur in the carotid and cerebral arteries. Progression of these lesions to complete occlusion almost never occurs.

The second most common variety is perimedial fibroplasia (20%), where there is proliferation of fibrous tissue in the outer half of the media. Radiographically the appearance is also of beads, but they are not aneurysmal, so that they are of smaller diameter than the arterial lumen. The stenoses are often quite severe and may occasionally progress to complete occlusion (57).

Medial hyperplasia and intimal fibroplasia (5%) are angiographically indistinguishable and may produce a single proximal stenosis which can resemble atheroma. The former is characterized histologically by increased smooth muscle in the media; the latter is characterized by proliferation of mesenchymal cells and connective tissue in the intima.

TABLE 4. *Classification of fibromuscular dysplasia of the renal arteries*

	Intima	Media			Adventitia
Site of lesion type	Intimal fibroplasia	Medial fibroplasia	Perimedial fibroplasia	Medial hyperplasia	Periarterial fibroplasia
Frequency	5%	70%	20%	5%	1%
Angiographic appearance	Single smooth lesion	String of beads	Smaller beads	Single smooth lesion	Single lesion
Progressive	Yes	1/3	Yes	Yes	?
Occlusion of artery	Yes	No	Yes	Yes	?
Comments	Children	Also extrarenal	Young women	Teenagers	

The rarest type is periarterial fibroplasia, which is characterized by fibrosis encircling the renal artery.

Arteritis

Takayasu's arteritis is a rare disease affecting mainly young women; it can cause discrete stenosis of the aorta and major arteries, including the renal arteries.

Cholesterol Emboli

In patients who have diffuse atheroma, fragments of plaque may break off and cause embolization in the kidneys and other vascular beds. This may occur spontaneously, or it may occur following aortic surgery and renal arteriography (58). Pathologically, the lesions are characterized by microemboli of cholesterol crystals and amorphous debris, which are later replaced by foreign-body giant cells and fibrosis.

Clinically, the emboli are manifested by a deterioration of renal function and an exacerbation of the hypertension (59). Other features include gastrointestinal bleeding, acute pancreatitis, and gangrene or livedo reticularis in the feet. The diagnosis may be suspected if these manifestations develop after an invasive procedure in a patient over the age of 60 with known atheromatous disease, but it can only be established with certainty if the microemboli are visualized on a tissue biopsy.

CLINICAL FEATURES OF RENOVASCULAR HYPERTENSION

Prevalence

The prevalence of renovascular hypertension is unknown, but it is probably around 5% of the general hypertensive population (60); however, for patients with more severe hypertension, much higher figures have been reported. In a series of 123 patients with accelerated or malignant hypertension (grade III or IV retinopathy), Davis et al. (61) reported a prevalence of 43% in white patients and 7% in blacks. Other studies have also reported a lower prevalence in blacks. A recent survey of 7200 black hypertensive patients detected 0.65% with renovascular hypertension, but not all of these patients were fully screened (62). The majority of such cases were due to atheroma.

These results were all based on clinical studies, which, with one exception (61), did not utilize arteriography in all patients. The prevalence rates are therefore almost certainly an underestimate. However, the situation is complicated by the fact that the demonstration of an anatomical stenosis in the renal artery of a hypertensive patient does not imply that the lesion is causing the hypertension. In an autopsy series of 295 patients, Holley et al. (63) found moderate or severe renal artery stenosis in 49% of normotensives and in 77% of hypertensives. In another series of 500 aortograms performed for investigation of peripheral vascular disease or hypertension, renal artery stenosis was detected in 32% of normotensives and in 62% of hypertensives (64).

Clinical Signs and Symptoms

Because of its relative frequency and curability, it is important not to miss the diagnosis of renovascular hypertension, and there may be many clues to its presence from the history and clinical examination. Some of the most important features which distinguish it from essential hypertension are shown in Table 5; the table also shows the differences between the two most common types, atheroma and fibromuscular dysplasia.

In younger patients (particularly women), fibromuscular disease is the most common cause, but it is relatively rare in blacks. A family history of hypertension is less likely to be present than in cases of essential hypertension, although a familial occurrence of fibromuscular dysplasia has occasionally been described. Thus in a young white woman with a recent onset of hypertension and a negative family

TABLE 5. *Clinical characteristics of renovascular hypertension*[a]

	Essential hypertension	Renovascular hypertension: Atheroma	Renovascular hypertension: Fibromuscular dysplasia
Race (black)	29%	7%	10%
Family history	67%	58%	41%
Age at onset			
<20 years	12%	2%	16%
>50 years	7%	39%	13%
Duration <1 year	10%	23%	19%
Obese	38%	17%	11%
Abdominal bruit	7%	41%	57%
High renin profile	15%	80%	80%
Hypokalemia			
($K < 3.4$ mEq/liter)	7%	14%	17%
Smoking	42%	88%	71%

[a] Based on the U.S. Cooperative Study (65).

expensive (92). Its use as a routine screening procedure is therefore not recommended.

Another current technique is one that uses technetium diethylene triamine penta-acetic acid (Tc-DTPA), which measures glomerular filtration. The sensitivity and specificity are around 70% and 79%, which are not much better than for the IVP (93).

Captopril Renography

A potentially interesting development of the conventional renal scan is that we can compare the renograms obtained before and after a single dose of captopril. The rationale for this is that the glomerular filtration rate of an ischemic kidney is dependent on the effects of angiotensin on the efferent glomerular arterioles, so that converting-enzyme inhibition produces a marked fall in GFR. There are also less pronounced changes in renal blood flow. Thus the characteristic effect of captopril in a kidney with renal-artery stenosis is a decrease of DTPA uptake (a measure of GFR) with little change of Hippuran uptake (a measure of renal blood flow), although the excretion phase of Hippuran is delayed (94,95). It has been suggested that prior furosemide administration may augment the sensitivity of the test (96).

Exercise Renography

Another recent development of the conventional renal scan has been the recording of Hippuran scans before and after exercise (97,98). In normal subjects there is some delay in Hippuran transport during exercise, probably occurring as a result of hemogenically mediated renal vasoconstriction. In patients with essential hypertension there is a much more pronounced delay, which may be indicative of a transient cortical perfusion disturbance. The reasons for this situation are not clear, but it may possibly be due to structural changes occurring in the kidney. Patients with curable renovascular hypertension show a normal response to exercise. This test is potentially of interest, since it may be able to detect irreversible parenchymal changes; however, it requires further evaluation.

Ultrasound Scans

Another new technique currently being investigated is the use of Doppler ultrasound scanning to record velocity profiles from the renal arteries (99,100). In patients with renal artery stenosis the flow profile is more sluggish, but this is also seen in patients with advanced renal parenchymal disease (100).

Split Renal Function Studies

In 1953, Howard et al. introduced split renal function studies to identify patients with surgically correctable renovascular hypertension (101). This remains one of the most accurate and reliable tests, but it has fallen into disfavor because of its relative invasiveness—it necessitates cystoscopy and catheterization of both ureters.

The criteria for identifying an ischemic kidney were that there should be a 50% reduction of urine flow together with a 15% reduction of urine sodium concentration when the ischemic kidney was compared to the nonischemic kidney (102).

In patients with bilateral renal artery stenosis, the same degree of asymmetry of excretory function is seen as in patients with unilateral stenosis (51).

Arteriography

The demonstration of a stenosis in a renal artery in a hypertensive patient does not necessarily imply that the stenosis is causing the hypertension, particularly when it is atheromatous. Hypertension from any cause accelerates the development of atheroma, so that in some cases a stenosis in a renal artery may occur secondarily to essential hypertension. To cause renal ischemia and hypertension, a stenosis must occlude at least 75% of the arterial lumen, but the correlation between the arteriographic appearance and the degree of ischemia is poor (103,104).

In one series where the accuracy of arteriography in diagnosing the pathology of the renal arteries was estimated by comparison with the pathologic specimens removed at surgery, the sensitivity for distinguishing fibromuscular disease from atheroma was 82% (105). The absence of abdominal aortic atherosclerosis was a reliable predictor of fibromuscular disease. Separation of the different types of fibromuscular disease could not be reliably assessed from the arteriogram, however.

Proposed Schema for Evaluation of Patients with Suspected Renovascular Hypertension

Our own schema for the evaluation of hypertensive patients for renovascular hypertension is shown in Fig. 7. We perform renin–sodium profiling after discontinuation of all antihypertensive medications whenever possible. If the patient has complications such as cardiovascular or cerebrovascular disease it may not be possible to do this, in which case the diagnosis can be evaluated by renal sonography, renal-vein renins, or digital intravenous angiography. Another very promising diagnostic test is provided by giving the patient a single 25-mg oral dose of captopril and measuring the response of PRA and blood pressure (see above). Patients with renovascular hypertension show a much larger rise of renin than do those with essential hypertension, although the differences in the blood pressure response is less pronounced (79,93). The captopril tests can be performed while patients are taking beta blockers. For those patients with high renin–sodium profiles or a positive captopril test, we would next proceed to perform renal-vein renin tests, which can be done as an outpatient procedure, preferably while on no medication. These are usually done before and after acute administration of captopril or in conjunction with digital intravenous angiography. If these

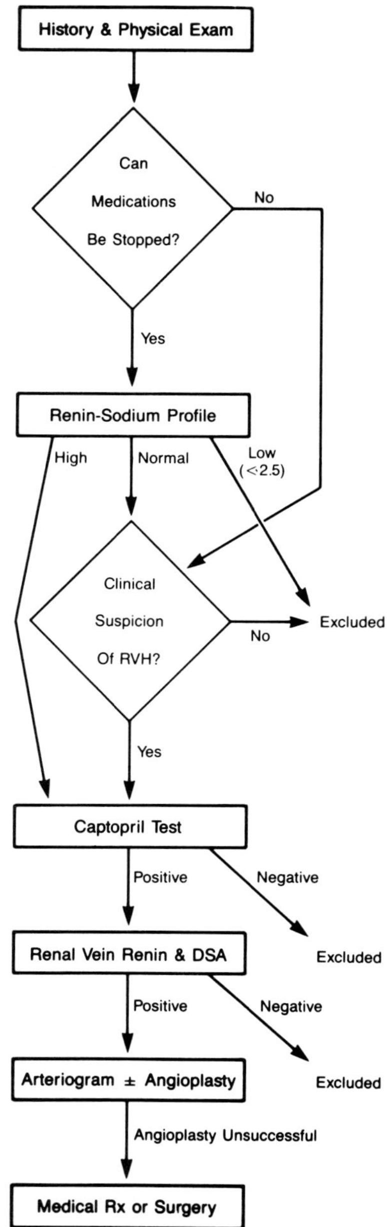

FIG. 7. Schema for evaluation of patients with renovascular hypertension.

tests are suggestive of renovascular hypertension, the patient is admitted to hospital for arteriography; if arteriography confirms the diagnosis, angioplasty can be performed at the same session.

NON-SURGICAL TREATMENT OF RENOVASCULAR HYPERTENSION

Renal Angioplasty

The technique of transluminal balloon dilatation was pioneered by the work of Dotter, who in 1964 first used co-axial catheters to produce progressive dilation of stenosed arteries (106), but at that time it did not find much popularity. Ten years later Grüntzig introduced the first successful balloon catheter (107), which has subsequently been further developed for use in several different arterial regions. In many centers, such as our own, renal angioplasty has become the treatment of first choice for patients with renovascular hypertension, particularly when the lesions are due to fibromuscular dysplasia. The fact that angioplasty can be performed at the same time as arteriography has led us to regard the arteriogram as a therapeutic rather than a diagnostic procedure. This means that the diagnosis should be reasonably certain before the arteriogram is performed.

Techniques

Before angioplasty is contemplated, it is our custom to consult a vascular surgeon. In a small proportion of cases emergency surgery is required, either to repair a bleeding femoral artery at the site of the catheterization, or to perform a renal bypass operation.

The procedure is performed under local anesthesia, in patients whose diastolic pressure should be less than 110 mmHg. The femoral approach is generally preferred (108), although some authors have favored using the axillary artery in patients whose renal artery comes off the aorta at a very acute angle. After the aortogram has been done to define the anatomy of the lesion, the patient is heparinized, and nitroglycerine is infused into the renal artery; then a thin guide wire is advanced across the stenosis. The guide wire is changed to a stiffer one which will support the balloon catheter, which is then passed over the guide wire so that the mid-portion of the balloon straddles the stenosis. When this has been accomplished the balloon is inflated with contrast medium to a pressure of 4–10 atmospheres for about 60 sec. Spot films are then taken to assess the adequacy of the dilation. This can also be assessed by measuring the pressure gradient across the stenosis before and after the procedure, bearing in mind the fact that the size of the catheter used to make this measurement may partially occlude the artery, and hence overestimate the gradient.

Mechanisms of Angioplasty

It used to be thought that in atheromatous lesions the effect of angioplasty was to compress the plaque. Subsequent studies using animal models and cadaver arteries showed that it caused endothelial desquamation and intimal splitting of the plaque, with separation of the plaque from the tunica media (109,110). There is stretching and often rupture of the media of the arterial wall, with bulging of the adventitia, and an increase in the outer diameter. This may explain why better long-term results are produced by using the largest possible balloon diameter.

The angiogram taken immediately following angioplasty often shows an intimal flap or dissection. This usually gets reabsorbed with time, and long-term follow-up often shows remodeling of the arterial lumen, with a smoother appearance.

Results with Angioplasty

There are now several published series of clinical results obtained with angioplasty, but as with surgery, it is appropriate to consider the results with atheroma and fibromuscular dysplasia separately. Success of the procedure can be gauged in two ways: First, the degree to which the lesion can be dilated, and second, the effects on the blood pressure. The criterion which we have used (111) for the former is that there should be a stenosis of at least 75% of the arterial lumen diameter on the arteriogram before angioplasty, and a successful dilation is one where the residual stenosis is less than 50%. Partial success is defined as a residual stenosis of 50–70%, and failure if no dilation of the lesion can be achieved. It should be emphasized that these criteria are somewhat crude, since the lumen is commonly eccentric, and angiography is performed in only one plane.

The blood pressure response to angioplasty or surgery is usually classified as Cured (that is a diastolic pressure below 90 mmHg without medication), Improved (a decrease of at least 15% but still requiring medication), or Failed (a decrease of less than 15%), according to the criteria originally developed for the US Cooperative Study of surgery for renovascular hypertension (65).

The results of some of the larger published series are summarized in Table 9. The results with the fibromuscular patients are uniformly good, and comparable to those obtained with surgery. Restenosis is very rare in these patients, and follow-up angiograms (up to 5 years after angioplasty) often show no trace of any stenosis at all. In the atheromatous group the results are not nearly so good, and there is a much wider scatter of the success rates in the published series. There are at least three possible reasons for this. One is the anatomy of the lesions: Ostial lesions can rarely be successfully dilated, presumably because they are an extension of large aortic plaques, as opposed to plaques originating within the renal artery, which usually can be dilated. A second reason for the variability of the results relates to the technique of the radiologist: It is important to use as large a balloon as possible. This would be in accordance with the anatomical postmortem findings which indicate that a functionally successful angioplasty usually results in tearing of the media, and bulging of the adventitia of the stenosed artery (110). Thirdly, in many cases of atheromatous renal artery stenosis it is likely that the stenosis was not the original cause of the hypertension. Thus, essential hypertension accelerates the formation of atheromatous plaques in the renal arteries just as in other regions. When the plaque reaches a critical size it may begin to add a renovascular component to the hypertension, and it is only this component that would be reversed by angioplasty or surgical revascularization. This is in contrast to fibromuscular dysplasia, where the patients are typically younger, the duration of the hypertension often shorter, and where there is a much greater degree of certainty that the stenosis is the original cause of the hypertension.

In those patients in whom the procedure is technically successful there is usually a prompt fall of blood pressure, which is maximal within 6 hr. In the atheromatous patients with unilateral stenoses in our series, the eventual benefit rate (judged at 3 months after angioplasty, and defined as an improvement or cure of the hypertension) was 87%, and 92% in the fibromuscular patients. Others have reported that there is a high incidence of restenosis in patients with atheromatous disease (119), but our own experience is that this is comparatively rare if a successful dilatation is achieved in the first place.

Angioplasty for the Preservation of Renal Function

In a smaller number of patients with renal failure we have also found that angioplasty can cause a significant improvement in renal function. We have seen this either in patients who have a critical stenosis of a solitary kidney, or in patients who have severe bilateral stenoses. Such patients are notoriously difficult to treat with medications, because a reduction of blood pressure is associated with a dramatic deterioration of renal function. This is most common when angiotensin-converting-enzyme inhibitors are used (120). If angioplasty can be achieved in this situation it is particularly rewarding, because it can both improve renal function and make the blood pressure easier to control. However, we have seen other patients in whom renal function has not improved or has deteriorated despite a successful angioplasty. These patients almost always have atheromatous disease, and may have an irreversible component to their azotemia, either from nephrosclerosis or cholesterol emboli (121). In other patients, with grossly normal renal function, angioplasty can result in an increase in size of the kidney. In our own series of 55 patients (122), all of whom had baseline serum creatinine above 2 mg/dl, 43 (75%) could be successfully dilated; 27 (63%) of these showed a decrease of creatinine, 5 (17%) no change, and 11 (26%) an increase. In those patients whose renal function improved, the changes were maintained for up to 3 years, whereas many of the other patients subsequently required dialysis. Somewhat similar results have been reported by Bell et al. (123). In 20 patients with atheromatous renovascular hypertension, renal function was improved in 7 (35%), unchanged in 10 (50%), and worsened in 3 (15%). As a group, these patients

TABLE 9 *Results of angioplasty series for treatment of renovascular hypertension*

	Number of patients	Successfully dilated (%)	Cured (%)	Improved (%)	Failed (%)	Mortality (%)
Fibromuscular dysplasia (Refs. 111–117)	132	91	57	35	8	0
Atheroma: Focal (Refs. 111,113,115,117,118)	196	91	35	49	16	0

had also shown a significant increase in serum creatinine during the six months preceding angioplasty. These results may be compared with those of a surgical series done for the same purpose (124), in which renal function was improved in 58% of patients, unchanged in 31%, and worsened in 11%.

Others have had less favorable results with angioplasty in these patients. Luft et al. (125) attempted angioplasty in 12 azotemic patients with severe hypertension who had stenoses of both renal arteries or a solitary kidney, and reported improved renal function in only three. Another 12 patients had surgery, with improvement in 10. Two of the surgical patients died, whereas none of the angioplasty patients did. The patients were not randomly allocated to the two forms of treatment, however, so it is probable that the angioplasty patients had more extensive disease.

Another advantage of angioplasty over surgery is that it can be undertaken in patients who would be turned down for surgery because of associated conditions such as coronary artery disease or cerebrovascular disease, both of which are of course common in patients with atheromatous renovascular hypertension.

Complications of Angioplasty

In all patients, the potential benefits of angioplasty must be carefully weighed against the risks. It is our belief that the main risks are those of arteriography rather than of the angioplasty itself. Thus the commonest complications have been hematoma (in 4% of patients), and transient worsening of renal function from the dye load (in 2%). The latter has been much less common since the advent of digital subtraction angiography, with which much less dye is needed. Both of these complications have been seen only in patients with atheromatous renal artery stenosis, who had extensive arterial disease. The main complication associated with the angioplasty itself is dissection of the renal artery, which occurred in about 5% of our cases (111), in both atheromatous and fibromuscular lesions. This is not a catastrophic complication, however, because surgical revascularization is normally possible in such cases. Only two of our patients (out of several hundred) have needed a nephrectomy following angioplasty, and 30 day mortality has been zero. One patient in Geyskes' series died of cholesterol emboli, and another required a leg amputation (113). One of our patients also required an amputation as a result of cholesterol emboli. This complication is only seen in patients with diffuse atheroma, who would also be at very high risk for surgery. It is potentially the most serious complication, and may be the reason why some patients with diffuse atheroma show an acute but sustained deterioration of renal function following angioplasty.

Angioplasty Versus Surgery

There has so far been no controlled randomized trial of surgery versus angioplasty, although some published studies (126,127) have attempted to compare the results of the two procedures. In general, the results with angioplasty are as good as with surgery for patients with fibromuscular dysplasia, and at a fraction of the cost and inconvenience to the patient. For patients with atheroma, the overall success rate is somewhat better with surgery, but against this must be weighed the higher mortality and rate of nephrectomy.

It should be emphasized that both angioplasty and surgical revascularization are procedures that should be performed only in centers where there are teams experienced in their performance. With the possible exception of the very high-risk patients with diffuse atheroma, we believe that when renovascular hypertension is diagnosed, one or another form of revascularization should be attempted, because in patients with fibromuscular dysplasia there is a high probability of a permanent cure, and in patients with atheromatous stenoses there may be progression of the lesion to complete occlusion of the renal artery if the patient is treated medically.

It is often stated that a clinical trial is needed to define the relative roles of angioplasty and surgery for the treatment of renovascular hypertension. We do not, however, regard the two forms of treatment as being mutually exclusive. Since, in skilled hands, angioplasty can be performed at the same time as the diagnostic arteriogram, and with relatively little trauma, we usually prefer to attempt an angioplasty before going on to surgery.

For patients with fibromuscular dysplasia, the results with angioplasty are as good as any of the published surgical series. There also seems to be little doubt that the benefit is long lasting in these patients and therefore angioplasty is the treatment of choice. For patients with localized atheroma, e.g., non-ostial unilateral lesions, the benefit rate is somewhat lower than with surgery, but when angioplasty is successful, the savings of cost and trauma as compared to surgery certainly make it worthwhile. If it is unsuccessful, there is still the option of a second attempt or of surgical revascularization. The greatest dilemma at the present time concerns the high-risk patients with diffuse atheroma and renal insufficiency (see above). Surgical morbidity in these patients is high, and these are also the patients most likely to develop complications after angioplasty. Nevertheless, we believe that angioplasty can benefit some of these patients, both from the point of view of their renal function and their blood pressure control. Further work is needed, however, to define which patients are the best candidates.

Medical Management

While revascularization of the ischemic kidney by either surgery or angioplasty is the preferred method of treatment, there are some patients in whom these procedures are either unsuccessful or cannot be undertaken. In such patients medical management must be relied on.

The two main concerns with medical treatment of such patients are the progression of the renal artery stenosis, and the hemodynamic effects of blood pressure reduction on renal function. In 1974 Hunt et al. (128) compared the results of medically and surgically treated patients and reported mortality over 7 to 14 years of 70% in the medically treated and 30% in the surgically treated patients. Most of the deaths were due to complications of atheroma, such as

27. Lucas J, Floyer MA. Changes in body fluid distribution and interstitial tissue compliance during the development and reversal of experimental renal hypertension in the rat. *Clin Sci Mol Med* 1974;47:1–11.
28. Liard JF, Cowley AW, McCaa RE, McCaa CS, Guyton AC. Renin, aldosterone, body fluid volumes, and the baroreceptor reflex in the development and reversal of Goldblatt hypertension in conscious dogs. *Circ Res* 1974;34:549–560.
29. Katholi RE, Winternitz SR, Oparil S. Decrease in peripheral sympathetic nervous system activity following renal denervation or unclipping in the one-kidney one-clip Goldblatt hypertensive rat. *J Clin Invest* 1982;69:55–62.
30. Thurston H, Bing RF, Swales JD. Reversal of two-kidney one-clip hypertension in the rat. *Hypertension* 1980;2:256–265.
31. Hallbäck-Nordlander M, Noresson E, Lundgren Y. Haemodynamic alterations after reversal of renal hypertension in rats. *Clin Sci* 1979;57:15s–17s.
32. Russell GI, Brice JM, Bing RF, Swales JD, Thurston H. Haemodynamic changes after surgical reversal of chronic two-kidney, one-clip hypertension in the rat. *Clin Sci* 1981;61:117s–119s.
33. Muirhead EE, Byers LW, Pitcock JA, Desiderio DM, Brooks B, Brown P, Brosius WL. Denervation of neutral antihypertensive lipid from renal venous effluent in rats. *Clin Sci* 1981;61:331s–333s.
34. Russell GI, Bing RF, Tavener D, Thurston H, Swales JD. The role of the renal medulla in experimental renovascular hypertension. In: Glorioso N, et al, eds. *Renovascular hypertension.* New York: Raven Press, 1987;53–60.
35. Russell GI, Bing RF, Thurston H, Swales JD. Surgical reversal of two-kidney one clip hypertension during inhibition of the renin-angiotensin system. *Hypertension* 1982;4:69–76.
36. Brown JJ, Davies DL, Lever AF, Robertson JIS. Plasma renin concentration in human hypertension. II. Renin in relation to aetiology. *Br Med J* 1965;2:144–148.
37. Fiorentini C, Guazzi M, Olivari MT, Bartorelli A, Necchi G, Magrini F. Selective reduction of renal perfusion pressure and blood flow in man: humoral and hemodynamic effects. *Circulation* 1981;63:973–978.
38. Bianchi G, Campolo L, Vegeto A, Pietra V, Piazza U. The value of plasma renin concentration per se, and in relation to plasma and extracellular fluid volume in diagnosis and prognosis of human renovascular hypertension. *Clin Sci* 1970;39:559–576.
39. Davies DL, McElroy K, Atkinson AB, Brown JJ, Cumming AMM, Fraser R, Leckie BJ, Lever AF, Mackay A, Morton JJ, Robertson JIS. Relationship between exchangeable sodium and blood pressure in different forms of hypertension in man. *Clin Sci* 1979;57:69s–75s.
40. McCann WS, Romansky MJ. Orthostatic hypertension: effect of nephroptosis on renal blood flow. *JAMA* 1940;115:573–578.
41. Braasch WF, Greene LF, Goyanna R. Renal ptosis and its treatment. *JAMA* 1948;138:399–403.
42. DeZeeuw D, Danker AJM, Burema J, Van der Hem GK, Mandema E. Nephroptosis and hypertension. *Lancet* 1977;1:213–215.
43. Kaufman JJ, Hanafee W, Maxwell MH. Upright renal arteriography in the study of renal hypertension. *JAMA* 1964;187:977–980.
44. Bianchi C, Bonadio M, Andriole VT. Influence of postural changes on the glomerular filtration rate in nephroptosis. *Nephron* 1976;16:161–172.
45. Derkx RHM, Tan-Tjiong HL, Wenting GJ, Man in't Veld AJ, Van Seyen AJ, Schalekamp JADH. Captopril test for diagnosis of renal artery stenosis. In: Glorioso N, et al, eds. *Renovascular hypertension.* New York: Raven Press, 1987;295–315.
46. Pickering TG, Sos TA, James GD, Vaughan ED, Sealey JE, Laragh JH. Comparison of renal vein renin activity in hypertensive patients with stenosis of one or both renal arteries. *J Hypertens* 1985;3(Suppl 3):S291–S293.
47. Vensel LA, Devereux RB, Pickering TG, Herrold EM, Borer JS, Laragh JH. Cardiac structure and function in renovascular hypertension produced by unilateral and bilateral renal artery stenosis. *Am J Cardiol* 1986;58:575–582.
48. Pickering TG, Herman L, Sotelo JE, Sos TA, James GD, Laragh JH. Recurrent pulmonary edema as a manifestation of renovascular hypertension and its treatment by renal revascularization. *Circulation* 1987;76(Suppl IV):274.
49. Sutters M, Al-Kutoubi MA, Mathias CJ, Peart S. Diuresis and syncope after renal angioplasty in a patient with one functioning kidney. *Br Med J* 1987;295:527–528.
50. Keeton TK, Campbell WB. The pharmacologic alteration of renin release. *Pharm Rev* 1980;32:81–227.
51. Poutasse EF, Donnelly A, Dustan JP. Separated kidney function tests in hypertensive patients. *Surg Forum* 1958;9:826–830.
52. Capponi AM, Aguilea G, Fakunding JL, Catt KJ. Angiotensin II: receptors and mechanisms of action. In: Soffer RL, ed. *Biochemical regulation of blood pressure.* New York: Wiley, 1981;205–262.
53. Maslowski AH, Nicholls MG, Espiner EA, Ikram H, Bones PJ. Mechanisms in human renovascular hypertension. *Hypertension* 1983;5:597–602.
54. Lake CR, Chernow B, Goldstein DS, Glass DG, Coleman M, Ziegler MG. Plasma catecholamine levels in normal subjects and in patients with secondary hypertension. *Fed Proc* 1984;43:52–56.
55. Pick JW, Anson EJ. The renal vascular pedicle: anatomical study of 430 body-halves. *J Urol* 1940;44:411–434.
56. Schreiber MJ, Pohl MA, Novick AC. The natural history of atherosclerotic and fibrous renal artery disease. *Urol Clin North Am* 1984;11:383–392.
57. Goncharenko V, Gerlock AJ, Schaff MI, Hollifield SW. Progression of renal artery fibromuscular dysplasia in 42 patients as seen on angiography. *Radiology* 1981;139:45–51.
58. Harrington JT, Sommers SC, Kassirer JP. Atheromatous emboli with progressive renal failure. Renal arteriography as the probable inciting factor. *Ann Intern Med* 1968;68:152–160.
59. Kassirer JP. Atheroembolic renal disease. *N Engl J Med* 1969;280:812–817.
60. Gifford R. Evaluation of the hypertensive patient with emphasis on detecting curable causes. *Millbank Mem Fund Q* 1969;47:170–186.
61. Davis BA, Crook JE, Vestal RE, Oates JA. Prevalence of renovascular hypertension in patients with Grade III or IV hypertensive retinopathy. *N Engl J Med* 1979;301:1273–1276.
62. Keith TA. Renovascular hypertension in black patients. *Hypertension* 1982;4:438–443.
63. Holley KE, Hunt JC, Brown AL, Kincaid OW, Sheps SG. Renal artery stenosis. A clinical–pathologic study in normotensive and hypertensive patients. *Am J Med* 1964;37:14–22.
64. Eyler WR, Clark MD, Garman JE, Rian RL, Meininger DE. Angiography of the renal areas including a comparative study of renal arterial stenoses in patients with and without hypertension. *Radiology* 1962;78:879–891.
65. Maxwell MH, Bleifer KH, Franklin SS, Varady P. Cooperative study of renovascular hypertension. Demographic analysis of the study. *JAMA* 1972;220:1195–1204.
66. Goldman AG, Varady PD, Franklin SS. Body habitus and serum cholesterol in essential hypertension and renovascular hypertension. Cooperative study of renovascular hypertension. *JAMA* 1972;221:378–383.
67. Vetrovec GW, Cowley MJ, Landwehr DM, Parker VE. High prevalence of renal artery stenosis in hypertensive patients with coronary artery disease. *J Am Coll Cardiol* 1984;3:518.
68. Nicholson JP, Teichman SL, Alderman MH, Pickering TG, Sos TA, Laragh JH. Cigarette smoking and renovascular hypertension. *Lancet* 1983;2:765–766.
69. Simon N, Franklin SS, Bleifer KH, Maxwell MH. Clinical characteristics of renovascular hypertension. *JAMA* 1972;220:1209–1218.
70. Berlyne GW, Tarill AS, Baker SBC. Renal artery stenosis and the nephrotic syndrome. *Q J Med* 1964;33:325–335.
71. Zimbler MS, Pickering TG, Sos TA, Laragh JH. Proteinuria in renovascular hypertension and the effects of renal angioplasty. *Annu J Cardiol* 1987;59:406–408.
72. Elkik F, Corvol P, Idatte J-M, Mernard J. Renal segmental infarction: a cause of reversible malignant hypertension. *J Hypertens* 1984;2:149–156.
73. Stanley JC, Fry WJ. Pediatric renal artery occlusive disease and

renovascular hypertension. Etiology, diagnosis, and operative treatment. *Arch Surg* 1981;116:669–676.
74. Novick AL, Straffon RA, Stewart BH, Benjamin S. Surgical treatment of renovascular hypertension in the pediatric patient. *J Urol* 1978;119:794–799.
75. Vaughan ED Jr, Bühler FR, Laragh JH, Sealey JE, Baer L, Bard RH. Renovascular hypertension: renin measurements to indicate hypersecretion and contralateral suppression, estimate renal plasma flow, and score for surgical curability. *Am J Med* 1973;55:402–414.
76. Vaughan ED Jr, Carey RM, Ayers CR, et al. A physiologic definition of blood pressure response to renal revascularization in patients with renovascular hypertension. *Kidney Int* 1979;15:S83–S92.
77. Sealey JE, Buhler FR, Laragh JH, Vaughan ED Jr. The physiology of renin secretion in essential hypertension: estimation of renin secretion rate and renal plasma flow from peripheral and renal vein renin levels. *Am J Med* 1973;55:391–401.
78. Case DB, Laragh JH. Reactive hyperreninemia in renovascular hypertension after angiotensin blockade with saralasin or converting enzyme inhibitor. *Ann Intern Med* 1979;91:153–160.
79. Muller FB, Sealey JE, Case CB, Atlas SA, Pickering TG, Pecker M, Priebisz J, Laragh JH. The captopril test for identifying renovascular disease in hypertensive patients. *Am J Med* 1986;80:633–644.
80. Judson WE, Helmer OM. Diagnostic and prognostic values of renin activity in renal venous plasma in renovascular hypertension. *Hypertension* 1965;13:79–89.
81. Marks LS, Maxwell MH. Renal vein renin valve and limitations in the prediction of operative results. *Urol Clin North Am* 1975;2:311–325.
82. Woods JW, Michelakis AM. Renal vein renin in renovascular hypertension. *Arch Intern Med* 1968;122:392–393.
83. Pickering TG, Sos TA, Vaughan ED Jr, Case DB, Sealey JE, Harshfield GA, Laragh JH. Predictive value and changes of renin secretion in hypertensive patients with unilateral renovascular disease undergoing successful renal angioplasty. *Am J Med* 1985;76:398–404.
84. Atkinson AB, Kellet RJ. Value of intravenous urography in investigating hypertension. *J R Coll Physicians Lond* 1974;8:175–181.
85. Bailey SM, Evans DW, Fleming HA. Intravenous urography in investigation of hypertension. *Lancet* 1975;2:57–58.
86. Block PC, Myler R, Sterzer S. Morphology after transluminal angioplasty in human beings. *N Engl J Med* 1981;305:382–385.
87. Thornbury JR, Stanley JL, Fryback DG. Limited use of hypertensive excretory urography. *Urol Radiol* 1982;3:209–211.
88. Buonocore E, Meaney TF, Borkowsky GP, Pavlicek W, Gallagher J. Digital subtraction angiography of the abdominal aorta and renal arteries. *Radiology* 1981;139:281–286.
89. Clark RA, Alexander ES. Digital subtraction angiography of the renal arteries—prospective comparison with conventional arteriography. *Invest Radiol* 1983;18:6–10.
90. Hillman BJ, Ovitt TW, Capp MD, Prosnitz EH, Osborne RW, Goldsteone J, Zukowski CF, Malone JM. The potential impact of digital video subtractions angiography on screening for renovascular hypertension. *Radiology* 1982;142:577–579.
91. Zabbo A, Novick AC. Digital subtraction angiography for noninvasive imaging of the renal artery. *Urol Clin North Am* 1984;11(3):409–416.
92. Maxwell MH, Lupu AN, Taplin GV. Radioisotope renogram in renal arterial hypertension. *J Urol* 1968;100:376–383.
93. Schalekamp MADH, Derkx FHM. Functional diagnosis of renovascular hypertension, with special reference to renin measurements. In: Schilfgaarde RV, et al, eds. *Clinical aspects of renovascular hypertension.* Boston: Martinus Nijhoff, 1983;62–73.
94. Geyskes GG, Oei HY, Puylaert CBAJ, Dorhout Mees EJ. Unilateral renal failure after captopril in patients with renovascular hypertension. In: Glorioso N, et al, eds. *Renovascular hypertension.* New York: Raven Press, 1987;281–294.
95. Fommei E, Ghione S, Palla L, Mosca F, Ferrari M, Palombo C, Giaconi S, Gazzetti P, Donato L. Renal scintigraphic captopril test in the diagnosis of renovascular hypertension. *Hypertension* 1987;10:212–220.
96. Kopecky RT, Thomas FD, McAfee JG. Furosemide augments the effects of captopril on nuclear studies in renovascular stenosis. *Hypertension* 1987;10:181–188.
97. Clorius JH, Allenberg J, Hupp T, Strauss LG, Schmidlin P, Irngartinger G, Wagner R, Mukhopadhyay C. Predictive value of exercise renography for presurgical evaluation of nephrogenic hypertension. *Hypertension* 1987;10:280–286.
98. Clorius JH, Mann J, Schmidlin P, Strauss LG, Savr T, Irngartinger G. Clinical evaluation of patients with hypertension and exercise-induced renal dysfunction. *Hypertension* 1987;10:287–293.
99. Jenni R, Vieli A, Lüscher TF, Schneider E, Vetter W, Anliker M. Combined two-dimensional ultrasound doppler technique. New possibilities for the screening of renovascular and parenchymatous hypertension? *Nephron* 1986;44(Suppl 1):2–4.
100. Kohler TR, Zierler E, Martin RL, Nicholls SC, Bergelin RO, Kazmers A, Beach KW, Strandness DE. Noninvasive diagnosis of renal artery stenosis by ultrasonic duplex scanning. *J Vasc Surg* 1986;4:450–456.
101. Howard JE, Berthrong M, Sloan RD, Yendt ER. Relief of malignant hypertension by nephrectomy in four patients with unilateral renal vascular disease. *Trans Assoc Am Physicians* 1953;66:164–169.
102. Stamey TA, Nudelman IJ, Good PH, Schwentker FN, Hendricks F. Functional characteristics of renovascular hypertension. *Medicine* 1961;40:347–394.
103. Shipley RE, Gregg DE. The effect of external constriction of a blood vessel on blood flow. *Am J Physiol* 1944;141:289–296.
104. Levin DC, Beckmann CF, Serur JR. Vascular resistance changes distal to progressive arterial stenosis: a critical re-evaluation of the concept of vasodilator reverse. *Invest Radiol* 1980;14:120–128.
105. Scott JA, Rabe FE, Becker GJ, Yum MN, Yune HY, Holden RW, Richmond DB, Klatte EC, Grim CE, Weinberger NJ. Angiographic assessment of renal artery pathology: how reliable? *AJR* 1983;141:1299–1303.
106. Dotter CT, Judkins MP. Transluminal treatment of arteriosclerotic obstruction: description of a new technique and a preliminary report of its applications. *Circulation* 1964;30:654–670.
107. Grüntzig A, Kuhlmann U, Vetter W. Treatment of renovascular hypertension with percutaneous transluminal dilatation of a renal artery stenosis. *Lancet* 1978;1:801–802.
108. Sos TA, Sniderman KW. Percutaneous transluminal angioplasty. *Semin Reontgenol* 1981;16:26–41.
109. Block PC, Myler R, Sterzer S. Morphology after transluminal angioplasty in human beings. *N Engl J Med* 1981;305:382–385.
110. Zarins CK, Chien-Tai L, Gewertz B. Arterial disruption and remodeling following balloon dilatation. *Surgery* 1982;92:1086–1095.
111. Sos TA, Pickering TG, Sniderman K, Saddekni S, Case DB, Silane MF, Vaughan ED, Laragh JH. Percutaneous transluminal renal angioplasty in renovascular hypertension due to atheroma or fibromuscular dysplasia. *N Engl J Med* 1983;309:274–279.
112. Tegtmeyer CJ, Elson J, Glass TA. Percutaneous transluminal angioplasty: the treatment of choice for renovascular hypertension due to fibromuscular dysplasia. *Radiology* 1982;143:631–637.
113. Geyskes GG, Puylaert CBAJ, Dei HY, Dorhout Mees EJ. Follow-up study of 70 patients with renal artery stenosis treated by percutaneous transluminal dilatation. *Br Med J* 1983;287:333–336.
114. Martin ED, Mattern RF, Baer L. Renal angioplasty for hypertension: predictive factors for long-term success. *Amer J Radiol* 1981;137:921–924.
115. Grim CE, Luft FC, Yune HY. Percutaneous transluminal dilatation in the treatment of renal vascular hypertension. *Ann Intern Med* 1981;95:439–442.
116. Millan VG, McCauley J, Kopelman RI, Madias NE. Percutaneous transluminal renal angioplasty in nonatherosclerotic renovascular hypertension. Long-term results. *Hypertension* 1985;7:674–688.
117. Kuhlmann U, Gramminger P, Grüntzig A, Schneider E, Pouliadis G, Lüscher T, Stevrer J, Siegenthaler W, Vetter W. Long-term experience in percutaneous transluminal dilatation of renal artery stenosis. *Am J Med* 1985;79:692–698.

These generally become manifest clinically by the sudden onset of pain that simulates renal colic. In some patients, the dissection in the wall of the vessel may re-enter the lumen more distally. In other patients, total arterial occlusion with renal infarction may ensue.

Intrarenal arterial aneurysms are of mixed origin and may be congenital, post-traumatic, iatrogenic, neoplastic, or associated with polyarteritis nodosa. Intrarenal aneurysms that follow blunt trauma or closed renal biopsy will occasionally resolve spontaneously with expectant management.

Renal Arteriovenous Fistula

Renal arteriovenous fistulas are relatively uncommon lesions that are generally discovered during the course of angiographic evaluation for suspected renal or renovascular disease (7). The most common clinical symptoms, when present, are hematuria, high-output cardiac failure, and diastolic hypertension. Congenital or cirsoid fistulas comprise approximately 25% of these lesions and are the result of a developmental anomaly of the involved renal vessels. The angiographic appearance is of multiple small interconnecting arterial and venous channels with impaired distal renal parenchymal vascularity and early filling of the renal vein. Idiopathic fistulas comprise only 3–5% of these lesions and have no apparent cause. They are thought to develop as a result of venous erosion from a preexisting arterial aneurysm. Acquired fistulas are the most common type, accounting for 70–75% of all renal arteriovenous fistulas. The most common cause is iatrogenic trauma resulting from needle biopsy of the kidney. The majority of these will close spontaneously under simple observation. Fistulas may also be acquired through blunt or penetrating trauma, tumor, inflammation, or previous renal surgery.

Middle Aortic Syndrome

The middle aortic syndrome, also termed aortic hypoplasia, is a rare disorder occurring in children or young adults (8). This disease is characterized by nonspecific stenosing arteritis that affects the aorta and its major branches, including the renal arteries. This may be a form of Takayasu's disease, and an autoimmune pathogenesis is suspected. This disease can extensively involve the subdiaphragmatic aorta, or in some cases there may be only focal aortic involvement. The iliac arteries are generally spared in this disease.

Neurofibromatosis

Neurofibromatosis affecting the renal artery is a congenital hereditary disorder characterized by café-au-lait cutaneous pigmentation, cutaneous neurofibromas, tumors of the central nervous system, skeletal disorders, and occasional gigantism. Hypertension in patients with neurofibromatosis is most often due to renal artery stenosis (9,10); less commonly, this may be the result of an associated pheochromocytoma or aortic coarctation. Vascular pathology occurs in the kidneys, heart, and gastrointestinal tract and consists of fibrosis and thickening of the intima, proliferation of neural tissue within the arterial wall, perivascular nodular proliferations, and occasional aneurysmal dilatation. In the kidney, arterial stenosis usually occurs at the origin or in the proximal third of the main renal artery. The angiographic appearance may be indistinguishable from that of intimal fibroplasia.

Renal Artery Thrombosis or Embolism

Acute occlusion of the renal artery or its branches may result from thrombosis or embolism. Embolic occlusions may occur as a complication of rheumatic heart disease, subacute bacterial endocarditis, cardiac operations, saccular aneurysm of the renal artery, or renal artery catheterization. Thrombosis of the renal artery is somewhat less common and is associated with a variety of diseases such as intimal fibroplasia, segmental arteritis, polycythemia vera, tumors, trauma, or umbilical arterial catheterization. Blunt trauma to the renal artery may result in disruption of the intima, with subsequent dissection and thrombotic occlusion.

Extrinsic Obstruction of the Renal Artery

Extrinsic obstruction of the renal artery has been observed but is extremely rare (11). Neural tissue, musculocutaneous fibers, and diaphragmatic crura have been suggested as etiologic factors. Other possible causes of extrinsic perivascular fibrosis include inflammation, trauma, tumor, or prior radiation.

CLINICAL SCREENING AND EVALUATION

It is important to differentiate between renovascular disease and renovascular hypertension, since lesions of the renal artery do not always result in hypertension. The diagnosis of renovascular disease depends on angiographic demonstration of a lesion in the renal artery or its branches, whereas the diagnosis of renovascular hypertension can be confirmed only in retrospect and connotes permanent relief of hypertension after surgical treatment or PTA. The medical evaluation of patients with renovascular hypertension is the subject of a separate chapter in this text and need not be reviewed herein. In our experience at the Cleveland Clinic, the most helpful clinical clues to the diagnosis of renovascular hypertension are: (a) a systolic/diastolic bruit in the epigastrium or flank (12); (b) an abrupt onset or exacerbation of hypertension with rapid progression (13); (c) onset of hypertension before age 30 or after age 55 (14); and (d) evidence of retinopathy (14). In patients with suspected renovascular hypertension, intravenous digital subtraction angiography is an excellent radiographic screening test (15–18). Differential renal-vein plasma renin assays can confirm the presence of renin-mediated hypertension with 90% accuracy, when there is lateralization to the affected kidney with a ratio greater than 2:1; unfortunately, there is a high incidence of false-negative results with this test (19,20). More recently, the peripheral plasma renin response to a single dose of oral captopril has proven to be a useful screening test for identifying patients with renovascular hypertension (21). Differential isotope renographic changes following captopril administration also appear to be useful in demonstrating functional renal artery stenosis (22).

There has been increasing concern in recent years with the threat to overall renal function posed by advanced high-grade atherosclerotic renal artery disease. Intervention with surgery or PTA is now being undertaken more often solely to preserve renal function in such patients. Angiographic screening for advanced atherosclerotic renal artery disease that threatens overall renal function is indicated for patients with the following clinical clues: (a) evidence of generalized atherosclerosis, (b) a unilateral small kidney, (c) mild to moderate azotemia, and (d) hypertension. Concerning the last, these patients may not have significant hypertension, and this should not influence the decision to perform angiography. Following angiographic diagnosis of atherosclerotic renal artery disease, and with knowledge of the natural history of this disease, one can identify patients for whom the risk of renal functional impairment from progressive arterial obstruction is greatest with a view toward renal revascularization for preservation of renal function.

INDICATIONS FOR SURGICAL TREATMENT

Renovascular Hypertension

In patients with renovascular hypertension due to fibrous dysplasia, the need for intervention (i.e., surgery or PTA) is guided by the specific type of disease based on angiographic findings and the associated natural history (2). Medical management of hypertension is the preferred initial treatment for patients with medial fibroplasia, since loss of renal function from progressive obstruction is uncommon with this disease. Interventive treatment is reserved for patients whose blood pressure is difficult to control with multiple-drug antihypertensive therapy. Conversely, renal artery stenosis due to intimal or perimedial fibroplasia generally progresses and often culminates in ischemic renal atrophy. Furthermore, these lesions tend to occur in younger patients and cause hypertension that is extremely difficult to control. Early interventive therapy in affected patients is therefore indicated, both to preserve renal function and to minimize the need for long-term antihypertensive medication.

In selecting patients with fibrous dysplasia for surgical renal revascularization, the efficacy of PTA must also be considered. The results of PTA for fibrous dysplasia of the main renal artery have been excellent and equal to those obtained with surgical revascularization (23–26); therefore, PTA is the initial treatment of choice in such cases. However, up to 30% of patients with fibrous dysplasia have branch renal arterial involvement, which increases the technical difficulty of PTA and often renders it impossible to perform; therefore, surgical renal revascularization is the primary interventive treatment method in this category (27).

In patients with atherosclerotic renovascular hypertension, more vigorous attempts at medical management are warranted, since these patients are older and often have extrarenal vascular disease. Therefore, multiple-drug regimens which control the blood pressure are often the preferred approach, particularly in patients with generalized atherosclerosis. Indeed, the advent of new beta-blocking agents and converting-enzyme inhibitors has enhanced the current efficacy of medical antihypertensive therapy. Intervention with surgery or PTA is best reserved for patients whose hypertension cannot be adequately controlled or wherein renal function is threatened by advanced vascular disease. In this regard, recent experience has shown that PTA can provide excellent therapy for the minority of patients with atherosclerotic renal artery stenosis who have unilateral nonostial lesions (24–26,28). The results of PTA in the more common ostial lesions have been poor, and surgical revascularization remains the treatment of choice in this catetory (27).

Renal Artery Aneurysm

Renal artery aneurysms may require surgical treatment when they are the cause of significant hypertension or to obviate the risk of rupture (7). The latter is of greatest concern with aneurysms that are larger than 2 cm in diameter and noncalcified, particularly when they occur in premenopausal females because of the predisposition for aneurysmal rupture during pregnancy. Saccular aneurysms can cause hypertension through several mechanisms. These include the following: (a) compression or displacement of the renal artery or its branches, with resulting ischemia; (b) aneurysmal erosion into a renal vein, with formation of an arteriovenous fistula; (c) mural thrombus formation within the aneurysm, with peripheral renal embolization; and (d) the association of some aneurysms with stenosing fibrous renal artery disease. Saccular aneurysms may also cause hypertension, in the absence of any of the above mechanisms, through relative renal ischemia caused by the turbulent flow of blood as it passes through an aneurysmally dilated arterial segment.

Preservation of Renal Function in Atherosclerotic Renal Artery Disease

Knowledge of the natural history of atherosclerotic renal artery disease has made it possible to define those patients in whom such disease poses a major threat to overall renal function (2). This designation applies to patients with high-grade (>75%) arterial stenosis affecting the entire renal mass, namely, where such stenosis is present bilaterally or involves a solitary kidney. In such patients, the risk of developing complete renal arterial occlusion is significant; if this type of occlusion occurs, the clinical outcome is a critical decrease in functioning renal mass, with resulting renal failure. It is in such patients that intervention to restore normal renal blood flow is indicated for the purpose of preserving renal function (29). Clinical experience has shown that these are generally older patients with diffuse atherosclerosis and ostial renal artery lesions. This description encompasses a group in which the results of PTA have been poor and where surgical revascularization provides optimum therapy (27–30). It has been well demonstrated that surgical revascularization can now be safely and successfully done even in older patients with diffuse extrarenal vascular disease.

In considering potential candidates for revascularization to preserve renal function, a determination must be made of the potential for salvageable renal function. Total occlusion of the renal artery does not necessarily imply irreversible ischemic parenchymal damage; furthermore, it is well accepted that with gradual arterial occlusion, the viability of the kidney can be maintained through the development of collateral arterial supply. Helpful clinical clues suggesting renal salvability include the following: (a) a kidney size greater than 9 cm, (b) function of the involved kidney upon intravenous urography or isotope renography, (c) angiographic demonstration of retrograde filling of the distal renal arterial tree from collateral vessels on the side of total renal arterial occlusion, and (d) a renal biopsy demonstrating well-preserved tubules and glomeruli with minimal arteriolar sclerosis. When such criteria indicative of renal salvageability are present, successful revascularization can lead to reversal of renal failure (31,32).

It is also important to emphasize that revascularization to preserve renal function is generally not worthwhile in patients with severe azotemia (serum creatinine greater than 4.0 mg/dl), because advanced underlying renal parenchymal disease inevitably is present and obviates improvement in renal function with restored perfusion. The single exception to this admonition is presented by patients with chronic bilateral total renal arterial occlusion, where, fortuitously, the viability of one or both kidneys is maintained through an abundant collateral supply. The degree of preoperative renal functional impairment in such patients often is severe, and the improvement following revascularization may be dramatic (33). Unfortunately, this clinical presentation is rare, and a less favorable outcome of bilateral arterial occlusion on renal viability is far more common.

PREPARATION FOR SURGICAL TREATMENT

When surgical revascularization is indicated for renal artery disease, it is important to accurately define the general medical condition of the patient, since this will determine the risk of undertaking a major vascular operation. Most patients with renal arterial fibrous dysplasia are young and otherwise healthy, and the operative risk is minimal in this group. In patients with atherosclerotic renovascular disease, evidence of generalized atherosclerosis should be carefully sought (34). Particularly important are a history of angina pectoris, congestive heart failure, myocardial infarction, transient ischemic attacks, cerebrovascular accidents, or intermittent claudication. On physical examination, careful attention should be paid to the presence of (a) carotid bruits, (b) focal neurologic deficits suggesting a prior cerebral infarct, (c) third and fourth heart sounds, (d) precordial left ventricular heave, (e) arterial pulsations in the extremities, and (f) an aortic aneurysm on examination of the abdomen.

The preoperative evaluation should include a thorough search for coronary artery disease, because this has been the leading cause of operative mortality following surgical treatment for atherosclerotic renovascular disease (35). In addition to a careful history, physical examination, and electrocardiogram, all operative candidates in this category should undergo a cardiac stress test. If any of the latter assessments suggest the presence of coronary artery disease, our policy is to then perform coronary cine angiography and left ventriculography. Coronary artery bypass grafting is recommended for patients with significant correctable coronary artery disease before renal revascularization. Patients with either mild to moderate or advanced but compensated coronary artery disease can safely undergo renal revascularization without prior coronary artery bypass grafting. For patients with severe noncorrectable coronary artery disease, major operative intervention for renovascular disease carries a significantly increased risk and is best deferred except for the most dire of circumstances.

Cerebrovascular accident has also been a major cause of death after renal revascularization in patients with atherosclerosis, albeit a less common complication than myocardial infarction. The approach to patients whose history or examination suggests the presence of extracranial cerebrovascular disease is analogous to that employed for patients with suspected coronary artery disease. In such patients, carotid arteriography is obtained preoperatively; if significant occlusive disease is found, endarterectomy is recommended before renal revascularization (35).

In most patients with generalized atherosclerosis and renal artery disease, cardiac function is compromised to varying degrees. In these patients, hypertension increases the workload on the left ventricle, which decreases cardiac reserve and renders the heart less efficient. In addition to an impaired myocardium, these patients also often have a decreased intravascular volume due to prior treatment with diuretic agents. These patients can benefit from a careful hemodynamic assessment in an intensive care unit for 12–24 hr prior to surgical revascularization. Swan–Ganz, arterial, and urethral catheters are placed for measurement of blood pressure, pulmonary capillary wedge pressure, pulmonary artery pressure, cardiac output, total peripheral resistance, and urinary output. While these parameters are being monitored, intravenous vasodilators can be administered to control the blood pressure and decrease cardiac afterload while, at the same time, the intravascular space is carefully expanded with isotonic fluid. Afterload reduction and fluid repletion in this manner optimizes perioperative cardiac function by increasing cardiac output and decreasing cardiac work. This approach can help to enhance the safety of surgical renal revascularization in patients with generalized atherosclerosis (36).

SURGICAL METHODS OF TREATMENT

Nephrectomy

Total or partial nephrectomy is rarely done today, since it is now possible to achieve successful renovascular reconstruction in most cases. These operations are occasionally indicated in patients with renal infarction, severe arteriolar nephrosclerosis, severe renal atrophy, and noncorrectable renovascular lesions. Nephrectomy may also be indicated in the elderly, poor-surgical-risk patient with a normal contralateral kidney or following a failed revascularization procedure, where extensive renal hilar fibrosis precludes satisfactory secondary revascularization.

Aortorenal Bypass

Although many renal revascularization operations are available for treating renovascular hypertension, aortorenal bypass with autogenous saphenous vein or arterial grafts is the preferred method (Figs. 1 and 2). Although excellent clinical results have been obtained with both types of bypass grafts (37–39), long-term studies of aortorenal saphenous vein grafts have shown a large number of dilated grafts on follow-up angiography (40). The clinical significance of these observations remains uncertain, since most of these patients continue to be normotensive with excellent renal function. Nevertheless, these findings have led to preferential use of arterial autografts when these are available. The viscoelastic properties of arterial grafts, unlike those of the saphenous vein, match those of the renal artery, and postoperative graft dilation has not been observed. We have used the hypogastric artery, and occasionally the splenic artery, as a free bypass graft with cure or improvement of hypertension in 96% of patients postoperatively (39); similar results have been reported by other authors with regard to aortorenal arterial grafts (38). Currently, aortorenal bypass with a synthetic material is indicated only when autogenous vascular grafts are not available, and polytetrafluorethylene is the preferred synthetic graft in these cases (41).

Revascularization is more complicated when vascular disease extends into the branches of the renal artery or when reconstruction is required for a kidney supplied by multiple renal arteries. Microvascular techniques now enable successful revascularization *in situ* with an aortorenal bypass operation when the diseased renal vessels are located outside the hilus of the kidney (42). The most useful technique for *in situ* revascularization of multiple segmental renal arteries is aortorenal bypass with a branched autogenous vascular graft (43). Extracorporeal branch arterial repair and autotransplantation are indicated either when there is intrarenal extension of vascular disease or if the diseased branches are extremely small in caliber.

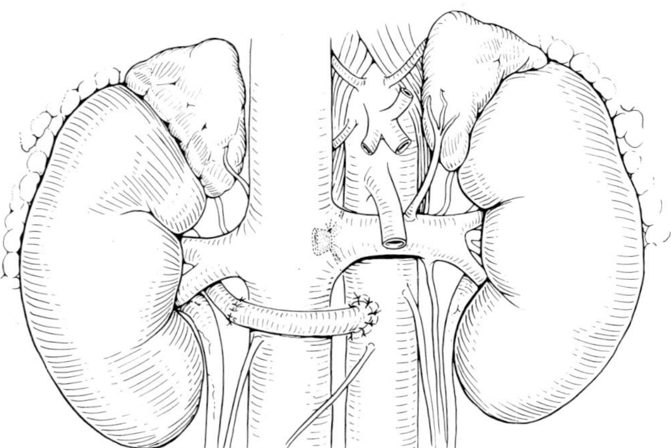

FIG. 1. Sketch illustrating the technique of aortorenal bypass. The graft is anastomosed end-to-side to the aorta and end-to-end to the distal renal artery.

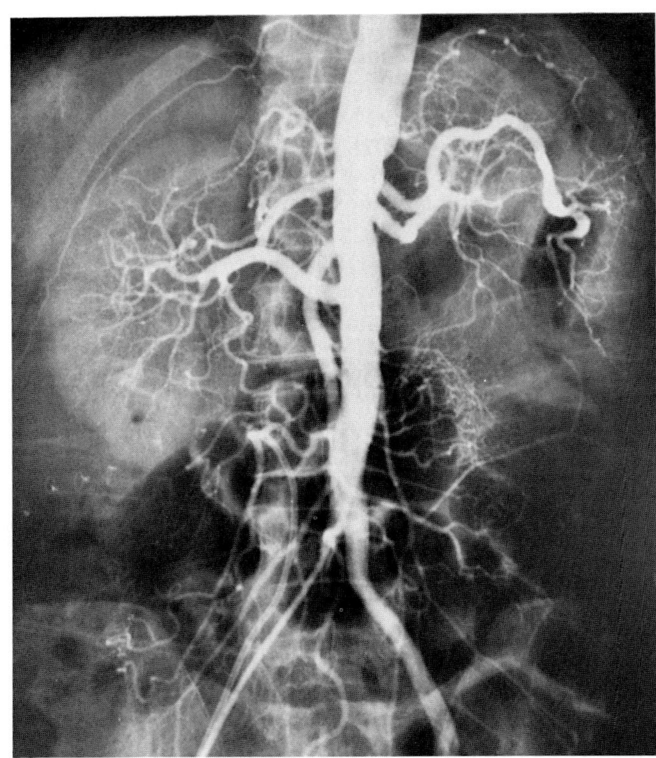

FIG. 2. Aortogram in a patient who underwent right aortorenal revascularization, demonstrating a patent bypass graft.

Techniques in the Surgically Difficult Aorta

In some patients with renal artery disease, severe atherosclerosis or a previous operation on the abdominal aorta may preclude safe performance of aortorenal bypass. These patients present difficult clinical problems, since they frequently have intractable hypertension and failing renal function and may possess only a solitary functioning kidney. Fortunately, alternative methods of revascularization are available that may be safely and effectively employed in such patients (44) (Fig. 3).

Splenorenal bypass provides an excellent method of performing left renal revascularization when preoperative aortography with selective celiac angiography demonstrates a healthy splenic artery (Fig. 4A). The advantages of this procedure are that it can be carried out in untouched vascular tissues at a distance from the aorta, and it involves performance of only a single vascular anastomosis (45). Since the liver receives dual vascular supply from the hepatic artery and portal vein, hepatorenal saphenous vein bypass represents the optimum method of achieving right

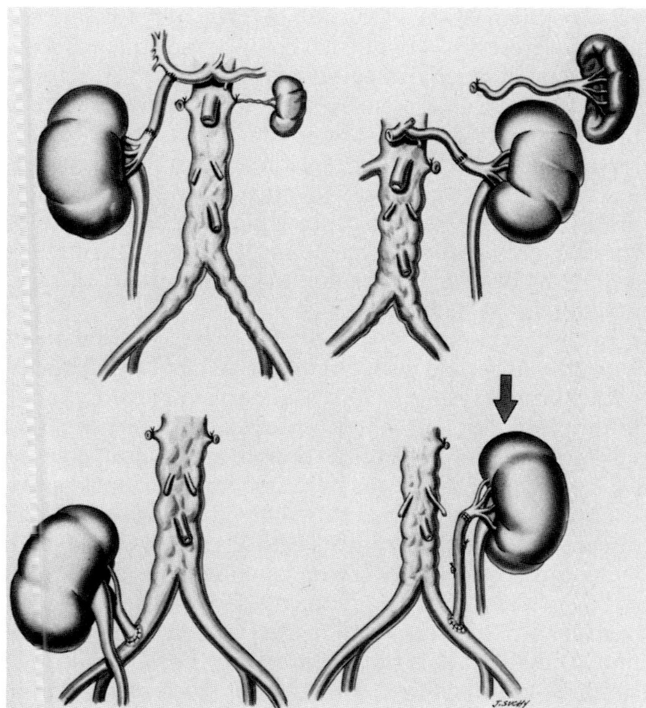

FIG. 3. Methods of renal revascularization for patients with a surgically difficult aorta. These include hepatorenal bypass (**top left**), splenorenal bypass (**top right**), autotransplantation (**bottom left**), and iliorenal bypass (**bottom right**).

renal revascularization in such patients (46) (Fig. 4B). In unusual cases, when aortography reveals an enlarged superior mesenteric artery, mesenterorenal bypass has been performed (47) (Fig. 5). Unfortunately, this artery either will usually be of normal caliber or will itself be involved in the disease process. Finally, renal autotransplantation or iliorenal bypass may be employed to treat renovascular hypertension in patients with severe aortic atherosclerosis when both good flow through the aorta and disease-free iliac vessels are present (48).

Complete excision of the aorta and replacement with a prosthesis may be done but, when combined with renal revascularization, has been associated with operative mortality rates ranging from 6% to 30% (49–52). This approach should therefore be limited to patients with an abdominal aortic aneurysm or symptomatic aortoiliac occlusive disease. Transaortic endarterectomy is also an extensive operation with a significant potential morbidity, and the techniques described above are more effective and less hazardous.

Extracorporeal Microvascular Renal Revascularization and Autotransplantation

Extracorporeal microvascular repair and autotransplantation are indicated in patients with extensive branch renal artery disease where intrarenal vascular extension and/or small vessel size preclude a satisfactory *in situ* repair (53,54). Prior to the advent of extracorporeal surgery, such patients would have been considered either inoperable or candidates for nephrectomy. The advantages of performing extracorporeal revascularization include optimum exposure and illumination, a bloodless surgical field, greater protection from prolonged renal ischemia, and more facile employment of microvascular techniques and optical magnification.

The removed kidney is flushed with an intracellular electrolyte solution and is then submerged in ice slush saline to

A

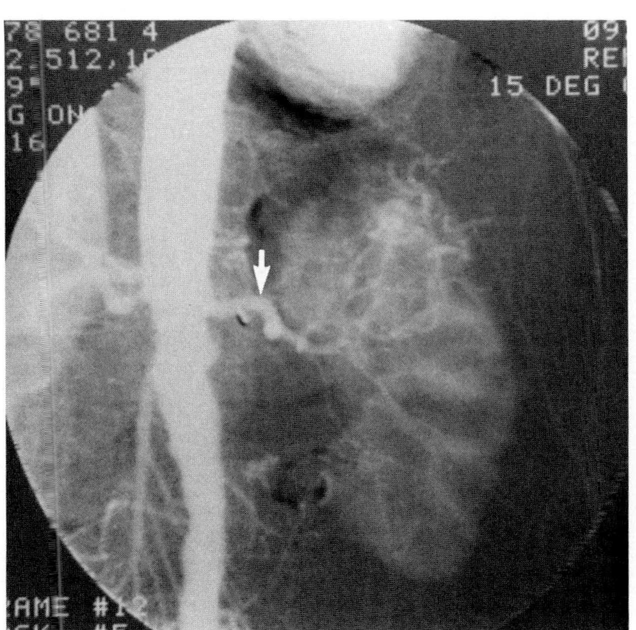

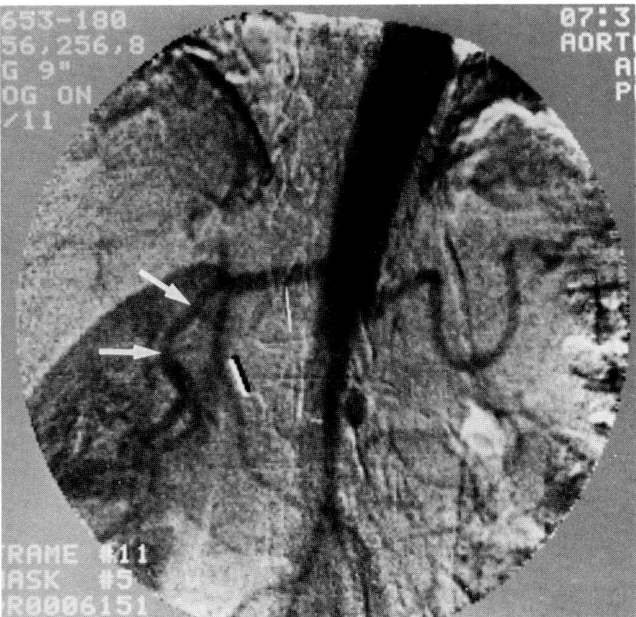

B

FIG. 4. A: Digital subtraction angiogram in a patient who underwent splenorenal bypass, demonstrating a patent anastomosis (*arrow*). **B:** Digital subtraction angiogram in a patient who underwent hepatorenal bypass; the arrows indicate the interposition saphenous vein graft.

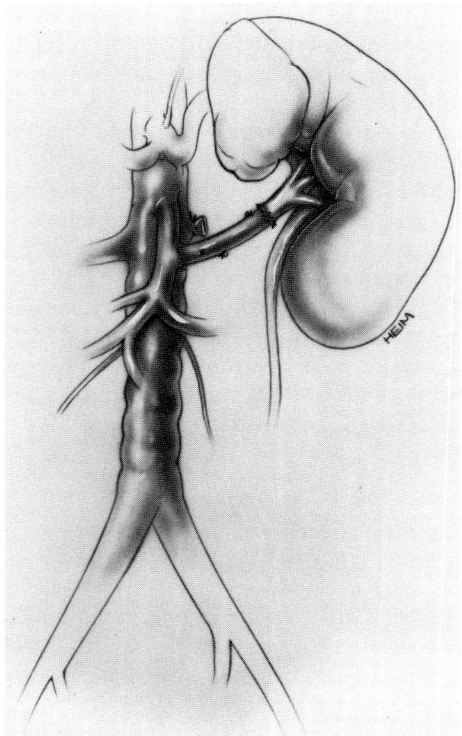

FIG. 5. Sketch illustrating the technique of superior mesenterorenal bypass with an interposition saphenous vein graft.

maintain hypothermia. Under these conditions, the kidney can safely tolerate periods outside the body far in excess of those required to perform even the most complex arterial repair. Extracorporeal revascularization is accomplished with a branched autogenous vascular graft of the hypogastric artery, saphenous vein, or inferior epigastric artery. Autotransplantation of the repaired kidney into the iliac fossa is then done, using the same technique as in renal allotransplantation (Fig. 6).

RESULTS OF SURGICAL TREATMENT

The results of surgical treatment for renovascular hypertension have always been excellent in patients with fibrous dysplasia (37–39,55). Traditionally, however, less satisfactory results have been observed in patients with atherosclerosis (56). During the past decade, refinements in establishing a preoperative diagnosis of renin-mediated hypertension and an enhanced technical efficacy of vascular reconstruction have led to improved surgical results in the latter category. There are now several reports of an 85–90% cure or improvement rate following renal revascularization for atherosclerotic renovascular hypertension (35,57,58).

We recently reviewed the Cleveland Clinic experience with surgical revascularization for renal artery disease from January 1975 to December 1984 (27). During this 10-year period, a total of 380 surgical revascularization operations were performed in 361 patients with renal artery disease; 19 patients underwent simultaneous or staged bilateral surgical revascularization. The cause of renal artery disease was atherosclerosis in 241 patients, fibrous dysplasia in 104 patients, and an arterial aneurysm in 16 patients. The indication for surgical revascularization in all patients with fibrous dysplasia or an aneurysm was to treat severe renovascular hypertension. The indications for surgical revascularization in patients with atherosclerotic renal artery disease were treatment of renovascular hypertension in 80 patients, preservation of renal function in 61 patients, and both control of hypertension and preservation of renal function in 100 patients.

In this series, operative mortality was 2.1% in patients with atherosclerotic renal artery disease and 0% in patients with fibrous dysplasia or an aneurysm. Postoperative thrombosis or stenosis of the repaired renal artery occurred following 17 of 380 surgical revascularization operations (4.5%). Hypertension was cured or improved postoperatively in 91.7% of patients with atherosclerotic renal artery disease and in 93% of patients with fibrous dysplasia or an aneurysm. Postoperative renal function was improved or stable in 88.8% of patients with atherosclerosis who underwent surgical revascularization (SR) to preserve renal function. These data illustrate the excellent clinical results that continue to be achieved with surgical revascularization in properly selected patients with renal artery disease.

RENOVASCULAR HYPERTENSION IN CHILDREN

The exact incidence of hypertension in children is not known but is estimated at 1.5–2.5%. Children and adults differ significantly in the spectrum of causative factors that may lead to an elevated blood pressure, with a secondary etiology being much more common in children. Among pediatric patients, renal artery disease is second in frequency only to coarctation of the thoracic aorta as a cause of surgically correctable hypertension.

Renal artery disease in children is generally caused by one of the fibrous dysplasias, most commonly intimal or perimedial fibroplasia. Other causes include an arterial aneurysm, arteriovenous malformation, Takayasu's arteritis, neurofibromatosis, thromboembolic disease, and trauma (59). The typical clinical presentation for most of these disorders is an asymptomatic patient with recently discovered hypertension upon a routine physical examination. Bilateral and/or branch renal artery involvement are frequently observed, particularly with the fibrous dysplasias; extrarenal vascular disease may also be present.

Surgical treatment of renal artery disease in children is generally directed at relief of hypertension, although preservation of renal function is of equal concern with diseases that are known to cause progressive vascular obstruction, such as intimal or perimedial fibroplasia. Although new medical agents have proven very effective in treating renin-mediated hypertension, they have no place in the definitive treatment of young patients, since their use would mean lifelong commitment to drug therapy with the significant risk of losing renal function from progressive disease. Percutaneous transluminal angioplasty is technically more difficult in children as a result of small vessel

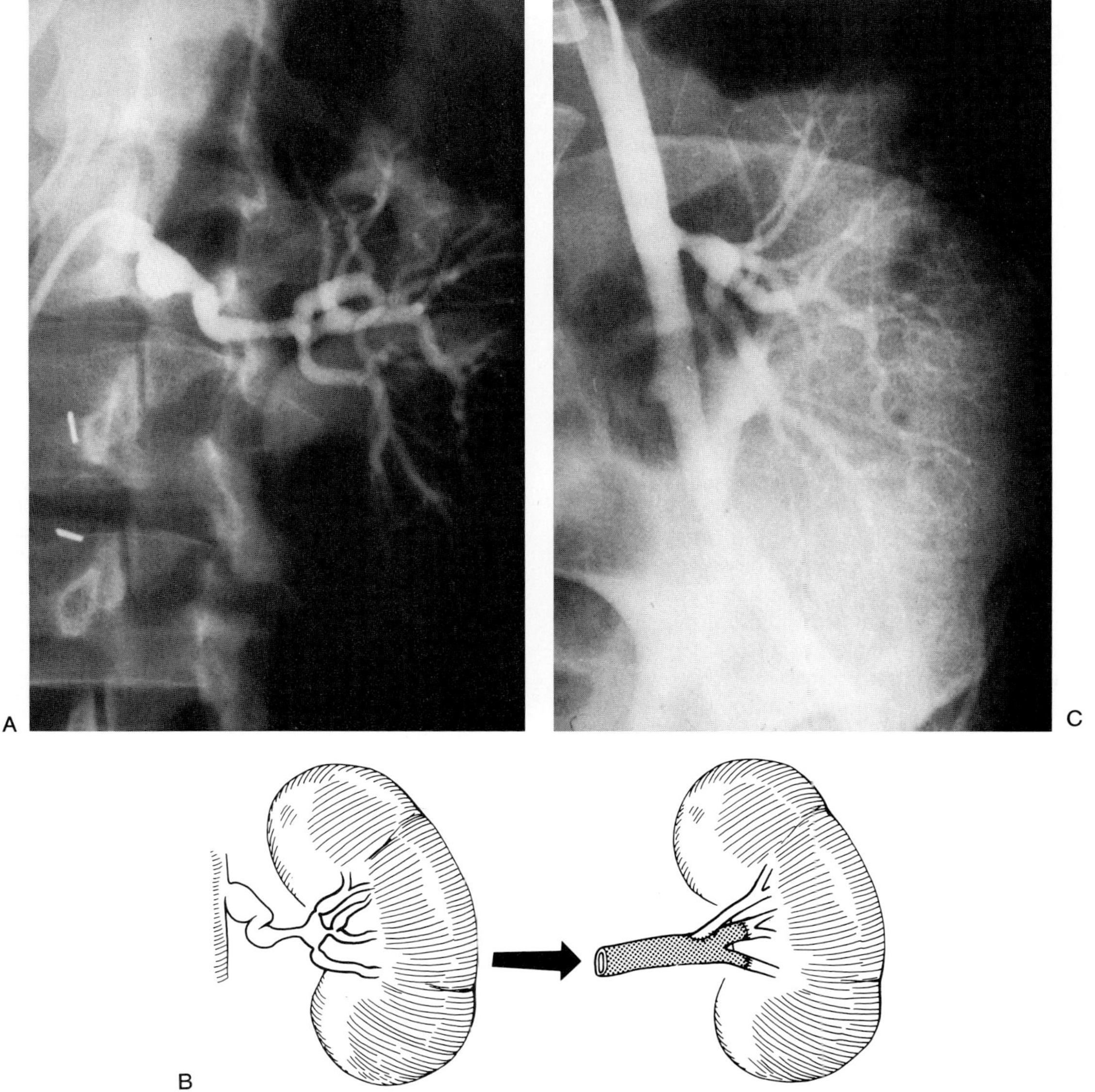

FIG. 6. A: Selective left renal arteriogram in a young woman, demonstrating aneurysmal and stenosing fibrous disease involving the main renal artery and three branches. **B:** Sketch illustrating the extent of vascular disease in this patient (*left*) and also illustrating the method of extracorporeal revascularization employing a branched graft of the hypogastric artery (*right*). **C:** Postoperative arteriogram following renal autotransplantation, demonstrating patent main renal artery and repaired branches. (From ref. 72.)

size, but it may be suitable for some patients with a focal lesion in the main renal artery.

In general, the cure rates following surgical treatment of renovascular hypertension have been better in children than in adults, probably because of a shorter duration of hypertension in the former (60–68). Yet, prior to 1972, surgical cure of this disease in children was most often achieved through nephrectomy rather than by revascularization. More recently, during the past decade, it has become possible to achieve successful renal vascular reconstruction in most pediatric patients. This evolution has occurred because of (a) the development of microvascular techniques and (b) a better appreciation of specific operative approaches that are most efficacious in children. It is important to emphasize that pediatric renal artery disorders should be repaired as soon as the diagnosis is made —rather than waiting until the child is older and the vessel becomes larger, as some have advocated. The latter approach carries the risk of developing (a) secondary nephrosclerosis from suboptimally controlled hypertension or (b) ischemic atrophy of the involved kidney caused by progressive renal artery obstruction.

The special problems associated with renovascular reconstruction in children relate primarily to the small size of the diseased vessels and frequent branch renal artery involvement. In addition, the available surgical options for performing revascularization are more limited because some techniques that have proven effective in adults are contraindicated in children. For example, splenorenal bypass is a satisfactory operation in selected adult patients but has yielded very poor results in children and is best avoided in this age group (65). Also, the problem of aneurysmal expansion of aortorenal saphenous vein grafts has been observed more frequently in small children (40,70). This may reflect an enhanced susceptibility to mural ischemia of vein segments procured from younger patients; regardless, it would seem prudent not to use saphenous vein grafts in the prepubertal age group.

Aortorenal bypass with an autogenous vascular graft is currently the mainstay technique for performing renal revascularization in the pediatric patient. A graft of autogenous hypogastric artery is preferred, however, in older children; a saphenous vein graft is also acceptable. In some children with proximal renal artery disease and an adequate amount of disease-free distal artery, direct aortorenal reimplantation may be performed (71). Renal autotransplantation alone, without an *ex vivo* repair, is indicated in children with aortic hypoplasia; it is also indicated in small prepubertal children when aortorenal bypass with a hypogastric arterial graft is not possible. Extracorporeal microvascular reconstruction and autotransplantation are indicated for disease involving branches of the renal artery that are either intrarenal or small in caliber (69). Renovascular hypertension in children is a potentially curable disease, and the results of surgical revascularization can be most gratifying.

SUMMARY

The role of surgical revascularization in the management of patients with renal artery disease has changed in recent years. This has occurred because of (a) the advent of PTA as an effective method of treatment for certain patients, (b) improved results of surgical revascularization in older patients with atherosclerosis, (c) an enhanced appreciation of advanced atherosclerotic renal artery disease as a correctable cause of renal failure, and (d) the development of more effective surgical techniques for patients with severe aortic atherosclerosis and branch renal artery disease. Surgical revascularization is presently the treatment of choice for patients who require intervention as a result of ostial atherosclerotic renal artery disease, branch renal artery disease, or a renal artery aneurysm; it is also the treatment of choice for small children. At the present time, excellent clinical results continue to be achieved with surgical revascularization in properly selected patients.

REFERENCES

1. Novick AC, Stewart BH. Surgical treatment of renovascular hypertension. *Curr Probl Surg* 1979;16(8):1–79.
2. Schreiber MJ, Pohl MA, Novick AC. The natural history of atherosclerotic and fibrous renal artery disease. *Urol Clin North Am* 1984;11:383.
3. Harrison HG, McCormack LJ. Pathologic classification of renal artery disease in renovascular hypertension. *Mayo Clin Proc* 1971;46:161.
4. Meaney TF, Dustan HP, McCormack LJ. Natural history of renal arterial disease. *Radiology* 1968;91:881.
5. Rybka SJ, Novick AC. Concomitant carotid, mesenteric and renal artery stenosis due to primary intimal fibroplasia. *J Urol* 1983;129:798.
6. Poutasse EF. Renal artery aneurysms. *J Urol* 1975;113:433.
7. Novick AC. Renal artery aneurysm and arteriovenous malformation. In: Novick AC, Straffon RA, eds. *Vascular problems in urologic surgery.* Philadelphia: WB Saunders, 1982.
8. Kaufman JJ. The middle aortic syndrome: report of a case treated by renal autotransplantation. *J Urol* 1973;109:711.
9. Grad E, Rance CP. Bilateral renal artery stenosis in association with neurofibromatosis (Recklinghausen's disease): report of two cases. *J Pediatr* 1972;80:804.
10. Tilford DL, Kelsch RC. Renal artery stenosis in childhood neurofibromatosis. *Am J Dis Child* 1973;126:665.
11. Silver D, Clements JB. Renovascular hypertension from renal artery compression by congenital bands. *Ann Surg* 1976;183:161.
12. Eipper DF, Gifford RW, Stewart BH, Alfidi JR, McCormack LJ, Vidt DG. Abdominal bruits in renovascular hypertension. *Am J Cardiol* 1976;13:48.
13. Hughes JS, Dove HG, Gifford RW, Feinstein AR. Duration of blood pressure elevation in accurately predicting surgical cure of renovascular hypertension. *Am Heart J* 1981;101:408.
14. Simon F, Franklin SS, Bleifer KH, Maxwell MH. Clinical characteristics of renovascular hypertension. *JAMA* 1972;220:1209.
15. Buonocore E, Meaney TF, Borkowski GP, et al. Digital subtraction angiography of the abdominal aorta and renal arteries: comparison with conventional aortography. *AJR* 1981;139:281.
16. Hillman BJ, Ovitt TW, Capp MP, et al. The potential impact of digital video subtraction angiography on screening for renovascular hypertension. *Radiology* 1982;142:577.
17. Smith CW, Winfield AC, Price RR, et al. Evaluation of digital venous angiography for the diagnosis of renovascular hypertension. *Radiology* 1982;144:51.
18. Zabbo A, Novick AC. Digital subtraction angiography for non-invasive imaging of the renal artery. *Urol Clin North Am* 1987;11:409.
19. Mark LS, Maxwell MH, Varady PD, et al. Renovascular hypertension: Does the renal vein renin ratio predict operative results? *J Urol* 1976;115:365.
20. Couch NP, Sullivan J, Crane C. The predictive accuracy of renal vein renin activity in the surgery of renovascular hypertension. *Surgery* 1976;79:70.
21. Muller FB, Seeley JE, Case DB, et al. The captopril test for identifying renovascular disease in hypertensive patients. *Am J Med* 1986;80:633.
22. Geyskes GG, Oei HY, Puylaert C, Mees EJ. Renovascular hypertension identified by captopril-induced changes in the renogram. *Hypertension* 1987;9:451.
23. Flechner SM. Percutaneous transluminal dilatation: a realistic appraisal in patients with stenosing lesions of the renal artery. *Urol Clin N Am* 1984;11:515.
24. Sos TA, Pickering PG, Sniderman KW, et al. Percutaneous transluminal renal angiography in renovascular hypertension due to atheroma or fibrous dysplasia. *N Engl J Med* 1983;309:274.
25. Council on Scientific Affairs. Percutaneous transluminal angioplasty. *JAMA* 1984;251:764.
26. Hayes J, Risius B, Novick AC, et al. Experience with percutaneous transluminal angioplasty for renal artery stenosis at the Cleveland Clinic. *J Urol* 1989;in press.
27. Novick AC: Ziegelbaum M, Vidt DG, Gifford RW, Pohl MA, Goormastic M. Trends in surgical revascularization for renal artery disease: ten years' experience. *JAMA* 1987;257:498.
28. Cicuto KP, McLean GK, Oleaga J, et al. Renal artery stenosis: anatomic classification for percutaneous angioplasty. *AJR* 1981;137:599.
29. Novick AC, Pohl MA, Schreiber MJ, Gifford RW, Vidt DG. Renal revascularization for preservation of kidney function in patients with atherosclerotic renovascular disease. *J Urol* 1983;129:907.
30. Ziegelbaum M, Novick AC, Hayes J, et al. Management of renal arterial disease in the elderly patient. *Surg Gynecol Obstet* 1987;165:130.
31. Scheft P, Novick AC, Stewart BH, Straffon RA. Renal revascular-

hypertension in which there is no activation of the renin–angiotensin system.

In general, most endocrine tumors are characterized by a relative degree of secretory autonomy. Inhibition of angiotensin II action by saralasin or lowering of angiotensin II by converting-enzyme blockade is accompanied by an increase of PRA resulting from the suppression of the negative feedback exerted by angiotensin II on renin secretion. The degree of plasma renin is directly related to the circulating basal level of angiotensin II. Therefore, it could be expected in cases of tumoral renin secretion that the suppression of angiotensin II action or of its plasma level by pharmacologic renin blockade would not alter renin secretion, contrary to what is observed in normal renin regulation. Indeed, in two cases, renin failed to increase after saralasin infusion (2,16) or did not vary during converting-enzyme treatment (Table 2), suggesting that the physiological feedback of angiotensin II on renin secretion was not present in these tumors. However, in other cases (Table 2), PRA increased during an acute captopril test. Similarly, renin secretion by these tumors may or may not be regulated by physiological factors such as orthostatism, sodium depletion, beta-adrenergic blockade, or the nyctohemeral cycle (29). The fact that some tumors may normally respond to well-established renin stimuli emphasizes that there is no physiological or pharmacological test which is likely to demonstrate the renin secretory autonomy of the juxtaglomerular tumoral tissue. It is also likely that there is a high degree of differentiation of these tumors which we have recently shown, *in vitro,* to possess functional angiotensin II, beta-adrenergic receptors, and ANP receptors (31); in general, renin juxtaglomerular tumoral cells must possess the normal membrane receptors which are efficiently coupled to the second messengers involved in renin release and biosynthesis. The absence in some juxtaglomerular cell tumors of a response to renin stimuli may be due to desensitization of their surface receptors or to the fact that the doses used were too low, or not administered for a sufficient time to significantly affect renin production with regard to the increased number of renin-secreting cells.

TABLE 2. *Effect of acute blockade of the renin–angiotensin system on diastolic blood pressure and plasma renin activity*

Case	Acute blockade of the renin–angiotensin system	Percent decrease in diastolic blood pressure	PRA (ng/Al/ml/h) Before	After[a]
1	Saralasin[b]	34	76	56
2	Captopril[c]	22	10	22
3	Captopril	40	28	22
4	Captopril	36	14	21
5	Captopril	34	57	104
6	Captopril	15	5	32
7	Captopril	37	35	32

[a] Plasma renin activity (PRA) was measured 1 hr after intravenous administration of saralasin (case no. 1) and 3 hr after captopril (case no. 2 through case no. 7).

[b] Saralasin: 1 μg/kg/min for 10 min.

[c] Captopril (1 mg/kg) was given orally, and the blood pressure was automatically measured. PRA was measured before and 1 hr after captopril administration.

TABLE 3. *Methods used for localization of the juxtaglomerular cell tumors*

Case	Renal arteriogram	CT scanner	Increase of renin in a renal vein[a]	Diameter of the tumor (mm)
1	Negative (3)[b]	ND[c]	Negative (3)[b]	50
2	Positive (1) Negative (2)	ND	Positive (1) Negative (2)	30
3	Positive	Positive	Negative	30
4	Negative	Positive	Positive	15
5	Negative	Positive	Positive	13
6	Negative	Positive	Positive	10
7	Positive (1) Negative (1)	Positive	Negative (3)	30

[a] A renin ratio of 1.5 between the affected side and the nonaffected side was considered to be significant.

[b] Numbers in parentheses indicate the number of different renal arteriograms and renin measurements performed in renal veins.

[c] ND, not done.

Tumor Localization

The diagnosis of a juxtaglomerular cell tumor is therefore based largely on the absence of other causes of high blood pressure in cases of severe hypertension with marked hyperreninism and hyperaldosteronism. In order to eliminate the possibility of renal artery disease or renal infarction, a renal arteriogram is mandatory. The direct diagnosis of the juxtaglomerular tumor can be made by several methods:

1. *Selective and segmental renin measurements in renal veins.* This procedure has been performed in most of the published cases of the literature, with varying success. Indeed, a clear increase in PRA in a renal vein or one of its branches is not always observed, as shown by a failure in four of seven cases in our own department (Table 3). In most cases, the renin concentration is only slightly elevated on the affected side. This may result from the tumor being located at the surface of the kidney and because most of the venous blood is collected by the pericapsular veins and not drained into the main renal vein. Selective catheterization of the branches of the renal vein has sometimes helped in localizing the tumor (15), but it can also be misleading. Another explanation for the difficulty in localizing the tumor by selective renin measurements in the renal vein is the possible high level of angiotensin II within the tumor, as detected by immunohistochemistry (2), which affects the vascularization of the tissue. Finally, in one case, previous captopril therapy obscured the renal-vein renin measurements (26).

2. *Selective renal arteriography.* On selective renal arteriograms, a small avascular zone, characteristic of the presence of the tumor, can be seen at the external contour of the kidney. Since the tumor may be located on the anterior or posterior side of the kidney, it can only be visualized if right and left anterior oblique views are performed. In any

case, the tumor, which may be as small as 0.8 cm in diameter, may not be seen.

3. *Computerized tomography (CT) scanning.* Because the two preceding diagnostic procedures can fail or be inaccurate, a kidney CT scan should be systematically performed where a renin juxtaglomerular tumor is suspected. The CT scan was positive in all of the five renin tumors explored in our department as well as in the recent cases in the literature (Table 3; Fig. 1). A small hypodense tumor is seen at the periphery of the kidney. In the last case of our series, a nuclear magnetic resonance imaging confirmed the CT scan diagnosis.

4. *Surgical exploration.* Because of the difficulty in localizing these tumors, most of them have been detected in the past by surgical exploration, as was the case in our first renin tumor (3). Careful palpation of the surface of the two kidneys may reveal the presence of a superficial tumor. Since the half-life of renin is about 30–40 min, clamping of the kidney pedicle induced a drop in blood pressure and helped in the localization of the tumor in one case (16), although no blood pressure decrease occurred in one of our cases because the tumor remained vascularized and drained by the perirenal vascular bed (3).

When localized at surgery, excision of the tumor can be achieved because the juxtaglomerular tumors are superficial and can be easily dissected from the adjacent kidney tissue. Nephrectomy is not necessary, since these tumors are benign and no case of malignant transformation has yet been reported.

The diagnosis of juxtaglomerular renin tumor is difficult to make and is certainly underestimated, although during the last years an increasing number of new cases have been reported. As already pointed out in this review, this diagnosis should be systematically evoked in a young patient with severe hypertension, hyperreninism, and hyperaldosteronism. The kidney CT scan is the most reliable diagnostic procedure for the localization of the tumor, after elimination of a renovascular disease by renal arteriography. The diagnosis is important to make, since excision of the tumor relieves hypertension and the associated hyperreninism. In all of the cases observed in our department, the patients had normal blood pressure after removal of the tumor; in the first case, there was a follow-up of 10 years. It is interesting to note that this normalization of blood pressure occurred even after 10 years of exposure to high blood pressure and extremely high levels of renin and angiotensin II. At the same time, left cardiac hypertrophy, lesions of optic fundi, and renal alterations disappeared. Pregnancy has occurred in two of our patients since the operation. In both cases, the patients carried through to full-term pregnancy; in one case, however, a mild antihypertensive treatment was required toward the end of the pregnancy. In both cases, ischemic lesions of the placenta were observed. After delivery, blood pressure returned to normal in the patient with pregnancy-induced hypertension and remained normal for more than 2 years of follow-up.

HISTOGENESIS AND HISTOLOGY

The natural history of juxtaglomerular tumors is not known, and therefore their nosology is confusing. If such tumors originate and develop only from the afferent arterioles of the glomeruli, then the term *tumor of the juxtaglomerular apparatus* is justified. However, if these tumors develop upstream from the juxtaglomerular apparatus, on the interlobular arteries which may contain renin secreting cells, the term *tumor of the juxtaglomerular apparatus* would be inappropriate.

The word *hemangiopericytoma* should be reserved only for tumors which have developed from Zimmermann pericytes, which are known to be contractile elements devoid of endocrine-type morphological characteristics unlike the epithelioid cells of the afferent glomerular arteriole.

The term *hamartoma,* which refers to an abnormal congenital development of the juxtaglomerular apparatus, has been suggested by some authors. This term would imply that the tumor contains elements belonging to the juxtaglomerular apparatus—in particular, the tubular elements of the macula densa. Indeed, several of these tumors contain tubular elements besides the vascular smooth muscle cells differentiated into renin-secreting cells.

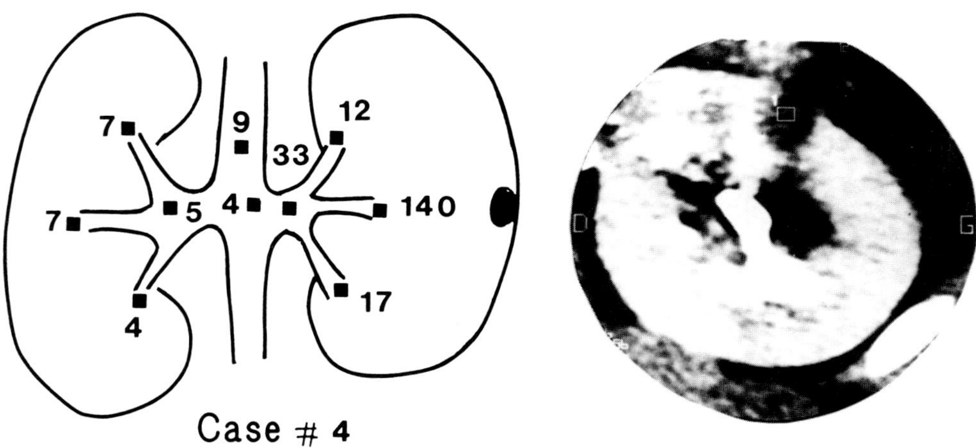

FIG. 1. Renal-vein renin measurements and computerized tomographic scan of a juxtaglomerular renin tumor. The hypodense tumor is located at the surface of the left kidney (case no. 4).

A

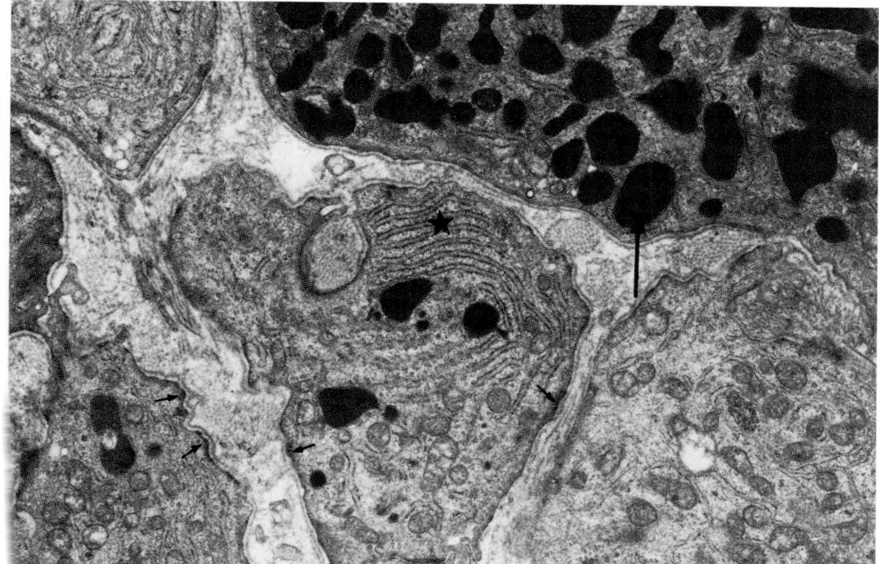

B

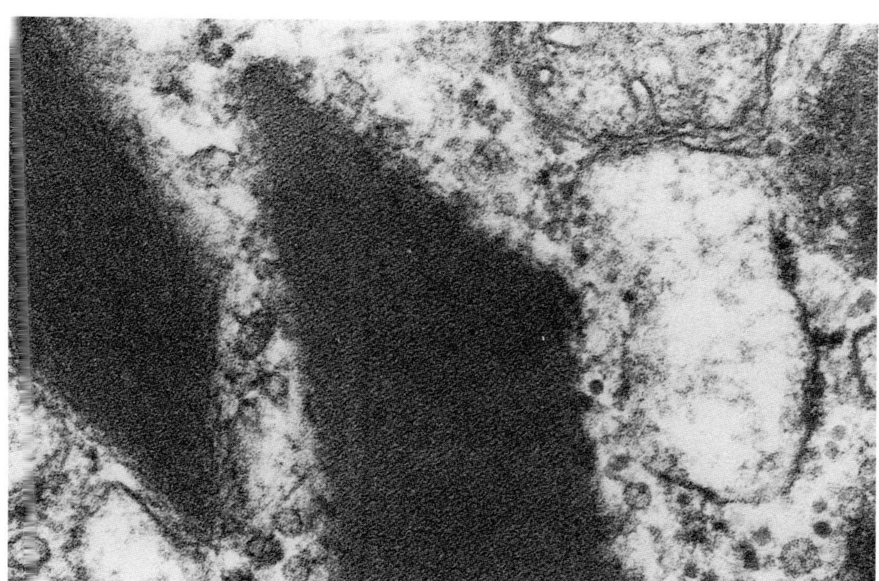

FIG. 2. Electron microscopy of a renin juxtaglomerular cell tumor. **A:** In the tumoral juxtaglomerular cells, we can observe numerous spherical mature granules (*long arrow*), a well-developed rough endoplasmic reticulum (*star*), and myofilaments with attachment bodies (*short arrow*). ×7200. **B:** Paracrystalline protogranules with characteristic periodic striation. ×85,000.

Light-microscopic, Electron-microscopic, and *In Situ* Hybridization Studies

Light- and electron-microscopic studies revealed the presence of (a) endocrine and vascular smooth muscle cells with neural components (32) and (b) transitional cells containing secretory granules, myofilaments, and attachment bodies (2,16,33). The ultrastructure of these cells is very similar to those of normal renin-producing cells, since we can observe the presence of secretory paracrystalline protogranules and round, amorphous, dense, mature granules (Fig. 2). These granules contained renin, as revealed by immunohistochemistry at the electron-microscopic level (33,34). *In situ* hybridization performed in two cases yielded a signal in all tumoral cells, even in those which were not positively stained by the renin antibody (35). However, the tumoral cells were not labeled by indirect immunofluorescence with human angiotensin-I-converting enzyme and human angiotensinogen antiserum (2). In addition, the tumoral renin-secreting cells did not produce angiotensinogen or converting enzyme in culture (36), which makes the presence of a functional intracellular renin–angiotensin system within these cells unlikely, in contrast to what has been described in other species (37). In three cases, a comparison was made between prorenin and active renin content in tumor extracts, and ultrastructural findings were also compared (33). The tumor with the highest total renin content per gram of tissue contained more mature renin granules and proportionately more active renin than the two others, suggesting a relationship between renin storage and renin processing (Table 4). The opposite situation was that of a pulmonary metastasis from an epithelioid sarcoma of the soft tissue where more than 95% of the plasma renin was prorenin (38). In this case, renin antibody detected few positive cells; this suggests that in such cells, newly synthesized renin was probably released

TABLE 4. *Plasma renin levels, renin tumoral content, and presence of renin granules in tumoral cells from four juxtaglomerular cell tumors and in one case of lung metastasis of a malignant tumor of vascular origin*[a]

Case	Plasma renin: Active renin (pg/ml)	Plasma renin: Prorenin (pg/ml)	Plasma renin: Percentage of prorenin	Tumoral tissue: Total renin (μg/g tissue)	Tumoral tissue: Presence of renin granules
1	11,100	21,000	66	1,018	++++
2	180	1,900	91	180	++
3	90	640	88	204	++
4	370	738	67	—	++
Epithelioid sarcoma of soft tissue (lung metastasis)	200	7,300	97	4	None

[a] Renin and prorenin were measured by direct assays (60).

without storage within the cell and incompletely processed, accounting for the very high levels of plasma prorenin (7300 pg/ml) compared to active renin (200 pg/ml) observed in this patient (Table 4). At the electron-microscopic level, pulmonary metastasis showed scanty intracytoplasmic granules in scarce tumoral cells. *In situ* hybridization showed that sparse tumor cells contained renin mRNA (35).

Another interesting and presently unexplained finding is the constant presence of mast cells in juxtaglomerular cell tumors, which may account for up to 25% of the total number of cells (2,16). These cells were cocultured with the renin tumoral cells (36) and released histamine during the primary culture. No mast cells are found in the normal or pathological juxtaglomerular apparatus, and there is no known relationship between these two types of cells. This raises the possibility that the juxtaglomerular tumoral cells produce a factor which could attract and favor the growth of mast cells.

PRIMARY RENINISM ASSOCIATED WITH RENAL TUMORS OTHER THAN THOSE OF THE JUXTAGLOMERULAR APPARATUS

In some cases of renal tumors, hypertension associated with hyperreninism and hyperaldosteronism can be observed. The renin production occurs therefore in cells other than the epithelioid cells which normally secrete renin and therefore can be considered as an ectopic renin secretion, even though it originates from kidney cells.

In nearly 60% of cases of *Wilms' tumors* (nephroblastoma), a renin-dependent hypertension can be noted (39–43). These tumors are curable by radiotherapy and surgical excision, but hypertension and renin hypersecretion resume with metastases. Renin can be easily localized by immunocytochemistry in these carcinomas. In some rare cases of *renal cell carcinomas*, hypertension associated with high renin secretion has been noted (44–46). Again, it has been shown that these carcinomas contain cells which stain positively for renin (47). Renin secreted in one case of renal carcinoma was mainly inactive, and its level was reduced to normal by nephrectomy (48). These cases should be distinguished from the renin secretion which occurs when the renal vessels are compressed by an expanding mass which, in itself, does not synthesize renin (47).

PRIMARY RENINISM ASSOCIATED WITH EXTRARENAL RENIN-SECRETING TUMORS

Excessive production of renin may also arise in a variety of other types of tumors. The derepression of the renin gene during cell multiplication may occur, resulting in the synthesis of a large amount of prorenin, the biosynthetic (and inactive) renin precursor. The processing of prorenin into active renin may be incomplete because of the absence of processing enzymes and specialized organelles in these neoplastic cells. The plasma levels of inactive renin can therefore be extremely high, compared to the high to normal plasma active renin values.

There are eight documented cases of ectopic renin-secreting cancers reported so far in the literature. Two were lung cancers (49,50). Two cases originated from the uterogenital tract: One was a paraovarian tumor (51), and one was a fallopian tube adenocarcinoma (52). The four other cases were an epithelial liver hamartoma (53), an orbital hemangiopericytoma (54), a pancreatic cancer (55), and an angiolymphoid hyperplasia with eosinophilia (56). We have observed recently in our department a new case of ectopic renin-secreting cancer, namely, an epithelioid sarcoma of soft tissue with lung metastasis (35,38).

All these cases possessed the same clinical features of severe hypertension with hypokalemia—with the surprising exception of the liver hamartoma, where a normal plasma potassium was noted (53). These patients had relatively higher values of prorenin than did patients suffering from renal tumors, as has been well described by Ruddy et al. (55). In our case of malignant hemangioreninoma, plasma prorenin detected by direct immunoradiometric assay or after prorenin activation by trypsin treatment was extremely high, and then the prorenin/renin ratio was higher than in high-plasma-renin patients. As discussed previously, these ectopic renin-secreting cancers do not process, to a normal extent, prorenin into renin; thus a large amount of prorenin is released into the blood. Similar findings have been made with other ectopic endocrine-secreting tumors.

Here again, it is possible that the prevalence of renin-secreting cancers might be underestimated. The development of hypertension, especially when associated with hypokalemia during the course of a malignant disease, should systematically evoke this diagnosis. The systematic measurement of prorenin, and not only of active renin, in the plasma of patients suffering from cancer might reveal that some cancers are associated with abnormal levels of prorenin. The absence or the abnormal processing of prorenin into renin within the tumoral tissue would account for the lack of clinical and biological syndrome of primary reninism.

BIOLOGICAL STUDIES IN THE PRIMARY RENINISM SYNDROME

The discovery of renin-secreting tumors has led to biological studies of major importance. Because of the extremely low concentration of renin and of renin-secreting cells in normal human kidney, the purification of renin and the study of its biosynthesis in this tissue are extremely difficult. The renin juxtaglomerular cell tumors represent an invaluable source of material, since they are considerably enriched in renin-secreting cells and in renin. They have been used in recent years for (a) the complete purification of renin, (b) biosynthesis and processing of prorenin and renin, (c) culture of renin-secreting cells, and (d) the characterization of the tumoral renin mRNA.

Purification of Tumoral Renin and Prorenin

A 400,000-fold purification is necessary for purifying renin from normal human kidneys. A renin-containing tumor permitted total purification of 5.3 mg of human renin in three stages with a purification factor of 40 times (57). The physicochemical characteristics of the renin from this tumor are identical to those of active renal renin from a normal kidney, including the presence, during migration on a polyacrylamide gel under denaturing conditions, of two forms of low-molecular-weight renin (25,000 and 20,000).

Production of polyclonal and monoclonal antibodies (57,58) by using this purified renin from a tumor has led to (a) the development of a direct assay of human tissue and plasma renin (59,60), (b) the intrarenal localization of renin in normal and pathological (61) human kidneys, and (c) the study of the role of renin in maintaining arterial pressure in normotensive and hypertensive monkeys (62).

Human prorenin has been characterized from several ectopic renin-producing cancers; these tissues produce mainly prorenin instead of renin. In a patient with Wilms' tumor (39), a high-molecular-weight renin (60,000) was found in tissue and plasma. It could be activated *in vitro* without undergoing any noteworthy loss in molecular weight. The higher molecular weight of inactive renin (46,000) found in two tumoral tissues (of the lung and the paraovarian region), when compared to that of active renin (42,500) separated on carboxybenzylpepstatin by affinity chromatography, suggests that cancer tissue, like the kidney, synthesizes a proenzyme similar to hormone precursors (63). The characteristics of active and inactive tumoral renin are comparable to those of renin extracted from normal kidney, both in molecular weight and migration, on Affigel-Blue (which retains the inactive renin) and, with affinity chromatography, on pepstatin (which retains active renin) (64). *In vitro* activation of tumoral renin is possible with trypsin, plasmin, and kallikrein (65). Finally, active and inactive tumoral renin from three tumors was recognized by antirenin antibodies in a manner identical to that for normal human prorenin from plasma, amniotic fluid, and the brain (64).

Historically speaking, the discovery of cases of ectopic production of renin in an inactive form and with a higher molecular weight was one of the fundamental arguments for the existence of a renin precursor which was termed *prorenin.*

Biosynthesis of Human Renin in Juxtaglomerular Cell Tumors

Endocrine tumors permit the study of hormone biosynthesis and of the processing of hormone precursor into the mature hormone, as was elegantly shown by Steiner et al., who first demonstrated the existence of an insulin precursor in a pancreatic insulinoma (66). Using a renin juxtaglomerular cell tumor, the biosynthesis of renin in tissue slices and in primary cell cultures was studied by incorporation of ^{35}S-methionine into immunoreactive renin and prorenin (67). Renin was biosynthesized as prorenin (mol. wt. 55,000) and then converted into renin (mol. wt. 44,000) in tissue slices. However, when the same experiment was performed in primary cell cultures, only prorenin was synthesized: No conversion of prorenin into renin occurred even after 24 hr, a phenomenon coincident with the disappearance of renin granules within the cells during the culture. From these experiments, the existence of two pathways for the processing, packaging, and secretion of renin in juxtaglomerular tumoral cells was postulated (67): (i) a regulated pathway where renin is processed, stored in granules, and released during stimulation and (ii) a constitutive pathway where prorenin is neither stored nor processed into renin but is released directly into plasma (Fig. 3). Such a pathway has subsequently been demonstrated to exist in infarcted and in normal human kidney tissues (68).

Recently, the primary amino acid sequence of human preprorenin was deduced from the structure of its cDNA (69). By analogy with the model described for processing of preprorenin into renin in the mouse submandibular gland (70), human prorenin is converted into renin after cleavage of a prosegment. This model also strongly suggested that the inactive renin found in tumoral tissues or in plasma was prorenin. However, this model could not establish with certainty the exact length of the signal peptide of renin. Again, using a human renin-secreting tumor, Murakami and co-workers (71) studied, *in vitro,* the processing of human renin precursor. Using radioactive microsequenc-

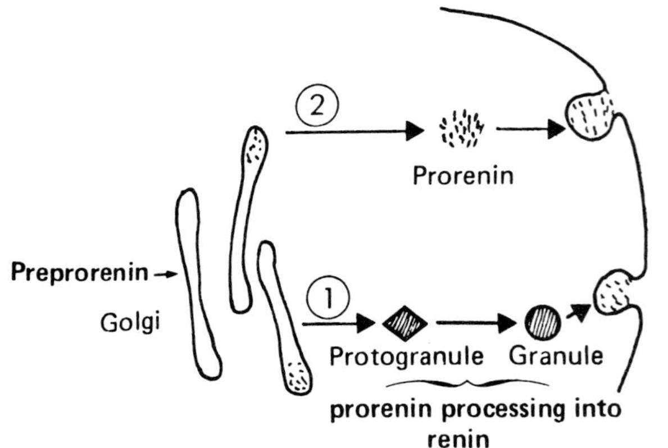

FIG. 3. Proposed model of two pathways for the release of renin as deduced from renin biosynthesis studies in a juxtaglomerular cell tumor. Pathway 1 is a regulated pathway leading to the release of active renin (mol. wt. 44,000). Pathway 2 would be a constitutive pathway leading to the release of prorenin (mol. wt. 55,000); this pathway is predominant in the renin-producing cells in culture. (From ref. 67.)

ing, they could locate the exact site of processing between pre- and prorenin and could show that renin prosegment was 43 amino acids long. The same tumoral source allowed them to demonstrate the *in vitro* glycosylation of renin.

Finally, the size of the mRNA coding for renin in one juxtaglomerular tumor has been shown to be similar to that of normal human kidney renin (1.6 kb) (72). The transcription starting point has been determined in this tumor by S_1 nuclease mapping, since two TATA boxes exist in the 5′ flanking region of the human gene and could be used by RNA polymerase. In both cases, the more proximal TATA box was used, and there was therefore no suggestion of abnormal transcription of the renin message.

Culture of Renin-Secreting Tumoral Cells

Renin production is influenced by multiple factors *in vivo,* and therefore *in vitro* models are needed for studying its biosynthesis and regulation. In humans, such models are particularly difficult to establish because of the scarcity of the renin-secreting cells and the difficulty in culturing them. Two attempts were made to maintain renin-producing cells from renin juxtaglomerular tumors in culture (1,67). However, in both cases, renin production declined and the cells could not be maintained for more than 1 month in primary and secondary cultures. In addition, these cells lost their ability to process prorenin into renin. An attempt to immortalize renin-producing cells from renin tumors was recently made.

Cells from a human juxtaglomerular cell tumor were transfected by three mutants of simian virus 40 (SV40) in order to establish renin-secreting cells which would maintain their differentiated state (36). Two types of cells were transfected: (i) mast cells which lost their ability to produce histamine after several passages but which kept some of their morphological features and (ii) renin-producing cells. Renin produced by these cells was almost exclusively prorenin and was not stored within the cells. After activation, renin had biochemical, enzymatic, and immunologic properties similar to those of pure human standard renin. The renin production was stable, and the cell cultures have been maintained for more than 2 years. The secretion of renin in these cells can be influenced by agents acting by activation of adenylate cyclase (forskolin, beta agonists) or by altering the intracellular Ca^{2+} content (angiotensin II) (31). This stable human juxtaglomerular cell line provides a unique model for studying (a) the different factors affecting renin secretion and (b) the specific second messengers involved in renin release.

Another attempt to culture human tumoral cells was made from the patient with pulmonary metastases from an epithelioid sarcoma of the soft tissue (38). These cells were maintained in culture for more than five passages and produced a low level of prorenin. Prorenin secretion could be stimulated by forskolin but not by dexamethasone, suggesting that the glucocorticoid regulatory element present in the 5′ flanking region of the human renin gene (72) does not play a functional role.

CONCLUSIONS

Analysis of the literature describing renin-secreting tumors suggests diagnosis of juxtaglomerular cell tumor should be routinely considered in a young patient with severe hypertension and hypokalemia when a diagnosis of renovascular lesion has been eliminated by arteriography. A very high PRA is usually observed, and blood pressure falls during converting-enzyme treatment. Under acute administration of captopril, plasma renin may or may not increase, showing the inconsistency of the secretory autonomy of the tumor. The most useful examination for the localization of the tumor is the CT scan. Excessive renin production may provoke vascular lesions, left ventricular hypertrophy, and impairment of renin function, which all disappear after surgical treatment, i.e., at the time when blood pressure returns to normal.

Primary reninism has great physiological importance for the hypothesis that favors the essential role of the kidney in determining the level of blood pressure. It can be considered as a unique, purely renin-dependent form of hypertension. This syndrome has no experimental equivalent and is the most caricatural form of other renin-dependent hypertension (such as renovascular disease and probably some other types of essential hypertension).

The discovery of a renin-secreting tumor thus constitutes (a) a life-saving diagnosis for the patient, (b) a subject of reflection for the specialist, and (c) a useful tool for studies of the general mechanisms involved in enzyme biosynthesis and tumoral endocrine cell function.

REFERENCES

1. Conn JW, Cohen EL, Lucas CP, McDonald WJ, Mayor GH, Blough WM, Eveland WC, Bookstein JJ, Lapides J. Hypertension, hyperreninemia and secondary aldosteronism due to renin-producing juxtaglomerular cell tumors. *Arch Intern Med* 1972;130:682–696.
2. Baruch D, Corvol P, Alhenc-Gelas F, Dufloux MA, Guyenne TT, Gaux JC, Raymond A, Brisset JM, Duclos JM, Menard J. Diagnosis and treatment of renin secreting tumors. Report of three cases. *Hypertension* 1984;6:760–766.
3. Corvol P, Kreft C, Safar M, Brisset JM, Camilleri JP, Menard J, Bariety J, Milliez P. Hypertension artérielle et tumeur à rénine. In: Sandoz C, ed. *Acquis Med Recent.* Paris: Louis Masson, 1979; 161–168.
4. Robertson PW, Klidjian A, Harding LK, Walters G, Lee MR, Robb-Smith AHT. Hypertension due to a renin-secreting renal tumour. *Am J Med* 1967;43:963–976.
5. Kihara T, Kitamura S, Hoshino T, Seida H, Watanabe T. A hitherto unreported vascular tumor of the kidney: a proposal of juxtaglomerular cell tumor. *Acta Pathol Jpn* 1968;18:197–206.
6. Conn JW. Primary reninism. In: Genest J, ed. *Hypertension.* New York: McGraw-Hill, 1978;840–847.
7. Lee MR. Renin secreting kidney tumours. A rare but remediable cause of serious hypertension. *Lancet* 1971;2:254–255.
8. Eddy RL, Sanchez SA. Renin-secreting renal neoplasm and hypertension with hypokalemia. *Ann Intern Med* 1971;75:725–729.
9. Bonnin JM, Hodge RL, Lumbers ER. A renin-secreting renal tumour associated with hypertension. *Aust NZ J Med* 1972;2:178–181.
10. Brown JJ, Fraser R, Lever AF, Morton JJJ, Robertson JIS, Tree M, Bell PRF, Davidson JK, Ruthven IS. Hypertension and secondary hyperaldosteronism associated with a renin-secreting renal juxtaglomerular cell tumour. *Lancet* 1973;2:1228–1231.
11. Shambellan M, Howes EL, Stockgit JR, Noakes CA, Biglieri EG. Role of renin and aldosterone in hypertension due to a renin secreting tumor. *Am J Med* 1973;55:86–92.
12. Hirose M, Arakawa K, Kikuchi M, Kawasaki T, Omoto T, Kato H, Nagayama T. Primary reninism with renal hamartomatous alteration. *JAMA* 1974;230:1288–1292.
13. Guerardi JG, Arya S, Hickler RB. Juxtaglomerular body tumor: a rare occult but curable cause of lethal hypertension. *Hum Pathol* 1974;5:236–240.
14. Orjavik OS, Aas M, Fauchald P, Hovig T, Oystese B, Brodwall EK, Flatmark A. Renin secreting renal tumour with severe hypertension. Case report with tumour renin analysis, histopathological and ultrastructural studies. *Acta Med Scand* 1975;197:329–335.
15. Bonnin JM, Cain MD, Jose JS, Mukherjee TT, Perret LV, Scropp GC, Seymour AE. Hypertension due to a renin-secreting tumour localised by segmental renal vein sampling. *Aust NZ J Med* 1977;7:630–636.
16. Mimran A, Leckie BJ, Fourcade JC, Barlet P, Navratil H, Barjon E. Blood pressure, renin–angiotensin system and urinary kallikrein in a case of juxtaglomerular cell tumor. *Am J Med* 1978;65:527–536.
17. Warshaw BL, Anand SK, Olson DL, Grushkin CM, Heuser ET, Lieberman E. Hypertension secondary to a renin-producing juxtaglomerular cell tumor. *J Pediatr* 1979;94:247–250.
18. Hanna W, Tepperman B, Logan AG, Robinette MA, Colapinto R, Philips MJ. Juxtaglomerular cell tumour (reninoma) with paroxysmal hypertension. *Can Med Assoc J* 1979;120:957–959.
19. El Matri A, Slim R, Hamida CH, Chadli A, Ben Maiz H, Haddad S, Milliez P, Camilleri JP, Zmerli S, Ben Ayed H. Hypertension artérielle secondaire à une tumeur à rénine. Une observation. *Nouv Presse Med* 1980;9:157–159.
20. Valdes G, Lopez JM, Martinez P, Rosenberg H, Barriga P, Rodriguez JA, Otipka N. Renin-secreting tumor. Case report. *Hypertension* 1980;2:714–718.
21. Moss AH, Peterson LJ, Scott WC, Winter K, Olin DB, Garber RL. Delayed diagnosis of juxtaglomerular cell tumor hypertension. *NC Med J* 1982;43:705–707.
22. Furusato M, Hayashi H, Kawaguchi N, Yokota K, Saito K, Aizawa S, Ishikawa E. Juxtaglomerular cell tumor. *Acta Pathol Jpn* 1983;33:609–618.
23. Tetu B, Totovic V, Bechtelsheimer H, Smerid J. Tumeur rénale à sécrétion de rénine. *Ann Pathol* 1984;4:55–59.
24. Squirres JP, Ulbright TM, Deschryver-Kreeskmeti K, Engleman W. Juxtaglomerular cell tumor of the kidney. *Cancer* 1984;53:516–523.
25. Dennis RT, MacDougal WS, Glick AD, MacDonnell RC. Juxtaglomerular cell tumor of the kidney. *J Urol* 1985;134:334–338.
26. Brand G, Vandongen R, Berlin LJ, Matz L. Juxtaglomerular tumour: diagnostic renal vein renin measurements obscured by chronic captopril therapy. *Aust NZ J Med* 1985;15:755–757.
27. Hermus ARMM, Pieters GFFM, Lamers APM, Sinals AGH, Hanselaar AGJM, Van Haelst UJG, Kloppenborg PWC. Hypertension and hypokaliemia due to a renin secreting kidney tumour. *Neth J Med* 1986;29:84–91.
28. Handa N, Fukunaga R, Yoneda S, Kimura K, Kamada T, Ichikawa Y, Takaha M, Sonoda T, Tokunaga K, Kuroda C, Onishi S. State of systemic hemodynamics in a case of juxtaglomerular cell tumor. *Clin Exp Hypertens [A]* 1986;8:1–19.
29. Ménard J, Soubrier F, Bariety J, Camilleri JP, Corvol P. Primary reninism. In: Genest J, ed. *Hypertension.* New York: McGraw-Hill, 1983;1034–1040.
30. Thibonnier M, Aldigier JC, Soto ME, Sassano P, Menard J, Corvol P. Abnormalities and drug-induced alterations of vasopressin in human hypertension. *Clin Sci* 1981;61:149s–151s.
31. Pinet F, Mizrahi J, Laboulandine I, Menard J, Corvol P. Regulation of prorenin secretion in cultured human transfected juxtaglomerular cells. *J Clin Invest* 1987;80:724–731.
32. Barajas L, Bennett CM, Connor G, Lindstrom RR. Structure of a juxtaglomerular cell tumor: the presence of a neural component. A light and electron microscopic study. *Lab Invest* 1977;37:357–368.
33. Camilleri JP, Hinglais N, Bruneval P, Bariety J, Tricottet V, Rouchon M, Mancilla-Jimenez R, Corvol P, Menard J. Renin storage and cell differentiation in juxtaglomerular cell tumors: study of three cases. *Hum Pathol* 1984;15:1069–1079.
34. Lindop GBM, Stewart JA, Moronie TT. The immunocytochemical demonstration of renin in a juxtaglomerular cell tumour by light and electron microscopy. *Histopathology* 1983;7:421–431.
35. Bruneval P, Fournier JG, Soubrier F, Belair MF, DaSilva JL, Guettier C, Pinet F, Tardivel F, Corvol P, Bariety J, Camilleri JP. Detection and localization of renin messenger RNA in human pathological tissues using *in situ* hybridization. *Am J Pathol* 1988;131:320–330.
36. Pinet F, Corvol MT, Dench F, Bourguignon J, Feunten J, Menard J, Corvol P. Isolation of renin-producing cells by transfection with three simian virus 40 mutants. *Proc Natl Acad Sci USA* 1985;82:8503–8507.
37. Taugner R, Hackenthal E, Rix E, Nobiling R, Poulsen K. Immunocytochemistry of the renin–angiotensin system: renin, angiotensinogen, angiotensin I, angiotensin II and converting enzyme in the kidneys of mice, rats and tree shrews. *Kidney Int* 1982;22(Suppl 12):S33–S43.
38. Morris BJ, Pinet F, Michel JB, Soubrier F, Corvol P. Renin secretion from a malignant pulmonary metastatic tumour cells of vascular origin. *Clin Exp Pharmacol Physiol* 1987;14:227–231.
39. Mitchell JD, Baxter TJ, Blair-West JR, McCredie DA. Renin levels in nephroblastoma (Wilms' tumour). Report of a renin secreting tumour. *Arch Dis Child* 1970;45:376–384.
40. Day RP, Luetscher JA. Big renin, a possible prohormone in kidney and plasma of a patient with Wilms' tumour. *J Clin Endocrinol Metab* 1974;38:923–926.
41. Sheth KJ, Tang TT, Blaedel ME, Good TA. Polydipsia, polyuria and hypertension associated with renin-secreting Wilms' tumour. *J Pediatr* 1978;92:921–924.
42. Luciani JC, Baldet P, Dumas R, Jean R. Etude du système rénine–angiotensine dans deux cas de tumeur de Wilms avec hypertension sévère. *Arch Fr Pediatr* 1979;36:240–249.
43. Spahr J, Demers LM, Shochat SJ. Renin producing Wilms' tumor. *J Pediatr Surg* 1981;16:32–34.

44. Hollifield JW, Page DL, Smith C, Michelakis AM, Staab E, Rhamy R. Renin-secreting clear cell carcinoma of the kidney. *Arch Intern Med* 1975;135:859–864.
45. Lebel M, Talbot J, Grose J, Morin J. Adenocarcinoma of the kidney and hypertension: report of 2 cases with special emphasis on renin. *J Urol* 1977;118:923–927.
46. Leckie BJ, Brown JJ, Frarer R, Kyle K, Lever AF, Morton JJ, Robertson JIS. A renal carcinoma secreting inactive renin. *Clin Sci Mol Med* 1978;55:159s–161s.
47. Lindop GM, Millan DWM, Murray D, Gibson AAM, McIntyre GD, Leckie BJ. Immunocytochemistry of renin in renal tumors. *Clin Exp Hypertens [A]* 1987;9:1305–1323.
48. Leckie BJ, McIntyre GD, Millan WD, Lindop GBM, Carachi R. Renin and inactive renin (prorenin) in the plasma of patients with malignant renal tumors. *Clin Exp Hypertens [A]* 1987;9:1325–1332.
49. Hauger-Klevene JH. High plasma renin activity in an oat cell carcinoma: a renin secreting carcinoma. *Cancer* 1970;26:1112–1114.
50. Genest J, Rojo-Ortega JM, Kuchel O, Boucher R, Nowaczinski W, Lefebvre R, Chretien M, Cantin J, Granger P. Malignant hypertension associated with hypokalemia in a patient with renin-producing pulmonary carcinoma. *Trans Assoc Am Phys* 1975;88:192–200.
51. Aurell M, Rudin A, Tisell LE, Kindblom LG, Sandberg G. Captopril effect on hypertension in patient with renin producing tumour. *Lancet* 1979;2:149–150.
52. Corvol P. Tumor-dependent hypertension. *Hypertension* 1984;6:593–596.
53. Cox JN, Pannier L, Vallotton MB, Humbert JR, Rohner A. Epithelial liver hamartoma, systemic arterial hypertension and renin hypersecretion. *Virchows Arch [A]* 1975;336:15–26.
54. Yokozama H, Yarmane Y, Takahara J, Yoschinouchi T, Ofuji T. A case of ectopic renin secreting orbital hemangiopericytoma associated with juvenile hypertension and hypokalemia. *Acta Med Okayama* 1979;33:315–322.
55. Ruddy MC, Atlas SA, Salerno FG. Hypertension association with a renin-secreting adenocarcinoma of the pancreas. *N Engl J Med* 1982;307:993–997.
56. Fernandez LA, Olsen GT, Barwick KW, Sanders M, Kaliszewski C, Inagami T. Renin in angiolymphoid hyperplasia with eosinophilia. *Arch Pathol Lab Med* 1986;110:1131–1135.
57. Galen FX, Devaux C, Guyenne TT, Menard J, Corvol P. Multiple forms of human renin. Purification and characterization. *J Biol Chem* 1979;254:4848–4855.
58. Galen FX, Devaux C, Atlas S, Guyene TT, Menard J, Corvol P, Simon D, Cazaubon C, Richer P, Badouaille C, Richaud JP, Gros P, Pau B. New monoclonal antibodies directed against human renin. *J Clin Invest* 1984;74:723–735.
59. Guyene TT, Galen FX, Devaux C, Corvol P, Menard J. Direct radioimmunoassay of human renin. Comparison with renin activity in plasma and amniotic fluid. *Hypertension* 1980;2:465–470.
60. Simon D, Badouaille G, Pau B, Guyene TT, Corvol P, Menard J. Measurement of active renin by the 4G1 anti-human renin monoclonal antibody. *Clin Exp Hypertens [A]* 1987;9:1333–1340.
61. Camilleri JP, Phat VN, Bariety J, Corvol P, Menard J. Use of a specific antiserum for renin detection in human kidney. *J Histochem Cytochem* 1980;28:1343–1346.
62. Michel JB, Wood J, Hofbauer K, Corvol P, Menard J. Blood pressure effects of renin inhibition by human renin antiserum in normotensive marmosets. *Am J Physiol* 1984;246:F309–F316.
63. Soubrier F, Devaux C, Galen FX, Skinner SL, Aurell M, Genest J, Ménard J, Corvol P. Biochemical and immunological characterization of ectopic tumoral renin. *J Clin Endocrinol Metab* 1982;54:139–144.
64. Atlas SA, Sealey JE, Hesson TE, Kaplan AP, Menard J, Corvol P, Laragh JH. Biochemical similarity of partially purified inactive renins from human plasma and kidney. *Hypertension* 1982;4 (Suppl II):II-86–II-95.
65. Leckie BJ, McGhee NK, Lever AF, Robertson JIS. The action of trypsin, glandular kallikrein and plasmin on inactive renin from a human renal tumour. In: Shambi MP, ed. *Heterogeneity of renin and renin substrate.* Amsterdam: Elsevier/North Holland, 1981;159–174.
66. Steiner DF, Cunningham D, Spigelman L, Aten B. Insulin biosynthesis: evidence for a precursor. *Science* 1967;157:697–700.
67. Galen FX, Devaux C, Houot AM, Menard J, Corvol P, Corvol MT, Gubler MC, Mounier F, Camilleri JP. Renin biosynthesis by human juxtaglomerular cells. Evidence for a renin precursor. *J Clin Invest* 1984;73:1144–1155.
68. Pratt RE, Carleton JE, Richie JP, Heusser C, Dzau VJ. Human renin biosynthesis and secretion in normal and ischemic kidneys. *Proc Natl Acad Sci* 1987;84:7837–7840.
69. Imai T, Miyazaki H, Hirose S, Hori H, Hayashi T, Kageyama R, Ohkubo H, Nakanishi S, Murakami K. Cloning and sequence analysis of cDNA for human renin precursor. *Proc Natl Acad Sci USA* 1983;80:7405–7409.
70. Panthier JJ, Foote S, Chambraud B, Strosberg AD, Corvol P, Rougeon F. Complete amino acid sequence and maturation of the mouse submaxillary gland renin precursor. *Nature* 1982;298:90–92.
71. Hirose S, Kim SJ, Miyazaki H, Park YS, Murakami K. *In vitro* biosynthesis of human renin and identification of plasma inactive renin as an activation intermediate. *J Biol Chem* 1985;260:16400–16405.
72. Soubrier F, Panthier JJ, Houot AM, Rougeon F, Corvol P. Segmental homology between the promoter region of the human renin gene and the mouse Ren-1 and Ren-2 promoter region. *Gene* 1986;41:85–92.

Hypertension: Pathophysiology, Diagnosis, and Management, edited by J. H. Laragh and B. M. Brenner. Raven Press, Ltd., New York © 1990.

CHAPTER 98

Hypertension in Renal Parenchymal Disease

Michael C. Smith and Michael J. Dunn

Unilateral Renal Disease, 1583
Renin-Secreting Tumors, 1583
Hydronephrosis, 1584
Unilateral Renal Parenchymal Disease, 1584
Miscellaneous Lesions, 1584
Bilateral Renal Parenchymal Disease, 1585
Pathophysiology, 1585
The Effect of Systemic Hypertension on Renal Function, 1588
Clinical Therapy, 1589
Hypertension After Renal Transplantation, 1591
Pathophysiology, 1591
Treatment of Post-Transplant Hypertension, 1593
References, 1595

The kidney plays a central, and perhaps dominant, role in the regulation of arterial blood pressure. Various hormones, autacoids, and divalent cations directly regulate the renal excretion of sodium chloride or indirectly influence salt balance by altering intrarenal hemodynamics (1–3). Moreover, significant decrements in functional renal mass not only can initiate and sustain hypertension (4) but also can subject the remaining renal parenchyma to the adverse hemodynamic consequences of elevated systemic pressure (5). It is not surprising, then, that renal parenchymal disease is the most common cause of secondary hypertension.

In this chapter we will discuss the pathophysiology, clinical features, and treatment of hypertension due to both unilateral and bilateral renal parenchymal disease. This will not be an exhaustive review but will emphasize key advances within the last decade and integrate them into a cohesive approach to the management of renal parenchymal hypertension.

UNILATERAL RENAL DISEASE

Renin-Secreting Tumors

Since Robertson's initial report (6), approximately 40 cases of primary hyperreninism due to benign juxtaglomerular (JG) cell tumors have been described in the literature (7–10). These tumors are important. Not only do they represent an eminently curable form of hypertension, but also they prove that hypersecretion of renin, independent of renal vascular disease, can cause sustained high blood pressure. Renin-secreting JG cell tumors occur predominantly in the second or third decade of life and result in (a) moderate to severe hypertension, (b) hypokalemia, (c) increased peripheral plasma renin activity (PRA), and (d) hyperaldosteronism. In patients with typical clinical characteristics, renal artery stenosis or renal infarction should be excluded by angiography. Although angiography can often detect a suspicious lesion, computerized axial tomography is the more sensitive diagnostic test for exact localization of the tumor (10).

Renin secretion is autonomous in some JG cell tumors, whereas in others it is responsive to postural changes and alteration in sodium balance (7,10). Similar to renovascular hypertension, lateralizing renal-vein renins are found in many, but not all, patients with renin-secreting JG cell tumors. Histologic examination of these tumors shows light- and electron-microscopic characteristics typical of JG cells. Recent studies utilizing primary cell cultures have demonstrated that these tumors secrete both renin and prorenin but lack angiotensin-converting enzyme (ACE) and the ability to synthesize angiotensinogen (10). Surgical management is preferable to medical therapy because blood pressure control with antihypertensive agents other than ACE inhibitors is problematic. Moreover, medical therapy implies long-term pharmacologic treatment in young patients. Local excision or unilateral nephrectomy, whether or not ipsilateral renal-vein renin concentration is increased, promptly reduces blood pressure and peripheral PRA.

Hypertension has frequently been described in association with Wilms' tumor (11,12). In some cases the increased arterial pressure is due to renin secretion consequent to compression of normal renal parenchyma or vasculature by the tumor. However, other Wilms' tumors actively synthesize and secrete renin. In either case, blood pressure and PRA normalize following resection of the tumor.

Hydronephrosis

Experimental and clinical studies suggest that acute unilateral ureteral obstruction is associated with the development of hypertension (13–18). Vaughn et al. demonstrated that acute ureteral occlusion in dogs resulted in hypertension that was temporally related to an increase in peripheral PRA. With chronic obstruction, however, both blood pressure and PRA returned to basal levels (13,14). Isolated case reports and small series similarly support the concept that, in humans, acute unilateral ureteral occlusion causes a hyperreninemic form of hypertension. Several investigators have documented elevated peripheral PRA and lateralizing renal-vein renins in patients with hypertension and unilateral hydronephrosis (15–20). Relief of the ureteral obstruction simultaneously normalized both blood pressure and PRA. Klein et al. have provided the most persuasive evidence regarding the etiologic role of the renin–angiotensin system in the hypertension associated with unilateral obstruction (18). They measured systemic blood pressure, renal-vein renin activity, and renal pelvis pressure in a patient with traumatic ureteral occlusion and hypertension. Increases in renal pelvis pressure above 50 mmHg resulted in systemic hypertension and an increase in ipsilateral renal-vein renin, whereas ureteral decompression normalized all three parameters. Not all patients with unilateral hydronephrosis and hypertension, however, have increased peripheral PRA and enhanced renin release from the obstructed kidney. In this regard, some workers (17) have found renal-vein renin ratios of the hydronephrotic/contralateral kidney $\geq$ 1.5 highly predictive of a favorable blood pressure response to surgical intervention. In contrast, others have found this test to lack sensitivity and specificity (21).

Recently, two large-scale studies have examined the prevalence of hypertension in patients with unilateral hydronephrosis (21,22). Wanner et al. (21) found that 20% of 101 consecutive patients with unilateral hydronephrosis were hypertensive, whereas the prevalence of hypertension in a control population was 23%. Similarly, Clark and Malek (22) found that only 10 of 110 patients with congenital ureteropelvic junction obstruction were hypertensive. Interestingly, over 80% of hypertensive subjects were cured or improved following surgical intervention in the former study (21), whereas only 20% became normotensive in the latter (22). The reason for these discrepant results is unclear but may reflect differences in (a) duration of obstruction, (b) etiology, or (c) other unknown factors. Thus, even though acute ureteral occlusion can cause experimental and clinical hypertension primarily, if not exclusively, mediated by the renin–angiotensin system, it is an uncommon cause of secondary hypertension. The coexistence of hypertension and unilateral hydronephrosis frequently represents two diseases, namely, essential hypertension and ureteral obstruction. Decisions regarding surgical intervention should be based primarily on preservation of renal function as a result of relief from the obstruction and not cure of hypertension. Nevertheless, if surgery is contemplated for control of blood pressure, lateralizing renal-vein renin ratios are highly predictive of an excellent response; nonlateralizing values, however, do not preclude cure or improvement in blood pressure.

Unilateral Renal Parenchymal Disease

The link between unilateral renal disease and hypertension was first described over 50 years ago (23), but the precise incidence of this form of secondary hypertension still remains unknown (24). Early enthusiasm for unilateral nephrectomy in patients with hypertension and unilateral renal parenchymal disease was tempered by a disappointing cure rate of only 26% (25). However, a large body of recent data suggests that an identifiable subset of patients clearly benefits from operative intervention. Initial work suggested that patients whose hypertension would respond favorably to nephrectomy could be distinguished from unresponsive subjects by split renal function studies or clinical characteristics (25,26). Renal-vein renin ratios, however, have proved more reliable in separating responders from nonresponders. Vaughn et al. (27) found that 13% of patients with hypertension and unilateral renal parenchymal disease had increased peripheral PRA, whereas 30% demonstrated evidence of unilateral hypersecretion of renin. Furthermore, other investigators demonstrated cure or improvement of hypertension in 90% of patients with lateralizing renal-vein renin ratios $\geq$ 1.5 (28,29). Finally, Gordon et al. studied 20 patients with hypertension and unilateral renal disease, measured recumbent and stimulated renal-vein renin ratios, and subjected all patients to nephrectomy irrespective of the renin values (30). The results of this small but important study suggest that recumbent lateralizing renal-vein renin ratios $\geq$ 1.5 identify those patients with hypertension and unilateral renal disease who are likely to benefit from nephrectomy with a sensitivity of 100%, a specificity of 84%, and a positive predictive value of 100%. Therefore, it is reasonable to restrict surgical intervention or renal arterial embolization to patients with unilateral renal parenchymal involvement and hypertension who demonstrate lateralizing renal-vein renin ratios. Patients with apparent unilateral renal disease and nonlateralizing renins probably represent subjects with essential hypertension or occult bilateral renal involvement.

Miscellaneous Lesions

Renal tuberculosis (31), intrarenal cysts (32), segmental hypoplasia of the kidneys (33,34), renal arteriovenous fistulae (35), unilateral reflux nephropathy (36), and renal infarction (37) have all been linked to the development of hypertension. In some instances (31,32,34,37), unilateral hypersecretion of renin has been documented and hypertension has resolved following surgical intervention. In other cases, nonlateralizing renal-vein renins ratios have provided little support for a primary role of the renin–angiotensin system in the genesis of hypertension (33,35,36).

BILATERAL RENAL PARENCHYMAL DISEASE

Hypertension occurs frequently in both acute and chronic renal parenchymal disease. In the former it is primarily volume-mediated, responsive to salt removal, and transient, whereas in the latter the pathogenesis is complex and the long-term sequelae are more problematic. Therefore, the following discussion will address exclusively the pathophysiology, consequences, and management of hypertension due to chronic renal disease.

Chronic renal parenchymal disease is the most common cause of secondary hypertension and accounts for 5% of all patients with high blood pressure (38). Hypertension often occurs with modest reductions of glomerular filtration rate (GFR) (i.e., even with normal serum creatinine concentrations) and increases in frequency as renal function declines (39–41). By the time end-stage renal disease (ESRD) develops, the prevalence of hypertension approaches 75–80% (42). Even among patients with chronic renal parenchymal disease, the frequency of hypertension varies. Elevated blood pressure is more frequent in patients with chronic glomerulonephritis than in subjects with polycystic kidney disease or chronic interstitial nephritis (40,43). Moreover, among patients with chronic glomerulonephritis, the prevalence of hypertension differs according to the histologic lesion. Patients with focal glomerulosclerosis and membranoproliferative glomerulonephritis have the highest prevalence of hypertension, whereas those with minimal change disease and IgA nephropathy have the lowest. Table 1 depicts the approximate frequency of hypertension in different renal parenchymal diseases. These data are summarized from several series in the literature (39–41), but they coincide with estimates based on our own clinical experience.

Pathophysiology

It is conceptually convenient to regard hypertension in patients with renal parenchymal disease as a spectrum with volume-mediated hypertension at one end and vasoconstrictor-related hypertension at the other. Clearly, there are isolated examples of each; however, most hypertensive patients reflect a combination of both volume and vasoconstrictor elements. Furthermore, at any point in time, arterial blood pressure represents the interactions of multiple factors (Table 2) that influence cardiac output or total peripheral resistance (TPR), or both. Although all of these factors have been implicated in the hypertension of renal disease, we will discuss only those for which there is substantial support. It is important to realize that the relative contribution of each of these elements to the development of hypertension probably varies depending on the underlying disease, dietary salt intake, and genetic predisposition to hypertension. For the sake of clarity we will discuss each separately.

TABLE 1. *Prevalence of hypertension in renal parenchymal disease*[a]

Disease	Percent of patients with hypertension
Glomerular disease	
Focal glomerulosclerosis	75–80
Membranoproliferative glomerulonephritis	65–70
Diabetic nephropathy	65–70
Membranous nephropathy	40–50
Mesangioproliferative glomerulonephritis	35–40
IgA nephropathy	30
Minimal change disease	15–20
Polycystic kidney disease	50–60
Chronic interstitial nephritis	30

[a] Based on estimates from references 39–41.

TABLE 2. *Factors that influence regulation of arterial blood pressure*

Cardiac output	TPR
Extracellular fluid volume–salt	Pressors
Angiotensin II	Angiotensin II
Aldosterone	Norepinephrine
Norepinephrine	Vasopressin
Atrial natriuretic peptides	Intracellular calcium
Glomerular filtration rate	Depressors
Sympathetic nervous system	PGE_2, PGI_2
Baroreceptor sensitivity	Kinins
	Atrial natriuretic peptides

Salt Balance

Several lines of evidence strongly suggest that salt balance is important in the genesis of human renal parenchymal hypertension. Patients with mild to moderate renal insufficiency demonstrate increased total exchangeable sodium compared to patients with essential hypertension or normotensive controls (44,45). Although early in the course of chronic renal disease the plasma and extracellular fluid volumes are generally normal (46,47), most (48,49), but not all (50), investigators have found expanded blood or extracellular fluid volumes in patients with ESRD. In addition, the preferential distribution of ingested salt to the intravascular volume rather than to the interstitial space in ESRD may further aggravate hypertension (51). Finally, arterial blood pressure directly correlates with both plasma volume and exchangeable sodium in mild to moderate renal insufficiency (47,52) and with exchangeable sodium and extracellular fluid volume in ESRD (48,53,54).

Consequently, alterations in salt balance exert a major influence on blood pressure in most patients with chronic renal insufficiency. Koomans et al. studied the relation between increased salt intake and changes in extracellular fluid volume and blood pressure in two groups of patients with chronic renal disease (54). In one group the creatinine clearance was less than 22 ml/min, whereas in the other it was greater than 32 ml/min. Increased dietary salt expanded the extracellular volume and increased arterial pressure in both groups; however, the increment in blood pressure was greater for any given increase in extracellular volume in the patients with more severe renal insufficiency. Conversely, restriction of dietary salt decreases exchangeable sodium, plasma volume, extracellular fluid volume, and blood pressure in hypertensive patients with chronic renal failure (55,56). The fact that salt subtraction by hemodialysis normalizes blood pressure in the majority of patients with ESRD, without requirement for pharmacologic therapy, provides further support for the importance of salt in the hypertension of renal parenchymal disease (57). Not all investigators, however, have concluded that salt balance is directly related to blood pressure in chronic renal disease. Some have found no correlation between plasma, blood, or extracellular fluid volume and arterial pressure (50), whereas others have shown a relation between salt and blood pressure only in renoprival hypertension (58). Nevertheless, the bulk of evidence strongly implicates salt as a central contributing factor in renal parenchymal hypertension. Positive salt balance expands the extracellular fluid volume and causes hypertension by increasing cardiac output or TPR, or both (see section entitled "Hemodynamic Patterns").

Neurogenic Factors

Neurogenic factors, particularly the sympathetic nervous system, contribute importantly to the regulation of blood pressure. Activation of the sympathetic nervous system directly increases cardiac output and TPR and indirectly increases vascular resistance by β-adrenergic-mediated stimulation of the renin–angiotensin system (59–61). Angiotensin II, in turn, reciprocally increases central and peripheral sympathetic activity (60). Finally, stimulation of the renal nerves directly increases reabsorption of sodium in the proximal tubule. Thus, there are several potential mechanisms by which increased sympathetic outflow could cause hypertension in patients with renal disease.

Plasma norepinephrine (NE) and PRA are increased in hypertensive patients with mild renal insufficiency as compared to normal controls or normotensive subjects with similar renal dysfunction (62,63). In one study, blood pressure correlated directly with plasma NE levels and inversely with estimates of renal blood flow (63). Moreover, Beretta-Piccoli et al. (64) demonstrated a decreased threshold for the pressor response to an infusion of NE in both normotensive and hypertensive patients with mild renal parenchymal disease. In patients with ESRD, plasma concentrations of NE are normal (65) or increased (66). Schohn et al. administered debrisoquin, a postganglionic sympathetic blocker, to hypertensive and normotensive patients on long-term dialysis and to normal subjects (65). Debrisoquin significantly decreased blood pressure in the hypertensive patients but not in the latter two groups. These investigators concluded that hypertension in ESRD is dependent not only on salt balance and the renin–angiotensin system but also on NE.

Hence, in mild to moderate renal insufficiency, both the circulating concentrations of NE and the vascular reactivity to exogenous NE are increased. Overactivity of the sympathetic nervous system contributes to hypertension by increasing TPR, stimulating PRA, and enhancing sodium reabsorption. In ESRD, despite the development of autonomic insufficiency (62), normal or increased plasma levels of NE are important in supporting arterial pressure in hypertensive patients.

Pressor Compounds

Several vasoconstrictors, including vasopressin and endogenous opiates, have been investigated with regard to their role in the control of blood pressure (67–70). However, there are few data to implicate these compounds in the control of arterial pressure under physiologic, let alone pathologic, circumstances. On the other hand, there is substantial evidence linking the renin–angiotensin–aldosterone system to the hypertension of renal parenchymal disease (71).

In hypertensive patients with mild to moderate renal insufficiency, PRA (62,63) and angiotensin II concentrations are increased (72) and correlate with arterial blood pressure. Exogenous NE increases vascular reactivity, but infusions of angiotensin II do not (64). Nevertheless, Wong et al. administered saralasin to hypertensive patients with early renal disease and noted a significant decrease in blood pressure that was proportional to basal PRA (73). Taken together, these data suggest that the renin–angiotensin system is etiologically involved in the hypertension of mild to moderate renal disease.

The majority of hypertensive patients with ESRD are salt sensitive and achieve adequate blood pressure control with attainment of dry weight during dialysis (74). In these patients, PRA and angiotensin II levels are within the normal range but are inappropriately elevated in relation to exchangeable sodium (75). However, 10–20% of patients on long-term dialysis clearly have a renin-dependent form of hypertension. Many (74,76), but not all, investigators (77) have found increased peripheral PRA in hypertensive patients with ESRD whose blood pressure does not respond to salt subtraction. In this subset of patients there is a significant correlation between arterial pressure and PRA (58,78). Before the advent of minoxidil and ACE inhibitors, binephrectomy, which normalized PRA and blood pressure, was often required to control hypertension (74,76,78). Lifschitz et al. showed that patients whose blood pressure normalized after binephrectomy demonstrated a sharp decline in blood pressure with saralasin administration and markedly increased PRA preoperatively (79). Predictably, administration of ACE inhibitors also normalizes arterial pressure in patients with dialysis-resistant hypertension and increased PRA (80,81).

Thus, there is persuasive evidence strongly linking the renin–angiotensin–aldosterone system to hypertension in renal parenchymal disease. In early renal insufficiency, this system exerts its hypertensive effect by directly increasing TPR and limiting renal excretion of salt. On the other hand, in ESRD the vasoconstrictor action of angiotensin II predominates, and hormonally mediated changes in sodium balance are less important. It should not be concluded, however, that alterations in volume or renin are exclusively responsible for hypertension in renal disease. Several investigators have found no correlation between blood pressure and either PRA or extracellular fluid volume and have correctly suggested that other factors must be implicated (50,77).

Depressor Compounds

The kidney is not only a source of prohypertensive compounds but is also a source of potentially antihypertensive substances. Renal prostaglandins (PGs), kallikrein, and vasodepressor medullary lipids, by virtue of their potentially important effects on salt excretion and renal vascular resistance (3,82,83), could be etiologically related to the development of hypertension in patients with renal parenchymal disease. Muirhead has extensively investigated the antihypertensive properties of nonprostaglandin renomedullary lipids (82,84). However, although renal medullary transplants reduce blood pressure in some forms of experimental hypertension (84), and, in rats, chemical renal medullectomy results in systemic hypertension (83), the precise role of these lipids in human renal parenchymal hypertension is unknown.

Levy et al. have shown that urinary kallikrein activity correlates directly with renal blood flow in patients with essential hypertension (85) and that whites with renal parenchymal hypertension have reduced urinary kallikrein excretion (86). In addition, plasma kininogen concentration is decreased in patients with malignant hypertension and moderate renal insufficiency as compared to subjects with essential hypertension or to normotensive individuals (87). Interestingly, these values do not normalize despite 3 months of adequate blood pressure control. Even though prolonged intrarenal infusion of bradykinin has no effect on long-term control of blood pressure in dogs (88), these data still suggest that, in humans, decreased activity of the kallikrein–kinin system could be causally related to the hypertension of renal disease.

Renal synthesis of PGE_2 is decreased in approximately one-third of patients with essential hypertension (89). In hypertensive patients with renal parenchymal disease, however, urinary excretion of PGE_2 is normal (90) or elevated (91) and increases with salt loading (92). Further, Niwa et al. found increased urinary excretion of both vasodilator and natriuretic PGs (PGE_2, PGI_2) and vasoconstrictor and antinatriuretic PGs ($PGF_2\alpha$, TXA_2) in patients with severe renal dysfunction (91). Thus, most studies have been unable to clearly demonstrate a decrease in renal PG production in hypertensive patients with renal insufficiency. Rather, it is more likely that normal or enhanced PG synthesis attenuates the vasoconstrictor and hypertensive effects of angiotensin II, NE, and other pressor compounds. In this regard, administration of nonsteroidal anti-inflammatory drugs (NSAID) to hypertensive patients with renal parenchymal disease often increases blood pressure and decreases GFR concomitant with a reduction in urinary PG excretion (89).

Atrial natriuretic peptide (ANP) has multiple effects on renal function, vascular tone, and hormone secretion. Numerous studies have shown that ANP increases urinary sodium excretion, relaxes vascular smooth muscle, and inhibits the release of renin, aldosterone, and AVP (93). Several investigators have measured ANP concentrations in hypertensive patients with renal disease and have reached similar conclusions. Plasma ANP levels are elevated in mild to moderate renal insufficiency (94) and in ESRD (95,96). In the latter group, ANP levels increase appropriately with volume expansion and decrease with volume contraction. Moreover, infusion of synthetic human ANP decreases blood pressure in a dose-related fashion (94). Therefore it is probable that, like the PGs, ANP modulates the vasoconstrictor action of pressor hormones in patients with renal disease, and it is also probable that reduced ANP production is not etiologically related to renal parenchymal hypertension.

Hemodynamic Patterns

Salt retention with extracellular fluid volume expansion, increased activity of the sympathetic nervous system, elevated concentrations of pressor hormones, or decreased production of vasodilator substances ultimately cause hypertension by increasing cardiac output or elevating TPR, or both. Cross-sectional studies in patients with early-stage (97–99) and late-stage (100,101) renal disease have demonstrated that hypertension is maintained primarily by an increased TPR. Valvo et al. found both increased blood volumes and elevated TPR in hypertensive patients with polycystic kidney disease or IgA nephropathy compared to normotensive patients with renal disease or compared to control subjects (98,99). Despite the significant increase in blood volume, however, cardiac index was normal and the increased arterial pressure was attributed to an elevated vascular resistance. Other investigators have reached similar conclusions in patients with ESRD. Kim et al. showed that cardiac index was similar in hypertensive and normotensive patients on maintenance dialysis but that TPR was significantly increased in the hypertensive group (100). Moreover, binephrectomy or salt removal during dialysis normalized blood pressure and TPR without changing cardiac output (100,101).

Longitudinal studies in patients with mild to moderate renal insufficiency (102,103), combined with hemodynamic measurements taken during volume expansion in subjects with ESRD (104,105), suggest that changes in cardiac output may antedate an increase in TPR or, in some cases, may even maintain hypertension. Brod et al. sequentially measured blood pressure, cardiac output, and TPR in patients with early renal disease over a period of 2–8 years (102,103). Thirty-two patients were initially normotensive but demonstrated an expanded blood volume, an increased cardiac output, and a decreased TPR. Ultimately 11 of the 12 developed hypertension. Patients with mild to moderate hypertension were characterized by an increase in cardiac output and normal vascular resistance, whereas those with more severe hypertension had an increase in TPR. Thus, early in the course of renal parenchymal hypertension, blood pressure is maintained by volume expansion and an increase in cardiac output; in the established phase, however, cardiac output is normal and vascular resistance is increased. Clinical studies utilizing salt loading in anephric patients or subjects with ESRD suggest

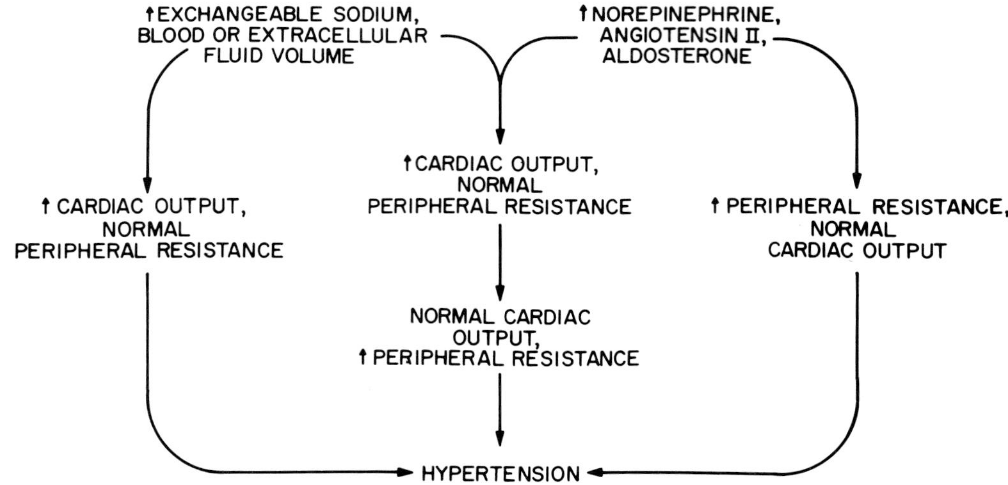

FIG. 1. Mechanisms that initiate hypertension, along with hemodynamic patterns that maintain it, in renal parenchymal disease.

that complex hemodynamic events initiate and sustain renal parenchymal hypertension (104,105). Kim et al. (105) demonstrated four hemodynamic patterns in patients with ESRD after volume expansion: (i) no change in arterial pressure; (ii) hypertension caused by a primary increase in cardiac output; (iii) hypertension consequent to a primary increase in TPR; and (iv) hypertension initiated by an increase in cardiac output but maintained by an elevated TPR.

Consequently, several hemodynamic patterns exist in patients with renal parenchymal hypertension (Fig. 1). According to our current understanding, an increase in total exchangeable sodium, blood volume, or extracellular fluid volume or an abnormal volume–renin relation will initiate a sequence of events resulting in hypertension. In patients with a low PRA or in anephric subjects, hypertension is sustained by an increased cardiac output. When the underlying renal disease is associated with increased levels of vasoconstrictors (e.g., NE, angiotensin II), hypertension is primarily mediated by an increase in TPR. In many instances, however, an elevated cardiac output precedes the rise in TPR that eventually maintains the increase in blood pressure. The latter sequence conforms to the autoregulation theory of arterial pressure control proposed by Guyton and co-workers and by Ledingham (106–108). The mechanism by which an initial increase in cardiac output is translated into increased vascular reactivity is unclear. However, alterations in the electrolyte or divalent cation content of vascular smooth muscle may mediate the increase in TPR (109,110).

The Effect of Systemic Hypertension on Renal Function

The concept that systemic hypertension adversely affects renal function has been recognized for over 40 years (111,112). Renal dysfunction is unusual in benign essential hypertension but progresses more rapidly in hypertensive patients with renal disease. For example, poorly controlled hypertension accelerates the loss of renal function in diabetic nephropathy (113) and contributes to progressive renal insufficiency in other glomerular diseases (114,115). Previously, it was believed that hypertension caused arteriolar nephrosclerosis and ischemic renal injury superimposed on primary renal parenchymal disease. Recently, however, numerous studies have suggested that alternative mechanisms might be responsible for the accelerated decline in kidney function in renal parenchymal hypertension.

Azar et al. were the first to conclusively demonstrate that in some forms of experimental hypertension, systemic increases in hydraulic pressure were transmitted directly to the glomerulus (116,117). They showed, using micropuncture, significantly elevated glomerular capillary pressures in rats with one-kidney post-salt hypertension as compared to normotensive controls. Elevated glomerular capillary pressures (P_{GC}) were associated with (a) decreased afferent arteriolar resistance (R_A), (b) significant increases in transcapillary hydraulic pressure differences, and (c) glomerular, rather than arteriolar, sclerosis (117). Subsequent work confirmed and extended these findings. Olson et al. showed greater glomerular damage in models of experimental hypertension with decreased R_A as compared to models with normal or increased R_A (118). Several lines of evidence suggest that similar pathophysiologic mechanisms are responsible for a progressive decline in GFR when hypertension coexists with renal parenchymal disease. The superimposition of hypertension in experimental, immunologically mediated renal disease increases proteinuria and accelerates glomerular sclerosis (119,120). In addition, nephrotoxic serum nephritis or partial renal ablation in rats impairs renal autoregulation, thus increasing both renal plasma flow and GFR as arterial pressure rises (121,122). Finally, direct measurements of glomerular plasma flow rates and P_{GC} in hypertensive rats subjected to a reduction in renal mass clearly demonstrate that elevated systemic pressure is transmitted to glomerular capillaries because of

(159,186). However, the sensitivity and specificity of converting-enzyme inhibition under these circumstances, either alone or combined with radioisotope renography, remain to be determined. Nevertheless, a significant increase in serum creatinine temporally associated with administration of ACE inhibitors should alert the physician to the possibility of an underlying TRAS.

Chronic Rejection

Repeated acute rejection episodes, culminating in chronic progressive allograft dysfunction, correlate strongly with hypertension in the post-transplant period (156, 157,170). Several investigators have clearly shown a direct correlation between blood pressure and serum creatinine concentration in renal transplant recipients (172,173). In addition, hypertensive transplant recipients have sustained more acute rejection episodes (156) and have higher serum creatinines (170,172) than normotensive transplant recipients. Finally, Bennett et al. obtained renal biopsies in 13 hypertensive transplant recipients; eight of the 13 demonstrated histologic evidence of chronic rejection (171). The mechanism by which chronic rejection results in hypertension is multifactoral and includes many of the same pathogenetic factors which cause hypertension in other forms of renal parenchymal disease. Post-transplant hypertensive patients exhibit significantly reduced renal blood flow with subsequent cortical ischemia as compared to normotensive recipients (167,171). In some studies (171) but not others (167), renin secretion from the allograft was increased. Taken together, these data suggest that chronic rejection causes hypertension by hemodynamic and hormonal factors that limit salt excretion, as well as by direct vasoconstrictor mechanisms.

Treatment of Post-Transplant Hypertension

There is no single orthodox approach to the treatment of the hypertensive transplant recipient. The urgency and mode of therapy depend, in part, upon (a) the tempo and severity of the hypertension, (b) significant co-morbid conditions, and (c) suspected pathophysiologic mechanisms. Nevertheless, general recommendations can be made based on four important considerations: (i) whether or not the patient has "normal" renal function (i.e., serum creatinine less than 2 mg/dl); (ii) the presence of multiple kidneys; (iii) whether or not the patient is receiving cyclosporine; and (iv) whether or not the patient is a candidate for surgery or percutaneous transluminal angioplasty (PTA).

With these principles in mind, our approach to the diagnosis and management of post-transplant hypertension in the patient with normal renal function is shown in Fig. 3. In the hypertensive transplant recipient with multiple kidneys and normal renal function, the diseased kidneys frequently sustain the hypertension (156,164–166,169). If these patients are receiving cyclosporine, a trial of salt depletion is worthwhile. When salt depletion fails or if cyclosporine is not part of the immunosuppressive regimen, we begin an ACE inhibitor or calcium channel blocker because of their efficacy and favorable hemodynamic profile

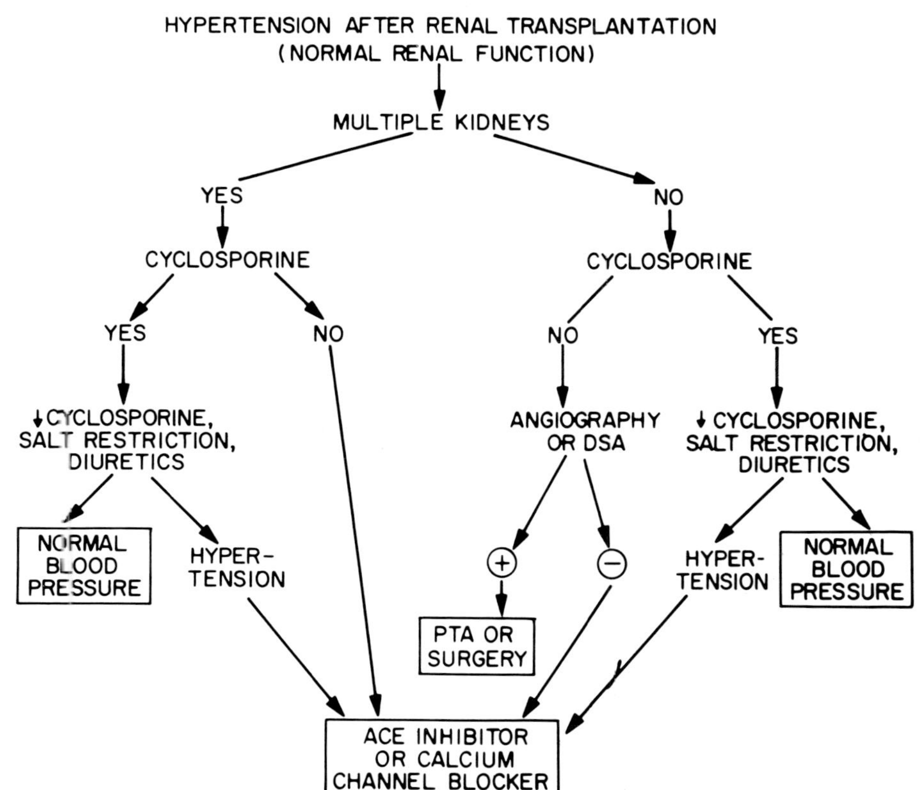

FIG. 3. An approach to the diagnosis and initial management of hypertensive transplant recipients with normal renal function (i.e., serum creatinine less than 2 mg/dl).

(124–126,144). Salt depletion does not usually reduce blood pressure in these patients (166,187), and administration of a converting-enzyme inhibitor can be a provocative test to diagnose unsuspected TRAS (179,186).

In hypertensive patients with a solitary kidney who are treated with cyclosporine, it is reasonable to reduce the dose of cyclosporine if plasma levels are elevated. In the face of normal cyclosporine concentrations, these patients should be treated with dietary salt restriction or with diuretics, or with both. Treatment with diuretics is often effective because cyclosporine-associated hypertension is sensitive to salt depletion (177–179). If salt depletion does not improve arterial pressure, we prefer an ACE inhibitor or calcium channel antagonist. Patients who have a solitary kidney and normal renal function and who are not receiving cyclosporine should be suspected of having TRAS, particularly if they develop accelerated hypertension. We usually proceed to arterial DSA or conventional angiography under these circumstances because the prior probability of TRAS is high. Demonstration of a significant lesion generally warrants consideration of PTA (181,185,188) or surgical revascularization (180,183,184) in a young recipient with severe hypertension. In older subjects or those with less severe hypertension, medical management with careful follow-up may be appropriate because of the possibility of permanent loss of allograft function with surgical intervention. Patients with a normal renal artery should receive pharmacologic therapy.

Chronic rejection must always be suspected of causing hypertension in transplant recipients with abnormal allograft function. Figure 4 outlines our approach to these patients. In hypertensive patients with renal insufficiency and multiple kidneys, the native kidneys may be responsible for both the hypertension and mild impairment of allograft function by virtue of the ability of angiotensin II to increase allograft vascular resistance and decrease GFR (166). In cyclosporine-treated patients, salt depletion or a reduction in the dose of cyclosporine often decreases blood pressure. If this maneuver is unsuccessful or cyclosporine has not been administered, we again treat the patient with a converting-enzyme inhibitor. Normalization of blood pressure, together with a stable or decreased creatinine, implies that the patient's own kidneys were causing the hypertension (159,166). If the serum creatinine increases as the blood pressure normalizes, then the possibility of TRAS should be considered. Identification of a significant arterial stenosis merits consideration of PTA or surgery, whereas a normal angiogram warrants pharmacologic therapy with

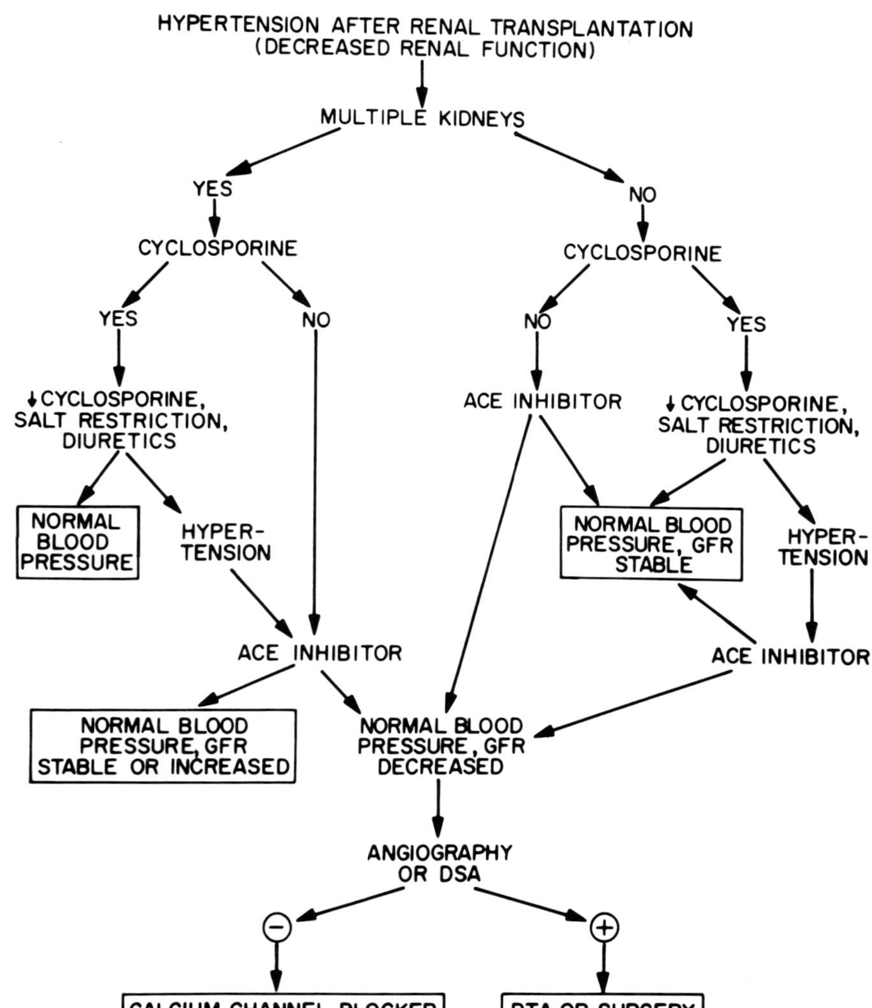

FIG. 4. An approach to the diagnosis and initial management of hypertensive transplant recipients with impaired renal function (i.e., serum creatinine greater than 2 mg/dl).

an alternative antihypertensive agent. In the latter instance, it should be noted that treatment with a converting-enzyme inhibitor has occasionally caused renal failure in patients with chronic rejection (159).

In those with a solitary kidney not receiving cyclosporine, it is reasonable to treat the hypertension with an ACE inhibitor. If blood pressure normalizes without an increase in serum creatinine, no further treatment is required. However, normalization of blood pressure with a concomitant decrease in renal function should prompt an investigation for TRAS. On the other hand, patients who have a solitary kidney and who receive cyclosporine should have the dose decreased if elevated plasma levels are found, or they should be given a trial of salt depletion. If they remain hypertensive, we again favor administration of an ACE inhibitor. Once again, normalization of blood pressure, along with a decrease in GFR, suggests the possibility of TRAS which should be appropriately evaluated.

In any hypertensive allograft recipient with multiple kidneys in whom TRAS has been excluded, consideration should be given to binephrectomy or renal ablation. These approaches normalize blood pressure in appropriately selected patients (164,168). We reserve these procedures, however, for patients requiring multidrug antihypertensive therapy in whom converting-enzyme inhibition has significantly improved blood pressure without reducing GFR.

REFERENCES

1. Guyton AC, Coleman TG, Cowley AW, Scheel KW, Manning RD, Norman RA. Arterial pressure regulation. Overriding dominance of the kidneys in long-term regulation and in hypertension. *Am J Med* 1972;52:584–594.
2. Ferris TF. The kidney and hypertension. *Arch Intern Med* 1982;142:1889–1895.
3. Smith MC, Dunn MJ. Renal kallikrein, kinins and prostaglandins in hypertension. In: Brenner BM, Stein JH, eds. *Contemporary issues in nephrology: hypertension.* New York: Churchill Livingstone, 1981;168–202.
4. Guyton AC. Renal function curve—a key to understanding the pathogenesis of hypertension. *Hypertension* 1987;10:1–6.
5. Klahr S, Schreiner G, Ichikawa I. The progression of renal disease. *N Engl J Med* 1988;318:1657–1666.
6. Robertson PW, Klidjian A, Harding LK, Waeters G, Lee MR, Robb-Smith AHT. Hypertension due to a renin-secreting renal tumour. *Am J Med* 1967;43:963–976.
7. Conn JW, Cohen EL, Lucas CP, et al. Primary reninism. Hypertension, hyperreninemia, and secondary aldosteronism due to renin-producing juxtaglomerular cell tumors. *Arch Intern Med* 1972;130:682–696.
8. Schambelan M, Howes EL, Stockigt JR, Noakes CA, Biglieri EG. Role of renin and aldosterone in hypertension due to a renin-secreting tumor. *Am J Med* 1973;55:86–92.
9. Mimran A, Leckie BJ, Fourcade JC, Baldet P, Navratil H, Barjou P. Blood pressure, renin–angiotensin system and urinary kallikrein in a case of juxtaglomerular cell tumor. *Am J Med* 1978;65:527–536.
10. Corvol P, Pinet F, Galen FX, et al. Seven lessons from seven renin secreting tumors. *Kidney Int* 1988;34:S38–S44.
11. Mitchell JD, Baxter TJ, Blair-West JR, McCredie DA. Renin levels in nephroblastoma (Wilms' tumour): report of a renin-secreting tumour. *Arch Dis Child* 1970;45:376–384.
12. Ganguly A, Gribble J, Tune B, Kempson RL, Luetscher JA. Renin-secreting Wilms' tumor with severe hypertension. Report of a case and a brief review of renin secreting tumors. *Ann Intern Med* 1973;79:735–837.
13. Vaughn ED, Sweet RC, Gillenwater JY. Peripheral renin and blood pressure changes following complete unilateral ureteral occlusion. *J Urol* 1970;104:89–92.
14. Vaughn ED, Shenasky JA, Gillenwater JY. Mechanism of acute hemodynamic response to ureteral occlusion. *Invest Urol* 1971;9:109–118.
15. Belman AB, Kropp KA, Simon NM. Renal-pressor hypertension secondary to unilateral hydronephrosis. *N Engl J Med* 1968; 278:1133–1136.
16. Wise HM. Hypertension resulting from hydronephrosis. *JAMA* 1975;231:491–492.
17. Weidmann P, Beretta-Piccoli C, Hirsch D, Reubi FC, Massry SG. Curable hypertension with unilateral hydronephrosis. Studies on the role of circulating renin. *Ann Intern Med* 1977;87:437–440.
18. Klein LA, Lupu A, Brosman SA. Hypertension due to traumatic ureteral occlusion. *Invest Urol* 1973;10:327–330.
19. Nemoy NJ, Fichman MP, Sellers A. Unilateral ureteral obstruction. A cause of reversible high renin content hypertension. *JAMA* 1973;225:512–513.
20. Vaughn ED, Bühler FR, Laragh JH. Normal renin secretion in hypertensive patients with primarily unilateral chronic hydronephrosis. *J Urol* 1974;112:153–156.
21. Wanner C, Lüscher TF, Schollmeyer P, Vetter W. Unilateral hydronephrosis and hypertension: cause or coincidence? *Nephron* 1987;45:236–241.
22. Clark WR, Malek RS. Uretero-pelvic junction obstruction. I. Observations on the classic type in adults. *J Urol* 1987;138:276–279.
23. Butler AM. Chronic pyelonephritis and arterial hypertension. *J Clin Invest* 1937;16:889–897.
24. Pfau A, Rosenmann E. Unilateral chronic pyelonephritis and hypertension: coincidental or causal relationship? *Am J Med* 1978;65:499–506.
25. McDonald DF. Renal hypertension without main arterial stenosis. Function tests predict cure. *JAMA* 1968;203:932–936.
26. Luke RG, Kennedy AC, Briggs JD, Struthers NW, Barr Sterling W. Results of nephrectomy in hypertension associated with unilateral renal disease. *Br Med J* 1968;3:764–768.
27. Vaughn ED, Bühler FR, Sealey JE, Gavras H, Baer L. Hypertension and unilateral renal parenchymal disease. Evidence for abnormal vasoconstriction–volume interaction. *JAMA* 1975; 233:1177–1183.
28. Siamopoulos K, Sellars L, Mishra SC, Essenhigh DM, Robson V, Wilkenson R. Experience in the management of hypertension with unilateral chronic pyelonephritis: results of nephrectomy in selected patient. *Q J Med* 1983;52:349–362.
29. Pujadas JO, Novello R, Ferré J, et al. Small kidney and hypertension: selection of patients for surgery. *Urol Int* 1986;41:95–101.
30. Gordon RD, Tunny TJ, Evans EB, Fisher PM, Jackson RV. Unstimulated renal venous renin ratio predicts improvement in hypertension following nephrectomy for unilateral renal disease. *Nephron* 1986;44:S25–S28.
31. Marks LS, Poutasse EF. Hypertension from renal tuberculosis. Operative cure predicted by renal vein renin. *J Urol* 1973;109:149–151.
32. Babka JC, Cohn MS, Sode J. Solitary intrarenal cyst causing hypertension. *N Engl J Med* 1974;291:343–344.
33. Godard C, Valloton MB, Broyer M. Plasma renin activity in segmental hypoplasia of the kidneys with hypertension. *Nephron* 1973;11:308–317.
34. Zezulka AV, Arkell DG, Beevers DG. The association of hypertension, the Ask-Upmark kidney and other congenital abnormalities. *J Urol* 1986;135:1000–1001.
35. Ullian ME, Molitoris BA. Bilateral congenital renal arteriovenous fistulas. *Clin Nephrol* 1987;27:293–297.
36. Bailey RR, McRae CU, Maling MJ, Tisch G, Little PJ. Renal vein renin concentration in the hypertension of unilateral reflux nephropathy. *J Urol* 1978;190:21–23.
37. Stockigt JR, Sacharias N, Wood AS, Dugdale LM. Segmental renal sampling and partial nephrectomy in renal hypertension. *Arch Intern Med* 1976;136:1297–1298.
38. Sinclair AM, Isles CG, Brown I, Cameron H, Murray BD, Rob-

ertson JWK. Secondary hypertension in a blood pressure clinic. *Arch Intern Med* 1987;147:1289–1293.
39. Danielson H, Kornerup HJ, Olsen S, Posborg V. Arterial hypertension in chronic glomerulonephritis. An analysis of 310 cases. *Clin Nephrol* 1983;19:284–287.
40. Blythe WB. Natural history of hypertension in renal parenchymal disease. *Am J Kidney Dis* 1985;5:A50–A56.
41. Orofino L, Quereda C, Lamas S, et al. Hypertension in primary chronic glomerulonephritis: analysis of 288 biopsied patients. *Nephron* 1987;45:22–26.
42. Acosta JH. Hypertension in chronic renal disease. *Kidney Int* 1982;22:702–712.
43. D'Amico G, Vendemia F. Hypertension in IgA nephropathy. *Contrib Nephrol* 1987;54:113–118.
44. Davies DL, Schalekamp MA, Beevers DG, et al. Abnormal relation between exchangeable sodium and the renin–angiotensin system in malignant hypertension and in hypertension with chronic renal failure. *Lancet* 1973;1:683–686.
45. Feldt-Rasmussen B, Mathieson ER, Deckert T, et al. Central role for sodium in the pathogenesis of blood pressure changes independent of angiotensin, aldosterone and catecholamines in type 1 (insulin-dependent) diabetes mellitus. *Diabetologia* 1987; 30:610–617.
46. Blumberg A, Nelp WB, Hegstrom RM, Scribner BH. Extracellular volume in patients with chronic renal disease treated for hypertension by sodium restriction. *Lancet* 1967;2:69–73.
47. Tarazi RC, Dustan HP, Frohlich ED, Gifford RW, Hoffman GC. Plasma volume and chronic hypertension: relationship to arterial pressure levels in different hypertensive diseases. *Arch Intern Med* 1970;125:835–342.
48. dePlanque BA, Mulder E, Dorhout Mees EJ. The behaviour of blood and extracellular volume in hypertensive patients with renal insufficiency. *Acta Med Scand* 1969;186:75–81.
49. Cannella G, Castellani A, Mioni G, et al. Blood pressure control in end-stage renal disease in man: indirect evidence of a complex pathogenetic mechanism besides renin or blood volume. *Clin Sci Mol Med* 1977;52:19–21.
50. Schultze G, Piefke S, Malzahn M. Blood pressure in terminal renal failure: fluid spaces and the renin–angiotensin system. *Nephron* 1980;25:15–24.
51. Koomans HA, Geere AB, Boer P, Roos JC, Dorhout Mees EJ. A study on the distribution of body fluids after rapid saline expansion in normal subjects and in patients with renal insufficiency: preferential intravascular deposition in renal failure. *Clin Sci* 1983;64:153–160.
52. Beretta-Piccoli C, Weidmann P, de Chatel R, Reubi F. Hypertension associated with early stage kidney disease. Complementary roles of circulating renin, the body sodium/volume state and duration of hypertension. *Am J Med* 1976;61:739–746.
53. Dathan JRE, Johnson DB, Goodwin FJ. The relationship between body fluid compartment volumes, renin activity and blood pressure in chronic renal failure. *Clin Sci Mol Med* 1973;45:77–88.
54. Koomans HA, Roos JC, Boer P, Geyskes GG, Dorhout Mees EJ. Salt sensitivity of blood pressure in chronic renal failure. Evidence for renal control of body fluid distribution in man. *Hypertension* 1982;4:190–197.
55. Bianchi G, Ponticelli C, Bardi U, et al. Role of the kidney in "salt and water dependent hypertension" of end-stage renal disease. *Clin Sci* 1972;42:47–55.
56. Chrysanthakopoulos SG, Kastagir BK, Jubiz W, Kolff W. Hypertension in patients on maintenance hemodialysis: evaluation of peripheral renin activity and bilateral nephrectomy. *Am J Med Sci* 1972:264:9–21.
57. Vertes V, Cangiano JL, Berman LB, Gould A. Hypertension in end-stage renal disease. *N Engl J Med* 1969;280:978–981.
58. Wilkinson R, Scott DF, Uldall PR, Kerr DNS, Swinney J. Plasma renin and exchangeable sodium in the hypertension of chronic renal failure. *Q J Med* 1970;39:377–394.
59. Frye RL, Braunwald E. Studies on Starling's law of the heart. I. The circulating response to acute hypervolemia and its modification by ganglionic blockade. *J Clin Invest* 1960;39:1043–1050.
60. DeQuattro V, Miura Y. Neurogenic factors in human hypertension: mechanism or myth? *Am J Med* 1973;55:362–378.
61. Textor SC, Gavras H, Tifft CP, Bernard DB, Idelson B, Brunner HR. Norepinephrine and renin activity in chronic renal failure. Evidence for interacting roles in hemodialysis hypertension. *Hypertension* 1981;3:294–299.
62. Levitan D, Massry SG, Romoff M, Campese V. Plasma catecholamines and autonomic nervous system function in patients with early renal insufficiency and hypertension: effect of clonidine. *Nephron* 1984;36:24–29.
63. Ishii M, Ikeda T, Takagi M, et al. Elevated plasma catecholamines in hypertensives with primary glomerular diseases. *Hypertension* 1983;5:545–551.
64. Beretta-Piccoli C, Weidmann P, Schiffl H, Cottier C, Reubi FC. Enhanced cardiovascular pressor reactivity to norepinephrine in mild renal parenchymal disease. *Kidney Int* 1982;22:297–303.
65. Schohn D, Weidmann P, Jahn H, Beretta-Piccoli C. Norepinephrine-related mechanism in hypertension accompanying renal failure. *Kidney Int* 1985;28:814–822.
66. Zucchelli P, Zuccola A, Degli Esposti E, Santoro A, Sturani A. Pathophysiology and management of hypertension in hemodialysis patients. *Contrib Nephrol* 1987;54:209–217.
67. Padfield PL, Brown JJ, Lever AF, Morton JJ, Robertson JIS. Blood pressure in acute and chronic vasopressin excess. *N Engl J Med* 1981;304:1067–1070.
68. Thibonnier M. Vasopressin and blood pressure. *Kidney Int* 1988;34:S52–S56.
69. Szilagyi JE, Chelly J, Doursout M-F. Suppression of renin release by antagonism of endogenous opiates in the dog. *Am J Physiol* 1986;250:R633–R637.
70. Dzau VJ. Significance of the vascular renin–angiotensin pathway. *Hypertension* 1986;8:553–559.
71. Smith MC, Dunn MJ. Renovascular and renal parenchymal hypertension. In: Brenner BM, Rector FC Jr, eds. *The kidney*. Philadelphia: WB Saunders, 1986;1221–1251.
72. Catt KJ, Cain MD, Coghlan JP, Zimmet PZ, Cran E, Best JB. Metabolism and blood levels of angiotensin II in normal subjects, renal disease and essential hypertension. *Circ Res* 1970;26–27(Suppl II):177–193.
73. Wong SF, Mitchell MI, Robson V, Wilkinson R. Sodium and renin in the hypertension of early renal disease. *Clin Sci Mol Med* 1978;55:301s–303s.
74. Stokes GS, Mani MK, Stewart JH. Relevance of salt, water, and renin to hypertension in chronic renal failure. *Br Med J* 1970;3:126–129.
75. Schalekamp MA, Beevers DG, Briggs JD, et al. Hypertension in chronic renal failure. An abnormal relation between sodium and the renin-angiotensin system. *Am J Med* 1973;55:379–390.
76. Weidmann P, Maxwell MH, Lupu AN, Lewin AJ, Massry SG. Plasma renin activity and blood pressure in terminal renal failure. *N Engl J Med* 1971;285:757–762.
77. Boer P, Koomans HA, Mees EJD. Renin and blood volume in chronic renal failure: a comparison with essential hypertension. *Nephron* 1987;45:7–15.
78. Verniory A, Potvliege P, Van Geertruyden JJ, et al. Renin and control of arterial blood pressure during terminal renal failure treated by haemodialysis and transplantation. *Clin Sci* 1972;42:685–700.
79. Lifschitz MD, Kirschenbaum MA, Rosenblatt SG, Gibney R. Effect of saralasin in hypertensive patients on chronic hemodialysis. *Ann Intern Med* 1978;88:23–27.
80. Vaughn ED, Carey RM, Ayers CR, Peach MJ. Hemodialysis, resistant hypertension: control with an orally active inhibitor of angiotension-converting enzyme. *J Clin Endocrinol Metab* 1979;48:869–871.
81. Wauters J-P, Waebner B, Brunner HR, Guignard J-P, Turini GA, Gavras H. Uncontrollable hypertension in patients on hemodialysis: long-term treatment with captopril and salt subtraction. *Clin Nephrol* 1981;16:86–92.
82. Muirhead EE. Vasodepressor renal medullary lipids. In: Dunn MJ, ed. *Renal endocrinology*. Baltimore: Williams and Wilkins, 1983;75–97.
83. Bing RF, Russell GI, Thurston H, et al. Chemical renal medul-

lectomy. Effect on urinary prostaglandin E_2 and plasma renin in response to variations in sodium intake in relation to blood pressure. *Hypertension* 1983;5:951–957.

84. Muirhead EE. Antihypertensive functions of the kidney. *Hypertension* 1980;2:444–464.

85. Levy SB, Lilley JJ, Frigon RP, Stone RA. Urinary kallikrein and plasma renin activity as determinants of renal blood flow. The influence of race and dietary sodium intake. *J Clin Invest* 1977;60:129–138.

86. Mitas JA, Levy SB, Holle R, Frigon RP, Stone RA. Urinary kallikrein in the hypertension of renal parenchymal disease. *N Engl J Med* 1978;299:162–165.

87. Almeida FA, Stella RCR, Voos A, Ajzen H, Ribeiro AB. Malignant hypertension: a syndrome associated with low plasma kininogen and kinin potentiating factor. *Hypertension* 1981;3:II46–II49.

88. Granger JP, Hall JE. Acute and chronic actions of bradykinin on renal function and arterial pressure. *Am J Physiol* 1985; 248:F87–F92.

89. Smith MC, Dunn MJ. The role of prostaglandins in human hypertension. *Am J Kidney Dis* 1985;5:A32–A39.

90. Ruilope L, Robles RG, Bernis C, et al. Role of renal prostaglandin E_2 in chronic renal disease hypertension. *Nephron* 1982;32:202–206.

91. Niwa T, Maeda K, Shibata M. Urinary prostaglandins and thromboxane in patients with chronic glomerulonephritis. *Nephron* 1987;46:281–287.

92. Schneider M, Rathaus M, Shapira J, Bernheim J. Urinary prostaglandins E_2 and F_2 in chronic renal failure. Influence of chronic and acute changes in Na balance. *Nephron* 1985;40:152–154.

93. Blaine EH. Role of atriopeptin in blood pressure regulation. *Am J Med Sci* 1988;31:293–298.

94. Suda S, Weidmann P, Saxenhofer H, Cottier C, Shaw SG, Ferrier C. Atrial natriuretic factor in mild to moderate chronic renal failure. *Hypertension* 1988;11:483–490.

95. Walker RG, Swainson CP, Yandle TG, Nicholls MG, Espiner EA. Exaggerated responsiveness of immunoreactive atrial natriuretic peptide to saline infusion in chronic renal failure. *Clin Sci* 1987;72:19–24.

96. Deray G, Maistre G, Cacoub P, et al. Plasma levels of atrial natriuretic peptide in chronically dialyzed patients. *Kidney Int* 1988;34:S86–S88.

97. Frolich ED, Tarazi RC, Dustan HP. Hemodynamic and functional mechanisms in two renal hypertensions: arterial and pyelonephritis. *Am J Med Sci* 1971;261:189–195.

98. Valvo E, Gammaro L, Bedogna V, et al. Hypertension in polycystic kidney disease. *Contrib Nephrol* 1987;54:95–102.

99. Valvo E, Gammaro L, Bedogna V, et al. Hypertension in primary immunoglobulin A nephropathy (Berger's disease): hemodynamic alterations and mechanisms. *Nephron* 1987;45:219–233.

100. Kim KE, Onesti G, Schwartz AB. Hemodynamics of hypertension in chronic end-stage renal disease. *Circulation* 1972; 46:456–464.

101. Cangiano JL, Ramirez-Muxo O, Ramirez-Gonzalez R, Trevino A, Campos JA. Normal renin uremic hypertension. Study of cardiac hemodynamics, plasma volume, extracellular fluid volume and the renin-angiotensin system. *Arch Intern Med* 1976;136:17–23.

102. Brod J, Bahlmann J, Cachovan M, Hubrich W, Preschner PD. Mechanisms for the elevation of blood pressure in human renal disease. *Hypertension* 1982;4:839–844.

103. Brod J, Bahlmann J, Cachovan M, Pretschner P. Development of hypertension in renal disease. *Clin Sci* 1983;64:141–152.

104. Coleman TG, Bower JD, Langford HG, Guyton AC. Regulation of arterial pressure in the anephric state. *Circulation* 1970;42:509–514.

105. Kim KE, Onesti G, DelGuercio ET, et al. Sequential hemodynamic changes in end-stage renal disease and the anephric state during volume expansion. *Hypertension* 1980;2:102–110.

106. Guyton AC, Coleman TG, Young DB, Lohmeier TE, DeClue JW. Salt balance and long-term blood pressure control. *Annu Rev Med* 1980;31:15–27.

107. Coleman TG, Samar RE, Murphy WR. Autoregulation versus other vasoconstrictors in hypertension. *Hypertension* 1979; 1:324–329.

108. Ledingham JM. Mechanisms in renal hypertension. *Proc R Soc Med* 1971;64:409–418.

109. Brod J, Schaeffer J, Hengstenberg JH, Kleinschmidt TG. Investigations on the Na^+,K^+-pump in erythrocytes of patients with renal hypertension. *Clin Sci* 1984;66:351–355.

110. Hamlyn JM, Blaustein MP. Sodium chloride, extracellular fluid volume, and blood pressure regulation. *Am J Physiol* 1986;251:F563–F575.

111. Wilson C, Byrom FB. Renal changes in malignant hypertension. *Lancet* 1939;1:136–139.

112. Ellis A. Natural history of Bright's disease. *Lancet* 1942;1:1–7, 35–37, 72–76.

113. Aubia J, Hojman L, Chine M, et al. Hypertension and nephrotoxicity in the rate of decline in kidney function in diabetic nephropathy. *Clin Nephrol* 1987;27:15–20.

114. Tu WH, Petitti DB, Biava CG, Tulunay O, Hopper J. Membranous nephropathy: predictors of terminal renal failure. *Nephron* 1984;36:118–124.

115. D'Amico G, Minetti L, Ponticelli C, et al. Prognostic indicators in idiopathic IgA mesangial nephropathy. *Q J Med* 1986;59:363–378.

116. Azar S, Tobian L, Johnson MA. Glomerular, efferent arteriolar, peritubular and tubular pressures in hypertension. *Am J Physiol* 1974;227:1045–1050.

117. Azar S, Johnson MA, Hertel B, Tobian L. Single-nephron pressures, flows and resistances in hypertensive kidneys with nephrosclerosis. *Kidney Int* 1977;12:28–40.

118. Olson JL, Wilson SK, Heptinstall RH. Relation of glomerular injury to preglomerular resistance in experimental hypertension. *Kidney Int* 1986;29:849–857.

119. Neugarten J, Feiner H, Schacht RG, Gallo GR, Baldwin DS. Aggravation of experimental glomerulonephritis by superimposed clip hypertension. *Kidney Int* 1982;22:257–263.

120. Raij L, Azar S, Keane W. Mesangial immune injury, hypertension, and progressive glomerular damage in Dahl rats. *Kidney Int* 1984;26:137–143.

121. Bidani AK, Schwartz MM, Lewis EJ. Renal autoregulation and vulnerability to hypertensive injury in remnant kidney. *Am J Physiol* 1987;252:F1003–F1010.

122. Baldwin DS, Neugarten J. Hypertension and renal diseases. *Am J Kidney Dis* 1987;10:186–191.

123. Dworkin LD, Feiner HD. Glomerular injury in uninephrectomized spontaneously hypertensive rats. A consequence of glomerular capillary hypertension. *J Clin Invest* 1986;77:797–809.

124. Anderson S, Rennke HG, Brenner BM. Therapeutic advantage of converting enzyme inhibitors in arresting progressive renal disease associated with systemic hypertension in the rat. *J Clin Invest* 1986;77:1993–2000.

125. Jackson B, Debrevi L, Cubela R, Whitty M, Johnston CI. Preservation of renal function in the rat remnant kidney model of chronic renal failure by blood pressure reduction. *Clin Exp Pharmacol Physiol* 1986;13:319–323.

126. Teschner M, Bahner V, Schaeffer RM, Möslein J, Heidland A. Early functional effects of various antihypertensive drugs in chronically uremic rats. *Kidney Int* 1988;34:S156–S159.

127. Mogensen CE. Long-term antihypertensive treatment inhibiting progression of diabetic nephropathy. *Br Med J* 1982;285:685–688.

128. Parving HH, Smith UM, Anderson AR, Sveendsen PAA. Early aggressive antihypertensive treatment reduces rate of decline in kidney function in diabetic nephropathy. *Lancet* 1983;1:1175–1179.

129. Kajiwara N. Therapy and prognosis of hypertension in chronic nephritis. *Jpn Circ J* 1975;39:779–786.

130. Fujise Y, Miyahara M. Comparison of the prognosis of hypertension associated with chronic glomerulonephritis with that of essential hypertension. *Jpn Circ J* 1974;39:793–798.

131. Pohl JEF, Thurston H, Swales JD. Hypertension with renal im-

pairment: influence of intensive therapy. *Q J Med* 1974;43:569–581.
132. Maiorca R, Scolari F, Cancarini G, Brunori G, Camerini C. Management of hypertension in chronic renal failure. *Contrib Nephrol* 1987;54:190–201.
133. Bank N, Lief PD, Piczon O. Use of diuretics in treatment of hypertension secondary to renal disease. *Arch Intern Med* 1978;138:1524–1529.
134. Finnerty FA, Davidov M, Mroczek WR, Gavrilovich L. Influence of extracellular fluid volume on response to antihypertensive drugs. *Circ Res* 1970;26–27(Suppl I):71–82.
135. Dustan HP, Tarazi RC, Bravo EL. Dependance of arterial pressure on intravascular volume in treated hypertensive patients. *N Engl J Med* 1972;286:861–866.
136. Ghose RR, Gupta SK. Synergistic action of metolazone with "loop" diuretics. *Br Med J* 1981;282:1432–1433.
137. Wollam GL, Tarazi RC, Bravo EL, Dustan HP. Diuretic potency of combined hydrochlorothiazide and furosemide therapy in patients with azotemia. *Am J Med* 1982;72:929–938.
138. Weber MA, Drayer JIM. Renal effects of beta-adrenoreceptor blockade. *Kidney Int* 1980;18:686–699.
139. Bauer JH. Effects of propranolol therapy on renal function and body fluid composition. *Arch Intern Med* 1983;143:927–931.
140. Bauer JH, Jones LB, Gaddy P. Effects of prazosin on BP, renal function and body fluid composition. *Arch Intern Med* 1984;144:1196–1200.
141. Bailey RR, Nairn PL, Walker RJ. Effect of doxazosin on blood pressure and renal hemodynamics of hypertensive patients with renal failure. *NZ Med J* 1986;99:942–945.
142. Textor SC, Bravo EL, Fouad FM, Tarazi RC. Hyperkalemia in azotemic patients during angiotensin-converting enzyme inhibition and aldosterone reduction with captopril. *Am J Med* 1982;73:719–725.
143. Coratelli P, Buongiorno E, Giannattasio M, Passavanti G. Antihypertensive efficacy of enalapril maleate in impaired renal function. *Kidney Int* 1988;34:S204–S206.
144. Pelaya JC, Harris DCH, Shanley PF, Miller GJ, Schrier RW. Glomerular hemodynamic adaptations in remnant nephrons: effects of verapamil. *Am J Physiol* 1988;254:F425–F431.
145. Nicholson JB, Resnick LM, Laragh JH. The antihypertensive effect of verapamil at extremes of dietary sodium intake. *Ann Intern Med* 1987;107:329–334.
146. Hull AR, Long DL, Prati RC, Pettinger WA, Parker TF. The control of hypertension in patients undergoing regular maintenance hemodialysis. *Kidney Int* 1975;2:S184–S187.
147. Sulková S, Válek A. Role of antihypertensive drugs in the therapy of patients on regular dialysis treatment. *Kidney Int* 1988;34:S198–S200.
148. Mion C, Slingeneyer A, Canaud B. Pathophysiology and management of hypertension in continuous ambulatory peritoneal dialysis patients. *Contrib Nephrol* 1987;54:202–209.
149. Keeton GR, Morrison S. Effects of frusemide in chronic renal failure. *Nephron* 1981;28:169–173.
150. Maggiore Q, Zoccali C, Monzani G, Contini C. Chronic hemodynamic effects of propranolol treatment in dialysis-refractory hypertension. *Nephron* 1978;22:391–398.
151. Hulter HN, Licht JH, Ilnicki LP, Singh S. Clinical efficacy and pharmacokinetics of clonidine in hemodialysis and renal insufficiency. *J Lab Clin Med* 1979;94:223–231.
152. Harter HR, Delmey JA. Effects of prazosin in the control of blood pressure in hypertensive dialysis patients. *J Cardiovasc Pharmacol* 1979;1:S43–S55.
153. Heidland A, Riegel W, Hörl W, Weipert J, Geiger H, Heidbreder E. Calcium antagonists: hypotensive and humoral actions in different forms of hypertension. *Contrib Nephrol* 1985;49:201–218.
154. Lindner A, Douglas SW, Adamson JW. Propranolol effects in long-term hemodialysis patients with renin-dependent hypertension. *Ann Intern Med* 1978;88:457–462.
155. Battle DC, von Riotte A, Lang G. Delayed hypotensive response to dialysis in hypertensive patients with end-stage renal disease. *Am J Nephrol* 1986;6:14–20.
156. Kasiske BL. Possible causes and consequences of hypertension in stable renal transplant patients. *Transplantation* 1987;44:639–643.
157. Bachy C, Alexandre GPJ, Van Ypersele de Strihou C. Hypertension after renal transplantation. *Br Med J* 1976;2:1287–1289.
158. Whelton PK, Russell P, Harrington DP, Williams GM, Walker WG. Hypertension following renal transplantation: causative factors and therapeutic implications. *JAMA* 1979;241:1128–1131.
159. Curtis JJ. Hypertension and kidney transplantation. *Am J Kidney Dis* 1986;7:181–196.
160. Gunnells JC, Stickel DC, Robinson RR. Episodic hypertension associated positive renin assays after renal transplantation. *N Engl J Med* 1966;274:543–547.
161. West TH, Turcotte JG, Vander A. Plasma renin activity, sodium balance, and hypertension in a group of renal transplant recipients. *J Lab Clin Med* 1969;73:564–573.
162. Popovtzer MM, Pinnggera W, Katz FH, et al. Variations in arterial blood pressure after kidney transplantation: relation to renal function, plasma renin activity, and the dose of prednisone. *Circulation* 1973;47:1297–1305.
163. Blaufox MD, Birbari AE, Hickler RB, Merrill JP. Peripheral plasma renin activity in renal-homotransplant recipients. *N Engl J Med* 1966;275:1165–1168.
164. Cohen SL. Hypertension in renal transplant recipients: role of bilateral nephrectomy. *Br Med J* 1973;3:78–81.
165. Pollini J, Guttmann RD, Beaudoin JG, Morehouse DD, Klassen J, Knaack J. Late hypertension following renal allotransplantation. *Clin Nephrol* 1979;11:202–212.
166. Curtis JJ, Luke RG, Jones P, Diethelm AG, Whelchel JD. Hypertension after successful renal transplantation. *Am J Med* 1985;79:193–200.
167. Grunfeld JP, Kleinknecht D, Moreau JF, et al. Permanent hypertension after renal homotransplantation in man. *Clin Sci Mol Med* 1975;48:391–403.
168. Curtis JJ, Luke RG, Diethelm AG, Whelchel JD, Jones P. Benefits of removal of native kidneys in hypertension after renal transplantation. *Lancet* 1985;2:739–742.
169. Linas SL, Miller PD, HcDonald KM, et al. Roles of the renin–angiotensin system in post-transplantation hypertension in patients with multiple kidneys. *N Engl J Med* 1978;298:1440–1444.
170. Jacquot C, Idatte J-M, Bedrossian J, Weiss Y, Safar H, Bariety J. Long-term blood pressure changes in renal homotransplantation. *Arch Intern Med* 1978;138:233–236.
171. Bennett WH, McDonald WJ, Lawson RK, Porter GA. Post-transplant hypertension: studies of cortical blood flow and the renal pressor mechanism. *Kidney Int* 1974;6:99–108.
172. Rao TKS, Gupta SK, Butt KMH, Kountz SL, Friedman EA. Relationship of renal transplantation to hypertension in end-stage renal failure. *Arch Intern Med* 1978;138:1236–1241.
173. Van Ypersele de Strihou C, Vereerstraeten P, Wauthier M, et al. Prevalence, etiology and treatment of late post-transplant hypertension. *Adv Nephrol* 1983;12:41–60.
174. McHugh MI, Tanboga H, Wilkinson R. Alternate-day steroids and blood pressure control after renal transplantation. *Proc Eur Dial Transplant Assoc* 1980;17:496–500.
175. Thompson ME, Shapiro AP, Johnson A-M, et al. The contrasting effects of cyclosporin-A and azathioprine on arterial blood pressure and renal function following cardiac transplantation. *Int J Cardiol* 1986;11:219–229.
176. Ringe B, Bechstein WO, Bunzendahl H, Wonigeit K, Frei V, Pichlmayr R. Chronic renal dysfunction and hypertension after hepatic transplantation in adults treated with cyclosporine A. *Transplant Proc* 1988;20:639–641.
177. Bennett WM, Porter GA. Cyclosporine-associated hypertension. *Am J Med* 1988;85:131–133.
178. Bantle JP, Boudreau RJ, Ferris TF. Suppression of plasma renin activity by cyclosporine. *Am J Med* 1987;83:59–64.
179. Curtis JJ, Luke RG, Jones P, Diethelm AG. Hypertension in cyclosporin-treated renal transplant recipients is sodium dependent. *Am J Med* 1988;85:134–138.
180. Kaufman HM, Sampson D, Fox PS, Doyle TJ, Maddison FE. Prevention of transplant renal artery stenosis. *Surgery* 1977;81:161–167.

181. Whiteside CI, Cardella CJ, Yeung H, deVeber GA, Cook GT. The role of percutaneous transluminal dilatation in the treatment of transplant renal artery stenosis. *Clin Nephrol* 1982;17:55–59.
182. Smellie WAB, Vinik M, Hume DM. Angiographic investigation of hypertension complicating human renal transplantation. *Surg Gynecol Obstet* 1969;128:963–968.
183. Doyle TJ, McGregor WR, Fox PS, Maddison FE, Rodgers RE, Kauffman HM. Homotransplant renal artery stenosis. *Surgery* 1975;77:53–60.
184. Margules RM, Belzer FO, Kountz SL. Surgical correction of renovascular hypertension following renal allotransplantation. *Arch Surg* 1973;106:13–16.
185. Gerlock AJ, MacDonell RC, Smith CW, et al. Renal transplant arterial stenosis: percutaneous transluminal angioplasty. *AJR* 1983;40:325–331.
186. Curtis JJ, Luke RG, Welchel JD, Diethelm AG, Jones P, Dustan HP. Inhibition of angiotensin-converting enzyme in renal-transplant recipients with hypertension. *N Engl J Med* 1983;308:377–381.
187. Kalbfleisch JH, Hebert LA, Piering WF, Beres JA. Habitual excessive dietary salt intake and blood pressure levels in renal transplant recipients. *Am J Med* 1982;73:205–210.
188. Etheredge SB, Mahoney JF, Savdie E, Waugh RG, Sheil AGR. Treatment of renal transplant artery stenosis by percutaneous transluminal dilatation. *Clin Nephrol* 1982;17:217–221.

Hypertension: Pathophysiology, Diagnosis, and Management, edited by J. H. Laragh and B. M. Brenner. Raven Press, Ltd., New York © 1990.

CHAPTER 99

Hypertension and Hydronephrosis

E. Darracott Vaughan, Jr. and R. Ernest Sosa

Definitions, 1601
Incidence, 1602
Unilateral Ureteral Obstruction, 1602
Hemodynamic Effects, 1602
Tubular Effects, 1603
Bilateral Ureteral Obstruction, 1603
Hemodynamic Effects, 1603
Tubular Effects, 1603
Mechanisms of Hypertension in Models of Hydronephrosis, 1603
Unilateral Ureteral Obstruction, 1603
Bilateral Ureteral Obstruction, 1604
Human Observations, 1604
Unilateral Ureteral Obstruction, 1604
Bilateral Ureteral Obstruction, 1605
Conclusions, 1606
References, 1606

The relationship between obstruction to the urinary tract, hydronephrosis, and hypertension has intrigued both investigators and clinicians since the studies of Goldblatt et al. (1) rekindled interest in the relationship between the kidney and increased blood pressure. Soon thereafter, in fact, increased pressor activity was found in renal extracts from rats with acute unilateral ureteral ligation (2,3). However, it is apparent that although obstruction to the urinary tract is relatively common, hypertension is the exception rather than the rule; furthermore, hypertension is often coexistent and not causal, and it persists following correction of the obstructive lesion.

Moreover, it is also clear that the mechanism of hypertension that can result from obstructive uropathy differs depending upon the experimental or clinical setting. For example, there are multiple case reports showing increased renin secretion following acute unilateral ureteral obstruction, with reversal of the hypertension following correction of obstruction. This phenomenon is quite similar to unilateral renovascular hypertension accompanied by an angiotensin-II-dependent, vasoconstrictor type of hypertension (4). In contrast, bilateral renal obstruction accompanied by azotemia and by sodium and water retention is a prototypic example of volume hypertension (5), with prompt return of blood pressure to normal in most cases following the diuresis and natriuresis that occur after relief of obstruction (6).

The understanding of these two examples of hypertension and hydronephrosis requires a review of the basic pathophysiology of nephron injury induced by obstruction. This review will serve as a foundation to explain some of the conflicting experimental and clinical observations found in the current literature. Moreover, the complex and evolving hormonal interactions currently under investigation (7) in models of obstructive injury may eventually explain some of the clinical observations which now escape rational explanation.

DEFINITIONS

Unfortunately, several different terms are utilized interchangeably when obstruction to the urinary tract is discussed. *Hydronephrosis* is basically an anatomical term describing dilatation to the upper urinary tract, ureter, and renal pelvis and does not necessarily signify either renal injury or even a lesion necessitating surgical correction. For example, adults with the diagnosis of congenital megaureter with resultant hydronephrosis due to a defective distal ureteral segment do not show progressive renal deterioration (8). However, in most cases, hydronephrosis secondary to mechanical, intrinsic or extrinsic, or functional obstruction is due to impaired outflow of urine (obstructive uropathy) and may lead to obstructive nephropathy, actual nephron injury, and loss of renal function.

Hence from a clinical standpoint, hydronephrosis signifies the potential for nephron injury; appropriate tests are warranted to define the "clinical significance" of a structural lesion (7,9). It follows that the relationship between the hydronephrotic state and associated hypertension will be dependent on (a) the further definition of the etiology of the hydronephrosis, (b) the duration of the hydronephrosis, (c) the extent of the renal injury, and (d) the status of the total renal function.

TABLE 1. *Classification of urinary tract obstruction*[a]

Duration
Acute (hours to days)
Subacute (days to weeks)
Chronic (months to years)
Location
Renal tubule
Upper urinary tract (most frequently unilateral, but may be bilateral)
Renal infundibulum and pelvis
Ureteropelvic junction
Ureter
Ureterovesical junction
Lower urinary tract (by definition, bilateral in nature)
Bladder and posterior urethra
Urethra
Degree
Complete (total) obstruction
Incomplete (partial) obstruction

[a] From ref. 7.

Hence, before continuing with an overview of nephron injury due to obstructive uropathy it is important to classify the types of obstruction which may be encountered, since both systemic and renal effects due to obstruction differ in the various settings (Table 1) (7). First, the duration of the obstruction is critical. Acute obstruction to a previously normal kidney results in the classical symptom complex of urinary colic. Obviously the intense pain associated with acute colic may impact on any blood pressure readings taken at that point. Subacute obstruction is a vague term, since in this setting the duration of obstruction is often unknown. However, the patient often has minimal symptoms, and the degree of renal damage depends on the degree of obstruction. Chronic obstruction is often silent, with complete renal atrophy eventually occurring secondary to complete obstruction (10) and variable damage occurring following partial obstruction (11). The location of obstruction is primarily of relevance in the present context as a causation of unilateral or bilateral hydronephrosis.

INCIDENCE

The incidence of hydronephrosis at autopsy varies from 3.5% to 3.8% (12). Below age 20 there is no difference between sexes; females show a higher frequency during child-bearing years as a result of pregnancy, and males over age 60 show a preponderance due to benign prostatic hypertrophy. Although it appears that the clinical frequency of meaningful obstruction to the kidney is less than reported in autopsy series, accurate data are not available. The most common cause of acute hydronephrosis is calculus disease, which necessitates hospitalization of one in every 1000 Americans each year (13). The incidence of hydronephrosis in children appears to be lower (about 2%), with a high preponderance in young children (14).

The incidence of hypertension associated with hydronephrosis is a much harder number to determine. Obviously the incidence will depend upon underlying renal function. For example, most patients with azotemia due to bilateral ureteral obstruction have hypertension with a reversible component which resolves following natriuresis and diuresis (6). In contrast, Brasch et al. (15) evaluated 372 patients with hydronephrosis and found that only 13.7% had a systolic blood pressure higher than 145 mmHg and that only 5.6% had a systolic pressure greater than 160 mmHg. Moreover, following corrective surgery in 29 patients, only 35% normalized their blood pressure over a 5-year follow-up period. A later study (16) found the incidence of hypertension with acute unilateral ureteral occlusion to be 30% (9 of 30), whereas hypertension was rare (1.35%, i.e., 3 of 222) in patients with chronic unilateral obstruction. However, these retrospective studies of selected patients may not truly reflect the incidence of hypertension in either setting. In the most comprehensive study to date, Wanner et al. (17) found 20% of 101 patients with unilateral hydronephrosis to have blood pressure greater than 140/90. Moreover, of 26 patients operated upon and followed 4 years, the hypertension was cured in 62%, improved in 19%, and unchanged in 19%. In 73% of cured patients, renin indices predicted curability.

The incidence of hypertension in children with unilateral hydronephrosis may be even lower than that described in adults. In a series of 238 hydronephrotic kidneys due to ureteropelvic junction obstruction, only one of 219 children was found to be hypertensive (18). However, again it should be emphasized that the study was retrospective and that hypertension was not a primary focus during the initial care of the patients.

Taken altogether, it appears that hypertension is most likely to accompany either acute unilateral obstruction or chronic bilateral obstruction with azotemia. It appears to be relatively uncommon in patients with established chronic unilateral obstruction. The explanation for these observations can be at least partially derived from experimental observations.

UNILATERAL URETERAL OBSTRUCTION

Hemodynamic Effects

The hallmark of acute total unilateral ureteral obstruction (UUO) is decreased renal blood flow and increased renal vascular resistance (19,20). Prior to this phase there is initial vasodilatation, which is thought to be an attempt to maintain glomerular filtration rate (GFR) in the face of increased tubular pressure (21). This reduction in afferent arteriolar tone may be due to the release of vasodilatory prostaglandins, since increased urinary prostaglandin E (PGE) has been reported at this time period (22); moreover, the increase in renal blood flow (RBF) can be prevented by the administration of indomethacin or meclofenamate (23–25). More important in the present context is the observation that there is increased renin secretion (19,24–26) during this early phase; in addition, systemic hypertension has been observed in some of these studies.

However, within 2–5 hr following UUO there is a gradual fall in RBF which persists as long as the occlusion is present (19,20). This increased renovascular resistance has been shown by micropuncture and microsphere techniques (27–29) to be the consequence of increased afferent arteriolar resistance. The mediator of this increased arteriolar tone remains unclear. There is evidence for both increased renin release (see above) and increased renal production of the vasoconstrictor prostaglandin thromboxane A_2 (30,31). However, although there is evidence that converting-enzyme inhibitors partially block the decrease in RBF in several species (32–35), the response is only partial; in addition, other studies with saralasin (36) or renin depletion by sodium loading (19,37) did not prevent the predicted falls in RBF and GFR. Similarly, and perhaps more clearly, inhibition of thromboxane A_2 production by synthetase inhibitors (34,38,39) or receptor blockers (40) in several species fail to improve RBF. Taken altogether, UUO activates several intrarenal hormonal systems which could influence RBF; however, there are other, presently unexplained factors that appear to be more important.

Tubular Effects

Interestingly, with acute elevation of ureteral pressure creating partial obstruction, the tubular response resembles that found with renovascular hypertension. In this setting the segmental reabsorption of solute and water are enhanced (41–43). In an excellent study, Suki et al. (43) also demonstrated that in this setting there was "nephron under perfusion," or a decreased GFR/nephron, again similar to the dynamics seen with acute renal arterial stenosis. It is also in this acute experimental setting that increased renin release has been demonstrated.

Chronically, the more typical clinical picture appears (43) with a decrease in concentrating ability, decrease of TmPAH, increased fractional excretion of sodium, decreased distal hydrogen ion production, and variable changes in the excretion of other electrolytes (44). In this setting, Suki et al. have shown "nephron over perfusion." The reduction in GFR limits the loss of solute and water. Accordingly, the so-called post-obstructive diuresis phenomenon is not seen following UUO (45–47). Inappropriate water loss reaching clinical importance can occur if there is preservation of GFR (48).

BILATERAL URETERAL OBSTRUCTION

Hemodynamic Effects

Bilateral ureteral obstruction (BUO) leads to a similar reduction in total blood flow as seen with UUO (49). However, there is evidence that increased afferent arteriolar tone is not as increased as in UUO. Evidence includes persistent increased ureteral pressure (49), better cortical perfusion (45), normal stop-flow pressure (47), and normal glomerular plasma flow (50). Taken altogether, these observations suggest that the increased renal vascular resistance is due to persistent increased tubular pressure and not due to increased afferent arteriolar tone as seen in UUO. Circulating vasodilatory factors in BUO such as atrial natriuretic peptide (51,52), shown to be elevated with BUO, may play a role in preventing the increased afferent arteriolar tone.

Tubular Effects

In general the specific tubular effects found in BUO resemble those found in UUO. However, in experimental animals and selected patients the release of BUO results in a dramatic increase in sodium and water excretion (47,50,53–57). This so-called "post-obstructive diuresis" is due to several factors. A limited diuresis and natriuresis is commonly seen and is most likely due to the physiologic excretion of retained sodium, water, and urea (6). However, animal studies with restriction of salt and water (55) during BUO did not prevent natriuresis and diuresis, thereby indicating nephron injury. Moreover, the marked increase in fractional excretion of both sodium and water suggests an effect upon multiple segments of the nephron. Again the collective data suggests the effect of a natriuretic factor on the kidneys in this setting; however, the site(s) of action of such a factor on the nephron is unclear.

MECHANISMS OF HYPERTENSION IN MODELS OF HYDRONEPHROSIS

Unilateral Ureteral Obstruction

In early studies of functional and anatomical changes in the dog following UUO, the development of hypertension was mentioned (58). Subsequently, Levy et al. also noted the hypertension (59). Additionally, after Goldblatt et al. published their initial studies (1), they combined renal artery stenosis (RAS) with ureteral ligation and found that there was actually a protective effect (i.e., amelioration of the hypertension) in this model (60). These observations have more recently been confirmed and expanded with demonstration of lower renal renin content in animals with RAS and UUO than in those with RAS alone (61).

However, despite variable findings at this time, the critical observation from two groups was that injection of renal extracts from hydronephrotic animals elicited an exaggerated pressor effect (2,3). Indeed, in 1964 Vander and Miller (62) demonstrated an increase in renin release following UUO and postulated the stimulus to be activation of the macula densa mechanism. This hypothesis seems logical in view of functional data showing nephron under perfusion (43) early in partial UUO. The increase in renal vascular resistance occurs during the early period of vasodilatation, so there is clearly increased renin secretion (19).

Taken altogether, there is convincing evidence for the activation of renin secretion following acute UUO. The unresolved issue is the participation of other factors in any resultant hypertension. It is also apparent that there is increased synthesis of intrarenal prostaglandins following UUO (30,31). However, because of the rapid systemic inactivation of the known vasoconstrictor prostaglandin thromboxane A_2, it is the consensus that prostaglandin activation may effect intrarenal hemodynamics and function but not systemic blood pressure.

Finally, in an elegant study based on earlier reports, it was shown that acute UUO stimulation of renal mechanoreceptors activates afferent cells of origin in the spinoreticular pathway, with resultant hypertension (63). In addition, renal denervation abolishes the hypertensive response. As previously mentioned, clinical reviews have shown the greatest incidence of hypertension following acute UUO secondary to ureteral calculi (16). It is most likely that this central effect, combined with renin release, is operative in this acute setting, thereby causing the observed hypertension. Clinically, the presence of afferent nerve stimulation or central effects on systemic hemodynamics have not been studied (64).

In chronic UUO there is progressive renal destruction which is irreversible by 6 weeks of total occlusion in the dog (10). In contrast, in partial UUO there is an initial decrease in function, followed by stabilization (11,65). The renin response to chronic UUO is not well studied, but limited bioassay data showed a return of peripheral PRA to normal in dogs with chronic UUO, a fall that paralleled a return of blood pressure to normal (66). Similarly, other studies suggest that blood pressure following total or partial chronic UUO falls or remains normal (67,68).

Bilateral Ureteral Obstruction

Total BUO has been extensively utilized as an animal model of post-obstructive diuresis (see previous discussion). Obviously, studies are short and there is little information concerning systemic effects. However, the acute model is one characterized by salt and water expansion, activation of atrial natriuretic factor, azotemia, and weight gain, all characteristics of patients with chronic partial BUO and sodium/volume excess hypertension (6,52,69). In studies of partial BUO there has been a variable response in systemic blood pressure, probably because of a variable degree of obstruction and resulting renal damage. In fact, BUO is an area where clinical studies have given more useful information concerning the mechanism of observed hypertension.

One interesting, albeit confusing, model is the rat with hereditary hydronephrosis. The degree of hydronephrosis is variable and can be unilateral or bilateral. Most of the studies have come from one laboratory which has shown that the animals are salt sensitive and that 1% saline accentuates the blood pressure while suppressing a high basal plasma renin activity (PRA). Sodium loading also caused a higher plasma volume and extracellular volume than in normal controls, thereby demonstrating an impairment of sodium excreting ability (70–72). Salt loading has also been found to elevate blood pressure in animals following UUO (73) and in rats with hereditary diabetes insipidus (74). In the latter study, unilateral nephrectomy was also required and only young females were affected. The authors postulate both an impairment in excretory function and the deficiency of a nonprostaglandin antihypertensive renomedullary factor, since renomedullary autotransplants protected the animals from developing the hypertension (71). The translation of this information to other models or to human hydronephrosis is difficult, since the usual observation is the absence of hypertension when there is the greatest medullary loss or damage—not the opposite, as the hypothesis would suggest.

HUMAN OBSERVATIONS

Unilateral Ureteral Obstruction

The major point to be emphasized is that most patients with unilateral hydronephrosis are normotensive (15–18). Hence when a patient with hydronephrosis is found to be hypertensive, it is most likely coincidental unless proven otherwise. The burden of proof is placed on the clinician to prove that the hydronephrotic kidney is causing the hypertension. Obviously if the cause of the renal obstruction itself requires surgical repair or nephrectomy, then the question is only of academic interest. However, if intervention is not otherwise required, then appropriate studies are necessary to prove a cause-and-effect relationship.

The literature is replete with cases of reversible hypertension following correction of hydronephrosis or nephrectomy (Table 2). Although these cases are in the minority, they do confirm observations made in the acute UUO animal model. Studies of renin secretory patterns and responses will accurately identify these patients (17,75,76). The approach (Table 3) is the same as the one used to identify patients with renovascular hypertension, and the same characteristics apply. These curable patients usually exhibit (a) hypersecretion of renin solely from the hydronephrotic kidney, (b) contralateral renin suppression, and (c) a positive captopril test (77–79).[1] In the collective literature, if these renin indicators are present, then it is likely that the hypertension will be cured following correction of the hydronephrosis. However, in studies of patients with a variety of unilateral parenchymal renal diseases, increased renin secretion is the exception and most patients exhibit normal or low peripheral PRA (80,81). A similar finding is reported in patients with chronic hydronephrosis (80–82). In addition, renal renin content has been shown to be inversely proportional to renal damage. In 18 patients the values were very low in thin-walled hydronephrotic kidneys; the highest level was found in a patient with acute obstruction (83). Finally, in a group of children followed after corrective surgery, the supine PRA remained normal throughout the period (84).

Taken altogether, it appears that most patients with unilateral hydronephrosis are normotensive. Of those who are hypertensive, chronic hydronephrosis is usually not the cause of the hypertension. In these patients, operative intervention should be performed only when indicated in order to preserve renal function, correct symptoms, or avoid later complications. If there is no other indication for repair or nephrectomy except possible correction of the hypertension, then appropriate studies of renin secretory patterns and of the blood pressure response to angiotensin-converting enzyme inhibition should be performed. If these studies indicate angiotensin II dependency of the blood pressure due to unilateral renin secretion from the hydronephrotic kidney, then there is a high probability that the

[1] For details of these renin criteria, see the chapter by Pickering, entitled "Renovascular Hypertension: Medical Evaluation and Non-Surgical Treatment."

TABLE 2. *Reported cases of correctable hypertension and hydronephrosis*

Author	Number of patients	Renin data[a]	Reference
Belman et al.	1	+	*N Engl J Med* 1968; 278:1133
Garrett et al.	2	ND	*Am J Med* 1970; 49:271
Kluge et al.	1	ND; trauma also	*Scand J Urol Nephrol* 1972; 6:304
Greenhalf and DeVere	1	ND	*J Obstet Gynecol Br Commonwealth* 1973; 80:754
Nemoy et al.	1	ND	*JAMA* 1973; 225:512
Andaloro	1	+	*Urology* 1975; 5:367
Chapman et al.	2	ND	*J Pediatr Surg* 1975; 10:281
Schiff et al.	3	2/3 +; 1/3 ND	*Urology* 1975; 5:178
Wise	1	+	*JAMA* 1975; 231:491
Carella and Silber	1	+	*J Pediatr* 1976; 88:987
Ribeiro and Quartey	1	ND	*Br J Urol* 1976; 48:107
Munoz et al.	2	ND	*Am J Dis Child* 1977; 131:38
Weidman et al.	8	5/8 +	*Ann Intern Med* 1977; 87:437
Squitieri et al.	3	1/3 +; 2/3 ND	*J Urol* 1978; 111:284
Uhari et al.	1	+; also RAS	*J Pediatr* 1978; 92:458
Bruckstein et al.	1	+	*Am J Med* 1979; 66:358
Pak et al.	1	+	*Urology* 1980; 16:499
Pranikoff et al.	1	+	*J Urol* 1980; 124:701
Lusher et al.	3/6 cured	+	*Clin Nephrol* 1981; 15:314
Riehle and Vaughan	1	+	*J Urol* 1981; 126:243
Abramson and Jackson	2	+	*J Urol* 1984; 132:746
Vrata et al.	1	+	*Jpn J Med* 1985; 24:44
Kawano et al.	1	+	*Eur Urol* 1986; 12:357
Warner	26; 21/26 helped	18/21 +	*Nephron* 1987; 45:236

[a] ND, not done; RAS, renal artery stenosis; +, positive renin indices.

elevated blood pressure will be lowered following correction of the hydronephrosis.

Bilateral Ureteral Obstruction

The relationship between hypertension and BUO is easier to understand and to manage in the clinical setting. Chronic bilateral hydronephrosis can result in decreased renal function, azotemia, weight gain, congestive heart failure, edema, and generalized signs and symptoms of volume overload (6,85). In addition, both increased exchangeable sodium and a sodium diuresis after relief of obstruction have been documented (69). These patients have normal sodium secretory patterns prior to the relief of obstruction but can have marked increased fractional excretion of sodium post-operatively (85). Following this period of "post-obstructive diuresis" the blood pressure usually returns to normal (6,85). Accordingly, this phenomenon would appear to be an excellent example of "volume" hypertension (5).

Further evidence supporting this concept comes from a few patients with UUO of a solitary kidney. An azotemic patient with a solitary kidney, a ureteropelvic junction obstruction, and hypertension was found to have a normal PRA without lateralization. Post-operatively, there was a massive post-obstructive diuresis, with a return of renal function and normalization of blood pressure (86). This

TABLE 3. *Renin values for predicting curability of renovascular hypertension*

Collection of samples (moderate sodium intake ± 100 mEq/day)	
Ambulatory peripheral renin and 24-hr urine sodium excretion under steady-state conditions (i.e., not on day of arteriography)	
Collection of blood for PRA before and after converting-enzyme blockade	
Collection of supine:	
Renal-vein renin from suspect kidney (V_1) and inferior vena caval renin (A_1)	
Renal-vein renin from contralateral kidney (V_2) and inferior vena caval renin (A_2)	
Enhancement of renin secretion by converting-enzyme blockade if initial renin sampling is inconclusive	
Criteria for predicting cure	
High PRA in relation to UNaV	Measurement of hypersecretion of renin
Contralateral kidney: $(V_2 - A_2) = 0$	An indicator of absent renin secretion from the contralateral kidney
Suspect kidney: $(V_1 - A_1)/A_1 = 0.50$	Measurement of reduced renal blood flow
$\frac{(V-A)}{A} + \frac{(V-A)}{A} = 0.50$ in patients with high PRA means	
Incorrect sampling	
Segmental disease	Repeat with segmental sampling

phenomenon has been confirmed (87), although one case with elevated peripheral and renal renin has been reported; both the PRA and blood pressure returned to normal post-operatively (88).

CONCLUSIONS

In summary, the experimental data show that there are increases in renin secretion, thromboxane A_2 production, afferent nerve traffic, and hypertension following acute UUO. The chronic setting is less defined, but it appears that with progressive renal injury the hypertension is not sustained, a finding which argues against the loss of any "anti-hypertensive" factor. BUO is characterized by salt and water retention, azotemia, increase in circulating natriuretic factor, and a prompt post-obstructive diuresis and natriuresis which restores homeostasis.

Clinical observations parallel these experimental findings. The highest incidence of hypertension associated with hydronephrosis occurs with acute renal colic, and reversible hypertension associated with activation of the renin–angiotensin–aldosterone system is well documented in select patients with unilateral hydronephrosis. However, most patients with established hydronephrosis are normotensive or have coexistent hypertension not caused by these renal lesions. Accordingly, surgical intervention is predicated on either (a) traditional urological indications or (b) renin values showing unilateral hypersecretion from the hydronephrotic kidney, along with a positive captopril test.

In contrast to the acute setting, chronic BUO resulting in azotemia as well as volume and sodium expansion is associated with a volume/sodium form of hypertension that is usually self-correcting following a post-obstructive diuresis and natriuresis.

REFERENCES

1. Goldblatt H, Lynch J, Hanzal RF, Summerville WW. Studies on experimental hypertension: the production of persistent elevation of systolic blood pressure by means of renal ischemia. *J Exp Med* 1934;59:347.
2. Williams JR, Wegria R, Harrison JR. Relation of renal pressor substance to hypertension in hydronephrotic rats. *Arch Intern Med* 1938;62:805.
3. Beckwith JR. The effect of the time factor on the amount of pressor material in kidney after unilateral ligation of renal pedicle and after unilateral ligation of ureter. *Am J Physiol* 1941;132:1.
4. Vaughan ED Jr, Buhler FR, Laragh JH, Sealey JE, Baer L, Bard RH. Renovascular hypertension; renin measurements to indicate hypersecretion and contralateral suppression, estimate renal plasma flow and score for surgical curability. *Am J Med* 1973;55:402.
5. Laragh JH, Sealey JE, Buhler FR, Vaughan ED Jr, Bruner HR, Gavras H, Baer L. Renin access and vasoconstriction of volume analysis for understanding and treatment of renovascular and renal hypertension. *Am J Med* 1975;58:4.
6. Vaughan ED Jr, Gillenwater JY. Diagnosis, characterization and management of post-obstructive diuresis. *J Urol* 1973;109:286.
7. Klahr S, Buerkert J, Morrison A. Urinary tract obstruction. In: Brenner BM, Rector FC, eds. *The Kidney.* Philadelphia: WB Saunders, 1986;1443.
8. Pitts WR Jr, Muecke EC. Congenital megaloureter: a review of 80 patients. *J Urol* 1974;111:468.
9. Gillenwater JY. The pathophysiology of urinary obstruction. In: Walsh PC, Gittes RF, Perlmutter AT, Stamey TA, eds. *Urology.* Philadelphia: WB Saunders, 1986;542.
10. Vaughan ED Jr, Gillenwater JY. Recovery following complete chronic unilateral ureteral occlusion: functional radiographic and pathologic alterations. *J Urol* 1971;106:27.
11. Stecker JR Jr, Gillenwater JY. Experimental partial ureteral obstruction: alteration in renal function. *Invest Urol* 1971;8:377.
12. Bell ET. *Renal diseases.* Philadelphia: Lea and Febiger, 1946.
13. Boyce WH, Strawcutter HE. Incidence of urinary calculi in general hospitals, 1948–1952. *JAMA* 1956;161:1437.
14. Campbell MF. Urinary obstruction. In: Campbell MF, Harrison JH, eds. *Urology,* 3rd edition. Philadelphia: WB Saunders, 1970; 227.
15. Brasch WF, Walters W, Hammer HJ. Hypertension and the surgical kidney. *JAMA* 1940;115:1837.
16. Schwartz DT. Unilateral upper urinary tract obstruction and arterial hypertension. *NY J Med* 1969;69:668.
17. Wanner C, Luscher TF, Schollmeyer P, Vetter W. Unilateral hydronephrosis and hypertension: cause or coincidence? *Nephron* 1987;45:236.
18. Johnston JH, Evans JP, Glassberg KI, Shapiro SR. Pelvic hydronephrosis in children: a review of 219 personal cases. *J Urol* 1977;117:97.
19. Vaughan ED Jr, Shenasky JH II, Gillenwater JY. Mechanism of acute hemodynamic response to ureteral occlusion. *Invest Urol* 1971;9:109.
20. Moody TE, Vaughan ED Jr, Gillenwater JY. Relationship between renal blood flow and ureteral pressure during eighteen hours of total unilateral occlusion. *Invest Urol* 1975;13:246.
21. Navar LG, Baer PG. Renal autoregulatory and glomerular filtration responses to graduated ureteral obstruction. *Nephron* 1970;7:301.
22. Olsen UB, Magnussen MP, Eilertsen E. Prostaglandins: a link between renal hydronephrosis and hemodynamic in dogs. *Acta Physiol Scand* 1976;97:369.
23. Allen JT, Vaughan ED Jr, Gillenwater JY. The effect of indomethacin on renal blood flow and ureteral pressure in unilateral ureteral obstruction in awake dogs. *Invest Urol* 1978;15:324.
24. Blackshear JL, Wathen RL. Effects of indomethacin on renal blood flow and renin secretory responses to ureteral occlusion in the dog. *Miner Electrolyte Metab* 1978;1:271.
25. Cadnapaphornchai P, Aisenbrey G, McDonald KM, Burke DJ, Schrier RW. Prostaglandin-mediated hyperemia and renin-mediated hypertension during acute ureteral obstruction. *Prostaglandins* 1978;16:965.
26. Vander AJ, Miller R. Control of renin secretion in anesthetized dog. *Am J Physiol* 1964;207:537.
27. Arendshorst WJ, Finn WF, Gottschalk CW. Nephron stop-flow pressure response to obstruction for twenty-four hours in rat kidney. *J Clin Invest* 1974;53:1497.
28. Dal Canton A, Corradi A, Stanziale R, Maruccio G, Migone L. Effect of twenty-four hour unilateral obstruction on glomerular hemodynamics in rat kidney. *Kidney Int* 1979;15:757.
29. Tanner GA. Effects of kidney tubule obstruction on glomerular filtration in rats. *Am J Physiol* 1979;237:F379.
30. Nishikawa K, Morrison AR, Needleman P. Exaggerated prostaglandin biosynthesis and its influence on renal resistance in isolated hydronephrotic rabbit kidney. *J Clin Invest* 1977;59:1143.
31. Morrison AR, Nishikawa K, Needleman P. Unmasking of thromboxane A_2 synthesis by ureteral obstruction in rabbit kidney. *Nature* 1977;267:259.
32. Carmines PK, Tanner GA. Angiotensin in the hemodynamic response to chronic nephron obstruction. *Am J Physiol* 1983;245:F75.
33. McDougal WS. Pharmacologic preservation of renal mass and function in obstructive uropathy. *J Urol* 1982;128:418.
34. Chevalier RL, Jones CE. Contribution of endogenous vasoactive compounds to renovascular resistance in neonatal chronic partial ureteral obstruction. *J Urol* 1986;136:532.
35. Chevalier RL, Peach MJ, Broccoli AV. Hemodynamic effects of enalapril on neonatal chronic partial ureteral obstruction. *Kidney Int* 1985;28:891.
36. Moody TE, Vaughan ED Jr, Wyker AT, Gillenwater JY. The role of intrarenal angiotensin II in the hemodynamic response to unilateral obstructive uropathy. *Invest Urol* 1977;14:390.
37. Huguenin M, Ott CE, Romero JC, Knox FG. Influence of renin depletion on renal function after release of twenty-four hour ureteral obstruction. *J Lab Clin Med* 1976;87:58.

38. Loo MH, Marion DN, Vaughan ED Jr, Felsen D, Albanesc CT. Effect of thromboxane inhibition on renal blood flow in dogs with complete unilateral ureteral obstruction. *J Urol* 1986;136:1343.
39. Loo MH, Egan D, Vaughan ED Jr, Marion D, Felsen D, Weisman S. The effect of the thromboxane A_2 synthesis inhibitor OKY-046 on renal function in rabbits following release of unilateral ureteral obstruction. *J Urol* 1987;137:571.
40. Loo MH, Marion D, Vaughan ED Jr, Moody TE, Felsen D, Weisman SM. Thromboxane A_2 receptor blockade fails to reverse the increased renovascular resistance following unilateral ureteral occlusion. *Surg Forum* 1986;37:650.
41. Selkurt EE. Effect of ureteral blockade on renal blood flow and urinary concentrating ability. *Am J Physiol* 1963;205:286.
42. Suki WN, Guthrie AG, Martinez-Maldonado M, Eknoyan G. Effects of ureteral pressure elevation on renohemodynamics and urine concentration. *Am J Physiol* 1971;220:38.
43. Suki WN, Eknoyan G, Rector FC Jr, Seldin DW. Patterns of nephron perfusion in acute and chronic hydronephrosis. *J Clin Invest* 1966;45:122.
44. Gillenwater JY, Westervelt FB Jr, Vaughan ED Jr, Howards SS. Renal function after release of chronic unilateral hydronephrosis in man. *Kidney Int* 1975;7:179.
45. Harris RH, Yarger WE. Renal function after release of unilateral ureteral obstruction in rats. *Am J Physiol* 1974;227:806.
46. Buerkert J, Martin D, Head M, Prasad J, Klahrs D. Nephron function after release of acute unilateral ureteral obstruction in young rat. *J Clin Invest* 1978;62:1228.
47. Safirstein R, Wright FS. Renal vessel and tubule pressures during and after obstruction of one or both ureters. *Fed Proc* 1975;34:393.
48. Schlossberg SM, Vaughan ED Jr. The mechanism of unilateral post-obstructive diuresis. *J Urol* 1984;131:534.
49. Moody TE, Vaughan ED Jr, Gillenwater JY. Comparison of the renal hemodynamic response to unilateral and bilateral ureteral obstruction. *Invest Urol* 1977;14:455.
50. Dal Canton A, Corradi A, Stanziale R, Maruccio G, Migone L. Glomerular hemodynamics before and after release of twenty-four hour bilateral ureteral obstruction. *Kidney Int* 1980;17:491.
51. Fried TA, Lau AT, Ayon MA, Stein JH. Elevation of atrial natriuretic peptide (ANP) levels in ureteral obstruction in the rat. *Clin Res* 1986;34:596A.
52. Gulmi FA, Mooppan UMM, Chou S-Y, Kim H. Atrial natriuretic peptide (ANP) in patients with obstructive uropathy. *J Urol* 1988;submitted for publication.
53. Yarger WE, Hynedjian HS, Bank N. A micropuncture study of post-obstructive diuresis in rat. *J Clin Invest* 1972;51:625.
54. Jaenike JR. The renal functional defect of post-obstructive nephropathy: the effects of bilateral ureteral obstruction in the rat. *J Clin Invest* 1972;51:2999.
55. Sonnenberg H, Wilson DR. The role of medullary collecting ducts in post-obstructive diuresis. *J Clin Invest* 1976;57:1564.
56. McDougal WS, Wright FS. Defect in proximal and distal sodium transport in post-obstructive diuresis. *Kidney Int* 1972;2:304.
57. Harris RH, Yarger WE. The pathogenesis of post-obstructive diuresis: the role of circulating natriuretic and diuretic factors, including urea. *J Clin Invest* 1975;56:880.
58. Keith NM, Snowden RR. Functional changes in experimental hydronephrosis. *Arch Intern Med* 1915;15:239.
59. Levy SE, Mason MF, Harrison TR, Blalock A. The effects of ureteral occlusion on the blood flow and oxygen consumption of the kidneys of unanesthetized dogs. *Surgery* 1937;1:238.
60. Goldblatt H, Kahn JR, Lewis HA. Studies on experimental hypertension. XV. Experimental observations on hypertension associated with unilateral renal disease: effects of occlusion of the ureter on experimental hypertension due to unilateral renal ischemia. *Arch Surg* 1941;43:327.
61. Jelinek J, Gross F. Effects of differently induced renal ischemia and of ureteral ligation on kidney renin and blood pressure. *Cardiovasc Res* 1970;4:84.
62. Vander AJ, Miller R. Control of renin secretion in the anesthetized dog. *Am J Physiol* 1964;207:537.
63. Ammons WS. Spinoreticular cell responses to renal venous and ureteral occlusion. *Am J Physiol* 1988;254:R268.
64. Oparil S. Hypertension in a 74-year-old man with hydronephrosis and coronary disease. *Hypertension* 1985;7:824.
65. Ryan PC, Maher KP, Murphy B, Hurley GD, Fitzpatrick JM. Experimental partial ureteric obstruction: pathophysiological changes in upper tract pressure and renal blood flow. *J Urol* 1987;138:674.
66. Vaughan ED Jr, Sweet RC, Gillenwater JY. Peripheral renin and blood pressure changes following complete unilateral ureteral occlusion. *J Urol* 1970;104:89.
67. Silk MR. Hypertension secondary to hydronephrosis in adult and young animals. *Invest Urol* 1967;5:30.
68. Classon J, Josephson S, Robertson B. Experimental partial ureteric obstruction in newborn rats: Do the morphological effects progress continuously? *J Urol* 1983;130:1217.
69. Muldowney FP, Duffy GJ, Kelly DG, Duff FA, Harrington C, Freaney R. Sodium diuresis after relief of obstructive uropathy. *N Engl J Med* 1966;274:1294.
70. Susic D, Sparks JC, Machado EA. Renomedullary deficiency: a contributory factor in the pathogenesis of experimental renal hypertension. *Experientia* 1976;32:354.
71. Susic D, Sparks JC, Machado EA. Salt-induced hypertension in rats with hereditary hydronephrosis: the effect of renomedullary transplant. *J Lab Clin Med* 1976;87:232.
72. Sparks JC, Susic D. Rapid onset of salt-induced hypertension in rats with hereditary hydronephrosis. *Res Commun Chem Pathol Pharmacol* 1975;11:425.
73. Rao NR, Hettinstall RH. Experimental hydronephrosis: a study of the response of glomeruli and arteries to hypertension. *Nephron* 1969;6:598.
74. Dlouha H, Krecek J, Zicha J. Hypertension in rats with hereditary diabetes insipidus: the role of the age. *Pflugers Arch* 1977;369:177.
75. Weidmann P, Beretta-Piccoli C, Hirsch D, Reuby FC, Massry SG. Curable hypertension with unilateral hydronephrosis: studies on the role of circulating renin. *Ann Intern Med* 1977;87:437.
76. Riehle RA, Vaughan ED Jr. Renin participation in hypertension associated with unilateral hydronephrosis. *J Urol* 1981;126:243.
77. Urata H, Masui S, Ideishi M, Kato Y, Ikada M, Arakawa K. A case of hyperreninemic hypertension with unilateral hydronephrosis. *Jpn J Med* 1985;24:44.
78. Abramson M, Jackson B. Hypertension and unilateral hydronephrosis. *J Urol* 1984;132:746.
79. Muller FB, Sealey JE, Case DB, Atlas SA, Pickering TG, Pecker MS, Preibisz JJ, Laragh JH. The captopril test for identifying renovascular disease in hypertensive patients. *Am J Med* 1986;80:633.
80. Armanini D, Fallo F, Opocher G, Boscaro M, Scaroni C, Mantero F. Peripheral and renal vein plasma renin activity in hypertensive urological patients. *Br J Urol* 1982;54:348.
81. Vaughan ED Jr, Buhler FR, Laragh JH, Sealey JE, Gavras H, Baer L. Hypertension and unilateral parenchymal renal disease. *JAMA* 1975;233:1177.
82. Vaughan ED Jr, Buhler FR, Laragh JH. Normal renin secretion in hypertensive patients with primary unilateral chronic hydronephrosis. *J Urol* 1974;112:153.
83. Kawabe K, Sokabe H. Renin content of kidney in renal and adrenal diseases associated with hypertension. *Surgery* 1966;60:986.
84. Eke FU, Winterborn MH, Currie ABM, Gosling P, Clogher L, Das VK. Plasma renin activity in children after surgical relief of hydronephrosis. *Int J Pediatr Nephrol* 1983;4:177.
85. Jones DA, O'Reilly PH, George NJR, Barnard RJ. Reversible hypertension associated with unrecognized high pressure chronic retention of urine. *Lancet* 1987;1:1052.
86. Palmer JM, Zweiman FG, Assaykeen TA. Renal hypertension due to hydronephrosis with normal plasma renin activity to age 3. *J Urol* 1970;10:32.
87. Whiting JC, Stanisic TH, Drach JW. Congenital ureteral valves: report of two patients including one with a solitary kidney and associated hypertension. *J Urol* 1983;129:1222.
88. Davis RS, Manning JA, Branch GL Jr, Cockett ATK. Renovascular hypertension secondary to hydronephrosis in a solitary kidney. *J Urol* 1973;110:724.

Hypertension: Pathophysiology, Diagnosis, and Management, edited by J. H. Laragh and B. M. Brenner. Raven Press, Ltd., New York © 1990.

CHAPTER 100

Adrenocortical Forms of Human Hypertension

Edward G. Biglieri, Ilan Irony, and Claudio E. Kater

Normal Adrenal Cortex: Steroidogenesis and Zonation, 1609
Mechanism of Mineralocorticoid Hormone Hypertension, 1610
Mineralocorticoid Hormones, 1610
Hormonal Action, 1611
Mineralocorticoid Hypertension, 1611
Mechanism of Glucocorticoid Hypertension, 1612
Cortisol Regulation, 1612
Hypertension in Cushing's Syndrome, 1612
Hypertensive Disorders of the Zona Glomerulosa, 1613
Syndromes of Aldosterone Excess, 1613
Subsets of Primary Aldosteronism, 1614
Hypertensive Disorders of the Zona Fasciculata, 1618
Syndromes of Cortisol Excess, 1618
Syndromes of Deoxycorticosterone Excess, 1620
Hypertensive Disorders of the Zona Reticularis, 1621
Androgen- and Estrogen-Producing Adrenocortical Tumors, 1621
References, 1622

NORMAL ADRENAL CORTEX: STEROIDOGENESIS AND ZONATION

The adrenal cortex synthesizes steroid hormones derived from a common precursor, cholesterol. The majority of cholesterol substrate is obtained from circulating lipoproteins through the cell membranes by specific receptors. Limited amounts of cholesterol can be synthesized by the adrenocortical cells themselves. The initial cleavage of the cholesterol side chain leads to the formation of Δ-5-pregnenolone, the initial step in steroid synthesis. The enzymes involved in this action are the desmolases (side-chain cleavage enzymes).

The adrenocortical tissue originates in the subcapsular cells, which gradually migrate centripetally. During this process the cells become identified with specific steroid mixtures by the relative distance they travel from the capsular area. Thus the older, heavily pigmented cells are in the zona reticularis (ZR) and the newer cells are in the zona glomerulosa (ZG). As these cells migrate, their characteristics change, probably due, in part, to the distance from capsular arterial supply and decreasing oxygen concentration from the outer zones to centrally located cells. The milieu of steroids in different zones of the adrenal must also have a significant influence on the final mix of steroids that are secreted by each physiological zone. Thus the outermost zone, the ZG, produces aldosterone and 18-hydroxycorticosterone as its major steroids. There is an orderly biosynthetic pathway in the ZG which, through a series of hydroxylations of progesterone, results in the formation of deoxycorticosterone (DOC), corticosterone (B), 18-hydroxycorticosterone (18-OHB), and finally aldosterone. The unique enzyme of this zone is corticosterone methyloxidase type II (18-dehydrogenase), which is instrumental in the formation of aldosterone from B and 18-OHB (Fig. 1).

The principal regulator of the ZG is the renin–angiotensin system (RAS). Renin is released from the juxtaglomerular cells of the kidney in response to (a) decreased pressure in efferent arterioles, (b) decreases in tubular fluxes of sodium at the macula densa, and (c) increases in prostaglandin secretion, primarily PGE_2 and PGA. This enzyme converts angiotensinogen to angiotensin I, an inactive decapeptide. The decapeptide is transformed into the octapeptide, angiotensin II, by converting enzymes located in the vasculature beds, especially in the pulmonary vascular bed. Angiotensin II is the most important stimulator of the aldosterone pathway. Potassium concentration also has an important effect on the regulation of aldosterone through its effect in varying the intracellular calcium concentration. Hyperkalemia usually increases aldosterone production whereas hypokalemia reduces it (1). The role of total body sodium or exchangeable sodium on aldosterone excretion can be demonstrated only when extreme reductions of sodium content or sodium concentration occur (2). Other, less effective substances can affect aldosterone secretion, but their physiological roles and mechanisms remain unclear. These include prostaglandins (3), serotonin (4), proopiomelanocortin-derived peptides (5), acidosis (6), and the luteal phase of the menstrual cycle. On the other hand, the dopaminergic system (7), atrial natriuretic peptide

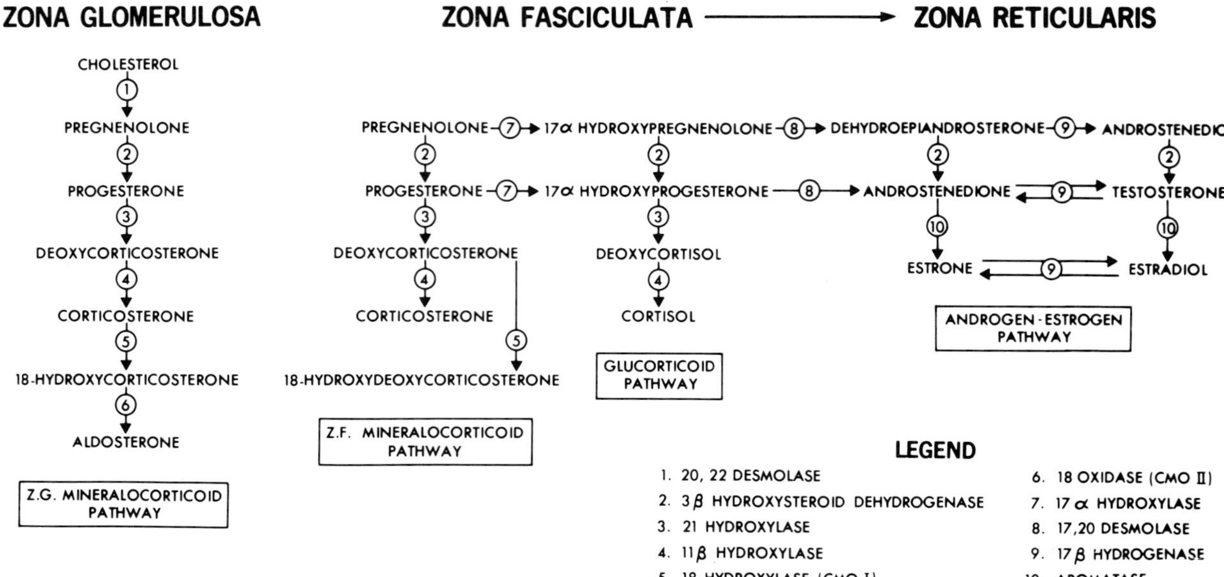

FIG. 1. Biosynthetic pathways of steroid hormones.

(8,9), somatostatin (2), and age reduce aldosterone production.

The intermediate zone, zona fasciculata (ZF), is the site of formation of the major adrenocortical steroid, cortisol. The late biosynthetic pathway involves the hydroxylation (cytochrome P-450) of progesterone to 17α-hydroxyprogesterone to 11-deoxycortisol and finally to cortisol. This pathway is referred to as the *glucocorticoid pathway* or the *17-hydroxy pathway.* There also exists a 17-deoxy pathway where progesterone is converted to DOC by the 21-hydroxylase, and then 18-hydroxylation follows to form 18-hydroxyDOC while 11-hydroxylation leads to the formation of B. All products of the late biosynthetic pathways in the ZF appear in the peripheral blood and can be used for the diagnosis of hypertension due to enzymatic deficiencies and adrenal tumors (Fig. 1). 11-Hydroxylation and 18-hydroxylation occur in the mitochondria and may represent a single enzyme function. 18-Hydroxylation also occurs in the 17-hydroxysteroid pathway, with the formation of 18-hydroxycortisol. However, oxidation of the 18-hydroxylated compounds to synthesize aldosterone does not occur in the ZF.

ACTH is the regulator of steroidogenesis as well as being an adrenal growth factor. Its action is exerted through increments of adenylcyclase activity, with subsequent activation of desmolase complexes which transform cholesterol into pregnenolone. Continued ACTH administration or chronic endogenous overproduction results in sustained stimulation of ZF steroids. ACTH is regulated by the hypothalamic hormone corticotropin-releasing hormone (CRH) and has a circadian rhythm. Although ACTH is the principal regulator of both the 17-deoxysteroids (DOC) and the 17-hydroxysteroids (cortisol), there is growing indirect evidence that other factors may be required for the normal ACTH regulation of the 17-deoxysteroids (10,11).

The most centrally located zone is the ZR. These pigmented older cells, although concentrated in the central area of the adrenal cortex, do appear in other various zones. In fact, cells from all zones appear throughout the adrenal gland. Adrenal androgen and estrogen production occurs here, and these are regulated by ACTH.

MECHANISM OF MINERALOCORTICOID HORMONE HYPERTENSION (FIG. 2)

Mineralocorticoid Hormones

The principal mineralocorticoids that enter the peripheral circulation from the adrenal cortex are aldosterone and DOC. Aldosterone binds, to a limited extent, to corticosteroid-binding globulin (CBG) and albumin. Approximately 30% of the measured circulating aldosterone concentration is free. Consequently, aldosterone has a relatively short half-life of 15–20 min. It is rapidly inactivated by the liver in a single passage, with the formation of tetrahydroaldosterone. Another metabolite of aldosterone, aldosterone-18-glucuronide, is formed by the kidney and usually represents 5–10% of the secreted aldosterone. A small amount of free aldosterone appears in the urine and can easily be quantitated. It is a particularly useful measurement when studying patients with low aldosterone production rates. The secretion of aldosterone varies from 50 to 250 μg/day on relatively normal sodium intake (7–10 g of sodium chloride per day).

DOC, a ZF mineralocorticoid, is secreted at approximately the same rate as aldosterone. However, it does not share some of the physical properties of aldosterone. It is virtually totally bound to corticosteroid-binding globulin, with only 5–8% appearing as free DOC in plasma, similar to cortisol. It is metabolized in the liver to tetrahydroDOC, conjugated with glucuronic acid, and excreted in the urine. There is virtually no detectable free DOC in the urine.

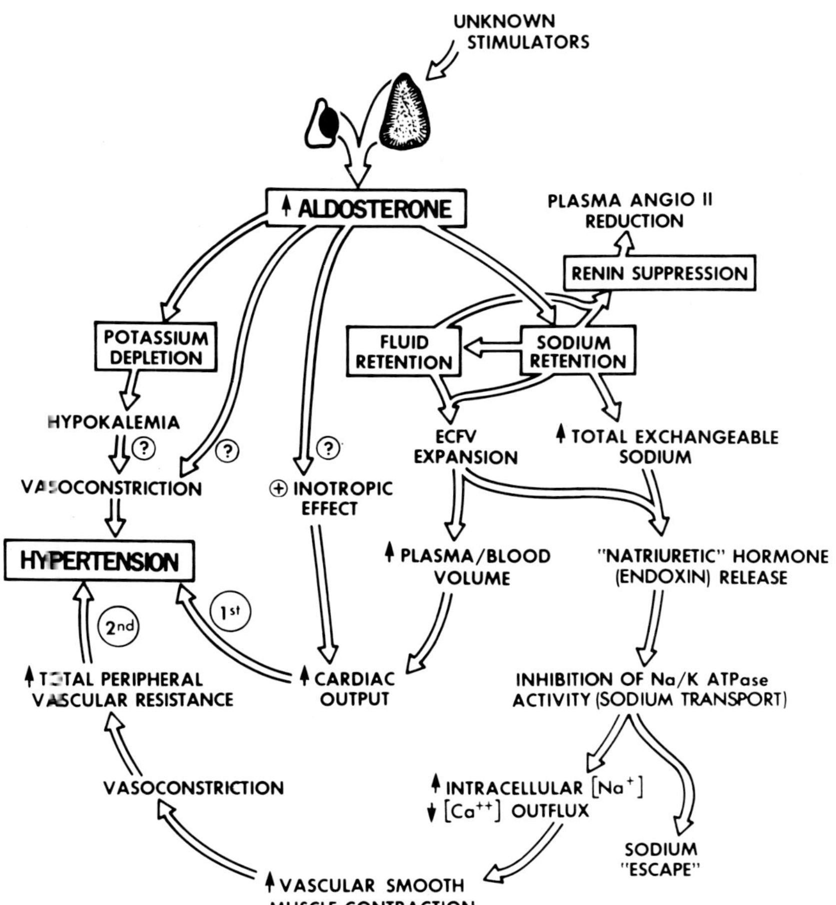

FIG. 2. Pathogenesis of hypertension due to mineralocorticoid excess.

Hormonal Action

A mineralocorticoid can exert an influence in virtually any cell that has Na^+,K^+-ATPase activity. Quantitatively, the most important target organs for the mineralocorticoids are the kidney, gastrointestinal mucosa, salivary glands, and sweat glands. The hormone crosses the cell membrane and binds to specific cytoplasmic receptor. The receptor–hormone complex is transported to the nucleus, where it acts with chromatin to promote synthesis of a specific mRNA with new protein formation for energy. The metabolic effect of aldosterone in the distal tubule results from its activation of the Na^+,K^+ ATPase in the serosal membrane to pump passively diffused sodium ions from the luminal side into the extracellular fluid. An alternate hypothesis suggests activation of the permease in the luminal membrane, thereby favoring sodium transport into the tubular cell and subsequently into the extracellular fluid. With either hypothesis, potassium and hydrogen ions are passively secreted into the luminal fluid as a result of the negative gradient created by sodium absorption.

Mineralocorticoid Hypertension

Mineralocorticoid hormones (MCHs) produce hypertension by several mechanisms. In long-standing mineralocorticoid hypertension, peripheral vascular resistance is increased. However, the initiating effects that lead to this increase in peripheral vascular resistance are most likely due to the early plasma volume and extracellular fluid expansion. The best insight into these early mechanisms comes from studies on the withdrawal of spironolactone treatment (aldosterone-receptor antagonist) from patients with a benign aldosterone-secreting adenoma. First, sodium and water retention occurred with an increase in body weight and extracellular fluid volume. After gaining approximately 1.5 kg, "sodium escape" followed, but renal potassium wasting and blood pressure increased. The hypertension was sodium- and volume-dependent. Sodium restriction did not prevent it (12). Normal subjects, given superphysiologic doses of fludrocortisone, became hypertensive because of an increase in stroke volume and cardiac output. Chronic MCH excess eventually results in an increase in peripheral vascular resistance along with normalization of stroke volume and cardiac output. The elevation of peripheral vascular resistance is also related, in part, to increased sensitivity to catecholamines, even without an increment in epinephrine or norepinephrine plasma levels. An additional mechanism may be the direct central action of aldosterone. Intracerebroventricular infusion of aldosterone produced hypertension in rats which could be reversed by infusion in the same site of a competitive aldosterone antagonist (13).

MECHANISM OF GLUCOCORTICOID HYPERTENSION (FIG. 3)

Cortisol Regulation

Ninety-five percent of cortisol is bound to CBG and albumin. The remaining free cortisol enters target cells to exert its metabolic effect. The liver is the major site for cortisol metabolism. Cortisol is reduced to dihydrocortisol and tetrahydrocortisol and is then conjugated with glucuronic acid, which is the major urinary metabolite. Free cortisol (40–100 μg/day) is also excreted in the urine and can be a useful measurement of cortisol production.

Although glucocorticoids exert a variety of effects in almost all body systems, the focus of this chapter will be on the mechanisms of hypertension. The most important glucocorticoid is cortisol, but increased B in some morbid conditions will also exhibit glucocorticoid activity.

Cortisol is a relatively weak mineralocorticoid. On a molecular basis, it has 1/400th the potency of aldosterone. However, its circulating concentrations are 1000 times higher than those of aldosterone or DOC, so that cortisol can exert mineralocorticoid effects when secretion is increased. In addition, cortisol acts in the proximal tubule to increase sodium reabsorption and plasma volume.

Hypertension in Cushing's Syndrome

Moderate to severe elevation of arterial blood pressure is associated with endogenous cortisol excess in spontaneous Cushing's syndrome. More than 80% of patients with Cushing's syndrome due to adrenocortical carcinoma or to ectopic ACTH secretion are hypertensive (14). Cortisol and other glucocorticoid hormones (e.g., corticosterone) are linked to hypertension in humans and in experimental animals. In contrast, potent synthetic glucocorticoids such as prednisone or dexamethasone are only occasionally associated with elevations in arterial blood pressure even when administered in pharmacological doses for long periods of time. Approximately 20% of patients who receive these hormones for certain medical disorders are prone to develop hypertension, but many of these patients may have hypertension as part of their disease process (e.g., renal or autoimmune disorders). The reason for these differences is not apparent, but synthetic glucocorticoids appear to be less "hypertensinogenic" than cortisol. They are almost completely devoid of mineralocorticoid activity.

In ACTH-dependent Cushing's syndrome (hypothalamic–pituitary Cushing's disease, ectopic production of ACTH or ACTH-like material by a nonendocrine tumor) several other ZF and/or ZR steroids are produced (e.g., DOC, B, and androgens) that can contribute to the development and/or maintainance of hypertension. Cortisol-producing adrenocortical tumors may also produce other steroids that could influence blood pressure.

The daily secretory rate of cortisol is 20–30 mg/24 hr. Its plasma concentration has a circadian rhythm, with higher levels in the morning (10–20 μg/dl) and gradually decreasing to 2–5 μg/dl in the late evening and early morning hours. Cortisol is approximately 95% bound to CBG. CBG is a readily saturable carrier protein. With the increased cortisol production in Cushing's syndrome, free cortisol is high and available to target organs. Many organs, tissues,

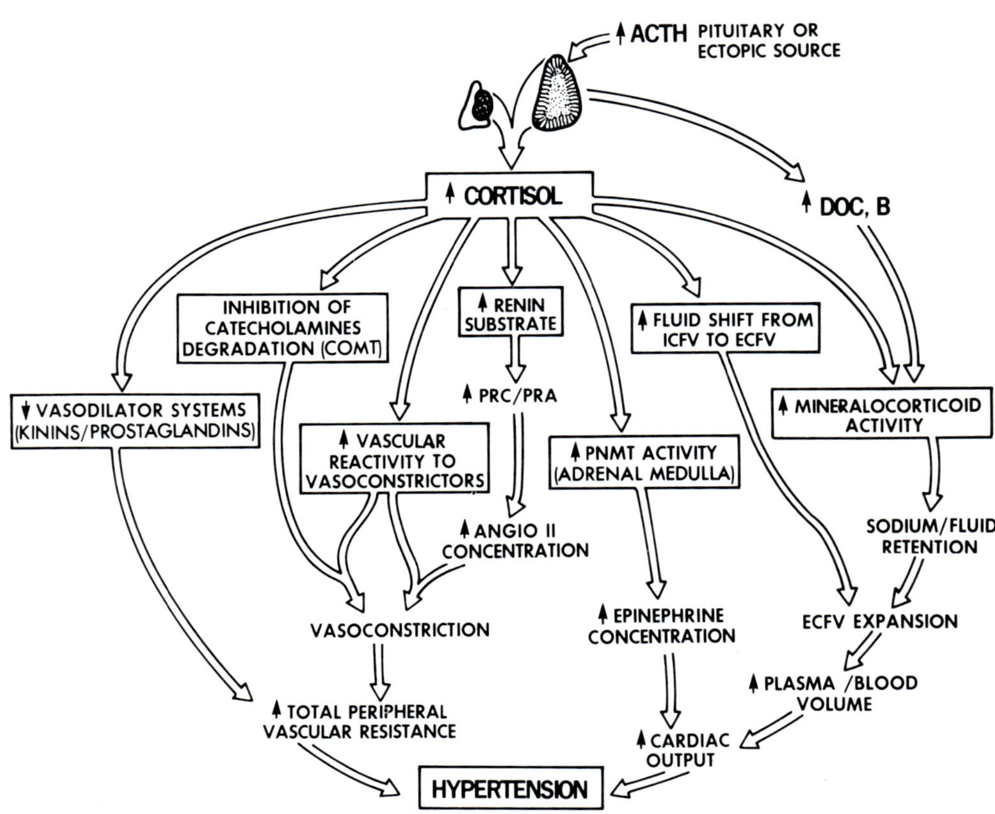

FIG. 3. Pathogenesis of hypertension due to glucocorticoid excess.

and systems are directly or indirectly affected by the increased amounts of free cortisol that will contribute to the development of hypertension. The cardiovascular hemodynamics of hypertension in Cushing's syndrome result in increased total peripheral vascular resistance and increased cardiac output. The following mechanisms may concurrently be involved in the pathogenesis of glucocorticoid-induced hypertension in Cushing's syndrome:

1. Increased concentrations of circulating angiotensin II resulting from an increase in hepatic production of angiotensinogen; acceleration of the renin–angiotensin reaction (15).
2. Inhibition of normal catecholamine metabolism, particularly norepinephrine, by interfering with its extraneuronal uptake and subsequent degradation by COMT (catechol-*O*-methyltransferase).
3. Glucocorticoid-mediated enhanced vascular reactivity to vasoconstrictor substances.
4. Inhibition of vasodilator systems (such as kinins and prostaglandins) thereby diminishing the counterregulatory forces on arteriolar tone, favoring vasoconstriction.
5. Possible increased production of the so-called "hypertensinogenic" steroids (17-hydroxyprogesterone; 17- and 20-dihydroxyprogesterone) in the ACTH-dependent Cushing's syndrome, similar to the experimental animal model in the sheep (16). As a result of all these effects, increased total peripheral resistance occurs.

Increases in cardiac output can be better associated with the following manifestations of glucocorticoid excess.

6. Increased plasma and/or blood volume following extracellular fluid volume expansion (ECF). The mineralocorticoid activity of cortisol contributes, in part, to these increases. In the ACTH-dependent Cushing's syndrome and the adrenocortical carcinoma, simultaneous production of mineralocorticoids like DOC and B contributes to sodium and fluid retention. In this unusual situation, plasma renin activity is reduced or suppressed, reflecting the expanded ECF.
7. Glucocorticoid hormones cause a shift of sodium and fluids from the intra- to extracellular compartment, increasing plasma volume even in the presence of a negative or unchanged sodium balance. This effect may explain the volume-expanded state in the presence of increased sodium excretion resulting from an increased glomerular filtration rate induced by cortisol.
8. A contributing mechanism to the elevated cardiac output may be increased epinephrine formation resulting from enhanced phenylethanolamine-*N*-methyl transferase (PNMT) activity in the adrenal medulla and probably the myocardium.

HYPERTENSIVE DISORDERS OF THE ZONA GLOMERULOSA

Syndromes of Aldosterone Excess

Primary aldosteronism accounts for less than 1% of the hypertensive population. Nevertheless, its recognition is important because patients can be cured by subtotal or unilateral adrenalectomy in a majority of cases. Primary aldosteronism is most prevalent between the ages of 30 and 50 and is slightly more common in females. Blood pressure levels are variable. Accelerated hypertension is rare. Funduscopic examination reveals only mild retinopathy, and, in the authors' experience, retinal hemorrhages have not been observed. The occurrence of orthostatic falls in blood pressure without reflex tachycardia, as well as the absence of the hypertensive overshoot and bradycardia following Valsalva's maneuver in a hypokalemic hypertensive patient, strongly suggests an aldosterone excess. Weakness, loss of stamina, nocturia, and paresthesia are common. A positive Chvostek's or Trousseau's sign during the clinical examination may be extremely relevant and may indicate hypokalemic alkalosis.

Serum potassium concentration is the most important screening test for aldosteronism in the hypertensive patient population, with a reliability of 75–90%. To be a reliable measurement it must be obtained after the patient has been off diuretics for at least 3 weeks and while he or she is in a fasting–resting state, avoiding prolonged venous stasis during collection. The patient should be on a sodium intake greater than 6 g of sodium chloride per day to reduce the chances of false-negative results. Additional salt tablets may be necessary to ensure that the sodium intake is elevated. Sodium restriction can retard potassium secretion by reducing sodium delivery to the distal tubule, masking a borderline potassium concentration. Increased renal potassium excretion in the face of hypokalemia is a constant characteristic of hyperaldosteronism (17).

Hypertension is initially related to increased sodium–volume expansion. This property of aldosterone suppresses plasma renin activity. There are many ways to address the measurement of plasma renin activity. If the diagnosis is primary aldosteronism, plasma renin activity measurements are invariably suppressed. Thus, posture, activity, and dietary sodium intake may not be essential in establishing a suppressed plasma renin activity in this disorder. A reduced level in the face of hypokalemia provides strong presumptive evidence of the hypermineralocorticoid state. The failure of renin to increase in the upright posture (endogenous volume depletion) or after the administration of the diuretic can also be used to magnify the degree of suppression. We feel that a suppressed plasma renin activity, with all the other metabolic consequences of aldosterone excess, is sufficient to confirm a diagnosis (18). If an elevated renin is obtained in a hypertensive patient, then renovascular hypertension, diuretic therapy, the use of converting-enzyme-inhibitor drugs, low-salt diet, and the rare renin-secreting tumors must be considered (17). Low-renin hypertension may be present (a) in 10–55% of the elderly population, (b) in endogenous or exogenous Cushing's syndrome, (c) following licorice excess, and (d) following the administration of exogenous mineralocorticoids other than aldosterone, such as DOC and fludrocortisone (19).

The 24-hr urinary aldosterone level is the most clinically reliable method for assessing production (17). In one series it showed a 96% sensitivity and 93% specificity in detecting patients with primary aldosteronism. Nomograms to correct for age and sodium intake may further improve the sensitivity.

A single measurement of plasma aldosterone can also provide information about a diagnosis but not about the aldosterone production. Multiple circadian plasma levels are required to calculate production rates. A valid and interpretable level requires control of meals, activity, posture, and circadian rhythm. Plasma aldosterone levels are the most important criteria in identifying the type of primary aldosteronism.

Hypokalemia with renal potassium wasting, suppressed plasma renin activity, and elevated 24-hr urinary aldosterone are the hallmarks of primary aldosteronism. The 24-hr integrated concentration of plasma aldosterone as well as suppression tests with intravenous saline, converting-enzyme inhibitors, DOC acetate, or fludrocortisone are more sophisticated maneuvers (but they do not increase the diagnostic sensitivity) as compared to the basal measurements. We feel that these tests should not be routinely performed but, instead, should be reserved for cases where borderline or unclear results are found in the basal measurements.

Subsets of Primary Aldosteronism (Tables 1 and 2)

The subsets of primary aldosteronism determine management. Two-thirds to three-fourths of the patients can be cured, or their hypertension can be significantly ameliorated, by unilateral adrenalectomy. These patients are identified by a combination of localization (anatomical) and biochemical testing procedures.

Idiopathic Hyperaldosteronism (IHA)

This subset is characterized by micro- or macronodular hyperplasia of both adrenals and rarely as unilateral disease. About one-fourth of patients have this form of hyperaldosteronism (19).

After establishing the presence of hyperaldosteronism, noninvasive localization procedures are indicated. The two recommended methods are abdominal computerized tomography (CT scan) and magnetic resonance imaging (MRI). Current high-resolution CT scanners can detect tumors of 0.5 cm in diameter (20). Results with MRI are as good as those with CT scanning. Scintigraphic localizations using ^{131}I-6β-iodomethyl-nor-cholesterol are noninvasive but require more time and expense, as well as concomitant use of high doses of dexamethasone and iodide. Ultrasound is restricted to very large abdominal lesions (17).

If imaging shows normal glands or bilateral nodular hy-

TABLE 1. *Basal values in primary aldosteronism*[a]

	IndHA	IHA	AP-RA	PAH	APA	NV
Age:	40.1	47.0	41.7	40.2	42.1	28
Range:	30–46	32–68	31–55	12–55	19–64	21–52
n:	7	40	4	5	94	55
K^+ (mEq/liter):	3.9	3.2	3.1	3.1	2.8	4.1
Range:	3.6–4.4	2.5–4.2	2.7–3.5	2.6–3.4	1.5–4.8	3.8–4.5
n:	7	40	4	5	90	55
PRA (ng/ml/hr):	2.3	1.2	0.26	0.62	0.19	1.37
Range:	2.3	0.1–2.34	0.1–0.5	0.1–1.9	0.1–0.6	0.5–2.5
n:	1	40	4	4	97	56
Urinary Aldo (μg/dl):	24.1	27.1	29.3	37.5	45.2	10.3
Range:	18.1–29.0	13.1–51.7	17.8–45.0	12.4–88.9	16.3–222	5–21
n:	7	41	4	5	94	27
Plasma Aldo (ng/dl):	12.4	16.7	12.3	37.9	49.6	8.2
Range:	6.3–16.1	5.9–50.5	7.0–14.2	19.8–58.7	14.7–338	4–12
n:	6	35	4	5	73	55
18-OHB (ng/dl):	12.5	39.8	38.4	129	162	23.5
Range:	12.5	17.8–139	30.0–50.9	31.8–318	50.6–507	15–35
n:	1	23	4	3	44	55
DOC (ng/dl):	10.8	7.6	7.4	17.7	20.9	5.4
Range:	15.6–28.8	1.3–22.8	4.5–12.3	8.5–29.9	3.4–53.4	4–12
n:	5	25	4	5	44	49
B (ng/dl):	141	250	239	514	432	368
Range:	100–171	90–825	90–458	124–921	53–1720	100–400
n:	3	18	4	5	35	49
18-OHDOC:	5.05	6.0	4.95	8.42	8.3	7.8
Range:	3.8–6.3	1.2–17.3	3.4–7.3	2.8–16.3	1.5–18.6	4–12
n:	2	18	4	5	41	49

[a] IndHA, indeterminate hyperaldosteronism; IHA, idiopathic hyperaldosteronism; AP-RA, aldosterone-producing renin-responsive adenoma; PAH, primary adrenal hyperplasia; APA, aldosterone-producing adenoma; NV, normal values; PRA, plasma renin activity; Aldo, aldosterone; 18-OHB, 18-hydroxycorticosterone; DOC, deoxycorticosterone; B, corticosterone; 18-OHDOC, 18-hydroxyDOC.

TABLE 2. *Plasma aldosterone (ng/dl) responses to discriminating maneuvers in primary aldosteronism*[a]

	DOCA		Posture		Saline		Ratio		Spironolactone	
					18-OHB/F	18-OHB/F	18-OHB/F			
	A	P	S	U	A	P	A	P	A	P
IndHA:	19.2	10.1	14.3	37.7	24.0/10.7	22.6/9.2	2.2	2.4	—	—
Range:	14.3–24.1	4.3–13.9	6.3–27.7	19.4–61.4						
n:	7	7	6	6	1	1				
IHA:	23.9	21.8	15.5	35.4	33.6/11.2	20.8/7.4	3.1	2.7	27.1	41.1
Range:	8.2–40.8	7.8–55.2	6.7–50.5	11.7–176					13.1–51.7	21.0–76.0
n:	25	25	35	35	10	10			17	17
AP-RA:			12.3	26.3	51.9/10.1	38.5/4.7	5.36	9.5	29.3	112
Range:			7.0–14.2	22.1–30					17.8–45.0	29.6–175
n:			4	4	2	2			4	4
PAH:	24.3	23.0	37.9	32.2	140.0/12.2	82.3/6.0	11.5	13.7	37.5	48.4
Range:	12.4–32.7	11.7–38.5	19.8–58.7	17.4–56.4					12.4–88.9	25.0–88.9
n:	4	4	5	5	1	1			4	4
APA:	35.1	34.4	49.6	47.5	178.5/12.5	123.8/7.7	15.4	17.6	45.2	48.1
Range:	16.3–95.4	14.2–114	18.4–338	13.5–351					16.3–222	12.9–134
n:	56	56	73	73	19	19			43	43

[a] A, before; P, after; S, supine; U, upright; Ratio, ratio before and after saline; 18-OHB in ng/dl; F, cortisol in μg/dl; AP-RA, aldosterone-producing responsive adenoma. Spironolactone, 150–200 mg/day for 6 weeks.

perplasia, additional biochemical maneuvers are necessary to identify the subsets with curable lesions. The following tests examine steroid patterns and autonomy.

Postural Study

Plasma aldosterone and/or its precursor 18-OHB, as well as cortisol, are obtained after overnight recumbency. A second sample is obtained after 2 hr in the upright posture. In patients with IHA, the 800 h aldosterone plasma levels are usually minimally elevated, rarely higher than 25 ng/dl, and plasma renin activity is suppressed but not to the same degree as in other subsets. The overlap of plasma renin activity among the subsets does not offer adequate discrimination for diagnosis. After 2 hr in the upright posture, plasma aldosterone concentrations are usually two- to threefold higher than the baseline value. This is due to a higher sensitivity to minor increases in renin activity during postural stimulation. The rise in plasma aldosterone concentration occurring with a decrease in cortisol, due to the circadian rhythm of the latter, is the typical response seen in patients with IHA. This type of response is considered an amplification of a normal response, similar to the response in healthy volunteers during low salt intake (21).

Saline Infusion

Saline infusion test for autonomy is useful in identifying subsets. It separates patients with essential hypertension from those with primary aldosteronism. Suppression of plasma aldosterone values to less than 8 ng/dl occurs in essential hypertension. The test can provide additional information by taking advantage of the combination of the circadian variation of all adrenocortical steroids and suppression of renin-sensitive steroids by saline in IHA. A basal plasma sample is collected at 800 h, followed by an intravenous infusion of 1.25–2 liters of normal saline over a period of 90 min. A second sample is then collected. The aldosterone/cortisol ratio—or, even better, the 18-OHB/cortisol ratio—after the infusion is always less than 3 in patients with IHA, whereas all other subsets have a ratio greater than 3 (22). Renin is "less suppressed" in IHA and can be further suppressed by volume expansion. In IHA, aldosterone and 18-OHB (renin-dependent) decrease more than cortisol, because the latter is influenced only by the circadian rhythm, whereas aldosterone and 18-OHB have the additional decrease in plasma renin activity as a result of a hypersensitive gland.

Urinary Steroids

The 24-hr urinary aldosterone level is elevated but is still lower than that of other subsets, but it is not of discriminatory value. Two cortisol metabolites, 18-hydroxycortisol and 18-oxocortisol, are now being measured in urine. Both are in the normal range in IHA and may prove to be of value.

Spironolactone Trial

Spironolactone is a competitive antagonist of aldosterone at the receptor level. An average daily dose of 200 mg usually normalizes serum potassium levels, but normalization of blood pressure is infrequently achieved in IHA. Effective second drugs are required, such as calcium-channel blockers. Although intracellular calcium modulates aldosterone production, its effect may be the result of its actions in other hypertension-related mechanisms. The response of plasma and urinary aldosterone levels to treatment with spironolactone in IHA is typically an increment two to three times the basal levels as a result of normalization of renin and potassium levels (23).

If doubt about the diagnosis persists after these maneuvers, bilateral adrenal vein catheterization with sampling of aldosterone and precursors is indicated. A patient with bilateral hyperplasia will have elevated levels of aldosterone in both adrenal veins.

Patients with IHA do not show autonomy to the various maneuvers described but do exhibit the expected responses at a different set of aldosterone production.

Some patients in this group have an unusual characteristic after suppression tests of saline infusion, DOC acetate, or fludrocortisone administration. Aldosterone levels can be suppressed to normal levels (less than 8 ng/dl). These patients are considered to have indeterminate hyperaldosteronism, a type not universally accepted. Some authors classify this subset as a type of idiopathic hyperaldosteronism and, therefore, primary aldosteronism; others, however, feel it is a subset of essential hypertension, possibly a continuum between essential hypertension and IHA.

Earlier articles reported that patients with IHA responded well to partial or total adrenalectomy. Between 80% and 85% of the patients diagnosed with IHA fail to respond to surgery, with recurrence of symptoms accompanied by hypertension and hypokalemia within 1–2 weeks after operation. Blood pressure was not normalized. Subsequently, additional and compelling evidence indicated that surgery was not curative in IHA and led to the virtual abandonment of surgery as a form of therapy (20). A strong suspicion remains that a hypertensinogenic and aldosterone-stimulating factor may be the cause of IHA. Others feel that this may represent a form of essential hypertension.

Primary Adrenal Hyperplasia (PAH)

Surgery is rarely used as treatment for IHA. Earlier reports included the occasional patient that had sustained reductions of blood pressure after subtotal or total adrenalectomy. There has now emerged a type of autonomous adrenal hyperplasia that may have accounted for blood pressure improvement of the few. The maneuvers previously described have been used as a means to test for autonomy and have helped identify this new subset, PAH. PAH is a subset of primary aldosteronism that combines the morphology of bilateral hyperplasia with biochemical and physiologic autonomy and therapeutic responses typical of adenoma (24). This hyperaldosterone state has the same findings on an abdominal CT scan as does IHA, namely, bilateral but occasionally unilateral hyperplasia or even normal-appearing adrenals.

A recumbent plasma sample for concentrations of aldosterone and its precursors will show levels higher than those found in typical patients with IHA. The response to the upright posture shows a minimal increase or decrease in aldosterone levels.

Saline infusion has proven to be a useful discriminator of this subset. The 18-OHB/cortisol ratios are elevated, with values higher than 3 (in our series, 13–30) (25). This could be due to (a) the degree of renin suppression found even before the infusion and (b) the relative "insensitivity" or autonomy of hyperplastic tissue.

Mean 24-hr urinary aldosterone levels are higher in PAH than in IHA, but there is great overlap between these two hyperplastic forms. The 24-hr urinary 18-hydroxycortisol and 18-oxocortisol levels in preliminary observations appear to be higher than those found in IHA but closer to those found in tumors (*unpublished observations*).

Treatment with spironolactone is usually successful in normalizing potassium and significantly reducing hypertension, a common finding with adenomas but unusual in IHA. After spironolactone treatment, aldosterone levels show little or no increase, as in patients with tumors. These patients can be adequately treated with low doses of spironolactone, but a surgical alternative can be offered in PAH. Reduction of adrenal mass can be achieved by subtotal or total adrenalectomy of the hyperplastic gland. This procedure has resulted in persistent normokalemia and normotension in the majority of these patients and significant amelioration of blood pressure in others (25). In the absence of unilateral disease, bilateral adrenal vein catheterization was required to eliminate the possibility of small adenomas.

Aldosterone-Producing Renin-Responsive Adenoma (AP-RA)

This subset of primary aldosteronism is the result of a unilateral adenoma exhibiting all the biochemical features of IHA. Confirmation of a unilateral source of aldosterone excess by adrenal vein analysis was initially required. The unusual feature of these adenomas is their sensitivity to changes in renin; they are not autonomous (26). The frequency of AP-RA is approximately 5% of the tumors and 3% of all patients with primary aldosteronism. Two distinguishing features of AP-RA require further confirmation. 18-Hydroxycortisol and 18-oxocortisol were normal in a small group of patients (26). Also, the result of the saline infusion test suggests some degree of autonomy because of its high aldosterone/cortisol ratio.

Aldosterone-Producing Adenoma (APA)

This subset of primary aldosteronism comprises 75% of patients. It occurs more often in females (3:1), especially between 30 and 50 years of age, a somewhat younger average than that of patients with IHA. CT scan or MRI will reveal a unilateral tumor—although in 2% of the cases, bilateral tumors are found (19).

Plasma and urinary aldosterone levels are higher than in all other subsets, as are 18-OH cortisol and 18-oxocortisol. Plasma DOC and 18-OHB (aldosterone precursors) are also higher than in other subsets, probably due to the overactivity of this pathway in adenomatous cells. Although helpful in suggesting the diagnosis, these basal levels do not reveal the full characteristics of APA.

Adenomas are characterized by their autonomy to the renin–angiotensin system. However, they still maintain some degree of ACTH dependency, as seen by the circadian variation shown in plasma aldosterone levels. Aldosterone and cortisol levels fall or show no change during the postural stimulation test. During saline infusion, aldosterone and 18-OHB decrease only to the same extent as cortisol, and the postinfusion 18-OHB/cortisol ratio remains much higher (mean = 17.6) than in IHA (22).

Plasma and urine aldosterone concentrations show limited changes with spironolactone treatment. A slight decrease is usually observed in the aldosterone values. In view of the normalization of serum potassium and renin, this fact is still unexplained. A current hypothesis suggests that intracellular spironolactone or its metabolites interfere with the oxidations in the late pathway of aldosterone synthesis. Intracellular spironolactone bodies are very common in the adenoma, more so than in contiguous tissue, which could support this proposal.

Spironolactone therapy results in normalization of blood pressure and potassium levels. Some patients in our research center have been treated with 100 mg spironolactone daily for more than 12 years and remain completely asymptomatic. Patients who do not respond with normalization of blood pressure are likely to have other causes for the hypertension (e.g., "background" essential hypertension).

Since the advent of high-resolution CT scan, the need for invasive procedures to localize the source of aldosterone, such as adrenal vein catheterization, has been progressively reduced. It is always advisable to treat these patients to normalization of serum potassium concentration and blood pressure before surgical removal of the adenoma.

Aldosterone-Producing Carcinoma (AP-Ca)

Among large series of patients with primary aldosteronism, the incidence of these malignant tumors is about 3–5%. However, excessive amounts of aldosterone can be secreted from cortisol or androgen-producing adrenocortical carcinomas, contributing to hypertension, hypokalemia, and suppression of renin. Malignant tumors can be suspected by the presence of very high levels of plasma and urinary aldosterone as well as high levels of precursor steroids.

The CT scan usually reveals a large adrenal mass (greater than 3 cm), often with local invasion, metastasis, and/or calcifications (27). A unique feature in our series is the early absence of a circadian rhythm for aldosterone, accompanied by the presence of normal cortisol rhythm. Aldosterone levels are unresponsive to ACTH stimulation, even though cortisol responses are adequate (28). However, a single patient was reported to have plasma aldosterone and precursor concentrations abnormally sensitive to infusions of ACTH (29).

We observed no responses in aldosterone levels to stimulatory or suppressive maneuvers. Taylor et al. reported the occurrence of angiotensin II receptors in one tumor (30).

Ectopic Aldosterone-Producing Tumors

Ectopic tumors causing primary aldosteronism are rare. Aldosterone can be secreted in minute amounts from undifferentiated carcinomas, along with other steroids and peptide hormones. The ovaries are the most common site of ectopic aldosterone production (31,32). The prevalent histologic type reported is arrhenoblastoma. An ectopic adrenocortical adenoma (namely, an APA) was also described in the kidney (33).

Although spironolactone can ameliorate the symptom of hypertension and hypokalemia, treatment is best provided by surgical removal of the original tumor. Prognosis is dependent upon the tumor origin and biological behavior.

Dexamethasone-Suppressible Hyperaldosteronism (DSH)

DSH is a rare type of hyperaldosteronism with an autosomal dominant mode of inheritance. Over 50 cases have been reported in the literature. The patients typically present with mineralocorticoid hypertension even though normal blood pressures have been recorded. The plasma renin activity (PRA) levels usually are suppressed and unresponsive to the usual stimulatory maneuvers. Aldosterone levels are usually high, but many have been reported to be normal because of the level of hypokalemia. The failure of inadequate postural increase in aldosterone levels is similar to that in patients with APA. An unusual and unique feature in patients with DSH is the sustained suppression of aldosterone secretion by dexamethasone and other glucocorticoids (34). Prolonged treatment with dexamethasone usually leads to reversal of the features of mineralocorticoid excess, even leading to the restoration of a normal increase in aldosterone after assuming the upright posture. A singular study might indicate the eventual outcome of patients with this disease. DSH is usually identified in childhood, but the sensitivity to glucocorticoid hormone suppression may eventually be dissipated, and hypertension will be of the renin hypertension type (35). There appears to be an unusual sensitivity of aldosterone to ACTH, which may partially explain the sustained elevations of its production. However, ACTH levels are normal, and there appears to be no evidence of another mineralocorticoid hormone causing the mineralocorticoid excess syndrome. Steroids such as DOC, B, and 18-OHDOC are normal. Another peculiar abnormality of aldosterone production is that prolonged treatment with ACTH may accentuate the hypertension and produce sustained increases in aldosterone without the expected "turnoff" in production after 24 hr. This could possibly be due to the unusual sensitivity of aldosterone to ACTH in these individuals. Recently, two steroids, 18-hydroxycortisol and 18-oxocortisol, presumably of ZF origin or from transitional cells between the ZF and ZG, have been found in large quantities in this form of hypertension

(36). Their exact role is not clear except that 18-oxocortisol has potent mineralocorticoid properties. There has been testing with putative aldosterone-stimulating factors (such as β-lipoprotein, γ-MSH, and α-MSH) in these individuals, but without any evidence of excessive sensitivity to these substances. Because the patients do extremely well on treatment with small doses of dexamethasone, surgery is rarely performed. Treatment consists of dexamethasone (0.5–2.0 mg/day) and could require other agents such as spironolactone, amiloride, or triamterene.

When such a patient is identified, a careful study of all family members is essential. The mechanism for this hypertensive disorder is still unresolved. ACTH increases blood pressure and produces sustained elevation of aldosterone. The number of mineralocorticoid receptors in mononuclear leukocytes is not depressed, suggesting that if there are other mineralocorticoids being produced, they are not down-regulating the receptor. Dexamethasone works, most likely, through the suppression of ACTH, because it seems to have no direct effect on aldosterone in this syndrome. An emerging hypothesis suggests that there may exist transitional cells or cells in the ZG and ZF areas that are capable of making both aldosterone, cortisol, 18-hydroxycortisol, and 18-oxocortisol (36,37). Thus, the failure to turn off aldosterone may represent a genetic abnormality whereby cortisol, acting as a substrate for 18-hydroxylation, does not influence aldosterone as normally seen with chronic ACTH administration. These 18-hydroxylated cortisol products may then contribute to the hypertension that is observed.

HYPERTENSIVE DISORDERS OF THE ZONA FASCICULATA

Syndromes of Cortisol Excess

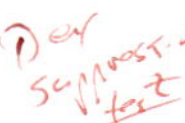

Cushing's Syndrome

Excessive cortisol production or prolonged glucocorticoid administration leads to the stigmata of Cushing's syndrome in humans: central or truncal obesity, moon-facies, plethora, purple striae, muscle atrophy, increased bruisability, menstrual abnormalities, diabetes, and hypertension. Hypertension is a common finding in endogenous hypercortisolism (more than 80% of cases) but occurs only among 10–20% of patients receiving exogenous synthetic glucocorticoid.

Increased cortisol levels may result from (a) autonomous adrenocortical tumors, (b) benign adenoma or carcinoma, or (c) bilateral ZF–ZR cell hyperplasia secondary to chronic (and usually excessive) adrenocorticotropin (ACTH) stimulation. Increased ACTH production may result from either (a) the corticotroph itself (pituitary micro/macroadenoma), (b) an abnormal regulation of the hypothalamic (CRH)–pituitary (ACTH) axis (Cushing's disease), or (c) an extrapituitary source, usually a malignancy of the lung, thymus, or pancreas (ectopic ACTH syndrome) (38–40). Rarely, ectopic CRH production by a nonendocrine malignancy can result in corticotrophic hyperplasia and Cushing's syndrome. The net result is an excessive, nonrhythmic, and nonsuppressible cortisol production which produces the clinical syndrome and forms the basis for the laboratory diagnostic tests of Cushing's syndrome.

Hypertension in Cushing's syndrome is usually more frequent in the adrenocortical hyperplasia (when ACTH excess is present). This implies that other ACTH-dependent steroids, such as DOC, B, or 18-OHDOC, may contribute to the development and/or maintenance of hypertension, in addition to cortisol itself. In addition, renal production of 19-nor-DOC by conversion from DOC is elevated in both the primary (adrenal) and secondary (pituitary) forms of Cushing's syndrome (41,42).

The diagnosis of Cushing's syndrome in the clinically suspected patient is established by determining elevated plasma cortisol levels, especially during the afternoon and evening hours, and increased 24-hr urinary excretion of free cortisol (usually more than 100 μg/24 hr). Cortisol production follows a circadian rhythmicity established by hypothalamic nuclei which produce higher levels of CRH (and consequently higher levels of ACTH) during the early morning hours, with a gradual decrease during the day and reaching its nadir in the early morning. Plasma cortisol levels above 15–20 μg/dl in the afternoon/evening hours in an otherwise unstressed patient are therefore suggestive of Cushing's syndrome. Concurrent urinary free cortisol excretion of above 100 μg/24 hr also supports the diagnosis.

Types and Diagnosis

Suppression of elevated plasma cortisol levels should be attempted by giving the outpatient a single 1-mg oral dose of dexamethasone (2300 h), followed by an 800 h morning sample. Post-dexamethasone cortisol levels of more than 6 μg/dl are suggestive of Cushing's syndrome if no causes for false-positive results are entertained (such as: the use of barbiturates and diphenylhydantoin, which accelerate hepatic metabolism of dexamethasone; acute or chronic depressive illnesses or other stressful situations; ethanol abuse; etc.) (43). Failure to suppress plasma or urinary free cortisol levels following a more prolonged suppression with 0.5 mg orally every 6 hr for 2 days (Liddle's low-dose dexamethasone suppression test) is pathognomonic of Cushing's syndrome, and the differential diagnosis should be undertaken. Three procedures are used for this purpose:

1. Failure to suppress cortisol levels to below 50% of the baseline control after either an overnight single 8-mg dose or the standard high-dose test (2 mg orally every 6 hr for two consecutive days) supports the diagnosis of a primary or autonomous adrenal disease or the ectopic ACTH syndrome (44). Patients with ACTH-dependent Cushing's disease reduce plasma cortisol levels to below 50% of the baseline values in 90% of the cases.
2. The diagnosis of ACTH-dependent Cushing's disease is also supported by the significant increases in both plasma ACTH levels (to values higher than 200 pg/ml) and 11-deoxycortisol (compound "S") (to values higher than 7 μg/dl) following the administration of a single overnight

dose (3.0 g orally) or the standard dose (750 mg orally every 4 hr for 24 hr) of the 11β-hydroxylase inhibitor, metyrapone (Metopirone).

3. More recently, administration of synthetic ovine CRH has been used to improve the accuracy in the differential diagnosis of Cushing's syndrome. The intravenous bolus injection or 60-min infusion of 100 μg (approximately 1 μg/kg of body weight) of ovine CRH significantly increases plasma ACTH (100–300%) in Cushing's disease but not in primary adrenal tumors or (only rarely) in the ectopic ACTH syndrome (45).

Plasma Steroid Profile (Table 3)

The determination of other ACTH-dependent steroids (ZF DOC, B, and 18-OHDOC) or even the ZR androgens [androstenedione, dehydroepiandrosterone (DHEA), and its sulfate (DHEA-S)], when simultaneously elevated, is corroborative for ACTH-dependent Cushing's disease (including the ectopic ACTH syndrome). However, adrenocortical carcinoma frequently produces, in addition to cortisol, a host of steroids, especially androgens, that may suggest the diagnosis. Although excess mineralocorticoid activity is frequently present in Cushing's syndrome as expressed by hypertension and hypokalemia, the ZG steroids aldosterone and its immediate precursor, 18-OHB, are consistently normal or reduced in the plasma of such patients. Table 3 shows the average plasma levels of cortisol, B, DOC, 18-OHB, 18-OHDOC, and aldosterone in hypertensive patients with Cushing's syndrome by their etiology. Hypertension may be due, in part, to the gluco- and/or mineralocorticoid activities resulting from the combination of these elevated products, including cortisol. Urinary excretion of 19-nor-DOC glucuronide is also elevated in patients with Cushing's syndrome, regardless of the etiology.

Imaging Procedures

Laboratory evaluation must be complemented by imaging procedures to validate the diagnosis and to offer supplementary information for the surgeon. Usually, primary adrenal tumors are best diagnosed and located by CT scan or MRI. Abdominal ultrasound can be diagnostic, especially in non-obese patients. When imaging procedures are equivocal, an adrenal vein catheterization should be performed to ascertain the source of adrenocorticosteroid excess, with determination of cortisol levels from both adrenal veins. Investigation for the suspected ACTH-producing pituitary (micro/macro) adenoma is best accomplished by MRI. Bilateral catheterization and sampling of the inferior petrosal venous sinus can be helpful to confirm and to lateralize the source of ACTH in the absence of a discrete pituitary microadenoma (46). Multiple samples along the thoracoabdominal vena cava are usually necessary to determine the source of an ectopic ACTH secretion when other procedures have failed.

Treatment

Adrenocortical tumors are treated by surgery. Removal of the pathologic adrenal gland resolves the state of hypercortisolism resulting from an adenoma. Carcinomas may need a more extensive surgical intervention and may not be fully resectable when local invasion or distant metastases occur (47).

Pituitary microadenomas are usually resectable by transphenoidal surgery (48). Whenever a discrete pituitary tumor cannot be found at surgery, the neurosurgeon may consider the cuneiform resection of the intermediate lobe (pars intermedia). Cure is obtained in 80–90% of cases following surgery in specialized centers. Alternatively, conventional or proton-beam particle radiotherapy should be attempted when surgery is not contemplated or in addition to a partially successful or incomplete surgical removal.

Pharmacological treatment of the hypercortisolism in Cushing's syndrome should be considered for a period of weeks or months prior to surgery to ameliorate the patient's clinical conditions, prevent excessive and easy bleeding, and improve postoperative prognosis. For this purpose, inhibitors of adrenocortical steroid biosynthesis can be used alone or in combination: metyrapone (doses of 2–3 g/day block 11β-hydroxylation), aminoglutethimide (to block cholesterol side chain cleavage), or trilostane (a 3β-hydroxysteroid dehydrogenase inhibitor) (49). More re-

TABLE 3. *Basal plasma steroid concentrations in patients with Cushing's syndrome*

	Cortisol (μg/dl)	DOC (ng/dl)	Aldo (ng/dl)	18-OHB (ng/dl)	B (ng/dl)	18-OHDOC (ng/dl)
Cushing's disease (n = 17):	19.7	12.3	4.9	21.6	475	6.1
SEM	1.3	2.4	0.8	3.2	53	0.8
Ectopic ACTH syndrome (n = 4):	60.5	68.5	6.6	23.0	1573	22.2
SEM	17.5	27.7	1.1	11.5	506	9.4
Adrenal adenoma (n = 3):	24.5	21.2	4.1	15.8	448	7.6
SEM	6.5	5.2	1.4	0.8	190	2.0
Adrenal carcinoma (n = 6):	25.8	115.8	3.4	13.6	693	5.5
SEM	4.2	47.6	1.1	7.8	211	3.4
Normal controls (n = 24):	10.8	8.6	7.9	24.8	343	7.4
SEM	0.5	1.3	0.5	1.6	34	0.8

[a] DOC, deoxycorticosterone; Aldo, aldosterone; 18-OHB, 18-hydroxycorticosterone; B, corticosterone; 18-OHDOC, 18-hydroxydeoxycorticosterone.

cently, the imidazolic derivative and broad spectrum antifungal drug ketoconazole has been demonstrated to inhibit, both *in vitro* and *in vivo,* several enzymatic steps in the biosynthesis of both cortisol and androgens in the adrenal cortex and testes (50). Its transient use in the treatment of Cushing's syndrome can be helpful in reducing the consequences of cortisol excess. The antiprogesterone and antiglucocorticoid (receptor antagonist) drug RU-486 (mifepristone) has been shown to block glucocorticoid activity in experimental animals and humans. It may emerge as a potential therapeutic agent to reverse excess cortisol effects in patients with Cushing's syndrome.

The adrenolytic agent mitotane (o,p′-DDD) is used primarily to treat unresectable adrenal cancer or is used when metastases are present. Doses of 4–6 g/day or greater for periods of up to 8 months have also been used with some success to destroy adrenocortical cells and reverse hypercortisolism in secondary (ACTH-dependent) Cushing's syndrome (51).

When CRH–ACTH imbalance results from a postulated primary hypothalamic–pituitary neurosecretory dysfunction or when pharmacologic inhibition of ACTH secretion is considered in Cushing's disease, certain drugs that interfere with neurotransmitters responsible for the CRH–ACTH control can be tentatively used to correct the abnormality [e.g., serotonin antagonist agents such as cyproheptadine (52), dopamine agonist agents such as bromocriptine, or GABA-decarboxylase inhibitors such as sodium valproate (valproic acid) (53)]. Therapeutic advantages from such drugs are limited.

Apparent Mineralocorticoid Excess Syndrome (Defect in Cortisol Metabolism)

Apparent mineralocorticoid excess syndrome is another unusual form of mineralocorticoid hypertension that has prompted great interest because of a potentially new mechanism for producing mineralocorticoid hypertension. In this disorder, excessive mineralocorticoid production is not observed by biological or chemical assay. These patients present with a mineralocorticoid-excess-type syndrome, with hypokalemia, suppressed renin activity, and low levels of aldosterone. The only known abnormality is in the peripheral metabolism of cortisol (54). There is decreased degradation of cortisol, with a prolonged half-disappearance time and a delay in the oxidation of cortisol to cortisone (55). In fact, the diagnosis is made by showing an increased cortisol/cortisone ratio of its metabolites. The hypertension is mineralocorticoid in character because salt restriction improves and spironolactone controls hypertension. The abnormal cortisol/cortisone ratio or the reduced ability to convert cortisol to cortisone, presumably at kidney sites, no longer protects the kidney mineralocorticoid receptor from cortisol (which has a high affinity, similar to that of aldosterone). Normally, the conversion to cortisone permits the mineralocorticoid receptor to accept aldosterone as the mineralocorticoid of consequence. Support for these observations comes from the observation that exogenous cortisol and ACTH increase hypertension whereas dexamethasone reduces blood pressure (56). This is a lethal disease. It is invariably detected in children with severe hypertension, and while management can be successful, none of the reported cases have survived into their twenties, except for a recent case (56).

Syndromes of Deoxycorticosterone Excess

Adrenal Tumors: Primary Hyperdeoxycorticosteronism (Table 4)

Hyperdeoxycorticosteronism results from increased DOC production with elevated plasma DOC levels but normal cortisol production. Hypokalemia and the suppression of renin and aldosterone accompany the mineralocorticoid hypertension (11).

Excessive production of DOC results from adrenal tumors (benign and malignant) or bilateral hyperplasia (57). Tumors producing excessive amounts of 17-deoxysteroids are rare (usually adenomas) and may be sensitive to ACTH stimulation. Spironolactone treatment is effective in treating the hypertension and potassium wasting, but cure requires surgery. A unique observation has been made in a patient after the removal of a benign tumor. Preoperatively, ACTH increased the elevated levels of all 17-deoxysteroids as well as the normal cortisol level. One week after surgery, the 1-hr cosyntropin test failed to stimulate 17-deoxysteroids from the contralateral gland, despite normal cortisol response. After 8 weeks the 17-deoxysteroids from the contralateral gland responded normally to ACTH. This supports the existence of an additional, non-ACTH regulator, specific for the 17-deoxysteroids, which, in this case, has been suppressed by the chronic tumor-produced DOC (11).

Adrenal carcinomas producing DOC are not sensitive to ACTH, although one report suggested suppression of metastatic production of DOC by dexamethasone (58). If corticosterone production is extremely high, ACTH suppression may occur with subsequent decreases in cortisol levels.

TABLE 4. *Basal steroid values in primary DOC excess*

Parameter	DOC adenoma	DOC carcinoma
Age (years)	30	55
Potassium (mEq/liter)	2.3	2.8
PRA (ng/ml/hr) (1.3 ± 0.3)[a]	0.1	0.4
Urinary aldosterone (μg/24 hr)	2.1	5.0
Plasma steroids (ng/dl)		
Aldosterone (8.5 ± 0.9)	0.6	2.0
18-hydroxyB (25.9 ± 2.4)	20.0	538.0
DOC (5.4 ± 0.5)	187	381
B (308 ± 57)	1988	37,200
18-hydroxyDOC (5.2 ± 0.9)	39.8	131.0
Cortisol (μg/dl) (10.8 ± 0.8)	7.2	1.1

[a] Normal values (mean ± SEM) are given in parentheses.

Enzymatic Deficiencies

11β-Hydroxylase Deficiency Syndrome

11β-Hydroxylation is the immediate biosynthetic step before cortisol formation. Its deficiency results in reduced cortisol levels and subsequent ACTH elevation. This stimulates secretion of both 11-deoxycortisol (the immediate precursor in cortisol formation in the glucocorticoid pathway of the ZF) and DOC, from the ZF 17-deoxy pathway. Virilization occurs as a result of a diversion of steroid synthesis to androgen production because of intact 17-hydroxylation. Aldosterone levels are low because of plasma expansion and renin suppression by high levels of DOC. ZG function is suppressed, and there is no evidence to suggest that 11β-hydroxylation is deficient. Special precautions must be taken when glucocorticoid treatment is initiated. A delay in aldosterone production due to prolonged suppression is the rule, which can result in hyperkalemia and hypovolemic crisis early in glucocorticoid treatment. If this occurs, sodium replacement and/or mineralocorticoids are required (59).

17α-Hydroxylase Deficiency Syndrome

This autosomal recessive disorder is characterized by mineralocorticoid hypertension without virilization, since the enzymatic defect prevents 17α-hydroxylation, a required step for 17-20-desmolase action to cleave the side chain permitting androgen and estrogen formation. This deficiency also occurs in the gonads. The clinical findings include primary amenorrhea and sexual infantilism in females and pseudohermaphroditism in males. This is treated with glucocorticoid hormone in doses to suppress ACTH and DOC excess. In the female patient, estrogen therapy is also recommended (60,61).

HYPERTENSIVE DISORDERS OF THE ZONA RETICULARIS (TABLE 5)

Androgen- and Estrogen-Producing Adrenocortical Tumors

The adult adrenocortical ZR produces mostly C-19 steroids (androstanes) with weak androgen activity, i.e., dehydroepiandrosterone (and its sulfate, DHEA-S) and androstenedione. Although aromatase activity is also present in cells of the ZR, estrogen formation (C-18 steroids, estranes) is minimal under physiologic conditions. Disturbances in both internal ZR-regulatory mechanisms and ZR's extra-adrenal regulators (ACTH and a putative androgen stimulating peptide) may lead to excessive sex-steroid production resulting in syndromes of hirsutism and virilization in the female or feminization in male adult patients.

Although the ZR has no intrinsic capacity to synthesize any effective gluco- or mineralocorticoid hormone, under conditions of chronic stimulation by ACTH, it has the potential to resume production of hormones of the ZF type.

ZR malignancies may be associated with clinical signs and symptoms that resemble a mineralocorticoid excess state with hypertension, hypokalemia, and even renin suppression. However, aldosterone levels are not necessarily elevated and are often reduced. Urinary or plasma steroid profiling in some of these patients suggests that inhibition of 11β-hydroxylase activity has occurred, presumably due to local production of androgen or estrogen by the malignancies. In addition, administration of methylandrostanediol to experimental animals and of testosterone to humans also suggests that exogenous androgen excess could, in fact, block the conversion of compound S (11-deoxycortisol) and DOC to their respective 11β-hydroxylated relatives cortisol and corticosterone. Excessive secretion of DOC could then act as an effective mineralocorticoid resulting in hypertension and hypokalemia. This syndrome can be reproduced in humans and animals by the administration of the synthetic 11β-hydroxylase inhibitor metyrapone.

Some patients with androgen- or estrogen-producing adrenocortical carcinomas with hypertension and hypokalemia have elevated urinary DOC metabolites or plasma DOC concentrations. We studied six adult patients with proven androgen-producing adrenocortical carcinomas (four women and two men, ranging from 28 to 51 years of age). Signs and symptoms of virilization were striking in the female patients. Retroperitoneal masses and inferior vena cava compression were present. All but one patient were hypertensive, and two had hypokalemia with potassium levels of 2.3 and 2.5 mEq/liter, respectively. Their baseline plasma steroid profile disclosed elevated androgen production, with androstenedione (494 ± 74 ng/dl, mean ± SEM) being the most consistent. Noteworthy was the elevation of 11-deoxycortisol in all six (971 ± 193 ng/dl, mean ± SEM) and of DOC in five of six (74.8 ± 37 ng/dl, mean ± SEM) (Table 5). The highest DOC levels (233 and 162 ng/dl) occurred in the two patients with hypokalemia (62).

Steroid levels were fixed and unresponsive to dexamethasone administration (2 or 8 mg/day for 2 days). In addition, the levels of the steroids distal to the block (cortisol, B, and 18-OHDOC) were normal or low and unresponsive to acute stimulation with exogenous ACTH. In the ZG, both aldosterone and 18-OHB were subnormal and did not respond to stimulation with ACTH or the upright posture. This probably was due to the combined effect of renin suppression, some degree of hypokalemia, and the enzymatic blockade [11β- and 18-hydroxylases (corticosterone methyloxidase)] in the ZG.

The steroid profile observed in these patients closely resembles that seen in the 11β-hydroxylase deficiency syndrome. The enzyme complex may be inhibited by intra-adrenal cortisol and androstenedione concentrations.

ACKNOWLEDGMENTS

This work was supported, in part, by U.S. Public Health Service grants from the National Institute of Arthritis, Me-

TABLE 5. *Plasma steroid concentrations in patients with androgen-producing adrenocortical carcinoma*[a]

	Cortisol (μg/dl)	S (ng/dl)	DOC (ng/dl)	Aldo (ng/dl)	18-OHB (ng/dl)	B (ng/dl)	18-OHDOC (ng/dl)
Basal values (*n* = 6, averaged):	18.6	971	74.8	3.0	14.6	537	5.7
SEM	4.2	193	36.8	1.0	7.5	235	3.4
Control values (*n* = 4):	13.9	985	67.5	2.5	7.3	343	2.3
SEM	2.8	214	49.5	1.1	3.7	181	1.3
Postural stimulation (*n* = 4):	15.0	787	82.8	3.6	8.7	352	3.8
SEM	3.8	222	64.9	1.0	3.8	193	1.8
ACTH stimulation (*n* = 4):	16.7	1107	85.0	9.8	24.7	572	7.0
SEM	5.2	169	57.9	4.5	3.8	205	1.6
Dex suppression (*n* = 4):	16.6	878	73.8	2.9	8.0	366	3.1
SEM	2.7	112	63.6	1.6	3.9	242	2.4
Normal range:	5.0–20.0	20–50	4.0–12.0	4.0–12.0	15.0–40.0	100–500	0–10.0

[a] S, 11-deoxycortisol; DOC, deoxycorticosterone; Aldo, aldosterone; 18-OHB, 18-hydroxycorticosterone; B, corticosterone; 18-OHDOC, 18-hydroxydeoxycorticosterone.

tabolism, and Digestive Diseases (AM-06415), the National Heart, Lung, and Blood Institute (HL-11046), and the Division of Research Resources, National Institutes of Health, General Clinical Research Center at San Francisco General Hospital Medical Center (RR00083C).

I. Irony is the recipient of a fellowship from CNPq, Conselho Nacional de Desenvolvimento Cientifico e Tecnologico, Brazil, under contract 20.0871/86.2-CL.

C. E. Kater is an established investigator in CNPq, Conselho Nacional de Desenvolvimento Cientifico e Tecnologico, Brazil, under contract 30.0449/81-CL.

REFERENCES

1. Schambelan M, Sebastian A, Biglieri EG, Hernandez R. Interaction potassium and the renin–angiotensin system in the control of aldosterone excretion in normal and pathophysiologic states. *Excerpta Med Int Congr* 1984;655:217–220.
2. Aguilera G, Kah KJ. Regulation of the sensitivity of the adrenal glomerulosa cell during altered sodium intake. In: Mantero F, Biglieri EG, Funder JW, Scoggins BA, eds. *The adrenal gland and hypertension,* vol 27. New York: Raven Press, 1986;33–53.
3. Zipser RD, Zia P, Stone RA, Horton R. The prostaglandin and kinin-kallikrein systems in mineralocorticoid escape. *J Clin Endocrinol Metab* 1978;47(5):996–1001.
4. Maestri E, Camellini L, Montanari R, et al. Aldosterone regulation: a role for serotonin. In: Mantero F, Biglieri EG, Funder JW, Scoggins BA, eds. *The adrenal gland and hypertension,* vol 27. New York: Raven Press, 1986;97–100.
5. Lis M, Hamet P, Gutowska J, et al. Effect of N-terminal portion of proopiomelanocortin on aldosterone release by human adrenal adenoma *in vitro. J Clin Endocrinol Metab* 1981;52:1052–1055.
6. Schambelan M, Sebastian A, Katuna BA, Arteaga E. Adrenocortical secretory response to chronic NHCl-induced metabolic acidosis. *Am J Physiol* 1987;252:454–460.
7. Carey RM. Acute dopaminergic inhibition of aldosterone secretion is independent of angiotensin II and adrenocorticotropin. *J Clin Endocrinol Metab* 1982;54:463–469.
8. Laragh JH. Atrial natriuretic hormone, renin–aldosterone axis and blood pressure electrolyte homeostasis. *N Engl J Med* 1985;313:1341–1346.
9. Richards AM, Ikram H, Yandlet G, et al. Renal, hemodynamic, and hormonal effects of human alpha atrial natriuretic peptide in healthy volunteers. *Lancet* 1985;1:545.
10. Biglieri EG, Schambelan M, Slaton PE. Effect of adrenocorticotropin on desoxycorticosterone, corticosterone and aldosterone excretion. *J Clin Endocrinol Metab* 1969;29:1090–1101.
11. Irony I, Biglieri EG, Perloff D. Pathophysiology of adrenal tumors with primary deoxycorticosterone excess. *J Clin Endocrinol Metab* 1987;65(5):836–840.
12. Wenting GJ, Man in't Veld AJ, Verhoeven RP, Derkx FH, Schalekamp MADH. Volume–pressure relationships during development of mineralocorticoid hypertension in man. *Circ Res* 1977;40(Suppl 1):163–170.
13. Gomez-Sanchez EP. Intracerebroventricular infusion of aldosterone induces hypertension in rats. *Endocrinology* 1986;819–823.
14. David SD, Griego MH, Cushman P. Adrenal glucocorticoids after twenty years: a review of their clinically relevant consequences. *J Chronic Dis* 1970;22:637–711.
15. Krakoff LR. Measurement of plasma renin substrate by radioimmunoassay of angiotensin I: concentration in syndromes associated with steroid excess. *J Clin Endocrinol Metab* 1973;37:110–117.
16. Scoggins BA, Butkus A, Denton DA, et al. ACTH dependent hypertension in sheep: a review of mechanisms involved in its production and modulation. In: Mantero BA, Biglieri EG, Funder JW, Scoggins BA, eds. *The adrenal gland and hypertension,* vol 27. New York: Raven Press, 1985;117–130.
17. Noth RH, Biglieri EG. Primary aldosteronism. *Med Clin North Am* 1988;72(5):1117–1131.
18. Biglieri EG. Syndrome of primary aldosteronism. In: Mantero F, Biglieri EG, Edwards CRW, eds. *Endocrinology of hypertension,* vol 50. New York: Academic Press, 1982;85.
19. Drury PL. Disorders of mineralocorticoid activity. *Clin Endocrinol Metab* 1985;14:175–202.
20. Lim RC, Nakayama DK, Biglieri EG, Schambelan M, Hunt TK. Primary aldosteronism: changing concepts in diagnosis and management. *Am J Surgery* 1986;152:116–121.
21. Schambelan M, Brust NL, Chang B, Slater K, Biglieri EG. Circadian rhythm and effects of posture in plasma aldosterone concentration in primary aldosteronism. *J Clin Endocrinol Metab* 1976;43:115–131.
22. Arteaga E, Klein RF, Biglieri EG. Use of saline infusion test to diagnose the cause of primary aldosteronism. *Am J Med* 1985;79:722–729.
23. Kater CE, Biglieri EG, Schambelan M, Arteaga E. Studies of impaired aldosterone response to spironolactive-induced renin and potassium elevations in adenomatosis but not hyperplastic primary aldosteronism. *Hypertension* 1983;5V-115–V-121.
24. Banks WA, Kastin AJ, Ruiz AE, Biglieri EG. Primary adrenal hyperplasia: a new subset of primary aldosteronism. *J Clin Endocrinol Metab* 1984;58:783–785.
25. Irony I, Kater CE, Arteaga E, Biglieri EG. Characteristics of correctable subtypes of primary aldosteronism. *Am J Hypertens* 1988;1(3, Pt 2):50A.
26. Gordon RD, Gomez-Sanchez CE, Hamlet SM, Tunny TJ, Klemm SA. Angiotensin-responsive aldosterone producing adenoma masquerades as idiopathic hyperaldosteronism of low renin essential hypertension. *J Hypertens* 1987;5(Suppl 5):S103–S106.

27. Farge D, Chatellier G, Pagny JY, Jeunemaitre X, Plouin PF, Corvol P. Isolated clinical syndrome of primary aldosteronism in four patients with adreno-cortical carcinoma. *Am J Med* 1987; 83(4):635–640.
28. Arteaga E, Biglieri EG, Kater CE, Lopez JM, Schambelan M. Aldosterone producing adrenocortical carcinoma; preoperative recognition and course in three cases. *Ann Intern Med* 1984;101(3):316–321.
29. Isles CG, MacDougall IC, Lever AF, Fraser R. Hypermineralocorticoidism due to adrenal carcinoma: plasma corticosteroids and their response to ACTH and angiotensin II. *Clin Endocrinol (Oxf)* 1987;26(2):239–251.
30. Taylor HC, Douglas JG, Berg GJ, Bravo EL. Primary aldosteronism caused by adrenal cortical carcinoma. *Endocrinol Jpn* 1982;29(6):701–708.
31. Jackson B, Valentine R, Wagner G. Primary aldosteronism due to a malignant ovarian tumor. *Aust NZ J Med* 1986;16(1):69–71.
32. Todesco S, Mantero F, Terribile V, Guarnieri GF, Borsati A. Ectopic aldosterone production. *Lancet* 1973;2(826):443.
33. Flanagan MJ, MacDonald JH. Heterotopic adrenocortical adenoma producing primary aldosteronism. *J Urology* 1967;98:133–139.
34. Ganguly A. New insights and questions about glucocorticoid-suppressible hyperaldosteronism. *Am J Med* 1982;72:851–854.
35. Stockight JR, Scoggins BA. Evolution of dexamethasone suppressible to idiopathic hyperaldosteronism. In: New M, Borrelli P, eds. *Dexamethasone-suppressible hyperaldosteronism,* Review #10. Rome: Ares-Serono Symposia.
36. Gomez-Sanchez CE, Gill JR, Ganguly A, Gordon RD. Glucocorticoid-suppressible aldosteronism: a disorder of the transitional zone. *J Clin Endocrinol Metab* 1988;67:444–448.
37. Ulick S. Evidence for defective functional zonation in adrenocortical hypertensive syndromes in man. In: Mantero F, Biglieri EG, Funder FW, Scoggins BD, eds. *The adrenal gland and hypertension.* Serono Symposium #27. New York: Raven Press, 1987; 357–361.
38. Richardson RL, Greco FA, Oldham RK, Liddle GW. Tumor products and potential markers in small cell lung cancer. *Semin Oncol* 1978;5:253.
39. Mason AMS, Ratcliff JB, Buckle RM, Mason AS. ACTH secretion by bronchial carcinoid tumors. *Clin Endocrinol (Oxf)* 1972;1:3.
40. Pimstone BL, Uys CJ, Vogelpoel L. Studies in a case of Cushing's syndrome due to an ACTH-producing thymic tumor. *Am J Med* 1972;53:251.
41. Shackleton CHL, Biglieri EG, Winter J, Gomez-Sanchez C. Evidence supporting the renal synthesis of 19-nor-DOC. *Clin Exp Hypertens* 1983;A6:939–949.
42. Griffing GT, Dale SL, Holbrook MM, Melby JC. The regulation of urinary free 19-nor deoxycorticosterone and its relation to systemic blood pressure in normotensive and hypertensive subjects. *J Clin Endocrinol Metab* 1983;56:99–103.
43. Aron DC, Tyrrell JB, Fitzgerald PC, Findling JW, Forsham PH. Cushing's syndrome: problems in diagnosis. *Medicine* 1981; 160:25.
44. Tyrrell JB, Fingling JW, Aron DC, Fitzgerald PA, Forsham PH. An overnight high dose dexamethasone suppression test for rapid differential diagnosis of Cushing's syndrome. *Ann Intern Med* 1986;104(2):180–186.
45. Boscaro M, Rampazzo A, Sonino N, Merola G, Scanarini M, Mantero F. Corticotropin releasing hormone stimulation test: diagnostic aspects in Cushing's syndrome. *J Endocrinol Invest* 1987;10(3):297–302.
46. Kindling JR, Aron DE, Tyrrell JB, et al. Selective venous sampling for ACTH in Cushing's syndrome: differentiation between Cushing's disease and the ectopic ACTH syndrome. *Ann Intern Med* 1981;94:647.
47. Hunt TD, Roizen MF, Tyrrell JB, Biglieri EG. Current achievements and challenges in adrenal surgery. *Br J Surg* 1984;71:983–985.
48. Bigos ST, Somma M, Rasio E, Eastman RC, Lanthier A, Johnston HH, Hardy J. Cushing's disease: management by transphenoidal pituitary microsurgery. *J Clin Endocrinol Metab* 1980;50:348.
49. Temple TE, Liddle GW. Inhibitors of adrenal steroid biosynthesis. *Annu Rev Pharmacol* 1970;10:199.
50. Sonino N, Boscaro M, Merola G, Mantero F. Prolonged treatment of Cushing's disease by ketoconazole. *J Clin Endocrinol Metab* 1985;61(4):718–722.
51. Becker D, Schumacher OP. O,p'DDD therapy in invasive adrenocortical carcinomas. *Ann Intern Med* 1975;82:677.
52. Krieger DT. Cyproheptadine for pituitary disorders. *N Engl J Med* 1976;295:394.
53. Lamberts SWJ, Klijn GJM, de Quijada M, et al. The mechanism of the suppressive action of bromocriptine on adrenocorticotropin secretion in patients with Cushing's disease and Nelson's syndrome. *J Clin Endocrinol Metab* 1980;51:307.
54. Ulick S, Ramirez LC, New MI. An abnormality in steroid reductive metabolism in a hypertensive syndrome. *J Clin Endocrinol Metab* 1977;44:799–802.
55. Ulick S, Levine LS, Gunczler P, et al. A syndrome of apparent mineralocorticoid excess associated with defects in the peripheral metabolism of cortisol. *J Clin Endocrinol Metab* 1979;49:757–764.
56. Stewart PM, Corrie JET, Shackleton CHL, Edwards CRW. The syndrome of "apparent mineralocorticoid excess." A defect in the cortisol-cortisone shuttle. *J Clin Invest* 1988;82:340–349.
57. Kondo K, Saruta T, Saito I, Yoshida R, Maruyama H, Matsuki S. Benign deoxycorticosterone producing adrenal tumor. *JAMA* 1976;236:1042–1044.
58. Powell-Jackson JD, Calin A, Fraser R. Excess deoxycorticosterone secretion from adrenocortical carcinoma. *Br Med J* 1974;2:32–44.
59. Levine LS, Rauh W, Gottesdiner H, et al. New studies of the 11beta-hydroxylation of 18-hydroxylase enzymes in hypertensive forms of congenital adrenal hyperplasia. *J Clin Endocrinol Metab* 1980;50:258–262.
60. Biglieri EG, Herron MA, Brust N. 17-Alpha hydroxylation deficiency in man. *J Clin Invest* 1966;45:1946–1954.
61. D'Armiento, Reda G, Kater CE, Biglieri EG. 17-Hydroxylase deficiency: mineralocorticoid hormone profiles in an affected family. *J Clin Endocrinol Metab* 1983;56:697–701.
62. Kater CE, Czepielewski MA, Biglieri EG, Irony I. Hypertension with deoxycorticosterone excess in androgen producing adrenocortical carcinoma. *J Hypertens* 1986;4(Suppl 6):S604–606.

Hypertension: Pathophysiology, Diagnosis, and Management, edited by J. H. Laragh and B. M. Brenner. Raven Press, Ltd., New York © 1990.

CHAPTER 101

The Syndrome of Hypertension with Hyperkalemia and Normal Glomerular Filtration Rate

A Rare Form of Hypertension

Richard D. Gordon, Terence J. Tunny, Shelley A. Klemm, and Stephen M. Hamlet

The Causes of Hyperkalemia, 1625
Internal Potassium Shifts, 1626
External Potassium Balance, 1626
Case Descriptions, 1627
Clinical Features, 1628
Hypertension, 1628
Short Stature, 1628
Muscle Weakness, 1629
Intellectual Impairment, 1629
Dental Abnormalities, 1630
Biochemical Features, 1630
Hyperkalemia, Hyperchloremia, and Acidemia, 1630
Renin and Aldosterone, 1630
Catecholamine Levels, 1630
Atrial Natriuretic Peptide (ANP) Levels, 1631
Effect of Prior Treatment, 1631
Renal Function, 1632
Glomerular Filtration Rate, 1632
Urinary Concentrating Ability, 1632
Urinary Acidification, 1632
Proximal Tubular Function: Clearance of Phosphate, Bicarbonate, and Lithium, 1632
Pathophysiology, 1632
Proposed Basic Mechanisms, 1632
Dynamic Testing to Elucidate the Pathophysiology, 1634
Relationships with Other Renal Tubular Disorders, 1636
Treatment, 1636
Dietary Salt Restriction, 1636
Diuretics, 1637
Cation-Exchange Resins, 1637
Conclusions and Unanswered Questions, 1637
References, 1637

Interest in the rare syndrome of hypertension and hyperkalemia despite normal glomerular filtration rate (H&H) centers around renal tubular mechanisms causing sodium/volume overload, hyperkalemia, and acidemia. As new patients with the syndrome are recognized, carefully studied, and reported, the database and our understanding both grow. With widespread screening for hypertension, routine autoanalyzer biochemical screening (regardless of presenting problem), and less use of thiazide diuretics as first-step therapy in uninvestigated hypertension, the syndrome of H&H may be more frequently recognized. Undoubtedly a rare form of hypertension, its recognition contributes to the continuing erosion of the large heterogeneous group of patients labeled "essential" or "primary" hypertensives.

THE CAUSES OF HYPERKALEMIA

The causes of hyperkalemia act through two distinct, but sometimes complementary, mechanisms. These mechanisms bring about an increase in total body potassium (external balance) on the one hand, or they produce an intracellular to extracellular shift of potassium (internal balance) on the other (Table 1). Only 1–2% of total body potassium is extracellular. The rest is held intracellularly by sodium/potassium-activated adenosine triphosphatase (Na^+/K^+ ATPase) at the cell membrane, responsible for the cell's resting transmembrane electrical potential. Disordered potassium balance can affect neuromuscular function (1) and, eventually, the function of all cells (2,3).

TABLE 1. *Factors affecting plasma K^+ levels*

1. Potassium flux across cell membranes
   a. Increased K^+ shift into cells, thereby lowering plasma K^+
      - Aldosterone
      - Beta-adrenoceptor agonists
      - Alpha-adrenoceptor antagonists
      - Metabolic alkalosis (H^+ out of cells, K^+ into cells)
      - Insulin action
      - Familial hypokalemic periodic paralysis (unknown mechanism)
   b. Increased K^+ release from cells, thereby raising plasma K^+
      - Cellular breakdown (e.g., red cells in circulation or gut)
      - Metabolic acidosis (H^+ into cells, K^+ out of cells)
      - Extracellular hypertonicity (H_2O out, K^+ out of cells)
      - Insulin deficiency
      - Beta-adrenoceptor antagonists
      - Alpha-receptor agonists
      - Familial hyperkalemic periodic paralysis (unknown mechanism)
2. External potassium balance
   a. Decreased intake or increased losses, thereby lowering plasma K^+
      - Anorexia, vomiting, diarrhea
      - Hyperaldosteronism
      - Metabolic alkalosis
      - Renal tubular acidosis (proximal or distal)
      - Diuretic therapy (thiazides, loop diuretics, acetazolamide)
      - Bartter's syndrome
      - Pseudohyperaldosteronism (Liddle's syndrome)
   b. Increased intake or reduced losses, thereby raising plasma K^+
      - Oral potassium supplements (if GFR reduced)
      - "Potassium-sparing" diuretics (spironolactone, amiloride, triamterene)
      - Hypoaldosteronism
        - Addison's disease
        - Isolated hypoaldosteronism
        - Hyporeninemic hypoaldosteronism
        - Chronic renal disease (lowers renin)
        - NSAIDs (lower renin)
      - Tubular resistance to aldosterone
        - Congenital (pseudohypoaldosteronism)
        - Acquired (lupus nephritis; amyloidosis; sickle cell nephropathy; obstructive uropathy; cyclosporine nephritis)
      - Critically reduced nephron population (CRF)
      - Distal renal tubular acidosis

Rapid movement of only a small fraction of total body potassium between the intracellular and extracellular compartments can cause potentially fatal changes in plasma potassium levels. Chronic hyper- or hypokalemia, on the other hand, is often very well tolerated.

Internal Potassium Shifts

Acidemia tends to cause hyperkalemia by driving hydrogen ions into the cell and driving potassium ions out of the cell (4). By a similar mechanism, hyperkalemia predisposes to acidemia by driving hydrogen ions out of the cell. Conversely, alkalemia draws hydrogen ions out of the cell, and their replacement by potassium ions predisposes to hypokalemia. Extracellular hypertonicity draws water out of the cell, and the higher resulting intracellular potassium concentration promotes diffusion of potassium out of the cell. Insulin stimulates Na^+/K^+ ATPase, and the administration of insulin and glucose is a method used to reduce hyperkalemia. Conversely, insulin deficiency promotes hyperkalemia. Beta-2-adrenoceptor agonists such as naturally secreted adrenaline, or salbutamol administered in the treatment of asthma, also stimulate Na^+/K^+ ATPase and tend to lower potassium levels. Conversely, beta-adrenoceptor blockers can raise potassium levels. Alpha-adrenoceptor agonists tend to raise plasma potassium by stimulating its release from liver cells and probably also from other cells. As well as its renal effects on external potassium balance, aldosterone is capable of stimulating potassium shift across many cell membranes, thereby promoting K^+ entry into cells and lowering plasma potassium. Breakdown of body cells, including red blood cells, releases large amounts of potassium into the extracellular compartment and is a potent cause of hyperkalemia, which is usually transient but potentially dangerous.

External Potassium Balance

Normal stool contains only 5–10 mEq of potassium, but vomiting or diarrhea can cause hypokalemia. In the absence of vomiting or diarrhea, the only significant route for potassium excretion is the kidney, and chronic hyperkalemia usually implies a defect in renal potassium excretion. The normal kidney has an enormous capacity to excrete potassium, and it is difficult to cause hyperkalemia by oral potassium loading in normal subjects. The filtered load of potassium is almost completely reabsorbed before the filtrate reaches the early distal tubule. In the distal tubule, some of the remaining sodium ions are reabsorbed, but this section of the nephron appears to be relatively impermeable to chloride. Although usually representing only a few percent of sodium ions filtered, sodium reabsorption at this point is a powerful mechanism for the fine control of sodium balance. Reabsorption of sodium without chloride generates luminal electronegativity; this promotes potassium and hydrogen ion excretion, depending on the availability of either. The number of potassium ions so excreted depends on (a) the delivery of sodium and chloride ions to the distal tubule, (b) the action of aldosterone, which promotes sodium reabsorption (and hence potassium excretion) at this site, and (c) the relative availability of potassium and hydrogen ions, as well as on other factors (5).

The most common cause of chronic hyperkalemia is diminished renal excretion of potassium secondary to critically reduced nephron population (6). In addition, the acidemia of chronic renal failure reduces potassium excretion, increases diffusion of potassium out of all cells, and promotes hyperkalemia. An important cause of reduced renal excretion of potassium is either (a) a deficiency of aldosterone or (b) a resistance to its action. In Addison's disease, deficient aldosterone action in the renal tubule causes hyperkalemia. The secondary effect of renal sodium wasting, which leads to hypovolemia and reduced glomerular filtration rate, is also important. Hyperkalemia also develops in isolated aldosterone deficiency (7) when cortisol secretion is intact. When there is a congenital tubular resistance to aldosterone action in the distal tubule, with secondary hyperreninemia and hyperaldosteronism (pseudohypoaldosteronism), hyperkalemia is again a feature (8). There are, as well, a number of acquired conditions in which the action of aldosterone in the distal tubule is defective. All these conditions are usually associated with both hyperkalemia and acidemia and are frequently referred to as *type 4 renal tubular acidosis* (9). Since "type 3" is generally considered the early childhood presentation of "type 1," a simpler classification, in which these are referred to as "hyperkalemic distal renal tubular acidosis," has been proposed (10). They can be theoretically divided into two groups, but the properties of the groups are sometimes shared. In one group, there is primarily aldosterone deficiency secondary to hyporeninemia (destruction of the juxtaglomerular apparatus or volume expansion suppressing renin production, or both); in the other group, there is primarily a tubular resistance to aldosterone and other mineralocorticoids (11,12). In the first group the urine can be acidified normally under appropriate conditions, whereas in the second group it cannot (13–15). Conditions in the second group include (a) diabetes mellitus, (b) interstitial nephritis due to infections or drugs such as methicillin and cyclosporine, (c) lupus nephritis, (d) amyloidosis, (e) sickle cell nephropathy, (f) obstructive uropathy, and (g) probably many other conditions associated with damage to the distal renal tubule (10), especially if there is some concomitant reduction in glomerular filtration rate resulting in an inability to excrete the prevailing dietary sodium load.

In patients with moderate reduction in nephron numbers, not in itself enough to cause hyperkalemia under normal circumstances, potentially dangerous hyperkalemia can be precipitated by a variety of circumstances, including (a) oral potassium supplements, (b) potassium-sparing diuretics, which either competitively inhibit aldosterone (spironolactone) or act at the same site independently of aldosterone to impair potassium excretion (amiloride, triamterene), (c) nonsteroidal anti-inflammatory drugs (NSAIDs), such as indomethacin, ibuprofen, and piroxicam, which inhibit renal prostaglandins, renin production, and renal sodium excretion, (d) sodium depletion (by reducing sodium load in the distal tubule), (e) dehydration (by reducing glomerular filtration rate), and (f) sodium loading (by further suppressing renin and aldosterone). Some of these patients are hypertensive and share with the disorder under discussion the features of hypertension and hyperkalemia (H&H).

Finally, the rare disorder that is the subject of this report is distinguished from most of the above conditions by the absence of any reduction in glomerular filtration rate (16–38). It is also distinguished by the severity of the hyperkalemia, which has exceeded 8 mEq/liter in some patients (16,17,25,29), and by the complete lack of symptoms in most mildly to moderately affected patients. Hypertension due to salt and water retention is usually present (16,17,20–23,26,28–34,36–38). Renin levels are low, as are aldosterone levels if hyperkalemia is corrected (17,21,28, 34), so that some degree of hyporeninemic hypoaldosteronism usually exists. In some patients, tubular responsiveness to mineralocorticoids can be demonstrated (17, 20,26,29,30,36,37), although, as in many other examples of hyporeninemic hypoaldosteronism and in contrast to Addison's disease, supernormal doses may be required. In others, in whom tubular resistance to aldosterone, DOCA, or fludrocortisone acetate has been demonstrated (18,21, 28,34), a chloride shunt in the distal tubule has been proposed (28). The syndrome of H&H can be classified in the group of disorders labeled "hyperkalemic distal renal tubular acidosis" (10).

CASE DESCRIPTIONS

The syndrome of hypertension and hyperkalemia (H&H) was first reported from Australia by Paver and Pauline (16) in 1964. A 15-year-old boy whose only complaints were headaches and enuresis presented requesting a medical certificate of fitness to commence factory work. The patient and his younger brother had absent maxillary lateral incisor teeth. His blood pressure was 180/120 mmHg and rose to unrecordable levels during cold pressor testing. Serum potassium ranged from 7.0 to 8.2 mEq/liter, and plasma phosphate was elevated at 5.6 mg%. Serum bicarbonate was reduced at 20 mEq/liter. Serum creatinine and urea, urea clearance, urinary concentrating ability, intravenous pyelography, renal angiography, and renal biopsy were all normal. Urine pH fell to 4.8 following oral ammonium chloride. Urinary sodium fell to 21 mEq/day on a Kempner low-sodium diet, but no other changes were observed during short-term dietary sodium restriction. Aldosterone excretion studies were attempted but were "unsatisfactory." His brother's blood pressure and serum biochemistry were normal. Paver and Pauline recognized that they were dealing with a new syndrome; thus they postulated that there existed a congenital renal tubular abnormality causing hyperkalemia, which then caused hypertension by stimulating aldosterone secretion. This same patient was later restudied by two other groups (39,40), but not before he had received treatment which included thiazide diuretics. Plasma renin activity levels were low, while plasma aldosterone levels were normal or raised, as compared to those of normokalemic subjects (39). Long-term treatment with chlorothiazide and sodium polystyrene sulfonate cation-exchange resin (and sometimes spironolactone as well) resulted in normal potassium and blood pressure levels (40). Hyperchloremia and acidemia, a renal defect in potassium excretion (appropriate balance studies), normal GFR, and pressor hyperresponsiveness to angiotensin were demonstrated (40). The patient's capacity to excrete potassium in response to oral acetazolamide and sodium sulfate infusion was normal only after low-sodium diet and oral fludrocortisone, but not before (40). A significant relationship between serum potassium and diastolic blood pressure was noted and was thought to be possibly causal (40). Now aged 21, the patient complained of attacks of muscle weakness when untreated. His mother was normokalemic, and his father was dead.

The second patient with H&H despite normal renal glomerular function was also Australian, with no evidence of other affected family members (17). A girl aged 10, she presented with short stature, attacks of muscle weakness following food or exercise, intellectual impairment, absent lateral maxillary incisor teeth, hypertension (160/110 mmHg), hyperkalemia (8.5 mEq/liter), hyperchloremia (117 mEq/liter), and acidemia (bicarbonate 14 mEq/liter, arterial pH 7.30). Creatinine clearance, urinary concentrating ability, intravenous pyelography, renal arteriography, and renal biopsy were all normal. Urinary pH was 5.15 when arterial pH was 7.30. Unlike the first patient, renin and aldosterone were measured before any treatment was commenced. Plasma renin activity was undetectable, whereas aldosterone excretion was in the lower part of the normal range, falling to very low levels when hyperkalemia was corrected using sodium polystyrene sulfonate, while maintaining sodium balance (17). Like the first patient, extreme pressor hyperresponsiveness to pressor stimuli (cold, norepinephrine, and angiotensin II) was present. Unlike the first patient, there was well-documented correction of this hyperresponsiveness by short-term dietary sodium restriction, which also caused (a) lowering of basal blood pressure and (b) cessation of attacks of weakness. Her mother used unusually large quantities of salt in cooking, and this practice was modified. Long-term (5 months) dietary sodium restriction resulted in (a) correction of expanded plasma volume, (b) elevation of renin and aldosterone levels to normal for an unrestricted diet, and (c) correction of hypertension, hyperkalemia, hyperchloremia, and acidemia. During 2 years of dietary sodium restriction as sole therapy, attacks of weakness ceased and she grew 3.8 in. taller. While she was receiving a 10 mEq/day sodium diet, a single dose of 0.5 mg cyclopenthiazide lowered plasma potassium to 2.8 mEq/liter. Moderate dietary sodium restriction and thiazide diuretic proved to be effective long-term treatment over the next 20 years. Renin and aldosterone rose to levels which were supernormal for an unrestricted diet, and plasma potassium levels were in the low-normal range and, occasionally, subnormal.

The low pretreatment aldosterone (allowing for potassium levels) and striking response to low-salt diet led the authors to conclude that this was yet another new syndrome. They postulated that this syndrome involves excessive renal sodium retention (proximal to where aldosterone acts), resulting in sodium/volume expansion, hypertension, suppression of renin/aldosterone, and impaired potassium excretion. It was this syndrome of hypertension, expanded extracellular fluid volume, and hyperkalemia—correctable by dietary sodium restriction and possibly due to excess sodium reabsorption by the proximal tubule—which de Wardener labeled *Gordon's syndrome* (41). The full syndrome consists of hypertension, hyperkalemia, hyperchloremic acidosis, muscle weakness, short stature, and intellectual impairment. Muscle weakness, impaired skeletal growth, and intellectual impairment are probably consequences of the severe biochemical derangement and might be expected to be lacking in less severely affected patients. Since all adults, but not all children, with the biochemical syndrome were hypertensive (42,43), and hyperkalemic patients with and without hypertension (Table 1) were seen in the same family (20,22,24,26,30,35,37,38), it seems likely that the syndrome minus hypertension represents an earlier stage in its development. The appearance of hypertension could depend on factors such as dietary salt and an inherited inability to resist it.

A second example of the full syndrome was reported in 1986, again from Australia (33), this time a girl aged 14 at presentation. The three Australian patients (16,17,33) had no other affected family members, nor were they blood relatives. By the close of 1988, at least 40 patients (23 males) with H&H had been reported from Australia, Israel, the United States, Japan, England, Scotland, Finland, France, and the Netherlands (Table 2). Twenty-eight of these patients belonged to seven families from Australia (seven in two generations), Israel (seven in three generations), the United States (six in three generations and two in two generations), England (two in two generations), Japan (two in one generation), and Finland (two in one generation). We have recently investigated a family from Brisbane (Australia) with H&H (Fig. 1), with at least seven living affected members in two generations, suggesting a high degree of penetrance (37). The three Australian sporadic cases all had missing maxillary lateral incisor teeth, but this feature is not present in the Brisbane family. This type of congenital dental abnormality is present in up to 1.7% of the normal population (44,45).

It is doubtless that other patients with the syndrome have been studied and that even more remain unrecognized. A patient with the syndrome given thiazide diuretic as treatment for hypertension might simply be regarded as a good responder. The published findings in 28 patients with the syndrome were reviewed in 1986 (42,43).

CLINICAL FEATURES

Hypertension

In patients older than 20 years with H&H, blood pressure has usually been raised before treatment with low-salt diet or diuretic. Often of severe degree (16,20–22,29,31–33), the hypertension was complicated by stroke in one patient (32). Children reported with the hyperkalemic syndrome aged 11, 10, 9, 9, 9, 6, 5, 4, 3, 2, and 1 years were normotensive, whereas others aged 15, 15, 14, 14, 13, and 10 years were hypertensive, suggesting that hypertension may develop with increasing age. Dietary salt restriction improved or removed the hypertension in some patients (17,20,21,29,36). Time of onset of hypertension, as well as the severity of hypertension, may be influenced by (a) age, (b) habitual dietary sodium intake, and (c) genetic factors predisposing to, or protecting from, hypertension.

Short Stature

The prime reason for presentation was short stature in four patients first seen during childhood (17–19,27), and short stature was present as an incidental finding in seven others (25,26,29,30,32,33) (Table 2). The hyperkalemia was severe in many of these, accompanied by severe acide-

TABLE 2. *Reported cases of hyperkalemia and acidemia with normal GFR*

Features	Case no.	Hyperkalemia and acidemia	Short stature	Hypertension	Sex[a]	Age	Familial[b]	Country	Reference
Hyperkalemia, acidemia, short stature, hypertension	1	+	+	+	F	10	No	Australia	17
	2	+	+	+	M	52	Yes (a)	USA	26
	3	+	+	+	F	13	Yes (b)	USA	29
	4	+	+	+	M	26	Yes (a)	USA	30
	5	+	+	+	M	24	Yes (a)	USA	30
	6	+	+	+	F	14	No	Australia	33
	7	+	+	+	M	33	No	Scotland	32
Hyperkalemia, acidemia, short stature	1	+	+	−	M	11	No	USA	18
	2	+	+	−	M	9	No	USA	19
	3	+	+	−	M	3	Yes (c)	Japan	25
	4	+	+	−	M	13	No	USA	27
Hyperkalemia, acidemia, hypertension	1	+	−	+	M	15	No	Australia	16
	2	+	−	+	M	29	Yes (d)	Israel	20
	3	+	−	+	M	21	Yes (d)	Israel	20
	4	+	−	+	M	52	Yes (d)	Israel	21
	5	+	−	+	F	28	Yes (d)	Israel	21
	6	+	−	+	F	23	Yes (d)	Israel	21
	7	+	−	+	M	33	Yes (e)	England	22
	8	+	−	+	F	17	No	USA	23
	9	+	−	+	M	54	Yes (a)	USA	26
	10	+	−	+	M	23	No	USA	28
	11	+	−	+	F	15	No	Finland	31
	12	+	−	+	M	17	No	France	34
	13	+	−	+	M	14	No	Netherlands	36
	14	+	−	+	M	40	Yes (f)	Australia	37
	15	+	−	+	M	38	Yes (f)	Australia	37
	16	+	−	+	F	19	Yes (g)	Finland	38
Hyperkalemia, acidemia	1	+	−	−	M	10	Yes (d)	Israel	20
	2	+	−	−	F	4	Yes (d)	Israel	20
	3	+	−	−	F	9	Yes (e)	England	24
	4	+	−	−	F	2	Yes (c)	Japan	25
	5	+	−	−	M	5	Yes (a)	USA	30
	6	+	−	−	F	5	Yes (a)	USA	30
	7	+	−	−	F	Birth	Yes (b)	USA	35
	8	+	−	−	F	37	Yes (f)	Australia	37
	9	+	−	−	F	9	Yes (f)	Australia	37
	10	+	−	−	F	6	Yes (f)	Australia	37
	11	+	−	−	M	5	Yes (f)	Australia	37
	12	+	−	−	F	1	Yes (f)	Australia	37
	13	+	−	−	M	18	Yes (g)	Finland	38

[a] F, female; M, male.
[b] The letters a through g represent seven different families.

mia, and these biochemical abnormalities may be responsible (9). An increase in growth rate was observed in three children during treatment which corrected hyperkalemia and acidemia (17,18,27).

Muscle Weakness

Although it is a striking feature of conditions associated with rapid changes in plasma potassium (such as hyperkalemic and hypokalemic familial periodic paralysis), muscle weakness was complained of infrequently by the patients afflicted by the chronic, stable hyperkalemia of H&H and was noted in only five patients (16,17,25,36,40), often after exercise or meals, and vanished after correction of hyperkalemia by low-salt diet (17) or thiazide diuretic (17,40). In each of these patients, plasma potassium had been observed to exceed 7.8 mEq/liter on several occasions. Since the resting transmembrane electrical potential depends primarily on the maintenance of the intracellular to extracellular potassium concentration gradient by sodium/potassium-activated ATPase, it is not surprising that severe hyperkalemia is associated with disordered muscle function. The beneficial effect of low-salt diet on muscle weakness was repeatedly observed within days in the severely affected (potassium 8.5 mEq/liter) patient described by Gordon et al. (17), before any significant changes in external sodium or potassium balance could have occurred.

Intellectual Impairment

Only two patients were significantly mentally retarded (17,33). Both had severe hyperkalemia (up to 8.5 and 7.4

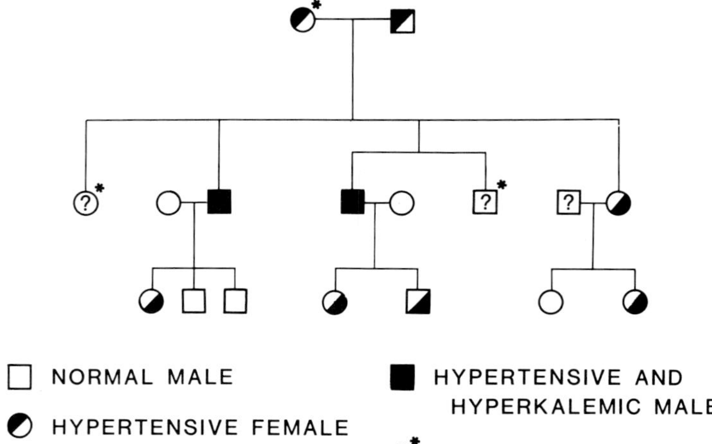

FIG. 1. Pedigree of a Brisbane family with at least seven members in two generations affected by the syndrome of H&H.

mEq/liter, respectively), acidemia, and short stature. The effects on intellectual function of treatment which lowered potassium to normal have not been documented, in these or other patients, but one of them (17) has been gainfully employed during treatment for 14 years in a clothing factory which caters to the intellectually handicapped.

Dental Abnormalities

Failure of development of permanent teeth is not an uncommon abnormality in otherwise healthy individuals (44,45), and the maxillary lateral incisors are absent in up to 1.7% of the normal population. It may therefore be simply a coincidence that this particular abnormality was present in three unrelated, but severely affected, Australian patients (16,17,33). It was looked for and was not present in the family reported by Bravo et al. (26), in the Brisbane family (37), and in several other sporadic cases, and so it is an inconsistent feature and is not a useful clinical marker.

BIOCHEMICAL FEATURES

Hyperkalemia, Hyperchloremia, and Acidemia

Hyperkalemia was always present, but it varied in severity, falling to 5.2 and 5.3 mEq/liter without treatment on various occasions in some patients (28,34), but never falling below 7.0 mEq/liter without treatment in others (16–18). Hyperchloremia ranging from 105 to 117 mEq/liter was noted in every patient in whom it was measured. Plasma bicarbonate was reduced in 33 of 36 patients for whom levels were reported, ranging as low as 14 mEq/liter (17,18,29) and 13 mEq/liter (19). Arterial pH was measured in nearly every case and was consistently reduced.

In general the hyperkalemia and acidemia were very well tolerated, with some patients asymptomatic despite potassium levels of 6.5–7.5 mEq/liter. Some complained of muscle weakness and growth failure, which were corrected by treatment; in one patient, nerve conduction velocity increased after correction of hyperkalemia (17). One patient with plasma potassium of 9.6 mEq/liter presented with cardiac arrhythmia and disturbed consciousness (25).

Renin and Aldosterone

Renin levels were consistently low, and often very low, at presentation. Aldosterone levels were usually normal or elevated when compared with those of normokalemic subjects, but they fell to very low levels if plasma potassium was lowered to normal with a cation-exchange resin (17,21,28,34). During treatment with low-salt diet or thiazide diuretic, levels of renin and aldosterone increased into the normal range for unrestricted diet and sometimes much higher. If diuretic treatment was ceased, they slowly returned toward pretreatment levels. Thus, levels on presentation were influenced by previous treatment.

In the patients studied by Farfel et al. (20) and Brautbar et al. (21), and in three patients with H&H studied by us, aldosterone was briskly responsive to infused angiotensin. In the three patients we studied, saline infusion caused further suppression of renin, but the response of aldosterone was influenced also by concurrent changes in plasma potassium, which tended to rise (Fig. 2). In their patient with H&H, Nahum et al. (34) found a close correlation between plasma potassium and aldosterone. It is clear that aldosterone responds to the stimuli of rising angiotensin and potassium levels in the syndrome of H&H, and we observed a brisk response of plasma aldosterone to ACTH in two patients studied recently.

Catecholamine Levels

Normal plasma and urinary catecholamine levels were reported in the patient described by Wayne et al. (33), and normal urinary catecholamines were reported in the patient discussed by Sanjad et al. (29). Basally, and after the stimuli of isometric exercise, mental arithmetic, and cold pressor, plasma adrenaline and noradrenaline were normal

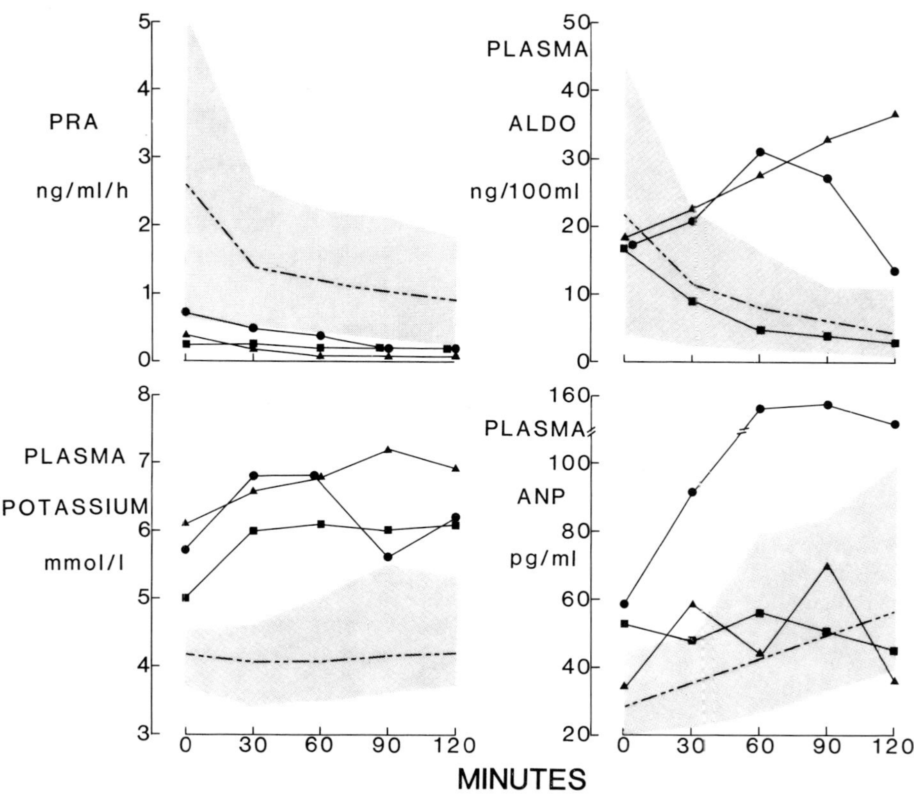

FIG. 2. Responses of plasma renin activity (PRA), plasma potassium, plasma aldosterone, and plasma atrial natriuretic peptide (ANP) to infusion of normal saline (2 liters in 2 hr) in three patients with the syndrome of H&H. The patients whose data are shown by triangles and circles are brothers. The range of normal responses is shown by the shaded area and the mean response by the broken line.

in a patient (17) restudied by us, and basal plasma catecholamines were normal in two hypertensive and hyperkalemic brothers (Fig. 1). Because of observed hyperresponsiveness to infused noradrenaline and to cold stimulation, normal levels of circulating catecholamines do not exclude a role for the sympathetic nervous system in the hypertension which these patients exhibit.

Atrial Natriuretic Peptide (ANP) Levels

Modestly elevated levels of ANP have been reported by us in H&H (37,46,47), but they are lower than those seen in primary aldosteronism, another condition with sodium/volume overload (Fig. 3). However, levels in the lower part of the normal range have recently been found in two patients with H&H (38).

EFFECT OF PRIOR TREATMENT

Because of its potential to mislead, the important effect of prior treatment on clinical and biochemical features must be stressed. Thus the patient studied by Licht et al. (30) who had been hypertensive and hyperkalemic 5 years earlier, and then treated with thiazide diuretic ceasing 5 months before re-presentation, was still normotensive. The patient studied by Farfel et al. (20) had a diastolic blood pressure (BP) of 120–140 mmHg and a potassium level of

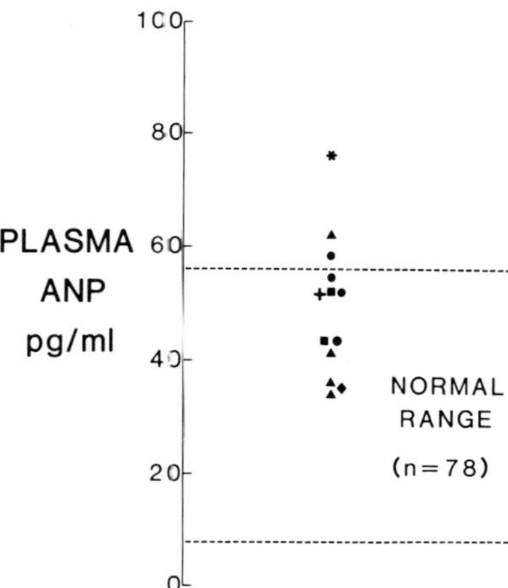

FIG. 3. Plasma atrial natriuretic peptide (ANP) levels in six patients with the syndrome of H&H, all taking moderately restricted sodium diets. The circles and triangles show data from two brothers, and the asterisk and cross show data from the two children of one of them.

6.4–6.7 mEq/liter before any treatment, but, after ceasing treatment with thiazide diuretic for 1 month, the BP was 170/90 mmHg and the potassium was 5.4–6.4 mEq/liter. When treatment with bendrofluazide was withdrawn for 3 weeks in the patient reported by Gordon and Hodsman (32), plasma potassium was 3.9–5.5 mEq/liter compared with 5.0–7.0 mEq/liter before treatment; the BP, which had been 240/140 mmHg before treatment, remained normal.

RENAL FUNCTION

Glomerular Filtration Rate

All patients had normal plasma creatinine, and many had clearance measurements of creatinine, inulin, or ^{51}Cr-EDTA which were normal. This is an essential ingredient of the syndrome of H&H; it serves to distinguish this syndrome from many otherwise similar conditions, in which moderate or severe reduction in GFR contributes to the development of hyperkalemia.

Urinary Concentrating Ability

This has invariably been normal when tested (16–19,21,22,25,26,28,29,34,36), consistent with normal vasopressin secretion and renal responsiveness.

Urinary Acidification

Basal urinary pH in the face of prevailing acidemia was usually appropriately reduced (17,28,30,32), and urine pH fell below 5.0 in many patients (16,19,21,22,26,28–30,32,34,38) subjected to the ammonium chloride loading test of Wrong and Davies (48). Net secretion of acid and ammonium was normal (29,34), rather than raised to the high levels expected in acidemia, but could be stimulated by low-sodium diet (29), presumably by significantly increasing aldosterone levels. These findings are consistent with significant mineralocorticoid activity in the distal tubule, both basally and after stimulation by low-salt diet (13–15).

Proximal Tubular Function: Clearance of Phosphate, Bicarbonate, and Lithium

The renal regulation of phosphate excretion is complex (49), but volume expansion, as occurs in the syndrome of H&H, tends to reduce phosphate reabsorption in the proximal tubule (50,51). The unexpected finding of elevated plasma phosphate levels in two patients (16,22), as well as levels at the upper limit of normal in two others (18,19), raises the possibility of deranged proximal tubular function, but there are many other possible explanations. Lithium is thought to be almost completely reabsorbed in the proximal tubule by mechanisms similar to those regulating sodium reabsorption, and so lithium clearance in the syndrome of H&H is of interest. Basal lithium clearance in the girl with H&H described by Gordon et al. (17) was reduced compared with normal subjects (*unpublished observations*), consistent with hyperactive sodium reabsorption in the proximal tubule.

Bicarbonate clearance is normally close to zero, due to complete reabsorption in the proximal tubule (10,11,13). However, both volume expansion (52) and hyperkalemia (53) can reduce bicarbonate reabsorption in the proximal tubule. Not surprisingly, therefore, the renal threshold for bicarbonate was reduced to 18–21 mEq/liter (normal range 24–30 mEq/liter) in a number of patients with H&H (18–20,25,29,30,34) but was restored to normal (34) by reduction of hyperkalemia. The bicarbonaturia seen was mild and was not in the range seen in proximal renal tubular acidosis.

PATHOPHYSIOLOGY

Proposed Basic Mechanisms

Tubular Avidity for Sodium and Chloride as Sole Mechanism

Proposed by Gordon et al. (17) after detailed study of a severely affected patient, the basic mechanism would be excessive sodium and chloride reabsorption occurring in the nephron proximal to where aldosterone acts. The volume expansion would then, through suppression of renin and aldosterone and a reduced fraction of filtered sodium reabsorbed in the distal tubule, lead to reduced excretion of potassium and hydrogen ions. A new equilibrium would be established, utilizing those forces which cause proximal tubular rejection of sodium ions once volume expansion had developed. The excessive sodium reabsorption could occur in the proximal tubule, loop of Henle, or early distal tubule. This hypothesis, which depends on the presence of relative hypoaldosteronism (given potassium levels) secondary to hyporeninemia, was confirmed in a number of patients when potassium was lowered to normal (17,21,28,34). This excessive potassium reabsorption then causes hyperkalemia and acidemia (11,42,43). The response to low-salt diet and to diuretics is explained by reduction of hypervolemia stimulating renin and aldosterone. The tubule must be capable of responding to mineralocorticoid for this hypothesis to be correct.

Chloride Shunt in the Distal Tubule

Proposed by Schambelan et al. (28,54) after detailed study of a mildly affected patient, the basic mechanism would be failure of the normal barrier to chloride reabsorption in the distal tubule. When sodium reabsorption is accompanied by chloride, the electrical gradient necessary for excretion of potassium and hydrogen ions cannot be developed. Hyperkalemia and acidemia result. Why should such patients become volume expanded and hypertensive? The hypothesis suggests that "increased reabsorptive avidity for chloride" augments distal sodium reabsorption. An alternative explanation would be that hyperkalemia stimu-

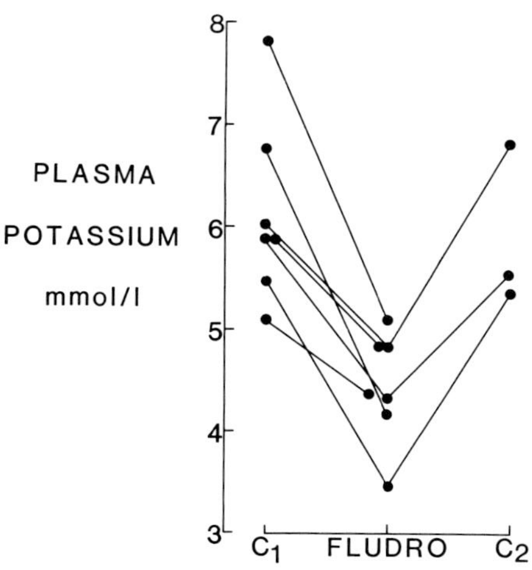

FIG. 4. Response of plasma potassium to oral fludrocortisone acetate (approximately 6 μg/kg/day in four divided doses) for 5–7 days in seven patients with the syndrome of H&H. Pre- and post-treatment control observations are shown as C_1 and C_2, respectively.

lates aldosterone, which then increases reabsorption of sodium and chloride. Volume expansion would reduce proximal sodium reabsorption, increase sodium delivery to the distal tubule, and eventually swamp the distal tubular sodium reabsorptive mechanism, thereby restoring balance. According to this hypothesis, aldosterone cannot promote excretion of potassium and hydrogen ions, and plasma potassium does not fall in response to mineralocorticoids. However, such a fall has been observed in many patients with H&H (Table 3) and in all patients studied by us (Fig. 4). Thiazide diuretics could presumably swamp the distal sodium reabsorptive site (with sodium being rejected more proximally), thereby reducing plasma volume and hypertension. Although thiazide diuretics might increase distal delivery of potassium, how they could so rapidly reduce plasma potassium is not readily explained by this theory, since no matter how much sodium is being reabsorbed distally, an electrical gradient to favor potassium excretion could not be established. A well-developed chloride shunt would permanently limit distal excretion of hydrogen ion. Ability to reduce urinary pH "normally" in response to an NH_4Cl load (48) would not be expected, but it has usually been observed in H&H (16,19,21,22,26,28–30,32,34,38).

The dichotomous responses to mineralocorticoids (Table 3) suggest that either of the two mechanisms just described, rather than a combination of both, is present in a given patient, since responsiveness is mandatory in the first case but could not occur in the second case. Administration of spironolactone during thiazide treatment of H&H would test the response of the tubule to endogenous aldosterone and would be most informative in apparently mineralocorticoid-resistant patients.

Generalized Membrane Defects

Proposed by Farfel et al. (20,55) after study of a mildly affected Jewish family (plasma K^+ 5.2–6.2 mEq/liter), the basic mechanism would be inability to transport potassium into the cell as a result of faulty membrane function. The intravenous infusion of four units of insulin over a period of 1 hr (with and without infusion of glucose) had little effect on plasma potassium. The affected family studied by Bravo et al. (26) responded normally, as did the patient described by Nahum et al. (34); also responding normally were two patients recently studied by us (37), whose plasma K^+ fell normally after intravenous infusion of 0.12 units/kg insulin (56). It is quite feasible that a cell permeability problem affecting sodium or chloride transfer in the kidney

TABLE 3. *Response to mineralocorticoid hormone*

Group no.	Patient no.	Sex[a]	Age	Familial	Test medication	Plasma K^+ Basal	Plasma K^+ Test	Urine Na^+/K^+ Basal	Urine Na^+/K^+ Test	Reference
Group 1, responsive	1	F	10	No	Aldosterone	7.7–8.5	—	51/21	10/25	17
	1	F	10	No	Spironolactone	7.7–8.5	—	65/20	81/11	17
	2	M	48	Yes	Fludrocortisone	5.4–6.4	—	189/71	88/97	20
	3	M	54	Yes	Fludrocortisone	5.8	4.9	—	—	26
	4	M	52	Yes	Fludrocortisone	5.7	4.6	—	—	26
	5	F	13	No	Fludrocortisone	6.1–8.6	—	147/12	111/33	29
	6	M	26	Yes	DOCA	5.2	4.2	—	—	30
	6	M	26	Yes	Fludrocortisone	5.1	4.4	—	—	30
	7	M	14	No	DOCA	—	—	180/18	105/28	36
	8	M	40	Yes	Fludrocortisone	6.0	4.8	—	—	37
	9	M	38	Yes	Fludrocortisone	5.9	3.7	—	—	37
	10	F	9	Yes	Fludrocortisone	6.1	4.9	—	—	37
	11	F	6	Yes	Fludrocortisone	6.8	4.2	—	—	37
	12	M	5	Yes	Fludrocortisone	7.7	5.1	—	—	37
Group 2, unresponsive	1	M	11	No	Fludrocortisone	7.3–7.7	6.1–6.9	—	—	18
	1	M	11	No	Aldosterone	6.0	5.8	—	—	18
	2	M	15	Yes	Fludrocortisone	6.0	6.0	—	—	21
	3	M	23	No	Fludrocortisone	5.0	5.0	—	—	28
	4	M	22	No	Fludrocortisone	5.3–6.9	5.8–7.0	—	—	34

[a] F, female; M, male.

could affect all cells. Problems with transmembrane transfer of sodium and potassium are unlikely to affect only one organ. As with the other proposed mechanisms, this deficiency could be partial. Soppi et al. (31) studied the red-cell sodium–potassium pump and the red-cell sodium–lithium countertransport in their affected Finnish patient, but found no abnormality.

Deficiency of Vasodilator Prostaglandins

After studying a patient with the syndrome of H&H (22), reviewing the literature, and considering H&H as the opposite of Bartter's syndrome, Tormey and Morgan (57) proposed as a mechanism causing hypertension and hyperkalemia a switch in intrarenal synthesis of prostaglandins from PGE_2 (vasodilator) to PGF_2 (vasoconstrictor). When they elaborated this hypothesis in 1980, prostaglandins had not been measured in the syndrome of H&H. Three years later, Sanjad et al. (58) reported markedly subnormal excretion of urinary prostaglandin E_2 in their patient with H&H (29), which increased 20-fold during treatment with furosemide, with correction of the biochemical abnormalities and the hypertension. Sanjad et al. then proposed (58) that renal hypoprostaglandism might have a pathogenetic role in the syndrome of H&H by enhancing chloride reabsorption in the ascending limb of the loop of Henle. Since salt restriction did not elevate prostaglandins in their patient but did improve the hypertension and the biochemical abnormalities, hypoprostaglandism does not appear to be a sole and sufficient explanation for the syndrome. Furthermore, normal levels of prostaglandins have recently been reported in a 14-year-old boy with H&H (36).

Deficient Chloriuretic or Natriuretic Hormone Secretion

While briefly reporting a young woman with H&H (23), Grekin et al. proposed a deficiency of "chloriuretic hormone" as the mechanism; they also proposed an excess of this hormone to explain Bartter's syndrome. This was before the natriuretic hormone secreted by the atria had been described, along with its action, and Grekin et al. postulated that chloriuretic hormone acted in the thick ascending limb of Henle's loop, with an action similar to that of loop diuretics. Such a chloriuretic hormone has yet to be isolated and synthesized. Basal levels of ANP so far reported in the syndrome of H&H have not been clearly subnormal (37,38,46,47).

In a similar vein, it could be said that patients with Bartter's syndrome behaved as though exposed to too much, and with Gordon's syndrome to too little, thiazide diuretic. The site of action of thiazides deserves special attention.

Renal Resistance to ANP

Recently, based on studies in a 14-year-old boy with H&H, it has been proposed that lack of sensitivity of the kidney to ANP is an important pathophysiological mechanism in H&H (36).

Dynamic Testing to Elucidate the Pathophysiology

Pressor Sensitivity to Cold, Angiotensin, and Noradrenaline

Pressor hypersensitivity has been consistently present, lies in the range seen in primary aldosteronism, and presumably reflects sodium/volume overload. It changed rapidly toward normal following institution of dietary sodium restriction (17).

Response of the Renal Tubule and of Other Tissues to Mineralocorticoid Hormones

The ability of the renal tubule to respond to mineralocorticoid hormones is crucial to an examination of the first two proposed mechanisms. In one proposal the ability is there, but it is exercised subnormally because of suppressed renin–angiotensin levels. In the other, it is absent.

Measurable aldosterone, often in the normal range for normokalemia but low for hyperkalemia, was indeed exerting an effect which could be unmasked by administration of spironolactone in one patient (17), demonstrating that the tubule was already responding to endogenous aldosterone. If the chloride shunt hypothesis were correct for this patient, no effect would be expected. Administered aldosterone or fludrocortisone acetate exerted the expected effect on plasma potassium or on urinary Na/K ratio in most patients (Table 3). This has been so in all patients studied by us (Fig. 4). We also observed, in a severely affected girl with potassium 8.5 mEq/liter (17), directional changes in salivary and sweat sodium and potassium consistent with a response to administered aldosterone. It is difficult to say if renal tubular responsiveness is normal, since the dosage of fludrocortisone has varied from twice to four times the usual replacement dose for Addison's disease. It is only possible to say that the tubule is capable of responding.

In what appears to be a distinct subset of patients, more or less complete resistance to administered fludrocortisone acetate has been observed (Table 3). The dose of fludrocortisone administered was similar (0.2–0.4 mg daily) in both groups shown in Table 3; the exception was the dose given by Nahum et al. (34), who administered 200 mg daily for 2 weeks without changing plasma potassium level (5.8–7.0 mEq/liter).

Response to Infusions of Mannitol, Sodium Chloride, Sodium Bicarbonate, Sodium Sulfate

Farfel et al. (55) observed a 30- to 60-fold increase in urinary sodium during infusion of 1000 ml of 20% mannitol over a period of 2.5 hr, as well as during infusion of 750 ml of 4% sodium sulfate over a period of 3 hr. The mannitol induced a 25-fold increase in urinary potassium and the sulfate induced a 13-fold increase. The mannitol exerts an effect by increasing (a) distal delivery of potassium, (b) flow rate, and (c) sodium load in the distal tubule. The very large kaliuresis suggests that the normal kaliuretic mechanism (luminal electronegativity due to sodium reabsorption without chloride) was operative in that patient, and this is evidence against a significant chloride shunt. A powerful kaliuresis following a sodium sulfate load is normal and has no bearing on the presence of a chloride shunt. This matter was explored by several workers (28–30,34,40), who compared kaliuretic responses to sodium chloride and sodium sulfate in patients with H&H and in a small number of normal subjects. Arnold and Healy (40) observed a markedly subnormal kaliuretic effect of sodium sulfate in their patient with H&H, which (a) was increased to normal when endogenous mineralocorticoid activity was stimulated by prior salt depletion and (b) was augmented by administration of fludrocortisone acetate. This suggests an initially hypofunctioning mineralocorticoid mechanism. Sanjad et al. (29) also found no increase in urinary potassium excretion when sulfate was infused during a high-salt diet, but they observed a fourfold increase when it was infused after prior sodium depletion. Both these findings are consistent with the basal potassium retention being due to inadequate mineralocorticoid activity, as a result of either inadequate levels or a partial tubular resistance to mineralocorticoid hormones. Stimulation of aldosterone secretion by either low-salt diet (17,29) or diuretics (16–20,22,24,28–30,33,34) appears to restore the kaliuretic mechanism to normal, favoring inadequate aldosterone action in the basal state as the fundamental abnormality. We observed a doubling of urinary potassium excretion during saline infusion (2 liters in 2 hr) in two brothers with H&H habitually taking a sodium restricted diet (37), and Valimaki et al. also observed a normal kaliuresis during saline infusion in a brother and sister with H&H (38). Sodium bicarbonate infusion trebled the fractional excretion of potassium in one study (34), and doubled it in another (29), presumably because more potassium reached the distal tubule and because bicarbonate is poorly absorbed there. Schambelan et al. (28) and Licht et al. (30) also reported a normal kaliuretic response to sodium sulfate plus bicarbonate (28) or to sodium sulfate alone (30) in their patients, after mineralocorticoid activity was stimulated by dietary sodium restriction or DOCA administration. Schambelan et al. (28) and Licht et al. (30) both employed dietary sodium restriction before infusing sodium sulfate, but not before infusing sodium chloride, and then compared the kaliuretic response. For 12–24 hr before both infusions, DOCA was administered. The kaliuretic response to sulfate was, of course, much higher than that to chloride infusion and was closer to that seen in normal subjects. With such small subject numbers, it is difficult to make sound quantitative, or even qualitative, comparisons with normal. If the mechanism of variable and usually incomplete resistance to mineralocorticoids is a chloride shunt, then this may represent a common mechanism with a wide spectrum of severity. Against this concept is the fact that two of the patients with extreme mineralocorticoid resistance had modest hyperkalemia (28,34) while others showing definite responses to mineralocorticoid had much more severe hyperkalemia (17,29,37). This favors two distinct mechanisms.

Response to Sodium Restriction

The habitual dietary sodium intake was known to be very high in some patients (17,33); furthermore, a lowering of elevated blood pressure in response to dietary salt restriction was dramatic in some patients (17,20,21,29,36), falling to normal within days or weeks. In some, the biochemical abnormalities also improved. Gordon et al. kept their patient on long-term dietary salt restriction before instituting any other therapy (17). After 5 months, all the biochemical abnormalities were corrected, and normal growth rate was restored. These responses are consistent with the manifestations of the syndrome all being secondary to salt overload. During sodium restriction, plasma renin and aldosterone increased; this would explain enhanced distal tubular kaliuretic activity. Correction of the biochemical abnormalities by salt restriction alone is not easily explained on the basis of a chloride shunt. It is difficult to see how a reduced distal sodium chloride load could enhance kaliuresis in the presence of a chloride shunt.

Response of Atrial Natriuretic Peptide to Various Stimuli

In patients under study with H&H, we have found ANP levels to vary from normal to slightly elevated in the basal state (Fig. 3). The response to saline infusion (Fig. 2) has been variable in our patients (37), and sometimes absent. A subnormal response has also been seen by Valimaki et al. (38). The response to pressor infusion of angiotensin II, a reliable stimulator of ANP levels in our experience (59,60),

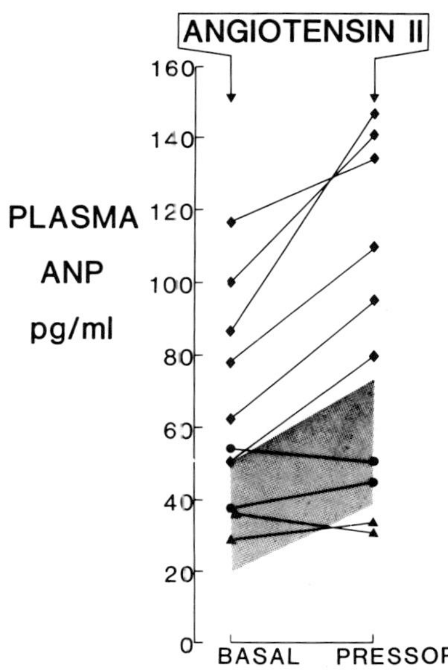

FIG. 5. The response of plasma atrial natriuretic peptide (ANP) to angiotensin II infusion at a rate sufficient to raise diastolic blood pressure 20 mmHg in normal subjects (*shaded area*), in six patients with primary aldosteronism (♦), and in two patients with the syndrome of H&H (●, ▲).

was negligible in two brothers with H&H (Fig. 5) and in an unrelated female with H&H (37). This is consistent with an abnormality in ANP regulation in H&H, or an abnormal response to angiotensin in some tissues but not others, in view of the normal aldosterone response to angiotensin already described. A brisk response of ANP to a maximal exercise test was seen in the brothers with H&H, rising from 62.2 to 143.2 pg/ml in one and from 54.3 to 141.7 pg/ml in the other. Hence ANP secretion achieves variable basal levels and responds briskly to some stimuli but not to others. Further studies are required before these results can be interpreted in relation to the pathophysiology of H&H.

Renal Tubular Resistance to ANP

Absence of the normal natriuretic response to ANP has been reported in a 14-year-old boy with H&H (36). If confirmed, this finding is of great importance in the pathophysiology of H&H.

Response to Diuretics

Thiazide diuretics rapidly lower blood pressure to normal and correct all the biochemical abnormalities in the syndrome of H&H (16–20,22,24,28–30,33,34). In some patients, their continued long-term efficacy has been reported for periods of many years (17,20,24,32). Cessation of diuretics leads to a prompt reappearance of the biochemical abnormalities in milder form, while hypertension redevelops more slowly. Following commencement of diuretics, renin and aldosterone are briskly stimulated to high levels which are sometimes associated with subnormal potassium levels. It is possible that patients with H&H are supersensitive to thiazide diuretics, and, if so, this may be a clue to the site of the renal tubular disorder in this syndrome. The brisk biochemical response to thiazide diuretics is consistent with correction of relative hypoaldosteronism secondary to volume overload. Lee et al. (22) considered the response to thiazides to be superior to the response to furosemide in their patient but added bendrofluazide to furosemide. Wayne et al. (33) regarded furosemide as ineffective, but it did, in fact, correct the hyperkalemia. A satisfactory long-term response to furosemide (58) has been reported, but no careful dose–response comparisons have been made between various diuretics. This might help to identify the site of the tubular lesion in H&H.

Response to Cation-Exchange Resins

Although a failed response was reported in one patient (19), hyperkalemia has been corrected in several patients using cation-exchange resins for short periods (17,20,21). The other biochemical abnormalities did not change, however. Perhaps with long-term correction of hyperkalemia, an improvement in acidemia would also be seen.

Response to Vasopressin

There is evidence for stimulation of potassium secretion by vasopressin (61,62). Vasopressin levels have not been reported in H&H, but they would be expected to be raised because of volume expansion in the presence of normal serum sodium levels. A hypokalemic response to vasopressin has recently been reported by Nahum et al. (34) in a mildly affected patient with H&H. This patient was undergoing forced water diuresis at the time vasopressin was administered intranasally as dDAVP, and plasma volume expansion with stimulation of ANP would be expected. No changes in plasma potassium levels were reported in other patients given vasopressin in order to assess tubular responsiveness. This observation requires confirmation and further study and may have implications for the pathophysiological mechanism in H&H.

RELATIONSHIPS WITH OTHER RENAL TUBULAR DISORDERS

Gordon et al. (17) pointed out that many of the features of the syndrome of H&H were the opposite of those seen in *Bartter's syndrome* (63), another congenital, occasionally familial condition first described in 1962 in which there appears to be disordered renal regulation of sodium and potassium excretion. The biochemical abnormalities in *Bartter's syndrome* are partially corrected by inhibitors of prostaglandin synthesis, but it is uncertain whether the high prostaglandin levels seen in *Bartter's syndrome* are a primary or a secondary event (64,65). The two disorders could result from renal tubular mechanisms affecting the same site or sites.

Another congenital, familial disorder affecting renal tubular physiology was first described in 1963 (66) and is known as *pseudohyperaldosteronism* or *Liddle's syndrome.* Presenting with hypertension and hypokalemia, renin is suppressed (as in primary aldosteronism) but aldosterone levels are also low. The tubule behaves as though it is constantly stimulated by aldosterone. As far as potassium and hydrogen ion secretion by the distal tubule is concerned, this condition is the opposite of the syndrome of H&H, but hypertension is present in both conditions. Thus a second site, in addition to the potassium secretory site, may be involved in the pathophysiology of H&H.

As already discussed, the syndrome of H&H can be included under the heading of hyperkalemic distal renal tubular acidosis. This heterogeneous group of congenital and acquired disorders share the characteristic of inadequate mineralocorticoid activity, either due to underproduction of aldosterone or to congenital or acquired resistance to its action. In many of these conditions, glomerular filtration rate is reduced, due either to destruction of nephrons (which may also cause sodium retention) or to volume contraction secondary to the sodium wasting of mineralocorticoid deficiency. The syndrome of H&H tends to stand apart because of normal glomerular filtration rate.

TREATMENT

Dietary Salt Restriction

As already discussed, most patients have improved during short-term dietary salt restriction; in one patient who was followed during dietary salt restriction for many months (17), all the abnormalities were eventually corrected. Adherence to low-salt diet must be checked by 24-hr urine sodium estimations. Because of its widespread use in the treatment of essential hypertension, doctors, dieticians, and patients are becoming more skillful at achieving long-term palatable dietary salt restriction, which thus represents a practical alternative to lifelong drug therapy.

Diuretics

As already discussed, patients with H&H appear to be very responsive to thiazide diuretics, and all the abnormalities are rapidly corrected. Hypokalemia can result, and careful dosage adjustment is essential. Effective long-term therapy with thiazide diuretics has been established in this condition.

Cation-Exchange Resins

While effective in treating hyperkalemia, cation-exchange resins cannot simultaneously correct sodium/volume overload, and the incidence of gastrointestinal side-effects makes them unsuitable for long-term use.

CONCLUSIONS AND UNANSWERED QUESTIONS

Although the syndrome of H&H superficially resembles some other forms of hyperkalemic distal renal tubular acidosis, it is distinguished by (a) normal glomerular filtration rate, (b) the severity of the hyperkalemia in some patients, and (c) sodium/volume overload leading to hypertension.

Study of the distribution of the various manifestations of the syndrome (Table 2), particularly since they vary within the same family, suggests very strongly that the only essential ingredient for the syndrome is hyperkalemic distal renal tubular acidosis. Probably renal sodium retention is another universal feature, leading eventually to hypertension unless dietary sodium restriction or treatment with diuretics is exhibited. Manifestations such as short stature, muscle weakness, and mental retardation probably depend on the severity of the hyperkalemia and acidemia, but short stature and mental retardation could result from additional genetic defects.

The major unanswered questions are: (a) Is more than one renal tubular site involved? (b) Where is this site or sites? (c) Is it the same site in all patients? (d) Why are most patients quite responsive to mineralocorticoids, whereas some are totally unresponsive? (e) When endogenous aldosterone secretion is stimulated by long-term thiazide therapy, is administration of spironolactone followed by the expected changes in plasma and urinary potassium? (f) Is there normal regulation of renin, aldosterone, and ANP? (g) Is there renal tubular resistance to ANP? (h) Is there increased sensitivity to thiazide diuretics, and is this the site of the lesion?

In many respects, patients with Bartter's syndrome behave as if exposed to too much, and patients with the syndrome of H&H as if exposed to too little, thiazide diuretic. Perhaps herein lies a clue to their respective renal tubular lesions.

Precise definition of the pathophysiological mechanisms operating in the rare subgroup of hypertensive patients with the syndrome of H&H may contribute to the further understanding of normal renal tubular physiology.

REFERENCES

1. Knochel JP. Neuromuscular manifestations of electrolyte disorders. *Am J Med* 1982;72:521–535.
2. Giebisch G, Malnic G, Berliner RW. Renal transport and control of potassium excretion. In: Brenner BM, Rector FC, eds. *The kidney,* 3rd edition. Philadelphia: WB Saunders, 1986;177–205.
3. Sterns RH, Narins RG. Disorders of potassium balance. In: Stein JH, ed. *Internal medicine,* 2nd edition. Boston: Little, Brown and Company, 1987;814–824.
4. Adrogue HJ, Madias NE. Changes in plasma potassium concentration during acute acid–base disturbances. *Am J Med* 1981;72:456–467.
5. DeFronzo RA, Bia M, Smith D. Clinical disorders of hyperkalemia. *Annu Rev Med* 1982;33:521–554.
6. van Ypersele de Strihou C. Potassium homeostasis in renal failure. *Kidney Int* 1977;11:491–504.
7. Perez G, Siegel L, Schreiner GE. Selective hypoaldosteronism with hyperkalemia. *Ann Intern Med* 1972;76:757–763.
8. Oberfield SE, Levine LS, Carey RM, Bejar R, New MI. Pseudohypoaldosteronism: multiple target organ unresponsiveness to mineralocorticoid hormones. *J Clin Endocrinol Metab* 1979;48:228–234.
9. McSherry E. Renal tubular acidosis in childhood. *Kidney Int* 1981;20:799–809.
10. Rocher LL, Tannen RL. The clinical spectrum of renal tubular acidosis. *Annu Rev Med* 1986;37:319–331.
11. DeFronzo RA. Hyperkalemia and hyporeninemic hypoaldosteronism. *Kidney Int* 1980;17:118–134.
12. Narins RG, Jones ER, Stom MC, Rudnick MR, Bastl CP. Diagnostic strategies in disorders of fluid, electrolyte and acid–base homeostasis. *Am J Med* 1982;72:496–520.
13. Halperin ML, Goldstein MB, Richardson RMA, Stinebaugh BJ. Distal renal tubular acidosis syndromes: a pathophysiological approach. *Am J Nephrol* 1985;5:1–8.
14. Batlle DC, Arruda JAL. Renal tubular acidosis syndromes. *Miner Electrolyte Metab* 1981;5:83–89.
15. Kurtzman NA. Acquired distal renal tubular acidosis. *Kidney Int* 1983;24:807–819.
16. Paver WKA, Pauline GJ. Hypertension and hyperpotassaemia without renal disease in a young male. *Med J Aust* 1964;2:305–306.
17. Gordon RD, Geddes RA, Pawsey CGK, O'Halloran MW. Hypertension and severe hyperkalaemia associated with suppression of renin and aldosterone and completely reversed by dietary sodium restriction. *Aust Ann Med* 1970;4:287–294.
18. Spitzer A, Edelmann CM, Goldberg LD, Henneman PH. Short stature, hyperkalemia and acidosis: a defect in renal transport of potassium. *Kidney Int* 1973;3:251–257.
19. Weinstein SF, Allan DME, Mendoza SA. Hyperkalemia, acidosis and short stature associated with a defect in renal potassium excretion. *J Pediatr* 1974;85:355–358.
20. Farfel Z, Iaina A, Rosenthal T, Waks U, Shibolet S, Gafni J. Familial hyperpotassemia and hypertension accompanied by normal plasma aldosterone levels: possible hereditary cell membrane defect. *Arch Intern Med* 1978;138:1828–1832.
21. Brautbar N, Levi J, Rosler A, Leitesdorf E, Djaldeti M, Epstein M, Kleeman CR. Familial hyperkalemia, hypertension and hyporeninemia with normal aldosterone levels: a tubular defect in potassium handling. *Arch Intern Med* 1978;138:607–610.
22. Lee MR, Ball SG, Thomas TH, Morgan DB. Hypertension and hyperkalaemia responding to bendrofluazide. *Q J Med* 1979;48:245–258.

23. Grekin RJ, Nichols MG, Padfield PL. Disorders of chloriuretic hormone secretion. *Lancet* 1979;i:1116–1118.
24. Lee MR, Morgan DB. Familial hyperkalaemia responsive to benzothiadiazine diuretic [Letter]. *Lancet* 1980;i:879.
25. Iitaka K, Watanabe N, Asakura A, Kasai N, Sakai T. Familial hyperkalemia, metabolic acidosis and short stature with normal renin and aldosterone levels. *Int J Pediatr Nephrol* 1980;1:242–245.
26. Bravo E, Textor S, Mujais S, Cotton D. Chronic hyperkalemia in siblings associated with enhanced renal chloride absorption [Abstract]. *Clin Res* 1980;28:782A.
27. Sauder SE, Kelch RP, Grekin RJ, Kelsch RC. Suppression of plasma renin activity in a boy with chronic hyperkalemia. *Am J Dis Child* 1987;141:922–927.
28. Schambelan M, Sebastian A, Rector FC. Mineralocorticoid-resistant renal hyperkalemia without salt wasting (type II pseudohypoaldosteronism): role of increased renal chloride reabsorption. *Kidney Int* 1981;19:716–727.
29. Sanjad SA, Mansour FM, Hernandez RH, Hill LL. Severe hypertension, hyperkalemia and renal tubular acidosis responding to dietary sodium restriction. *Pediatrics* 1982;69:317–324.
30. Licht JH, Amundson D, Hsueh WA, Lombardo JV. Familial hyperkalaemic acidosis. *Q J Med* 1985;54:161–176.
31. Soppi E, Viikari J, Seppala P, Lehtonen A, Saarinen R, Miilunpalo S. Unusual association of hyperkalemia and hypertension. *Hypertension* 1986;8:174–177.
32. Gordon RD, Hodsman GP. The syndrome of hypertension and hyperkalaemia without renal failure: long term correction by thiazide diuretic. *Scott Med J* 1986;31:44–45.
33. Wayne VS, Stockigt JR, Jennings GL. Treatment of mineralocorticoid-resistant renal hyperkalemia with hypertension (type II pseudohypoaldosteronism). *Aust NZ J Med* 1986;16:221–223.
34. Nahum H, Paillard M, Prigent A, Leviel F, Bichara M, Gardin J, Idatte J. Pseudohypoaldosteronism type II: proximal renal tubular acidosis and dDAVP-sensitive renal hyperkalemia. *Am J Nephrol* 1986;6:253–262.
35. Kirshon B, Edwards J, Cotton DB. Gordon's syndrome in pregnancy. *Am J Obstet Gynecol* 1987;156:1110–1111.
36. Semmekrot B, Monnens L, Theelen BGA, Rascher W, Gabreels F, Willems J. The syndrome of hypertension and hyperkalemia with normal glomerular function (Gordon's syndrome). A pathophysiological study. *Pediatr Nephrol* 1987;1:473–478.
37. Gordon RD, Ravenscroft PJ, Klemm SA, Tunny TJ, Hamlet SM. A new Australian kindred with the syndrome of hypertension and hyperkalemia have dysregulation of atrial natriuretic peptide. *J Hypertens* 1988;6(Suppl 4):S323–S326.
38. Valimaki M, Pelkonin R, Tikkanen I, Fyhrquist F. A deficient response of atrial natriuretic peptide to volume overload in Gordon's syndrome. *Acta Endocrinol* 1989;120;331–336.
39. Stokes GS, Gentle JL, Edwards KDG, Stewart JH, Scoggins BA, Coghlan JP. Syndrome of idiopathic hyperkalaemia and hypertension with decreased plasma renin activity: effects on plasma renin and aldosterone of reducing the serum potassium level. *Med J Aust* 1968;2:1050–1053.
40. Arnold JE, Healy JK. Hyperkalemia, hypertension and systemic acidosis without renal failure associated with a tubular defect in potassium excretion. *Am J Med* 1969;47:461–472.
41. De Wardener HE. Selective defects of tubular function. In: *The kidney: an outline of normal and abnormal structure and function,* 4th edition. London: Churchill Livingstone, 1973;230–243.
42. Gordon RD. Syndrome of hypertension and hyperkalemia with normal glomerular filtration rate. *Hypertension* 1986;8:93–102.
43. Gordon RD. The syndrome of hypertension and hyperkalemia with normal GFR. A unique pathophysiological mechanism for hypertension? *Clin Exp Pharmacol Physiol* 1986;13:329–333.
44. Gorlin RJ, Pindborg JJ. *Syndromes of the head and neck,* 1st edition. New York: McGraw-Hill, 1964;546.
45. Grahnen H. Hypodontia in the permanent dentition. A clinical and genetical investigation. *Odont Rev* 1956;7(Suppl 3):1–100.
46. Tunny TJ, Gordon RD. Plasma atrial natriuretic peptide in primary aldosteronism (before and after treatment) and in Bartter's and Gordon's syndromes. *Lancet* 1986;1:272–273.
47. Tunny TJ, Gordon RD, Klemm SA, Hamlet SM. Effects of acute volume expansion on atrial natriuretic peptide levels in normal subjects, primary aldosteronism and low renin essential hypertension. *J Hypertens* 1986;4(Suppl 6):S509–S511.
48. Wrong D, Davies HEF. The excretion of acid in renal disease. *Q J Med* 1959;28:259–313.
49. Knox FG, Haramati A. Renal regulation of phosphate excretion. In: Seldin DW, Giebisch G, eds. *The kidney: physiology and pathophysiology.* New York: Raven Press, 1985;1381–1396.
50. Massry SG, Coburn JW, Kleeman CR. The influence of extracellular volume expansion on renal phosphate reabsorption in the dog. *J Clin Invest* 1969;48:1237–1245.
51. Suki WN, Martinez-Maldonado M, Rouse D, Ting A. Effect of expansion of extracellular fluid volume on renal phosphate handling. *J Clin Invest* 1969;48:1888–1894.
52. Kurtzman NA. Regulation of renal bicarbonate reabsorption by extracellular volume. *J Clin Invest* 1970;49:586–595.
53. Kurtzman NA, White MG, Rogers PW. The effect of potassium and extracellular volume on renal bicarbonate reabsorption. *Metabolism* 1973;22:481–492.
54. Sebastian A, Hernandez RE, Schambelan M. Disorders of distal handling of potassium. In: Brenner BM, Rector FC, eds. *The kidney,* 3rd edition. Philadelphia: WB Saunders, 1986:519–549.
55. Farfel Z, Iaina A, Levi J, Gafni J. Proximal renal tubular acidosis: association with familial normaldosteronemic hyperpotassemia and hypertension. *Arch Intern Med* 1978;138:1837–1840.
56. Guerra SMO, Kitabchi AE. Comparison of the effectiveness of various routes of insulin injection: insulin levels and glucose response in normal subjects. *J Clin Endocrinol Metab* 1976; 42:869–874.
57. Tormey WP, Morgan DB. Etiological considerations in Gordon's syndrome: possible role of prostaglandins. *Prostaglandins Med* 1980;4:107–112.
58. Sanjad SA, Keenan BS, Hill LL. Renal hypoprostaglandism, hypertension and type IV renal tubular acidosis reversed by furosemide. *Ann Intern Med* 1983;99:624–627.
59. Klemm SA, Tunny TJ, Gordon RD. Atrial natriuretic peptide levels during angiotensin infusion and indomethacin administration are consistent with angiotensin-mediated regulation in man. *J Hypertens* 1987;5(Suppl 5):S75–S78.
60. Klemm SA, Gordon RD, Tunny TJ, Hamlet SM. Altering angiotensin levels by administration of captopril or indomethacin, or by angiotensin infusion, contributes to an understanding of atrial natriuretic peptide regulation in man. *Clin Exp Pharmacol Physiol* 1988;15:349–355.
61. Field MJ, Stanton BA, Giebisch GH. Influence of ADH on renal potassium handling: a micropuncture and microperfusion study. *Kidney Int* 1984;25:502–511.
62. Guggino SE, Suarez-Isle BA, Guggino WB, Sacktor B. Forskolin and antidiuretic hormone stimulate a Ca^{2+}-activated K^+ channel in cultured kidney cells. *Am J Physiol* 1985;249:F448–F455.
63. Bartter FC, Pronove P, Gill JR, MacCardle RC, Diller E. Hyperplasia of the juxta-glomerular complex with hyperaldosteronism and hypokalemic alkalosis: a new syndrome. *Am J Med* 1962;33:811–828.
64. Bowden RE, Gill JR, Radfar N, Taylor AA, Keiser HR. Prostaglandin synthetase inhibitors in Bartter's syndrome. Effect on immunoreactive prostaglandin E excretion. *JAMA* 1978;239:117–121.
65. Gill JR, Bartter FC. Evidence for a prostaglandin-independent defect in chloride reabsorption in the loop of Henle as a proximal cause of Bartter's syndrome. *Am J Med* 1978;65:766–772.
66. Liddle GW, Bledsoe T, Coppage WS. A familial renal disorder simulating primary aldosteronism but with negligible aldosterone secretion. *Trans Assoc Am Physicians* 1963;76:199–213.

Hypertension: Pathophysiology, Diagnosis, and Management, edited by J. H. Laragh and B. M. Brenner. Raven Press, Ltd., New York © 1990.

CHAPTER 102

Pheochromocytoma

William M. Manger and Ray W. Gifford, Jr.

Catecholamine Biosynthesis, 1639
Receptors, 1640
Uptake and Catabolism, 1640
Origin, 1640
Pathophysiology, 1641
Clinical Presentation, 1641
Pathologic Entities Sometimes Associated with Pheochromocytoma, 1645
Apudomas and Neurocrestopathies, 1646
Differential Diagnosis, 1647
Diagnosis, 1648
Laboratory and ECG Abnormalities, 1648
Biochemical Tests, 1650
Clonidine Suppression Test, 1650
Urinary Catecholamines and Their Metabolites, 1651
Pharmacologic Tests, 1652
Preoperative Localization of Pheochromocytomas, 1652
Radiography, 1652
Central Venous Blood Sampling, 1653
Treatment, 1653
Preoperative Evaluation and Management, 1653
Adrenergic Blockade, 1655
Operative and Postoperative Management and Follow-Up, 1656
Chronic Medical Management, 1657
References, 1657

There is no more important cause of hypertension to recognize than pheochromocytoma, since it can be successfully removed in 90% of cases, whereas if left untreated it will almost always be lethal. The peril of an unrecognized tumor is strikingly evident in a report from the Mayo Clinic: Of 40,078 autopsies performed from 1928 to 1977, 54 patients had pheochromocytomas which were not suspected in 76% and which contributed to the death of 55% of the patients (1)! (These data do not reflect the large number of cases accurately diagnosed since 1928 at the Mayo Clinic but emphasize that diagnosis can sometimes be exceptionally elusive.)

CATECHOLAMINE BIOSYNTHESIS

A knowledge of the metabolic, physiologic, and pharmacologic effects of catecholamines secreted by pheochromocytomas is basic to understanding the pathophysiology of these amines. The catecholamines present in humans (i.e., dopamine, norepinephrine, and epinephrine) are important in neural and endocrine function.

Dopamine serves as a neurotransmitter in the central nervous system (CNS), in peripheral sympathetic nerves, and in some sympathetic ganglia. Activation of dopaminergic nerves and their receptors exert unique effects in the brain and elsewhere. Dopamine stimulation of dopaminergic receptors in the splanchnic and renal vascular beds causes vasodilatation. Dopamine enhances myocardial contractility (probably via β-receptors), and it appears to exert a diuretic and natriuretic action. Dopamine is also the precursor for norepinephrine and can modulate some adrenergic nerve activity.

Catecholamine biosynthesis occurs in sympathetic neurons (mainly nerve endings), in the brain, and in chromaffin tissue. Some chromaffin cells in the adrenal medulla, the organs of Zuckerkandl, and certain cells in the brain are capable of converting norepinephrine to epinephrine through the action of the enzyme phenylethanolamine-*N*-methyltransferase (PNMT). Norepinephrine, epinephrine, and dopamine are synthesized in some chromaffin cells and in parts of the brain, but only norepinephrine and dopamine are synthesized in postganglionic sympathetic nerves. Norepinephrine serves the important function of neurotransmitter (mediator of nerve activity) at most postganglionic sympathetic endings in the autonomic nervous system. Epinephrine and norepinephrine are of major importance in affecting metabolism and cardiovascular physiology. Neurons that liberate catecholamines are called "sympathetic" or "adrenergic" neurons. (The term "adrenergic system" is used to indicate the entire sympathoadrenal system.)

Our experience with normal humans at rest indicates that plasma dopamine accounts for about 13% of the free catecholamines, whereas epinephrine and norepinephrine account for roughly 14% and 73%, respectively. These are almost identical to the concentrations found by Buu and Kuchel (*personal communication*). In human peripheral plasma, about 76% of epinephrine and norepinephrine and 98% of dopamine are conjugated by sulfate (2–4).

RECEPTORS

Catecholamines exert their cardiovascular and metabolic effects by stimulating specific cellular receptors (adrenoceptors) which are protein-binding sites; when activated by an agonist (i.e., a substance that interacts with a receptor and evokes a biologic response), a series of events occur which cause a response in the cells stimulated. Catecholamines can activate a wide variety of cells. Receptors recognizing catecholamines have been designated α- and β-adrenergic receptors and dopaminergic receptors; they have been identified and classified on the basis of rank order of potency of their responses (i.e., the relative magnitude of response) to agonists and antagonists (5,6).

The β-adrenergic receptors can be subdivided into β_1 receptors [i.e., those which, when stimulated, cause (a) a positive inotropic and chronotropic effect on the myocardium, (b) lipolysis of fat cells, and (c) an increased renin secretion] and β_2 receptors [i.e., those which, when stimulated, cause (a) bronchodilatation, (b) vasodilatation in some vessels, (c) glycogenolysis, (d) myometrial and intestinal smooth muscle relaxation, and (e) an increased neurotransmitter release from sympathetic nerves]. Epinephrine and norepinephrine are approximately equipotent in eliciting β_1 responses, whereas epinephrine is much more potent than norepinephrine in eliciting β_2 responses.

The α-adrenergic receptors can be subdivided into α_1 receptors (i.e., those on vascular smooth muscle which, when stimulated, cause vasoconstriction and thereby increase blood pressure; stimulation of other α_1 receptors can also cause glycogenolysis) and α_2 receptors (i.e., those on presynaptic nerves which, when stimulated, inhibit norepinephrine secretion, those on vascular smooth muscle which, when stimulated, cause vasoconstriction, and those in the brain which, when stimulated, decrease sympathetic nerve activity; stimulation of those in the pancreas, in adipocytes, and in the intestine, respectively, inhibit insulin secretion, inhibit lipolysis, and cause smooth muscle relaxation).

Dopaminergic receptors have been identified in the brain and peripheral nervous system and also in renal, mesenteric, and cerebral vascular beds, where dopamine causes vasodilatation. Some evidence indicates that coronary vessels contain dopaminergic receptors which, when stimulated, can cause vasodilatation. The dopaminergic receptors have been subdivided into DA_1 receptors (i.e., those in certain vascular regions which, when stimulated, cause vasodilatation) and DA_2 receptors (i.e., those on presynaptic sympathetic nerve endings which, when stimulated, inhibit the release of norepinephrine). There is evidence that dopamine can also activate β_1 and α receptors and possibly β_2 and serotonin receptors.

Prolonged exposure to excess catecholamines can decrease cell responsiveness to these amines. This process of desensitization or down-regulation may result from disappearance (internalization) of receptors from the cell surface and/or an impaired ability of catecholamines to bind (couple) with their receptors.

Figure 1 reveals the pathways of biosynthesis and metabolism of catecholamines and indicates the enzymes catalyzing the various reactions.

UPTAKE AND CATABOLISM

Inactivation of catecholamines occurs in several ways. The neuronal reuptake process is of major importance in terminating the physiologic action of norepinephrine released at sympathetic nerve terminals. Approximately 80% of the norepinephrine liberated from these nerves may be taken up by adjacent sympathetic nerves (via a high-affinity membrane uptake process that is sodium-dependent and probably non-stereospecific) and stored (by an exchange of catecholamine for hydrogen ions) in synaptic vesicles for future use. This neuronal uptake mechanism (termed "$uptake_1$") can also be used for other structurally similar amines (e.g., epinephrine, dopamine, tyramine, α-methylnorepinephrine, metaraminol, amphetamine), and it can be inhibited by certain drugs (e.g., cocaine, tricyclic antidepressants). Catecholamines are also taken up (via a low affinity, non-sodium-dependent, non-stereospecific process) by non-neuronal tissues (termed "$uptake_2$") such as smooth muscle, collagen, elastic tissue, and even blood cells and platelets.

Catecholamines that are free in the tissues or circulation are also converted to inactive metabolites by monoamine oxidase (MAO) plus aldehyde dehydrogenase and/or catecholamine-*O*-methyltransferase (COMT). In addition, the free catecholamines may be converted by phenol sulfotransferase to sulfoconjugates in humans. The catecholamine metabolites may also be conjugated as indicated in Fig. 1.

Small amounts of free epinephrine and norepinephrine (about 5% of catecholamines entering the circulation) are excreted in the urine; the relatively larger amount of urinary free dopamine results from conversion of dopa to dopamine in the kidney. Catecholamines are mainly eliminated in the urine as their metabolites and conjugates.

A more detailed account of catecholamine metabolism, as well as current concepts regarding receptor subtypes and their responses to agonists and antagonists, can be found elsewhere (4,5,7–14).

ORIGIN

Pheochromocytomas arise from chromaffin cells of the adrenal medullae (90% of tumors) and the organ of Zuckerkandl and from chromaffin cells occurring in association with sympathetic nerves and plexuses in extra-adrenal sites in the abdomen, chest (<2% of tumors), and neck (<0.1% of tumors) (Fig. 2). A number of intrapericardial and cardiac pheochromocytomas have been reported; these are frequently located in the left atrial region (15,16). Multiple tumors (adrenal and/or extra-adrenal) are more common in children (35% of cases) than in adults (8%). About 10% of pheochromocytomas are familial, and at least 70% of these tumors are bilateral.

PATHOPHYSIOLOGY

Severe morbidity and lethal complications (e.g., cerebrovascular and cardiovascular accidents, cardiomyopathy, cardiac decompensation, arrhythmias) from the effects of hypertension and excessive circulating catecholamines almost invariably result if the disease is not controlled.

The average pheochromocytoma is roughly 5 cm in diameter, and 70% weigh less than 70 g; however, they may be microscopic or weigh up to 4000 g. Most are quite vascular, although some are relatively avascular or cystic; rarely they contain calcium. Usually these tumors are encapsulated.

Benign as well as malignant pheochromocytomas may contain cells with hyperchromatic nuclei, mitotic figures, and giant cells. Only 10% of pheochromocytomas are malignant, as evidenced by metastases or invasion of adjacent structures. Histological determination of malignancy is not possible, since cells of malignant or benign tumors appear identical. However, recent reports indicate that nuclear deoxyribonucleic acid patterns of pheochromocytomas studied by flow cytometry may provide useful prognostic information for patients with these tumors (17,18).

Some have claimed that pheochromocytomas containing dopamine are malignant; however, although the incidence of malignancy is significantly greater in tumors containing dopamine and its precursor (dopa) (19) than in those containing only epinephrine and norepinephrine, the presence of dopamine or its precursor does not establish malignancy. The incidence of malignancy in extra-adrenal pheochromocytomas (30–40%) is reportedly somewhere between 3 and 15 times more common than that in adrenal tumors (2.4–1_%) (20,21).

Pheochromocytoma cells tend to be larger than those of the normal adrenal medulla and are generally pleomorphic and polygonal or spheroidal, with eosinophilic and/or basophilic cytoplasm harboring multiple minute catecholamine-containing granules. The number of these granules (storage vesicles) seen in electron micrographs appears to correlate with the catecholamine content of pheochromocytomas. In some tumors there is a good correlation between the morphology of the granules (epinephrine being diffusely dense and norepinephrine containing a central or eccentrically situated dense core) and the biochemical character of these tumors; however, no strong correlation exists in most patients between (a) catecholamines in their pheochromocytomas and (b) elevation of plasma catecholamine levels due to actively secreting tumors (8). Furthermore, no good correlation exists between (a) the size of a tumor or its catecholamine concentrations and (b) the clinical or laboratory manifestations. Severity of symptomatology depends mainly on the amount of catecholamine liberated into the circulation and whether this liberation is sustained or episodic. Small tumors frequently have a rapid turnover of catecholamines and liberate large amounts of norepinephrine and epinephrine into the circulation. In contrast, turnover is often slow in large tumors, with relatively large amounts of catecholamines metabolized within the tumor and only small amounts of active biogenic amines reaching the circulation.

Pheochromocytomas have the enzymes necessary to convert tyrosine to catecholamines. Most tumors secrete both norepinephrine and epinephrine, but norepinephrine is usually the predominant amine. Some secrete only norepinephrine or, rarely, only epinephrine; very rarely, dopamine, dopa, and even serotonin (22) may also be secreted.

In contrast to the calcium-dependent exocytotic mechanism of catecholamine secretion (i.e., discharge of the contents of the catecholamine storage vesicle to the cell's exterior) in the normal innervated adrenal medulla, secretion from pheochromocytomas (none of which appear innervated) is thought to occur mainly by diffusion. However, reports indicating simultaneous elevations of dopamine-β-hydroxylase (8,23), chromogranin A (24), and catecholamines in the plasma of some patients with pheochromocytoma suggest that these substances (all present in catecholamine storage vesicles) are released simultaneously by exocytosis from some tumors.

Some pheochromocytomas have also been found to contain vasoactive intestinal peptide (VIP, a potent vasodilator), opioid peptides (e.g., enkephalins, β-endorphin, dynorphin), α-MSH, somatostatin, parathyroid-like hormone, calcitonin, serotonin, ACTH, and neuropeptide Y (a potent vasoconstrictor) and its "flanking" peptide. These substances may be released into the circulation and may play a role in the symptomatology of some patients with pheochromocytoma (8,25–31). The diverse manifestations and syndromes caused by excess ACTH, serotonin, and VIP may confuse the diagnosis. Opioid peptides may be synthesized by adrenomedullary or pheochromocytoma cells, co-stored with catecholamines, and released into the circulation in large amounts (27,32). Apparently, opioid peptides are markers of neuroendocrine differentiation in many tumors, including pheochromocytoma (27).

Pheochromocytoma probably occurs in less than 0.05% of persons with sustained diastolic hypertension; however, in estimating total prevalence it must be appreciated that about 45% of these tumors cause only paroxysmal hypertension.

CLINICAL PRESENTATION

Pheochromocytoma often presents dramatically and explosively. Manifestations are so diverse and numerous that the tumor can mimic a variety of disease entities. The occurrence of hypertension is of great diagnostic importance, since "attacks" or symptoms suggesting excess circulating catecholamines without sustained or episodic hypertension are most atypical if due to pheochromocytoma. An exception to this latter statement applies to familial pheochromocytoma, where hypertension may occasionally be ab-

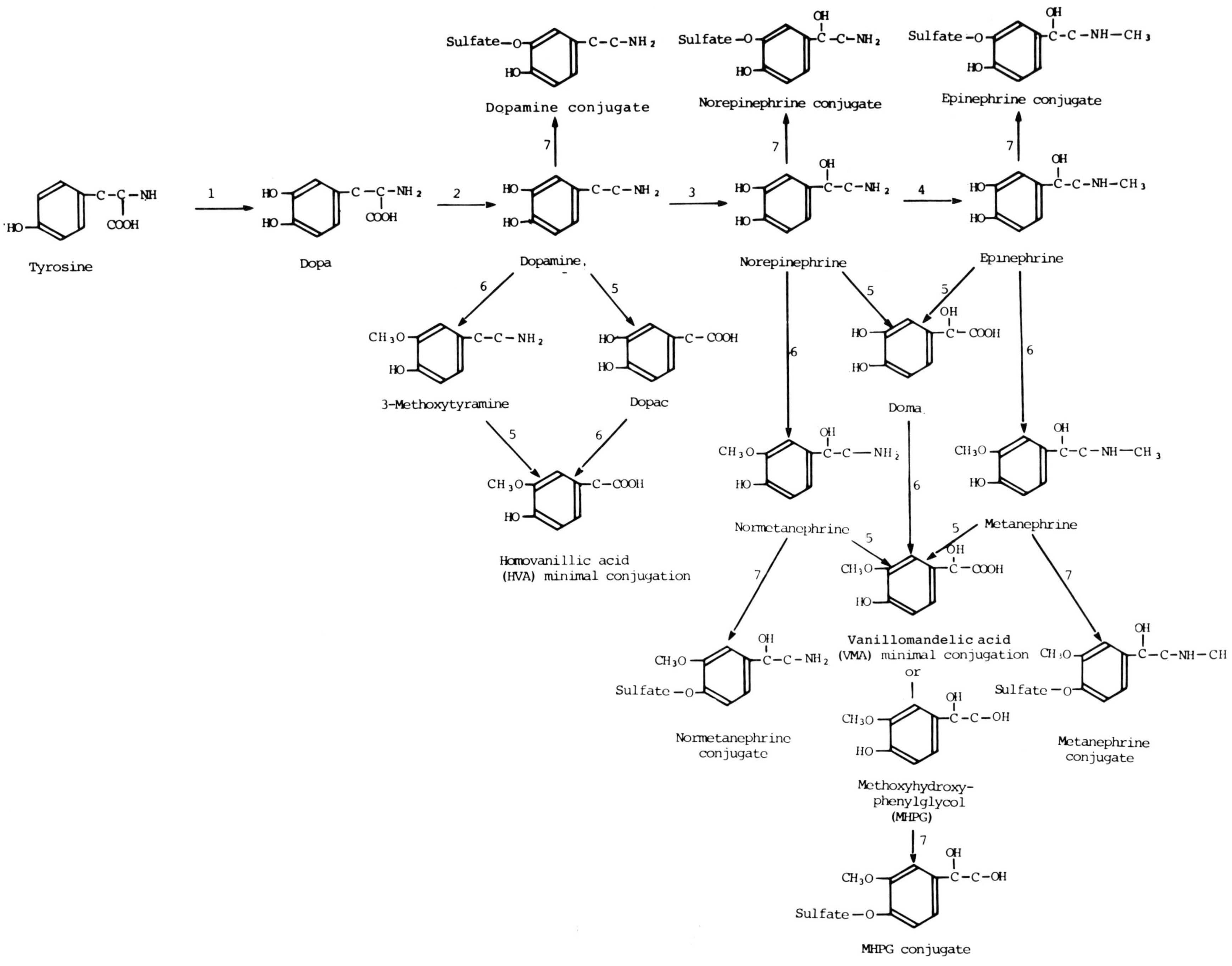

Sulfate–O– / HO– ring –C–C–NH₂

Dopamine conjugate

Sulfate–O– / HO– ring –C(OH)–C–NH₂

Norepinephrine conjugate

Sulfate–O– / HO– ring –C(OH)–C–NH–CH₃

Epinephrine conjugate

Tyrosine → (1) → Dopa → (2) → Dopamine → (3) → Norepinephrine → (4) → Epinephrine

Dopamine → (7) → Dopamine conjugate

Norepinephrine → (7) → Norepinephrine conjugate

Epinephrine → (7) → Epinephrine conjugate

Dopamine → (6) → 3-Methoxytyramine

Dopamine → (5) → Dopac

3-Methoxytyramine → (5) → Homovanillic acid

Dopac → (6) → Homovanillic acid

Homovanillic acid (HVA) minimal conjugation

Norepinephrine → (6) → Normetanephrine

Norepinephrine → (5) → Doma

Epinephrine → (5) → Doma

Epinephrine → (6) → Metanephrine

Doma → (6) → Vanillomandelic acid

Normetanephrine → (5) → Vanillomandelic acid

Metanephrine → (5) → Vanillomandelic acid

Normetanephrine → (7) → Normetanephrine conjugate

Metanephrine → (7) → Metanephrine conjugate

Vanillomandelic acid (VMA) minimal conjugation

or

Methoxyhydroxy-phenylglycol (MHPG)

MHPG → (7) → MHPG conjugate

Normetanephrine conjugate

Metanephrine conjugate

MHPG conjugate

sent and where plasma and urinary concentrations of catecholamines and their metabolites may be normal or only slightly elevated.

Seventy-five percent of patients experience one or more symptomatic hypertensive attacks weekly. However, one or more attacks may occur daily or once every few months; with time they tend to increase in frequency. Attacks are abrupt in onset but subside more slowly; in 80% of patients they last less than 1 hr, but they may last less than a minute or continue for a week. Attacks may sometimes be precipitated by pressure in the region of the tumor, postural changes, various forms of exertion, anxiety, trauma, pain, micturition or bladder distension, ingestion of foods or beverages containing tyramine (e.g., cheese, beer, and wine), or synephrine (e.g., citrus fruits), administration of certain drugs (e.g., histamine, glucagon, tyramine, phenothiazines, metoclopramide, and possibly ACTH), intubation, anesthesia, or operative manipulation (33).

Clinical manifestations are mainly due to the effects of excess circulating catecholamines or to complications of hypertension. Table 1 cites the symptoms in 76 patients with paroxysmal or persistent hypertension and pheochromocytoma as well as manifestations due to complications or coexisting diseases or syndromes.

Headache, the most common symptom, can occur in any part of the head and is usually very severe and throbbing during a paroxysmal attack. Patients may be awakened by severe headache and may experience nausea and vomiting. With persistent hypertension, headache may be moderate or mild.

Sweating (generalized and sometimes drenching) and palpitations, accompanied by tachycardia (or, occasionally, reflex bradycardia), occur frequently. Severe anxiety and fear of death are often experienced, but patients with pheochromocytoma do not exhibit chronic anxiety unless they are neurotic.

Significant weight loss may result from the hypermetabolism caused by excessive catecholamines, but some patients, particularly those with paroxysmal hypertension, may remain obese. Severe constipation or even pseudo-obstruction (34) (due to catecholamine inhibition of peristalsis) occurs in some patients with persistent hypertension; very rarely, ischemic enterocolitis with intestinal necrosis has complicated the intense mesenteric artery vasoconstriction caused by excessive circulating catecholamines. On rare occasions, secretion of VIP, serotonin, or calcitonin by some pheochromocytomas (or secretion of calcitonin, serotonin, and prostaglandin from a coexisting medullary thyroid carcinoma) may cause diarrhea. A severe, watery diarrhea may be accompanied by hypokalemia and hypo- or achlorhydria (the Verner–Morrison WDHH or WDHA syndrome) (29).

Signs observed in patients with pheochromocytoma are listed in Table 2.

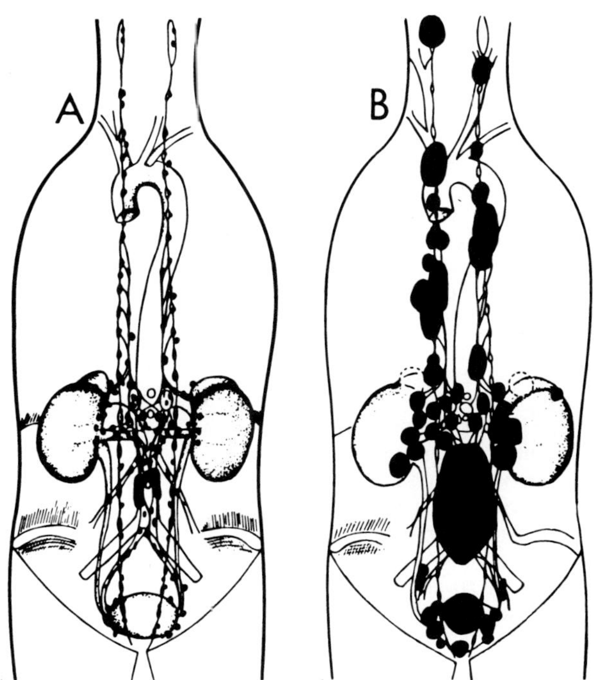

FIG. 2. A: Anatomic distribution of extra-adrenal chromaffin tissue in the newborn. **B:** Location of extra-adrenal pheochromocytomas reported in the literature up to 1965. (From ref. 77.)

Usually, marked increases of both systolic and diastolic pressures occur in patients having paroxysmal attacks (45% of patients); in those with sustained hypertension (50% of patients), pressures may fluctuate widely as a result of variations in circulating catecholamines. About 5% of patients may remain normotensive. Some patients have paroxysms superimposed on their hypertension. Very rarely, some patients may have attacks of hypertension alternating with hypotension (especially when tumors secrete mainly epinephrine). Occasionally, patients with paroxysms become permanently hypertensive; rarely, patients remain normotensive. In familial pheochromocytoma (with multiple endocrine neoplasia) the pattern of hypertension appears to be consistent; i.e., all family members have either sustained or paroxysmal hypertension. Very rarely, a fulminating progression with a rapid increase in both the severity and frequency of hypertensive attacks (sometimes alternating with hypotension) may require emergency surgery.

No close correlation exists between levels of systolic or diastolic pressures and plasma catecholamine concentrations (8); it appears that the sympathetic nervous system is involved in the maintenance of hypertension in clinical (35) as well as experimental pheochromocytoma (36).

Orthostatic hypotension in the untreated hypertensive

←

FIG. 1. Pathway of synthesis and metabolism of catecholamines with enzymes catalyzing various reactions: (1) tyrosine hydroxylase; (2) aromatic amino acid decarboxylase; (3) phenylamine-β-hydroxylase; (4) phenylethanolamine-*N*-methyltransferase; (5) monoamine oxidase plus aldehyde dehydrogenase; (6) catechol-*O*-methyltransferase; (7) conjugating enzymes (phenol sulfotransferase in humans). (Modified from ref. 8.)

TABLE 1. *Symptoms reported by 76 patients (almost all adults) with pheochromocytoma associated with paroxysmal or persistent hypertension*[a]

Symptoms presumably due to excessive catecholamines or hypertension	Paroxysmal (37 patients), %[b]	Persistent (39 patients), %[b]
Headaches (severe)	92	72
Excessive sweating (generalized)	65	69
Palpitations ± tachycardia	73	51
Anxiety or nervousness (± fear of impending death, panic)	60	28
Tremulousness	51	26
Pain in chest, abdomen (usually epigastric), lumbar regions, lower abdomen or groin	48	28
Nausea ± vomiting	43	26
Weakness, fatigue, prostration	38	15
Weight loss (severe)	14	15
Dyspnea	11	18
Warmth ± heat intolerance	13	15
Visual disturbances	3	21
Dizziness or faintness	11	3
Constipation	0	13
Paresthesia or pain in arms	11	0
Bradycardia (noted by patient)	8	3
Grand mal seizures	5	3
Miscellaneous (A larger number of miscellaneous symptoms have been reported. Especially noteworthy are painless hematuria, frequency, nocturia, and tenesmus in pheochromocytoma of the urinary bladder)		
Manifestations due to complications		
Congestive heart failure ± cardiomyopathy		
Myocardial infarction		
Cerebrovascular accident		
Ischemic enterocolitis ± megacolon		
Azotemia		
Dissecting aneurysm		
Encephalopathy		
Shock		
Hemorrhagic necrosis in a pheochromocytoma		
Manifestations due to coexisting diseases or syndromes		
Cholelithiasis		
Medullary thyroid carcinoma ± effects of secretions of serotonin, calcitonin, prostaglandin, or ACTH-like substance		
Hyperparathyroidism		
Mucocutaneous neuromas with characteristic facies		
Thickened corneal nerves (seen only with slit lamp)		
Marfanoid habitus		
Alimentary tract ganglioneuromatosis		
Neurofibromatosis and its complications		
Cushing's syndrome (rare)		
Von Hippel–Lindau disease (rare)		
Virilism, Addison's disease, acromegaly, duodenal carcinoid (extremely rare)		
Symptoms caused by encroachment on adjacent structures or by invasion and pressure effects of metastases		

[a] From ref. 83.
[b] Approximate percent.

patient should suggest pheochromocytoma. This hypotension may be related to desensitization of adrenergic receptors (caused by excess circulating catecholamines) and a depression of the sympathetic reflex response to upright posture; a reduced blood volume, which occurs in some patients with pheochromocytoma and sustained hypertension, may contribute to orthostatic hypotension. The pressure decrease is usually to normotensive (but rarely to shock) levels (Fig. 3) and is accompanied by tachycardia. Resistance to antihypertensive therapy, paradoxic blood pressure (BP) increases following ingestion of certain antihypertensive drugs (e.g., β-blockers, guanethidine, ganglionic blockers), or marked pressor responses to intubation or anesthetic induction should suggest pheochromocytoma.

Tachycardia and pallor commonly occur, especially during hypertensive paroxysms. Flushing is occasionally observed in patients with paroxysms, but it has not been reported when hypertension is sustained. Group 3 or 4 retinopathy (Fig. 4) (indistinguishable from that occurring in essential hypertension) is not infrequently seen with sustained hypertension but infrequently occurs with paroxysmal hypertension. A fine tremor is not uncommon, and Raynaud's phenomenon is occasionally noted. Slight temperature elevations are often present; rarely, severe hyperpyrexia occurs.

TABLE 2. *Signs observed in patients with pheochromocytoma*[a]

- Blood pressure changes
  - ± Hypertension ± wide fluctuations (rarely, paroxysmal hypotension or hypertension alternating with hypotension)
  - Hypertension induced by physical maneuver such as exercise, postural change, or palpation and massage of flank or mass elsewhere
  - Orthostatic hypotension ± postural tachycardia
  - Paradoxic blood pressure response to certain antihypertensive drugs; marked pressor response with induction of anesthesia
- Other signs of catecholamine excess
  - Hyperhidrosis
  - Tachycardia or reflex bradycardia, very forceful heartbeat, arrhythmia
  - Pallor of face and upper part of body (rarely flushing; mottled cyanosis)
  - Anxious, frightened, troubled appearance
  - Hypertensive retinopathy
  - Dilated pupils (very rarely exophthalmos, lacrimation, scleral pallor, or injection; pupils may not react to light)
  - Leanness or underweight
  - Tremor (± shaking)
  - Raynaud's phenomenon or livedo reticularis (occasionally puffy, red, cyanotic hands in children); skin of extremities wet, cold, clammy, pale, gooseflesh; occasionally cyanotic nail beds
  - Fever
- Mass lesion (rarely palpable)
  - Tumor in abdomen or neck [pheochromocytoma, chemodectoma, thyroid carcinoma, or thyroid swelling (very rare and only during hypertensive paroxysm)]
- Signs caused by encroachment on adjacent structures or by invasion and pressure effects of metastases
- Manifestations related to complications or to coexisting diseases or syndromes[b]

[a] Observed in some of the 76 patients cited in Table 1. From ref. 33.
[b] See Table 1.

Atypical manifestations may be evident in children (e.g., polydipsia, polyuria, and convulsive seizures are not uncommon and, rarely, a puffy, red, cyanosis of the hands appears). Pheochromocytoma attacks may be aggravated or may subside during pregnancy, and clinical manifestations may be confused with eclampsia or preeclampsia, or with a ruptured uterus if shock occurs during or immediately following labor.

Paroxysmal attacks induced by micturition or bladder distension suggest pheochromocytoma of the urinary bladder; about 65% of these tumors cause painless hematuria.

PATHOLOGIC ENTITIES SOMETIMES ASSOCIATED WITH PHEOCHROMOCYTOMA

Approximately 10% of pheochromocytomas are familial; their coexistence with multiple endocrine neoplasms, or with hyperplasia of the thyroid and sometimes parathyroid, is designated multiple endocrine neoplasia (MEN) type 2. Recently, this inherited (autosomal dominant) endocrinopathy has been assigned a locus on chromosome 10 (37). Coexistence of pheochromocytomas, medullary thyroid carcinoma, mucosal neuromas, thickened corneal nerves, alimentary tract ganglioneuromatosis and, frequently, a marfanoid habitus constitutes still another entity, MEN type 3 (Fig. 5). Hyperparathyroidism occurs in about 50% of patients with MEN type 2 but rarely occurs in MEN type 3.

In MEN syndromes, medullary thyroid carcinoma is multicentric, involves both lobes of the thyroid, and frequently spreads to cervical and mediastinal nodes. Serotonin, prostaglandin (E_2 and $F_{2\alpha}$), and calcitonin secretions from these thyroid carcinomas may cause moderate or severe diarrhea; secretion of ACTH-like substances from medullary thyroid carcinomas or from pheochromocytomas may, rarely, cause Cushing's syndrome. Patients with pheochromocytoma should be screened for evidence of medullary thyroid carcinoma or premalignant C-cell hyperplasia as well as for the presence of hyperparathyroidism. These thyroid carcinomas may be detected first and sometimes occur years before the pheochromocytoma (8,38).

Demonstration of hypercalcitonemia (which sometimes requires pentagastrin stimulation) suggests the presence of medullary thyroid carcinoma or C-cell hyperplasia; however, it is not pathognomonic, since hypercalcitonemia may occur in a number of miscellaneous conditions and occasionally pheochromocytoma may produce calcitonin

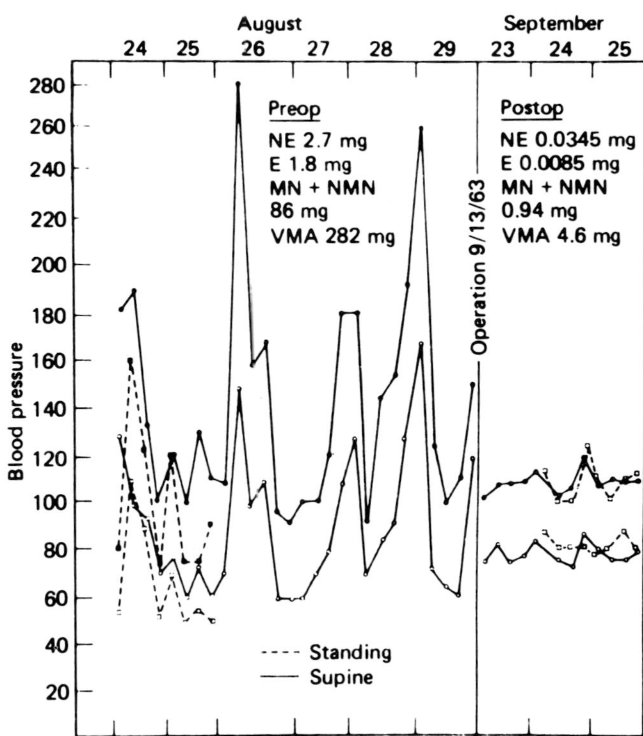

FIG. 3. Typical blood pressure pattern in a patient with pheochromocytoma. Note the orthostatic hypotension and the paroxysmal pressor episodes during the preoperative period. Twenty-four-hour urinary catecholamines and their metabolites preoperatively and postoperatively are also recorded. (From ref. 78.)

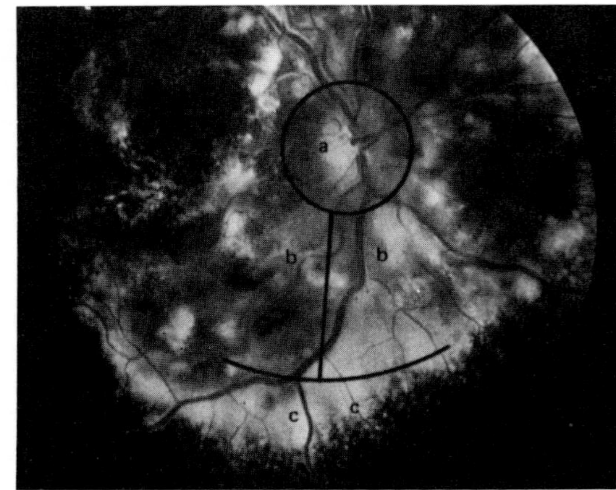

A

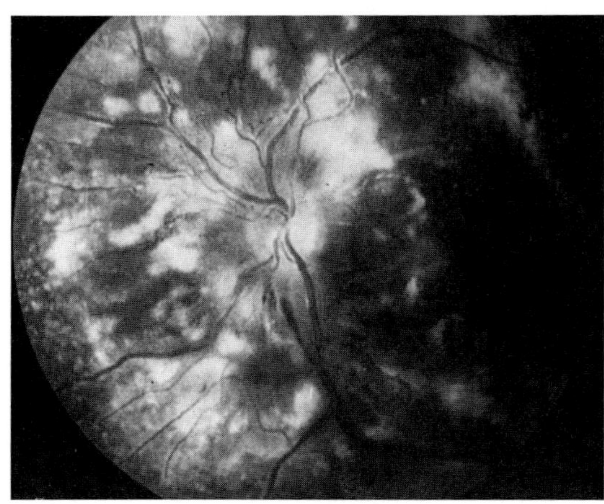

B

FIG. 4. A: Right fundus: (a) zone of papilledema, (b) zone of hard and soft exudates, (c) zone of hard exudates (high molecular weight lipoproteins). **B:** Left fundus of a 22-year-old man with sustained hypertension (250/150 mmHg) due to a large pheochromocytoma of the right adrenal. One year previously he had been given electroshock therapy by a psychiatrist. Blood pressure had been normal 5 months before. Initially he had been hospitalized because of markedly blurred vision (only able to count fingers) for 3 months. Treatment with cortisone started 7 months before admission brought little visual improvement. Photographs A and B [wide-angle (45°) Nikon camera] reveal an acute group-4 hypertensive retinopathy with bilateral papilledema, many hemorrhages, hard and soft exudates (extending along the arcades and involving the macular zones), neovascularization in the peripapillary areas, and severe arteriolar narrowing. The marked degree of retinal edema extended 30° from the optic discs (i.e., even beyond the limits of these funduscopic photographs). Following extirpation of a 165-g pheochromocytoma, the BP and catecholamine metabolites normalized. The retinopathy completely resolved within 10 months, leaving only residual fibrous sheathing along some of the arterioles near the discs, pigment epithelial disruption, and glial tissue along former areas of edema. Vision improved to 20/40 OS and 20/80 OD within 1 year but did not return to normal because of residual gliotic changes. Photographs were obtained through the courtesy of Dr. F. A. L'Esperance, Jr., Professor of Ophthalmology, Columbia Medical Center, New York, New York. (From ref. 8.)

(39,40). Similarly, hypercalcemia in a patient with pheochromocytoma may not indicate the presence of multiple endocrine neoplasia. The cause of non-parathyroid-hormone-mediated hypercalcemia remains unclear, but secretion of calcitonin by some sporadic pheochromocytomas may be implicated (41). Therefore, reevaluation of patients for evidence of a thyroid C-cell hyperplasia (or carcinoma) and hyperparathyroidism should be performed following pheochromocytoma removal; these conditions can be appropriately treated at a later date without risk of hypertensive crises.

Neurofibromatosis (Fig. 6) (von Recklinghausen's disease), often with café-au-lait spots, occurs in 5% of patients with pheochromocytoma; the incidence of pheochromocytoma in persons with neurofibromatosis is 1%. Recently, the rare association of neurofibromatosis, pheochromocytoma, and somatostatin-rich duodenal carcinoid tumor has been reported (42). Rarely, pheochromocytoma coexists with von Hippel–Lindau disease (cerebellar hemangioblastoma and retinal angioma) or acromegaly.

The fact that pheochromocytoma and associated lesions of the thyroid and neural tissues are all of neuroectodermal origin suggests that these entities arise from maldevelopment of the neural crest.

The high incidence of cholelithiasis in patients with pheochromocytoma and paroxysmal (30%) or sustained (10%) hypertension remains unexplained.

APUDOMAS AND NEUROCRESTOPATHIES

Pearse introduced the concept of the "APUD" cell system. He delineated a group of cells that have certain cytochemical and ultrastructural features in common. These cells, which are present in a variety of endocrine as well as nonendocrine tissues, appear to have a neuroendocrine function and probably arise from the neural crest. They produce low-molecular-weight polypeptide hormones or hormone precursors. The term "APUD" is an acronym derived from the initial letters of the most characteristic cytochemical behavior of these cells [i.e., *a*mine (amino acid) and amine *p*recursor *u*ptake and *d*ecarboxylation]. Thus, these cells produce amines by taking up amine precursors, which they then decarboxylate. Pearse proposed that the APUD cell system constitutes "a peripheral neuroendocrine system, analogous to the central neuroendocrine system of the hypothalamus" (43).

Subsequently, Bolande (44) presented a unifying concept of disease arising from neural crest maldevelopment. He coined the term "neurocrestopathies" to designate the constellation of embryogenetically related disease entities such as pheochromocytoma, neuroblastoma, neurofibromatosis, medullary thyroid carcinoma, carcinoid tumors, Hirschsprung's disease, nonchromaffin paragangliomas (chemodectomas), melanotic progonoma, multiple endocrine neoplasia, and neurocutaneous melanosis. The pathogenic common denominator in these conditions appeared to be an aberrant neural crest development (44). The finding that some of these conditions cause the production of catecholamines supports this concept.

An immunochemical technique has identified neuron-

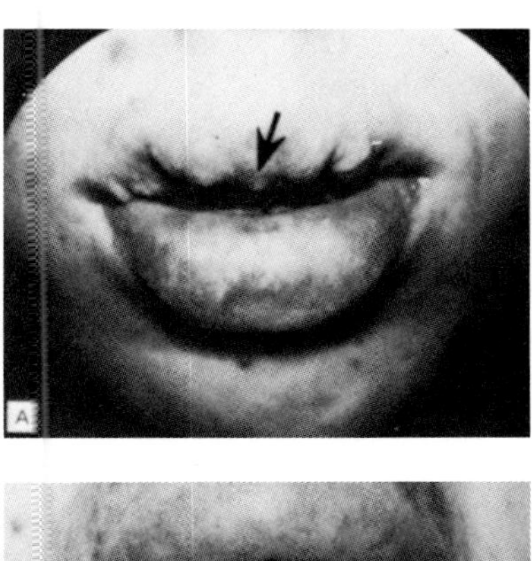

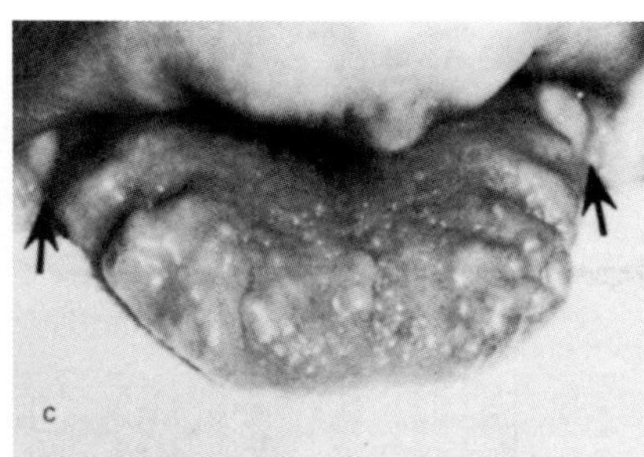

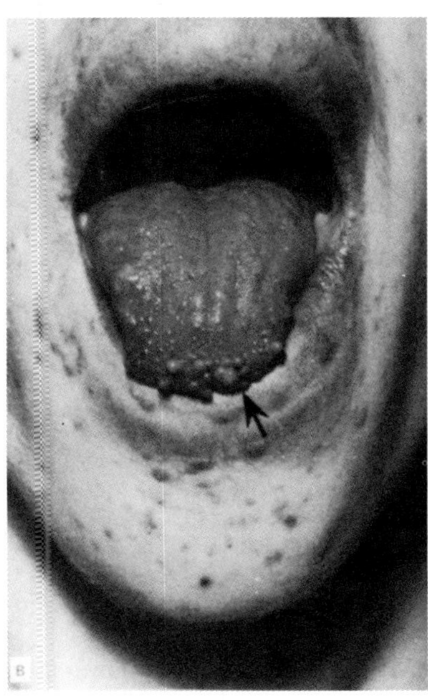

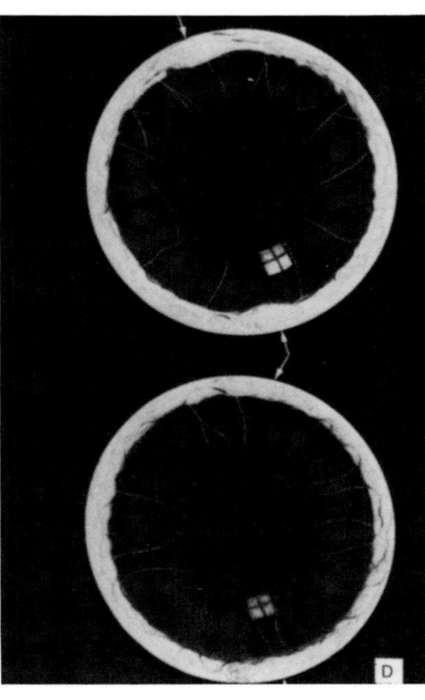

FIG. 5. Lesions of the lips, tongue, and corneas, observed in four patients with multiple endocrine neoplasia, type 3. **A:** Diffuse thickening of lower lip, which is everted and patulous. Thickening of upper lip is less prominent but is irregular and accentuated centrally (*arrow*) and produces a bumpy appearance. Medullary thyroid carcinomas and pheochromocytomas occurred in this patient. **B:** Multiple sessile confluent nodules stud tip of tongue. Slightly elevated plaque-like lesions, more evident on right (*arrow*), are present along margins of tongue. Upper lip is diffusely thickened. Similar alteration of lower lip is concealed by tongue. Medullary thyroid carcinoma was present without evidence of pheochromocytoma. **C:** Several large nodules are present on anterior third of tongue. Lateral margin exhibits a coarse undulating (*left*) and bumpy (*right*) appearance. Intraoral conical projections at angles of mouth are just visible bilaterally (*arrows*). Upper lip is diffusely thickened and exhibits characteristic central accentuation of thickening. Medullary thyroid carcinoma was present without pheochromocytoma. (From ref. 79.) **D:** Thickened corneal nerve of right and left eyes of a patient with MEN, type 3. Thickened perilimbal neuromas are visible on either side of each limbus (*arrows*). This drawing by Dr. Dennis M. Robertson was based on the precise location of corneal nerves and neuromas determined by sequential slit-lamp examination of the entire cornea. (From ref. 80.)

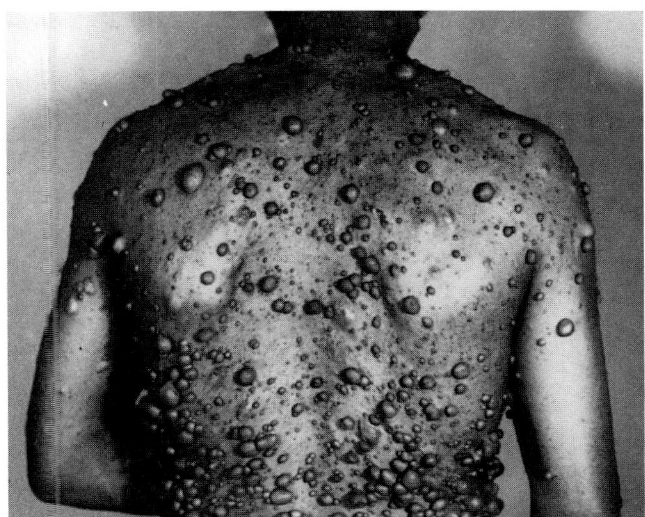

FIG. 6. Neurofibromatosis in a patient without pheochromocytoma. These lesions, which probably arise from neurilemma of peripheral nerves, are subcutaneous, freely mobile, and may be tender. They seldom interfere with nerve function. Rarely, sarcomatous degeneration occurs. Courtesy of Dr. A. Doronkos, late Professor of Dermatology, Columbia Medical Center, New York. (From ref. 8.)

specific enolase in all pheochromocytomas studied. Enolase, a common neuroendocrine marker, was demonstrated in melanomas and peripheral nerve tumors (in addition to nerves and normal adrenal medullae). The presence of enolase in these tumors (45), as well as the presence of chromogranin A in normal and neoplastic polypeptide hormone-producing tissues (46), is evidence in support of the neuroendocrine nature of the APUD system.

Potential ramifications of the neuroectodermal cell, along with its transformation into diverse tumors, are illustrated in Fig. 7.

DIFFERENTIAL DIAGNOSIS

No disease causes more diverse manifestations than pheochromocytoma. The differential diagnosis includes a long list of conditions which may produce manifestations suggesting pheochromocytoma (Table 3); those in italics in Table 3 may be accompanied by increased urinary concentrations of catecholamines and their metabolites. Most of these conditions can be excluded on clinical grounds. [Differential diagnosis is discussed in detail elsewhere (8,47).] The preoperative diagnosis of pheochromocytoma must be

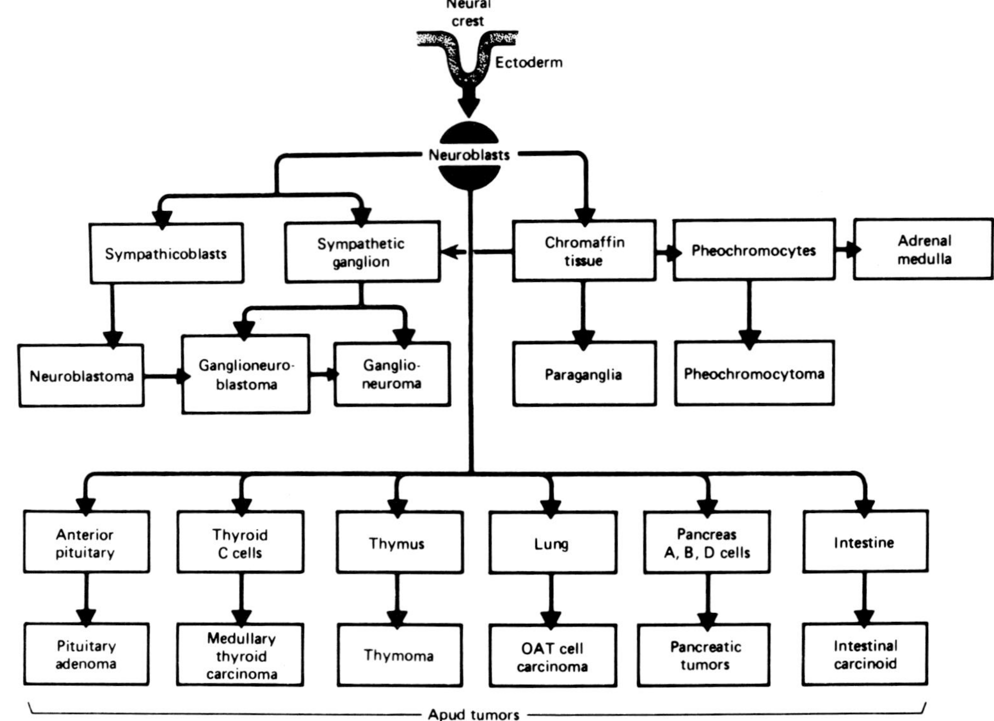

FIG. 7. Ectodermal origin of APUD tumors. (From ref. 81. Modified by Dr. M. M. Melicow, Columbia University Medical Center, New York.)

established by demonstrating substantial elevations of catecholamines and/or their metabolites in the urine or plasma.

Consumption of certain illegal drugs [e.g., amphetamine, cocaine, phencyclidine (PCP), lysergic acid diethylamide (LSD)] and some prescription and nonprescription drugs (e.g., decongestants, Comtrex, Contac, Acutrim, Dexatrim, Anorexin) which contain phenylpropanolamine (PPA) may cause hypertensive crises and symptoms mimicking pheochromocytoma. Factitious production of symptoms (pseudopheochromocytoma) by an emotionally disturbed person having access to drugs should be considered.

Rarely, hemorrhagic necrosis occurs in a pheochromocytoma and presents as an acute abdomen or cardiovascular catastrophe; without early recognition, prompt treatment, and tumor extirpation, the patient will almost certainly die.

DIAGNOSIS

Since 95% of patients are symptomatic, a detailed history and physical examination is essential in deciding who should be screened for pheochromocytoma.

All symptomatic patients with sustained or paroxysmal hypertension should be screened unless the cause of their hypertension is known. Even asymptomatic patients with hypertension of unknown cause should be screened if they have (a) abnormal laboratory or electrocardiographic (ECG) findings that may be caused by increased circulating catecholamines, (b) radiologic evidence suggesting pheochromocytoma, or (c) diseases known to occasionally coexist with pheochromocytoma (Table 1).

The indications for screening patients for pheochromocytoma are listed in Table 4. Screening can be reliably performed in the great majority of cases by quantitating 24-hr urinary metanephrines or determining plasma catecholamines. Measurement of urinary catecholamines and VMA is less reliable.

A point of extreme importance is that manifestations of pheochromocytoma occasionally first appear during pregnancy and, if not lethal, may remit, only to return at a later date, sometimes in association with a subsequent pregnancy. Pregnancy and childbirth in the presence of an unsuspected pheochromocytoma carry a high risk of maternal and fetal mortality.

Table 5 contains facts ("pheochromocytoma pearls") that are helpful in evaluating patients for evidence of pheochromocytoma.

LABORATORY AND ECG ABNORMALITIES

Laboratory abnormalities that may be observed in patients with pheochromocytoma and some associated conditions are enumerated in Table 6 and are discussed in detail elsewhere (8).

Hyperglycemia, hypermetabolism, and increased free fatty acids may result from elevated circulating catecholamines and should suggest pheochromocytoma. Rarely, patients may develop (a) lactic acidosis from altered intermediary metabolism and (b) impaired peripheral circulation due to excess circulating catecholamines (48). Hypovolemia is present in the majority of patients—primarily those with sustained hypertension. Rarely, polycythemia

TABLE 3. *Differential diagnosis*[a]

All hypertensives (sustained and paroxysmal)
Anxiety, tension states, psychoneurosis, psychosis
Hyperthyroidism
Paroxysmal tachycardia
Hyperdynamic β-adrenergic circulatory state
Menopause
Vasodilating headache (migraine and cluster headaches)
Coronary insufficiency syndrome
Acute hypertensive encephalopathy
Diabetes mellitus
Renal parenchymal or renal arterial disease with hypertension
Focal arterial insufficiency of the brain
Intracranial lesions (with or without ↑ intracranial pressure)
Autonomic hyperreflexia
Diencephalic seizure and syndrome
Toxemia of pregnancy (*or eclampsia with convulsions*)
Hypertensive crises associated with monoamine oxidase inhibitors
Carcinoid
Hypoglycemia
Mastocytosis
Familial dysautonomia
Acrodynia
Neuroblastoma; ganglioneuroblastoma; ganglioneuroma
Neurofibromatosis (with or without renal arterial disease)
Adrenocortical carcinoma
Acute infectious disease
Rare causes of paroxysmal hypertension (*acute medullary hyperplasia; acute porphyria; lead poisoning;* tabetic crisis; encephalitis; *clonidine withdrawal;* hypovolemia with inappropriate vasoconstriction; pulmonary artery fibrosarcoma; pork hypersensitivity; dysregulation of hypothalamus; *tetanus; Guillain–Barré syndrome; factitious*)
Fortuitous circumstances simulating pheochromocytoma
Conditions sometimes associated with pheochromocytoma
- Coexisting disease or syndromes
  - Cholelithiasis
  - Medullary thyroid carcinoma
  - Hyperparathyroidism
  - Mucosal neuromas
  - Thickened corneal nerves
  - Marfanoid habitus
  - Alimentary-tract ganglioneuromatosis
  - Neurofibromatosis
  - Cushing's syndrome
  - Von Hippel–Lindau disease
  - Polycythemia
  - Virilism, Addison's disease, acromegaly
- Complications
  - Cardiovascular disease[b]
  - Cerebrovascular disease
  - Renovascular disease
  - Circulatory shock
  - Renal insufficiency
  - Hemorrhagic necrosis of pheochromocytoma[b]
  - Dissecting aneurysm[b]
  - Ischemic enterocolitis with or without intestinal obstruction[b]

[a] Conditions in italics may have increased excretion of catecholamines and/or metabolites. From ref. 8.
[b] May present as an abdominal or cardiovascular catastrophe.

(due to erythropoietin secretion by some pheochromocytomas) may occur. Cushing's syndrome, rarely observed in patients with sporadic or familial pheochromocytoma, may result from excess production of ACTH-like substance by the pheochromocytoma or by an associated thyroid carcinoma.

Severe catecholamine-induced ischemia involving multiple organ systems may result in plasma elevations of pancreatic, liver, and cardiac enzymes (49). Plasma renin elevations may result from catecholamine stimulation of β_1-adrenergic receptors in the kidneys. Rarely, renal artery stenosis due to renal artery spasm or to compression by the pheochromocytoma or a coexisting neurofibroma may elevate plasma renin, angiotensin II, and aldosterone and contribute to the hypertension (8,50).

A wide variety of ECG changes have been observed (e.g., disorders of rhythm or abnormalities suggesting myocardial ischemia, damage, or strain); although nonspecific,

TABLE 4. *Indications for screening patients for pheochromocytoma*

1. Hypertension (sustained or paroxysmal) with the following:
   a. Symptoms (Table 1) and signs (Table 2) or coexisting disease or syndromes (Table 3)
   b. Group 3 or 4 retinopathy of unknown cause
   c. Weight loss
   d. Hyperglycemia
   e. Hypermetabolism without hyperthyroidism
   f. Cardiomyopathy
   g. Resistance to antihypertensive therapy
   h. Orthostatic hypotension (without antihypertensive drugs)
   i. Unexplained fever
2. Persons with marked hyperlability of blood pressure
3. Recurrent attacks of symptoms and signs of pheochromocytoma, even if hypertension not demonstrated
4. Severe pressor response during or induced by the following:
   a. Anesthesia induction
   b. Intubation
   c. Surgery
   d. Angiography
   e. Parturition
   f. Antihypertensive therapy
   g. Precipitating factors listed under "Clinical Presentation" in text
5. Unexplained circulatory shock
   a. During anesthesia
   b. During pregnancy, delivery, or in puerperium
   c. During operation or postoperatively
   d. Following administration of phenothiazine drugs
6. Family history of pheochromocytoma, especially if hypertensive (also screen siblings and children)
7. Hypertension with disease or complications sometimes associated with pheochromocytoma (Table 1)
8. Hyperlabile BP or severe hypertension during pregnancy or apparent preeclampsia or eclampsia
9. Transient abnormal electrocardiogram during hypertensive episodes
10. X-ray evidence of suprarenal mass

[a] Adapted from ref. 84.

TABLE 5. *Pheochromocytoma "pearls" (facts worth memorizing)*[a]

6 H's[b]:	Hypertension Headache Hyperhidrosis Heart consciousness Hypermetabolism Hyperglycemia
95% will have:	Headache or hyperhidrosis or palpitation
Rough rule of 10:	10% familial 10% bilateral (adrenal)[c] 10% malignant 10% multiple (other than bilateral adrenal)[c] 10% extra-adrenal 10% occur in children
MEN, type-2 triad:	Medullary thyroid carcinoma Bilateral-familial pheochromocytoma (frequent) Hyperparathyroidism (~50%)
MEN, type-3 sextet:	Medullary thyroid carcinoma Bilateral-familial pheochromocytoma (frequent) Mucosal neuromas Thickened corneal nerves Marfanoid habitus Alimentary-tract ganglioneuromatosis (very rarely hyperparathyroidism)
4 C's:	Cholelithiasis Cushing's syndrome (very rare) Cutaneous lesions Cerebellar hemangioblastoma (very rare)
Pheochromocytoma manifestations may appear during pregnancy.	

[a] Adapted from ref. 8.
[b] The term "triad of H's" was used by Dr. John E. Howard and refers to hypertension, hyperglycemia, and hypermetabolism (without hyperthyroidism) occurring in patients with pheochromocytoma. We have extended this category to include 6 H's.
[c] Adults and children combined.

their transient appearance during a paroxysm suggests pheochromocytoma, especially in the absence of other causes. Permanent ECG changes may result from hypertension, coronary atherosclerosis, and catecholamine myocarditis and cardiomyopathy. The latter may result from myocarditis due to excess circulating catecholamines and can occur in patients with sustained or only paroxysmal hypertension or, rarely, in some with normotension (51). With appropriate treatment, marked improvement—and even reversibility—of catecholamine cardiomyopathy has been reported (52).

BIOCHEMICAL TESTS

Plasma and urinary catecholamines and their metabolites are almost invariably elevated in patients with sustained hypertension due to pheochromocytoma; however, with pheochromocytomas causing only paroxysmal hypertension, plasma and urinary catecholamines and metabolites may be normal when the BP is relatively normal. When evaluating these latter patients, it is imperative either to obtain blood during a hypertensive period (spontaneous or provoked) or to collect urine following a hypertensive episode to establish the preoperative diagnosis.

Clonidine Suppression Test

A small percentage of patients with essential hypertension and symptoms and signs suggesting pheochromocy-

TABLE 6. *Laboratory findings sometimes present in pheochromocytoma*[a]

Fasting hyperglycemia (two-thirds of sustained hypertensives)
Glycosuria
Impaired glucose tolerance
↑ BMR (>20%) (three-fourths of sustained hypertensives)
↑ Plasma FFA (mainly sustained hypertensives) (? ↑ glycerol)
Hypercholesterolemia
Anemia or polycythemia; ↑ WBC and ESR normal (? ↑ platelets)
↓ Plasma and/or total blood volume
↑ Blood urea < 60 mg/dl in 95%; with or without proteinuria (rarely slight serum creatinine ↑)
Hyperreninemia ± aldosteronism
Hypokalemia
↑ Serum glucagon
Hypercalcemia (caused by pheochromocytoma)
Hypoinsulinemia (rarely hyperinsulinemia + hypoglycemia)
Hyperamylasemia
Lactic acidosis (↓ pH, ↓ Po_2, ↑ phosphorus)
↑ Serum PTH-like substance, ACTH, VIP, calcitonin, serotonin, gastrin, opioids, MSH, ? ANP, somatostatin (all rarely elaborated by pheochromocytoma)
If associated with:
Cushing's syndrome
↑ Serum ACTH (from pheochromocytoma or medullary thyroid carcinoma)
↑ Plasma cortisol
↑ Urinary steroids
Hyperparathyroidism
↑ Serum calcium
↑ Serum parathyroid hormone
↓ Serum phosphate
Medullary thyroid carcinoma
↑ Serum thyrocalcitonin
↑ Serum prostaglandin (E_2 and $F_{2\alpha}$)
↑ Serum serotonin
↑ Urinary 5-HIAA
↑ Serum histaminase
↑ Serum ACTH

[a] Modified from ref. 8. BMR, basal metabolic rate; FFA, free fatty acids; WBC, white blood cells; ESR, erythrocyte sedimentation rate; PTH, parathyroid hormone; ACTH, adrenocorticotropic hormone; VIP, vasoactive intestinal polypeptide; MSH, melanocyte-stimulating hormone; ANP, atrial natriuretic peptide.

toma have borderline or modest elevations of plasma (i.e., between 500 and 2000 pg/ml under basal conditions) or urinary catecholamines and their metabolites.

The clonidine-suppression test has proved exceptionally reliable in differentiating neurogenic from pheochromocytic hypertension (53,54). [Although the suppression test is safe, clonidine's vagotonic effect, particularly in the presence of β-blockade, can cause marked hypotension, which may transiently aggravate symptoms of peripheral vascular ischemia. (observed by W.M.M.)] The ability of clonidine to suppress the sympathetic nervous system and thereby reduce plasma concentrations of norepinephrine (by 50% and to within normal limits) in patients with neurogenic hypertension and normal subjects but not in those with pheochromocytoma (Fig. 8) confers diagnostic specificity. Changes in epinephrine concentrations are a less reliable diagnostic guide; however, significant increases in epinephrine, consistent with pheochromocytoma, have been observed during clonidine suppression (54). Since β-blockers may prevent significant clonidine suppression of plasma catecholamines in patients with neurogenic hypertension and thus falsely suggest the presence of pheochromocytoma (E. L. Bravo, *personal communication*), β-blockers should be discontinued 48 hr before the test. Very few drugs (e.g., isoproterenol, methyldopa, levodopa) cause spurious elevations of plasma catecholamines determined radioenzymatically; drugs which interfere with neuronal uptake of catecholamines or alter their storage may cause minor changes in plasma catecholamines.

Some have reported elevated concentrations of platelet catecholamines in patients with pheochromocytoma (but not in those with neurogenic hypertension) to be of diagnostic value (55). A decrease in β-adrenoceptors on leukocytes may also be of value in detecting patients with pheochromocytoma (56,57).

Urinary Catecholamines and Their Metabolites

Measurement of 24-hr urinary total metanephrines (metanephrine plus normetanephrine) is a highly reliable method of screening, since more than 95% of patients with pheochromocytoma have elevated levels.

Table 7 gives the upper limits of normal concentrations for catecholamine and metabolites and indicates substances that can interfere with their determination. We are unaware of drugs (except for metyrosine) that lower the urinary concentration of catecholamines or their metabolites to a normal range in patients with pheochromocytomas. However, radiopaque media containing methylglucamine can lead to false-negative results for metanephrines. [Conditions that alter excretion of catecholamines and their metabolites are listed in detail elsewhere (8).]

If a significant fraction of urinary catecholamines is epinephrine or its metabolite (metanephrine), or if plasma epinephrine is elevated, it is very likely that the pheochromocytoma is in the adrenal area or, rarely, in the organs of Zuckerkandl.

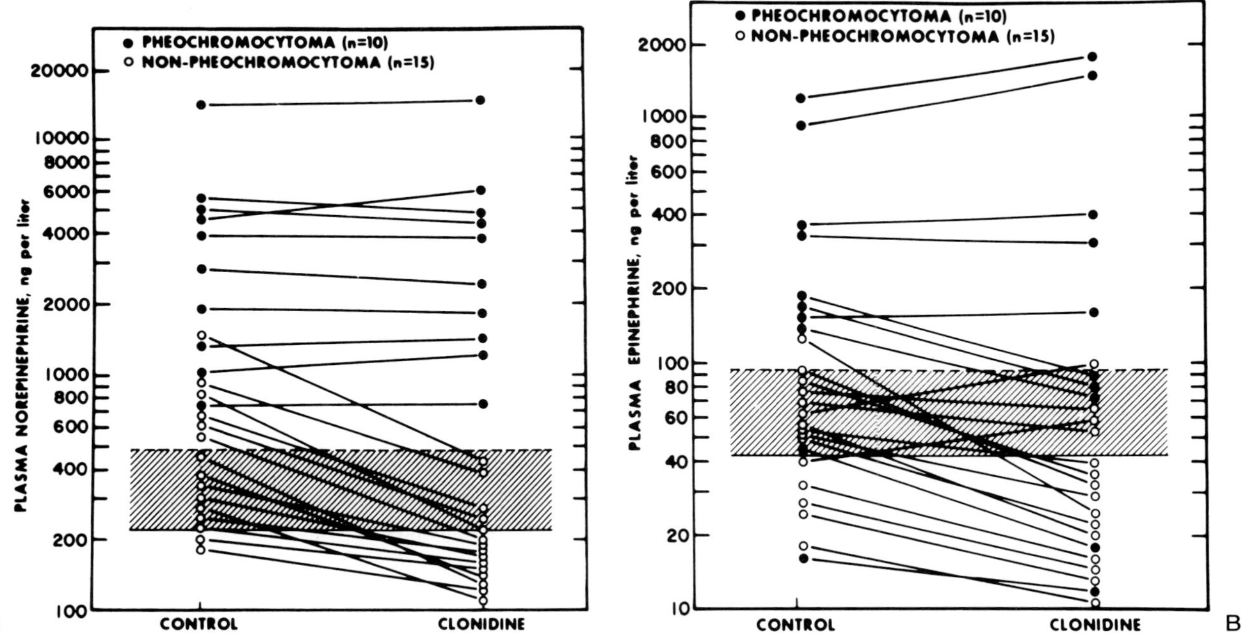

FIG. 8. Plasma norepinephrine (**A**) and epinephrine (**B**) values in individual patients before and 3 hr after a single oral dose of clonidine (0.3 mg). With the patient in a recumbent position, control samples are collected from a catheter placed in a peripheral vein at least 30 min earlier. Samples are then collected 2 and 3 hr after clonidine administration, since the peak suppression of plasma norepinephrine in patients with neurogenic hypertension usually occurs 2 or 3 hr after clonidine ingestion. The hatched area represents the mean of values obtained from 60 healthy, adult subjects (±3 SD). To convert values to nanomoles per liter, multiply by 0.006. (From ref. 53.)

TABLE 7. *Effects of drugs and interfering substances on concentrations of urinary catecholamines and metabolites*[a]

Upper limit of normal (Adult) (mg/24 hr)		Effects	
		Increases apparent value	Decreases apparent value
Catecholamines		Catecholamines	Fenfluramine (large doses)
Epinephrine	0.02	Drugs containing catecholamines	
Norepinephrine	0.08	Isoprenolol (isoproterenol)[b]	
Total	0.10	Levodopa	
Dopamine	0.20	Methyldopa	
		Labetalol[b]	
		Tetracyclines[b]	
		Erythromycin[b]	
		Chlorpromazine[b]	
		Other fluorescent substances[b] (e.g., quinine, quinidine, bile in urine)	
		Rapid clonidine withdrawal	
		Ethanol	
Metanephrines		Catecholamines	Methylglucamine (in Renovist, Renografin, etc.)
Metanephrine	0.4	Drugs containing catecholamines	
Normetanephrine	0.9	Monoamine oxidase inhibitors	Fenfluramine (large doses)
Total	1.3	Benzodiazepines	
		Rapid clonidine withdrawal	
		Ethanol	
Vanillomandelic acid	6.5	Catecholamines (minimal increase)	Clofibrate
		Drugs containing catecholamines (minimal increase)	Disulfiram
			Ethanol
		Levodopa	Monoamine oxidase inhibitors
		Nalidixic acid[b]	Fenfluramine (large doses)
		Rapid clonidine withdrawal	

[a] As determined by most reliable assays. Modified from ref. 83.
[b] Probably spurious interference with fluorescence assays.

PHARMACOLOGIC TESTS

In rare instances, a provocative test with glucagon, when combined with quantitation of plasma catecholamines, can prove indispensable in establishing the presence of a paroxysmally secreting pheochromocytoma. A provocative test is safe if performed correctly and with proper precautions to counteract hypertensive crises, arrhythmias, or hypotension; it is contraindicated in hypertensives (BP of 170/110 mmHg or greater) or in patients with any condition in which a sudden elevation of BP could be hazardous.

PREOPERATIVE LOCALIZATION OF PHEOCHROMOCYTOMAS

As mentioned above, elevation of plasma or urine epinephrine or its metabolite (metanephrine) suggests an adrenal pheochromocytoma; however, radiography can usually identify tumor location.

Radiography

Computerized axial tomography (CAT) can identify about 95% of pheochromocytomas; it is extremely accurate in revealing lesions 1 cm or greater in the adrenals and 2 cm or greater in extra-adrenal locations of the abdomen. A CAT scan is usually initially performed without contrast media; if a tumor is not evident, the scan should be repeated with contrast (both intravenous and oral) in order to permit optimal interpretation of areas being examined. CAT scanning is superior to angiography (now rarely indicated) and has the additional advantage of being noninvasive (Fig. 9); it is also highly reliable in identifying pheochromocytomas of the chest; however, experience in demonstrating these tumors in the neck is limited. Preoperative localization will prevent the possibility of an unnecessary abdominal exploration when the tumor is located in the thorax or neck.

If there is hematuria or a suggestion that hypertensive attacks occur with micturition or bladder distension, cystoscopy should be performed under α-adrenergic blockade in order to prevent a potentially serious hypertensive crisis resulting from the procedure. Cystoscopy will almost always determine whether a bladder pheochromocytoma is present.

Any patient suspected of having a malignant pheochromocytoma (about 10% of cases) should have bone and liver isotopic scans to detect evidence of metastatic disease. Metastases frequently appear in lymph nodes, liver, lung, and bone; however, interestingly, we are not aware of pheochromocytoma metastasizing to the brain. CAT liver scan with intravenous contrast is an excellent method of demonstrating liver metastases and has largely replaced liver isotopic scans. Since one cannot exclude the presence of metastases to the spine by conventional x-rays, a CAT scan or MRI (magnetic resonance imaging) should be uti-

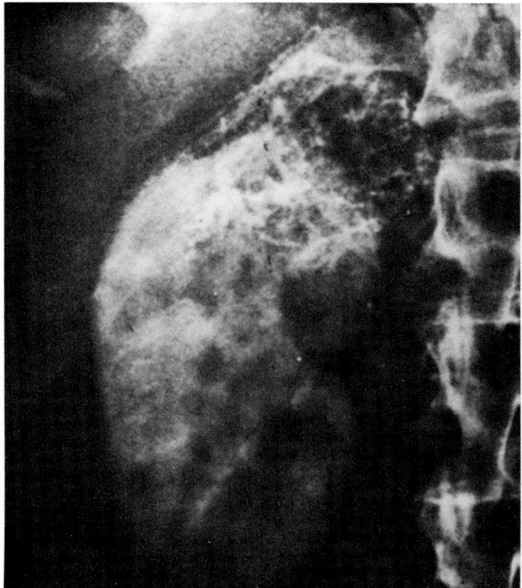

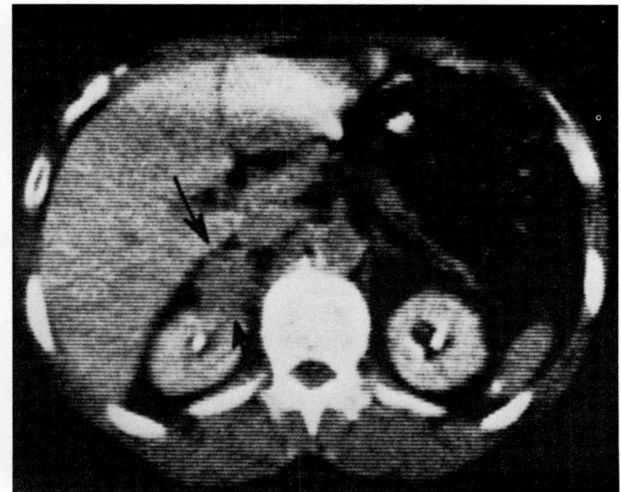

A B

FIG. 9. Demonstration of a pheochromocytoma in the right adrenal gland by (**a**) angiography (note vascularity of tumor above right kidney) and (**b**) computed axial tomography (arrows indicate tumor location). (Courtesy of Dr. Thomas Meaney, Cleveland Clinic Foundation. From ref. 82.)

lized if metastatic malignancy is suspected. Presence of metastases should not necessarily prevent surgical removal (debulking) of as much of the primary tumor as possible to reduce circulating catecholamines.

The use of the radiopharmaceutical agent ^{131}I-metaiodobenzylguanidine (^{131}I-MIBG) provides a fairly sensitive and specific technique for the diagnosis and localization of pheochromocytomas, since ^{131}I-MIBG has a propensity to concentrate in these tumors (Fig. 10) (58). Nevertheless, experience indicates that up to 15% of tumors are not recognized by this technique; only about 50% of malignant pheochromocytomas appear to concentrate ^{131}I-MIBG. Uniquely, ^{131}I-MIBG uptake establishes that tumors or metastatic lesions are pheochromocytomas. This modality can be invaluable when the identity of a tumor or metastasis is uncertain.

Recently, MRI has provided another valuable modality for demonstrating the presence of a pheochromocytoma. Although not providing the resolution of CAT scan, the behavior of the signal intensity observed on MRI scan appears to be characteristic for malignancy, pheochromocytoma, and certain other endocrine tumors (Fig. 11) (59); however, rarely, other benign adrenal lesions may mimic malignancy or pheochromocytoma on MRI (60).

Central Venous Blood Sampling

When all preoperative attempts to localize a pheochromocytoma have failed, sampling blood from various levels of the vena cava in the abdomen and chest may be very helpful in localizing abdominal tumors and in excluding intrathoracic and cervical pheochromocytomas. (Sampling blood from the left renal vein can be helpful in locating a pheochromocytoma in the left adrenal gland, since drainage from the latter almost always empties into the renal vein; however, we do not usually catheterize the adrenal veins, since catheterization of these veins may stimulate catecholamine secretion from normal adrenal glands and falsely suggest the presence of a tumor.) It is important to closely monitor pressure and pulse during sampling from various levels of the vena cava; significant alterations of these vital signs could result from fluctuations in the secretion rate of a pheochromocytoma and from changes in the levels of circulating catecholamines which could negate the reliability of localization by this procedure.

The algorithm in Fig. 12 can be used as a diagnostic guide in investigating patients suspected of harboring a pheochromocytoma.

TREATMENT

Successful management of pheochromocytoma requires expertise. Surgical removal, the only curative procedure, should be performed expeditiously in all patients for whom surgery is not contraindicated.

Preoperative Evaluation and Management

Medullary thyroid carcinoma and hyperparathyroidism should be excluded in all patients with pheochromocytoma and in relatives of patients known to have familial pheochromocytoma (61,62). Diagnosis and treatment of these conditions should be delayed until after pheochromocytoma removal.

Before surgery, it is prudent to establish the presence of bilateral renal function, in the event that the surgeon is faced with sacrificing a kidney during tumor removal.

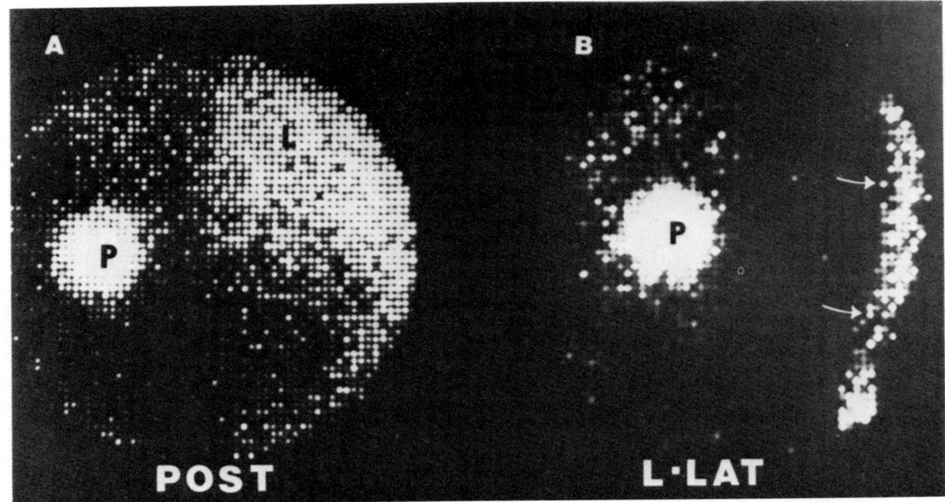

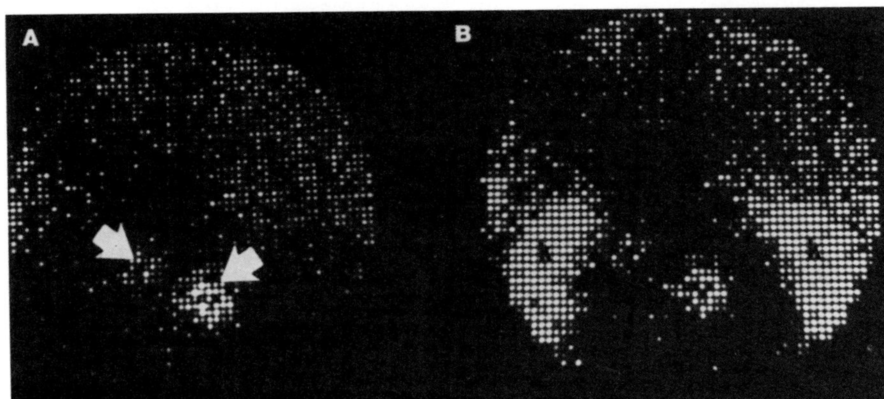

FIG. 10. Top: Scintigrams made 1 day after injection of ^{131}I-MIBG in a patient who had a 24-g tumor in the left adrenal gland. The pheochromocytoma (P) is readily identified in panel A (POST, posterior view) and panel B (L-LAT, left lateral view). The liver (L) is seen in panel A. Arrows in panel B point to a radioactive marker on the patient's back. **Bottom:** Posterior view of a patient two days after injection of ^{131}I-MIBG. Panel A shows concentrations of radioactivity near the midline (*arrows*). The radioactivity on the upper right is in the liver. Panel B shows kidney images (k), made with ^{99m}Tc-pentetic acid, superimposed on the scintigram shown in panel A. The concentrations of radioactivity produced by ^{131}I-MIBG correspond to the pheochromocytomas removed from the periaortic region; the larger one weighed 7.4 g, and the smaller one weighed 0.2 g. (From ref. 58.)

Rarely, patients with pheochromocytoma may have (a) a hypertensive crisis, (b) malignant hypertension, or (c) acute abdominal or cardiovascular complications requiring immediate medical and/or surgical therapy. Acute hypertensive crises (before or during surgery, or induced by angiography or a provocative test) can usually be controlled by a rapid intravenous bolus of phentolamine (3–5 mg); if there is no response within 1 or 2 min, an additional 5 mg can be given and repeated until the BP is adequately reduced. Since the effect of phentolamine is transient, it is preferable to control some hypertensive crises, especially those occurring during surgery, by infusing sodium nitroprusside or phentolamine (usually 100 mg of either drug mixed with 500 ml of 5% dextrose in water) at a rate sufficient to keep the BP relatively normal. (With impaired renal function or prolonged nitroprusside infusion, thiocyanate levels should be monitored because concentrations of greater than 10 mg/dl can cause thiocyanate toxicity, psychosis, and, very rarely, cyanide poisoning.) Caution in acutely lowering BP should be observed because of possible myocardial ischemia or damage (63).

If immediate operation is indicated, the presence of a significantly contracted blood volume should be corrected with whole blood or infusion of appropriate fluid within 18 hr preceding operation in order to minimize postoperative hypotension.

Abdominal palpation or diagnostic procedures that entail any trauma or stress should be performed with caution and with drugs available to treat hypertensive crises, arrhythmias, or hypotension.

Morphine and phenothiazines should be avoided because they may precipitate hypertensive crises or hypoten-

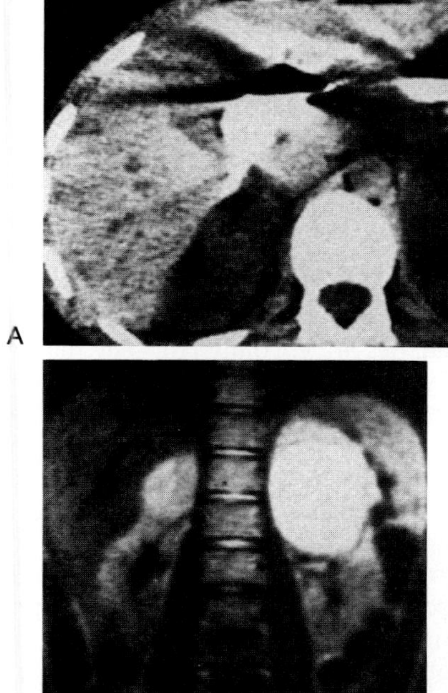

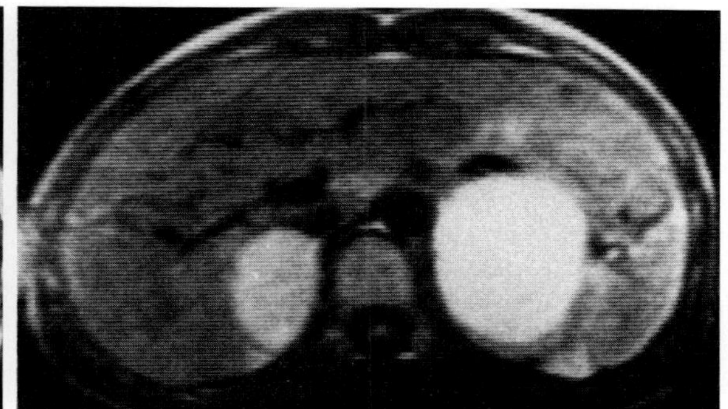

FIG. 11. A: Noncontrast CAT scan shows bilateral adrenal masses. The left adrenal pheochromocytoma has a large central cavity of lower attenuation. The margin of the right adrenal mass is poorly distinguished from the right kidney. **B:** Axial MR image [spin echo (SE) 40/1700] shows both pheochromocytomas as regions of high signal intensity. The higher signal intensity of the left tumor is due to the markedly increased T2 of its necrotic center. The margins of the pheochromocytomas are easily distinguished from the kidneys posterior to the masses. **C:** Coronal image from SE 40/1700 sequence shows relationship of both adrenal masses to the kidneys, liver, and spine. (From ref. 59.)

sion. If bilateral adrenalectomy is contemplated, steroid replacement should be instituted before surgery.

Adrenergic Blockade

Preoperative α-adrenergic blockade with phenoxybenzamine (10–20 mg twice daily) or prazosin (starting with 1 mg and increasing to 1 or 2 mg two or three times daily) for a week or more and continued to the time of surgery usually prevents severe preoperative clinical manifestations, reverses hypovolemia, and promotes smooth induction of anesthesia and relatively stable BP during surgery. However, in patients with pheochromocytoma who do not have severe hypertension or hypertensive crises or cardiovascular complications, preoperative blockade is optional

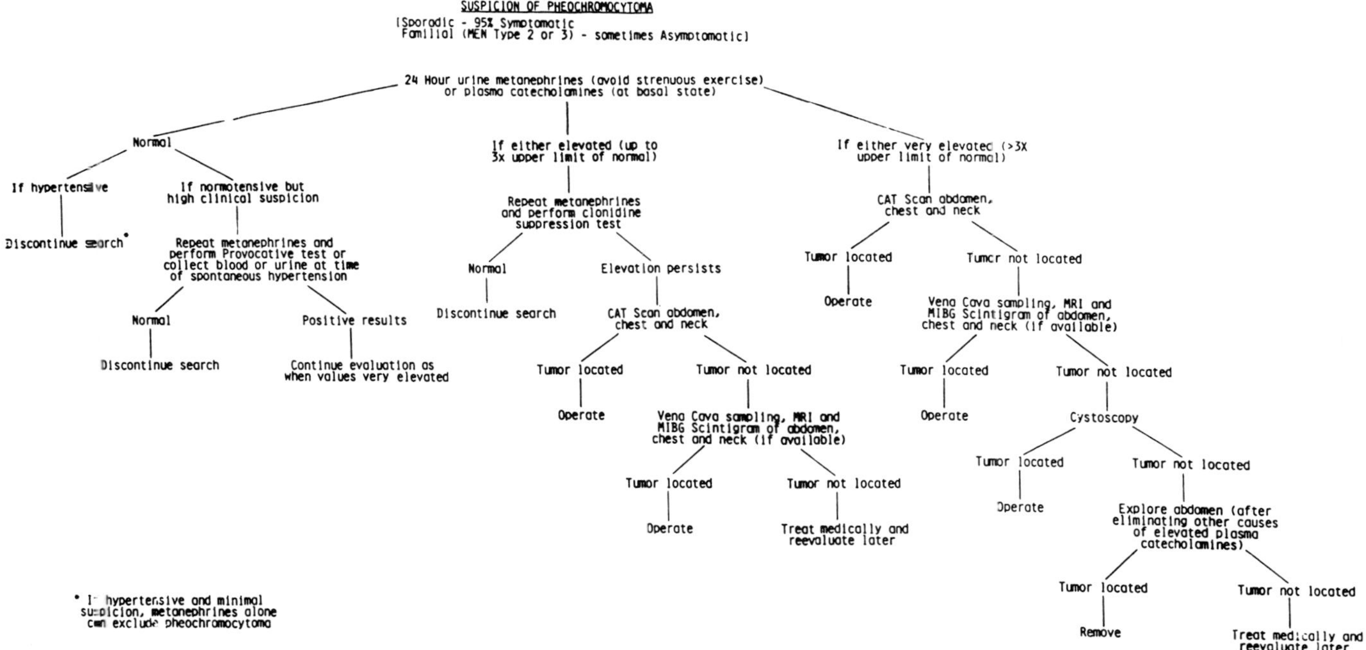

FIG. 12. Algorithm guide for the diagnosis of pheochromocytoma.

and not routinely employed in some of the leading medical centers. Complete blockade (to the point of marked orthostatic hypotension) is contraindicated, since with total blockade the surgeon will not have the advantage of utilizing increases in BP (caused by palpation in the vicinity of the tumor during intra-abdominal exploration) as a guide to tumor location or of immediately recognizing, by persistence of hypertension following tumor removal, that another tumor may be present.

Preoperative β-adrenergic blockade is indicated for persistent supraventricular tachycardia or arrhythmias that appear hazardous, or if angina occurs, provided that there are no contraindications. *The β-blockers should never be given without first creating α-adrenergic blockade, since β-blockade alone can cause a marked elevation in BP.* The latter phenomenon is particularly apt to occur if a β-blocker such as propranolol or nadolol is used, since these nonselective blockers would inhibit any vasodilating effect of the catecholamines (by blocking β_2 receptors) and thus enhance their vasoconstrictor effect; a relative cardioselective β-blocker (e.g., metoprolol) would be more appropriate. Ventricular arrhythmias should be treated with lidocaine.

Labetalol, an α- and β-adrenergic blocker, was reported effective in controlling BP and clinical manifestations in some patients with pheochromocytoma (64); however, its safety is controversial, since it sometimes causes hypertension (65,66).

The operative mortality (0–3.3%) has been relatively low in several medical centers with a wide experience in treating pheochromocytoma; expertise is the key to successful management.

OPERATIVE AND POSTOPERATIVE MANAGEMENT AND FOLLOW-UP

Preoperatively, a tranquilizer (e.g., diazepam) or a barbiturate premedication (e.g., secobarbital) or meperidine (Demerol) is given routinely to allay anxiety, which could trigger catecholamine release. Fentanyl and droperidol should be avoided because they may cause tumor secretion of catecholamines. Atropine should also be avoided, since it could cause severe tachycardia in the presence of excess circulating catecholamines.

Appropriate monitoring of arterial BP and ECG as well as preparation with muscle relaxants are important before endotracheal intubation. Isoflurane has gained popularity, although enflurane and halothane are suitable anesthetic agents.

During intubation and surgery, prompt control of hypertensive crises with intravenous phentolamine and/or nitroprusside and of arrhythmias with propranolol (newer short-acting cardioselective β-adrenergic blockers, such as esmolol, would be preferable) and/or lidocaine is critical and is discussed in detail elsewhere (8). Preoperative and intraoperative correction of blood volume deficits is essential in preventing postoperative hypotension.

Intra-abdominal pheochromocytomas should be removed through an anterior transperitoneal incision, since tumors may be multiple and extra-adrenal. Although controversial, it has been recommended that bilateral adrenalectomy be performed in patients with multiple endocrine neoplasia because of the great likelihood that both adrenals are, or will be, involved.

Patients with hypercalcitonemia and/or hypercalcemia should be reevaluated after pheochromocytoma removal, since the tumor may cause these biochemical elevations; return of the latter to normal eliminates the presence of multiple endocrine neoplasia as the cause.

If cholelithiasis, intra-abdominal neurofibromatosis, and vascular abnormalities are encountered, they may require additional surgery.

Pheochromocytomas of the neck, chest, and urinary bladder require special surgical techniques; otherwise, management is the same as with intra-abdominal tumors. Removal of cardiac pheochromocytomas can prove particularly difficult; apparently, MRI may be superior to CAT scanning in assessing some cardiac and pericardial lesions (15). Arteriography and ^{131}I-MIBG scintigraphy may be of additional value in identifying and defining these tumors. If pheochromocytoma is discovered during pregnancy, it is probably preferable to remove the tumor; however, if pregnancy is carried to term, cesarean section and tumor extirpation is advisable to avoid the stress of labor and vaginal delivery.

Postoperatively, close monitoring should be continued until the patient's condition is stable. Hemorrhage at operative sites and a blood volume deficit may cause hypotension; hypertension, on the other hand, may result from fluid overload, pain, urinary retention, hypoxia, hypercarbia, or residual pheochromocytoma. Inadvertent renal artery ligation can cause hypertension if residual circulation to the ischemic kidney resulted in hyperreninemia; however, hypertension due to renal ischemia would likely not occur immediately after renal ligation but would probably appear at least a few days or weeks later. Postoperative hypotension usually requires volume replacement.

Severe hypoglycemia with CNS manifestations and coma has been reported in several patients within 2 hr postoperatively; it is a transient phenomenon caused by a reactive rise in insulin which may be augmented by α-adrenergic blockers (by reducing the inhibitory effect of catecholamines on insulin secretion). Beta-adrenergic blockers may also impair hypoglycemic recovery (by reducing release of gluconeogenic substances and inhibiting glycogenolysis) and can mask signs of hypoglycemia by preventing tachycardia and sweating (67). Hypoglycemia should be treated promptly with infusion of dextrose and water. The initiation of an infusion of 5% dextrose in water immediately following tumor removal and continuing it for about 24 hr will prevent the potentially serious hazards of hypoglycemia (68,69). Transient hyperinsulinemia and reactive hypoglycemia have been reported in two patients with pheochromocytoma following glucose tolerance tests (51).

About 75% of patients become normotensive after tumor removal; the cause of persistent hypertension in the remainder is unclear but may be due to coexisting essential hypertension. Five-year survival for patients with benign tumors is 95%, whereas it varies from 36% to 50% if the tumor is malignant.

CHRONIC MEDICAL MANAGEMENT

When a malignant pheochromocytoma cannot be totally removed, as much as possible should be resected (debulked) to minimize functioning tissue. Radiotherapy has sometimes proved effective, especially with bone metastases.

Although irradiation with large doses of ^{131}I MIBG (two or three courses over 12–15 months) can cause partial tumor regression and decrease catecholamine secretion and symptomatology in about 25% of malignant pheochromocytomas, a 2-year follow-up study revealed that all patients relapsed. Because of these discouraging results and the expense and time required for treatment, this form of therapy with ^{131}I MIBG has been temporarily discontinued by those who introduced this therapeutic approach (James Sisson, University of Michigan, *personal communication*). Combination intravenous chemotherapy with cyclophosphamide, vincristine, and decarbazine has proved helpful in reducing tumor mass, catecholamine excretion, and symptomatology in some patients with malignant pheochromocytomas (70).

Prolonged treatment with α- and β-adrenergic blockade has effectively controlled BP and symptomatology for many years. Beta-blockade may also prove valuable in preventing catecholamine cardiomyopathy (71).

Metyrosine (Demser) can markedly decrease catecholamine synthesis and reduce or abolish manifestations of excess circulating catecholamines; it may be useful in the treatment of catecholamine-induced cardiomyopathy (52). It should be used cautiously and with adequate fluid intake. Increasing experience indicates it can be used safely and effectively in preoperative (as well as in chronic) medical management of pheochromocytoma (72).

Nifedipine, a calcium channel blocker, was recently reported to suppress clinical symptoms and plasma and urinary catecholamine levels in patients with pheochromocytoma (73,74). Verapamil was also reported to control hypertension in patients with pheochromocytoma without reducing plasma catecholamine concentrations (75). Experience indicates that calcium channel blockers can be helpful in the management of pheochromocytoma.

Somatostatin may be useful in controlling hypersecretory disorders (76); only with large intravenous doses of this hormone was it possible to partially control very severe secretory diarrhea in one of our patients who had marked elevations of plasma VIP and calcitonin, produced by extensive metastatic pheochromocytoma.

ACKNOWLEDGMENTS

Grateful acknowledgment for assistance in preparation of this manuscript is expressed to Florence Ling, Mildred C. Hulse, Tom Brown, Rev. Don A. Bundy, and Dr. Irvine H. Page.

Mildred C. Hulse also provided excellent technical assistance.

The preparation of this report was supported by the National Hypertension Association, Inc.

Note: Many of the views expressed above have been reported in detail in refs. 8 and 33.

REFERENCES

1. St. John Sutton MG, Sheps SG, Lie JT. Prevalence of clinically unsuspected pheochromocytoma: review of a 50-year autopsy series. *Mayo Clin Proc* 1981;56:354–360.
2. Buu NT, Kuchel O. A new method for the hydrolysis of conjugated catecholamines. *J Lab Clin Med* 1977;90:680–684.
3. Kuchel O, Buu NT, Fountaine A, et al. Free and conjugated plasma catecholamines in the venous effluent of various organs of hypertensive patients. *Eur J Clin Invest* 1977;7:75–76.
4. Snider SR, Kuchel O. Dopamine: an important neurohormone of the sympathoadrenal system. Significance of increased dopamine release for the human stress response and hypertension. *Endocr Rev* 1983;4:291–309.
5. Williams LT, Lefkowitz RJ. *Receptor binding studies in adrenergic pharmacology.* New York: Raven Press, 1978.
6. Weinshilboum RM. Clinical pharmacology: series on pharmacology in practice and antihypertensive drugs that alter adrenergic function. *Mayo Clin Proc* 1980;55:1390–1402.
7. Manger WM. *Catecholamines in normal and abnormal cardiac function.* New York: S Karger, 1982.
8. Manger WM, Gifford RW Jr. *Pheochromocytoma.* New York: Springer-Verlag, 1977.
9. Hoffman BB, Lefkowitz RJ. Alpha-adrenergic receptor subtypes. *N Engl J Med* 1980;302:1390–1396.
10. Weiner N, Taylor P. Neurohumeral transmission: the autonomic and somatic motor nervous system. In: Gilman AG, Goodman LS, Rall TW, Mural F, eds. *The pharmacological basis of therapeutics,* 7th edition. New York: Macmillan, 1985;66–99.
11. Goldberg LI, Kohli JD, Kotake AN, et al. Characteristics of the vascular dopamine receptor: comparison with other receptors. *Fed Proc* 1978;37:2396–2402.
12. Creese I, Fraser CM, eds. *Dopamine receptors in receptor biochemistry and methodology,* vol 8 (Venter JC, Harrison LC, series eds.) New York: Alan R Liss, 1987;261.
13. Goldberg LI, Volkman PH, Kohli JD. A comparison of the vascular dopamine receptor with other dopamine receptors. *Annu Rev Pharmacol Toxicol* 1978;18:57–79.
14. Axelrod J. *The fate of noradrenaline in the sympathetic neurone.* Harvey Lectures, series 67. New York: Academic Press, 1972;187–197.
15. Stowers SA, Gilmore P, Stirling M, et al. Cardiac pheochromocytoma involving the left main coronary artery presenting with exertional angina. *Am Heart J* 1987;114:423–427.
16. Shimoyama Y, Kawada K, Imamura H. A functioning intrapericardial paraganglioma (pheochromocytoma). *Br Heart J* 1987;57:380–383.
17. Hosaka Y, Rainwater LM, Grant CS, Farrow GM, Van Heerden JA, Lieber MM. Pheochromocytoma: nuclear deoxyribonucleic acid patterns studied by flow cytometry. *Surgery* 1986;100:1003–1010.
18. Klein AF, Kay S, Ratliff JE, White FKH, Newsome HH. Flow cytometric determinations of ploidy and proliferation patterns of adrenal neoplasms: an adjunct to histological classification. *J Urol* 1985;134:862–866.
19. Goldstein DS, Stull R, Eisenhofer G, Session JC, Weder A, Averbuch SD, Keiser HR. Plasma 3,4-dihydroxyphenylalanine (dopa) and catecholamines in neuroblastoma or pheochromocytoma. *Ann Intern Med* 1986;105:887–888.
20. Van Heerden JA, Sheps SG, Hamberger B, et al. Pheochromocytoma: current status and changing trends. *Surgery* 1982;91:367–373.

21. Melicow MM. One hundred cases of pheochromocytoma (107 tumors) at the Columbia–Presbyterian Medical Center, 1926–1976: a clinicopathological analysis. *Cancer* 1977;40:1987–2004.
22. Winkler H, Smith AD. Pheochromocytoma and other catecholamine-producing tumors. In: Blaschko H, Muscholl E, eds. *Catecholamines.* New York: Springer, 1972;900–933.
23. Wocial B, Januszewicz W, Siedlecki L, et al. Alterations in plasma dopamine-beta-hydroxylase and catecholamine concentrations during removal of pheochromocytoma. *Endocrinologie* 1982; 79:131–139.
24. O'Connor DT, Bernstein KN. Radioimmunoassay of chromogranin A in plasma as a measure of exocytotic sympathoadrenal activity in normal subjects and patients with pheochromocytoma. *N Engl J Med* 1984;311:764–770.
25. Giraud P, Eiden LE, Audigier Y, et al. ACTH, α-MSH and β-endorphin in human pheochromocytoma. *Neuropeptides* 1981; 1:236–252.
26. Eiden LE, Giraud P, Hotchkiss A, et al. Enkephalins and VIP in human pheochromocytomas and bovine adrenal chromaffin cells. In: Trabucchi M, Costa E, eds. *Regulatory peptides from molecular biology to function: advances in biochemical psychopharmacology,* vol 33. New York: Raven Press, 1982;387–395.
27. Bostwick DG, Null WE, Holmes D, Weber E, Barchas JD, Bensch KG. Expression of opioid peptides in tumors. *N Engl J Med* 1987;317:1439–1443.
28. Sano T, Saito H, Inaba H, et al. Immunoreactive somatostatin and vasoactive intestinal polypeptide in adrenal pheochromocytoma: an immunochemical and ultrastructural study. *Cancer* 1983;52:282–289.
29. Viale F, Dell'orto P, Moro E, Gozzaglio L, Goggi G. Vasoactive intestinal polypeptide-, somatostatin- and calcitonin-producing adrenal pheochromocytoma associated with the watery diarrhea (WDHH) syndrome. *Cancer* 1985;55:1099–1106.
30. Garbini A, Mainardi M, Grimi M, Repaci G, Nanni G, Bragherio G. Pheochromocytoma and hypercalcemia due to ectopic production of parathyroid hormone. *NY State J Med* 1986;86:25–27.
31. Allen JM, Yeats JC, Causon R, Brown MJ, Loom SR. Neuropeptide Y and its flanking peptide in human endocrine tumors and plasma. *J Clin Endocrinol Metab* 1987;64:1199–1204.
32. Wilson SP, Cubeddu LX, Chang KJ, et al. Met-enkephalin, len-enkephalin and other opiate-like peptides in human pheochromocytoma tumors. *Neuropeptides* 1981;1:273–281.
33. Manger WM, Gifford RW Jr, Hoffman BB. Pheochromocytoma: a clinical and experimental overview. *Curr Probl Cancer* 1985;9:12–13.
34. Mullen JR, Cartwright RC, Tisherman SE, Misage JR, Shapiro AP. Case report: pathogenesis and pharmacologic management of pseudo-obstruction of the bowel in pheochromocytoma. *Am J Med Sci* 1985;290:155–158.
35. Bravo EL, Tarazi RC, Fouad FM, Textor SC, Gifford RW Jr, Vidt DG. Blood pressure regulation in pheochromocytoma. *Hypertension* 1982;4(Suppl II):II-193–II-199.
36. Prockocimer PG, Maze M, Hoffman BB. Role of the sympathetic nervous system in the maintenance of hypertension in rats harboring pheochromocytoma. *J Pharmacol Exp Ther* 1987; 241:870–874.
37. Simpson NE, Kidd KK, Goodfellow PJ, et al. Assignment of multiple endocrine neoplasia type 2A to chromosome 10 by linkage. *Nature* 1987;328:528–530.
38. Raue F, Frank K, Meybier H, Ziegler R. Pheochromocytoma in multiple endocrine neoplasia. *Cardiology* 1985;72(Suppl):147–149.
39. Sizemore GW. Medullary thyroid carcinoma. *Thyroid Today* 1982;5:106.
40. Weinstein RS, Ide LF. Immunoreactive calcitonin in pheochromocytomas. *Proc Soc Exp Biol Med* 1980;165:215–217.
41. Heath H III, Edis AJ. Pheochromocytoma associated with hypercalcemia and ectopic secretion of calcitonin. *Ann Intern Med* 1979;91:208–210.
42. Wheeler MH, Curley IR, Williams ED. The association of neurofibromatosis, pheochromocytoma, and somatostatin-rich duodenal carcinoid tumor. *Surgery* 1986;100:1163–1168.
43. Pearse AGE. Cytochemical evidence for the neural crest origin of mammalian ultimobranchial C cells. *Histochemie* 1971;27:96–102.
44. Bolande RP. The neurocrestopathies: a unifying concept of disease arising in neural crest maldevelopment. *Hum Pathol* 1974;5: 409–429.
45. Lloyd RV, Shapiro B, Sisson JC, et al. An immunohistochemical study of pheochromocytomas. *Arch Pathol Lab Med* 1984; 108:541–544.
46. O'Connor DT, Burton D, Deftos LJ. Immunoreactive human chromogranin A in diverse polypeptide hormone producing human tumors and normal endocrine tissue. *J Clin Endocrinol Metab* 1983;57:1084–1086.
47. Manger WM, Gifford RW Jr, Hoffman BB. Pheochromocytoma: a clinical and experimental overview. *Curr Probl Cancer* 1985;9:29–33.
48. Bornemann M, Hill SC, Kidd GS. Lactic acidosis in pheochromocytoma. *Ann Intern Med* 1986;105:880–882.
49. Case 6, 1986 Case Records of the Massachusetts General Hospital. *N Engl J Med* 1986;314:431–429.
50. Kohara K, Mikami H, Ogihara T, et al. Extra-adrenal pheochromocytoma manifesting renovascular hypertension. *J Clin Hypertens* 1987;3:303–309.
51. Heramalsu K, Takahashi K, Kanemoto N, Arimori S. A case of pheochromocytoma with transient hyperinsulinemia and reactive hypoglycemia. *Jpn J Med* 1987;26:88–90.
52. Imperato-McGinley J, Gautier T, Ehlers K, Zullo MA, Goldstein DS, Vaughan DE Jr. Reversibility of catecholamine-induced dilated cardiomyopathy in a child with a pheochromocytoma. *N Engl J Med* 1987;316:793–797.
53. Bravo EL, Tarazi RC, Fouad FM, et al. Clonidine-suppression test: a useful aid in the diagnosis of pheochromocytoma. *N Engl J Med* 1981;305:623–626.
54. Karlberg BE, Hedman L. Value of clonidine suppression test in the diagnosis of pheochromocytoma. *Acta Med Scand [Suppl]* 1986;714:15–21.
55. Zweifler AJ, Julius S. A diagnostic test in patients with elevated plasma catecholamines. *N Engl J Med* 1982;306:890–894.
56. Manger WM, Gifford RW Jr, Hoffman BB. Pheochromocytoma: a clinical and experimental overview. *Curr Probl Cancer* 1985;9:72–73.
57. Valet P, Damase-Michel C, Chamontin B, Durand D, Gaillard G, Salvador M, Montastruc JL. Adrenoceptors in the diagnosis of pheochromocytoma. *Lancet* 1987;2:337.
58. Sisson JC, Frager MS, Valk TW, et al. Scintigraphic localization of pheochromocytoma. *N Engl J Med* 1981;305:12–17.
59. Fink IJ, Reinig JW, Dwyer AJ, Doppman JL, Linehan WM, Keiser HR. MR imaging of pheochromocytomas. *J Comput Assist Tomogr* 1985;9:454–458.
60. Baker EM, Spritzer C, Blinder R, Herfkens RJ, Leight GS, Dunnick NR. Benign adrenal lesions mimicking malignancy on MR imaging: report of two cases. *Radiology* 1987;163:669–671.
61. Graze K, Spiler IJ, Tashjian AH, et al. Natural history of familial medullary thyroid carcinoma. *N Engl J Med* 1978;299:980–985.
62. Manger WM, Gifford RW Jr, Hoffman BB. Pheochromocytoma: a clinical and experimental overview. *Curr Probl Cancer* 1985;9:52.
63. Friedman E, Mandel M, Katznelson D, Sack J. Pheochromocytoma and hydralazine-induced myocardial ischaemia in a 14-year-old boy. *Eur J Pediatr* 1986;145:318–320.
64. Rosei EA, Brown JJ, Lever AF, et al. Treatment of pheochromocytoma and of clonidine withdrawal hypertension with labetalol. *Br J Clin Pharmacol* 1976;3(Suppl 3):809–815.
65. Briggs RSJ, Birtwell AJ, Pohl JEF. Hypertensive response to labetalol in pheochromocytoma. *Lancet* 1978;1:1045–1046.
66. Reach G, Thibonnier M, Chevillard CP, et al. Effect of labetalol on blood pressure and plasma catecholamine concentrations in patients with pheochromocytoma. *Br Med J* 1980;280:1300–1301.
67. Meeke RI, O'Keefe JD, Gaffney JD. Pheochromocytoma removal and postoperative hypoglycemia. *Anesthesia* 1985;40:1093–1096.
68. Pullerits J, Reynolds C. Pheochromocytoma: a clinical review with emphasis on pharmacologic aspects. *Clin Invest Med* 1982;5:259–265.
69. Manger WM, Gifford RW Jr, Hoffman BB. Pheochromocytoma:

a clinical and experimental overview. *Curr Probl Cancer* 1985;9:57–58.
70. Manger WM, Gifford RW Jr, Hoffman BB. Pheochromocytoma: a clinical and experimental overview. *Curr Probl Cancer* 1985;9:58.
71. Rosenbaum JS, Ginsburg R, Billingham ME, Hoffman BB. Effects of adrenergic receptor antagonists on cardiac morphological and functional alterations in rats harboring pheochromocytoma. *J Pharmacol Exp Ther* 1987;241:354–360.
72. Brogden RN, Heel RC, Speight TM, et al. Alpha methyl-L-tyrosine: a review of its pharmacology and clinical use. *Drugs* 1984;21:81–89.
73. Serfas D, Shoback DM, Lorell BH. Pheochromocytoma and hypertrophic cardiopathy: apparent suppression of symptoms and noradrenaline secretion by calcium-channel blockade. *Lancet* 1983;2:711–713.
74. Favre L, Vallotton MB. Nifedipine in pheochromocytoma [Letter to the Editor]. *Ann Intern Med* 1986;104:125.
75. Mannelli M, De Feo MU, Maggi M, Geppetti P, Baldi E, Pupilli C, Serio M. Effect of verapamil on catecholamine secretion by human pheochromocytoma [Letter to the Editor]. *Hypertension* 1986;8:811–814.
76. Moreau JP, De Feudis FV. Minireview—pharmacological studies of somatostatin and somatostatin-analogues: therapeutic advances and perspectives. *Life Sci* 1987;40:419–437.
77. Coupland R. *The natural history of the chromaffin cell.* Essex, England: Longman, Green & Co., 1965.
78. Engelman K. Principles in the diagnosis of pheochromocytoma. *Bull NY Acad Med* 1969;45:852.
79. Carney JA, Sizemore GW, Lovestedt SA. Mucosal ganglioneuromatosis, medullary thyroid carcinoma, and pheochromocytoma: multiple endocrine neoplasia, type 2b. *Oral Surg* 1976;41:746–747.
80. Robertson DM, Sizemore GW, Gordon H. Thickened corneal nerves as a manifestation of multiple endocrine neoplasia. *Trans Am Acad Ophthalmol Otolaryngol* 1975;79:733.
81. Baylin SB. Ectopic production of hormones and other proteins by tumors. *Hosp Pract* 1975;10:124.
82. Manger WM, Gifford RW Jr. Pheochromocytoma. In: Sleight P, Freist ED, eds. *Cardiology I: Hypertension.* London: Butterworth, 1982.
83. Manger WM, Gifford RW Jr. Current concepts of pheochromocytoma. *Cardiovasc Med* 1978;3:289–303.
84. Manger WM, Gifford RW Jr. Hypertension secondary to pheochromocytoma. *Bull NY Acad Med* 1982;58:139–158.

Hypertension: Pathophysiology, Diagnosis, and Management, edited by J. H. Laragh and B. M. Brenner. Raven Press, Ltd., New York © 1990.

CHAPTER 103

Thyroid Hormone and Blood Pressure Regulation

Irwin Klein

Mechanism of Action of Thyroid Hormone, 1661
Intracellular Effects, 1661
Stimulation of Thermogenesis, 1662
Direct Effects of Thyroid Hormone, 1663
Effects on Adrenergic Activity, 1663
Drug Metabolism, 1663
Effects of Thyroid Hormone on the Cardiovascular System, 1663
Vascular Resistance, 1664
Blood Volume, 1664
Cardiac Contractility, 1664
Cardiac Size, 1665
Thyroid Hormone and Blood Pressure Regulation, 1665
Catecholamines, 1666
Renin Synthesis and Release, 1666
Angiotensin Production, 1666
Aldosterone Metabolism, 1667
Atrial Natriuretic Factors: Synthesis and Release, 1667
Vasopressin Activity in Hypothyroidism, 1667
Hyperthyroidism, 1667
Prevalence of Hypertension, 1667
Cardiovascular Manifestations, 1668
Response to Therapy, 1668
Thyroid Storm, 1669
Hypothyroidism, 1669
Prevalence of Hypertension, 1669
Cardiovascular Manifestations, 1670
Mechanism of Hypertension in Hypothyroidism, 1670
Response to Therapy, 1670
Myxedema Coma, 1671
Thyroid-Associated Disease States, 1671
Addison's Disease, 1671
Systemic Lupus Erythematosus, 1671
Progressive Systemic Sclerosis (Scleroderma), 1671
Atherosclerotic Cardiovascular Disease, 1671
Summary, 1672
References, 1672

It is well recognized that thyroid hormone has profound effects on the cardiovascular system and blood pressure regulation. Dating back to the earliest clinical descriptions of thyrotoxicosis by Caleb Parry (1) and Robert Graves (2), a relationship between thyroid hormone and blood pressure regulation has been presumed. Thus, the increased cardiac output, widened pulse pressure, tachycardia, and hyperdynamic precordium of hyperthyroidism are frequent clinical findings (3–7) and stand in marked contrast to the decrease in cardiac work, narrow pulse pressure, and quiet precordium that are characteristic of myxedema (4,8–10) (Table 1).

Thyroid hormone exerts direct cellular effects on almost all tissues of the body (11–14). This explains, in part, the diverse symptoms associated with thyroid disease. Included in these cellular changes is the so-called thermogenic response to alterations in oxygen consumption (11,15–17). These changes, in turn, require adaptation of the cardiovascular system over both the short and long term. The clinical manifestations of these processes can result in changes in blood pressure.

It has been suggested that hypertension is a common accompaniment of thyroid disease; therefore it is important to address the role of thyroid hormone in blood pressure regulation. This chapter will review the possible mechanisms by which alterations in thyroid hormone action accompanying either hyperthyroidism or hypothyroidism can effect cardiovascular homeostasis. Understanding the cellular mechanisms of thyroid hormone action and resulting changes in the heart and cardiovascular system can facilitate a rational approach to the management of hypertension in the setting of thyroid disease.

MECHANISM OF ACTION OF THYROID HORMONE

Intracellular Effects

The profound effects of thyroid hormone on normal physiology arise as a result of the fact that both tetraiodothyronine (T_4) and triiodothyronine (T_3) exert effects upon

TABLE 1. *Cardiovascular manifestations of thyroid disease[a]*

	Peripheral vascular resistance	Blood volume	Cardiac output	Heart rate	Pulse pressure	Precordial examination	Cardiac contractility
Hyperthyroid	↓↓	↑	↑↑	↑	↑↑	Hyperdynamic	↑
Hypothyroid	↑↑	↓	↓↓	↓	↓↓	Quiet	↓

[a] Compared to euthyroid state: ↑, increased; ↓, decreased.

almost every organ system in the body (11) (Fig. 1). Similar to the steroid, but distinct from the polypeptide, hormones, thyroid hormones exert many of their biologic actions intracellularly and at the level of the cell nucleus rather than at the plasma membrane (12,14). Following the identification of discrete nuclear binding sites for T_3 in various organs (16), it was subsequently determined that thyroid hormone was capable of altering specific gene transcription (13,17). Just which proteins are under the control of thyroid hormone and can allow for increased thermogenesis is currently under investigation (11,17). The specificity that arises from the ability to regulate gene expression and the synthesis of certain proteins has led to a better understanding of the cellular effects of thyroid hormone.

To exert its cellular effect, T_3 (with a higher affinity than T_4) passes directly from the non-protein-bound pool of thyroid hormone in the serum, through the cell cytoplasm to nuclear receptor proteins (12). The cell then responds to an increase in T_3 nuclear receptor occupancy by promoting the transcription of specific messenger RNA (mRNA) sequences coding for selected proteins (17). Nonhistone protein nuclear receptors for T_3 which regulate the synthesis of growth hormone have been extensively studied, and the mechanism of this effect has been well characterized (13). In addition, thyroid hormones have been suggested to also effect the synthesis of various hepatic, cardiac enzymes (7,11,18,19) and other yet-to-be-identified mRNA species (11).

Stimulation of Thermogenesis

The biologic hallmark of abnormal thyroid function is a change in the basal metabolic rate (BMR). Various changes in cellular physiology have been postulated to account for these changes (11,17,20). Recent studies examining the direct nuclear action of thyroid hormone suggest a role for alterations in the synthesis, and possibly the activity, of various enzymes involved in oxidative metabolism and cellular respiration.

Edelman and co-workers have established that the activity of the membrane enzyme sodium–potassium-activated ATPase (Na/K ATPase) from liver of hypothyroid animals is acutely increased by T_3 treatment (15). In the resting individual, much of basal oxygen consumption results from the maintenance of cellular transmembrane gradients of Na^+ and K^+ (16). Thus it is apparently useful to explain thyroid-hormone-mediated changes in oxygen consumption as a result of alterations in the activity of this enzyme system (15,16). Recent work also points to an increase in the functional activity of Na/K ATPase to counteract T_3-induced changes in Na and K flux (21).

As a result of many different lines of investigation, it is possible to summarize that thyroid hormone increases energy utilization and heat production (thermogenesis) through a series of steps (Fig. 2). Thyroid hormone initially acts at the level of the cell nucleus to increase the transcription of the mRNA for a protein that, in some way, alters

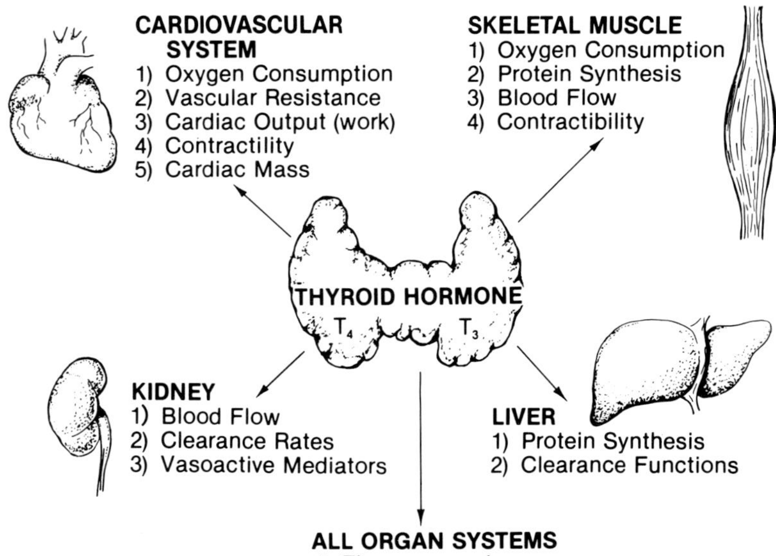

FIG. 1. The effects of thyroid hormone on the various organ systems.

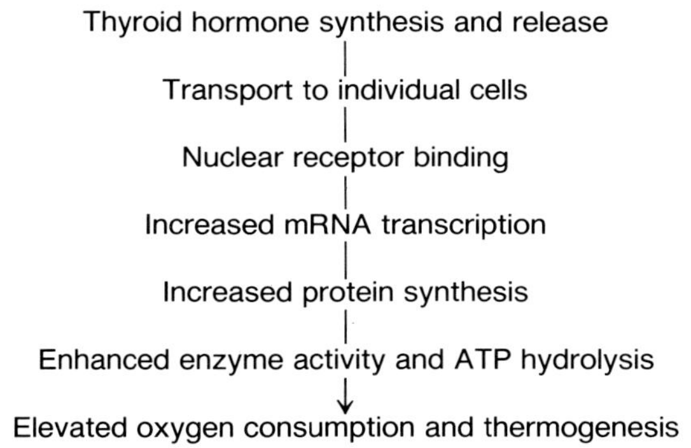

FIG 2. Sequence of events leading to thyroid-hormone-induced thermogenesis.

oxygen consumption (12). Increased synthesis leads to an increased cellular content of the enzyme along with enhanced catalytic activity. ATP hydrolysis is promoted and ADP levels rise, which, in turn, stimulate mitochondrial respiration, oxygen consumption, and heat production (11,15,18). The net effect of these steps is an increase in the BMR. Whether additional alterations in transmembrane Na^+ or K^+ currents contribute to the rise in Na/K-ATPase activity remains to be resolved (16). A role for the specific proteins in the process of thermogenesis seems inevitable (17) Oppenheimer et al. have postulated that as much as 8% of the genetic expression of hepatocytes may be under the control of T_3. One specific mRNA, referred to as S-14, is regulated by T_3 and may play a role in heat generation via an uncoupling of oxidative phosphorylation (17).

The net effect of these cellular processes on the cardiovascular system is to impose an increased need for oxygen and fuel delivery to peripheral tissues to provide for energy generation and for the efficient removal of the increased heat which is generated (3,22–24). This requires an increase in resting cardiac output. How this process is regulated will ultimately determine the changes in vascular resistance and blood pressure associated with thyroid disease.

Direct Effects of Thyroid Hormone

In addition to the effects of thyroid hormone, which are mediated via the cell nucleus, various other cellular organelles have been postulated to serve as a target for hormone action. These include the plasma membrane of erythrocytes (25) and of the sinoatrial node of the heart (26), the plasma membrane enzyme adenylate cyclase (6), sarcolemma membrane Ca^{2+}-ATPase (25), and specific T_3 receptors in the mitochondria (11,20). Since it is not yet possible to explain all of the biologic effects of thyroid hormone via changes in the transcription rate of specific proteins, it is tempting to implicate these additional direct effects of the hormone. Regardless of the site of action, the unifying feature of thyroid hormone on cells is to increase energy utilization and cellular respiration.

Effects on Adrenergic Activity

Many of the cardiovascular manifestations of hyperthyroidism are similar to the signs and symptoms of catecholamine excess that accompany disease states such as pheochromocytoma (5,18,27–30) or that occur after the administration of sympathomimetic drugs such as theophylline. These include tachycardia, widened pulse pressure, hyperdynamic precordium, and an increased cardiac output (3,7,31). It has been suggested that adrenal or free-nerve-ending catecholamine production and release is increased in hyperthyroidism and alternatively decreased in hypothyroidism (6,27–29,32–34). However, direct measures of serum catecholamines have been found to be *low* or normal in hyperthyroidism and *increased* in hypothyroidism (27,29,35,36).

In an attempt to resolve this apparent discrepancy, Lefkowitz and co-workers directly measured the myocardial content of beta-adrenergic receptors in hyperthyroid rats and found them to be increased (37). Similarly, acute T_3 administration can increase the mononuclear leukocyte density of beta-adrenergic receptors in humans (38). Other reports find no change in the beta-adrenergic receptor number in experimental hyperthyroidism (39).

Despite the increase reported for beta-adrenergic receptor number, the cardiac chronotropic response to infused isoproterenol is no different in an animal with experimental hyperthyroidism than in a euthyroid control. Thus while changes in beta-adrenergic receptor density do occur in thyrotoxic states, it is still not possible to account for the changes that are observed clinically (6,18,35).

Drug Metabolism

Drug metabolism varies as a function of thyroid status. The steady-state dosage, absorption, metabolism, and excretion of many drugs are increased by hyperthyroidism (22,40). Hypothyroidism has the reverse effect. This explains the observation that the therapeutic effect, as well as the serum level, of digoxin is lower in a hyperthyroid patient for any given dose of administered drug when compared to that in the euthyroid counterpart (4,40). As will be discussed below, other factors (including the tissue content of Na/K ATPase) may also play a role in this phenomenon (41). Hepatic metabolism of various drugs (including hypnotics, sedatives, and certain vitamins) are accelerated in hyperthyroidism (Fig. 1). Whether other endogenous vasoactive substances capable of altering vascular tone also have altered half-lives or biologic activity with varying thyroid disease states remains to be investigated.

EFFECTS OF THYROID HORMONE ON THE CARDIOVASCULAR SYSTEM

As noted above, the cardiovascular manifestations of thyroid disease states are some of the most profound clinical changes noted. The effects of thyroid hormone on the heart and circulation constitute a spectrum extending from severe hypothyroidism with myxedema to hyperthyroidism and thyroid storm. In this review, unless specifically noted, the pathophysiologic changes of hyperthyroidism will be assumed to be diametrically opposed to those occurring in hypothyroidism (Table 1).

Vascular Resistance

One of the earliest cardiovascular responses to thyroid hormone administration is a decrease in peripheral vascular resistance (42). This has been observed in hypothyroid patients, as well as in euthyroid animals, after acute thyroid hormone administration. Hyperthyroidism may be associated with as much as a 50% decline in systemic vascular resistance (SVR) (18,24,43,44); however, the mechanisms for the changes in SVR have not been completely elucidated (8,13,35,43,45). In animals, beta-adrenergic blockade with propranolol reversed the T_3-mediated acute drop in SVR (42) and also blunted the thyroid-hormone-mediated increase in cardiac output. We have observed that chronic propranolol treatment blocks the T_4-induced increase in heart rate, heart work, and cardiac hypertrophy associated with experimental hyperthyroidism (46).

Blood flow to the skin, kidneys, heart, and muscles is increased in hyperthyroidism. Kontos et al. have observed that the increase in blood flow could, in part, be abolished by atropine (47). However, the role of cholinergic tone or other local vasodilators in producing the changes in vascular resistance remains to be resolved. It is interesting to speculate that increased cellular respiration leads to the release of local vasodilators (15,44,48), which, in turn, mediate local resistance vessels (Fig. 3).

Thyroid hormone may primarily affect SVR, which, in turn, causes alterations in diastolic blood pressure and reflexly alters cardiac output. This postulate is supported by the studies of Theilen and Wilson (49), who observed a significant decrease in cardiac output after administration of phenylephrine in hyperthyroid but not in normal subjects. The ability to block the elevated cardiac output by pharmacologically reversing the changes in SVR of hyperthyroidism reinforces the possibility that many of the cardiovascular changes of hyperthyroidism occur in response to changes in peripheral tissues. However, Morkin et al. observed a much smaller decline in cardiac output after the administration of phenylephrine to thyrotoxic calves and also questioned the importance of changes in SVR (7).

An alternative hypothesis involves the ability of thyroid hormone to directly affect systemic vascular resistance via changes in arteriolar smooth muscle tone. Similar to the effects on erythrocytes, hepatocytes, and diaphragmatic muscle, T_3 may alter Na and K flux in smooth muscle cells, thereby leading to a decrease in contraction (16,41). More rapid calcium pumping by the sarcolemmal vesicles may also serve to relax arteriolar musculature (25,50). Thus the effect of thyroid on vascular resistance may occur by direct action on the peripheral circulation or in conjunction with (a) T_3-mediated changes in thermogenesis and (b) the generation of other vasodilators (Fig. 3).

Blood Volume

Hyperthyroidism is associated with an increase in blood volume, and the converse occurs with hypothyroidism (8,43,51). Gibson and Harris demonstrated a correlation between blood volume and BMR which resolved with appropriate therapy (51). Erythropoiesis and serum levels of erythropoietin vary directly with changes in serum levels of T_4 and can alter red blood cell mass (4). Hyperthyroid animals have increases of up to 25% in total blood volume, plasma volume, and erythrocyte mass.

Cardiac Contractility

Increased cardiac contractility and cardiac hypertrophy accompany both spontaneously occurring and experimentally induced hyperthyroidism (3,6,7,18,22,46,52). Treatment of animals with T_4 leads to an increase in heart weight as a result of an increased rate of cardiac protein synthesis (46,53). Organ culture studies suggest that the effects of T_4 on the heart are mediated by direct effects on protein metabolism (53). However, augmented rates of protein and ribosomal RNA synthesis also occur as a generalized and rapid response to increased cardiac work from various causes. Thus, thyroid hormone could promote the development of cardiac hypertrophy either by a direct effect on the rate of myocardial protein synthesis or indirectly through changes in cardiac work (18,22,46,52).

Hyperthyroidism is characterized by positive cardiac inotropism (24). Contractile parameters such as the rate of ventricular pressure development or velocity of contraction are uniformly increased (7,18). Hyperthyroid patients may have as much as a 100% increase in cardiac output and resting heart rate. Recent studies have suggested that there is a reversible form of cardiomyopathy in patients with hyperthyroidism. At rest, hyperthyroid patients had an elevated left ventricular ejection fraction that failed to normally increase with exercise. The response of left ventricular ejection fraction to exercise returned toward normal

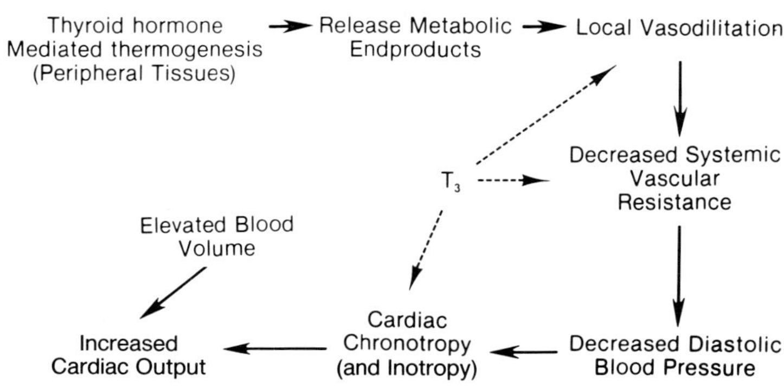

FIG. 3. Thyroid-hormone-mediated changes that produce alterations in cardiac output and cardiac work.

after the patients became euthyroid (54). No explanation was offered for this paradoxical finding of altered cardiac physiology in the setting of increased contractility.

The process of cardiac contraction is mediated via the interaction of the two major contractile proteins actin and myosin. Their interaction, a sliding of the thick myosin filament on the thin actin filament, requires myosin-mediated ATP hydrolysis and is regulated by other myofibrillar proteins and by the cytosolic concentration of calcium. One parameter of cardiac contractility is the maximum velocity of muscle fiber shortening which correlates with the activity of myosin ATPase.

Thyroid hormone can exert effects on cardiac contractility at several discrete points. Myosin ATPase enzymatic activity has been shown to vary with changes in serum levels of both T_4 and T_3. The myosin molecule is composed of two heavy chains which contain ATPase enzymatic activity in their globular head portion. There are two heavy-chain isomers with differing enzymatic activity (alpha and beta) (7,18). The intact myosin molecule exists in three isoenzymatic forms in a number of animal species. The alpha and beta heavy chains are under distinct genetic control, and the resulting dimeric combinations of these heavy-chain monomers (aa,aB,BB) constitute the three different myosin isoenzymes. The alpha homodimer is associated with the highest level of myosin ATPase, and the beta homodimer demonstrates the lowest level of myosin ATPase activity (7,11).

A number of investigators have suggested that the distribution of these isoenzymes in the rat and rabbit is under the control of thyroid hormone (7,11). In general, thyroid hormone stimulates the transcription of the α-myosin mRNA and inhibits β-myosin synthesis, whereas thyroxine deficiency gives rise to β-chain predominance. Thyroid hormone could directly increase muscle fiber shortening as a consequence of increased myosin ATPase activity (7,11). Conversely, it has been suggested that hemodynamic factors primarily alter alpha and beta heavy-chain expression and that thyroid-hormone-mediated changes in heart rate and cardiac output are the determinants of the isoenzyme shift (46,52).

It has not been conclusively demonstrated that myosin exists in isoenzymic forms in human heart. In normal postmortem human hearts and in human heart samples obtained from patients with severe cardiomyopathy, partially purified myosin appeared to be the low-enzyme-activity β-chain (5608H). It is interesting to speculate that, similar to the rabbit heart, human cardiac myosin exists in a relatively inactive ATPase form that can be shifted to a higher activity isoenzyme, either directly or indirectly, by an excess of thyroid hormone (7,18).

As noted above, thyroid hormone increases the activity of the enzyme Na/K ATPase (15). This enzyme is responsible for active sodium transport across the cardiac cell membrane and is inhibited by digitalis, with a resulting positive cardiac inotropic effect (41). Cardiac digitalis glycoside-binding sites have been shown by Kim and Smith to vary directly with the level of T_4 (41). This phenomenon predicts that the hyperthyroid heart and possibly other types of muscle and tissues are relatively insensitive to the positive inotropic effects of digitalis, which requires maximum receptor occupancy. In contrast, the hypothyroid heart and vascular contractile tissues should exhibit increased sensitivity (40).

Cardiac Size

The increase in left ventricular mass associated with hyperthyroidism represents an increase in all the major contractile proteins (46). As noted above, it was not previously possible to distinguish between (a) the potential direct nuclear effects of thyroid hormone on cardiac protein synthesis (12) and (b) the associated increases in cardiac work, which may independently serve as a stimulus for myocardial protein synthesis (52). Hyperthyroidism is associated with a volume overload similar to that of Paget's disease or chronic anemia or to that obtained with intracardiac shunts (18,52). In contrast to the hypertrophy that is produced by an increase in afterload (such as occurs with hypertension or aortic stenosis), the hypertrophy of volume overload is characterized by rapid rates of ventricular shortening. Thus, hyperthyroidism gives rise to a hyperdynamic, volume-overloaded form of cardiac hypertrophy (46).

To further explore the mechanism of hypertrophy in hyperthyroidism, we have employed the model of the syngeneic heterotopically transplanted rat heart. Heterotopic cardiac transplantation into the abdominal cavity allows for the long-term maintenance of a vascularly perfused, spontaneously beating, essentially nonworking heart exposed to the same hormonal milieu as the *in situ* heart (52). If T_4 directly affects the quantity of myocardial protein synthesis, then similar to the *in situ* heart the transplanted heart should hypertrophy with experimental hyperthyroidism. If, in contrast, T_4 stimulates heart growth through changes in cardiovascular hemodynamics, then only the *in situ,* not the transplanted, heart should increase in size. The results of those studies show that thyroid hormone caused a marked increase in the heart weight and protein content of the *in situ* working heart but not of the heterotopically transplanted nonworking heart (52). Direct measurements of protein synthesis were similarly increased in the *in situ* heart, but not in the transplanted heart, by thyroid hormone treatment. These results strongly support the concept that thyroxine-induced cardiac hypertrophy is mediated by changes in cardiac output and cardiac work (52).

THYROID HORMONE AND BLOOD PRESSURE REGULATION

Various hormonal systems have been implicated in both the normal and pathologic states of blood pressure regulation. The role of catecholamines, renin, mineralocorticoids, vasopressin, and atrial naturetic peptide are discussed elsewhere in this volume. In an attempt to explain the changes in blood pressure that accompany thyroid disease, alterations in the normal homeostasis of these related endocrine systems have been examined. It has been suggested that the hypertension of thyroid disease is mediated, in part, by alterations in other hormones.

Catecholamines

Because of the apparent similarities between excessive catecholamine secretion and the clinical presentation of patients with hyperthyroidism, it has been tempting to attribute the cardiovascular manifestations of hyperthyroidism to increased adrenergic stimulation (6,28–30). However, multiple investigators have directly measured the serum levels of norepinephrine and epinephrine in thyrotoxic patients and found them to be normal or decreased (27,29,34–36,55). To explain this seeming paradox, other components of the sympathoadrenal axis have been explored. These include (a) catecholamine turnover and excretion (32,33,36), (b) tissue sensitivity to adrenergic stimulation at the level of the beta receptor (37,39), and (c) the possibility of alternative adrenergic-like stimulators (56). The evidence for such mechanisms will be discussed.

When the turnover of catecholamines in the heart is directly measured, the results are normal or low (33). Similarly, the urinary excretion of adrenergic metabolites are either unchanged or less than that in euthyroid subjects (27,29,34,36). In contrast, both the serum levels and turnover rates of catecholamines are increased in hypothyroidism (6,29,36,55,57). The urinary excretion rates for norepinephrine, but not for epinephrine, vary inversely with thyroid function (34).

Failure to demonstrate the expected changes in serum levels of catecholamines in hyperthyroidism led to the postulate of an increased tissue sensitivity to adrenergic stimulation. However, critical review of the concept of a cardiovascular hypersensitivity to catecholamines fails to find support for this concept (6,18).

Beta-adrenergic agents exert their effects on heart muscle and other tissues by binding to beta-adrenergic receptors on the cell surface and activating adenylate cyclase, which, in turn, catalyzes the conversion of ATP to cyclic 3′,5′-adenosine monophosphate (cAMP) (58). Intracellular cAMP then initiates a series of reactions which characterize the cardiac response to catecholamines (58). Williams et al. have reported that membranes from hyperthyroid hearts contain a significantly greater number of beta-adrenergic binding sites when compared to those from the hearts of euthyroid animals (37). These data suggest that the increase in beta-adrenergic activity might arise from a direct thyroid-hormone-mediated increase in adrenergic receptor number. Alternatively, the lower tissue or plasma catecholamine levels of thyrotoxicosis might increase receptor number via the process of "up-regulation". In contrast to this postulate is the observation that isoproterenol produces a similar magnitude rise in heart rate in animals with experimental thyrotoxicosis when compared to controls (59). At present, the clinically apparent hyperadrenergic cardiovascular system of hyperthyroidism does not appear to result solely from the effects of adrenergic stimulation. It has been suggested that these changes are a result of a combination of the effects of both thyroid hormone and catecholamines upon the heart and upon the peripheral circulation (6,18). Thus, an additive effect of both thyroid hormone and beta-adrenergic stimulation to produce the tachycardia of thyrotoxicosis conforms to most experimental data (6). Multiple experimental systems have confirmed the ability of thyroid hormone to directly increase heart rate (26). Whether this is the predominant effect in hyperthyroid humans or whether the changes in heart rate and cardiac output are reflex in nature and involve other potentially vasoactive components remains to be resolved.

There exist structural similarities between thyroid hormone and catecholamines. This has led to the suggestion that some of the adrenergic signs of hyperthyroidism may be mediated by synaptic uptake and release of T_4 and T_3. Dratman et al. postulated a central nervous system role for iodocompounds as neurotransmitters, stemming from their ability to enhance heart rate when administered intrathecally (56). The magnitude of that effect, however, is not in keeping with the rise in heart rate observed with peripherally administered T_4 (46).

Renin Synthesis and Release

Renin is secreted by the juxtaglomerular cells of the kidney in response to various stimuli (60–62). One of these mediators is beta-adrenergic activity (61). Since, as discussed above, hyperthyroidism clinically appears as a state of heightened adrenergic activity, it is interesting to speculate that hyperthyroidism is associated with increased renin activity (104). Resnick and Laragh have directly measured plasma renin activity in hyperthyroid patients and found it to be increased compared to that in euthyroid controls (63). In contrast, hypothyroid patients have a lower-than-normal level of plasma renin (64–66).

When hypothyroid patients were studied before and after thyroid hormone replacement, it was observed that both basal and furosemide-stimulated plasma renin activity increased with treatment (66). Similar results for both plasma renin concentration and plasma renin activity were observed in the rat (67). Thus, the hypertension that accompanies hypothyroidism occurs in the setting of low levels of plasma renin.

Angiotensin Production

Plasma angiotensinogen is an α_2-globulin and serves as a substrate for the action of plasma renin (68). In perfused rat liver slices, angiotensinogen production was markedly and directly affected by prior *in vivo* concentrations of thyroid hormone. The release of angiotensinogen was inhibited by 60% in hypothyroid animals; this change was reversed by T_4 treatment. When *in vivo* plasma levels of angiotensinogen were measured, the effects were even greater (68). Similar to estrogens and cortisol, thyroid hormone appears to exert a direct effect to stimulate hepatic production of angiotensinogen. In the setting of increased plasma renin activity and with elevations of angiotensin-converting enzyme (ACE), it would be predicted that both angiotensin II and aldosterone would be increased by thyroid hormone (69).

Aldosterone Metabolism

Aldosterone is a mineralocorticoid formed almost entirely in the zona glomerulosa of the adrenal gland. The production of aldosterone is primarily regulated through a positive stimulation by angiotensin II or angiotensin III, but other factors also can modulate hormone synthesis and release (61,68). As noted above, serum levels of both renin and angiotensinogen vary directly with the levels of thyroid hormone, and therefore a similar relationship should exist for aldosterone. Serum aldosterone levels have been measured in various thyroid disease states and have uniformly been found to be low in hypothyroidism (66,69). The response to stimulation by furosemide, ACTH, angiotensin, and potassium is blunted when thyroid hormone is deficient and improves with thyroid hormone treatment (66). The 24-hr excretion rate of aldosterone, when measured on a fixed sodium intake, varies directly with the dose of thyroid hormone replacement (69).

In summary, there are marked variations in the renin–angiotensin–aldosterone axis accompanying thyroid disease (44). Almost all reports demonstrated a direct relationship between serum levels of thyroid hormone and the various components of this blood pressure autoregulatory system (61,64,66,69). Since both hypothyroidism and hyperthyroidism can give rise to high blood pressure, there does not appear to be a unifying mechanism to account for these changes based upon the measurable components of this system. A role for renin and aldosterone in the hypertension which accompanies hypothyroidism is quite unlikely.

Atrial Natriuretic Factors: Synthesis and Release

Atrial natriuretic peptide(s) (ANP, ANF) is a group of polypeptides produced by cardiac atrial cells that can affect sodium handling by the kidney. In an attempt to explain some of the blood pressure and blood volume changes associated with thyroid disease, serum levels of ANP were directly assayed in humans and in rats (70,71,106). In one study, ANP did not vary with thyroid status in humans, whereas in rats the serum levels were increased in hyperthyroid, as compared to euthyroid and hypothyroid, animals (621 versus 266 and 210 pg/ml) (52). A separate study of hypothyroid patients with normal serum sodium levels reported a decreased serum level of ANP compared to that in age-matched controls. After thyroid hormone replacement, ANP levels rose concurrently with a rise in T_4 (71). It is interesting to speculate that changes in ANP may play a role in the expanded extracellular fluid space of hypothyroidism.

In addition to reports of thyroid-mediated changes in serum levels of ANP, recent studies implicate ANP in the regulation of TSH-dependent steps of thyroid hormone biosynthesis. A specific set of high-affinity ANP receptors have been identified on human thyroid cells which interact with, and which are regulated by, TSH (107). Thus ANP can potentially play a role in the control of thyroid hormone release as a function of changes in blood volume sensed by cardiac atrial receptors.

Vasopressin Activity in Hypothyroidism

Hypothyroidism can be associated with a significant degree of hyponatremia in the setting of an inappropriately concentrated urine (4,73,74). Thus, hypothyroidism has been postulated as a cause of the syndrome of inappropriate antidiuretic hormone secretion (SIADH) (74). Various authors have measured increased serum levels of vasopressin (AVP) in hypothyroidism (74). In contrast, Derubertis and co-workers measured urinary concentrations of hypothyroid patients in response to a standard water load. In contrast to patients with SIADH, hypothyroid subjects were able to dilute their urine after free water injection, leading to the conclusion that the hyponatremic hypothyroidism was a result of alterations in renal free water clearance (73). Similar to other hypothyroid-mediated alterations in serum chemistries, adequate thyroid hormone replacement normalizes these changes over a predictable period of time (4).

Vasopressin can act as a powerful constrictor of certain vascular beds. It is interesting to speculate that the mild elevations of AVP reported in hypothyroidism may be partly responsible for the increase in peripheral vascular resistance observed in this diseased state (8,43,48).

HYPERTHYROIDISM

Hyperthyroidism is a fairly common endocrine disease. In cross-sectional studies, it has been estimated to affect approximately 2% of the female population and 0.2% of the male population. An annual incidence of 0.03% for females in the United States was reported in 1970, whereas an incidence of 0.3% was reported for English women (75). Hyperthyroidism has been diagnosed at all ages; however, thyrotoxicosis of the Graves' disease variety often occurs during the child-bearing years.

Hypertension is also a common disease (76). Depending upon the criteria used for diagnosis, the prevalence of this disease is as high as 25% and clearly increases with increasing age. Thus, in any study of the role of thyroid disease as a cause of high blood pressure, it is important to identify the age of the patients involved and the definitions used to establish hypertension. For the purpose of this discussion a systolic pressure greater than 150 mmHg or a diastolic blood pressure greater than 95 mmHg will be used. The validity of such criteria have been widely discussed. The increased risk of cardiovascular disease in patients meeting these criteria is well established (76).

Prevalence of Hypertension

There is no extensive study of blood pressure changes in hyperthyroidism. As noted above, thyrotoxicosis is characterized by an increase in cardiac output and blood volume and a decrease in systemic vascular resistance (3,18,24). Thus, a widened pulse pressure and possible increase in peak systolic pressure would be the expected findings. Hurxthal has reported that one-third of patients with diffuse toxic goiter have systolic hypertension (77). This finding is even more striking because it occurs in a relatively young patient population in whom the occurrence of hypertension is less common. In contrast, isolated systolic hypertension is being recognized with increasing frequency in patients 65 years and older (44). The development of elevated systolic blood pressure in hyperthyroidism presumably reflects the inability of the vascular tree to accommodate the marked increase in cardiac output and stroke volume. This also explains the infrequent finding of diastolic hypertension and the overall lower mean arterial pressures which have been reported in hyperthyroidism (18,24). The increase in pulse pressure and normal to low diastolic pressures are consistent with the pronounced fall in systemic vascular resistance (Table 1; Fig. 3) and the normal elastic (compliance) properties of the arterial tree in younger patients. With aging, a decrease in arterial compliance has been postulated and would contribute to the elevation of systolic pressure.

The prevalence of hypertension is somewhat greater when patients with toxic adenomas are studied (78). Perhaps this reflects the older age of the involved population. Since cardiovascular manifestations can be some of the sole clinical findings in older patients with thyrotoxicosis (23), the combination of persistent tachycardia and an elevated systolic blood pressure, accompanied by a normal diastolic pressure, should raise the possibility of hyperthyroidism as the etiology.

Cardiovascular Manifestations

As a result of the thyroid-hormone-mediated increase in total body oxygen consumption and perhaps, in part, through direct effects of thyroid hormone on the heart, hyperthyroidism has marked cardiovascular manifestations (6,7,18,24,29,43,54). In its full clinical expression, thyrotoxic patients uniformly manifest (a) cardiac outputs of two to three times normal and (b) increased left ventricular ejection fractions. All noninvasive measures of left ventricular function are increased but return to normal with reestablishment of a euthyroid state. It is only as a result of the ability of the arterial bed to accommodate these changes that not all hyperthyroid patients demonstrate systolic hypertension.

Increased cardiac work due to either hypertension or volume overload is an important stimulus, causing increased protein synthesis and growth of the heart (52). The hyperdynamic circulatory state of hyperthyroidism is a similar stress; as a result, the mass of the hyperthyroid heart is greater in humans and in animals than in euthyroid controls (24,52). Recent studies suggest that this growth is an adaptive response to the imposed workload rather than a direct protein synthetic response to excess thyroid hormone (46). Myocardial oxygen consumption also rises as a result of the increased cardiac work. In patients whose myocardial blood supply is limited (such as those with atherosclerotic vascular disease), ischemia and angina pectoris can result (3,6).

Forfar and colleagues have suggested that hyperthyroidism is associated with a reversible form of cardiomyopathy (54). They observed a failure of the left ventricular ejection fraction to increase with exercise in thyrotoxic patients as compared to normal subjects. This finding, which reversed with treatment, was taken as evidence for left ventricular dysfunction. However, in view of the supernormal ejection fraction recorded at rest in hyperthyroid patients, it is hard to attribute the symptoms of shortness of breath or fatigue to cardiac pump failure. In the absence of coexistent cardiovascular disease, heart failure should not develop solely as a result of hyperthyroidism. It is possible that the dyspnea, fatigue, and decreased exercise tolerance of hyperthyroidism is a result of skeletal muscle weakness rather than of cardiac dysfunction (5).

Atrial arrhythmias, including atrial fibrillation, are well known to accompany thyrotoxicosis (22,23). Thyroxine can directly stimulate the rate of depolarization of the sinus node pacemaker and increase the rate of atrioventricular nodal conduction (26). The postulated increased adrenergic activity of the hyperthyroid myocardium would be expected to produce similar changes. It has been observed that pulmonary congestion and classic signs of heart failure can occur in hyperthyroid patients with atrial fibrillation and rapid ventricular response rates. Older patients appear to be more susceptible (22).

Thyrotoxic patients classically have low serum levels of cholesterol. It is interesting to speculate that this metabolic side effect of hyperthyroidism may decrease the risk for the development of atherosclerosis.

Response to Therapy

Therapy in hyperthyroidism includes the acute management of the signs and symptoms of the disease coupled with the long-term, definitive treatment of the thyroid overactivity (79). As a result of the similarity between the cardiovascular manifestations of hyperthyroidism and a hyperadrenergic state, the therapeutic strategies have usually included antiadrenergic drugs (23). Prior to the advent of beta-adrenergic blocking drugs, the mainstays of this therapy were reserpine and guanethedine. Current treatment includes propranolol or one of the $beta_1$-selective blocking drugs. With doses of propranolol between 80 and 120 mg/day, it is possible to correct the tachycardia, increased cardiac output, elevated systolic pressure, widened pulse pressure, hyperdynamic precordium, tremor, emotional lability, and muscle weakness frequently observed (5,18,72). In contrast, beta-adrenergic blockade does not acutely alter the serum levels of T_4, the augmented cardiac contractility, or the increased basal oxygen consumption of hyperthyroidism (23).

Long-term therapy of thyrotoxicosis can be achieved with a variety of modalities. Most authors note the efficacy of ^{131}I to control thyroid overactivity and to restore serum levels of thyroxine to normal or below. The indications and side effects of the different definitive therapies have been discussed elsewhere (79).

It must be emphasized that if the clinical consideration is that hypertension is a result of hyperthyroidism, then a return to the euthyroid state should be associated with a normalization of blood pressure. A complete blood pressure response is more likely to result from therapy in younger patients because of the greater likelihood of other coexistent causes of hypertension being present in older patients (77,78).

Thyroid Storm

The clinical syndrome known as "thyroid storm" or "thyroid crisis" is one of the most dramatic and feared manifestations of hyperthyroidism. It occurs in a small percentage of hyperthyroid patients and accounts for much of the mortality associated with the disease. The pathogenesis of thyroid storm is poorly understood and occurs in patients with preexistent hyperthyroidism caused by Graves' disease who are previously untreated or inadequately treated (22).

The signs and symptoms of thyroid storm are frequently thought to represent an exaggerated or decompensated state of hyperthyroidism. Many consider fever to be the *sine qua non* for the diagnosis; other symptoms include extreme restlessness, emotional lability, confusion, psychosis, and, occasionally, coma. The heart rate is usually increased out of proportion to the extent of the fever. Although the tachycardia is generally sinus in nature, it is occasionally ectopic in origin, most commonly atrial fibrillation.

When the diagnosis of thyroid storm is suspected, therapy should be started promptly and is directed at decreasing the synthesis and release of thyroid hormones, blocking the apparent increased adrenergic activity, treating electrolyte abnormalities, and reducing fever. Systolic hypertension is the characteristic finding of hyperthyroidism, whereas hypotension, decreased organ perfusion, shock, and cardiovascular collapse signify decompensation of the normal physiologic regulatory mechanisms.

HYPOTHYROIDISM

Prevalence of Hypertension

Similar to hyperthyroidism, hypothyroidism is a common disease, affecting approximately 2% of the adult female population (63). Most cases arise from primary thyroid gland failure due to the pathologic process of chronic autoimmune lymphocytic thyroiditis (Hashimoto's disease) (4,80,81). It has been suggested that 10% of the overall female population have antithyroid antibodies measurable in their serum, confirming the high prevalence of autoimmune thyroid disease (75). Hypothyroidism resulting from prior treatment of Graves' disease by either surgery or radioactive iodine makes up an increasing segment of patients. In contrast to Graves' disease, which affects primarily a premenopausal population, hypothyroidism has an increasing prevalence with age beyond 40 years (75). This is similar to what has been reported for hypertension (76).

Review of the previously reported series reveals a wide variation for the prevalence of hypertension in hypothyroidism (9,10,44,64–66,78,82–86). Whereas some authors suggest a frequent concurrence (10,66,78), others do not find an association between these two diseases (84). In review of 12 of the previously published studies, it was possible to summarize the findings for 907 hypothyroid patients in whom the overall prevalence of hypertension was 21% (Table 2). This includes nonrandom patient samples, varying age groups, and varying degrees of both hypothyroidism and hypertension. This indicates that the prevalence rate of 21% is consistent with the estimates for hypothyroidism as a cause of secondary hypertension quoted by others (44,62,76,87).

Of the work reported to date, only two studies employed control groups and specified the prevalence with regard to age and/or degree of hypothyroidism. In the report of Endo et al. (84), 81 hypothyroid patients were categorized according to the degree of thyroid dysfunction and were compared to a large random control female population and to a smaller population of known euthyroid women of similar age. In both control groups, hypertension (defined as a systolic blood pressure greater than 160 mmHg and/or diastolic blood pressure greater than 95 mmHg) was increased in the fifth and sixth decades. By comparison, hypertension was more common in patients with mild hypothyroidism when compared to the large control group but not when compared to the age-matched euthyroid controls. For patients with moderate and severe hypothyroidism, there was no increase in the incidence of hypertension. In fact, the latter group had blood pressures that were *lower* than that of the control group. In those with severe hypothyroidism, blood pressure rose with T_4 replacement therapy. Thus, there was an overall prevalence of 16% for hypertension in hypothyroid patients as compared to 20% in the control group. These authors concluded that hypertension is not increased in Japanese women with hypothyroidism (84).

Saito et al. evaluated 477 patients with chronic thyroiditis in the age range of 20–69 years (85). Of the total group, 169 were chemically hypothyroid (35%). Hypertension (defined as blood pressure greater than 160/95 mmHg) was statistically more prevalent among hypothyroid patients (14.8%) than among euthyroid controls (5.5%). This differ-

TABLE 2. *Studies of hypertension in hypothyroidism*

Reference	Study population numbers	Percent affected
82	92	26
83	6	100
44	58	16
64	6	16
84	81	16
9	30	43
65	5	100
85	169	15
66	15	27
86	36	14
78	24	38
10	400	18
Total	907	21%

ence was especially striking for patients between the ages of 50 and 59, with prevalences of 29% versus 6.8% ($p < 0.01$). Of the 14 hypertensive hypothyroid patients who received adequate thyroid hormone replacement, the diastolic blood pressure decreased significantly—from a mean of 99 mmHg to 90 mmHg—without any additional therapy.

Cardiovascular Manifestations

In contrast to the high cardiac output and hyperdynamic circulatory state of hyperthyroidism, hypothyroidism is characterized by a low cardiac index, decreased stroke volume, decreased vascular volume, and increased systemic vascular resistance (Table 1) (4,8,10,43). In a comprehensive study of hemodynamics in patients with chronic myxedema, the cardiac index was decreased by 35% and remained subnormal, even with exercise (8). The mean arteriovenous (A-V) oxygen difference was within the normal range, suggesting that the cardiac output was appropriate for the total body oxygen consumption. This is also in marked contrast to that observed in patients with heart failure, in whom a decline in cardiac output is associated with an increase A-V O_2 difference. Thus there is no substantial evidence to suggest that hypothyroidism, in the absence of other coexistent medical problems, results in heart failure (9). Cardiac enlargement in hypothyroidism is often a result of pericardial effusions, and pleural effusions may similarly arise (4,8). However, as a result of the increased systemic vascular resistance and elevated diastolic blood pressure, myocardial hypertrophy may develop (44). Conversely, the fall in cardiac output and decreased cardiac work in normotensive patients can result in cardiac atrophy.

Total blood volume is decreased in hypothyroidism (43,51) and varies directly as a function of the basal metabolic rate (51). Renal perfusion, when measured by glomerular filtration, is also decreased (60,88,89). Whereas steady-state sodium excretion is normal (60,88), free water clearance is impaired and can lead to hyponatremia (73,90). In keeping with the development of high-protein-content effusions in many body cavities, total body albumin distribution is expanded in myxedema. (4).

Mechanism of Hypertension in Hypothyroidism

In experimental studies the plasma renin, plasma aldosterone, and aldosterone production rates are decreased in hypothyroid patients with hypertension (64–66). Thus, the secondary hypertension of myxedema falls into the Laragh classification of a low renin state (61). This finding is even more striking in view of the low plasma volumes that accompany hypothyroidism (51).

As discussed above, decreases in serum levels of thyroid hormone are accompanied by a decrease in tissue respiration but a normal A-V O_2 difference (8). This suggests that the fall in cardiac output is appropriate and compensatory. It has also been observed that total body sodium levels, and perhaps intracellular sodium levels, are increased (44). Whereas renal sodium handling appears normal, intrarenal blood flow and free water clearance are impaired (60,88,89). All of these observations are consistent with a rise in vascular resistance in specific organs and tissues. This change in peripheral resistance can lead to a decrease in cardiac output, but if the homeostasis is not complete the result would be a rise in diastolic blood pressure, elevated mean arterial pressure, and a narrowed pulse pressure. The latter is characteristic of the hypertension of hypothyroidism (4,8).

In addition to changes in basal oxygen consumption, hypothyroidism is associated with a decrease in the rate of drug metabolism and clearance (Fig. 1). An example of this change occurs in hypothyroid patients treated with digitalis who exhibit an enhanced biologic action and higher serum levels of the drug for any given administered dosage (4,40).

Recent studies have implicated a role for an endogenous digitalis-like factor in some cases of essential hypertension and in the hypertension of acromegaly (91,92). It is interesting to speculate that in hypothyroid patients with hypertension, such an endogenous factor is present in increased amounts. The biologic action of increased smooth muscle contraction would be enhanced within the resistance vessels of the peripheral circulation. A return to the euthyroid state would potentially correct both of these lesions and restore normotension with a decline in systemic vascular resistance. Further proof of this hypothesis would require direct measurements of this reputed factor.

Other authors have suggested that the increased systemic vascular resistance of hypothyroidism occurs as a result of myxedematous changes in the vessel walls (44,82,86). Although morphologic changes may occur with prolonged disease as a result of hypertension, this theory is not consistent with (a) the fall in SVR with exercise (8) or (b) the response to thyroid hormone replacement (105).

Response to Therapy

Although there remains some disagreement with regard to the prevalence of hypertension in hypothyroidism, most reports find that thyroid hormone replacement improves blood pressure control in approximately half of treated patients (44,45,56,62,83,90). In one study, Fuller et al. observed that one-third of patients treated with thyroid hormone alone had a return to normal blood pressure (45). Bing and Swales, when reviewing this response to therapy, emphasized the importance of achieving optimum hormone replacement to establish a euthyroid state and a prolonged time course of the response (44,83). The older the patient and the more long-standing the hypertension, the lesser the response that can be expected. In some cases, improved blood pressure control with lower doses of antihypertensive medications will signify a thyroid hormone effect (45). Patients with severe hypothyroidism whose blood pressure and cardiac output are low may respond to replacement therapy with a rise in these parameters (84).

In studies of both humans and animals, vascular resistance is one of the earliest cardiovascular parameters to return toward normal (2,42). This, in turn, is followed by changes in cardiac output and cardiac contractility. The time course for restoration of renal blood flow and clearance functions have not been characterized. Thus while acute changes in the factors regulating blood pressure may occur, the complete response may require periods of up to 2–4 months.

The proper dosage, preparation, and timing schedule for thyroid hormone (*l*-thyroxine) replacement therapy have been discussed elsewhere (18). It has been recently observed that euthyroidism is achieved in patients older than 50 years with lower doses of T_4 (approximately 0.1 mg/day) than those previously employed.

Myxedema Coma

Myxedema coma represents the end stage of undiagnosed primary hypothyroidism. This requires prompt and effective treatment. The predisposing factors that induce myxedema coma in the hypothyroid patient include exposure to cold, infection, trauma, drugs such as morphine or barbiturates, and general anesthesia. Patients with myxedema coma have (a) many of the signs noted in uncomplicated hypothyroidism and (b) the additional signs of hypothermia, hypotension, and hypoventilation with carbon dioxide retention. Hypothermia is considered to be the *sine qua non* for the diagnosis. After suspecting the diagnosis, replacement of thyroid hormone must be accomplished quickly (18). The initial loading dose of *l*-thyroxine is necessary in order to saturate the unoccupied thyroid-hormone-binding sites on thyroxine-binding globulin and within cells (12,13). Parenteral therapy is required because oral administration may be associated with incomplete absorption. Additional considerations, including the use of corticosteroids, have been discussed elsewhere (18).

THYROID-ASSOCIATED DISEASE STATES

The pathophysiology of the most common forms of hyperthyroidism (Graves' disease) and of hypothyroidism (chronic lymphocytic thyroiditis, Hashimoto's disease) is strongly linked to changes in the immune system. Specific defects in thymus-dependent lymphocyte suppressor cells (81), characteristic expression of histocompatibility (HLA) antigens (93), and the presence of serum autoantibodies in genetically susceptible individuals have been demonstrated. Similar findings have been reported for juvenile onset (Type I) diabetes mellitus, adrenal insufficiency (Addison's disease), primary ovarian failure, lymphoid hypophysitis (93–96), and other endocrine diseases. Since the expression of a coexistent autoimmune process is more common in affected individuals, patients with thyroid disease must be suspect for other forms of endocrine gland failure or for other autoimmune vascular diseases (81,96).

Addison's Disease

Addison's disease has been described in association with autoimmune thyroid disease (95,97). Alterations in cortisol metabolism have been reported to accompany changes in thyroid hormone levels (98). Adrenal gland failure leads to a loss of corticoid production (aldosterone) as well as deficient glucocorticoid production. Thus such patients are characterized by hypotension, cardiac atrophy, hyperkalemia, and signs of volume depletion. The finding of a low diastolic blood pressure with accompanying orthostatic changes suggesting volume depletion should alert the physician to the possibility of adrenal insufficiency. Similarly, if a patient treated with *l*-thyroxine for hypothyroidism should experience worsening clinical symptoms or develop any of the above findings, the possibility that the therapy "unmasked" Addison's disease exists (95,97,98).

Systemic Lupus Erythematosus

Systemic lupus erythematosus (SLE) is a disease characterized by specific autoimmune markers and multiple organ system involvement. In a retrospective analysis of a large series, it was reported that 45% of patients with SLE had hypertension. In the majority of patients, this occurred in the absence of overt renal failure or proteinuria (94). As noted above, hypothyroidism also has an autoimmune etiology; moreover, in a recent study there was an increased prevalence of hypothyroidism in patients with SLE. Thus it is interesting to speculate that in a subgroup of patients with autoimmune systemic vasculitis, hypothyroidism and its attendant changes in systemic vascular resistance may be playing a role in the development of hypertension. This may be especially true in patients without evidence of renal involvement, and routine thyroid function studies should be obtained in all such affected individuals.

Progressive Systemic Sclerosis (Scleroderma)

Progressive systemic sclerosis (PSS) is a connected tissue disease in which a number of immune reactions have been identified (99). Although earlier reports questioned any association between PSS and hypothyroidism, recent retrospective and prospective studies using standard thyroid function studies have established the presence of thyroid dysfunction in as many as 25% of affected patients (99,100). Since untreated hypothyroidism and PSS share many signs and symptoms (including hypertension), it is important to routinely screen patients with PSS for thyroid disease and institute treatment as indicated. Whether other clinical manifestations of PSS will improve with *l*-thyroxine therapy remains to be resolved.

Atherosclerotic Cardiovascular Disease

Much has been written concerning the prevalence of atherosclerotic cardiovascular disease (ASCVD) in patients with hypothyroidism. Studies have suggested that the disorders of lipid metabolism, including elevations in serum cholesterol as well as other changes in cellular metabolism, are significant risk factors for the development of ASCVD (4,80,101,102). Bastenie and co-workers have described an association between serum markers of autoimmune thyroid disease and an increased prevalence of coronary artery disease (CAD) in women (80). Hypertension is a well-established risk factor for the development of ASCVD; moreover, with the blood pressure changes that accompany hypothyroidism, there are a number of clinical parameters to link thyroid disease with ischemic vascular disease and CAD.

In a case-controlled autopsy series, Steinberg (86) found that while CAD was more prevalent in hypothyroid patients, this association occurred only in patients with coexistent hypertension; furthermore, hypothyroidism alone did not lead to the same pathologic vascular changes.

The hypothyroid heart, as a result of decreased cardiac work, has a lower oxygen consumption and will, in theory, tolerate various degrees of CAD and result in a decrease in myocardial blood flow. Taken together, these observations have led to the clinical practice of avoiding or limiting thyroid hormone replacement in patients known to have, or suspected of having, CAD (102). In view of the systemic effects of thyroid hormone, the appropriateness of thyroid hormone therapy in this clinical setting can be reevaluated.

In 1961, Keating reported on the results of thyroid hormone replacement in 1501 hypothyroid patients with regard to the *de novo* expression or apparent worsening of clinical symptoms of ASCVD and CAD (103). In that report there were 55 patients with preexisting angina (mean age 62 years) and 35 patients who developed angina or a myocardial infarction (mean age 71 years) after thyroid hormone therapy was instituted. Of the former group, more than one-third had a resolution or significant improvement of their anginal syndrome coincident with thyroid hormone therapy. Unless the systemic effects of thyroid hormone with a fall in mean blood pressure and SVR predominate, this effect cannot be explained solely by a direct effect of thyroid hormone on the myocardium. In the group of patients who developed new anginal syndrome, only one-third did so within 1 year of initiating therapy. Since the denominator for the prevalence of cardiac events (angina and myocardial infarction) is some proportion of the total population of 1501 treated patients and not only the 90 patients with clinical symptoms (102), the incidence of myocardial infarction in cardiac-related deaths in this patient population does not appear untoward. In fact, the potential beneficial role for *l*-thyroxine in this clinical setting would suggest the desirability of establishing a euthyroid stage and, if necessary, treating the symptoms of CAD and ASCVD concomitantly with a conventional medical routine using the currently available drugs (4,18,22). The potential for thyroid hormone to decrease afterload and optimize myocardial work and cardiac output can then be realized. Whether institution of thyroid hormone treatment with a lowering of serum cholesterol also leads to a documented improvement in the extent of coronary artery atherosclerosis requires further study.

SUMMARY

1. Thyroid hormones have profound effects on the heart and cardiovascular system. In response to the increased oxygen in metabolic demands of hyperthyroidism, there is a decreased systemic vascular resistance accompanied by an increase in cardiac output and left ventricular stroke volume. In hypothyroidism, opposite hemodynamic alterations are observed.

2. Systolic hypertension has been recorded in as many as one-third of hyperthyroid patients. The prevalence of hypertension in hypothyroidism is approximately 20% and involves both diastolic and systolic blood pressure elevations.

3. Measurements of the renin–angiotensin–aldosterone system reveal a direct correlation between serum levels of thyroid hormone and the excretion and production rates of renin and aldosterone. Thus, the hypertension of hypothyroidism is characterized as a low-renin state.

4. In response to treatment of hyperthyroidism with beta-adrenergic blocking drugs, it can be anticipated that systolic blood pressures will improve. Following definitive therapy, most patients will return to normotensive. As a result of treatment of hypothyroidism, the most common observation is an improvement or a complete resolution of the previously recorded increases in diastolic blood pressure.

5. Various hypotheses for the hypertension of hypothyroidism have been discussed. These include the presence of an endogenous digitalis-like factor which directly stimulates the contractility of arterial smooth muscle and increases systemic vascular resistance. The role of the kidney in sodium and water retention has also been implicated in hypothyroidism.

6. Thyroid disease is most commonly the result of an autoimmune process. Therefore other autoimmune diseases such as Addison's disease and systemic lupus erythematosus, which have their own associated changes in blood pressure, are observed with increased frequency.

ACKNOWLEDGMENT

These studies were supported in part by NIH Grant HL 41304.

REFERENCES

1. Parry CH. Collections from the unpublished papers of the late Caleb Hilliel Parry. *Dis Heart* 1825;2:111–165.
2. Graves RJ. Newly observed affection of the thyroid gland in females. *Lond Med Surg J* 1835;7:516–517.
3. Grossman W, Robin NI, Johnson IW, et al. Effects of beta-blockade on peripheral manifestations of thyrotoxicosis. *Ann Intern Med* 1971;74:875–879.
4. Klein I, Levey GS. Unusual manifestations of hypothyroidism. *Arch Intern Med* 1984;144:123–128.
5. Klein I, Trzepacz P, Roberts M, Levey GS. Symptom rating scale for assessing hyperthyroidism. *Arch Intern Med* 1988;148:387–390.
6. Levey GS. Catecholamine sensitivity, thyroid hormone and the heart. *Am J Med* 1971;50:413–420.
7. Morkin E, Flink IL, Goldman S. Biochemical and physiologic effects of thyroid hormone on cardiac performance. *Prog Cardiovasc Dis* 1983;25:435–464.
8. Graettinger JS, Muenster JJ, Checchia CS, Grissom RL, Campbell JA. A correlation of clinical and hemodynamic studies in patients with hypothyroidism. *J Clin Invest* 1957;37:502–510.
9. Lerman J, Clark RJ, Means JH. The heart in myxedema: electrocardiograms and roentgen-ray measurements before and after therapy. *Ann Intern Med* 1933;6:1251–1271.

10. Watanakunakorn C, Hodges RE, Evans TC. Myxedema—a study of 400 cases. *Arch Intern Med* 1965;116:183–190.
11. Dillman WH. Mechanism of action of thyroid hormones. *Med Clin North Am* 1985;69:849–861.
12. Oppenheimer JH. Thyroid hormone action at the cellular level. *Science* 1979;203:971–979.
13. Samuels HH, Tsai JS. Thyroid hormone action in cell culture: demonstration of nuclear receptors in intact cells and isolated nuclei. *Proc Natl Acad Sci USA* 1973;70:3488–3491.
14. Tata JR, Ernster L, Lindberg O. The action of thyroid hormones at the cell level. *Biochem J* 1963;86:408–413.
15. Guernsey DL, Edelman IS. Regulation of thermogenesis by thyroid hormones. In: Oppenheimer J, Samuels H, eds. *Molecular basis of thyroid hormone action.* New York: Academic Press, 1983;293–324.
16. Haber RS, Loeb JN. Effect of 3,5,3′-triiodothyronine treatment on potassium efflux from isolated rat diaphragm: role of increased permeability in the thermogenic response. *Endocrinology* 1982;3:1217–1223.
17. Oppenheimer JH, Schwartz HL, Mariash CN, et al. Advances in our understanding of thyroid hormone at the cellular level. *Endocr Rev* 1987;8:288–308.
18. Klein I, Levey GS. New perspectives on thyroid hormone catecholamines and the heart. *Am J Med* 1981;76:167–171.
19. Salata R, Klein I, Levey GS. Thyroid hormone and the liver. *Semin Liver Dis* 1985;5:29–34.
20. Sterling, K. Thyroid hormone action at the cell level. *N Engl J Med* 1979;300:117–119.
21. Ismail-Beigi F, Haber RS, Loeb JN. Stimulation of active Na and K transport by thyroid hormone in a rat liver cell line: role of enhanced Na entry. *Endocrinology* 1986;119:2527–2536.
22. Klein I, Levey GS. Thyroid emergencies: thyroid storm and myxedema coma. *Top Emerg Med* 1984;5:33–40.
23. Levey GS. The adrenergic nervous system in hyperthyroidism: therapeutic role of beta adrenergic blocking drugs. *Pharmacol Ther* 1:431–442.
24. Merillon JP, Passa P, Chastre J, Wolf A, Gourgon R. Left ventricular function and hyperthyroidism. *Br Heart J* 1981;46:137–143.
25. Davis PJ, Davis FB. Blas SD. Studies on the mechanism of thyroid hormone stimulation *in vitro* of human red cell Ca^{2+}-ATPase activity. *Life Sci* 1982;30:675–682.
26. Arnsdorf MF, Childers RW. Atrial electrophysiology in experimental hyperthyroidism in rabbits. *Circ Res* 1970;26:575–581.
27. Coulombe P, Dussault JH, Walker P. Plasma catecholamine concentrations in hyperthyroidism and hypothyroidism. *Metabolism* 1976;25:973–978.
28. Kuschke HJ, Wernze H, Becker G. Sympatho-adrenal activity in thyrotoxicosis. *Br Med J* 1960;ii:1656.
29. Landsberg L. Catecholamines and hyperthyroidism. *Clin Endocrinol Metab* 1977;6:697–713.
30. Manger WM, Hulse MC, Forsyth MS, Chute RN, Brown CE, Webb K, Sussman R, Warren, S. Pheochromocytoma and hypophysectomy: effects on blood pressure and catecholamines [Abstract]. *Life Sci* 1982;30:601–602.
31. Dratman MB. Thyroid function and high blood pressure. *Cardiovasc Med* 1976;1:319–331.
32. Bayliss RIS, Edwards OM. Urinary excretion of free catecholamines in Graves' disease. *Endocrinology* 1971;49:167–173.
33. Beaven MA, Costa E, Brodie BB. The turnover of norepinephrine in thyrotoxic and nonthyrotoxic mice. *Life Sci* 1963;4:241–246.
34. Coulombe P, Dussault JH, Letarte J, Simard SJ. Catecholamines metabolism in thyroid diseases. I. Epinephrine secretion rate in hyperthyroidism and hypothyroidism. *J Clin Endocrinol Metab* 1976;42:125–131.
35. Bilezikian JP, Loeb JN. The influence of hyperthyroidism and hypothyroidism on α- and β-adrenergic receptor systems and adrenergic responsiveness. *Endocr Rev* 4:378–396.
36. Coulombe P, Dussault JH, Walker P. Catecholamine metabolism in thyroid disease. II. Norepinephrine secretion rate in hyperthyroidism and hypothyroidism. *J Clin Endocrinol Metab* 1977;44:1185–1192.
37. Williams LT, Lefkowitz RJ, Watanabe AM, et al. Thyroid hormone regulation of β-adrenergic number. *J Biol Chem* 1977;252:2787–2789.
38. Ginsberg AM, Clutter WE, Shah SD, Cryer PE. Triiodothyronine-induced thyrotoxicosis increases mononuclear leukocyte β-adrenergic receptor density in man. *J Clin Invest* 1981;67:1785–1791.
39. Bilezikian JP, Loeb JN. Mechanisms of altered beta-adrenergic responsiveness in the hyperthyroid and hypothyroid turkey erythrocyte. *Life Sci* 1982;30:663–674.
40. Croxson MS, Ibbertson HK. Serum digoxin in patients with thyroid disease. *Br Med J* 1975;3:566–568.
41. Kim D, Smith TW. Effects of thyroid hormone on sodium pump sites, sodium content, and contractile responses to cardiac glycosides in cultured chick ventricular cells. *J Clin Invest* 1984;74:1481–1488.
42. Kapitola J, Vilimovska D. Inhibition of the early circulatory effects of triiodothyronine in rats by propranolol. *Physiol Bohemoslov* 1981;30:347–352.
43. Anthonisen P, Holst E, Thomsen AA. Determination of cardiac output and other hemodynamic data in patients with hyper- and hypothyroidism, using dye dilution technique. *Scand J Clin Lab Invest* 1960;12:472–480.
44. Bing RF, Swales JD. Thyroid disease and hypertension. In: Robertson JIS, ed. *Handbook of hypertension, vol. 2: Clinical aspects of secondary hypertension.* Amsterdam: Elsevier, 1983;276–290.
45. Fuller H Jr, Spittell JA Jr, McConahey WM, Schirger A. Myxedema: a cause of reversible hypertension. *Circulation* 1965;31:91–92.
46. Klein I, Hong C. Role of thyroid hormone in the regulation of cardiac hypertrophy. In: Dhalla N, ed. *Pathophysiology of heart disease.* The Hague: Martinus Nijhoff, 1987;73–82.
47. Kontos HA, Shapiro W, Mauck P Jr, et al. Mechanism of certain abnormalities of the circulation to the limbs in thyrotoxicosis. *J Clin Invest* 1965;41:947–956.
48. Zsoter T, Tom H, Chappel C. Effect of thyroid hormones on vascular response. *J Lab Clin Med* 1964;64:433–441.
49. Theilen EO, Wilson WR. Hemodynamic effects of peripheral vasoconstriction in normal and thyrotoxic subjects. *J Appl Physiol* 1967;22:207–210.
50. Rodgers RL, Black S, Katz S, et al. Thyroidectomy of SHR: effect on ventricular relaxation and on SR calcium uptake activity. *Am J Physiol* 1986;250:H361–865.
51. Gibson JG, Harris AW. Clinical studies of the blood volume. V. Hyperthyroidism and myxedema. *J Clin Invest* 1938;18:59–65.
52. Klein I, Hong C. Effects of thyroid hormone on the myosin content and myosin isoenzymes of the heterotopically transplanted heart. *J Clin Invest* 1986;77:1694–1698.
53. Sanford CF, Griffon EE, Wildenthal K. Synthesis and degradation of myocardial protein during the development and regression of thyroxine-induced cardiac hypertrophy in rats. *Circ Res* 1978;43:688–694.
54. Forfar JC, Muir AL, Sawers SA, et al. Abnormal left ventricular function in hyperthyroidism. *N Engl J Med* 1982;307:1165–1170.
55. Stoffer SS, Jiang MS, Gorman CA, Pikler GM. Plasma catecholamines in hypothyroidism and hyperthyroidism. *J Clin Endocrinol Metab* 1973;36:587–589.
56. Dratman MB, Goldman M, Crutchfield FL, Gordon JT. Nervous system role of iodocompounds in blood pressure regulation. *Life Sci* 1982;30:611–622.
57. Christensen NJ. Increased levels of plasma noradrenaline in hypothyroidism. *J Clin Endocrinol Metab* 1972;35:359–363.
58. Sutherland EW, Robinson GA, Butcher, RW. Some aspects of the biological role of adenosine 3′5′-monophosphate (cyclic AMP) *Circulation* 1968;37:279–306.
59. Liggett SB, Shah SD, Cryer PE. Increased fat cell and skeletal muscle β-adrenergic receptor densities but unattended lipolytic, glycemic and cardiac chronotropic *in vivo* in experimental human thyrotoxicosis. *J Clin Invest* 1989;83:803–809.
60. Bradley SE, Coelho JB, Sealey JE, Edwards KDG, Stephan F. Changes in glomerulotubular dimensions, single nephron glomerular filtration rates and the renin–angiotensin system in hypothyroid rats. *Life Sci* 1982;30:633–640.

61. Laragh JH, Sealey JE, Brunner HR. The control of aldosterone secretion in normal and hypertensive man: abnormal renin–aldosterone patterns in low-renin hypertension. In: Laragh JH, ed. *Hypertension manual.* New York: Yorke Medical Books, 1975;197–225.
62. Strong CG, Northcutt RC, Sheps SG. Clinical examination and investigation of the hypertensive patient. In: Genest J, Koiw E, Kuchel O, eds. *Hypertension.* New York: McGraw-Hill, 1977;112–133.
63. Resnick LM, Laragh JH. Plasma renin activity in syndromes of thyroid hormone excess and deficiency. *Life Sci* 1982;30:585–588.
64. Elias AN, Kyaw T, Valenta LJ, Meshkinpour H. The renin–angiotensin system in hypothyroidism of short duration. *Horm Metab Res* 18:349–351.
65. Richards AM, Nicholls MG, Espiner EA, Ikram H, Turner JG, Brownlie BEW. Hypertension in hypothyroidism: arterial pressure and hormone relationships. *Clin Exp Theory Practice* 1985;11:1499–1514.
66. Saruta T, Kitajima W, Hayashi M, Kato E, Matsuki S. Renin and aldosterone in hypothyroidism: relation to excretion of sodium and potassium. *Clin Endocrinol* 1980;12:483–489.
67. Ganong WF. Thyroid hormones and renin secretion. *Life Sci* 1982;30:561–570.
68. Dzau VJ, Herrmann HC. Hormonal control of angiotensinogen production. *Life Sci* 1982;30:577–584.
69. Marks P, Anderson J, Vincent R. Aldosterone in myxedema. *Lancet* 1978;ii:1277–1278.
70. Kohno M, Murtkawa K, Yasunari K, et al. Circulating atrial natriuretic peptides in hyperthyroidism and hypothyroidism. *Am J Med* 1987;83:648–652.
71. Zimmerman RS, Gharib H, Zimmerman D, et al. Hypothyroidism: the first metabolic abnormality associated with decreased atrial natriuretic peptide. *Endocrinology* 119 (Suppl Am Thyroid Assoc Mtg) T-42.
72. Trzepacz P, McCue M, Klein I, Levey FS. Psychiatric and neuropsychiatric response to propranolol in Graves' disease. *Biol Psychol* 1988;23:678–688.
73. Derubertis FR Jr, Michelis MF, Bloom ME, Mintz DH, Field JB, Davis BB. Impaired water excretion in myxedema. *Am J Med* 1971;51:41–53.
74. Skowsky RW, Kikuchi TA. The role of vasopressin in the impaired water excretion of myxedema. *Am J Med* 1978;64:613–621.
75. Tunbridge WMG, Evered DC, Hall R, Appleton D, Brewis M, Clark F, Grimley Evans J, Young E, Bird T, Smith PA. Lipid profile and cardiovascular disease in the Wickham area with particular reference to thyroid failure. *Clin Endocrinol* 1977;7:481–495.
76. Kaplan NM, Lieberman E. Hypertension in the population at large. In: Collins N, ed. *Hypertension.* Baltimore, MD: Williams & Wilkins, 1986;1–28.
77. Hurxthal LM. Blood pressure before and after operation in hyperthyroidism. *Arch Intern Med* 1931;47:167–174.
78. Thompson WO, Dickie LFN, Morris AE, Hilkevitch BH. The high incidence of hypertension in toxic goiter and in myxedema. *Endocrinology* 1931;15:265–272.
79. Braverman LE. Therapeutic considerations. *Clin Endocrinol Metab* 1978;7:221–240.
80. Bastenie PA, Bonnyns M, VanHaelst L. Natural history of primary myxedema. *Am J Med* 1985;79:91–100.
81. Volpe R. The role of autoimmunity in hypoendocrine and hyperendocrine function. *Ann Intern Med* 1977;87:86–99.
82. Attarian E. Myxedema and hypertension. *NY State J Med* 1963;63:2801–2804.
83. Bing RF, Briggs SJ, Burden AC, Russell GI, Swales JD, Thurston H. Reversible hypertension and hypothyroidism. *Clin Endocrinol* 1980;13:339–342.
84. Endo T, Komiya I, Tsukui T, Yamada T, Izumiyama T, Nagata H, Kono S, Kamata K. Re-evaluation of a possible high incidence of hypertension in hypothyroid patients. *Am Heart J* 1979;98:684–688.
85. Saito I, Kunihiko I, Saruta T. Hypothyroidism as a cause of hypertension. *Hypertension* 1983;5:112–115.
86. Steinberg AD. Myxedema and coronary artery disease—a comparative autopsy study. *Ann Intern Med* 1968;68:338–344.
87. Sowers JR, Tuck ML. Hypertension associated with diabetes mellitus, hypercalcaemic disorders, acromegaly and thyroid disease. *Clin Endocrinol Metab* 1981;10:631–651.
88. Katz AI, Emmanoel DS, Lindheimer MD. Thyroid hormones and the kidney. *Nephrology* 1975;15:223–249.
89. Yount E, Little MJ. Renal clearance in patients with myxedema. *J Clin Endocrinol Metab* 1955;15:343–346.
90. Castleden CM, Williams AJ. Hypothyroidism—classic symptoms plus the unexpected. *Geriatrics* 1982;37:133–138.
91. Deray G, Rieu M, Devynck MA, Pernollet MG, Chanson P, Luton JP, Meyer P. Evidence of an endogenous digitalis-like factor in the plasma of patients with acromegaly. *N Engl J Med* 1987;316:575–580.
92. Haddy FJ, Pamnani M, Clough D, Huot S. Role of a humoral sodium–potassium pump inhibitor in experimental low renin hypertension. *Life Sci* 1982;30:571–576.
93. Davies TF. Thyroid cell major histocompatibility antigens in autoimmune thyroid disease. *Thyroid Today* 1987;10(3):1–8.
94. Budman DR, Steinberg AD. Hypertension and renal disease in systemic lupus erythematosus. *Arch Intern Med* 1976;136:1003–1007.
95. Parker M, Klein I, Fishman L, et al. Silent thyrotoxic thyroiditis in association with chronic adrenocortical insufficiency. *Arch Intern Med* 1980;1108–1109.
96. Portoccarrero C, Robinson AG, Klein I. Lymphoid hypophysitis. *JAMA* 1981;246:1811–1812.
97. Carpenter CJ, Solomon N, Silvenberg SG, et al. Schmidt's syndrome (thyroid and adrenal insufficiency): a review of the literature and a report of 15 new cases including ten cases of co-existent diabetes mellitus. *Medicine* 1964;43:153–180.
98. Hellman D, Bradlow HL, Zumoff B, et al. The influence of thyroid hormone on hydrocortisone production and metabolism. *J Clin Endocrinol Metab* 1961;21:1231–1247.
99. Gordon MB, Klein I, Dekker A. Thyroid disease in progressive systemic sclerosis: increased frequency of glandular fibrosis and hypothyroidism. *Ann Intern Med* 1981;95:431–435.
100. Kahl L, Medsger TA, Klein I. Prospective evaluation of thyroid function in patients with systemic sclerosis (scleroderma). *J Rheumatol* 1986;13:103–107.
101. Barnes BO. On the genesis of atherosclerosis. *J Am Geriatr Soc* 1973;21:350–358.
102. Becker C. Hypothyroidism and atherosclerotic heart disease: pathogenesis, medical management and the role of coronary artery bypass surgery. *Endocr Rev* 1985;6:432–440.
103. Keating FR Jr, Parkin TW, Selby JB, et al. Treatment of heart disease associated with myxedema. *Prog Cardiovasc Dis* 1961;3:364–381.
104. Hauger-Klevene JH, Brown H, Zavaleta J. Plasma renin activity in hyper- and hypothyroidism: effect of adrenergic blocking agents. *J Clin Endocrinol Metab* 1972;34:625–629.
105. Kaptein EM, Quion-Verde H, Swinney RS, Egodage PM, Massry SG. Acute hemodynamic effects of levothyroxine loading in critically ill hypothyroid patients. *Arch Intern Med* 1986;146:662–666.
106. Ladenson PW, Langevin H, Michener M. Plasma atriopeptin in hyperthyroid, euthyroid and hypothyroid man and rat. *Endocrinology* 1986;119(Suppl Am Thyroid Assoc Mtg) T-26.
107. Tseng YC, Sellitti DF, Wartofsky L. TSH modulated atriopeptin receptors on intact human thyroid cells. *Clin Res* 1988;36(3):555A.

PART B

Diabetes and Obesity

Hypertension: Pathophysiology, Diagnosis, and Management, edited by J. H. Laragh and B. M. Brenner. Raven Press, Ltd., New York © 1990.

CHAPTER 104

Experimental Diabetes and Hypertensive Vascular Disease

Sharon Anderson and Barry M. Brenner

Hemodynamic Abnormalities in Experimental Diabetes, 1677
Systemic Hypertension in Diabetes, 1680
Hypertension and Experimental Diabetic Glomerulopathy, 1680
Effects of Antihypertensive Therapy in Experimental Diabetic Glomerulopathy, 1682
Role of Hemodynamic Factors in Extrarenal Diabetic Microangiopathy, 1683
Summary and Implications, 1684
References, 1684

Diabetes mellitus is characterized by numerous metabolic and hormonal abnormalities, which, together, result in early functional changes as well as late morphologic injury in multiple target organs. Microangiopathy remains a major cause of morbidity and mortality in both insulin-dependent (Type I) and non-insulin-dependent (Type II) diabetic patients. Although there is optimism that recent technologic advances in glycemic control will ultimately abrogate the devastating natural history of this disease, maintenance of normoglycemia is currently not feasible in many patients, and the efficacy of tight blood glucose control in preventing microvascular complications remains unproven (1). Accordingly, much investigative attention has been focused on (a) risk factors for progressive microangiopathy, (b) identification of patients at risk for such complications, and (c) potentially beneficial dietary and pharmacologic interventions.

Systemic hypertension is a serious adverse consequence of diabetes mellitus, contributing appreciably to cardiovascular morbidity and mortality by acceleration of diabetic micro- and macrovascular complications (2,3). Both hypertension and the diabetic state contribute to vascular injury. Elevated arterial pressure enhances shear stress on endothelial cells and leads to increased transcapillary pressure gradients. Nonenzymatic protein glycosylation, induced by hyperglycemia, contributes as well (4), since glycosylation of hemoglobin impairs oxygen delivery to vascular tissues, whereas glycosylation of low-density lipoprotein enhances atherogenicity. Glycosylation of collagen stimulates binding of low-density lipoprotein, and nonenzymatic glycosylation of capillary basement membranes may contribute to thickening and increased permeability (4). Thus, hypertension and metabolic abnormalities, together, render the hypertensive diabetic patient at extreme risk for vascular complications.

HEMODYNAMIC ABNORMALITIES IN EXPERIMENTAL DIABETES

Abnormalities of regional hemodynamics characterize the early diabetic state and are evident long before the development of systemic hypertension. These changes are most readily apparent in the renal circulation. Paradoxically, in view of their striking representation in contemporary hemodialysis units, markedly elevated values for glomerular filtration rate (GFR) are frequently found at the time diabetes is diagnosed in Type I (5–7) and (in some cases) Type II (8,9) diabetic patients. This glomerular hyperfiltration is usually accompanied by increments in renal plasma flow and by a substantial increase in kidney size (10,11).

In the 1950s, Stalder and Schmid (7) suggested that these early functional changes might relate to the morphologic injury which eventuates in diabetic patients. These investigators further suggested that the increased GFR and filtration fraction were associated with increased filtration pressure or increased permeability of the glomerular capillary wall, which, in turn, contributed to morphologic injury. Indeed, Mogensen and Christensen (12) have subsequently confirmed that those patients with the highest GFRs in the early stages of diabetes are more likely to progress to persistent proteinuria or overt diabetic glomerulopathy than those patients whose values for GFR are closer to the normal range.

That renal hyperperfusion and hyperfiltration might contribute to the development of diabetic glomerulopathy has been further suggested by observations in diabetic patients with unilateral renal artery stenosis, in whom morphologic evidence of diabetic nephropathy was confined to the nonstenosed kidney (13,14). Since abnormal metabolic conditions would be expected to affect both kidneys equally, it seems likely that the stenosis protected the ipsilateral kidney from hemodynamic influences such as hyperperfusion and hyperfiltration. Animal studies indicate that uninephrectomy, which enhances renal perfusion and filtration in the remaining kidney, markedly accelerates such markers of diabetic glomerulopathy as mesangial matrix thickening and fractional volume expansion, glomerular basement membrane thickening, and mesangial deposition of circulating plasma proteins (15,16).

Recent experimental studies have elucidated the importance of hemodynamic factors in the initiation and pathogenesis of diabetic microangiopathy (17,18). Animal models wherein diabetes develops spontaneously or is induced chemically or surgically offer the opportunity to study the role of altered hemodynamics in the development of diabetic glomerulopathy. In the rat, a clinically relevant model of conventionally treated diabetes mellitus can be developed as a result of chemical induction of diabetes and administration of insulin in doses sufficient to maintain moderate hyperglycemia. In this model, Hostetter et al. (19) found increases of approximately 40% in whole-kidney and single-nephron glomerular filtration rates as compared to those in normal rats. Reductions in intrarenal vascular resistances resulted in elevation of the glomerular capillary plasma flow rate, Q_A. Because the decrease in afferent arteriolar resistance was proportionately greater than that in efferent resistance, mean glomerular capillary hydraulic pressure ($\bar{P}_{GC}$) was also elevated. Together, glomerular capillary hyperperfusion and hypertension accounted for the observed single-nephron hyperfiltration. Though glomerular capillary pressures cannot be measured in humans, the observed increases in renal plasma flow account for only about 50–60% of the increase in GFR (20,21). This increase in filtration fraction has been taken to suggest that intraglomerular pressure may be elevated (22), implying that the hemodynamic pattern in moderately hyperglycemic rats is analogous to that in human diabetics.

Rats with long-standing diabetes develop familiar renal morphologic changes, including renal (23) and glomerular (24,25) hypertrophy, glomerular basement-membrane thickening (25), mesangial matrix thickening (24), and hyaline deposition and glomerular sclerosis (24,26,27). Of note, experimental diabetes in the rat is not accompanied by systemic hypertension (19,26,27); these renal hemodynamic and morphologic abnormalities thus occur in the absence of systemic hypertension. Thus, as discussed below, hypertension may accelerate both clinical and experimental glomerulopathy but is not a prerequisite for experimental (or, in fact, clinical) diabetic glomerulopathy.

Experimentally, maneuvers which increase glomerular capillary perfusion, filtration, and hypertension accelerate the development of glomerular injury in the diabetic rat. Uninephrectomy, which increases single-nephron glomerular filtration rate (SNGFR), Q_A and $\bar{P}_{GC}$ in normal rats (28), accelerates the degree of mesangial expansion (15,29), as well as the development of albuminuria and glomerular sclerosis (29), in diabetic rats. Diabetic renal injury is also amplified by augmentation of dietary protein content (26,30,31), which increases renal perfusion and filtration (26). These studies involved aggravation of renal hemodynamics without alterations in metabolic control, thereby strongly implicating hemodynamic factors as important contributors to the development of diabetic glomerulopathy.

Dietary protein restriction, which limits glomerular capillary pressures and flows in normal rats (32) and in other models of progressive renal disease characterized by hyperfiltration (33,34), was utilized by Zatz et al. (26) to clarify the role of hemodynamic factors in the pathogenesis of diabetic glomerulopathy. Rats that were made diabetic with streptozotocin and that were kept moderately hyperglycemic with daily insulin injections were fed diets containing 6%, 12%, or 50% protein, representing severe protein restriction, moderate protein restriction, and a high-protein diet, respectively. As is depicted in Fig. 1, values for SNGFR and Q_A clearly rose with increasing dietary protein content, in both normal and diabetic rats. In the high-protein-diabetic rats, values for SNGFR were overtly elevated as a result of increases in both Q_A and $\bar{P}_{GC}$. Both reduced-protein diets limited single-nephron hyperfiltration in the diabetic rats to near-normal levels by reducing the supranormal glomerular capillary pressures and flows. After 14 months of diabetes, protein-restricted rats exhibited virtually no albuminuria or glomerular morphologic injury. In contrast, diabetic rats that were fed the high-protein diet and that had overt glomerular hemodynamic abnormalities exhibited striking increases in albuminuria over the long duration of this study, together with significant glomerular morphologic injury (26).

Of note, there were no differences in metabolic control, as assessed by blood glucose or glycosylated hemoglobin levels, in the various groups, suggesting that amelioration of abnormal hemodynamic factors may confer protection, even in the absence of improved metabolic control. Abnormalities in hemodynamic and metabolic parameters may be difficult to differentiate, since correction of hyperglycemia also generally reverses hyperfiltration. Thus, this study was the first to clearly dissociate hemodynamic from metabolic abnormalities in diabetes and provided strong evidence that amelioration of the altered glomerular hemodynamics could prevent diabetic renal disease, even in the presence of continued hyperglycemia.

Although long-term well-controlled clinical correlates of such a study remains to be performed, restriction of dietary protein intake has already shown great promise in preventing the progression of nondiabetic renal disease (35). Furthermore, recent short-term studies in small numbers of diabetic patients have provided encouraging preliminary evidence that dietary protein restriction may be associated with reduction in albuminuria (36–39) as well as with slowing of progression of diabetic nephropathy (38,39).

Of interest, hemodynamically mediated glomerular in-

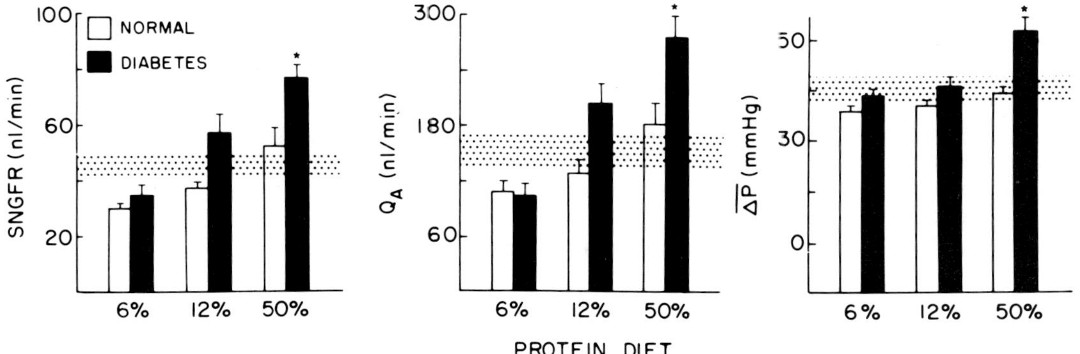

FIG. 1. Effects of dietary protein intake on single-nephron glomerular filtration rate (SNGFR), plasma flow rate (Q_A), and glomerular transcapillary hydraulic pressure gradient ($\overline{\Delta P}$) in normal and diabetic rats. Open bars represent normal rats, and solid bars represent diabetic rats. Horizontal bands represent normal ranges. Note that only diabetic rats fed the 50% protein diet exhibit increases in all three parameters. *$p < 0.05$ versus normal. (From ref. 26.)

jury also eventuates in nondiabetic conditions in which metabolic or neurohumoral abnormalities produce renal vasodilatation and, hence, glomerular hyperfiltration. For example, early hyperfiltration, possibly due to elevated serum lactate levels, precedes the development of glomerular sclerosis and renal failure in patients with Type I glycogen storage disease (40). Similarly, the potent renal vasodilatory properties of glucocorticoids may contribute to the relatively poor renal prognosis (41) of patients with lupus nephritis treated with these agents. Experimentally, vasodilator glucocorticoids augment single-nephron hyperfiltration by aggravating both Q_A and $\bar{P}_{GC}$, and also accelerate glomerular sclerosis, in rats with chronic renal failure (42). Thus, renal vasodilatation and subsequent hyperfiltration appear to play a role in the eventual glomerular destruction which characterizes diabetes and other metabolic diseases.

Numerous metabolic and hormonal abnormalities have been proposed as mediators of diabetic hyperfiltration (Table 1); it seems likely that while each of these may contribute, the etiology is multifactorial and related to the stage of diabetes. One obvious candidate is hyperglycemia, which sometimes, (11,43) but not always (44), raises GFR when artificially induced in normal subjects. Although initial institution of insulin therapy reduces GFR and renal plasma flow rates in Type I diabetics, normalization of blood glucose may precede normalization of renal function by days or even weeks, suggesting that diabetic hyperfiltration consists of a rapidly reversible element, possibly associated with hyperglycemia, and a more slowly reversible component of unknown etiology, of approximately the same magnitude (45). Similarly, reduction of blood glucose to normal levels with a constant subcutaneous insulin infusion pump normalizes GFR, but, again, not until long after normoglycemia is achieved (46). When compared to moderately hyperglycemic diabetic rats, animals that are kept normoglycemic with chronic insulin therapy exhibit fairly normal values for SNGFR, due primarily to lower values for $\bar{P}_{GC}$ than those seen in hyperglycemic rats (47–49). Of note, acute infusion of insulin does not appear to reduce GFR in diabetic patients (21) or rats (50) but has recently been reported to reduce $\bar{P}_{GC}$ in moderately hyperglycemic diabetic rats, even when hyperglycemia is maintained with concurrent dextrose infusion (50). Thus, insulinopenia may play a role in the glomerular capillary hypertension which contributes to glomerular hyperfiltration.

However, these observations cannot implicate hyperglycemia or insulinopenia as the sole culprits in view of (a) the time course discrepancy and (b) the multiple hormonal derangements which characterize untreated diabetes. For instance, ketone body infusion results in a dramatic increase in GFR in normal subjects and, in diabetic subjects, is accompanied by a rise of 29% in renal plasma flow and 14% in filtration fraction (51). Elevated levels of plasma glucagon and growth hormone have been noted in some diabetic patients, and each of these hormones may raise GFR in the normal kidney under certain conditions (52,53). However, plasma levels of these hormones are comparably elevated in Type I diabetics with normal and elevated values for GFR (54). Furthermore, increments in GFR induced by infusion of these agents in nondiabetic subjects fail to reproduce diabetic hyperfiltration, even when plasma levels comparable to those found in diabetic patients are attained (53,55,56).

TABLE 1. *Potential mediators of diabetic hyperfiltration*

Hyperglycemia
Insulinopenia
Extracellular fluid volume expansion; atrial natriuretic peptide
Imbalance between production of prostaglandin and of thromboxane
Abnormalities in kinin metabolism
Increased plasma ketone bodies
Increased plasma glucagon levels
Increased plasma growth hormone levels
Excessive dietary protein intake
Renin deficiency
Hyporesponsiveness to catecholamines/angiotensin II
Altered cellular *myo*-inositol metabolism
Blunting of tubuloglomerular feedback mechanism
Abnormalities in calcium metabolism
Tissue hypoxia; abnormalities in local vasoregulatory factors

The moderately hyperglycemic diabetic state is also characterized by chronic plasma volume expansion (43,57) with consequent elevation of plasma atrial natriuretic peptide (ANP) levels (58–60) and a reduction in atrial ANP content (60), suggesting enhanced ANP release. In diabetic rats, moderate hyperglycemia is associated with elevated values for both plasma ANP levels and GFR, whereas maintenance of normoglycemia with intensive insulin administration limits both ANP and GFR to normal levels. Moreover, infusion of a specific anti-ANP antiserum reduces the excessively high values for GFR in moderately hyperglycemic diabetic rats to the normal range, suggesting that this hormone may play a role in diabetic hyperfiltration (58). In support of this concept, dietary sodium restriction, which would be expected to prevent plasma volume expansion and enhanced ANP release, prevents hyperfiltration in diabetic rats (61).

Enhanced activity of vasodilator prostaglandins, as well as an imbalance between prostaglandin and thromboxane production, has been implicated in diabetic hyperfiltration. Glomerular production of the vasodilator prostaglandins PGE_2 and PGI_2 is increased in diabetic rats (62–64), and increased levels of urinary vasodilator prostaglandins are sometimes (65,66), though not consistently (67), found in Type I diabetics. Effects of short-term prostaglandin synthetase inhibition on GFR are similarly conflicting (65,66,68), though a recent comparative study found elevated prostaglandin levels, as well as a reduction of GFR with indomethacin, only in patients with established nephropathy (65). In diabetic rats, administration of aspirin (69) or indomethacin (64,70) in doses which suppress PGE_2 production ameliorates early hyperfiltration; furthermore, aspirin prevents glomerular basement thickening and late deterioration of renal function in diabetic rats (69). Studies in the isolated perfused kidney have suggested that administration of indomethacin prevents glucose-induced increases in GFR in this model (71). In a micropuncture study of diabetic rats, Jensen et al. (70) noted that chronic administration of indomethacin resulted in significant reductions in SNGFR, Q_A, and $\bar{P}_{GC}$ in diabetic rats, although a slight decrease in blood glucose levels also occurred during indomethacin administration. However, a recent report of acute indomethacin infusion into untreated diabetic rats found no effect on glomerular hemodynamics (72). Although these studies suggest that enhanced activity of vasodilator prostaglandins may be involved in diabetic hyperfiltration, other factors must also be invoked. In diabetic rats, the very early stages of hyperfiltration (2 weeks) are associated with increased prostaglandin synthesis; however, after a month of diabetes, prostaglandin production is no longer enhanced whereas hyperfiltration persists (64), suggesting that other mechanisms support the chronic hyperfiltration state. Moreover, increased prostaglandin production is not found in spontaneously diabetic BB rats (73). Though hemodynamic effects were not specifically measured, Donadio et al. (74) have reported, in a 10-year prospective study, that administration of aspirin and dipyridamole may afford some degree of renal protection in patients with early nephropathy, though not in those with more advanced disease. Taken together, these somewhat disparate findings suggest that although abnormalities in prostaglandin/thromboxane metabolism may be involved, their contribution varies significantly in different stages of diabetes or in different levels of diabetic control.

Increased activity of the polyol pathway, as well as related disturbances in cellular *myo*-inositol metabolism, has been implicated in the pathogenesis of several diabetic microangiopathic complications (75). Aldose reductase inhibitors have been reported to limit hyperfiltration (76,77), renal hypertrophy (78), and proteinuria (79) in short-term studies in diabetic rats. However, a recent long-term study of these agents found no effect on blood pressure, GFR, albuminuria, or glomerular injury in diabetic rats, though the incidence of cataracts was appreciably reduced (80).

Many other features of the diabetic state could theoretically influence intrarenal hemodynamics, including depression of plasma or intrarenal renin activity (81,82), reduced numbers of glomerular angiotensin II receptors (83), vascular hyporesponsiveness to catecholamines and angiotensin II (82), blunting of the tubuloglomerular feedback mechanism (83), abnormalities of calcium metabolism (84), tissue hypoxia (85), hemorrheologic factors (86), and abnormalities in kinin production or action (72,87,88). Clearly, elucidation of the complex mechanisms which contribute to diabetic hyperfiltration remains a challenging investigative task.

SYSTEMIC HYPERTENSION IN DIABETES

Systemic hypertension is a frequent complication of both Type I and Type II diabetes and has proven to be an important risk factor for development of microangiopathy (89). Once present, hypertension accelerates the rate at which diabetic complications worsen. Elevation of blood pressure shortens the time interval between onset of diabetes and occurrence of both renal failure and retinopathy (90,91). The incidence of retinopathy is increased in diabetic patients with hypertension (91), but definitive data regarding the potential beneficial effect of blood pressure reduction on diabetic retinopathy is lacking. Of the microvascular complications of diabetes, the impact of systemic hypertension on glomerulopathy has been the most extensively studied. The most convincing evidence for the role of systemic hypertension in the acceleration of diabetic nephropathy comes from studies, primarily in Scandinavia, demonstrating that blood pressure control slows the progression of diabetic renal disease (92,93).

HYPERTENSION AND EXPERIMENTAL DIABETIC GLOMERULOPATHY

Animal studies have provided insight into the mechanisms by which systemic hypertension accelerates diabetic glomerulopathy and by which therapeutic interventions afford protection. Specifically, these studies suggest that the adverse effects of systemic hypertension on progression of renal disease may depend upon the intraglomerular hemodynamic consequences. Afferent arteriolar resistance determines the fraction of systemic arterial pressure which is transmitted to the glomerular capillary network. In some models, such as the spontaneously hypertensive rat (SHR), relative afferent arteriolar vasoconstriction prevents glomerular capillary hypertension (94), and the kidney is relatively protected from the development of glomerular sclerosis (95). In other models, however, including experimental diabetes, relative afferent arteriolar vasodilation allows the development of glomerular capillary hypertension, which, in turn, is associated with progressive proteinuria and glomerular sclerosis (26,27).

Systemic hypertension appears to contribute to diabetic glomerulopathy by aggravation of the abnormal glomerular microcirculatory hemodynamics. With the institution of two-kidney Goldblatt hypertension, a striking intensification of glomerular lesions is observed in the unclipped kidney of diabetic rats, whereas the clipped kidney is substantially protected from glomerular injury (96). Though renal hemodynamics were not studied, unilateral renal artery clipping intensifies glomerular hypertension in the intact, contralateral kidney (97), suggesting that enhanced glomerular capillary hypertension produced this acceleration of diabetic renal injury.

Experimental diabetic glomerulopathy is also accelerated when diabetes is induced in the SHR; glomerular injury in hypertensive diabetic rats is greater than that seen in rats with hypertension alone (98–100) (Table 2). Albuminuria and mesangial expansion were enhanced in each of these studies, though they correlated more with diabetes than with hypertension per se (99). Micropuncture studies have reported conflicting results in this model. In one study, elevation of $\bar{P}_{GC}$ was noted in diabetic hypertensive rats, though not in rats with diabetes or hypertension alone (98), whereas others did not document glomerular hypertension in the diabetic SHR with either moderate or severe hyperglycemia (101). In the latter study, however, evidence of glomerular injury was found only in the deep glomeruli (101), which are presumed to exhibit higher glomerular

TABLE 2. *Effects of superimposed hypertension and of antihypertensive therapy in experimental diabetes*[a]

Group	Duration	SBP (mmHg)	$\bar{P}_{GC}$ (mmHg)	AER (mg/day)	Mesangial expansion	Other morphology	Reference
C	4 months	127 ± 4	—	—	~0.2		96
DM		135 ± 4	—	—	~0.6^{b}		
DM/GH		234 ± 6^{b,c}	—	—	~1.8^{c}		
SHR	6 months	181 ± 2	—	28 ± 1	↑1/12		100
SHR/DM		168 ± 2^{b}	—	74 ± 17^{b}	↑4/9		
SHR/DM/TRX		140 ± 2^{b,c}	—	23 ± 2^{b,c}	Normal		
WKY	6 months	109 ± 2	43 ± 1	Normal	15 ± 3		98
WKY/DM		114 ± 1	48 ± 1^{b}	Normal	27 ± 1^{b}		
SHR		159 ± 4^{d}	44 ± 1	Normal	22 ± 2		
SHR/DM		168 ± 3^{d}	53 ± 1^{b,d}	Normal	26 ± 2^{b}		
SHR/DM/TRX		112 ± 3^{b,c}	47 ± 1^{c}	Normal	16 ± 2^{c}		
WKY	8 months	136 ± 5	—	3	↑ by DM but not by ↑SBP	GBM thickening ↑ by both DM and ↑SBP	99
WKY/DM		128 ± 4	—	3			
SHR		224 ± 7^{b}	—	20^{d}			
SHR/DM		194 ± 7^{d}	—	70^{b,d}			
SHR/DM/CEI		~145^{c}	—	8^{c}			
C	14 months	119 ± 3^{e}	53 ± 1	25 ± 6	—	Glomerular sclerosis ↑ only in untreated DM rats	27
DM		117 ± 4	63 ± 2^{b}	111 ± 22^{b}	—		
DM/CEI		98 ± 2^{b,c}	50 ± 1^{c}	18 ± 3^{c}	—		
C	3 months	117 ± 3		8 ± 0.2	—		102
DM		133 ± 3^{b}		71 ± 18^{b}	—		
DM/CEI		108 ± 3^{c}		36 ± 3^{c}	—		
DM/CCB		114 ± 2^{c}		58 ± 10	—		
C	9 months	117 ± 3	—	12 ± 3	—		108
DM		130 ± 3	—	45 ± 10^{b}	—		
DM/CEI		106 ± 5^{b,c}	—	41 ± 9^{b,c}	—		
DM/H		114 ± 3^{b,c}	—	2 ± 1^{c}	—		
C	16 months	126 ± 4	—	14 ± 3	—		107
DM		147 ± 4	—	57 ± 9^{b}	—		
DM/TRX		114 ± 4^{c}	—	42 ± 13^{b,c}	—		
DM/CEI		124 ± 5^{c}	—	3 ± 0.4^{c}	—		

[a] Values are means ± SEM. SBP, systolic blood pressure; $\bar{P}_{GC}$, glomerular capillary pressure; AER, urinary albumin excretion rate; C, nondiabetic control; DM, diabetic; GH, Goldblatt hypertension; SHR, spontaneously hypertensive rat. TRX, triple therapy; WKY, Wistar-Kyoto rat. CEI, converting-enzyme inhibitor; CCB, calcium channel blocker; H, hydralazine. ↑, increased.

[b] $p < 0.05$ versus nondiabetic control.

[c] $p < 0.05$ versus untreated diabetes.

[d] $p < 0.05$ versus comparable WKY.

[e] Mean arterial pressure under anesthesia.

capillary pressures and flows than are the superficial glomeruli accessible to micropuncture.

EFFECTS OF ANTIHYPERTENSIVE THERAPY IN EXPERIMENTAL DIABETIC GLOMERULOPATHY

Studies in the diabetic rat have also elucidated the mechanisms by which antihypertensive therapy slows the progression of diabetic glomerulopathy (Table 2). In the normotensive, moderately hyperglycemic Munich–Wistar rat, the angiotensin I-converting-enzyme inhibitor (CEI) enalapril was administered in a dose which modestly lowered systemic arterial pressure by about 15 mmHg (27). Despite this modest effect, as well as the absence of any changes in glycemic control, CEI therapy selectively controlled glomerular capillary hypertension without affecting the supranormal SNGFR and Q_A (Fig. 2). Control of glomerular hypertension was associated with limitation of albuminuria and glomerular injury to levels seen in nondiabetic control rats (27). Thus, these findings confirm the earlier results with dietary protein restriction (26) that amelioration of hemodynamic abnormalities affords protection even in the absence of any changes in metabolic control. Moreover, they suggest that of the hemodynamic determinants of hyperfiltration, glomerular capillary hypertension is the critical factor in the pathogenesis of structural injury. Though glomerular hemodynamics were not studied, CEI therapy has also been shown to (a) limit albuminuria, mesangial expansion, and glomerular basement-membrane thickening in the diabetic SHR (99) and (b) reduce blood pressure, filtration fraction (possibly reflecting $\bar{P}_{GC}$), and proteinuria in uninephrectomized diabetic rats (102).

In relatively short-term studies, administration of reserpine, hydralazine, and hydrochlorothiazide ("triple therapy") lowers blood pressure (98,100) and $\bar{P}_{GC}$ (98), and it also limits mesangial expansion (98,100) and proteinuria (100) in the diabetic SHR. Bank et al. (98) reported that moderately hyperglycemic diabetic SHRs and Wistar–Kyoto (WKY) rats both exhibited increases in SNGFR, Q_A, and $\bar{P}_{GC}$ as compared to nondiabetic controls, with values for $\bar{P}_{GC}$ being slightly, though significantly, higher in the diabetic SHR than in the diabetic WKY rat. Unfortunately, the study was terminated prior to the development of proteinuria or glomerular sclerosis. At the time of sacrifice, mesangial expansion was comparable in the diabetic SHR and WKY rat, and it was ameliorated in a third group of diabetic SHRs in which antihypertensive therapy lowered $\bar{P}_{GC}$ toward, but did not cause it to reach, the normal range. Thus, within the scope of this study, both diabetic groups exhibited glomerular hypertension and mesangial expansion, whereas the group receiving antihypertensive therapy exhibited lower values for both $\bar{P}_{GC}$ and mesangial expansion.

Whether the group receiving antihypertensive therapy which does not completely normalize $\bar{P}_{GC}$ will truly be protected, or perhaps demonstrate slightly delayed development of injury, remains to be determined. Other evidence suggests that triple therapy may not prove ultimately effective in protecting against morphologic injury. In the partially nephrectomized rat, values for proteinuria are significantly reduced very early in the course of the disease, but they later increase to values comparable to those in untreated hypertensive rats (103). In the nondiabetic SHR, long-term studies have established that this regimen only delays, but does not prevent, glomerular injury (95). Studies in other, nondiabetic models of progressive renal disease have indicated that effective antihypertensive control with triple therapy prevents glomerular hypertension and injury in some models (104,105) but limits neither in others (103,106). More recently, a comparison study performed in moderately hyperglycemic diabetic rats suggests that although reduction of blood pressure with triple therapy slows the development of albuminuria in this model, the effect is only to delay the development of injury, whereas comparable blood pressure control with CEI appears to prevent the development of diabetic glomerulopathy (107).

In contrast, however, hydralazine alone affords no protection against development of diabetic glomerulopathy, despite reduction of blood pressure to levels comparable to those achieved with CEI; monotherapy with hydralazine

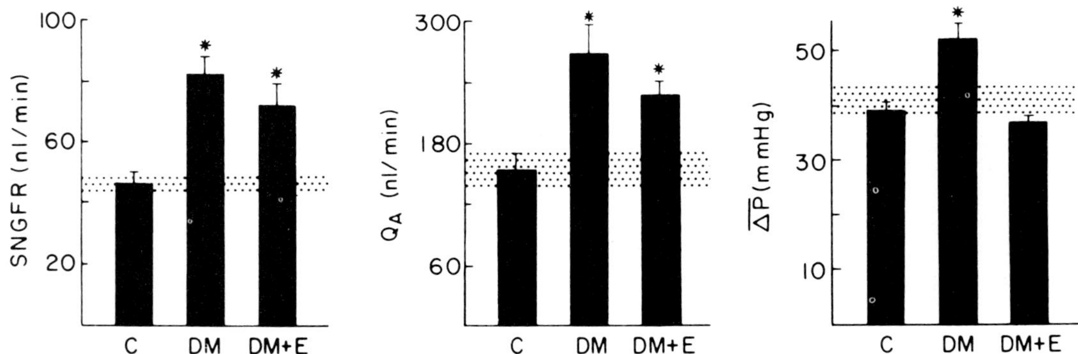

FIG. 2. Effects of converting-enzyme inhibitor (CEI) therapy on single-nephron glomerular filtration rate (SNGFR), plasma flow rate (Q_A), and glomerular transcapillary hydraulic pressure gradient ($\overline{\Delta P}$) in diabetic rats. Values for all parameters were increased above the normal range (horizontal band) in diabetic rats (D) as compared to normal rats (C). Diabetic rats treated with CEI (DM + E) exhibited comparable single-nephron filtration and perfusion rates, but the glomerular transcapillary hydraulic pressure gradient ($\overline{\Delta P}$) was selectively normalized by CEI treatment. *$p < 0.05$ versus C. (From ref. 27.)

fails to normalize $\bar{P}_{GC}$ in diabetic rats (108). In the uninephrectomized diabetic rat, excellent control of systemic blood pressure with verapamil results in no reduction in filtration fraction or proteinuria (102). Taken together, these studies suggest that reduction in blood pressure per se may afford protection in the presence of severe hypertension but that a substantial beneficial effect on slowing the progression of diabetic glomerulopathy may be most successfully achieved when antihypertensive therapy results in control of glomerular capillary hypertension.

Numerous clinical studies have established that control of systemic hypertension slows the development of diabetic glomerulopathy. However, the observations in diabetic rats, as well as in other models of progressive glomerulopathy, suggest that all antihypertensive agents may not prove equally efficacious in slowing glomerular injury. In patients with nondiabetic renal disease, several recent studies suggest that CEI therapy may be superior to conventional combination regimens in reducing proteinuria and in preventing renal functional deterioration (109–111). Long-term, prospective clinical studies of this issue are currently lacking in diabetic, as well as in nondiabetic, renal disease. However, several recent observations suggest that interventions which reduce $\bar{P}_{GC}$ in the rat may have comparable glomerular hemodynamic effects in patients as well. In patients with severe diabetic nephropathy, a substantial decrease in proteinuria was noted after an 8-week course of therapy with the CEI captopril. In this study, captopril was added to the existing antihypertensive regimen in doses which did not further reduce systemic blood pressure (112). Moreover, CEI therapy reduces albuminuria in normotensive diabetic patients with minimal evidence of renal disease (113,114). In each of these studies, absence of a marked reduction in systemic arterial pressure strongly suggests that the reduction in albuminuria resulted from a decrease in $\bar{P}_{GC}$, most likely due to inhibition of angiotensin II formation and subsequent relaxation of efferent (postglomerular) arteriolar tone.

ROLE OF HEMODYNAMIC FACTORS IN EXTRARENAL DIABETIC MICROANGIOPATHY

Vascular hemodynamic abnormalities in diabetes are not limited to the renal circulation (18). As with the glomerulus, a remarkably similar correlation between functional and morphologic alterations is found in the retinal microcirculation. Indeed, the development of albuminuria in diabetic patients signals risk not only of nephropathy but also of proliferative retinopathy, and vice versa (115). In analogy with the glomerulus, hemodynamic abnormalities may be detected in the retina a number of years before retinopathy becomes overt. Retinal hyperperfusion (116,117), as well as dilatation of the retinal arteries and veins (118), is found in patients with early Type I diabetes, at a stage when there is little or no evidence of retinopathy. The presence of dilated retinal veins has been correlated with the subsequent development of severe retinal lesions (119). More recent studies, using bidirectional laser Doppler velocimetry techniques, confirm that retinal blood flow is increased, and autoregulation impaired, in Type II diabetics as well; achieving normoglycemia with an insulin infusion corrects these hemodynamic abnormalities (120). Elevated retinal capillary pressures may also contribute to eventual structural injury, since normal or even elevated flows have been noted by ophthalmodynamometry only in the morphologically damaged eyes of patients with unilateral diabetic retinopathy. In a series of 10 such patients, reduced retinal hydraulic pressures were found in the contralateral, unaffected retina, which was presumably protected from elevated pressure by the presence of an ipsilateral partial carotid arterial stenosis or ipsilateral glaucoma (121). As in the glomerular capillary, retinal capillary barrier function is disrupted in the early stages of diabetes, at which time there is (a) extravasation of macromolecules, along with the deposition of these macromolecules into the basement membrane, and (b) focal retinal capillary basement-membrane thickening (122). More advanced stages include marked capillary basement-membrane thickening, endothelial proliferation, microaneurysm formation, and intracapillary thrombosis. Of note, dietary protein restriction is associated not only with limitation of glomerular basement-membrane thickening (123) but also with limitation of retinal basement-membrane thickening (124). In this study, reduction of dietary protein content in moderately hyperglycemic diabetic rats resulted in limitation of both glomerular and retinal basement-membrane thicknesses to values seen in nondiabetic control rats, in the absence of any improvement in metabolic control (26). These findings lend further support to the hypothesis that hemodynamic factors may contribute to diabetic retinopathy as they do to glomerulopathy (18).

Similarly, hyperperfusion is found in forearm, skin, and adipose tissue capillaries in diabetes (18). Autoregulation of peripheral capillary blood flow is impaired (125), with exaggerated increases in capillary blood flow occurring in response to exercise (126). These peripheral capillaries exhibit increased permeability to plasma proteins, which are deposited in the capillary wall, leading to basement-membrane thickening (127). The end result is progressive capillary wall hyalinization and proliferation, with consequent intracapillary thrombosis and luminal obliteration. Increased muscle capillary basement-membrane thickness correlates with widening of the glomerular capillary basement membrane (128). Indeed, recent studies confirm that intestinal capillary blood flow and hydraulic pressure are increased in diabetic rats (129,130) and that diabetes induces thickening of intestinal capillary basement membranes in diabetic hamsters (131). Of note, cross-perfusion experiments wherein intestinal preparations of normal rats were perfused with arterial blood from diabetic rats resulted in intestinal hyperperfusion in the normal rats, suggesting that a circulating humoral factor contributed to the hyperperfusion (130).

An integrated mechanism whereby hemodynamic factors may constitute a major pathogenetic mechanism in the development of diabetic microangiopathic complications is schematized in Fig. 3 (132). Chronic moderate hyperglycemia leads to extracellular fluid volume expansion and also leads to abnormalities in various vasoactive neurohormonal modulators. These factors lead to sustained vasodi-

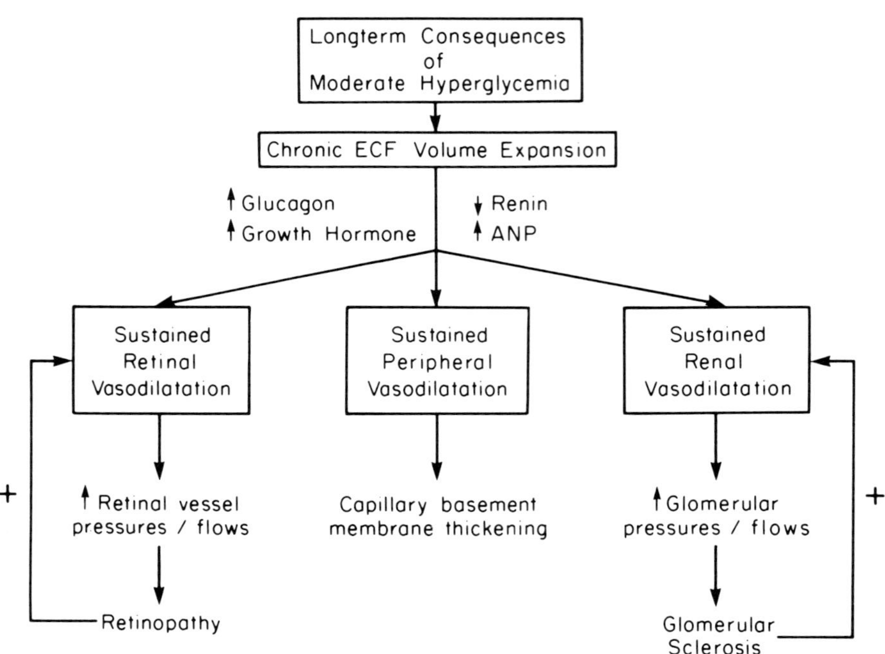

FIG. 3. Mechanism of generalized hyperperfusion in the pathogenesis of retinal, peripheral, and renal microangiopathic complications of diabetes. The long-term consequences of moderate hyperglycemia include chronic ECF (extracellular fluid) volume expansion, leading to decreased plasma renin and increased plasma atrial natriuretic peptide (ANP) levels which, in conjunction with altered levels of other vasoactive hormones, lead to generalized sustained vasodilatation. This generalized vasodilatation promotes basement-membrane thickening in all capillary beds and, in the case of the retina and the kidney, elevation of capillary pressures and flows. These hemodynamic maladaptations cause structural damage, which, in turn, contributes to a vicious cycle as the remaining intact capillaries receive a higher proportion of the total blood flow, resulting in further augmentation of pressures and flows. (From ref. 132.)

latation of the retinal, peripheral, and renal capillary microcirculatory beds. This generalized vasodilatation promotes basement-membrane thickening in all capillary beds and, in the case of the retina and the kidney, elevation of capillary pressures and flows. Together, these abnormalities lead to structural damage, including retinopathy and glomerular sclerosis, which, in turn, contribute to a vicious cycle as the remaining intact capillaries receive a higher proportion of the total blood flow, resulting in further augmentation of pressures and flows.

SUMMARY AND IMPLICATIONS

Recent advances in the treatment of hyperglycemia and hypertension have not yet begun to have a substantial impact on the incidence of end-stage renal disease in patients with diabetes mellitus. Nonetheless, enhanced understanding of the risk factors for development of diabetic complications, together with improved hypoglycemic technology, recognition of optimal dietary therapies, and an expanded antihypertensive pharmacopoeia, generate optimism that the diabetic state need not lead to devastating microvascular complications. These newer strategies will require validation with long-term, prospective, controlled clinical trials. In addition, several important questions will need to be addressed in future studies. Firstly, how can we identify those patients at risk for diabetic complications, who are perhaps candidates for earlier and more aggressive intervention? The recent demonstration that patients who develop diabetic renal disease are more likely to have a parent with essential hypertension (133,134) suggests a genetic susceptibility, and reported abnormalities in red blood cell sodium–lithium countertransport (134,135) offer a promising avenue of investigation of this question. Secondly, at what point should preventive measures be instituted? Although it may be imprudent to wait until renal function is severely compromised, universal application of these interventions at the time diabetes is diagnosed will prove inappropriate, unnecessary, and possibly perilous for those patients not destined to suffer serious complications of the disease. Though short-term studies of CEI therapy in normotensive diabetic patients show promise, currently available data do not yet justify the widespread use of antihypertensive therapy in normotensive patients. Finally, the suggestion from animal studies that antihypertensive agents (such as CEIs) which reduce $\bar{P}_{GC}$ afford superior protection to other antihypertensive regimens requires careful comparison studies in diabetic patients. These caveats notwithstanding, further investigation into the mechanisms of hemodynamic injury may reveal nutritional and pharmacologic strategies which will provide successful, and readily achievable, means for conferring protection against the debilitating complications of diabetes mellitus.

ACKNOWLEDGMENT

Studies in the authors' laboratory were supported by U.S. Public Health Service grants AM 35930, AM 07206, AM 30410, and TW 03263-01S1.

REFERENCES

1. DCCT Research Group. Diabetes control and complications trial (DCCT): results of feasibility study. *Diabetes Care* 1987;10:1–19.
2. Kannel WB. Diabetes and cardiovascular disease: the Framingham Study: 18-year follow-up. *Cardiol Digest* 1976;11:11–15.
3. Janka HU, Dirschedl P. Systolic blood pressure as a predictor for

cardiovascular disease in diabetes. A 5-year longitudinal study. *Hypertension* 1985;7(Suppl II):II-90–II-94.
4. Brownlee M, Cerami A, Vlassara H. Advanced glycosylation end products in tissue and the biochemical basis of diabetic complications. *N Engl J Med* 1988;318:1315–1321.
5. Cambier P. Application de la theorie de Rehberg a l'étude clinique des affections renales et du diabete. *Ann Med* 1934;35:273–299.
6. Ditzel J, Junker K. Abnormal glomerular filtration rate, renal plasma flow and renal protein excretion in recent and short-term diabetes. *Br Med J* 1972;2:13–19.
7. Stalder G, Schmid R. Severe functional disorders of glomerular capillaries and renal hemodynamics in treated diabetes mellitus during childhood. *Ann Paediatr* 1959;193:129–138.
8. Palmisano J, Sachrechi I, Lebovitz HE. Hyperfiltration in patients with Type 2 diabetes mellitus [Abstract]. *Clin Res* 1987;35:636A.
9. Berionade V. Creatinine clearance in non-insulin-dependent diabetes mellitus [Abstract]. *Kidney Int* 1986;31:179.
10. Mogensen CE, Andersen MJF. Increased kidney size and glomerular filtration rate in early juvenile diabetes. *Diabetes* 1973;22:706–712.
11. Christiansen JS, Gammelgaard J, Frandsen M, Parving H-H. Increased kidney size, glomerular filtration rate, and renal plasma flow in short term insulin-dependent diabetics. *Diabetologia* 1981;20:451–456.
12. Mogensen CE, Christensen CK. Predicting diabetic nephropathy in insulin-dependent patients. *N Engl J Med* 1984;311:89–93.
13. Berkman J, Rifkin H. Unilateral nodular diabetic glomerulosclerosis (Kimmelstiel–Wilson). Report of a case. *Metabolism* 1973;22:715–722.
14. Berionade VC, Legevre R, Falardeau P. Unilateral nodular diabetic glomerulosclerosis: recurrence of an experiment of nature. *Am J Nephrol* 1987;7:55–59.
15. Steffes MW, Brown DM, Mauer SM. Diabetic glomerulopathy following unilateral nephrectomy in the rat. *Diabetes* 1978;27:35–41.
16. Steffes MW, Buchwald H, Wigness BD, Groppoli TJ, Rupp WM, Rohde TD, Blackshear PJ, Mauer SM. Diabetic nephropathy in the uninephrectomized dog: microscopic lesions after one year. *Kidney Int* 1982;21:721–724.
17. Hostetter TH, Rennke HG, Brenner BM. The case for intrarenal hypertension in the initiation and progression of diabetic and other glomerulopathies. *Am J Med* 1982;72:375–380.
18. Zatz R, Brenner BM. Pathogenesis of diabetic microangiopathy: the hemodynamic view. *Am J Med* 1986;80:443–453.
19. Hostetter TH, Troy JL, Brenner BM. Glomerular hemodynamics in experimental diabetes mellitus. *Kidney Int* 1981;19:410–415.
20. Mogensen CE, Andersen MJF. Increased kidney size and glomerular filtration rate in untreated juvenile diabetes: normalization by insulin treatment. *Diabetologia* 1975;11:221–224.
21. Christiansen JS, Frandsen M, Parving H-H. The effect of intravenous insulin infusion on kidney function in insulin-dependent diabetes mellitus. *Diabetologia* 1981;20:199–204.
22. Mogensen CE. Renal function changes in diabetes. *Diabetes* 1976;25:872–879.
23. Seyer-Hansen K, Hansen J, Gundersen HSG. Renal hypertrophy in experimental diabetes. A morphometric study. *Diabetologia* 1980;18:501–505.
24. Mauer SM, Michael AF, Fish AJ, Brown DM. Spontaneous immunoglobulin and complement deposition in glomeruli of diabetic rats. *Lab Invest* 1972;27:488–494.
25. Rasch R. Studies on the prevention of glomerulopathy in diabetic rats. *Acta Endocrinol [Suppl] (Copenh)* 1981;242:43–44.
26. Zatz R, Meyer TW, Rennke HG, Brenner BM. Predominance of hemodynamic rather than metabolic factors in the pathogenesis of diabetic glomerulopathy. *Proc Natl Acad Sci USA* 1985;82:5963–5967.
27. Zatz R, Dunn BR, Meyer TW, Anderson S, Rennke HG, Brenner BM. Prevention of diabetic glomerulopathy by pharmacological amelioration of glomerular capillary hypertension. *J Clin Invest* 1986;77:1925–1930.
28. Deen WM, Maddox DA, Robertson CR, Brenner BM. Dynamics of glomerular ultrafiltration in the rat. VII. Response to reduced renal mass. *Am J Physiol* 1974;227:556–562.
29. O'Donnell MP, Kasiske BL, Daniels FX, Keane WF. Effect of nephron loss on glomerular hemodynamics and morphology in diabetic rats. *Diabetes* 1986;35:1011–1015.
30. Neugarten J, Liu D, Feiner H, Schacht R, Chuba J, Baldwin DS. Aggravation of experimental diabetic nephropathy by high dietary protein [Abstract]. *Clin Res* 1983;31:438A.
31. Wen S-F, Huang T-P, Moorthy AV. Effects of low-protein diet on experimental diabetic nephropathy in the rat. *J Lab Clin Med* 1985;106:589–597.
32. Ichikawa I, Purkerson ML, Klahr S, Troy JL, Martinez-Maldonado M, Brenner BM. Mechanism of reduced glomerular filtration rate in chronic malnutrition. *J Clin Invest* 1980;65:982–988.
33. Brenner BM, Meyer TW, Hostetter TH. Dietary protein intake and the progressive nature of renal disease. The role of hemodynamically mediated glomerular injury in the pathogenesis of progressive glomerular sclerosis in aging, renal ablation, and intrinsic renal disease. *N Engl J Med* 1982;307:652–659.
34. Meyer TW, Anderson S, Rennke HG, Brenner BM. Reversing glomerular hypertension stabilizes established glomerular injury. *Kidney Int* 1987;31:752–759.
35. Maschio G, Oldrizzi L, Rugiu C. The effects of dietary protein restriction on the course of early chronic renal failure. In: Mitch WE, Brenner BM, Stein JH, eds. *The progressive nature of renal disease. Contemporary issues in nephrology,* vol 14. New York: Churchill Livingstone, 1986;203–218.
36. Cohen D, Dodds R, Viberti GC. Effect of protein restriction in insulin dependent diabetics at risk of nephropathy. *Br Med J* 1987;294:795–798.
37. Ciavarella A, Di Mizio G, Stefoni S, Borgnino LC, Vannini P. Reduced albuminuria after dietary protein restriction in insulin-dependent diabetic patients with clinical nephropathy. *Diabetes Care* 1987;10:407–413.
38. Evanoff GV, Thompson CS, Brown J, Weinman EJ. The effect of dietary protein restriction on the progression of diabetic nephropathy. A 12-month follow-up. *Arch Intern Med* 1987;147:492–495.
39. Zeller KR, Jacobson H, Raskin P. The effect of dietary protein modification on renal function in diabetic nephropathy—preliminary report of an ongoing study [Abstract]. *Kidney Int* 1987;31:225.
40. Chen Y-T, Coleman RA, Scheinman JI, Kolbeck PC, Sidbury JB. Renal disease in Type I glycogen storage disease. *N Engl J Med* 1988;318:7–11.
41. Steinberg AD. The treatment of lupus nephritis. *Kidney Int* 1986;30:769–787.
42. Garcia DL, Rennke HG, Brenner BM, Anderson S. Chronic glucocorticoid therapy amplifies glomerular injury in rats with renal ablation. *J Clin Invest* 1987;80:867–874.
43. Brochner-Mortensen J. Glomerular filtration rate and extracellular fluid volumes during normoglycemia and moderate hyperglycaemia in diabetics. *Scand J Clin Lab Invest* 1973;32:311–316.
44. Mogensen CE. Glomerular filtration rate and renal plasma flow in normal and diabetic man during elevation of blood sugar levels. *Scand J Clin Lab Invest* 1971;28:177–182.
45. Christiansen JS, Gammelgaard J, Tronier B, Svendsen PA, Parving H-H. Kidney function and size in diabetics before and during initial insulin treatment. *Kidney Int* 1982;21:683–688.
46. Wiseman MJ, Saunders AJ, Keen H, Viberti GC. Effect of blood glucose control on increased glomerular filtration rate and kidney size in insulin-dependent diabetes. *N Engl J Med* 1985;312:617–621.
47. Daniels FX, O'Donnell MP, Kasiske BL, Keane WF. Insulin therapy normalizes glomerular function in long-term experimental diabetes mellitus [Abstract]. *Kidney Int* 1986;29:316A.
48. Hostetter TH, Meyer TW, Rennke HG, Brenner BM. Influence of strict control of diabetes on intrarenal hemodynamics [Abstract]. *Kidney Int* 1983;23:215A.
49. Jensen PK, Christiansen JS, Steven K, Parving H-H. Strict metabolic control and renal function in the streptozotocin diabetic rat. *Kidney Int* 1987;31:47–51.
50. Scholey JW, Meyer TW. Insulin infusion normalizes glomerular

capillary pressure in experimental diabetes mellitus [Abstract]. *Kidney Int* 1987;31:426A.
51. Trevisan R, Nosadini R, Fioretto P, Velussi M, Avogaro A, Duner E, et al. Metabolic control of kidney hemodynamics in normal and insulin-dependent diabetic subjects. Effects of aceto-acetic, lactic, and acetic acids. *Diabetes* 1987;36:1073–1081.
52. Courvilain J, Abramow M. Some effects of human growth hormone on renal hemodynamics and on tubular phosphate transport in man. *J Clin Invest* 1962;41:1230–1235.
53. Parving H-H, Noer J, Kehlet H, Mogensen CE, Svendsen PA, Heding L. The effect of short-term glucagon infusion on kidney function in normal man. *Diabetologia* 1977;13:323–325.
54. Wiseman MJ, Redmond S, House F, Keen H, Viberti GC. The glomerular hyperfiltration of diabetes is not associated with elevated plasma levels of glucagon and growth hormone. *Diabetologia* 1985;28:718–721.
55. Christiansen JS, Gammelgaard J, Orskov H, Andersen AR, Telmer S, Parving H-H. Kidney function and size in normal subjects before and during growth hormone administration for one week. *Eur J Clin Invest* 1981;11:487–490.
56. Parving H-H, Christiansen JS, Noer I, Tronier B, Mogensen CE. The effect of glucagon infusion on kidney function in short-term insulin-dependent juvenile diabetes. *Diabetologia* 1980;19:350–354.
57. Illstrup KM, Keane WF, Michels LD. Intravascular and extracellular volumes in the diabetic rat. *Life Sci* 1981;29:717–724.
58. Ortola FV, Ballermann BJ, Anderson S, Mendez RE, Brenner BM. Elevated plasma atrial natriuretic peptide in diabetic rats: a potential mediator of hyperfiltration. *J Clin Invest* 1987;80:670–674.
59. Heinemann L, Sawicki P, Rave K, Hohmann A, Berger M. Increased plasma concentrations of natriuretic peptide in Type I diabetic patients with different stages of diabetic nephropathy [Abstract]. *Proc 2nd World Congr Biol Active Atrial Peptides* 1987:196.
60. Chua BHL, Chua CC, Rose SL. Atrial natriuretic factor production in diabetes and in press-overload hypertrophied hearts [Abstract]. *Proc 2nd World Congr Biol Active Atrial Peptides* 1987:195.
61. Bank N, Lahorra MAG, Aynedjian HS, Wilkes BM. Sodium restriction corrects hyperfiltration of diabetes. *Am J Physiol* 1988;254:F668–F676.
62. Kreisberg JI, Patel PY. The effects of insulin, glucose and diabetes on prostaglandin production by rat kidney glomeruli and cultured glomerular mesangial cells. *Prostaglandins Leukotrienes Med* 1983;11:431–442.
63. Schambelan M, Blake S, Sraer J, Bens M, Nivez MP, Wahbe F. Increased prostaglandin production by glomeruli isolated from rats with streptozotocin-induced diabetes. *J Clin Invest* 1985;75:404–412.
64. Craven PA, Caines MA, DeRubertis FR. Sequential alterations in glomerular prostaglandin and thromboxane synthesis in diabetic rats: relationship to the hyperfiltration of early diabetes. *Metabolism* 1987;36:95–103.
65. Hommel E, Mathiesen E, Arnold-Larsen S, Edsberg B, Olsen UB, Parving H-H. Effects of indomethacin on kidney function in Type I (insulin-dependent) diabetic patients with nephropathy. *Diabetologia* 1987;30:78–81.
66. Stirati G, Gambardella S, Pietravalle P, et al. Effect of piroxicam, an inhibitor of cyclooxygenase activity, on the glomerular hyperfiltration of type I newly diagnosed diabetic patients [Abstract]. *Kidney Int* 1986;29:611A.
67. Esmatjes E, Fernandez MR, Halperin I, et al. Renal hemodynamic abnormalities in patients with short term insulin-dependent diabetes mellitus: role of renal prostaglandins. *J Clin Endocrinol Metab* 1985;60:1231–1236.
68. Christiansen JS, Rasmussen BF, Parving H-H. Short-term inhibition of prostaglandin synthesis has no effect on the elevated glomerular filtration rate of early insulin-dependent diabetes. *Diabet Med* 1985;2:17–20.
69. Moel DI, Safirstein RL, McEvoy RC, Hsueh W. Effect of aspirin on experimental diabetic nephropathy. *J Lab Clin Med* 1987;110:300–307.
70. Jensen PK, Steven K, Blaehr H, Christiansen JS, Parving H-H. Effects of indomethacin on glomerular hemodynamics in experimental diabetes. *Kidney Int* 1986;29:490–495.
71. Kasiske BL, O'Donnell MP, Keane WF. Glucose induced increases in renal hemodynamic function. Possible modulation by renal prostaglandins. *Diabetes* 1985;34:360–364.
72. Bank N, Lahorra MAG, Aynedjian HS, Schlondorff D. Vasoregulatory hormones and the hyperfiltration of diabetes. *Am J Physiol* 1988;254:F202–F209.
73. Barnett R, Scharschmidt L, Ko Y-H, Schlondorff D. Comparison of glomerular and mesangial prostaglandin synthesis and glomerular contraction in two rat models of diabetes mellitus. *Diabetes* 1987;36:1468–1475.
74. Donadio JV, Ilstrup DM, Holley KE, Romero JC. Platelet-inhibitor treatment of diabetic nephropathy: a 10-year prospective study. *Mayo Clin Proc* 1988;63:3–15.
75. Kador PF, Kinoshita JH. Role of aldose reductase in the development of diabetes-associated complications. *Am J Med* 1985;79(Suppl 5A):8–12.
76. Kern EO, Simmonds D, Goldfarb S. Dietary inositol supplement lowers glomerular hyperfiltration and normalizes glomerular response to captopril in acute experimental diabetes [Abstract]. *Kidney Int* 1987;31:387A.
77. Goldfarb S, Kern E, Simmons D. Differential effects of supplementary dietary inositol on glomerular hyperfiltration due to early diabetes and high protein diet [Abstract]. *Clin Res* 1987;35:623A.
78. Cohen MP, Dasmahapatra A, Shapiro E. Reduced glomerular sodium/potassium adenosine triphosphatase activity in acute streptozotocin diabetes and its prevention by oral sorbinil. *Diabetes* 1985;34:1071–1074.
79. Beyer-Mears A, Cruz E, Edelist T, Varagiannis E. Diminished proteinuria in diabetes mellitus by sorbinil, an aldose reductase inhibitor. *Pharmacology* 1986;32:52–60.
80. Daniels BS, Hostetter TH. Aldose reductase inhibitor does not ameliorate glomerular damage in diabetic rats [Abstract]. *Clin Res* 1988;36:594A.
81. Ballermann BJ, Skorecki KL, Brenner BM. Reduced glomerular angiotensin II receptor density in early untreated diabetes mellitus in the rat. *Am J Physiol* 1984;247:F110–F116.
82. Christlieb AR. Renin, angiotensin and norepinephrine in alloxan diabetes. *Diabetes* 1974;23:962–970.
83. Woods LL, Mizelle HL, Hall JE. Control of renal hemodynamics in hyperglycemia: possible role of tubuloglomerular feedback. *Am J Physiol* 1987;252:F65–F73.
84. Hough S, Russell JE, Teitelbaum SL, Avioli LV. Calcium homeostasis in chronic streptozotocin-induced diabetes mellitus in the rat. *Am J Physiol* 1982;242:E451–E456.
85. Ditzel J, Standl E. The problem of tissue oxygenation in diabetes mellitus. II. Evidence of disordered oxygen release from the erythrocytes of diabetics in various conditions of metabolic control. *Acta Med Scand [Suppl]* 1975;578:59–68.
86. McMillan DE. The effect of diabetes on blood flow properties. *Diabetes* 1983;32(Suppl 2):56–63.
87. Harvey JN, Jaffa AA, Margolius HS, Mayfield RK. Relation of renal kallikrein to the glomerular hyperfiltration of experimental diabetes [Abstract]. *Diabetes* 1987;36:85A.
88. Jaffa AA, Miller DH, Bailey GS, Chao J, Margolius HS, Mayfield RK. Abnormal regulation of renal kallikrein in experimental diabetes. Effects of insulin on prokallikrein synthesis and activation. *J Clin Invest* 1987;80:1651–1659.
89. Ritz E, Hasslacher C, Tschope W, Koch M, Mann JFE. Hypertension in diabetes mellitus. *Contrib Nephrol* 1987;54:77–85.
90. Hasslacher C, Ritz E, Terpstra J, Gallasch G, Kunowski G, Rall C. Natural history of nephropathy in Type I diabetes. Relationship to metabolic control and blood pressure. *Hypertension* 1985;7(Suppl II):II-74–II-78.
91. Knowler WC, Bennett PH, Ballantin EJ. Increased incidence of retinopathy in diabetics with high blood pressure. *N Engl J Med* 1980;302:645–650.
92. Mogensen CE. Long-term antihypertensive treatment inhibiting progression of diabetic nephropathy. *Br Med J* 1982;285:685–688.
93. Parving H-H, Andersen AR, Smidt UM, Hommel E, Mathiesen ER, Svendsen PA. Effect of antihypertensive treatment on kid-

Impaired renal function could also be an obvious contributor to sodium retention and hypervolemia in diabetes, as suggested by the findings that the highest levels of exchangeable sodium are found in diabetic patients with severe proteinuria and significant reductions in creatinine clearance (8,42). The suppression of PRA and aldosterone in patients with diabetic nephropathy is consistent with the expected response of these hormones to volume expansion (8), as is the fact that reductions in volume with diuretic therapy can restore the levels of PRA and aldosterone towards normal (3,43).

Thus, hypervolemia in diabetes may have important sequelae. Hypervolemia per se may lead to increased arterial pressure, particularly in susceptible individuals. The observed strong correlation between total exchangeable body sodium and mean arterial pressure in diabetic subjects (8), as well as the normalization of volume status and blood pressure in response to diuretics (3), would support this volume–pressure relationship.

Another consequence of hypervolemia in diabetes could be augmented secretion of atrial natriuretic peptide (ANP). Increased circulating ANP levels have been observed in animals with experimental diabetes (44). Since ANP is known to directly increase glomerular filtration rate, the high circulating ANP levels may promote the glomerular hyperfiltration found in diabetes mellitus (45,46). Hyperfiltration may, in turn, contribute to increased intraglomerular pressure, thus accelerating glomerulosclerosis and diabetic nephropathy (44,47). Since overt diabetic nephropathy is, in turn, almost invariably accompanied by elevated arterial pressure, this mechanism might offer further insight into the interrelationships among hypervolemia, hypertension, and nephropathy in the diabetic patient.

RENIN–ANGIOTENSIN SYSTEM AND DIABETIC HYPERTENSION

Levels of PRA have been found to be low, normal, and high in patients with diabetes mellitus. Low PRA levels have been reported in diabetic patients with established autonomic neuropathy (48,49), thus suggesting that the neural control of renin release mediated predominantly by beta-adrenergic activation (50,51) is altered in this disorder. The presence of microvascular complications also appears to be a determinant of renin release, since patients with both diabetic nephropathy and retinopathy display reduced PRA levels (52–54). However, this issue is not settled, since Drury et al. have actually reported high levels of PRA in IDDM patients with proliferative retinopathy (16,17). Most observations show that diabetic patients without evidence of microvascular disease or with only mild nephropathy have normal PRA levels (2,16,22,55). However, in a study where PRA was evaluated in NIDDM patients who were without microvascular complications and who were under controlled high and low sodium intake, there was a trend for lower PRA levels in normotensive diabetics (compared to controls) and even lower levels in hypertensive diabetics (Fig. 1). These findings suggest that the presence of both diabetes and hypertension can alter the activity of the renin–angiotensin system.

The majority of circulating renin is in the form of a high-molecular-weight, inactive molecule that can be activated to the active form of renin by certain *in vitro* physicochemical processes. This inactive renin may be identical to prorenin, which is the biosynthetic precursor of renin. Levels of inactive renin are elevated in some patients with diabetes. The presence of microvascular disease in diabetes is associated with increases in circulating levels of inactive renin (56,57). In fact, Luetcher et al. (56) have proposed that the finding of elevated inactive renin levels in diabetic subjects may be an indicator for the presence of microvascular complications. However, one recent study could not identify increased inactive renin in diabetic subjects with renal and retinal microangiopathy but could identify it only in diabetics with coexisting neuropathy (58). Since inactive renin may be the precursor for active renin, increased inactive renin levels may reflect a suboptimal activation of renin as another potential explanation for the reduced PRA levels described in diabetic subjects (59).

Several other factors could influence the activity of the

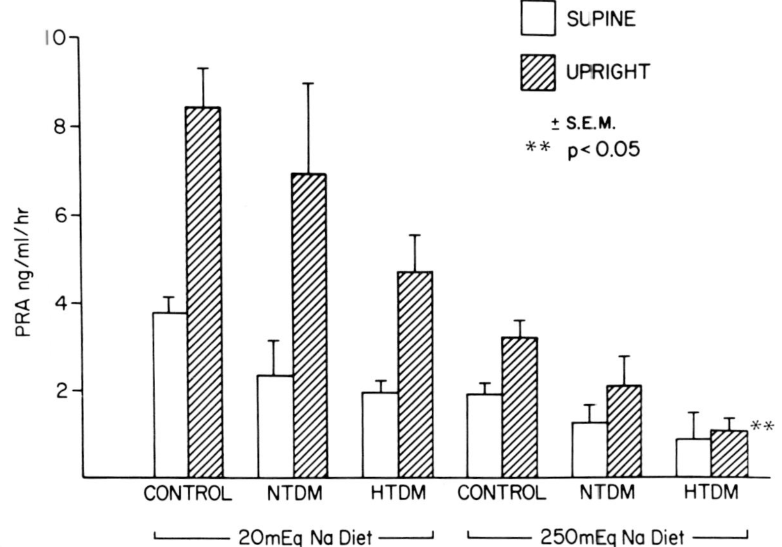

FIG. 1. Mean levels of supine and upright plasma renin activity in controls, normotensive diabetic patients (NTDM), and hypertensive diabetic patients (HTDM) studied in balance on a low-sodium (20 mEq/day) and high-sodium (250 mEq/day) diet. Diabetic patients had Type II diabetes mellitus without evidence of microvascular complications.

renin–angiotensin system in diabetes mellitus. PRA declines with age, and this process appears to be accelerated in the presence of arterial hypertension (60,61). Age and hypertension have not always been controlled for in studies of the renin–angiotensin system in diabetes. Dietary intake of sodium is another determinant of renin secretion, but most studies of renin in diabetics were not carried out under dietary sodium balance. Thus, the level of activity of the renin–angiotensin system in diabetes mellitus may reflect multiple factors such as hypervolemia, diabetic neuropathy, microvascular complications of nephropathy and retinopathy, renin activation capacity, patient age, presence of hypertension, and dietary intake of salt. Regardless of the level of renin in diabetes mellitus, most investigators would agree that the renin–angiotensin system is not a major factor contributing to the hypertension of diabetes mellitus.

INSULIN AND DIABETIC HYPERTENSION

Epidemiologic studies have demonstrated several common metabolic and hemodynamic factors that overlap between the essential hypertensive population and patient populations with glucose intolerance (62). Hypertension is associated with hyperinsulinemia in both obese diabetic and obese nondiabetic subjects as well as in patients with essential hypertension where hyperinsulinemia occurs independent of obesity or glucose intolerance. Hyperinsulinemia reflects resistance to insulin's action and is a complex process representing a compensatory response to diminished target tissue sensitivity to insulin's effects, predominantly on glucose handling. The high circulating insulin levels may further perpetuate insulin resistance by downregulation of insulin receptor number (63). In some obese and NIDDM subjects, even supermaximal doses of insulin fail to enhance receptor-mediated peripheral glucose utilization, suggesting the existence of insulin resistance at the postreceptor level (64,65). Hyperglycemia may also contribute to a post-receptor resistance, since intensive insulin treatment in NIDDM ameliorates this defect following attainment of euglycemia (66,67).

There are multiple biologic effects of insulin, so that peripheral resistance to this hormone can be different in various tissues. Several types of insulin-resistant states have been described with distinctly different resistance profiles. If insulin excess is to be linked to hypertension, one must identify potential insulin effects (such as retention of sodium or stimulation of the sympathetic nervous system) that could lead to elevated blood pressure. Several potential areas of how insulin might lead to hypertension will be considered. These areas include identification of patterns of insulin resistance in the hypertensive population, effects of insulin on amino acid transport and on the sympathetic nervous system, and potential direct effects of insulin on the vascular bed and on sodium transport.

Patterns of Insulin Resistance

The biologic actions of insulin include effects on carbohydrate, lipid, protein, and potassium metabolism. Insulin increases peripheral uptake and utilization of glucose, particularly in the liver and skeletal muscle, and suppresses hepatic gluconeogenesis. The lipogenic and antilipolytic properties of insulin lead to a reduction in plasma free fatty acids. Insulin also facilitates skeletal muscle uptake of branched-chain amino acids, many of which are of the large neutral amino acid (LNAA) group (68). Finally, insulin promotes tissue uptake of potassium.

Ferrannini et al. (31) have recently reported on the patterns of insulin resistance in three hypertensive study groups: nonobese essential hypertensive subjects, patients with Type II diabetes, and obese nondiabetic subjects (Table 2). All three conditions are characterized by diminished insulin-mediated effects on glucose utilization and on the nonoxidative glucose disposal pathway. However, obese individuals and patients with NIDDM also show reduced glucose oxidation. In addition, obesity is associated with a reduced effect of insulin to normally attenuate hepatic glucose output and to alter tissue uptake of potassium. In both NIDDM and essential hypertension there is a diminished effect of insulin to inhibit lipolysis associated with exaggerated increases in plasma free fatty acids in the postabsorptive state (29). The variable patterns of insulin action in these three conditions may translate into relatively different roles for insulin in the etiology of hypertension in these disorders.

Insulin and Plasma Amino Acids

The effect of insulin on amino acid handling may have a potential link to blood pressure control through central nervous system effects on the regulation of neurogenic activity. Obese individuals display reduced insulin dependent uptake of LNAAs (69). The availability of tryptophan to the brain depends on the plasma concentration of this

TABLE 2. *Characteristics of insulin resistance in obesity, non-insulin-dependent diabetes mellitus (NIDDM), and essential hypertension*[a]

	Obesity	NIDDM	Hypertension
Whole-body glucose uptake	↓	↓	↓
Suppression of glucose output	↓	±	±
Glucose oxidation	↓	↓	±
Lipid oxidation	↑	±	±
Nonoxidative glucose disposal	↓	↓	↓
Suppression of lipolysis	±	↓	±
Promotion of potassium uptake	↓	±	±

[a] From ref. 31. ↓, reduced; ↑, increased; ±, more or less unchanged.

amino acid relative to the concentration of other LNAAs, and the ratio tryptophan/LNAA is important in this process (70). With diminished insulin-induced uptake of LNAAs in obesity, the availability of tryptophan to the brain is also decreased (69–71). Since tryptophan is the main precursor for the biosynthesis of serotonin, individuals with diminished LNAA uptake may have reduced central release of serotonin following the insulin rise after a carbohydrate-rich meal. Serotonin generation in the brain acts as a central feedback mechanism that suppresses appetite, especially carbohydrate intake (71). Serotonin agonists selectively suppress carbohydrate intake (72), and tryptophan administration reduces overall nutrient intake in humans (73,74). Since carbohydrate ingestion leads to stimulation of sympathetic activity (75,76) and elevation of arterial pressure (77,78), defective feedback inhibition of carbohydrate intake based on abnormal amino acid handling in insulin-resistant obese individuals may contribute to the development of hypertension. This defect has been demonstrated in some obese individuals (69,71) and may well be applicable to obese NIDDM patients.

Insulin and Sympathetic Nervous System Activity

Nutrient intake has been shown to modulate sympathetic nervous system activity. Restricted caloric intake leads to a reduction in plasma catecholamines in humans (79–81) and to diminished tissue norepinephrine turnover in the rat (82,83). Conversely, sucrose overfeeding enhances norepinephrine turnover in rat cardiac, pancreatic, and hepatic tissues (75,83). Landsberg and Young (84) have formulated the concept that glucose and/or insulin may be the signals that couple alterations in diet to changes in sympathetic outflow. Insulin infusion leads to increased release of catecholamines. Studies in humans using insulin and glucose clamp techniques which allow the attainment of steady-state hyperinsulinemia with normal glucose levels (euglycemic clamp) show that insulin can increase plasma norepinephrine levels (85). These changes occur independent of alterations in norepinephrine metabolic clearance rate, thus indicating that insulin directly enhances sympathetic outflow (85). Experimental data have localized the insulin-generated signal to activate sympathetic outflow to the ventromedial area of the hypothalamus, a center which regulates food intake (86,87). Thioglucose treatment destroys this brain center and allows the development of uncontrolled feeding and, eventually, marked obesity. In this model, alterations in carbohydrate intake with the ensuing insulin responses have no effect on sympathetic activity (87). In laboratory animals, acute and chronic sucrose feeding is accompanied by sympathetic hyperactivity, tachycardia, and a mild to moderate increase in arterial blood pressure (77,78,88,89). At the same time, insulin resistance (as indicated by hyperinsulinemia and hypertriglyceridemia) also evolves (78,90).

Obese individuals may have increased sympathetic nervous system activity, especially as demonstrated in the close relationship between reductions in plasma catecholamine levels and blood pressure during weight loss (80,81,91,92). In contrast, most studies evaluating sympathetic nervous system activity in diabetic patients have found normal levels of plasma catecholamines (3,4,8). However, many of the studies in diabetic patients did not control for age, body weight, type of diabetes, or level of blood pressure. Thus, the issue of sympathetic hyperactivity in association with insulin resistance, obesity, and diabetes cannot be resolved until it is addressed in reference to more adequate control groups.

Insulin and the Vascular Bed

Hyperinsulinemia appears to be a potential factor in the enhanced atherosclerosis observed in diabetes mellitus, and hyperglycemia itself may also alter vascular wall function. These effects on the vasculature could contribute to hypertension, since structural and functional abnormalities in the arterial bed are well-established factors contributing to the development of hypertension (93).

A basic model for the initiating event in the evolution of the atherosclerotic plaque has been proposed by Ross and Glomset (94). In brief, a variety of offensive processes such as hypertension, hyperglycemia, hyperlipidemia, or immune reactions may cause endothelial cell injury (94,95). Exposure of subendothelial collagen due to disruption of the normal endothelial lining may precipitate platelet aggregation, which, in turn, results in the release of platelet-derived vasoconstrictor and vasodilatory prostaglandins as well as growth factors. Released growth factors can enhance macrophage migration as well as smooth muscle and fibroblast proliferation, effects which are further abetted by circulating insulin. Local deposition of lipids is facilitated by (a) distortion of the normal vascular surface, (b) the lipotrophic effect of insulin, and (c) hyperlipidemia. This process of vascular damage is further accentuated by hyperglycemia, hyperinsulinemia, and perhaps other determinants prevailing in diabetes (96,97). The production of prostacyclin, a platelet-derived vasodilator which is also a potent antiaggregant, is diminished in human and experimental diabetes (98–100). On the other hand, the synthesis of thromboxane, which promotes aggregation and vasoconstriction, is increased (101–103). Correction of hyperglycemia may normalize the imbalance between prostacyclin and thromboxane (104,105). The biosynthesis of von Willebrand factor (a component of factor VIII) by endothelial cells is enhanced in Type II diabetics with macroangiopathy (106). Plasminogen activator, the platelet-derived enzyme which promotes thrombolysis via the generation of plasmin, may be depressed in diabetes (107), whereas plasmin inhibitors may be increased (108). Collectively, these multiple abnormalities could promote local hypercoagulability and platelet aggregation (97,100), thus leading to increased release of endothelial-derived growth factors (109) which could facilitate cell growth and replication and ultimately result in arterial wall thickening (110). Of particular interest is the diabetic serum growth factor (DSGF), a potent platelet-derived promoter of smooth muscle cell proliferation and migration (111) which is enhanced during poor diabetic control, with levels normalizing with improved glucose concentration (112). Insulin itself can enhance proliferation of cultured smooth muscle cells (113,114), so that hyperinsulinemia could contribute to subendothelial vascular smooth muscle cell replication. In addition, supernatant obtained from platelets of insulin-treated patients was 83% more active in promoting growth of rat vascular smooth muscle cells than was the platelet-derived supernatant from normal subjects (115). Finally, vascular wall lipid deposition is enhanced, especially in poorly controlled diabetics, because of elevations in low-density lipoprotein (LDL) cholesterol (95,116) and reductions in high-density lipoprotein (HDL) cholesterol (117,118); this enhancement is secondary to increases in apoproteins B and E (119). Systemic hyperinsulinemia may further accelerate fat deposition into the vasculature via the lipogenic effect of insulin (120).

Epidemiologic and clinical studies reinforce the relationship between insulin and vascular disease. Atherosclerotic conditions such as macrovascular disease (121), coronary artery disease (122–124), cerebrovascular disease (125), and hypertension (62) all show strong, independent correlations with hyperinsulinemia. Thus, enhancement of atherogenesis by insulin in the resistance vessels in patients with diabetes may well contribute to the pathogenesis of hypertension in this disease.

Insulin and Sodium Homeostasis

Clinical and experimental studies show that insulin can alter sodium transport and can promote renal sodium reabsorption. Insulin administration to normal subjects leads to a reduction in sodium excretion (126), and the natriuresis associated with fasting has been attributed to acute lowering of circulating insulin levels (127–129). Conversely, carbohydrate refeeding following protracted fasting results in significant sodium retention secondary to concomitant rises in plasma insulin (127,128,130). In a series of studies, DeFronzo et al. (24,25) and Nizet et al. (131) have provided evidence that insulin directly enhances sodium retention independent of changes in (a) the filtered load of glucose, (b) glomerular filtration rate, (c) renal blood flow, or (d) circulating aldosterone levels. This effect of insulin takes place at the renal level, as suggested by observations with direct insulin infusion to the renal artery *in situ* (25) or to the isolated perfused kidney (131). Studies with micropipettes in the dog proximal tubule suggest that the site where insulin enhances sodium reabsorption is the more distal part of the nephron (25). Studies in cells derived from aldosterone-sensitive segments of the nephron [i.e., the distal tubule (39)] and from other aldosterone-responsive cells (amphibian skin and bladder) (40,132,133) show that insulin stimulates active sodium transport as determined by short-circuit current or cation transport methods. The finding that these effects of insulin display spatial preference to the basolateral aspects of epithelial cells (39) suggests both specificity and physiologic relevance to net transepithelial cation uptake.

Insulin could also indirectly alter sodium reabsorption by effects on the renin–angiotensin–aldosterone system (134–137). Recently, Petrasek et al. (134) have demonstrated that insulin directly stimulates the secretion of aldosterone in rat glomerulosa cells *in vitro*. Insulin could also act via the potassium ion to change aldosterone secretion. Aldosterone secretion *in vivo* is tightly controlled by plasma potassium, so that even small insulin-induced changes in extracellular potassium could affect the release of aldosterone (135). Thus, insulin may enhance sodium retention by a direct effect on the distal nephron as well as by indirect mechanisms involving various components of the renin–angiotensin–aldosterone system.

METABOLIC CONTROL AND DIABETIC HYPERTENSION

There is some evidence that changes in blood glucose and metabolic control in diabetes mellitus may influence the level of blood pressure. Epidemiologic surveys involving both diabetic and nondiabetic subjects show a positive correlation between blood pressure and plasma glucose (138–140). Both systolic and diastolic arterial pressures are positively related to plasma glucose response to oral glucose load; this relationship occurs independent of age, body weight, and heart rate. The correlation between glucose and blood pressure may be related to coexisting hyperinsulinemia (62), suggesting a further relationship between metabolic control and blood pressure in diabetes mellitus. O'Hare et al. (5,141) have observed small but significant reductions in systolic and diastolic blood pressures following improvement in metabolic control in diabetic patients. Surprisingly, the reductions in blood pressure with better metabolic control were accompanied by actual increases in plasma volume and exchangeable sodium but were also accompanied by reductions in PRA, angiotensin II, and aldosterone concentrations. Similar correlations between metabolic control and blood pressure were observed by Gunderson (142), who studied IDDM subjects during controlled insulin withdrawal. With the worsening of metabolic control, blood pressure increased. In this study, changes in blood pressure were correlated with increases in serum bicarbonate and fatty acid levels as well as with increasing glucose concentrations. In animal studies, insulin treatment ameliorates the increased arterial pressure in the streptozotocin-induced hypertensive diabetic rat (143). These observations offer some evidence that tight metabolic control in patients with diabetes mellitus may provide beneficial effects on blood pressure levels.

VASCULAR REACTIVITY AND DIABETIC HYPERTENSION

Several studies have demonstrated that the sensitivity to pressor hormones is enhanced in subjects with diabetes mellitus (Table 3). Despite differences in patient selection with regard to the type of diabetes (IDDM versus NIDDM), age, presence of complications, presence or absence of hypertension, and control of sodium intake, all the studies have found a consistent increase in vascular responses to both angiotensin II and norepinephrine. Vascular hyperreactivity could be secondary to hypervolemia and increased exchangeable sodium in diabetes mellitus (148), since normalization of vascular responses to angiotensin II and norepinephrine are noted following short-term treatment with diuretics (3). It is well established that vascular responsivity to angiotensin II is modulated by sodium homeostasis (149): High sodium levels enhance, whereas low

50. Campbell IW, Ewing DJ, Anderton JL, Thompson JH, Horin DB, Clark BF. Plasma renin activity in diabetic autonomic neuropathy. *Eur J Clin Invest* 1976;6:381–385.
51. Tuck ML, Sambhi MP, Levin L. Hyporeninemic hypoaldosteronism in diabetes mellitus: studies of the autonomic nervous system control of renin release. *Diabetes* 1979;28:237–241.
52. Christlieb AR. Nephropathy, the renin system and hypertensive vascular disease in diabetes mellitus. *Cardiovasc Med* 1978;2:417–431.
53. Perez GO, Lespier L, Jacobi J, et al. Hyporeninemia and hypoaldosteronism in diabetes mellitus. *Arch Intern Med* 1977;137:852–855.
54. Manchandia MR, Gossian VV, Michelakis AM, Rovner DR. Plasma cryoactivated renin and active renin in diabetes mellitus. *J Clin Endocrinol Metab* 1982;53:1025–1029.
55. Tomita K, Matsudu O, Ideura T, Shiigai T, Taeuchi J. Renin–angiotensin–aldosterone system in mild diabetic nephropathy. *Nephron* 1982;31:361–366.
56. Luetcher JA, Kraemer FB, Wilson DM, Schwartz HC, Bryer-Ash M. Increased plasma inactive renin in diabetes mellitus: a marker of microvascular complications. *N Engl J Med* 1985;312:1412–1417.
57. Hsueh WA, Carlson EZ, Luetscher JA, Grislis G. Activation and characterization of inactive big renin in plasma of patients with diabetic nephropathy and unusual active renin. *J Clin Endocrinol Metab* 1980;51:535–543.
58. Misbin R, Grant MB, Pecker MS, Atlas S. Elevated levels of plasma prorenin (inactive renin) in diabetic and nondiabetic patients with autonomic dysfunction. *J Clin Endocrinol Metab* 1987;64:964–968.
59. Bryer-Ash M, Froze EB, Luetscher JA. Plasma renin and prorenin (inactive renin) in diabetes mellitus: effects of intravenous furosemide. *J Clin Endocrinol Metab* 1988;66:454–458.
60. Tuck ML, Williams GH, Cain JP, Sullivan JM, Dluhy RB. Relation of age, diastolic pressure and known duration of hypertension to presence of low renin hypertension. *Am J Cardiol* 1973;32:637–641.
61. Stern N, Sowers JR, McGinty D, Beahm E, Littner M, Catania R, Eggena P. Circadian rhythm of plasma renin activity in older men: relation with inactive renin, aldosterone, cortisol and REM sleep. *J Hypertens* 1986;4:550–553.
62. Modan M, Halkin H, Almog S, Lusky A, Eshkol A, Shefi M, Shitrit A, Fuchs Z. Hyperinsulinemia: a link between hypertension, obesity and glucose intolerance. *J Clin Invest* 1985;75:809.
63. Kobayashi M, Olefsky J. Effect of experimental hyperinsulinemia on insulin binding and glucose transport in isolated rat adipocytes. *Am J Physiol* 1978;234:E53–62.
64. Olefsky JM. Insulin resistance and insulin action in obesity and noninsulin-dependent (type II) diabetes mellitus. In: Brodoff BN, Bleicher SJ, eds. *Diabetes mellitus and obesity.* Baltimore: Williams & Wilkins, 1982;250–260.
65. Kolterman OG, Gray RS, Griffin J, Burstein P, Insel J, Scarlett JA, Olefsky JM. Receptor and postreceptor defects contribute to the insulin resistance in noninsulin-dependent diabetes mellitus. *J Clin Invest* 1981;68:957–969.
66. Scarlett JA, Gray RS, Griffin J, Olefsky JM, Kolterman OG. Insulin treatment reverses the insulin resistance of type II diabetes mellitus. *Diabetes Care* 1982;5:353–363.
67. Ginsberg H, Rayfield EJ. Effect of insulin therapy on insulin resistance in type II diabetic subjects. Evidence for heterogeneity. *Diabetes* 1981;30:739–745.
68. Fukagawa NK, Minaker KL, Young VR, Rowe JW. Insulin dose-dependent reductions in plasma amino acids in man. *Am J Physiol* 1986;250:E13–E17.
69. Felig P, Marliss E, Cahill GF. Plasma amino acid levels and insulin secretion in obesity. *N Engl J Med* 1969;281:811–816.
70. Pardridge WM. Regulation of amino acid availability to the brain. In: Wurtman RJ, Wurtman JJ, eds. *Nutrition and the brain.* New York: Raven Press, 1977;141–204.
71. Caballero B. Insulin resistance and amino acid metabolism in obesity. *Ann NY Acad Sci* 1987;499:84–93.
72. Wurtman JJ, Wurtman RJ, Growdon JH, Henry P, Lipscomb S, Zeisel H. Carbohydrate craving in obese people: suppression by treatments affecting serotoninergic neurotransmission. *Int J Eating Disord* 1981;1:2–15.
73. Hrboticky N, Leiter LA, Anderson GH. Effects of *l*-tryptophan on short term food intake in lean men. *Nutr Res* 1985;5:595–607.
74. Blundell JE, Mavjee V, Williams CJ, Hill AY. Interactive effects of tryptophan and macronutrients on hunger motivation and dietary preferences. *J Cell Metab* [*Suppl*] 1986;6:461–472.
75. Young JB, Landsberg L. Stimulation of the sympathetic nervous system during sucrose feeding. *Nature* 1977;269:615–617.
76. Welle S, Lilavivanthana U, Campbell RG. Increased plasma norepinephrine concentrations and metabolic rates following glucose ingestion in man. *Metabolism* 1980;29:806–809.
77. Young JB, Landsberg L. Effect of oral glucose on blood pressure in the spontaneously hypertensive rat. *Metabolism* 1981; 30:421–424.
78. Hwang SI, Ho H, Hoffman B, Reaven GM. Fructose induced insulin resistance and hypertension in rats. *Hypertension* 1987;10:512–516.
79. Jung RT, Shetty PS, Barrand M, Callingham BA, James WPT. Role of catecholamines in hypotensive responses to dieting. *Br Med J* 1979;1:12–13.
80. DeHaven J, Sherwin R, Hendler R, Felig P. Nitrogen and sodium balance and sympathetic-nervous system activity in obese subjects treated with low-caloric protein or mixed diet. *N Engl J Med* 1980;302:477–482.
81. Sowers JR, Nyby M, Stern N, Beck FWJ, Baron S, Catania R, Vlachakis N. Blood pressure and hormone changes associated with weight reduction in the obese. *Hypertension* 1982;4:686–691.
82. Young JB, Landsberg L. Suppression of sympathetic nervous system during fasting. *Science* 1977;196:1465–1473.
83. Young JB, Landsberg L. Effect of diet and cold exposure on norepinephrine turnover in pancreas and liver. *Am J Physiol* 1979;236:E524–533.
84. Landsberg L, Young JB. Caloric intake and sympathoadrenal activity: implications for thermogenesis, obesity and hypertension. In: Ziegler MG, Lake CR, eds. *Norepinephrine.* Baltimore: Williams & Wilkins, 1983;217–226.
85. Rowe JW, Young JB, Minaker KL, Stevens AL, Pallota J, Landsberg L. Effect of insulin and glucose infusions on sympathetic nervous system activity in normal man. *Diabetes* 1981;30:219–225.
86. Debons AF, Krimsky I, From A, Cloutier RJ. Rapid effects of insulin on the hypothalamic satiety center. *Am J Physiol* 1969; 217:1114–1118.
87. Young JB, Landsberg L. Impaired suppression of sympathetic activity during fasting in the gold thioglucose-treated mouse. *J Clin Invest* 1980;65:1086–1094.
88. Fournier RD, Chineh CC, Kopin IJ, Knapka JJ, Dipette D, Preuss HG. Refined carbohydrate increases blood pressure and catecholamine excretion in SHR and WKY. *Am J Physiol* 1986;250:E381–385.
89. Bunag RD, Tomita T, Sasaki S. Chronic sucrose ingestion induces mild hypertension and tachycardia in rats. *Hypertension* 1983;5:218–225.
90. Reaven GM, Risser TR, Chen Y-DIK, Reaven EP. Characterization of a model of dietary induced hypertriglyceridemia in young, nonobese rats. *J Lipid Res* 1979;20:371–378.
91. James WP, Haraldsdottir J, Liddel F, Jung TR, Shefty PS. Autonomic responsiveness in obesity with and without hypertension. *Int J Obes* 1981;5:73–78.
92. Sowers JR, Whitfield LA, Catania RA, Stern N, Tuck ML, Dornfeld L, Maxwell M. Role of the sympathetic nervous system in blood pressure maintenance in obesity. *J Clin Endocrinol Metab* 1982;54:1181–1186.
93. Folkow B. Cardiovascular structural adaptation: its role in the initiation and maintenance of primary hypertension. The fourth Volhard lecture. *Clin Sci Mol Med* 1978;55(Suppl):3s–22s.
94. Ross R, Glomset JA. The pathogenesis of atherosclerosis. *N Engl J Med* 1976;295:369–377, 420–425.
95. Ruderman NA, Haudenschild C. Diabetes as an atherogenic factor. *Prog Cardiovasc Dis* 1984;26:373–412.
96. Colwell JA, Halushka PV, Sarji KE, et al. Diabetic vascular dis-

ease. Pathophysiological mechanisms and therapy. *Arch Intern Med* 1979;139:225–230.

97. Stolar MW. Atherosclerosis in diabetes: the role of hyperinsulinemia. *Metabolism* 1988;37(Suppl 1):1–9.
98. Schernthaner G, Sinizinger H, Silberbauer K, et al. Vascular prostacyclin and platelet-specific proteins in diabetes mellitus. *Horm Metab Res* 1981;13(Suppl 11):33–43.
99. Harrison HE, Reece AH, Johnson M. Decreased vascular prostacyclin in experimental diabetes. *Life Sci* 1978;23:351–355.
100. Halushka PV, Mayfield R, Colwell JA. Insulin and arachidonic acid metabolism in diabetes mellitus. *Metabolism* 1985;34(Suppl 1):32–36.
101. Halushka PV, Roger RC, Loadholt CB, et al. Increase platelet thromboxane synthesis in diabetes mellitus. *J Lab Clin Med* 1981;97:87–96.
102. Roth DM, Reibel DK, Lefer AM. Vascular responsiveness and eicosanoid production in diabetic rats. *Diabetologia* 1983;24:372–376.
103. Colwell JA, Winocour PD, Halushka PV. Do platelets have anything to do with diabetic microvascular disease? *Diabetes* 1983;32(Suppl 2):14–19.
104. Gerrard JM, Stuart MJ, Rao GHR, et al. Alteration in the balance of prostaglandin and thromboxane synthesis in diabetic rats. *J Lab Clin Med* 1980;95:950–958.
105. Valentovic M, Lubawy W. Impact of insulin or tolbutamide on ^{14}C-arachidonic acid conversion to prostacyclin and/or thromboxane in lungs, aortas and platelets of streptozotozin induced diabetic rats. *Diabetes* 1983;32:846–851.
106. Rak K, Beck P, Udvardy M, et al. Plasma levels of betathromboglobulin and factor VIII-related antigen in diabetic children and adults. *Thromb Res* 1983;29:155–162.
107. Almer LO, Pandolfi M, Nilson IM. Diabetic retinopathy and the fibrinolytic system. *Diabetes* 1975;24:529–534.
108. Almer LO. Vascular fibrinolytic activity in long term treatment with second generation sulfonylurea compounds *Acta Endocrinol* 1980;239(Suppl):53–55.
109. Koschinsky T, Buntin CE, Rutter R, et al. Vascular growth factors and the development of macrovascular disease in diabetes mellitus. *Horm Metab Res* 1985;17(Suppl):23–27.
110. King GL. Cell biology as an approach to the study of the vascular complications of diabetes. *Metabolism* 1985;34(Suppl 1):17–24.
111. Koschinsky T, Bunting CE, Schuippert B, et al. Increased growth stimulation of fibroblasts from diabetics by diabetic serum factors of low molecular weight. *Atherosclerosis* 1980;37:311–317.
112. Koschinsky T, Bunting CE, Schuippert B, et al. Regulation of diabetic serum growth factors for human vascular cells by the metabolic control of diabetes mellitus. *Atherosclerosis* 1981;39:313–319.
113. King GL, Goodman AD, Buzngy S, et al. Receptors and growth promoting effects of insulin and insulin-like growth factors on cells from bovine retinal capillaries and aorta. *J Clin Invest* 1985;75:1028–1036.
114. Pfeile B, Dischaneit H. Effects of insulin on growth of cultured human arterial smooth muscle cells. *Diabetologia* 1981;20:155–158.
115. Hamet P, Sugimoto H, Umeda, Lecavalier L, Franks DJ, Orth DN, Chiasson K. Abnormalities of platelet-derived growth factors in insulin-dependent diabetes. *Metabolism* 1985;34(Suppl 1):25–31.
116. Goldberg RB. Lipid disorders in diabets. *Diabetes Care* 1981;4:561–577.
117. Sosenko JM, Breslow JL, Miettinen OS, et al. Hyperglycemia and plasma lipid levels: a prospective study of young insulin-dependent diabetic patients. *N Engl J Med* 1980;302:650–654.
118. Nikkila EA. High density lipoproteins in diabetes. *Diabetes* 1981;30(Suppl 2):82–87.
119. Fielding CJ, Reaven GM, Fielding PE. Human noninsulin dependent diabetes: identification of a defect in plasma cholesterol transport normalized *in vivo* by insulin and *in vitro* by selective immunoadsorption of apolipoprotein E. *Proc Natl Acad Sci USA* 1982;79:6365–6369.
120. Stout RW. The effect of insulin and glucose on sterol synthesis in cultured rat arterial smooth muscle cells. *Atherosclerosis* 1977;27:271–278.
121. Sloan JM, Mackay JS, Sheridian B. The incidence of plasma insulin, blood sugar and serum lipid abnormalities in patients with atherosclerotic disease. *Diabetologia* 1971;7:431–433.
122. Pyorala K. Relationship of glucose tolerance and plasma insulin to the incidence of coronary artery disease: results from two population studies in Finland. *Diabetes Care* 1979;2:131–141.
123. Welborn TA, Wearne K. Coronary heart disease incidence and cardiovascular mortality in Busselton with reference to glucose and insulin concentrations. *Diabetes Care* 1979;2:154–160.
124. Ducimetiere P, Eschwege E, Papoz L, et al. Relationship of plasma insulin levels to the incidence of myocardial infarction and coronary heart disease mortality in a middle-aged population. *Diabetologia* 1980;19:205–210.
125. Gerther MM, Leetma HE, Saluste E, et al. Covert diabetes mellitus in ischemic heart and cerebrovascular disease. *Geriatrics* 1972;2:105–120.
126. Miller JH, Bogdonoff MD. Antidiuresis associated with administration of insulin. *J Appl Physiol* 1954;6:509–512.
127. DeFronzo RA. Insulin and renal sodium handling: clinical implications. *Int J Obes* 1981;5(Suppl 1):93–104.
128. Kolanowski J. Influence of insulin and glucagon on sodium balance in obese subjects during fasting and refeeding. *Int J Obes* 1981;5(Suppl 1):105–114.
129. Weinsier RL. Fasting—a review with emphasis on the electrolytes. *Am J Med* 1970;50:233–240.
130. Kolanowski J, DeGasparo M, Desmecht P, Grabbi J. Further evolution of the role of insulin in sodium retention associated with carbohydrate administration after a fast in the obese. *Eur J Clin Invest* 1972;2:439–444.
131. Nizet A, Lefebre P, Crabbe J. Control by insulin of sodium, potassium and water excretion by the isolated dog kidney. *Pflugers Arch* 1971;323:11–20.
132. Anders R, Crabbe J. Stimulation by insulin of active sodium transport by toad skin: influence of aldosterone and vasopressin. *Arch Int Physiol Biochem* 1966;74:538–540.
133. Herrera FC. Effect of insulin on short circuit current and sodium transport across toad urinary bladder. *Am J Physiol* 1965; 209:819–824.
134. Petrasek D, Tuck ML, Jensen G, Stern N. Direct and bimodal effect of insulin on aldosterone secretion in rat glomerulosa cells. *Clin Res* 1988;36:126A.
135. Himathongkam T, Dluhy RG, Williams GH. Potassium–aldosterone–renin interrelationships. *J Clin Endocrinol Metab* 1975;41:153–159.
136. Vierhapper H. Effect of exogenous insulin on blood pressure regulation in healthy and diabetic subjects. *Hypertension* 1985;7(Suppl II):II49–II53.
137. Pratt JH, Parkinson CA, Weinberger MH, Duckworth WC. Decreases in renin and aldosterone secretion in alloxan diabetes: an effect of insulin deficiency. *Endocrinology* 1985;116:1712–1716.
138. Stamler J, Rhomberg P, Schoenberger JA, et al. Multivariate analysis of the relationship of seven variables to blood pressure. *J Chronic Dis* 1975;28:527–548.
139. Jarret RJ, Keen H, McCartney M, et al. Glucose tolerance and blood pressure in two populations: their relation to diabetes mellitus and hypertension. *Int J Epidemiol* 1978;7:15–24.
140. Florey CduV, Uppal S, Lowy C. Relation between blood pressure, weight and plasma sugar and serum insulin levels in school children aged 9–12 years in Westland, Holland. *Br Med J* 1976;1:1368–1371.
141. Ferris JB, O'Hare JA, Kelleher CCM, Sullivan PA, Cole MM, Ross HF, O'Sullivan DJ. Diabetic control and the renin angiotensin system, catecholamines and blood pressure. *Hypertension* 1985;7(Suppl II):II58–II63.
142. Gunderson HJG. Peripheral blood flow and metabolic control in juvenile diabetes. *Diabetologia* 1974;10:225–231.
143. Sasaki S, Bunag RD. Insulin reverses hypertension and hypothalamic depression in streptozotocin diabetic rats. *Hypertension* 1983;5:34–40.
144. Barnay FR. Abnormal vascular reaction in diabetes mellitus. *Acta Med Scand* 1955;304(Suppl):152–155.

145. Christlieb AR, Janka HU, Kraus B, et al. Vascular reactivity to angiotensin II and norepinephrine in diabetic subjects. *Diabetes* 1976;25:268–274.
146. Beretta-Piccoli C, Weidmann P. Exaggerated pressor responsiveness to norepinephrine in nonazotemic diabetes mellitus. *Am J Med* 1981;71:829–835.
147. Drury PL, Smith GM, Ferris JB. Increased vasopressor responsiveness to angiotensin II in type I (insulin dependent) diabetic patients without complications. *Diabetologia* 1983;27:174–179.
148. Weidman P, Beretta-Piccoli C, Trost BN. Pressor factors and responsiveness in hypertension accompanying diabetes mellitus. *Hypertension* 1985;7(Suppl II):II33–II42.
149. Hollenberg NK, Chenitz WR, Adams DF, Williams GH. Reciprocal influence of salt intake on adrenal glomerulosa and renal vascular responses to angiotensin II in normal man. *J Clin Invest* 1977;54:34–42.
150. Faris I, Agerskov K, Henrikenson O. Decreased distensibility of a passive vascular bed in diabetes mellitus: an indicator of microangiopathy. *Diabetologia* 1982;23:411–414.
151. Zatz R, Brenner BM. Pathogenesis of diabetic microangiopathy: the hemodynamic view. *Am J Med* 1986;80:443–453.
152. Hostetter TH, Rennke HG, Brenner BM. The case for intra-renal hypertension in the initiation and progression of diabetic and other glomerulopathies. *Am J Med* 1982;72:375–380.
153. Butterfield WJH, Wichelow MJ. Peripheral glucose metabolism in control subjects and diabetic patients during glucose, glucose–insulin and insulin sensitivity tests. *Diabetologia* 1965;1:42–53.
154. Christensen NJ. A reversible vascular abnormality associated with diabetic ketosis. *Clin Sci* 1970;39:539–548.
155. Chazan BI, Balodimos MC, Lavine RL, Koncz L. Capillaries of the nailbed of the toe in diabetes mellitus. *Microvasc Res* 1970;2:504–507.
156. Landau J, Davis E. The small blood vessels of the conjunctiva and nailbed in diabetes mellitus. *Lancet* 1960;2:731–734.
157. Gitelson S, Wertheimer-Kaplinski N. Color of the face in diabetes mellitus. *Diabetes* 1965;14:201–208.
158. Bohlen HG, Hankins KD. Early arteriolar and capillary changes in streptozotocin-induced diabetic rats and in intraperitoneal hyperglycemic rats. *Diabetologia* 1982;22:344–348.
159. McCuskey PA, McCuskey RS. *In vivo* and electron microscopic study of the development of cerebral diabetic microangiopathy. *Microcirc Endothel Lymphat* 1983;1:221–244.
160. Halushka PV, Lurie D, Colwell JA. Increased synthesis of prostaglandin-E-like material by platelets from patients with diabetes mellitus. *N Engl J Med* 1977;297:1306–1310.
161. Rosen P, Schror K. Increased prostacyclin release from perfused hearts of acutely diabetic rats. *Diabetologia* 1980;18:391–394.
162. Schamblan M, Blake S, Sraer J, et al. Increased prostaglandin production by glomeruli isolated from rats with streptozotocin-induced diabetes mellitus. *J Clin Invest* 1985;75:404–412.
163. deChatel R, Toth M, Barna I. Exchangeable sodium: its relationship with blood pressure and ANP in patients with diabetes mellitus. *J Hypertens* 1986;4(Suppl 6):S526–528.
164. Horstman P. The oxygen consumption in diabetes mellitus. *Acta Med Scand* 1951;139:326–330.
165. Nair KS, Halliday D, Garrow JS. Increased energy expenditure in poorly controlled type I (insulin-dependent) diabetic patients. *Diabetologia* 1984;27:13–16.
166. Ross JM, Fairchild HM, Weldy S, Guyton AC. Autoregulation of blood flow by oxygen lack. *Am J Physiol* 1962;202:21–24.
167. Ditzel J, Standl E. The problem of tissue oxygenation in diabetes mellitus. II. Evidence of disordered oxygen release from the erythrocytes of diabetics in various conditions of metabolic control. *Acta Med Scand* 1975;578(Suppl)59–68.
168. Tarazi RC. The hemodynamics of hypertension. In: Genest J, Kuchel O, Hamet P, Cantin M, eds. *Hypertension,* 2nd edition. New York: McGraw-Hill, 1983;15–42.
169. DeiCas L, Zuliani J, Manca C, Zonca A, Bernardini B, Mansour M. Noninvasive evaluation of left ventricular performance in 294 diabetic patients without clinical heart disease. *Acta Diabetol Lat* 1980;17:145–152.
170. Sykes CA, Wright AD, Malins JM, Pentecost BL. Changes in systolic time intervals during treatment of diabetes mellitus. *Br Heart J* 1977;39:255–259.
171. Zelinske BA. The effect of insulin on the functional site of the cardiovascular system in patients with diabetes mellitus. *Probl Endokrinol (Mosk)* 1975;21:16–21.
172. Hasslacher C, Ritz E, Terpstra J, Gallasch G, Kunowski G, Rall C. Natural history of nephropathy in type I diabetes: relationship to metabolic control and blood pressure. *Hypertension* 1985;7(Suppl II):II74–II78.
173. Christlieb AR, Warram JH, Krolewski AS, et al. Hypertension —the major risk factor in insulin dependent diabetics with juvenile onsets. *Diabetes* 1981;30(Suppl 2):90.
174. Reubi F, Franz KA, Horber F. Hypertension as related to renal function in diabetes mellitus. *Hypertension* 1985;7(Suppl II):II21–II28.
175. Mogensen CE, Christensen CK. Blood pressure changes and renal function in incipient and overt diabetic nephropathy. *Hypertension* 1985;7(Suppl II):II64–II73.
176. Parving HH, Anderson AR, Smidt UM, Svendsen PA. Early aggressive antihypertensive treatment reduces rate of decline in kidney function in diabetic nephropathy. *Lancet* 1983;1:1175–1178.
177. Mogensen CE. Long term antihypertensive treatment inhibits the progression of diabetic nephropathy. *Br Med J* 1982; 285:685–688.
178. Christensen CK, Mogensen CE. Effects of antihypertensive treatment on progression of incipient diabetic nephropathy. *Hypertension* 1985;7(Suppl II):II109–II113.
179. Bjorck S, Nyberg G, Mulec H, Granerus G, Herlitz H, Aurell M. Beneficial effects of angiotensin converting enzyme inhibition on renal function in patients with diabetic nephropathy. *Br Med J* 1986;293:471–474.
180. Goldstein D, Massry SG. Diabetic nephropathy: clinical course and effects of hemodialysis. *Nephron* 1988;20:286–296.
181. Parving HH, Andersen AR, Smidt UM, Oxenboll B, Edsberg B, Christiansen JS. Diabetic nephropathy and arterial hypertension. *Diabetologia* 1983;24:10–12.
182. Christiansen JS, Gammelgaard J, Frandsen M, Parving HH. A prospective study of glomerular filtration rate and arterial blood pressure in insulin dependent diabetics with diabetic nephropathy. *Diabetologia* 1981;20:457–461.
183. Wiseman M, Viberti G, Mackintosh D, Jarret RJ, Keen H. Glycemia, arterial pressure and microalbuminuria in type I (insulin-dependent) diabetes mellitus. *Diabetologia* 1984;26:401–405.
184. Mathiesen ER, Oxenball B, Johnasen K, Svendsen PA, Decker T. Incipient nephropathy in type I (insulin-dependent) diabetes. *Diabetologia* 1984;26:406–410.
185. Feldt-Rasmussen B, Borch-Johnson K, Mathiesen ER. Hypertension in diabetes as related to nephropathy: early blood pressure changes. *Hypertension* 1985;7(Suppl II):II18–II20.
186. Fabre J, Balant LP, Dayer PG, Fox HM, Vernet AT. The kidney in maturity onset diabets mellitus: a clinical study of 510 patients. *Kidney Int* 1982;21:730–738.
187. Krolewski AS, Warram JH, Christlieb AR, Busick EJ, Kahn CR. The changing natural history of nephropathy in type I diabetes. *Am J Med* 1985;78:785–794.
188. Seaquist E, Goetz F, Barbosa J, Rich S. Evidence for genetic susceptibility to diabetic nephropathy. *Diabetes* 1987;36(Suppl I):105A. [Abstract].
189. Viberti GC, Keen H, Wiseman MJ. Raised arterial pressure in parents of proteinuric insulin dependent diabetics. *Br Med J* 1982;295:515–517.
190. Borch-Johnsen K, Nissen H, Nerup J. Blood pressure after 40 years of insulin-dependent diabetes. *Diabetic Nephrop* 1985;4:11–12.
191. Oakley WG, Pyke DA, Tattersall RB, Watkins PJ. Long term diabetes: a clinical study of 92 patients after 40 years. *Q J Med* 1973;43:145–156.
192. Trevisan M, Vaccaro O, Laurenzi M, DeChiara F, DiMuro M, Iacone R, Franzese A. Hypertension, non-insulin-dependent diabetes and intracellular sodium metabolism. *Hypertension* 1988;11:264–268.
193. Ostfeld AM. Epidemiologic overview. In: Horan MJ, Steinberg GM, Dunbar JB, Hadley EC, eds. *Blood pressure regulation and aging: NIH symposium.* New York: Biomedical Information Corporation, 1986;3–10.
194. Kannel WB, Brand N, Skinner JJ. The relation of adiposity to

blood pressure and development of hypertension: the Framingham Study. *Ann Intern Med* 1967;67:48.
195. Drury PL. Diabetes and arterial hypertension. *Diabetologia* 1983;24:1–9.
196. Fuller JH. Epidemiology of hypertension associated with diabetes mellitus. *Hypertension* 1985;7(Suppl II):II3–II7.
197. Berntorp K, Lindgarde F. Familial aggregation of type II diabetes mellitus as an etiological factor in hypertension. *Diabetes Res* 1986;1:307–313.
198. Drury PL. Hypertension in diabetic mellitus. In: Edwards CRW, Carey RM, eds. *Essential hypertension as an endocrine disease.* London: Buttersworth, 1985;301–332.

Hypertension: Pathophysiology, Diagnosis, and Management, edited by J. H. Laragh and B. M. Brenner. Raven Press, Ltd., New York © 1990.

CHAPTER 106

Hypertension and Vascular Disease as Complications of Diabetes

Eberhard Ritz, Christoph Hasslacher, Johannes Mann, and Ji-Zhen Guo

Mechanisms of Hypertension in Diabetes, 1703
Changes in Sodium and Volume, 1703
Atrial Natriuretic Peptide, 1704
The Sympathetic System and the Renin System, 1704
Particular Mechanisms of Hypertension in the Type II Diabetic, 1705
Epidemiology of Hypertension in Diabetes, 1705
Relationship Between Hypertension and Stage of Nephropathy, 1705
Secondary Hypertension in the Diabetic, 1706
Hypertension as a Factor in Progression of Diabetic Nephropathy, 1707
Experimental Observations, 1707
Epidemiologic Findings on the Relationship Between Blood Pressure and the Evolution of Nephropathy, 1707
Intervention Studies: Effect of Blood Pressure Control on the Evolution of Nephropathy, 1707
Hypertension and Macroangiopathy, 1708
Antihypertensive Therapy in the Diabetic, 1710
ACE Inhibitors, 1710
Calcium Antagonists, 1711
References, 1712

Ever since the demonstration of the high prevalence of hypertension in diabetics by Hitzenberger (1) in 1921, hypertension has been recognized as a major complication of diabetes. However, to some extent it has remained a neglected aspect of diabetology. Recently, this has changed dramatically: (i) The mechanisms involved in the genesis of hypertension have been studied, (ii) the influence of hypertension on the progression of nephropathy has been recognized, and (iii) the necessity of rigorous blood pressure control has been widely appreciated. Although considerable information on hypertension in Type I diabetes has accumulated in the past few years, there is still a relative lack of information concerning Type II diabetes. Based on our local experience in Heidelberg and Shanghai, respectively, this chapter will review the above issues and will deal subsequently with recent progress in antihypertensive treatment.

MECHANISMS OF HYPERTENSION IN DIABETES

Hypertension in the diabetic is generally viewed as the result of the combined presence of two abnormalities, namely, excess sodium and increased pressor responsiveness (2,3).

Changes in Sodium and Volume

An increase of exchangeable sodium (4–8), measured with the ^{24}Na dilution technique, and of total body sodium (9), measured by neutron activation analysis, is demonstrated in both insulin-dependent and non-insulin-dependent normotensive diabetic patients without overt nephropathy. On the other hand, on the average, plasma and blood volumes are normal in normotensive diabetics and low in hypertensive diabetics (4–6), suggesting that fluid is sequestered in the extravascular space with a tendency for blood volume contraction when diabetes mellitus is complicated by hypertension. Sodium retention is even more increased in the stage of overt nephropathy (8). In nonazotemic hypertensive diabetics, systolic blood pressure correlates with exchangeable sodium (5); moreover, the sodium renin product is significantly elevated (6). Finally, the natriuretic response to water immersion is blunted in diabetics (10), as is the ability to excrete a sodium load (11).

The causes for sodium retention in prehypertensive diabetics are unknown. Factors discussed in its pathogenesis include the following: (a) an extravascular shift of fluid in parallel with increased capillary permeability and fluid extravasation into the interstitial space (12); (b) primary renal retention of sodium (10,11) related, or not, to the antinatriuretic action of insulin (13); (c) altered volume sensing secondary to disturbed compliance in the low-pressure compartment; and (d) deficiency of vasodilator prostaglandins (14) or kinins (15). The above sodium abnormality is unique to diabetes, since in uncomplicated essential hypertension, exchangeable sodium is normal; furthermore, it changes only minimally in response to diuretic therapy in patients with essential hypertension (16).

Atrial Natriuretic Peptide

Atrial natriuretic peptide (ANP) has recently been studied extensively, particularly with respect to its potential role with regard to volume expansion and glomerular hyperfiltration. In mildly hyperglycemic streptozotocin Sprague–Dawley rats, Ortola et al. (17) found significantly increased ANP levels. A role of enhanced endogenous ANP release with regard to the rise in glomerular filtration rate (GFR) was suggested by the observation that specific ANP antiserum, but not control nonimmune serum, obliterated the rise in GFR. With respect to humans, evidence is conflicting. No increase in immunoreactive ANP (iANP) levels was reported in diabetics without autonomic neuropathy (18); other authors reported normal basal ANP levels with an exaggerated increment in response to a volume load. ANP levels were increased in incipient nephropathy, and even more so in clinically overt nephropathy (19).

The Sympathetic System and the Renin System

Under baseline conditions, but not in the metabolically unstable state (20), the following indices of activity of the adrenergic and renin systems are normal or low: (a) plasma total catecholamines (21); (b) plasma and urinary norepinephrine or epinephrine (22); and (c) plasma renin, angiotensin II (Ang II), and aldosterone (8,22–24).

Whereas in the past there was agreement that the renin system was consistently suppressed in experimental and clinical diabetes (25,26), it has emerged recently that the abnormalities of the renin system are more complex (27,28). This is well documented in Type I diabetics, whereas Type II diabetics have been less well studied. In non-nephropathic Type I diabetics, plasma renin activity (PRA) and Ang II levels are in the upper normal range (29,30), with the exception of one report of inexplicably low Ang II despite normal PRA (31). Burden and Thurston (32) found higher PRA when diabetics were compared with matched controls with similar blood pressures. No difference was noted, however, between (a) diabetic patients with hypertension or complications and (b) those without. Interestingly, one group (33) noted elevated PRA in diabetic patients with increased GFR, implicating a role of the renin–aldosterone system (RAS) in the genesis of hyperfiltration. In patients with nephropathy (34) or retinopathy (30), most [but not all (35,36)] authors reported elevated PRA values, with PRA being higher than in other forms of renal failure of similar severity (34); the product of exchangeable sodium × log PRA was significantly higher in nephropathic patients than in other groups. Walker et al. (37) found a correlation between blood pressure and Ang II levels in nephropathic diabetics; in a prospective study, Ang II and hypertension were independent risk factors for progression of nephropathy. This applied also to Type II diabetics (38). It is of note that low PRA was found in nephropathic diabetics on a low-sodium diet (35); this may reflect reduced sodium loss and persistent volume expansion. Evaluation of the activity of the renin system certainly must take sodium balance into consideration; moreover, it is evident that in diabetic patients receiving an unrestricted sodium intake, plasma levels of renin, Ang II, and aldosterone are not appropriately suppressed (6,29,30,39). Bryer-Ash et al. (36) considered elevated prorenin as a risk factor for the later development of nephropathy. Drury et al. (40) found significantly higher PRA in patients with Type I diabetes and proliferative retinopathy than in matched diabetic subjects without complications; in these patients, PRA was higher but blood pressure was elevated, illustrating that such elevation was clearly inappropriate. More recently, Franken et al. (41) found increased prorenin levels in patients with proliferative retinopathy, independent of nephropathy; prorenin levels decreased after panretinal laser photocoagulation, suggesting retinal production of prorenin. Only a few investigators dealt specifically with Type II diabetics (6) and found low PRA in patients with and without late complications. This was accompanied by elevated exchangeable sodium and unchanged intravascular volume. Others found low renin in patients with autonomic polyneuropathy and orthostatic hypotension (22,27). It is also of note that a considerable proportion of elderly Type II diabetics had very low or very much elevated PRA, respectively. This may reflect the high prevalence of hyporeninemic hypoaldosteronism, on the one hand, and of atherosclerotic renal artery stenosis, on the other hand, in this age group. In our clinic we noted that diabetes mellitus was present in 30% of the 83 consecutive patients referred for percutaneous transluminal arterioplasty. The pressor response to infusion of Ang II is increased (relative to controls) in diabetic patients under no dietary sodium restriction (22,29) as well as in Type I diabetics both without (22) and with late complications. This may be related to sodium retention, since sodium sensitizes the vasculature to the pressor effects of Ang II. Indeed, unchanged pressor response to Ang II was found in uncomplicated Type I diabetics on a low-sodium diet (42); furthermore, Ang II pressor responsiveness was normalized by diuretic therapy (3,22). Of great interest is one recent preliminary report stating that, in diabetics, one finds not only increased pressor response (43,44) but also a greater increment of GFR in response to low doses of Ang II (45). This complements findings of elevated PRA in patients with glomerular hyperfiltration (33) and suggests a role of the renin system in glomerular hyperfiltration.

Increased Ang II pressor responsiveness may also be related to our recent demonstration that despite the presence of high-normal Ang II levels, platelet Ang II receptors tended to be higher in normotensive Type I diabetics without proteinuria or retinal complications (46). In previous studies, a good correlation has been noted between platelet receptors and Ang II pressor responsiveness (47,48). Previously, in severely hyperglycemic insulinopenic rats (49), diminished glomerular Ang II receptors had been found, and this was normalized by administration of low doses of insulin (49–51). Consequently, animal data do not directly bear on the insulin-treated near-normoglycemic Type I diabetic.

In a similar fashion, blood pressure responsiveness to norepinephrine tends to be increased relative to concomitant plasma norepinephrine concentrations (52,53). Norepinephrine hyperresponsiveness was seen in nonhypertensive diabetics without microvascular complications (both Type I and Type II), irrespective of age and type (or duration) of treatment. Pressor hyperresponsiveness to norepinephrine, and later to Ang II, is also a feature in prehypertensive offspring in hypertensive families; it has been emphasized (5) that the defect is more pronounced in diabetics than in essential hypertensives.

Both we (54) and others (55) have been unable to identify Type I diabetics who develop nephropathy (as a result of their blood pressures) at the time of diagnosis or at the time of first consultation, respectively; however, the sensitivity of this approach may be limited. More recently, raised arterial pressures were found in parents of proteinuric insulin-dependent diabetics (56); moreover, increased sodium–lithium countertransport activity, as a putative marker for primary hypertension, has been noted in nephropathic Type I diabetics (57,58). This suggestion is intuitively plausible in light of recent evidence that abnormal intrarenal hemodynamics are found in prehypertensive offspring of families with primary hypertension.

In addition, a strong genetic element for the risk of the Type I diabetic to develop nephropathy is also suggested by the preliminary observation that the risk of nephropathy is considerably higher for the diabetic sibling of a diabetic propositus with nephropathy than for the diabetic sibling of a diabetic propositus without nephropathy (59).

Particular Mechanisms of Hypertension in the Type II Diabetic

The relationship between diabetes and hypertension is more complex in the Type II diabetic. The study of Pell and D'Alonzo (60) noted a higher prevalence of hypertension in diabetic employees of the Dupont Company. Hypertension was more prevalent even prior to the diagnosis of diabetes. More recently, the Bedford survey (61) and other studies showed that systolic blood pressures were significantly higher in individuals with newly detected and borderline diabetes than in normoglycemic controls, even after adjustment for age and degree of obesity (62). Although the pathogenesis appears to be complex, several new findings shed light on potential pathogenetic mechanisms. The study by Modan et al. (63) suggested that high blood pressure was associated with impaired glucose tolerance independently of obesity. It has been proposed that the feature common to obesity, non-insulin-dependent diabetes, and hypertension was hyperinsulinemia or insulin resistance, or both. Insulin in itself may be a hypertensinogenic factor. Insulin has been shown to promote sodium retention in studies using the euglycemic clamp technique (13). Insulin also stimulates volume absorption in isolated tubules (64). Furthermore, insulin has been shown to stimulate release of norepinephrine (65) and to affect catecholamine responsiveness in a complex fashion.

Therefore it is of interest that even in nondiabetic patients with primary hypertension, past studies showed impaired glucose tolerance (66) and, more recently, insulin resistance (67). Insulin resistance was restricted to nonoxidative pathways of glucose disposal in peripheral tissue and did not concern lipid or potassium metabolism. A possible etiologic role is suggested by the observation that a correlation existed between insulin resistance and severity of hypertension.

EPIDEMIOLOGY OF HYPERTENSION IN DIABETES

Hypertension is a grave complication of diabetes, both of Type I and of Type II. In the past it was regarded as an indicator of advanced nephropathy. More recently, elevated blood pressure, as well as a rise of blood pressure within the normotensive range, has been shown even in early stages of nephropathy (55,68). The dire prognostic implications of nephropathy involve risks other than that of renal failure: Recently, Borch-Johnsen et al. (69) demonstrated that cardiovascular mortality in Type I diabetics relative to the general population was also markedly increased in proteinuric Type I diabetics but not in nonproteinuric Type I diabetics. The relationship between hypertension and nephropathy is complex: On the one hand, renal impairment is an important cause of hypertension in the microalbuminuric or proteinuric diabetic (55,68,69); on the other hand, hypertension, in itself, accelerates evolution of nephropathy.

Relationship Between Hypertension and Stage of Nephropathy

The prevalence and severity of blood pressure increase with progressively advancing stages of nephropathy, both in Type I (54) and Type II (70) diabetes. The prevalence of hypertension at various stages of nephropathy in Type I and Type II diabetics in our own patients (54,70–73) is summarized in Table 1. It is of interest that despite marked sociocultural differences, a high overall prevalence of hypertension (i.e., 35% versus 13.9% in healthy controls) was also noted in 411 diabetics studied in Beijing, half of whom had proteinuria (74). Increasing prevalence of hypertension with advancing stages of nephropathy is in agreement with the impressive Scandinavian experience (55,68). Of note in Table 1 is the high prevalence of hypertension in nonproteinuric Type II diabetics which exceeds the prevalence in the age-, sex-, and body-mass-index-matched local population in southern Germany (Dr. Keil, *personal communication*). This observation is in agreement with other studies (61,62) and may point to pressor mechanisms related to obesity or to an endogenous excess of insulin independent of nephropathy (63–67). Furthermore, the common isolated systolic hypertension of the elderly diabetic may, in part, explain the finding. In Type II diabetics, prevalence

TABLE 1. *Prevalence of hypertension[a] and median blood pressures as a function of nephropathy in Type I and Type II diabetics who developed nephropathy*

	Parameter	Stage of nephropathy: No proteinuria	Persistent proteinuria	Elevated serum creatinine
Type I (n = 52) (ref. 56)	Prevalence of hypertension (%)	44%	67%	92%
	Systolic BP (mmHg)	140 (105–196)	148 (118–202)	158 (115–198)
	Diastolic BP (mmHg)	84 (75–105)	88 (76–122)	92 (82–118)
Type II (n = 63) (ref. 57)	Prevalence of hypertension (%)	70%	83%	100%
	Systolic BP (mmHg)	164 (105–215)	166 (127–203)	168 (130–200)
	Diastolic BP (mmHg)	78 (70–106)	88 (72–122)	93 (76–116)

[a] Hypertension is defined as blood pressure (BP) greater than 140/90 mmHg, taken on three occasions while sitting.

and severity of hypertension further increased with more advanced stages of nephropathy, but less so than in Type I diabetics.

The natural history of nephropathy in Type II diabetes is not well characterized. In agreement with studies in Pima Indians (75), we were recently able to show (76) that the cumulative incidence of proteinuria and renal failure, respectively, is similar in Type II diabetics (Fig. 1). We also noted higher blood pressures in nonproteinuric patients who subsequently developed proteinuria (70).

Secondary Hypertension in the Diabetic

As recently emphasized by the Working Group on Hypertension in Diabetes (77), several forms of secondary hypertension may be present in the diabetic. *Primary hypertension* (57,58) may, by genetic association, be related to the risk of nephropathy in the Type I diabetic. Whether primary hypertension is also more common in the Type II diabetic has not been clarified. *Isolated systolic hypertension* is frequently found in the elderly Type II diabetic; it may be related, at least in part, to diminished vascular compliance. Advanced glycosylation products have been shown to increase vascular stiffness. Pseudohypertension (i.e., elevated blood pressure upon sphygmomanometric measurement, with normotension upon intra-arterial blood pressure measurement) may be noted in the elderly diabetic. The discrepant results are due to diminished compressibility of vessels. This artifact may be suspected when Osler's sign is positive (i.e., when the artery is palpable even though the cuff has been inflated above systolic

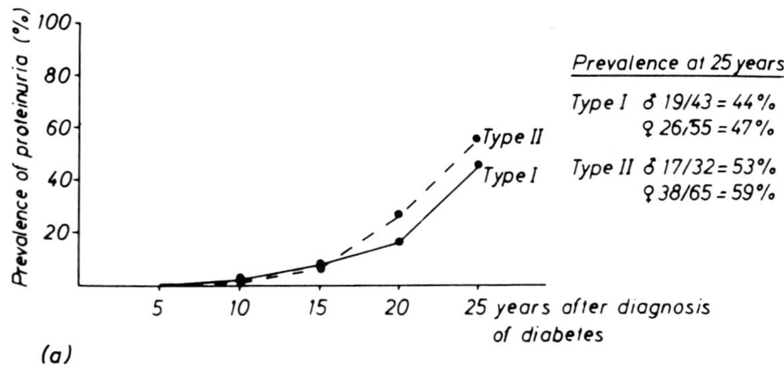

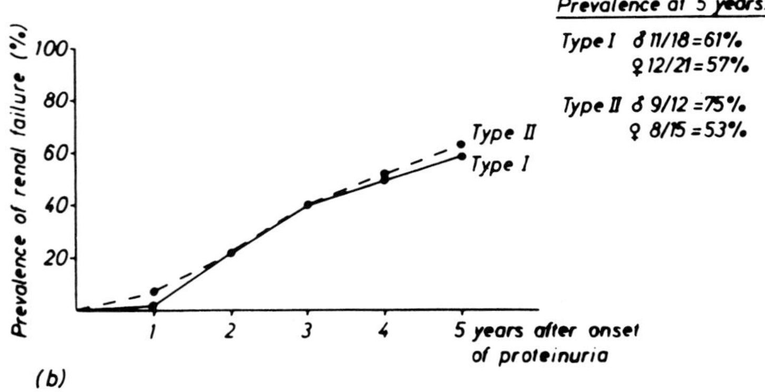

FIG. 1. Cumulative prevalence of proteinuria (**a**) and renal failure (**b**) as a function of duration of diabetes in type I and type II diabetics, respectively. (From ref. 75.)

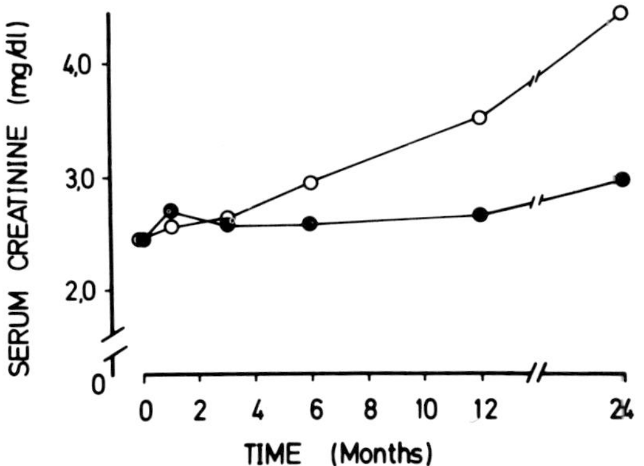

FIG. 4. Time course of median serum creatinine concentration in patients with renal failure and hypertension (ref. 128). (●) Thirty-nine patients treated with ACE inhibitors. (○) Forty-one patients treated with alternative antihypertensive agents. Note more pronounced rise of serum creatinine on alternative antihypertensive agents despite similar blood pressure control.

relation between circulating renin and antihypertensive efficacy of ACE inhibitors would not be surprising.

Two aspects of ACE inhibitors in diabetics—their action on proteinuria (96–99) and their action on blood pressure control (129–132)—deserve special comment. In normotensive, but microalbuminuric, Type I and Type II diabetics, Marre et al. (96) administered 20 mg enalapril or placebo over a period of 6 months. Median fractional albumin clearance decreased in the enalapril group and increased in the placebo group. In the enalapril group, blood pressure decreased but glomerular filtration rose. Taguma et al. (97) administered captopril to 10 azotemic diabetics with heavy proteinuria. Urinary protein excretion decreased, but changes in filtration rate were not thoroughly excluded. Hommel et al. (132) administered captopril to hypertensive diabetics with persistent albuminuria. No significant changes were seen in placebo-treated patients. However, in captopril-treated patients, albuminuria fell, associated with a minor decrease in GFR; blood pressure decreased in parallel. The authors tentatively ascribed diminished proteinuria to a decrease in glomerular capillary pressure. Numerous studies document that ACE inhibitors permit excellent control of blood pressure, even in diabetic patients with renal failure (129–132). Of more specific interest is the claim (130) that ACE inhibitors exert a renoprotective action. Indeed, in the study of Björck et al. (130), no correlation was found between (a) the reduction in blood pressure after administration of captopril and (b) the reduction of the rate of decline of GFR. Qualitatively similar observations on ACE inhibitors in patients with renal failure of various causes, including diabetes mellitus, were also made in the study of Reisch et al. (128). The results of ongoing controlled trials are eagerly awaited.

The following results have been described in captopril-treated diabetics: (a) improved metabolic control with decreased HbA_{1c}, (b) improvement of glucose tolerance despite no change in immunoreactive insulin, and (c) appearance of hypoglycemic episodes (133). Hypoglycemia was initially ascribed to the penicillamin-like SH group of captopril, but similar lowering of blood glucose has recently also been shown for enalapril (134). Using glucose clamp techniques, Jauch et al. (135) demonstrated similar improvement of glucose consumption after bradykinin and after ACE inhibition; this suggests that the mechanism of ACE action on muscular glucose consumption is mediated by kinins.

Calcium Antagonists

Calcium antagonists have several advantages which make them uniquely suited for antihypertensive treatment (136). However, insulin secretion is calcium-dependent, and calcium channel blockers may interfere with it (137). The possibility was raised that metabolic control could deteriorate under the influence of calcium antagonists. This concern was reinforced by uncontrolled anecdotal reports (138). Acute administration of nifedipine has been shown to cause abnormalities of carbohydrate metabolism in normal individuals and, particularly, in Type II diabetics (139,140). In early studies, acutely elevated fasting plasma glucose levels occurred after sublingual administration of nifedipine (140). Charles et al. (141) administered 60 mg nifedipine per day for 3 days to nondiabetic probands and noted increased glucose concentrations and insulin secretion rates under fasting conditions as well as after glucose loading. In contrast, again in nondiabetic patients, lower doses of nifedipine (30 mg/day) for 10 days improved glucose tolerance despite lower insulin secretion (142). Several considerations are pertinent with respect to the acute and chronic effects of calcium antagonists on metabolic control. First, there are important species differences to consider (143): In rats, dose-dependent impairment of glucose tolerance and insulin secretion was noted, whereas no consistent major abnormalities of HbA_{1c} and various indices of glucose metabolism were noted in a large number of carefully controlled, mostly randomized double-blind placebo-controlled studies on long-term treatment with moderate therapeutic doses of nifedipine or verapamil (144–148). Indeed, out of nine studies, five showed unchanged glucose tolerance and insulin secretion, three showed improvement, and only one showed modest impairment. Furthermore, seven studies showed no change in HbA_1 profile; in some studies, observation periods extended up to 3 years. It has also been noted that blood pressure is lowered more efficaciously in diabetic patients; this may be due to decreased reflex tachycardia, presumably as a result of autonomic polyneuropathy (149). Thus, it appears that the initially elevated glucose levels, particularly after administration of nifedipine, might result from transient activation of the sympathoadrenal system (147) without further adverse long-term metabolic consequences.

The use of calcium antagonists in diabetic patients with nephropathy does present some problems. Jackson et al. (150), when studying uninephrectomized (streptozotocin) diabetic rats with elevated blood pressure, elevated GFR, and progressive proteinuria, found no effect on increasing proteinuria with the use of verapamil. In contrast, enalapril (which caused equivalent lowering of blood pressure) decreased proteinuria. Similarly, in humans, increased fractional albuminuria with the use of calcium antagonists was noted in diabetic (99) and nondiabetic patients (100). Consequently, the long-term renal consequences of calcium antagonists require further study.

ACKNOWLEDGMENT

Ji-Zhen Guo is the recipient of a scholarship from the Shanghai High Blood Pressure Institute.

REFERENCES

1. Hitzenberger K. Über den Blutdruck bei Diabetes mellitus. *Wien Arch Inn Med* 1921;2:461.
2. Hasslacher CH, Rambausek M, Ritz E. Genesis and management of hypertension in diabetic nephropathy. In: Keen H, Legrain M, eds. *Prevention and treatment of diabetic nephropathy.* Boston: MTP Press, 1983;177–189.
3. Weidmann P. Recent pathogenetic aspects in essential hypertension and hypertension associated with diabetes mellitus. *Klin Wochenschr* 1980;58:1071.
4. De Châtel R, Weidmann P, Flammer J, Ziegler WH, Beretta-Piccoli C, Vetter W, Reubi FC. Sodium, renin, aldosterone, catecholamines, and blood pressure in diabetes mellitus. *Kidney Int* 1977;12:412–421.
5. Weidmann P, Beretta-Piccoli C, Trost BN. Pressor factors and responsiveness in hypertension accompanying diabetes mellitus. *Hypertension* 1985;7(Suppl II):33–42.
6. O'Hare JA, Ferriss JB, Brady D, Twomey B, O'Sullivan DJ. Exchangeable sodium and renin in hypertensive diabetic patients with and without nephropathy. *Hypertension* 1985;7(Suppl II):II43–II48.
7. De Châtel R, Toth M, Barna I. Exchangeable body sodium: its relationship with blood pressure and atrial natriuretic factor in patients with diabetes mellitus. *J Hypertens* 1986;4(Suppl 6):S526–S528.
8. Feldt-Rasmussen B, Mathiesen ER, Deckert T. Central role for sodium in the pathogenesis of blood pressure changes independent of angiotensin, aldosterone and catecholamines in type 1 (insulin-dependent) diabetes mellitus. *Diabetologia* 1987; 30:610–617.
9. Brennan BL, Roginsky MS, Cohn S. Increased total body sodium as a mechanism for suppressed plasma renin activity in diabetes mellitus. *Clin Res* 1979;27:591A.
10. O'Hare JP, Roland JM, Walters G, Corrall RJM. Impaired sodium excretion in response to volume expansion induced by water immersion in non-insulin-dependent diabetes mellitus. *Clin Sciences* 1986;71:403–409.
11. Roland JM, O'Hare JP, Walters G, Corrall RJM. Sodium retention in response to saline infusion in uncomplicated diabetes mellitus. *Diabetic Res* 1986;3:213–215.
12. O'Hare JA, Ferriss JB. Transcapillary escape rate of albumin and extracellular fluid volume in diabetes. *Diabetologia* 1985; 28:937–938.
13. DeFronzo RA. The effect of indulin on renal sodium metabolism. *Diabetologia* 1981;21:165–171.
14. Katayama S, Lee JB. Hypertension in experimental diabetes mellitus: renin-prostaglandin interaction. *Hypertension* 1985;7:554–561.
15. Olshan AR, O'Connor DT, Cohen IM. Hypertension in adult onset diabetes mellitus: abnormal renal hemodynamics and endogenous vasoregulatory factors. *Am J Kidney Dis* 1982;2:271–280.
16. Weidmann P, Beretta-Piccoli C, Meier A. Antihypertensive mechanism of diuretic treatment with chlorthalidone. Complementary roles of the sympathetic axis and sodium. *Kidney Int* 1983;23:320–326.
17. Ortola FV, Ballermann BJ, Anderson S, Mendez RE, Brenner BM. Elevated plasma atrial natriuretic peptide levels in diabetic rats. *J Clin Invest* 1987;80:670–674.
18. Kahn JK, Grekin RJ, Shenker Y, Vinik AI. Plasma levels of immunoreactive atrial natriuretic hormone in patients with diabetes mellitus. *Regul Pept* 1986;15:323–332.
19. Sawicki PT, Heinemann L, Rave K. Atrial natriuretic factor in various stages of diabetic nephropathy. *J Diabetic Complications* 1989;in press.
20. Ferriss JB, O'Hare JA, Kelleher CCM, Sullivan PA, Cole MM, Ross HF, O'Sullivan DJ. Diabetic control and the renin–angiotensin system, catecholamines, and blood pressure. *Hypertension* 1985;7(Suppl II):II-58–II-63.
21. Christensen NJ. Plasma catecholamines in long-term diabetics with and without nephropathy and in hypophysectomized subjects. *J Clin Invest* 1972;51:779–787.
22. Beretta-Piccoli C, Weidmann P, de Châtel R. Plasma catecholamines and renin in diabetes mellitus: relationships with age, posture, sodium and blood pressure. *Klin Wochenschr* 1979;57:681–691.
23. Christlieb AR. Nephropathy, the renin system, and hypertensive vascular disease in diabetes mellitus. *Cardiovasc Med* 1978;3:417–432.
24. Ferriss JB, Sullivan PA, Gonggrijp H. Plasma angiotensin II and aldosterone in unselected diabetic patients. *Clin Endocrinol* 1982;17:261–269.
25. Hsueh WA, Carlson EJ, Luetscher JA. Activation and characterization of inactive big renin in plasma of patients with diabetic nephropathy and unusual active renin. *J Clin Endocrinol Metab* 1980;51:535–543.
26. Christlieb AR, Kaldany A, D'Elia JA. Aldosterone responsiveness in patients with diabetes mellitus. *Diabetes* 1978;27:732–737.
27. Weidmann P, Reinhart R, Maxwell MH. Syndrome of hyporeninemic hypoaldosteronism and hyperkalemia in renal disease. *J Clin Endocrinol Metab* 1973;36:965–977.
28. Mann E, Ritz E. Renin–angiotensin system beim diabetischen Patienten. *Klin Wochenschr* 1989;in press.
29. Drury PL, Smith GM, Ferriss JB. Increased vasopressor responsiveness to angiotensin II in type 1 (insulin-dependent) diabetic patients without complications. *Diabetologia* 1984;27:174–179.
30. Drury PL, Bodansky HJ. The relationship of the renin-angiotensin system in type I diabetes to microvascular disease. *Hypertension* 1985;7(Suppl II):II-84–II-89.
31. Feldt-Rasmussen B, Mathiesen ER, Deckert T, Giese J, Christensen NJ, Bent-Hansen L, Nielsen MD. Central role for sodium in the pathogenesis of blood pressure changes independent of angiotensin, aldosterone and catecholamines in type 1 (insulin-dependent) diabetes mellitus. *Diabetologia* 1987;30:610–617.
32. Burden AC, Thurston H. Plasma renin activity in diabetes mellitus. *Clin Sci* 1979;56:255–259.
33. Wiseman MJ, Drury PL, Keen H, Viberti GC. Plasma renin activity in insulin-dependent diabetes with raised glomerular filtration rate. *Clin Endocrinol* 1984;21:409–414.
34. Bjorck S, Delin K, Herlitz H, Larsson O, Aurell M. Renin secretion in advanced diabetic nephropathy. *Scand J Urol Nephrol [Suppl]* 1984;79:53–57.
35. Manchandia MR, Grossain VV, Michelakis AM, Rovner DR. Plasma cryoactivated renin and active renin in diabetes mellitus. *J Endocrinol Metab* 1981;53:1025.
36. Bryer-Ash M, Ammon RA, Luetscher JA. Increased inactive renin in diabetes mellitus without evidence of nephropathy. *J Endocrinol Metab* 1983;56:557–561.
37. Walker WG, Hermann J, Murphy R, Patz A. Elevated blood pressure and angiotensin are associated with accelerated loss of renal function in diabetic nephropathy. *4th Int Congr Nutr Metab Renal Disease, Williamsburg* 1985:Abstract 80.
38. Codd T, Hermann J, Walker G. Elevated blood pressure is associated with rapid loss of renal function in non-insulin dependent (NIDDM) diabetes mellitus. *18th Int Ann Meet Am Soc Nephrol, New Orleans* 1985:Abstract 34.
39. Ferriss JB, Sullivan PA, Gonggrijp H, Cole M, O'Sullivan DJ. Plasma angiotensin II and aldosterone in unselected diabetic patients. *Clin Endocrinol* 1982;17:261–269.
40. Drury PL, Bodansky HJ, Oddie CJ, Cudworth AG, Edwards

the organ (the kidney) is important; and (d) the system should relate to other vascular abnormalities that are characteristic of the disease or its complications. Importantly, the system should also be clinically action-oriented, such that clinical decisions can be made on the basis of classifying the individual patient: For instance, should the patient be put on another diet (e.g., low-protein diet), should blood pressure be monitored more closely (and possibly treated more effectively), or should insulin and general diabetes treatment be optimized?

A classification system for IDDM patients has been elaborated during the last few years (18,19) and is presented in Table 2. To some extent, it fulfills the criteria for the classification system indicated above. On the other hand, there are presently no other alternatives in classifying patients. Renal biopsy does not help the clinician in clarifying the situation in diabetic patients. However, it should also be stressed that patients with a normal albumin excretion rate are not necessarily protected against diabetic nephropathy throughout their lifetimes, although their prognosis concerning development of overt nephropathy with clinical proteinuria and hypertension over the next decade is much better than the prognosis for patients with microalbuminuria. With a normal albumin excretion rate the risk may be around 5% over the next decade, whereas the risk in patients with microalbuminuria may be around 80%, provided that no intervention is given (Fig. 1). Indeed, new intervention modalities have appeared since these retrospective studies were published, and the risk of subsequent nephropathy at present, with proper metabolic control and effective antihypertensive treatment and possibly low dietary protein, is likely to be considerably less than 80% over the next 10 years.

STAGES OF RENAL INVOLVEMENT AS RELATED TO BLOOD PRESSURE ELEVATION

Figure 1 summarizes the course of urinary albumin excretion (UAE) in IDDM, both in patients developing complications and in those free of renal disease, in spite of a long duration of diabetes. Table 2 provides more detailed information on renal changes and blood pressure involvement in the stages of renal change in diabetes.

Stage I is the early hyperfunction–hypertrophy stage found at diagnosis. Increases in glomerular and kidney size are common findings (20). Microalbuminuria may be present at diagnosis but is readily reversible by insulin treatment. Glomerular filtration rate (GFR) is high in these patients; this abnormality is also reversible, but in most cases only partially. At the clinical diagnosis, elevated blood pressure is not found (or very rarely found) in IDDM patients.

Stage II is the silent stage, where there are renal lesions without clinical and laboratory signs of disease. One hallmark of diabetic glomerulopathy, basement membrane thickening, is detectable after about 2–3 years of diabetes (21). Some years later, a relative expansion of mesangial regions (mesangium as percent of tuft) becomes evident. By definition, UAE is normal. A number of patients continue in this stage throughout their lifetimes. Usually, blood pressure is completely normal.

Stage III is the stage of incipient diabetic nephropathy, typically found after 10–15 years and lasting, without intervention, 5–10 years. Microalbuminuria increases steadily over the years (20 to >200 μg/min). However, GFR is still high or normal in this stage, but it starts to decline as microalbuminuria increases. Blood pressure also starts to increase in this stage, in parallel with the increase in UAE (22,23). Structural lesions are more advanced, and glomerular closure probably starts at this stage (21).

Stage IV is the well-known stage, with clinical nephropathy, and is eventually found in 30–40% of patients, often after 15–25 years of diabetes. It is characterized by the classical morphological lesions (24,25), but the diagnosis is most often made on clinical grounds. Hypertension is often present; with treatment, blood pressure increases considerably. Microalbuminuria has now become clinical proteinuria, and GFR has declined further. The fall in GFR can often be reduced by effective antihypertensive treatment (9,10).

Stage V is end-stage renal failure (ESRF), occurring after many years of diabetes and characterized by generalized glomerular closure and a very low GFR. ESRF in diabetics represents a major health problem throughout the world (26,27).

Renal involvement can thus be traced throughout the course of diabetes, either by renal function tests or by biopsy. It is important to stress that control and evaluation of diabetic nephropathy, including blood pressure monitoring, have to start very early. If delayed until advanced overt nephropathy appears, the game is already lost; furthermore, treatment must be directed at renal supportive measures with dialysis and transplantation.

Associated Abnormalities of Microalbuminuria in Incipient Diabetic Nephropathy (Renal and Nonrenal)

Incipient diabetic nephropathy is a very decisive stage and is important to diagnose because treatment at this stage (including antihypertensive treatment) is likely to be much more effective than treatment in established overt nephropathy. Patients with microalbuminuria are in the process of developing multiple vascular lesions, and since vascular changes may be related to blood pressure and may therefore interfere with treatment, these changes will be discussed in some detail (19).

Blood Pressure Elevation

Many studies have shown that some degree of blood pressure elevation, of the order of 10% (22,23,28–36), is present in patients with microalbuminuria, although there is a considerable overlap between normoalbuminuric and microalbuminuric patients. In a 2-year follow-up study, a significant increase in blood pressure was found which was significantly correlated to rise in UAE rate (31). This correlation was also found in another study on the progression of

TABLE 2. *Microalbuminuria and diabetic nephropathy stages in diabetic renal involvement and nephropathy (DN) in IDDM patients*

Stage and time sequence	Designation	Main characteristics	Main structural changes	GFR (ml/min)	Urinary albumin excretion (UAE)	Blood pressure	Suggested main pathophysiologic change
Stage I							
At clinical diagnosis	Hyperfunction and hypertrophy stage[a]	Large kidneys and glomerular hyperfiltration	Glomerular hypertrophy; normal basement membrane and mesangium	~150	May be increased, but readily reversible	Normal	Glomerular volume expansion and increased intraglomerular pressure
Stage II							
In short-term diabetes (1–15 years)	"Silent" stage with normal UAE, but structural lesion present	Normal UAE	Increasing basement membrane (BM) thickness and mesangial expansion	With or without hyperfiltration[a,b]	Normal (often increased in stress situations)	Normal	Changes as indicated above but quite variable (dependent on metabolic control?); in addition, increased accumulation of basement-membrane and basement-membrane-like material
In long-term diabetes (>15 years)	Same as above	Normal UAE	No (or few) studies	With or without hyperfiltration[a,b]	Normal (often increased in stress situations)	Normal or slightly elevated	
Stage III							
Early	Incipient DN (or "at-risk patient")	Persistently elevated UAE (20–200 μg/min)	Severity probably in between II and IV	~160	20–70 μg/min	Often elevated compared to healthy subjects[c]; also blood pressure elevated during exercise	Glomerular closure probably starts in this stage; in some patients, high intraglomerular pressure
Late	Same as above	Same as above	Same as above	~130 (considerable range)	70–200 μg/min		
Stage IV							
Early	Overt DN	Clinical proteinuria or UAE > 200 μg/min	Further increase in basement membrane thickening and mesangial expansion	~130–70	>200 μg/min, increasing clinical proteinuria	Often frank hypertension[d]	High rate of glomerular closure and advancing mesangial expansion; hyperfiltration in remaining glomeruli (deleterious?)
Intermediate	Overt DN	Same as above	Increasing rate of glomerular closure Hypertrophy of remaining glomeruli	~70–30	Same as above	Hypertension in almost all patients	
Advanced	Overt DN	Same as above	Same as above	~30–10	Same as above	Hypertension in almost all patients	
Stage V	Uremia	End-stage renal failure	Generalized glomerular closure	0–10	Decreasing (due to nephron closure)	High but often controlled by dialysis treatment	Advanced lesions and glomerular closure

[a] Changes present probably in all stages when control is imperfect.
[b] Possible marker of future nephropathy (if GFR > 150 ml/min).
[c] Increase by ~3–4 mmHg per year without treatment.
[d] Increase by ~7 mmHg per year without treatment.

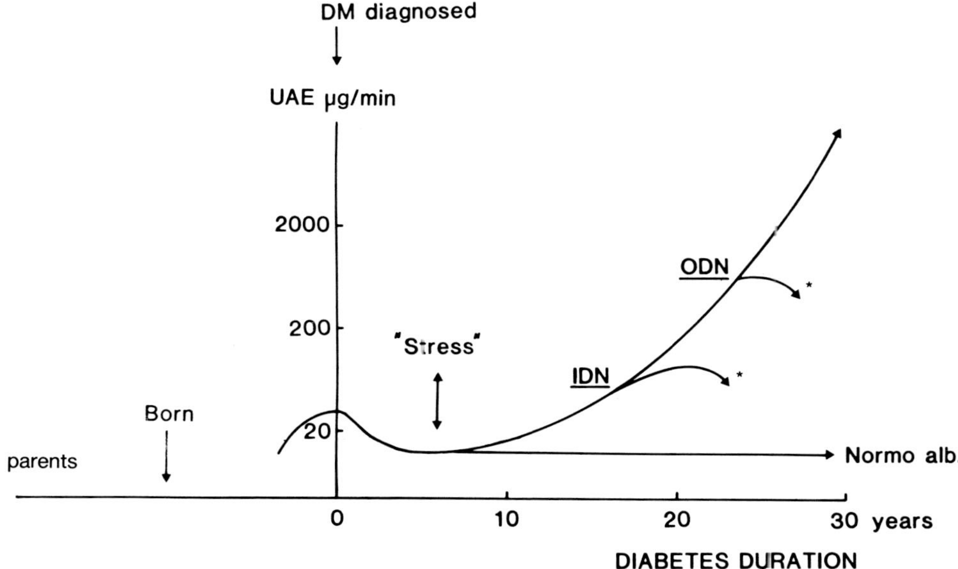

FIG. 1. Urinary albumin excretion (UAE) rate in the course of diabetes. DM, diabetes mellitus; Normo alb., normoalbuminuria; IDN, incipient diabetic nephropathy; ODN, overt diabetic nephropathy. Parents of diabetic patients developing nephropathy may or may not have increased blood pressure. Otherwise, blood pressure starts to increase in the insulin-dependent diabetic patient along with an increase in UAE rate or as a result of incipient diabetic nephropathy, characterized by persistent and increasing microalbuminuria. Overt diabetic nephropathy is characterized by proteinuria and, often, considerable increase in blood pressure. *Effect of antihypertensive treatment.

microalbuminuria (22). The blood pressure elevation is systolic and diastolic, but diastolic elevation is particularly characteristic in these patients. An increase in blood pressure develops in parallel with the rise in UAE rate; therefore it is difficult to sort out which abnormality comes first, increase in blood pressure or increase in UAE rate. A close description of development of blood pressure elevation in the whole course of diabetes will be given later.

Renal Structure and Function

A recent study from Japan (37) reports that glomerular lesions, diffuse and nodular, as well as arteriolar hyalinosis, are common in patients with microalbuminuria. Even patients with a normal UAE rate show abnormalities, but patients with microalbuminuria are in between the normoalbuminuric and the proteinuric patients.

Hyperfiltration is often found in the early stage of microalbuminuria, but GFR starts to decline during the phase of incipient diabetic nephropathy (22,29). Acute reduction of arterial blood pressure in incipient diabetic nephropathy reduces UAE rate, without normalization, suggesting that microalbuminuria is partly pressure-dependent and partly associated with structural lesions (38).

Retinal Changes

It has been shown that microalbuminuria also predicts proliferative diabetic nephropathy (39), but it should be stressed that there is an inconsistent relationship between retinopathy and nephropathy (40,41). Patients with a normal UAE rate may show rather advanced retinal lesions, although there is usually a correlation, not only to UAE but also to blood pressure level (39). The opposite situation—that is, the presence of completely normal eye backgrounds, nephropathy, and associated hypertension—is more uncommon and suggests a nondiabetic renal disease, and therefore a biopsy procedure may be required.

Cardiac Changes

It has recently been shown that patients with some degree of microalbuminuria show increased contractility as measured by ultrasound technique (42). The patients also have somewhat increased blood pressure if microalbuminuria is present. Thereafter, with an increasing UAE rate and overt nephropathy, contractility decreases, probably because of advancing cardiac diseases in patients with nephropathy and hypertension. These findings are compatible with a state of hyperperfusion and some hypertension early on in patients prone to development of generalized vascular disease (42).

General Vascular Changes

There is also evidence of more generalized vascular disease and leakage of albumin in patients with microalbuminuria and associated increase in blood pressure. Thus, the transcapillary escape rate of albumin is increased in patients with microalbuminuria and borderline hypertension (43). They also show impaired aerobic work capacity (44) and a high blood pressure increase during physical exercise (28). New studies suggest adverse lipid abnormalities not only in overt nephropathy but also in incipient nephropathy.

Sodium Retention

It is quite characteristic that patients with incipient diabetic nephropathy show some sodium retention (45), and this may be due to peripheral hyperinsulinism, either endogenous in NIDDM patients or exogenous in IDDM patients (45–47). In the case of incipient diabetic nephropathy and overt diabetic nephropathy of IDDM patients, blood pressure is correlated to the level of exchangeable sodium (45).

Blood Pressure Changes in the Course of Diabetes and Its Complications

New interesting results have appeared during the last few years regarding blood pressure changes in the course of diabetes mellitus; these results confirm that blood pressure elevation—in some cases only slight increases—is closely associated with development of diabetic renal disease, as expressed by changes in the UAE rate, as outlined in Fig. 1.

Although development of diabetic nephropathy is, to some extent, associated with poor metabolic control, there seems to be a huge overlap in levels of HbA_{1c} in patients with and without microalbuminuria/proteinuria. Therefore, genetic determinants for susceptibility to nephropathy have been suspected. It has been suggested that raised blood pressure may not be a consequence of renal disease, but rather an independent marker of liability to hypertension, conferring susceptibility to renal disease, if diabetes is present. This hypothesis has recently been tested by Viberti et al. (48), who examined parents of proteinuric diabetics and matched diabetic controls. Indeed, blood pressure was significantly elevated in parents of proteinuric diabetics, as shown in Table 3. Krolewski et al. (49) recently reported similar findings. Having a parent with hypertension tripled the risk of nephropathy, and the risk was even higher in patients who also had poor glycemic control during the first decade of diabetes. Krolewski et al. (49) and Mangili et al. (50) also found significantly higher values for maximal velocity of lithium–sodium countertransport in red blood cells of diabetics as compared to those of controls. Mediation of blood pressure increases through sharing of environmental factors cannot be excluded. However, new studies from Copenhagen did not confirm these results (T. Deckert, *personal communication*). The Copenhagen study was very well planned. The number of patients required to document differences, not only with regard to blood pressure elevation in parents of diabetic patients with and without nephropathy, but also with regard to the level of sodium lithium counter transport activity in erythrocytes, was determined before the start of study. The reason for discrepancies is not clear, but no trend at all was observed in the Copenhagen study. Therefore, widespread clinical consequences should not be taken from the London and Boston studies.

TABLE 3. *Blood pressure (mmHg) in parents of diabetic patients*

Group of patients	Parents of normoalbuminuric controls	Parents of proteinuric patients
Blood pressure in parents	146/86 (n = 17)	161/94[a] (n = 17)
Blood pressure in patients	125/82	135/87

[a] Significant increase.

TABLE 4. *Blood pressure (mmHg) prior to nephropathy*[a]

Group of patients	Normoalbuminuric controls (n = 58)	Patients with subsequent nephropathy (n = 58)
>10 years before proteinuria	125/79	124/78
6–10 years before proteinuria	127/80	130/85[b]
1–5 years before proteinuria	129/80	138/87[b]
At onset of proteinuria	131/80	140/90[b]

[a] Patients were studied at the Steno Hospital.
[b] Significant increase.

Still, it might be thought that proteinuric diabetics would show higher blood pressure values very early on, before the onset of clinical proteinuria or even before the onset of microalbuminuria. However, this is not the case, as documented by Jensen et al. (51). Blood pressure more than 10 years prior to nephropathy appeared to be very similar in proteinuric diabetics and their controls (Table 4). Only 6–10 years before the onset of proteinuria (i.e., in the period of time where microalbuminuria and incipient diabetic nephropathy prevails) did blood pressure appear to be slightly elevated, and it increased thereafter until the onset of proteinuria. These findings suggest that the increase in blood pressure is a consequence of renal abnormalities (or is parallel to renal changes) and is not the course prior to renal damage. On the other hand, increase in blood pressure may certainly accelerate development of diabetic nephropathy and glomerular hypertension, thus constituting an important aggravating factor in the progression of renal disease rather than being the initiating factor. Figures 2 and 3 summarize blood pressure levels in patients with increasing renal damage, as indicated by level of UAE.

Longitudinal studies (10,31) have shown that a considerable rise in blood pressure is seen in both incipient and overt diabetic nephropathy, with a rise in blood pressure of around 4% and 7% per year, respectively (Table 5). This rise is quite considerable and is also associated with progression of nephropathy (6,31). Blood pressure can readily be normalized by standard treatment (beta-blockers and diuretics), as shown in Table 5.

Quite interestingly, comparatively low blood pressure values are a very characteristic finding among long-term survivors of diabetes. Diastolic pressure in diabetic patients surviving more than 40 years of diabetes appeared to be significantly lower than that in a comparable Danish background population group (52,53) (Table 6).

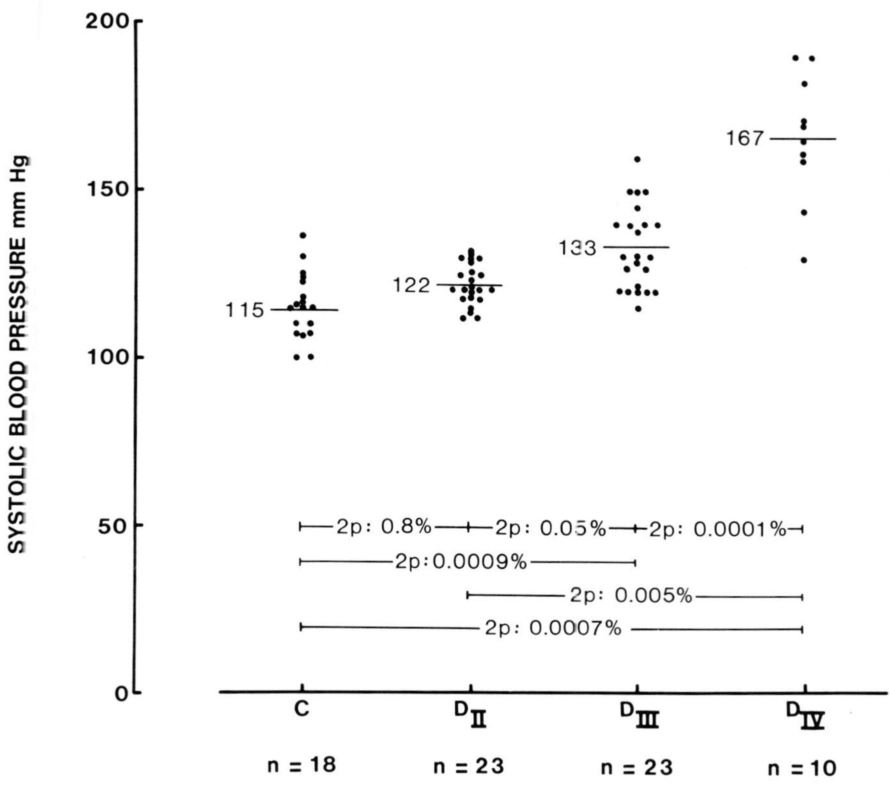

FIG. 2. Systolic blood pressure in IDDM patients with varying degrees of renal involvement. C, controls; D_{II}, normoalbuminuric patients; D_{III}, patients with incipient diabetic nephropathy; D_{IV}, patients with overt diabetic nephropathy.

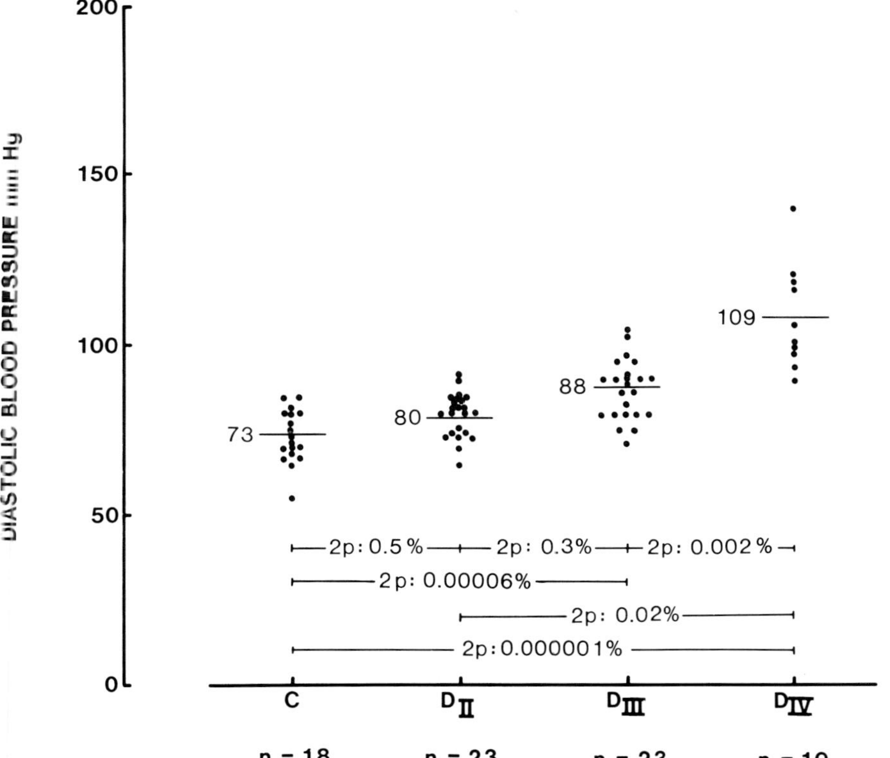

FIG. 3. Diastolic blood pressure in IDDM patients with varying degrees of renal involvement. C, controls; D_{II}, normoalbuminuric patients; D_{III}, patients with incipient diabetic nephropathy; D_{IV}, patients with overt diabetic nephropathy.

TABLE 5. *Rise in mean arterial blood pressure (mmHg) in a 2-year period, and reversal by standard antihypertensive treatment*

Group of patients	Normoalbuminuria	Micro/macroalbuminuria
Spontaneous rise in BP in incipient DN (Steno)	No change anticipated	128/82 to 133/90 (S)
Fall during AHT treatment (Aarhus)	—	135/93 to 122/79 (S)
Spontaneous rise in BP in overt DN (Hvidøre)	—	101 MAP to 115 MAP
Fall during AHT treatment (Hvidøre)	—	143/96 to 129/84 (S)

BP, blood pressure; DN, diabetic nephropathy; AHT, antihypertensive; MAP, mean arterial pressure; (S), significant change.

ESSENTIAL HYPERTENSION IN IDDM AS COMPARED WITH DIABETIC NEPHROPATHY

The data discussed above are very much in line with the study of Christensen et al. (54,55), which showed increasingly elevated blood pressure in incipient and overt diabetic nephropathy. Comparing blood pressure elevation and UAE rate, these authors were able to identify diabetic patients likely to have essential hypertension and diabetes (54), and not diabetic nephropathy with associated blood pressure increase (Figs. 4 and 5). Essential hypertension is probably much more common in NIDDM patients (13–16), but quantitative data are presently not available.

BLOOD PRESSURE ELEVATION AS AN AGGRAVATING FACTOR IN THE PROGRESSION OF NEPHROPATHY

The first study to quantify progression of diabetic nephropathy also observed a correlation with rate of progression, as measured by fall in GFR (ml/min/month) (6). Subsequently, such a correlation was further documented in other studies (55–57), including nondiabetic renal disease (7,8). In incipient diabetic nephropathy, too, progression is most rapid in those patients with the highest blood pressure or with the greatest increase in blood pressure (23,31). Figures 6 and 7 show increases in UAE rate in incipient diabetic nephropathy as a function of HbA_{1c} level and blood pressure increase. These early observations (6) appeared to be extremely important for therapy. Indeed, subsequent studies have shown that antihypertensive treatment delays the development of uremia in such patients (9,10).

TABLE 6. *Blood pressure and long-term survival*

Diabetes duration	*n*	Systolic	Diastolic
2–10 years	184	115 (75–190)	70 (40–110)
42–66 years (median age 60 years)	184	135 (100–190)	70 (50–110)
Nondiabetic controls (age 60 years)	665	136 (95–225)	85 (55–130)
		NS	$p < 0.001$

From ref. 53.

COMPARISON OF HYPERTENSION IN IDDM AND NIDDM PATIENTS

The major part of this chapter deals with data from patients with IDDM because most studies on hypertension have been carried out in patients with insulin-dependent diabetes. However, there also appears to be an increased prevalence of hypertension among NIDDM patients (13–16), and, indeed, raised blood pressure may be found at the time diabetes is detected (14–16). The genesis of blood pressure elevation in NIDDM is not well understood, although sodium retention and exaggerated pressure response to norepinephrine and angiotensin II probably play a role (58,59). It is likely that a variety of causes operate, including obesity, coexistent essential hypertension (which is more prominent in patients in older age), and, of course, diabetic nephropathy and other glomerulopathies. It has also been proposed that hyperinsulinism may play a role in the genesis of hypertension in NIDDM patients (46,47); hyperinsulinism may also play a role in patients with IDDM diabetes resulting from administration of large doses of insulin injected subcutaneously and not via the physiologic route with intraportal delivery. Interestingly, insulin resistance may be found in nondiabetics with essential hypertension, correlated to severity of hypertension (60).

The management of hypertension in NIDDM patients does not differ from that in IDDM patients, although of course one would accept a higher blood pressure level in these patients than in the young patients with insulin-dependent diabetes. Of course, NIDDM patients with newly diagnosed diabetes may show glucose intolerance (i.e., low-serum-potassium-induced glucose intolerance or even diabetes) resulting from diuretic administration.

PATHOGENESIS OF HYPERTENSION IN DIABETES, AND ITS RELATIONSHIP TO TREATMENT MODALITIES (ESPECIALLY EARLY IN THE COURSE OF DIABETES)

The pathophysiologic background for development of hypertension in diabetic patients is incompletely understood, although renal involvement is a major determinant (61–63), at least in insulin-dependent patients. A detailed discussion is given in chapter 105. Which structural lesions

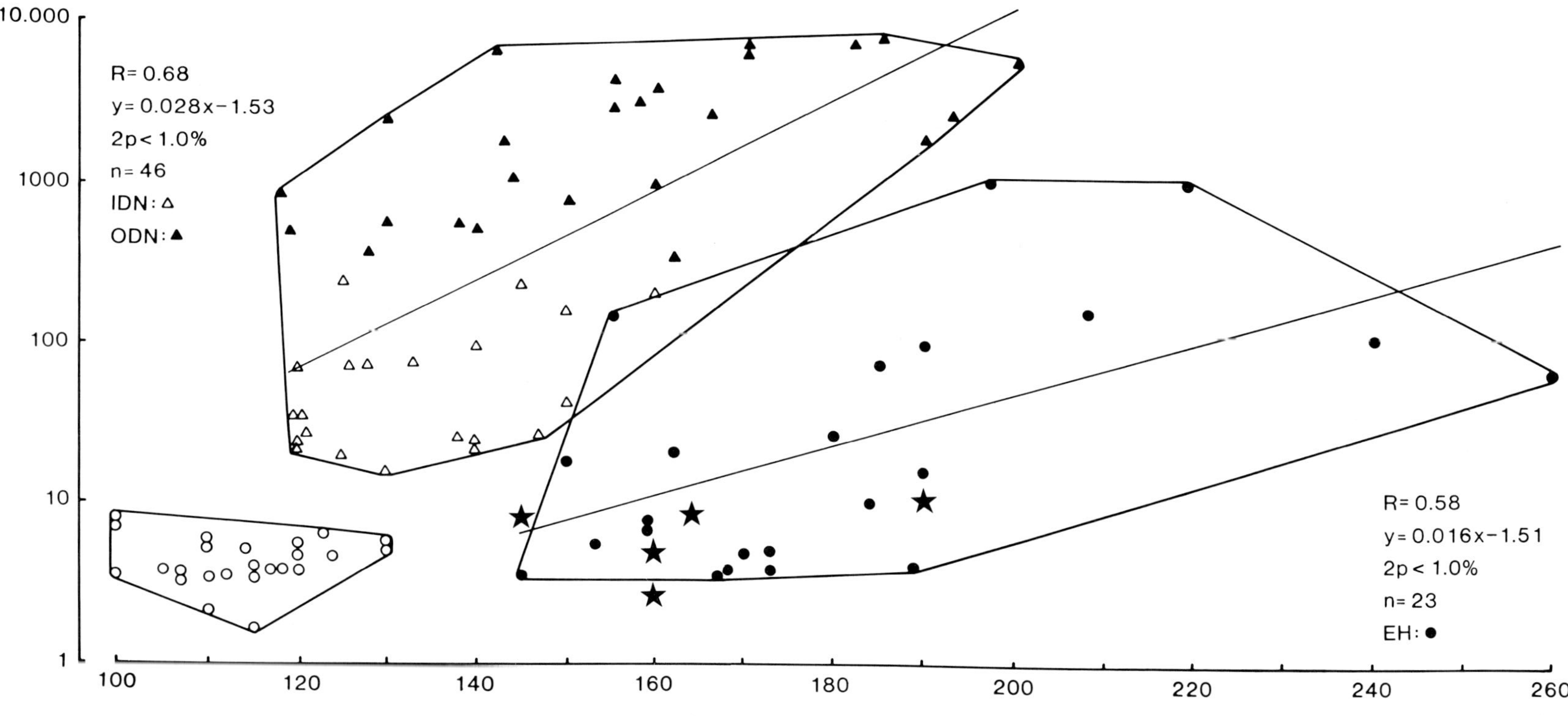

FIG. 4. Correlation between systolic blood pressure and urinary albumin excretion in: diabetic patients with incipient diabetic nephropathy (IDN) (△, $n = 21$) and overt diabetic nephropathy (ODN) (▲, $n = 25$); patients with essential hypertension (EH) (●, $n = 23$); healthy controls (○, $n = 24$); and diabetics with essential hypertension (★, $n = 5$).

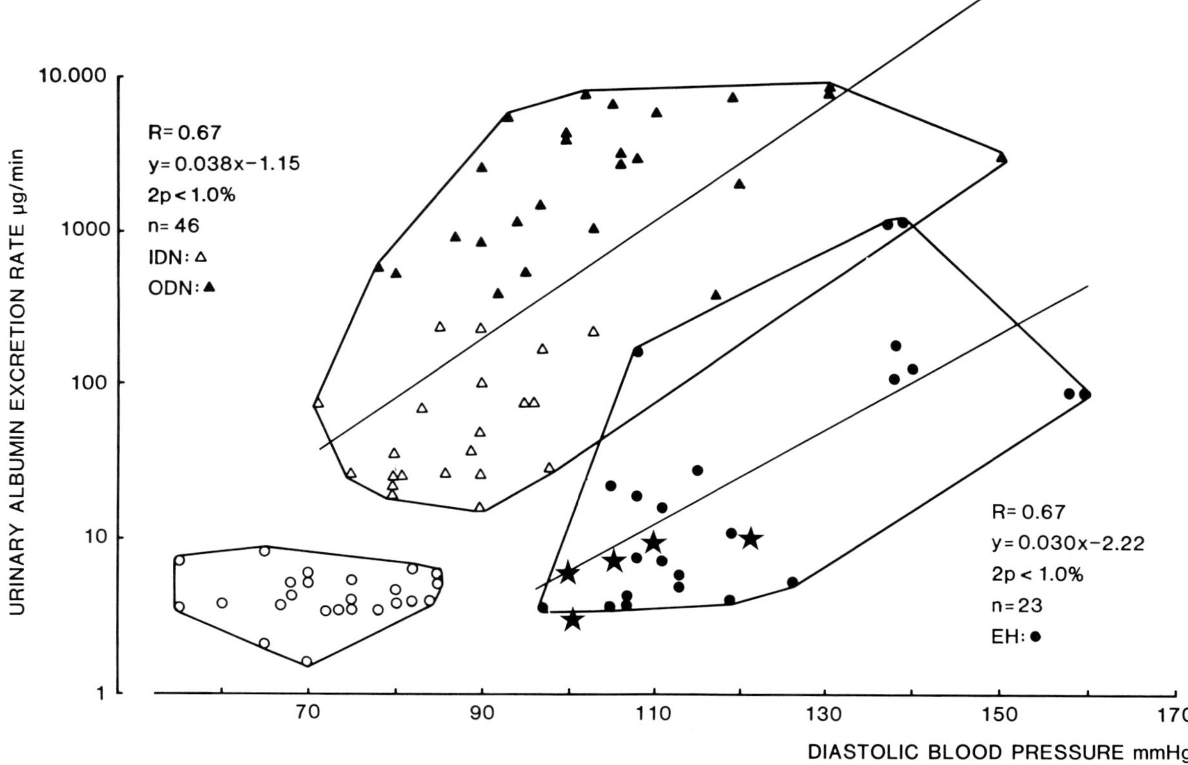

FIG. 5. Correlation between diastolic blood pressure and urinary albumin excretion in: diabetic patients with incipient diabetic nephropathy (IDN) (△, n = 21) and overt diabetic nephropathy (ODN) (▲, n = 25); patients with essential hypertension (EH) (●, n = 23); healthy controls (○, n = 24); and diabetics with essential hypertension (★, n = 5).

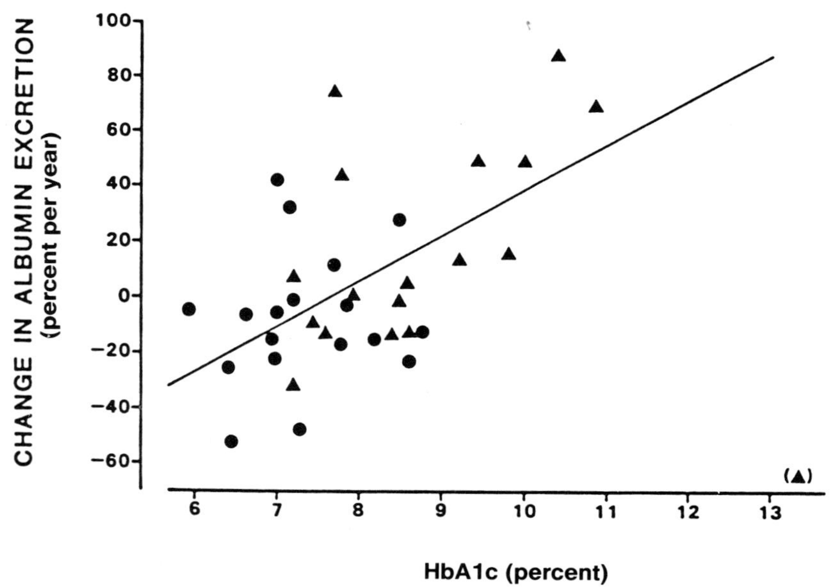

FIG. 6. Steno Study II. Yearly change in urinary albumin excretion rate (percent per year) as a function of glycated hemoglobin (HbA_{1c}) in a 2-year follow-up study. (▲) Conventional treatment; (●) insulin pump treatment. (From ref. 31, with permission.)

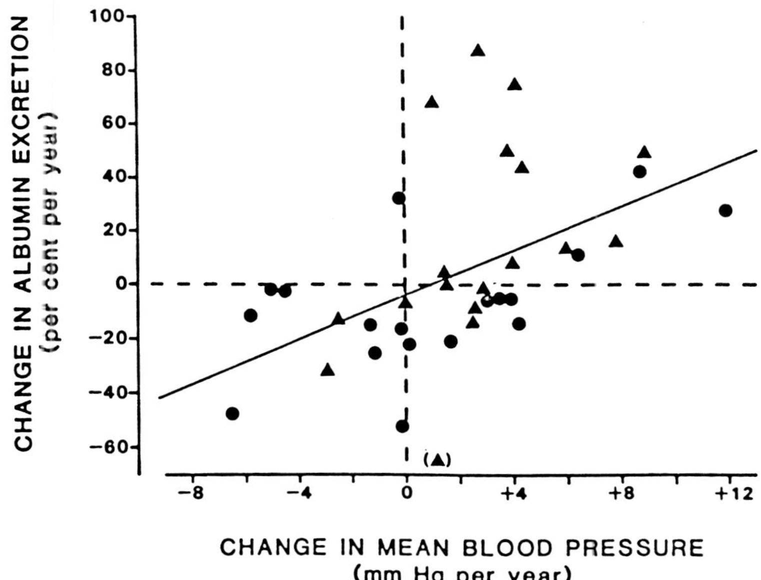

FIG. 7. Yearly change in urinary albumin excretion rate (percent per year) as a function of change in mean arterial blood pressure in a 2-year follow-up study in a patient with incipient diabetic nephropathy. (▲) Conventional treatment; (●) insulin pump treatment. (From ref. 31, with permission.)

in the glomeruli are responsible for the high blood pressure is not clear. However, mesangial expansion seems to be closely associated with elevated blood pressure (64), and it is also possible that structural lesions in both the afferent and efferent glomerular vessels play a role (24,37). Microscopic lesions in the glomerulus, of both diffuse and nodular nature, are also characteristic of hypertensive diabetes (24,65).

Sodium retention seems to be important in the genesis of hypertension in diabetes, particularly in patients with proteinuria and severe urinary protein loss but also in nonazotemic patients (58) and in microalbuminuric patients (45). Surprisingly, exchangeable sodium also showed rather high values in uncomplicated diabetes, and an abnormal UAE rate may disclose a susceptibility factor toward elevation of blood pressure and nephropathy. In this study on sodium retention (45), the blood values of aldosterone, angiotensin II and catecholamines were suppressed in patients with the early rise in blood pressure, associated with diabetic renal disease. Renal arterial stenosis does not seem not to be more frequent in diabetics as compared with nondiabetics (66). Abnormal increases in blood pressure are seen during physical exercise (28,67).

These mechanisms may be important from a therapeutic point of view. If sodium retention is involved in the pathogenesis of raised blood pressure, diuretic therapy would be indicated. The abnormal renal pathophysiologic pattern in diabetes suggests that angiotensin-converting enzyme (ACE) inhibitors might be important agents in treatment modality. Beta-blockers may also be effective by reducing cardiac output, which can even be elevated in patients with early microalbuminuria (42).

WHAT IS GOOD GLYCEMIC CONTROL, AND WHAT IS ITS IMPORTANCE FOR PROGRESSION OF RENAL DISEASE IN COMPARISON WITH ANTIHYPERTENSIVE TREATMENT?

Although this chapter deals with management of hypertension in diabetes, it is important also to briefly discuss glycemic control. There is presently no evidence that glycemic indices need to be totally normalized in order to avoid late microvascular complications such as nephropathy. If reliable and specific methods are used (e.g., high-pressure liquid chromatography procedures), the reference glycated hemoglobin is at a mean value of 5.5%, with a standard deviation of 0.5 and a range from approximately 4.4 to 6.4; these reference values are found in most centers. Increasing evidence suggests that risk of nephropathy or progression of nephropathy is low, provided that glycemic control corresponds to a HbA_{1c} level of less than 7.5–8%, that is, 4 standard deviation units above the mean reference for HbA_{1c} (4,68). These figures are valid, provided that the glycated hemoglobin was measured by specific methods. It should be pointed out that there is still some skepticism regarding the role of improved metabolic control in preventing the development of vascular lesions, especially in the United States (69); a large trial is still in progress and will continue for many years (70).

The relative importance of improved glycemic control and effective antihypertensive treatment remains poorly defined (4). However, an important clinical fact is that it is usually much easier to reduce blood pressure effectively (often with an immediate effect on renal function) than to obtain sufficiently good metabolic control ($HbA_{1c} \leq 7.5\%$) on a long-term or even lifelong basis. Antihypertensive treatment is most important when incipient and overt nephropathy are developing, although in the future it may be used much earlier (71,72).

CLINICAL INTERVENTION TRIALS, WITH SPECIAL REFERENCE TO ANTIHYPERTENSIVE TREATMENT

A number of review articles on different intervention modalities are available (4,11,68–70,73–75). This is a rapidly expanding area, and new large studies are in progress [e.g., the large DCCT trial (69,70) and the British multicenter microalbuminuria trial (35), both aiming at better metabolic control]. Large multicenter trials of antihypertensive treatment [e.g., those including ACE inhibitors] are also in progress. Table 7 shows an outline of the natural history of diabetic nephropathy, including a summary of results of (a) already-published clinical trials within the area of intensified insulin treatment, (b) blood pressure intervention, and (c) trials with low-protein diet. Antihypertensive treatment cannot be considered isolated but has to be considered in conjunction with other intervention modalities. In this context, however, only antihypertensive trials will be considered.

When incipient diabetic nephropathy is developing, elevation of blood pressure becomes important, and, indeed, studies suggest that rate of progression of renal disease is associated with blood pressure elevation as well as with metabolic control (Figs. 6 and 7). Therefore, antihypertensive treatment is an important area of intervention in these patients. Tables 8 and 9 summarize results of new intervention trials. Blood pressure is not elevated in patients with normal UAE rates, or, rather, not more so than in nondiabetic populations. However, treatment with ACE inhibitors may be interesting, because renal hemodynamics may be altered by these agents. Indeed, a new 3-month intervention study reports that fractional albumin clearance and filtration fraction can be reduced by ACE inhibition in such patients (71). These findings are compatible with the idea that filtration pressure can be reduced by ACE inhibition in these patients, as would be expected. The authors also conclude that treatment with an ACE inhibitor in normoalbuminuric diabetics, with the perspective of preventing overt diabetic nephropathy, cannot of course, be recommended at the present time. We have to await results of very-long-term trials in such patients, and such trials are not even planned.

In patients with persistent microalbuminuria and normal or borderline elevation of blood pressure, ACE inhibition in a 12-month study was shown to reduce microalbuminuria, whereas microalbuminuria continued to increase in the control group (76). Glomerular filtration rate (GFR) increased by active treatment. In a 10-year follow-up study in patients with microalbuminuria, a reversal of the increase in microalbuminuria was seen in the 5-year treatment period in these patients, again underlining the important role of antihypertensive treatment (Fig. 8). In this study a combination of cardioselective beta-blockers and diuretics was used (77). Exercise-induced changes in blood pressure can also be normalized by beta-blocking therapy (Fig. 9A and B) (72).

In patients with overt diabetic nephropathy it has been shown that conventional treatment with cardioselective beta-blockers and diuretics—in some cases, supplemented with vasodilators—induces a dramatic reduction in the progression of nephropathy (10) in accordance with the original observation made some years ago (9) (Fig. 10). Indeed, the new, long-term follow-up study of Parving et al. (10) suggests that progression is very slow in diabetics on long-term antihypertensive treatment (Fig. 11 and Table 10). Björck et al. were able to show that addition of ACE inhibitors to other antihypertensive agents was able to slow down the progression of diabetic nephropathy (78). Proteinuria can also be considerably reduced with this treatment modality, along with extracellular volume reduction (79). At the present time it may be concluded that cardioselective beta-blockers and ACE inhibitors, both most often combined with diuretics, are useful in slowing down the progression of renal disease in diabetic patients with overt nephropathy. Triple treatment may also be useful (4). In most studies, patients were included irrespective of the blood pressure level. Rate of progression was reduced considerably when mean blood pressure during intervention was reduced to a level of around 135/85.

DIAGNOSIS AND TREATMENT OF HYPERTENSION IN DIABETES

As in the management of patients with essential hypertension, it is important to have an established program in the evaluation of patients with hypertension in diabetes. Throughout the course of their disease, patients with diabetes should be regularly checked for development of hypertension and should also undergo evaluation of renal function (e.g., by yearly measurement of UAE and blood pressure). Blood pressure elevation usually develops very slowly, and with such a program there are seldom urgent problems; repeated measurement can easily be done before treatment is required.

Evaluation Before Pharmacologic Treatment

Table 11 outlines a diagnosis and treatment program. Before treatment, the following points are to be clarified: (a) What is the exact level of blood pressure at repeated measurements? It is extremely important that over a period of time (e.g., 3 months) a number of measurements of blood pressure are done (three to six) under peaceful circumstances, to avoid overtreatment. (b) What is the underlying cause of hypertension? (Secondary causes should be excluded, preferably on the basis of simple clinical and laboratory examination.) (c) Are there contributory or modulating factors present, such as high salt intake, heavy smoking, or a stressful lifestyle? (d) What is the extent of damage to the kidneys, eyes, heart, and peripheral vessels? General measures should be taken, such as encouraging weight loss, modifying smoking habits, reducing salt intake, altering a stressful lifestyle, and encouraging the best possible control of diabetes, including modern dietary treatment.

Antihypertensive Effect of Diabetic Diets

A modern diabetes diet with low-fat, high-carbohydrate, and moderately low-protein content plus reduced sodium content has been shown to lower blood pressure in diabetic patients with moderate levels of hypertension (80). The effect of diet was, in fact, comparable to the effect of thiazide diuretics or a cardioselective beta-blocking agent. No control group without treatment was included (Table 12). The dietary treatment was associated with a fall in (a) glycated hemoglobin, (b) serum triglyceride, and (c) body weight. On the other hand, treatment with diuretics in-

TABLE 7. *Natural history of renal functional changes and nephropathy in insulin-dependent diabetes in the situation without intervention*[a]

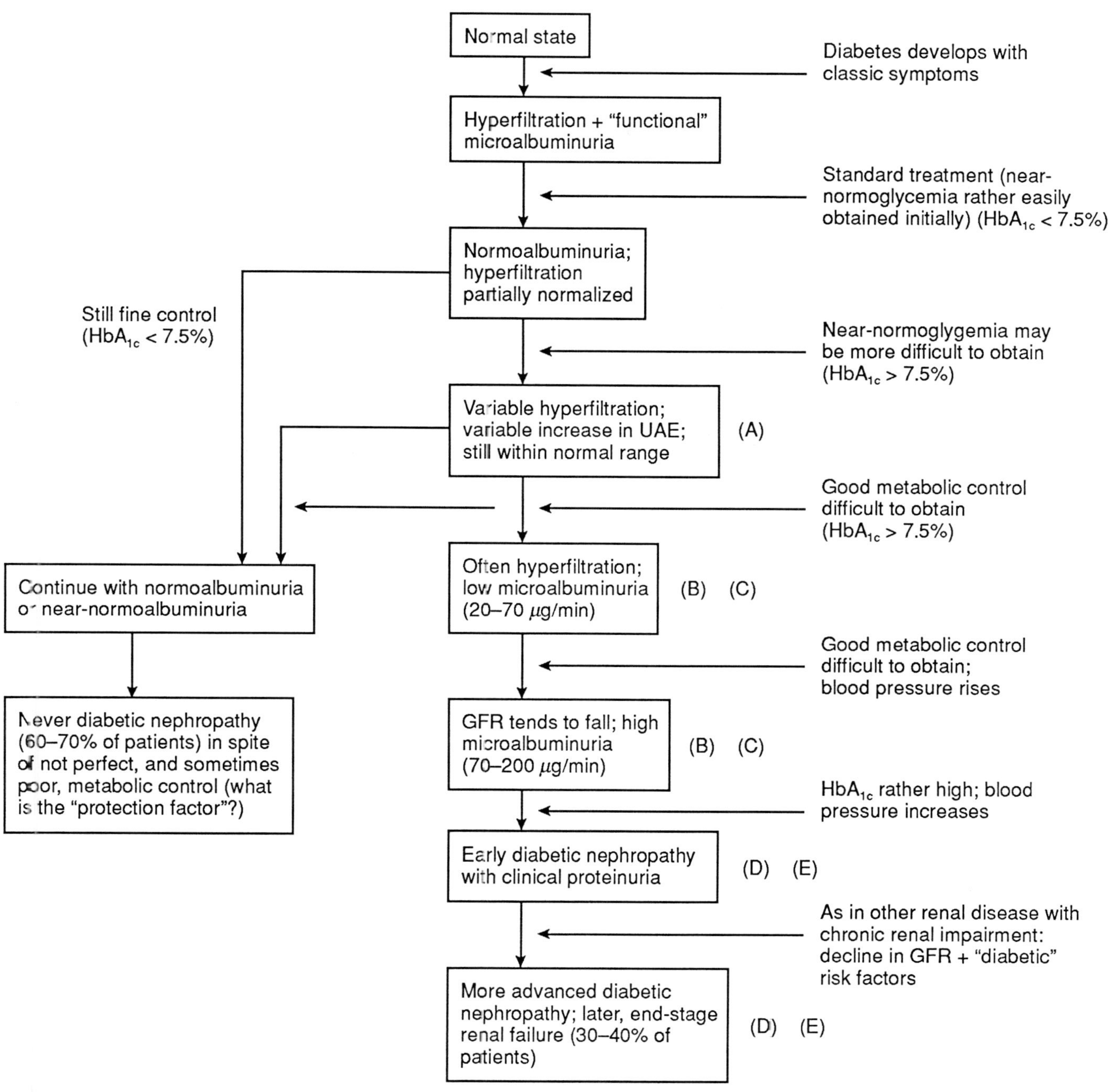

Trials already undertaken:

(A) "High-normal" UAE and hyperfiltration relatively normalized
(B) Microalbuminuria reduced or stabilized by insulin pump treatment
(C) Microalbuminuria reduced by antihypertensive treatment
(D) Proteinuria and rate of decline in GFR reduced by antihypertensive treatment
(E) Proteinuria and possibly rate of decline in GFR reduced by low-protein diet

[a] Adapted from ref. 4. UAE, urinary albumin excretion; GFR, glomerular filtration rate.

TABLE 8. *Effect of long-term antihypertensive treatment on progression of DN (not ACE inhibition)[a]*

	UAE	GFR	Blood pressure
Normoalbuminuria	No study	No study	(In acute studies: reduction of exercise-induced BP increase)
Microalbuminuria (IDN)	↓; 20% reduction per year	Small fall	Relative normalization
Overt nephropathy	↓	Fall rate reduced by 60%	Relative normalization

[a] DN, diabetic nephropathy; ACE, angiotensin-converting enzyme; UAE, urinary albumin excretion; GFR, glomerular filtration rate; BP, blood pressure; IDN, incipient diabetic nephropathy; ↓, decrease.

TABLE 9. *Effect of long-term antihypertensive treatment on progression of DN (ACE inhibition alone, or combined with other antihypertensive agents)[a]*

	UAE	GFR/FF	Blood pressure
Normoalbuminuria	↓	FF: ↓	—
Microalbuminuria (IDN)	↓	GFR: —/↑	↓ or —
Overt nephropathy	↓	Fall rate of GFR reduced	↓ or —

[a] DN, diabetic nephropathy; ACE, angiotensin-converting enzyme; UAE, urinary albumin excretion; FF, filtration fraction; IDN, incipient diabetic nephropathy; ↓, decrease; ↑, increase; —, no change.

creased glycated hemoglobin values, but no change was seen with metropolol. Therefore, modern diabetes diets should be included in all treatment programs; patients should, of course, be put on such diets immediately following the diagnosis of diabetes. The preventative effect of such diets is unknown. So far, the effect of a diabetes diet on blood pressure has been shown only by Dodson et al. (80).

A low-protein diet may be of special value in diabetic patients with incipient and overt nephropathy, owing to a reduction in microalbuminuria, proteinuria, and, possibly, rate of decline in GFR (74,75). Blood pressure is generally not changed by the low-protein diet.

Pharmacologic Treatment of Hypertension in Diabetes with the Use of Specific Antihypertensive Agents: Advantages and Disadvantages

It is usually possible to control hypertension in diabetic patients with relatively few agents (three or four); and a

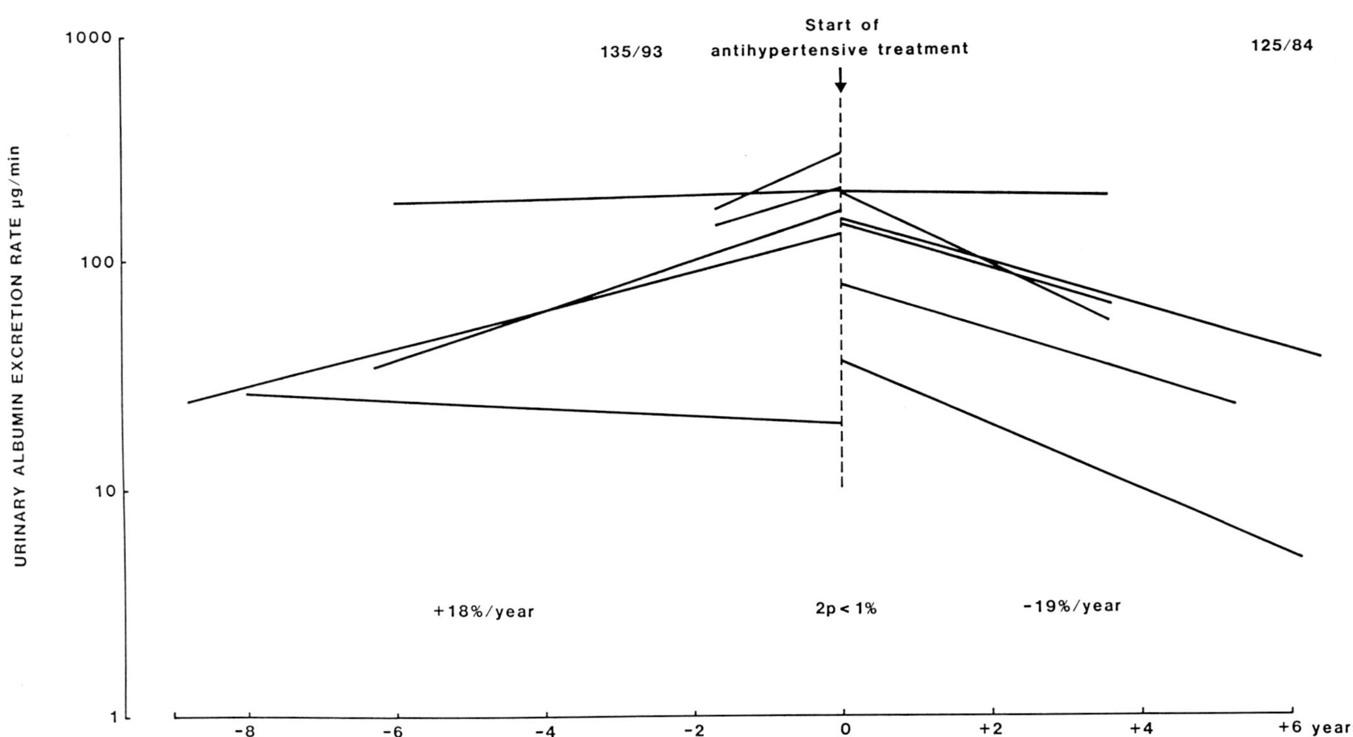

FIG. 8. Urinary albumin excretion rate in the course of incipient diabetic nephropathy prior to, as well as during, antihypertensive treatment in six patients. A significant reduction in blood pressure is found, along with a reduction in urinary albumin excretion rate.

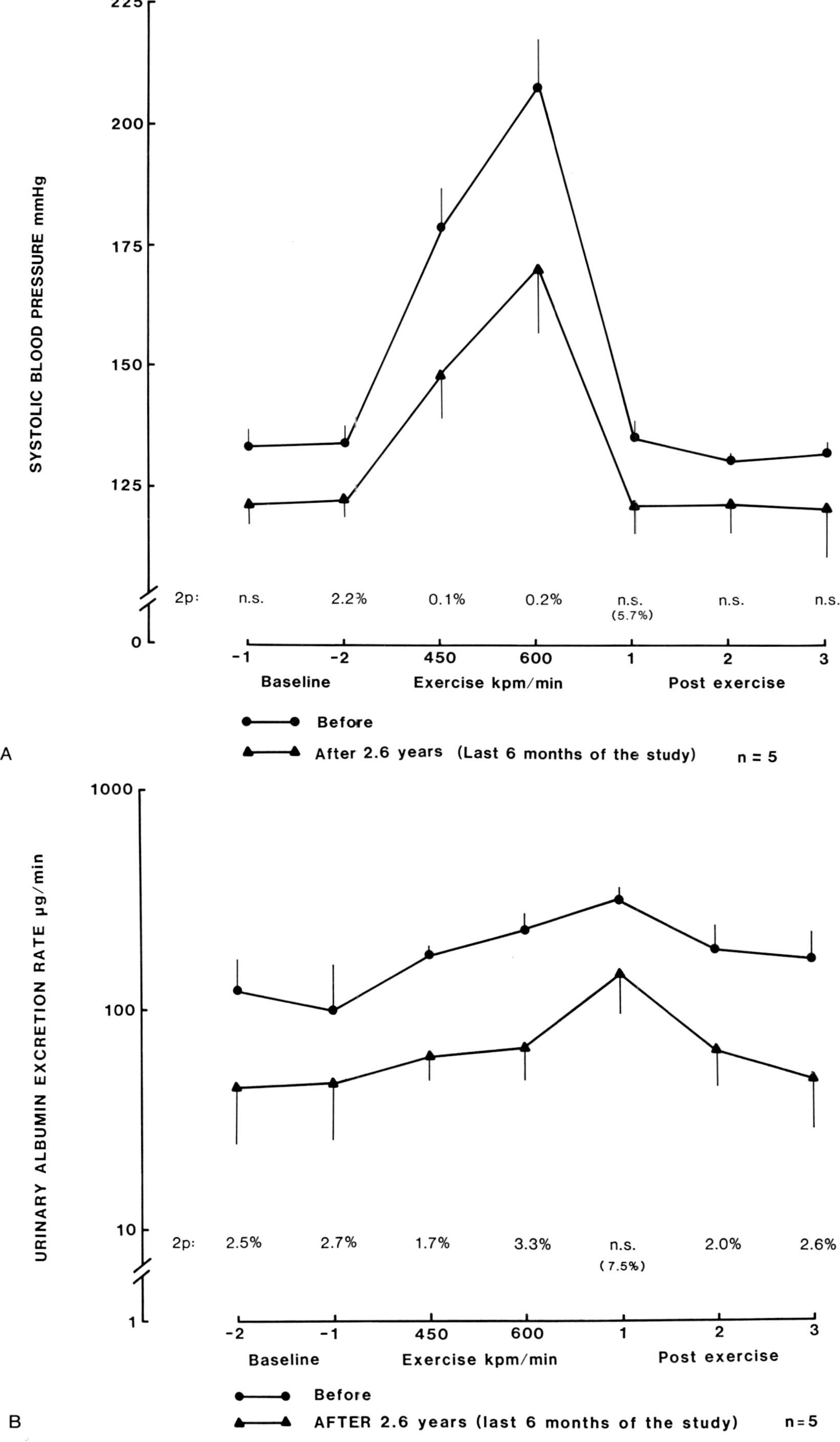

FIG. 9. Increase in systolic blood pressure (**A**) and in urinary albumin excretion rate (**B**) during physical exercise in IDDM patients (n = 5) prior to, as well as 2.6 ± 1.0 (SD) years after, antihypertensive treatment. (●) Before; (▲) after 2.6 years (last 6 months of the study).

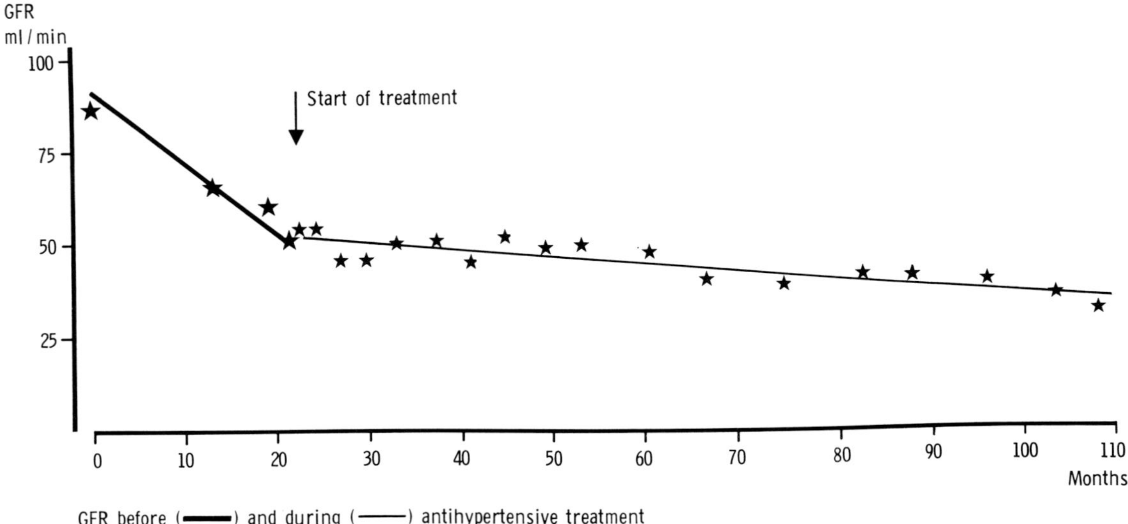

FIG. 10. Glomerular filtration rate (GFR) before (▬) and during (—) antihypertensive treatment in a patient with overt diabetic nephropathy. The patient was treated with cardioselective beta-blockers combined with diuretics and vasodilators. (From ref. 6, with permission.)

simple, conventional scheme of antihypertensive treatment, with some modification, should be used. Treatment may be started with either beta-blockers, diuretics, or ACE inhibitors. Only limited experience is available with calcium antagonists; however, in the case of impaired peripheral circulation, they may be advantageous, especially in NIDDM patients. Cardioselective beta-blockers, in contrast to nonselective blockers, should strongly be recommended, since problems with hypoglycemic unawareness seldom occur with these agents, provided that a moderate dosage is used. Masking of hypoglycemia is occasionally found in propranolol-treated patients, and this drug should be avoided. The relative safety of cardioselective beta-blockers in diabetics has recently been further established, at least when used in moderate dosages (9,10,81). However, some patients still experience problems with hypoglycemic unawareness, and also with selective blockers, and it may be necessary to reduce the dosage or discontinue the drug. When diuretics are used in the treatment of diabetic patients, one should bear in mind the possible aggravation of the diabetic state in non-insulin-dependent patients (82). This may be related to potassium loss, and therefore serum potassium should be monitored regularly along with evaluation of kidney function and clinical status. In diabetic nephropathy, loop diuretics (often in high dosages) are useful for eliminating edema as well as for reduction of blood pressure. Subsequently, vasodilators such as hydralazine or prazosin have been used widely; with these programs a fair reduction in blood pressure may be obtained, although normalization is not always achieved.

ACE inhibitors are likely to prove very useful in diabetics (76,78,79,83–86), even after many years of treatment with other agents (78). ACE inhibitors may be used as first-line drugs, often along with diuretics. The arguments for the use of ACE inhibitors are twofold. First of all, they seem to be free of diabetes-related side effects. Secondly, their administration is likely to reduce intraglomerular pressure, perhaps more so than the agents mentioned above. ACE inhibition may be used in conjunction with cardioselective beta-blockers and diuretics, and with calcium antagonists. A considerable reduction in blood pressure is usually seen with such a combination.

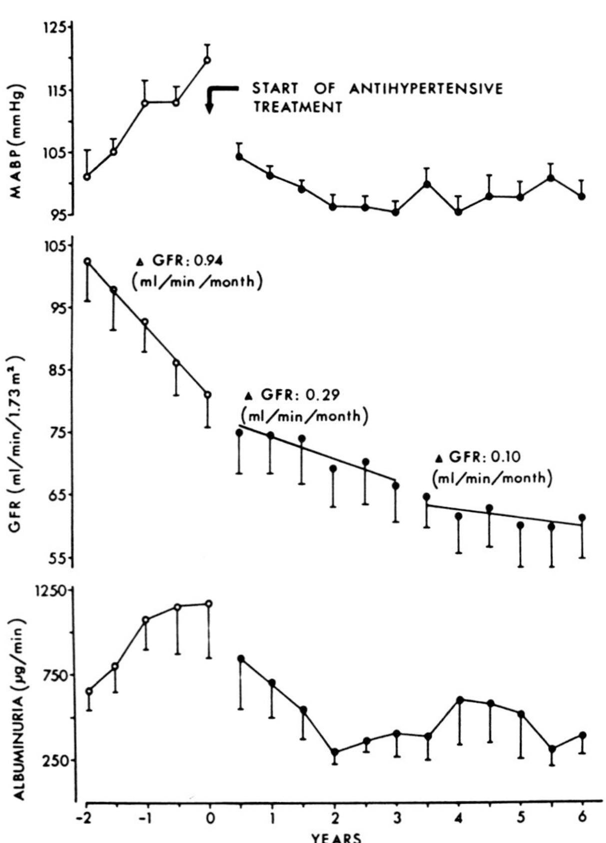

FIG. 11. Average course of mean arterial blood pressure (MABP), glomerular filtration rate (GFR), and albuminuria before (○) and during (●) long-term effective antihypertensive treatment of nine insulin-dependent diabetic patients who had nephropathy. (From ref. 10, with permission.)

TABLE 10. *Effect of antihypertensive treatment on blood pressure and renal function in diabetic nephropathy*

Authors (reference)	Treatment	Number of subjects	Age (years)	Duration of diabetes (years)	Observation period (months)	Glomerular filtration rate before treatment (ml/min)	Blood pressure before and during treatment (mmHg)	Decrease in glomerular filtration rate (ml/min/month)	Albumin excretion (yearly increase)
Mogensen (9)	Before treatment	6	30	18	28	86	162/103	1.23	107%
	During treatment	6	30	18	73		144/95	0.49	5%
Parving et al. (10)	Before treatment	11	29	16	32	80	143/96	0.89	Further increase
	During treatment	11	29	16	72		124/84	0.22	Reversed

Table 13 provides an outline of side effects during antihypertensive treatment which are specifically relevant for diabetic patients.

Overtreatment

It is a general problem within the field of hypertension that too many patients are undergoing treatment, even though many do not actually need it. This may also be a problem in diabetes. With the above program, overtreatment should not take place. It is of special importance to measure blood pressure repeatedly before the start of treatment. Also, it should be borne in mind that antihypertensive treatment (e.g., with ACE inhibitors) has no indication in normoalbuminuric normotensive diabetics, with a perspective of prevention of late nephropathy. There are no studies to document such a possible beneficial effect, and of course it is not permissible to extrapolate from studies on animals with experimental diabetes to human diabetes. Although it has been shown that ACE inhibition can prevent structural lesions and proteinuria in diabetic rats, such studies do not, by any means, support the idea of preventative treatment with ACE inhibition in normoalbuminuric and normotensive diabetic patients.

Special Problems

Special problems may arise in evaluation of patients with isolated systolic hypertension. No interventional studies regarding isolated systolic hypertension in diabetic patients are available; therefore, indications for treatment as advocated for nondiabetic patients with isolated elevated systolic blood pressure may be recommended.

The problem with increased supine blood pressure and postural hypotension presents a complicated situation, which may be present in some diabetic patients, especially if the patient shows autonomic diabetic neuropathy and advanced long-term diabetic lesions in general. Treatment in such a patient is difficult, and medication as outlined above must be adjusted to what can be tolerated by the patient. Today, there is no specific choice of drugs, but the general proposals as outlined in Table 11 may be explored, possibly with ACE inhibitors as the first choice, along with diuretics.

What Is the Optimal Blood Pressure Level During Treatment?

The optimal blood pressure level during antihypertensive treatment in patients with diabetic nephropathy is not clearly defined. Rate of fall in GFR and blood pressure level during antihypertensive treatment is shown in Table 10 (9,10). The smallest decline in renal function is found in patients with blood pressure levels around 130/85, a level also easily obtainable during treatment in incipient diabetic nephropathy, before the decline in GFR has started (76,77). As a practical guideline it is therefore proposed that in patients below the age of 45, blood pressure during antihypertensive treatment should be reduced to 120–140/75–90. Too low a pressure (e.g., 110/65–70 mmHg) is not advisable, since GFR may be reduced (while UAE may be increased) by such an aggressive reduction of blood pressure resulting in renal ischemia.

MORTALITY IN IDDM PATIENTS AFTER IMPLEMENTATION OF SYSTEMATIC ANTIHYPERTENSIVE TREATMENT PROGRAMS

Mortality rates in the first 6–8 years after the appearance of proteinuria have been reduced considerably, as shown in Table 14. These patients did not develop end-stage renal failure. The reduction in mortality in these patients as compared with that in historical controls is closely related to (a) the implementation of screening for hypertension and (b) subsequent effective and systematic antihypertensive treatment in these patients, as earlier outlined (9). Other factors may also be involved, but modality of diabetes treatment (diet and insulin) has not changed radically in these patients. In addition, control in patients with nephropathy is usually not very satisfactory, with mean values of HbA_{1c} ranging from 9.5% to 10%.

TABLE 11. *Diabetes and hypertension: evaluation and treatment program*[a]

I. Evaluation:

Elevated casual blood pressure (for patients aged less than 40–45 years, BP > 140/90 mmHg) →	Observation, measurement of UAE; repeated measurements of BP and UAE under peaceful circumstances (possibly at hospital) →	Consider screening for secondary hypertension; evaluation of renal function

II. No pharmacologic intervention

	Relative normalization, <140/90 If not, continue program	Relative normalization, <140/90 If not, pharmacologic intervention (step III)
Still high blood pressure. Information on the nature of elevated BP ("Blood Pressure School") observation →	Ensure modern dietary treatment of diabetes (low-fat diet, high amount of complex carbohydrate). Low salt intake and good diabetes control. →	Weight reduction; reduced smoking; alter stressful lifestyle; no heavy exercise

III. Pharmacologic intervention:
If no satisfactory decrease, continue program

	Relative normalization, <140/90 If not, continue program	Relative normalization, <140/90 If not, go to step IV

Alternatives:

Diuretics →	+ Cardioselective β-blockers/ ACE inhibitors →	+ ACE inhibitors/ cardioselective β-blockers
Cardioselective β-blockers/ ACE inhibitor →	Diuretics (in case of impaired renal function, use loop diuretics) →	+ ACE inhibitors/ cardioselective β-blockers
Calcium antagonists (e.g., if contraindication against β-blocker) →	+ Diuretics →	+ ACE inhibitors

IV. No or insufficient effect:

BP > 140–160/90–95

Consider compliance (does the patient actually take the drugs?) →	Reevaluation of genesis of hypertension →	If renal function is stable, accept slight elevation of BP on diuretics + cardioselective β-blockers + ACE inhibitors (treat until one has unacceptable side effects); other drugs are not likely to be more effective without side effects

[a] UAE, urinary albumin excretion; BP, blood pressure; ACE, angiotensin-converting enzyme.

70. The DCCT Research Group. Are continuing studies of metabolic control and microvascular complications in insulin-dependent diabetes justified? *N Engl J Med* 1988;318:246–250.

71. Pedersen MM, Schmitz A, Pedersen EB, Christiansen JS. Acute and long-term renal effects of angiotensin converting enzyme inhibition in normotensive, normoalbuminuric insulin-dependent diabetics. *Diabetic Medicine* 1988;5:562–569.

72. Christensen CK, Mogensen CE. Acute and long-term effect of antihypertensive treatment on exercise-induced albuminuria in incipient diabetic nephropathy. *Scand J Clin Lab Invest* 1986;46:553–559.

73. Dahl-Jørgensen K. Near-normoglycemia and late diabetic complications. The Oslo study. *Acta Endocrinol (Copenh)* 1987; 114(Suppl 284):1–38.

74. Wiseman MJ, Dodds R, Bending JJ, Viberti GC. Dietary protein and the diabetic kidney. *Diabetic Med* 1987;4:144–146.

75. Viberti GC, Dodds RA, Bending JJ, Bognetti E. Nonglycemic intervention in diabetic nephropathy: the role of dietary protein intake. In: Mogensen CE, ed. *The kidney and hypertension in diabetes mellitus.* Boston: Martinus Nijhoff, 1988;205–216.

76. Marre M, Chatellier G, Leblanc H, Guyenne T-T, Ménard J, Passa P. Prevention of diabetic nephropathy with enalapril in normotensive diabetics with microalbuminuria. *Br Med J* 1988; 297:1092–1095.

77. Christensen CK, Mogensen CE. Antihypertensive treatment: long-term reversal of progression of albuminuria in incipient diabetic nephropathy. A longitudinal study of renal function. *J Diabetic Complications* 1987;1:45–52.

78. Björck S, Nyberg G, Mulec H, Granerus G, Herlitz H, Aurell M. Beneficial effects of angiotensin converting enzyme inhibition on renal function in patients with diabetic nephropathy. *Br Med J* 1986;293:471–474.

79. Hommel E, Parving H-H, Mathiesen E, Edsberg B, Damkjær Nielsen M, Giese J. Effect of captopril on kidney function in insulin-dependent diabetic patients with nephropathy. *Br Med J* 1986;293:467–470.

80. Dodson PM, Pacy PJ, Ball P, Kuniki AJ, Fletcher RF, Taylor KG. A controlled trial of a high-fibre, low-fat and low-sodium diet for mild hypertension in type II (non-insulin-dependent) diabetic patients. *Diabetologia* 1984;27:522–526.

81. Kølendorf K, Bonnevie-Nielsen V, Borch-Møller B. A trial of metoprolol in hypertensive insulin-dependent diabetic patients. *Acta Med Scand* 1982;211:175–178.

82. Struthers AD, Murphy MB, Dollery CT. Glucose tolerance during antihypertensive therapy in patients with diabetes mellitus. *Hypertension* 1985;7(Suppl II):II-95–II-101.

83. Gambaro G, Morbiato F, Cicerello E, Del Turco, Sartori L, D'Angelo A, Crepaldi G. Captopril in the treatment of hypertension in type I and type II diabetic patients. *J Hypertens* 1985;3(Suppl 2):149–151.

84. Parving HH, Hommel E, Smidt UM. Protection of kidney function and decrease in albuminuria by captopril in insulin dependent diabetics with nephropathy. *Br Med J* 1988;297:1086–1091.

85. Kisch ES. Captopril and proteinuria in diabetes mellitus. *Isr J Med Sci* 1987;23:833–834.

86. Christensen CK, Pedersen MM, Mogensen CE. Long-term effect of ACE-inhibition on albumin excretion (UAE), blood pressure and renal hemodynamics in type 1 IDDM patients with early diabetic nephropathy, already treated with selective beta-blocker and diuretics [Abstract]. Second International Symposium on Hypertension Associated with Diabetes Mellitus (Passa P, ed). 1988;19.

87. Goldstein DE, Little RR, Wiedmeyer H-M, England JD, McKenzie EM. Glycated hemoglobin: methodologies and clinical applications. *Clin Chem* 1986;32:B64–B70.

88. Ellis G, Diamandis EP, Giesbrecht EE, Daneman D, Allen LC. An automated "high-pressure" liquid-chromatographic assay for hemoglobin A1c. *Clin Chem* 1984;30:1746–1752.

89. Jarrett RJ, Keen H. Hyperglycaemia and diabetes mellitus. *Lancet* 1976;II:1009–1012.

90. Svendsen PAA, Jørgensen J, Nerup J. HbA_{1c} and the diagnosis of diabetes mellitus. *Acta Med Scand* 1981;210:313–317.

91. Nyberg G, Nordén G, Attman P-O, Aurell M, Uddebom G, Lenner RA, Isaksson B. Diabetic nephropathy: is dietary protein harmful? *J Diabetic Complications* 1987;1:37–40.

92. Dodson PM, Pacy PJ. The effect of diet on blood pressure in hypertensive type II diabetic patients. *Diabetic Nephropathy* 1985;4:43–45.

Hypertension: Pathophysiology, Diagnosis, and Management, edited by J. H. Laragh and B. M. Brenner. Raven Press, Ltd., New York © 1990.

CHAPTER 108

Obesity and Hypertension

Diane R. Krieger and Lewis Landsberg

Overweight Versus Obesity, 1741
Significance of Obesity-Related Hypertension, 1742
Cuff Artifact Hypertension, 1742
Epidemiology, 1742
Body Weight and Blood Pressure Through the Life Cycle, 1743
Change in Weight and Blood Pressure, 1744
Reciprocity of the Weight–Blood Pressure Relationship, 1744
Importance of Body Fat Distribution, 1744
Pathogenesis of Obesity-Related Hypertension, 1744
Dietary Salt and Obesity Hypertension, 1744
Hemodynamics and Cardiac Function in the Obese, 1745
Overweight Versus Obesity, 1745
Body Fat Distribution, 1746
Hyperinsulinemia in Obesity-Related Hypertension, 1747
Insulin and Hypertension, 1749
Hyperinsulinemia and Hypertension in the Nonobese, 1749
Insulin and Blood Pressure, 1749
Insulin and the Sympathetic Nervous System: Potential Roles in the Pathogenesis of Obesity-Related Hypertension, 1750
Metabolic Role of Insulin Resistance, Hyperinsulinemia, and Sympathetic Stimulation in the Obese, 1750
Treatment of Hypertension in Obesity, 1752
Caloric Restriction, 1752
Weight Loss, 1753
Sodium Restriction, 1753
Nutrient Composition of the Diet, 1753
Exercise, 1754
Summary, 1754
References, 1754

Obesity and hypertension are both complex regulatory disturbances. Although the association between obesity and hypertension is well recognized, the interrelationship remains poorly understood. Trivial attributions previously in vogue, such as sphygmomanometer cuff size artifact and excessive dietary salt intake, do not suffice as explanations for the association. Recent epidemiologic and clinical investigations, however, have highlighted particular features of obesity-related hypertension that implicate neurohumoral mechanisms in the pathogenesis of hypertension in the obese. These observations suggest that the hypertension associated with obesity can be best understood as the consequence of metabolic alterations imposed by the obese state. This chapter will review the epidemiology, pathogenesis, and treatment of obesity-related hypertension.

OVERWEIGHT VERSUS OBESITY

It is important to note that overweight and obesity, though often used interchangeably, are not synonymous. Overweight indicates increased size compared with an established standard, whereas obesity connotes excess body fat. At any body weight the proportions of fat and lean tissue depend on age, activity level, diet, and other factors (1). Only at extremes of weight are muscle and fat contents closely correlated (2). As a result, moderate "overweight" does not necessarily imply "obesity". Similarly, an individual can have excess body fat without being overweight.

Controversy has surrounded the relative importance of overweight versus obesity as risk factors for hypertension (2–4). Some of the problem results from the imprecision of the anthropometric tools used to estimate body fat in epidemiologic and clinical studies. The two most commonly used methods to compare weight across height groups are *body mass index* (BMI) and *relative weight* (Table 1). These measures control for the contribution of height to weight and are well correlated with each other. BMI, also called *Quetelet's index,* is determined by dividing body weight (in kilograms) by height (in meters) squared. In some studies, height to the 1.5 power is used for calculation in females (2). Although BMI has been correlated with percent body fat (5), at moderately elevated levels of BMI an excess of fat is not always present (6).

Relative weight expresses the individual's weight as a percentage of an age-, sex-, and height-specific standard.

TABLE 1. *Commonly used anthropometric measures*

Measure	Calculation	Comment
Body mass index (Quetelet's index)	$\frac{\text{Weight (kg)}}{(\text{Height})^2 \text{ (meters)}}$	>30 indicates "obesity"; 25–30 indicates "overweight" in males; 24–30 indicates "overweight" in females
Relative weight	$\frac{\text{Observed weight}}{\text{Desirable weight for age- \& height-matched group}} \times 100$	Overweight > 120
Ponderal index	$\sqrt[3]{\frac{\text{Weight (kg)}}{\text{Height (meters)}}}$	Least reliable measure

This measure is less correlated with body fat than is BMI; moderate increases in relative weight could represent increases in lean tissue or fat tissue, or both (1). Furthermore, the validity of the reference weights, usually derived from life insurance data, has been questioned. The ponderal index, or the cube root of weight divided by height, is a less reliable measure because it varies with height.

Skin-fold thickness is frequently used to measure adiposity. Using the thumb and forefinger, the investigator separates the subcutaneous fat from muscle in the subscapular, triceps, biceps, or iliac areas and pinches the separated tissue with a caliper calibrated to measure thickness at a constant pressure (7). In some studies, the sum of individual thicknesses—triceps and subscapular, for example—is used. The results can be quite variable for a number of reasons such as the skill of the examiner. The skin-fold technique assumes, furthermore, that total body fat can be estimated from subcutaneous fat and that triceps and subscapular measurements are representative of other sites; the validity of these assumptions has been questioned (7).

Because most studies do not distinguish the independent contributions of lean body mass and adiposity, it is often difficult to distinguish the role of excess fat from that of body mass in the pathogenesis of hypertension. In this chapter, distinctions between overweight and obesity are made whenever possible; frequently, however, overweight and adiposity cannot be distinguished and are considered together to constitute "obesity."

SIGNIFICANCE OF OBESITY-RELATED HYPERTENSION

Obesity confers a widely recognized increase in cardiovascular risk (8,9). In the Framingham population a distinct excess incidence of cardiovascular disease and death was evident in those who were overweight (10). In the Build and Blood Pressure Study, male individuals who were 30% above average weight had a 44%-higher-than-average risk of death from coronary heart disease. Overweight females, similarly, had a 34%-higher-than-average risk (9). Much of this effect has been thought to be mediated through the well-recognized obesity-related risk factors of hypertension, hyperlipidemia, and diabetes mellitus (11). Reanalysis of the Framingham data, however, suggests that obesity also contributes independently to cardiovascular risk (12). The peculiar recent assertion that obesity may actually be "protective" against cardiovascular disease (13), since hypertension associated with obesity has less impact on mortality as compared with that associated with leanness (14,15), has been questioned with regard to study bias (16) and must be viewed in light of the above evidence that obesity and its consequences have well-established untoward cardiovascular effects (8–10).

Cuff Artifact Hypertension

It is clear that the distinct relationship between obesity and hypertension is real and not a measurement of artifact (17). Erroneous "cuff hypertension" resulting from the loss of cuff pressure through the thick soft tissue in the obese arm can be corrected with the use of a cuff large enough so that the bladder width is 40% of the arm circumference (18). When an appropriately large cuff is used, there is a high correlation between auscultatory and intra-arterial measurements (19). If a large cuff is unavailable, the small cuff should be placed around the forearm while the radial artery is auscultated (18).

EPIDEMIOLOGY

The association between obesity and hypertension has been amply documented in a wide array of socioeconomic, racial, and ethnic groups (9,10,17,20,21). The exact prevalence of obesity hypertension varies with the definitions used for "obesity" and "hypertension". Of one million individuals surveyed in the multicenter Community Hypertension Evaluation Clinic Study (CHECS), the prevalence of hypertension in those who reported being overweight was 50–300% higher than in those who reported normal or low weights (22). In the Framingham population (23), the likelihood of hypertension increased with increases in body weight (Fig. 1). In the most obese group, 46% were hypertensive (23). Conversely, in the Framingham population the prevalence of obesity was much greater in hypertensives than in normotensives (Fig. 2). In a large Norwegian study, each 10-kg increase in body weight was responsible for a 3-mm rise in systolic and a 2-mm rise in diastolic blood pressure (24). For reasons that remain obscure, body

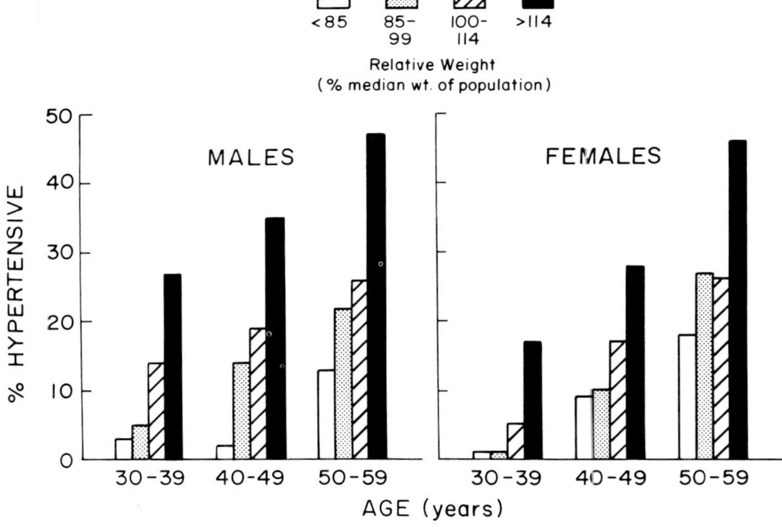

FIG. 1. Prevalence of hypertension (systolic > 160 mmHg or diastolic 95 mmHg) by age and sex in four relative weight groups at the first Framingham Heart Study examination. All trends are significant at $p = 0.05$. (Adapted from ref. 23.)

weight has been reported to have a greater influence on systolic blood pressure in some studies (17,25) but on diastolic blood pressure in others (2).

The association between body weight and blood pressure is not uniform and varies with sex, race, and age. Body weight appears to have a greater impact on blood pressure in females than in males (17). In the National Health and Nutrition Examination Survey (NHANES), obese women were four times more likely to have diastolic hypertension than were nonobese females (2), whereas overweight conferred less risk for obese males (2). Weight gain, on the other hand, had a stronger relationship with blood pressure in males than in females in the Framingham population (26), and, as noted below, clinical studies suggest that males suffer more from the "metabolic" complications of obesity.

The high prevalence of hypertension in black Americans is widely recognized. The contribution of body weight to hypertension in this group is less clear. In the CHECS survey, blacks had higher blood pressures than did whites in each weight class (22), making differences in weight an unlikely explanation for the higher prevalence of hypertension in blacks. Overweight did, however, contribute importantly to excess cases of hypertension in blacks in that study (22). In the Evans County cardiovascular study of a biracial community in Georgia, adiposity was associated with blood pressure and predictive of hypertension in all groups except black males, an observation not readily explainable (25). The second National Health and Nutrition Evaluation Study (NHANES II) data suggest that whites have a greater risk of hypertension from overweight than do blacks (2).

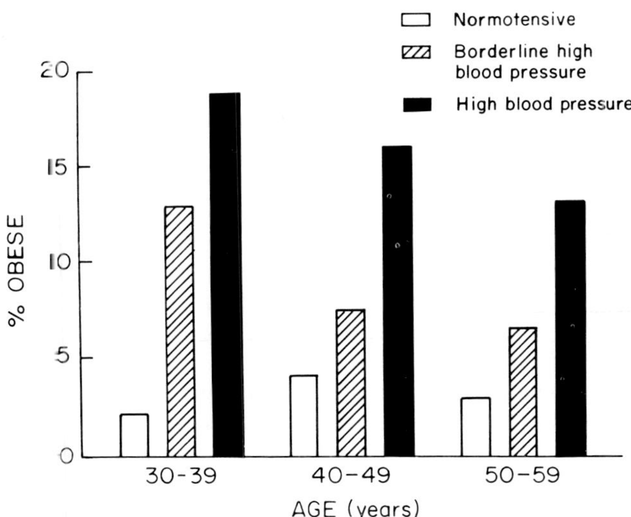

FIG. 2. Prevalence of obesity (relative weight > 120) in males according to blood pressure status at the first Framingham Heart Study examination. All trends are significant at $p = 0.05$. (Adapted from ref. 23.)

Body Weight and Blood Pressure Through the Life Cycle

The relationship between body size and blood pressure begins in childhood. In the Bogalusa Heart Study of 3500 children aged 5–14 years, body mass and height correlated strongly with blood pressure and were more predictive of blood pressure than was age (27). In early adulthood, increased body weight is associated with elevated blood pressure (25). In the Evans County population, overweight was a definite risk factor for hypertension in those under 30 years of age. Body weight in young adulthood is also predictive of the subsequent development of hypertension (25). A retrospective analysis of middle-aged hypertensive college graduates showed that they were significantly heavier as students than were normotensive alumni (28).

Although the relationship between hypertension and obesity persists throughout the life cycle, the association appears to decrease with age (10,22). Data analysis from NHANES II revealed that the relative risk of hypertension dropped from 5.6 in overweight 20- to 45-year-olds to 1.9 in overweight 45- to 75-year-olds (2). It has been suggested, however, that at least part of the increase in blood pressure associated with aging in Westernized societies is due to age-related weight gain (20), a phenomenon less evident in nonindustrialized societies. When tribal South Africans were compared with urbanized members of the same ethnic group, the members of the urban group were heavier and had higher blood pressures (29). Although blood pressure correlated with age and weight in both populations, only in the urban group was the age-related rise in blood pressure significant (29).

Change in Weight and Blood Pressure

Weight gain may have an even more potent impact on blood pressure than does weight itself. In the Framingham population, weight gain after age 25 distinctly increased the risk of developing hypertension (26) (Fig. 3). In the already obese young adult, weight gain increases the risk of subsequent hypertension to eight times the normal risk (26). Weight loss, on the other hand, has been repeatedly demonstrated to reduce blood pressure (30,31).

Reciprocity of the Weight–Blood Pressure Relationship

Interestingly, the relationship between hypertension and obesity appears to operate in both directions. Just as overweight normotensives are at risk to develop hypertension, lean hypertensives are at increased risk of becoming obese (17,23). Hypertensives who were lean at the outset of the Framingham Study had twice the likelihood of becoming overweight than did normotensives (23,26) (Fig. 4).

Importance of Body Fat Distribution

As considered in detail below, recent epidemiologic evidence demonstrates that fat distribution plays an important role in the relationship between hypertension and obesity. Fat deposition in the upper body segments, particularly the abdomen, is uniquely associated with hypertension and cardiovascular risk (32,33).

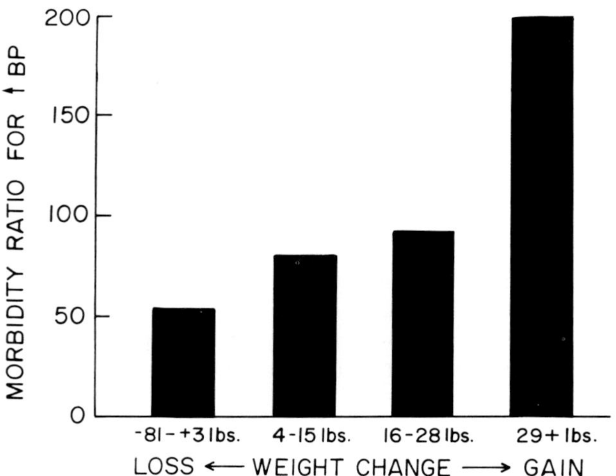

FIG. 3. Risk of developing hypertension in 11 years based on weight change since age 25 in subjects aged 35–74. $p = 0.05$ for the (−81 to +3 lbs) and (29+ lbs) groups.

Morbidity ratio

$$= \frac{\text{Observed cases of hypertension}}{\text{Expected cases of hypertension in age group}} \times 100$$

(Adapted from ref. 23.)

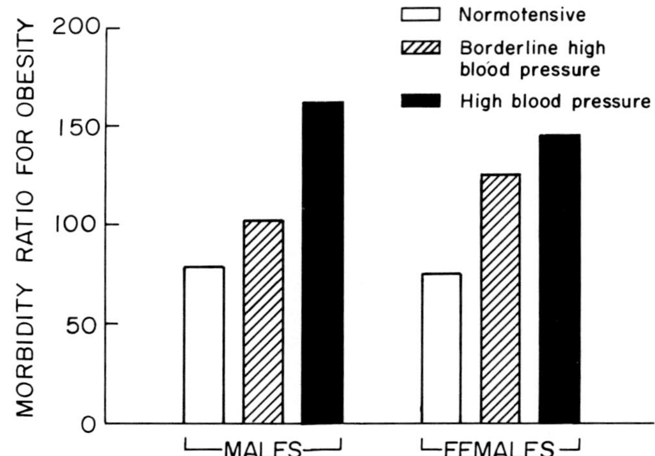

FIG. 4. Risk of developing obesity in 10 years based on initial blood pressure in subjects aged 30–59 at entry.

Morbidity ratio

$$= \frac{\text{Observed cases of obesity}}{\text{Expected cases of obesity in age group}} \times 100$$

$p = 0.05$ for hypertensive males and for normotensive females. (Adapted from ref. 23.)

PATHOGENESIS OF OBESITY-RELATED HYPERTENSION

Although the association between obesity and hypertension is firmly established, the mechanisms involved are only poorly understood. Dietary salt, hemodynamic factors, and neuroendocrine mechanisms have all been considered to play a role in the pathogenesis of obesity-related hypertension.

Dietary Salt and Obesity Hypertension

The relationship between dietary salt intake and hypertension is complex and controversial (34). Salt consumption in the obese has been considered excessive, an inference derived from the presumed increase in caloric intake that accompanies obesity. Some studies, moreover, have actually demonstrated generous salt consumption in the obese (35). Sodium chloride intake per se, however, is an unlikely cause of hypertension in and of itself, in either lean or obese individuals. In obese hypertensives, marked reductions in blood pressure have been demonstrated to accompany caloric restriction (36) and weight loss (37) without reduction in salt consumption, and in spite of continued high salt intake (36). This is not to say, however, that salt intake is without significance in the pathogenesis of obesity-related hypertension. A subset of patients with essential hypertension are known to be particularly sensitive to salt intake (38). The available evidence suggests that obesity-related hypertension is, in fact, a salt-sensitive form of the disease (36,39). It seems likely that endocrine and autonomic nervous system adaptations to obesity enhance renal sodium reabsorption, as discussed below, thereby altering the relationship between blood pressure and sodium excretion and imposing a "natriuretic handicap." Under these circumstances, excessive salt intake would be expected to increase blood pressure.

Hemodynamics and Cardiac Function in the Obese

Both obesity and hypertension affect the cardiovascular system. In obese hypertensives the hemodynamic pattern that emerges appears to reflect the independent contributions of obesity on the one hand and hypertension on the other.

Cardiac Output and Blood Volume

Increased body size is associated with elevated oxygen consumption (40) and expanded blood volume (35,41). These observations are readily explicable in terms of the additional metabolic demands imposed by the expanded mass of metabolizing tissue and are supported by the correlation of body size and cardiac output (42). Moreover, both cardiac output (35) and blood volume (43) normalize when expressed per unit of body size (35,43,44). Whether the size-corrected values are more meaningful than measured values is not clear, an issue that confounds the comparison of lean and obese with regard to many physiologic variables. Since heart rate is usually not increased in obesity per se, it is the increase in stroke volume (35,40,41) that accounts for the increased cardiac output.

Peripheral Vascular Resistance

Systemic vascular resistance (SVR) is calculated from mean arterial pressure (MAP) and cardiac output (CO) (SVR = MAP/CO). Since the larger size of the obese individual necessitates a higher cardiac output at any level of blood pressure, it is tautological that calculated SVR in the obese at a given blood pressure is low (41) when compared with that in lean individuals at the same blood pressure. Like blood volume and cardiac output, SVR normalizes when the calculation is adjusted for size using cardiac index (cardiac output/body surface area) instead of cardiac output (35).

Left Ventricular Hypertrophy and Cardiac Failure

Obesity is associated with cardiac hypertrophy (45), even in the absence of hypertension. An "eccentric" left ventricular hypertrophy of obesity has been described, characterized by increased wall thickness and increased chamber size and occurring, perhaps, in response to elevated blood volume and stroke volume (46). Established essential hypertension, on the other hand, is associated with "concentric" left ventricular hypertrophy, with increased wall thickness and contracted chamber size developing in response to elevations in systemic vascular resistance. The combination of obesity and hypertension exerts the double burden of increased preload (stroke volume and blood volume) and afterload (SVR). Weight reduction in the obese hypertensive is associated with decreases in left ventricular mass independent of changes in blood pressure (45). Despite the frequent finding of left ventricular hypertrophy in obesity, ventricular function is not always impaired. The degree of obesity determines its impact on ventricular function. Morbidly obese individuals display diminished ventricular function and compliance (40), whereas the moderately overweight do not (46). The expanded central blood volume in the morbidly obese (42) is thought to contribute to the high incidence of heart failure in this group.

Obese Normotensives Versus Obese Hypertensives

Comparison of the hemodynamic features of obese normotensives and obese hypertensives is helpful in evaluating the contribution of altered hemodynamics per se to the pathogenesis of obesity hypertension (Table 2). Hypertensive and normotensive obese do not differ in cardiac output (44) (Table 2), despite the fact that obese hypertensives have been reported to have greater extracellular and intracellular fluid volumes than do obese normotensives (44). SVR is higher in obese hypertensives than in obese normotensives (41,44), and it is higher in lean hypertensives than in lean normotensives. The calculated SVR at a given level of blood pressure in lean and obese hypertensives differ in magnitude as a consequence of the higher cardiac output in obesity noted above. This relationship between SVR and blood pressure is critical in evaluating the assertion that the lower SVR in obese hypertensives could be protective against some of the end-organ complications of hypertension (47). While the SVR in obese hypertensives is lower than in lean hypertensives, it is higher than in obese normotensives. Thus both lean and obese hypotensives have higher SVR when compared with weight-matched normotensives; the relationship between SVR and blood pressure in hypertensive subjects persists independent of body weight. As shown in Table 2, obese hypertensives have the hemodynamic features associated with obesity (high cardiac output) and hypertension (high SVR). The combination is not unique and does not provide an explanation for the increased blood pressure in and of itself.

Overweight Versus Obesity

In the NHANES II study the relative contributions of overweight (estimated with BMI) and obesity (estimated by skin-fold thickness) to blood pressure were compared (2). Using these measures, overweight was predictive of blood pressure whereas adiposity was not. In contrast, other studies show a relationship between skin-fold and blood pressure (4). Studies employing underwater weighing and isotope dilution (time-consuming and expensive methods of

TABLE 2. *Hemodynamic findings in matched lean and obese patients*[a]

	Normotensives		Hypertensives	
	Lean	Obese	Lean	Obese
Heart rate (beats/min)	70.6 ± 2.1	68.8 ± 2.3	74.2 ± 2.1	71.1 ± 3.1
Cardiac output (liters/min)	5.51 ± 0.19	7.32 ± 0.40	5.04 ± 0.22	6.26 ± 0.26
Cardiac index $\left(\frac{\text{Cardiac output}}{\text{Body surface area}}\right)$	3.24 ± 1.8	3.25 ± 0.26	2.95 ± 0.21	3.01 ± 0.19
Total peripheral resistance (mmHg/liters/min)	16.4 ± 0.8	13.0 ± 0.8	25.5 ± 1.0	20.3 ± 0.9
Total blood volume (liters)	4.4 ± 0.2	5.4 ± 0.3	4.0 ± 0.3	5.0 ± 0.3
Central blood volume (liters)	2.3 ± 0.2	3.0 ± 0.2	2.4 ± 0.1	2.5 ± 0.1

[a] Values represent means ± 1 SEM. Note: (a) Significant differences in cardiac output between lean and obese ($p = 0.001$) are not evident when cardiac index is used. (b) Total peripheral resistance: $p = 0.001$ for differences between (i) normotensives and hypertensives, (ii) lean and obese, and (iii) obese hypertensives and obese normotensives. (c) Blood volume: $p = 0.01$ for lean versus obese. (d) Central blood volume: $p = 0.02$ for lean versus obese. Adapted from ref. 41.

assessing body composition) have not clarified this issue. In one study, fat mass was more important than lean body mass (4); however, in another study, the opposite was found (3). The individual contributions of "body size" and "adiposity" to hypertension in the obese have not been established.

Heterogeneity of Obesity

Obesity is not a homogeneous disorder; it appears that specific characteristics of obesity may have an important impact on blood pressure. Anthropometric, humoral, and histologic measurements have all been used to differentiate distinct subgroups within the obese population. Since not all obese individuals are hypertensive, the comparison between normotensive and hypertensive obese individuals has provided important potential clues to the pathogenesis of obesity hypertension.

Body Fat Distribution

In the 1950s, Jean Vague, a French physician, suggested that the distribution of body fat was important in predisposing to complications of obesity, including hypertension (48). He observed that compared with normal-weight males, normal-weight females had more body fat and thicker subcutaneous fat tissue in all areas of the body except over the first three cervical vertebrae. He noted, furthermore, that gluteal and femoral (lower body) fat was thicker than trunk (upper body) fat in females. In males, on the other hand, upper-body fat was thicker than lower-body fat. These gender differences are evident in early infancy (49). Using what he referred to as an "index of masculine differentiation" derived from skin-fold thicknesses and limb circumferences, Vague classified obese subjects by their pattern of fat distribution. Females typically had a lower-body or "gynoid" pattern of fat distribution, and males had a preponderance of upper-body fat, a pattern he called "android." However, there was gender overlap in this classification, since some females had an android pattern while (less commonly) some males had a gynoid distribution. He noted that males, in general, had more metabolic complications of obesity than did females; he also noted that women with the android pattern had a higher incidence of hypertension and other complications when compared with women demonstrating the typical gynoid pattern.

Waist/Hip Ratio

More recently, studies using other measures of fat distribution have supported Vague's general conclusions (49,50). The anthropomorphic measure that best predicts hypertension is the ratio of waist circumference to hip circumference, known as the *waist/hip ratio* (49). The latter measure is more strongly related to blood pressure than to BMI or percentage body fat (51). Furthermore, computerized tomography (CT) scans have revealed that the waist/hip ratio is related more to intra-abdominal fat than to subcutaneous fat (52): A high waist/hip ratio reflects abdominal fat predominance, whereas a low waist/hip ratio indicates more gluteal fat. Males have higher waist/hip ratios than do weight-matched females, along with higher blood pressures, despite the greater amount of body fat in females. Unfortunately, waist/hip ratio is not a well-standardized measurement (51). The methods for determining waist and hip circumferences vary, depending upon the investigator, so that absolute values are less meaningful than comparisons made within individual studies. Waist/hip ratio provides, nonetheless, a convenient method of quickly assessing body fat distribution.

The results of a large longitudinal study of males and females support the association of upper-body fat distribution and hypertension (32,33). In both men and women, a relationship between waist/hip ratio and cardiovascular morbidity and mortality has been demonstrated (Fig. 5). In middle-aged males (33) observed over a period of 13 years, baseline waist/hip ratio was a better predictor of stroke and ischemic heart disease than were skin-fold thicknesses and BMI. Within each tertile of BMI, increasing waist/hip ratio was associated with higher rates of cardiovascular morbid-

however, is the effect of insulin on the sympathetic nervous system and sympathetically mediated thermogenesis.

Role of Insulin in Sympathetically Mediated Thermogenesis

The sympathetic nervous system is of major importance in the regulation of the adaptive or regulatory portion of metabolic rate (108,109). The changes in metabolic rate that accompany changes in dietary intake (decreased with fasting and caloric restriction; increased with overfeeding) are mediated, at least in part, by diet-induced changes in sympathetic nervous system activity (110). During fasting, sympathetic nervous system suppression has obvious survival value; by conserving calories during a period of limited caloric intake, survival during famine is potentiated. The increase in metabolic rate with overfeeding may have its origins in the thermogenic response to low-protein diets, which increase sympathetic activity (111). The high carbohydrate and fat content of these diets enhances sympathetic activity, since the latter nutrients are both stimulatory (112) whereas protein is not (113). From an evolutionary standpoint, this mechanism would allow an organism to consume increased quantities of a low-protein diet, thereby providing adequate supplies of nitrogen for growth and development, while permitting the dissipation of the excess calories as heat and avoiding increased energy storage as fat (110).

Insulin appears to function as a major signal in the relationship between dietary intake and sympathetic activity (82) Evidence has been developed that insulin-mediated glucose metabolism within neurons of the ventromedial hypothalamus (82,114) relates sympathetic outflow to nutritional status (84–86). Since the obese are not resistant to the stimulatory effects of insulin on the sympathetic nervous system (93), the possibility exists that the hyperinsulinemia of obesity is associated with stimulation of the sympathetic nervous system. Sympathetically mediated thermogenesis, recruited in the obese by hyperinsulinemia, would therefore limit weight gain and restore energy balance at the expense of increased sympathetic activity.

Thermogenesis and Energy Balance in the Obese

Until recently, it was generally believed that obesity was the consequence of excessive dietary intake and physical inactivity ("gluttony and sloth"), despite well-substantiated observations that individuals differ appreciably in the range of caloric intakes over which energy balance can be maintained (115–117). It is now recognized that the capacity for thermogenesis is an inherited trait (118) and that low metabolic rates may predispose to the development of obesity (119). Whether obesity is secondary to increased dietary intake or secondary to a thermogenic defect (low metabolic rate), or secondary to both (Fig. 7) the recruitment of sympathetically mediated thermogenesis would limit weight gain, thereby restoring energy balance. According to this formulation, hyperinsulinemia and sympathetic stimulation results in hypertension via effects on the kidney and

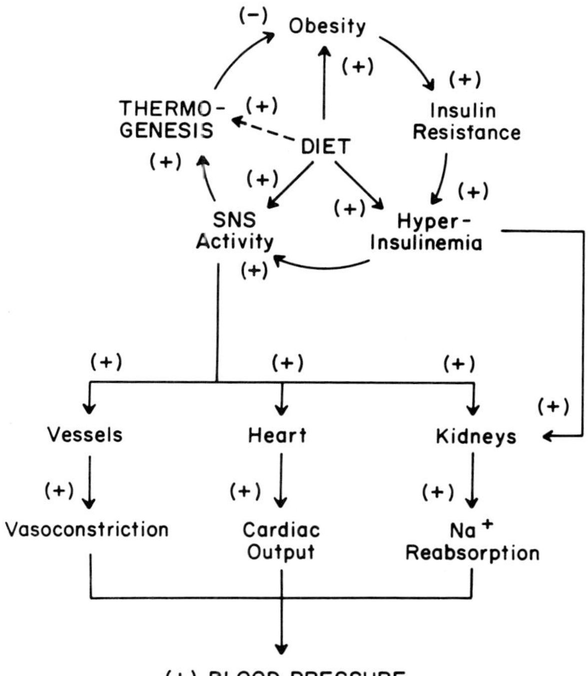

FIG. 7. Relationship between diet, thermogenesis, and blood pressure. The plus sign (+) indicates stimulation or elevation; the minus sign (−) indicates antagonism. The rationale behind the model proposed is provided in detail in the text. Obesity is seen to be the consequence of excessive dietary intake and a defect in dietary thermogenesis; in individual cases, one or the other may predominate. Stimulation of insulin by diet favors the development of large hypertrophic adipocytes distributed in the upper-body regions and abdomen, since these fat cells are most sensitive to the antilipolytic effects of insulin. Insulin resistance develops as obesity progresses, thereby augmenting the development of hyperinsulinemia, which, in turn (down-regulation), may increase resistance. Hyperinsulinemia stimulates the sympathetic nervous system (SNS) because the obese are not resistant to this action of insulin; hyperinsulinemia also restores glucose uptake and utilization, which are impaired by insulin resistance at the level of skeletal muscle. Diet may also stimulate sympathetic activity by mechanisms unrelated to hyperinsulinemia. The increased sympathetic activity stimulates thermogenesis, which antagonizes further weight gain and, in some cases, limits weight gain despite dietary excess. However, in addition to stimulating thermogenesis, the hyperinsulinemia and heightened sympathetic nervous system activity increase blood pressure by enhancing renal sodium reabsorption and by stimulating the heart and blood vessels. In the diagram, the dashed line between diet and thermogenesis represents the obligatory heat produced by the processes of digestion, absorption, and assimilation (nonadaptive), in distinction to the adaptive or regulatory stimulation of thermogenesis that results from hyperinsulinemia and activation of the sympathetic nervous system. With a decrease in dietary intake, fat stores diminish and the stimulatory effects on thermogenesis and blood pressure are reversed, leading to a decrease in metabolic rate and a fall in blood pressure. This model is not intended to describe the totality of the relationship between hypertension and obesity; undoubtedly, other blood-pressure-regulating systems are involved as well. (From ref. 106.)

the cardiovascular system. Viewed in this light, the hypertension of obesity is the unfortunate by-product of physiologic mechanisms evolved to limit weight gain.

This hypothesis addresses the association between hyperinsulinemia and hypertension in the nonobese and may explain the poorly understood observation that hypertension predisposes to the development of obesity as described above (23). Increased dietary intake, if accompanied by sufficient thermogenic capacity to dissipate the excess calories (Fig. 7), would not be associated with weight gain. The compensatory increase in insulin levels and sympathetic activity, while conferring protection against the development of obesity, would predispose to hypertension. However, as thermogenic capacity declines with age, the increase in caloric intake would progressively manifest itself as obesity.

Sympathetic Activity in Obese Hypertensives: Impact of Caloric Restriction

The relationships depicted in Fig. 7 predicts an increase in sympathetic activity in obese hypertensives. Decisive data on this point are not available, partly because of the difficulty of assessing sympathetic nervous system activity in humans (120,121). Some (122,123), but not all (39), studies employing plasma NE measurements support this prediction. The sequence of hormonal and blood pressure changes following marked caloric restriction in obese hypertensives is consistent with the schema shown in Fig. 7. Plasma NE levels and blood pressure fall promptly and in parallel (124) after the institution of very-low-energy diets. The time course of this reduction parallels the known decrease in insulin secretion during fasting in the obese (125).

TREATMENT OF HYPERTENSION IN OBESITY

The magnitude of the clinical problem posed by obesity-related hypertension has directed considerable attention to treatment strategies. A focus on nonpharmacologic therapies is particularly relevant in obese hypertensives, since many of the current antihypertensive agents can exacerbate obesity-related disturbances of carbohydrate and lipid metabolism (126). Caloric restriction, weight loss, exercise, and salt restriction have proved somewhat successful; the role of diet composition is more controversial (Table 3).

Caloric Restriction

The hypotensive effect of caloric restriction is distinct from, and is observed prior to, that of weight loss (127). One study indicated that it is a more potent hypotensive force than is weight loss itself (128). The most likely explanation for the diminution of blood pressure is the combined effect of (a) fasting-induced natriuresis (129) and (b) reductions in sympathetic nervous system tone (130).

Natriuresis of Fasting

The first few days of modified or total starvation is accompanied by a natriuresis that is reversed by carbohydrate refeeding (129). This "natriuresis of fasting" is due, in part, to the sodium excretion required to maintain electroneutrality in the setting of ketonuria (129). Other mediators of this phenomenon have been proposed, including alterations in sensitivity to aldosterone (131), increases in glucagon, decreases in insulin (125), and diminished sympathetic nervous system tone (124).

The diminished insulin secretion that accompanies fasting has three potential effects on natriuresis: (i) a direct tubular effect via changes in insulin-mediated renal sodium reabsorption, (ii) indirect effects via stimulation of ketonemia and ketonuria, and (iii) diminished sympathetic nervous system tone. The last is supported by decreases in postural and exercise responses of plasma NE in obese hypertensives during 2 weeks of severe caloric restriction (124). Thus, decreases in insulin, combined with decreases in sympathetic nervous system activity, stimulate sodium excretion and may reverse the natriuretic handicap imposed by these factors in the obese.

Sympathetic Nervous System

Fasting-induced decreases in sympathetic nervous system activity may affect blood pressure independent of the sympathetic nervous system effect on natriuresis. Within 48 hr of a low-carbohydrate low-calorie diet, obese normotensives demonstrate decreases in systolic and diastolic blood pressure paralleled by decreases in urinary catecholamines (127). This phenomenon has been observed during sodium balance (127) and prior to a maximum sodium diuresis (130). The parallel decreases in blood pressure and in indices of sympathetic nervous system function point to decreased cardiovascular stimulation by the sympathetic nervous system.

TABLE 3. *Nonpharmacologic treatment of obesity-related hypertension*[a]

	Blood pressure	Insulin secretion/sensitivity	Sympathetic nervous system activity
Caloric restriction	↓	↓/↑	↓
Weight loss	↓	↓/↑	↓
Exercise leading to conditioning	↓	↓/↑	↓
High-fiber diet	↓	↓/↑	?

[a] ↓, decreased; ↑, increased.

Weight Loss

Weight loss results in decreases in blood pressure in both normotensives and hypertensives (132). Weight loss can diminish or replace drug therapy for hypertension (126,133). When compared with beta blockade in the treatment of overweight hypertensives, weight loss produced a greater decrease in diastolic blood pressure along with a more favorable lipid profile (134). The distinct contribution of weight loss to the reduction in blood pressure can be difficult to separate from that of caloric restriction, since even modest weight loss influences blood pressure. Blood pressure became normalized in two-thirds of a group of obese hypertensives once 50% of their excess body weight was lost (31). A 5% decrease in body weight over a period of 5 years has been shown to influence blood pressure in overweight men (30); as long as weight loss was maintained, blood pressure reductions persisted. An average weight loss of 4 kg in a group of overweight hypertensives withdrawn from medicines and instructed in a diet moderately restricted in calories, salt, and alcohol allowed 39% to remain off medicine over a 4-year period (133).

Three factors have been implicated in the hypotensive effect of weight loss: (i) decreased sodium intake, (ii) diminished insulin levels, and (iii) reduced sympathetic nervous system activity (124). The decreased insulin levels and increased insulin sensitivity that accompany weight loss could suppress sympathetic nervous system activity, thereby altering the pressure–natriuresis relationship. Associations between weight-loss-lowered blood pressure and diminished insulin levels support this hypothesis (30). A causal link still needs to be demonstrated.

Diminished Sympathetic Nervous System Activity

The hemodynamic changes that accompany weight loss (decreased cardiac output, decreased total blood volume, and cardiopulmonary blood volume) (123) may be due to parallel decreases in sympathetic nervous system activity. Reduced sympathetic nervous system tone usually produces a redistribution of blood volume away from the central circulation, and the resultant decreases in cardiac output lead to diminished blood pressure. Furthermore, total peripheral resistance does not increase with weight loss (123,135) despite the fall in blood pressure and cardiac output, suggesting diminished sympathetic nervous system tone as a mechanism. The fall in heart rate that accompanies weight loss (19,123,124) in obese hypertensives is also consistent with diminished sympathetic nervous system activity. Decreases in plasma renin activity and aldosterone accompany weight loss (36) despite natriuresis and diminished blood pressure. Decreased sympathetic tone would explain these changes (124).

The decreases in left ventricular wall thickness and left ventricular mass in obese hypertensives after a 50% reduction in excess weight is not entirely dependent upon decreases in blood pressure (45). Since sympathetic nervous system activity contributes to the development of cardiac hypertrophy (136), it is plausible that diminished sympathetic nervous system activity could explain the decrease in cardiac hypertrophy as well (45).

Sodium Restriction

Recommendations that dietary salt restriction accompanies weight loss have been the subject of debate. In some studies, caloric restriction alone was sufficient to diminish blood pressure (31,105); in others, diminished caloric intake did not produce a hypotensive effect without concomitant sodium restriction (19,135). The discrepancies probably reflect the different degrees of caloric restriction in these studies. When calories are extremely restricted, sodium restriction is not required (31). Moderately restricted diets (1200 kcal), however, do appear to need adjunctive sodium restriction in order to achieve lowered blood pressure (19,135), supporting the assertion that salt sensitivity is present in obesity-related hypertension.

Nutrient Composition of the Diet

Dietary Carbohydrates

Carbohydrate intake influences insulin secretion (55) and sympathetic nervous system activity (137) in the obese. In hyperinsulinemic obese adults, weight-maintaining high-carbohydrate diets increased basal levels and stimulated insulin levels, whereas low-carbohydrate diets had the opposite effect (55). Carbohydrate feeding also stimulates sympathetic nervous system activity in laboratory rodents (137–139). In obese subjects, very-low-calorie mixed diets suppressed the sympathetic nervous system to a lesser extent than did low-carbohydrate diets (137). Refined carbohydrates appear to have a specific blood-pressure-elevating effect. When the spontaneously hypertensive rat (140) and other rat strains (141) are fed sucrose, rises in blood pressure are observed. A hypertensive response to high-carbohydrate feeding has not been demonstrated in humans (142), but normal men fed short-term high-carbohydrate diets did exhibit transient decreases in urinary sodium. Further studies on the effect of high-carbohydrate feeding on blood pressure in the obese are required before specific recommendations can be established, but it would appear prudent to modestly restrict refined sugars.

Dietary Fat

Epidemiologic data links monosaturated and polyunsaturated fatty acid intake with lower blood pressure (51). Linoleic (polyunsaturated) and oleic (monosaturated) acids are precursors for vasodilating prostaglandins, suggesting a possible mechanism for the blood-pressure-lowering effects of these fatty acids. Further work is required, however, before specific recommendations can be made.

Dietary Fiber

A hypotensive response to high-fiber diets has been demonstrated by some investigators (143). Furthermore, high levels of dietary fiber may supplement the blood-pressure-lowering effect of caloric restriction (144). When obese subjects consuming high-fiber low-calorie diets were compared with those ingesting lower-calorie liquid diets, blood pressure reductions were greater in the group eating fiber despite equivalent weight loss. Reduced insulin levels may be involved in the fiber effect on blood pressure, since improved peripheral insulin sensitivity has been attributed to high-fiber diets (145).

Exercise

Long-term physical training can result in blood pressure reduction even in the absence of weight loss (146). Training appears to have a greater effect on blood pressure in hypertensives than in normotensives (146), as well as a greater effect in those with the highest insulin levels (147).

Exercise and conditioning affect both insulin and the sympathetic nervous system. Fasting and stimulated serum insulin levels are decreased by acute exercise as well as by long-term conditioning. Training increases sensitivity to endogenous insulin (71). Therefore, reductions in insulin levels and in sympathetic nervous system tone may contribute to the hypotensive effect of training.

SUMMARY

Obesity-related hypertension imposes a double hemodynamic burden and contributes importantly to the increases in cardiovascular morbidity and mortality noted in obesity. Nonetheless, the pathogenesis of obesity-related hypertension remains poorly understood. The importance of the distribution of body fat in the metabolic abnormalities of obesity, such as hypertension, has been well demonstrated. Upper-body-fat predominance is more strongly associated with hypertension than is the concentration of fat in the lower body. Hyperinsulinemia, a well-known feature of obesity, is also more prominent in upper-body obesity than in lower-body obesity. High levels of insulin have been linked to sympathetic nervous system stimulation and enhanced sodium reabsorption. These observations, combined with other clinical and laboratory data reviewed in this chapter, suggest a neurohumoral mechanism for obesity-related hypertension. Further work is required in order to confirm this hypothesis.

The treatment of hypertension in the obese remains a vexing clinical problem. Treating the underlying obesity with caloric restriction (achieving even a limited weight loss), combined with an exercise program, is often effective at reducing blood pressure. Each of these nonpharmacologic treatments leads to lowered insulin levels and diminished sympathetic nervous system tone, supporting the mechanism proposed above. Unfortunately, difficulties in compliance with these treatment regimens frequently necessitate drug treatment, which may, in turn, exacerbate the existing metabolic disturbances of obesity.

ACKNOWLEDGMENTS

This work was supported, in part, by USPHS grants DK20378, HL36568, HL37871, AG00599.

REFERENCES

1. Grande F. Assessment of body fat in man. In: Bray A, ed. *Obesity in perspective.* Washington, DC: US Government Printing Office, 1973;189–203.
2. Van Itallie TB. Health implications of overweight and obesity in the United States. *Ann Intern Med* 1985;103:983–988.
3. Weinsier RL, Norris DJ, Birch R, Bernstein RS, Wang J, Yang M-U, Pierson RN Jr, Van Itallie TB. The relative contribution of body fat and fat pattern to blood pressure level. *Hypertension* 1985;7:578–585.
4. Siervogel RM, Roche AF, Chumlea WC, Morris JG, Webb P, Knittle JL. Blood pressure, body composition, and fat tissue cellularity in adults. *Hypertension* 1982;4:382–386.
5. Haffner SM, Stern MP, Hazuda HP, Pugh J, Patterson JK, Malina R. Upper body and centralized adiposity in Mexican Americans and non-Hispanic whites: relationship to body mass index and other behavioral and demographic variables. *Int J Obes* 1986;10:493–502.
6. Palombo JD, Hayward E, Bistrian BR, Blackburn GL. Nutritional assessment of the obese patient. In: Levenson SM, ed. *Nutritional assessment—present status, future directions and prospects.* Columbus, OH: Ross Laboratories, 1981;3–10.
7. Lukaski HC. Methods for the assessment of human body composition: traditional and new. *Am J Clin Nutr* 1987;46:537–556.
8. Grundy SM, Greenland P, Herd A, Huebsch JA, Jones RJ, Mitchel JH, Schlant RC. Cardiovascular and risk factor evaluation of healthy American adults. *Circulation* 1987;75(6):1340A–1362A.
9. Havlik RJ, Hubert HB, Fabsitz RR, Feinleib M. Weight and hypertension. *Ann Intern Med* 1983;98:855–859.
10. Gordon T, Kannel WB. Obesity and cardiovascular disease: the Framingham Study. *Clin Endocrinol Metab* 1976;5(2):367–375.
11. Keys A, Aravanis C, Blackburn H, Van Buchem FSP, Buzina R, Djordjevic BS, Fidanza F, Karvonen MJ, Menotti A, Puddu V, Taylor HL. Coronary heart disease: overweight and obesity risk factors. *Ann Intern Med* 1972;77:15–27.
12. Hubert HB, Feinleib M, McNamara PM, Castelli WP. Obesity as an independent risk factor for cardiovascular disease: a 26-year follow-up of participants in the Framingham Heart Study. *Circulation* 1983;67(5):968–977.
13. Messerli FH. Letter to the editor re obesity, hypertension, and cardiovascular risk. *JAMA* 1987;257(12):1598.
14. Barrett-Connor E, Khaw K-T. Is hypertension more benign when associated with obesity? *Circulation* 1985;72(1):53–60.
15. Bloom E, Reed D, Yano K, MacLean C. Does obesity protect hypertensives against cardiovascular disease? *JAMA* 1986; 256(21):2972–2975.
16. Manson JE, Stampfer MJ, Hennekens CH, Willett WC. Body weight and longevity: a reassessment. *JAMA* 1987;257(3):353–358.
17. Chiang BN, Perlman LV, Epstein FH. Overweight and hypertension. *Circulation* 1969;39:403–421.
18. Kirkendall WM, Feinleib M, Freis ED, Mark AL. Recommendations for human blood pressure determination by sphygmomanometers. *Circulation* 1980;65(2):1146A–1155A.
19. Fagerberg B, Andersson OK, Isaksson B, Bjorntorp P. Blood pressure control during weight reduction in obese hypertensive men: separate effects of sodium and energy restriction. *Br Med J* 1984;288:11–14.
20. Berchtold P, Jorgens V, Finke C, Berger M. Epidemiology of obesity and hypertension. *Int J Obes* 1981;5(Suppl 1):1–7.
21. Reed D, McGee D, Yano K. Biological and social correlates of blood pressure among Japanese men in Hawaii. *Hypertension* 1982;4:406–414.
22. Stamler R, Stamler J, Riedlinger WF, Algera G, Roberts RH. Weight and blood pressure; findings in hypertension screening of 1 million Americans. *JAMA* 1978;240:1607–1610.
23. Kannel WB, Brand N, Skinner JJ Jr, Dawber TR, McNamara PM. The relation of adiposity to blood pressure and development of hypertension. *Ann Intern Med* 1967;67(1):48–59.
24. Boe J, Humerfelt S, Wedervang F, Oecon C. The blood pressure in a population: blood pressure readings and height and weight determinations in the adult population of the city of Bergen. *Acta Med Scand* 1957;157:202–206.

25. Johnson AL, Cornoni JC, Cassel JC, Tyroler HA, Heyden S, Hames CG. Influence of race, sex and weight on blood pressure behavior in young adults. *Am J Cardiol* 1975;35:523–530.
26. Tobian L. Hypertension and obesity. *N Engl J Med* 1978; 298(1):46–47.
27. Voors AW, Webber LS, Frerichs RR, Berenson GS. Body height and body mass as determinants of basal blood pressure in children—the Bogalusa Heart Study. *Am J Epidemiol* 1977; 106(2):101–108.
28. Paffenbarger RS Jr, Thorne MC, Wing AL. Chronic disease in former college students: characteristics in youth predisposing to hypertension in later years. *Am J Epidemiol* 1968;88(1):25–32.
29. Sever PS, Gordon D, Peart WS, Beighton P. Blood-pressure and its correlates in urban and tribal Africa. *Lancet* 1980;2:60–64.
30. Berchtold P, Jorgens V, Kemmer FW, Berger M. Obesity and hypertension: cardiovascular response to weight reduction. *Hypertension* 1982;4(Suppl II):II50–II55.
31. Eliahou HE, Iaina A, Gaon T, Shochat J, Modan M. Body weight reduction necessary to attain normotension in the overweight hypertensive patient. *Int J Obes* 1981;5:157–163.
32. Lapidus L, Bengtsson C, Larsson B, Pennert K, Rybo E, Sjostrom L. Distribution of adipose tissue and risk of cardiovascular disease and death: a 12 year follow up of participants in the population study of women in Gothenburg, Sweden. *Br Med J* 1984;289:1257–1261.
33. Larsson B, Svardsudd K, Welin L, Wilhelmsen L, Bjorntorp P, Tibblin G. Abdominal adipose tissue distribution, obesity, and risk of cardiovascular disease and death: 13 year follow up of participants in the study of men born in 1913. *Br Med J* 1984;288:1401–1404.
34. Einhorn D, Landsberg L. Nutrition and diet in hypertension. In: Shils ME, Young VR, eds. *Modern nutrition in health and disease.* Philadelphia: Lea & Febiger, 1988;1269–1282.
35. Messerli FH, Christie B, DeCarvalho JGR, Aristimuno GG, Suarez DH, Dreslinski GR, Frohlich ED. Obesity and essential hypertension: hemodynamics, intravascular volume, sodium excretion, and plasma renin activity. *Arch Intern Med* 1981;141:81–85.
36. Tuck ML, Sowers J, Dornfeld L, Kledzik G, Maxwell M. The effect of weight reduction on blood pressure, plasma renin activity, and plasma aldosterone levels in obese patients. *N Engl J Med* 1981;304(16):930–933.
37. Reisin E, Abel R, Modan M, Silverberg DS, Eliahou HE, Modan B. Effect of weight loss without salt restriction on the reduction of blood pressure in overweight hypertensive patients. *N Engl J Med* 1978;298:1–6.
38. Kawasaki T, Delea CS, Bartter FC, Smith H. The effect of high-sodium and low-sodium intakes on blood pressure and other related variables in human subjects with idiopathic hypertension. *Am J Med* 1978;64:193–198.
39. Yamaji I, Kikuchi K, Shibata S, Nishimura M, Acki K, Nozawa A, Honma C, Kobayakawa H, Komura H, Iimura O. Sympathetic nerve activity, plasma renin activity and water-sodium balance in obese patients with essential hypertension. *Jpn Circ J* 1986;50:155–1157.
40. De Divitiis O, Fazio S, Petitto M, Maddalena G, Contaldo F, Mancini M. Obesity and cardiac function. *Circulation* 1981;64(3):477–482.
41. Messerli FH, Sundgaard-Riise K, Reisin E, Dreslinski G, Dunn FG, Frohlich E. Disparate cardiovascular effects of obesity and arterial hypertension. *Am J Med* 1983;74:808–812.
42. Kaltman AJ, Goldring RM. Role of circulatory congestion in the cardiorespiratory failure of obesity. *Am J Med* 1976;60:645–653.
43. Dustan HP, Tarazi RC, Mujais S. A comparison of hemodynamic and volume characteristics of obese and non-obese hypertensive patients. *Int J Obes* 1981;5:19–25.
44. Raison J, Achimastos A, Asmar R, Simon A, Safar M. Extracellular and interstitial fluid volume in obesity with and without associated systemic hypertension. *Am J Cardiol* 1986;57:223–226.
45. MacMahon SW, Wilcken DEL, Macdonald GJ. The effect of weight reduction on left ventricular mass: a randomized controlled trial in young, overweight hypertensive patients. *N Engl J Med* 1986;314:334–339.
46. Messerli FH, Sundgaard-Riise K, Reisin ED, Dreslinski GR, Ventura HO, Oigman W, Frohlich ED, Dunn FG. Dimorphic cardiac adaptation to obesity and arterial hypertension. *Ann Intern Med* 1983;99:757–761.
47. Schmieder RE, Messerli F. Obesity hypertension. *Med Clin North Am* 1987;71(5):991–1001.
48. Vague J. The degree of masculine differentiation of obesities: a factor determining predisposition to diabetes, artherosclerosis, gout, and uric calculous disease. *Am J Clin Nutr* 1956;4:20–34.
49. Krotkiewski M, Bjorntorp P, Sjostrom L, Smith U. Impact of obesity on metabolism in men and women. Importance of regional adipose tissue distribution. *J Clin Invest* 1983;72:1150–1162.
50. Kissebah AH, Vydelingum N, Murray R, Evans DJ, Hartz AJ, Kalkhoff RK, Adams PW. Relation of body fat distribution to metabolic complications of obesity. *J Clin Endocrinol Metab* 1982;54:254–259.
51. Williams PT, Fortmann SP, Terry RB, Garay SC, Vranizan KM, Ellsworth N, Wood PD. Associations of dietary fat, regional adiposity, and blood pressure in men. *JAMA* 1987;257(23):3251–3256.
52. Ashwell M, Cole TJ, Dixon AK. Obesity: new insight into the anthropometric classification of fat distribution shown by computed tomography. *Br Med J* 1985;290:1692–1694.
53. Berglund G, Ljungman S, Hartford M, Wilhelmsen L, Bjorntorp P. Type of obesity and blood pressure. *Hypertension* 1982;4:692–696.
54. Smith U. Regional differences in adipocyte metabolism and possible consequences *in vivo.* In: Hirsch J, Van Itallie TB, eds. *Recent advances in obesity research. IV. Proceedings of the 4th International Congress on Obesity.* London: John Libbey, 1983;33–36.
55. Grey N, Kipnis DM. Effect of diet composition on the hyperinsulinemia of obesity. *N Engl J Med* 1971;285:827–831.
56. Olefsky JM. Decreased insulin binding to adipocytes and circulating monocytes from obese subjects. *J Clin Invest* 1976; 57:1165–1172.
57. Olefsky JM. The insulin receptor: its role in insulin resistance of obesity and diabetes. *Diabetes* 1976;25:1154–1162.
58. Cushman SW, Wardzala LJ, Hissin PJ, Karnieli E, Simpson IA, Salans LB. Mechanism of insulin resistant glucose transport in the isolated rat adipose cell. In: Angel A, Hollenberg CH, Roncari DAK, eds. *The adipocyte and obesity: cellular and molecular mechanisms.* New York: Raven Press, 1983;105–111.
59. Kalkhoff RK, Hartz AH, Rupley D, Kissebah AH, Kelber S. Relationship of body fat distribution to blood pressure, carbohydrate tolerance, and plasma lipids in healthy obese women. *J Lab Clin Med* 1983;102(4):621–627.
60. Ohlson L-O, Larsson B, Svardsudd K, Welin L, Eriksson H, Wilhelmsen L, Bjorntorp P, Tibblin G. The influence of body fat distribution on the incidence of diabetes mellitus: 13.5 years of follow-up of the participants in the study of men born in 1913. *Diabetes* 1985;34:1055–1058.
61. Salans L, Knittle J, Hirsch J. The role of adipose cell size and adipose tissue insulin sensitivity in the carbohydrate intolerance of human obesity. *J Clin Invest* 1968;47:153–165.
62. Sjostrom L. Adult human adipose tissue cellularity and metabolism. *Acta Med Scand [Suppl]* 1972;544:1–52.
63. Stern J, Batchelor B, Hollander N, Cohen C, Hirsch J. Adipose-cell size and immunoreactive insulin levels in obese and normal weight adults. *Lancet* 1972;2:948–951.
64. Randle PJ, Hales CN, Garland PB, Newsholme EA. The glucose fatty-acid cycle role in insulin sensitivity and the metabolic disturbances of diabetes mellitus. *Lancet* 1963;1:787–789.
65. Peiris AN, Mueller RA, Smith GA, Struve MF, Kissebah AH. Splanchnic insulin metabolism in obesity. *J Clin Invest* 1986;78:1648–1657.
66. Bjorntorp P. Fat cell distribution and metabolism. *Ann NY Acad Sci* 1987;499:66–72.
67. Evans DJ, Hoffmann RG, Kolkhoff RK, Kissebah AH. Relationship of androgenic activity to body fat topography, fat cell morphology, and metabolic aberrations in premenopausal women. *J Clin Endocrinol Metab* 1983;57(2):304–310.
68. Krotkiewski M, Blohme B, Lindholm N, Bjorntorp P. The effects

of adrenal corticosteroids on regional adipocyte size in man. *J Clin Endocrinol Metab* 1976;42(1):91–97.
69. Christlieb AR, Krolewski AS, Warram JH, Soeldner JS. Is insulin the link between hypertension and obesity? *Hypertension* 1985;7(Suppl II):II-54–II-57.
70. Manicardi V, Camellini L, Bellodi G, Coscelli C, Ferrannini E. Evidence for an association of high blood pressure and hyperinsulinemia in obese man. *J Clin Endocrinol Metab* 1986; 62:1302–1304.
71. Rose HG, Yalow RS, Schweitzer P, Schwartz E. Insulin as a potential factor influencing blood pressure in amputees. *Hypertension* 1986;8:793–800.
72. Modan M, Halkin H, Almog S, Lusky A, Eshkol A, Shefi M, Shitrit A, Fuchs Z. Hyperinsulinemia: a link between hypertension obesity and glucose intolerance. *J Clin Invest* 1985;75:809–817.
73. Ferrannini E, Buzzigoli G, Bonadonna R, Giorico MA, Oleggini M, Graziadei L, Pedrinelli R, Brandi L, Bevilacqua S. Insulin resistance in essential hypertension. *N Engl J Med* 1987; 317(6):350–356.
74. Francois B, de Gasparo M, Crabbe J. Interaction between isolated amphibian skin and insulin. *Arch Int Physiol Biochim* 1969;77:527–530.
75. Herrera FC. Effect of insulin on short-circuit current and sodium transport across toad urinary bladder. *Am J Physiol* 1965;209:819–824.
76. Herrera FC, Whittembury G, Planchart A. Effect of insulin on short-circuit across isolated frog skin in the presence of calcium and magnesium. *Biochim Biophys Acta* 1963;66:170–172.
77. DeFronzo RA. Insulin and renal sodium handling: clinical implications. *Int J Obes* 1981;5(Suppl 1):93–104.
78. Kurokawa K, Lerner R. Binding and degradation of insulin by isolated renal cortical tubules. *Endocrinology* 1980;106:655–662.
79. Fidelman L, Watlington CO. Insulin and aldosterone interaction on Na^+ and K^+ transport in cultured kidney cells (A6). *Endocrinology* 1984;115:1171–1178.
80. Saudek CD, Boulter PR, Knopp RH, Arky RA. Sodium retention accompanying insulin treatment of diabetes mellitus. *Diabetes* 1974;23:240–246.
81. Nizet A, Lefebvre P, Crabbe J. Control by insulin of sodium potassium and water excretion by the isolated dog kidney. *Pflugers Arch* 1971;323:11–20.
82. Landsberg L, Young JB. Insulin-mediated glucose metabolism in the relationship between dietary intake and sympathetic nervous system activity. *Int J Obes* 1985;9:63–68.
83. Christensen NJ, Gundersen HJG, Hegedus L, Jacobsen F, Mogensen CE, Osterby R, Vittinghus E. Acute effects of insulin on plasma noradrenaline and the cardiovascular system. *Metabolism* 1980;29:1138–1145.
84. Rowe JW, Young JB, Minaker KL, Stevens AL, Pallotta JA, Landsberg L. Effect of insulin and glucose infusions on sympathetic nervous system activity in normal man. *Diabetes* 1981;30:219–225.
85. Acheson K, Jequier E, Wahren J. Influence of beta-adrenergic blockade on glucose-induced thermogenesis in man. *J Clin Invest* 1983;72:981–986.
86. Acheson KJ, Ravussin E, Wahren J, Jequier E. Thermic effect of glucose in man. *J Clin Invest* 1984;74:1572–1580.
87. Liang C-S, Doherty JU, Faillace R, Maekawa K, Arnold S, Gavras H, Hood WB Jr. Insulin infusion in conscious dogs: effects on systemic and coronary hemodynamics, regional blood flows, and plasma catecholamines. *J Clin Invest* 1982;69:1321–1336.
88. Pereda SA, Eckstein JW, Abboud FM. Cardiovascular responses to insulin in the absence of hypoglycemia. *Am J Physiol* 1962;202:249–252.
89. Page MM, Smith RBW, Watkins PJ. Cardiovascular effects of insulin. *Br Med J* 1976;1:430–432.
90. Landsberg L, Greff L, Gunn S, Young JB. Adrenergic mechanisms in the metabolic adaptation to fasting and feeding: effects of phlorizin on diet-induced changes in sympathoadrenal activity in the rat. *Metabolism* 1980;29:1128–1137.
91. Rappaport EB, Young JB, Landsberg L. Effects of 2-deoxy-D-glucose on the cardiac sympathetic nerves and the adrenal medulla in the rat: further evidence for a dissociation of sympathetic nervous system and adrenal medullary responses. *Endocrinology* 1982;110:650–656.
92. Young JB, Landsberg L. Sympathoadrenal activity in fasting pregnant rats: dissociation of adrenal medullary and sympathetic nervous system responses. *J Clin Invest* 1979;64:109–116.
93. O'Hare JA, Minaker K, Young JB, Rowe JW, Pallotta JA, Landsberg L. Insulin increases plasma norepinephrine (NE) and lowers plasma potassium equally in lean and obese men. *Clin Res* 1985;33:441A.
94. Landsberg L, Young JB. Sympathetic nervous system in hypertension. In: Brenner B, Stein JH, eds. *Hypertension: contemporary issues in nephrology,* vol 8. New York: Churchill Livingstone, 1981;100–141.
95. Landsberg L, Young JB. Catecholamines and the adrenal medulla. In: Foster DW, Wilson JD, eds. *Williams textbook of endocrinology,* 7th edition. Philadelphia: WB Saunders, 1985;891–965.
96. Grimm M, Weidmann P, Keusch G, Meier A, Gluck Z. Norepinephrine clearance and pressor effect in normal and hypertensive man. *Klin Wochenschr* 1980;58:1175–1181.
97. Philipp TH, Distler A, Cordes U. Sympathetic nervous system and blood-pressure control in essential hypertension. *Lancet* 1978;2:959–963.
98. DiBona GF. Neural mechanisms in body fluid homeostasis. *Fed Proc* 1982;45:2871–2884.
99. Rubenstein AH, Mako ME, Horwitz DL. Insulin and the kidney. *Nephron* 1975;15:306–326.
100. Katholi RE, Carey RM, Ayers CR, Vaughan ED Jr, Yancey MR, Morton CL. Production of sustained hypertension by chronic intrarenal norepinephrine infusion in conscious dogs. *Circ Res* 1977;40(Suppl I):I118–I126.
101. Kleinjans JCS, Smits JFM, Kasbergen CM, Vervoort-Peters HTM, Poudier HAJS. Blood pressure response to chronic low-dose intrarenal noradrenaline infusion in conscious rats. *Clin Sci* 1983;65:111–116.
102. Guyton AC, Coleman TG, Cowley AW Jr, Scheel KW, Manning RD Jr, Norman RA Jr. Arterial pressure regulation: overriding dominance of the kidneys in long-term regulation and in hypertension. *Am J Med* 1972;52:584–594.
103. Hall JE. Arterial pressure and body fluid homeostasis. *Fed Proc* 1986;45:2862–2863.
104. Hall JE, Guyton AC, Coleman TG, Mizelle HL, Woods LL. Regulation of arterial pressure: role of pressure natriuresis and diuresis. *Fed Proc* 1986;45:2897–2903.
105. Roman RJ. Pressure diuresis mechanism in the control of renal function and arterial pressure. *Fed Proc* 1986;45:2878–2884.
106. Landsberg L. Diet, obesity and hypertension: an hypothesis involving insulin, the sympathetic nervous system, and adaptive thermogenesis. *Q J Med* 1986;236:1081–1090.
107. Landsberg L. Insulin and hypertension—lessons from obesity. *N Engl J Med* 1987;317:378–379.
108. Landsberg L, Young JB. The role of the sympathoadrenal system in modulating energy expenditure. In: James WPT, ed. *Clinics in endocrinology and metabolism obesity,* vol 13. London: WB Saunders, 1984;475–499.
109. Landsberg L, Saville ME, Young JB. The sympathoadrenal system and regulation of thermogenesis. *Am J Physiol* 1984; 247:E181–E189.
110. Landsberg L, Young JB. The influence of diet on the sympathetic nervous system. In: Muller EE, MacLeod RM, Frohman LA, eds. *Neuroendocrine perspectives.* Amsterdam: Elsevier, 1985:191–218.
111. Young JB, Kaufman LN, Saville ME, Landsberg L. Increased sympathetic nervous system activity in rats fed a low-protein diet. *Am J Physiol* 1985;248:R627–R637.
112. Schwartz JH, Young JB, Landsberg L. Effect of dietary fat on sympathetic nervous system activity in the rat. *J Clin Invest* 1983;72:361–370.
113. Kaufman LN, Young JB, Landsberg L. Effect of protein on sympathetic nervous system activity in the rat: evidence for nutrient-specific responses. *J Clin Invest* 1986;77:551–558.
114. Young JB, Landsberg L. Impaired suppression of sympathetic

activity during fasting in the gold thioglucose-treated mouse. *J Clin Invest* 1980;65:1086–1094.

115. Miller DS, Mumford P. Gluttony 1. An experimental study of overeating on high protein diets. *Am J Clin Nutr* 1967;20:1212–1222.
116. Miller DS, Mumford P, Stock MJ. Gluttony 2. Thermogenesis in overeating man. *Am J Clin Nutr* 1967;20:1223–1229.
117. Sims EAH, Danforth E, Horton ES, Bray G, Glennon JA, Salans LB. Endocrine and metabolic effects of experimental obesity in man. *Recent Prog Horm Res* 1973;29:457–496.
118. Bogardus C, Lillioga S, Ravussin E, Abbott W, Zawadzki JK, Young A, Knowler WC, Jacobowitz R, Moll PP. Familial dependence of the resting metabolic rate. *N Engl J Med* 1986;315:96–100.
119. Jequier E, Schutz Y. Does a defect in energy metabolism contribute to human obesity? In: Hirsch J, Van Itallie TB, eds. *Recent advances in obesity research: IV.* London: John Libbey, 1985;76–81.
120. Hjemdahl P. Measurements of plasma catecholamines by HPLC and the relation of their concentrations to sympathoadrenal activity. In: Fillenz M, Macdonald IA, Marsden CA, eds. *Monitoring neurotransmitter release during behaviour.* Chichester, England: Ellis Horwood, 1986;17–32.
121. Landsberg L, Young JB. Assessment of sympathetic nervous activity from measurements of noradrenaline turnover in rats. In: Joseph MH, ed. *Monitoring neurotransmitter release during behavior.* Chichester, England: Ellis Horwood, 1986;33–47.
122. Sowers JR, Whitfield LA, Catania RA, Stern N, Tuck ML, Dornfeld L, Maxwell M. Role of the sympathetic nervous system in blood pressure maintenance in obesity. *J Clin Endocrinol Metab* 1982;54:1181–1186.
123. Reisin E, Frohlich ED, Messerli FH, Dreslinski GR, Dunn FG, Jones MM, Batson HM Jr. Cardiovascular changes after weight reduction in obesity hypertension. *Ann Intern Med* 1983;98:315–319.
124. Sowers JR, Nyby M, Stern N, Beck F, Baron S, Catania R, Vlachis N. Blood pressure and hormone changes associated with weight reduction in the obese. *Hypertension* 1982;4:686–691.
125. Kolanowski J. Influence of insulin and glucagon on sodium balance in obese subjects during fasting and refeeding. *Int J Obes* 1981;5(Suppl 1):105–114.
126. Sims EA. Mechanisms of hypertension in the overweight. *Hypertension* 1983;4(Suppl III):III43–III49.
127. Jung RT, Shetty PS, Barrand M, Callingham BA, James WPT. Role of catecholamines in hypotensive response to dieting. *Br Med J* 1979;1:12–13.
128. Weinsier R, Liu C, Norris D, Birch R, Darnell B, Hunter G, Dustan H. The relative effects of calorie restriction and weight loss on blood pressure in moderately hypertensive obese women. *Clin Res* 1987;35(3):781A.
129. Kolanowski J, Bodson A, Desmicht P, Bemelmans S, Stein F, Crabbe J. On the relationship between ketonuria and natriuresis during fasting and upon refeeding in obese patients. *Eur J Clin Invest* 1978;8:277–282.
130. Koppeschaar HPF, Meinders AE, Schwarz F. The effects of modified fasting on blood pressure and sympathetic activity: a correlation? *Int J Obes* 1983;7:569–574.
131. Barney CC, Wuertz KE, Katovich MJ. Effects of thyroid replacement on beta-adrenergic responsiveness of food-deprived rats. *Am J Physiol* 1986;250:R861–R867.
132. Dustan HP. Obesity and hypertension. *Ann Intern Med* 1985;103(6 Pt 2):1047–1049.
133. Stamler R, Stamler J, Grimm R, Gosch FC, Elmer P, Dyer A, Berman R, Fishman J, Van Heel N, Civinelli J, McDonald A. Nutritional therapy for high blood pressure: final report of a four-year randomized controlled trial—the Hypertension Control Program. *JAMA* 1987;257(11):1484–1491.
134. MacMahon SW, MacDonald GJ, Bernstein L, Andrews G, Blackett RB. Comparison of weight reduction with metoprolol in treatment of hypertension in young overweight patients. *Lancet* 1985;1:1233–1236.
135. Andersson OK, Fagerberg B, Hedner T. Importance of dietary salt in the hemodynamic adjustment to weight reduction in obese hypertensive men. *Hypertension* 1984;6:814–819.
136. Ostman-Smith I. Cardiac sympathetic nerves as the final common pathway in the induction of adaptive cardiac hypertrophy. *Clin Sci* 1981;61:265–272.
137. DeHaven J, Sherwin R, Hendler R, Felig P. Nitrogen and sodium balance and sympathetic-nervous-system activity in obese subjects treated with a low-calorie protein or mixed diet. *N Engl J Med* 1980;302:477–482.
138. Walgren MC, Kaufman LN, Young JB, Landsberg L. The effects of various carbohydrates on sympathetic activity in heart and interscapular brown adipose tissue (IBAT) of the rat. *Metabolism* 1987;36(6):585–594.
139. Young JB, Landsberg L. Stimulation of the sympathetic nervous system during sucrose feeding. *Nature* 1977;269:615–617.
140. Young JB, Mullen D, Landsberg L. Caloric restriction lowers blood pressure in the spontaneously hypertensive rat. *Metabolism* 1978;27:1711–1714.
141. Preuss MS, Preuss HG. The effects of sucrose and sodium on blood pressures in various substrains of Wistar rats. *Lab Invest* 1980;43:101–107.
142. Affarah HB, Hall WD, Heymsfield SB, Kutner M, Wells JO, Tuttle EP Jr. High-carbohydrate diet: antinatriuretic and blood pressure response in normal men. *Am J Clin Nutr* 1986;44:341–348.
143. Anderson JW, Tietyen-Clark J. Dietary fiber: hyperlipidemia, hypertension, and coronary heart disease. *Am J Gastroenterol* 1986;81:907–919.
144. Anderson JW. High-fiber, hypocaloric vs very-low-calorie diet effects on blood pressure of obese men. *Am J Clin Nutr* 1986;43:695.
145. Anderson JW, Bryant CA. Dietary fiber: diabetes and obesity. *Am J Gastroenterol* 1986;81:898–906.
146. Horton ES. The role of exercise in the treatment of hypertension in obesity. *Int J Obes* 1981;5:165–171.
147. Krotkiewski M, Mandroukas K, Sjostrom L, Sullivan L, Wetterqvist H, Bjorntorp P. Effects of long-term physical training on body fat, metabolism, and blood pressure in obesity. *Metabolism* 1979;28:650–658.

PART C

Hypertension in Special Situations

Hypertension: Pathophysiology, Diagnosis, and Management, edited by J. H. Laragh and B. M. Brenner. Raven Press, Ltd., New York © 1990.

CHAPTER 109

The Renin–Angiotensin System in Normal and Hypertensive Pregnancy and in Ovarian Function

Phyllis August and Jean E. Sealey

The Renin–Angiotensin–Aldosterone System in Normal Physiology, 1761
The Circulating Renin–Angiotensin System, 1761
Prorenin: The Ovarian and Placental Prorenin–Renin–Angiotensin System, 1762
The RAAS in Normal Pregnancy, 1764
Hemodynamic Changes, 1764
Renal Changes, 1764
Endocrine Changes, 1765
The Functional Significance of the RAAS in Normal Pregnancy, 1769
Blood Pressure Regulation, 1770
Vascular Responsiveness, 1770
Sodium Balance, 1770
Maintenance of Uteroplacental Blood Flow, 1771
The Renin–Angiotensin System in Pregnancy Hypertension, 1772
Preeclampsia, 1772
Chronic Hypertension, 1773
Essential Hypertension, 1773
Renovascular Hypertension, 1774
Primary Aldosteronism, 1774
Conclusions, 1775
References, 1775

The renin–angiotensin–aldosterone system (RAAS) plays a major role in blood pressure regulation and in fluid and electrolyte balance. The renal secretion of renin causes a cascade of events that results in the generation of angiotensin II. Angiotensin II causes vasoconstriction and elevation in blood pressure, and it stimulates the adrenal gland to secrete aldosterone, which then increases sodium reabsorption and kaliuresis. The rise in blood pressure, which is due to angiotensin-II-mediated vasoconstriction and aldosterone-induced expansion of blood volume, results in lowering of plasma renin activity, and the system is thus kept in check (Fig. 1) (1).

Normal pregnancy is associated with profound alterations in cardiovascular and renal physiology. These alterations are accompanied by striking adjustments of the RAAS Currently under active investigation is the precise nature of the interrelationship between (a) the cardiovascular and renal alterations in pregnancy and (b) the RAAS. A new dimension to the field has been added with the recognition that in the ovary and placenta there may be locally active renin–angiotensin systems that play a role in the physiology of pregnancy (2). It is hoped that further clarification of the interactions between the RAAS and reproductive events should shed light on the pathophysiology of major clinical disorders such as hypertension in pregnancy. Meanwhile, an awareness of the state of the art may provide the foundation for the care of such patients and for the design of future studies.

THE RENIN–ANGIOTENSIN–ALDOSTERONE SYSTEM IN NORMAL PHYSIOLOGY

The Circulating Renin–Angiotensin System

Renin, a proteolytic enzyme (MW 40,000) with highly restricted substrate specificity, is secreted into the circulation by the kidney. Renin is synthesized and stored in the renal juxtaglomerular cells which are found at the pole of the glomerulus. Renin-secreting cells are also found along the afferent arteriole. Changes in renin secretion occur with changes in renal perfusion pressure, posture, and extracellular fluid volume. These responses may be mediated by (a) a baroreceptor mechanism within the afferent arteriole (b) changes in the concentration of sodium chloride in renal tubular fluid which are sensed at the macula densa region

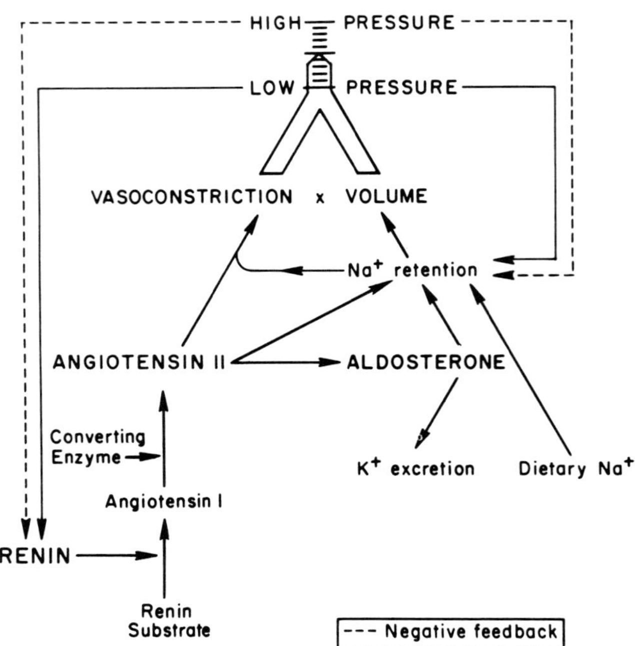

FIG. 1. The circulating renin–angiotensin–aldosterone system. (From ref. 125.)

of the distal tubule, (c) the sympathetic nervous system, (d) angiotensin-II-mediated feedback inhibition, and (e) other humoral and locally active agents such as vasopressin, atrial natriuretic factors, adenosine, and prostaglandins (1). Evidence suggests that these mechanisms operate via changes in intracellular calcium and cyclic AMP. Both prostacyclin (PGI_2) and PGE_2 directly stimulate renin release (3–5).

Once renin is released into the circulation, it acts on circulating angiotensinogen (renin substrate), which is of hepatic origin. The concentration of angiotensinogen in blood is normally at K_m; therefore, increases in renin substrate, without a concurrent fall in renin, could increase the rate of angiotensin formation by a maximum of twofold. Angiotensinogen is cleaved by renin, and the resulting decapeptide angiotensin I is subsequently converted to the active octapeptide hormone angiotensin II by angiotensin-converting enzyme (ACE). This last step is thought to take place primarily in the pulmonary circulation, where ACE is bound to the vascular endothelium.

The renin–angiotensin system, by its dual effects on arteriolar vasoconstriction and fluid volume via aldosterone, is a primary regulator of arterial blood pressure. Wherever systemic blood pressure falls, the rate of renin release increases, a phenomenon mediated by activation of the renal baroreceptor mechanism, the macula densa mechanism, and the sympathetic nervous system. The increase in circulating renin leads to (a) an increased rate of angiotensin II formation and (b) restoration of blood pressure. The increased angiotensin II also promotes renal sodium conservation and expansion of extracellular fluid volume by direct renal effects and by stimulation of aldosterone secretion by the adrenal cortex. The resulting volume expansion helps to maintain blood pressure and tissue perfusion. The resulting increased renal perfusion pressure, expansion of fluid volume, and increased levels of circulating angiotensin II, in turn, serve to return renin secretion toward normal.

Prorenin: The Ovarian and Placental Prorenin–Renin–Angiotensin System

Renin has been identified in several extrarenal tissues, many of which are involved in reproductive function, including the placenta, uterus, testes, ovary, and anterior pituitary. Other sources include the adrenal gland and perhaps also the pineal gland, brain, heart, and vascular system. Current evidence suggests that the extrarenal renin–angiotensin systems may be controlled by changes in prorenin rather than by changes in active renin (2).

In the kidney, prorenin functions as the biosynthetic precursor of active renin. It has a molecular weight of approximately 50,000. Close to 90% of the renin in the circulation is normally inactive and is present as prorenin. In the plasma, prorenin is measured by converting it to active renin by limited proteolysis with trypsin, and then the total renin is measured. Prorenin is then calculated by subtracting active renin from total renin. The kidney is the only known source of active renin; the kidney also secretes most of the circulating prorenin, but, after nephrectomy, when active renin has disappeared from the circulation, small amounts of prorenin remain.

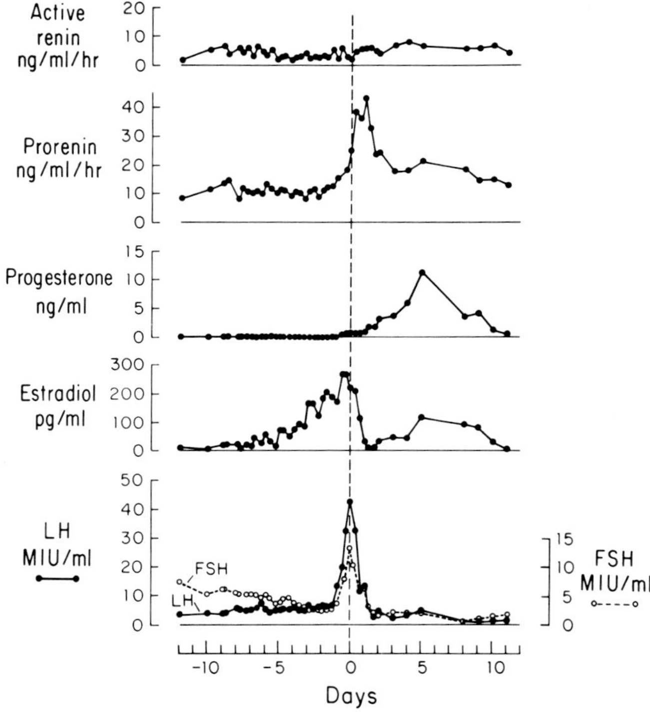

FIG. 2. Hormonal changes throughout the menstrual cycle in one normal woman. Day zero represents LH (luteinizing hormone) peak. FSH, follicle-stimulating hormone. Note that the peak of prorenin immediately follows the LH surge and is not accompanied by any change in active renin. (From ref. 12.)

Current evidence suggests that the renal secretion of active renin and prorenin are linked. In general, any stimulus to renin secretion usually also results in an increase in the blood level of prorenin. Changes in plasma prorenin are slower (measured in terms of days rather than minutes) and usually are proportionally less (6).

Two extrarenal tissues have very high concentrations of prorenin but relatively low levels of active renin; they are the placenta (7,8) and the ovaries at mid-menstrual cycle or during pregnancy (9). Placental prorenin will be discussed in the section entitled "The RAAS in Normal Pregnancy," since it is only present during pregnancy; however, changes in ovarian prorenin secretion occur in normal women during the menstrual cycle and will be reviewed here.

The ovaries appear to synthesize prorenin for 2 or 3 days during each menstrual cycle at the time of ovulation. Prorenin is found in the ovarian follicular fluid that surrounds the mature egg in concentrations close to 100 times the normal blood level (approximately 3000 ng/ml/hr) (10). The ovary secretes prorenin, but not active renin, into the blood within 8 hr after the beginning of the luteinizing hormone (LH) surge, and the blood level remains high until about 24 hr after LH has returned to baseline (i.e., just after ovulation) (Fig. 2) (11,12). In normal women, who usually have only one mature follicle per month, a twofold rise in plasma prorenin occurs at mid-menstrual cycle. Women who have undergone ovarian hyperstimulation and who have several mature follicles may have a much greater rise, to as much as 20 times the baseline level (13). In fact, the magnitude of the mid-cycle rise is directly related to the number of mature follicles. Sometimes the blood level of prorenin in ovarian-hyperstimulated women is transiently as high as that found in patients with renin-secreting tumors (Fig. 3).

Ovarian prorenin secretion is under gonadotropin control. It is stimulated by the exogenous administration of human chorionic gonadotropin (hCG) (Fig. 3) (14). The ovary will continue to secrete prorenin during the luteal phase of the menstrual cycle if hCG is administered at mid-cycle in lieu of a spontaneous LH surge because the half-life of hCG is very long (36 hr) compared to that of LH; furthermore, the blood level of hCG remains detectable well into the luteal phase.

The role of prorenin in ovarian function has yet to be discovered. Pellicar et al. (15) have reported a reduction in the number of eggs found in rat fallopian tubes after administration of an angiotensin II antagonist to hyperstimulated rats. This demonstrates that angiotensin may be required for successful ovulation, but it does not define the mechanism. Prorenin appears to function via angiotensin II, since angiotensin II receptors and angiotensin II itself are present in the ovary (16,17). We do not know how

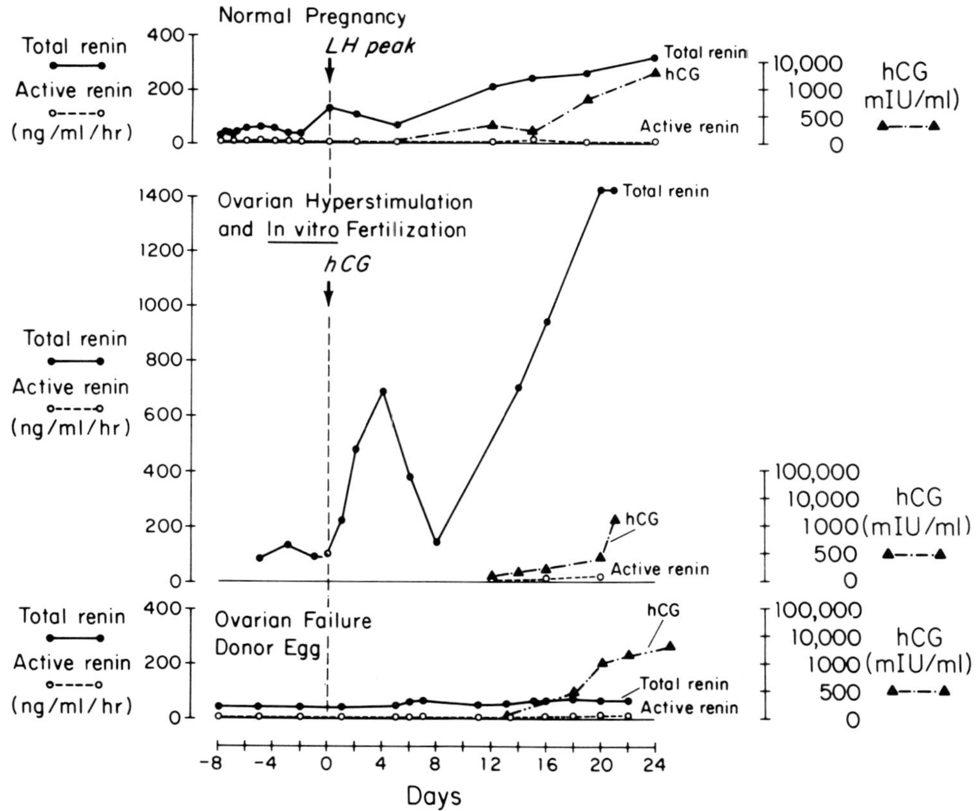

FIG. 3. Plasma total renin, active renin, and hCG measurements during early pregnancy in a normal pregnant patient (**upper panel**), in an ovarian-stimulated patient who conceived following *in vitro* fertilization (IVF) and embryo transfer (**middle panel**), and in a patient with ovarian failure who conceived after induction of an artificial cycle and IVF of a donated oocyte (**lower panel**). She received exogenous estrogen and progesterone during the first trimester. (From ref. 127.)

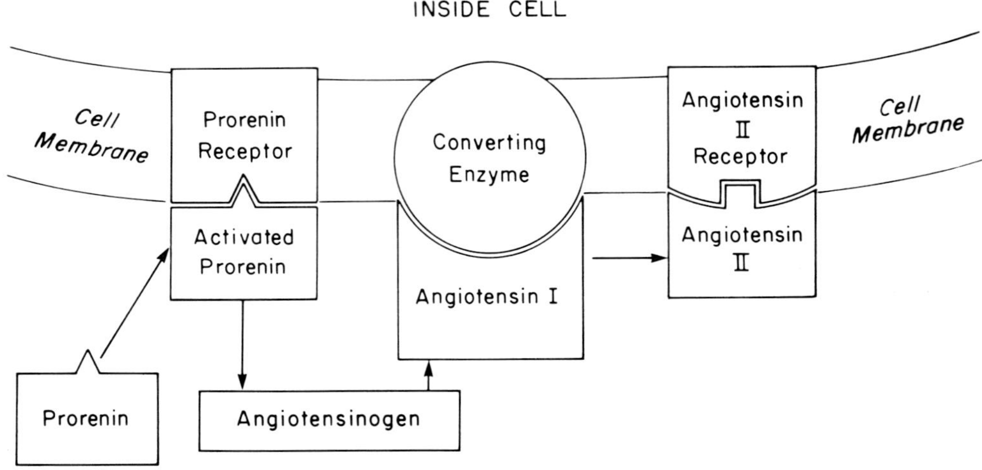

FIG. 4. Hypothetical mechanism of action of a local prorenin–renin–angiotensin system which may function in tissues where the renin gene is expressed and in which prorenin has a receptor and where binding to the receptor results in exposure of the active site. The enzyme would be active only for as long as prorenin was bound to its receptor. Thus, the prorenin–angiotensin system would function only where there are prorenin receptors, and it would function independently of circulating active renin. (From ref. 9.)

prorenin can form angiotensin without the concurrent formation of active renin in appreciable amounts. Our current working hypothesis is that there are prorenin receptors which recognize only the prosequence of prorenin; when prorenin binds to its receptor, the active site of renin may be exposed, resulting in a locally active prorenin and a locally active prorenin–angiotensin system which does not require the formation of active renin (Fig. 4) (2,9).

Current studies are aimed at defining the physiological role of the ovarian prorenin–angiotensin system. Possibilities include steroid biosynthesis, ovulation, angiogenesis, and prostaglandin biosynthesis. Since angiotensin II can affect intracellular calcium and can also inhibit adenylate cyclase activity, there are many potential roles for angiotensin II in cells which have angiotensin receptors. Of course, one must also entertain the possibility that prorenin may function independently of renin.

THE RAAS IN NORMAL PREGNANCY

By mid-pregnancy, the normal pregnant woman has an increased cardiac output, lower blood pressure, decreased systemic vascular resistance, increased blood volume, and increased renal blood flow and glomerular filtration rate (GFR) (18). The specific hemodynamic and hormonal adjustments that result in these changes are still incompletely understood as is the precise time course of their development.

Hemodynamic Changes

During pregnancy the cardiac output rises 30–40% relative to the nonpregnant resting state (19,20). The increase in cardiac output occurs as early as the 12th week and is a result of increased heart rate and stroke volume (20). The increased stroke volume is believed to be due to the increase in plasma volume (up to 50%) that occurs beginning in the first trimester and is sustained until term.

Despite the increased cardiac output and increased plasma volume, blood pressure falls during normal pregnancy in association with a decrease in peripheral vascular resistance (21,22). The decrease in blood pressure is apparent by the end of the first trimester, and it reaches a nadir in the second trimester (Fig. 5). Blood pressure then increases gradually in the third trimester and often approaches prepregnancy levels at term. The reasons for the fall in peripheral vascular resistance are not established, but they are presumed to be the consequence of increased vasodilatory substances such as prostaglandins, estrogens, and possibly progesterone (23,24). The time course of all these physiologic changes, as well as their relationship to each other, has not been conclusively established. Very few studies of hemodynamics have been done in humans before the end of the first trimester. Of interest is a recent study of serial hemodynamic changes in baboon pregnancy in which it was shown that cardiac output rose, blood pressure fell, and vascular resistance fell prior to the increase in plasma volume (25).

Renal Changes

Renal blood flow (measured by *p*-amino hippurate clearance) increases markedly during pregnancy with mid-pregnancy increments of 60–80%. This is followed by a fall in the third trimester. GFR is increased by about 50% throughout pregnancy (26). Significant elevation of the creatinine clearance is apparent as soon as 4 weeks after conception (27). The basis for these striking changes is not known but has been attributed to the increased cardiac output and fluid volume, as well as to concurrent endocrine changes, although many of these changes are appar-

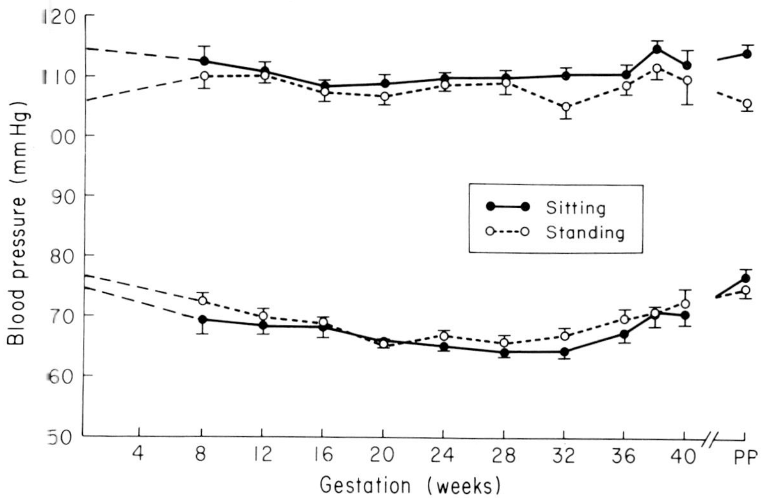

FIG. 5. Serial changes in sitting and standing blood pressure during pregnancy. (From ref. 22.)

ent only after GFR has already risen. Micropuncture studies of single-nephron GFR in the pregnant rat indicate that the increase in GFR is due to increased glomerular plasma flow, which, in turn, is a result of renal vasodilation (28).

In addition to the alterations in renal hemodynamics, many other renal adaptations to pregnancy have been reported, including increased uric acid clearance, decrease in plasma osmolality, and a cumulative retention of sodium.

Endocrine Changes

The endocrine adaptations to pregnancy are the most dramatic physiologic adjustments that occur. The fetus, placenta, and maternal ovary and adrenal gland participate in the production of large amounts of estradiol-17β, estriol, progesterone (Fig. 6), aldosterone, deoxycorticosterone, human placental lactogen, and hCG, as well as other pregnancy-specific peptide hormones and prostaglandins (29). Although considerable progress has been made in our understanding of the synthesis and metabolism of these substances, less is known regarding the precise ways in which these hormones maintain a normal pregnancy. Both estrogens and progesterone have been shown to have hemodynamic and renal effects; therefore, it is quite likely that these hormones interact with other regulatory systems in the control of blood pressure during pregnancy. For example, elevated levels of estrogens during pregnancy are, in part, responsible for the elevations in renin substrate (see below). Progesterone is natriuretic and appears to inhibit the renal tubular effect of aldosterone.

It is against this background of massive changes in fluid and electrolyte homeostasis and in hormonal levels, during pregnancy, that the alterations in the RAAS must be considered.

Prorenin

One of the first components of the RAAS to change during pregnancy is prorenin (Fig. 3). The rise in plasma prorenin parallels the increase in hCG and occurs within 2 weeks after conception (30). It reaches a peak (approximately 10 times the normal blood level) within 20 days after conception and remains high until parturition. There is a slight fall in plasma prorenin during the second and third trimester. Plasma prorenin falls slowly post-partum but is back to pre-pregnancy levels after about 3 weeks.

These changes in prorenin during early pregnancy are exaggerated in women who conceive after ovarian hyper-

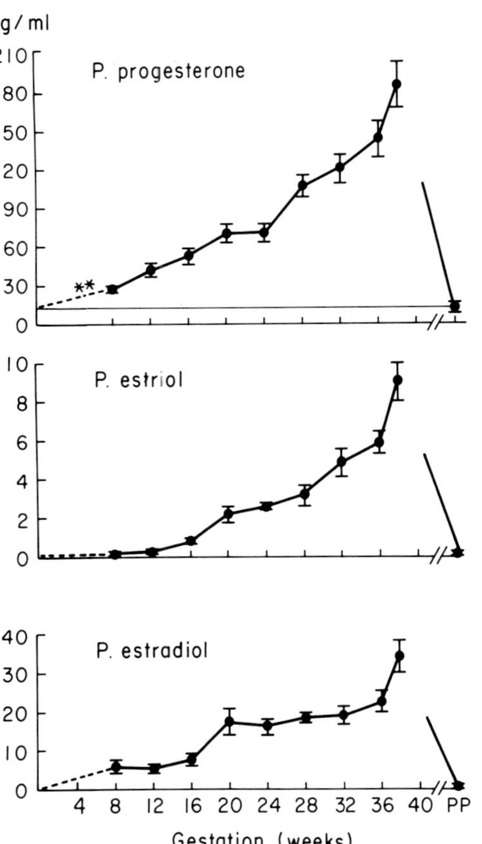

FIG. 6. Sequential changes, throughout pregnancy, in plasma progesterone, plasma estriol, and plasma estradiol (mean ± SE) (**$p < 0.01$). (From ref. 22.)

stimulation (Fig. 3). In these individuals the height of the prorenin rise is related to (a) the number of mature follicles at the time of aspiration and (b) the number of corpora lutea that are formed (13). When the number of follicles is high, the rise in prorenin can be very striking, as illustrated in Fig. 3, middle panel (31).

The 10-fold rise in plasma prorenin that occurs early in normal pregnancy does not occur in women with ovarian failure who conceive with donor eggs and whose pregnancy is maintained with exogenous estrogen and progesterone replacement (Fig. 3) (9,32). Thus, this early rise in prorenin is from the ovaries. Nonetheless, women with ovarian failure do exhibit a small increase in prorenin early in pregnancy, and prorenin rises further during the second and third trimesters. At no time, however, does it reach the levels found in women with normal ovaries. The first-trimester rise in prorenin in women with ovarian failure may be due to renal secretion of prorenin in response to the diuretic effect of progesterone, which is given to such patients in the first trimester to maintain the pregnancy. As gestation proceeds, this effect may be magnified as the placenta produces more and more progesterone. Alternatively, the rise could be the result of uterine secretion of prorenin.

In the second and third trimesters, prorenin may also be secreted from uterine and placental tissues (33). The contribution of these organs to circulating prorenin levels is currently under study. Decidual tissue from the uterus can synthesize renin (34), but so far there are no studies that reveal whether uterine secretion of prorenin occurs. From *in vivo* and *in vitro* studies, there is evidence that the placenta secretes prorenin into the maternal circulation, but the magnitude of this contribution is unknown (33,35). The placenta cannot account for most of the prorenin in the maternal circulation in third-trimester pregnancy; this is because the postpartum fall in plasma prorenin takes many days, yet the half-life of prorenin is quite short (close to an hour) (6). Nonetheless, the uterus could be an important source of prorenin.

It is likely that placental prorenin acts locally. The highest prorenin concentrations in the placenta are found in the chorion laeve (36,37), which has a poor vascular supply and is therefore unlikely to secrete prorenin into the maternal circulation. Very high concentrations of prorenin are also found in amniotic fluid. It is likely that the chorion laeve is the source of amniotic fluid prorenin; this is because the amnion also has a high prorenin content, yet there is no evidence that the amnion can synthesize renin. Prorenin, like prolactin, may pass through the amnion into the amniotic fluid.

We do not know if ovarian, uterine, or placental prorenin plays a role in cardiovascular regulation during pregnancy or if it contributes to the pathophysiology of toxemia of pregnancy. The answers to these questions should become clearer during the next few years as we learn more about the prorenin–angiotensin system in reproductive tissues.

Angiotensinogen

Angiotensinogen increases gradually throughout pregnancy to about five times pre-pregnancy levels by the end of the third trimester in response to increasing estrogen levels (Fig. 7) (8,22,38,39). This change could double the rate of angiotensin formation, thereby doubling plasma renin activity; however, feedback inhibition of renin secretion occurs, thereby effectively maintaining a physiologically appropriate level of angiotensin II production. Therefore, during pregnancy, elevation in angiotensinogen cannot entirely account for the increased plasma renin activity. The placenta synthesizes a high-molecular-weight form of renin substrate (40), and this is the major form in amniotic fluid. High-molecular-weight angiotensinogen is also secreted into the circulation from the placenta, and it comprises close to 20% of the total plasma renin substrate of pregnant women. It is reported to be abnormally high in

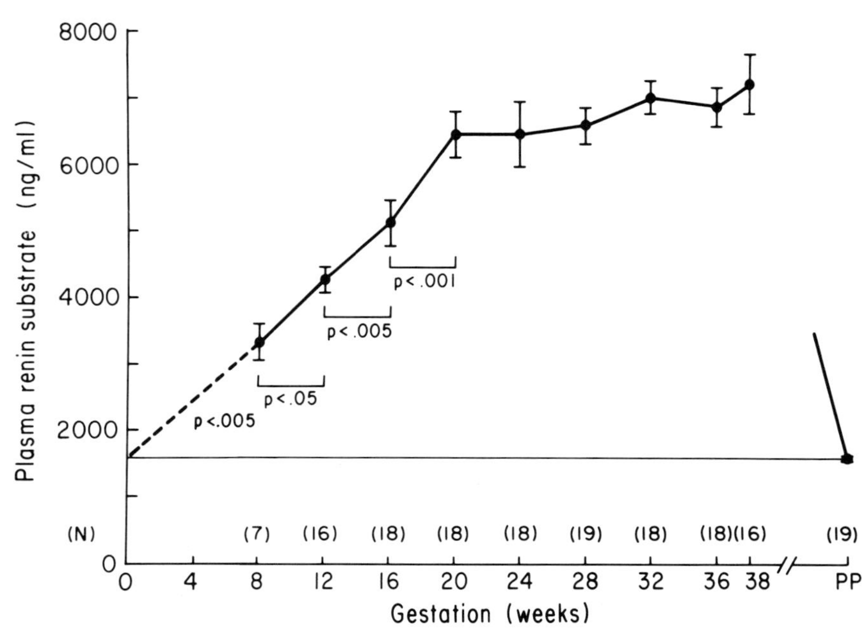

FIG. 7. Sequential changes in plasma renin substrate (angiotensinogen) throughout normal pregnancy. (From ref. 22.)

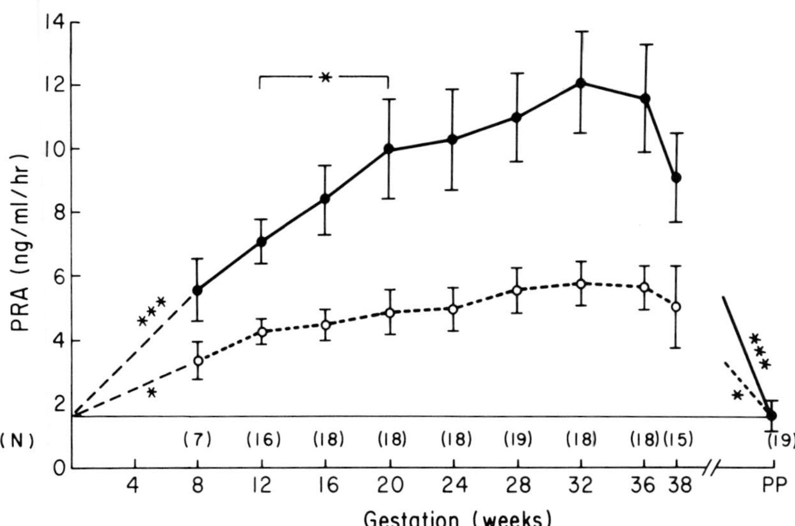

FIG. 8. Sequential changes in PRA (●) and in PRA normalized to the postpartum substrate values (○) (mean ± SE) throughout pregnancy (*$p < 0.05$; ***$p < 0.001$). (From ref. 22.)

the plasma of hypertensive pregnant women (41). Tewksbury has shown that high-molecular-weight angiotensinogen has a molecular weight of close to 350,000. This is made up of a dimer, each half of which is about 170,000; this, in turn, is comprised of low-molecular-weight angiotensinogen and unidentified protein (D. Tewksbury, *personal communication*).

Active Renin

As shown in Fig. 8, plasma renin activity (PRA) rises during the first few weeks of pregnancy; there is, on average, close to a fourfold increase by the end of the first trimester, with a further rise until at least 20 weeks (22). The initial rise in active renin may be caused by the same hormonal changes that occur during the luteal phase of the menstrual cycle. Active renin is higher during the luteal phase than during the follicular phase, and this may be due to the diuretic effect of increased plasma progesterone levels (11). During the follicular phase the progesterone level is less than 1 ng/ml, and it increases to a peak of 15–25 ng/ml during the luteal phase. Following conception, this level of progesterone is maintained for several weeks until the placental progesterone appears in the circulation; then the levels increase further, up to a peak of around 200 ng/ml during the third trimester. The hypothesis that the rise in PRA early in pregnancy may be related to increased progesterone levels is supported by our observation that active renin can be very high in early pregnancy after ovarian hyperstimulation (13). These women have very high progesterone levels, and in individual subjects the relationship between plasma renin and plasma progesterone is strong (Fig. 9).

The changes in PRA during late pregnancy follow different patterns in different individuals (Fig. 10). Sealey et al. (42) studied PRA in 14 women throughout gestation. In eight women, PRA continued to rise during the second and third trimesters, while in six it remained constant after 20 weeks. There were no apparent differences between the groups with respect to blood pressure, 24-hr urine sodium, or renin substrate. However, the women in whom active

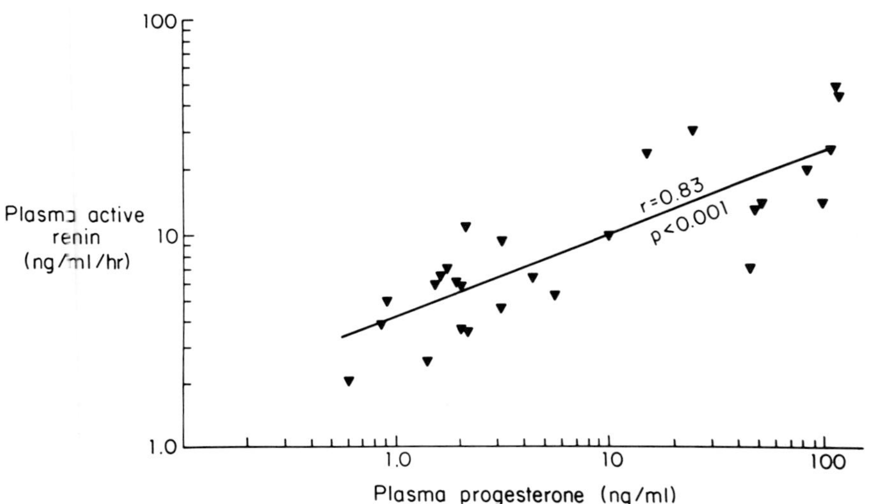

FIG. 9. The relationship between plasma progesterone and plasma renin before and during first-trimester pregnancy in one woman after ovarian hyperstimulation. She received FSH and pergonal for 8 days and then was given hCG on the next day, day 0 (10,000 IU, intramuscularly), day 2 (5000 IU), day 5 (2500 IU), and day 8 (2500 IU). Bloods were collected daily until day 2, every 2nd or 3rd day until day 29, then weekly until day 64. Following conception, active renin increased to levels as high as those seen at term in normal pregnancy (Fig. 8), in association with plasma progesterone levels similar to those seen in the third trimester (From ref. 126.)

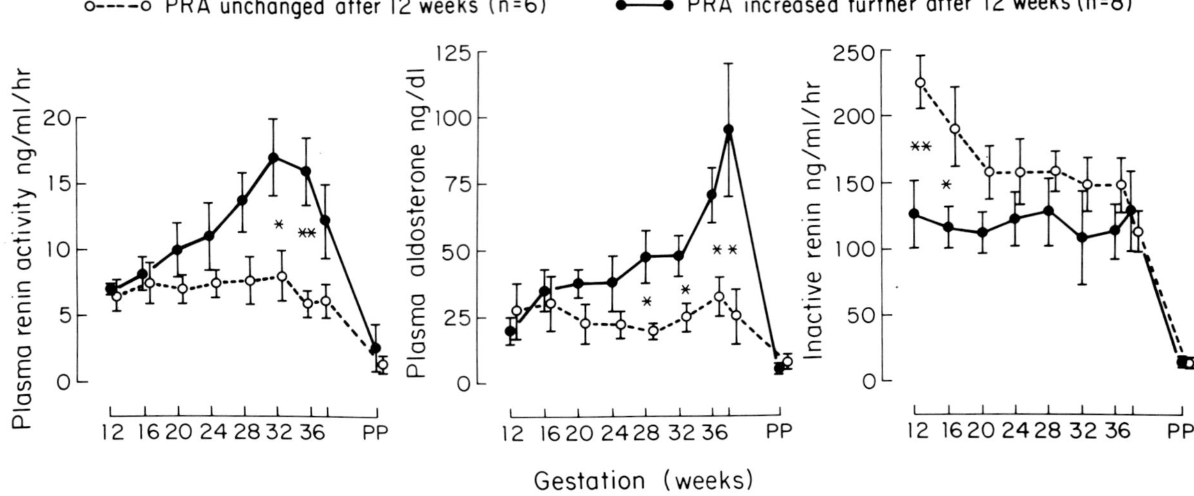

FIG. 10. Changes in active renin, plasma aldosterone, and inactive renin in two groups of normal pregnant women separated according to changes in active renin after 16 weeks gestation. PRA increased further in Group A (●), whereas it remained unchanged in Group B (○). Group A was 6 years younger (24 ± 1.8 years) and had lower plasma prorenin levels at 12 and 16 weeks. (From ref. 42.)

renin continued to rise were younger (24 ± 1.8 years compared to 30 ± 2, $p < 0.05$) and had higher inactive renin (prorenin) levels during early pregnancy.

In vitro cryoactivation of plasma prorenin has led to false reports of PRA levels in pregnancy (6). Cryoactivation of prorenin can occur in plasma at temperatures between +6°C and freezing. Cryoactivation of prorenin occurs because endogenous inhibitors of plasma serine proteases cannot work properly at cold temperatures and therefore endogenous plasma proteases, such as plasmin and plasma kallikrein, can slowly cleave the prosegment of prorenin, which itself undergoes a conformational change when cold (43). Cryoactivation is especially a problem in pregnancy when the plasma prorenin level can be 100-fold higher than active renin. If as little as 10% of this prorenin is activated *in vitro,* the reported level of active renin could be 10-fold higher than it should be. Lack of recognition of this problem has led to some of the confusion about the changes in active renin that occur in pregnancy and about their relation to angiotensin II levels.

In nonpregnant subjects, total nephrectomy leads to a disappearance of active renin from the blood. This suggests that circulating active renin is exclusively of renal origin (44). In pregnancy the issue of the source of active renin is not resolved, since uterine and fetal–placental tissue are also a potential source. Nonetheless, since changes in sodium intake during pregnancy affect active renin in the same way as in normal subjects, the kidneys are the most likely source of most of the active renin in human plasma (45–47). However, studies of nephrectomized rabbits have raised the possibility that, in some species, active renin may be secreted by the uterus or the fetoplacental unit and may help to maintain blood pressure (48–51). These studies were not confirmed in the dog, suggesting that major species differences may occur (52). Since the hormonal changes that occur in pregnancy are different in various species, one must be cautious in assuming that the hormonal regulation of rabbit and human pregnancy is the same. For example, the ovaries are essential for maintaining pregnancy in the rabbit but are only required during the first trimester in humans (53).

The possible effect of uteroplacental renin on uteroplacental blood flow will be discussed below.

Angiotensin II

The increased PRA that occurs during pregnancy would be expected to cause increased angiotensin II levels as well. Although it is technically difficult to measure circulating angiotensin II, the few studies that have been done confirm that angiotensin II is elevated during gestation (38). Moreover, the fact that pregnancy is characterized by a decreased pressor response to angiotensin II (54) is consistent with increased circulating angiotensin II levels (see below). Furthermore, when pregnant animals are given converting-enzyme inhibitors, blood pressure falls (55,56). We have recently demonstrated a similar angiotensin II dependency of blood pressure in pregnant women (Fig. 11) (57).

Aldosterone

Changes in renin and angiotensin in the circulation are associated with commensurate changes in the secretory rate of aldosterone (1). Like active renin, aldosterone is high during the luteal phase of the menstrual cycle; this high level is sustained into early pregnancy. Elevations in the secretory rate of aldosterone have been reported during pregnancy by several investigators (22,38,58). Wilson et al. (22) measured plasma and urine aldosterone levels sequentially in 69 pregnant women (Fig. 12). Plasma aldosterone increased significantly by 8 weeks and continued to rise during the next 2 months. A further increase in aldosterone

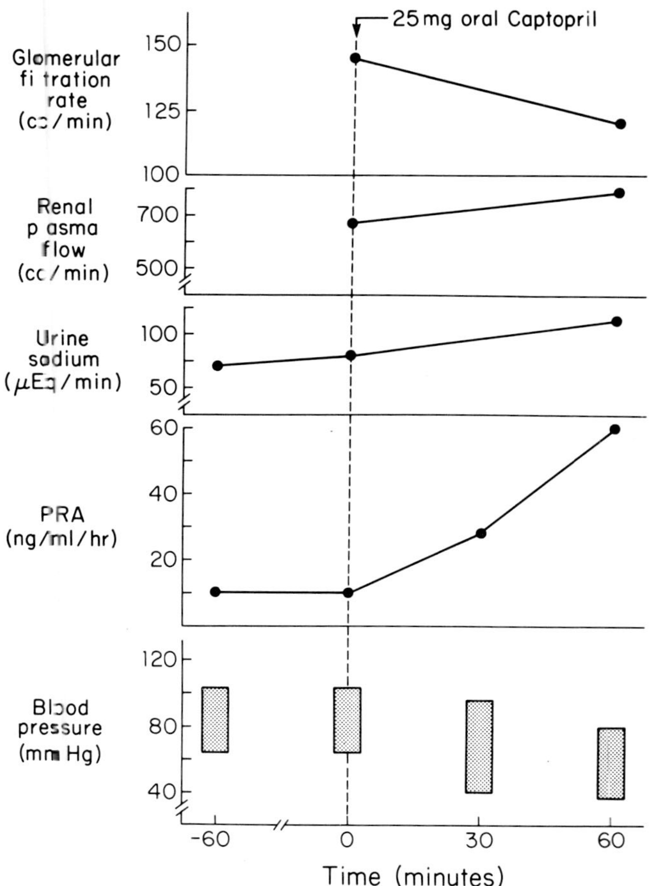

FIG. 11. Renal hemodynamics, PRA, and blood pressure response to oral captopril in a normal pregnant woman at 11 weeks gestation. Glomerular filtration rate (inulin clearance), renal plasma flow (*p*-amino hippurate clearance), urine sodium, plasma renin activity (PRA), and blood pressure were determined before and after administration of 25 mg captopril (time 0). (From ref. 126.)

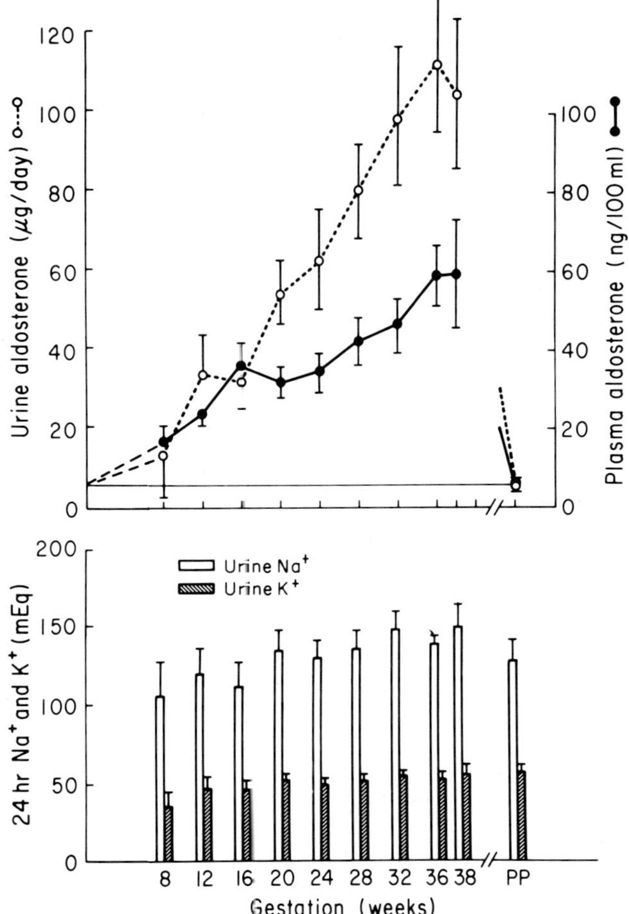

FIG. 12. Sequential changes throughout pregnancy in plasma aldosterone, urine aldosterone, urinary sodium, and potassium (mean ± SE). (From ref. 22.)

occurred in the last trimester, so that by 38 weeks the level was 10 times that measured at 6 weeks post-partum. There was a weak correlation between plasma aldosterone and PRA during pregnancy ($r = 0.37$; $p < 0.001$). Nonetheless, in individual patients the relationship was more striking. This is illustrated in Fig. 10, in which it can be seen that plasma aldosterone failed to rise further in those patients in whom plasma renin reached a plateau after 20 weeks gestation, but plasma aldosterone rose significantly after 20 weeks gestation in those in whom active renin increased further (43).

In general, the changes in urinary aldosterone paralleled those of plasma aldosterone (Fig. 12). By 12 weeks, the urinary aldosterone (34.5 ± 9.6 μg/day) was sevenfold higher than baseline. It rose steeply and progressively, to a peak of 112 ± 17 μg/day at 36 weeks; this was not associated with any trend away from normal in the 24-hr urinary sodium and potassium excretion (Fig. 12). Between 16 and 38 weeks gestation, there appeared to be a greater proportional increase in urinary aldosterone than in plasma aldosterone. This may reflect an increased production of the 3-oxo conjugate of aldosterone (the urinary metabolite that is measured) as compared to the production of other metabolites of aldosterone.

THE FUNCTIONAL SIGNIFICANCE OF THE RAAS IN NORMAL PREGNANCY

The physiologic consequences of the stimulated RAAS in pregnancy are incompletely understood at the present time. The limitations of our knowledge are due, in part, to (a) a paucity of data in early pregnancy and (b) insufficient longitudinal studies throughout pregnancy relating PRA levels to other hormonal and hemodynamic parameters. Because of the importance of the RAAS in the physiology of blood pressure control, and the prevalence of hypertensive disorder of pregnancy, the field remains one of great importance.

Before we discuss the possible role of the RAAS in hypertensive disorders of pregnancy, it is worthwhile reviewing what is known about how this system operates during normal pregnancy.

Blood Pressure Regulation

As mentioned, during normal pregnancy the blood pressure falls while cardiac output, plasma volume, GFR, and renal blood flow increase. The decrease in blood pressure is associated with a decreased systemic vascular resistance, which is presumably a result of an increased production of vasodilatory substances such as prostacyclin (PGI_2), PGE_2, or steroid hormones (23,24). It would appear, then, that one basis for the stimulated PRA during pregnancy is vasodilatation with consequent decreased renal perfusion pressure and that, in this setting, angiotensin II is necessary to maintain blood pressure. Indeed, when pregnant animals are given converting-enzyme inhibitors, blood pressure drops—demonstrating the need for angiotensin to maintain the blood pressure. We have recently demonstrated a similar response in humans (Fig. 11) (57). There is considerable controversy surrounding this issue, however. For example, it is argued that pregnancy is a volume-expanded state and that the increases in GFR and renal plasma flow are secondary to progressive volume expansion which occurs as a result of primary renal sodium retention (59). If the volume status of a pregnant woman is sensed by baroreceptors as expanded or normal, this would not support a baroreceptor-mediated mechanism for increased PRA. Rather, one would have to invoke the direct effect of elevated prostacyclin on renin secretion—or possibly an extrarenal source of renin—to explain the stimulated RAAS.

A study by Phippard et al. (25) of serial changes in hemodynamics in the pregnant baboon has shed light on some of these issues. These authors made sequential observations of cardiac output, blood pressure, systemic vascular resistance, blood volume, PRA, and aldosterone concentrations throughout gestation, beginning at 4 weeks. Their results showed systemic vasodilation and a synchronous fall in arterial pressure very early in pregnancy, and from the outset the fall in arterial pressure was entirely due to a fall in peripheral resistance. Indeed, the most striking point of this investigation was that these hemodynamic changes and the increase in PRA occurred prior to any volume expansion, thereby supporting the notion that the stimulated RAAS in pregnancy is a consequence of vasodilation and lower blood pressure. These measurements need to be confirmed in humans.

Vascular Responsiveness

In 1961, Abdul-Karim and Assali (54) observed that the pressor response to angiotensin II was much less during pregnancy than in nonpregnant individuals. This observation has been repeatedly confirmed over the years (reviewed in ref. 60). Gant et al. (61) prospectively studied the pressor responses to angiotensin II in 192 primigravid females and confirmed that normal pregnant women are relatively refractory to the pressor effects of angiotensin II but that pregnant women with preeclampsia regain sensitivity to this pressor substance. Brown et al. (62) recently documented that this phenomenon is apparent early in pregnancy, by the end of the first trimester. Possible mechanisms for the decreased pressor responsiveness in pregnancy are as follows: increased levels of angiotensin II, resulting in greater occupancy of vascular angiotensin II receptors; a decrease in angiotensin II receptor number or affinity; a generalized defect in the vascular smooth muscle contraction; and/or the need to overcome the effect of an angiotensin-II-induced vasodilator substance such as prostacyclin. Studies in animals and women have not resolved this issue. Pregnant rats given the converting-enzyme inhibitor captopril (to decrease angiotensin II levels) still demonstrated blunted pressor responses to angiotensin II, suggesting that prior occupancy of vascular angiotensin II receptors is probably not entirely responsible for the decreased pressor response (63). In the pregnant ewe, however, acute elevation of circulating angiotensin II levels did indeed decrease the pressor responses to angiotensin II (64). Studies of vascular reactivity in pregnant women in response to various volume loads (and a significant decrease in circulating renin and angiotensin II) have shown that pressor responsiveness to angiotensin II was unchanged (60). Gant et al. (60) hypothesized that the increased refractoriness to angiotensin II in pregnancy may be a direct result of the action of prostaglandins on vascular smooth muscle. In fact, these authors have shown that prostaglandin synthesis inhibitors restore vascular sensitivity to angiotensin II, although this has not been consistently observed in experimental animals (65). Other investigators have suggested that 17β-estradiol or prolactin might mediate the altered vascular responsiveness in pregnancy (63,66). Altogether, we think that the bulk of the evidence favors the idea that the blunted pressor response to angiotensin II during pregnancy is the result of increased activity of the renin–angiotensin system together with an augmented ability of angiotensin II to stimulate vasodilatory substances, most likely prostaglandins.

Sodium Balance

One of the most striking physiologic changes in pregnancy is the kidneys' ability to increase sodium reabsorption. Despite the large increase in the filtered load of sodium, the normal pregnant woman has a slightly positive sodium balance, estimated at 950 mEq during gestation (18).

During pregnancy, several factors lead to increased natriuresis. These include: increased GFR, increased renal blood flow, and increased plasma progesterone. Progesterone enhances sodium excretion in humans by its ability to competitively inhibit the salt-retaining effect of aldosterone in the distal nephron (67,68). In addition, it has been suggested that progesterone may directly inhibit proximal sodium reabsorption (69). We have studied hormonal changes in women who conceived after ovarian hyperstimulation. In this setting, estrogen and progesterone levels during the first trimester are similar in magnitude to those which are normally seen in the third trimester (22). Active renin and urinary aldosterone are increased as well. The correlation between renin and progesterone (Fig. 9) suggests that the stimulation of the RAAS is responsive to (a) the hormonal changes of pregnancy and (b) the presence of the fetoplacental unit per se. In these hyperstimulated women, despite extremely high levels of urinary aldosterone (over 100 μg/day compared to a normal of 5 μg/day) there were no apparent changes in urinary excretion of sodium and potassium. This suggests that (a) the aldosterone level was high in order to overcome the effect of progesterone binding to the aldosterone receptor, (b) the effective aldosterone level was appropriate to the physiological situation, and (c) aldosterone was necessary to maintain sodium balance in the setting of increased natriuretic stimuli.

Aldosterone secretion in late pregnancy has been shown to respond readily to changes in salt balance and to postural stimuli, and these responses are associated with parallel changes in PRA (70–72). Brown et al. (47) have recently documented that both renin and aldosterone levels respond appropriately (and in parallel) to changes in dietary sodium intake in normal women in the second and third trimester. PRA and plasma and urinary aldosterone levels rose in response to salt depletion. When pregnant women were fed a high-salt diet, PRA was suppressed—although not to the degree seen in nonpregnant individuals.

Pregnant women are quite sensitive to the sodium-retaining activity of administered mineralocorticoids, in spite of the baseline elevation of plasma aldosterone (73). Thus, when Ehrlich et al. (73) administered deoxycorticosterone acetate (DOCA) to pregnant women, they found that these women retained sodium, gained weight, and demonstrated the normal mineralocorticoid "escape". In addition, blockade of aldosterone secretion in normal pregnant subjects by administration of heparinoid resulted in natriuresis and weight loss (74).

In nonpregnant individuals, angiotensin II contributes to sodium balance by its role in the control of aldosterone secretion and by its local intrarenal effects which modulate tubular reabsorption of salt and water (75). There is evidence that angiotensin II stimulates proximal tubular sodium reabsorption and that it may also increase the sensitivity of the tubuloglomerular feedback mechanism (75). Most of these data have been obtained from experimental animals or from isolated perfused kidney models. There is very little data on the intrarenal effects of angiotensin II on sodium balance in pregnancy. Chesley (76) infused *pressor* doses of angiotensin II into pregnant women and found that, compared to nonpregnant women, they had less of a drop in sodium excretion, GFR, and renal blood flow, as measured by inulin and PAH clearance, suggesting that during pregnancy there is a blunted renal response to angiotensin II (76). Subsequently, Brown et al. (62) infused angiotensin II into normal first-trimester women and found that fractional excretion of sodium decreased, but less so than in nonpregnant women (62). In both studies, the renal effects of exogenously administered angiotensin II were studied. The role of physiologic levels of angiotensin II on salt balance in pregnancy has yet to be investigated.

Maintenance of Uteroplacental Blood Flow

In addition to maintaining normal blood pressure and regulating sodium balance, there is evidence that the renin–angiotensin system, in conjunction with vasodilatory prostaglandins (PGI_2, PGE_2), modulates uteroplacental blood flow (77–82). The maternal circulation interfaces with the placenta at the level of the spiral arteries, which end in the lacuna which form the intervillous space. The maternal blood bathes the chorionic villi of the placenta and then flows back to the mother via the uterine veins. The fetal circulation consists of the umbilical artery, which branches into multiple small capillary networks in the placental chorionic villi and then returns to the fetus via the umbilical vein. Factors that influence the uteroplacental circulation may therefore be of fetal, placental, or maternal origin. In this chapter we have considered, so far, the physiological effects of the maternal renin–angiotensin system in pregnancy. However, the fetus has a functionally active renin–angiotensin system, and at least some components of the renin–angiotensin system can be localized to placental tissue. Therefore, the modulation of uteroplacental blood flow by angiotensin II or other vasoactive substances may represent a combination of local (fetal, placental) and circulating (maternal) effects.

It is technically difficult to measure uteroplacental blood flow in humans; therefore, much of what is known so far has been from animal studies. In 1972, Ferris et al. (49) reported that angiotensin II caused paradoxical vasodilation in the uterine circulation of nephrectomized pregnant rabbits. In addition, administration of the converting-enzyme inhibitor captopril to pregnant rabbits significantly reduced uterine blood flow and uterine vein PGE levels without changing cardiac output or renal blood flow (83). Of interest is the observation that when captopril was administered to pregnant ewes and rabbits in one study, there was a high incidence of stillbirths (55). The suggestion has been made that the mechanism might be angiotensin blockade, with resulting reduction of uterine PGE synthesis and decreased uteroplacental blood flow. However, it is difficult to interpret this effect of captopril in rabbits, since it has not been observed in sheep or in humans (56,84–86). Franklin et al. (78) subsequently showed that in monkeys, intravenous infusion of angiotensin II led to increased concentrations of PGE_2 in uterine vein, decreased uterine vascular resistance, and increased uterine blood flow. Since angiotensin II stimulates arachidonic acid release from phospholipids of cell membranes and promotes prostaglandin synthesis, it is likely that the vasodilating effects of angiotensin II are mediated by prostaglandins (87,88).

In contrast, Seino et al. (51) gave captopril to nephrectomized pregnant rabbits and demonstrated an increase in uteroplacental blood flow; they suspected that the effect was due to increased generation of kinins.

It appears that although angiotensin II may sometimes have a vasodilatory effect on uterine blood flow, it consistently has a vasoconstricting effect on the fetal circulation. Experiments performed on the isolated perfused placental cotyledon have shown that the fetal circulation is highly sensitive to angiotensin II and responds to pharmacologic doses of angiotensin I or angiotensin II by vasoconstriction (89,90). Angiotensin-converting enzyme is known to be present in the capillary vessels of the placental villi and in the trophoblast tissue (91). Furthermore, the placenta has the functional capacity for conversion of angiotensin I to angiotensin II. Additional studies of isolated placental cotyledons have confirmed the vascular responsiveness to the renin–angiotensin system in the fetoplacental circuit and have identified and characterized human placental angiotensin II receptors (92).

It is assumed that the renin measured in the fetal circulation is of fetal kidney origin and that the renin measured in the maternal circulation is of maternal origin. A role for the large amounts of prorenin synthesized in chorionic or trophoblast tissue has not yet been identified. An effect on either maternal or fetal circulations has not been ruled out.

THE RENIN–ANGIOTENSIN SYSTEM IN PREGNANCY HYPERTENSION

Hypertension in pregnancy is not one clinical entity. Multiple clinical diagnostic categories, each with somewhat different pathophysiology, are recognized by the American College of Obstetrics and Gynecology: (i) preeclampsia/eclampsia, (ii) chronic hypertension with or without superimposed preeclampsia, and (iii) transient hypertension.

Preeclampsia

Preeclampsia is defined clinically as elevated blood pressure and proteinuria occurring after 20 weeks gestation. The clinical expression of preeclampsia is very variable, ranging from (a) mild elevations in blood pressure at term to (b) early-onset severe disease. A multitude of hemodynamic and hormonal alterations occur, including increased peripheral vascular resistance, failure to develop the physiologic hypervolemia of pregnancy, reduction(s) in GFR and renal blood flow, abnormalities in sodium excretion, increased vascular sensitivity to pressor substances, and, occasionally, coagulopathy.

Recent studies have documented that preeclampsia is characterized by abnormal placentation, in which the trophoblast does not properly invade the muscular wall of the maternal spiral arteries (93). These arteries abnormally retain their ability to vasoconstrict in response to vasoactive substances and to neural stimuli, resulting in inadequate blood flow to the fetal placental unit. It is hypothesized that the clinical features of preeclampsia, such as hypertension, are a consequence of this abnormal placentation process. Women with chronic hypertension appear more likely to develop inadequate uteroplacental blood flow.

There is a tremendous amount of controversy regarding what role, if any, the renin–angiotensin system plays in preeclampsia. Unfortunately, most of the currently available data on the renin–angiotensin system in hypertensive pregnancy have been obtained in women in the third trimester of pregnancy. Very few longitudinal studies have been conducted. Although it is probable that some (or even all) forms of pregnancy hypertension *are not* directly mediated by excess angiotensin II, an understanding of the alterations in the RAAS that occur in these conditions may clarify the pathophysiology.

Most authors have observed that in established preeclampsia, PRA and aldosterone are usually lower than in normal pregnancy but are higher than in nonpregnancy (94–96). Moreover, in kidney biopsies taken several days after delivery from women with pregnancy-induced hypertension, the juxtaglomerular cells contained less immunoreactive renin than did the normal kidney (97).

There are a few studies in which angiotensin II levels have been measured in hypertensive pregnancy, and the results of these studies are inconclusive (98,99). This may be due to the great difficulty in measuring angiotensin II accurately in the circulation. Symonds and Broughton-Pipkin (100) measured angiotensin II levels in 50 primigravid women at term and found a positive correlation between diastolic blood pressure and angiotensin II levels. They also found that preeclamptics had higher levels of angiotensin II despite lower PRA levels. The authors suggested that angiotensin II is secreted from the placental bed. Additional studies have shown that angiotensin II levels in cord venous blood are higher in infants born to mothers with pregnancy hypertension (101). It has been suggested that the raised levels of angiotensin II originating from the fetoplacental unit may be the cause of suppression of maternal renin secretion (due to feedback inhibition) in addition to being responsible for the elevations in blood pressure. This explanation is not supported by another study, in which different investigators infused angiotensin into second-trimester women with pregnancy-induced hypertension and found that raised levels of angiotensin II did not result in suppression of PRA (102).

The uteroplacental renin–angiotensin system has been implicated in the pathogenesis of preeclampsia. In a rabbit model of preeclampsia, angiotensin II levels were reported to be higher in vessels draining the uterus, despite lower maternal arterial levels of angiotensin II (103). Brar et al. (104) reported that cord venous and arterial active renin were higher in women with pregnancy-induced hypertension than in normal pregnant women. They suggest that the *fetal* renin–angiotensin system plays a role in maintaining placental perfusion in the face of inadequate uteroplacental circulation.

In addition to having lower PRA, women with preeclampsia are more sensitive to the pressor effects of angiotensin II than are normal pregnant women (60,61,105). The increase in sensitivity, which precedes the hypertension, begins as early as the 18th week of gestation in women destined to develop preeclampsia (61). As mentioned above, the pressor response to angiotensin II is diminished in normal pregnancy—a phenomenon that has been attributed to the effects of elevated levels of angiotensin II. It has been hypothesized that a reduction in vasodilatory prostaglandins is responsible for both the decrease in PRA and the increased sensitivity to angiotensin II that is characteristic of preeclampsia. Remuzzi et al. (106) first reported that umbilical arteries from preeclamptic pregnancies synthesized less PGI_2. Subsequently, both cross-sectional and longitudinal studies (during pregnancy) of urinary PGI_2 metabolites (6-keto $PGF_{1\alpha}$ and 2,3-dinor 6-keto $PGF_{1\alpha}$) support the observation that prostacyclin synthesis is reduced in preeclampsia (107,108). In *in vitro* studies of perfused placentas obtained from preeclamptics, impaired PGI_2 generation has been reported in umbilical artery and vein (109,110).

Because PGI_2 stimulates renal renin release, the lower levels of this substance may explain the decreased PRA in preeclampsia. Similarly, lower levels of prostacyclin may

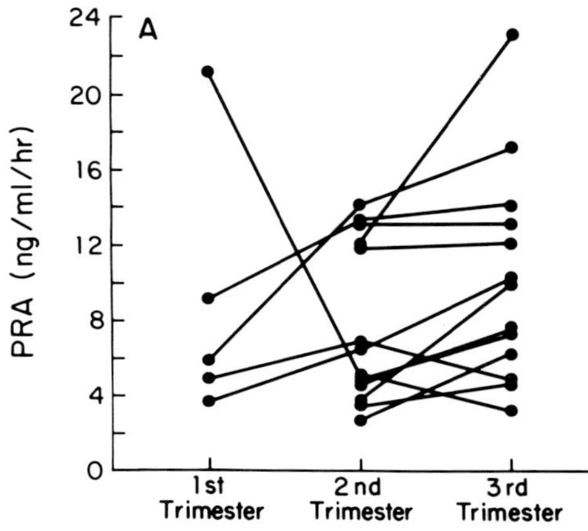

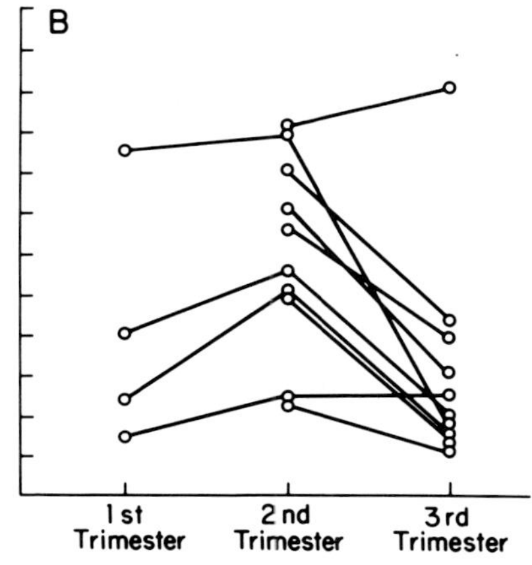

FIG. 13. Serial changes in plasma renin activity (PRA) in each trimester in pregnant women with chronic hypertension. **A:** Demonstration of serial PRA in women with uncomplicated chronic hypertension; **B:** Demonstration of serial PRA in chronic hypertensive women who developed superimposed preeclampsia in the third trimester. (From ref. 126.)

be responsible for the increased sensitivity to angiotensin II. This is supported by the data in normal pregnant women documenting that prostaglandin synthesis inhibitors restore vascular sensitivity to angiotensin II (65).

Although it is generally agreed that plasma volume is lower in preeclampsia than in normal pregnancy, it is uncertain whether this decreased plasma volume is sensed by the renal baroreceptor mechanisms as "hypovolemia" or whether the increased peripheral resistance (and therefore smaller circulatory capacity) leads to a smaller measured plasma volume. The lower PRA in preeclampsia is more consistent with a volume-expansed state than with a volume-contracted state. Indeed, it has been shown that women with preeclampsia abnormally retain sodium, an observation which is compatible with lower PRA (111). Additionally, preeclamptic women have been reported to show reduced sodium excretion, particularly after saline infusion (112–114). One interpretation of the data is that angiotensin II sensitivity is increased by sodium retention, leading to suppressed PRA—with hypertension ensuing as a result of a combination of sodium retention and increased angiotensin II sensitivity. Others have interpreted the suppressed PRA in preeclampsia in the setting of sodium retention as an inadequate renal response to plasma volume contraction (114).

We have observed that in some patients with severe preeclampsia, atrial natriuretic peptide (ANP) levels are increased and PRA is suppressed (115). A higher ANP/PRA ratio is often seen in clinical settings characterized by volume expansion; however, it is possible that in pregnancy, volume status may not be the primary determinant of ANP secretion. Further studies are needed to clarify the relationship between plasma volume, renin, and ANP in pregnancy.

The bulk of evidence is that maternal PRA is lower in preeclampsia, although the reason for PRA suppression is unclear. There is evidence that serial changes in PRA in high-risk pregnancies reflect subsequent clinical events such as development of preeclampsia or poor fetal outcome (116,117). In pregnant chronic hypertensive women, we have found that PRA decreases prior to, or at the time of, development of superimposed preeclampsia, while in uncomplicated pregnancies it rises or stays the same (Fig. 13) (116). Moreover, we have found that in hypertensive pregnancy, an abnormally low PRA prior to delivery is frequently associated with growth-retarded infants or with small-for-gestational-age infants (117).

One of the major difficulties in establishing the role of the renin–angiotensin system in preeclampsia has been the reluctance to administer converting-enzyme inhibitors to pregnant women because of the adverse experience in rabbits. Recently, reports on their use have begun to appear in the literature. The data are not conclusive regarding their safety or efficacy (84–86,118). Dramatic improvements or definitive adverse effects have not been reported.

Chronic Hypertension

In women with chronic hypertension due to essential hypertension or secondary hypertension, the changes in the RAAS may be similar to those observed in normal pregnancy; or deviations may be present, depending on the underlying diagnosis.

ESSENTIAL HYPERTENSION

There are only a few studies of the RAAS in women with essential hypertension in pregnancy (119,120). Broughton-Pipkin et al. (119) reported serial measurements and found them to be similar to values observed in normotensive women. Weinberger et al. (120) reported serial PRA and plasma aldosterone levels in 26 chronic hypertensive women throughout pregnancy and found that these parameters were similar to those observed in normal pregnancy —except in the third trimester, when PRA and plasma aldosterone decreased. These authors did not correlate the third-trimester PRA with clinical outcome, and it is possible that suppression of PRA was associated with the devel-

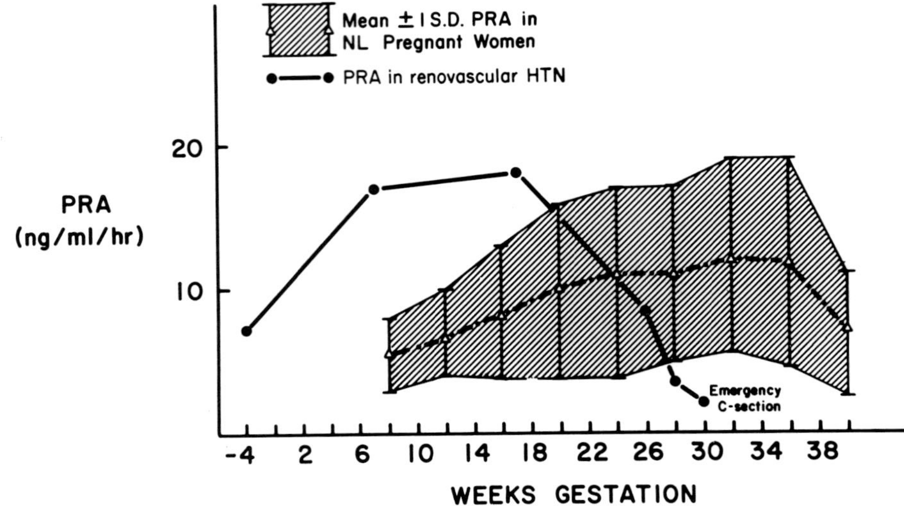

FIG. 14. Plasma renin activity (PRA) throughout pregnancy in a woman with renovascular hypertension. The patient developed superimposed preeclampsia at 30 weeks, and an emergency C-section was performed. A drop in PRA was apparent at 26 weeks. The shaded area represents the mean ± one standard deviation of PRA in normal pregnant women (n = 69). (From ref. 126.)

opment of superimposed preeclampsia. Results from our laboratory show that in pregnant women with chronic hypertension, PRA decreases prior to, or at the time of, development of superimposed preeclampsia. In our patients with uncomplicated essential hypertension during pregnancy, PRA was similar to that observed in normotensive pregnant women (Fig. 13) (116).

RENOVASCULAR HYPERTENSION

Renovascular hypertension due to fibromuscular dysplasia of the renal artery is a common cause of secondary hypertension in young women, and it frequently presents in the second and third decades. It would therefore be expected that women with this condition would often become pregnant without being aware of the diagnosis. Indeed, in one series of patients who developed severe preeclampsia, postpartum renal angiography showed an incidence of renal artery stenosis of 12% (121), suggesting that this diagnosis may be frequently missed. Renovascular hypertension is associated with elevated PRA in nonpregnant individuals; however, it is not known whether the RAAS behaves differently during pregnancy. We have followed serial PRA in a woman with fibromuscular dysplasia throughout pregnancy and observed that her PRA was in the high range of normal throughout most of the pregnancy. Shortly before she developed severe superimposed preeclampsia, her PRA precipitously dropped to a level that was lower than her prepregnancy value (Fig. 14).

PRIMARY ALDOSTERONISM

Rarely, a pregnant woman with chronic hypertension may have primary aldosteronism. Several cases have been reported (122–124). Gordon et al. (122) were the first to document that during pregnancy, women with primary aldosteronism will have a suppressed PRA despite a high aldosterone secretion rate—in contrast to normal pregnant women, in whom both PRA and aldosterone are elevated. In most of the reported cases of primary aldosteronism in

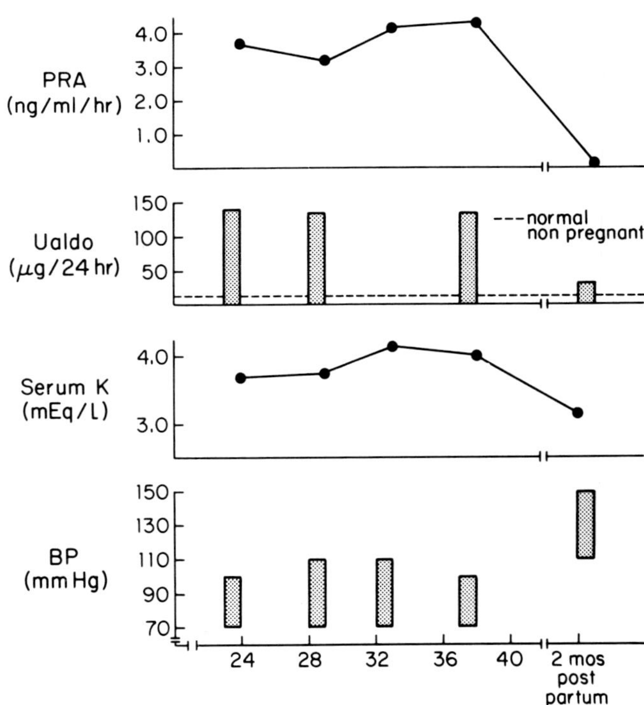

FIG. 15. Plasma renin activity (PRA), urine aldosterone excretion, serum potassium, and blood pressure during pregnancy and 2 months post-partum in a woman with primary aldosteronism. Hypertension and hypokalemia disappeared during pregnancy on no therapy and recurred after delivery. (From ref. 126.)

pregnancy, hypertension and hypokalemia persist; however, this is not always the case. Biglieri and Slaton (123) reported a patient with primary aldosteronism in whom metabolic and blood pressure abnormalities were improved during pregnancy, an effect attributed to elevated progesterone levels. We have followed blood pressure, PRA, serum potassium, and urine aldosterone in a pregnant woman with primary aldosteronism and observed a similar phenomenon. As shown in Fig. 15, PRA was lower than expected during pregnancy, blood pressures and serum potassium were normal, and urinary aldosterone was elevated. It appears that, in primary aldosteronism during pregnancy, suppressed PRA may be a useful diagnostic criterion, as it is in nonpregnant individuals.

CONCLUSIONS

The RAAS plays an integral role in the physiology of pregnancy and ovarian function. A hypothetical scheme of events related to the circulating RAAS in pregnancy is shown in Fig. 16. During pregnancy, PRA is stimulated, probably in response to prostaglandin and hormonally mediated vasodilation and progesterone-induced natriuresis. The elevated levels of angiotensin and aldosterone are necessary for the maintenance of blood pressure and salt balance. It is likely that the RAAS and prostaglandins participate in the regulation of fetal–uteroplacental blood flow.

In preeclampsia, PRA is lower, possibly because of either (a) decreased levels of prostaglandins or (b) renal disease with concomitant sodium retention. Since preeclamptics are more sensitive to the pressor effects of angiotensin II despite a lower PRA, it is possible that increased angiotensin II sensitivity may, in part, be responsible for the elevated blood pressure in this condition. Changes in the RAAS during pregnancy may aid in the diagnosis of different hypertensive disorders such as primary aldosteronism, renovascular hypertension, and superimposed preeclampsia.

The ovary and the placenta both express the renin gene throughout gestation but do not process prorenin to renin. The uterus also synthesizes prorenin. So far, only the ovary has been shown to have regulated secretion of prorenin. The role of these tissue prorenin systems in reproductive function is unknown and is the focus of current research into the function of locally active renin–angiotensin systems.

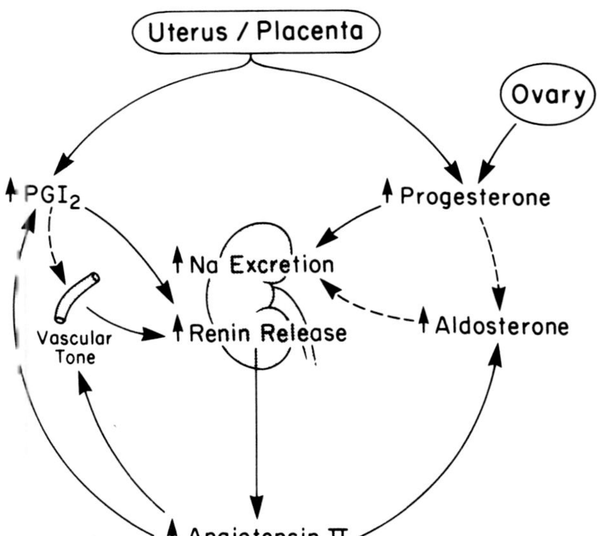

FIG. 16. A point of view concerning the circulating renin–angiotensin system in pregnancy. During pregnancy, increased levels of ovarian and placental progesterone result in natriuresis. Increases in prostacyclin (PGI_2) result in vasodilation. The natriuresis, vasodilation, and a direct effect of prostaglandins can all increase plasma renin activity. The resulting elevated levels of angiotensin II and aldosterone, in turn, help to maintain blood pressure and salt balance. Broken arrows denote inhibitory effects, whereas solid arrows denote stimulatory effects.

REFERENCES

1. Laragh JH, Sealey JE. The renin–angiotensin–aldosterone hormonal system and regulation of sodium, potassium, and blood pressure homeostasis. In: Orloff J, Berliner RW, eds. *American Physiological Society handbook of physiology: renal physiology.* Chapter 26, Baltimore: Waverly Press, 1973;831–908.
2. Sealey JE, Glorioso N, Itskovitz J, Laragh JH. Prorenin as a reproductive hormone; new form of the renin system. *Am J Med* 1986;81:1041–1046.
3. Churchill P. Second messengers in renin secretion. *Am J Physiol* 1985;F175–F184.
4. Whorton AR, Misono K, Hollifield J, Frolich JC, Inagami T, Oates JA. Prostaglandins and renin release: I. Stimulation of renin release from rabbit rena cortical slices by PGI_2. *Prostaglandins* 1977;14:1095–1104.
5. Gerber JG, Branch RA, Nies AS, Gerkens JF, Shand DG, Hollifield J, Oates JA. Prostaglandins and renin release. II. Assessment of renin secretion following infusion of PGI_2, E_2 and D_2 into the renal artery of anesthetized dogs. *Prostaglandins* 1978;15:81–87.
6. Sealey JE, Atlas SA, Laragh JH. Prorenin and other large molecular weight forms of renin. *Endocr Rev* 1980;1:365–391.
7. Lenz T, Sealey JE, August P, James GD, Laragh JH. Tissue levels of active and total renin, angiotensinogen, human chorionic gonadotropin, estradiol, and progesterone in human placentas from different methods of delivery. *J Clin Endocrinol Metab* 1989;69:in press.
8. Skinner SL, Cran EJ, Givson R, Raylor R, Walters WAW, Catt KJ. Angiotensin I and II, renin-substrate, renin activity, and angiotensinase in human liquor amnii and plasma. *Am J Obstet Gynecol* 1975;121:625.
9. Sealey JE, Glorioso N, Itskovitz J, Atlas SA, Pitarresi TM, Preibisz JJ, Troffa C, Laragh JH. Ovarian prorenin. *Clin Exp Hypertens* 1987;A9(8&9):1435–1454.
10. Glorioso N, Atlas SA, Laragh JH, Jewelewicz R, Sealey JE. Prorenin in high concentrations in human ovarian follicular fluid. *Science* 1986;233:1411–1424.
11. Sealey JE, Atlas SA, Glorioso N, Manapat H, Laragh JH. Cyclical secretion of prorenin during the menstrual cycle: synchronization with luteinizing hormone and progesterone. *Proc Natl Acad Sci USA* 1985;82:8705–8709.
12. Sealey JE, Cholst I, Glorioso N, Troffa C, Weintraub ID, James G, Laragh JH. Sequential changes in plasma LH and plasma prorenin during the menstrual cycle. *J Clin Endocrinol Metab* 1987;63:1–5.
13. Itskovitz J, Sealey JE, Glorioso N, Rosenwaks Z. Plasma prorenin response to hCG in ovarian hyperstimulated women: correlation with the number of ovarian follicles and steroid hormone concentrations. *Proc Natl Acad Sci USA* 1987;84:7285–7289.
14. Sealey JE, Glorioso N, Toth A, Atlas SA, Laragh JH. Stimulation of plasma prorenin by gonadotropic hormones [Letter]. *Am J Obstet Gynecol* 1985;153:596.
15. Pellicar A, Palumbo A, DeCherney AH, Naftolin F. Blockage of

ovulation by an angiotensin antagonist. *Science* 1988;240:1660–1661.
16. Husain A, Bumpus FM, DeSilva P, Speth RC. Localization of angiotensin II receptors in ovarian follicles and the identification of angiotensin II in rat ovaries. *Proc Natl Acad Sci USA* 1987;84:2498–2493.
17. Culler MD, Tarlatzis BC, Lightman A, Fernandez LA, Decherney AH, Negro-Vilar A, Naftolin F. Angiotensin II-like immunoreactivity in human ovarian follicular fluid. *J Clin Endocrinol Metab* 1986;62:613–615.
18. Lindheimer MD, Katz AI. The kidney in pregnancy. In: Brenner BM, Rector FC, eds. *The kidney.* Philadelphia: WB Saunders, 1986;1253–1295.
19. Bader ME, Bader RA. Cardiovascular hemodynamics in pregnancy and labor. *Clin Obstet Gynecol* 1968;11:924–939.
20. Wallenberg HCS. Hemodynamics in hypertensive pregnancy. In: Rubin PC, ed. *Handbook of hypertension,* vol 10. Amsterdam: Elsevier, 1988;66–101.
21. Chesley LC. *Hypertensive disorders in pregnancy.* New York: Appleton-Century-Crofts, 1978.
22. Wilson M, Morganti AA, Zervoudakis I, Letcher RL, Romney BM, Von Oeyon P, Papera S, Sealey JE, Laragh JH. Blood pressure, the renin–aldosterone system and sex steroids throughout normal pregnancy. *Am J Med* 1980;68:97.
23. Terragno NA, McGiff JC, Murray S, Terragno A. Patterns of prostaglandin production in the bovine fetal and maternal vasculature. *Prostaglandins* 1978;16:847–855.
24. Tamai T, Matsuura S, Tatsumi N, Nunotani T, Sagawa N. Role of sex steroid hormones in relative refractoriness to angiotensin II during pregnancy. *Am J Obstet Gynecol* 1984;149:177.
25. Phippard AF, Horvath JS, Glynn EM, Garner MG, Fletcher PJ, Duggin GG, Tiller DJ. Circulatory adaptation to pregnancy—serial studies of hemodynamics, blood volume, renin and aldosterone in the baboon (*Papio hamadryas*). *J Hypertens* 1966;4:773–779.
26. Davison JM, Dunlop M. Renal hemodynamics and tubular function in normal human pregnancy. *Kidney Int* 1980;18:152–161.
27. Davison JM, Noble MCB. Serial changes in 24 hour creatinine clearance during normal menstrual cycles and the first trimester of pregnancy. *Br J Obstet Gynecol* 1980;88:10.
28. Baylis C. Effect of early pregnancy on glomerular filtration rate and plasma volume in the rat. *Renal Physiol* 1980;2:333–339.
29. Pritchard JA, MacDonald PC, Gant NF, eds. *Williams Obstetrics,* 17th ed. East Norwalk, CT: Appleton–Century–Crofts, 1985.
30. Sealey JE, McCord D, Taufield PA, Ales KA, Druzin ML, Atlas SA, Laragh JH. Plasma prorenin in first trimester pregnancy: relationship to changes in human chorionic gonadotropin. *Am J Obstet Gynecol* 1985;153:514–519.
31. Sealey JE, Glorioso N, Itskovitz J, Troffa C, Cholst I, Rosenwaks Z. Plasma prorenin during early pregnancy: ovarian secretion under gonadotropin control? *J Hypertens* 1986;4(Suppl 5):S92–S95.
32. Derkx FH, Alberda AT, DeJong FH, Zeilmaker FH, Makovitz JW, Schalekamp MADH. Source of plasma prorenin in early and late pregnancy: observations in a patient with primary ovarian failure. *J Clin Endocrinol Metab* 1987;65:349–354.
33. Brar HS, Do Y-S, Tam HB, Valenzuela GJ, Murray RD, Longo LD, Yonekura ML, Hsueh WA. Uteroplacental unit as a source of elevated circulating prorenin levels in normal pregnancy. *Am J Obstet Gynecol* 1986;155(6):1223–1226.
34. Hsueh W, Kios S, Anderson PW, Maccaulay L, Sherrod A, Koss M, Shinagawa T, Do YS. Human decidua is a major extrarenal source of prorenin [Abstract]. In: *Program of the Council for High Blood Pressure Research 41st Annual Fall Conference and Scientific Sessions,* New Orleans, 1987;368.
35. Lenz T, Sealey JE, Laragh JH. Prorenin in perfusate of human placenta: evidence for secretion into maternal circulation. In: *Third European Meeting on Hypertension,* Milan, Italy, 1987.
36. Poisner AM, Words GW, Poisner R, Inagami T. Localization of renin in trophoblasts in human chorion laeve at term pregnancy. *Endocrinology* 1981;109:1150–1154.
37. Acker GM, Galen FX, Devaux C, Foote S, Papernik E, Pesty A, Menard J, Corvol P. Human chorionic cells in primary culture: a model for renin biosynthesis. *J Clin Endocrinol Metab* 1982;55:902–909.
38. Weir RJ, Brown JJ, Fraser R, Lever AF, Logan RW, MacIlwaine GM, Morton JJ, Robertson JIS, Tree M. Relationship between plasma renin, renin substrate, angiotensin II, aldosterone and electrolytes in normal pregnancy. *J Clin Endocrinol Metab* 1975;40:108–115.
39. Tree M. Measurement of plasma renin substrate in man. *J Endocrinol* 56:159–171.
40. Tewksbury DA, Tryon ES, Burrill RE, Dart RA. High molecular weight angiotensinogen: a pregnancy associated protein. *Clin Chim Acta* 1986;158:7–12.
41. Tewksbury DA, Dart RA. Elevated high molecular weight angiotensinogen levels in hypertensive pregnant women. *Hypertension* 1982;4:729–734.
42. Sealey JE, Wilson M, Morganti AA, Zervoudakis I, Laragh JH. Changes in active and inactive renin throughout normal pregnancy. *Clin Exp Hypertens* 1982;4A:2372–2384.
43. Sealey JE, Rubattu S. Prorenin and renin as separate medicators of tissue and circulatory systems. *Am J Hypertens* 1989;2:in press.
44. Sealey JE, Moon C, Laragh JH, Atlas SA. Plasma Prorenin in normal, hypertensive and anephric subjects and its effect on renin measurements. *Circ Res* 1977;40(Suppl I):41–45.
45. Weinberger MH, Kramer NJ, Grim CE, Petersen LP. The effect of posture and saline loading on plasma renin activity and aldosterone concentration in pregnant, non-pregnant and estrogen-treated women. *J Clin Endocrinol Metab* 1977;44:69.
46. Bay WH, Ferris TF. Factors controlling plasma renin and aldosterone during pregnancy. *Hypertension* 1979;1:410–415.
47. Brown MA, Nicholson E, Ross MR, Norton HE, Gallery EDM. Progressive resetting of sodium–renin–aldosterone relationship in human pregnancy. *Clin Exp Hypertens* [*B*] 1986/1987; B5(3):349–375.
48. Gorden P, Ferris TF, Mulrow PJ. Rabbit uterus as a possible site of renin synthesis. *Am J Physiol* 1967;212:703–706.
49. Ferris TF, Stein JH, Kauffman J. Uterine blood flow and uterine renin secretion. *J Clin Invest* 1972;51:2827–2833.
50. Albertini R, Seino M, Scicli AG, Carretero OA. Uteroplacental renin in regulation of blood pressure in the pregnant rabbit. *Am J Physiol* 1980;239:H266–H271.
51. Seino M, Carretero OA, Albertini R, Scicli AG. Kinins in regulation of uteroplacental blood flow in the pregnant rabbit. *Am J Physiol* 1982;242:H142–H147.
52. Carretero OA, Polomski C, Piwonska A, Afsari A, Hodgkinson CP. Renin release and the uteroplacental–fetal complex. *Am J Physiol* 1972;223:561–564.
53. Hilliard J, Scaramuzzi RJ, Parcardi R, Sawyer CH. Progesterone, estradiol and testosterone levels in ovarian venous blood of pregnant rabbits. *Endocrinology* 1973;93:1235.
54. Abdul-Karim R, Assali NS. Pressor response to angiotensin in pregnant and nonpregnant women. *Am J Obstet Gynecol* 1961;82:246–251.
55. Broughton-Pipkin F, Symonds EM, Turner SR. The effect of captopril upon mother and fetus in the chronically cannulated ewe and in the pregnant rabbit. *J Physiol* 1982;323:415.
56. Olsson K, Fyhrquist F, Benlamlih K. Effects of captopril on arterial blood pressure, plasma renin activity and vasopressin concentration in sodium-repleted and sodium-deficient goats: a serial study during pregnancy, lactation and anestrus. *Acta Physiol Scand* 1984;121:73–80.
57. August Taufield P, Mueller FB, Edersheim TG, Druzin ML, Laragh JH, Sealey JE. Blood pressure regulation in normal pregnancy: unmasking the role of the renin angiotensin system with captopril. *Clin Res* 1988;35:433A.
58. Watanabe M, Meeker CI, Gray MJ, Sims EAH, Solomon S. Aldosterone secretion rates in abnormal pregnancy. *J Clin Endocrinol* 1965;25:1665.
59. Lindheimer MD, Katz AI. Renal physiology in pregnancy. In: Seldin DW, Giebesch G, eds. *The kidney: physiology and pathophysiology.* New York: Raven Press, 1985;2017–2041.
60. Gant NF, Whalley PJ, Everett RB, Worley RJ, MacDonald PC. Control of vascular reactivity in pregnancy. *Am J Kidney Dis* 1987;IX(4):303–307.

61. Gant NF, Daley GL, Chand S, Whalley PJ, MacDonald PC. A study of angiotensin II pressor response throughout primigravid pregnancy. *J Clin Invest* 1973;52:2682–2689.
62. Brown MA, Boughton Pipkin F, Symonds EM. The effects of intravenous angiotensin II upon blood pressure and sodium and urate excretion in human pregnancy. *J Hypertens* 1988;6:457–464.
63. Paller MS. Mechanism of decreased pressor responsiveness to ANG II NE and vasopressin in pregnant rats. *Am J Physiol* 1984;247:H100–H108.
64. Clark KE. Effects of circulating levels of vasoconstrictors on systemic pressor responsiveness to angiotensin II and norepinephrine. *Am J Obstet Gynecol* 1984;149:480–484.
65. Everett RB, Worley RJ, MacDonald PC, et al. Effect of prostaglandin synthetase inhibitors on pressor response to angiotensin II in human pregnancy. *J Clin Endocrinol Metab* 1978;46:1007–1010.
66. Rosenfeld CR, Jackson GM. Estrogen-induced refractoriness to the pressor effects of infused angiotensin II. *Am J Obstet Gynecol* 1984;148:429–435.
67. Landau RL, Lugibihl K. Inhibition of the sodium retaining influence of aldosterone by progesterone. *J Clin Endocrinol Metab* 1958;18:1237–1245.
68. Wambach G, Higgens JR. Antimineralocorticoid action of progesterone in the rat: correlation of the effect on electrolyte excretion and interaction with renal mineralocorticoid receptors. *Endocrinology* 1978;102:1686–1693.
69. Oparil S, Ehrlich EN, Lindheimer MD. Effects of progesterone on renal sodium handling in man: relation to aldosterone excretion and plasma renin activity. *Clin Sci Mol Med* 1975;49:139–147.
70. Watanabe M, Meeker CI, Gray MJ, Sims EAH, Solomon S. Secretion rate of aldosterone in normal pregnancy. *J Clin Invest* 1963;42:1619–1631.
71. Ehrlich EN, Lugibihl K, Taylor C, Janulis M. Reciprocal variations in urinary cortisol and aldosterone in response to the sodium depletion influence of hydrochlorothiazide and ethacrynic acid in humans. *J Clin Endocrinol* 1967;27:836–842.
72. Lindheimer MD, DelGreco F, Ehrlich EN. Postural effects on Na and steroid excretion and serum renin activity during pregnancy. *J Appl Physiol* 1973;35:343–348.
73. Ehrlich EN, Lindheimer MD. Effect of administered mineralocorticoids or ACTH in pregnant women: attenuation of kaliuretic influence of mineralocorticoids during pregnancy. *J Clin Invest* 1972;51:1301–1309.
74. Ehrlich EN. Heparinoid-induced inhibition of aldosterone secretion in pregnant women: the role of augmented aldosterone secretion in sodium conservation during normal pregnancy. *Am J Obstet Gynecol* 1971;109:963–970.
75. Navar GL, Carmines PK, Huang WC, Mitchell EK. The tubular effects of angiotensin II. *Kidney Int* 1987;31(2):S81–S88.
76. Chesley LC. Renal responses of pregnant and nonpregnant women to isopressor doses of angiotensin II. *Am J Obstet Gynecol* 1963;87:410–412.
77. Terragno NA, Terragno DA, Pacholczyk D, McGiff JC. Prostaglandins and the regulation of uterine blood flow in pregnancy. *Nature* 1974;249:57–58.
78. Franklin GO, Dowd AJ, Caldwell BV, Speroff L. The effect of angiotensin II intravenous infusion on plasma renin activity and prostaglandin A, E, and F levels in the uterine vein of the pregnant monkey. *Prostaglandins* 1974;6:261–280.
79. Venuto RC, O'Dorisio T, Stein JH, Ferris TF. Uterine prostaglandin E secretion and uterine blood flow in the pregnant rabbit. *J Clin Invest* 1975;55:193–197.
80. Ferris TF, Weir EK. Effect of captopril on uterine blood flow and prostaglandin E synthesis in the pregnant rabbit. *J Clin Invest* 1983;71:809–815.
81. Elder MG, Glance DG, Rose M, Myatt L. Arachidonic acid metabolites in human placental tissue: their role in controlling placental blood flow. *Adv Prostaglandin Thromboxane Leukotriene Res* 1985;15:627.
82. Parisi VM, Rankin JHG. The effect of prostacyclin on angiotensin II-induced placental vasoconstriction. *Am J Obstet Gynecol* 1985;151:444–449.
83. Ferris TF, Weir F. Effect of captopril on uterine blood flow and prostaglandin E synthesis in the pregnant rabbit. *J Clin Invest* 1983;71:809–815.
84. Tchobroutsky C, Kreft-Jais C, Plouin PF. Angiotensin converting enzyme inhibitors during pregnancy. *Clin Exp Hypertens [B]* 1987;B6(I):71.
85. Scanferla F, Coli U, Landini S, Fracasso A, Morachiello P, Righetto F, Gendi R, Bazzato G. Treatment of pregnancy-induced hypertension (PIH) with ACE inhibitor enalapril. *Clin Exp Hypertens [B]* 1987;B6(I):45.
86. Mochizuki M, Marao T, Motoyama S. Treatment of hypertension in pregnancy by a combined drug regimen including captopril. *Clin Exp Hypertens [B]* 1986;B5(I):69–78.
87. Dusting GJ, Mullins EM. Stimulation by angiotensin of prostacyclin biosynthesis in rats and dogs. *Clin Exp Pharmacol* 1980;7:545–550.
88. Grodzinska L, Gryglewski RJ. Angiotensin-induced release of prostacyclin from perfused organs. *Pharmacol Res Commun* 1980;12:339–347.
89. Gautieri RF, Mancini RT. Effect of certain drugs on perfused human placenta. VII. Serotonin versus angiotensin II. *J Pharm Sci* 1967;56:296.
90. Glance DG, Elder MG, Bloxam DL, Myatt L. The effects of the components of the renin-angiotensin system on the isolated perfused human placental cotyledon. *Am J Obstet Gynecol* 1984;149:450–454.
91. Alhenc-Gelas F, Tache A, Saint-Andre JP, Milliez J, Sureau C, Corvol P, Menard J. The renin–angiotensin system in pregnancy and parturition. *Adv Nephrol* 1986;15:25–33.
92. Wilkes BM, Krim E, Mento PF. Evidence for a functional renin–angiotensin system in full-term fetoplacental unit. *Am J Physiol* 1985;249:E366–E373.
93. Fox H. Pathology of the placenta. *Clin Obstet Gynecol* 1986;13:501–519.
94. Brown JJ, Davies DL, Doak PB, Lever AF, Robertson JIS, Trust P. Plasma renin concentration in hypertensive disease of pregnancy. *Lancet* 1965;ii:1219.
95. Tapia HR, Johnson CE, Strong CE. Renin–angiotensin system in normal and in hypertensive disease of pregnancy. *Lancet* 1972;ii:847–850.
96. Weir RJ, Doig A, Fraser R, Morton JJ, Parboosingh J, Robertson JIS, Wilson A. Studies of the renin–angiotensin–aldosterone system, cortisol, DOC, and ADH in normal and hypertensive pregnancy. In: Lindheimer M, Katz A, Zuspan F, eds. *Hypertension in pregnancy.* New York: John Wiley & Sons 1976;251–258.
97. Nochy D, Bariety J, Camilleri JP, Corvol P, Menard J. Diminished number of renin-containing cells in kidney biopsy samples from hypertensive women immediately postpartum. An immunomorphometric study. *Kidney Int* 1984;26:85–87.
98. Symonds EM, Broughton-Pipkin F, Craven DJ. Changes in the renin–angiotensin system in primigravidae with hypertensive disease of pregnancy. *Br J Obstet Gynaecol* 1975;83:643–650.
99. Weir RJ, Brown JJ, Fraser R, et al. Plasma renin, renin substrate, angiotensin II, and aldosterone in hypertensive disease of pregnancy. *Lancet* 1973;I:291–294.
100. Symonds EM, Broughton-Pipkin F. Pregnancy hypertension, pariety, and the renin–angiotensin system. *Am J Obstet Gynecol* 1978;132:473–479.
101. Broughton-Pipkin F, Craven DJ, Symonds EM. The uteroplacental renin–angiotensin system in normal and hypertensive pregnancy. *Contrib Nephrol* 1981;25:49–52.
102. Ruilope L, Paya C, Alcazar JM, Sancho RJ, Garcia-Robles R, Rodico J, Hammond TG, Knox FG, Romero JC. Failure of angiotensin II to reduce plasma renin activity in hypertensive pregnant women. *J Hypertens* 1984(Suppl 2)3:S251–254.
103. Losonczy G, Todd H, Almer DC, Hertelendy F. Prostaglandins, norepinephrine, angiotensin II and blood pressure changes induced by uteroplacental ischemia in rabbits. *Clin Exp Hypertens [B]* 1986/1987;B5(3):271–293.
104. Brar HS, Kjos SL, Dougherty W, Do Y, Tam HB, Hsueh WA. Increased fetoplacental active renin production in pregnancy-induced hypertension. *Am J Obstet Gynecol* 1987;157:363–368.
105. Gant NF, Worley RJ, Everett RB, MacDonald PC. Control of vascular responsiveness during human pregnancy. *Kidney Int* 1980;18:253–258.
106. Remuzzi G, Marchesi D, Zoja C, et al. Reduced umbilical and

placental vascular prostacyclin in severe preeclampsia. *Prostaglandins* 1980;20:105.

107. Pedersen EB, Christensen NJ, Christensen P, Johnanesen P, Kornerup HJ, Kristensen S, Lauritsen JG, Leyssac PP, Rasumussen A, Wohlert M. Preeclampsia—a state of prostaglandin deficiency. Urinary prostaglandin excretion, the renin–aldosterone system, and circulating catecholamines in preeclampsia. *Hypertension* 1983;5:105–111.
108. Fitzgerald DJ, Entman SS, Mulloy K, Fitzgerald GA. Decreased prostacyclin biosynthesis preceding the clinical manifestation of pregnancy-induced hypertension. *Circulation* 1987;75(5):956–963.
109. Stuart MJ, Clark DA, Sunderji SG, Allen JB, Yombo T, Elrad H, Slott JH. Decreased prostacyclin production: a characteristic of chronic placental insufficiency syndrome. *Lancet* 1981;i:1126.
110. Walsh SW, Behr MJ, Allen NH. Placental prostacyclin production in normal and toxemic pregnancies. *Am J Obstet Gynecol* 1985;151:110–115.
111. Dieckmann WJ, Pottinger RE, Rynkiewicz LM. Etiology of preeclampsia-eclampsia. *Am J Obstet Gynecol* 1952;63:783–791.
112. Chesley LC, Valenti C, Rein H. Excretion of sodium loads by nonpregnant and pregnant normal, hypertensive and preeclamptic women. *Metabolism* 1958;7:575–588.
113. Sarles HE, Hill SS, Le Blanc AL, Smith GH, Canales CO, Remmers AR. Sodium excretion patterns during and following intravenous sodium chloride loads in normal and hypertensive pregnancies. *Am J Obstet Gynecol* 1968;102:1–7.
114. Brown MA, Gallery EDM, Ross MR, Esber RP. Sodium excretion in normal and hypertensive pregnancy: a prospective study. *Am J Obstet Gynecol* 1988;159:297–307.
115. Bond AL, Druzin ML, Atlas SA, Sealey JE, Laragh JH, August PA. Atrial natriuretic factor in normal and hypertensive pregnancy. *Am J Obstet Gynecol* 1989;in press.
116. Taufield PA, Druzin ML, Sealey JE, Laragh JH. Serial plasma renin activity in normal and hypertensive pregnancy. *Kidney Int* 1988;33:306.
117. Taufield PA, Druzin ML, Edersheim TE, Sealey JE, Laragh JH. Correlation between plasma renin activity and birthweight in hypertensive pregnancy. *J Hypertens* 1986;4(Suppl 5):S96–S98.
118. Coen G, Gugini P, Gerlini G, Finistauri D, Cinotti GA. Successful treatment of long-lasting severe hypertension with captopril during a twin pregnancy. *Nephron* 1985;40:498–500.
119. Broughton-Pipkin F, Symonds EM, Lamming GD, Jadoul FAC. Renin and aldosterone concentration in pregnant essential hypertensives—a prospective study. *Clin Exp Hypertens* 1983;B2(2):255–269.
120. Weinberger MH, Kramer NJ, Petersen LP et al. Sequential changes in the renin–angiotensin–aldosterone system and plasma progesterone concentrations in normal and abnormal pregnancy. In: Lindheimer MD, Katz A, Zuspan FP, eds. *Hypertension in pregnancy.* New York: John Wiley & Sons, 1976;263–270.
121. Koskela O, Kaski P. Renal angiography in the follow-up examination of toxemia of late pregnancy. *Acta Obstet Gynecol Scand* 1971;50:41.
122. Gordon RD, Fishman LM, Liddle GW. Plasma renin activity and aldosterone secretion in a pregnant woman with primary aldosteronism. *J Clin Endocrinol* 1967;27:385.
123. Biglieri EG, Slaton PE. Pregnancy and primary aldosteronism. *J Clin Endocrinol* 1967;27:1628.
124. Lotgering FK, Derkx FMH, Wallenburg HCS. Primary hyperaldosteronism in pregnancy. *Am J Obstet Gynecol* 1986;155:986–988.
125. Laragh JH, Letcher RL, Pickering TG. Renin profiling for diagnosis and treatment of hypertension. *JAMA* 1979;241:151–156.
126. August Taufield P, Sealey JE. The renin system in normal and hypertensive pregnancy and in ovarian function. In: Brenner BM, Kaplan NM, Laragh JH, eds. *Endocrine mechanism in hypertension: perspectives in hypertension.* New York: Raven Press, 1989;129–155.
127. Itskovitz J, Sealey JE. Ovarian prorenin in women undergoing ovarian stimulation with gonadotropins and during pregnancy. In: Hodgen GD, Rosenwaks Z, Spieler JM, eds. *Nonsteroidal gonadal factors: physiological roles and possibilities in contraceptive development.* Norfolk: Jones Institute Press, 1988;355–363.

Hypertension: Pathophysiology, Diagnosis, and Management, edited by J. H. Laragh and B. M. Brenner. Raven Press, Ltd., New York © 1990.

CHAPTER 110

Abnormal Placentation in Hypertensive Disorders of Pregnancy

Frederick P. Zuspan

General Considerations for Hypertensive Diseases of Pregnancy, 1779
Classifications of Hypertensive Disorders of Pregnancy, 1780
The Vascular and Neurovascular Anatomy of the Nonpregnant Uterus, 1780
Adrenergic Uterine Nerves, 1781
The Vascular and Neurovascular Anatomy of the Pregnant Uterus, 1781
Uterine Nerve Changes, 1783
Changes in the Uteroplacental Bed in Preeclampsia/Eclampsia, 1784
Clinical Implications, 1786
Changes in the Uteroplacental Bed in Chronic Hypertension, 1786
Clinical Implications, 1787
References, 1787

GENERAL CONSIDERATIONS FOR HYPERTENSIVE DISEASES OF PREGNANCY

The hypertensive disorders of pregnancy, both acute and chronic, regardless of cause, are among the most serious medical complications seen in pregnancy. The incidence of hypertensive problems in pregnancy is remarkably constant among developed countries, but it varies in different patient population groups within these countries. The hypertensive diseases of pregnancy complicate 8–10% of all pregnancies: Preeclampsia/eclampsia accounts for 6–8%, and the remaining 2–4% account for other hypertensive diseases of pregnancy, most notably chronic hypertension. The hypertensive diseases of pregnancy constitute a potential for death to both mother and fetus. The problems for the fetus relate mostly to premature delivery necessitated by both maternal and fetal considerations. Maternal vascular disease may also cause fetal growth retardation, which is usually seen after the 30th week of gestation.

The clinical problems seen in patients who have hypertension during pregnancy depend upon several factors—most notably the severity of the hypertension and the amount of placental reserve or functioning placenta that is present. If placental reserve is diminished, then the effects on the fetus are clinically seen in the third trimester of pregnancy, notably by the presence of (a) a small-for-gestational-age fetus or (b) overt intrauterine growth retardation of more than 10% below the mean for a particular gestational age. Clinical generalizations include the presence of chronic hypertension in the mother and is usually associated with a smaller and less functional placenta.

One of the significant problems for the fetus is the presence of an abruptio placenta in an already-compromised uteroplacental bed. This further compromises fetal circulation and results in fetal distress. The retroplacental bleed may be small in magnitude, or it may be acute, sudden, and large in amount, often resulting in death of the fetus. It is more significant in women who have mild or severe chronic hypertension, since this further impedes the already compromised placental function. Our studies at the Chicago Lying-In Hospital identified the following:

Incidence of Abruptio Placenta at the Chicago Lying-In Hospital (1)

Normal patients	0.8%
Preeclampsia	
Mild	1.5%
Severe	1.0%
Chronic hypertensive disease	
Mild	3.0%
Severe	6.3%

Preeclampsia occurs only in the presence of placental tissue. Therefore, it is logical to consider the causative factor of preeclampsia to originate in either the placenta or the uteroplacental bed. This chapter will devote attention to these considerations.

CLASSIFICATIONS OF HYPERTENSIVE DISEASES OF PREGNANCY

Vascular derangements may accompany or antedate pregnancy, and all are manifested by elevation in maternal blood pressure. The International Society for the Study of Hypertension in Pregnancy has proposed the following definitions for hypertension in pregnancy: Hypertension in pregnancy is defined on the basis of the measurement of the diastolic blood pressure by sphygmomanometry using the "point of muffling" (Phase IV Korotkoff sounds) in women lying on their side at 15–30° horizontal with two consecutive measurements of 90 mmHg or more 4 or more hours apart, or one measurement of 110 mmHg or more. The diastolic blood pressure of 90 mmHg corresponds to approximately three standard deviation units above the mean in mid-pregnancy. Previous suggestions include using a rise of 15 mmHg in the diastolic blood pressure from low mid-trimester readings. Previous definitions also included the use of the systolic blood pressure of an increase of 30 mmHg or more from the lowest mid-pregnancy reading. However, the systolic pressure does not appear to be significant, does not add to the prognostic significance, and is more complicated than measurement of the diastolic blood pressure. Re-classification of the hypertensive disorders of pregnancy is based upon clinical findings of hypertension and/or proteinuria during pregnancy (2):

1. *Gestational hypertension.* The presence of diastolic hypertension and the absence of proteinuria.
2. *Preeclampsia.* The presence of gestational hypertension and the presence of proteinuria (more than 300 mg/day).
3. *Chronic hypertension.* When hypertension is either diagnosed and present before pregnancy, diagnosed during pregnancy, or persisting after pregnancy, it can be subdivided into the following categories:
   a. Chronic hypertension (without proteinuria).
   b. Chronic renal disease (proteinuria with or without hypertension).
   c. Chronic hypertension with superimposed preeclampsia.

It is noted that the previous considerations of a >30-mmHg increase in the systolic blood pressure and the 15-mmHg increase in the diastolic blood pressure have not been recommended. The Committee on Terminology of the American College of Obstetricians and Gynecologists, however, continues to use the change in systolic and diastolic blood pressure as evidence of the onset of preeclampsia. Two problems have existed in past studies and in data collected in that the patient has not had her blood pressure taken in the lateral recumbent position, eliminating the hemodynamic changes due to the pregnant uterus and eliminating the use of the Korotkoff fourth sound, since most individuals use the fifth sound for the diastolic reading. It is therefore difficult to equate one group's data to another, except to state that the new proposed recommendations hopefully will eliminate some of the ambiguity of the past.

THE VASCULAR AND NEUROVASCULAR ANATOMY OF THE NONPREGNANT UTERUS

The uterine artery and its branches, along with those of the ovarian arteries, penetrate the lateral margins of the uterine wall at an oblique angle and proceed to the middle layer of the myometrium, where they are joined and form an arcuate wreath (Fig. 1) (3).

Projecting from the arcuate wreath are radial arteries that penetrate the endometrium and course perpendicularly to the uterine lumen. The first branch of the radial artery is the basal artery; this finally becomes the spiral artery, which it courses to the endometrium. The basal arteries supply the stratum basale and are unaffected by hormonal stimuli and maintain their integrity through all phases of the menstrual cycle. The spiral arteries supply the stratum functionale and are sensitive to the hormonal endocrine environment in the female. The spiral arteries undergo fluctuations during the menstrual cycle as a result of the hormone stimuli from estrogen and progesterone (Fig. 2). Constriction associated with the radial artery during the menstrual cycle was described by Bartelmez in the monkey (4). This constriction took place near the myoendometrial junction, and the cause was never determined (Fig. 3) (4,5). The veins of the uterus and the endometrium do not undergo the same dramatic alterations as seen in the arteries during the menstrual cycle or in pregnancy. Markee transplanted endometrium into the anterior chamber of the eye

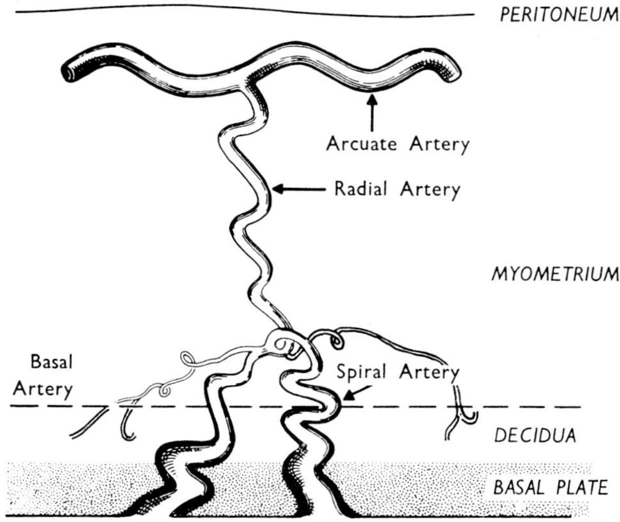

FIG. 1. Diagramatic illustration of the arterial blood supply to the intervillous space and the placental bed. Note the arcuate artery, the branching radial artery, the basal arteries, and the spiral arteries. The spiral arteries course through the decidua and myometrium. (From ref. 15.)

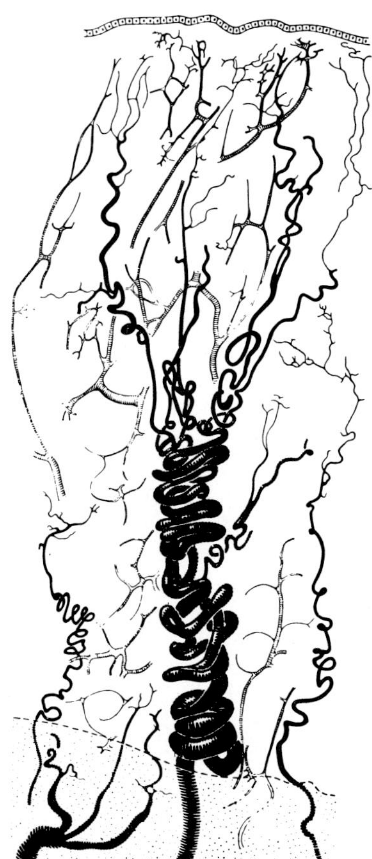

FIG. 2. Projection drawing of an endometrial spiral artery in a monkey uterus. Coils extend into the mid-endometrium. Apical rami of the vessel connect with the subepithelial capillary network but do not intercommunicate. The uterus was injected on the 17th day of the menstrual cycle, and the corpus luteum was 6–7 days old. ×25.1. (From ref. 5.)

of the Rhesus monkey and showed intermittent vasoconstriction in the radial artery during the menstrual cycle (6).

The classic descriptions of the uterine vascular anatomy do not usually include the role of nerves in the myoendometrial junction, either during pregnancy or during nonpregnancy. We believe the neurovascular innervation is important in the physiologic and pathophysiologic function of these arteries during pregnancy, especially in the hypertensive diseases of pregnancy.

Adrenergic Uterine Nerves

The classic work of Frankenhauser in 1897 identified the nerve innervation of the uterus and cervix (7).

Langley and Anderson were the first to suggest that parts of the sympathetic postganglionic nerves to the uterus did not originate from the ordinary para- and prevertebral ganglia situated near the effector organ (8).

The concern for the adrenergic uterine nerves remained dormant for many years until the Swedish group from the Institute of Histology at the University of Lund identified and unraveled the questions to many of these problems. The methodology used was a specific histochemical fluorescent method devised by Falk, Hillarp, and Thime to visualize the adrenergic neurotransmitter utilizing a freeze-dried tissue specimen that was exposed to gaseous paraformaldehyde under dry conditions (9–11).

It was later shown by Sjoberg and others in his group that the distribution of the terminal adrenergic innervation of the uterus varies from species to species (12). The Swedish group was able to show that uterine vessels, as well as uterine smooth muscles, are innervated to a varying extent by adrenergic nerve fibers. The human cervix contains significantly larger numbers of adrenergic nerves than does the fundus or the corpus. It has now been established that in the human the sympathetic ganglia formations are in the immediate vicinity of the uterus, namely, near the uterovaginal junction (12).

THE VASCULAR AND NEUROVASCULAR ANATOMY OF THE PREGNANT UTERUS

The intimate, but separate, circulations between mother and fetus necessary for mammalian reproduction is

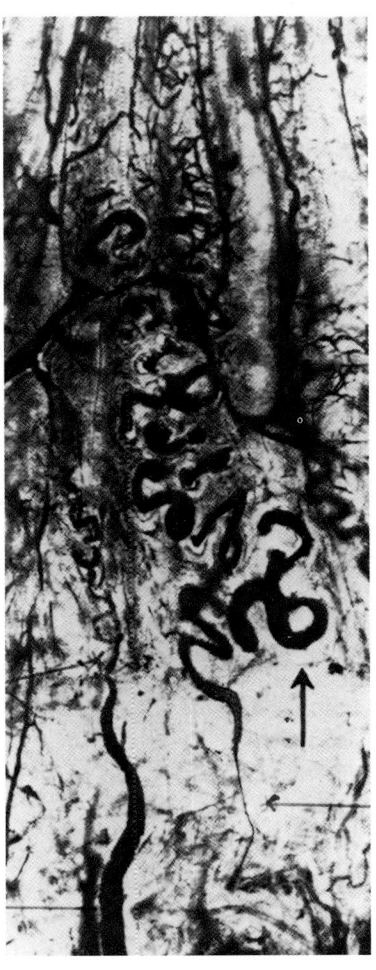

FIG. 3. Myoendometrial junction shown in a monkey uterus during the 11th day of the menstrual cycle, showing the basal portion of the spiral artery and the constriction of the associated radial artery. The segment of the radial artery that is out of focus has been strengthened. ×45. (From ref. 5.)

achieved in the human by hemochorial placentation. In the hemochorial placenta, the maternal epithelium, connective tissue, and capillary endothelium have disappeared and maternal blood bathes the trophoblasts directly. The function of the placental bed depends, to a large extent, upon its vascular anatomy and the behavior of the invading trophoblasts, along with their interaction and the presence or absence of maternal disease. The relationship between maternal and fetal vessels in the placenta has been controversial since ancient times, when Galen described connections between the uterine vessels and the fetal vessels of the placenta. Later anatomists, including William Harvey, doubted this theory. The Hunters from England, working with Collin MacKenzie, an obstetrician, demonstrated the existence of what we now call the intervillous space or the functional area between the mother and fetus. They injected molten wax into the uterine arteries and found that it passed through the placental bed, then lodged in the area of the placenta, but was not found in the umbilical cord or the fetus, thereby identifying two separate circulations. This technique allowed the Hunters to observe (13) that "The arteries of the uterus . . . passed through the decidua without ramifying it; just before they enter the placenta, making two or three close spiral turns upon themselves, they open at once into its spongy substance without any diminution in size. . . . The intention of the spiral turns would appear to be that of diminishing the force of the circulation as it approaches the spongy substance of the placenta . . . for quick motion of the blood is not wanted."

The investigation of the Hunters preceded the use of the compound microscope, and the so-called hunterian "Curling Arteries" thus became even more important in subsequent years of investigation and sophistication of science. The pathologist-anatomist Elizabeth Ramsey culminated her meticulous studies of the morphology and the physiology of placental circulation in her book, *Placental Vasculature and Circulation* (14).

The physiologic changes occurring in the spiral arteries in normal gestation, as well as the pathologic changes seen in the spiral arteries in hypertensive disorders of pregnancy, have been clarified by Brosens et al. (15) (Fig. 4).

Most recently, the work of their colleagues, DeWolf and Pijnenborg, as well as of Sheppard and Bonnar, has provided us with an understanding of the placental ultrastructure (16–19).

When conception occurs, the development of the endometrium and its blood vessels continues under the influence of the hormones of the corpus luteum of pregnancy. The blastocyst first attaches to the endometrium by simple adhesion 6–7 days after fertilization. Electron micrographs show that this adhesion involves interdigitation between microvilli of the cytotrophoblasts and those of the maternal epithelium (20,21).

Subsequently, individual cytotrophoblast cells penetrate between maternal epithelial cells. This initial nidation always occurs near the subepithelial capillaries (22). After attachment, the advancing margin of trophoblastic tissue becomes a syncytiotrophoblast (23).

Placentation in the human is interstitial, with the entire blastocyst becoming imbedded in the endometrial straw.

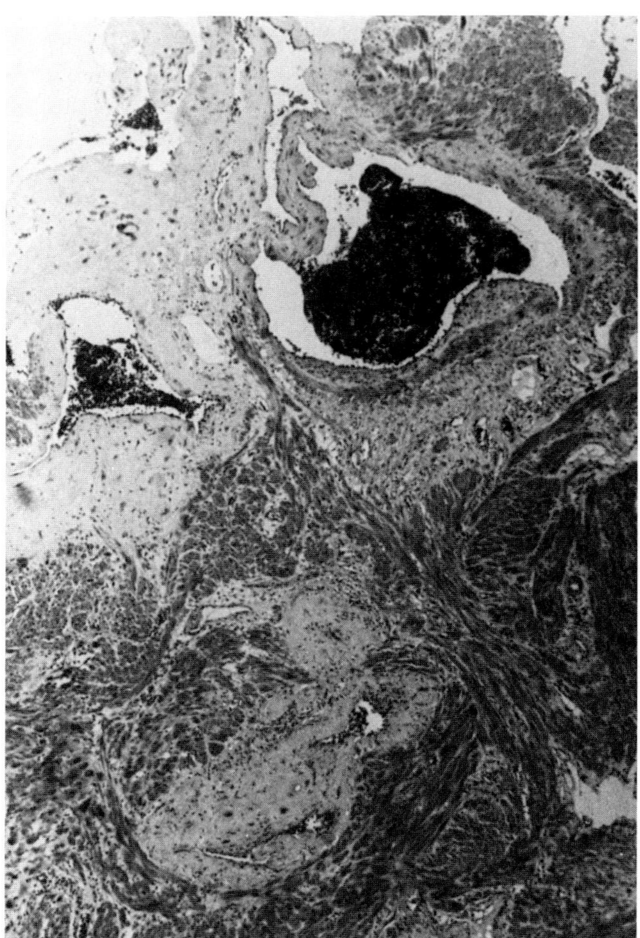

FIG. 4. A uteroplacental-bed biopsy oriented with the decidua at the top and the myometrium below. Myometrial and decidual segments of the uteroplacental (spiral) artery with physiologic changes are shown. Hematoxylin and eosin, ×37.5. (From ref. 29.)

There is no noticeable proliferation of the maternal uterine epithelium, although there is marked decidual reaction with swelling of stromal cells (24).

The interaction between the advancing trophoblasts and maternal vessels is similar in all primates. The trophoblast grows around maternal capillaries and gradually erodes through the endothelium, thereby creating an irregular boundary between maternal and fetal tissues. This establishes communication between the trophoblastic interstitial spaces and the endometrial capillaries. These blood-filled interstitial spaces, called *lacunae,* are lined by syncytiotrophoblasts and represent the earliest "intervillous space". As the trophoblast invades more deeply into the endometrium, it encounters vessels of progressively larger size. The spiral arteries, as well as major endometrial veins, are eventually opened, allowing blood to enter the intervillous space with the higher pressure, and then drain into the maternal systemic veins at a low pressure. Early in this process, plugs of trophoblastic tissue can be seen filling the vascular lumen. As cells progress proximally ("like wax drippings down the side of a candle"), there is less filling of the vascular lumen (22).

The cells which invade vessels have now been shown to be cytotrophoblasts by sex chromatin studies (25), electromicroscopy studies (26,27), and immunologic techniques (28).

When human pregnancy has advanced to at least 12 weeks' gestation, intraluminal cytotrophoblasts have advanced to the level of the myometrial segments of the spiral arteries. This is known as the *first invasion of the trophoblasts into the spiral arteries* (18,24).

The trophoblast begins to enter the arterial wall after the initial intraluminal phase and replaces the normal muscle and elastic tissue. Finally the intramural cytotrophoblast is replaced by fibrous connective tissue. This replacement of muscular and elastic tissue extends in the human to the myometrial segments of the spiral arteries and may occasionally involve the terminal segments of the radial arteries. These changes have been termed the *physiologic changes of pregnancy* by Brosens, Robertson, and Dixon as well as by others. These findings have been confirmed by electron-microscopic studies of DeWolf et al. and of Sheppard and Bonnar (17,19,29) (Fig. 5). This loss of muscular and elastic tissue from the coiled spiral artery converts them to dilated tortuous vessels, permitting the delivery of greater volumes of blood at a lower flow rate than before; hence, a high-resistance system is converted to a low-resistance system to promote the maximum exchange of nutrients and gases. These physiologic changes are most pronounced at the center of the placental bed, presumably at the original implantation site, and are less apparent at its periphery. Remarkably, they disappear at the end of the first menstrual period post-partum.

Uterine Nerve Changes

The short adrenergic neurons are dependent upon hormonal influence of steroids and can serve as a model system for the study of neuroendocrine regulation in the peripheral adrenergic nervous system. The use of electron microscopy (30) and of fluorescent histochemical (11,31) and biochemical (30–32) determinations indicate that norepinephrine is the predominate catecholamine in these reproductive nerves. It would be assumed that the norepinephrine content of these organs is generally believed to be proportional to the amount of adrenergic innervation and can be used as an index of the neuronal state.

The original thesis that tissue levels were reliable indices of neuronal activity has not been substantiated, since there is turnover and metabolism of norepinephrine that may be directly related to sympathetic activity (33,34). The turnover rate of norepinephrine in the heart is unaffected by pregnancy or ovarian steroids, but the turnover rate in the reproductive organs is indeed affected by ovarian steroids. The turnover is the net result of synthesis, degradation, release, and re-uptake of the neurotransmitter. The ovarian steroids affect the activity of tyrosine hydroxylase (TH), which is the rate-limiting enzyme for catecholamine biosynthesis. If ovariectomy is done in the rabbit, a fall in TH activity occurs. The administration of estrogen without progesterone restores TH activity to normal levels (30,31).

Many studies have utilized the guinea pig, since it is well suited for study, has a placenta similar to that in humans, and carries fetuses in only one uterine horn; hence, the empty nongravid horn can also be studied because there is no effect of stretch by the fetal placental unit in the nongravid horn. Thorbert and his group from Sweden were

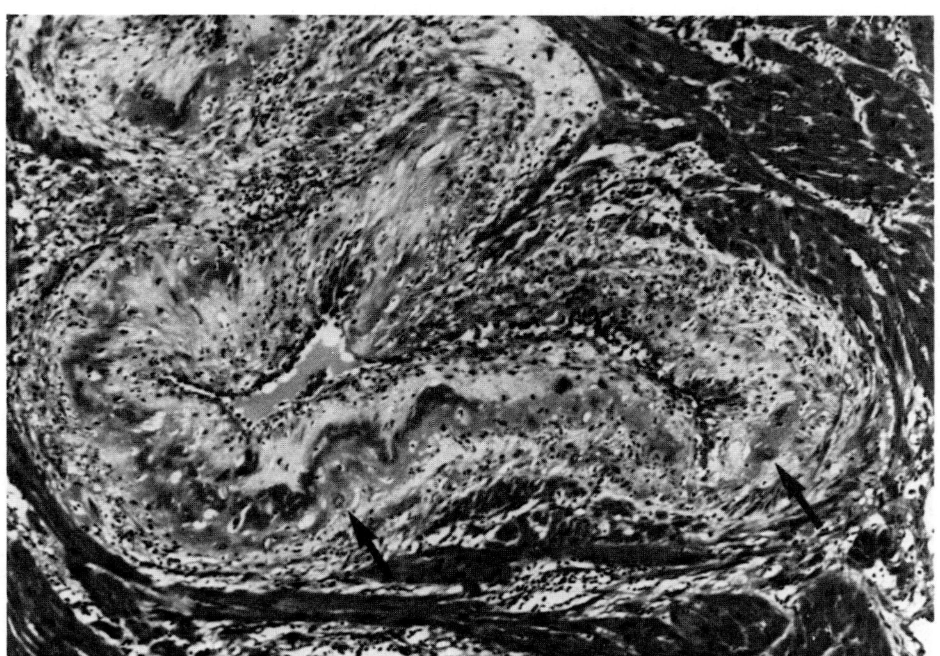

FIG. 5. Uteroplacental bed biopsy indicating a fully developed physiologic change in the myometrial segment of the spiral artery. The prominent convoluted layers of the fibrinoid in which discrete trophoblastic cells are imbedded are arrowed. The vessel is artificially collapsed. Hematoxylin and eosin, ×93.7. (From ref. 29.)

able to show that during pregnancy, adrenergic nerves undergo extensive reduction in the number and intensity of their characteristic fluorescence and that by the end of pregnancy, almost all fluorescent nerves disappear (31). This fluorescence cannot be restored by the administration of the transmitter analogue alpha-methylnorepinephrine and suggests actual nerve degeneration, which has been confirmed by ultrastructural studies. The norepinephrine content of the pregnant uterus near the end of the pregnancy is near zero, and the uptake to tritiate norepinephrine, as well as TH activity, falls to 10% that of the nonpregnant animal (31). Functionally speaking, the only parts of the uterus where normal adrenergic transmission occurs at the end of pregnancy would be the tube and cervix, but certainly not in the body of the uterus, where the short adrenergic neurons reside. The mechanisms that result in a disappearance of adrenergic activity in pregnancy were first thought to be due to the mechanical stretch–strain and muscular hypertrophy associated with the growing fetus. These may well be one of the factors. However, Bell and Malcolm were able to show that the decrease in fluorescence is due to progesterone (35). A progesterone pellet was implanted into the lumen of one uterine horn of the nonpregnant guinea pig, and they observed a subsequent decrease in the nerve fluorescence in both horns. This change takes approximately 10 days to begin. The effects could not be duplicated by uterine implantation of estradiol or by the subcutaneous or intramuscular injections of progesterone; hence, a local progesterone effect from the placenta is most likely the major reason for the decrease in adrenergic activity (35).

The pregnancy and denervation changes in the adrenergic nervous system persists for at least 6 months post-partum in the guinea pig (36). We have been able to show the adrenergic innervation of the uterine vasculature in human term pregnancy in some selected patients, but the norepinephrine was diminished (32).

CHANGES IN THE UTEROPLACENTAL BED IN PREECLAMPSIA/ECLAMPSIA

Early studies of the uteroplacental bed involved the concern for hypertensive diseases in pregnancy. Actually, we knew about pathology before we were aware of normal physiology in the uteroplacental bed. Friedlander, in 1870, studied the spiral arteries in the uteroplacental bed and described large basophilic cells in these arteries. He suggested that they may be trophoblastic tissue with the power to invade and perforate the arterial wall (37).

Hertig, in 1945, first described a lesion now thought to be pathognomonic of preeclampsia, consisting of fibrinoid necrosis of the walls of decidua arteries by infiltration with lipophages (38).

Zeek and Assali later called this abnormality "acute atherosis" because of the prominent lipid component and the resemblance to atheroma elsewhere in the vasculature (39).

There has been much controversy about the nature and pathogenesis of these lesions. The debate has centered around whether they were (a) the effect of hypertension or (b) primary lesions leading to other changes of preeclampsia. The most recent workers in the field are Robertson, Dickson, Brosens, and their associates, whose work has lead to a general accepted premise that a uteroplacental lesion, known as *acute atherosis,* occurs in preeclampsia. This change is not seen in all patients with preeclampsia but is usually found as the disease becomes more severe, and it is associated with a lack of invasion of trophoblastic tissue down the spiral arteries into the myometrial segment. This lack of myometrial invasion is the lesion seen in preeclampsia/eclampsia.

The electron-microscopic studies of acute atherosis in the spiral arteries have enabled DeWolf and colleagues to compare the pathogenesis of these lesions to those of hypertensive arterial lesions elsewhere in the vasculature (29). The early lesions show a proliferation of smooth muscle cells leading to intimal hyperplasia with an expanded, extracellular space containing fibrin aggregates between these myointimal cells. Focal disruption of the endothelium, along with the chronic changes in the media of the vessel, is also present. DeWolf and colleagues postulate that the disruption of the endothelial lining allowed the infiltration of plasma components into the damaged arterial wall; they also postulate that the medial necrosis was due principally to vasospasm, the primary component seen in preeclampsia. A progressive accumulation of fat droplets in the myointimal cells was then observed, giving them the appearance of foam cells under light microscopy. The ultrastructural features have verified that these were smooth muscle cells. The more advanced lesions of acute atherosis show fat droplets in the intracellular space and also show the existence of a separate population of lipid-laden cells, this time having the fine structure of microphages. The prominent changes in the preeclamptic lesions of the placental bed consist of fat accumulation in myointimal cells, and necrosis of the vessel walls can also be observed in the systemic vessels of patients with essential vascular hypertension. Rolled strips of placental membranes are a valuable source of decidua vera containing spiral arteries showing acute atherosis but no physiologic changes. Robertson identifies that this is the easiest and clearest area for differential diagnosis (Fig. 6) (29). Figure 7 is a typical example of acute atherosis in a spiral artery.

Our study involved patients who have preeclampsia. The study consisted of studying both normal and hypertensive women and measuring catecholamines in uterine tissue. Myometrial samples were obtained from 10 nonpregnant and menstruating women following hysterectomy. Fifteen normal pregnant women at repeat cesarean section and eight preeclamptic patients all had cesarean section. The full-wedge biopsy was taken at the placental and anti-placental sites. Uterine tissue concentrations of catecholamines per gram of wet weight were used along with concentrations per milligram of protein for samples from the placental-bed and nonplacental-bed myometrium. Observations include a significant decrease in uterine content of norepinephrine per gram of tissue during normal pregnancy when compared to that during nonpregnancy. This confirms the work from Sweden, in which an adrenergic denervation was shown. Patients with preeclampsia have significantly increased uterine tissue norepinephrine when compared to that of women with normal pregnancy. More-

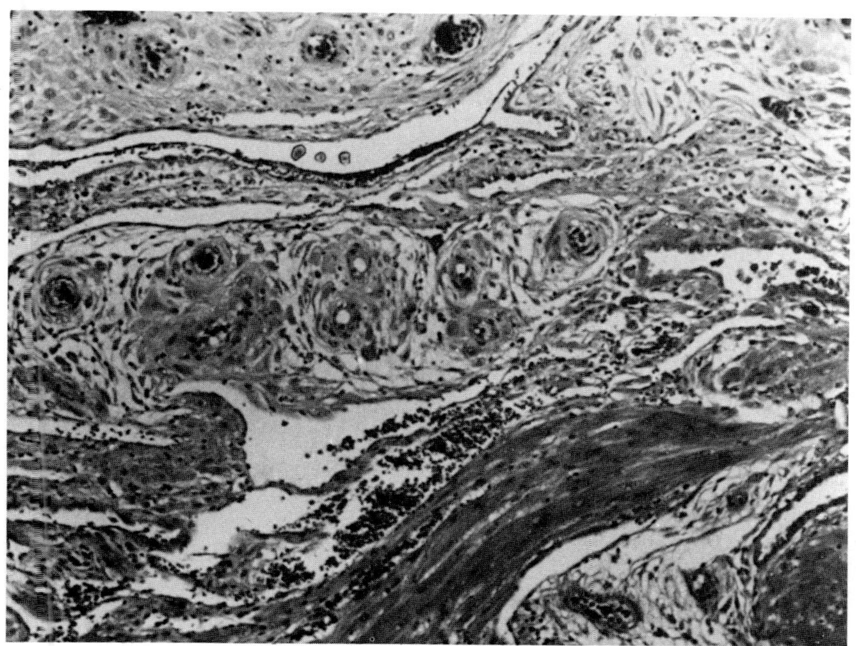

FIG. 6. Biopsy from the nonplacental bed including decidua vera and underlying myometrium. There are no trophoblastic cells, and the spiral arteries show no evidence of physiologic changes. Hematoxylin and eosin, ×93.7.

over, a significant difference between placental-bed and nonplacental-bed myometrium was noted. Plasma catecholamines were drawn at the time of uterine biopsy and did not reflect the changes seen in the uterus (40).

The changes in normal and preeclamptic hypertensive pregnancies are summarized as follows:

1. Spiral arteries which supply blood to the intervillous space are invaded by cytotrophoblasts soon after nidation. The spiral arteries are progressively converted to large, tortuous channels by the replacement of its normal musculoelastic wall with a mixture of fibrinoid and fibrous tissue. This invasion takes place in two phases, the last being completed by the 20th week of gestation, at which time the invasion extends into the myometrial segment of the spiral artery.

2. The replacement of the musculoelastic wall permits the spiral arteries to dilate and to convert a high-resistance system to a low-resistance system, affording better exchange of gases and nutrients.

3. The changes in these vessels allow for a greater volume of blood to be delivered and carried to the intervillous space, which is estimated to be 10 times greater than if no dilatation took place.

4. The basal arteries show no physiologic pregnancy changes. They do not communicate with the intervillous

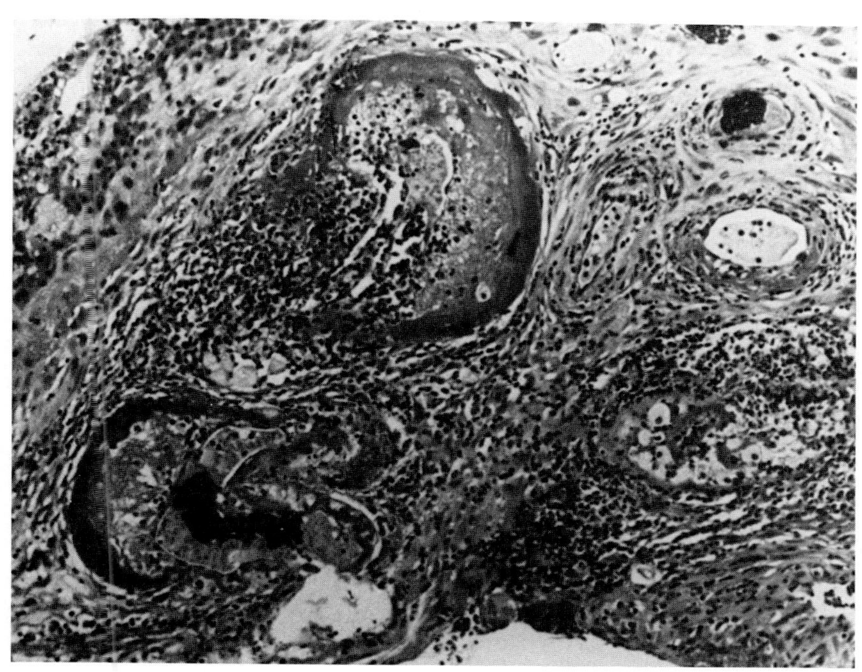

FIG. 7. A uteroplacental-bed biopsy showing a typical example of acute atherosis in the spiral artery. This is in a fragment of decidua attached to the placental membranes. The wall of the artery has undergone fibrinoid necrosis, and there are numerous foam cells plus extensive paravascular round-cell infiltration. Hematoxylin and eosin, ×93.7. (From ref. 29.)

space but do supply blood to the decidua and superficial myometrium. Only the spiral arteries react to the changing hormonal milieu—most likely involving progesterone, as seen in pregnancy.

5. Our studies of catecholamines in the uteroplacental bed have identified an increased amount of norepinephrine in the uterus in patients who have preeclampsia.

These data suggest that there is hyperactivity of the uterine adrenergic nervous system in preeclampsia, with a local modification at the site of implantation. These findings are compatible with our previous hypothesis of an increase of sympathetic nervous system activity in preeclampsia that reflects alterations in the adaptive mechanisms seen in normal pregnancy. The schematic representation is proposed, identifying less decrease in the number of nerves in the uteroplacental bed in patients with preeclampsia, which makes this associated with more vasoconstriction (Fig. 8).

During normal pregnancy the placenta produces equivalent amounts of thromboxane and prostacyclin, which produces a balance with regard to biologic action on vascular tone and platelet aggregation. Walsh has been able to show that in preeclampsia the placenta produces seven times more thromboxane than prostacyclin (41). This leads to an increase in vasoconstriction, an increase in platelet aggregation, an increase in uterine activity, and a decrease in uteroplacental blood flow. His study, utilizing fresh human placentas from normal and preeclamptic patients, measured thromboxane B_2 (a stable metabolite) and 6-ketoprostaglandin $F_{1\alpha}$ (a stable metabolite of prostacyclin). These products come from major enzymatic pathways of the arachidonic acid metabolism.

Clinical Implications

The clinical implications of alterations in placental physiology with lack of dilatation of the spiral arteries should make the clinician reconsider the salutary effects of drugs in the disease. Preeclampsia may well be an inappropriate immunologic adaptation between trophoblastic tissue (fetal) and maternal spiral arteries. If adaptation is normal, appropriate invasion of trophoblastic cells provides physiologic dilatation of the spiral arteries in the absence of hypertensive diseases of pregnancy. This misadaptation occurs shortly after the implantation and continues throughout pregnancy. The amount of placental reserve dictates whether or not the effect will be seen on the fetus. The lack of adrenergic denervation makes possible the theoretic constriction at the base of the spiral arteries with enhancement of vasoconstriction, in which there is an associated decreased production of prostacyclin (dilation) and an increased production of thromboxane (constriction) which further aggravate the problem. Studies by Wallenburg et al. are encouraging, since they have been able to show that a low-dose aspirin given chronically may be effective in preventing the progression of preeclampsia through this mechanism (42). A multicenter study is now under consideration in the United States in an attempt to substantiate this work.

CHANGES IN THE UTEROPLACENTAL BED IN CHRONIC HYPERTENSION

The difference between chronic hypertension and preeclampsia is the acute necrosis of the vessel wall which occurs in the basal arteries that are unaffected by the normal physiologic changes of pregnancy. The most extensive pathologic changes seen in the placental bed show almost total disruption of spiral arteries, occlusive thrombosis, and necrosis of the decidua with occasional secondary thrombosis of veins. Decidual hemorrhage may also occur, and these combinations are the ones that are seen in essential hypertension with preeclampsia.

Essential hypertension causes fibrinoid necrosis of the vessel wall and later leads to damaged vessel endothelium with foam cells and, subsequently, to fibrinoid necrosis and plasmatic vasculosis. If essential hypertension is present, there is usually a combination of necrotizing and proliferative lesions in the placental-bed arteries (Fig. 9). Our studies of the uteroplacental bed, in which we measured catecholamines, show no difference in catecholamines between normal patients and hypertensives. This means that the

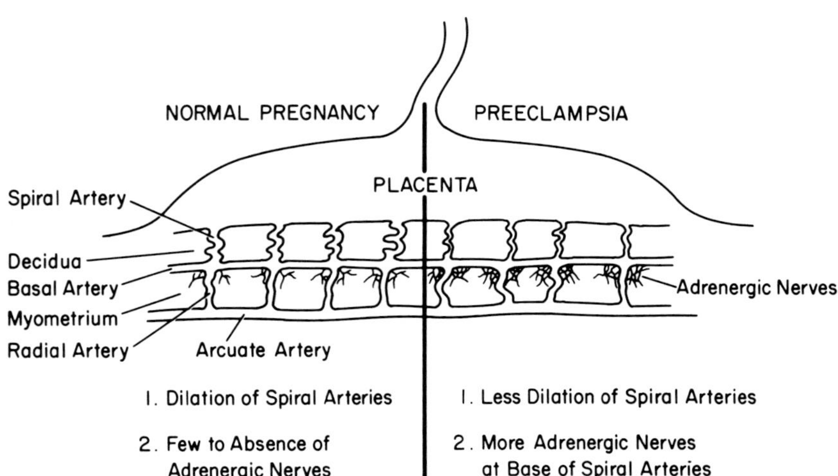

FIG. 8. Schematic of our theory, which postulates that preeclampsia not only has a lesion of constriction at the base of the spiral artery with less dilatation of the spiral artery, but also has a greater number of adrenergic nerves at the base of the spiral artery that may well account for the vasoconstriction present. Preeclampsia is associated with an incomplete denervation of the adrenergic nerves during pregnancy. Normal pregnancy is depicted schematically on the left, and preeclampsia is shown on the right.

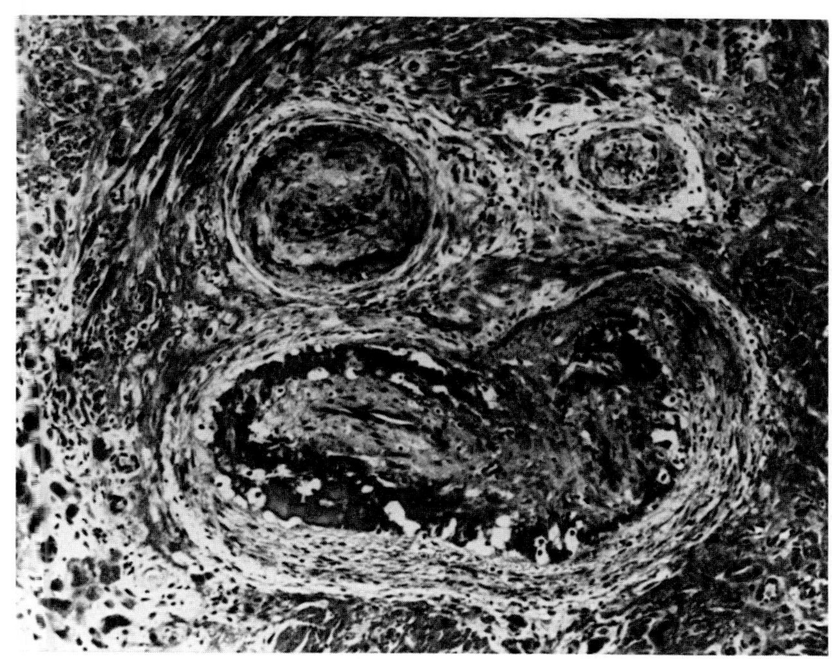

FIG. 9. Uteroplacental-bed biopsy in a patient with essential vascular hypertension and superimposed preeclampsia. Myometrial segments of the uteroplacental artery (spiral artery) show hyperplastic changes relating to the preexisting hypertension, and the largest segment shows superimposed acute atherosis due to preeclampsia. Hematoxylin and eosin, ×93.7. (From ref. 29.)

increase in catecholamines found in the uteroplacental bed is specific for preeclampsia. There is no increased adrenergic nervous component in patients who have essential vascular hypertension in the absence of preeclampsia.

Clinical Implications

The physiologic changes that occur in the uteroplacental bed with dilation of the spiral arteries promotes fetal welfare. There is a generalization that patients who have chronic hypertension have placentas that are smaller than normal, but weight does not necessarily mean that functional reserve is not present. The dilatation of the spiral arteries, along with adrenergic denervation, promotes maximum exchange of nutrients and gases in the intervillous space and promotes increased blood flow in this area. The pregnancy with essential vascular hypertension in the absence of preeclampsia does not have the profound vasoconstriction seen in preeclampsia but is associated with an increase in uterine tissue norepinephrine. Most likely, the production of thromboxane and prostacyclin are balanced in the chronic essential hypertensive patient who is pregnant. When preeclampsia intercedes in the patient who has chronic hypertension, this is one of the most profound problems seen for the fetus. An additional clinical concern is the fact that patients with chronic hypertension have a sixfold-greater chance of having abruptio placenta when compared to women with normal pregnancy.

REFERENCES

1. Zuspan FP. Hypertension and renal diseases in pregnancy. *Clin Obstet Gynecol* 1984;27:861.
2. Davey DA, MacGillivray I. The classification and definition of the hypertensive disorders of pregnancy. *Clin Exp Hypertens Pregnancy* 1986;5(1):97–133.
3. Okkels H, Engle EP. Studies on the finer structure of the uterine blood vessels of the Macacus monkey. *Acta Pathol Microbiol Scand* 1938;15:150–168.
4. Bartelmez GW. The phases of the menstrual cycle and their interpretation. *Am J Obstet Gynecol* 1957;74:931–955.
5. Ramsey EM. Vascular anatomy. In: Wynn RM, ed. *Biology of the uterus.* New York: Plenum Press, 1977;59–76.
6. Markee JE. Menstruation in intraocular endometrial transplants in the Rhesus monkey. *Carnegie Contrib Embryol* 1940;28:279–308.
7. Frankenhauser F. *Nerven der gebarmutter wund ihre endigund in glatten muskelfasern.* Jena: Mauke, 1867.
8. Langley JN, Anderson HK. The innervation of the pelvic and adjoining viscera, part V. Position of the nerve-cells on the course of the efferent nerve-fibers. *J Physiol (London)* 1895;19:131.
9. Falk B, Hillarp NA, Thime G. Fluorescence of catecholamines and related compounds condensed with formaldehyde gas. *J Histochem Cytochem* 1962;10:348.
10. Owman CH, Rosengren E, Sjoberg NO. Adrenergic innervation of the human female reproductive organs: a histochemical and chemical investigation. *Obstet Gynecol* 1967;30:763–773.
11. Owman CH, Falk ED, Johansson E, Rosengren E, Sjoberg NO, Sporrung B, Svennson KG, Walles B. Autonomic nerves and related amine receptors mediating motor activity in the oviduct of monkeys and man: a histochemical and chemical pharmacologic study. In: Harper MJK, et al, eds. *Ovum transport and fertility regulation.* Silver Spring, MD: Scripta Publishers, 1976;256–275.
12. Sjoberg NO. New considerations on the adrenergic innervation of the cervix and uterus. *Acta Physiol Scand* [*Suppl*] 1967:305.
13. Corner GW. Exploring the placental maze. *Am J Obstet Gynecol* 1963;86(3):408.
14. Ramsey EM, Donner MW. *Placental vasculature and circulation.* Philadelphia: WB Saunders, 1980.
15. Brosens I, Robertson WB, Dixon HG. The physiologic response of the vessels of the placental bed to normal pregnancy. *J Pathol Bacteriol* 1967;93:569–579.
16. DeWolf F, DeWolf-Peters C, Brosens I. Ultrastructures of the spiral arteries of the human placental bed at the end of normal pregnancy. *Am J Obstet Gynecol* 1973;117:833–848.

17. DeWolf F, Robertson WB, Brosens I. The ultrastructure of acute atherosis in hypertensive pregnancy. *Am J Obstet Gynecol* 1975;123:164–174.
18. Pijnenborg R, Bland JM, Robertson WB, Dixon HG, Brosens I. The pattern of interstitial trophoblastic invasion of the myometrium in early pregnancy. *Placenta* 1981;2:303–316.
19. Sheppard BL, Bonnar J. The ultrastructure of the arterial supply of the human placenta in pregnancy complicated by fetal growth retardation. *Br J Obstet Gynaecol* 1976;83:948–959.
20. Enders AC, Schlafke S. Cytological aspects of trophoblastic uterine interaction and early implantation. *Am J Anat* 1969;125:1–30.
21. Enders AC. Cytology of human early implantation. *Res Reprod* 1976;8:1–2.
22. Ramsey EM, Donner MW. *Placental vasculature and circulation.* Philadelphia: WB Saunders, 1980.
23. Wynn RM. Cytotrophoblastic specializations: an ultrastructural study of the human placenta. *Am J Obstet Gynecol* 1972; 114:339–355.
24. Ramsey EM, Houston ML, Harris JW. Interactions of the trophoblast and maternal tissues in three closely related primate species. *Am J Obstet Gynecol* 1976;124:647–652.
25. Harris JWS. Intravascular trophoblast in human baboon and monkey uteri. *Anat Rec* 1971;169:334.
26. DeWolf F, DeWolf-Peters C, Brosens I. Ultrastructures of the spiral arteries in the human placental bed at the end of normal pregnancy. *Am J Obstet Gynecol* 1973;117:833–848.
27. Wynn RM, Panigel M, MacLennan AH. Fine structure of the placenta and fetal membranes of the baboon. *Am J Obstet Gynecol* 1971;109:638.
28. Tuttle SE, O'Toole RV, O'Shaughnessy RW, Zuspan FP. Immunohistochemical evaluation of human placental implantation: an initial study. *Am J Obstet Gynecol* 1985;153:239–244.
29. Robertson WB, Khong TH, Brosens I, DeWolf F, Sheppard BL, Bonnar J. The placental bed biopsy: review from three European centers. *Am J Obstet Gynecol* 1986;155:401–412.
30. Sporrung B, Alm P, Owman C, Sjoberg NO, Thorbert G. Ultrastructural evidence for adrenergic denervation in a guinea pig uterus during pregnancy. *Cell Tissue Res* 1978;195:188–192.
31. Thorbert G, Alm P, Owman C, Sjoberg NO, Sporrung B. Regional changes in structural and functional integrity of the myometrial adrenergic nerves in the pregnant guinea pig, and their relationship to localization. *Acta Physiol Scand* 1978;103:120–131.
32. Zuspan FP, O'Shaughnessy RW, Vinsel J, Zuspan M. Adrenergic innervation of uterine vasculature in human and term pregnancy. *Am J Obstet Gynecol* 1981;139:678–690.
33. Marshall JM. Effects of ovarian steroids in pregnancy on adrenergic nerves of the uterus and oviduct. *Am J Physiol* 1981;240:C165–C174.
34. Kennedy DR, Marshall JM. Effects of ovarian steroids *in vitro* kinetic properties of tyrosine hydroxylase from rabbit oviducts. *Biol Reprod* 1978;19:824–829.
35. Bell C, Malcolm SJ. Observations on the loss of catecholamine fluorescence from intrauterine adrenergic nerves during the pregnancy in human and guinea pig. *J Reprod Fertil* 1978;53:51–58.
36. Gardmark SC, Owman C, Sjoberg NO. Recovery of the transmitter content of uterine adrenergic nerves after pregnancy. *Am J Obstet Gynecol* 1971;109:997–1002.
37. Friedlander C. Physiologisch-Anatomische. *Untersuchingen uber den uterus.* Leipzig, 1870;32.
38. Hertig AT. The vascular pathology in the hypertensive albuminuric toxemias of pregnancy. *Clinics* 1945;4:602–614.
39. Zeek PM, Assali NS. Vascular changes in the decidua associated with eclamptogenic toxemia of pregnancy. *Am J Clin Pathol* 1950;20:1099–1109.
40. O'Shaughnessy RW, O'Toole R, Tuttle S, Zuspan FP. Uterine catecholamine in normal and hypertensive human pregnancy. *Clin Exp Hypertens Pregnancy* 1983;B3:447–457.
41. Walsh SW. Preeclampsia: an imbalance in placental prostacyclin and thromboxane production. *Am J Obstet Gynecol* 1985; 152:335–340.
42. Wallenburg HCS, Makovitz JW, Dekker GA, et al. Low-dose aspirin prevents pregnancy-induced hypertension in preeclampsia in angiotensin-sensitive primigravidae. *Lancet* 1986;1:1–3.

Hypertension: Pathophysiology, Diagnosis, and Management, edited by J. H. Laragh and B. M. Brenner. Raven Press, Ltd., New York © 1990.

CHAPTER 111

Eicosanoids in the Pathogenesis of Preeclampsia

Desmond J. Fitzgerald and Garret A. FitzGerald

Biology of Prostaglandins and Thromboxane A_2, 1789
Formation of Prostaglandins and Thromboxane by Reproductive Tissues, 1790
***In Vivo* Formation of Prostaglandins in Pregnancy, 1791**
Functional Relevance of Altered Eicosanoid Formation in Normal Pregnancy, 1794
Prostaglandin Formation in Preeclampsia, 1795
Thromboxane A_2 in Preeclampsia, 1798
Modulation of Eicosanoid Biosynthesis and the Incidence of Preeclampsia, 1800
Conclusion, 1802
References, 1803

Eicosanoids are a diverse group of products generated by oxidative metabolism of polyunsaturated 20-carbon fatty acids. Their most abundant precursor in humans is arachidonic acid, which has four double bonds; the double bond closest to the carboxyl end is at carbon 6 (20:4, $n - 6$). Depending on the dietary fat intake, eicosanoids generated from eicosapentaenoic acid (20:5, $n - 3$) may also achieve biologically significant concentrations in humans. Arachidonic acid is esterified into the phospholipid fractions of cell membranes. Specific stimuli activate phospholipases, which release the free fatty acid for subsequent metabolism. Three major enzymatic pathways of arachidonic acid metabolism have been described (Fig. 1): (i) cyclooxygenase metabolism to the prostaglandins (PGD_2, PGE_2, $PGF_{2\alpha}$, and prostacyclin) and thromboxane (Tx) A_2; (ii) lipoxygenase metabolism to the hydroxyeicosatrienoic acids (HETEs), leukotrienes (LTB_4, LTC_4, LTD_4, and LTE_4), and lipoxins; and (iii) metabolism (by cytochrome P450) to the epoxyeicosatrienoic acids (EETs).

This chapter will focus largely on cyclooxygenase products—in particular, TxA_2 and prostacyclin (PGI_2). The increase in vascular tone and platelet activity in preeclampsia has focused interest on these products, which have potent effects on platelets and vascular smooth muscle cells. Recent studies on their formation in pregnancy and preeclampsia support the hypothesis that these eicosanoids play a role in the pathogenesis of pregnancy hypertension. This is further supported by early clinical trials with the Tx inhibitor, aspirin. In this chapter we examine the pathophysiology of eicosanoids in preeclampsia and explore the pharmacology of TxA_2 inhibition. Little is known about the role of lipoxygenase and P450 products in pregnancy or in preeclampsia. However, in view of their *in vitro* effects on smooth muscle tone, vascular permeability, platelet function, and sodium/water balance, these products may be of importance in both the physiology and pathophysiology of pregnancy.

BIOLOGY OF PROSTAGLANDINS AND THROMBOXANE A_2

Prostaglandins are not stored but are generated upon activation of the cell and intracellular release of arachidonic acid (Fig. 2) (1). Membrane-associated cyclooxygenase converts arachidonate to the 15S-hydroperoxy compound, PGG_2, by the introduction of two molecules of oxygen; this, in turn, is enzymatically converted to the 15S-hydroxy compound PGH_2 (2). These prostaglandin endoperoxides have biologic activity in that they activate a receptor which they are thought to share with TxA_2 and which mediates platelet activation and vasoconstriction (3). However, in tissues, they are rapidly and enzymatically converted to prostaglandins and TxA_2 (4,5). The enzymes for this final step—and, therefore, the products that are formed—tend to be specific for a particular tissue. The major enzyme in platelets is TxA_2 synthase, which converts PGH_2 to TxA_2. Two molecules of PGH_2 react with the enzyme and result in the formation of one molecule each of TxA_2, malondialdehyde (a three-carbon compound) and 12-hydroxyheptadecatrienoic acid (6). In endothelial cells, two enzymes are relatively abundant: PGI_2 synthase and PGH-PGE isomerase, which result in the formation of PGI_2 and PGE_2, respectively (7).

Release of arachidonic acid (and its subsequent metabolism) follows activation of the cell by specific stimuli, and the products formed are, in general, short-lived. For example, TxA_2 and PGI_2 (with half-lives of seconds to minutes) are rapidly inactivated in tissues and biologic fluids by hy-

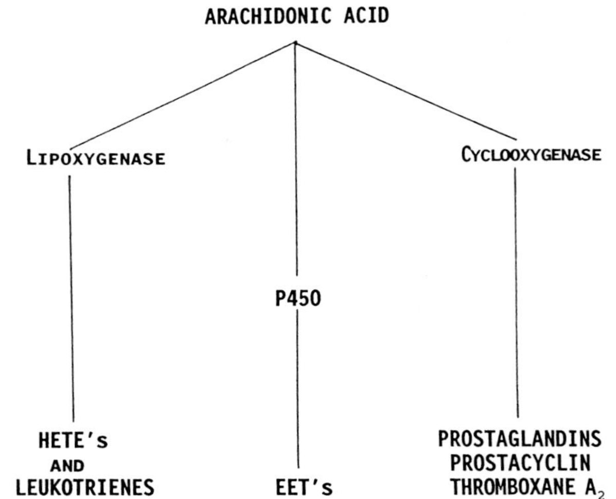

FIG. 1. Major pathways of metabolism of arachidonic acid.

drolysis, and both PGE_2 and $PGF_{2\alpha}$ are metabolized rapidly by a nicotinamide adenine dinucleotide (NAD)-linked 15-dehydrogenase (8). This suggests that prostaglandins act as local modulators of the response to cell stimulation. An example of this is the formation of PGI_2 and PGE_2 by vascular tissue upon stimulation with angiotensin II, which, in turn, blunts the response to this vasoconstrictor (9,10). Similarly, TxA_2, a potent platelet activator, is released by, as well as amplifies, the response to a number of platelet agonists (4).

Specific binding of radiolabeled analogs of PGI_2 and TxA_2 has been demonstrated in a variety of tissues, including vascular smooth muscle and endothelial cells (11,12) and platelets (13,14). Specific binding has also been described for PGE_2 and $PGF_{2\alpha}$ (15). This suggests that prostaglandins activate specific membrane receptors. These, in turn, transduce a signal via specific guanyl-nucleotide-binding regulatory (G) proteins. Distinct signal transduction mechanisms have been identified for different prostaglandins in the same tissue. Thus, PGI_2 stimulates adenylate cyclase, which mediates hydrolysis of cytosolic ATP to cyclic AMP, resulting in inhibition of vascular smooth muscle cells and platelets (16). In contrast, TxA_2 activates phospholipase C, resulting in phosphoinositide turnover and the subsequent activation of these tissues (17).

FORMATION OF PROSTAGLANDINS AND THROMBOXANE BY REPRODUCTIVE TISSUES

Reproductive tissues have long been recognized as a rich source of, and as a target organ for, prostaglandins. Indeed,

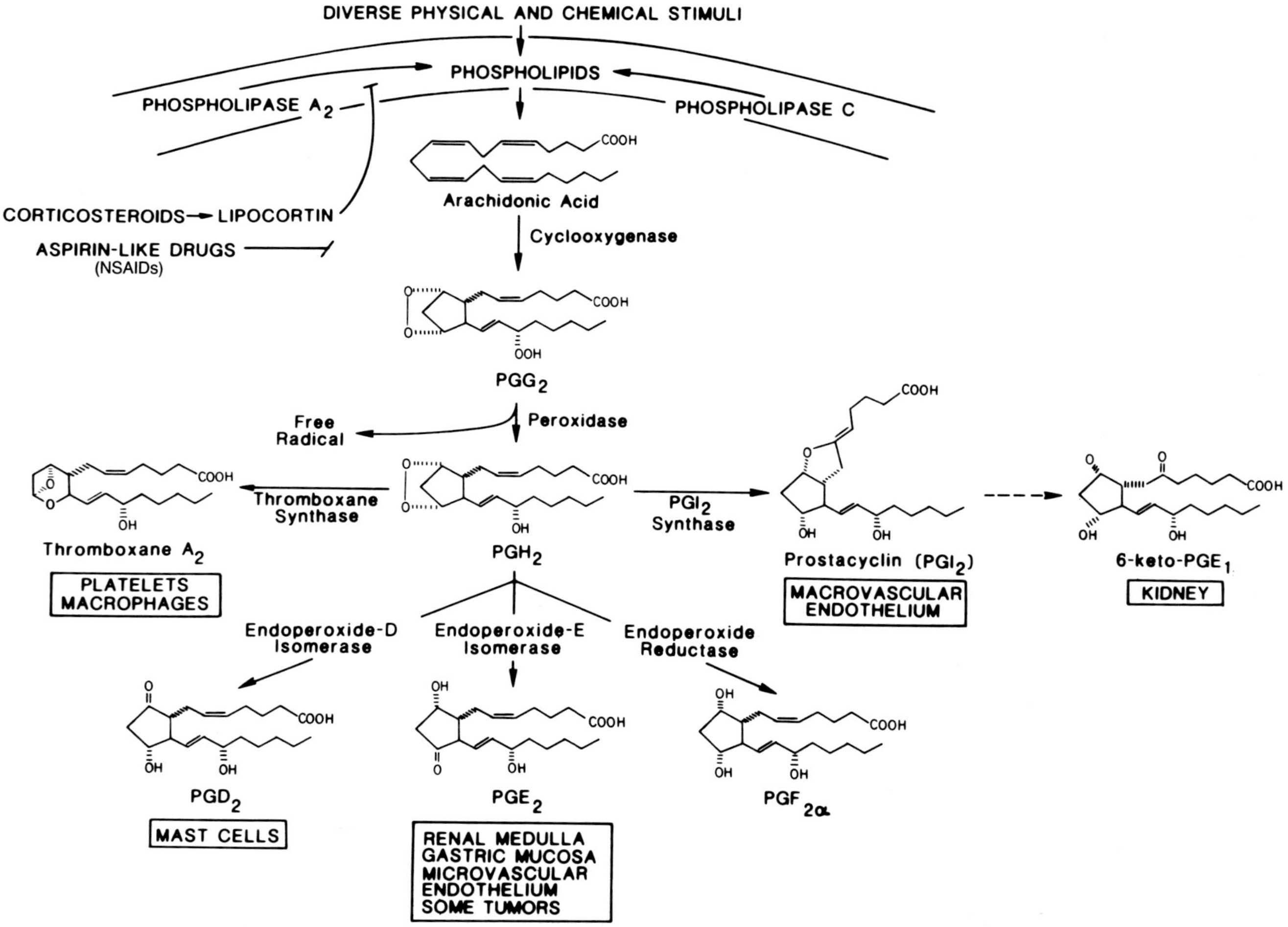

FIG. 2. Cyclooxygenase metabolism of arachidonic acid to prostaglandins, PGI_2 and TxA_2. (From ref. 189.)

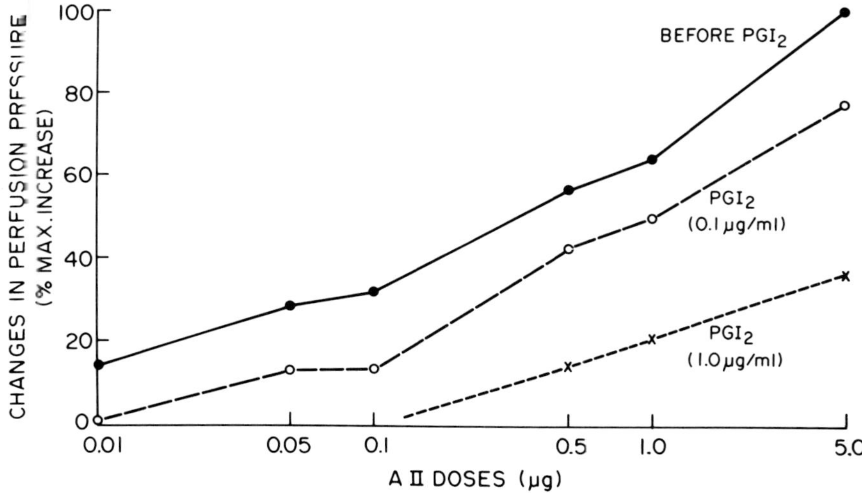

FIG. 7. Effect of PGI_2 on the pressor response to angiotensin II (A II) in the isolated, perfused human cotyledon. Note that at the lower dose, PGI_2 had no effect on resting vascular tone.

(92,106) and increases resistance in the isolated perfused human cotyledon (88,89,93). That this is mediated through a specific TxA_2/prostaglandin endoperoxide receptor is suggested by two findings. Firstly, the response to U46619 is inhibited by TxA_2/prostaglandin endoperoxide receptor antagonists (107). Secondly, specific binding of a radiolabeled TxA_2/prostaglandin endoperoxide receptor antagonist to human placental membranes has been demonstrated (108). Endogenous TxA_2, like PGI_2, may modulate the response to angiotensin II during pregnancy. Thus, aspirin, at a dose which selectively inhibits TxA_2 biosynthesis, decreased the pressor response to angiotensin II in normal pregnant subjects (109). Whether this is a direct result of diminished TxA_2 formation or is due to a reduction in another platelet product, serotonin, which enhances the response to angiotensin II (110), is unknown.

In addition to their effects on vascular smooth muscle, PGI_2 and TxA_2 exert opposite effects on platelets. PGI_2 is a potent platelet inhibitor (111), preventing platelet activation in response to all recognized agonists. In contrast, TxA_2 is generated by platelets in response to many platelet activators and, in turn, induces platelet activation (5). The increase in TxA_2 biosynthesis is consistent with other evidence of mild platelet activation during pregnancy (112–114). The increase in PGI_2 formation is unlikely to achieve significant systemic inhibition of platelets, since, based on the rate of metabolite excretion (68) and plasma 6-keto-$PGF_{1\alpha}$ (67) in pregnant subjects, this is below the threshold for antiplatelet activity (95). However, if confined to the placental vascular bed, the enhanced PGI_2 biosynthesis may play an important role in modulating platelet activity and preventing thrombosis in the placenta.

It has been postulated that prostaglandins also play a role in the altered renal function of gestation. Glomerular filtration and renal blood flow both increase in pregnant subjects (115). The kidney is a rich source of PGE_2 and $PGF_{2\alpha}$ (42). In addition, these prostaglandins increase blood flow to the renal medulla and inner cortical region, promote water excretion and are natriuretic. Consistent with this concept, urinary PGE_2 and 6-keto-$PGF_{1\alpha}$, which reflect renal production of the parent compounds, are increased in pregnant rats (42); furthermore, excretion of PGE_2 is increased in human pregnancy (116). However, cyclo-oxygenase inhibition has no effect on renal function in the pregnant rat (42) or rabbit (117). Moreover, the increase in renal excretion of these products may be a reflection of the altered renal function per se (41,118), since renal medullary tissue from pregnant rats does not generate increased amounts of PGE_2 or PGI_2 (42). Thus, it seems unlikely that an alteration in prostaglandin formation is a major mechanism of altered renal function in pregnancy. On the other hand, PGE_2 and PGI_2 are potent renin secretagogues (119) and may be important mediators of the increased renin production of pregnancy. Consistent with this, plasma renin activity correlates with PGE_2 (116) and is decreased by cyclooxygenase inhibition (117) during pregnancy.

PROSTAGLANDIN FORMATION IN PREECLAMPSIA

Abnormalities in prostaglandin formation have been consistently demonstrated in patients with preeclampsia. The most frequently noted abnormality is a reduction in PGI_2 formation by placental and umbilical vessels (120–124), first reported by Remuzzi et al. (120). A diminished capacity to form PGI_2 was also demonstrated in dermal vessels from hypertensive subjects (125). Although it has been suggested that abnormal PGI_2 formation is specific for preeclampsia as distinct from essential hypertension in pregnancy (68,123), studies demonstrate a similar defect in other obstetrical conditions, including intrauterine growth retardation (126). A marked reduction in PGE_2 formation by placental tissues has also been shown to occur in patients with preeclampsia (127,128), suggesting that the abnormality may be a nonspecific alteration in prostaglandin biosynthesis.

To explore this further, PGI_2 biosynthesis was compared in normotensive pregnant subjects and in patients with preeclampsia by measuring excretion of the enzymatic metabolite, 2,3-dinor-6-keto-$PGF_{1\alpha}$, in the third trimester (64). Excretion of this metabolite was lower in preeclamptic patients than in normotensive pregnant subjects in the third trimester (Table 1). Although this was consistent with a reduction in the formation of the parent compound, it may also have reflected an alteration in its metabolism. Thus, placental prostaglandin 15-dehydrogenase is increased in patients with preeclampsia (129), and this may result in a reduction in beta-oxidation to 2,3-dinor-6-keto-PGF$_{1\alpha}$. However, urinary excretion of 6,15-diketo-13,14-dihydro-2,3-dinor-PGF$_{1\alpha}$, reflecting the prostaglandin 15-dehydrogenase pathway, was also decreased in preeclamptic patients, indicating that prostacyclin biosynthesis was, indeed, impaired (64). In a subsequent study (68), urinary 2,3-dinor-6-keto-PGF$_{1\alpha}$ excretion was determined in each trimester in 67 pregnant subjects. Twelve patients subsequently developed pregnancy-induced hypertension, defined as either a blood pressure of greater than 140/90 mmHg, an increase of 30 mmHg in systolic blood pressure, or a 15-mmHg rise in diastolic blood pressure. Nine patients had a history of chronic hypertension. Urinary 2,3-dinor-6-keto-PGF$_{1\alpha}$ increased markedly in the first trimester in normotensive subjects and remained elevated throughout gestation (Fig. 8). A smaller increase occurred in patients who subsequently developed pregnancy-induced hypertension. This difference was present in the first trimester, long before there was clinical evidence of the disease, and persisted throughout pregnancy. In contrast, there was a normal gestational increase in excretion of 2,3-dinor-6-keto-PGF$_{1\alpha}$ in chronic hypertensives.

The mechanism of the decrease in PGI_2 formation in preeclamptic subjects is uncertain. *In vitro* studies demonstrate a reduction in the capacity of placental tissue and umbilical vessels from preeclamptic subjects to generate PGI_2 and PGE_2 (120–128). This may reflect endothelial injury, since both are major products of vascular endothelium. Histologic evidence of endothelial denudation in the placenta supports this hypothesis (130). Alternatively, the decrease in PGI_2 formation may reflect a reduction in substrate availability (131). A reduction in the arachidonic acid content of cell membranes from umbilical vessels has been reported in patients with this condition (131). Interestingly, arachidonic acid (20:4, $n - 6$) was replaced by another fatty acid, Mead's acid (20:3, $n - 9$), which fails to form prostaglandins. Accumulation of Mead's acid has been reported to occur only in the setting of essential fatty acid deficiency, where the substrate for arachidonic acid formation is missing from the diet (132). Furthermore, a condition similar to preeclampsia has been induced in rats by feeding them a diet deficient in essential fatty acids (133).

Although the work of Dadak et al. (122) and Makila et al. (123) suggested that the reduction in PGI_2 formation was unique for preeclampsia, a similar defect has been demonstrated in other obstetrical conditions. In particular, PGI_2 formation by umbilical vessels and placental tissue is reduced in patients with intrauterine growth retardation (126,134). This suggests that the reduction in biosynthesis of this eicosanoid may reflect placental insufficiency. However, PGI_2 biosynthesis is decreased even in patients with mild preeclampsia with no clinical evidence of placental insufficiency or intrauterine growth retardation (68). Furthermore, in two patients who developed severe IUGR without hypertension, PGI_2 biosynthesis was normal (68).

The reduction in PGI_2 biosynthesis early in the course of preeclampsia suggests that it may play a role in the pathogenesis of this disease. It is unlikely that the increase in blood pressure directly reflects a loss of the vasodilator effect of PGI_2. Measurement of urinary 2,3-dinor-6-keto-PGF$_{1\alpha}$ excretion predicts a plasma level in the range of 8–10 pg/ml and a biosynthetic rate of 0.5–1.0 ng/kg/min (68). This is below the threshold for systemic hemodynamic effects. Furthermore, the changes in PGI_2 formation

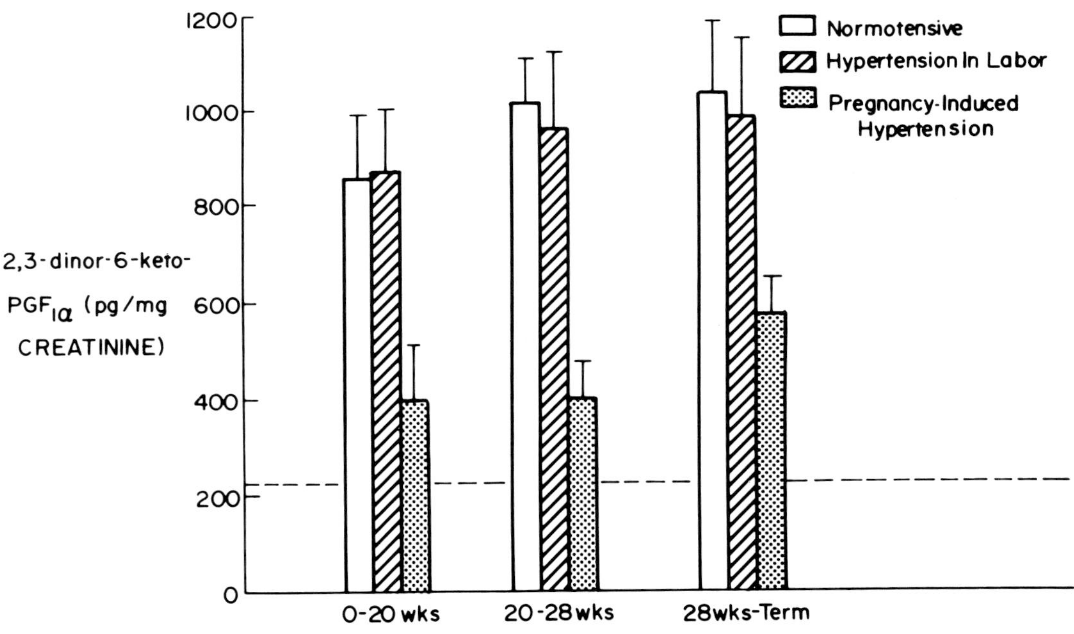

FIG. 8. Excretion of 2,3-dinor-6-keto-PGF$_{1\alpha}$ throughout pregnancy in normotensive subjects, in patients who developed pregnancy-induced hypertension, and in patients exhibiting increased blood pressure only during labor. In this latter group the increased blood pressure was probably a normal response to labor. The hatched bar represents the upper limit of normal in nonpregnant subjects. (From ref. 68.)

in preeclampsia long precede the rise in blood pressure. An alternative hypothesis is that the loss of PGI_2 enhances the effects of angiotensin II and other endogenous vasoconstrictors. Plasma angiotensin II is increased in both normotensive and, to a lesser extent, hypertensive pregnant subjects (104). Patients destined to develop preeclampsia demonstrate increasing sensitivity to angiotensin II prior to the development clinical signs (102). The increased sensitivity to angiotensin II can be reversed by infusions of PGE_1 (135) and PGI_2 (100). Furthermore, the response to angiotensin II *in vivo* (136,137) and in isolated tissues (138) is exaggerated by inhibition of cyclooxygenase and deprivation of prostaglandin precursors (139), suggesting that endogenous vasodilator prostaglandins generated by the target tissue modulate the response to this hormone.

To determine if the reduction in PGI_2 biosynthesis resulted in an alteration in the sensitivity to angiotensin II, angiotensin sensitivity was examined in 33 normotensive pregnant subjects in the third trimester and was compared with excretion of 2,3-dinor-6-keto-$PGF_{1\alpha}$ (68). Angiotensin II sensitivity was determined as the intravenous dose required to increase diastolic blood pressure by 20 mmHg. Six patients developed pregnancy-induced hypertension, only two of whom exhibited an abnormal sensitivity to angiotensin II. There was no correlation between the excretion of the prostacyclin metabolite and the dose of angiotensin II required to increase diastolic blood pressure by 20 mmHg (Fig. 9). Thus, the reduction in prostacyclin biosynthesis appears unrelated to increased systemic sensitivity to angiotensin II.

As discussed earlier, the gestational increase in PGI_2 may be largely derived from the placenta, where it may achieve a concentration sufficient to regulate vascular tone. Thus, prostacyclin may play a major role in regulating placental blood flow during pregnancy. In preeclampsia, placental blood flow is decreased by as much as 50% (140,141) and may be a major mechanism of the placental insufficiency which characterizes this condition. In addition, a primary reduction in placental blood flow can induce a syndrome similar to human preeclampsia in animal models of pregnancy (142,143). What regulates placental blood flow *in vivo* is unknown. *In vitro* studies using the isolated perfused human cotyledon demonstrate the presence of angiotensin receptors and a functional renin–angiotensin system (105). Furthermore, angiotensin is a potent vasoconstrictor in the placental vascular bed (144). The response to angiotensin in this system is blunted by PGI_2, even at concentrations which fall below threshold for a vasodilator effect (Fig. 7). Thus, decreased PGI_2 biosynthesis in the placental vascular bed may allow unopposed vasoconstriction by angiotensin and other endogenous pressors.

In addition to its effects on vascular tone, PGI_2 may play a pathogenic role in preeclampsia through its effects on platelet activity. There is strong evidence that platelet activity is increased in patients with preeclampsia as compared to that seen in normotensive pregnant subjects (145–148). Thus, platelet turnover, measured as recovery of platelet cyclooxygenase activity after the administration of aspirin, is increased (146). Furthermore, there is a marked fall in platelet count, accompanied by evidence of disseminated intravascular coagulation, in patients with severe forms of the disease (147). Based on pathologic findings, a major site of this platelet activation appears to be the placenta (149). What induces the increased platelet activity in preeclamptic patients is uncertain, but studies in other syndromes of platelet activation suggest that prostacyclin is a potent regulator of platelet activity in humans. Formation of this eicosanoid is increased in a variety of conditions associated with platelet activation, including severe atherosclerosis (150), unstable angina (151), and systemic sclerosis (152). Furthermore, there is evidence that doses of aspirin that preserve prostacyclin formation are more effective in preventing platelet activation in experimental models (153). These data suggest that endogenous prostacyclin limits platelet activity *in vivo*. Therefore, the reduction in prostacyclin formation early in the course of preeclampsia may induce or amplify platelet activation in this condition.

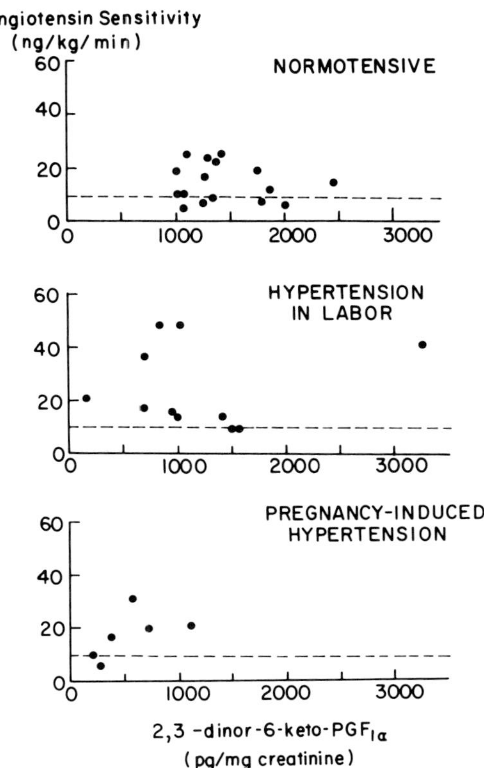

FIG. 9. Comparison of angiotensin sensitivity and urinary 2,3-dinor-6-keto-$PGF_{1\alpha}$ in normotensive and hypertensive pregnancies. There was no relationship between the pressor response to angiotensin and PGI_2 biosynthesis. (From ref. 68.)

Irrespective of its role in the pathogenesis of preeclampsia, failure to increase prostacyclin formation may identify a population at risk of developing the disease. Indeed, in a prospective study of 67 pregnant subjects, excretion of less than 400 pg/mg creatinine of 2,3-dinor-6-keto-$PGF_{1\alpha}$ was associated with a 65% risk of developing the disease (68). This compares favorably with demographic markers, which are predictive in 4–15% of cases (154–156), and may allow targeting of interventions to populations most likely to benefit.

THROMBOXANE A_2 IN PREECLAMPSIA

The increase in TxA_2 biosynthesis in normal pregnancy is consistent with an increase in platelet activity. TxA_2 is released by platelets upon activation (5), and increased TxA_2 biosynthesis has been demonstrated in a variety of conditions associated with platelet activation, including unstable angina (151) and severe atherosclerosis (157). Platelet activation is further enhanced in patients with clinical evidence of preeclampsia (144–148), although it is not known at what point in the course of the disease that this phenomenon is initiated. If the reduction in PGI_2 formation mediates its effects through increased platelet activity, it would be expected that evidence of platelet activation would be apparent in the first trimester. To address this hypothesis, we determined TxA_2 biosynthesis prospectively in pregnant subjects by measuring urinary 2,3-dinor-TxB_2 excretion in 24-hr samples collected in each trimester (158). Urinary 2,3-dinor-TxB_2 was increased in these patients throughout gestation but was not significantly different from levels in normotensive pregnant subjects (Fig. 10).

Patients who develop pregnancy-induced hypertension, therefore, do not demonstrate evidence of increased platelet activity prior to development of the disease as compared to that seen in normal pregnancy. However, these findings do not exclude increased platelet activation and TxA_2 biosynthesis with progression of the disease to a more severe form. To address this possibility, we examined TxA_2 biosynthesis in patients presenting to the hospital in florid preeclampsia (159). These patients had severe hypertension and proteinuria, and all but one had thrombocytopenia. In addition, plasma LDH, SGOT, and uric acid were elevated in the majority of patients. For comparison, normal pregnant subjects admitted for delivery were also studied. Urinary 2,3-dinor-TxB_2 and 11-dehydro-TxB_2 were elevated in the normal group (Fig. 11), as demonstrated previously (70). A further (and, in some cases, massive) increase in the excretion of both metabolites occurred in patients with preeclampsia, demonstrating that TxA_2 biosynthesis is greatly increased in this condition. The rapid fall in metabolite excretion following delivery (Fig. 11) suggests that the increase in TxA_2 formation is derived from the placenta and is consistent with the hypothesis that it reflects platelet activation within the placental vascular bed. This, in turn, may be responsible for the pathologic findings of thrombosis and infarction in placentae from patients with preeclampsia (149).

The increase in TxA_2 formation in preeclampsia may exert a number of effects. In particular, because it is a potent vasoconstrictor, it may mediate the reduction in placental blood flow which is characteristic of preeclampsia. To determine the response to TxA_2 on the placental vasculature, we examined the effect of the TxA_2/prostaglandin endoperoxide analog U46619 (160) in the isolated, perfused human cotyledon (Fig. 12). In this preparation, a branch of the umbilical artery supplying one to two cotyledons is perfused with cold modified Krebs solution soon after delivery. The isolated segment is mounted in a twin chamber system which allows independent perfusion of the maternal and fetal circulations. The vein corresponding to the isolated artery is also cannulated, and a closed system is used to perfuse the tissue with oxygenated buffer. The maternal side is also cannulated directly, with a system of six perfusion catheters. Flow is maintained constant so that alterations in vascular tone are detected as changes in perfusion pressure. Infusion of U46619 increased perfusion pressure more markedly and with a lower IC_{50} than did angiotensin II (Fig. 13). Furthermore, the dose–response curve for U46619 was shifted to the right by EP045, an antagonist of the shared TxA_2/prostaglandin endoperoxide receptor on vascular smooth muscle (Fig. 14) (161). These data demonstrate evidence of a functional TxA_2/prosta-

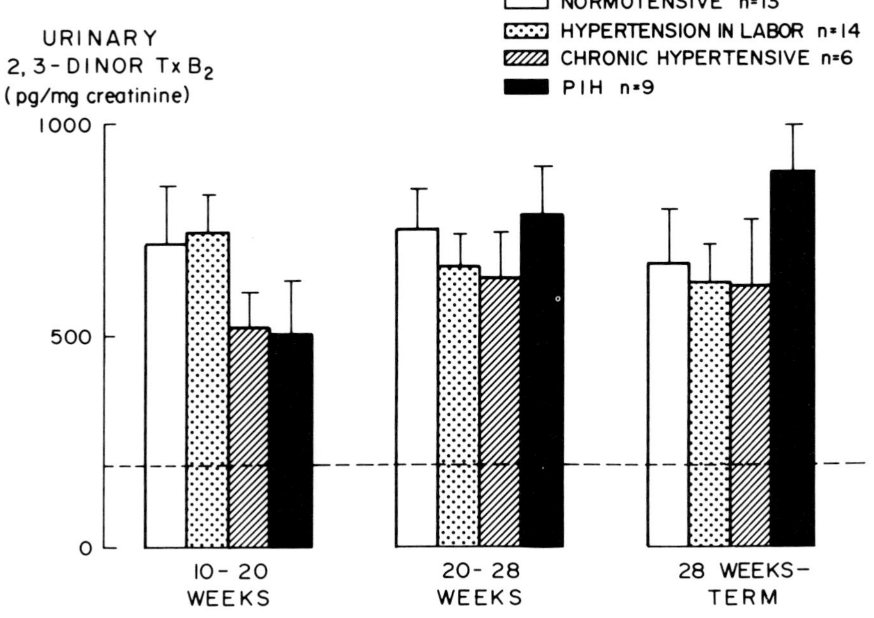

FIG. 10. Excretion of 2,3-dinor-TxB_2 in normotensive and hypertensive pregnancy. The hatched bar represents the upper limit of normal for nonpregnant subjects. Note that TxA_2 was increased in pregnancy and was not significantly higher in patients who subsequently developed pregnancy-induced hypertension (PIH).

lation which would inhibit maternal, but not fetal, platelet cyclooxygenase, thereby reducing the risk of fetal bleeding.

ACKNOWLEDGMENTS

This research was supported by grants from the National Institutes of Health (HL30400, HD17414). Dr. G. A. FitzGerald is an Established Investigator of the American Heart Association. We are indebted to Mrs. Esther Stuart for editorial assistance.

REFERENCES

1. Flower RJ, Blackwell GJ. The importance of phospholipase A_2 in prostaglandin biosynthesis. *Biochem Pharmacol* 1976;25:285–291.
2. Miyamoto T, Ogina N, Yamamoto S, Hayaishi O. Purification of prostaglandin endoperoxide synthetase from bovine vesicular gland microsomes. *J Biol Chem* 1976;251:2619–2636.
3. Hamberg M, Svensson J, Wakabayashi T, Samuelsson B. Isolation and structure of two prostaglandin endoperoxides that cause platelet aggregation. *Proc Natl Acad Sci USA* 1974;71:345–349.
4. Hamberg M, Svensson J, Samuelsson B. Thromboxanes: a new group of biologically active compounds derived from prostaglandin endoperoxides. *Proc Natl Acad Sci USA* 1975;72:2994–2298.
5. Granstrom E, Diczfalusy U, Hamberg M, Malmsten C, Samuelsson B. Thromboxane A_2; biosynthesis and effect on platelet. *Adv Prostaglandin Thromboxane Leukotriene Res* 1982;10:15–58.
6. Hammarstrom S, Falardeau P. Resolution of prostaglandin endoperoxide synthase and thromboxane synthase of human platelets. *Proc Natl Acad Sci USA* 1977;63:3691–3695.
7. Gerristen ME, Cheli CD. Arachidonic acid and prostaglandin endoperoxide metabolism in isolated and cultivated coronary microvessel endothelial cells. *J Clin Invest* 1983;72:1658–1671.
8. Pike JE, Fitzpatrick FA, Lincoln FH, Sun FF. Metabolism of prostaglandins with cardiovascular and platelet effects. In: Johnsson Hegyeli R, ed. *Prostaglandins and cardiovascular diseases.* New York: Raven Press, 1981;39–52.
9. Grodzinska L, Gryglewski R. Angiotensin-induced release of prostacyclin from perfused organs. *Pharmacol Res Commun* 1980;12:339–347.
10. Barrow SE, Dollery CT, Heavey DJ, Hickling NE, Ritter JM, Vial J. Effect of vasoactive peptides on prostacyclin synthesis in man. *Br J Pharmacol* 1986;87:243–247.
11. Hanasaki K, Nakano K, Kasai H, Kurihara H, Arita H. Identification of thromboxane A_2 receptor in cultured vascular endothelial cells of rat aorta. *Biochem Biophys Res Commun* 1988;151:1352–1357.
12. Hanasaki K, Nakano K, Arita H, Ohtari K, Doteuchi M. Specific receptor for thromboxane A_2 in cultured vascular smooth muscle cells of rat aorta. *Biochem Biophys Res Commun* 1988;130:1170–1175.
13. Armstrong RA, Jones RL, Wilson NH. Ligand binding to thromboxane receptors on human platelets: correlation with biological activity. *Br J Pharmacol* 1983;79:953–964.
14. Saussey DL, Mais DE, Burch RM, Halushka PV. Identification of a putative thromboxane A_2/prostaglandin H_2 receptor in human platelet membranes. *J Biol Chem* 1986;261:3025–3029.
15. Smith WL, Sonnenburg WK, Watanabe T, Umegaki K. Mechanism of action of prostaglandin E_2 and prostaglandin $F_{2\alpha}$, PGE and PGF_α receptors. In: Halushka PV, Mais DE, eds. *Eicosanoids in the cardiovascular and renal systems.* Norwell, MA: MTP Press, 1984;232–248.
16. Gorman RR, Bunting S, Miller OV. Modulation of human platelet adenylate cyclase by prostacyclin (PGX). *Prostaglandins* 1977;13:377–388.
17. Brass LF, Shaller CC, Belmonte EJ. Inositol 1,4,5-triphosphate-induced granule secretion in platelets. *J Clin Invest* 1987;79:1269–1275.
18. von Euler US. On the specific vasodilating and plain muscle stimulating substance from accessory genital glands in man and certain animals (prostaglandin and vesiglandin). *J Physiol (Lond)* 1936;88:213–234.
19. Levitt MJ, Tobon H, Josimovich JB. Prostaglandin content of human endometrium. *Fertil Steril* 1975;26:296–300.
20. Brown CG, Poyser NL. Further studies on prostaglandin and thromboxane production by the rat uterus during the oestrous cycle. *J Reprod Fertil* 1985;73:391–399.
21. Bloch MH, McLaughlin LL, Martin SA, Needleman P. Prostaglandin production by the pregnant and non-pregnant rabbit uterus. *Prostaglandins* 1983;26:33–46.
22. Fenwick L, Jones RL, Naylor B, Poyser NL, Wilson NH. Production of prostaglandins by the pseudopregnant rat uterus, *in vitro,* and the effect of tamoxifen with the identification of 6-keto-prostaglandin $F_{1\alpha}$ as a major product. *Br J Pharmacol* 1977;59:191–199.
23. Tsang BK, Oi TC. Prostaglandin secretion by human endometrium *in vitro. Am J Obstet Gynecol* 1982;142:626–633.
24. Mitchell MD, Bibby JG, Hicks BR, Turnbull AC. Possible role for prostacyclin in human parturition. *Prostaglandins* 1978;16:931–937.
25. Williams KI, Dembinska-Kiec A, Zmuda A, Gryglewski RJ. Prostacyclin formation by myometrial & decidual fractions of the pregnant rat uterus. *Prostaglandins* 1978;15:343–350.
26. Liggins GC, Campos GA, Roberts CM, Skinner SJ. Production rates of prostaglandin $F_{2\alpha}$, 6-keto-$PGF_{1\alpha}$ and thromboxane B_2 by perifused human endometrium. *Prostaglandins* 1980;19:461–477.
27. Phillips CA, Poyser NL. Prostaglandins, thromboxanes and the pregnant rat uterus at term. *Br J Pharmacol* 1981;73:75–80.
28. Terragno NA, McGiff JC, Smigel M, Terragno A. Patterns of prostaglandin production in the bovine fetal and maternal vasculature. *Prostaglandins* 1978;16:847–855.
29. Remuzzi G, Misiani R, Muratore D, Marchesi D, Livio M, Schieppati A, Mecca G, de Gaetano G, Donati MB. Prostacyclin and human foetal circulation. *Prostaglandins* 1979;18:341–348.
30. Kwano M, Mori N. Prostacyclin producing activity of human umbilical, placental and uterine vessels. *Prostaglandins* 1983;26:645–662.
31. Bjoro K, Hovig T, Stokke KT, Stray-Pedersen S. Formation of prostanoids in human umbilical vessels. *Prostaglandins* 1986;31:683–697.
32. Walsh SW, Parisi VM. The role of arachidonic acid metabolites in preeclampsia. *Semin Perinatol* 1986;10:334–355.
33. Bjoro K. Prostacyclin and thromboxane formation in human umbilical arteries following stimulation with vasoactive autacoids. *Prostaglandins* 1986;31:701–715.
34. Dubin NH, Ghodgaonkar RB, Blake DA. Thromboxane production in the pregnant rat: differential recovery by platelets and uterus following aspirin administration. *Biol Reprod* 1983; 29:743–749.
35. Moodley J, Norman RJ, Reddi K. Central venous concentrations of immunoreactive prostaglandins E, F, and 6-keto-prostaglandin $F_{1\alpha}$ in eclampsia. *Br Med J* 1984;288:1487–1489.
36. Valenzuela G, Harper MJK, Hayashi RH. Uterine venous, peripheral venous, and radial arterial levels of prostaglandins E and F in women with pregnancy-induced hypertension. *Am J Obstet Gynecol* 1983;145:11–14.
37. Keirse MJNC, Mitchell MD, Turnbull AC. Changes in prostaglandin F and 13,14-dihydro-15-keto-prostaglandin F concentrations in amniotic fluid at the onset of and during labour. *Br J Obstet Gynaecol* 1977;84:743–746.
38. Willman EA, Collins WP. The concentrations of prostaglandin E_2 and prostaglandin $F_{2\alpha}$ in tissues within the fetoplacental unit after spontaneous or induced labour. *Br J Obstet Gynaecol* 1976;83:786–789.
39. Bay WH, Ferris TF. Factors controlling plasma renin and aldosterone during pregnancy. *Hypertension* 1979;1:410–415.
40. Frolich JC, Wilson TW, Sweetman BJ, Smigel M, Nies AS, Carr K, Watson JT, Oates JA. Urinary prostaglandins: identification and origin. *J Clin Invest* 1975;55:763–770.
41. Lifschitz MD, Epstein M, Larios O. Relationship between urine

flow rate and prostaglandin E excretion in human beings. *J Lab Clin Med* 1985;105:234–238.
42. Conrad KP, Dunn MJ. Renal synthesis and urinary excretion of eicosanoids during pregnancy in rats. *Am J Physiol Soc* 1987;253:F1197–F1205.
43. Mitchell MD, Keirse MJNC, Anderson ABM, Turnbull AC. Thromboxane B_2 in amniotic fluid before and during labour. *Br J Obstet Gynaecol* 1978;85:442–445.
44. Mitchell MD, Keirse MJNC, Brunt JD, Anderson ABM, Turnbull AC. Concentrations of the prostacyclin metabolite, 6-keto-prostaglandin $F_{1\alpha}$, in amniotic fluid during late pregnancy and labour. *Br J Obstet Gynaecol* 1978;86:350–353.
45. MacKenzie IZ, MacLean DA, Mitchell MD. Prostaglandins in the human fetal circulation in mid-trimester and term pregnancy. *Prostaglandins* 1980;20:649–654.
46. Ylikorkala O, Makarainen L, Viinikka L. Prostacyclin production increases during human parturition. *Br J Obstet Gynaecol* 1981;88:513–516.
47. Bolton PJ, Jogee M, Myatt L, Elder MG. Maternal plasma 6-oxo-prostaglandin $F_{1\alpha}$ levels throughout pregnancy: a longitudinal study. *Br J Obstet Gynaecol* 1981;88:1101–1103.
48. Ylikorkala O, Jouppila P, Kirkinen P, Viinikka L. Maternal prostacyclin, thromboxane, and placental blood flow. *Am J Obstet Gynecol* 1983;145:730–732.
49. Roy AC, Karim SMM, Kottegoda SR, Ratnam SS. Thromboxane A_2 and prostacyclin levels in molar pregnancy. *Br J Obstet Gynaecol* 1984;91:908–912.
50. Greer IA, Walker JJ, McLaren M, Bonduelle M, Cameron AD, Calder AA, Forbes CD. Immunoreactive prostacyclin and thromboxane metabolites in normal pregnancy and the puerperium. *Br J Obstet Gynaecol* 1985;92:581–585.
51. Ylikorkala O, Viinikka L. Maternal plasma levels of 6-keto-prostaglandin $F_{1\alpha}$ during pregnancy and puerperium. *Prostaglandins Med* 1981;7:95–99.
52. Koullapis EN, Nicolaides KH, Collins WP, Rodeck CH, Campbell S. Plasma prostanoids in pregnancy-induced hypertension. *Br J Obstet Gynaecol* 1982;89:617–621.
53. FitzGerald GA, Pedersen AK, Patrono C. Analysis of prostacyclin and thromboxane A_2 biosynthesis in cardiovascular disease. *Circulation* 1983;67:1174–1177.
54. Roy L, Knapp H, Robertson RM, FitzGerald GA. Endogenous biosynthesis of prostacyclin during cardiac catheterization and angiography in man. *Circulation* 1985;71:434–440.
55. Blair IA, Barrow SE, Waddell KA, Lewis PJ, Dollery CT. Prostacyclin is not a circulating hormone in man. *Prostaglandins* 1982;23:579–589.
56. Pedersen AK, Watson M, FitzGerald GA. Inhibition of thromboxane synthase in serum: limitations of the measurement of immunoreactive 6-keto-$PGF_{1\alpha}$. *Thromb Res* 1983;33:99–103.
57. Roberts LJ, Sweetman BJ, Oates JA. Metabolism of thromboxane B_2 in man: identification of twenty urinary metabolites. *J Biol Chem* 1981;256:8384–8387.
58. Lawson J, Patrono C, Ciabattoni G, FitzGerald GA. Long lived enzymatic metabolites of thromboxane B_2 in the human circulation. *Anal Biochem* 1986;155:198–205.
59. Patrono C, Ciabattoni G, Pugliese F, Pierucci A, Blair IA, FitzGerald GA. Estimated rate of thromboxane secretion into the circulation of normal humans. *J Clin Invest* 1986;77:590.
60. Brash AR, Jackson EK, Sagasse CA, Lawson JA, Oates JA, FitzGerald GA. The metabolic disposition of prostacyclin in man. *J Pharmacol Exp Ther* 1983;166:78–87.
61. FitzGerald GA, Brash AR, Falardeau P, Oates JA. Estimated rate of prostacyclin secretion into the circulation in normal man. *J Clin Invest* 1981;68:1272–1276.
62. Schweer H, Kammer J, Seyberth HW. Simultaneous determination of prostanoids in plasma by gas chromatography–negative ion chemical ionization–mass spectrometry. *J Chromatogr* 1985;338:273–280.
63. Catella F, Healy D, Lawson J, FitzGerald GA. 11-Dehydro-TxB_2: a quantitative index of thromboxane A_2 biosynthesis in the human circulation. *Proc Natl Acad Sci USA* 1986;83–5861.
64. Brash AR, Goodman RP, FitzGerald. Endogenous prostaglandin biosynthesis in human pregnancy. In Lewis PJ, Moncada S, O'Grady J, eds. *Prostacyclin in pregnancy.* London: Raven Press, 1983;71–77.
65. Vesterqvist O, Green K. Urinary excretion of 2,3-dinor-thromboxane B_2 in man under normal conditions, following drugs and during some pathological conditions. *Prostaglandins* 1984;27:627–644.
66. Fischer S, Bernutz C, Meier H, Weber C. Formation of prostacyclin and thromboxane in man as measured by the main urinary metabolites. *Biochim Biophys Acta* 1986;876:194–199.
67. Barrow SE, Blair IA, Waddell KA, Shepherd GL, Lewis PJ, Dollery CT. Prostacyclin in late pregnancy: analysis of 6-oxo-prostaglandin $F_{1\alpha}$ in maternal plasma. In: Lewis PJ, Moncada S, O'Grady J, eds. *Prostacyclin in pregnancy.* London: Raven Press, 1983;79–85.
68. Fitzgerald DJ, Entmann SS, Mulloy K, FitzGerald GA. Decreased prostacyclin biosynthesis preceding the clinical manifestations of pregnancy-induced hypertension. *Circulation* 1987;75:956–963.
69. Gerber JG, Payne NA, Murphy RC, Nies AS. Prostacyclin produced by the pregnant uterus in the dog may act as a circulating vasodepressor substance. *J Clin Invest* 1981;67:632–636.
70. Fitzgerald DJ, Mayo G, Catella F, Entmann SS, FitzGerald GA. Increased thromboxane biosynthesis in normal pregnancy is mainly derived from platelets. *Am J Obstet Gynecol* 1987;157:325–330.
71. Roth GJ, Stanford A, Majerus PW. Acetylation of prostaglandin synthase by aspirin. *Proc Natl Acad Sci USA* 1976;72:3073.
72. FitzGerald GA, Oates JA, Hawiger J, Maas RL, Roberts LJ II, Brash AR. Endogenous synthesis of prostacyclin and thromboxane and platelet function during chronic aspirin administration in man. *J Clin Invest* 1983;71:676–688.
73. Reilly IAG, FitzGerald GA. Aspirin in cardiovascular disease. *Drugs* 1988;35:154–176.
74. MacDonald PC, Schultz FM, Duenhoelter JH, et al. Initiation of human parturition. *Obstet Gynecol* 1974;44:629–636.
75. Lindberg BO. The induction of labour by the intravenous infusion of prostaglandin $F_{2\alpha}$. *Prostaglandins* 1977;14:993–1004.
76. Laudanski T, Akerlund M. Interaction of vasopressin and prostaglandin on myometrial activity *in vivo* in the first trimester of human pregnancy. *Br J Obstet Gynaecol* 1980;87:132–138.
77. Alsat E, Cedard. The simulatory action of the prostaglandins on the production of oestrogens by the human placenta perfused *in vitro. Prostaglandins* 1973;3:145–153.
78. Bygdeman M. The effect of different prostaglandins on the human myometrium *in vitro. Acta Physiol Scand* [*Suppl*] 1964;242:5.
79. Brummer HC. Interaction of E prostaglandins and syntocinon on the pregnant human myometrium. *J Obstet Gynaecol Br Commonwealth* 1971;78:305–309.
80. Green K, Bygdeman M, Toppozada M, Wiqvist N. The role of prostaglandin $F_{2\alpha}$ in human parturition. *Am J Obstet Gynecol* 1974;120:25–31.
81. Lewis RB, Schulman JD. Influence of acetylsalicylic acid, an inhibitor of prostaglandin synthesis, on the duration of human gestation and labour. *Lancet* 1973;i:1159–1161.
82. Wiqvist N, Kjellmer I, Thiringer K, Ivarsson E, Karlsson K. Treatment of premature labor by prostaglandin synthetase inhibitors. *Acta Biol Med Germ* 1978;37:923.
83. Dyer DC. Comparison of the constricting actions produced by serotonin and prostaglandins on isolated sheep umbilical arteries and veins. *Gynecol Invest* 1970;1:204–209.
84. Hillier K, Karim SMM. Effects of prostaglandins E_1, E_2, $F_{1\alpha}$, and $F_{2\alpha}$ on isolated human umbilical and placental blood vessels. *J Obstet Gynaecol Br Commonwealth* 1968;75:667–673.
85. Willman EA, Rodeck CH, Collins WP, Clayton SG. The relation between umbilical cord tissue prostaglandin E_2 levels, mode of onset of labour, fetal distress and method of delivery. *Br J Obstet Gynaecol* 1977;83:605–607.
86. Willman EA, Collins WP. The concentrations of prostaglandin E_2 and prostaglandin $F_{2\alpha}$ in tissues within the fetoplacental unit after spontaneous or induced labor. *Br J Obstet Gynaecol* 1976;83:786–789.
87. Novy MJ, Piasecki G, Jackson BT. Effect of prostaglandins E_2 and $F_{2\alpha}$ on umbilical blood flow and fetal hemodynamics. *Prostaglandins* 1974;5:543–555.
88. Tulenko TN. The actions of prostaglandins and cyclo-oxygenase

inhibition on the resistance vessels supplying the human fetal placenta. *Prostaglandins* 1981;21:1033–1043.

89. Howard RB, Hosokawa T, Maguire MH. Pressor and depressor actions of prostanoids in the intact human fetoplacental vascular bed. *Prostaglandins Leukotrienes Med* 1986;21:323–330.
90. Terragno NA, Terragno DA, Pacholczyk D, McGiff JC. Prostaglandins and the regulation of uterine blood flow in pregnancy. *Nature* 1974;249:57–58.
91. Glance DG, Elder MG, Myatt L. Prostaglandin production and stimulation by angiotensin II in the isolated perfused human placental cotyledon. *Am J Obstet Gynecol* 1985;151:387–391.
92. Bjoro K. Effects of angiotensin I and II and their interactions with some prostanoids in perfused human umbilical arteries. *Prostaglandins* 1985;30:989.
93. Mak KKW, Gude NM, Walters WAW, Boura ALA. Effects of vasoactive autacoids on the human umbilical-fetal placental vasculature. *Br J Obstet Gynaecol* 1984;91:99–106.
94. O'Brien PMS, Filshie GM, Pipkin FB. The effect of prostaglandin E_2 on the cardiovascular response to angiotensin II in pregnant rabbits. *Prostaglandins* 1977;13:171–181.
95. FitzGerald GA, Friedman LA, Miyamori I, O'Grady J, Lewis PJ. A double blind, placebo controlled, cross-over study of prostacyclin in man. *Life Sci* 1979;25:665–672.
96. de Moura RS. Effect of prostacyclin on the perfusion pressure and on the vasoconstrictor response of angiotensin II in the human isolated foetal placental circulation. *Br J Clin Pharmacol* 1987;23:765–768.
97. Landauer M, Phenetton TM, Parisi VM, Clark KE, Rankin JHG. Ovine placental vascular response to the local application of prostacyclin. *Am J Obstet Gynecol* 1985;151:460–464.
98. Jouppila P, Kirkinen P, Koivula A, Ylikorkala O. Failure of exogenous prostacyclin to change placental and fetal blood flow in preeclampsia. *Am J Obstet Gynecol* 1985;151:661–665.
99. Tuvemo T. Role of prostaglandins, prostacyclin, and thromboxanes in the control of the umbilical–placental circulation. *Seminars in Perinatology* 1980;4:91–95.
100. Broughton-Pipkin F, Morrison R, O'Brien PMS. Effects of prostacyclin on the pressor response to angiotensin II in human pregnancy. *Eur J Clin Invest* 1984;14:3.
101. Abdul-Karim R, Assali RS. Pressor response to angiotensin in pregnant and non-pregnant women. *Am J Obstet Gynecol* 1961;82:246–251.
102. Gant NF, Daley GL, Chand S, Whorley RJ, MacDonald PC. A study of angiotensin II pressor response throughout primigravid pregnancy. *J Clin Invest* 1973;52:2682–2689.
103. Bruce NW, Abdul-Karim RW. Mechanisms controlling maternal placental circulation. *Clin Obstet Gynecol* 1974;17:135–151.
104. Symonds EM, Broughton Pipkin F. Pregnancy hypertension, parity and the renin–angiotensin system. *Am J Obstet Gynecol* 1978;132:473–479.
105. Wilkes BM, Krim E, Mento PF. Evidence for a functional renin–angiotensin system in the full-term fetoplacental unit. *Am J Physiol* 1985;249:E366–E373.
106. Tuvemo T, Standberg K, Hamberg M. Contractile action of a stable prostaglandin endoperoxide analogue on the human umbilical artery. *Acta Physiol Scand* 1978;102:495–496.
107. Rocki W, Fitzgerald DJ, Entman SS, FitzGerald GA. Thromboxane A_2: a potent regulator of vascular tone in the human placental circulation. *Circulation* 1986;74(Suppl II):11–498.
108. Mento P, Hedberg A, Liu E, Hollander A, Wilkes B. Evidence for TxA_2 receptor sites linked to modulation of fetoplacental vascular resistance in the human placenta. *Clin Res* 1988;36:387A.
109. Sanchez-Ramos L, O'Sullivan MJ, Garrido-Calderon. Effect of low-dose aspirin on angiotensin II pressor response in human pregnancy. *Am J Obstet Gynecol* 1987;156:193–194.
110. Weiner C, Hdez M, Chestnut D, Wang JP, Herrig J. The interaction between serotonin and angiotensin II in the chronically instrumented guinea pig and its alteration by indomethacin. *Am J Obstet Gynecol* 1987;156:869–875.
111. Bunting SR, Gryglewski R, Moncada AS, Vane JR. Arterial walls generate from prostaglandin endoperoxides a substance (prostaglandin X) which relaxes strips of mesenteric and coeliac arteries and inhibits platelet aggregation. *Prostaglandins* 1976;12:897–913.
112. Wallenburg HCS, van Kessel PH. Platelet lifespan in normal pregnancy as determined by a nonradioisotopic technique. *Br J Obstet Gynaecol* 1978;85:33–36.
113. Inglis TCM, Stuart J, George AJ, Davies AJ. Haemostatic and rheological changes in normal pregnancy and pre-eclampsia. *Br J Haematol* 1982;50:461–465.
114. O'Brien WF, Saba HI, Knuppel RA, Scerbo JC, Cohen GR. Alterations in platelet concentration and aggregation in normal pregnancy and preeclampsia. *Am J Obstet Gynecol* 1986; 155:486–490.
115. Sims EAH, Krantz KE. Serial studies of renal function during pregnancy and the puerperium in normal women. *J Clin Invest* 1958;31:1764.
116. Pedersen EB, Christensen NJ, Christensen P, et al. Preeclampsia —a state of prostaglandin deficiency? Urinary prostaglandin excretion, the renin–aldosterone system, and circulating catecholamines in preeclampsia. *Hypertension* 1983;5:105–111.
117. Venuto RC, Donker AJM. Prostaglandin E_2, plasma renin activity, and renal function throughout rabbit pregnancy. *J Lab Clin Med* 1982;99:239–246.
118. Kaye Z, Zipser R, Hahn J, Zia P, Horton R. Is urinary flow rate a major regulator of prostaglandin E excretion in man? *Prostaglandins Med* 1980;4:303–309.
119. Oates JA, Whorton AR, Gerkens JF, Branch RA, Hollifield JW, Frolich JC. The participation of prostaglandins in the control of renin release. *Fed Proc* 1979;38:72–74.
120. Remuzzi G, Marchessi D, Capetta P, et al. Reduced umbilical and placental vascular prostacyclin in severe pre-eclampsia. *Prostaglandins* 1980;20:105–110.
121. Downing I, Shepherd GL, Lewis PJ. Kinetics of prostacyclin synthetase in umbilical artery microsomes from normal and pre-eclamptic pregnancies. *Br J Clin Pharmacol* 1982;13:195–198.
122. Dadak C, Kefalides A, Sinzinger H, Weber G. Reduced umbilical artery prostacyclin formation in complicated pregnancies. *Am J Obstet Gynecol* 1982;144:792–795.
123. Makila U-M, Viinikka L, Ylikorkala O. Evidence that prostacyclin deficiency is a specific feature in preeclampsia. *Am J Obstet Gynecol* 1984;148:772–774.
124. Walsh SW, Behr MJ, Allen NH. Placental prostacyclin production in normal and toxemic pregnancies. *Am J Obstet Gynecol* 1984;151:110–115.
125. Bussolino F, Benedetto C, Massobrio M, Camussi G. Maternal vascular prostacyclin activity in pre-eclampsia. *Lancet* 1980; ii:702.
126. Stuart MJ, Sunderjii SG, Yambo T, Clark DA, Allen JB, Elrad H, Slott JH. Decreased prostacyclin production: a characteristic of chronic placental insufficiency syndromes. *Lancet* 1981;i:1126–1128.
127. Demers LM, Gabbe SG. Placental prostaglandin levels in pre-eclampsia. *Am J Obstet Gynecol* 1976;126:137–139.
128. Hillier K, Smith MD. Prostaglandin E and F concentrations in placentae of normal, hypertensive and pre-eclamptic patients. *Br J Obstet Gynaecol* 1981;88:274–277.
129. Jarabak J, Watkins JD, Lindheimer M. In vitro activity of nicotinamide adenine dinucleotide- and nicotinamide adenine dinucleotide phosphate-linked 15-hydroxyprostaglandin dehydrogenases in placentas from normotensive and preeclamptic/eclamptic pregnancies. *J Clin Invest* 1987;80:936–940.
130. de Wolf F, Robertson WB, Brosens I. The ultrastructure of acute atherosis in hypertensive pregnancy. *Am J Obstet Gynecol* 1975;123:164–174.
131. Ongari MA, Ritter JM, Orchard MA, Waddell KA, Blair IA, Lewis PJ. Correlation of prostacyclin synthesis by human umbilical artery with status of essential fatty acid. *Am J Obstet Gynecol* 1984;149:455–460.
132. Holman R. Essential fatty acid deficiency: a long scaly tail. *Prog Chem Fats Other Lipids* 1968;9:279–348.
133. McKay DG, Goldenberg V, Kaunitz H, Csavossy I. Experimental eclampsia (an electron microscope study and review). *Arch Pathol* 1967;84:557–597.
134. Jogee M, Myatt L, Elder MG. Decreased prostacyclin production by placental cells in culture from pregnancies complicated by fetal growth retardation. *Br J Obstet Gynaecol* 1983;90:247–250.
135. Pipkin FB, Hunter JC, Turner SR, O'Brien PMS. The effect of prostaglandin E_1 upon the biochemical response to infused angiotensin II in human pregnancy. *Clin Sci* 1984;66:399–406.

136. McLaughlin MK, Brennan SC, Chez RA. Effects of indomethacin on sheep uteroplacental circulations and sensitivity to angiotensin II. *Am J Obstet Gynecol* 1978;132:430–435.
137. Everett RB, Whorley RJ, MacDonald PC, Gant NF. Effect of prostaglandin synthetase inhibitors on the pressor response to angiotensin II in human pregnancy. *J Clin Endocrinol Metab* 1978;46:1007–1010.
138. Glance DG, Elder MG, Myatt L. The actions of prostaglandins and their interactions with angiotensin II in the isolated perfused human placental cotyledon. *Br J Obstet Gynaecol* 1986;93:488–494.
139. O'Brien PMS, Broughton-Pipkin F. The effect of deprivation of prostaglandin precursors on vascular sensitivity of angiotensin II and on the kidney in the pregnant rabbit. *Br J Pharmacol* 1979;65:29–34.
140. Browne JCM, Veall N. The maternal placental blood flow in normotensive and hypertensive women. *J Obstet Gynaecol Br Commonwealth* 1953;60:141–145.
141. Kaar K, Jouppila P, Kuikka J, Luotola H, Toivanen J, Rekonen A. Intervillous blood flow in normal and complicated late pregnancy measured by means of an intravenous ^{133}Xe method. *Acta Obstet Gynecol Scand* 1980;59:7–10.
142. Kumar D. Chronic placental ischemia in relation to toxemia of pregnancy. *Am J Obstet Gynecol* 1985;151:987–999.
143. Cavanagh D, Rao PS, Knuppel RA, Desai U, Balis JU. Pregnancy-induced hypertension: development of a model in the pregnant primate (*Papio anubis*). *Am J Obstet Gynecol* 1962;84:1323–1324.
144. Glance DG, Elder MG, Bloxam DL, Myatt L. The effects of the components of the renin–angiotensin system on the isolated perfused human placental cotyledon. *Am J Obstet Gynecol* 1984;149:450–454.
145. Redman CWG, Bonnar J, Beilin L. Early platelet consumption in pre-eclampsia. *Br Med J* 1978;1:467–469.
146. Rakoczi I, Tallian F, Bagdany S, Gati I. Platelet life-span in normal pregnancy and pre-eclampsia as determined by a non-radioisotope technique. *Thromb Res* 1979;15:553–556.
147. McKay D. Chronic intravascular coagulation in normal pregnancy and preeclampsia. *Contrib Nephrol* 1981;25:108–119.
148. Socol ML, Weiner CP, Louis G, Rehnberg K, Rossi EC. Platelet activation in preeclampsia. *Am J Obstet Gynecol* 1985;151:494–497.
149. Wallenburg HC, Stolte LA, Janssens J. The pathogenesis of placental infarction. 1. A morphological study in the human placenta. *Am J Obstet Gynecol* 1973;116:835–840.
150. FitzGerald GA, Smith B, Pedersen AK, Brash AR. Prostacyclin biosynthesis is increased in patients with severe atherosclerosis and platelet activation. *N Engl J Med* 1984;310:1065–1068.
151. Fitzgerald DJ, Roy L, Catella C, FitzGerald GA. Platelet activation in unstable coronary disease. *N Engl J Med* 1986;315:983–989.
152. Reilly IAG, Roy L, FitzGerald GA. Biosynthesis of thromboxane in patients with systemic sclerosis. *Br Med J* 1986;292:1037–1039.
153. Wu KK, Chem YC, Fordham E, Ts'Ao CH, Rayudu G, Matayoshi D. Differential effects of two doses of aspirin on platelet-vessel wall interaction *in vivo*. *J Clin Invest* 1981;68:382–387.
154. Lindheimer MD, Motz AI. Hypertension and pregnancy. In: Genest J, Kuchel O, Hamet P, Cantin M, eds. *Hypertension*, 2nd edition. New York: McGraw-Hill, 1983;889.
155. Editorial. Genetics of preeclampsia. *Lancet* 1988;2:778.
156. Beaufils M, Densimons R, Uzan S, Colon JC. Prevention of pre-eclampsia by early antiplatelet therapy. *Lancet* 1985;1:840–842.
157. Reilly IAG, Doran JB, Smith B, FitzGerald GA. Increased thromboxane biosynthesis in human preparation of platelet activation: biochemical and functional consequences of selective inhibition of thromboxane synthase. *Circulation* 1986;73:1300–1309.
158. Fitzgerald DJ, Entman SS, Catella F, FitzGerald GA. Thromboxane (Tx) A_2 biosynthesis in normotensive and hypertensive pregnancies. In: *Proceedings of the 5th Congress of the International Society for the Study of Hypertension in Pregnancy*, Nottingham, England. 1986;84.
159. Fitzgerald DJ, Catella F, Rocki W, Entman SS, FitzGerald GA. Increased thromboxane A_2 biosynthesis in severe pregnancy-induced hypertension. *Clin Res* 1988;36:425A.
160. Bundy G. The synthesis of prostaglandin endoperoxide analogs. *Tetrahedron Lett* 1975;24:1957–1960.
161. Jones RI, Peesapati V, Wilson NH. Antagonism of the thromboxane-sensitive contractile systems of the rabbit aorta, dog saphenous vein and guinea-pig trachea. *Br J Pharmacol* 1982;76:423–428.
162. Hedberg A, Hall SE, Ogletree ML, Harris DH, Liu ECK. Characterization of [5,6-^{3}H]SQ29,548 as a high affinity radioligand, binding to thromboxane A_2/prostaglandin H_2-receptors in human platelets. *J Pharmacol Exp Ther* 1988;245:786–792.
163. Murray R, FitzGerald GA. Regulation of thromboxane receptor activation in human platelets. *Proc Natl Acad Sci USA* 1989;86:124–128.
164. Mais DE, Burch RM, Saussy DL, Kochel PJ, Halushka PV. Binding of a thromboxane A_2/prostaglandin H_2 receptor antagonist to washed human platelets. *J Pharmacol Exp Ther* 1985;235:729–734.
165. Thatcher CD, Keith JC. Pregnancy-induced hypertension: development of a model in the pregnant sheep. *Am J Obstet Gynecol* 1986;155:201–207.
166. Keith JC, Thatcher CD, Schaub RG. Beneficial effects of U-63,557A, a thromboxane synthetase inhibitor, in an ovine model of pregnancy-induced hypertension. *Am J Obstet Gynecol* 1987;157:199–203.
167. Fitzgerald DJ, Fragetta J, FitzGerald GA. Prostaglandin endoperoxides modulate the response to thromboxane synthase inhibition during coronary thrombosis. *J Clin Invest* 1988;82:1708–1713.
168. Wallenburg HCS, Dekker GA, Makovitz JW, Rotmans P. Low-dose aspirin prevents pregnancy-induced hypertension and pre-eclampsia in angiotensin-sensitive primigravidae. *Lancet* 1986;1:1–3.
169. Jaspers WJ, de Jang IA, Molder AW. Decrease of angiotensin sensitivity after bed rest and strongly sodium-restricted diet in pregnancy. *Am J Obstet Gynecol* 1983;145:792–796.
170. Lubbe WF, Liggins GC. Lupus anticoagulant and pregnancy. *Am J Obstet Gynecol* 1985;132:322–327.
171. Elder MG, deSwiet M, Robertson A, Elder MA, Flloyd E, Hawkins DF. Low-dose aspirin in pregnancy [Letter]. *Lancet* 1988;i:410.
172. Capetta P, Airoldi ML, Tasca A, Bertulessi C, Rossi E, Polvani F. Prevention of preeclampsia and placental insufficiency [Letter]. *Lancet* 1986;i:919.
173. Trudinger B, Cook C-M, Thompson R, Giles W, Connelly A. Low-dose aspirin improves fetal weight in umbilical placental insufficiency [Letter]. *Lancet* 1988;ii:214–215.
174. Stuart MJ, Cross SJ, Elrad H, Graeber JE. Effects of acetylsalicylic-acid ingestion on maternal and neonatal hemostasis. *N Engl J Med* 1982;307:909–912.
175. Heymann MA, Rudolph AM. Effects of salicylic acid on the ductus arteriosus and circulation in fetal lambs *in utero*. *Circ Res* 1976;38:418–423.
176. Silver MM, Freedom RM, Silver MD, Olley PM. The morphology of the human ductus arteriosus: a reappraisal of its structure and closure with special reference to prostaglandin E_1 therapy. *Hum Pathol* 1981;12:1123–1131.
177. Rumack CM, Guggenheim MA, Rumack BH, Peterson RG, Johnson ML, Braithwaite WR. Neonatal intracranial hemorrhage and maternal use of aspirin. *Obstet Gynecol* 1981;58:52–56.
178. Patrignani P, Filabozzi P, Patrono C. Selective cumulative inhibition of platelet thromboxane production by low-dose aspirin in healthy subjects. *J Clin Invest* 1982;69:1366–1372.
179. Rowland M, Riegelman S, Haris PA, Sholkoff SB. Absorption kinetics of aspirin in man following oral administration of an aqueous solution. *J Pharm Sci* 1982;61:379–385.
180. Pedersen AK, FitzGerald GA. Dose-related kinetics of aspirin. *N Engl J Med* 1984;311:1206–1211.
181. Cerletti C, Gambino MC, Garattini S, de Gaetano G. Biochemical selectivity of oral versus intravenous aspirin in rats. Inhibition

by oral aspirin of cyclooxygenase activity in platelets and presystemic but not systemic vessel. *J Clin Invest* 1986;78:323–326.
182. Ritter JM, Farquhar C, Rodin A, Thom MH. Low dose aspirin treatment in late pregnancy differentially inhibits cyclooxygenase in maternal platelets. *Prostaglandins* 1987;34:717–722.
183. Husslein P, Gitsch E, Pateisky N. Prostacyclin does not influence placental blood pool *in vivo. Gynecol Obstet Invest* 1985;19:78–81.
184. Kuhn DC, Stuart MJ. Cyclooxygenase inhibition reduces placental transfer: Reversal by carbacyclin. *Am J Obstet Gynecol* 1987;157:194–198.
185. England MJ, Atkinson PM, Sonnendecker EWW. Pregnancy induced hypertension: will treatment with dietary eicosapentaenoic acid be effective? *Med Hypotheses* 1987;24:179–186.
186. O'Brien PMS, Morrison R, Pipkin FB. The effect of dietary supplementation with linoleic and gammalinolenic acids on the pressor response to angiotensin II—a possible role in pregnancy-induced hypertension? *Br J Clin Pharmacol* 1985;19:335–342.
187. Olsen SF, Sorensen TIA, Secher NJ, Hansen HS, Jensen B, Sommer S, Knudsen LB. Intake of marine fat, rich in ($n - 3$)-polyunsaturated fatty acids, may increase birthweight by prolonging gestation. *Lancet* 1986;ii:367–369.
188. Knapp HR, FitzGerald GA. The hypotensive effects of fish oil: a controlled study in human essential hypertension. *N Engl J Med* 1989;in press.
189. FitzGerald GA. Prostaglandins and related compounds. In: Wyngaarden JS, Smith LH, eds. *Cecil Loeb textbook of medicine.* Philadelphia: WB Saunders, 1988;154–176.
190. FitzGerald GA. The clinical pharmacology of prostacyclin. In: Wu KK, Rossi E, eds. *Prostaglandins in clinical medicine: cardiovascular and thrombotic disorders.* Chicago: Year Book Medical Publishers, 1982;141–150.

Hypertension: Pathophysiology, Diagnosis, and Management, edited by J. H. Laragh and B. M. Brenner. Raven Press, Ltd., New York © 1990.

CHAPTER 112

Management of Hypertension During Pregnancy

William M. Barron, Michael B. Murphy, and Marshall D. Lindheimer

Blood Pressure in Normal Pregnancy, 1809
Measurement of Blood Pressure, 1809
Epidemiologic Studies, 1809
Classification of Hypertensive Disorders in Pregnancy, 1810
Preeclampsia–Eclampsia, 1811
Chronic Hypertension of Whatever Cause, 1811
Chronic Hypertension with Superimposed Preeclampsia, 1811
Late or Transient Hypertension, 1812
Pathophysiology of Preeclampsia, 1812
Cardiovascular Hemodynamics, 1812
Placental Perfusion, 1813
Renal Function, 1813
Coagulation, 1813
Eicosanoid Metabolism, 1813
Prevention of Preeclampsia, 1813
Management of the Hypertensive Gravida, 1814
Rationale for Treatment of Hypertension in Pregnancy, 1814
Preeclampsia–Eclampsia: General Approach, 1815
Drug Therapy of Acute Hypertension, 1816
Volume Expansion Therapy, 1818
Antieclamptic Therapy, 1819
Management of Chronic Hypertension, 1819
Summary and Conclusions, 1822
References, 1823

This chapter focuses on hypertension during gestation, a common clinical problem which remains one of the major causes of maternal and perinatal morbidity and mortality (1–4). As we shall see, treatment of elevated blood pressure in pregnant patients is controversial, reflecting, in part, our lack of understanding of both normal gestational cardiovascular physiology and the pathogenesis of a form of hypertension unique to pregnancy, namely, preeclampsia. This chapter, therefore, begins with a brief review of the course of normal blood pressure during gestation, followed by short descriptions of (a) the various hypertensive disorders which complicate pregnancy and (b) the pathophysiology of preeclampsia, since awareness of these issues underlies a rational approach to therapy. The majority of the chapter will then be devoted to the clinical management of hypertensive gravidas, wherein it will become apparent that many unique aspects of high blood pressure in pregnancy necessitate an approach which differs in many important ways from that employed in nonpregnant patients.

BLOOD PRESSURE IN NORMAL PREGNANCY

Measurement of Blood Pressure

Review of the literature relating to blood pressure in pregnancy reveals numerous methodologic difficulties. For example, investigators often neglect or fail to note if the blood pressure cuff is maintained at the level of the heart, especially when gravidas are studied in lateral recumbency (the posture of choice for many physiologic investigations during gestation). In addition, there is confusion concerning the recording of diastolic levels: Investigators in the United States focus on Korotkoff Phase V (5), while others use Korotkoff Phase IV (6–8). Use of the latter makes sense because, during pregnancy, sounds are often audible to very low levels. However, since Phase V remains the standard measurement in the United States, we recommend continued use of this value in order to avoid confusion; we utilize Phase IV only when the discrepancy between muffling and disappearance of sound becomes large.

Epidemiologic Studies

There are few adequate investigations of how gestation influences basal blood pressure (9,10). Initial measurements are usually not recorded until after the 8th gestational week, and determinations made 6 weeks post-partum are often equated with pre-pregnant values, an assumption which may be incorrect (11). In 1969, MacGillivray et al. (12) reported a meticulously performed prospective investigation of 226 primigravidae in whom blood pressure, measured with the London School of Hygiene random-zero sphygmomanometer, was noted to decrease early in pregnancy and to reach a nadir at 16–20 weeks, at which time the decrements in systolic and diastolic pressures averaged 9 and 17 mmHg, respectively. Thereafter, blood pressure increased gradually to values which, at term, approached those measured post-partum. In contrast, Christianson (13) observed maximal decrements at gestational week 22, with systolic and diastolic pressure decreasing only 5 and 6 mmHg, respectively; moreover, Wilson et al. (14) noted nadir values at 28 weeks, with diastolic levels falling approximately 12 mmHg while systolic pressures were only minimally changed.

Alterations in arterial pressure during pregnancy raise the question of whether the upper limits of normal differ from those in nongravid populations. In this regard, two large epidemiologic studies have demonstrated that even modest elevations in arterial pressure may be associated with impaired pregnancy outcome. Friedman and Neff (4), analyzing data from 38,636 women, observed that fetal mortality rose abruptly when diastolic blood pressure was greater than 84 mmHg at any stage of gestation (Fig. 1). In another large prospective study (14,833 singleton births), Page and Christianson (3) noted increases in perinatal mortality and intrauterine growth retardation when second and third trimester mean arterial pressures exceeded 90 and 95 mmHg, respectively. Together these reports establish that levels of blood pressure which would be considered entirely normal in nongravid individuals may have a significant adverse impact on pregnancy outcome, and therefore we consider diastolic levels of 75 mmHg in the second and 85 mmHg in the third trimester as the upper limit of normal.

Further analysis of data from these epidemiologic studies reveals that the cause of the hypertension appears to be much more important to perinatal outcome than is elevated blood pressure per se. For example, the appearance of elevated blood pressure alone late in pregnancy does not appear to adversely influence fetal outcome; however, the combination of significant proteinuria and hypertension, which suggests preeclampsia, is associated with increases in both intrauterine growth retardation and perinatal mortality (3,4).

CLASSIFICATION OF HYPERTENSIVE DISORDERS IN PREGNANCY

Students of gestational hypertension will readily perceive that the mere classification of these disorders is an area of concern and confusion. One finds a multitude of schemas, each utilizing different nomenclature; for example, pregnancy-induced hypertension, pregnancy-associated hypertension, gestosis, and toxemia are among the terms used to describe the disease discussed below as preeclampsia. This

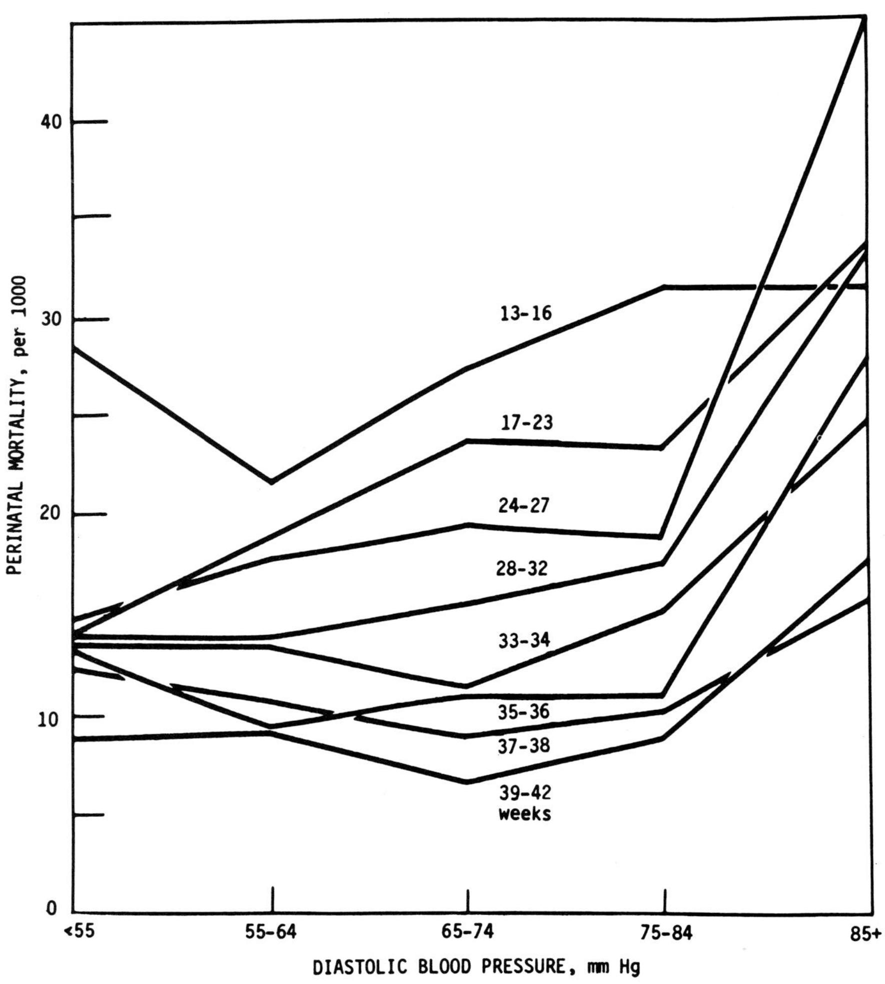

FIG. 1. Trends in perinatal mortality rates as a function of diastolic pressure for gestational ages 13 weeks to term. Note the significant increase in perinatal mortality associated with pressures exceeding 84 mmHg. (From ref. 4.)

confusion relates, in part, to the difficulty in distinguishing, by clinical criteria alone, between preeclampsia, essential or secondary hypertension, chronic renal disease, and combinations thereof. This dilemma has been convincingly demonstrated by the results of several clinical–pathologic correlation studies where renal biopsy was used to determine the definitive diagnosis. Fisher et al. (15) reported that the clinical diagnosis of preeclampsia was wrong in over 60% of multigravidas, and Katz et al. (16) failed to find renal histologic evidence of preeclampsia in 40% of gravidas with underlying renal disease who were given a clinical diagnosis of superimposed preeclampsia.

Of the numerous classifications in current use (8,17–19), we continue to prefer that suggested in 1972 by the Committee on Terminology of the American College of Obstetricians and Gynecologists (17), since it remains the most concise and practical:

1. Preeclampsia–eclampsia
2. Chronic hypertension of whatever cause
3. Chronic hypertension with superimposed preeclampsia–eclampsia
4. Transient or late hypertension

Preeclampsia–Eclampsia

Preeclampsia, a disorder specific to pregnancy, is characterized by hypertension, proteinuria, generalized edema, and, at times, coagulation or liver function abnormalities or both. It occurs in 5–10% of all pregnancies, primarily in primigravidas after the 20th gestational week and most frequently near term. Preeclampsia may progress rapidly without warning to the convulsive phase known as *eclampsia*—one of the most dramatic and life-threatening complications of pregnancy.

Hypertension is defined by most authorities as (a) a blood pressure of ≥140/90 (but we consider diastolic pressure >85 abnormal) or (b) increases in systolic and/or diastolic levels of ≥15 and 30 mmHg, respectively. The criterion of a rise in blood pressure is important, since an increase in diastolic pressure from 50 mmHg to 80 mmHg in a young primigravida may signal serious disease. On the other hand, use of such increments may lead to "overdiagnosis," since studies cited previously (12–14) suggest that diastolic blood pressure increases approximately 10 mmHg during the third trimester in normal gestation.

Although the Committee on Terminology did not require the presence of significant proteinuria for the clinical diagnosis of preeclampsia, the diagnosis is suspect in its absence (20). The third major traditional criterion, edema, is no longer used by many authorities (7,20), since up to 30% of normal gravidas may have generalized edema (21,22); furthermore, in the large epidemiologic survey of Friedman and Neff (4), neither edema nor maternal weight gain alone was associated with any adverse fetal outcome. The lack of utility of this sign is further underscored by a report in which 26 of 67 eclamptics had no edema (23).

Attempts have been made to distinguish "mild" from "severe" preeclampsia, with the latter being defined by systolic or diastolic pressures of 160 and 110 mmHg or greater, respectively, or by the presence of heavy proteinuria, oliguria, cerebral or visual disturbances, pulmonary edema, or cyanosis. Other evidence of severe disease includes epigastric pain, abnormal liver function tests, microangiopathic hemolytic anemia, and thrombocytopenia, the so-called HELLP syndrome (*h*emolysis, *e*levated *l*iver enzymes, *l*ow *p*latelets) (24,25). Another subtle sign of severe disease is marked hemoconcentration. It should be stressed, however, that *differentiating mild from severe preeclampsia may be dangerously misleading because although the risks of eclampsia are greater when markers of severity are present, as many as one-quarter of eclamptics have so-called "mild" disease and minimal elevations of blood pressure prior to convulsing* (9,23).

Chronic Hypertension of Whatever Cause

This diagnosis rests on the presence of hypertension prior to or following pregnancy. In addition, levels of ≥140/85 mmHg prior to the 20th gestational week may be taken as presumptive evidence of chronic hypertension, although preeclampsia may rarely present at this early stage, especially when gestation is complicated by hydatidiform mole or hydrops fetalis (9).

The vast majority of patients in this category will have mild to moderate, uncomplicated essential hypertension, and most will have a benign course during pregnancy (26), with blood pressures often falling well into the normal range during the second trimester (26,27). It is of note that such an exaggeration of the normal decrement in blood pressure may obscure the presence of chronic hypertension if the patient is seen for the first time in midtrimester. The subsequent, expected increase in blood pressure during the third trimester may then lead to an erroneous diagnosis of preeclampsia.

One factor which appears to predict a more complicated course in gravidas with chronic hypertension is a failure of blood pressure to decrease in midgestation. Poorer prognoses are also associated with certain secondary causes of hypertension, especially pheochromocytoma (28,29), scleroderma (30), periarteritis nodosa (31), and moderate or severe renal functional impairment antedating pregnancy (32,33).

Chronic Hypertension with Superimposed Preeclampsia

This category contains patients with the most severe disease, who often present in midgestation or in the early third trimester. It is in such cases that maternal complications (i.e., stroke, heart failure, or renal failure) are most likely and that fetal jeopardy is the greatest. It should be stressed, however, that the diagnosis of superimposed preeclampsia can be difficult and is often erroneous (16). The classical criteria are increments of 30 mmHg or more in systolic pressure and 15 mmHg or more in diastolic pressure, together with the development of proteinuria or generalized edema or both. More recently it has been suggested that abundant proteinuria (at least 3+) be present, since the blood pressure of many chronically hypertensive gravidas will increase substantially at the end of pregnancy in the absence of other evidence of preeclampsia.

The older literature suggests that preeclampsia is more common in gravidas with chronic hypertension; however, the variability of criteria used for diagnosis of the former makes interpretation of such reports difficult. Of interest is a study of 211 chronically hypertensive pregnant women in whom the incidence of preeclampsia was no different than that in the general obstetrical population (26).

Late or Transient Hypertension

This disorder is characterized by the development of hypertension alone during the latter stages of pregnancy or in the early puerperium, accompanied by the subsequent return to normal blood pressure within 10 days after delivery. This category will necessarily include several groups of women, including many nulliparas who may have had early preeclampsia but failed to manifest other evidence of the disease. Also included is a group of women who have hypertension in the absence of proteinuria during two or more pregnancies and who become normotensive shortly after delivery. Such recurrent hypertension appears to be a marker for the development of chronic hypertension (15,34) in much the same way that the development of gestational glucose intolerance predicts an increased risk for the occurrence of diabetes mellitus later in life.

PATHOPHYSIOLOGY OF PREECLAMPSIA

The pathophysiology of preeclampsia is detailed elsewhere (35) as well as in other chapters of this book, and this section will focus mainly on those aspects relevant to management. Hypertension in preeclampsia is extremely labile and may be associated with reversal of the normal circadian rhythm, in which case the highest blood pressures may be recorded at night (36,37). Additional characteristic features include the following: marked vasoconstriction, reflecting an increased vascular sensitivity to all pressor systems (angiotensin, catecholamines, and vasopressin); hemoconcentration; increased vascular permeability to macromolecules; decrements in placental and renal perfusion; and coagulation abnormalities ranging from subtle to severe.

Cardiovascular Hemodynamics

Studies using Swan–Ganz technology to measure central hemodynamics in hypertensive gravidas have yielded conflicting data because investigators have combined results from heterogeneous populations, often neglecting to distinguish between preeclampsia and chronic hypertension. In addition, measurements were often made after therapeutic interventions such as volume loading and magnesium sulfate administration. A major exception to these shortcomings is the studies of Wallenburg and colleagues (38,39), from which a clearer picture of the undisturbed hemodynamics of preeclampsia can be obtained. In their study of 44 untreated nulliparous preeclamptics, cardiac output was reduced, pulmonary capillary wedge and right atrial pressure were low normal, and systemic vascular resistance was markedly elevated (Fig. 2). Others have demonstrated that this intravascular volume contraction occurs prior to overt hypertension (40,41), an observation which may be due, in part, to increased vascular permeability (42). Thus, while blood volume decreases, the interstitial space expands and edema may occur. These perturbations in hemodynamics and volume regulation are important to keep in mind when

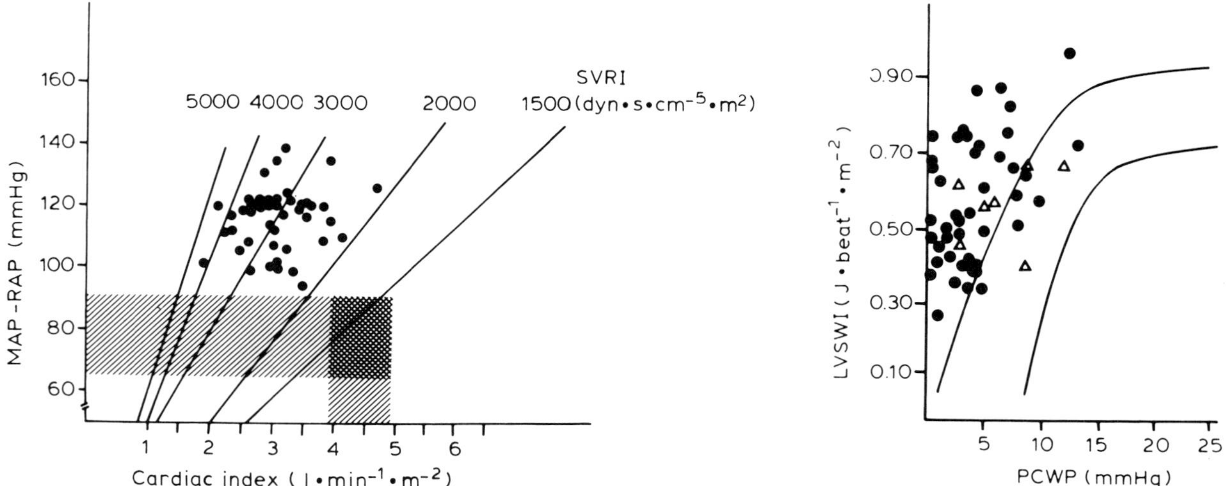

FIG. 2. Left: Relationship between systemic perfusion pressure, cardiac index, and systemic vascular resistance index in 44 untreated nulliparous preeclamptics. Values for normotensive pregnant women fall within the crosshatched area. Note that preeclamptic women have decreased cardiac output and increases in systemic arterial pressure due to markedly elevated peripheral vascular resistance. **Right:** Left ventricular stroke work index plotted against pulmonary capillary wedge pressure in these same 44 patients compared to data from seven normotensive controls (△). Solid lines represent the normal range in nonpregnant subjects. Note that left ventricular filling pressures are lower in the hypertensive gravidas. (Modified from ref. 38.)

one assesses ongoing controversies regarding the use of diuretics and/or sodium restriction on the one hand and volume expansion on the other (see below).

Placental Perfusion

In normal pregnancy, implantation of the embryo is followed by migration of trophoblastic cells into the walls of the uterine spiral arteries. These vessels thereby lose their muscular media and appear as passive conduits which serve to accommodate a 10-fold increase in uterine blood flow. This process fails to occur normally in preeclampsia and, in combination with later vascular lesions termed *acute atherosis*, leads to diminished placental blood flow which may, in turn, cause intrauterine growth retardation and fetal loss. Observations that such reductions in placental perfusion occur prior to the onset of clinical disease are supportive of the view that uteroplacental ischemia may cause the elevated blood pressure (as well as other manifestation of preeclampsia). If true, treatment of hypertension in this disorder might not be expected to prevent the disease or to halt its progression. Equally important, the influence of any therapeutic intervention on an already-compromised placental perfusion must be taken into account if fetal jeopardy is to be avoided.

Renal Function

Glomerular filtration rate (GFR) and renal plasma flow decrease in preeclampsia (35). These decrements may be due to vasoconstriction but also reflect glomerular capillary endothelial swelling. The combination of a reduced intravascular volume and an ischemic renal lesion may lead to reduced urine volumes. Oliguria, especially in acute clinical situations, often concerns the physician and has led some to recommend volume expansion. However, such a maneuver is rarely necessary, since acute renal failure is a very unusual complication of preeclampsia (43) (see section entitled "Volume Expansion Therapy," below).

Coagulation

Preeclampsia is associated with coagulation abnormalities, but controversy has existed as to how often this occurs and to what extent such perturbations contribute to the pathogenesis of the disease. It appears that standard tests of coagulation activity are normal in the majority of preeclamptic patients (44); however, a number of recent investigations employing more sensitive assays such as factor VIII-related antigen, antithrombin III, fibrinopeptide A, platelet survival, serum iron, and carboxyhemoglobin indicate that subtle abnormalities are typical features of even mild disease (45).

Eicosanoid Metabolism

One current theory suggests that decrements in vasodilatory prostaglandins (e.g., PGE_2, prostacyclin) and/or increases in vasoconstrictor products (e.g., thromboxane A_2, leukotrienes) may be causally related to much of the pathophysiology of preeclampsia, including (a) coagulation abnormalities, (b) increased vascular reactivity, (c) alterations in placental perfusion, and (d) injury in the kidneys, brain, and liver (46,47). The unifying aspect of this postulate is appealing, appears to be supported by a considerable body of data, and underlies increasing enthusiasm for the use of low-dose aspirin in the prevention of preeclampsia (see below).

PREVENTION OF PREECLAMPSIA

Several approaches to the prevention of preeclampsia have been proposed, including administration of diuretics, antihypertensives, low-dose aspirin, and calcium supplementation. Prophylactic administration of diuretics was actively investigated in the 1960s, based on the theory that sodium retention was etiologically related to the disorder. Collins et al. (48) recently analyzed nine prospective, randomized trials of diuretic therapy administered primarily for edema and/or rapid weight gain. When the data of all studies were combined, there appeared to be a significant reduction in the incidence of "preeclampsia" in the drug-treated group as compared to the control group. However, as noted by the authors, at least two major methodologic difficulties preclude a firm conclusion. First, the criteria used to establish the diagnosis of preeclampsia were varied, unreliable, and, in at least one series, not stated. Second, since diuretics can be expected to decrease blood pressure and reduce edema, such therapy may simply mask two of the diagnostic signs of preeclampsia without altering the presence of the underlying disease and its adverse impact.

Therefore, a more direct assessment of the potential benefit of diuretic therapy was performed. In the nine studies analyzed, rates of stillbirth and neonatal death were 1.9% in controls and 1.7% in diuretic-treated women, a nonsignificant difference (48). Further evaluation of potential adverse drug effects failed to reveal significant differences between treated and control groups, although careful laboratory evaluations were not performed in many studies. Of note, however, are several case reports of diuretic-induced neonatal thrombocytopenia and jaundice as well as maternal electrolyte imbalance and pancreatitis, including four fatal instances of the latter (49).

In summary, the above data fail to support a clear benefit for diuretics in the prevention of preeclampsia. In addition, although prospective trials fail to demonstrate a major adverse effect, there are rare reports of serious (and sometimes fatal) complications associated with such therapy. Thus, the balance of risk–benefit considerations contraindicates the use of prophylactic diuretic treatment during pregnancy.

Another approach is based on the premise that early treatment of hypertension may forestall appearance of other manifestations of preeclampsia. There is, however, little reason to believe this to be the case, since the placental, cerebral, renal, hepatic, and coagulation abnormalities of preeclampsia do not appear to be a direct consequence of elevated blood pressure. While one study (50) has demonstrated a reduced incidence of proteinuria in hypertensive gravidas treated with atenolol, this report has been criticized in part because of an excessive incidence of proteinuria in the control group. Furthermore, results of other studies fail to support this observation (51–53).

A more recent strategy for the prevention of preeclampsia involves the administration of low-dose aspirin. The premise is that small amounts of aspirin (30–60 mg/day) produce a greater inhibition of thromboxane production compared to that of prostacyclin in both pregnant women and their fetuses (54–56), thus preventing or reversing the vasodilator–vasoconstrictor eicosanoid imbalance which may underlie much of the pathophysiology of preeclampsia. In favor of this are observations by Crandon and Isherwood (57), who reported a reduced incidence of third-trimester hypertension in women with history of regular aspirin ingestion. Subsequently, low-dose aspirin (150 mg/day) in combination with dipyridamole (300 mg/day) was shown to reduce the incidence of preeclampsia and to improve perinatal outcome in women with clinical risks for intrauterine growth retardation and/or preeclampsia (58). Most recently, Wallenburg et al. (59) randomized 46 normotensive women who had enhanced pressor responsiveness to angiotensin II and who were thus judged to be at increased risk of developing preeclampsia; these subjects either received 60 mg of aspirin per day or were given placebo. The incidence of preeclampsia and cesarean section was significantly reduced in the treated gravidas, and, similar to results of others (58), no increase in maternal or neonatal hemorrhage was observed. In summary, these early results are most promising; moreover, if safety and efficacy are confirmed in several ongoing multicenter trials, the use of aspirin for the prevention of preeclampsia may become an important addition to standard prenatal care.

Finally, dietary calcium deficiency has been suggested to underlie hypertension in both nonpregnant and pregnant populations (60). In this regard, Taufield et al. (61) noted hypocalciuria in most women with pure and superimposed preeclampsia, while Kawasaki et al. (62) reported that 600 mg of calcium supplement per day enhanced pressor resistance to infused angiotensin II in 22 normal gravidas as compared to nonsupplemented controls chosen in a nonrandomized manner. In addition, two randomized trials have demonstrated small decrements in the blood pressure of healthy gravidas receiving calcium supplementation of 1–2 g/day; however, the incidence of pregnancy-induced hypertension was similar in control and supplemented groups (60). In contrast, in a recent preliminary report, Montanaro et al. (63) claimed that calcium supplementation reduces the occurrence of preeclampsia.

MANAGEMENT OF THE HYPERTENSIVE GRAVIDA

Rationale for Treatment of Hypertension in Pregnancy

The decision to treat elevated blood pressure during gestation is more complex and controversial than in nongravid patients. This is because of the relatively short duration of the problem and the need to consider a second patient, the fetus. In addition, the majority of data bearing on this issue come from nonrandomized, uncontrolled (often retrospective) observations of gravidas with various types of hypertension, an approach which serves only to add confusion to an already-difficult clinical problem (64). Current controversies in this area are underscored by an extraordinary divergence of opinion among physicians regarding the management of hypertension in pregnancy (65).

Maternal Considerations

In the pregnant patient, the major risks of severe hypertension are cardiac decompensation and cerebrovascular accidents. In contrast, the hazards of mild to moderately elevated blood pressures, over a period of several weeks to months, are less clear. Therefore, the rationale used to treat such levels of blood pressure in nonpregnant populations (i.e., prevention of vascular pathology, which requires years to develop) cannot reasonably be applied during gestation. Yet another consideration is that the treatment of mild to moderately elevated blood pressure during pregnancy may reduce the progression to severe hypertension and/or the need for hospitalization; there are some data to support this (50,66).

Fetal Considerations

Although fetal risks associated with even minimally elevated blood pressure during pregnancy appear clear (Fig. 1) (3,4), whether or not they can be altered by drug therapy remains to be established. In this regard, Fletcher and Bulpitt (67) have reviewed five randomized, controlled trials of drug therapy versus no treatment (50–52,68,69) for hypertension complicating pregnancy. Although four of the five failed to demonstrate a significant reduction in perinatal mortality, the pooled relative risk of fetal or neonatal loss for all five studies showed a significant benefit favoring treatment. Of note is that in the largest trial in which the reduction in perinatal mortality was the greatest (52), the improved outcome was due to a reduction in the incidence of midtrimester stillbirths, leading the authors to suggest that the mechanism of any potential benefit may be independent of a reduction in blood pressure per se (see discussion of methyldopa therapy, below).

Another potential positive effect of antihypertensive therapy is the prevention of premature delivery necessitated by severe maternal hypertension. Although early studies (52,68) suggested that this might be the case, gestational age at delivery in more recent trials was similar in treated and untreated subjects (50,51).

The above maternal and fetal benefits of antihypertensive treatment must be weighed carefully against possible adverse effects, both immediate and long-term, on the offspring. This area has been particularly poorly studied in large part because there are no standards for animal and/or human drug testing which include (a) effects of the agent on the fetus' ability to withstand hypoxic stress, (b) a thorough analysis of morphologic and physiologic variables in the

eclampsia (43). On the other hand, administration of large volumes of fluid appears to increase the risk of pulmonary (144,145) or cerebral edema (146), particularly in the immediate puerperium. These complications may be partially explained by (a) increased vascular permeability (42), (b) decrements in colloid oncotic pressure which are most marked post-partum and are aggravated by crystalloid administration (147,148), and (c) increases in central filling pressures following delivery (149). Therefore, our current recommendation is to minimize crystalloid infusions (75–125 ml/hr) in preeclamptic women during labor and following delivery until a diuresis is established. Finally, in the unusual preeclamptic patient in whom volume expansion is deemed essential, right heart catheterization should be considered as a guide to therapy, since central venous pressure measurements do not accurately reflect pulmonary capillary wedge pressures in hypertensive pregnant women (150).

Antieclamptic Therapy

The cause of seizures in pregnant women with eclampsia is unknown; however, there is a mistaken tendency to equate them with hypertensive encephalopathy. The fact that approximately 20% of gravidas have minimally elevated blood pressure shortly before convulsing is proof that control of blood pressure will not entirely prevent eclamptic convulsions. In the United States, parenteral magnesium sulfate is the drug of choice for both the prevention and treatment of eclampsia (86); and although prospective, randomized trials comparing this drug with other agents have not been reported, maternal mortality decreased dramatically following its introduction into clinical use (9). It should be emphasized that magnesium sulfate is not used as an antihypertensive agent, since blood pressure reductions following parenteral administration are modest and transient (151).

Use of magnesium sulfate in preeclampsia–eclampsia has been criticized as archaic and empiric. Nonetheless, the excellent results of Pritchard et al. (86) remain the standard against which other antieclamptic regimens must be judged. In their series of 245 cases of eclampsia, there was only a single maternal mortality, this being the consequence of administration of five times the recommended dose. Alternate anticonvulsant drugs such as diazepam, dilantin, or phenobarbital have been recommended (70), but there are few studies documenting the relative safety and efficacy of such agents. Indeed, available data suggest that neonatal depression is more common following maternal administration of diazepam than after magnesium sulfate (152,153).

The mechanism of action of magnesium remains enigmatic. Some believe its primary action lies at the myoneural junction blocking the peripheral motor responses to cerebral cortical dysfunction. However, Borges and Gucer (154) have reported that magnesium sulfate in doses mimicking those used clinically suppresses penicillin-induced seizures in several animal models, although these results have been criticized (155). Recently, evidence has been presented that magnesium stimulates prostacyclin synthesis *in vivo* (156) and *in vitro* (157), raising the possibility that a salutary effect on cerebral vasospasm and/or platelet aggregation may be responsible for its beneficial effects in the prevention and treatment of eclampsia.

Management of Chronic Hypertension (Table 3)

As noted previously, our general approach to the pregnant patient with uncomplicated chronic hypertension is to initiate drug therapy when diastolic blood pressures are >95 mmHg. If a woman with treated mild to moderate hypertension becomes pregnant, we make an attempt to stop all drugs because little is known about the teratogenicity of hypotensive agents. If continued drug therapy is deemed necessary, we prefer to replace current medication with methyldopa for reasons detailed below.

Central Adrenergic Inhibitors

Methyldopa has a long history of effective use in pregnancy and has been prospectively evaluated in randomized clinical trials (52,68), one of which included periodic evaluation of offspring to the age of 7 (158). The most complete is that of Redman et al. (52), which involved 242 gravidas with diastolic blood pressures 90–110 mmHg who were randomized to receive either methyldopa or no treatment. There were nine pregnancy losses in the control group, four of which were midtrimester stillbirths; there was only one fetal loss in the treated group. Based on these results, which were similar to those of a previous study by Leather et al. (68), the authors concluded that the benefits could not be attributed to the control of hypertension per se and suggested that some presently undefined action of methyldopa may have been responsible.

Although use of methyldopa as a single agent has been criticized on the basis of limited efficacy (70), several studies suggest otherwise. Redman et al. (66) reported that the frequency of severe hypertension occurring antenatally or in labor was significantly reduced by methyldopa treatment; additional reports have demonstrated that this drug is as effective as a beta-blocker (159–162) or clonidine (163) for hypertension during pregnancy.

The well-documented side-effect profile of methyldopa indicates that maternal adverse effects are generally mild and well tolerated (66). Rigorous assessment of the offspring in the study of Redman et al. (52,158,164,165) has provided reassuring data regarding the fetal and neonatal safety of this drug. Birthweights, neonatal complications, and progress in the first year of life were similar in methyldopa-treated and control groups (164,165); however, in one other uncontrolled investigation, neonatal tremors were associated with maternal ingestion of the drug (166). Studies in animals (167) have demonstrated that antenatal administration of methyldopa is associated with depletion of neonatal cardiac catecholamine levels, raising the possibility that the ability of the fetus or newborn to mount an adequate cardiovascular response to stress may be impaired; however, such observations have not been reported in humans.

TABLE 3. *Drug therapy of chronic hypertension in pregnancy*[a]

Drug	Dose	Adverse effects and comments
Agent of choice:		
Methyldopa	500–3000 mg in 2–4 divided doses	Safety for mother and fetus (after 1st trimester) is well documented.
Second-line agents:		
Hydralazine	50–300 mg in 2–4 divided doses	Few controlled trials but extensive experience with few serious adverse effects documented; several reports of neonatal thrombocytopenia.
Beta-adrenergic inhibitors (and the combined alpha–beta-blocker, labetalol)	Dependent on specific agent used	May cause fetal bradycardia and impair fetal responses to hypoxia. Risk of intrauterine growth retardation remains unclear.
Third-line agents:		
Thiazide diuretics	Dependent on agent used	Most controlled studies in normotensive gravidas; little data in hypertensive gestation. Implicated in volume depletion, electrolyte imbalance, pancreatitis, and thrombocytopenia.
Clonidine	0.1–0.8 mg in 2 divided doses	Limited data.
Nifedipine	30–120 mg in 3–4 divided doses	Limited data; may inhibit labor; potential for severe hypotension in patients receiving $MgSO_4$.
Prazosin	1–30 mg in 2–3 divided doses	Limited data.
Contraindicated:		
Angiotensin-converting-enzyme inhibitors	Dependent on agent used	High rates of fetal loss in animals. Several cases of neonatal anuric acute renal failure in humans.

[a] Note that safety during the first trimester has not been established for any antihypertensive agent.

Long-term follow-up of offspring whose mothers received methyldopa while pregnant also attests to the drug's safety. Among children of women who entered the above methyldopa trial between weeks 16 and 20, head circumference at 4 (168) and 7 (158) years of age was slightly but significantly less in the sons of methyldopa-treated women; however, mean intelligence quotients and performance on tests from the British Ability Scales were similar in the two groups of children.

Thus, because methyldopa has been extensively studied and has a well-documented record of safety, we believe it to be the agent of choice for the treatment of chronic hypertension during gestation.

Clonidine, another alpha-2 agonist, has been compared with methyldopa in a randomized, double-blind trial: There were no significant differences between the drugs in terms of efficacy or adverse effects (163). One long-term follow-up study comparing 22 children whose mothers had received clonidine during pregnancy with matched controls found no effect of the drug on head circumference, neurological development, or school performance; however, there was some excess sleep disturbance in the clonidine group (169). These observations led the authors to question whether this drug is a behavioral teratogen, thereby serving as a reminder that prenatal drug administration may have subtle, remote adverse effects. Animal studies have failed to identify teratogenic effects of clonidine; however, some embryotoxicity was observed at doses comparable to those used in humans (170).

Vasodilators

Hydralazine has been used in pregnancy, primarily as a parenteral agent in the therapy of acute, severe hypertension (see above). It has also been employed successfully in the chronic setting as a second-line agent in combination with either methyldopa or a beta-blocker (53,160,161,171, 172). In a small, prospective, randomized trial, Rosenfeld et al. (173) found hydralazine monotherapy to be as effective as hydralazine plus pindolol; however, a much higher incidence of palpitations, dizziness, and headache was observed in subjects not receiving a beta-blocker. Hydralazine appears reasonably safe for the fetus, although thrombocytopenia of uncertain etiology has been reported in a few infants whose mothers were treated with this drug (100). Furthermore, we are unaware of any long-term follow-up studies on children exposed to this drug *in utero.* Animal studies have shown hydralazine to be teratogenic in mice but not in rats (170). Our practice is to use oral hydralazine as a second-line agent in patients whose blood pressure is inadequately controlled on methyldopa.

Calcium Channel Blockers

The use of oral nifedipine for chronic hypertension during pregnancy has scarcely been reported (108,174); moreover, given the paucity of patients and the uncontrolled nature of the observations, its safety remains unclear. Furthermore, nifedipine has been shown to be teratogenic and embryotoxic when administered to rodents in amounts severalfold greater than the maximum recommended human dose (170).

Beta-Adrenergic Blockers

There have been numerous studies of beta-blockers in animal pregnancy, and their use in humans has been extensively reported (50,51,53,159–161,172,173,175–190); nonetheless, the safety and precise indication for use of these antihypertensives are still unclear. These agents cross the placenta (175,181,183,190,191), and studies in animals have suggested potential adverse maternal and fetal effects. For instance, decreased uteroplacental blood flow (192–194) and altered fetal cardiovascular responses to hypoxia (135,137,138) have been observed in sheep subjected to beta-adrenoreceptor blockade. Another, albeit theoretical, concern is that since beta-agonists have a relaxant effect on the myometrium, beta-blocking drugs might induce premature labor (192,193).

Initial reports of retrospective, uncontrolled observations associating maternal propranolol use with intrauterine growth retardation, neonatal respiratory depression, bradycardia, and hypoglycemia (175–177,179,180) were disturbing; however, more recent results of prospective randomized comparisons of atenolol (50) and metoprolol (51,53), each versus no drug therapy, failed to document significant adverse maternal or fetal effects of these drugs. Modest decreases in fetal and neonatal heart rates in drug-treated groups were reported (195,196); however, this did not appear to be associated with any significant morbidity. Further evidence of safety has been provided by a 1-year follow-up study which failed to find any adverse effect of *in utero* exposure to atenolol on later development (197).

Oxprenolol, a nonselective beta-blocker (currently unavailable in the United States) has been compared with methyldopa in two randomized trials (160,161). Control of hypertension as well as measures of perinatal outcome were comparable with the two drugs, although Fidler et al. (160) observed more intrapartum fetal bradycardia in women treated with oxprenolol. Also of note is the study of Gallery et al. (77,161) in which plasma volume and birthweight were significantly greater in oxprenolol-treated patients as compared to methyldopa-treated patients; however, this was not confirmed in a similar study by Fidler et al. (160).

Despite the above reassuring results of controlled trials (50,51,53,159–161,185), the data should be interpreted with caution. Each study was relatively small, and gestational age at entry was generally 29–33 weeks, leaving unanswered the possibility that treatment of larger numbers of patients and/or a longer duration of drug administration may reveal heretofore unrecognized adverse effects. In this regard, in a preliminary report (187) of a placebo-controlled trial in which atenolol was initiated for chronic hypertension between 12 and 24 weeks of pregnancy, a clinically significant reduction in infant and placental weights was observed in the drug-treated group. These data emphasize that the safety of beta-blockers in pregnancy has not been fully established, and therefore we use these agents only when blood pressure is not adequately controlled with methyldopa.

Labetalol, a beta-blocker with some alpha-adrenoreceptor-blocking activity, has been claimed to be superior to other agents in the treatment of hypertension in pregnancy (189,198); however, data from well-designed randomized trials do not support this view. Redman observed no difference in maternal side effects or pregnancy outcome in 74 gravidas treated with labetalol or methyldopa (199); moreover, in a study of 211 preeclamptics remote from term, Sibai et al. (200) found that labetalol treatment was associated with a higher incidence of intrauterine growth retardation when compared with no drug therapy. Thus, this agent requires further study before its use for chronic hypertension in pregnancy can be recommended.

Alpha-Adrenergic Blockers

Prazosin, an alpha-1-receptor antagonist, has been used in uncontrolled studies of chronic hypertension (201–203) and pheochromocytoma (204,205) complicating gestation. No specific untoward effects have been identified; however, given the limited data and the lack of benefit over other, better-studied agents, there is little reason to use this drug for hypertension during pregnancy.

The one clear indication for alpha-adrenoreceptor blockade during pregnancy is pheochromocytoma. Although rare, this tumor is associated with maternal and fetal mortality rates exceeding 50% when undiagnosed prior to delivery (28,29). For this reason, we recommend obtaining urine and/or plasma catecholamine levels in any gravida in whom there is any suspicion of a pheochromocytoma. Magnetic resonance imaging is the procedure of choice to visualize the tumor, since it spares the fetus from being exposed to ionizing radiation (206). Pharmacologic management is similar to that used in nonpregnant patients (i.e., alpha-blockade alone or in combination with beta-blockade), and failure to employ the former has been associated with a much worse pregnancy outcome (29). With regard to surgical management, most recommend a combined procedure of cesarean section followed by tumor resection when the disease is identified in the third trimester. Appropriate timing of surgical intervention for tumors identified in early gestation is less clear. The traditional approach is resection in the second trimester following adequate pharmacologic blockade; however, postponement of surgical treatment until the time of cesarean delivery may be accomplished in selected cases (206).

Angiotensin-Converting-Enzyme (ACE) Inhibitors

We are unaware of any controlled trials of the use of ACE inhibitors in human pregnancy; however, several reports of anuric renal failure in human neonates exposed to the drug *in utero* (207,208), combined with high rates of fetal wastage in animal studies (209,210), lead us to conclude that these drugs are contraindicated during gestation (even though some are listed by their manufacturer as risk category C).

Diuretics and Sodium Restriction

Although there have been many trials of the effect of prophylactic diuretic treatment in pregnancy (see section entitled "Prevention of Preeclampsia," above), there are few data concerning the use of these agents in established hypertension. In one study (211), preeclampsia actually became worse, with blood pressure rising in 11 of 24 gravidas on chlorothiazide. In another (212) study, gravidas receiving bendrofluazide plus a low-sodium diet lost an average of 3 kg, but blood pressure was unchanged, proteinuria increased, and plasma sodium decreased. More recently, Sibai et al. (213) randomized 20 gravidas with mild to moderate chronic hypertension who were taking diuretics to continue their medication or to stop treatment. Blood pressure in the two groups was similar at every stage of gestation; the addition of methyldopa was required in two of 10 subjects continued on diuretics and in one of 10 in whom the medication was stopped. Of potential importance was the observation that plasma volume expansion was considerably greater and more physiologic in the group whose diuretic therapy was stopped (+52%) than in the group whose treatment was continued (+18%).

The primary rationale for the use of diuretics in preeclampsia is that the disorder is associated with rapid weight gain, edema, and an expanded extracellular volume (9). However, the excessive sodium retention which accompanies preeclampsia is confined primarily to the interstitial space, since plasma volume and cardiac filling pressures are typically reduced (9,38). There is no evidence that diuretics favorably affect this fundamental volume disturbance or improve pregnancy outcome in preeclampsia. In addition, there are several reports of severe extracellular volume depletion, azotemia, and electrolyte disturbances in hypertensive gravidas treated with diuretics (212,214–217); placental perfusion may also be adversely affected (93,218). Maternal fatalities secondary to hemorrhagic pancreatitis (219), as well as neonatal thrombocytopenia and hemorrhage (220), have been associated with diuretic administration during gestation. Finally, these drugs commonly cause hyperuricemia, thereby obscuring an important diagnostic sign of preeclampsia.

Because diuretics have not yet been proved to be beneficial and may be associated with a number of adverse effects, we caution against their routine use in either preeclampsia or chronic hypertension during gestation. The only gravidas for whom we prescribe saliuretics unhesitatingly are those with pulmonary edema and/or left ventricular failure.

Dietary restriction of sodium in the management of preeclampsia was advocated more than 50 years ago, and, despite its abandonment by the majority of the obstetric community (19,49,78), some continue to recommend its use (70,221). Jaspers et al. (221) observed that the dose of angiotensin II required to increase diastolic pressure by 20 mmHg was increased (i.e., decreased pressor responsiveness) following severe sodium restriction in hypertensive and normal near-term gravidas; however, no effect on basal blood pressure or on course of the hypertension was reported. Mengert and Tacchi (222) randomized 48 consecutive patients with "toxemia" to either a 6–7-g/day or 0.5–1.0-g/day sodium diet and observed no difference in the clinical course of the two groups. Bower (223) reported similar results, observing no differences among a total of 243 preeclamptics treated with 2, 10, or 25 g of salt per day.

Sodium restriction during pregnancy has been associated with severe volume depletion, azotemia, and electrolyte disturbance (216,217,224). In view of such reports and the lack of documented benefit, we do not employ sodium restriction in the management of elevated blood pressure during gestation. If, however, a patient with chronic hypertension enters pregnancy on a moderately restricted sodium intake, we do not recommend alteration in dietary habits.

SUMMARY AND CONCLUSIONS

Hypertension during pregnancy affects ~10% of gravidas and remains a major cause of maternal and fetal morbidity and mortality. These adverse events, however, can be drastically reduced by vigilant and aggressive prenatal care, an approach which requires familiarity with (a) the normal cardiovascular alterations of gestation and (b) the pathophysiology of conditions causing hypertension in gestation. Importantly, diastolic blood pressure is ~10 mmHg lower than nonpregnant values through much of pregnancy; moreover, levels greater than 85 mmHg, which are associated with a poorer outcome, should be considered abnormal.

Diseases which cause hypertension during gestation may be similar to those of nonpregnant patients; in addition, there are two forms of hypertension peculiar to the gravid woman, namely, *preeclampsia* and *transient hypertension of pregnancy.* The former is the most serious of the common hypertensive complications and may present in an explosive manner, progressing rapidly to a convulsive stage termed *eclampsia,* even when blood pressure is only minimally elevated and few other warning signs are present.

There are many gaps in our knowledge of the pathophysiology of preeclampsia, but what is known does allow a rational approach to management. The disease is characterized by marked increases in peripheral vascular resistance, enhanced reactivity to vasopressors, and decreased intravascular volume. Accompanying disturbances include varying degrees of coagulation and/or liver function abnormalities as well as decreased renal and placental perfusion. An imbalance between vasoconstrictor and vasodilator eicosanoid synthesis may underlie many of these observations; in this respect, prophylactic use of low-dose aspirin has produced promising results in several preliminary studies.

Ambulatory treatment has little place in the management of preeclampsia, and patients suspected of having the disease should be hospitalized for further evaluation. In general, if preeclampsia or severe hypertension occurs beyond the 36th gestational week, delivery is the therapy of choice. When problems arise earlier, delivery may be delayed in selected patients with mild disease, but this must be done under strict supervision. Delivery is, however, indicated regardless of gestational age, if there is evidence of advanced disease (especially thrombocytopenia or abnormal liver function tests) or signs and/or symptoms of impending eclampsia, since temporization in such instances places both mother and fetus in considerable jeopardy.

For acute, severe hypertension in preeclampsia we recommend intravenous hydralazine and initiate treatment when diastolic pressure is ≥105 mmHg, aiming for gradual reduction to levels of 90–100 mmHg. Magnesium sulfate remains the treatment of choice to prevent eclamptic convulsions. We caution against the use of either volume expansion therapy (especially crystalloid) or potent diuretics.

The former increases the risk of pulmonary edema, and since preeclampsia is accompanied by reduced intravascular volume the latter approach may aggravate hemodynamic abnormalities. Furthermore, neither of these therapeutic modalities has been demonstrated to be of significant benefit when compared with more conventional therapy. Finally, central hemodynamic monitoring is only rarely required in the management of preeclampsia.

Drug therapy of chronic hypertension in pregnancy remains controversial. We tend to discontinue antihypertensives (including diuretics) in women with mild, uncomplicated hypertension who conceive, and we institute methyldopa if diastolic pressures exceed 95 mmHg. Oral hydralazine is used as a second-line agent; however, beta-blockers (i.e., atenolol) also appear safe when used in the third trimester (although they may cause fetal growth retardation when used over a more prolonged period). We rarely prescribe diuretics except when (a) blood pressure is difficult to control and (b) temporization is required for fetal reasons. We also do not recommend sodium-restricted diets. ACE inhibitors are contraindicated because they have been associated with serious fetal and neonatal complications, some of which have been fatal. Nonetheless, our philosophy concerning the treatment of poorly controlled hypertension is that the mother's well-being takes precedence over the fetus; when the above approach fails, we treat the patient as if she were not pregnant.

Finally, the practice of indiscriminate prescription of newer, inadequately studied antihypertensive medication to pregnant women is to be condemned. Instead, the physician should rely on those few drugs with a well-documented history of efficacy and safety, a philosophy which underlies the recommendations presented in this chapter.

REFERENCES

1. Sachs BP, Brown DAJ, Driscoll SG, et al. Maternal mortality in Massachusetts. *N Engl J Med* 1987;316:667–672.
2. Rochat RW, Koonin LM, Atrash HK, Jewett JF. Maternal mortality in the United States: report from the Maternal Mortality Collaborative. *Obstet Gynecol* 1988;72:91–97.
3. Page EW, Christianson R. The impact of mean arterial pressure in the middle trimester upon the outcome of pregnancy. *Am J Obstet Gynecol* 1976;125:740–746.
4. Friedman EA, Neff RK. *Pregnancy hypertension: a systematic evaluation of clinical diagnostic criteria.* Littleton, MA: PSG Publishing Co., 1977.
5. The 1988 report of the Joint National Committee on detection, evaluation, and treatment of high blood pressure. *Arch Intern Med* 1988;148:1023–1038.
6. Rubin PC. Hypertension in pregnancy: clinical features. In: Rubin PC, ed. *Hypertension in pregnancy.* New York: Elsevier, 1988;10–15.
7. Redman CWG. The definition of pre-eclampsia. In: Sharp F, Symonds EM, eds. *Hypertension in pregnancy: proceedings of the Sixteenth Study Group of the Royal College of Obstetricians and Gynaecologists.* Ithaca, NY: Perinatology Press, 1987;3–13.
8. Davey DA, MacGillivray I. The classification and definition of the hypertensive disorders of pregnancy. *Am J Obstet Gynecol* 1988;158:892–898.
9. Chesley LC. *Hypertensive disorders in pregnancy.* New York: Appleton-Century-Crofts, 1978.
10. De Swiet M. The cardiovascular system. In: Hytten F, Chamberlain G, eds. *Clinical physiology in obstetrics.* Oxford: Blackwell, 1980;3–42.
11. Walters BNJ, Thompson ME, Lee A, De Swiet M. Blood pressure in the puerperium. *Clin Sci* 1986;71:589–594.
12. MacGillivray M, Rose GA, Rowe B. Blood pressure survey in pregnancy. *Clin Sci* 1969;37:395–407.
13. Christianson RE. Studies on blood pressure during pregnancy. *Am J Obstet Gynecol* 1976;125:509–513.
14. Wilson M, Morganti AA, Zervoudakis I, et al. Blood pressure, the renin–aldosterone system and sex steroids throughout normal pregnancy. *Am J Med* 1980;68:97–104.
15. Fisher KA, Luger A, Spargo BH, Lindheimer MD. Hypertension in pregnancy: clinical–pathological correlations and remote prognosis. *Medicine* 1981;60:267–276.
16. Katz AI, Davison JM, Hayslett JP, Singson E, Lindheimer MD. Pregnancy in women with kidney disease. *Kidney Int* 1980;18:192–206.
17. Hughes EC. *Obstetric gynecologic terminology.* Philadelphia: Davis, 1972.
18. Nelson TR. A clinical study of pre-eclampsia. *J Obstet Gynaecol* 1955;62:48–57.
19. Management of preeclampsia. *Am Coll Obstet Gynecol Tech Bull* 1986;91:1–6.
20. Chesley LC. Diagnosis of preeclampsia [Editorial]. *Obstet Gynecol* 1985;65:423–425.
21. Thomson AM, Hytten FE, Billewicz WZ. The epidemiology of oedema during pregnancy. *J Obstet Gynaecol Br Commmonw* 1967;74:1–10.
22. Robertson EG. The natural history of oedema during pregnancy. *J Obstet Gynaecol Br Commmonw* 1971;78:520–529.
23. Sibai BM, McCubbin JH, Anderson GA, Lipshitz J, Dilts PV Jr. Eclampsia. I. Observations from 67 recent cases. *Obstet Gynecol* 1981;58:609–613.
24. Killam AP, Dillard SH Jr, Patton RC, Pederson PR. Pregnancy induced hypertension complicated by acute liver disease and disseminated intravascular coagulation. *Am J Obstet Gynecol* 1975;823–828.
25. Weinstein L. Syndrome of hemolysis, elevated liver enzymes, and low platelet count: a severe consequence of hypertension in pregnancy. *Am J Obstet Gynecol* 1982;142:159–167.
26. Sibai BM, Ardella TN, Anderson GD. Pregnancy outcome in 211 patients with mild chronic hypertension. *Obstet Gynecol* 1983;61:571–576.
27. Chesley LC, Annitto JE. Pregnancy in the patient with hypertensive disease. *Am J Obstet Gynecol* 1947;53:372–381.
28. Mulcahy D, O'Dwyer WF, Carmody M, Walsh A, O'Callaghan J, Garrett PJ. Phaeochromocytoma presenting in pregnancy. *Ir J Med Sci* 1984;153:389–391.
29. Burgess GE III. Alpha blockade and surgical intervention of pheochromocytoma in pregnancy. *Obstet Gynecol* 1979;53:266–270.
30. Ballou SP, Morley JJ, Kushner I. Pregnancy and systemic sclerosis. *Arthritis Rheum* 1984;27:295–298.
31. Burkett G, Richards R. Periarteritis nodosa and pregnancy. *Obstet Gynecol* 1982;59:252–254.
32. Hou SH, Grossman SD, Madias NE. Pregnancy in women with renal disease and moderate renal insufficiency. *Am J Med* 1985;78:185–193.
33. Lindheimer MD, Katz AI. Gestation in women with kidney disease: prognosis and management. *Clin Obstet Gynecol (Baillere's)* 1987;1:921–937.
34. Chesley LC. Hypertension in pregnancy: definitions, familial factor, and remote prognosis. *Kidney Int* 1980;18:234–240.
35. Lindheimer MD, Katz AI. Preeclampsia: pathophysiology, diagnosis and management. *Annu Rev Med* 1989;40:233–250.
36. Sawyer MM, Lipshitz J, Anderson GD, Dilts PV Jr, Halperin L. Diurnal and short-term variation of blood pressure: comparison of preeclamptic, chronic hypertensive, and normotensive patients. *Obstet Gynecol* 1981;58:291–296.
37. Redman CWG, Beilin LJ, Bonnar J. Variability of blood pressure in normal and abnormal pregnancy. In: Lindheimer MD, Katz AI, Zuspan FP, eds. *Hypertension in pregnancy.* New York: John Wiley & Sons, 1976;53–59.
38. Wallenburg HCS. Hemodynamics in hypertensive pregnancy. In: Rubin PC, ed. *Hypertension in pregnancy.* New York: Elsevier, 1988;66–101.

39. Groenendijk R, Trimbos JBMJ, Wallenburg HCS. Hemodynamic measurements in preeclampsia: preliminary observations. *Am J Obstet Gynecol* 1984;150:232–236.
40. Blekta M, Hlavaty V, Trnkova M, Bendl J, Bendova L, Chytil M. Volume of whole blood and absolute amount of serum proteins in the early stage of late toxemia of pregnancy. *Am J Obstet Gynecol* 1970;106:10–13.
41. Gallery EDM, Hunyor SN, Gyory AZ. Plasma volume contraction: a significant factor in both pregnancy-associated hypertension (preeclampsia) and chronic hypertension in pregnancy. *Q J Med* 1979;192:593–602.
42. Øian P, Maltau JM, Noddeland H, Fadnes HO. Transcapillary fluid balance in pre-eclampsia. *Br J Obstet Gynaecol* 1986;93:235–239.
43. Grünfeld J-P, Pertuiset N. Acute renal failure in pregnancy: 1987. *Am J Kidney Dis* 1987;IX:359–362.
44. Pritchard JA, Cunningham FG, Mason RA. Coagulation changes in eclampsia: their frequency and pathogenesis. *Am J Obstet Gynecol* 1976;124:855–864.
45. Weiner CP. Clotting alterations associated with the pre-eclampsia/eclampsia syndrome. In: Rubin PC, ed. *Hypertension in pregnancy.* New York: Elsevier, 1988;241–256.
46. Friedman SA. Preeclampsia: a review of the role of prostaglandins. *Obstet Gynecol* 1988;71:122–137.
47. Ferris TF. Prostanoids in normal and hypertensive pregnancy. In: Rubin PC, ed. *Hypertension in pregnancy.* New York: Elsevier, 1988;102–117.
48. Collins R, Yusuf S, Peto R. Overview of randomised trials of diuretics in pregnancy. *Br Med J* 1985;290:17–23.
49. Chesley LC. The control of hypertension in pregnancy. *Obstet Gynecol Annu* 1981;10:69–84.
50. Rubin PC, Butters L, Clark DM, et al. Placebo-controlled trial of atenolol in treatment of pregnancy-associated hypertension. *Lancet* 1983;1:431–434.
51. Wichman K, Ryden G, Karlberg B. A placebo controlled trial of metoprolol in the treatment of hypertension in pregnancy. *Scand J Clin Lab Invest* 1984;44(Suppl 169):90–95.
52. Redman CWG, Beilin LJ, Bonnar J, Ounsted MK. Fetal outcome in trial of antihypertensive treatment in pregnancy. *Lancet* 1976;2:753–756.
53. Hogstedt S, Lindeberg S, Axelsson O, et al. A prospective controlled trial of metoprolol-hydralazine treatment in hypertension during pregnancy. *Acta Obstet Gynecol Scand* 1985;64:505–510.
54. Ylikorkala O, Makila UM, Kaapa P, Viinikka L. Maternal ingestion of acetylsalicylic acid inhibits fetal and neonatal prostacyclin and thromboxane in humans. *Am J Obstet Gynecol* 1986;155:345–349.
55. Wallenburg HCS, Rotmans N. Prevention of recurrent idiopathic fetal growth retardation by low-dose aspirin and dipyridamole. *Am J Obstet Gynecol* 1987;157:1230–1235.
56. Spitz B, Magness RR, Cox SM, Brown CEL, Rosenfeld CR, Gant NF. "Low dose aspirin". I. Effect on angiotensin II pressor responses and blood prostaglandin concentrations in angiotensin II-sensitive pregnant women. *Am J Obstet Gynecol* 1988;159:1035–1043.
57. Crandon AJ, Isherwood DM. Effect of aspirin on incidence of pre-eclampsia. *Lancet* 1979;1:1356.
58. Beaufils M, Uzan S, Donsimoni R, Colau JC. Prevention of pre-eclampsia by early antiplatelet therapy. *Lancet* 1985;1:840–842.
59. Wallenburg HCS, Dekker GA, Makovitz JW, Rotmans P. Low-dose aspirin prevents pregnancy-induced hypertension and pre-eclampsia in angiotensin-sensitive primigravidae. *Lancet* 1986;1:1–3.
60. Belizan JM, Villar J, Repke J. The relationship between calcium intake and pregnancy-induced hypertension: up-to-date evidence. *Am J Obstet Gynecol* 1988;158:898–902.
61. Taufield PA, Ales KL, Resnick LM, Druzin ML, Gertner JM, Laragh JH. Hypocalciuria in preeclampsia. *N Engl J Med* 1987;316:715–718.
62. Kawasaki N, Matsui K, Ito M, et al. Effect of calcium supplementation on the vascular sensitivity to angiotension II in pregnant women. *Am J Obstet Gynecol* 1985;153:576–582.
63. Montanaro D, Bascutti G, Antonucci F, et al. Prevention of pregnancy-induced hypertension (PIH) and preeclampsia (PE) by oral calcium supplementation [Abstract]. *10th Int Congr Nephrol* 1987:291.
64. Chalmers TC. The clinical trial. *Milbank Mem Fund Q* 1981;59:324–339.
65. Lewis PJ, Bulpitt CJ, Zuspan FP. A comparison of current British and American practice in the management of hypertension in pregnancy. *J Obstet Gynaecol* 1980;1:78–82.
66. Redman CWG, Beilin LJ, Bonnar J. Treatment of hypertension in pregnancy with methyldopa: blood pressure control and side effects. *Br J Obstet Gynaecol* 1977;84:419–426.
67. Fletcher AE, Bulpitt CJ. A review of clinical trials in pregnancy hypertension. In: Rubin PC, ed. *Hypertension in pregnancy.* New York: Elsevier, 1988;186–201.
68. Leather HM, Baker P, Humphreys DM, Chadd MA. A controlled trial of hypotensive agents in hypertension in pregnancy. *Lancet* 1968;488–490.
69. Walker JJ, Crooks A, Erwin L, Calder AA. Labetalol in pregnancy-induced hypertension: fetal and maternal effects. In: Riley A, Symonds EM, eds. *The investigation of labetalol in the management of hypertension in pregnancy.* Amsterdam: Excerpta Medica, 1982;148–160.
70. Ferris TF. Toxemia and hypertension. In: Burrow GN, Ferris TF, eds. *Medical complications during pregnancy,* 3rd edition. Philadelphia: WB Saunders, 1988;1–33.
71. Briggs GG, Freeman RK, Yaffe SJ. *Drugs in pregnancy and lactation. A reference guide to fetal and neonatal risk,* 2nd edition. Baltimore: Williams & Wilkins, 1986.
72. Mallie JP, Coulon G, Billery C, Faucourt A, Morin JP. *In-utero* aminoglycoside induced nephrotoxicity in rat neonates. *Kidney Int* 1988;33:36–44.
73. Venuto RC, Cox JW, Stein JH, Ferris TF. The effect of changes in perfusion pressure on uteroplacental blood flow in the pregnant rabbit. *J Clin Invest* 1976;57:938–941.
74. Ladner C, Brinkman CR III, Weston P, Assali NS. Dynamics of uterine circulation in pregnant and nonpregnant sheep. *Am J Physiol* 1970;218:257–263.
75. De Swiet M, Hoffbrand BI. Effect of bethanidine on placental blood flow in conscious rabbits. *Am J Obstet Gynecol* 1971;111:374–378.
76. Greiss FC Jr. Uterine pressure-flow relationships. In: Moawad AH, Lindheimer MD, eds. *Uterine and placental blood flow.* New York: Masson, 1982;67–71.
77. Gallery EDM, Saunders DM, Hunyor SN, Györy AZ. Randomised comparison of methyldopa and oxprenolol for treatment of hypertension in pregnancy. *Br Med J* 1979;1:1591–1594.
78. Pritchard JA, MacDonald PC, Gant NF. *Williams obstetrics,* 17th edition. Norwalk, CT: Appleton-Century-Crofts, 1985.
79. Naden RP, Redman CWG. Antihypertensive drugs in pregnancy. *Clin Perinatol* 1985;12:521–538.
80. Gant NF Jr, Worley RJ. *Hypertension in pregnancy. Concepts and management.* New York: Appleton-Century-Crofts, 1980.
81. Whalley PJ, Everett RB, Gant NF, Cox K, MacDonald PC. Pressor responsiveness to angiotensin II in hospitalized primigravid women with pregnancy-induced hypertension. *Am J Obstet Gynecol* 1983;145:481–483.
82. Assali NS, Suyemoto R. The place of the hydrazinophthalazine and thiophanium compounds in the management of hypertensive complications of pregnancy. *Am J Obstet Gynecol* 1952;64:1021–1036.
83. Vink GJ, Moodley JH, Philpott RH. Effect of dihydralazine on the fetus in the treatment of maternal hypertension. *Obstet Gynecol* 1980;55:519–522.
84. Mabie WC, Gonzalez AR, Sibai BM, Amon E. A comparative trial of labetalol and hydralazine in the acute management of severe hypertension complicating pregnancy. *Obstet Gynecol* 1987;70:328–333.
85. Kuzniar J, Skret A, Piela A, Szmigiel Z, Zaczek T. Hemodynamic effects of intravenous hydralazine in pregnant women with severe hypertension. *Obstet Gynecol* 1985;66:453–458.
86. Pritchard JA, Cunningham FG, Pritchard SA. The Parkland Memorial Hospital protocol for treatment of eclampsia: evaluation of 245 cases. *Am J Obstet Gynecol* 1984;148:951–963.
87. Assali NS, Kaplan S, Oighenstein S, Suyemoto R. Hemodynamic effects of 1-hydrazinophthalazine (apresoline) in human preg-

nancy: results of intravenous administration. *J Clin Invest* 1953;32:922–930.
88. Lipshitz J, Ahokas RA, Reynolds SL. The effect of hydralazine on placental perfusion in the spontaneously hypertensive rat. *Am J Obstet Gynecol* 1987;156:356–359.
89. Ring G, Krames E, Shnider SM, Wallis KL, Levinson G. Comparison of nitroprusside and hydralazine in hypertensive pregnant ewes. *Obstet Gynecol* 1977;50:598–602.
90. Ladner CN, Weston PV, Brinkman CR III, Assali NS. Effects of hydralazine on uteroplacental and fetal circulations. *Am J Obstet Gynecol* 1970;108:375–381.
91. Suonio S, Saarikoski S, Tahvanainen K, Paakkonen A, Olkkonen H. Acute effects of dihydralazine mesylate, furosemide, and metoprolol on maternal hemodynamics in pregnancy-induced hypertension. *Am J Obstet Gynecol* 1986;155:122–125.
92. Jouppila P, Kirkinen P, Koivula A, Ylikorkala O. Effects of dihydralazine infusion on the fetoplacental blood flow and maternal prostanoids. *Obstet Gynecol* 1985;65:115–118.
93. Gant NF, Madden JD, Siiteri PK, MacDonald PC. The metabolic clearance rate of dehydroisoandrosterone sulfate. IV. Acute effects of induced hypertension, hypotension, and naturesis in normal and hypertensive pregnancies. *Am J Obstet Gynecol* 1976;124:143–148.
94. Lunell NO, Lewander R, Nylund L, Sarby B, Thornstrom S. Acute effect of dihydralazine on uteroplacental blood flow in hypertension during pregnancy. *Gynecol Obstet Invest* 1983;16:274–282.
95. Girard H, Brun J-L, Muffat-Joly M. An angiographic study of the sensitivity to epinephrine of the uterine arteries of the guinea pig: a comparison with angiotensin. *Am J Obstet Gynecol* 1971;111:687–691.
96. Wallenburg HCS, Hutchinson DL. A radioangiographic study of the effects of catecholamines on uteroplacental blood flow in the Rhesus monkey. *J Med Primatol* 1979;8:57–65.
97. Jansson T. Responsiveness to norepinephrine of the vessels supplying the placenta of growth-retarded fetuses. *Am J Obstet Gynecol* 1988;158:1233–1237.
98. Redman CWG. The management of hypertension in pregnancy. *Semin Nephrol* 1984;4:270–282.
99. Cotton DB, Gonik B, Dorman KF. Cardiovascular alterations in severe pregnancy-induced hypertension seen with an intravenously given hydralazine bolus. *Surg Gynecol Obstet* 1985;161: 240–244.
100. Widerlov E, Karlman I, Storsater J. Hydralazine-induced neonatal thrombocytopenia. *N Engl J Med* 1980;303:1235.
101. Brazy JE, Grimm JK, Little VA. Neonatal manifestations of severe maternal hypertension occurring before the thirty-sixth week of pregnancy. *J Pediatr* 1982;100:265–271.
102. Walters BNJ, Redman CWG. Treatment of severe pregnancy-associated hypertension with the calcium antagonist nifedipine. *Br J Obstet Gynaecol* 1984;91:330–336.
103. Rubin PC, Butters L, McCabe R. Nifedipine and platelets in preeclampsia. *Am J Hypertens* 1988;1:175–177.
104. Veille JC, Bissonnette JM, Hohimer AR. The effect of a calcium channel blocker (nifedipine) on uterine blood flow in the pregnant goat. *Am J Obstet Gynecol* 1986;154:1160–1163.
105. Harake B, Gilbert RD, Ashwal S, Power GG. Nifedipine: effects on fetal and maternal hemodynamics in pregnant sheep. *Am J Obstet Gynecol* 1987;157:1003–1008.
106. Read MD, Wellby DE. The use of a calcium antagonist (nifedipine) to suppress preterm labour. *Br J Obstet Gynaecol* 1986;93:933–937.
107. Golichowski AM, Hathaway DR, Fineberg N, Peleg D. Tocolytic and hemodynamic effects of nifedipine in the ewe. *Am J Obstet Gynecol* 1985;151:1134–1140.
108. Constantine G, Beevers DG, Reynolds AL, Luesley DM. Nifedipine as a second line antihypertensive drug in pregnancy. *Br J Obstet Gynaecol* 1987;94:1136–1142.
109. Iseri LT, French JH. Magnesium: nature's physiologic calcium. *Am Heart J* 1984;108:188–193.
110. Waisman GD, Mayorga LM, Camera MI, Vignolo CA, Martinotti A. Magnesium plus nifedipine: potentiation of hypotensive effect in preeclampsia? *Am J Obstet Gynecol* 1988;159:308–309.
111. Neuman J, Weiss B, Rabello Y, Cabal L, Freeman RK. Diazoxide for the acute control of severe hypertension complicating pregnancy: a pilot study. *Obstet Gynecol* 1979;53:50S–55S.
112. Morris JA, Arce JJ, Hamilton CJ, et al. The management of severe preeclampsia and eclampsia with intravenous diazoxide. *Obstet Gynecol* 1977;49:675–680.
113. Thien Th, Koene RAP, Schijf Ch, Pieters GFFM, Eskes TKAB, Wijdeveld PGAB. Infusion of diazoxide in severe hypertension during pregnancy. *Eur J Obstet Gynecol Reprod Biol* 1980;10:367–374.
114. Ram CV, Kaplan NM. Individual titration of diazoxide dosage in the treatment of severe hypertension. *Am J Cardiol* 1979;43:627–630.
115. Sankar D, Moodley J. Low-dose diazoxide in the emergency management of severe hypertension in pregnancy. *S Afr Med J* 1984;65:279–280.
116. Dudley DKL. Minibolus diazoxide in the management of severe hypertension in pregnancy. *Am J Obstet Gynecol* 1985;151:196–200.
117. Nuwayhid B, Brinkman CR III, Katchen B, Symchowicz S, Martinek H, Assali NS. Maternal and fetal hemodynamic effects of diazoxide. *Obstet Gynecol* 1975;46:197–203.
118. Caritis SN, Morishima HO, Stark RI, James LS. The effect of diazoxide on uterine blood flow in pregnant sheep. *Obstet Gynecol* 1976;48:464–468.
119. Wallenburg HCS, Kuijken JPJA. Effects of diazoxide on maternal and fetal circulations in normotensive and hypertensive pregnant sheep. *J Perinatal Med* 1984;12:85–95.
120. Landesman R, de Souza JA, Coutinho EM, Wilson KH, de Souza MB. The inhibitory effect of diazoxide in normal term labor. *Am J Obstet Gynecol* 1969;103:430–433.
121. Morishima HO, Caritis SN, Yeh MN, James LS. Prolonged infusion of diazoxide in the management of premature labor in the baboon. *Obstet Gynecol* 1976;48:203–207.
122. Boulos BM, Davis LE, Almond CH, Jackson RL. Placental transfer of diazoxide and its hazardous effect on the newborn. *J Clin Pharmacol* 1971;11:206–210.
123. Paull J. Clinical report of the use of sodium nitroprusside in severe preeclampsia [Abstract]. *Anaesth Intensive Care* 1975;III:72.
124. Stempel JE, O'Grady JP, Morton MJ, Johnson KA. Use of sodium nitroprusside in complications of gestational hypertension. *Obstet Gynecol* 1982;60:533–538.
125. Shoemaker CT, Meyers M. Sodium nitroprusside for control of severe hypertensive disease of pregnancy: a case report and discussion of potential toxicity. *Am J Obstet Gynecol* 1984;149: 171–173.
126. Naulty J, Cefalo RC, Lewis PE. Fetal toxicity of nitroprusside in the pregnant ewe. *Am J Obstet Gynecol* 1981;139:708–711.
127. Ellis SC, Wheeler AS, James FM III, et al. Fetal and maternal effects of sodium nitroprusside used to counteract hypertension in gravid ewes. *Am J Obstet Gynecol* 1982;143:766–770.
128. Lieb SM, Zugaib M, Nuwayhid B, et al. Nitroprusside-induced hemodynamic alterations in normotensive and hypertensive pregnant sheep. *Am J Obstet Gynecol* 1981;139:925–931.
129. Wheeler AS, James FM III, Meis PJ, et al. Effects of nitroglycerin and nitroprusside on the uterine vasculature of gravid ewes. *Anesthesiology* 1980;52:390–394.
130. Walker JJ, Greer I, Calder AA. Treatment of acute pregnancy-related hypertension: labetalol and hydralazine compared. *Postgrad Med J* 1983;59(Suppl 3):168–170.
131. Davey DA, Dommisse J, Garden A. Intravenous labetalol and intravenous dihydralazine in severe hypertension in pregnancy. In: Riley A, Symonds EM, eds. *The investigation of labetalol in the management of hypertension in pregnancy.* Amsterdam: Excerpta Medica, 1982;51–61.
132. Ashe RG, Moodley J, Richards AM, Philpott RH. Comparison of labetalol and dihydrallazine in hypertensive emergencies of pregnancy. *S Afr Med J* 1987;71:354–356.
133. Lunell NO, Nylund L, Lewander R, Sarby B. Acute effect of an antihypertensive drug, labetalol, on uteroplacental blood flow. *Br J Obstet Gynaecol* 1982;89:640–644.
134. Jouppila P, Kirkinen P, Koivula A, Ylikorkala O. Labetalol does not alter the placental and fetal blood flow or maternal prostanoids in pre-eclampsia. *Br J Obstet Gynaecol* 1986;93:543–547.

135. Joelsson I, Barton MD. The effect of blockade of the beta receptors of the sympathetic nervous system of the fetus. *Acta Obstet Gynecol Scand* 1969;48(Suppl 3):75–79.
136. Reuss ML, Parer JT, Harris JL, Krueger TR. Hemodynamic effects of alpha-adrenergic blockade during hypoxia in fetal sheep. *Am J Obstet Gynecol* 1982;142:410–415.
137. Cottle MKW, Van Petten GR, van Muyden P. Maternal and fetal cardiovascular indices during fetal hypoxia due to cord compression in chronically cannulated sheep. *Am J Obstet Gynecol* 1983;146:678–685.
138. Kjellmer I, Dagbjartsson A, Hrbek A, Karlsson K, Rosen KG. Maternal beta-adreneceptor blockade reduces fetal tolerance to asphyxia. *Acta Obstet Gynecol Scand* 1984;118(Suppl):75–80.
139. Sehgal NN, Hitt JR. Plasma volume expansion in the treatment of pre-eclampsia. *Am J Obstet Gynecol* 1980;138:165–168.
140. Gallery EDM, Delprado W, Gyory AZ. Antihypertensive effect of plasma volume expansion in pregnancy-associated hypertension. *Aust NZ J Med* 1981;11:20–24.
141. Gallery EDM, Mitchell MDM, Redman CWG. Fall in blood pressure in response to volume expansion in pregnancy-associated hypertension (pre-eclampsia): why does it occur? *J Hypertens* 1984;2:177–182.
142. Joyce JH III, Debnath KS, Baker EA. Preeclampsia—relationship of cvp & epidural analgesia. *Anesthesiology* 1979;510:S297.
143. Clark SL, Greenspoon JS, Aldahl D, Phelan JP. Severe preeclampsia with persistent oliguria: management of hemodynamic subsets. *Am J Obstet Gynecol* 1986;154:490–494.
144. Sibai BM, Mabie BC, Harvey CJ, Gonzalez AR. Pulmonary edema in severe preeclampsia–eclampsia: analysis of thirty-seven consecutive cases. *Am J Obstet Gynecol* 1987;156:1174–1179.
145. Benedetti TJ, Kates R, Williams V. Hemodynamic observations in severe preeclampsia complicated by pulmonary edema. *Am J Obstet Gynecol* 1985;152:330–334.
146. Benedetti TJ, Quilligan EJ. Cerebral edema in severe pregnancy-induced hypertension. *Am J Obstet Gynecol* 1980;137:860–862.
147. Zinaman M, Rubin J, Lindheimer MD. Serial plasma oncotic pressure levels and echoencephalography during and after delivery in severe pre-eclampsia. *Lancet* 1985;1:1245–1247.
148. Gonik B, Cotton D, Spillman T, Abouleish E, Zavisca F. Peripartum colloid osmotic pressure changes: effects of controlled fluid management. *Am J Obstet Gynecol* 1985;151:12–15.
149. Hankins GDV, Wendel GD Jr, Cunningham G, Leveno KJ. Longitudinal evaluation of hemodynamic changes in eclampsia. *Am J Obstet Gynecol* 1984;150:506–512.
150. Cotton DB, Gonik B, Dorman K, Harrist R. Cardiovascular alterations in severe pregnancy-induced hypertension: relationship of central venous pressure to pulmonary capillary wedge pressure. *Am J Obstet Gynecol* 1985;151:762–764.
151. Cotton DB, Gonik B, Dorman KF. Cardiovascular alterations in severe pregnancy-induced hypertension: acute effects of intravenous magnesium sulfate. *Am J Obstet Gynecol* 1984;148:162–165.
152. Cree JE, Meyer J, Hailey DM. Diazepam in labour: its metabolism and effect on the clinical condition and thermogenesis of the newborn. *Br Med J* 1973;251–255.
153. Stone SR, Pritchard JA. Effect of maternally administered magnesium sulfate on the neonate. *Obstet Gynecol* 1970;35:574–577.
154. Borges LF, Gucer G. Effect of magnesium on epileptic foci. *Epilepsia* 1978;19:81–91.
155. Koontz WL, Reid KH. Effect of parenteral magnesium sulfate on penicillin-induced seizure foci in anesthetized cats. *Am J Obstet Gynecol* 1985;153:96–99.
156. Watson KV, Moldow CF, Ogburn PL, Jacob HS. Magnesium sulfate: rationale for its use in preeclampsia. *Proc Natl Acad Sci USA* 1986;83:1075–1078.
157. Nadler JL, Goodson S, Rude RK. Evidence that prostacyclin mediates the vascular action of magnesium in humans. *Hypertension* 1987;9:379–383.
158. Cockburn J, Moar VA, Ounsted M, Redman CWG. Final report of study on hypertension during pregnancy: the effects of specific treatment on the growth and development of the children. *Lancet* 1982;2:647–649.
159. Livingstone I, Craswell PW, Bevan EB, Smith MT, Eadie MJ. Propranolol in pregnancy—three year prospective study. *Clin Exp Hypertens—Hypertens Pregnancy* 1983;B2:341–350.
160. Fidler J, Smith V, Fayers P, De Swiet M. Randomised controlled comparative study of methyldopa and oxprenolol in treatment of hypertension in pregnancy. *Br Med J* 1983;286:1927–1930.
161. Gallery EDM, Ross MR, Gyory AZ. Antihypertensive treatment in pregnancy: analysis of different responses to oxprenolol and methyldopa. *Br Med J* 1985;291:563–566.
162. Fidler J, Smith V, De Swiet M. A randomized study comparing timolol and methyldopa in hospital treatment of puerperal hypertension. *Br J Obstet Gynaecol* 1982;89:1031–1034.
163. Horvath JS, Phippard A, Korda A, Henderson-Smart DJ, Child A, Tiller DJ. Clonidine hydrochloride—a safe and effective antihypertensive agent in pregnancy. *Obstet Gynecol* 1985;66:634–638.
164. Mutch LMM, Moar VA, Ounsted MK, Redman CWG. Hypertension during pregnancy, with and without specific hypotensive treatment. II. The growth and development of the infant in the first year of life. *Early Hum Dev* 1977;1:59–67.
165. Mutch LMM, Moar VA, Ounsted MK, Redman CWG. Hypertension during pregnancy, with and without specific hypotensive treatment. I. Perinatal factors and neonatal morbidity. *Early Hum Dev* 1977;1:47–57.
166. Bodis J, Sulyok E, Ertl T, Varga L, Hartmann G, Csaba IF. Methyldopa in pregnancy hypertension and the newborn. *Lancet* 1982;2:498–499.
167. Hoskins EJ, Friedman WF. Influence of maternal alpha-methyldopa on sympathetic innervation in the newborn rabbit heart. *Am J Obstet Gynecol* 1980;137:496–498.
168. Ounsted MK, Moar VA, Good FJ, Redman CWG. Hypertension during pregnancy with and without specific treatment: the development of the children at the age of four years. *Br J Obstet Gynaecol* 1980;87:19–24.
169. Huisjes HJ, Hadders-Algra M, Touwen BCL. Is clonidine a behavioural teratogen in the human? *Early Hum Dev* 1986;14:43–48.
170. *Physicians' desk reference,* 42nd edition. Oradell, NJ: Medical Economics Co., 1988.
171. Sandstrom B. Adrenergic beta-receptor blockers in hypertension of pregnancy. *Clin Exp Hypertens—Hypertens Pregnancy* 1982;1:127–141.
172. Bott-Kanner G, Schweitzr A, Reisner SH, Joel-Cohen SJ, Rosenfeld JB. Propranolol and hydrallazine in the management of essential hypertension in pregnancy. *Br J Obstet Gynaecol* 1980;87:110–114.
173. Rosenfeld J, Bott-Kanner G, Boner G, et al. Treatment of hypertension during pregnancy with hydralazine monotherapy or with combined therapy with hydralazine and pindolol. *Eur J Obstet Gynecol Reprod Biol* 1986;22:197–204.
174. Ulmsten U. Treatment of normotensive and hypertensive patients with preterm labor using oral nifedipine, a calcium antagonist. *Arch Gynecol* 1984;236:69–72.
175. Cottrill CM, McAllister RG Jr, Gettes L, Noonan JA. Propranolol therapy during pregnancy, labor, and delivery: evidence for transplacental drug transfer and impaired neonatal drug disposition. *J Pediatr* 1977;91:812–814.
176. Gladstone GW, Hordof AL, Gersony WM. Propranolol administration during pregnancy: effects on the fetus. *Pediatrics* 1975;86:962–964.
177. Lieberman BA, Stirrat GM, Cohen SL, Beard RW, Pinker GD. The possible adverse effect of propranolol on the fetus in pregnancies complicated by severe hypertension. *Br J Obstet Gynaecol* 1978;85:678–683.
178. Eliahou HE, Silverberg DS, Reisin E, Romem I, Mashiach S, Serr DM. Propranolol for the treatment of hypertension in pregnancy. *Br J Obstet Gynaecol* 1978;85:431–436.
179. Habib A, McCarthy JS. Effects on the neonate of propranolol administered during pregnancy. *J Pediatr* 1977;91:808–811.
180. Pruyn SC, Phelan JP, Buchanan GC. Long-term propranolol therapy in pregnancy: maternal and fetal outcome. *Am J Obstet Gynecol* 1979;135:485–489.
181. Taylor EA, Turner P. Anti-hypertensive therapy with propranolol during pregnancy and lactation. *Postgrad Med J* 1981;57:427–430.
182. Tcherdakoff PH, Colliard M, Berrard E, Kreft C, Dupay A, Ber-

naille JM. Propranolol in hypertension during pregnancy. *Br Med J* 1978;2:670.
183. O'Hare MF, Murnaghan GA, Russell CJ, Leahey WJ, Varma MPS, McDevitt DG. Sotalol as a hypotensive agent in pregnancy. *Br J Obstet Gynaecol* 1980;87:814–820.
184. Dumez Y, Tchobroutsky C, Hornych H, Amiel-Tison C. Neonatal effects of maternal administration of acebutolol. *Br Med J* 1981;283:1077–1079.
185. Williams ER, Morrissey JR. A comparison of acebutolol with methyldopa in hypertensive pregnancy. *Pharmatherapeutica* 1983;3:487–491.
186. Sandstrom B. Antihypertensive treatment with the adrenergic beta-receptor blocker metoprolol during pregnancy. *Gynecol Obstet Invest* 1978;9:195–204.
187. Butters L, Kennedy S, Rubin P. Atenolol and fetal weight in chronic hypertension [Abstract]. *Int Soc Study Hypertens Pregnancy* 1988;265.
188. Rubin PC. Beta-blockers in pregnancy. *N Engl J Med* 1981;305:1323–1326.
189. Riley AJ. Clinical pharmacology of labetalol in pregnancy. *J Cardiovasc Pharmacol* 1981;3(Suppl 1):S53–S59.
190. Lardoux H, Gerard J, Blazquez G, Chouty F, Flouvat B. Hypertension in pregnancy: evaluation of two beta blockers atenolol and labetalol. *Eur Heart J* 1983;4(Suppl G):35–40.
191. Melander A, Niklasson B, Ingemarsson I, Liedholm H, Scherstein B, Sjoberg N-O. Transplacental passage of atenolol in man. *Eur J Clin Pharmacol* 1978;14:93–94.
192. Barden TP, Stander RW. Myometrial and cardiovascular effects of an adrenergic blocking drug in human pregnancy. *Am J Obstet Gynecol* 1968;101:91–99.
193. Mahon WA, Reid DWJ, Day RA. The in vivo effects of beta adrenergic stimulation and blockade on the human uterus at term. *J Pharmacol Exp Ther* 1967;156:178–185.
194. Harbert GM Jr, Spisso KR. Effect of adrenergic blockade on dynamics of the pregnant primate uterus (*Macaca mulatta*). *Am J Obstet Gynecol* 1981;139:767–780.
195. Rubin PC, Butters L, Clark D, et al. Obstetric aspects of the use in pregnancy-associated hypertension of the β-adrenoceptor antagonist atenolol. *Am J Obstet Gynecol* 1984;150:389–392.
196. Wichman K. Metoprolol in the treatment of mild to moderate hypertension in pregnancy—effects on fetal heart activity. *Clin Exp Hypertens—Hypertens Pregnancy* 1986;B5:195–202.
197. Reynolds B, Butters L, Evans J, Adams T, Rubin PC. First year of life after the use of atenolol in pregnancy associated hypertension. *Arch Dis Child* 1984;59:1061–1063.
198. Michael CA, Potter JM. A comparison of labetalol with other antihypertensive drugs in the treatment of hypertensive disease of pregnancy. In: Riley A, Symonds EM, eds. *The investigation of labetalol in the management of hypertension in pregnancy.* Amsterdam: Excerpta Medica, 1982;111–122.
199. Redman CWG. A controlled trial of the treatment of hypertension in pregnancy: labetalol compared with methyldopa. In: Riley A, Symonds EM, eds. *The investigation of labetalol in the management of hypertension in pregnancy.* Amsterdam: Excerpta Medica, 1982;101–110.
200. Sibai BM, Gonzalez AR, Mabie WC, Moretti M. A comparison of labetalol plus hospitalization versus hospitalization alone in the management of preeclampsia remote from term. *Obstet Gynecol* 1987;70:323–327.
201. Lubbe WF, Hodge JV. Combined α- and β-adrenoceptor antagonism with prazosin and oxprenolol in control of severe hypertension in pregnancy. *NZ Med J* 1981;94:169–172.
202. Dommisse J, Davey DA, Roos PJ. Prazosin and oxprenolol therapy in pregnancy hypertension. *S Afr Med J* 1983;64:231–233.
203. Rubin PC, Butters L, Low RA, Reid JL. Clinical pharmacological studies with prazosin during pregnancy complicated by hypertension. *Br J Clin Pharmacol* 1983;16:543–547.
204. Devoe LD, O'Dell BE, Castillo RA, Hadi HA, Searle N. Metastatic pheochromocytoma in pregnancy and fetal biophysical assessment after maternal administration of alpha-adrenergic, beta-adrenergic, and dopamine antagonist. *Obstet Gynecol* 1986;68(Suppl):15S–18S.
205. Venuto R, Burstein P, Schneider R. Pheochromocytoma: antepartum diagnosis and management with tumor resection in the puerperium. *Am J Obstet Gynecol* 1984;150:431–432.
206. Greenberg M, Moawad AH, Wieties BM, et al. Extraadrenal pheochromocytoma: detection during pregnancy using MR imaging. *Radiology* 1986;161:475–476.
207. Schubiger G, Flury G, Nussberger J. Enalapril for pregnancy-induced hypertension: acute renal failure in a neonate. *Ann Intern Med* 1988;108:215–216.
208. Rosa FW, Bosco LA, Graham CF, Milstein JB, Dreis M, Creamer J. Neonatal anuria with maternal angiotensin converting enzyme inhibition. *Obstet Gynecol* 1989, in press.
209. Broughton-Pipkin F, Symonds EM, Turner SR. The effect of captopril (SQ14,225) upon mother and fetus in the chronically cannulated ewe and in the pregnant rabbit. *J Physiol* 1982;323:415–422.
210. Ferris TF, Weir EK. Effect of captopril on uterine blood flow and prostaglandin E synthesis in the pregnant rabbit. *J Clin Invest* 1983;71:809–815.
211. Salerno LJ, Stone ML, Ditchik P. A clinical evaluation of chlorothiazide in the prevention and treatment of toxemia of pregnancy. *Obstet Gynecol* 1959;14:188–192.
212. MacGillivray I, Hytten FE, Taggart N, Buchanan TJ. The effect of a sodium diuretic on total exchangeable sodium and total body water in pre-eclamptic toxaemia. *J Obstet Gynaecol Br Commmonw* 1962;69:458–462.
213. Sibai BM, Grossman RA, Grossman HG. Effects of diuretics on plasma volume in pregnancies with long-term hypertension. *Am J Obstet Gynecol* 1984;150:831–835.
214. Miller JN Jr. Hyponatremia: a complication of the treatment of the edema of pregnancy. *Obstet Gynecol* 1960;16:587–590.
215. Pritchard JA, Walley PJ. Severe hypokalemia due to prolonged administration of chlorothiazide during pregnancy. *Am J Obstet Gynecol* 1961;81:1241–1244.
216. Mule JG, Tatum HJ, Sawyer RE. "Nitrogenous retention" in patients with toxemia of pregnancy—an unusual complication of salt restriction. *Am J Obstet Gynecol* 1957;74:526–537.
217. Palomaki JF, Lindheimer MD. Sodium depletion simulating deterioration in a toxemia pregnancy. *N Engl J Med* 1970;282:88–89.
218. Gant NF, Madden JD, Siiteri PK, MacDonald PC. The metabolic clearance rate of dehydroisoandrosterone sulfate. III. The effect of thiazide diuretics in normal and future preeclamptic pregnancies. *Am J Obstet Gynecol* 1975;123:159–163.
219. Minkowitz S, Soloway HB, Hall JE, Yermakov V. Fatal hemorrhagic pancreatitis following chlorothiazide administration in pregnancy. *Obstet Gynecol* 1964;24:337–342.
220. Rodriquez SUI, Leikin SL, Hiller MC. Neonatal thrombocytopenia associated with ante-partum administration of thiazide drugs. *N Engl J Med* 1964;270:881–884.
221. Jaspers WJM, deJong PA, Mulder AW. Decrease of angiotensin sensitivity after bed rest and strongly sodium-restricted diet in pregnancy. *Am J Obstet Gynecol* 1983;145:792–796.
222. Mengert WF, Tacchi DA. Pregnancy toxemia and sodium chloride. *Am J Obstet Gynecol* 1961;81:601–605.
223. Bower D. The influence of dietary salt intake on pre-eclampsia. *J Obstet Gynaecol Br Commmonw* 1964;71:123–125.
224. Schewitz LJ. Hypertension and renal disease in pregnancy. *Med Clin North Am* 1971;55:47–69.

Hypertension: Pathophysiology, Diagnosis, and Management, edited by J. H. Laragh and B. M. Brenner. Raven Press, Ltd., New York © 1990.

CHAPTER 113

Cyclosporine-Induced Hypertension

John J. Curtis

Clinical Complication of Hypertension, 1829
Cyclosporine Vasoconstriction, 1830
Possible Nonrenal Mechanisms, 1830
Cyclosporine Nephrotoxicity, 1831
Mechanisms of Nephrotoxicity, 1831
Clinical Investigations of Cyclosporine-Associated Hypertension, 1832
Antihypertensive Therapy, 1833
Summary, 1833
References, 1833

Cyclosporine is an immunosuppressant agent in widespread clinical use in the United States; since 1984 it has gained "first drug of choice" status in solid-organ transplant centers. Cyclosporine, unlike many of the previously used immunosuppressive agents, is not myelosuppressive (1). Furthermore, its mechanism of action involves the interleukin-mediated system of communication between T lymphocytes and is reversible (2). It is, therefore, a more specific form of immunosuppression than were the previously employed agents. Despite more powerful immunosuppression against allograft rejection episodes, opportunistic infections appear not to be increased (3). Before release for human use, the drug was found to be remarkably safe in animals (4). Most studies in rats, even when extremely high doses are given, have been associated with hypotension rather than hypertension (5).

CLINICAL COMPLICATION OF HYPERTENSION

It is thus surprising that, in humans, cyclosporine was quickly identified to have major undesirable effects (6). In humans, cyclosporine causes both nephrotoxicity and hypertension (along with numerous other side effects). Cyclosporine-induced hypertension is a new form of drug-induced hypertension that has not yet been fully investigated. It has been suggested that the nephrotoxicity and hypertension may not be mediated via the same mechanism. Since neither mechanism is understood, however, it may be premature to suggest that they are either identical or independent in mechanism.

The hypertension associated with cyclosporine occurs both in organ transplant recipients and in individuals who have not received organ transplants but have been prescribed cyclosporine for other conditions in which immunosuppression is felt to be indicated (7,8). It appears that the hypertension associated with cyclosporine is dose dependent; however, not all patients given cyclosporine develop hypertension, and some patients whose blood levels are clearly in the toxic range remain normotensive.

While, by far, the greatest number of patients exposed to cyclosporine are recipients of kidney transplants, centers that perform cardiac and bone marrow transplants were among the first to document the serious side effect of hypertension. Kidney transplant recipients have always had an extremely high rate of hypertension, even before the widespread use of cyclosporine. Most reviews of the subject of hypertension in kidney transplant recipients were performed prior to cyclosporine use (pre-1983) and suggest that at least 50% of kidney transplant patients were hypertensive 1 year after successful transplantation (9).

Controlled trials of cyclosporine (as compared to trials using "standard immunosuppression," namely, azathioprine and prednisone) carried out in Canada and Europe did not clearly identify hypertension as being markedly increased in the cyclosporine-treated groups. These two large, randomized, controlled trials are in modest disagreement: The European trial found the standard therapy group to "require" antihypertensive medications at a rate of 66% as compared to only 45% in the cyclosporine group. The Canadian trial, on the other hand, reported that "hypertension occurred" in 41% of the cyclosporine group and in only 30% of the standard group. Two of the cyclosporine-treated patients in the Canadian trial developed malignant hypertension associated with seizures, whereas none did in the control group. To be fair, neither of these large multicenter studies was primarily designed to look at the incidence or severity of hypertension but rather at graft survival (which was clearly improved in both studies in the cyclosporine-treated patients). Jarowenko et al. (10) reported on 200 concurrent (not randomized) kidney transplant recipients who were treated with cyclosporine and prednisone ($n = 150$) or azathioprine and prednisone ($n = 50$). By 12 months, 63% of the cyclosporine group was hypertensive, as opposed to 42% of the azathioprine group ($p < 0.05$). The authors believed the hypertension was more difficult to treat in the cyclosporine group. Hamilton et al. (11), in a retrospective chart review, reported an incidence of hypertension of 67% for cyclosporine-treated patients compared to 46% for azathioprine-treated renal transplant patients. Both Chapman et al. (12) and Curtis et al. (13) have reported that conversion of renal transplant patients on cyclosporine to azathioprine results in significant decreases in blood pressure. In these studies the patients served as their own control groups. The study by Chapman et al. also had a randomized control group of patients on azathioprine throughout the entire study period and could be another control comparison group to eliminate the effect of time elapsed after conversion on blood pressure. These studies, in aggregate, suggest that use of cyclosporine is associated with an increased rate of hypertension in kidney transplant patients, but it is of interest that other solid-organ transplant experience came to this conclusion quicker and with less need of such rigorous studies.

Historically, unlike kidney transplant patients, cardiac transplant patients did not have a high rate of hypertension after transplantation when azathioprine and prednisone were standard immunosuppression. Thus, conversion to widespread use of cyclosporine, along with the simultaneous onset of the nearly universal complication of hypertension in these cardiac transplant recipients, was a more dramatic change for these centers than for the kidney transplant centers. The heart transplant group at Stanford (14) reported a retrospective analysis of the first 109 patients in whom cyclosporine was employed as compared to a control group of 65 patients in whom azathioprine was used. The average systolic and diastolic blood pressure for the control group (azathioprine) was 115/80 mmHg, whereas it was 137/95 mmHg for the cyclosporine group (both at 1 year from transplantation). Moreover, with longer follow-up the cyclosporine group increased their blood pressure while the control remained stable. Hakim et al. (15) reported an 88% incidence of cyclosporine-associated hypertension in cardiac transplant recipients in England. Thompson et al. (16) made a comparison between (a) 18 cardiac transplant patients treated with cyclosporine and (b) 12 azathioprine (control group) cardiac transplant patients; their study revealed (a) nearly universal hypertension in the cyclosporine group and (b) normal pressures in the control group. Indeed, the hypertension seen in cardiac, bone marrow, and liver transplant programs has been described as more severe than that usually described by kidney transplant groups. These groups have reported very-difficult-to-control blood pressure along with malignant forms of pressure elevation (17).

Although all groups that use cyclosporine are impressed that the drug induces hypertension, at least two suggestions as to the seemingly different descriptions reported by kidney transplant programs and other organ transplant programs are the following: (a) Kidney transplant programs generally use a lower total exposure to cyclosporine because such patients have a much safer "fall-back position" (dialysis) if they reject their allografts as a result of a lack of adequate immunosuppression. This "fall-back position" allows those who manage such patients the option of reduced dosage of immunosuppression. (b) Unlike the other forms of solid-organ transplantation, kidney transplant patients have denervated renal tissue. It is possible that denervation of the kidney mitigates the hypertension induced by cyclosporine. On the other hand, since hypertension had been so prevalent in kidney transplant clinics before the advent of cyclosporine, it is possible that the complication received more emphasis among other groups of transplant physicians because it was new.

CYCLOSPORINE VASOCONSTRICTION

The evidence that cyclosporine decreases renal blood flow despite increasing mean arterial pressure—increased renal vascular resistance—is strong. Murray et al. (5) were the first to demonstrate this effect in rats, whereas Curtis et al. (13) demonstrated increased renal vascular resistance in humans. The most graphic demonstration of cyclosporine-induced changes in renal vascular diameter was reported by English et al. (18), using photographs of renal microcirculation with and without cyclosporine. Since increases in renal vascular resistance are characteristic of most hypertensive states (19), and this change in renal hemodynamics can be induced quickly by cyclosporine, it has been suggested that cyclosporine induces hypertension via its renal hemodynamic effects (acute toxicity). It should be noted, however, that not all investigators are convinced that cyclosporine-induced hypertension is mediated by renal mechanisms (20).

Thus far, then, clinical researchers have noted a marked increase in the prevalence of hypertension among patients taking cyclosporine. The increase has been less striking in kidney transplant follow-up clinics, which may be due to comparison to a prevalence which was already quite high before the introduction of cyclosporine. On the other hand, the possibility exists that the clinical observations that differ between kidney transplant groups and others may provide important clues as to the mechanism of cyclosporine-induced hypertension. Clinical observations also suggest that the hypertension is dose dependent and can be reversed by discontinuation of the drug. Severe hypertension has been observed among cardiac (21), bone marrow, (22,23), and liver transplant (24) groups, and most have suggested that cyclosporine-induced hypertension is difficult to control with most antihypertensive drugs currently available. It is likely that the same mechanisms involved in causing cyclosporine nephrotoxicity are involved in causing hypertension, although this is not firmly established.

POSSIBLE NONRENAL MECHANISMS

Cyclosporine may be a general vasoconstrictor of smooth muscles and may affect the systemic circulation and total peripheral resistance independent of its effects on renal tissue (25). It has also been shown that cyclosporine therapy results in mild hypomagnesemia (26). Hypomagnesemia could contribute to hypertension. Effects of cyclosporine on intracellular calcium binding proteins may also be of significance in that vascular tone and blood pressure may be directly affected without need to implicate the kidney (27).

Effects of cyclosporine on the sympathetic nervous system, aldosterone metabolism, and vasopressin and atrial natriuretic factor have all been investigated, with no firm conclusions yet reached. It does appear that cyclosporine tends to synergistically augment other known vasoconstrictors.

Clinical evidence that hypertension can occur without renal involvement comes from observation in which patients with "normal renal function" developed hypertension on cyclosporine. Unfortunately, most of these studies have not included measurement of renal function in any more sophisticated manner than serum creatinine. Perhaps the best experimental data to suggest that renal impairment is not essential to cyclosporine-induced hypertension come from Whitworth et al. (28), who have reported that the hypertension in sheep occurs despite no change in either renal blood flow or glomerular filtration rate (GFR).

CYCLOSPORINE NEPHROTOXICITY

Cyclosporine nephrotoxicity has received even more attention than has hypertension. Although it was initially believed that the impairment of renal function associated with cyclosporine was similar to the renal impairment caused by aminoglycoside antibiotics [i.e., acute tubular necrosis (ATN)], clinical researchers noted several features that were quite different with regard to cyclosporine-induced nephrotoxicity: (a) The nephrotoxicity is often quite easily and immediately reversed with discontinuation of the drug. With tubular toxins, recovery from injury is usually much slower. (b) Impaired renal function with cyclosporine appears to be relatively stable. If the drug dosage is maintained in the face of severely impaired function (e.g., serum creatinine of 2.0 mg/dl), serum creatinine does not rapidly increase as it would with continued dosage of aminoglycoside or other tubular toxins. Eventually, prolonged maintenance of a toxic dose may lead to permanent and irreversible damage, but even this has not been as clearly demonstrated as it has for tubular toxins.

Thus the clinical features of cyclosporine toxicity are different than those observed with more classical nephrotoxins. Clinical investigators using cyclosporine have noted at least three different types of nephrotoxicity: (i) immediate toxicity with nonfunction of the allograft; (ii) acute episodic toxicity; and (iii) chronic irreversible toxicity.

The early use of cyclosporine in kidney transplant centers was associated with an increased frequency of nonfunction of allografts. Calne et al. (29) recommended that renal transplant recipients not be exposed to cyclosporine until a diuresis was established. Others have noted that recovery from the ATN-like syndrome that accompanies cadaveric transplantation is often prolonged when cyclosporine is given (30). This observation has led many to changes in immunosuppressive protocols that omit cyclosporine until the allograft has fully recovered from the ischemic damage of harvesting and artificial perfusion. Moreover, it has been noted that most nephrotoxic exposures that an allograft experiences become worse in the setting of cyclosporine. The so-called acute episodic toxicity usually occurs after the new allograft has functioned well for at least a brief period of time. It is usually, but not always, associated with high blood levels of cyclosporine but has proven quite difficult to differentiate from acute allograft rejection. It does, however, respond (usually within 24–48 hr) to holding or decreasing the dose of cyclosporine. Unfortunately, acute rejection and acute cyclosporine toxicity are not mutually exclusive events. Finally, and perhaps most important clinically, is the chronic form of nephrotoxicity that has been well described by Myers et al. (31) and that can result in end-stage renal failure. Unlike the acute episodes of toxicity, chronic toxicity results in clear-cut fibrosis of the kidney and does not reverse when cyclosporine is discontinued. It should be noted that other investigators have reported lack of progressive chronic renal failure in renal transplant recipients exposed to cyclosporine therapy for 5 or more years (32). Investigators are not certain whether acute toxicity eventually leads to chronic toxicity or whether the chronic scarring that eventually occurs requires more than chronic vasoconstriction as a mechanism. It is possible that the mechanisms involved in acute and chronic toxicity differ.

MECHANISMS OF NEPHROTOXICITY

All of the three clinically observed forms of nephrotoxicity are associated with decreased renal blood flow and increased renal vascular resistance. The most frequently mentioned pathological description of cyclosporine nephrotoxicity involves afferent arteriolar narrowing (33). It is likely that chronic renal vasoconstriction eventually leads to renal fibrosis and the chronic lesions, although, as noted above, other mechanisms may be involved. While vasoconstriction appears to be a central feature of all forms of cyclosporine toxicity, the mechanisms that cause this vasoconstriction are not settled. There is evidence that favors involvement of the renal nerves, alterations in prostaglandin balance, and/or the renin–angiotensin system. It is possible that all three of these systems (or none) are involved in producing the renal hemodynamic effects of cyclosporine.

Moss et al. (34) reported that genitofemoral nerve traffic can be increased by infusion of cyclosporine into rats. Of special note in relation to the hypertensive effects of cyclosporine, Moss et al. demonstrated that this increased nerve traffic was associated with sodium retention via the kidneys of the rats. Even more supportive of the role of renal nerves is a report by Murray and Paller (35) demonstrating that cyclosporine-induced decreases in renal blood flow could be mitigated by denervation of the kidney or by an alpha-1 antagonist, prazosin. The fact that renal allografts are denervated could explain the seemingly more severe hypertension and nephrotoxicity seen in cardiac and other solid-organ transplantation as compared to those seen in renal transplantation.

Cyclosporine interferes with glomerular synthesis of prostaglandins (36). Cyclosporine also increases thromboxane synthesis (37) (thromboxane is a prostaglandin with potent vasoconstrictor effects). Thus, cyclosporine may act via alterations in the vasodilator/vasoconstrictor balance of the prostaglandin system. It should be noted, however, that prostaglandin inhibition via use of Indocin or other nonsteroidal anti-inflammatory agents usually exacerbates cyclosporine toxicity.

The role of the renin–angiotensin system in cyclosporine toxicity and hypertension is unsettled, especially when animal and human studies are compared. Renal vasoconstriction, low renal perfusion rates, and renal ischemia are usually associated with marked stimulation of the renin–angiotensin system. It might have been expected, then, that cyclosporine would be a stimulus to increase plasma renin activity. In the early animal investigations (38), this was found to be the case, with both plasma renin activity and cortical renal slices demonstrating marked elevation of renin levels. The study of Murray et al. (5), while demonstrating elevation of plasma renin, did not reveal any beneficial response to angiotensin-converting enzyme. In humans, however, Bantle et al. (39) suggested that plasma renin was suppressed by cyclosporine. Stanek et al. (40) also found that plasma renin was low and that cyclosporine patients, like the animal model of Murray and Paller (35), had relative unresponsiveness to converting-enzyme inhibitors. Bellet et al. (41) also were impressed that plasma renin was low in cardiac transplant patients treated with cyclosporine. Several reasons exist for this apparent conflict between animal experiments and the findings in humans: (a) Most of the animal work involved acute administration and cyclosporine, whereas the human reports involved the chronic use of cyclosporine. (b) The animal studies were done with larger doses of cyclosporine than those used clinically. (c) Much of the early animal work was done in non-pair-fed rats, which tend to become sick and volume depleted on high doses of cyclosporine, whereas man tends to become volume expanded on cyclosporine.

Recently, there have been at least two reports of investigations of cyclosporine toxicity employing micropuncture techniques in rats. Both the report of Barros et al. (42) and Thomson et al. (43) agree that renal vasoconstriction appears to be a marked feature of cyclosporine toxicity. Although Thomson's data suggested that the afferent arteriole was the prime site of vasoconstriction, the study of Barros et al. pointed toward efferent arteriole constriction. Neither report, however, was able to expand upon the cause of the glomerular hemodynamic abnormalities found, although Barros et al. believed the changes seen were consistent with vasoconstriction caused by activation of the renin–angiotensin system.

In summary, there is a general consensus that a consistent finding in the acute (reversible) form of cyclosporine nephrotoxicity is vasoconstriction. There is histological and micropuncture study confirmation of this concept. The exact mechanism of cyclosporine-induced vasoconstriction, however, remains unclear and may involve a direct effect of the drug itself or may be mediated via the sympathetic nervous system, alteration in prostaglandins, or stimulation of the renin–angiotensin system, or any combination of these possibilities. Less is known about the clinically more important chronic and irreversible toxicity except that it, too, is associated with decreased renal blood flow and hypertension; moreover, the afferent arteriole appears to be the predominant site of the increased resistance (44).

CLINICAL INVESTIGATIONS OF CYCLOSPORINE-ASSOCIATED HYPERTENSION

We have recently published data on 15 renal transplant patients treated with cyclosporine who were hypertensive and admitted to the Clinical Research Center at the University of Alabama Medical Center (45). In these studies the patients appeared to have a form of hypertension that was associated with extracellular volume expansion; these patients did not appear to be responsive to converting-enzyme inhibitors or to have elevated plasma renin activity. The cyclosporine patients appeared to avidly retain sodium on either a high- or low-sodium diet.

The tendency for cyclosporine-treated patients to have an expanded vascular volume has been previously reported by Bantle et al. (39), and Stanek et al. (40) have previously noted that cyclosporine-treated renal transplant patients do not appear to be responsive to captopril. Dubovsky et al. (46) suggested that the response of effective renal plasma flow (ERPF) to a captopril challenge was helpful in the diagnosis of post-transplantation hypertension; however, this was based on data obtained prior to the routine use of cyclosporine. Ever since the advent of cyclosporine, we have not been impressed that captopril therapy results in an increase in ERPF under most conditions (47).

Hypertension in renal transplant patients, however, is multifactorial in nature (48). As noted above, the high expected rate of hypertension even before routine use of cyclosporine makes this group of patients difficult to evaluate; however, Bellet et al. (41) examined hypertension among cardiac transplant recipients and reported (a) expansion of extracellular volume and (b) absence of any major abnormalities of the renin–angiotensin–aldosterone system. As in kidney transplant patients, these cardiac transplant patients did not appear to be responsive to converting-enzyme inhibition.

Thus most, but not all (49), reports of cyclosporine-associated hypertension in humans have de-emphasized the role of the renin–angiotensin system and have pointed to volume expansion and sodium retention as descriptive characteristics of this specialized form of hypertension. The tendency for volume expansion has consistently been in association with increased renal vascular resistance. Laskow et al. (50) have recently suggested that the proximal tubular reabsorption of sodium and urea is markedly enhanced with cyclosporine therapy. Indeed, cyclosporine appears to result in greater plasma levels of uric acid and an increased incidence of clinical gout, which also suggests that reabsorption in the proximal tubular is increased in a nonspecific fashion (51,52).

Thus, one view of the characteristics of the hypertension associated with cyclosporine therapy in humans suggests that the acute reversible vasoconstriction of the afferent renal arterioles results in decreased renal blood flow rates, decreased GFR, and propensity for the proximal tubule to retain sodium despite elevated systemic arterial pressure. Macroangiopathy has been observed in an important case report by Sawaya et al. (53), who demonstrated with serial arteriograms that cyclosporine can induce marked reversible vasoconstriction of the major renal arteries in an allograft. This emphasis on renal vasoconstriction, however, does not assign a role to the hypomagnesemia described with cyclosporine (54) or to its deleterious effects of serum lipid metabolism (55)—both factors which may ultimately prove to be of importance in the mechanism of cyclosporine-induced hypertension. The chronic toxicity described by Myers (56) is also associated with hypertension, and this hypertension is difficult to distinguish from other hypertension seen with any form of chronic renal insufficiency.

ANTIHYPERTENSIVE THERAPY

Clearly, hypertension caused by cyclosporine can be favorably treated by discontinuing the drug (12,13). Unfortunately, this approach is not practical in a number of settings, since acute rejection often follows discontinuation of cyclosporine (57). Some renal transplant groups have markedly decreased the dose of cyclosporine and have gone to so-called "triple-drug" immunosuppression with reinstitution of azathioprine in the hopes of decreasing both the azathioprine dose and the cyclosporine dose to minimize the side effects of both drugs. Few controlled trials are available comparing this approach to the one using cyclosporine and prednisone alone; however, among renal transplant groups in the United States, "triple-drug" immunosuppression appears to be becoming the standard.

If renal vasoconstriction is of prime importance in the mechanism of cyclosporine-associated hypertension, drugs that result in renovascular vasodilation may be of value. Most attention has been focused on calcium-channel blockers as being effective in therapy of cyclosporine-induced hypertension. Feehally et al. (58) noted in a retrospective review that hypertensive renal transplant patients on cyclosporine and treated with nifedipine had good blood pressure control and apparently less nephrotoxicity and fewer rejection episodes. Kwan et al. (59), however, were unable to document all these beneficial effects of nifedipine in a retrospective review of their clinic population. Recently, Curtis et al. (60) reported that nifedipine was significantly more effective in lowering renal vascular resistance than was captopril in renal transplant patients on cyclosporine therapy. It should be noted that different calcium-channel blockers have different effects on the metabolism of cyclosporine and may raise serum levels of cyclosporine (61); thus, cyclosporine levels should be monitored carefully when such agents are employed as antihypertensive therapy. On the other hand, calcium-channel blockers may add to the immunosuppressive benefits of cyclosporine (62). Thus, it is conceivable that calcium-channel blockers could decrease blood pressure, decrease the cyclosporine dose required, and increase immunosuppression. However, this potential for multiple benefits of combined therapy has yet to be demonstrated in human trials.

Converting-enzyme inhibitors appear not to be especially effective in cyclosporine hypertension, and there have been case reports of a possible interaction between converting-enzyme inhibitors and cyclosporine that may have resulted in reversible declines in renal function (63). In light of the volume expansion seen with cyclosporine, diuretic agents and sodium restriction seem appropriate. Other antihypertensive agents have not appeared to stand out as being especially more or less effective in the management of this form of hypertension.

SUMMARY

Cyclosporine hypertension is a newly described form of hypertension that is probably associated with cyclosporine nephrotoxicity. While seen among all groups that employ cyclosporine, renal transplant groups have not seen the complication as being as dramatic as have other groups.

The hypertension is associated with increases in renal vascular resistance; the site of this resistance increase appears to be the afferent renal arteriole. Sodium retention is another feature of the cyclosporine-induced hypertension; the proximal tubule appears to be the site of this sodium reabsorption and retention. Increased renal vascular resistance and increased sodium retention are probably linked, but the exact mechanism leading to these two events remains a subject of investigation.

Therapy with calcium-channel blockers and diuretics seems appropriate, but there is a great need for clinical trials in transplant recipients in order to determine the most appropriate form of therapy.

ACKNOWLEDGMENT

This work was supported, in part, by Grant 5 P50-HL-35051 from the Specialized Center of Research, Grant RR-0032 from the General Clinical Research Center, and Grant 1 P50 DK39258 from the Renal Center.

REFERENCES

1. Borel JF. Comparative study on *in vitro* and *in vivo* drug effects on cell mediated cytotoxicity. *Immunology* 1976;31:631.
2. Hess AD, Tutschka PJ, Santos GW. Effect of cyclosporine on the induction of cytotoxic T lymphocytes: role of interleukin-1 and interleukin-2. *Transplant Proc* 1983;15:32–42.
3. European Multicentre Trial Group. Cyclosporine in cadaveric renal transplantation: one-year follow-up of a multicentre trial. *Lancet* 1983;ii:986–989.
4. Ryffel B, Donatsch P, Madorin M, Matter BE, Ruttiman G, Schon H, Stoll R, Wilson J. Toxicological evaluation of cyclosporin A. *Arch Toxicol* 1983;53:107–141.
5. Murray BM, Paller MS, Ferris TF. Effect of cyclosporine administration on renal hemodynamics in conscious rats. *Kidney Int* 1985;28:767–774.
6. Bennett WM, Pulliam J. Cyclosporine nephrotoxicity. *Ann Intern Med* 1983;99(6):851–854.
7. Palestine AG, Nussenblatt RB, Chan CC. Side effects of cyclo-

sporine in patients not undergoing transplantation. *Am J Med* 1984;77:652–658.
8. Dieterle A, Abeywickrama K, von Graffenried B. Nephrotoxicity and hypertension in patients with autoimmune disease treated with cyclosporine. *Transplant Proc* 1988;20(Suppl 4):349–355.
9. Bachy C, Alexandre GPJ, van Ypersele de Strihou C. Hypertension after renal transplantation. *Br Med J* 1976;2:1287–1289.
10. Jarowenko MV, Flechner SM, Van Buren CT, Lorber MI, Kahan BD. Influence of cyclosporine on post transplant blood pressure response. *Am J Kidney Dis* 1987;10:98–103.
11. Hamilton DV, Carmichael DJS, Evans DB, Calnery RY. Hypertension in renal transplant recipients on cyclosporine A and corticosteroids and azathioprine. *Transplant Proc* 1982;14:597–600.
12. Chapman JR, Marcen R, Arias M, Rain AEG, Dunnill MS, Morris PJ. Hypertension after renal transplantation. *Transplantation* 1987;43:860–864.
13. Curtis JJ, Luke RG, Dubovsky E, et al. Cyclosporine in therapeutic doses increases renal allograft vascular resistance. *Lancet* 1986;ii:477–479.
14. First WH, Oyer PE, Shumway NE. Long-term hemodynamic results after cardiac transplantation. *J Thorac Cardiovasc Surg* 1987;94:685–693.
15. Hakim M, Spiegelhalter D, English TA, Caine N, Wallwork J. Cardiac transplantation with cyclosporine and steroids: medium- and long-term results. *Transplant Proc* 1988;20:327–332.
16. Thompson ME, Shapiro AP, Johnsen AM, et al. The contrasting effects of cyclosporin-A and azathioprine on arterial blood pressure and renal function following cardiac transplantation. *Int J Cardiol* 1986;11:219–229.
17. Textor SC, Forman SJ, Borer W, Bravo E, Carlson J. Blood pressure, hormonal and renal changes during cyclosporine administration in normotensive bone marrow transplant recipients with normal renal function [Abstract]. *Clin Res* 1986;34:487A.
18. English J, Evan A, Houghton DC, Bennett WM. Cyclosporine-induced renal dysfunction in the rat: evidence for arteriolar vasoconstriction with preservation of tubular function. *Transplantation* 1987;44:135–141.
19. Hollenburg NK, Adams DF, et al. Renal vascular tone in essential hypertension and secondary hypertension. *Medicine* 1975;54:29–35.
20. Bennett WM, Porter GA. Cyclosporine-associated hypertension. *Am J Med* 1988;85:131–133.
21. Goldman MH, Barnhart G, Mohanakumar T, Wetstein L, Szentpetery S, Wolfgang TC, Lower RR. Cyclosporine in cardiac transplantation. *Surg Clin North Am* 1985;65:637–659.
22. Textor SC, Forman SJ, Bravo EL, Carlson J. *De novo* accelerated hypertension during sequential cyclosporine and prednisone therapy in normotensive bone marrow transplant recipients. *Transplant Proc* 1988;20(Suppl 3):480–486.
23. Loughran TP, Deeg HJ, Dahlberg S, Kennedy MS, Strob R, Thomas ED. Incidence of hypertension after marrow transplantation among 112 patients randomized to either cyclosporine or methotrexate as graft-versus-host disease prophylaxis. *Br J Haematol* 1985;59:547–553.
24. Grant D, Wall W, Duff J, Stiller C, Ghent C, Keown P. Adverse effects of cyclosporine therapy following liver transplantation. *Transplant Proc* 1987;19:3463–3465.
25. Xue H, Bukowasi R, McCarron DA, Bennett WM. Cyclosporine A induces contraction in isolated rat aorta. *Transplantation* 1987;43:715–718.
26. June CH, Thompson CB, Kennedy MS, Nims J, Thomas ED. Profound hypomagnesemia and renal magnesium wasting associated with the use of cyclosporine for marrow transplantation. *Transplantation* 1985;39:620–624.
27. Handschmacher RE, Harding MW, Rice J, Drugge RJ, Speicher DW. Cyclophlin: a specific cytosolic binding protein for cyclosporine A. *Science* 1984;226:544–547.
28. Whitworth JA, Tresham J, McDougall JF, Scoggins BA, Bennett WM. Cyclosporine-induced hypertension in conscious sheep is modified by thromboxane synthesis inhibition [Abstract]. *Kidney Intl* 1989;35(1):510.
29. Calne RY, Rolles K, Thiru S, McMaster P, Craddock GN, Aziz S, White DJG, Evans DB, Dunn DC, Henderson RG, Lewis P. Cyclosporin A initially as the only immunosuppressant in 34 recipients of cadaveric organs. *Lancet* 1979;ii:1033–1036.
30. Hall BM, Tiller DJ, Duggin G, Horvath JS, Farnsworth A, May J, Johnson JR, Sheil AGR. Post-transplant acute renal failure in cadaver renal recipients treated with cyclosporine. *Kidney Int* 1985;28:178–186.
31. Myers BD, Ross J, Newton L, Luetscher J, Perlroth M. Cyclosporine-associated chronic nephropathy. *N Engl J Med* 1984; 311:699–705.
32. Lewis RM, Janney RP, Golden DL, Kerr NB, Van Buren CT, Kerman RH, Kahan BD. Stability of renal allograft function associated with long-term cyclosporine immunosuppressive therapy —five year follow-up. *Transplantation* 1989;47:266–272.
33. Mihatsch MJ, Theil G, Spichtin HP. Morphological findings in kidney transplants after treatment with cyclosporine. *Transplant Proc* 1983;15:2821–2835.
34. Moss NG, Powell SL, Falk WF. Intravenous cyclosporine activates afferent and efferent renal nerves and causes sodium retention in innervated kidneys in rats. *Proc Natl Acad Sci USA* 1985;82:8222–8226.
35. Murray BM, Paller MS. Beneficial effects of renal denervation and prazosin on GFR and renal blood flow after cyclosporine in rats. *Clin Nephrol* 1986;25(Suppl 1):S37–S39.
36. Perico N, Benigni A, Bosco E, Rossini M, Orisio S, Ghilardi F, Piccinelli A, Remuzzi G. Acute cyclosporine A nephrotoxicity in rats: which role for renin–angiotensin system and glomerular prostaglandins? *Clin Nephrol* 1986;25(Suppl 1):S83–S88.
37. Coffman TM, Carr DR, Yarger WE, Klotman PE. Evidence that renal prostaglandin and thromboxane production is stimulated in chronic cyclosporine nephrotoxicity. *Transplantation* 1986; 43:282–285.
38. Siegl H, Ryffel B, Petric R, Shoemaker P, Muller A, Donatsh P, Mihatsch M. Cyclosporine, the renin–angiotensin–aldosterone system, and renal adverse reactions. *Transplant Proc* 1983;15 (Suppl 1):2719–2725.
39. Bantle JP, Boudreau RJ, Ferris TF. Suppression of plasma renin activity by cyclosporine. *Am J Med* 1987;83:59–65.
40. Stanek SJ, Kovarik J, Rasoul-Rockenschaub S, Silberbauer K. Renin–angiotensin–aldosterone system and vasopressin in cyclosporine treated renal allograft recipients. *Clin Nephrol* 1987;28:186–189.
41. Bellet M, Cabrol C, Sassano P, Leger P, Corvol P, Menard J. Systemic hypertension after cardiac transplantation: effect of cyclosporine on the renin–angiotensin–aldosterone system. *Am J Cardiol* 1985;56:927–931.
42. Barros EJG, Boim MA, Ajzen H, Ramos OL, Schor N. Glomerular hemodynamics and hormonal participation on cyclosporine nephrotoxicity. *Kidney Int* 1987;32:19–25.
43. Thomson SC, Tucker BJ, Gabbai F, Blantz RC. Functional effects on glomerular hemodynamics of short-term chronic cyclosporine in male rats. *J Clin Invest* 1989;83(3):960–969.
44. Myers BD, Newton L, Boshkos C, Macoviak JA, Frist WH, Derby GC, Perlroth MG, Sibley RK. Chronic injury of human renal microvessels with low-dose cyclosporine therapy. *Transplantation* 1988;46:694–703.
45. Curtis JJ, Luke RG, Jones PA, Diethelm AG. Hypertension in cyclosporine-treated renal transplant patients is sodium dependent. *Am J Med* 1988;85:134–138.
46. Dubovsky EV, Curtis JJ, Luke RG, Jones P, Edwards M, Keller F, Whelchel JD, Diethelm AG. Captopril as a predictor of curable hypertension in renal transplant recipients. *Contrib Nephrol* 1987;56:117–123.
47. Curtis JJ. Hypertension in the renal transplant patient. In: Morris PJ, Tilney NL, eds. *Transplantation reviews,* vol 2. Philadelphia: W.B. Saunders, Harcourt Brace Jovanovich, 1988;17–27.
48. Luke RG. Hypertension in renal transplant recipients. *Kidney Int* 1987;31:1024–1037.
49. Saloman DR, Sadler LA, Carmichael MJ, Alexander JA. Hypertension following cardiac transplantation and cyclosporine therapy is dependent on the renin–angiotensin system [Abstract]. *Proc Int Congr Nephrol* 1987;10:300.
50. Laskow D, Curtis JJ, Jones P, Luke RG, Deierhoi M, Barber H, Diethelm A. Renal response to volume depletion in CSA and AZA TXPTS [Abstract]. *Am J Kidney Dis* 1988;XI(01):A11.
51. Tiller DJ, Hall BA, Horvarth JS, Duggin GC, Thompson JF, Sheil AGR. Gout and hyperuricaemia in patients on cyclosporin and diuretics. *Lancet* 1985;i:453.

pressures did not decline at night as early as they had in previous reports in white subjects). This observation may be especially important, since, as noted, it is likely that it is the total area under the pressure curve that leads to vascular damage and other target organ damage. Because the major determinant of glomerular filtration is arterial pressure, the observation that blood pressure did not decrease as early in the evening in black subjects may explain the observations by Luft et al. (21) that glomerular filtration rate (GFR) did not decrease at night in blacks as it did in whites. If the 24-hr pattern of blood pressure is found, on average, to be different in blacks, then it will be necessary in future studies to match black and white subjects for 24-hr blood pressure in order to examine the question of the greater sensitivity of the brain, the heart, or the kidney to blood pressure. Furthermore, it will be necessary to be certain that the subjects have been carefully matched for the level of pressure over several years as well as to carefully match the black/white groups for known factors that cause variations in renal function between individuals.

Early hemodynamic changes may occur in young black males (22). One explanation for the changes is that vascular reactivity to environmental factors may play a relatively important role in leading to a premature cycle of vascular hypertrophy and increased vascular tone. Folkow (23) hypothesized that the precapillary arterioles ("resistance vessels") throughout the body might play an important role, with vasoconstriction triggered initially by repeated exposures to environmental stressors. With repeated exposures, the functional changes are accompanied by structural vascular changes such as vascular smooth muscle hypertrophy that act as a ". . . forceful amplifying lever in transforming [smooth] muscle contraction to luminal reduction . . . [adding] a corresponding, nonspecific vascular hyperreactivity . . ." (23). Less potent environmental stimuli, including relatively minor irritations that occur from day to day, could lead to substantially greater vasoconstriction and subsequent blood pressure responses than would ordinarily occur (23).

A series of studies have documented greater blood pressure and vasoconstrictor responses to standardized stressors in young normotensive black males than in normotensive white males of similar age. Arensman et al. (24) have documented a greater systemic vascular resistance response to exercise in 10-year-old black schoolboys when compared to similar-aged white boys. Three other studies have documented greater blood pressure and peripheral vasoconstrictor responses to other standardized stressors in older black boys, adolescents, and young adults when compared to similar-aged white boys (25–27). Whether these are the earliest signs of vascular changes which become associated with hypertension and are followed by the premature cardiac hypertrophy in young black men remains to be determined. Adding more detailed evaluation with such tools as ambulatory blood pressure monitoring, echocardiography, and reactivity to standardized stressors, along with Doppler assessment of early vascular changes in a variety of black and white populations of varying demographic constitution, might help to explore this potential mechanism for the link between environmental factors and physiologic factors involved in the pathogenesis of hypertension; these added features might also help to explore the differences in hypertension between such black and white populations.

Hypertensive heart disease has been defined traditionally as the presence of both left ventricular hypertrophy (LVH) and hypertension. The advent of new sensitive approaches to diagnosis of LVH with substantial prognostic significance (28) has stimulated interest in whether such heart disease could help to explain the apparent paradox of a significant excess of heart disease death in the black population despite studies suggesting less obstructive epicardial coronary artery disease in the black population when compared to the white population (29,30). A brief, selective review of some old data, as well as some more recent data, on hypertensive heart disease suggests that exploring this possibility represents an important line of investigation.

The electrocardiogram (with or without the chest x-ray) has been used traditionally to assess the presence or absence of LVH in clinical and epidemiologic studies of hypertensive subjects. Such studies have shown black hypertensive subjects to have a higher prevalence of hypertensive heart disease when compared with white hypertensive subjects. For example, the black hypertensive men and women in the Hypertension Detection and Follow-up Program were three to four times more likely than white hypertensive men and women to have electrocardiographic LVH, with prevalences in the white men and women ranging from 1.7% to 3.1% and those in black men and women ranging from 7.8% to 9% (31). This excess of LVH in black hypertensive subjects persisted even after adjustment for age and blood pressure level. The Evans County, Georgia Study showed similar excess hypertrophy and cardiac enlargement in black subjects (compared to white subjects) on electrocardiograms and on chest x-rays, even after adjusting for blood pressure differences (32). The risk of subsequent morbidity and mortality escalates rapidly with the advent of electrocardiographic LVH. Electrocardiographic LVH confers a two- to ninefold increased risk of stroke, cardiac failure, overt coronary event, and symptomatic peripheral arterial disease in some populations (33). Electrocardiographic LVH is a marker of advanced hypertension, with 35% of men and 20% of women dead within 5 years of its appearance in one study (33).

In the Hypertension Detection and Follow-up Program, age-adjusted 5-year mortality in the stratum with mild hypertension at baseline (stratum I) was approximately double for (usual care) black males who had electrocardiographic LVH compared to those who did not have such LVH (31). Some subgroups of black subjects in the Hypertension Detection and Follow-up Program had even greater mortality associated with the presence of LVH than did comparable white subjects. For example, age-adjusted analyses of black men with less than a high-school education who were not receiving medications at baseline (usual care) indicated a 33.2% 5-year mortality in those with electrocardiographic LVH (34). White men with this similar education level who had LVH (and were not receiving medications at baseline) had a 12.4% 5-year mortality (35).

More sensitive and specific noninvasive diagnostic tools such as M-mode and two-dimensional echocardiography (35), as well as computerized electrocardiography (36), are increasingly being used to investigate prevalence, incidence, characteristics (including reversibility), and prognostic significance of hypertensive heart disease in black and white subjects. Only small studies of black subjects have been published to date, and these show the heterogeneity of heart findings in hypertensive subjects. Such studies have shown both structural (various degrees and forms of LVH) and functional heterogeneity (systolic and diastolic, or only diastolic, dysfunction) (35). Black subjects with mild hypertension have been shown to have as much as a twofold greater prevalence of LVH by echocardiography when compared to hypertensive subjects with a similar blood pressure level (16% versus 8%) (37). Other studies have shown greater left ventricular mass (38), greater left ventricular wall thickness (39), or no echocardiographic differences in small samples of black hypertensive patients when compared with white patients with similar blood pressure levels (40).

Echocardiographic LVH has been shown to be among the most powerful risk factors for coronary heart disease events (independent of the standard cardiovascular risk factors) in apparently healthy white subjects over age 60 years (41). For example, apparently healthy white men had a 66% greater risk of a coronary disease event in 4 years for each additional 50 g/m of echocardiographic left ventricular mass (41). This increased risk was independent of the standard cardiovascular disease risk factors, including office blood pressure. No such quantitative risk data are available for black subjects. However, a national sample of black men aged 35 years and older, and who were in the top quintile of left ventricular mass estimated from computerized electrocardiograms, had a 60% 12-year death rate from cardiovascular disease as compared to a less than 25% death rate for a similar-aged group of white men also with left ventricular mass in the top quintile (36). This raises the possibility that not only may black men have a greater incidence of hypertensive heart disease but also that such disease may be more malignant in black men than in white men.

Changes of increasing peripheral vascular resistance associated with hypertensive heart disease may start in young black men before office blood pressures reflect elevated blood pressure. Soto et al. (22), in a study of over 500 black and white children from a population sample in Bogalusa, Louisiana, found that black boys between the ages of 12 and 22 years showed, on average, increasing levels of peripheral vascular resistance whereas white boys and girls, as well as black girls, showed declining peripheral resistance between these ages (22). These findings were independent of blood pressure and body size and were inversely related to changes in cardiac output and stroke volume.

Data suggesting that black adolescents and young adults have patterns of increasing peripheral vascular resistance which is seen in middle-aged white men and women may represent a harbinger of premature hypertensive heart disease in black men (22). Prevention of hypertensive heart disease is important, but these early hemodynamic findings in black men and boys suggest that preventive actions may need to occur very early. Some antihypertensive interventions may be more effective than others with regard to reversal of changes associated with hypertensive heart disease despite similar efficacy in lowering blood pressure (42). This is under intense investigation because such information may ultimately have a profound impact not only on who is treated but also on how they should be treated. The new, sensitive tools for detecting hypertensive heart disease will help accelerate such studies.

Studies of middle-aged white patients with mild to moderate hypertension show a predominant pattern of increased peripheral vascular resistance and, consequently, concentric LVH (43). In the Framingham general population sample, concentric hypertrophy was rarely seen under age 30 years but evolved as a common form of hypertrophy in 40- to 49-year-old white men (44). The concentric form of hypertrophy emerged as a predominant form of LVH about 10 years later in white Framingham women (44). These patterns become particularly frequent in the elderly general population, with continued increases in peripheral resistance and concentric hypertrophy along with reduced cardiac output. Taken together, these observations and those in Bogalusa suggest that the hemodynamic patterns in young black men may represent "early aging"; that is, they resemble the patterns seen emerging in older white individuals.

The young black men and adolescents in Bogalusa were the leanest race–sex group. White boys and girls and black girls thus were more obese and had more of a volume load. Young black males and adolescents could, under these circumstances, have an office blood pressure that is similar to, or lower than, that of white males (see 18- to 24-year age group, Table 1) with a relatively low cardiac output but could still have increased peripheral vascular resistance and more vascular and cardiac changes related to this. An analogous situation might be reflected in the fact that Barrett-Connor and Khaw (45) reported greater cardiovascular morbidity in a prospective study of lean hypertensive men when compared to obese hypertensive men. On the other hand, Messerli et al. (46) highlighted the synergistic increases in left ventricular stroke work that can result (by disparate hemodynamic mechanisms) from arterial hypertension and obesity, which would be expected to accelerate development of left ventricular dysfunction and failure.

Renal Damage

As early as the 1930 U.S. mortality statistics, blacks were reported to have a greater mortality from nephritis. For acute nephritis, the rate was five times greater; for chronic nephritis, it was 1.3 times greater; and for nephritis—unspecified, it was 2.9 times greater (47). The Metropolitan Life Insurance Company reported in 1937 that from 1911 to 1935 the annual death rate due to acute nephritis for black males was 3.1 times greater than the rate in white policy holders (48). The advent of universal dialysis in the United States in 1973 has enabled a systematic collection of data from several regions; this reveals that the risk of black patients needing dialysis is greater for all forms of renal disease except polycystic disease. The greatest difference was a 17.7-fold greater renal failure rate due to hypertension in the black population as compared to the white population (49). A report from Los Angeles (50) suggests that there may be an increasing rate of the development of renal failure in blacks.

Additional evidence for black–white differences in renal function come from the observations made during the screening of 159,000 persons across the nation for the Hypertension Detection and Follow-up Program (51). Serum creatinine was higher in black men and women at all levels of blood pressure. However, because creatinine is produced in proportion to muscle mass, this higher blood level could be due to higher production rates in blacks, who tend to have a higher lean body mass than do whites of the same weight.

Whether the kidneys of black individuals with hypertension are more likely to be damaged by high blood pressure than the kidneys of white individuals with hypertension of similar severity has long been debated. The renal damage from arterial pressure appears to be primarily related to the vascular damage induced by the average level of systemic arterial pressure. The major sources of variance in renal function between individuals, as measured by GFR, include factors such as sex, body size (larger people have larger kidneys), percent muscle mass, systemic arterial pressure, age (GFR declines with age in blacks and whites), posture (GFR is higher in the recumbent position), time of day [Luft et al. (21) have reported that GFR declines at night in whites but not in blacks], sodium intake (low sodium intake lowers GFR), protein intake (high intake increases GFR), creatinine intake, physical exercise, and biobehavioral stress. Unfortunately, there have not been any systematic studies that carefully matched black and white subjects for these known factors; therefore, it is not yet possible to conclude that blacks are more susceptible than whites to renal damage due to the same level of pressure.

Luft et al. (21) have reported on studies of 94 black subjects and 94 white subjects matched for age, weight, body surface area, and sodium intake. They noted that although creatinine clearance decreased with age in both groups, the decrease in blacks was steeper. This was not correlated with blood pressure, and duration of hypertension was not analyzed. Radiographic studies of the renal arterial system were performed by Levy et al. (52) in 19 white and 8 black patients who underwent angiography for severe hypertension (average diastolic blood pressure: 117 mmHg). Despite the fact that the creatinine clearance was similar (59.4 ml/min in black subjects and 58.6 ml/min in white subjects), renal blood flow was lower in blacks than in whites (390 ml/min versus 473 ml/min). Examination of the peripheral renal vessels revealed that blacks had more nephrosclerosis characterized by disease in the arcuate arteries: Observed were (a) poor tapering tortuosity, (b) focal obstruction, and (c) small regions of nonperfusion. This radiographic picture would explain the hemodynamic observations by Frohlich et al. (53), who reported that the lower renal blood flow in blacks was associated with a higher renal vascular resistance.

Microscopic examinations of renal tissue obtained from black patients with malignant hypertension have been compared to autopsy data obtained in whites (54). In contrast to the expected findings of classic fibrinoid necrosis found in most white patients with malignant hypertension, Pitcock et al. (54) noted that in black patients the arterioles were strikingly thickened; also noted in blacks patients were (a) smooth muscle hyperplasia and (b) mucopolysaccharide deposited between smooth muscle cells. When advanced, this severe intimal hyperplasia led to complete obstruction of glomerular flow and, thus, to glomerular obsolescence. The shrunken glomeruli were surrounded by eosinophilic material which had the periodicity of collagen by electron microscopy. There have been few recent reports of renal microscopic morphology in matched black and white subjects.

Cerebrovascular Damage

In the United States, death rates for all cerebrovascular disease is 50% greater in blacks than in whites (55), and only Japan has a higher stroke death rate (209/100,000) than that of American blacks (165/100,000). The greatest decline in stroke that occurred from 1960 to 1975 was in black females, who have experienced a 48% decrease (55).

The mechanism by which high systemic pressure leads to vascular damage in the brain is not clear. The ability of the brain vascular bed to autoregulate probably plays a key role, since increasing systemic pressure leads to increasing vascular resistance in the cerebral vascular bed. However, when the pressure exceeds the ability of the brain to autoregulate, the vessels begin to dilate; this "breakthrough" increase in flow and transmission of systemic pressure leads to transudation of fluid or to leakage of blood, ultimately leading to stroke (55). Cerebral vascular pathology in blacks also differs in that there tends to be more intracranial (as opposed to extracranial) artery atherosclerosis (56). This observation has not been a universal one, since there are some geographical differences in the location of the atherosclerosis. In one study (57), Nigerians had less disease than did white Americans, who, in turn, had less disease than did black Americans.

The Hypertension Detection and Follow-up Program clearly demonstrated that lowering the blood pressure in blacks resulted in a 50% reduction in fatal and nonfatal stroke (58) and that this protective effect applies to all ages and to all levels of hypertension. It should be remembered that this program is the only controlled study that has demonstrated this in blacks. Standard therapy was chlorthalidone, to which reserpine was added if the blood pressure was not controlled.

POTENTIAL BASES FOR BLACK–WHITE DIFFERENCES

A number of studies have explored potential bases for black–white differences in prevalence and severity of hypertension, including psychosocial, socioeconomic, and related environmental factors (59), body weight, and genetic factors (60). Differences in a variety of physiologic measurements have been identified between black and white subjects, including differences in renal physiology such as renovascular responsiveness, sodium and potassium excretion (61), plasma renin (62), kallikrein levels (63), dopamine β-hydroxylase levels (64), response to norepinephrine

(65), and endocrine factors (66–68). The most consistent conclusion from these studies is that no single factor has emerged that adequately explains all the black–white differences. However, some leads that suggest some important contributors with implications for intervention have emerged.

Environmental Factors

James (59) has reviewed studies that investigated socioeconomic and environmental factors and that emphasized the socioeconomic differentials between black and white populations as well as the consistent inverse association of risk for hypertension and socioeconomic status. He cited information suggesting that black workers might be more likely to be in occupational settings of high psychosocial stress involving unfavorable decisions regarding hiring, retention, wages, apprenticeship, and promotional opportunities (69,70). He related such settings to significantly higher blood pressures (69). He also cited data which suggested that some measures of limited social support and social disorganization and/or low socioeconomic level might be more likely to be positively related to blood pressure in black populations than in white populations (71–73). Finally, he reviewed ecological data that showed associations between hypertension-associated mortality and social disorganization or instability (74,75).

These studies are limited in that the variables examined do not provide adequate specificity and pathophysiologic information to clarify the impact and mechanism of environmental factors as an explanation for black–white differences in hypertension. As suggested earlier, more direct links between environmental stressors and blood pressure differences in individuals may come from reviewing patient logs and findings of ambulatory blood pressure monitoring and linking them to other physiologic and anatomic characteristics in black and white individuals (76). Such studies may also provide insight into mechanisms linking environmental factors to the early appearance of hypertension in black populations. This would be particularly likely if exposures to environmental stressors that result in transient elevations of blood pressure prove to be quantitatively or qualitatively different, on average, in black populations.

Pathogenetic Hypotheses

If black populations are exposed, on average, to greater psychosocial and/or physical stresses than are white populations, the vascular changes as proposed by Folkow (23) (described above) provide a mechanism for translation of such repeated exposures to (a) stressors to vascular changes producing earlier elevations in total peripheral resistance and (b) stressors to localized changes in vascular resistance (e.g., in the kidneys). Structural and functional vascular changes in the kidneys as responses to repeated psychosocial and/or physical stressors could initiate a series of adaptive changes as outlined by Guyton et al. (77) which would explain how the kidney then contributes to a chronic elevation of blood pressure. Julius (78) described a blood-pressure-seeking property of the central nervous system and hypothesized how it could contribute to neurogenically initiated changes in cardiac output and peripheral vascular resistance, to maintain a "desired" pressure. He proposed that transition from neurogenic hypertension to a structurally mediated hypertension occurred which was associated with a subsequent decline in sympathetic overactivity. This process could be accelerated if there were substantially greater repeated exposures to stressors which triggered the adaptive responses. Denton (79) points to the evolutionary changes, over 20,000–40,000 generations, among black and white populations in Africa and Europe, respectively, with different environmental availability of salt prior to their arrival in the Americas and the Caribbean. On the one hand, he highlights the necessity of salt intake with regard to normal physiology, particularly under stress; on the other hand, he describes the excess of salt intake in black and white populations in the Americas. He suggests that this excess of salt intake relative to needs, perhaps coupled with a genetic functional "defect" in the kidney (particularly prominent in black populations), would be the best explanation of the excess of hypertension in black populations as compared to white populations. He cites the diverse influence of sodium (and sodium balance and distribution in the organism) on relevant parameters such as (a) modulation of response of excitable tissues and (b) effects of hormone secretion and action, including the renin–angiotensin system, antidiuretic hormone, catecholamines, and steroid hormones. He appropriately indicates that it is possible that ". . . the role of high sodium intake is permissive of the expression of other factors which might contrive the hypertensive state, including influence of obesity and psychogenic factors . . ." associated with lifestyle (79). On the other hand, since 60–85% of the individuals in each race–sex group in the United States have hypertension by the age of 65 years and older (3) (Table 1), there is the possibility that some permissive genetic predisposition to hypertension may be present in the majority of North Americans (black and white), becoming manifest at different ages; this is perhaps related to various other environmental and/or genetic factors.

Genetic Hypothesis

There is abundant evidence that blood pressure has a heritable component in both black and white populations (Table 2) and that the degree of genetic determination is not different between blacks and whites. Studies that have shown a portion of the variance of blood pressure level as heritable do not directly address the question of the cause of differences in blood pressure between black and white populations. Nonetheless, the studies assessing the heritable component of blood pressure in black and white subjects have yielded potentially valuable insights into blood pressure control systems. The heritable component of blood pressure must be due to genetic influences on one or more of the blood pressure control systems. In white subjects it has been shown that such a genetic influence is present in the renin system (for the renal excretion of sodium), in the blood-pressure-lowering effects of low-so-

TABLE 2. *Ethnic, familial, and genetic observations in normotensive and hypertensive subjects*[a]

Variable of interest	Black versus white		Family history		Genetic influence?	
	Normal	Hyper	Black	White	Black	White
Blood pressure						
Western Hemisphere (60,80)	B > W	B > W	+ > −	+ > −	Yes	
Africa (81)	B < W	B < W	?	?	?	Yes
Body weight						?
Males (81)	B < W	B < W	?	?	No	Yes
Females (82)	B > W	B > W	?	?	No	Yes
Diet						
Sodium (61a,62,86)	B = W	B = W	+ = −	+ = −	?	No
Potassium (61a,62,86)	B < W	B < W	+ = −	+ = −	?	No
Calcium (61)	B < W	B < W	?	?	?	?
Hematocrit (61a,62)	B < W	B < W	?	?	?	Yes
Plasma volume (83)	B = W	B = W	?	?	?	?
Kidney (83)						
Creatinine clearance	B = W	B < W	?	?	?	?
Renal blood flow	?	B < W	?	?	?	?
Excretion of Na^+ load	B < W	B < W	?	+ < −	?	Yes
Increase in BP with Na^+ load	B > W	?	?	?	?	?
Decrease in BP with Na^+ depletion	B > W	B > W	?	?	?	Yes
Fractional excretion Li^+ (84)	?	?	+ > −	?	?	?
Plasma renin activity (61a,85,86)	B < W	B < W	+ > −	+ > −	?	Yes
Other						
Aldosterone (61b)	B = W	B = W	?	?	?	?
Sympathetic nervous system (UNE or PNE) (65)	B = W	B = W	+ = −	+ < −	?	Yes
Response to stressors (86,92)	B = W	B > W	+ > −	+ > −	?	Yes
Dopamine β-hydroxylase (64)	B < W	B < W	?	?	?	?
Kallikrein (63)	B < W	B < W	+ < −	+ < −	?	?
Red-cell transport (87)	B < W	B < W	?	+ < −	?	Yes

[a] Normal, normotensive; Hyper, hypertensive; B, black; W, white; +, family history positive for hypertension; −, family history negative; >, greater than; <, less than; =, groups are similar; UNE, urinary norepinephrine; PNE, plasma norepinephrine.
From ref. 59, with permission.

dium diet (60), in the biochemical measures of the sympathetic nervous system, and in the blood pressure response to stress (60). In addition, there are black–white differences in each of these systems except for the biochemical measures of the activity of the sympathetic nervous system.

Physiologic differences have been found in the blood pressure control systems when comparing black and white subjects (Table 2). These differences relate to the vascular reactivity to stress (blacks are more reactive), to the renin system (blacks have lower values), to the ability to excrete sodium (blacks are slower), and to the blood pressure effects of increasing dietary sodium (blacks are more sensitive). Black–white differences in the reactivity to stressors (such as the cold pressor test) were identified as early as 1935 by Schwab (88), when he tested 172 white and 153 black subjects and measured blood pressure at 30, 90, and 150 sec. Blacks had a greater elevation of blood pressure, which suggested that there might be a racial difference in the vasomotor response to stress. Studies by Falkner et al. (89) and by Light et al. (26) have confirmed and expanded these earlier observations. Falkner et al.'s data suggest that the greater reactivity is brought out by salt-loading in those with the highest levels of blood pressure. Light et al. have likewise described greater reactivity to active coping tests in those with the greatest blood pressure levels. Dimsdale et al. (90) reported that hypertensive black subjects (but not normotensives) showed a greater sensitivity to the pressor effects of norepinephrine and that this was enhanced by a high-sodium diet. However, these responses should be viewed with some caution because the subjects compared were not carefully matched for 24-hr blood pressure. The suspicion is that those with the highest 24-hr blood pressure will have more hypertrophied blood vessels, which will respond better to any pressor stimulus.

Racial differences in the renin–angiotensin–aldosterone system were described by Helmer (85) in 1964. Helmer was also the first to suggest that this might be related to an evolutionary adaptation by blacks in Africa to the hot, humid environment which was low in sodium. Thus, he suggested that survival in such an environment required extremely efficient mechanisms to conserve sodium lost through (a) the sweat, (b) the urine, and (c) the stool. Aldosterone plays a key role in conserving sodium through all of these routes. However, systematic differences in blood or urinary aldosterone have not been demonstrated between whites and blacks. In contrast, a number of studies have demonstrated that renin levels, the major stimulus to aldosterone production, are lower in blacks and do not increase as much in response to sodium and volume depletion. Thus, suppression of the renin–angiotensin system has been detected in school children in Bogalusa (91) and in Charleston (86), in young adults in Indianapolis, and in older individuals in several other areas across the country (92). The distribution curve of renin in blacks in the United

States and in Africa is not a "normal" curve but is logarithmic. This is quite different than the "normal" distribution curve found in whites.

Genetic influences on blood pressure can be due to classical single-gene differences or, more likely, to multiple genes (polygenic trait) influencing the wide variety of blood pressure control systems. The single-gene problem occurs in families with glucocorticoid-responsive hyperaldosteronism (93) or with polycystic kidney disease. The first of these diseases has never been reported in a black patient, and the latter is less common in blacks.

Usually the earliest evidence that a disease may have a heritable component is that it tends to occur in families. The first study to demonstrate familial aggregation of hypertension in blacks was that of Miall et al. in Jamaica (94). The sib–sib and parent–sib correlations were significant and were similar (about 0.2) to those reported in studies on white subjects in England. Similar observations were made by McDonough et al. in Evans County, Georgia (82), by Prineas et al. in Minneapolis, Minnesota (95), and by Hohn et al. in Charleston, South Carolina (86). Parent–offspring studies on black subjects with and without a hypertensive parent have been performed by Hohn et al. (86). In their studies, blacks had lower renin levels than did whites. However, the offspring of hypertensive black parents had higher levels of plasma renin activity than did the offspring of normotensive parents. Another design to test the role of the environment on blood pressure is to study adopted children. If blood pressure is influenced by the family environment, the adopted children's blood pressure should resemble that of the adopted parents and this should increase with time. Elegant studies have been done in Canada with white adoptees in white families (96); these studies have shown that there is no correlation between blood pressure of the adoptee and the family. Such studies are not available for black children.

Another approach to the study of the inheritance of blood pressure has been to look for the association between blood pressure and traditional genetic markers. Such studies have been attempted in Belize (97). There was a tendency for the blood pressure to be higher in those blacks believed to have a greater percentage of African genetic heritage. Studies in Brazil have suggested that individuals with blood group O have a higher blood pressure than those with other blood types (98). Three studies have examined the relationship between skin color and blood pressure. In Charleston (99), Detroit (100), and Belize (97), skin color was used as a phenotypic marker for dilution of African genetic heritage. The first two cross-sectional studies (but not the Belize study) have all shown that the lighter the skin, the lower the blood pressure. Moreover, the longitudinal study from Charleston (101) did not show a relationship between skin color and the risk of developing elevated blood pressure. Studies from Brazil have demonstrated that those classified as mulatto have blood pressure levels that were lower than darker blacks but higher than whites (98). The intertwining of skin color, psychosocial stress, and socioeconomic status makes the interpretation of this association difficult at best.

It is very easy to demonstrate the environmental (diet, stress, sleep) effects on blood pressure in normotensive and hypertensive subjects by simply measuring blood pressure in the clinic or with the 24-hr device. There are several general approaches to answer the question, Does the average level of blood pressure have a heritable component? Variables that are strongly determined by inherited factors tend not to change over time. For example, if you measure height in an adult, you would find that this variable is very stable. Consequently, a simple way to get some useful information with regard to this question is to determine how variable the blood pressure is from day to day or from week to week. There have been no measures of the long-term stability of 24-hr blood pressure. However, as noted by Webber et al. (102), there have been long-term studies of the "tracking" of blood pressure rank in children in Iowa (103), and in Bogalusa (102) and of adults in Framingham, Massachusetts (104) and Evans County, Georgia (105). In general, it appears that blood pressure levels measured in the clinic will "track" relatively well. Because there are no known genetic markers for the tendency to have a blood pressure in the upper part of the distribution curve, one must rely on observational studies that examine genetic relatives to determine if the correlation of blood pressure in related pairs of subjects is greater than zero. If not, there is no reason to suspect a genetic basis for blood pressure level in blacks or whites. If the correlation is significantly greater than zero, one would also expect that the correlation will decrease as the closeness of the genetic relative decreases: parent–offspring > first cousins. If genetic factors were the major explanation for the correlation, you would not expect spouses or adopted children to be correlated with other family members. In studies in Evans County, Georgia, there was a significant correlation between white and black spouse's blood pressure (106), but others have not been able to verify this. The evidence for a strong genetic influence on blood pressure has been obtained in both white and black subjects, although the studies in blacks have not been as numerous nor have all methods been used.

A powerful method to test for the role of genetic factors is the study of twins. Of course, the ideal use of twins is to study identical twins raised apart, but these are so rare that they have never been reported in blacks. In the study of monozygotic (MZ) and dizygotic (DZ) twins, data are collected (e.g., blood pressure, renin, atrial natriuretic factor, or behavioral scales such as anger) on sets of MZ and DZ twins. The conditions for the twin method require that the mean value of the trait should not differ between MZ twins and DZ twins. A second requirement is that the variance in MZ twins should not differ significantly from the variance in DZ twins. If these two conditions are met, the twin model can then be used to assess the relative contribution of genetic versus environmental factors on the trait of interest. The next step is to calculate the difference of the variable within each twin pair. The mean within-pair differences of MZ and DZ pairs are then tested to determine if MZ twins are more alike than DZ twins. If so, then that trait is said to be under genetic control. Using these data, one can also calculate the so-called heritability of the trait. The heritability is considered as an estimate of the proportion of variance of that trait that is under genetic control.

A concern with all twin models is, How does one recruit an adequate number of twins? Because one in every 100 births is a twin birth, one in every 50 people in the population should be a twin. Given the high prevalence of hypertension, a significant number of the twins have hypertension, and there is a family history of hypertension in over half of the twins recruited in studies in the United States.

In preliminary studies using the analytic principles described above in black twins, it has been estimated that the variability in blood pressure related to genetic factors (80) is 60–80%. Obviously, there are important environmental components.

Grim et al. also studied the physiologic response to stress in identical and nonidentical white twins. They were interested in whether the blood pressure response to stress is influenced by genetic factors (i.e., a family history of hypertension). At Indiana University, twin pairs were studied simultaneously in separate rooms connected by a computer, which drove the protocol so that each received exactly the same stimulus at exactly the same time. The protocol alternated periods of relaxation and stress for 45 min. Stresses included mental arithmetic, Stroup color–word test, mirror drawing, isometric hand grip, and the cold pressor test. Blood pressure of identical twins tended to vary up and down very closely, much more so than for DZ twins.

Study of approximately 100 pairs of unrelated individuals revealed no concordance of blood pressure responses to stress, whereas blood pressure correlated within twins during the stress period. These data suggest that response to stress has a genetic determinant, at least to these types of stresses (60).

Differences Between Blood Pressure in Blacks in the Western Hemisphere and in Africa

As noted earlier, available data suggest that the blood pressure distribution curve is shifted to the right in Western Hemisphere blacks (10,107,108) compared to blacks in Africa or other populations; that is, blacks in the Western Hemisphere have higher blood pressure levels than do whites or blacks in other parts of the world. This may be mainly due to environmental differences between blacks and whites in the West or between American and African blacks. On the other hand, most blacks in the West are descended from survivors of the so-called "Slavery Period" of history (1500s–1800s), a period of forced migration unlike any other in the recorded history of mankind. Grim (109) has recently suggested, in line with previous related hypotheses (79,85), that selective survival during this period now contributes to the higher blood pressure in Western Hemisphere blacks who are descended from survivors of this ordeal.

During the slavery period, 11 million black people were transported against their will to the Western Hemisphere to provide slave labor in the agricultural enterprises (110–115). These people were young (average age 18, mostly between 10 and 30), and most were men.

A review of the extensive new and old research literature of the period has revealed conditions that must have imposed severe demands on sodium conservation and may have resulted in selective survival of those best able to conserve sodium. Estimated mortality in Africa after capture was 10% (range 4–50%), on board ship it averaged 15% (3–80%), and it was 5% (3–30%) while awaiting sale in the Americas. Conditions were crowded, access to water and food was limited, food consisted of mostly nonsalted products, seasickness was common and prolonged, and conditions of extreme heat and humidity were characteristic. The most common causes of death were diarrhea and febrile illnesses, both of which may result in severe sodium depletion. After arrival, work conditions were severe, and death rates averaged 10% per year (2–50%) for the first two years and were highest during the hottest parts of the year.

Grim (109) hypothesized that those individuals most efficient at retaining salt (sodium) were better able to maintain sodium and volume homeostasis and thus were better able to defend against fatal sodium depletion resulting from a combination of poor dietary sodium intake and excessive losses from sweat and diarrhea. Those who survived were the parents of future generations who were likewise forced to slave under severe conditions. The mortality was so severe that most areas had to continue to import more people as the death rate of adults and children exceeded the birth rate. The hypothesis predicts an inherited (genetic) increased prevalence of salt-sensitive hypertension (and biochemical markers) in present-day black Americans of this ancestry compared to present-day black Africans (or Americans) without this ancestry. In the presence of excess dietary salt intake characteristic of our society, these individuals may develop increases in blood pressure, subsequently leading to the health consequences of high blood pressure. Careful studies comparing present-day blacks of these two ancestries may yield information on the greater prevalence of hypertension in black Americans.

The adaptive mechanisms postulated as inherited may, of course, have components which are responses to hemodynamic and other current stresses in black and white individuals and should be explored for further understanding of genetic–environmental interactions. The finding that adolescent and young black men (in some age categories) in the United States have, on average, lower (not higher) prevalence of hypertension may give a false sense of security, since their relative thinness may mask (i.e., with lower blood volume and cardiac output) a premature increase in peripheral resistance which may be particularly malignant in contributing to premature target organ disease. This may have a component related to recurrent environmental stresses as discussed earlier. For example, if young black men are much more physically active, on average, than young white men (as some preliminary data suggest for some samples—G. Harshfield et al., *personal communication*), the hemodynamic stresses of a lower caloric intake and inadequate fluid intake could enhance mechanisms for conserving salt and maintaining blood pressure. Differential exposure to other recurrent stresses could also be associated with such changes. Such possibilities deserve exploration. In addition, heritable factors may interact with such recurrent environmental stressors in determining the level of physiologic response. The aspects of such interactions that are the main explanation for premature and more severe hypertension in some black populations could very well be mainly genetic or mainly environmental but appear to have a major modifiable component.

TREATMENT OF HYPERTENSION IN BLACK POPULATIONS

The absence or limited number of black patients in many of the major clinical trials of antihypertensive regimens, as well as the known differential degree of response of black hypertensive patients (on average) to some agents, emphasizes the need for careful evaluation of the data on the efficacy of various antihypertensive therapies in such patients. The Hypertension and Detection Follow-up Program demonstrated that antihypertension therapy with a special-care regimen (as opposed to usual care) was associated with an 18.5% and 28% reduction of 5-year total mortality in black men and women, respectively (116). The comparable reductions in total mortality in white men was 14.9% (116). There was a 2.7% greater total mortality in white women in the special-care group as compared to that in the usual-care group (116). These data suggest that for black subjects, the special-care treatment was particularly more effective than the usual-care treatment. Diuretic therapy was the cornerstone of this therapy, but there were a number of other considerations such as free therapy, transportation, etc., which might have been particularly beneficial for individuals of low socioeconomic level. Nonetheless, as Hall (117) points out, the results have been important because ". . . it is the only recent large-scale epidemiologic trial that applies directly to the risks and benefits of long-term treatment of hypertension in blacks."

Nonpharmacologic Therapy

Amery et al. (118) summarized data from a number of studies and showed that, on average, each kilogram of weight loss in hypertensive subjects is associated with a 3-mmHg decline in systolic blood pressure and a 2-mmHg decline in diastolic pressure up to 11 kg (118). One preliminary study confirmed these findings in 187 obese black women (119). However, other confounders such as sodium and potassium intake were not controlled in this study.

MacGregor et al. (120) studied 19 patients, seven of whom were black, and showed significant reductions in systolic and diastolic blood pressure with increased potassium intake. More information is needed about the role of salt restriction and increased potassium intake for blood pressure management in various black populations. The role of other dietary interventions in treatment of hypertension also needs further study in a variety of populations.

Klasky et al. (121) assessed data from a large Kaiser–Permanente database which included over 10,000 black patients and found substantially higher blood pressures in subjects who drank three to five alcoholic drinks per day than in those who drank less (11 mmHg/5 mmHg higher than in those that did not drink). They found that those who drank two or fewer drinks daily had slightly lower blood pressures than those who did not drink. Cause-and-effect relations are not proven; however, the consensus recommendations for limiting alcoholic drinks to the equivalent of 1 oz./day appear to be generally prudent for black, as well as white, populations (122).

The role and effectiveness of exercise, biofeedback, relaxation techniques, and stress reduction techniques are important areas for further study, both in general and particularly in regard to potential black–white differences in response to therapies (122).

Pharmacologic Therapy

The choice of any drug as first-line therapy or monotherapy, or as a component of therapy for hypertension in any patient group (especially in black patients), can be made rationally only if a number of conflicting factors are weighed. The drugs must be compared with respect to cost (123), effectiveness, side effects, and potential physiological benefits. In terms of cost (a determinant of adherence to therapy), it is clear that diuretics, especially generic products, have distinct advantages over beta-blockers and over most other pharmacologic antihypertensive agents. This is an important consideration for low socioeconomic status groups (in which black individuals are overrepresented). Side effects, especially nuisance symptoms, may result (to varying extents) from all antihypertensives and are another determinant of long-term adherence. Side effects of diuretics, such as alteration of lipid distributions during chronic therapy, deterioration of glucose tolerance, and alteration of potassium metabolism, have potentially adverse implications for cardiovascular disease outcomes. As discussed earlier in this chapter, increased left ventricular mass has emerged as an important risk factor for cardiovascular morbidity and mortality, and though physiological benefits attributable to regression of LVH have been demonstrated for some drugs, reduction of cardiovascular morbidity and mortality has not yet been demonstrated. Nonetheless, such structural changes, as well as related physiologic changes, may be a marker (or even an endpoint) of successful management in the future. This is particularly true in black populations, which tend to have a substantial excess of such changes. Hall (117,124) has reviewed the results of antihypertensive drug trials in black and white subjects and has summarized the findings for each class of agents in detail.

Diuretics

On average, black patients are more likely than white patients to respond to monotherapy with diuretics (125). In a Veterans Administration study, 71.3% of black patients, as compared with 55.3% of white patients, reached goal blood pressure in treatment with diuretics (125). In addition, a smaller dosage of hydrochlorothiazide was required to achieve the goal blood pressure in black, as compared with white, patients (average daily dose of 79 mg versus 114 mg, respectively) (125). Black subjects were more likely to attain a diastolic blood pressure of less than 90 mmHg with 50 mg of hydrochlorothiazide than were whites (62% versus 38%). In two other trials (126,127) in which the efficacy of diuretic therapy was compared, black patients had a similar greater decrease in blood pressure as compared with white patients (additional decrement of 5–7 mmHg systolic and 1–2 mmHg diastolic).

There was a 60–65% greater mortality from coronary heart disease in white male subjects with abnormal electrocardiograms who were treated with the special-care regimen (relatively high doses of diuretics) in the Multiple Risk Factor Intervention Trial (MRFIT) study (128) and in the Hypertension and Detection Follow-up Program (HDFP) (129) By contrast, there was a 36% lower mortality seen in a sample of black subjects with abnormal electrocardiograms who were treated with the HDFP special-care regimen as compared to those treated with the usual-care regimen (129). This sample was small (298 in the referred-care group and 232 in the usual-care group), with eight coronary heart disease deaths in the referred-care group and four such deaths in the special-care group. More data are needed to assess these findings.

Calcium-Channel Blockers

Blood pressure reductions in black patients with calcium-channel blockers as monotherapy approach those obtained with diuretic therapy (124–128,130). Moser et al. (126) documented comparable blood pressure responses to the calcium-channel blocker, diltiazem, and to hydrochlorothiazide in 20 black subjects with hypertension. The efficacy of diltiazem (120–360 mg/day) and propranolol (160–480 mg/day) in reducing supine diastolic blood pressure to levels of less than 90 mmHg has also been compared in a parallel-group, randomized, double-blind study of 196 patients with mild to moderate essential hypertension (101 black and 95 nonblack) (131). At the end of a 16-week monotherapy period, 57% of diltiazem patients and 60% of propranolol patients attained the treatment goal. Both agents produced blood pressure control in approximately 50% of black patients and 70% of nonblack patients, and no race–drug interaction was apparent. The authors noted that the study does not support earlier suggestions that demographic factors should be a major determinant of the choice between the two drug classes involved. Mohanty et al. (132) found that diltiazem virtually abolished forearm vascular resistance responses to lower-body negative pressure in 18 subjects (11 black), whereas hydrochlorothiazide did not abolish these responses despite similar levels of mean arterial pressure and basal forearm vascular resistance. They hypothesized that this type of agent might have greater efficacy than would diuretics in preventing large increases in arterial pressure that occur in response to environmental stresses and result in sympathoexcitation.

Fadayomi et al. (127) documented the efficacy of nifedipine in the treatment of black Nigerians with mild to moderate hypertension. Cubeddu et al. (130), in a study completed largely in Veterans Administration centers, evaluated the response of 118 patients (41 black and 77 white) to verapamil (240–480 mg/day) and propranolol (120–360 mg/day) during a 4-week double-blind trial (130). The effect of propranolol on diastolic blood pressure in white patients was significantly greater than in blacks. However, there was no significant difference in the effect of verapamil on blood pressures in white and black patients. Sitting diastolic blood pressures less than 90 mmHg were attained in 73% of patients. Age was not significantly related to verapamil efficacy.

Combined Alpha–Beta Blockers

Labetalol, a drug with selective alpha-1-adrenergic blocking properties and nonselective beta-blocking properties, has been compared to propranolol for the treatment of mild to moderate hypertension in black and white patients (133). In a double-blind multicenter clinical trial, labetalol (titrated from 100 to 600 mg b.i.d.) and propranolol (titrated from 40 to 240 mg b.i.d.) were compared. Hydrochlorothiazide was added as needed during the maintenance phase of the study. Labetalol was equally effective in black and white patients, whereas propranolol was significantly more effective in white patients than in black patients.

Beta-Blockers

Black patients, on average, do not respond as well as white patients to beta-blocker therapy (117). The most comprehensive data on effectiveness of beta-blockers in blacks as compared to their effectiveness in whites have been provided by the Veterans Administration Cooperative Study Group on antihypertensive agents (125,134). In a comparison of propranolol and hydrochlorothiazide in the initial treatment of hypertension, 6083 men (388 black) with initial diastolic blood pressures in the range of 95 to 114 mmHg were titrated, in a double-blind study, to diastolic blood pressures of less than 90 mmHg or to maximal daily doses of propranolol (640 mg) or hydrochlorothiazide (200 mg). In black subjects treated with propranolol, the goal diastolic blood pressure of less than 90 mmHg was attained in 53.5%. In white subjects treated with propranolol, Goal diastolic blood pressure was attained in 61.7%. The drug–drug (propranolol versus diuretic) difference was statistically significant only in black subjects. It is worthy of note that there was no racial difference in the dose response to propranolol.

A group of 394 of these patients entered a long-term treatment protocol for 12 months of further treatment (134). Statistically significant racial differences or race–drug interactions were not detected. This study demonstrated a more sustained effectiveness of hydrochlorothiazide than of propranolol in both races, and it also demonstrated a greater likelihood of adequate control with a lower dose of drug for hydrochlorothiazide (25 mg b.i.d.) than for propranolol (40 mg b.i.d.). The investigators stated (134): "The data suggested, but did not conclusively demonstrate, a racial difference in responsiveness to the two drugs. The mean reduction in blood pressure with propranolol was greater in whites than in blacks, while with hydrochlorothiazide the mean reduction was greater in blacks. However, the reductions in diastolic blood pressure with hydrochlorothiazide were greater than with propranolol in either race, and the differences between the drugs by race were not significant." The combination of beta-blockers and diuretic therapy is equally efficacious in black and white patients (117).

Plotnick et al. (135) provided data on the effect of pindolol (a beta-receptor antagonist with intrinsic sympathomimetic activity) on blood pressure in a predominately (75%) black group of 70 hypertensive men. The mean systolic and diastolic pretreatment blood pressures were, respectively, 151 mmHg and 102 mmHg, and the mean blood pressure was 119 mmHg. After therapy with 15, 30, 60 mg/day of pindolol in divided doses, the mean systolic and diastolic blood pressures were reduced, respectively, to 137 mmHg and 91 mmHg, and the mean blood pressure was reduced to 107 mmHg. There were 33 patients (47%) in whom the mean blood pressure was reduced by more than 10% of the pretreatment level.

Angiotensin-Converting-Enzyme Inhibitors

Angiotensin-converting-enzyme (ACE) inhibitors are less likely to be adequate monotherapy for black, as compared to white, hypertensive patients (117). When used in combination with diuretics, ACE inhibitors are as efficacious in black patients as in white patients (117).

The Veterans Administration Cooperative Study Group has provided data on the ACE inhibitor, captopril, in black and white patients (136). In a randomized study of 475 men with diastolic blood pressures in the range of 92 to 109 mmHg, captopril in daily doses of 37.5, 75, and 150 mg was compared to a placebo for 7 weeks of treatment. After 7 weeks, hydrochlorothiazide (50 mg daily) was added to the placebo group, as well as to two-thirds of each captopril group, for a further 7 weeks of observation. The 170 white patients had larger blood pressure reductions than did the 151 black patients (15/11 versus 9/8 mmHg). About 50% of black subjects and about 70% of white subjects were controlled by captopril alone. The racial difference in the percentages of patients attaining diastolic blood pressure of less than 91 mmHg was largely abolished by addition of hydrochlorothiazide. About 80–90% of both black and white subjects attained goal diastolic blood pressures with combination therapy. Similar data confirming lower efficacy of enalapril (another ACE inhibitor) as monotherapy in black subjects, as compared to that in white subjects, has been described (117,137,138). Race may be a more powerful predictor of response to enalapril than is plasma renin activity (139).

Other Antihypertensive Agents

Prazosin is a selective antagonist of peripheral postsynaptic alpha-receptors and has shown variable efficacy as monotherapy in black samples (140–145). Substantial efficacy has been demonstrated in studies in which prazosin has been used in combination therapy with diuretics (146,147).

Direct vasodilators such as hydralazine have been used as second-line agents in combination therapy in black and white patients (148). Black patients are substantially less likely than white patients to develop hydralazine-induced lupus erythematosus whether they are slow acetylators (have reduced activity of acetyl transferase) or not (149–152).

Centrally acting sympathetic inhibitors such as methyldopa, clonidine, and guanabenz have been shown to be similarly efficacious in hypertensive black patients (117,153–161). Black patients are substantially less likely than white patients to develop a positive direct Coombs' test when treated with methyldopa (162–166).

Reserpine was found to be less efficacious as monotherapy for hypertension in black patients as compared to polythiazide (167). However, reserpine had been documented as efficacious when used in combination with diuretic therapy (168). Hall (117) indicates that guanethidine and guanadrel may be useful in hypertensive blacks resistant to other therapy.

The studies reviewed indicate that diuretics, the calcium-channel blockers, and the alpha–beta blocker, labetalol, are more effective than the beta-blockers and ACE inhibitors in reducing blood pressures in blacks. Between one-third and one-half of blacks with mild to moderate hypertension treated with a beta-blocker alone have a satisfactory blood pressure response. Between one-half and three-quarters of black patients treated with diuretics in conventional doses will have an adequate blood pressure response. About 50% of black patients treated with an ACE inhibitor will have an adequate diastolic blood pressure response. The calcium-channel blockers will produce goal blood pressure in about 75% of black patients with mild to moderate hypertension. In addition, when a diuretic and beta-blocker or a diuretic and ACE inhibitor are used in combination, the effect is superior to that attained with either drug alone and may be comparable to that observed in whites.

There is little or no evidence of differential racial susceptibility to side effects of antihypertensive drugs. As noted earlier, the incidence (and hence the prevalence) of end-organ damage (both increased left ventricular mass and impaired renal function) are higher in blacks than in whites at similar levels of blood pressure. This may well be due to a longer duration of hypertension. There are some suggestive data on the impact of lower potassium intake in blacks on susceptibility to renal and cardiac dysfunction. Some beta-blockers, calcium-channel blockers, and ACE inhibitors appear to decrease left ventricular mass more effectively than other agents as blood pressure is reduced, and demonstration of improved outcomes associated with regression of LVH would strengthen the argument for their use.

REFERENCES

1. Cooper R. A note on the biologic concept of race and its application in epidemiologic research. *Am Heart J* 1984;108(Suppl.): 715–723.
2. Prineas RJ, Gillum RF. U.S. epidemiology of hypertension in blacks. In: Hall WD, Saunders E, Shulman N, eds. *Hypertension in blacks: epidemiology, pathophysiology and treatment.* Chicago: Yearbook Medical Publishers, 1985;17–36.
3. Joint National Committee on Detection, Evaluation and Treatment of Hypertension. Final report of the Subcommittee on Definition and Prevalence. *Hypertension* 1985;7:457–468.
4. Londe S, Goldring D, Gollub SW, Hernandez A. Blood pressure

and hypertension in children: studies, problems and perspectives. In: New MI, Levine MS, eds. *Juvenile hypertension.* New York: Raven Press, 1977;13–24.

5. Kotchen JM, Kotchen TA. Geographic effect on racial blood pressure differences in adolescents. *J Chronic Dis* 1978;31:581–586.
6. Kilcoyne MM. Adolescent hypertension. In: New MI, Levine MS, eds. *Juvenile hypertension.* New York: Raven Press, 1977;25–35.
7. Reed WL. Racial differences in blood pressure levels of adolescents. *Am J Public Health* 1981;71:1165–1167.
8. Voors AW, Foster TA, Frerichs RR, Webber LS, Berenson GS. Studies of blood pressures in children, ages 5–14 years, in a biracial community—the Bogalusa Heart Study. *Circulation* 1976;54:319–327.
9. Apostolides AY, Cutter G, Daugherty SA, et al. Three-year incidence of hypertension in thirteen U.S. communities. *Prev Med* 1982;11:487–499.
10. Akinkugbe OO. World epidemiology of hypertension in blacks. In: Hall WD, Saunders E, Shulman N, eds. *Hypertension in blacks: epidemiology, pathophysiology and treatment.* Chicago: Yearbook Medical Publishers, 1985;3–16.
11. Donnison CP. Blood pressure in the African native: the bearing upon the aetiology of hyperpiesia and arteriosclerosis. *Lancet* 1929;1:6–7.
12. Williams AW. Blood pressure of Africans. *East Afr Med J* 1941;18:109–117.
13. Shaper AG, Leonard PJ, Jones KW, Jones M. Environmental effects on the body build, blood pressure and blood chemistry of nomadic warriors serving in the army in Kenya. *East Afr Med J* 1969;46:282–289.
14. Interdepartmental Committee on Nutrition for National Defence (ICNND). *Ethiopia: nutrition survey, 1958.* Washington, DC: US Government Printing Office, 1959.
15. Truswell AS, Kennelly BM, Hansen JDL, Lee RB. Blood pressures of !Kung Bushmen in northern Botswana. *Am Heart J* 1972;84:5–12.
16. Mann GV, Shaffer RD, Anderson RS, Sandstead HH. Cardiovascular disease in the Masai. *J Atheroscler Res* 1964;4:289–312.
17. Akinkugbe OO. *High blood pressure in the African.* Edinburgh: Churchill Livingstone, 1972.
18. Akinkugbe OO, Ojo OA. Arterial pressures in rural and urban populations in Nigeria. *Br Med J* 1969;2:222–224.
19. Akinkugbe OO. Hypertensive disease in Ibadan, Nigeria: a clinical prospective study. *East Afr Med J* 1969;46:313–20.
20. Harshfield GA, Hwang C, Grim CE. Circadian variation of blood pressure during a normal day in normotensive blacks. *Circulation* 1988;78(Suppl):II-188.
21. Luft FC, Fineberg NS, Miller JZ, et al. The effects of age, race and heredity on glomerular filtration rate following volume expansion and contraction in normal man. *Am J Med Sci* 1980;279:15–24.
22. Soto LF, Kikuchi D, Arcilla RA, Savage DD, Berenson GS. Blood pressure levels and echocardiographic function in children: the Bogalusa Heart Study. *Am J Med Sci* 1989;297:271–279.
23. Folkow B. Physiological aspects of primary hypertension. *Physiol Rev* 1982;62:347–503.
24. Arensman WA, Gruber MP, Strong WB, Treiber FA. Doppler determination of exercise cardiac output and systemic vascular resistance in a biracial population of healthy ten-year-old males. *Am J Dis Child* 1989;in press.
25. Murphy JK, Alpert BS, Moes DM, Somes GW. Race and cardiovascular reactivity: a neglected relationship. *Hypertension* 1986;8:1075–1083.
26. Light KC, Obrist PA, Sherwood A, James SA, Strogatz D. Effect of race and marginally elevated blood pressure on responses to stress. *Hypertension* 1987;10:555–563.
27. Anderson NB, Lane JF, Muranaka M, Williams RB, Houseworth SJ. Racial differences in blood pressure and forearm vascular responses to the cold face stimulus. *Psychosom Med* 1988;50:57–63.
28. Savage DD. Significance of increased left ventricular mass in black and white hypertensive patients. *J Natl Med Assoc* 1988;80(Suppl):7–11.
29. Carryon P, Matthews MM. Clinical and coronary arteriographic profile of 100 black Americans: focus on subgroup with undiagnosed suspicious chest discomfort. *J Natl Med Assoc* 1987;79:265–71.
30. Maynard D, Fisher LD, Passamani ER. Survival of black persons compared with white persons in the Coronary Artery Surgery Study (CASS). *Am J Cardiol* 1987;60:513–518.
31. Taylor JO, Borhani NO, Entwisle G, Farber M, Hawkins CM on behalf of the HDFP Cooperative Group. Summary of the baseline characteristics of the hypertensive participants. *Hypertension* 1983;5(Suppl):IV-44–IV-50.
32. Beaglehole R, Tyroler HA, Cassel JC, Duebner DC, Bartel A, Hames CG. An epidemiological study of left ventricular hypertrophy in a biracial population of Evans County, Georgia. *J Chronic Dis* 1975;28:554–559.
33. Kannel WB, Dannenberg AL. Prevalence and natural history of electrocardiographic left ventricular hypertrophy. In: Messerli F, ed. *The heart and hypertension.* New York: Yorke Medical Books, 1987;53–61.
34. Tyroler HA. Overview of risk factors for coronary heart disease in black populations. *Am Heart J* 1984;108(Suppl):658–660.
35. Liebson PR, Savage DD. Echocardiography in hypertension: a review. I. Left ventricular wall mass, standardization, and ventricular function. *Echocardiography* 1986;3:181–218.
36. Rautaharju PM, et al. Electrocardiographic estimate of left ventricular mass versus radiographic cardiac size and the risk of cardiovascular disease mortality in the epidemiologic follow-up study of the first National Health and Nutrition Examination Survey. *Am J Cardiol* 1988;62:60–66.
37. Hammond IW, Devereux RB, Alderman MH, et al. The prevalence and correlates of echocardiographic left ventricular hypertrophy among employed patients with uncomplicated hypertension. *J A M Coll Cardiol* 1986;7:639–650.
38. Dunn FG, Oigman W, Sungard-Riise K, et al. Racial differences in cardiac adaptation to essential hypertension determined by echocardiographic indexes. *J Am Coll Cardiol* 1983;5(1):1348–1351.
39. Hammond IW, Devereux RB, Alderman MH, et al. Contrast in cardiac anatomy and function between black and white patients with hypertension. *J Natl Med Assoc* 1984;76:247–55.
40. Savage DD, Henry WL, Mitchell JR, et al. Echocardiographic comparison of black and white hypertensive subjects. *J Natl Med Assoc* 1979;71:709–712.
41. Levy D, Garrison RJ, Savage DD, Kannel WB, Castelli WP. Left ventricular mass and incidence of coronary heart disease in an elderly cohort: the Framingham Study. *Ann Intern Med* 1989;110:101–107.
42. Liebson PR, Savage DD. Echocardiography in hypertension: a review. II. Echocardiographic studies of the effects of antihypertensive agents on left ventricular wall mass and function. *Echocardiography* 1987;4:215–249.
43. Devereux RB, Savage DD, Sachs I, Laragh JH. Hemodynamic determinants of left ventricular geometry and function in hypertension. *Am J Cardiol* 1983;51:171–176.
44. Savage DD, Garrison RJ, Kannel WB, Levy D, Anderson SJ, Stokes J III, Feinleib M, Castelli WP. The spectrum of left ventricular hypertrophy in a general population sample—the Framingham Study. *Circulation* 1987;75(Suppl I):I-26–I-33.
45. Barrett-Connor E, Khaw KT. Is hypertension more beneficial when associated with obesity? *Circulation* 1985;72:53.
46. Messerli FH, Sundgard-Riise K, Reisin ED, Dreslinski GR, Ventura HO, Oigman W, Frohlich ED. Dimorphic cardiac adaptation to obesity and arterial hypertension. *Ann Intern Med* 1983;99:757–761.
47. Lewis JH. *The biology of the Negro.* Chicago: University of Chicago Press, 1942.
48. Metropolitan Life Insurance Co. Twenty years of health progress, New York, 1937.
49. Rostand SG, Kirk KA, Rutsky EA, et al. Racial differences in the incidence of treatment for end-stage renal disease. *N Engl J Med* 1982;306:1276–1279.
50. Ferguson R, Grim CE, Opgenorth TJ. The epidemiology of end-stage renal disease: the six-year South-Central Los Angeles experience, 1990–95. *Am J Pub Health* 1987;77:994–995.
51. Maxwell MH, Fitzsimmons E, Harrist R, et al. Baseline labora-

tory examination characteristics of the hypertensive participants. *Hypertension* 1983;5(Suppl 4):133–159.

52. Levy SB, Talner LB, Coel MN, et al. Renal vasculature in essential hypertension: racial differences. *Ann Intern Med* 1978;88:12–16.
53. Frohlich ED, Messerli FH, Dunn FG, et al. Greater renal vascular involvement in the black patient with essential hypertension. A comparison of systemic and renal hemodynamics in black and white patients. *Miner Electrolyte Metab* 1984;10:173–177.
54. Pitcock JA, Hohnson JG, Hatch RE, et al. Malignant hypertension in blacks. Malignant intrarenal arterial disease as observed by light and electron microscopy. *Human Pathol* 1976;7:333–346.
55. Cooper ES. Cerebrovascular disease in blacks. In: Hall WD, Saunders E, Shulman N, eds. *Hypertension in blacks.* Chicago: Yearbook Medical Publishers, 1985;83–105.
56. Resch JA. The epidemiology and geographic pathology of atherosclerotic cerebrovascular disease. *Curr Concepts Cerebrovasc Dis (Stroke)* 1970;5:33–37.
57. Williams AO, Resch JA, Loewenson RB. Cerebral atherosclerosis a comparative autopsy study between Nigerian Negroes and American Negroes and Caucasians. *Neurology* 1969;19:205–210.
58. Hypertension Detection and Followup Cooperative Group. Five year findings to the Hypertension Detection and Follow-up Program. III. Reduction in stroke incidence amount in persons with high blood pressure. *JAMA* 1982;247:633–638.
59. James SA. Psychosocial and environmental factors in black hypertension. In: Hall WD, Saunders E, Shulman N, eds. *Hypertension in blacks.* Chicago: Yearbook Medical Publishers, 1985;132–143.
60. Grim CE, Luft FC, Weinberger MH, et al. Genetic, familial and racial influences on blood pressure control systems in man. *Aust NZ J Med* 1984;14:453–457.
61. Langford HG, Langford FPJ, Tyler M. Dietary profile of sodium, potassium, and calcium in U.S. blacks. In: Hall WD, Saunders E, Shulman N, eds. *Hypertension in blacks.* Chicago: Yearbook Medical Publishers, 1985.

61a.Grim CE, Miller JZ, Luft FC, et al. Genetic influences on renin, aldosterone, and the excretion of sodium and potassium following volume expansion and contraction in normal man. *Hypertension* 1979;1:583–590.

61b.Luft FC, Rankin LI, Block R, et al. Cardiovascular and humoral responses to extremes of sodium intake in normal white and black men. *Circulation* 1979;60:697–706.

62. Grim CE, Luft FC, Miller JZ, et al. Racial differences in blood pressure in Evans County, Georgia: relationship to sodium and potassium intake and plasma renin activity. *J Chronic Dis* 1980;33:87–94.
63. Zinner SH, Margolius HS, Rosner B, et al. Familial aggregation of urinary kallikrein concentration in childhood: relation to blood pressure, race and urinary electrolytes. *Am J Epidemiol* 1976;104:124–132.
64. Levy SB, Frigon RF, Stone RA. Plasma dopamine-β-hydroxylase activity and blood pressure variability in hypertensive man. *Clin Endocrinol (Oxf)* 1979;11:187–199.
65. Miller JZ, Luft FC, Grim CE, et al. Genetic influences on plasma and urinary norepinephrine after volume expansion and contraction in normal man. *J Clin Endocrinol Metab* 1980;50:219–222.
66. Kotchen TA., Guthrie GP Jr. Renin–angiotensin–aldosterone and hypertension. *Endocr Rev* 1980;1:78–99.
67. Gillum RF. Pathophysiology of hypertension in blacks and whites: a review of the basis of racial blood pressure differences. *Hypertension* 1979;1:468–475.
68. Russell RP, Masi AT. Significant associations of adrenal cortical abnormalities with "essential" hypertension. *Am J Med* 1973;54:44.
69. James SA, Lacroix AZ, Kleinbaum DG, Strogatz DS. John Henryism and blood pressure differences among black men. II. The role of occupational stressors. *J Behav Med* 1984;7:259–75.
70. Harris W. *The harder we run: black workers since the Civil War.* New York: Oxford University Press, 1982.
71. Harburg E, Erfurt JC, Chape C, Hauenstein LS, Schull WJ, Schork MA. Socioecological stressor areas and black-white blood pressure: Detroit. *J Chronic Dis* 1973;26:595–611.
72. Harburg E, Erfurt JC, Hauenstein LS, Chape C, Schull WJ, Schork MA. Socioecological stress, suppressed hostility, skin color and black–white male blood pressure: Detroit. *Psychosom Med* 1973;35:276–296.
73. Harburg E, Gleibermann L, Roeper P, Schork MA. Schull WJ. Skin color, ethnicity, and blood pressure. I. Detroit blacks. *Am J Public Health* 1978;68:1177–1188.
74. James SA, Kleinbaum DG. Socioecologic stress and hypertension-related mortality rates in North Carolina. *Am J Public Health* 1976;66:354–358.
75. Neser WB, Tyroler HA, Cassel JC. Social disorganization and stroke mortality in the black population of North Carolina. *Am J Epidemiol* 1971;93:166–175.
76. Devereux RB, Pickering TG, Harshfield GA, Kleinert HD, Denby L, Clark L, Pregibon D, Jason M, Kleiner B, Borer JS, Laragh JH. Left ventricular hypertrophy in patients with hypertension: importance of blood pressure response to regularly occurring stress. *Circulation* 1983;68:470–476.
77. Guyton AC, Coleman TG, Cowley AW, Scheel KW, Manning RD Jr, Norman RA Jr. Arterial pressure regulation: overriding dominance of the kidneys in long-term regulation and in hypertension. *Am J Med* 1972;52:584–594.
78. Julius S. Transition from high cardiac output to elevated vascular resistance in hypertension. *Am Heart J* 1988;116:600–606.
79. Denton D. *Hunger for salt—an anthropological, physiological, and medical analysis.* Berlin:Springer-Verlag, 1982.
80. Grim CE, Harshfield GH, Savage DD, Anderson SJ, Hwang C. Genetic influences on blood pressure, body size, and left ventricular mass in blacks (Abstract). *Cardiovasc Epi Newsl,* 1987; 41:37.
81. Grim CE, Wilson TW. Blood pressure in blacks in Africa and in the western hemisphere: a metanalysis. Presented at: Proceedings, Fourth Conference of the International Society for Hypertension in Blacks, 1989.
82. McDonough JR, Garrison GE, Hames CG. Blood pressure and hypertensive disease among negroes and whites: a study in Evans County, Georgia. *Ann Intern Med* 1964;61:208–228.
83. Luft FC, Grim CE, Weinberger MH. Electrolyte and volume homeostasis in blacks. In: Hall WD, Saunders E, Shulman N, eds. *Hypertension in blacks.* Chicago: Yearbook Medical Publishers, 1985;115–131.
84. Weder AB. Red-cell lithium–sodium countertransport and renal lithium clearance in hypertension. *N Engl J Med* 1986;314:198–201.
85. Helmer OM. Renin activity in blood from patients with hypertension. *Can Med Assoc J* 1964;38:221–225.
86. Hohn AR, Piopel DA, Djeil JE, et al. Child familial and racial differences in physiologic and biochemical factors related to hypertension. *Hypertension* 1983;5:56–70.
87. Weder AB, Torretti BA, Julius S. Racial differences in erythrocyte cation transport. *Hypertension* 1984;6:115–123.
88. Schwab EH, Dolph L, Curb D, Matthews JL, Schultze DL. Blood pressure response to a standard stimulant in the white and Negro. *Proc Soc Exp Biol Med* 1935;32:583–585.
89. Falkner B, Kushner H, Onesti G, et al. Cardiovascular characteristics in adolescents who develop hypertension. *Hypertension* 1981;3:521–527.
90. Dimsdale JE, Graham RM, Ziegler MG, et al. Age, race, diagnosis, and sodium effects on the pressor response to infused norepinephrine. *Hypertension* 1987;10:564–569.
91. Berenson GS, Voors AW, Dalferes ER Jr. Creatinine clearance, electrolytes, and plasma renin activity related to blood pressure of white and black children—the Bogalusa Heart Study. *J Clin Med* 1979;93:535–548.
92. Miller JZ, Grim CE. Heritability of blood pressure. In: Kotchen TA, Kotchen JM, Wright J, eds. *High blood pressure in the young.* Boston: PSG, 1983;79–90.
93. Ganguly A, Grim CE, Bergstein J, et al. Genetic and pathophysiologic studies of a new kindred with glucocorticoid-suppressible hyperaldosteronism manifest in three generations. *J Clin Endocrinol Metab* 1981;53:1040–1046.
94. Miall WE, Kass EH, Ling J, et al. Factors influencing arterial pressure in the general population in Jamaica. *Br Med J* 1962;2:497–506.
95. Prineas RJ, Gillum RF, Gomez-Marin O. The determinant of blood pressure levels in children. In: Loggie JMH, Horan MJ,

Gruskin AB, et al, eds. *Workshop in juvenile hypertension.* New York: BMI, 1984.
96. Annest JL, Sing CF, Biron P, Mongeau JG. Familial aggregation of blood pressure and weight in adoptive families. II. estimation of the relative contributions of genetic and common environmental factors to blood pressure correlations between family members. *Am J Epidemiol* 1979;110:492–503.
97. Hutchinson J, Lin PM, Crawford MH. Factors influencing blood pressure level among the black caribs of St. Vincent Island. *Current Developments in Anthropological Genetics* 1984;3:215–239.
98. Cruze-Coke R, Covarrubias E. Blood pressure correlation between relatives in a endogamic population. *Acta Genet (Basel)* 1963;15:87–94.
99. Boyle E Jr. Biological patterns in hypertension by race, sex, body weight, and skin color. *JAMA* 1970;213:1637–1643.
100. Harburg E, Gleibermann L, Roeper P, et al. Skin color, ethnicity, and blood pressure. I. Detroit blacks. *Am J Public Health* 1978;68:1177–1188.
101. Keil JE. Skin color and education effects on blood pressure. *Am J Public Health* 1981;68:532–534.
102. Webber LS, Cresanta JL, Voors AW, Berenson GS. Tracking of cardiovascular disease risk factors variables in school-aged children. *J Chronic Dis* 1983;36:647–660.
103. Lauer RM, Clarke WR, Beaglehole R. Level, trend, and variability of blood pressure during childhood: the Muscatine Study. *Circulation* 1984;69:242–249.
104. Gordon T, Shurtleff D. *The Framingham Study: an epidemiologic investigation of cardiovascular disease.* DHEW Publication No. (NIH) 74-478, Section 29. Washington, DC: US Government Printing Office.
105. Heyden S, Bartel AG, Hames CG, McDonough JR. Elevated blood pressure levels in adolescents, Evans County, Georgia: seven-year follow-up of 30 patients and 30 controls. *JAMA* 1969;209:1683–1689.
106. Hayes CG, Tyroler HA, Cassel JC. Familial aggregation of blood pressure in Evans County, Georgia. *Arch Intern Med* 1971;128:965–975.
107. Schneckloth RE, Corcoran AC, Stuart KL, et al. Arterial pressure and hypertensive disease in a West Indian Negro population: Report of a survey in St. Kitts, West Indies. *Am Heart J* 1962;63:607–628.
108. Johnson BC, Remington RD. A sampling study of blood pressure levels in white and negro residents of Nassau, Bahamas. *J Chronic Dis* 1961;13:39–51.
109. Grim CE. On slavery, salt and the higher blood pressure in black Americans. *Clin Res* 1988;36:426A.
110. Galenson DW. *Traders, planters and slaves. Market behavior in early English America.* Cambridge: Cambridge University Press, 1986.
111. Engerman SL, Genovese ED. *Race and slavery in the Western Hemisphere: quantitative studies.* Princeton, NJ: Princeton University Press, 1975.
112. Harris JE. *Africans and their history.* New York: Mentor, NAL Penguin, 1987.
113. Franklin JH. *From slavery to freedom: a history of Negro Americans.* New York: Knopf, 1980.
114. *Human cargoes: the British slave trade to Spanish America, 1700–1739.* Urbana: University of Illinois Press, 1981.
115. Rawley JA. *The transatlantic slave trade: a history.* New York: WW Norton, 1981.
116. Hypertension Detection and Follow-up Cooperative Group. Five-year findings of the Hypertension Detection and Follow-up Program. II. Mortality by race–sex and age. *JAMA* 1979;242:2572–2577.
117. Hall D. Pharmacologic therapy of hypertension in blacks. In: Hall WD, Saunders E, Shulman NB, eds. *Hypertension in blacks: epidemiology, pathophysiology and treatment.* Chicago: Year Book Medical Publishers, 1985;182–208.
118. Amery A, Bulpitt C, Fagard R, et al. Does diet matter in hypertension? *Eur Heart J* 1980;1:299–308.
119. Kumanyika SK, Charleston J. A church-based weight loss program for blood pressure control among black women. Presented at: Proceedings of the National High Blood Pressure Control Conference, 1987.
120. MacGregor GA, Smith SJ, Markandu ND, Banks RA, Sagnella GA. Moderate potassium supplementation in essential hypertension *Lancet* 1982;2:567–570.
121. Klasky AL, Friedman GD, Siegelaub AB, Gerard MJ. Alcohol consumption and blood pressure: Kaiser–Permanente Multiphasic Health Examination data. *N Engl J Med* 1977;296:1194–1200.
122. Joint National Committee on Detection, Evaluation, and Treatment of High Blood Pressure. The 1988 report of the Joint National Committee on Detection, Evaluation, and Treatment of High Blood Pressure. *Arch Intern Med* 1988;148:1023–1038.
123. Shulman NB, Martinez B, Brogan D, et al. Financial cost as an obstacle to hypertension therapy. *Am J Public Health* 1986;76:1105–1108.
124. Hall WD. Hypertension in blacks: rationale for pharmacologic therapy. *J Natl Med Assoc* 1988;80(Suppl):17–22.
125. Veterans Administration Cooperative Study Group on Antihypertensive Agents. Comparison of propranolol and hydrochlorothiazide for the initial treatment of hypertension. I. Results of short-term titration with emphasis on racial differences in response. *JAMA* 1982;248:1996–2003.
126. Moser M, Lunn J, Materson BJ, et al. Comparative effects of diltiazem and hydrochlorothiazide in blacks with systemic hypertension. *Am J Cardiol* 1985;56:101H–104H.
127. Fadayomi MD, Akinroye KK, Ajao RD, et al. Monotherapy with nifedipine for essential hypertension in adult blacks. *J Cardiovasc Pharmacol* 1986;8:466–469.
128. Multiple Risk Factor Intervention Trial Research Group. Multiple Risk Factor Intervention Trial: Risk Factor changes and mortality results. *JAMA* 1982;248:1465–1477.
129. Hypertension Detection and Follow-up Program Cooperative Research Group. The effect of antihypertensive drug treatment on mortality in the presence of resting electrocardiographic abnormalities at baseline; the HDFP experience. *Circulation* 1984;70:996–1003.
130. Cubeddu LX, Aranda J, Singh B, et al. A comparison of verapamil and propranolol for the initial treatment of hypertension. Racial differences in response. *JAMA* 1986;256:2214–2221.
131. Massie B, McCarthy P, Romanatha K, et al. Diltiazem and propranolol in mild to moderate hypertension as monotherapy or with hydrochlorothiazide. *Ann Intern Med* 1987;107:150–157.
132. Mohanty PK, Sowers JR, Thames MD. Effects of hydrochlorothiazide and diltiazem on reflex vasoconstriction in hypertension. *Hypertension* 1987;10:35–42.
133. Flamenbaum W, Weber MA, McMahon FG, et al. Monotherapy with labetalol compared with propranolol: differential effects by race. *J Clin Hypertens* 1985;1:56–69.
134. Veterans Administration Cooperative Study Group on Antihypertensive Agents. Comparison of propranolol and hydrochlorothiazide for the initial treatment of hypertension. II. Results of long-term therapy. *JAMA* 1982;248:2004–2011.
135. Plotnick GD, Fisher ML, Wohl B, et al. Improvement in depressed cardiac function in hypertensive patients during pindolol treatment. *Am J Med* 1984;76:25–30.
136. Veterans Administration Cooperative Study Group on Antihypertensive Agents. Racial differences in response to low-dose captopril are abolished by the addition of hydrochlorothiazide. *Br J Clin Pharmacol* 1982;14(Suppl 2):97–101.
137. Wilkins LH, Dustan HP, Walker JF, et al. Enalapril in low-renin essential hypertension. *Clin Pharmacol Ther* 1983;34:297–302.
138. Weed SG, Reisin E, Robie NW, et al. Enalapril and hydrochlorothiazide in the treatment of essential hypertensive black patients [Abstract]. *Clin Res* 1983;31:878A.
139. Weinberger MH, Fineberg NS. Variables predicting blood pressure response to enalapril. *Clin Pharmacol Ther* 1984;35:281.
140. Mroczek WJ, Fotin S, Davidov ME, et al. Prazosin in hypertension: a double-blind evaluation with methyldopa and placebo. *Curr Ther Res* 1974;16:769–777.
141. Falase AO, Salako LA, Aminu JM, et al. Lack of effect of low doses of prazosin in hypertensive Nigerians. *Curr Ther Res* 1976;19:603–611.
142. Inouye I, Massie B, Benowitz N, et al. Monotherapy in mild to moderate hypertension: comparison of hydrochlorothiazide, propranolol and prazosin. *Am J Cardiol* 1984;53:24A–28A.
143. Warren SE, O'Conner DT. Does a renal vasodilator system medi-

ate racial differences in essential hypertension? *Am J Med* 1980;69:425–429.

144. Warren SE, O'Conner DT, Cervenka J. Racial differences during chronic prazosin (PZN) therapy of hypertension [Abstract]. *Am Soc Nephrol Abstracts* 1980:70A.
145. Kirkendall WM, Hammond JJ, Thomas JC, et al. Prazosin and clonidine for moderately severe hypertension. *JAMA* 1978; 240:2553–2556.
146. Graham RM. Selective alpha$_1$-adrenergic antagonists: Therapeutically relevant antihypertensive agents. *Am J Cardiol* 1984;53:16A–20A.
147. Kochar MS, Kalbfleisch JH, Blumenthal SS, et al. Prazosin versus propranolol plus prazosin: a comparison in diuretic-treated patients. *Am J Cardiol* 1984;53:55A–58A.
148. Veterans Administration Cooperative Study Group on Antihypertensive Agents. Comparison of prazosin with hydralazine in patients receiving hydrochlorothiazide. A randomized, double-blind clinical trial. *Circulation* 1981;64:772–779.
149. Perry HM Jr, Tan EM, Carmody S, et al. A relationship of acetyl transferase activity to antinuclear antibodies and toxic symptoms in hypertensive patients treated with hydralazine. *J Lab Clin Med* 1970;76:114–125.
150. Condemi JJ, Moore-Jones D, Vaughan JH, et al. Antinuclear antibodies following hydralazine toxicity. *N Engl J Med* 1967;276:486–491.
151. Hahn BH, Sharp GC, Irvin WS, et al. Immune responses to hydralazine and nuclear antigens in hydralazine-induced lupus erythematosus. *Ann Intern Med* 1972;76:365–374.
152. Hess EV, Litwin A, Foad BSI. Hydralazine therapy in idiopathic SLE [Letter]. *Arthritis Rheum* 1976;19:122–123.
153. Okanga JBO. Atenolol (Tenormin) compared with methyldopa (Aldomet) in the treatment of hypertension. *East Afr Med J* 1978;55:447–452.
154. Olatunde A, Aderounmu AF, Nbanefo CN, et al. A comparative double blind clinical trial of atenolol and methyldopa in the outpatients treatment of hypertension. *Trop Cardiol* 1979;5:143–151.
155. Wood M, Hall WD, Wollam GL, et al. Response rate of black hypertensives to methyldopa monotherapy over a twelve-month treatment period [Abstract]. *Clin Res* 1983;31:845A.
156. Yeh BK, Nantel A, Goldberg LI. Antihypertensive effect of clonidine: Its use alone and in combination with hydrochlorothiazide and guanethidine in the treatment of hypertension. *Arch Intern Med* 1971;127:233–237.
157. Onesti G, Schwartz AB, Kim KE, et al. Pharmacodynamic effects of a new antihypertensive drug, Catapres (ST-155). *Circulation* 1969;39:219–228.
158. Jain AK, Ryan JR, Vargos R, et al. Efficacy and acceptability of different dosage schedules of clonidine. *Clin Pharmacol* 1977;21:382–387.
159. Anderson RJ, Harg GR, Crumpler CP, et al. Oral clonidine loading in hypertensive urgencies. *JAMA* 1981;246:848–850.
160. Walker BR, Deitch MW, Schneider BE, et al. Comparative antihypertensive effects of guanabenz and methyldopa. *Clin Ther* 1981;4:275–284.
161. Walker BR, Hare LE, Deitch MW. Comparative antihypertensive effects of guanabenz and clonidine. *J Int Med Res* 1982;10:6–14.
162. Garratty G, Petz LD. *The investigation of drug-induced problems in the blood bank.* Washington, DC: American Association of Blood Banks, 1977;10.
163. Perry HM Jr, Chaplin H Jr, Carmody S, et al. Immunologic findings in patients receiving methyldopa: a prospective study. *J Lab Clin Med* 1971;78:905–917.
164. Grell GAC, Wilson WA, James O. Prevalence of drug-induced immunologic changes in hypertensive Jamaicans. *South Med J* 1980;73:1044–1045.
165. Brechenridge A, Dollery CT, Worlledge SM, et al. Positive direct Coombs' tests and antinuclear factor in patients treated with methyldopa. *Lancet* 1967;2:1265–1268.
166. Patel R, Johnson J, Ansari A. Immunogenetic studies in essential hypertension among black patients: correlative studies of serum autoantibody formation. *Int Arch Allergy Appl Immunol* 1982;67:145–148.
167. Talso PJ, Carballo AJ. Polythiazide in the management of hypertensive disease. II. Comparison of the effects of polythiazide and reserpine in the management of hypertension in ambulatory patients. *Curr Ther Res* 1974;6:169–179.
168. Smith WM, Bachman B, Galante JG, et al. Cooperative clinical trial of alpha-methyldopa. III. Double-blind control comparison of alpha-methyldopa and chlorothiazide, and chlorothiazide and rauwolfia. *Ann Intern Med* 1966;65:657–671.

Hypertension: Pathophysiology, Diagnosis, and Management, edited by J. H. Laragh and B. M. Brenner. Raven Press, Ltd., New York © 1990.

CHAPTER 115

Childhood Hypertension

Alan R. Sinaiko and Thomas G. Wells

Measurement of Blood Pressure in Children, 1854
Natural History of Blood Pressure in Children, 1854
Normal Blood Pressure, 1854
Blood Pressure Tracking in Children, 1856
Other Factors Influencing Blood Pressure in Children, 1858
Hypertension, 1859
Definition and Prevalence, 1859
Causes of Hypertension, 1860
Evaluation of the Hypertensive Child, 1863
Treatment of Childhood Hypertension, 1864
Nonpharmacologic Therapy, 1864
Antihypertensive Drug Therapy, 1865
References, 1865

Measurement of blood pressure in children has been an integral component of the pediatric physical examination for only two decades. Historically, hypertension was considered to be a disease of adults. It was rarely diagnosed in children and, when found, was almost always associated with some other primary condition, such as renal parenchymal disease, renal artery stenosis, or coarctation of the aorta (1). Reliable blood pressure distribution curves for children were not available, and adult reference standards were used to categorize childhood blood pressure. As a consequence, hypertension was rarely diagnosed, and only the most severe cases were recognized.

Hypertension as a health care concern in children began to surface in the 1960s (2). Shortly thereafter, comprehensive data from large-scale epidemiologic studies of blood pressure in children began to appear and established that mild hypertension is more common than previously acknowledged during childhood, particularly in adolescents (3–6). The 1977 NIH Task Force on Blood Pressure Control in Children was organized in response to the many questions raised by these studies. The report of this Task Force (7) did the following: (a) It established blood pressure measurement as a part of the routine pediatric examination and set standards for normal blood pressure distribution; (b) it defined hypertension as blood pressure greater than the 95th percentile of distribution for age and sex; and (c) it provided guidelines for evaluation and treatment of hypertensive children. The Second Task Force on Blood Pressure Control in Children—1987 (8) accomplished the following: (a) It evaluated new information published following the 1977 report; (b) it incorporated additional epidemiologic data on the distribution and natural history of blood pressure in children into more accurate normal standards; and (c) it refined previous definitions and recommendations to firmly reinforce the importance of blood pressure measurement in pediatrics.

The following generalizations have not changed over the years: (a) Blood pressure is lower in children than in adults but increases gradually throughout the first and second decades of life; (b) the diagnosis of hypertension in children is made at levels of blood pressure considerably lower than in adults; and (c) when hypertension at a level high enough to require antihypertensive therapy occurs in children, it is usually secondary in nature (i.e., the result of some identifiable cause such as renal disease, renal artery stenosis, etc.). However, there has been a change in the focus of interest in childhood blood pressure: It has gone from one of diagnosis and treatment of secondary hypertension to one of early identification of children with essential hypertension. Although the prevalence of hypertension is much lower in children than in adults, there is now highly persuasive evidence from familial and longitudinal studies that factors influencing the development of hypertension are operative during the childhood years. The challenge will be to isolate these factors and design intervention strategies that can be introduced safely early in life to reduce the high prevalence of adult hypertension.

Other chapters in this book are devoted to specific diseases, physiologic systems, classes of drug, etc., relating to hypertension. Consequently, these topics will be addressed in the present chapter only as they relate to childhood issues of blood pressure and hypertension. Normal blood pressure and the natural history of blood pressure during childhood and adolescence will be discussed. Hypertension will be presented according to age, etiology, diagnostic evaluation, and treatment. It is anticipated that the reader will gain an appreciation of the relevance of childhood blood pressure to cardiovascular risk, similar to its status in adults.

MEASUREMENT OF BLOOD PRESSURE IN CHILDREN

Blood pressure should be measured in children once each year after the age of 3 years, as recommended by the American Academy of Pediatrics (9) and the Task Force on Blood Pressure Control in Children (8). The basic methodology and instrumentation for blood pressure measurement is the same in children as in adults. However, there are certain factors unique to the pediatric blood pressure examination.

First, blood pressure measurement by conventional auscultation, while quite reliable in older children, is almost always impractical in children less than 3 years of age. This is due to the practical problem of keeping the infant and young child quiet and free from anxiety. Infant blood pressure was formerly measured by the "flush" method (10), in which the blood pressure cuff is inflated while blood drains from the limb distal to the cuff. The cuff is then deflated slowly, and blood pressure is defined as the point at which a flush of color is noted. The flush method is less accurate because of its subjectivity, and it is a measure of mean blood pressure. Rarely, if ever, is there any indication for its use.

Doppler and oscillometric automatic devices have been widely used in children, but the Doppler appears to be less accurate. The correlation coefficient between Doppler and simultaneously obtained intra-arterial measurements is 0.8 for systolic and 0.7 for diastolic blood pressure (11). The intra-arterial–oscillometric correlation is 0.97 for systolic and 0.9 for diastolic blood pressure (12). The accuracy of oscillometric devices is inversely correlated with infant size, and, in general, measurements in premature infants are not as well correlated to intra-arterial measurements as observed in older children (13).

Second, appropriate blood pressure cuff size is crucial for accurate blood pressure measurements. The blood pressure cuff (i.e., bladder) should be (a) long enough to completely encircle the upper arm and (b) wide enough to cover at least 75–80% of the arm between the antecubital fossa and axilla. Currently manufactured cuffs have been designed so that use of either circumference or width will provide the correct size. Occasionally, the widths of two adjacent-sized cuffs will both be close to the measured width of the arm. In that case, the cuff with the larger width should be used. A small cuff will cause inaccurately high readings, whereas use of a cuff slightly larger than suggested by the upper arm measurement rarely will lower blood pressure enough to prevent the recognition of true hypertension.

Third, diastolic blood pressure is recorded differently in children than in adults. In children 12 years of age and younger, it is defined as the fourth Korotkoff phase (D4); however, in children 13 years of age and older, the fifth Korotkoff phase (D5) is used (8). These recommendations are based on clinical experience recognizing that (a) D5 may not be present in infants and children (i.e., blood pressure sounds heard all the way to 0 mmHg), and (b) blood pressure measurement in larger children and adolescents is similar to, and should be evaluated in the same context as, that of adults.

TABLE 1. *Distribution of the difference between fourth-phase (D4) and fifth-phase (D5) diastolic blood pressures for 19,274 5th- to 8th-grade students in Minneapolis and St. Paul*[a]

Difference between D4 and D5 (mmHg)	N	%
0	9,682	50
1–4	2,837	15
5–10	3,908	20
11–77	2,847	15
Totals:	19,274	100

[a] From A. R. Sinaiko, O. Gomez-Marin, and R. P. Prineas. The Children and Adolescent Blood Pressure Program, *unpublished data.*

The use of D4 or D5 to define diastolic blood pressure has been a source of conflict in pediatrics (14,15). Neither of the Korotkoff phases represents true intra-arterial diastolic blood pressure in children, with D4 tending to be higher and D5 lower (16). An evaluation of D4 and D5 from a recent blood pressure screening of school children (Table 1) confirmed that there are substantial differences between D4 and D5. D4–D5 differences of 5 mmHg or greater were found in 20% of these children, and differences of 10 mmHg or greater were detected in another 15%. Because standard diastolic reference data published by the 1987 Task Force (see next section) use only D4 or D5, depending on age, the incorrect choice of D4 or D5 for diastolic blood pressure can have a potentially significant effect on the diagnosis of diastolic hypertension. When data from the above screening were analyzed according to Task Force criteria, the prevalence of significant diastolic hypertension varied by 2–3%, depending on whether D4 or D5 was used.

NATURAL HISTORY OF BLOOD PRESSURE IN CHILDREN

Normal Blood Pressure

Blood pressure in children is directly correlated with age from infancy through the second decade of life, and it appears to be directly correlated with gestational development in the premature newborn. The normal, healthy, full-term newborn has a systolic blood pressure of 60 mmHg and a diastolic blood pressure of 40 mmHg at birth. The adjustment to extrauterine life is characterized by a gradual increase in blood pressure during the first few hours after birth (17).

Data from the 1987 Task Force blood pressure curves (Figs. 1 and 2) show that systolic and diastolic blood pressure follow separate patterns during the first year of life. Systolic blood pressure increases on a daily basis the first week after birth (Table 2) and then increases more slowly until 2 months of age (18,19). From 2 to 12 months of age, systolic blood pressure remains stable. Diastolic blood

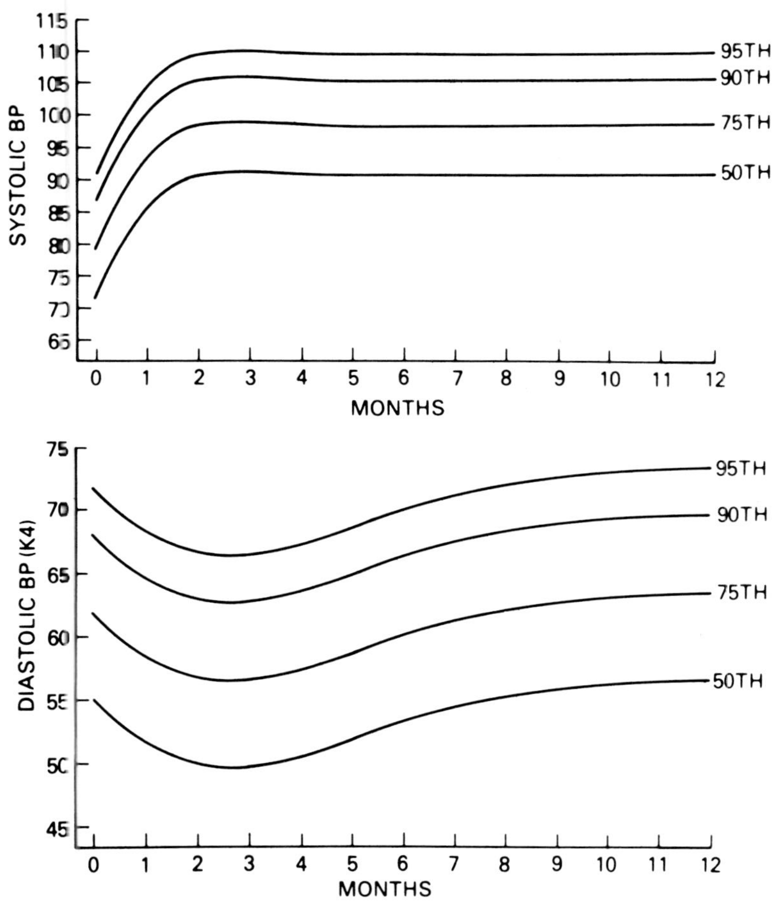

FIG. 1. Age-specific percentiles of blood pressure measurements in boys, birth to 12 months. (From ref. 8.)

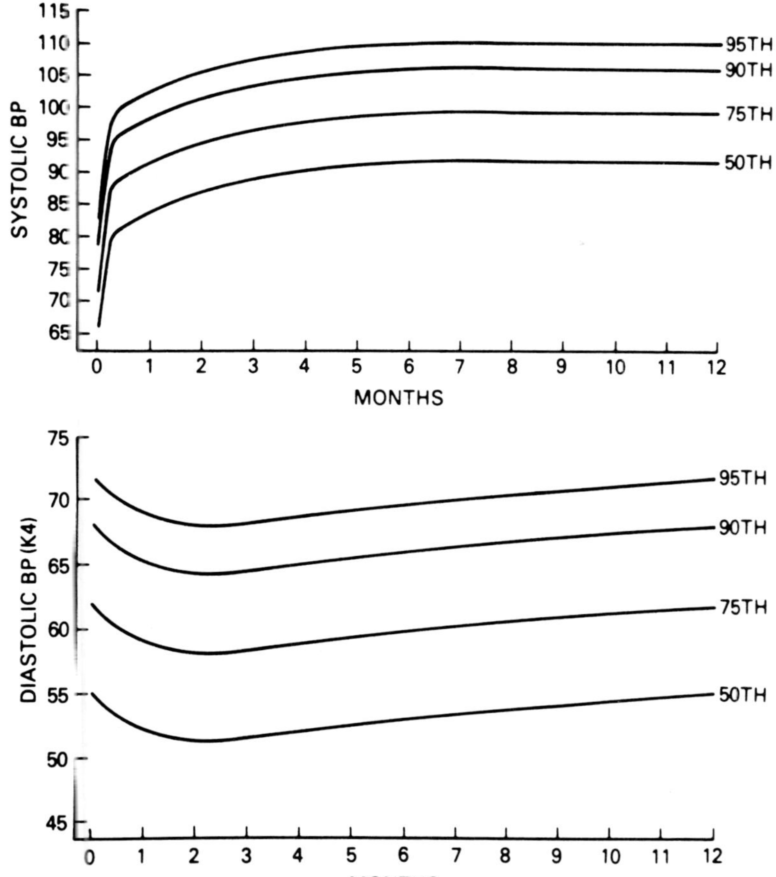

FIG. 2. Age-specific percentiles of blood pressure measurements in girls, birth to 12 months. (From ref. 8.)

TABLE 2. *Blood pressure (mean ± SD) during the first month of life*[a]

Age	Blood pressure (mmHg) Systolic	Diastolic
1 day	65 ± 6	48 ± 6
2 days	68 ± 6	50 ± 6
3 days	72 ± 7	53 ± 8
4 days	75 ± 8	56 ± 8
5 days	77 ± 10	55 ± 10
6 days	77 ± 10	55 ± 10
1 week	79 ± 10	55 ± 10
2 weeks	80 ± 10	50 ± 8
1 month	85 ± 10	46 ± 9

[a] Data from AR Sinaiko and from refs. 18 and 19.

pressure increases slightly during the first week of life and then declines steadily to reach a nadir at approximately 2–3 months. For the remainder of the first year, it increases slowly; however, it never exceeds the 1-week level.

Systolic blood pressure increases at a relatively steady rate from 1 year of age through adolescence (Fig. 3). There is very little change in diastolic blood pressure until 5–6 years of age; at that age it begins a gradual ascent, in parallel to systolic blood pressure. The developmental factors influencing the variability between systolic and diastolic blood pressure and in rates of change during childhood remain a mystery.

There are few published data on normal blood pressure in premature infants, primarily because most prematures are treated with volume expansion, pharmacologic agents, and/or respiratory support and are not in a basal physiologic condition. Nevertheless, it is clear that blood pressure in premature infants is even lower than that of full-term infants and is directly related to body weight and gestational age (20–22).

The data base for premature infant blood pressure is derived from direct arterial measurements. Systolic and diastolic blood pressure during the first 12 hr of life are correlated with both birth weight (20,21) and gestational age (20,22). However, body weight appears to be the better standard in small-for-gestational-age infants (20). Figure 4 represents approximate normal standards for blood pressure in infants during the first 12 hr of life, regardless of gestational age, based on birth weight.

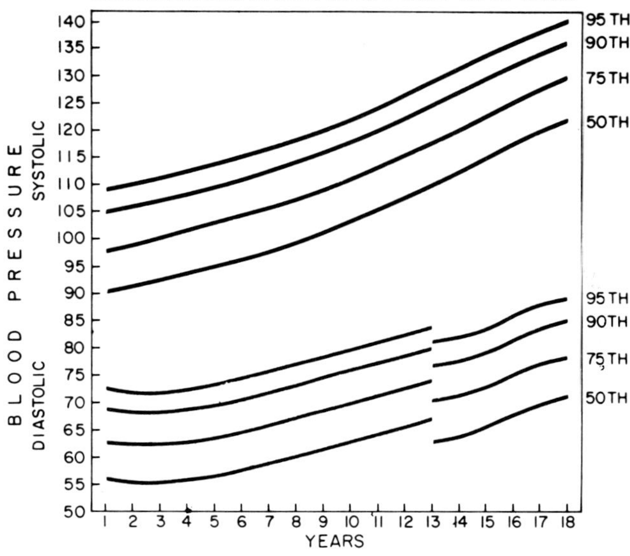

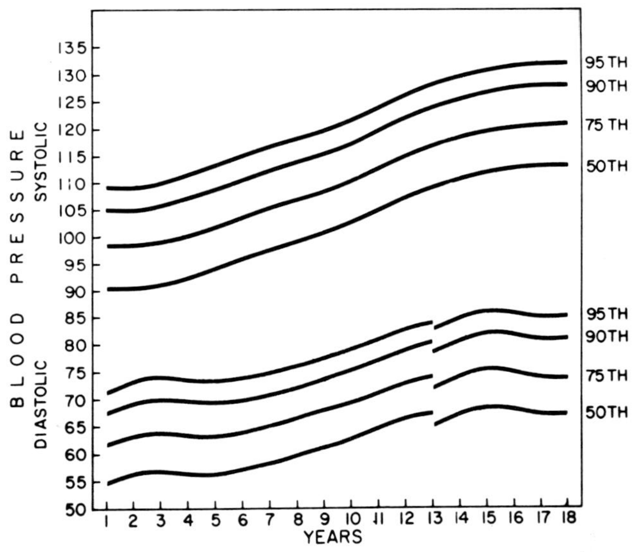

FIG. 3. Age-specific percentiles of blood pressure measurements in boys (**top**) and girls (**bottom**) aged 1 year to 18 years. The interruption in the diastolic blood pressure curves at age 13 is due to the use of the 4th Korotkoff phase (D4) to define diastolic blood in children ≤12 years and the 5th Korotkoff phase to define diastolic blood pressure in children ≥13 years. (Adapted from ref. 8.)

Blood Pressure Tracking in Children

"Tracking" refers to the tendency of children at a given percentile of blood pressure distribution to maintain that percentile relative to their peer group as they grow older. As an example, a child with a systolic blood pressure of 107 mmHg at age 5 and 120 mmHg at age 12 is tracking at a high-normal level of systolic blood pressure. The tracking phenomenon has been clearly established during childhood; however, the crucial piece of data linking tracking during childhood and adolescence with hypertension in adulthood has not been provided.

Tracking begins at some point during the first year of life. Newborn blood pressures are not significantly correlated (14,23) with measurements taken at a variety of ages during the first 2 years of life. However, beginning at 6 months of age, systolic blood pressure is correlated significantly with blood pressure measured over the ensuing 7 years (19,23,24). Diastolic blood pressure does not show a significant tracking pattern during this stage of development (24).

A number of analytical methodologies have been used to

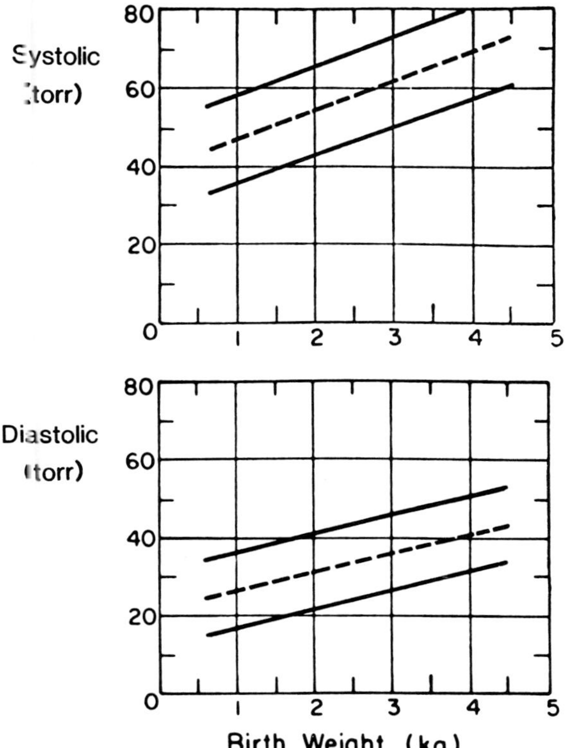

FIG. 4. Linear regression (*broken lines*) and 95% confidence limits (*solid lines*) of systolic (**top**) and diastolic (**bottom**) aortic blood pressures based on birth weight during the first 12 hr of life. (From ref. 20.)

evaluate tracking in older children. There is a high degree of variability between studies that may be accounted for by differences in the precision of blood pressure measurement, differences in sample size, age of the children, and duration of longitudinal blood pressure evaluation. In particular, the frequency of blood pressure measurement over the course of the study may be an important factor in the tracking analysis (25,26).

Correlation coefficients are probably the simplest measure of tracking over time. Regression analyses between baseline blood pressure and blood pressure at some later age show uniformly positive correlations, ranging from 0.30 to 0.66 for systolic and 0.12 to 0.57 for diastolic blood pressure (as summarized in ref. 25). The correlations are higher for systolic blood pressure, and there is a greater variability for diastolic blood pressure (D4 or D5).

Tracking can be demonstrated by examining changes in quartile or quintile distribution of blood pressure over time. In the U.S. Health Examination Surveys of children 6–12 years old (27), 41% of children in the lowest blood pressure quintile in 1963–1965 remained in the lowest quintile; another 27% had increased only to the next highest quintile at the second survey 3–4 years later. Conversely, of children in the highest quintile in 1963–1965, 45% remained in that quintile and 22% had fallen only to quintile 4 at the second survey. Almost identical data have come from the Minneapolis Children's Blood Pressure Study (25), in which 55% of children in the highest quartile at age 6–8 remained in the top quartile at ages 11–13 (i.e., after 5 years of follow-up), and from the Bogalusa Heart Study (26), in which 68% of children with three serial blood pressure measurements in the highest quartile during the 8-year longitudinal evaluation remained in the highest quartile at the end of the study.

Tracking has also been evaluated by dividing children into two cohorts (high and low blood pressure) and following their progress longitudinally with a series of blood pressure measurements (28). As seen in Fig. 5, tracking patterns are similar for the two cohorts. The mean blood pressures parallel one another but remain significantly different at each screening. Similar (but even more striking) differences

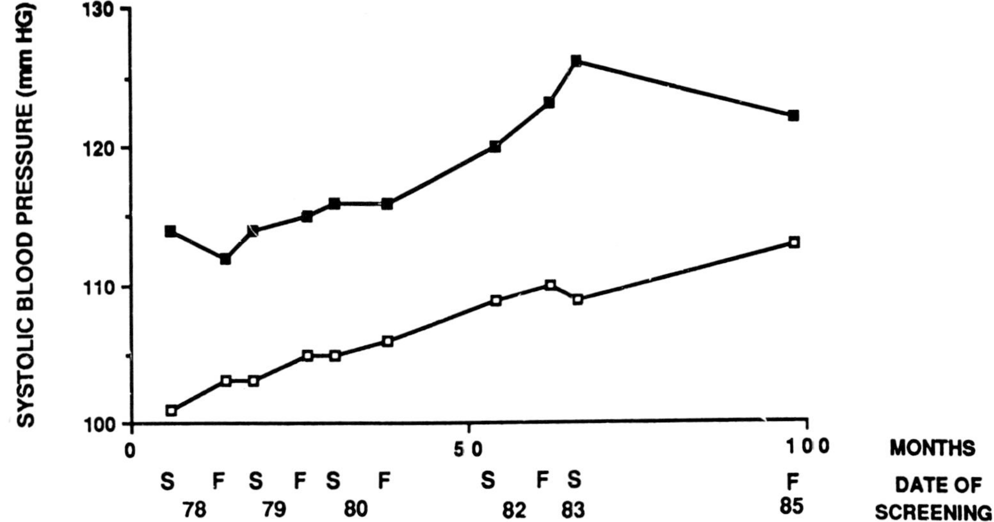

FIG. 5. Blood pressure tracking in two cohorts of children ($N = 630$) selected on the basis of systolic blood pressure ≥120 mmHg (■) or <120 mmHg (□) in the spring of 1983. Each box represents the group mean at the respective screening. S, spring; F, fall. The children were in grades 1, 2, and 3 at the first screening (spring, 1978) and grades 8, 9, and 10 at the 15th screening (fall, 1985). (Adapted from R. J. Prineas and O. Gomez-Marin. The Minneapolis Children's Blood Pressure Program, *unpublished data*.)

were observed in small cohorts of students in the Minneapolis study selected from the upper 1 percentile and lowest 5 percentiles at the first screening (29). After 7 years of evaluation with twice-yearly blood pressure measurements, the mean percentile distribution of the high blood pressure group fell from the 99th only to the 89th percentile, whereas the mean percentile distribution of the low blood pressure group increased from the 5th only to the 28th percentile.

Factors known to influence blood pressure also have an affect on tracking. The quintile of systolic blood pressure distribution after 5 years of observation is significantly correlated not only with the initial systolic blood pressure but also with height, weight, pulse rate, and maternal systolic blood pressure (30). In a unique analysis of tracking, blood pressure was examined according to the trend of change and variability over time (31). Using this methodology, approximately 12% of children are tracking toward future high blood pressure, because they have either a high percentile rank of blood pressure distribution at each examination or a persistent upward trend in their percentile distribution. Level and trend of blood pressure also were closely related to level and trend of body size measurements. Thus, blood pressure tracking is not an isolated phenomenon. It represents the integrated effect of body size, family history, race, and other factors known to influence blood pressure.

Other Factors Influencing Blood Pressure in Children

Race

Differences in blood pressure between blacks and whites are not pronounced during childhood and adolescence. There are some conflicting data from childhood epidemiologic studies, but differences between races are minor until sometime in the second decade. Blood pressure in blacks and whites is similar from birth through the first 2 years of life (23,32). There is general unanimity that blood pressure does not differ significantly between black and white older children and adolescents (5,6,33). In particular, racial differences were not noted in the nine studies used to compile the Task Force graphs (8). However, there are exceptions. In the Bogalusa Study of children 5–14 years old, blacks had significantly higher blood pressure when the analysis was limited to children from the upper 5 percentiles of distribution (5); and in a Houston study of children aged 3–17 years, whites had low systolic and diastolic blood pressure, even after adjustments were made for body size (34).

Other ethnic groups have not been studied as thoroughly. Blood pressure in Mexican-American children is similar to that in whites (33,34). Blood pressure of Southeast Asian children is significantly higher than that in white and black children, and these differences become more significant when blood pressure is adjusted for body size (R. Munger, O. Gomez-Marin, R. P. Prineas, and A. R. Sinaiko. The Children and Adolescent Blood Pressure Program, *unpublished data*).

Family History

Genetic factors begin to influence blood pressure at birth, if not earlier. Both systolic and diastolic blood pressures in mothers and their newborns are significantly correlated (19). This relationship, which is not found in father–infant pairs, is maintained between the mothers and infants through the first 2 years of life, during which time significant correlations are also found between infant and sibling blood pressures. Familial aggregation of blood pressure has also been used to document the genetic influence on blood pressure. In 6- to 18-year-old children from 163 separate families, the variance of blood pressure within families is significantly less than the variance observed when all children are studied together (35).

Studying families with both nonbiologic (or adopted) and biologic children offers the opportunity to investigate genetic influences under controlled environmental conditions. Correlations in these families are many times lower between parents and their adopted children than between the same parents and their biological children (36). Similar relationships were observed between parents and children in the Minneapolis study (25).

Children with normal blood pressure, but at the upper percentiles of distribution, tend to have parents with established hypertension or other forms of cardiovascular disease (26,30). This relationship can be identified in early childhood. A striking difference in family history was recorded between 8- and 9-year-old children selected from the upper 0.26% and lower 5% of blood pressure distribution (37). The high blood pressure group had a history of hypertension, stroke, or heart disease in 40% of first-degree family relatives, whereas only 18% of the low blood pressure group had a similar family history.

Body Size

Body size is the major factor accounting for blood pressure variability among children, but this relationship is not firmly established until the early grade-school years. There is a very low correlation between blood pressure and height, weight, body mass index, and body surface area during the first year of life (23). These correlations do not change appreciably during the pre-school years, a developmental period when blood pressure plateaus while body growth continues at a steady rate.

The positive relationship between body size and blood pressure is established by age 6 (25), and the two parallel one another thereafter (8,27,30,31). Not all overweight children will become hypertensive. Nevertheless, as one moves toward the extremes of the blood pressure distribution, the relationship becomes more pronounced. Average weight differences between 8- and 9-year-old children from the upper 0.26% and lower 5% of the blood pressure distribution have been reported to be 15.6 kg (37). Percent overweight in adolescents is correlated significantly with systolic and diastolic blood pressure (r = 0.64 and 0.41, respectively) (38), and systolic and diastolic blood pressure distributions in obese adolescents are skewed greater than 1 standard deviation to the right when compared to normal blood pressure distributions (39).

It is not clear whether fatness has an independent role in childhood hypertension. A small but significant correlation has been shown between central body fat (determined by subscapular skinfold measurements) and blood pressure (40). Data from the Health Examination Survey (41) suggest that weight–blood-pressure relationships are not related to fat but, instead, to other components of body mass.

Sex

Blood pressure in boys is virtually identical to that in girls during childhood (Fig. 3), and significant differences do not become apparent until the teenage years. Systolic blood pressure is significantly higher in teenage boys (33), and diastolic blood pressure tends to be significantly higher in girls in early adolescence. However, between the ages of 13 and 18, diastolic blood pressure also becomes significantly higher in boys. Attempts have been made to correlate the degree of sexual development with the level of blood pressure (27), but the reliability of this type of analysis is open to question. There is a confounding effect of growth and body size on sexual maturity. Moreover, blood pressure is independent of objective indicators of sexual development, such as serum follicle-stimulating hormone or luteinizing hormone (42).

HYPERTENSION

Definition and Prevalence

Childhood hypertension, with all the clinical and prognostic cardiovascular implications attributable to hypertension in adults, occurs at some upper level of blood pressure distribution. However, unlike the situation in adults in which natural history studies and therapeutic clinical trials have established prevalence and risk according to incremental changes in blood pressure, long-term experience on risk and outcome in children is not available. Current definitions of hypertension, as well as recommendations for evaluation and therapy, are based on clinical experience and limited published data (7,8). At the present time, the consensus report from the 1987 Task Force (8) is the acknowledged reference source for childhood and adolescent hypertension.

A major contribution of the 1977 Task Force (7) was its definition of hypertension as blood pressure equal to or greater than the 95th percentile of distribution for sex and age. This definition was reaffirmed in the 1987 report (8), and a new category of "high-normal" blood pressure was established to ensure that children with blood pressure at the upper end of the distribution have careful longitudinal evaluation (Table 3). A great deal of controversy continues to surround diagnosis, evaluation, and intervention in mild to moderate hypertension. Far fewer than 5% of children will be hypertensive, and fewer than 1% will ultimately require evaluation and treatment.

TABLE 3. *Definitions of blood pressure categories in children*[a]

Blood pressure category	Definition
Normal	Systolic and diastolic blood pressures less than the 90th percentile for sex and age.
High normal	Average systolic and/or diastolic blood pressure between the 90th and 95th percentiles for age and sex.
Hypertension	Average systolic and/or diastolic blood pressures equal to or greater than the 95th percentile for age and sex, with measurements obtained on at least three occasions.

[a] Adapted from the Report of the Second Task Force on Blood Pressure Control in Children—1987 (8).

The diagnosis of hypertension is made only after blood pressure is confirmed to be greater than the 95th percentile at three separate examinations. The average blood pressure from two or more measurements is calculated at each visit, and percentile distribution is determined from the graphs in Figs. 1–3. Despite the use of the 95th percentile on the Task Force curves, far fewer than 5% of children will have hypertension when the three-examination protocol is followed. With repeated blood pressure measurements, high blood pressure tends to fall as a result of (a) accommodation on the part of the child to the measurement procedure and (b) the statistical phenomenon of regression toward the mean. The Task Force distribution curves were constructed from single blood pressure measurements per child. Therefore, only after the initial measurement can the blood pressure of 5% of children be expected to be at the 95th percentile or above, and it is expected that the percentage of children with hypertension will decrease with each subsequent visit.

Childhood hypertension is divided into two categories (Table 4): "Significant" hypertension is defined as blood pressure between the 95th and 99th percentiles of distribution, and "severe" hypertension is defined as blood pressure at the 99th percentile or above. There is a limited amount of information published about the prevalence of hypertension. From all indications, prevalence is low in children. Only 26 of 10,000 6- to 8-year-olds (0.26%) in the Minneapolis study (6) had a systolic blood pressure of 130 mmHg or a diastolic blood pressure of 90 mmHg (37) at the time of the initial screening. In the Muscatine Study of children 5–18 years old, the prevalence of blood pressure 140/90 mmHg or greater was less than 1% (43); and in the Dallas screening of 8th- to 12th-grade students, the prevalence of significant hypertension was only 1.6%, 1.7%, and 1.9% in separate 8th-, 10th- and 12th-grade surveys (44). Using 1987 Task Force curves, data were analyzed from a recent screening of 20,000 5th-, 6th-, 7th-, and 8th-grade students (45). After only two separate examinations, using the average of two measurements at each examination, the prevalence of significant systolic, diastolic, and systolic

TABLE 4. *Classification of hypertension by age group*[a]

Age group	Hypertension[b] Significant	Severe
Newborn		
7 days	SBP ≥ 96 mmHg	SBP ≥ 106 mmHg
8–30 days	SBP ≥ 104 mmHg	SBP ≥ 110 mmHg
Infant	SBP ≥ 112 mmHg	SBP ≥ 118 mmHg
(<2 years)	DBP ≥ 74 mmHg	DBP ≥ 82 mmHg
Children	SBP ≥ 116 mmHg	SBP ≥ 124 mmHg
(3–5 years)	DBP ≥ 76 mmHg	DBP ≥ 84 mmHg
Children	SBP ≥ 122 mmHg	SBP ≥ 130 mmHg
(6–9 years)	DBP ≥ 78 mmHg	DBP ≥ 86 mmHg
Children	SBP ≥ 126 mmHg	SBP ≥ 134 mmHg
(10–12 years)	DBP ≥ 82 mmHg	DBP ≥ 90 mmHg
Adolescents	SBP ≥ 136 mmHg	SBP ≥ 144 mmHg
(13–15 years)	DBP ≥ 86 mmHg	DBP ≥ 92 mmHg
Adolescents	SBP ≥ 142 mmHg	SBP ≥ 150 mmHg
(16–18 years)	DBP ≥ 92 mmHg	DBP ≥ 98 mmHg

[a] From the Report of the Second Task Force on Blood Pressure Control in Children—1987 (8).
[b] SBP, systolic blood pressure; DBP, diastolic blood pressure.

and/or diastolic hypertension was 0.3%, 0.8%, and 1.1%, respectively.

The low prevalence of hypertension in children should not detract from current recommendations to monitor blood pressure yearly. The diagnosis of severe hypertension is most often associated with secondary, identifiable causes that may be amenable to specific forms of therapy. Of equal importance is the longitudinal evaluation of blood pressure to detect individuals tracking in the upper percentiles of blood pressure distribution.

Causes of Hypertension

It is generally recognized that the incidence of secondary hypertension [i.e., hypertension resulting from a disease process that is usually identifiable, in contrast to primary (or essential) hypertension] is directly related to the level of blood pressure and is inversely correlated with age. Thus, secondary hypertension is likely to be diagnosed in children with severe hypertension, particularly those of grade school age and younger, whereas it is far less likely that a secondary cause will be uncovered in an adolescent with blood pressure in the significant hypertension, or mildly elevated, range. There are many diseases that can cause hypertension in children. However, there are only a few of these that occur with any frequency, and they are responsible for the majority of cases.

Causes for hypertension vary according to age. The classifications in the tables are listed in approximate decreasing frequency, and this is discussed in detail in the text. In some cases, the age category for a specific disease is very clear. However, for most diseases there is overlap; for this reason, pre-school and grade-school age groups were combined. Despite its low prevalence, the finding of severe hypertension requires a thorough medical evaluation. A clear understanding of probable etiologies is required to formulate a rational, efficient plan for diagnostic investigation.

Neonate and Infant

Hypertension occurs in approximately 1–2% of all newborns admitted to neonatal intensive care nurseries (46,47). Neonates and infants in the first few months of life commonly present in extreme distress, particularly when hypertension develops after discharge from the hospital. The initial signs of hypertension (i.e., irritability, feeding problems, vomiting, cyanosis, and respiratory distress) are usually related to congestive heart failure (Table 5). This progresses steadily and rapidly to circulatory collapse with severe respiratory distress, oliguria, hypotension, and seizures, followed by cardiac arrest. Although it is rarely possible to distinguish, at the initial examination, between cardiac failure caused by hypertension and congenital heart disease, blood pressure in hypertensive infants may be in the upper normal range, a finding generally not consistent with overt cardiac failure from other causes. It is not clear why the adverse effect of systemic hypertension is so much more dramatic and precipitous in infants than in older children or adults.

Renal artery thrombosis has become the most common cause of neonatal hypertension (Table 6). This is directly attributable to the widespread use of umbilical artery catheters in distressed newborns (48). Despite recognition of this potential complication and attempts to maintain catheter placement at an aortic level below the renal arteries, the problem continues to be seen. Renal arterial thrombosis is the consequence of embolization of thrombotic plaques formed at the catheter tip, producing small areas of renal infarction. The resultant hypertension is usually mild or moderate in degree but can be severe. In either case, it rarely persists longer than a few weeks or months. The overall prognosis is excellent despite residual severe unilateral renal atrophy (48).

Renal artery stenosis is rare in young infants. Reviews of extended experience at major teaching hospitals (49,50) commonly do not include any cases younger than 1 year of age. At the University of Minnesota Hospital, four young infants, 1 week to 6 months old, have been treated for renal artery stenosis in the past 10 years. Each of these infants presented with severe cardiac failure, and hypertension was not recognized until cardiac function was reestablished. These patients were managed conservatively with antihypertensive drug therapy until the age of 4 or 5 years, at which time the lesions were corrected successfully by renal autotransplantation. The exception to this protocol was an infant with unilateral disease who underwent nephrectomy at 18 months of age because of nonfunction in the affected kidney.

TABLE 5. *Signs of hypertension in the newborn and infant*

Failure to grow
Irritability
Feeding problems
Vomiting
Cyanosis
Respiratory distress
Cardiac failure
Seizures

TABLE 6. *Causes of hypertension in the neonate and infant*

Renal artery thrombosis (following umbilical artery catheterization)
Coarctation of the aorta
Congenital renal structural or parenchymal disease
Renal artery stenosis
Bronchopulmonary dysplasia
Abdominal surgery (51)
Extracorporeal membrane oxygenation (ECMO)

Other causes of hypertension are listed in Table 6. It occurs in 100% of infants with autosomal recessive polycystic kidney disease (52) and tends to be more severe in early infancy. It is less frequent in infants with the dominant form of the disease (52). Hypertension can develop in infants with bronchopulmonary dysplasia (53). The etiology is unknown but may be related to hypoxia-mediated changes in vasoreactivity or to angiotensin-converting-enzyme activity (54). Hypertension has been reported as a frequent complication of extracorporeal membrane oxygenation (ECMO) (55), developing in 93% of infants and associated with intracranial hemorrhage.

Children Aged 1 Year to 10 Years

Hypertension in children after infancy is usually discovered during a routine physical examination, even in patients presenting with the most severe degrees of blood pressure elevation. However, certain clinical features are characteristic of hypertension and should draw the clinician's attention to the diagnosis (Table 7). Headache can be a sign of hypertension but may be difficult to evaluate because it is such a common, nonspecific complaint in this age group. Cardiac failure is less common, but cardiac enlargement may be an indication of chronic disease. The initial and only indication of illness may be a stroke. This can vary from transient localized neurologic findings to hemiplegia. In general, the prognosis for ultimate full neurologic recovery is good. An uncommon, unique sign of hypertension is facial or Bell's palsy (56). It is believed to be the result of a vascular lesion within the facial canal and is reversible with control of the hypertension.

The principal cause of hypertension in pre-school and grade-school children is renal disease (Table 8). It is diagnosed in approximately 43–84% of children with hypertension referred to major medical centers (59–61), and this percentage does not appear to be changing. The presence of hypertension can have important implications for severity and prognosis of the renal disease, and these vary according to the basic disease process (Table 9).

Hypertension is found in 75–80% of hospitalized patients with acute post-streptococcal glomerulonephritis and is reported to be the most common physical finding in this disease (62,63). It is the consequence of sodium and fluid retention. Analysis of fractional excretion of sodium (FE_{Na}) in patients who develop hypertension after hospitalization has shown that blood pressure does not increase to hypertensive levels when the FE_{Na} is greater than 0.5, whereas patients with a FE_{Na} of less than 0.5 develop hypertension (63).

TABLE 7. *Symptoms and signs of hypertension in children and adolescents*

Failure to thrive (i.e., growth retardation)
Nausea and/or vomiting
Lethargy
Irritability
Headache
Visual problems
Cardiac failure
Seizures
Stroke
Facial palsy

TABLE 8. *Causes of hypertension in children and adolescents*

From 1 year to 10 years of age
Renal disease
Coarctation of the aorta
Renal artery stenosis
Hypercalcemia
Neurofibromatosis
Neurogenic tumors
Pheochromocytoma
Mineralocorticoid excess
Primary hyperaldosteronism
11β-Hydroxylase deficiency
17α-Hydroxylase deficiency
Dexamethasone-suppressible hyperaldosteronism
Apparent mineralocorticoid excess
Hyperthyroidism
Transient hypertension following urologic surgery
Immobilization (traction)-induced hypertension (57)
Sleep-apnea-associated hypertension (58)
Essential hypertension (rare)
From 10 years of age until adolescence
Renal disease
Essential hypertension
Diagnoses listed above in 1- to 10-year category

TABLE 9. *Frequency of hypertension in selected renal diseases at time of initial presentation*

Renal disease	Percentage of patients with hypertension
Acute post-streptococcal glomerulonephritis	75–80
Nephrotic syndrome	26
Minimal change	21
Focal segmental glomerulosclerosis	36–50
Membranoproliferative glomerulonephritis	42–51
Membranous nephropathy	6–50
Hemolytic–uremic syndrome	49–73
Chronic pyelonephritis	14–35
Henoch–Schönlein purpura	14
IgA nephropathy	6

Hypertension is found during the initial examination in 26% of children presenting with the nephrotic syndrome (64,65). The presence of hypertension in this syndrome has important adverse prognostic implications, particularly for older children (64). Although 21% of children with minimal change nephrotic syndrome have hypertension, it is usually very mild. In contrast, approximately 50% of children with focal segmental glomerulosclerosis (64,65) and membranoproliferative glomerulonephritis (64,66) will have hypertension. In both diseases, hypertension persists long-term but does not accelerate the disease process. The incidence of hypertension in membranous nephropathy varies widely among referral centers (67,68). These children seem more likely to progress to chronic renal failure than do patients without hypertension.

Hypertension is extremely common in children with hemolytic–uremic syndrome, affecting 50% of children developing the disease in their first 3 years of life and approximately 75% of older children (69). Persistent hypertension is an ominous sign, indicating active disease or incomplete resolution of the renal lesion. Patients with hemolytic–uremic syndrome can have the most severe degrees of hypertension during the active phase of their disease, and some have required bilateral nephrectomy to control blood pressure, despite aggressive antihypertensive therapy.

Hypertension occurs in 14–35% of children with pyelonephritis (59–61) and is closely associated with renal cortical scar formation. Scarring and hypertension may appear months after active infection or after surgical correction of vesicoureteral reflux (VUR), suggesting that these children require careful long-term evaluation. Hypertension is infrequent in patients with Henoch–Schönlein purpura nephritis (70) and IgA nephropathy (71).

Renal artery stenosis is seen with a frequency of 1–2 per year at major referral centers (49,50). The physical examination of these children is usually unremarkable, with the exception of blood pressure. A careful search for abdominal bruits should be conducted, but these will be found in fewer than one-third of patients (49,50). Conventional laboratory tests are also not particularly helpful. Peripheral plasma renin activity (PRA) may be elevated but cannot be relied upon to establish the diagnosis. However, low serum potassium in the presence of normal PRA may be a clue to a hyperreninemic state. Radiographic studies other than arteriogram have been uniformly disappointing (49). Intravenous pyelogram, renal ultrasonography, and isotopic renograms have low sensitivity, with an excessive number of false-negative results. Administration of captopril prior to the renogram may increase the reliability of this procedure, but additional data are needed in children.

Renovascular hypertension may be the result of other disease processes. Children with abdominal aortic and/or other abdominal artery disease may have had undocumented intrauterine infection, e.g., rubella (72). Multiple artery involvement may also be seen in Takayasu arteritis (73). Somewhat more common are (a) neurofibromatosis, in which the pathogenesis for renal artery stenosis is a proliferation of Schwann cells within the arterial wall (74), and (b) Williams syndrome, a disorder of calcium metabolism in which hypertension is the clinical expression of hypercalcinemia, nephrocalcinosis, or renal artery stenosis (75).

The major nonrenal cause of hypertension in children and infants is coarctation of the aorta. The majority of children with this disease will be identified before they start school; however, the diagnosis is frequently missed, and detection may be delayed to later childhood (76). A careful physical examination is the key to diagnosis and characteristically includes hypertension in the arms, a reduction in blood pressure of 20 mmHg or more in the legs, and reduced or absent femoral pulses. The presence of an abdominal bruit is common and can misdirect the evaluation toward renal artery stenosis. Echocardiography will usually confirm the diagnosis.

The etiology for coarct-induced hypertension continues to be a matter of controversy. It is probably due, in part, to mechanical obstruction of aortic blood flow; however, the major etiologic relationship appears to be a reduction in renal perfusion pressure, similar to the effect of renal artery stenosis. A prerequisite for coarct hypertension is the presence of renal tissue distal to the arterial constriction (77), suggesting the involvement of a renal pressor agent. PRA increases after aortic coarctation is produced but returns to normal within a few weeks (78). PRA is not significantly higher in children with coarctation than in normal children. However, with volume depletion, PRA becomes significantly higher in coarct patients (79). Furthermore, PRA decreases significantly after surgical coarctation repair (80).

Hypertension is also a problem in the immediate postoperative period after coarctation repair (81). In its most exaggerated form, it is associated with a syndrome of mesenteric arteritis, characterized by abdominal pain, rebound tenderness, vomiting, fever, leukocytosis, and ileus (82). On rare occasions, bowel infarction occurs. The hypertension is thought to be related to activation of the sympathetic nervous (83) and renin–angiotensin systems (81). In support of this, administration of propranolol pre- and postoperatively will reduce the postcoarctectomy hypertensive response (83,84). Despite nonrecurrence of the coarctation, hypertension persists in 24% of patients (85). Clinical success appears to be related to the patient's age at the time of surgery, with repair after the age of 5–6 associated with a higher incidence of residual hypertension (85).

Other causes of hypertension occur infrequently in this age group. It is found in only 20% of children with neurogenic tumors (e.g., neuroblastoma) (86). Pheochromocytoma is an extremely rare tumor in childhood (60,61). Its clinical presentation differs from that in adults because of (a) the sustained, rather than intermittent, nature of the hypertension, (b) lower frequency of cardiovascular symptoms, and (c) higher incidence of extra-adrenal tumor sites (87).

Mineralocorticoid-induced hypertension is also extremely rare in childhood. A reliable clue is a significant reduction in PRA, whereas other tests (e.g., serum potassium) have a lower sensitivity. Primary hyperaldosteronism has been reported in only 21 children, and it is usually the result of bilateral adrenal hyperplasia rather than tumor (88). Other etiologies in children are: congenital deficiencies of 11β-hydroxylase or 17α-hydroxylase (89); dexamethasone-suppressible hyperaldosteronism (90), a rare familial syndrome in which aldosterone secretion is totally suppressible with dexamethasone or other glucocorticoid therapy; and "apparent mineralocorticoid excess" (91), a syndrome with severe hypertension, low renin, and hypokalemia but without an increase in steroid production. These children are treated successfully with spironolactone.

Early and Late Adolescence

Secondary causes for hypertension become less frequent beginning in late childhood and continuing through adolescence as more children are recognized with early, mild essential hypertension. However, in cases of secondary hypertension, renal-related diseases will be the predominant diagnosis (see above). It has become clear that mild to moderate elevations in blood pressure are more common than previously recognized, particularly in children of junior high school age and older. While the evaluation of children in this age range is designed to eliminate secondary causes of hypertension, attention should begin to focus on essential hypertension in the context of general cardiovascular risk.

Data on the prevalence of essential hypertension in children are scarce. Earlier reviews from major pediatric centers are influenced by referral, in most cases, of patients with severe hypertension (59–61). The consensus experience reflected in the 1987 Task Force Report (8) suggests that the percentage with primary hypertension is substantially increased when children in the significant hypertension range (i.e., 95th to 99th percentiles of distribution) are also considered.

Few attempts have been made to identify childhood factors influencing the development of essential hypertension: (a) In a small study of 8-year-olds with high and low blood pressure (37), plasma norepinephrine levels were not significantly different between the two groups at rest, after 2 hr of upright posture, or after vigorous exercise. PRA was significantly lower in the high blood pressure group under the same sampling conditions, and 24-hr urinary kallikrein excretion was also significantly lower in the high blood pressure group (92). (b) A role for sympathetic nervous system hyperactivity is suggested by the dramatic response to mental stress exhibited by adolescents with borderline hypertension and a family history of hypertension (93). Moreover, these individuals have a higher risk for the eventual development of fixed essential hypertension (94). (c) There is a positive correlation between blood pressure and insulin levels in obese adolescents (95). The significance of this finding is uncertain because of the confounding effect of weight on each of these variables. (d) A significant interrelationship between blood pressure and other cardiovascular risk factors early in development is suggested by the positive correlation between blood pressure, serum lipids, and arterial (aortic and coronary) fatty streaks in young subjects dying from noncardiovascular causes (96).

EVALUATION OF THE HYPERTENSIVE CHILD

There continues to be considerable controversy among pediatricians with regard to (a) which children with hypertension should be investigated with laboratory and other tests and (b) the extent to which investigation should be pursued. There is a difference between children with severe and mild hypertension. In the former group, particularly when symptoms are present or when there are signs of target organ involvement, there is general agreement that a diagnostic evaluation should be vigorously conducted. In the latter group, the disease-risk–investigation-benefit ratio is poorly defined. It is unreasonable to initiate investigation of a child suspected of having mild to moderate hypertension without confirmation from three separate examinations that the level of blood pressure falls under the definitions listed in Table 4. Investigation is not indicated for children with blood pressure in the high-normal range—even for those with an occasional reading above the 95th percentile—unless the medical history or physical examination suggests a specific disease entity.

Diagnostic evaluation should be designed to fit the clinical presentation and age of the child (see Tables 6 and 8). When there are not any clues to the etiology, the diagnostic plan should be directed in its early stages toward renal disease. Table 10 lists an outline for evaluation of hypertensive children. It is arranged to begin with general screening tests, proceeding in a stepwise fashion to more complicated procedures required to diagnose the less common causes of hypertension. This list is intended only as a guide. The medical history, family history, or physical examination may provide information enabling the clinician to move more rapidly toward investigation of specific disease entities.

The initial evaluation consists of (a) a complete blood count, (b) serum electrolytes, creatinine, urea nitrogen, calcium, uric acid, and cholesterol, and (c) urinalysis. A urine culture is also obtained because of the silent nature of chronic pyelonephritis. PRA is obtained primarily to look for suppression of activity, suggesting mineralocorticoid excess. PRA is less useful in the diagnosis of renal artery stenosis because of overlap in values between these patients and patients with other forms of hypertension. It is crucial that normal standards for PRA be established by the laboratory performing the test, since PRA values vary according to age in children (97). Serum cholesterol will not aid in the diagnosis but is important for the introduction of the broader concept of cardiovascular risk in the context of hypertension.

TABLE 10. *Diagnostic evaluation of the hypertensive child*

Complete blood count
Serum electrolytes, creatinine, urea nitrogen, calcium, uric acid, cholesterol
Urinalysis
Urine culture
Plasma renin activity (PRA)
Renal ultrasound
Isotopic renogram
Echocardiogram
Urine collection for catecholamines
Plasma and urinary steroids
Renal arteriography

Because of the high incidence of renal disease in children with hypertension, a detailed examination of the kidney is indicated. The intravenous pyelogram (IVP) is rarely used today, without a specific indication. Kidney size and anatomy are evaluated by renal ultrasound, and renal blood flow is evaluated by the renogram. Unfortunately, the sensitivity of the isotopic renogram in the diagnosis of renal artery stenosis is severely limited (49,50). This can be circumvented, in part, by the use of DTPA (diethylene triamine penta-acetic acid), which is excreted at the glomerulus and is not excreted or absorbed by the renal tubule. Pretreatment of the patient with captopril prior to administration of DTPA will enhance flow differences between the affected and normal kidney by further reducing glomerular filtration rate and clearance of DTPA on the stenotic side (98). Even this maneuver cannot be depended on to detect branch-arterial stenotic lesions, commonly missed without an arteriogram.

An echocardiogram should be obtained in children with severe hypertension and in any child considered for antihypertensive therapy (99,100). The chest x-ray is not a sensitive enough measure of early cardiac changes. Echocardiographic examination is not indicated for children with mild hypertension, even though early changes in left ventricular geometry have been shown to be present across the normal distribution of childhood blood pressure (101).

Catecholamine production is evaluated by measurement of 24-hr urinary excretion of catecholamines or catechol metabolites [i.e., vanillylmandelic acid (VMA)]. In some centers, plasma measurements are also used, but these do not appear to be as sensitive as urinary measurements (102). Measurement of VMA and homovanillic acid (HVA) in randomly collected urine specimens are now used for neuroblastoma detection but have not been tested in patients with pheochromocytoma (103). In the patient with a very low PRA, plasma samples for aldosterone and other steroids should be obtained to eliminate the possibility of mineralocorticoid excess.

In the severely hypertensive child, particularly in the infant and young child, renal arteriography should be performed when other causes for hypertension have been eliminated, even when the isotopic renogram is normal. This study should be done at an institution with the capability for transluminal angioplasty—although care must be taken with regard to patient selection and the angioplastic procedure itself, to prevent procedural mishaps. Renal-vein renin measurements have traditionally been obtained in children. The test was introduced in adults to assist in distinguishing between renovascular and essential hypertension, but this is not a problem in pediatric patients with hypertension. At the University of Minnesota Hospital, all children with renal artery stenosis have responded to angioplasty or corrective surgery, and renal-vein renin determinations are no longer part of the routine evaluation of renal artery stenosis.

TREATMENT OF CHILDHOOD HYPERTENSION

Issues relating to therapy for childhood hypertension are clouded by the lack of information about natural history, risk, and response to intervention, particularly during the critical developmental transition period between adolescence and adulthood. Antihypertensive therapy is indicated for severe hypertension, to prevent adverse cardiovascular events (104). It is less clear what approach is best for the child with mild to moderate hypertension.

The goal of treatment is reduction of blood pressure to a level below the 95th percentile. This may take a period of days or weeks to accomplish. The important factor is achievement of steady progress in blood pressure reduction, since there is no evidence that more rapid reduction of blood pressure, except for those patients with extreme hypertension, improves prognosis or well-being.

Nonpharmacologic Therapy

Children with blood pressure in the "significant" hypertension range should be started on a nonpharmacologic regimen, introduced in the context of cardiovascular risk (including family history, lipids, tobacco, overweight, and exercise). Nonpharmacologic therapy includes weight reduction, exercise, and diet adjustment. The effectiveness of each of these is related directly to (a) motivation on the part of the patient and (b) reinforcement on the part of the health care provider.

In successful weight loss programs, blood pressure decreases in response to weight reduction (38), and the reduction is greatest in the heaviest children. The reduction in blood pressure is not an isolated finding but occurs, instead, in conjunction with other components of cardiovascular risk (105).

Aerobic exercise reduces blood pressure in adolescents (39,106) and has a beneficial effect on serum lipids (105). Weight training (i.e., static exercise) also reduces blood pressure (107) but is not recommended over aerobic training because of its questionable effect on cardiovascular fitness.

An important issue for the older hypertensive child is strenuous exercise during participation in organized sports. Blood pressure increases significantly with exercise in normal children as well as in those with high blood pressure (108), and there is no evidence to suggest that children with mild hypertension are at increased risk (109). Without evidence of cardiac disease or an abnormality on the electrocardiogram or echocardiogram, participation in sports for these children is not contraindicated, provided that blood pressure is carefully monitored with regular examinations (110). The child with severe hypertension is likely to be at greater risk and should not participate in strenuous sports activity. Successful reduction of blood pressure with treatment probably reduces overall exercise risk, but there is no evidence to support this. Because exercise has a positive effect on blood pressure and cardiovascular risk, it should be unconditionally contraindicated only in those individuals with ongoing severe hypertension.

Dietary intervention in children has focused on modification of sodium or potassium intake. Blood pressure in normal children is not significantly affected by severe sodium restriction. The effect of low sodium on hypertensive children has been mixed, with a significant reduction seen by some (111) but not by others (112). Potassium supplements were not effective in children during short-term studies (113), but a significant reduction in blood pressure was seen when potassium was combined with sodium restriction (112).

Antihypertensive Drug Therapy

Drug therapy in childhood hypertension is based on the same basic principles established for adults. Drugs are added in a stepwise fashion until blood pressure control is achieved. When more than one drug is required, drugs acting on the same physiologic system are not used simultaneously.

Severe hypertension in children resulting from primary renal disease frequently requires aggressive therapy with multidrug regimens. These patients may experience a deterioration in renal function coincident with a reduction in blood pressure (114). With ongoing therapy, renal function should return to pretreatment levels.

Acute Hypertensive Emergency (Table 11)

Acute hypertensive emergencies are usually defined by blood pressure likely to cause some major vascular accident without immediate treatment. Sodium nitroprusside and labetalol are widely used in these children because they are effective and because they can control the rate of blood pressure reduction. Diazoxide is also a very effective drug, but its use is often accompanied by a precipitous fall in blood pressure that is best avoided. Hydralazine is less potent and has a short duration of action. It is useful over the short term, but it loses its effectiveness when frequent repeated dosing is required.

Chronic Antihypertensive Therapy (Table 12)

The availability of newer antihypertensive agents has greatly improved the management of children with severe hypertension. Converting-enzyme inhibitors and calcium antagonists are now included with diuretics and beta-blockers as options for initial therapy.

Converting-enzyme inhibitors have been widely used in children (115) with all degrees of renal function (116). They are particularly useful in newborn infants but should be initiated at 10% of the usual children's dose to avoid adverse effects (117,118).

Published experience with calcium antagonists in children has been limited to nifedipine (119). It is effective for rapid reduction of blood pressure, but its duration is short, precluding wider use for chronic therapy. A newer calcium antagonist, nitrendipine, is effective in severe childhood hypertension and has a longer duration of action (T. G. Wells and A. R. Sinaiko, *unpublished data*).

Diuretic therapy is an important component of therapy in children with renal disease. The thiazides have proven to be exceptionally free from adverse effects. Furosemide is generally reserved for patients with a reduction in renal function to 50% of normal or lower. All members of the class of beta-blocking drugs have been used safely in children, as have the remainder of the drugs listed in Table 12.

TABLE 11. *Antihypertensive drug therapy for hypertensive emergencies*

Drug	Dose
Sodium nitroprusside	0.5–8 μg/kg/min, intravenously
Labetalol	1–3 mg/kg, intravenously
Diazoxide	2–5 mg/kg, intravenously
Hydralazine	0.2–0.4 mg/kg, intravenously
Nifedipine	0.25–0.5 mg/kg, sublingually
Minoxidil	0.1–0.2 mg/kg, orally

TABLE 12. *Antihypertensive drugs for chronic therapy*

Drug	Dose (mg/kg/day) Initial	Dose (mg/kg/day) Maximum
Converting-enzyme inhibitors		
Captopril		
Neonates	0.03–0.15	2
Children	1.5	6
Enalapril	0.15	0.6
Calcium antagonists		
Nifedipine	0.25	3
Nitrendipine	0.25	2
Diuretics		
Hydrochlorothiazide	1	2–3
Metolazone	0.1	3
Furosemide	1	12
Bumetanide	0.02–0.05	0.3
Spironolactone	1	3
Triamterene	1	3
Beta-adrenergic blockers		
Propranolol	1	8
Atenolol	1	8
Alpha-blockers		
Prazosin	0.05–0.1	0.5
Vasodilators		
Hydralazine	0.75	7.5
Minoxidil	0.1–0.2	1

ACKNOWLEDGMENT

This work was supported by NHLBI grant HL-34659.

REFERENCES

1. Loggie JMH. Hypertension in children and adolescents. I. Causes and diagnostic studies. *J Pediatr* 1969;74:331–355.
2. Londe S. Blood pressure in children as determined under office conditions. *Pediatrics* 1966;5:71–78.
3. U.S. Department of Health, Education and Welfare. *Blood pressure levels of children 6–11 years.* DHEW publication No. (HRA) 74-1617, Vital and Health Statistics Series 11-135, 1973.
4. Lauer RM, Connor WE, Leaverton PE, Reiter MA, Clarke WR. Coronary heart disease risk factors in school children: the Muscatine Study. *J Pediatr* 1975;86:697–706.
5. Voors AW, Foster TA, Frerichs RR, Webber LS, Berenson GS. Studies of blood pressures in children ages 5–14 years, in a total biracial community. The Bogalusa Heart Study. *Circulation* 1976;54:319–327.
6. Prineas RJ, Gillum RF, Horibe H, Hannan PJ. The Minneapolis Children's Blood Pressure Study, Parts I & II. *Hypertension* 1980;2(Suppl I):I-18–I-28.

7. Report of the Task Force on Blood Pressure Control in Children —1977. *Pediatrics* 1977;59:797–820.
8. Report of the Second Task Force on Blood Pressure Control in Children—1987. *Pediatrics* 1987;79:1–25.
9. American Academy of Pediatrics. Guidelines for Health Supervision. News and comment, May 1982.
10. Moss AJ, Liebling W, Austin WO, Adams FH. An evaluation of the flush method for determining blood pressures in infants. *Pediatrics* 1957;20:53–62.
11. Reder RF, Dimich I, Cohen ML, Steinfeld L. Evaluating indirect blood pressure measurement techniques: a comparison of three systems in infants and children. *Pediatrics* 1978;62:326–330.
12. Park MK, Menard SM. Accuracy of blood pressure measurement by the Dinamap monitor in infants and children. *Pediatrics* 1987;79:907–914.
13. Wareham JA, Haugh LD, Yeager SB, Horbar JD. Prediction of arterial blood pressure in the premature neonate using the oscillometric method. *Am J Dis Child* 1987;141:1108–1110.
14. Moss AJ. Criteria for diastolic pressure. Revolution, counterrevolution and now a compromise. *Pediatrics* 1983;71:854–855.
15. Londe S. Fifth versus fourth Korotkoff phase. *Pediatrics* 1985;76:460–461.
16. Moss AJ, Adams FH. Index of indirect estimation of diastolic blood pressure. *Am J Dis Child* 1963;106:747–777.
17. Lagler U, Duc G. Systolic blood pressure in normal newborn infants during the first 6 hours of life: transcutaneous doppler ultrasonic technique. *Biol Neonate* 1980;37:243–245.
18. de Swiet M, Fayers P, Shinebourne EA. Systolic blood pressure in a population of infants in the first year of life: the Brompton Study. *Pediatrics* 1980;65:1028–1035.
19. Zinner SH, Rosner B, Oh W, Kass EH. Significance of blood pressure in infancy. Familial aggregation and predictive effect on later blood pressure. *Hypertension* 1985;7:411–416.
20. Versmold HT, Kitterman JA, Phibbs RH, Gregory GH, Tooley WH. Aortic blood pressure during the first 12 hours of life in infants with birth weight 610 to 4,220 grams. *Pediatrics* 1981;67:607–613.
21. Moscoso P, Goldberg RN, Jamieson J, Bancalari E. Spontaneous elevation in arterial blood pressure during the first hours of life in the very-low-birth weight infant. *J Pediatr* 1983;103:114–117.
22. Adams MA, Pasternak JF, Kupfer BM, Gardner TH. A computerized system for continuous physiologic data collection and analysis: initial report on mean arterial blood pressure in very-low-birth-weight infants. *Pediatrics* 1983;71:23–30.
23. Schacter J, Cutler LH, Perfetti C. Blood pressure during the first two years of life. *Am J Epidemiol* 1982;116:29–41.
24. Burke GL, Voors AW, Shear CL, Webber LS, Smoak CG, Cresanta JL, Berenson GS. Blood pressure: the Bogalusa Heart Study. *Pediatrics* 1987;80(Suppl):784–788.
25. Prineas RJ, Gillum RF, Gomez-Marin O. The determinants of blood pressure levels in children: the Minneapolis Children's Blood Pressure Study. In: Loggie JMH, Horan MJ, Gruskin AB, Hohn AR, Dunbar JB, Havlik RJ, eds. *NHLBI Workshop on Juvenile Hypertension.* New York: Biomedical Information Service, 1984;21–35.
26. Shear CL, Burke GL, Freedman DS, Berenson GS. Value of childhood blood pressure measurements and family history in predicting future blood pressure status: results from 8 years of follow-up in the Bogalusa Heart Study. *Pediatrics* 1986;77:862–869.
27. Lauer RM, Anderson AR, Beaglehole R, Burns TL. Factors related to tracking of blood pressure in children. U.S. National Center for Health Statistics Health Examinations Surveys Cycles II and III. *Hypertension* 1984;6:307–314.
28. Prineas RJ, Gomez-Marin O, Sinaiko AR. Electrolytes and blood pressure levels in childhood hypertension: measurement and change. *Clin Exp Hypertens [A]* 1986;8:583–604.
29. Sinaiko AR, Bass J, Gomez-Marin O, Prineas RJ. Cardiac status of adolescents tracking with high and low blood pressure since early childhood. *J Hypertens* 1986;4(Suppl 5):S378–S380.
30. Prineas RJ, Gomez-Marin O, Gillum RF. Tracking of blood pressure in children and nonpharmacological approaches to the prevention of hypertension. *Ann Behav Med* 1985;7:25–29.
31. Lauer RM, Clarke WR, Beaglehole R. Level, trend and variability of blood pressure during childhood: the Muscatine Study. *Circulation* 1984;69:242–249.
32. Schacter J, Kuller LH, Perkins JM, Radin ME. Infant blood pressure and heart rate: relation to ethnic group (black or white) nutrition and electrolyte value. *Am J Epidemiol* 1979;110:205–218.
33. Baron AE, Freyer B, Fixler DE. Longitudinal blood pressures in blacks, whites and Mexican Americans during adolescence and early adulthood. *Am J Epidemiol* 1986;123:809–817.
34. Gutgesell M, Terrell G, Labarthe D. Pediatric blood pressure: ethnic comparisons in a primary care center. *Hypertension* 1981;3:39–47.
35. Zinner SH, Martin LF, Sacks F, Rosner B, Kass EH. A longitudinal study of blood pressure in childhood. *Am J Epidemiol* 1974;100:437–442.
36. Biron P, Morgeau JG. Familial aggregation of blood pressure and its components. *Ped Clin No Am* 1978;25:29–33.
37. Sinaiko AR, Gillum RF, Jacobs DR, Sopko G, Prineas RJ. Renin-angiotensin and sympathetic nervous system activity in grade school children. *Hypertension* 1982;4:299–306.
38. Brownell KD, Kelaran JH, Stunkard AJ. Treatment of obese children with and without their mothers: changes in weight and blood pressure. *Pediatrics* 1983;71:515–523.
39. Rocchini AP, Katch V, Anderson J, Hinderliter J, Becque D, Martin M, Marks C. Blood pressure in obese adolescents: effect of weight loss. *Pediatrics* 1988;82:16–23.
40. Shear CL, Freedman DS, Burke GL, Harsha DW, Berenson GS. Body fat patterning and blood pressure in children and young adults. *Hypertension* 1977;9:236–244.
41. Stallones L, Mueller WH, Christensen BL. Blood pressure, fatness, and fat patterning among USA adolescents from two ethnic groups. *Hypertension* 1982;4:483–486.
42. Londe S, Johanson A, Kronemer NS, Goldring D. Blood pressure and puberty. *J Pediatr* 1975;87:896–900.
43. Rames LC, Clarke WR, Connor WE, Recher MA, Lauer RM. Normal blood pressures and the evaluation of sustained blood pressure elevation in childhood: the Muscatine Study. *Pediatrics* 1978;61:245–251.
44. Fixler DE, Laird WP. Validity of mass blood pressure screening in children. *Pediatrics* 1983;72:459–463.
45. Sinaiko AR, Gomez-Marin O, Prineas RJ. Prevalence of "significant" hypertension in junior high school-aged children: The Children and Adolescent Blood Pressure Program. *J Pediatr* 1989;114:664–669.
46. Skalina MEL, Kliegman RM, Fanaroff AA. Epidemiology and management of severe symptomatic neonatal hypertension. *Am J Perinatol* 1986;3:235–239.
47. Buchi KF, Siegler RL. Hypertension in the first month of life. *J Hypertens* 1986;4:525–528.
48. Adelman RD. Long-term follow-up of neonatal renovascular hypertension. *Pediatr Nephrol* 1987;1:35–41.
49. Daniels SR, Loggie JMH, McEnerny PT, Towbin RB. Clinical spectrum of intrinsic renovascular hypertension in children. *Pediatrics* 1987;80:698–704.
50. Watson AR, Balfe JW, Hardy BE. Renovascular hypertension in childhood: a changing perspective in management. *J Pediatr* 1985;106:366–372.
51. Adelman RD, Sherman MP. Hypertension in the neonate following closure of abdominal wall defects. *J Pediatr* 1980;97:642–644.
52. Cole BR, Conley SB, Stapleton FB. Polycystic kidney disease in the first year of life. *J Pediatr* 1987;111:693–699.
53. Abman SH, Warady BA. Lum GM, Koops BL. Systemic hypertension in infants with bronchopulmonary dysplasia. *J Pediatr* 1984;104:928–931.
54. Mattioli L, Zakheim RM, Mullis K, Molteri A. Angiotensin-I converting enzyme activity in idiopathic respiratory distress of the newborn infant and in experimental alveolar hypoxia in mice. *J Pediatr* 1978;87:97–101.
55. Sell LL, Cullen ML, Lerner GR, Whittlesey GC, Shanley CJ, Klein MD. Hypertension during extracorporeal membrane oxygenation: cause, effect and management. *Surgery* 1987;102:724–730.
56. Lloyd AVC, Jewett DE, Still JDL. Facial paralysis in children with hypertension. *Arch Dis Child* 1968;41:292–294.
57. Linshaw MA, Stapleton FB, Gruskin AB, Baluarte HJ, Harbin

GL. Traction-related hypertension in children. *J Pediatr* 1979;95:994–996.
58. Ross RD, Daniels SR, Loggie JMH, Meyer RA, Ballard ET. Sleep apnea-associated hypertension and reversible left ventricular hypertrophy. *J Pediatr* 1987;111:253–255.
59. Dillon MJ. Investigation and management of hypertension in children. *Pediatr Nephrol* 1987;1:59–68.
60. Uhari M, Kostinies O. A survey of 164 Finnish children and adolescents with hypertension. *Acta Paediatr Scand* 1979; 68:193–198.
61. Loirat C, Pillion G, Blum C. Hypertension in children: present data and problems. *Adv Nephrol* 1982;11:65–97.
62. Lieberman E, Donnell GN. Recovery of children with acute glomerulonephritis. *Medicine* 1965;109:398–407.
63. Mota-Hernandez F, Feiman R, Gordillo-Paniagua G. Predictive value of fractional excretion of filtered sodium for hypertension in acute post-streptococcal glomerulonephritis. *J Pediatr* 1984;104:560–563.
64. International Study of Kidney Disease in Children. Nephrotic syndrome in children: prediction of histopathology from clinical and laboratory characteristics at time of diagnosis. *Kidney Int* 1978;13:159–165.
65. Southwest Pediatric Nephrology Study Group. Focal segmental glomerulosclerosis in children with idiopathic nephrotic syndrome. *Kidney Int* 1985;27:442–449.
66. West CD. Childhood membranoproliferative glomerulonephritis: an approach to management. *Kidney Int* 1986;29:1077–1093.
67. Habib R, Kleinknecht C, Gubler MC. Extramembranous glomerulonephritis in children: report of 50 cases. *J Pediatr* 1973;82:754–756.
68. Ramirez F, Brouhard BH, Travis LB, Ellis EN. Idiopathic membranous nephropathy in children. *J Pediatr* 1982;101:677–681.
69. Habib R, Levy M, Gagnadoux MF, Broyer M. Prognosis of the hemolytic–uremic syndrome in children. *Adv Nephrol* 1982; 11:99–128.
70. Levy M, Broyer M, Arsan A, Levy-Bantolila D, Habib R. Anaphylactoid purpura nephritis in childhood: natural history and immunopathology. *Adv Nephrol* 1976;6:183–228.
71. Southwest Pediatric Nephrology Study Group. A multicenter study of IgA nephropathy in children. *Kidney Int* 1982;22:643–652.
72. Menser MA, Dorman DC, Reye RDK, Reid RR. Renal-artery stenosis in the rubella syndrome. *Lancet* 1966;1:790–792.
73. Wiggelinkhuizea J, Cremin BS. Takayasu arteritis and renovascular hypertension in childhood. *Pediatrics* 1978;62:209–217.
74. Fallman R, Roth FJ. Treatment of neurofibromatosis associated renal artery stenosis with hypertension by percutaneous transluminal angioplasty. *Clin Exp Hypertens* [*A*] 1986;A8:893–899.
75. Daniels SR, Loggie JMH, Schwartz DC, Strife JL, Kaplan S. Systemic hypertension secondary to peripheral vascular anomalies in patients with Williams syndrome. *J Pediatr* 1985; 106:249–251.
76. Stafford MA, Griffiths SP, Gersony WM. Coarctation of the aorta: a study in delayed detection. *Pediatrics* 1982;69:159–163.
77. Scott HW, Collins HA, Langa ASM, Olsen NS. Additional observations concerning the physiology of the hypertension associated with experimental coarctation of the aorta. *Surgery* 1954;36:445–459.
78. Yogi S, Kramsch DM, Madoff IM, Hollander W. Plasma renin activity in hypertension associated with coarctation of the aorta. *Am J Physiol* 1968;215:605–610.
79. Alpert BS, Baur HH, Balfe JW, Kidd BSL, Olley PM. Role of the renin–angiotensin–aldosterone system in hypertensive children with coarctation of the aorta. *Am J Cardiol* 1979;43:828–834.
80. Parker FB, Streeter DHP, Farrell B, Blackman MS, Sondheimer HM, Anderson GH. Preoperative and postoperative renin levels in coarctation of the aorta. *Circulation* 1982;66:513–514.
81. Rocchini AP, Rosenthal A, Barger AC, Castaneda AR, Nadas AS. Pathogenesis of paradoxical hypertension after coarctation resection. *Circulation* 1976;54:382–387.
82. Ho ECK, Moss AJ. The syndrome of "mesenteric arteritis" following surgical repair of aortic coarctation. *Pediatrics* 1972;49:40–45.
83. Leenen FHH, Balfe JA, Pelech AN, Barker GA, Balfe JW, Olley PM. Postoperative hypertension after repair of coarctation of aorta in children: protective effect of propranolol? *Am Heart J* 1987;5:1164–1173.
84. Gidding SS, Rocchini AP, Beekman R, Szounar CA, Moorehead C, Behrendt D, Rosenthal A. Therapeutic effect of propranolol on paradoxical hypertension after repair of coarctation of the aorta. *N Engl J Med* 1985;312:1224–1228.
85. Nanton MA, Olley PM. Residual hypertension after coarctectomy in children. *Am J Cardiol* 1976;37:769–772.
86. Weinblatt ME, Heisel MA, Siegel SE. Hypertension in children with neurogenic tumors. *Pediatrics* 1983;71:947–951.
87. Hodgkinson DJ, Telander RL, Sheps SG, Gilchrist GS, Crowe JK. Extra-adrenal intrathoracic functioning paraganglionic (pheochromocytoma) in childhood. *Mayo Clinic Proc* 1980; 55:271–276.
88. Rauh W, Oberfield SE. The adrenal cortex in childhood hypertension. *Pediatr Adolesc Endocrinol* 1984;13:210–230.
89. White PC, New MI, Dupont B. Congenital adrenal hyperplasia. *N Engl J Med* 1986;8:669–676.
90. Connell JMC, Kenyon CJ, Corrie JET, Fraser R, Watt R, Lever AF. Dexamethasone-suppressible hyperaldosteronism. *Hypertension* 1986;8:669–676.
91. Ulick S, Levine LS, Gunezler P, Zanconato G, Ramirez LC, Rank W, Rosler A, Bradlow HC, New MI. A syndrome of apparent mineralocorticoid excess associated with defects in the peripheral metabolism of cortisol. *J Clin Endocrinol Metab* 1979;449:757–764.
92. Sinaiko AR, Glasser RJ, Gillum RF, Prineas RJ. Urinary kallikrein excretion in grade school children with high and low blood pressure. *J Pediatr* 1982;100:938–940.
93. Falkner B, Onesti G, Angelakos ET, Fernandes M, Langman C. Cardiovascular response to mental stress in normal adolescents with hypertensive parents. *Hypertension* 1979;1:23–30.
94. Falkner B, Kushner H, Onesti G, Angelakos ET. Cardiovascular characteristics in adolescents who develop essential hypertension. *Hypertension* 1981;3:521–527.
95. Rocchini AP, Katch V, Schork A, Kelch RP. Insulin and blood pressure during weight loss in obese adolescents. *Hypertension* 1987;10:267–273.
96. Newman WP, Freedman DS, Voors AW, Gard PD, Srinivasan SR, Cresanta JL, Williamson GD, Webber LS, Berenson GS. Relation of serum lipoprotein levels and systolic blood pressure to early atherosclerosis. *N Engl J Med* 1986;314:138–144.
97. Dillon MJ, Ryness JM. Plasma renin activity and aldosterone concentration in children. *Br Med J* 1975;4:316–319.
98. Sfakianakis GN, Bourgoignie JJ, Jaffe D, Kyriakides G, Perez-Stable E, Duncan RC. Single-dose captopril scintigraphy in the diagnosis of renovascular hypertension. *J Nucl Med* 1987;28: 1383–1392.
99. Shieken RM, Clarke WR, Lauer RM. Left ventricular hypertrophy in children with blood pressures in the upper quintile of the distribution: the Muscatine Study. *Hypertension* 1981;3: 669–675.
100. Culpepper WS, Sodt PC, Messerli FH, Reschhaupt DG, Arcilla RA. Cardiac status in juvenile borderline hypertension. *Ann Intern Med* 1983;98:1–7.
101. Burke GL, Arcilla RA, Culpepper WS, Webber LS, Chiang LK, Berenson GS. Blood pressure and echocardiographic measures in children: the Bogalusa Heart Study. *Circulation* 1987;75:106–114.
102. Duncan MW, Compton P, Lazarus L, Smythe GA. Measurement of norepinephrine and 3,4-dihydroxyphenyl-glycol in urine and plasma for the diagnosis of pheochromocytoma. *N Engl J Med* 1988;319:136–142.
103. Tuchman M, Morris CL, Ramnaraine ML, Bowers LD, Krivit W. Value of random urinary homovanillic and vanillylmandelic acid levels in the diagnosis and management of patients with neuroblastoma: comparison with 24-hour urine collections. *Pediatrics* 1985;75:324–328.
104. Heyden S, Bartel AG, Hames CG, McDonough JR. Elevated blood pressure levels in adolescents, Evans County, Georgia. *JAMA* 1969;209:1683–1689.
105. Becque MD, Katch VL, Rocchini AP, Marks CR, Moorehead C.

Coronary risk incidence of obese adolescents: reduction by exercise plus diet intervention. *Pediatrics* 1988;81:605–612.

106. Hagberg JM, Goldring D, Ehsani AA, Heath GW, Hernandez A, Schechtman K, Halloszy JO. Effects of exercise training in the blood pressure and hemodynamic features of hypertensive adolescents. *Am J Cardiol* 1983;52:763–768.
107. Hagberg JM, Ehsani AA, Goldring D, Hernandez A, Sinacore DR, Holloszy JO. Effect of weight training on blood pressure and hemodynamics in hypertensive adolescents. *J Pediatr* 1984;104:147–151.
108. Wilson SL, Gaffney FA, Laird WP, Fixler DE. Body size, composition and fitness in adolescents with elevated blood pressures. *Hypertension* 1985;7:417–422.
109. Fixler DE, Laird WP, Browne R, Fitzgerald V, Wilson S, Vance R. Response of hypertensive adolescents to dynamic and isometric exercise stress. *Pediatrics* 1979;64:579–583.
110. Strong WB. Hypertension and sports. *Pediatrics* 1979;64:693–695.
111. Costa FV, Ambrosioni E, Montepugnoli L, Paccalmi L, Vasconi L, Magnani P. Effects of a low-salt diet and of acute salt loading on blood pressure and intra-lymphocyte sodium concentration in young subjects with borderline hypertension. *Clin Sci* 1981;61:215–235.
112. Grobbe DE, Hofman A, Roelandt JT, Boomsma F, Schalekamp MA, Valkenburg HA. Sodium restriction and potassium supplementation in young people with mildly elevated blood pressure. *J Hypertens* 1987;5:115–119.
113. Miller JZ, Weinberger MH, Christian JC. Blood pressure response to potassium supplementation in normotensive adults and children. *Hypertension* 1987;10:437–442.
114. Green TP, Nevins TE, Hauser MT, Sibley R, Fish AJ, Sinaiko AR. Renal failure as a complication of acute antihypertensive therapy. *Pediatrics* 1983;67:850–854.
115. Mirkin BL, Newman TJ. Efficacy and safety of captopril in the treatment of severe childhood hypertension. Report of the International Collaborative Study Group. *Pediatrics* 1985;75:1091–1100.
116. Sinaiko AR, Mirkin BL, Hendrick DA, Green TP, O'Dea RF. Antihypertensive effect and elimination kinetics of captopril in hypertensive children with renal disease. *J Pediatr* 1983;103:799–805.
117. Tack ED, Perlman JM. Renal failure in sick hypertensive premature infants receiving captopril therapy. *J Pediatr* 1988;112:805–810.
118. O'Dea RF, Mirkin BL, Alward CT, Sinaiko AR. Treatment of neonatal hypertension with captopril. *J Pediatr* 1988;113:403–406.
119. Siegler RL, Brewer ED. Effect of sublingual oral nifedipine in the treatment of hypertension. *J Pediatr* 1988;112:811–813.

Hypertension: Pathophysiology, Diagnosis, and Management, edited by J. H. Laragh and B. M. Brenner. Raven Press, Ltd., New York © 1990.

CHAPTER 116

Hypertension in the Elderly

Richard L. Byyny

Definitions, 1869
Epidemiology, 1870
Prevalence, 1870
Risk of Hypertension, 1871
Pathophysiology, 1872
Etiology of Hypertension in the Elderly, 1874
Obesity, 1874
Vascular Changes, 1874
Baroreceptor Sensitivity, 1875
Hormonal Changes, 1875
Sympathetic Nervous System, 1875
The Kidney, 1876
Cellular Sodium Transport, 1876
Physical Inactivity, 1876
Sleep Disorders, 1877
Diagnosis and Clinical Assessment, 1877
Measurement, 1877
Errors in Diagnosis, 1877
Clinical Assessment, 1877
Laboratory Evaluation, 1877
Secondary Causes of Hypertension, 1877
Left Ventricular Hypertrophy, 1878
Treatment, 1878
Clinical Trials, 1878
Nonpharmacologic Therapy, 1880
Drug Treatment, 1880
Diuretic Therapy, 1880
Nondiuretic Therapy, 1881
Compliance, 1883
Adverse Events, 1883
Reduction in Medications, 1883
Systolic Hypertension in the Elderly, 1883
Conclusions, 1884
References, 1884

The elderly (i.e., those over 65 years of age) represent the most rapidly growing group in the United States. It is estimated that 5000 individuals reach age 65 each day. This age group is increasing two and one-half times faster than the overall population. More than 25 million people over age 65 live independently, and the number is increasing by 20% each decade. The oldest group, those over 85, represent 2.7 million people and is growing even more rapidly and will increase about fivefold, to about 16 million, in the next 40 years. The elderly currently consume over one-third of all U.S. health care dollars, even though they represent 12% of the population. In 1985, a 65-year-old individual had an average life expectancy of 15.1 additional years for men and 19.5 years for women (1).

The elderly vary widely in (a) physical, behavioral, cognitive, and emotional characteristics, (b) independence, (c) severity of illness, and (d) choices for medical care. The major goals for this group are prevention of premature mortality, prevention of disability, and maintenance of function and independence.

Hypertension is the single most potent, common, and remediable risk factor for cerebrovascular disease, congestive heart failure, and coronary heart disease, which are the major causes of cardiovascular morbidity and mortality in the population over age 65 (2). However, there is good evidence that cardiovascular disease is not an inevitable part of aging. Prevention of cardiovascular disease in the elderly would decrease premature mortality, decrease chronic disability, and improve the quality of life.

This chapter reviews the subject of hypertension in the elderly. The review includes the following: definitions of hypertension in the elderly; epidemiology; pathophysiology; etiology; clinical assessment and diagnosis; treatment; and isolated systolic hypertension.

DEFINITIONS

Cardiovascular risk is independently related to both the systolic and diastolic blood pressure (3). The risk from blood pressure gradually increases, but the gradient of risk for each increment in blood pressure becomes much steeper with advancing age (4). Even though the risk continues with each increment in pressure, one must dichotomize blood pressure into hypertension and normotension in order to present epidemiologic data (for communication) and to make treatment choices.

What is the level of systolic and diastolic blood pressure that will define hypertension for this age group? Hypertension can be best defined as that level of blood pressure at which the benefits of therapy exceed the risks and costs of no treatment. This definition, however, has changed over time. The Framingham Study used a definition of hypertension as a blood pressure greater than 160/95 mmHg. The World Health Organization has used the same definition. The Joint National Committee on Detection, Evaluation, and Treatment of High Blood Pressure confirms the diagnosis of hypertension in adults when the average of two or more diastolic blood pressures on at least two subsequent visits is 90 mmHg or higher or when the average of multiple systolic blood pressures on two or more subsequent visits is consistently greater than 140 mmHg (5). Therefore, one makes the diagnosis of hypertension in the elderly when the systolic blood pressure is greater than 140 mmHg and the diastolic pressure is greater than 90 mmHg. According to the Working Group on Hypertension in the Elderly, "an average systolic blood pressure greater than 160 mmHg and/or average diastolic pressure greater than or equal to 90 mmHg on three consecutive visits constitute the diagnosis of hypertension, although the 140- to 160-mmHg range represents borderline isolated systolic hypertension when diastolic pressure is less than 90 mmHg" (6).

Table 1 illustrates a subclassification of hypertension which is applicable to the elderly. As will be discussed in later sections, most of the elderly with combined hypertension (i.e., blood pressure greater than 160/90 mmHg) will be treated. The patients with borderline hypertension (i.e., blood pressure 140–159/90 mmHg or more) require close observation, and many will be empirically treated with nonpharmacologic therapy; others, exhibiting clinical evidence of cardiovascular disease with mild elevation of systolic pressure, will be treated with drugs. The importance of the predominant systolic hypertensive group is still being debated. Those with isolated systolic hypertension are at increased risk of cardiovascular disease and mortality despite the normal diastolic blood pressure. They will be discussed in a separate section.

EPIDEMIOLOGY

Both systolic and diastolic blood pressure rise with age in industrialized societies. In the United States, systolic blood pressure increases 5–10 mmHg from age 40 to 70, and diastolic blood pressure rises 5–6 mmHg (7).

Systolic pressure rises progressively with age until the age of 70 or 80. However, diastolic pressure rises with age until the age of 50–60 and then tends to level or even decrease slightly with advancing age. Figure 1 illustrates the relationship between age and blood pressure for men and women in the United States and in three other communities (8). Peak blood pressure occurs at a slightly earlier age in males than in females.

Race also influences the rise in blood pressure with age. Both systolic and diastolic blood pressure are higher in blacks than in whites during each decade after age 30 (9).

Between the third and seventh decade, the increase in systolic blood pressure is 1–9 mmHg greater for women than for men; moreover, with advancing age, the increase in diastolic blood pressure is slightly greater for women than for men (9).

Individuals with the lowest blood pressures at younger ages have the least tendency for blood pressure to rise with advancing age, whereas those with higher blood pressures at younger ages have the greatest increase in blood pressure with increasing age (10).

The rise in blood pressure with age is not inevitable. Studies on several primitive populations in South America and the South Pacific have demonstrated no significant increase in blood pressure with advancing age (11–14). This suggests that sociocultural factors such as diet, stress, smoking, physical activity, obesity, alcohol, or other factors may be causative in the hypertension seen in the elderly in industrialized societies. Many elderly individuals retain normal or low blood pressures with increasing age and have lower cardiovascular mortality and morbidity rates than those with higher blood pressures (2).

Prevalence

The prevalence of hypertension in the elderly depends upon (a) the blood pressure criteria selected to define hypertension and (b) the number of blood pressure determinations and visits prior to the diagnosis of hypertension. The risk from increasing blood pressure is a continuum; however, in order to estimate rates for hypertension, the categories of normal, borderline, or high must be selected.

The 1976–1980 National Health and Nutrition Examination Survey (NHANES) evaluated an ambulatory population, aged 65–74, and selected the average of three blood pressure measurements obtained on a single visit in order to estimate prevalence. The overall prevalence of hypertension for this age group is 64.3% for a blood pressure greater than 140/90 mmHg. Using these blood pressure criteria, the prevalence in the subgroups was as follows: black women, 82.9%; black men, 67.1%; white women, 66.2%; white men, 59.2%. The overall prevalence was 45.1% when the blood pressure selected was greater than 165/95 mmHg. The prevalence in the subgroups was as follows: black women, 72.8%; black men, 42.9%; white women, 48.3%; white men, 37.5%. Even when one used multiple visits to establish continued elevation in blood

TABLE 1. *Classification of hypertension in the elderly, based upon the level of systolic and diastolic blood pressure*

Classification	Blood pressure (mmHg) Systolic	Diastolic
Combined hypertension	>160	>90
Borderline hypertension	140–159	>90
Predominant systolic hypertension	>(DBP − 15) × 2[a]	>90
Isolated systolic hypertension	>160	<90

[a] DBP, diastolic blood pressure.

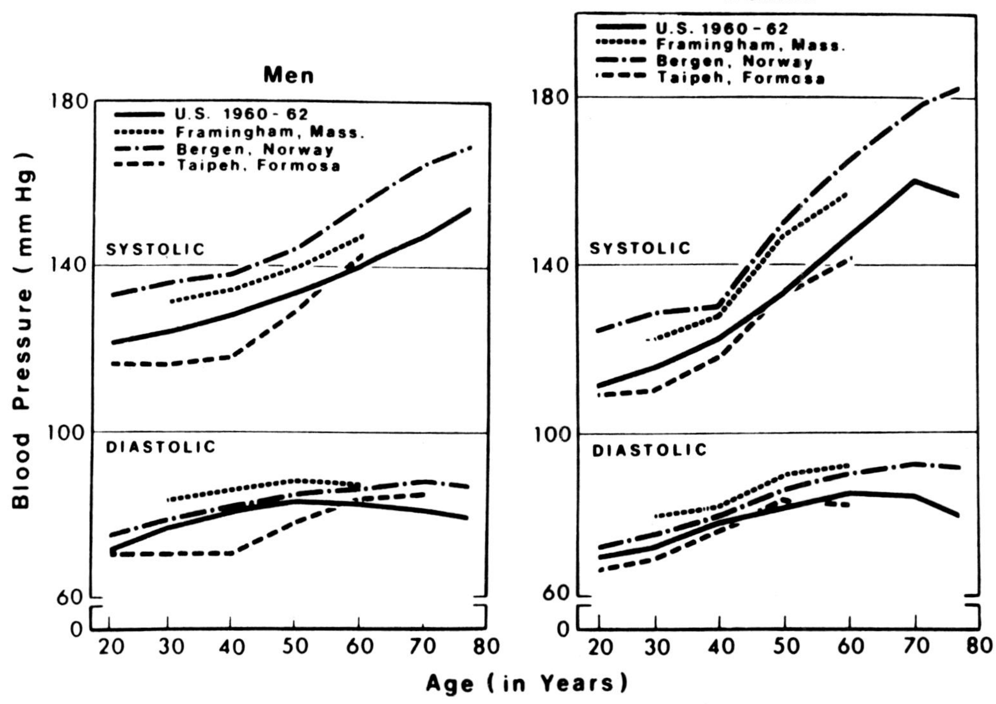

FIG. 1. Rise in systolic and diastolic blood pressure for men and women with increasing age in the United States and in three other communities.

pressure, the prevalence in this elderly population was very high (15). Similar prevalence rates were found in a 1982 probability survey of a smaller population in Connecticut (16). Sixty-eight percent of those aged 65–74 who were screened in the Systolic Hypertension in the Elderly Program (SHEP) were hypertensive (17).

Based upon data from large epidemiologic surveys, the prevalence of isolated systolic hypertension has been estimated to be 6.8–7.3%. The prevalence of isolated systolic hypertension in a population over age 60, using a systolic blood pressure equal to or greater than 160 mmHg and a diastolic pressure less than 90 mmHg after four visits, was as follows: males, 9%; females, 12%; whites, 11%; nonwhites, 13%; ages 60–69, 7%; ages 70–79, 11%; ages 80–89, 18%; over 90, 25% (18).

Risk of Hypertension

More than half of all mortality beyond age 65 is due to cardiac and cerebrovascular disease. Cardiovascular diseases are the most common cause of mortality in persons beyond age 65. Cardiovascular and renal diseases decrease life expectancy by about 10 years. Table 2 demonstrates the high incidence of cardiovascular events in elderly men and women from the Framingham Study.

Other studies have demonstrated a 40% prevalence of cardiac disease in those 65–74 years of age and a prevalence of more than 50% in those over 75. Between 40% and 60% of old people have electrocardiographic abnormalities (19,20). Advancing age significantly affects survival after the occurrence of a cardiovascular event. Mortality rates from myocardial infarction increase to 38% for ages 60–69, 43% for ages 70–79, and 58% for ages 80–89 (21). Only 20% of stroke patients over the age of 60 have a good recovery, as compared to 30–50% of younger stroke patients (22). The decreased rate of cardiovascular disease in young women, as compared to that in young men, decreases progressively with advancing age.

Hypertension stands out as the major risk factor for cardiovascular disease and mortality in the elderly. Table 3 illustrates the marked increase in cardiovascular risk in relation to hypertensive status for the elderly.

The increased attributable risk of hypertension for el-

TABLE 2. *Average annual incidence of cardiovascular events in elderly men and women in the Framingham Study: 20-year follow-up*

Coronary heart disease		Cerebrovascular disease		Peripheral arterial disease		Congestive heart failure	
Men	Women	Men	Women	Men	Women	Men	Women
20.4	14.5	8.4	8.6	6.3	3.8	8.2	6.8

[a] Rate per 1000 population (2).

TABLE 3. *Risk of cardiovascular disease in relation to hypertensive status in the elderly in the Framingham Study: 20-year follow-up[a]*

Hypertensive status[b]	Men, 65–74 years	Women, 65–74 years
Normal	17.1	8.6
Borderline	32.7	22.5
Hypertension	51.0	35.6

[a] Incidence per 1000 population.
[b] Normal, pressure < 140/90 mmHg; borderline, pressure of 140–160/90–95 mmHg; hypertension, pressure > 160/95 mmHg (2).

derly men and women is as follows: overall mortality for men and women, 8.4 and 14.9, respectively; cardiovascular mortality for men and women, 12.9 and 34.5, respectively; cardiovascular morbidity for men and women, 18.8 and 26.9, respectively (2). Cardiovascular mortality is increased eightfold in hypertensive (blood pressure ≥ 160/95 mmHg) women and twofold in hypertensive men aged 65–74 when compared to normotensive elderly subjects (23).

The risk from hypertension is due to elevation of both the systolic and diastolic blood pressure, but with advancing age the systolic blood pressure has a greater influence on the risk of stroke, left ventricular hypertrophy, and congestive heart failure than does diastolic pressure in both men and women (24).

Table 4 demonstrates the risk of cardiovascular events according to diastolic blood pressure in elderly men and women (25).

Figure 2 illustrates the probability of cardiovascular disease within 8 years in low-risk subjects according to systolic blood pressure for men and women at specified ages (26).

The probability of cardiovascular events increases dramatically for a 70-year-old with any level of systolic blood pressure when compared to the probability for a 35-year-old. The risk nearly doubles when the systolic blood pressure increases from 140 to 185 mmHg (26).

In the Framingham Study, 73% of men and 81% of women who died had blood pressure greater than 140/90 mmHg. Hypertension markedly increases the risk for congestive heart failure, atherothrombotic brain infarction, coronary heart disease, and intermittent claudication (27).

Mild hypertension (blood pressure of 140–160/90–95 mmHg) increases cardiovascular mortality fourfold for men and twofold for women aged 65–74 when compared to normotensive subjects aged 65–74 (2).

Isolated systolic hypertension increases the risk of cardiovascular morbidity and mortality in the elderly. In the Framingham Study, isolated systolic hypertension increased the risk of stroke in elderly men fourfold and more than twofold in elderly women when compared to those with normal systolic blood pressure (28). In this study, isolated systolic hypertension increased the risk of cardiovascular morbidity and mortality two- to fourfold. Isolated systolic hypertension increased mortality in the Chicago Blood Pressure Study, and the 3-year incidence of stroke was increased 2.5-fold in the Chicago Stroke Study (3,29).

It is estimated that hypertension in the elderly is responsible for 33% of all cases of cardiac disease, 42% of strokes in elderly men, and 70% of strokes in elderly women (30).

Therefore, both combined systolic and diastolic hypertension and isolated systolic hypertension are frequent in the elderly and markedly increase the risk of cardiovascular morbidity and mortality.

Other risk factors, such as a reduction in HDL cholesterol, an increase in LDL cholesterol, smoking, diabetes mellitus, and electrocardiographic evidence of left ventricular hypertrophy, are also associated with an increased risk of developing coronary heart disease in the elderly (2).

Pathophysiology

Despite the high incidence of hypertension in the elderly, a rise in blood pressure is not a normal part of the aging process. Some populations and many individuals do not have an increase in blood pressure with age. Rat models of aging do not demonstrate an increase in blood pressure with increasing age (31–34).

The normal aorta and its branches provide a distensible reservoir which modifies the pulsatile flow from the left ventricle to maintain a more continuous flow in order to perfuse vital organs and peripheral tissues (35). About half the pressure attenuation of the arterial system is provided by the thoracic aorta, and approximately 50% of the stroke volume is stored in the aorta during systole and is subsequently propelled in the vascular system during diastole in order to maintain the required mean perfusion pressure (36–38). The major effects of normal aging on the cardiovascular system involve alterations in (a) the anatomy and (b) the dynamic mechanical properties of the aorta and systemic vasculature. Aortic wall thickness increases with age, and aortic elasticity is reduced. The aorta becomes elongated and tortuous with increased diameter and volume. The increase in aortic cross-sectional area begins at the age of 20 and is linear with increasing age (38–41). These changes result in a linear increase in vascular stiffness and pulse wave velocity between 20 and 60 years of age. As the aorta loses its elasticity from aging, the left ventricle is required to pump against increased impedance. Aging increases impedance because of increased aortic

TABLE 4. *Risk of cardiovascular events according to diastolic blood pressure in men and women aged 65–74 in the Framingham Study: 18-year follow-up[a]*

Diastolic blood pressure (mmHg), men			Diastolic blood pressure (mmHg), women		
<90	90–109	≥110	<90	90–109	≥110
24.2	42.9	55.6	17.2	32.4	54.5

[a] Average annual incidence per 1000 population. From 1984 Report of the Joint National Committee on Detection (25).

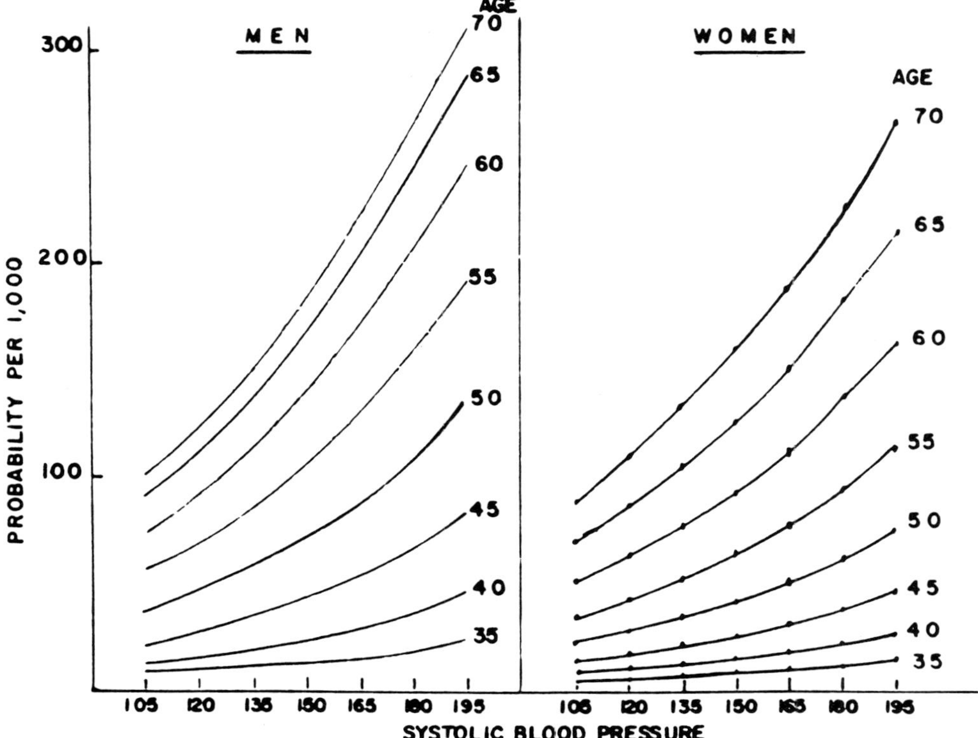

FIG. 2. Probability of cardiovascular disease within 8 years in low-risk subjects according to systolic blood pressure (mmHg) at specified ages in each sex: Framingham Study, 18-year follow-up. (Low-risk Framingham subjects have a serum cholesterol level of 185 mg per 100 ml, do not smoke, and have no glucose intolerance or left ventricular hypertrophy by electrocardiogram.) (From ref. 26.)

stiffness, which reduces diastolic recoil; in addition, the aortic contribution to forward flow decreases with a larger end-diastolic aortic volume, which increases impedance by requiring the left ventricle to work against a larger inertial force at the onset of systole. The effect of these changes includes the following: normal left ventricular end-diastolic pressure; normal heart rate; prolonged left ventricular ejection time; prolonged isovolemic relaxation time; and decreased cardiac output due to a reduced stroke volume. During maximal exercise, the following occur: an exaggerated rise in left ventricular end-diastolic pressure; decreased maximal oxygen consumption; decreased maximal heart rate; and higher arterial blood pressure and vascular resistance (42). There is also a rise in systolic blood pressure and systemic vascular resistance measured in these studies of older men, but all of the subjects are selected from industrialized societies.

Cardiac output and peripheral resistance determine the level of mean arterial pressure. The pulse pressure is a function of stroke volume and the arterial capacitance, with left ventricular ejection playing a lesser role (43). Arterial compliance is defined as the slope of the curve relating volume to pressure in the large arteries. The arterial compliance or rigidity is the ratio of pulse pressure to stroke volume. Even in normotensive individuals, aging displaces the arterial-pressure–volume curve downward and therefore decreases compliance. Because of the changes in the aorta and vasculature with age, any rise in mean arterial pressure will result in a greater increase in the pulse pressure. This increase in pulse pressure occurs regardless of whether mean arterial pressure is increased by raising cardiac output or peripheral resistance. Any patient with systolic hypertension, a normal cardiac output, and a normal diastolic blood pressure must have an increase in both total peripheral resistance and work of the heart. For each rise of 10 mmHg in systolic blood pressure, the diastolic blood pressure must fall 5 mmHg if the peripheral resistance remains normal. However, cardiac work remains elevated when the systolic blood pressure is elevated, even when peripheral resistance remains normal and the diastolic blood pressure decreases. The rise in systolic blood pressure resulting from a loss of elasticity in the larger arterial vessels should be accompanied by a compensatory decrease in diastolic blood pressure; however, this most often does not occur with aging, suggesting that other factors are causative in hypertension and aging (44).

Messerli et al. (45) evaluated the pathophysiologic characteristics of a carefully selected group of elderly hypertensive subjects and compared their systemic and regional hemodynamics, echocardiographic results, intravascular volumes, plasma renin activity, and circulating catecholamine levels to a younger group of hypertensive subjects. Table 5 illustrates the differences between the two groups (45).

Cardiac output, heart rate, stroke volume, intravascular volume, renal blood flow, and plasma renin activity were significantly lower in the elderly than in young hypertensives. Total peripheral and renal vascular resistance, left

TABLE 5. *Pathophysiologic differences in hypertensive patients*[a]

Parameter	Elderly	Young	*p* values
Age (years)	73.0	32.2	
Systolic pressure (mmHg)	182	153	$<10^{-5}$
Mean arterial pressure (mmHg)	114	113	
Diastolic pressure (mmHg)	80.7	93.2	$<10^{-5}$
Heart rate (beats/min)	67.1	72.4	<0.0186
Cardiac output (liters/min)	4.70	6.22	$<10^{-5}$
Cardiac index (liters/min/m^2)	2.60	3.38	$<10^{-5}$
Stroke volume (ml)	70.7	88.3	<0.0009
Mean LV[b] ejection rate (ml/sec)	213	292	$<10^{-5}$
Total peripheral resistance (units)	25.8	18.8	$<10^{-5}$
Ejection time (msec)	332	295	$<10^{-5}$
LV stroke work (units)	161	175	
Central blood volume (liters)	2.36	2.77	<0.0497
Total blood volume (liters)	4.10	4.64	<0.0327
Renal blood flow (ml/min)	674	1110	<0.0006
Renal vascular resistance (units)	1691	1012	$<10^{-5}$
Norepinephrine (pg/ml)	418	331	
Epinephrine (pg/ml)	95	98	
Dopamine (pg/ml)	63	62	
Plasma renin activity (μg/ml/min)	0.454	1.154	<0.047
LV diastolic diameter (mm)	51.4	49.3	
LV systolic diameter (mm)	29.8	33.2	
LV wall thickness (mm)	12.0	9.7	<0.0297
Septal thickness (mm)	11.2	10.5	<0.0444
LV mass (g)	311	222	<0.0340
LV mass index (g/m^2)	169	123	<0.0190
Velocity of circumferential fiber shortening (circ/sec)	123	107	
Radius/posterior wall thickness	224	243	

[a] From ref. 46.
[b] LV, left ventricular.

ventricular posterior wall and septal thicknesses, and left ventricular mass were higher in the elderly hypertensives. Peripheral vascular resistance was inversely related to intravascular volume in both groups. Hypertension in the elderly is characterized by increased total and peripheral resistance and decreased cardiac output and intravascular volume. There is concentric cardiac hypertrophy, accompanied by a slower heart rate and reduced stroke volume. Renal blood flow is disproportionately reduced (45,46).

Unfortunately, there are no studies comparing age-matched elderly hypertensives to elderly normotensives. It is therefore difficult to determine which of the above observations are related to hypertension and which are due to normal aging.

ETIOLOGY OF HYPERTENSION IN THE ELDERLY

The etiology of hypertension in the elderly is unknown; however, a number of important observations relating to possible etiologic factors will be reviewed.

Obesity

Body composition changes in the elderly, with a decrease in lean body mass and an increase in adipose tissue (47). There is a positive, but weak, association between increasing body mass index and increasing blood pressure in the elderly (48).

Vascular Changes

There is an increase in rigidity and a decrease in elasticity of the aorta and other large vessels with aging, caused by fracturing and uncoiling of the elastic fibers and deposition of calcium and collagenous matrix within the vessel walls (43,49). The hemodynamic effects of these changes have been discussed above. Because of these changes there is reduced compliance, and the pulse generated during systole results in a steeper rise in pressure per unit of stroke volume into the large arteries (50).

Aging arterioles have hyaline degeneration within the media, which decreases the lumen-to-wall ratio and the overall lumen cross-sectional area. Interlobular arteries exhibit intimal thickening and duplication of the elastic lamina along with hyaline changes in the media of arterioles, especially in small arteries and arterioles of the kidney. The arteries are thickened, accompanied by a decrease in cross-sectional area. Large and medium arteries (e.g., carotid, coronary, and renal arteries) demonstrate atherosclerosis (51). Hyaline changes in afferent glomerular arterioles of the kidney are common with advancing age, occurring in 16.5% of subjects over age 50 (52). Vessels which are already narrowed demonstrate increased resistance in response to vasoconstrictor agents (53).

The subsequent increment in systolic pressure results from loss of arterial distensibility and increased peripheral vascular resistance. The decrease in arterial distensibility accounts for about twice the increment in systolic pressure as compared to the rise in peripheral resistance. The natural history of essential hypertension is not characterized by further increase in peripheral resistance but, instead, by accelerated arterial stiffening, which further increases the systolic blood pressure more than the diastolic (54).

Baroreceptor Sensitivity

Baroreceptor sensitivity is decreased in the elderly (55,56). Baroreceptor reflexes are responsible for attenuating sudden increases or decreases in arterial blood pressure. One example is the drop in blood pressure with sudden standing; this activates carotid sinus and aortic baroreceptors which transmit afferent signals to the area of the nucleus tractus solitarius, resulting in (a) efferent adrenergic vasoconstrictor stimulation from the medulla and (b) cholinergic inhibition. The net effect is an increase in peripheral resistance and an increase in heart rate, resulting in stabilization of the blood pressure. Under normal circumstances, a rise in blood pressure will be attenuated by baroreceptor reflex mechanisms which decrease cardiac rate and cause peripheral vasodilation, thereby decreasing the arterial blood pressure.

Baroreflex sensitivity is commonly measured as (a) the tachycardia produced by a depressor agent or (b) the bradycardia produced by a pressor agent. When phenylephrine is administered to elderly normals or to hypertensive subjects, there is less bradycardia produced; and when vasodilators (e.g., nitroprusside, calcium-channel blockers) and other agents are administered, there is less tachycardia. The rise or fall in blood pressure with these agents is greater in older individuals than in young ones (57). Alterations in baroreceptor reflex mechanisms may have a role in the etiology of hypertension in the elderly. They may also explain the variability of blood pressure seen when the elderly hypertensives' blood pressure is monitored continuously (58). Diminished baroreceptor sensitivity results in an impairment of postural reflexes, making the elderly hypertensive more susceptible to orthostatic hypotension with or without treatment (59). Plasma norepinephrine response to upright posture rises steadily with increasing age, which suggests that the afferent limb of the baroreceptor reflex is responsive to stimuli. This suggests that the defect is in the efferent limb of the baroreceptor reflex pathways (60). Atherosclerosis in the carotid body and aortic arch, as well as changes in neural responses, have also been hypothesized to be responsible for the impairment of baroreceptor function (61).

Hormonal Changes

Renin–Angiotensin–Aldosterone

Most studies demonstrate a decrease in plasma renin with increasing age (62–66). Plasma renin activity is suppressed in the majority of elderly patients in basal circumstances when these individuals are on a fixed sodium intake and after administration of diuretics. The elderly have a decreased renin response at any given level of salt intake (67,68). The suppression of plasma renin is greater in elderly hypertensive subjects than in normotensive elderly subjects (65,69). The diminished response in plasma renin may be due to hyaline degeneration in the afferent arterioles of the kidney in the elderly, which makes the juxtaglomerular apparatus less responsive to normal stimuli, thereby decreasing renin release. Others have proposed that there is an age-related decrease in juxtaglomerular beta-adrenergic receptor response in the elderly (70). There is also diminished renin responsiveness to upright posture in the elderly, which may predispose to orthostatic hypotension (71). There is a decrease in the sensitivity of the adrenal zona glomerulosa to angiotensin II infusion in the elderly (72). Plasma aldosterone appears to be partially controlled by factors other than renin and angiotensin II in the elderly, since biologically active aldosterone does not appear to decrease in the elderly hypertensive (73).

Sympathetic Nervous System

Plasma norepinephrine levels increase with age and are independent of the age-related increase in obesity. Plasma norepinephrine averages 200 pg/ml at age 10 and 410 pg/ml at age 80 (74–77). The increase in plasma norepinephrine probably represents increased norepinephrine secretion in the elderly (78). Provocative stimuli, including upright posture and hand-grip isometric exercise, increase plasma norepinephrine to a greater extent in the elderly than in the young (77). However, the rise in norepinephrine is probably not causal for the hypertension but is, instead, an epiphenomenon. Plasma norepinephrine increases with age in both hypertensive and normotensive elderly subjects, but more in the normotensive subjects (75,79). There is an inverse relationship between blood pressure and norepinephrine in older hypertensive subjects, and continuous norepinephrine sampling in elderly subjects with essential hypertension demonstrates lower levels of norepinephrine, epinephrine, and dopamine when compared to that in age-matched normotensive individuals (80,81). The rise in norepinephrine with exercise is the same in the elderly as in the young, but the heart rate response to exercise is less in the elderly (78).

Reduced beta-1-adrenoreceptor sensitivity has been demonstrated in the elderly by a decreased heart rate response to isoproterenol infusions (82). Animal studies have demonstrated an age-related reduction in the ability of blood vessels to relax with beta-2-adrenergic stimulation (83). However, the vasodepressor response to beta-adrenergic agonists is unaffected by age in intact humans, suggesting that the beta-2-adrenoreceptors are normal (84). However, others have demonstrated a greater increase in forearm blood flow due to intra-arterial isoprenaline administration in young subjects as compared to older subjects (85). Drug sensitivity to propranolol, a nonselective beta-adrenoreceptor antagonist, is reduced in the elderly as compared to the young, despite higher plasma levels (82). However, propranolol is a racemate, and age-related changes in stereoselective metabolism could explain this finding. The elderly are not less sensitive to timolol—a nonracemate, nonselective beta-adrenoreceptor antagonist (86). There is no apparent decrease in beta-adrenoreceptor number or affinity in myocardial cells, lymphocytes, or pulmonary cells, but there is a 30% decrease in isoproterenol-stimulated adenylate cyclase activity in myocardial membranes in aged rat myocardium (87). The plasma cyclic-AMP response to infusion of salbutamol (a beta-2-adrenoreceptor-selective agonist) is less in the elderly than in young subjects.

Therefore, there is a decrease in beta-1 cardiac adrenoreceptor responsiveness in the elderly, which is probably due to decreased post-receptor mechanisms. Perhaps there is reduced beta-2-adrenoreceptor responsiveness in some vascular beds and in the kidney.

Alpha-1-adrenoreceptor response is probably unchanged by aging. Elliott et al. (88) demonstrated that the dose of phenylephrine needed to increase systolic blood pressure 20 mmHg in elderly volunteers was less than the dose needed in younger subjects. However, alpha-1-adrenoreceptor blockade with prazosin resulted in comparable orthostatic hypotension in the elderly, and a smaller dose of phenylephrine was required in order to overcome the same dosage of alpha-1-adrenoreceptor blockade with prazosin in the elderly (88). However, there is no age-related change in alpha-adrenoreceptor sensitivity in human blood vessels *in vitro* (89). There is no age-related change in response to the adrenoreceptor antagonist phentolamine when it was infused into normal forearm vessels (90). Simpkins et al. (91) and McAdams et al. (92) demonstrated decreased responsiveness to norepinephrine, but not to the alpha-1-selective agonist methoxamine in the aorta of old rats. Therefore, there is no definite abnormality in alpha-1-adrenoreceptor responsiveness with increased age.

Some authors have hypothesized that a decrease in alpha-2-adrenoreceptor responsiveness could increase blood pressure. Hyland and Docherty (93) observed that the alpha-2 agonist yohimbine was less potent in older rats. Featherstone et al. (94) administered oral clonidine to old and young subjects and demonstrated similar suppression of plasma norepinephrine, suggesting that alpha-2-adrenoreceptor-mediated suppression of norepinephrine is not diminished in elderly men.

The ability of the anticholinergic drug atropine to produce tachycardia is reduced with age in the rat and in humans (95,96). The bradycardia and negative inotropic response to muscarinic agonists is reduced in aged rats (95). There is evidence for reduced vasodilation with acetylcholine in older humans, and there is no change in vasodilation in old rats (97,98).

Therefore, reduced responsiveness with aging has been most consistent for cardiac beta-1-adrenoreceptors, cardiac muscarinic cholinergic receptors, vascular beta-adrenoreceptors and vascular alpha-2-adrenoreceptors. There is an age-related increase in norepinephrine, which is probably not related to the increase in blood pressure with age. This subject is reviewed by Docherty (32).

The role of vasopressin in hypertension is uncertain. However, elderly subjects fail to demonstrate the normal postural rise in vasopressin levels, even with symptomatic orthostatic hypotension (99).

The Kidney

The glomerular filtration rate (GFR) is approximately 140 ml/min/1.73 m^2 until age 30. Subsequently, there is a linear decline in GFR of about 8 ml/min/1.73 m^2 per decade (100,101). More recently it has been demonstrated that the decline in GFR with age is not inevitable. When subjects with hypertension, renal, or urinary tract disease or treatment with a diuretic are excluded, the mean decrease in GFR was 0.75 ml/min/year. One-third had no decrease in GFR, and a small group actually had an increase in GFR with advancing age (102).

Renal blood flow is maintained at about 350 ml/min until the fourth decade and then declines by about 10% per decade (97,103). This results in a decreased vasodilator responsiveness to acetylcholine and to a sodium load. The reduction in renal blood flow is not due solely to reduction in renal mass, since there is a progressive reduction in renal blood flow per unit of kidney mass. Cortical renal blood flow is reduced the most, and the redistribution of flow from the cortex to the medulla may account for the increase in filtration fraction. There is an increase in urinary protein and albumin excretion.

The number of functioning glomeruli declines with a reduction in renal weight; moreover, the incidence of sclerotic glomeruli increases with advancing age, from less than 5% at age 40 to about 40% by the eighth decade. Anderson and Brenner (104) have suggested that these changes are at least partly accounted for by increased renal blood flow and glomerular pressure from high dietary protein.

Elderly subjects require more time to excrete a sodium chloride load—31 hr for those over 60 years of age as compared to 18 hr for those under 25 years of age. However, after 6 days on a high- or low-salt diet, there is no difference in sodium balance. The elderly may also have more problems acutely conserving sodium when placed on a low-sodium diet (105,106). Furthermore, the elderly demonstrate a decreased ability to concentrate and dilute their urine in response to hypotonic or hypertonic solutions. Atrial natriuretic peptide is increased in aged men. This could be a result of sodium retention, atrial stretch due to other factors, or decreased peripheral receptor response. The latter seems most likely from the limited data. There are no data on elderly hypertensive subjects (107).

The relationship between these factors and hypertension in the elderly requires more investigation.

Cellular Sodium Transport

Na–K-ATPase activity declines with age in red blood cells and myocardium (108). Alterations in red-cell and white-cell sodium transport have been demonstrated in younger hypertensives and their relatives (109). However, erythrocyte Na^+–K^+ cotransport is similar in normotensive and hypertensive elderly subjects (110).

Physical Inactivity

Most elderly subjects demonstrate a decreased maximum oxygen consumption [Vo_2(max)]. The decline aver-

128. Topol EJ, Traile JA, Fortuin NJ. Hypertensive hypertrophic cardiomyopathy in the elderly. *N Engl J Med* 1985;312:277–283.
129. Veterans Administration Cooperative Study Group on Antihypertensive Agents. Effects of treatment on morbidity in hypertension III. Influence of age, diastolic pressure and prior cardiovascular disease; further analysis of side effects. *Circulation* 1982;XLV:991–1004.
130. Management Committee. Treatment of hypertension in the elderly. *Med J Aust* 1981;2:398–402.
131. Five year findings of the Hypertension Detection and Follow-up Program. Mortality by race, sex, and age. *JAMA* 1979; 141:2572–2577.
132. Langford HG, Stamler J, Wassertheil-Smoller S, Prineas RJ. All cause mortality in the HDFP Program. *Prog Cardiovasc Dis* 1986;XXIX:29–54.
133. Curb JD, Borhani NO, Schnaper H, Kass E, Entwisle G, Williams W, Berman R. Detection and treatment of hypertension in older individuals. *Am J Epidemiol* 1985;121:371–376.
134 Kuramota K, Matsushita S, Kuwajima I, Murakami M. Prospective study on the treatment of mild hypertension in the aged. Japanese mild hypertension trial. *Jpn Heart J* 1981;22:75–85.
135 Carter AB. Hypotensive therapy in smoke survivors. *Lancet* 1970;1:485–489.
136. Spackling ME, Mitchell JRA, Short AH, Walt G. Blood pressure reduction in the elderly: a randomized controlled trial of methyldopa. *Br Med J* 1981;283:1151–1153.
137. Amery A, Birkenhager W, Brixko P, et al. Mortality and morbidity results from the European Working Party on High Blood Pressure in the Elderly Trial. *Lancet* 1985;1:1349–1354.
138. Amery A, Brixko R, Clement L, et al. Efficacy of antihypertensive drug treatment according to age, sex, blood pressure and previous cardiovascular disease in patients over age 60. *Lancet* 1986;2:589–592.
139. Amery A, Berthaux P, Bulpitt C, et al. Glucose intolerance during diuretic therapy. Results from the European Working Party on Hypertension in the Elderly Trial. *Lancet* 1978;1:681–683.
140. Luft FC, Weinberger HH, Feinberg NS, Mitler JZ, Grim CE. Effects of age on renal sodium homeostasis and its relevance to sodium sensitivity. *Am J Med* 1987;82(1B):9–15.
141. Jeffery RW, Folsom AR, Luepker RV, Jacobs DR Jr, Gillum RF, et al. Prevalence of overweight and weight loss behavior in a metropolitan adult population: the Minnesota Heart Survey experience. *Am J Public Health* 1984;74(4):349–352.
142. Tabuchi Y, Ogihara T, Hashizume K, Saito H, Kumahara Y. Hypotensive effect of long term oral calcium supplementation in elderly patients with essential hypertension. *J Clin Hypertens* 1986;3:254–262.
143. Greenblatt DJ, Sellers EM, Shader RI. Drug disposition in old age. *N Engl J Med* 1982;306:1081–1087.
144. Strandgaard S. Autoregulation of cerebral blood flow in hypertensive patients. The modifying influence of prolonged antihypertensive treatment on the tolerance to acute drug induced hypotension. *Circulation* 1976;53:720–727.
145. Strandgaard S, Oleson J, Skinhoj E, et al. Autoregulation of brain circulation in severe arterial hypertension. *Br Med J* 1973;1:507–510.
146. Anderson RJ, Hart GR, Lee DK. Pitfalls in management of essential hypertension: diuretic therapy. *Prim Cardiol* 1979:63.
147. Thananopavarn C, Golub MS, Sambhi MP. Clonidine in the elderly hypertensive: monotherapy and therapy with a diuretic. *Chest* 1983;83:410–411.
148. Jeunemaitre X, Ged E, Ducrocq MB, Alhenc-Gelas F, Corvol P, Menard J. Effects of transdermal clonidine in young and elderly patients with mild hypertension: evaluation by three noninvasive methods of blood pressure measurement. *J Cardiovasc Pharmacol* 1987;10:162–167.
149. Niarchos AP, Laragh JH. Hypertension in the elderly. *Mod Concepts Cardiovasc Dis* 1980;XLIX:49–54.
150. Buhler FR, Burkart F, Lutold BE, Kung M, Marbet G, Pfister M. Antihypertensive beta blocking action as related to renin and age: a pharmacologic tool to identify pathogenetic mechanisms in essential hypertension. *Am J Cardiol* 1975;36:653–669.
151. Castledon CM, George CK. The effect of aging on the hepatic clearance of propranolol. *J Clin Pharmacol* 1979;7:49–54.
152. Kendall MJ, Brown D, Yates RA. Plasma metoprolol concentrations in young and old and hypertensive subjects. *Br J Clin Pharmacol* 1972;4:497–499.
153. Wikstrand J, Westergren G, Berglund G, et al. Antihypertensive treatment with metoprolol or hydrochlorothiazide in patients aged 60–75 years. *JAMA* 1986;255:1304–1310.
154. Down PF, Rao SK, Braverman AM, Poloniecki JD. Treatment of hypertension in the elderly with a low dose combination of beta-adrenoreceptor blocker and a thiazide diuretic: comparison with methyldopa. *Br J Clin Pract* 1983;371–374.
155. McNeil JJ, Drummer OH, Conway EL, Workman BS, Louis WJ. Effect of age on pharmacokinetics of and blood pressure responses to prazosin and terazosin. *J Cardiovasc Pharmacol* 1987;10:168–175.
156. Ramsay JWA, Scott GI, Whitfield HN. A double-blind controlled trial of a new alpha-1 blocking drug in the treatment of bladder outflow obstruction. *Br J Urol* 1985;57:657–659.
157. Eisalo A, Virta P. Treatment of hypertension in the elderly with labetalol. *Acta Med Scand* 1984;665S:129–133.
158. Abernathy DR, Schwartz JB, Plachetka JR, Todd EL, Egan JM. Comparison in young and elderly patients of pharmacodynamics and disposition of labetalol in systemic hypertension. *Am J Cardiol* 1987;60:697–702.
159. Erne P, Bolli P, Bertel O, et al. Factors influencing the hypotensive effects of calcium antagonists. *Hypertension* 1983;5(Suppl 2):II-97–II-102.
160. Muller FB, Bolli P, Erne P, Kiowski W, Buhler FR. Use of calcium antagonists as monotherapy in the management of hypertension. *Am J Med* 1984;77(Suppl 2B):11–15.
161. Ben-Ishay D, Leibel B, Stessman J. Calcium channel blockers in the management of hypertension in the elderly. *Am J Med* 1986;81(Suppl 6A):30–34.
162. Schnapp P, Hermann H, Cernak P, Kahay J. Nifedipine monotherapy in the hypertensive elderly. *Curr Med Res Opin* 1987;10:407–413.
163. Schwartz JB, Abernathy DR. Responses to intravenous oral diltiazem in elderly and younger patients with systemic hypertension. *Am J Cardiol* 1987;59:1111–1117.
164. Abernathy DR, Schwartz JB, Todd EL, Ludie R, Snow E. Verapamil pharmacodynamics and disposition in young and elderly hypertensive patients. *Ann Intern Med* 1986;105:329–336.
165. Adler AG, Leahy JJ, Cressman MD. Management of perioperative hypertension using sublingual nifedipine. *Arch Intern Med* 1986;146:1927–1930.
166. Jenkins AC, Knill, Dreslinski GR. Captopril in the treatment of the elderly hypertensive patient. *Arch Intern Med* 1985; 145:2029–2031.
167. Woo J, Wook S, Kin T, Vallance-Owen J. A single-blind randomized crossover study of angiotensin-converting enzyme inhibitor and triamterene and hydrochlorothiazide in the treatment of mild to moderate hypertension in the elderly. *Arch Intern Med* 1987;147:1386–1388.
168. Ajayi AA, Hockings N, Reid JL. Age and the pharmacodynamics of angiotensin converting enzyme inhibitor enalapril and enalaprilat. *Br J Clin Pharmacol* 1986;21:349–357.
169. Laher MS, Natin D, Rao SK, Jones RW, Carr P. Lisinopril in elderly patients with hypertension. *J Cardiovasc Pharmacol* 1987;9(Suppl 3):569–571.
170. Croog SH, Levine S, Testa MA, et al. The effects of antihypertensive therapy on the quality of life. *N Engl J Med* 1986;314:1657–1664.
171. Luxenberg J, Feigenbaum LZ. The use of reserpine for elderly hypertensive patients. *J Am Geriatr Soc* 1983;31(9):556–559.
172. Morgan TO, Nowson C, Murphy J, Snowden R. Compliance and the elderly hypertensive. *Drugs* 1986;31(Suppl 4):174–183.
173. Black DM, Brand RJ, Greenlick M, et al. Compliance to treatment for hypertension in elderly patients: the SHEP pilot study. *J Gerontol* 1987;42:552–557.
174. Herman KJ, Eisalo A. Possibility of reduction of antihypertensive therapy in hypertension [Abstract]. In: *Proceedings, Seventh Scientific Meeting of the International Society of Hypertension,* New Orleans, 1980;136.
175. Perry HM, McDonald RH, Hulley SB, McFale Smith W, et al. Systolic hypertension in the elderly program, pilot study: morbidity and mortality experience. *J Hypertens* 1986;4(Suppl 6):521–523.

Hypertension: Pathophysiology, Diagnosis, and Management, edited by J. H. Laragh and B. M. Brenner. Raven Press, Ltd., New York © 1990.

CHAPTER 117

Anesthesia in the Hypertensive Patient

Leroy D. Vandam

History of the Relation Between Anesthesia and Hypertension, 1889
Preanesthetic Considerations, 1890
- Hospital Records and the Interview, 1890
- The Physical Examination, 1891
- Laboratory Tests, 1892
- Abnormal Serum Potassium Levels During Anesthesia, 1892
- Discovery of Hypertension Before Elective Operation, 1892
- Choice of Anesthesia, 1893
- Anesthetic Risk Versus Physical Status, 1893
- Monitoring of Physiologic Function, 1893

Cardiovascular Effects of General Anesthetics, 1896
- Cerebral Circulation, 1896
- Coronary Circulation, 1896
- Splanchnic Circulation, 1896
- Renal Circulation, 1897
- Cardiac Effects, 1897
- Renal Effects, 1897
- Circulatory Effects of Opioids, 1897
- Circulatory Effects of Regional Anesthesia, 1897

Anesthesia and Antihypertensive Drugs, 1898
The Varieties of Hypertension Considered from the Standpoint of Anesthesia, 1898
- Primary Hypertension, 1899
- Endocrine Forms of Hypertension, 1899

Hypertensive Crises in the Perioperative Period, 1900
Operative Morbidity and Mortality in Hypertensive Patients, 1901
References, 1901

Since it is unlikely that an anesthesiologist would consult this text for information on the management of surgical anesthesia for hypertensive patients, the aim of this section is to acquaint other physicians with the anesthesiologist's role in this regard. Through explanation of how anesthesiologists view the problems of hypertension and their approach thereto, one might expect that referring physicians would be better able to collaborate in the preparation of patients for anesthesia and thereby provide relevant consultative opinion.

Anesthesia entails the use of highly potent drugs, which, in conjunction with the stressful response to surgery, accounts for the morbidity and mortality encountered in any kind of patient population. In spite of their growing identification with internal medicine, anesthesiologists are handicapped in providing optimal patient care as a result of their brief association with patients preoperatively and a lag in acquisition of recent knowledge in the field of hypertension, which comprises new concepts of etiology and therefore the latest treatments.

HISTORY OF THE RELATION BETWEEN ANESTHESIA AND HYPERTENSION

Anesthesiologists' concerns regarding hypertension as a symptom of disease have merely paralleled advances in medical practice in general. Even though Harvey Cushing, as a medical student in 1895, was the first to keep anesthetic records (1) and subsequently to advocate use of the Riva–Rocci method for measurement of blood pressure (2), anesthetists (as they were then known) were slow to adopt either monitoring device. At that time, patients with high blood pressure were not singled out as such. Nevertheless, from the beginning, anesthetists, through use of the senses, knew about the circulatory response to anesthetics. For example, chloroform could produce rapid collapse; whether it was cardiac or respiratory in origin was a matter of contention. Only after 1910 and the introduction of the electrocardiogram was it shown that chloroform, in the cat, sensitized the myocardium to catecholamines, with resulting ventricular fibrillation (3). Thus was born the classical hydrocarbon–epinephrine experiment which, to this day, is applicable to the use of anesthesia.

Aside from nitrous oxide, a weak anesthetic at best, and always beset by the prospect of hypoxia, diethylether (the second of the original anesthetics) must, in retrospect, be regarded as a safe anesthetic in view of its more than 100 years of usage under primitive conditions. This performance was a manifestation of sympathetic nervous stimulation and catecholamine release (4), so that respiration always ceased before the circulation in deep planes of anesthesia. In the 1930s, because of its sympathetic nervous system stimulation, cyclopropane was enthusiastically adopted because the blood pressure was usually maintained at higher-than-normal levels under many an adverse circumstance. Later on, in relation to tissue perfusion and cardiac work load, the sympathetic effects of cyclopropane were found to be deleterious rather than beneficial. Finally, both ether and cyclopropane were abandoned because of their flammability and were then succeeded by a class of nonflammable inhalation agents with lesser sympathomimetic properties.

The circulatory response to spinal anesthesia also implicated the sympathetic nervous system. From the beginning, around 1900, surgeons noticed the rapid onset of hypotension following induction of spinal anesthesia, and some routinely used a head-down position during operation. Since a cerebrovascular accident might happen in the older patient following a precipitous fall in pressure, prophylactic injection of ephedrine was introduced.

According to the above, anesthetists were merely concerned with maintenance of blood pressure at no particular level other than that it should be high enough. In defense of this attitude, one might recall that, until the 1940s, little was known of the factors that govern perfusion in the major vascular beds: brain, heart, liver, and kidneys.

In the 1940s, anesthesia's involvement with the hypertensive patient quickened as Smithwick began to perform lumbodorsal sympathectomy in an attempt to treat malignant hypertension. One can imagine what the resulting mortality was at that stage of medical knowledge. Also, surgical correction of pheochromocytoma and coarctation of the aorta had been instituted. In the late 1940s, deliberate hypotension was introduced by anesthesiologists to facilitate operation and diminish blood loss during prolonged and difficult dissections. Use of this technique had several important outcomes which eventually led to safer anesthetic practice, overall. First, unless patients were carefully evaluated beforehand for possible vascular impairment, morbidity and mortality could be high as a result of ischemic accidents in brain, heart, or kidneys. Second, the need for more accurate and consistent monitoring of blood pressure became evident. Thus, the oscillotonometer was adopted for this purpose, and routine electrocardiographic monitoring began. Finally, the pharmacologic agents used to induce hypotension—ganglionic blockers and peripheral vasodilators—were the forerunners of current antihypertensive medications, and one learned more about their actions in conjunction with anesthesia.

A climax was reached during this period of anesthetic involvement with hypertension, when reserpine was introduced for therapy, the first of many drugs to come. Although the mode of action of reserpine was still uncertain, anesthesiologists claimed that hypertensive patients treated with this drug experienced major declines in blood pressure during anesthesia, leading to cardiac arrest (5). When it became apparent that reserpine depleted norepinephrine at sympathetic nerve endings, they advocated withdrawal of the drug for at least 2 weeks before scheduled operation. This was the first encounter with drug–anesthetic interactions, not only among antihypertensive agents but among others as well. That this attitude was irrational and based on insufficient evidence was shown by the finding that untreated hypertensive patients manifested the same wide gyrations in blood pressure as did the treated subjects (6). Today we understand that adequately treated patients are far better candidates for anesthesia, in an era where the basis of essential hypertension is under scrutiny and where new drugs and combinations thereof are used therapeutically.

PREANESTHETIC CONSIDERATIONS

Under ideal circumstances, every surgical patient should be interviewed beforehand by the anesthesiologist assigned, no matter what the arrangements: inpatient status, morning admission, or outpatient surgery. Several studies have shown that an appropriate relationship between patient and anesthesiologist significantly diminishes the need for both sedative and analgesic medications during the perioperative period (7,8).

Hospital Records and the Interview

Review of previous and current hospital records is necessary to define the patient's present status. If an operation had been performed in the past, the record may reveal anesthetic complications sometimes unknown to the patient, to be avoided when possible—for example: (a) difficulty with tracheal intubation or administration of regional anesthesia and (b) serious incidents such as myocardial infarction, postoperative hepatic necrosis, or a major allergic reaction. If the operation had been performed at another hospital, the referring physician or surgeon may know of these complications and should transmit the information to the anesthesiologist. Records from other hospitals even in the same area are not readily obtained on the day before a projected operation.

During the interview, an experienced anesthesiologist can detect a patient's emotional attitude and background that determine the amount of sedation and analgesia required. In the hypertensive patient, attention is paid to contributory factors that might suggest the presence of vascular disease: obesity, smoking, physical activity, exercise tolerance, and diabetes. Information on familial disease and anesthetic experiences should also be elicited. An unexpected death of a family member during anesthesia might have been the result of a vascular accident or related to an inheritable syndrome such as malignant hyperthermia or a cholinesterase abnormality. Furthermore, a familial history of hypertension, coronary artery disease, myocardial infarction, or diabetes mellitus must be considered in relation to the patient's having occult vascular problems. In this respect, the referring physician may possess relevant information that should be transmitted to the anesthesiologist.

Current Drug Usage

Aside from documented allergic responses to drugs and the problems of drug abuse, anesthesiologists are confronted with many patients who receive specific medical therapies. Those most compelling are the vasoactive agents used in the treatment of hypertension, coronary artery disease, congestive heart failure, and cardiac dysrhythmias. Anesthesiologists now look upon use of these drugs with equanimity as they do improve the patient's condition and render them more suitable for anesthesia. However, there must be an understanding of how these medications act and how they interact with anesthetics, a subject considered later in the discussion of anesthetic actions on the circulation. Furthermore, the extent of a patient's compliance with treatment, as well as whether adequate plasma levels of drug exist, must be known.

Smoking

Smoking poses major problems for anesthesia. While referring physicians might advise their patients to stop smoking preoperatively, several weeks are required to reverse any tobacco-induced pathology. Moreover, abstinence is usually too much to ask of the inveterate smoker facing the anxieties of a major operation. Nicotine is a potent adrenergic stimulus, causing tachycardia and elevations in both systolic blood pressure and peripheral vascular resistance. During periods of heavy smoking, about 15% of the oxygen-carrying capacity of hemoglobin may be involved with carboxyhemoglobin, and therefore this portion of the hemoglobin reserve may not be available for oxygen transport. Consequently, during inhalation anesthesia, considerable amounts of carbon monoxide may accumulate in rebreathing systems (9). In addition to other factors such as elevated blood pressure, hypercholesterolemia, and obesity, smoking is said to be responsible for approximately half of the excess mortality relating to cardiovascular disease, whereas the risk of development of myocardial infarction or death from coronary artery disease is about doubled.

Chronic smoking is associated with development of airway disease in the form of bronchospasm, chronic bronchitis, and pulmonary emphysema, any of which can result in an appreciable increase in postoperative pulmonary complications. From the purely anesthetic standpoint, more subtle effects of smoking include impaired immunogenic responses, hepatic microsomal induction, gastric hyperacidity, peptic ulceration, and reflux, so that aspiration of gastric contents in the postoperative phase is more frequent and potentially lethal. A list of tobacco-related ailments appears in Table 1.

TABLE 1. *Increased risks for cigarette smokers*

Cardiovascular disease
Coronary artery disease
Peripheral vascular disease
Aortic aneurysm
Stroke (at younger ages)
Cancer
Lung
Larynx, oral cavity, esophagus
Bladder, kidney
Pancreas, stomach
Lung disorders
Cancer (as noted above)
Chronic bronchitis with air-flow obstruction
Emphysema
Complications of pregnancy
Infants: small for gestational age, higher perinatal mortality
Maternal complications: placenta previa, abruptio placentae
Gastrointestinal complications
Peptic ulcer
Esophageal reflux

From ref. 16.

The Physical Examination

While the anesthesiologist's examination need not be as extensive as in the customary general medical evaluation, attention should focus on conditions that might predispose toward anesthetic complications. Accordingly, the heart is examined for abnormal rhythms and murmurs as well as for enlargement, and the breath sounds are listened to. Blood pressure is measured in both arms and, when necessary, in the legs. Peripheral blood vessels are examined for their quality and presence of sclerosis, particularly if cannulation of veins and arteries is contemplated for circulatory monitoring. Body position of the patient, as might be required during operation, can be tested beforehand to ascertain if the head-up, head-down, prone, or lateral positions can be tolerated both physically and physiologically.

As examination proceeds, the able anesthesiologist employs all of the natural senses (as should also be done during the course of anesthesia) to detect evidence of complicating diseases. The clues are legion, as shown in Table 2.

Mouth and Airway

Few physicians other than anesthesiologists need to pay such careful attention to the mouth and airway, because the specific anatomy and presence of oral disease can pose considerable difficulty in administration of anesthesia. Can

TABLE 2. *Use of the senses: clues to disease*

Nutrition: distribution of body fat; tissue wasting
The skin: cyanosis; plethora; pigmentation; telangiectasia
The voice: arthritis; tobacco smoking; alcoholism; laryngeal carcinoma
Speech: pulmonary insufficiency; cerebrovascular accident
Cough: chronic bronchitis; COPD
The breath: uremia; ketoacidosis; alcoholism
Endocrine stigmata: Cushing's syndrome; acromegaly; hyper- and hypothyroidism; pituitary insufficiency; Addison's disease; Parkinson's disease
The eyes: exophthalmos, Horner's syndrome; arcus senilis; jaundice; strabismus
Extremities: pulmonary osteoarthropathy; nicotine stains; arthritis; nail-biting; intravenous drug use; tremor; edema
Posture and gait: lordosis; kyphosis; scoliosis; arthritis
Congenital syndromes

the patient flex the neck while extending the head to assume the "sniffing position," which is best for tracheal intubation? Can the mouth be opened fully, and are there symptoms of temporomandibular joint disease (pain, clicking sounds, crepitus, or a history of recurrent dislocation)? Is the tongue excessively large, thereby obstructing a view of the pharynx and faucial pillars and uvula, where structural changes can affect the ease of tracheal intubation? Finally, is there evidence of dental and periodontal disease accompanied by (a) loss of bony substance, (b) loose teeth, (c) caries, and (d) presence of prosthetic devices? Dentures are usually removed before anesthesia to avoid loss or damage to them, although retention of full dentures will provide a better facial contour and anesthetic mask fit. Because manipulation, even in the healthy mouth, can result in bacteremia and the threat of bacterial endocarditis, it is surprising that so many patients are permitted to approach anesthesia and operation with diseased mouths that should have been corrected beforehand.

Laboratory Tests

The tests routinely performed before operation relate to (a) the severity of a patient's illness, both medical and surgical, (b) the extent of operation contemplated, and (c) whether a major or minor anesthetic will be required. In any circumstance, the referring physician who has taken care of a patient for some time will know what is necessary —for example, whether to repeat a chest x-ray, whether to use the electrocardiogram (ECG), or whether to employ specific chemical tests pertaining to the kind of hypertension and its treatment. Usually the requirements are a hematocrit, a white-cell count and differential, and urinalysis, but an anesthesiologist may seek further information on the status of the vascular system—for example, a more recent ECG or noninvasive tests of myocardial function. A recently recorded ECG is necessary for intraoperative comparisons of tracings in patients with known heart disease such as: ischemia; conduction block in any degree; unusual syndromes such as the Wolff–Parkinson–White, sick sinus syndrome, prolapsed mitral valve, or idiopathic hypertrophic subaortic stenosis; and heart disease requiring drug therapy as in congestive heart failure, dysrhythmias, and hypertension—with possible alterations in serum electrolyte concentrations (potassium, calcium, and magnesium), as may be induced by diuretics.

A different set of problems arises when a patient's medical illness has not been adequately supervised beforehand or when, shortly before operation, an anesthesiologist believes that an essential laboratory datum is missing or that a medical consultation is necessary to establish the current status and project its course. Before embarking on a series of unnecessary actions that may lead to delay or cancellation of operation, the physicians concerned should arrive at a mutually agreeable decision on whether to perform the additional tests.

Abnormal Serum Potassium Levels During Anesthesia

Potassium concentrations in the intracellular and extracellular compartments are essential determinants of cardiac resting membrane potentials and cell excitability. Anesthesiologists have long contended that potassium imbalance can predispose to cardiac dysrhythmias during anesthesia. Respiratory alkalosis, elevations in plasma catecholamines, insulin injection, corticosteroids, digoxin, gastrointestinal losses, hypothermia, and diuretics all may lower serum potassium concentrations. Hyperkalemia commonly accompanies renal failure, hypoaldosteronism, use of potassium-sparing diuretics, extensive tissue damage, and acidosis. The fasciculations and varying degrees of skeletal muscle injury that occur with succinylcholine administration also result in a small (average 0.5 mEq/liter) increase in serum potassium. Severe hyperkalemia associated with succinylcholine administration is seen in patients with major burns or central nervous system disease of both recent and indeterminate duration. In these patients, use of succinylcholine is contraindicated, and muscle relaxation should be achieved with the use of noncompetitive neuromuscular blockers.

It is the intracellular–extracellular potassium ratio that determines resting membrane potential and excitability, so that attempts at rapid correction of chronic potassium imbalance are hazardous. This is particularly true when longstanding hypokalemia is vigorously treated with intravenous potassium, which may cause one in 200 patients to suffer life-threatening or fatal hyperkalemia. In mild to moderate chronic hypokalemia, the ratio is not so much disturbed; therefore, cardiac dysrhythmias are uncommon. During anesthesia of various kinds, it has been shown that the incidence of cardiac dysrhythmias is the same in both normal and chronically hypokalemic patients (serum potassium 2.6 to 3.4 mEq/liter). Thus, in patients at low risk for other kinds of cardiac complications, a modest reduction in serum potassium (3.0–3.5 mEq/liter) should not result in dysrhythmias and might not require potassium therapy. In acute hypokalemia or severe chronic hypokalemia, postponement of operation is prudent. Chronic hyperkalemia is well-tolerated by patients undergoing dialysis; but here too, unless serum potassium exceeds 6 mEq/liter, elective operations are not usually postponed. In both severe chronic hyperkalemia and acute hyperkalemia, appropriate therapy should be instituted before proceeding with anesthesia.

Discovery of Hypertension Before Elective Operation

Mild hypertension without symptoms, signs, or evidence of cardiovascular disease poses few problems; however, the initial discovery of major hypertension shortly before operation calls for delay, not only to find an unusual cause (e.g., pheochromocytoma) but also for thorough assessment of the circulation. Physical examination should therefore include examination of blood vessels (namely, vessels in the eyegrounds, extracranial vessels, peripheral arteries, and measurement of blood pressure in both arms and legs). In addition to the routine laboratory data, one might ask for the following: anterior and lateral chest x-rays; possibly a flat plate of the abdomen; multilead ECG tracings; and blood analysis for urea nitrogen, glucose, serum potassium, and uric acid. A diagnosis of pheochromocytoma can be established within 12 hr by urinary analysis for catecholamines and metabolites. Having eliminated the unusual causes, blood pressure should be returned toward a normal level by appropriate drug therapy, preoperatively.

Choice of Anesthesia

The anesthetic plan eventually chosen is a tripartite decision involving the patient (emotional and physical status), the surgeon and operation contemplated, and finally the anesthesiologist. With the variety of anesthetic agents and techniques available today, one can hardly conceive of a situation in which only one method should be the choice. A pertinent example in this regard is the current operative mortality in uncomplicated coronary artery bypass surgery, which is so low (below 2%) that a distinction cannot be made on the contributing role among several anesthetic techniques currently advocated. The reasons for this excellent record and the inability to select one anesthetic regimen over another are to be found in the far better preparation of patients pharmacologically, a better knowledge of cardiac performance before operation, improvement in surgical technique, more informed anesthetic management based on physiologic monitoring, and, finally, refinement in intensive care, postoperatively.

Anesthetic Risk Versus Physical Status

Risk assessment has been defined as a way of examining risks so that they may be better avoided, reduced, or otherwise managed (10): "Risk implies uncertainty, so that risk is largely concerned with uncertainty and, hence, with a concept of probability that is hard to grasp." Epidemiologically, insofar as anesthesia is concerned, risk may be assessed in terms of the following: the patient as host; the agents involved; with regard to the anesthesiologist, the anesthetic technique and the operation proposed; and, lastly, the environment, which may embrace socioeconomic and environmental factors, including hospital management and its operating-room discipline. Consequently, because of the many variables at play, the term *risk* is not applicable to predictions of anesthetic outcome.

A better way to assess the patient's encounter with anesthesia is to consider the elemental concept of physical status—as first conceived by the New York Heart Association—to prognosticate on the outcome of heart disease according to several categories ranging from disease associated with no disability to the totally incapacitated state. Subsequently this classification was utilized by the American Society of Anesthesiologists, but on a more comprehensive scale of physical status (PS) (11). Accordingly, as shown in Table 3, a patient in PS category 1 would have no complicating medical ailment, nor would the surgical condition add to the disability. In contrast, a patient listed in PS category 4 would have a major medical or surgical illness, or both, so that morbidity and mortality might be expected to be high. The PS category 5 suggests that an individual is close to being moribund and that anesthesia (minimal as it might be) and operation must be performed with the possibility that his or her life might be spared. Finally, in any PS category, the need for emergency operation implies that a patient is in poorer condition, in which case the letter E is affixed to the risk category.

TABLE 3. *New classification of physical status*

Classification of Physical Status
1: A normal healthy patient.
2: A patient with a mild systemic disease.
3: A patient with a severe systemic disease that limits activity but is not incapacitating.
4: A patient with an incapacitating systemic disease that is a constant threat to life.
5: A moribund patient not expected to survive 24 hr with or without operation.
In the event of emergency operation, the number should be preceded by an E.

According to this system, a patient with intermittent labile hypertension not requiring treatment and with no stigmata of vascular disease might fit into the PS 1 category, although some might elect status 2. On the other hand, a patient with uncontrollably high pressures in spite of expert pharmacologic management, as well as already having had a myocardial infarction and with evidence of renal failure, might be designated as PS 4.

The use of this system, even though there might not always be exact agreement on assignment of a category, permits (a) comparisons of anesthetic outcomes from one clinic to another and (b) assessment of anesthetic methods on the common basis of physical condition. Several studies on anesthetic mortality have shown a direct relation to physical status category (Table 4).

Monitoring of Physiologic Function

During anesthesia, continual evaluation of a patient's condition is necessary in order to detect deleterious changes in circulation and respiration. In the beginning, anesthetists relied solely on their senses to make such observations. As anesthetic techniques developed and new agents were introduced to keep pace with advances in surgery, while the patients treated were more seriously ill, the development of monitoring equipment proliferated. Today the galaxy of equipment necessary to maintain safe conditions during anesthetic administration is formidable, even for routine operations. The American Society of Anesthesiologists' Standards for Basic Intraoperative Monitoring, as shown in Table 5, have gone a long way toward satisfying the demands of risk management organizations. Nevertheless, the constant presence of anesthesiologists and nurse anesthetists during operation is obligatory in order to detect changes not otherwise detected by the devices, to discover failures in the equipment, and to establish diagnoses and immediately institute appropriate treatment. Because this chapter pertains to the hypertensive patient, we briefly discuss here only the elements of circulatory monitoring.

TABLE 4. *Anesthesia mortality (primary and contributory) and physical status*[a]

Authors	Total anesthetic deaths	Percentage of all anesthetic deaths by physical status class					Incidence by physical status class				
		1	2	3	4	5	1	2	3	4	5
Beecher and Todd	384	56			44		1:2,426			1:599	
Edwards et al.[b]	586	17	21	46		16					
Dripps et al.	80	0	15	34	41	10	0	1:1,013	1:151	1:22	1:11
Boba and Landmesser[b]	44 (cardiac arrests)	32			68						
Clifton and Hotten[b]	52	33			67						
Memery[b]	64	5	19	44	23	9					

[a] From ref. 17.
[b] Breakdown of total population at risk not available.

Circulatory Monitoring

Auscultation

Continuous auscultation of the chest allows monitoring of the cardiorespiratory system, and the quality of heart sounds provides information on the strength of cardiac contraction. During induction of anesthesia, a weighted stethoscope bell placed at the suprasternal notch or on the chest (anteriorly) permits cardiopulmonary monitoring. If the quality of sounds is inadequate, an esophageal stethoscope may be substituted once the trachea is protected against aspiration by a cuffed tracheal tube.

TABLE 5. *American Society of Anesthesiologists' Standards for Basic Intraoperative Monitoring*[a]

I: Qualified personnel present in room
II: Continual[b] evaluation of
- Oxygenation
- Ventilation
- Circulation
- Temperature

Oxygenation
- Breathing circuit O_2 concentration
- Skin and blood observed
- Pulse oximetry encouraged

Ventilation
- Continual
  - Clinical signs may be adequate
  - CO_2 and/or exhaled volume encouraged
- Tube placement verification
  - Clinical assessment essential
  - End-tidal CO_2 encouraged
- Mechanical
  - Device to detect disconnection mandatory
- Regional anesthesia
  - Qualitative clinical signs adequate

Circulation
- ECG continuously displayed
- Heart rate and blood pressure determined every 5 min
- Continual monitoring by clinical signs or devices

Body temperature
- Device available
- Monitor when indicated

Encouraged
- Pulse oximetry
- End-tidal CO_2
- Expired volume

[a] Does not apply to obstetric anesthesia or pain treatment.
[b] Continual: repeated regularly and frequently in steady, rapid succession.

Blood Pressure Measurement

Noninvasive Techniques. In addition to constant qualitative monitoring of the circulation, arterial blood pressure is assessed at least every 5 min by sphygmomanometry. Accurate sphygmomanometry necessitates that full cuff pressure be transmitted to the artery, so that the cuff width should be at least 20% greater than the mean diameter of the extremity. If the cuff is too narrow, the resulting pressure will be higher than true arterial pressure; if too wide, artifactually low pressures sometimes result.

Auscultation of Korotkoff sounds is the standard technique for blood pressure measurement according to the guidelines of the American Heart Association. Alternatively, blood pressure can be measured by other techniques that also employ a sphygmomanometer. Oscillotonometry (oscillometry) is utilized under some circumstances. Here, a second pressure-sensing bladder within the compression cuff is connected to a sensitive indicator of pulsatile pressure. As cuff pressure decreases from above systolic values, the indicator begins to bounce at systolic pressure. When pulsations reach a maximum, cuff pressure is equal to systolic arterial pressure; and when pulsations suddenly diminish or cease, cuff pressure equals diastolic pressure.

A third blood pressure measurement technique utilizes a flow detection device incorporating the Doppler principle, whereby the frequency of sound waves is increased or decreased by reflection from a surface that moves toward or away from the sound source, respectively. Depending on the relation between sound wave direction and the artery, the moving surface can comprise either the arterial wall or the wave-front of red blood cells within. The sound is of ultrahigh frequency (approximately 8 million cycles per second, or 8 MHz), known as *ultrasound.* The difference between transmitted and received frequencies is converted to sounds indicative of blood flow. The transducer is placed at the distal end of the pressure cuff, permitting determination of both systolic and diastolic pressures.

Systolic pressure can also be detected by sensing the pulse distal to a sphygmomanometer cuff, by the index finger placed over the radial artery, by an "optical" finger plethysmograph waveform as displayed by a pulse oximeter, or by an electronically transduced intra-arterial pressure waveform. Diastolic pressure cannot be assessed with occlusion techniques.

Automated Monitoring. Automated devices periodically measure blood pressure via one or more of the flow detection methods described; oscillometry is the most common. Measurements of systolic, diastolic, and mean blood pressure, in addition to heart rate, can be made as often as every 20 sec. Most commercial devices (Dinamap) can measure blood pressure accurately even during circulatory shock, perhaps less reliably below 70 mmHg. When these devices are programmed to make frequent measurements and to sound an alarm at abnormal conditions, they act as true circulatory monitors.

Invasive Techniques. Any patient requiring blood pressure measurement more frequently than from minute to minute requires intra-arterial monitoring. This recommendation includes patients who are critically ill, those with anticipated rapid blood loss, or those undergoing major procedures involving cardiopulmonary bypass, aortic cross-clamping, intracranial surgery, or carotid sinus manipulation. Arterial cannulation is also required when frequent blood gas sampling is necessary. Whenever an arterial cannula is required for respiratory gas analysis, blood pressure should also be monitored.

Electrocardiography

Although yielding information only on the electrical (not the mechanical) activity of the heart, the ECG is useful in diagnosing and quantifying bradycardia, tachycardia, and dysrhythmias. For an accurate diagnosis to be made, continual oscilloscopic display is required. An audible indicator of QRS complexes is useful whenever the activity of the heart is not under continual surveillance as with a stethoscope or pulse oximeter. This audible indicator allows the anesthesiologist to carry on other necessary activities while being prepared to observe the ECG trace should the sound suggest an arrhythmia or absent activity.

The ECG can also be a useful monitor of myocardial ischemia. Because ischemia most often involves the anterior, lateral, or inferior cardiac surfaces, ECG leads that are appropriately sensitive should be utilized. A modified lead II—from right shoulder to cardiac apex, as commonly used—is moderately and equally sensitive to ischemia arising in these locations. An additional advantage is that both P waves and QRS complexes are upright and of sufficient amplitude because the cardiac and monitoring axes are similar.

Central Venous Pressure

Right- and left-heart filling pressures provide useful indices of the adequacy of circulating blood volume and myocardial contractility. Central venous pressure (CVP) represents the hydrostatic pressure in the right atrium or intrathoracic vena cavae. A normal CVP ranges from 2 to 15 cm H_2O or from 1.5 to 11 mmHg. The pressure rises and falls with changes in intrathoracic pressure, an effect particularly pronounced during positive-pressure pulmonary ventilation. Therefore, CVP must always be measured at end-expiration or averaged over one or several breaths. The central location of the catheter must be verified by careful observation of the respiratory fluctuation of the CVP trace or by use of an electronic transducer. Cannulation of the central venous circulation can be accomplished via several routes. The internal and external jugular veins are most commonly chosen, with the antecubital and subclavian routes less often elected; none is without complications. Therefore, CVP monitoring is reserved for those patients who may undergo major alterations in blood volume or when central venous cannulation is required for other purposes.

When CVP is low, circulating blood volume may be inadequate or venous capacity may be enlarged—as a result of sympathetic blockade or vasodilation. In patients with normal cardiac function, a high CVP suggests an elevated circulating blood volume or decreased venous capacity owing to vasoconstriction or vasoactive drug therapy. Measurement of CVP is required whenever there is uncertainty over adequacy of circulating blood volume in relation to the need for fluid replacement.

Pulmonary Artery Pressure

When left-heart failure is present preoperatively, or when the potential for its onset exists during anesthesia, left-heart filling pressure should be measured. This is accomplished by use of a balloon-tipped, pulmonary artery flotation catheter (PA catheter), as first described by Swan and Ganz.

A plastic sheath with introducer is inserted percutaneously into the internal jugular vein; occasionally the external jugular or basilic vein is used. The sheath offers an internal diameter sufficient to pass a No. 8 French catheter with a side port for fluid infusion. The balloon at the catheter tip is inflated with 1 ml of air, and the catheter is advanced while the pressure waveform is visually monitored. Characteristic waveforms are identified as the catheter passes from right atrium through right ventricle into pulmonary artery. The catheter is then further advanced to the wedged position, where display of a venous waveform with the balloon inflated—as well as pulmonary artery waveform with the balloon deflated—is possible. When the balloon is wedged, a waveform with A (atrial) and V (ventricular) waves is observed because the catheter is in direct fluid-continuity with the left atrium in a system where there is no flow; pulmonary capillary wedge pressure (PCWP), therefore, accurately represents mean left atrial pressure (LAP). To avoid respiratory artifacts, PCWP should always be obtained at ambient pressure and at end-expiration, with employment of an electronic pressure transducer. In the absence of pulmonary disease, pulmonary artery diastolic pressure (PADP) closely approximates PCWP and can be continuously monitored.

If PCWP is high (above 23 mmHg), myocardial function is deemed inadequate regardless of CVP. If PCWP is normal (less than 12 mmHg) and simultaneous with a normal

CVP, circulating blood volume and myocardial function are probably adequate. With the balloon deflated, pulmonary artery pressure can be monitored—a useful measurement in patients with elevated pulmonary vascular resistance or right-heart failure.

Complications of pulmonary artery catheterization are common: Clot formation along the catheter surface as well as ventricular arrhythmias during insertion are the rule rather than the exception, whereas pulmonary infarction and hemorrhage are rare, but major complications.

Cardiac Output

An overall quantitative estimate of cardiovascular performance is provided by measurement of cardiac output (CO), since this represents total blood flow to all body tissues as well as to associated vascular shunts. Although alterations in peripheral vascular resistance can result in regional ischemia despite normal CO, total output is nevertheless a useful guide to cardiovascular assessment.

Cardiac output is most easily measured with thermodilution. A modification of the balloon-tipped pulmonary artery flotation catheter is used with a thermistor (temperature-sensing transducer) placed near the tip, just proximal to the balloon. Either a 10-ml bolus of iced solution or a solution at room temperature (normal saline or dextrose) is injected through the CVP port of the catheter. Thus, a thermal indicator, as quantified in negative calories, is carried through the right ventricle into the pulmonary artery and diluted as blood flows through the right heart. Temperature is sensed by the thermistor in the pulmonary artery. Cardiac output is inversely proportional to the area under the temperature–time curve, since blood flow is the source of "thermal dilution." Room temperature injectate can be used without significant decrease in overall measurement accuracy.

Thermodilution has several drawbacks: It provides only intermittent measurements; a pulmonary artery catheter is necessary; cold fluid administration is required; and sterility is not readily guaranteed. Thus, several techniques for continuous CO monitoring are available. The transthoracic impedance technique has had only limited success despite a several-decade trial. The trans-esophageal Doppler velocity technique shows promise as a quantitative monitor and appears, at least, to be a satisfactory circulatory trend indicator under many circumstances.

CARDIOVASCULAR EFFECTS OF GENERAL ANESTHETICS

As observed in the section on monitoring of physiologic function, in-depth recording of circulatory changes during anesthesia has become routine, with more probing techniques applied to patients with major disease. No longer is blood pressure measurement the sole criterion, since anesthesiologists attempt to assess the performance of the heart in terms of its oxygen demand and supply. Preload—through its effect on end-diastolic fiber length and, therefore, on stroke volume (SV)—can be assessed by determination of CVP and PCWP. Afterload, which affects systolic wall stress (force per cross-sectional area), is inferred from measurements of systolic, diastolic, and mean arterial pressures and calculation of peripheral vascular resistance (PVR). In addition to SV and PVR, the main determinants of myocardial work and oxygen demand comprise the pulse rate and contractile or inotropic state of the myocardium. In choosing anesthetic agents and techniques for patients with circulatory compromise, one attempts to minimize the workload while supporting the circulation in terms of its oxygen delivery capacity.

Effective concentrations of most general anesthetics significantly alter blood flow. The actions on several vascular beds are considered separately here, since alterations in flow result from both centrally and locally mediated mechanisms and cannot be predicted on the basis of changes in arterial pressure alone.

Cerebral Circulation

Aside from their influence on blood pressure, anesthetics affect the cerebral circulation, both directly and indirectly, and also affect the indirect actions mediated by respiratory ventilatory depression and accumulation of CO_2 (a potent cerebral vasodilator) as well as by depression of cerebral metabolism rate (CMR), which may affect local control over cerebral perfusion. Since inhalation anesthetics directly affect cerebrovascular smooth muscle and also depress CMR, they are direct cerebral vasodilators. The effect is most prominent with halothane, less so with enflurane or isoflurane. Increases in intracranial pressure taken as indices of cerebral vasodilation have been reported with all of the commonly used inhalation anesthetics. However, the direct effect on vascular smooth muscle may not be the principal cause of cerebral vasodilation but, rather, the result of uncoupling of metabolic control of the circulation. Cerebrovascular autoregulation is depressed by all of the commonly used volatile anesthetics.

Coronary Circulation

The interactions between coronary blood flow, mean arterial blood pressure, cardiac work, and myocardial metabolism are well known. Halothane, isoflurane, and enflurane all reduce coronary blood flow and myocardial oxygen consumption, apparently as a result of decreased myocardial need for oxygen; these effects are to some extent, counteracted by catecholamine secretion (apprehension, excitement, hypertension).

Splanchnic Circulation

The splanchnic circulation comprises the vessels of the gastrointestinal tract, liver, spleen, and pancreas. Halothane, enflurane, and isoflurane all reduce splanchnic blood flow in a dose-related manner, but not always by the same mechanism. For example, halothane leaves vascular resistance unaltered while reducing perfusion pressure;

however, nitrous oxide does not significantly alter splanchnic hemodynamics. Changes in hepatic blood flow can affect the metabolism of drugs and are probably responsible for the abnormal liver function tests observed postoperatively.

Renal Circulation

Renal blood flow is reduced by anesthetics independently of alterations in arterial pressure. Nitrous oxide, halothane, enflurane, and isoflurane all increase renal vascular resistance and decrease cortical blood flow. These effects are easily explained for agents that stimulate the sympathetic nervous system but hardly account for the renal vasoconstriction observed with halothane. Reductions in glomerular filtration rate (GFR), ranging from 19% to 55%, and in renal plasma flow (RPF; para-amino hippurate clearance), ranging from 36% to 67%, have been reported at surgical planes of anesthesia. In general, greater reductions in GFR and RPF are associated with deeper levels of anesthesia. The filtration fraction (GFR/RPF) and calculated renal vascular resistance are consistently increased, suggesting that augmented efferent arteriolar tone sustains glomerular filtration pressure. Changes in renal perfusion also activate the renin–angiotensin system, so that part of the vasoconstriction may be explained on that basis.

Cardiac Effects

All of the commonly used potent anesthetics exert a direct depressant effect on myocardial contractility. In the isolated heart, this depression is approximately equivalent to that seen in uncompensated congestive heart failure. During anesthesia with isoflurane, the patient's cardiac output, stroke volume, and mean arterial pressure are maintained at normal levels (or above) as a result of stimulation of sympathetic nervous activity. Nitrous oxide causes little change or only a minor increase in cardiac output as a result of minor sympathetic stimulation. By contrast, halothane and enflurane lack sympathetic stimulatory properties, and cardiovascular depression is evidenced by a dose-dependent decrease in arterial pressure, stroke volume, and cardiac output. Heart rate increases with enflurane and isoflurane but remains essentially unchanged with nitrous oxide and halothane. Isoflurane is unique among the commonly used volatile anesthetics in increasing the cardiac index. Prolonged anesthetic administration partially reverses the depressant effects of halothane and increases the stimulant effects of agents that activate the sympathetic nervous system. These changes may result from increased beta-sympathetic activity.

Renal Effects

General anesthesia results in an antidiuresis characterized by a marked reduction in urine volume (60–70%), increased urine osmolality, and reabsorption of water by the renal tubules in excess of solute, resulting in negative free water clearance. Partial reversal of the antidiuresis by intravenous administration of ethanol suggests that antidiuretic hormone (ADH) is released during general anesthesia, responsible, in part, for the antidiuresis. Reduction in GFR also contributes to the oliguria. Sodium and potassium excretion are reduced as a result of the reduction in GFR, possibly because of hormonal influences acting on the renal circulation. Increased amounts of plasma renin sampled from the renal vein during halothane anesthesia suggest that activation of the renin–angiotensin–aldosterone system may, in part, be responsible for renal vasoconstriction as well as sodium retention.

The antidiuresis resulting from anesthesia, together with that arising from operative trauma and the use of opioids, may result in persistent oliguria and postoperative fluid retention. Administration of large quantities of fluid in the immediate postoperative period may therefore result in dilutional hyponatremia and water intoxication, particularly in elderly patients.

In most patients with normal kidneys, changes in hemodynamics and water and electrolyte excretion are transitory and return to normal following anesthesia. Renal effects of general anesthesia in patients with preexisting renal disease have not been thoroughly assessed. A toxic effect of methoxyflurane to produce nephrogenic diabetes insipidus led to its abandonment.

Circulatory Effects of Opioids

With a subject in the supine position, little change in blood pressure or pulse results from intravenous injection of an opioid. E. Lowenstein found that large doses of morphine (1–3 mg per kg of body weight) given intravenously to cardiac surgical patients increased cardiac index, stroke index, central venous pressure, and pulmonary artery pressure while decreasing systemic vascular resistance. Thus, morphine or its congeners are now extensively used for analgesia and anesthesia in cardiovascular operations. However, with a subject in the erect position, morphine usually results in arterial hypotension because of a direct effect on smooth muscle of peripheral vessels, related to histamine release. Under these circumstances, elderly patients are particularly prone to develop hypotension and syncope, as are patients with diminished circulating blood volumes.

Under some circumstances, when patients respond to surgically induced activation of the sympathetic nervous system by becoming hypertensive and tachycardic, a volatile anesthetic such as isoflurane may be employed as a vasodilator to reduce systemic vascular resistance and to control blood pressure. This use of lesser amounts of an inhalation anesthetic to supplement large-dose opioid anesthesia contrasts with the former practice of using inhalation agents alone.

Circulatory Effects of Regional Anesthesia

Local anesthetics are utilized to provide regional anesthesia in isolated areas of the body, in contrast to general anesthesia. For any patient the advantages are many:

avoidance of the many adverse effects of general anesthesia; more rapid and uncomplicated recovery; simplicity of method; and low cost. Peripheral nerve blocks have little effect on the circulation except in the advent of overdosage and toxicity or possible systemic effects of epinephrine added to the anesthetic solution. Regional anesthesia also eliminates the hormonal stress response to surgery.

Spinal and epidural anesthesia, the two major kinds of regional anesthesia, affect the circulation by interruption of sympathetic nervous outflow to the vasculature in proportion to the spinal level of blockade. In spinal anesthesia, the small amount of local anesthetic injected into the subarachnoid space has no systemic consequences, but sympathetic blockade occurs rapidly. The diminution in preload resulting from an increase in venous capacitance, combined with the decrease in peripheral vascular resistance, decreases myocardial work load. However, and especially in the presence of sclerosis, the decline in mean arterial blood pressure should not be allowed to compromise perfusion in the major circulatory areas. Therefore, preliminary intramuscular or intravenous injection of a vasopressor drug is given either prophylactically or after the fact, to maintain an appropriate mean diastolic pressure. Ephedrine, with its mixed alpha- and beta-sympathetic agonistic properties, and phenylephrine (Neo-Synephrine), with its mainly alpha-type stimulation, are the two agents commonly used.

For epidural anesthesia, larger volumes of local anesthetic are required for a given level of blockade than for spinal anesthesia. Although the onset of hypotension is less rapid and less severe if epinephrine is added to the anesthetic solution, direct cardiac effects are not uncommon. The resulting depression of the circulation is qualitatively the same as in spinal anesthesia and is treated accordingly.

ANESTHESIA AND ANTIHYPERTENSIVE DRUGS

Nowadays, only the rare hypertensive patient is not treated by drugs (Table 6). In general, these compounds affect the central and peripheral components of the sympathetic nervous system by altering the synthesis, release, biotransformation, or action (at end-organs) of norepinephrine. Since the circulatory depressant effects of general anesthetics may be additive, the combination of antihypertensive drugs and anesthetics has caused concern and controversy.

As occurred with the introduction of reserpine, controversy arose over the preanesthetic use of beta-adrenergic blockers. These drugs, first used as antiarrhythmics and then for treatment of angina, are now adjuvants or the sole drugs employed in the treatment of hypertension. Propranolol (Inderal), the first of the compounds, exerts negative inotropic and chronotropic effects on the heart, has little influence on peripheral vascular resistance, and has a tendency to induce bronchospasm. Thus, anesthetists became concerned over the possibility of additive effects during administration of general anesthesia. It would have been necessary to discontinue the drug at least 8–12 hr preoperatively because the half-life of propranolol is approximately 4–6 hr after chronic use, while complete dissipation of effect requires about 48 hr. When this was done, however, some patients with angina who continued in their customary daily activities developed myocardial ischemia and infarction. Thus, adrenergic blockade is now considered essential during the perioperative period, and anesthesiologists regard the medically treated patient as a better candidate for anesthesia.

THE VARIETIES OF HYPERTENSION CONSIDERED FROM THE STANDPOINT OF ANESTHESIA

At one time or another, every anesthesiologist will be confronted by a patient with one of the hypertensive syndromes listed in Table 7. With the exception of primary or essential hypertension, the other categories frequently require surgical correction.

TABLE 6. *Drugs used in the treatment of hypertension*

Drugs	Frequent adverse effects
Diuretics	
Thiazide type	Hypokalemia, hyperuricemia, hyperglycemia,
Chlorothiazide (Diuril), others	hypomagnesemia, allergy
Loop diuretics	Above, plus dehydration
Furosemide (Lasix)	
Potassium-retaining	Hyperkalemia, hyponatremia
Spironolactone (Aldactone), others	
Peripheral sympatholytics	Bradycardia, fatigue, sedation, increased airway
Beta-adrenergic blockers	resistance, CHF, beware of sudden
Propranolol (Inderal)	withdrawal
Prazosin (Minipress)	
Reserpine (Serpasil), others	
Central sympatholytics	Major rebound hypertension, headache,
Clonidine (Catapres)	sedation, dry mouth
Methyldopa (Aldomet)	
Arteriolar dilators	Tachycardia, postural hypotension
Hydralazine (Apresoline)	

TABLE 7. *Etiology of hypertension*

1. Essential or primary hypertension
2. Primary renal disease: nephritis, renal arterial stenosis, congenital abnormalities
3. Toxemia of pregnancy
4. Endocrinopathy
   - A. Adrenal cortical hyperfunction
     - a. Hyperaldosteronism
     - b. Cushing's syndrome
     - c. Adrenogenital syndrome (hypertensive forms)
   - B. Chromaffinomata
     - a. Pheochromocytoma
     - b. Paraganglionoma (especially organ of Zuckerkandl)
   - C. Hyperthyroidism, acromegaly, hyperparathyroidism
5. Hemodynamic alterations
   - A. Coarctation of the aorta
   - B. Reduced elasticity of vascular system
   - C. Decreased peripheral resistance
6. Neurogenic hypertension
   - A. Rapidly elevated intracranial pressure
   - B. Seizures: grand mal, autonomic
   - C. Denervation of the carotid sinus
   - D. Polyneuritides, porphyria, bulbar poliomyelitis, tetanus

[a] From ref. 18.

Primary Hypertension

The discussions in this text have shown that the cause of essential hypertension is most likely multifold. Early in its course, the pressure may be elevated because of an increase in cardiac output or an elevation in peripheral vascular resistance, or both. The anesthesiologist recognizes this as labile hypertension, which is not of great concern unless it is drug-treated or possibly associated with early onset of vascular disease. In this regard, the statistics show that life expectancy relates inversely to elevations both in systolic and diastolic pressure, whereas the chief causes of death comprise cerebrovascular accidents, myocardial infarction, and renovascular sclerosis terminating in failure. Thus the goal in any kind of hypertension is the maintenance of adequate tissue perfusion in these vascular beds and application of measures to treat extremes of pressure, high or low as may be necessary. Upon entry to hospital, the pressure may be unduly elevated; moreover, during anesthesia there may be wide gyrations, with hypotension often a manifestation of a low plasma volume in the chronically hypertensive state.

Endocrine Forms of Hypertension

This category of hypertensive disease comprises about 5–10% of all cases of hypertension, most of them potentially curable by surgical means.

Pheochromocytoma

Fewer than 0.5% of hypertensive patients have a pheochromocytoma, a physiologic kind of malignancy which is a relatively easily diagnosed and treated disease but, when untreated, can result in malignant hypertension and death. Pheochromocytoma may be a component of one of the familial, multiple endocrine syndromes in association with medullary carcinoma of the thyroid and parathyroid adenoma. In patients with untreated pheochromocytoma undergoing routine surgical procedures, the mortality rate may exceed 10%. Thus, in taking a history from a hypertensive patient, one must be alert to detect the characteristic symptoms. The tumor, which arises from chromaffin tissue in the adrenal medulla or at other paraaortic sites and rarely intracranially, secretes excess amounts of the catecholamines (epinephrine and norepinephrine), which spill over into the circulation and cause the distinctive syndrome. Although the latter is usually typified by paroxysmal hypertension, headache, tachycardia, tremor, nervousness, ventricular arrhythmias, and sweating, in some patients the elevated blood pressure is sustained, with episodic elevations. The diagnosis is confirmed by analysis of urine or plasma for catecholamines and their metabolites: epinephrine, norepinephrine, metanephrine, normetanephrine, and vanillylmandelic acid.

Since there are both false positives and negatives, diagnostic tests for pheochromocytoma must be timed to coincide with hypertensive paroxysms. Provocative methods—namely, the cold pressor test or intravenous injection of glucagon (1–2 mg)—are now rarely employed. The tumor or multiple tumors may be located with x-ray, computerized tomography, or selective sampling for catecholamines from the vena cava.

Since extirpation of the tumor is the currently accepted treatment, meticulous preparation of patients is essential. An attempt is made to return blood pressure to normal via the action of phenoxybenzamine (Regitine), a short-acting alpha-1 blocker taken by mouth (10–20 mg, three to four times daily). Prazosin (Minipress), also an alpha-adrenergic blocker (2–5 mg, b.i.d.), has a longer duration of action. However, a prolonged hypotensive drug effect can conceal the blood pressure rise, thereby sometimes helping a surgeon to locate the tumor during exploration. Because of the contracted vascular bed in these chronically hypertensive patients, vasodilator therapy results in hemodilution, a decline in hematocrit, and a tendency toward postural hypotension. Thus, supplemental saline infusions may be necessary, or packed red-cell transfusion may be given if the hematocrit is too low before operation. Since tachycardia and ventricular arrhythmias may persist despite adrenergic blockade, they may be treated in the perioperative period with propranolol (Inderal), a beta-1-adrenergic blocker, or labetalol (Normodyne), a combined alpha- and beta-blocker.

After a satisfactory preoperative physiologic condition has been attained, anesthesia is currently given with isoflurane (Forane) the main agent, or a balanced combination of potent opioid (Fentanyl), nitrous oxide, and a neuromuscular blocking agent. Extensive monitoring of the circulation is practiced, with observance of intra-arterial, central venous, and pulmonary artery pressures, plus multiple channel electrocardiographic recording. The goal is to avoid wide swings in blood pressure. Thus, careful fluid and electrolyte replacement plays a major role, as does the use of (a) vasodilator drugs [sodium nitroprusside (Nipride)], nitroglycerin, or phentolamine to lower pressure or (b) a vasoactive drug (phenylephrine) to elevate pressure. Lidocaine (Xylocaine) and propranolol are on hand to treat arrhythmias. When an adrenal gland is removed, subsequent replacement with hydrocortisone may be necessary. This plan of management is carried out postoperatively until the circulation stabilizes. If the blood pressure does not return to normal within several days postoperatively, residual tumor or a metastasis may be present. Malignant tumor metastases may be responsive to radiation therapy, and the symptoms may be controlled by drugs which block the synthesis of catecholamines: metyrosine and alpha-methyltyrosine (Demser capsules), 0.25 mg, four times daily.

Cushing's Syndrome and Hyperadrenocorticism

Excess production of hydrocortisone—resulting from either adrenal hyperplasia, neoplasm, or a pituitary adenoma (classical Cushing's disease)—leads to hypertension in the majority of cases. Although the cause of the hypertension is not certain, administration of high doses of corticosteroids to laboratory animals results in hypertension. Furthermore, the vasopressor response to norepinephrine is potentiated while sodium and fluids are retained, thus increasing intravascular and extravascular volume. In some instances, hyperaldosteronism is an associated factor. Anesthesia is complicated to a lesser extent by the hypertension,which is handled in the usual manner, more so by altered sodium, potassium, and fluid balance and the need for steroid therapy when the adrenal glands are removed.

Primary Hyperaldosteronism

Adrenal cortical hypersecretion of aldosterone resulting from benign or malignant tumors or from hyperplasia leads to increased sodium reabsorption and potassium loss in the renal tubules. The clinical manifestations of hyperaldosteronism derive mainly from these biochemical alterations, with hypertension and hypokalemia being most prominent. Cardiac output is normal, peripheral vascular resistance is increased, and blood volume is expanded. Because the hypertension is usually moderate, except for the rare instance of progression to the malignant phase, problems in anesthesia concern alterations in the essential electrolytes, as well as replacement therapy with corticosteroids upon surgical removal of the adrenal glands.

Renovascular Hypertension

Renal arterial stenosis results in the most common form of potentially curable hypertension. For the anesthesiologist's information, the hypertension is caused by increased renin secretion from the juxtaglomerular apparatus as a result of diminished renal blood flow and also because of alterations of sodium content in the macula densa of the distal renal tubule. Renin output, as found during renal venous sampling, increases during cyclopropane (no longer employed) and halothane anesthesia, probably a manifestation of renal vasoconstriction. Increase in renin output is followed by elaboration through several enzymatic steps of the potent pressor substance, angiotensin II. Then, through the action of angiotensin on the glomerulosa layer of the adrenal cortex, hyperaldosteronism occurs to a modest degree in some cases, more so in the malignant phase of renovascular disease. From the anesthesia standpoint, the problems are very much like those encountered in other forms of endocrine hypertension, often with the additional factor of generalized arteriosclerosis. Today, many a hypertensive patient is treated with angiotensin-converting-enzyme-blocking drugs, with the reasons for the effectiveness not being clear.

HYPERTENSIVE CRISES IN THE PERIOPERATIVE PERIOD

Alarming elevations in blood pressure may occur in any patient in the perioperative period upon provocation by specific stimuli. A hypertensive crisis may be defined as a level of blood pressure considerably above the maximum to which a patient had been accustomed, perhaps above 30–50 mmHg systolic and 10–20 mmHg diastolic. A crisis exists because continuance of the hypertension, even for a brief period, might result in any of the following: cerebrovascular accident; aortic dissection; left-heart failure and development of pulmonary edema; S-T segment depression on the ECG; myocardial infarction; or operative hemorrhage. Thus, diagnosis and therapy must be prompt, using the pharmacologic approach outlined at the conclusion of this section.

Intraoperatively, it is the previously hypertensive individual who is most susceptible to the crisis; however, in any patient, the common precipitating causes are (a) failure to block the autonomic nervous system response to pain and (b) circulatory fluid overload. Less prevalent factors are (a) hypoxemia and CO_2 retention, (b) the malignant hyperthermia syndrome, (c) previously undetected pheochromocytoma or hyperthyroid crisis, (d) fluid transudation during transurethral prostatectomy, (e) toxemia of pregnancy, and (f) iatrogenic causes relating to use of vasoactive drugs or to prior treatment with monoaminoxidase inhibitors.

In the recovery room and intensive care unit, development of hypertension is common in those who have undergone cardiac, vascular, or intracranial operations. A rise in intracranial pressure represents a true emergency. Postoperatively, the common denominators that result in hypertension include the following: pain; delirium; hypoxemia and hypercapnia; hypothermia accompanied by shivering; circulatory fluid overload; and prolonged effects of vasoactive drugs. Geriatric patients are readily thrust in the hypertensive direction by these phenomena.

According to the cause of the hypertension, appropriate therapy would seem apparent: adequate pain relief with analgesics given intravenously at first; improvement of oxygenation and alveolar ventilation; warming for hypothermia; and induced diuresis for fluid overload. All the while, the ECG and blood pressure should be closely observed, the latter via a Dinamap (automatic oscillotonometry) or via an intra-arterial recording if already in use. In addition to specific measures, vasodilatory drugs are given to reduce mean arterial blood pressure and to reduce cardiac preload and afterload. One must not overshoot the mark, since this would lead to equally dangerous hypotension.

The direct- and indirect-acting vasodilators are given intravenously in the crisis. All of these compounds have advantages and disadvantages insofar as their vascular actions are concerned, so that any one of them should be given slowly and deliberately to avoid overshooting the mark; namely, an appropriate mean arterial pressure for the particular patient concerned.

OPERATIVE MORBIDITY AND MORTALITY IN HYPERTENSIVE PATIENTS

Aside from the anesthetic management of pheochromocytoma, few data exist that pertain to anesthetic and operative morbidity and mortality in other hypertensive syndromes. Goldman et al. (12) found little correlation between preoperative blood pressure levels and development of cardiovascular complications. Patients with asymptomatic hypertension, accompanied by diastolic blood pressures below 115 mmHg, were not at increased risk for cardiac complications regardless of whether blood pressure was adequately or inadequately treated. Moreover, although hypertension is usually associated with other circulatory abnormalities, when controlling for these conditions, mild to moderate hypertension per se was not a predictor of postoperative cardiac complications.

In a prospective epidemiologic study of 5127 men and women over a period of 14 years, Kannel et al. (13) found a well-established association between hypertension and coronary heart disease (CHD). The incidence of all manifestations of CHD (including angina, coronary insufficiency, myocardial infarction, and sudden death) was significantly related to antecedent, elevated levels of systolic and diastolic pressure. Furthermore, Frank et al. (14) found that the presence of hypertension prior to initial myocardial infarction was associated with an increased mortality.

In view of these findings, data on operative mortality in relation to coronary artery disease and myocardial infarction are relevant. Tarhan et al. (15), in a retrospective analysis of 32,877 patients (aged 30 years or over) who underwent some form of operation or diagnostic procedure, found evidence of myocardial infarction in 422 patients before operation. In this group, reinfarction, as suggested by symptoms, ECG and enzyme changes, or postmortem examination, occurred in 28, or 6.6%, during the first postoperative week. Furthermore, 43% with no prior suggestion of myocardial infarction developed infarction postoperatively. Thus, the incidence of myocardial infarction was 0.13% in all patients who were given anesthesia. Of the 28 patients with reinfarction, 15 died (54%); in 12 of these (80%) death occurred during the first 48 hr. Among those patients with no preoperative myocardial infarction, 16 had CHD with angina. In the other 27, there was no history of CHD; however, six had diabetes and 10 were being treated for hypertension. The shorter the interval between a previous myocardial infarction and a major operation, the greater the hazard of reinfarction; within 3 months, the mortality approached 16%. Overall, the kind of anesthetic and duration of operation had no influence on the incidence of reinfarction.

ACKNOWLEDGMENT

I wish to thank James H. Philip, M.D., for considerable aid in preparing the section on Monitoring of Physiologic Function.

REFERENCES

1. Beecher HK. The first anesthesia records. *Surg Gynecol Obstet* 1940;71:689–693.
2. Cushing H. On routine determination of arterial tension in operating room and clinic. *Boston Med Surg J* 1903;148:250–251.
3. Levy AG. Sudden death under light chloroform anaesthesia. *Proc R Soc Med* 1914;7:383–393.
4. Brewster WR Jr, Isaacs JP, Waino-Anderson T. Depressant effect of ether on myocardium of the dog and its modification by reflex release of epinephrine and norepinephrine. *Am J Physiol* 1953;175:399–414.
5. Coakley CS, Alpert S, Boling JS. Circulatory responses during anesthesia of patients on Rauwolfia therapy. *JAMA* 1956; 161:1143–1144.
6. Alper MH, Flacke W, Krayer O. Pharmacology of reserpine and its implications for anesthesia. *Anesthesiology* 1963;24:524–542.
7. Egbert LD, Battit GE, Turndorf H. The value of the preoperative visit by an anesthetist. *JAMA* 1963;185:553–555.
8. Leigh JM, Walker J, Janaganathan P. Effect of preanesthetic visit on anxiety. *Br Med J* 1977;2:987–989.
9. Middleton V, Van Poznak A, Artusio JF Jr, Smith SM. Carbon monoxide accumulation in closed circle anesthesia systems. *Anesthesiology* 1965;26:715–719.
10. Wilson R, Crouch EAC. Risk assessment and comparisons: an introduction. *Science* 1987;236:67.
11. American Society of Anesthesiologists. New classification of physical status. *Anesthesiology* 1963;24:111.
12. Goldman L, Caldera DL, Nussbaum SR, Southwick FS, Krogstad D, Murray B, et al. Multifactorial index of cardiac risk in noncardiac surgical procedures. *N Engl J Med* 1977;297:845–850.
13. Kannel WB, Schwartz MJ, McNamara PM. Blood pressure and risk of coronary heart disease: the Framingham Study. *Dis Chest* 1969;56:43–52.
14. Frank CW, Weinblatt E, Shapiro S, Sager RV. Prognosis of men with coronary heart disease as related to blood pressure. *Circulation* 1968;38:432–438.
15. Tarhan S, Moffitt EA, Taylor WF, Giuliani ER. Myocardial infarction after general anesthesia. *JAMA* 1972;220:1451–1454.
16. Burns DM. Tobacco and health. In: Wyngaarden JB, Smith LH Jr, eds. *Cecil textbook of medicine,* 17th edition. Philadelphia: WB Saunders, 1985;47.
17. Goldstein A Jr, Keats AS. The risk of anesthesia. *Anesthesiology* 1970;33:130–143.
18. Hickler R, Vandam LD. Hypertension. *Anesthesiology* 1970;33:214–228.

PART D

Iatrogenic Forms of Hypertension

Hypertension: Pathophysiology, Diagnosis, and Management, edited by J. H. Laragh and B. M. Brenner. Raven Press, Ltd., New York © 1990.

CHAPTER 118

Cyclo-oxygenase Inhibitors and Blood Pressure

Interaction with Antihypertensive Drugs

John A. Oates

Interaction Between Antihypertensive Drugs and Nonsteroidal Anti-Inflammatory Drugs, 1905
Biochemical Consequences of the Administration of Nonsteroidal Anti-Inflammatory Drugs, 1905
Participation of Prostanoids in the Regulation of Arterial Pressure: Diverse and Opposing Actions, 1905
The Clinical Effects of Nonsteroidal Anti-Inflammatory Drugs in Hypertensive Patients, 1907
Differences Between the Nonsteroidal Anti-Inflammatory Drugs, 1907
Interindividual Variation in the Effect of Nonsteroidal Anti-Inflammatory Drugs on Arterial Pressure, 1907
Conclusion, 1909
References, 1909

INTERACTION BETWEEN ANTIHYPERTENSIVE DRUGS AND NONSTEROIDAL ANTI-INFLAMMATORY DRUGS

The action of antihypertensive drugs may be blocked by certain nonsteroidal anti-inflammatory drugs (NSAIDs). This is an important consideration in the treatment of hypertensive patients because the elevation in blood pressure caused by these drug interactions may be severe and even catastrophic. Because approximately 30% of patients with arthritis have hypertension, the potential for concurrent administration of NSAIDs and antihypertensive drugs is considerable.

BIOCHEMICAL CONSEQUENCES OF THE ADMINISTRATION OF NONSTEROIDAL ANTI-INFLAMMATORY DRUGS

NSAIDs all act to inhibit the biosynthesis of prostaglandins and thromboxane A_2 (prostanoids), and this action is thought to mediate their effect on arterial pressure. The biotransformation of arachidonic acid into thromboxane A_2, prostacyclin, prostaglandin D_2 (PGD_2), PGE_2, and $PGF_{2\alpha}$ is initiated by a common enzyme, the *fatty acid cyclo-oxygenase* (Fig. 1). This cyclo-oxygenase enzyme is inhibited by aspirin, indomethacin, and other NSAIDs. The product of this cyclo-oxygenase is an unstable endoperoxide, PGG_2, which is converted by a hydroperoxidase to PGH_2. PGH_2 is a common precursor of PGD_2, PGE_2, $PGF_{2\alpha}$, thromboxane A_2, and prostacyclin. Whereas many cells contain the cyclo-oxygenase and metabolize arachidonic acid to PGH_2, the enzymes that catalyze the metabolism of PGH_2 to active prostanoids confer cellular specificity to the biosynthetic process.

PARTICIPATION OF PROSTANOIDS IN THE REGULATION OF ARTERIAL PRESSURE: DIVERSE AND OPPOSING ACTIONS

The effects of cyclo-oxygenase inhibition on the regulation of arterial pressure are predictable, in part, from knowledge of the actions and sites of biosynthesis of cyclo-oxygenase products. Prostacyclin is formed in human vessel walls, particularly in the endothelium (1). Capillary endothelial cells also produce PGE_2. Both PGE_2 and prostacyclin are vasodilators, and they are thought to contribute to the basal level of vasodilator tone in that portion of the splanchnic circulation that subserves the gut (2). Accordingly, NSAIDs will elevate the mesenteric vascular resistance. By such actions on regional basal vascular resistance, the vasodilator prostaglandins act to lower blood pressure (Fig. 2).

In addition to direct vasodilation, prostaglandins may lower vascular resistance indirectly by modulating the effect of neural and humoral influences on vascular tone. There is evidence suggesting that endogenous prostanoids can modulate the release of norepinephrine from sympathetic varicosities. Local administration of PGE_2 and PGD_2 (and, to a lesser extent, prostacyclin) reduces norepineph-

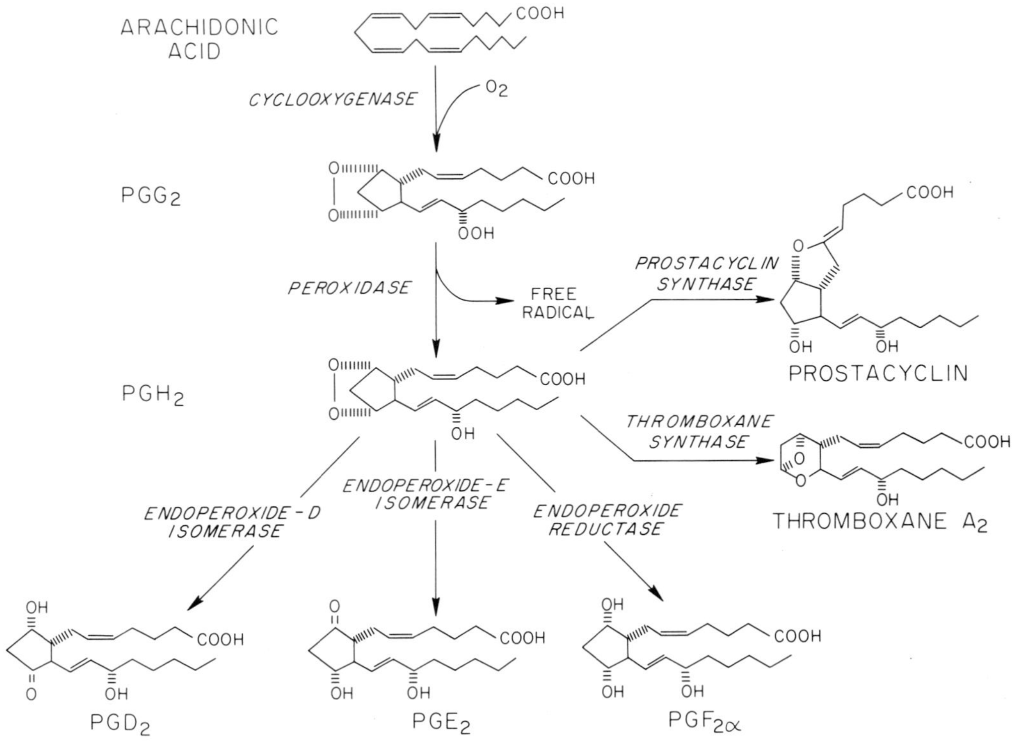

FIG. 1. Pathways of the biosynthesis of prostaglandins and thromboxane A_2.

rine release from adrenergic neurons (3,4). In addition, prostaglandin E_2 reduces the potentiation of noradrenergic neurotransmission by angiotensin II (5). However, the physiologic importance of prostanoid-induced attenuation of noradrenergic neurotransmission remains to be elucidated. The pressor responses to angiotensin II (6,7) and vasopressin (8) in humans are enhanced by inhibition of prostaglandin biosynthesis.

In the kidney, both PGE_2 and prostacyclin act at a tubular site to promote sodium excretion (9). These natriuretic prostaglandins are formed in the kidney. Indomethacin and other NSAIDs act to cause sodium retention in humans (10), implying a role for these natriuretic prostaglandins in sodium homeostasis. The natriuretic action of these prostaglandins would provide a second mechanism whereby they could reduce arterial pressure (Fig. 2).

In contrast to these actions of prostaglandins that lower blood pressure, prostacyclin and PGE_2 also act to stimulate the secretion of renin, which exerts a powerful pressor effect mediated by the action of angiotensin II to cause vasoconstriction, enhanced adrenergic neurotransmission, and aldosterone secretion. The secretion of renin is regulated by adrenergic reflex control and, at a local level, by prostaglandins (11–15). Both prostacyclin and PGE_2 are formed in the renal cortex. One, or both, of these prostaglandins transduces the intrarenal stimulation of renin release that is initiated by pressure changes in the afferent arterioles or by alterations in chloride reabsorption at the macula densa. Accordingly, inhibition of renal cyclo-oxygenase will inhibit that component of renin secretion that is prostaglandin dependent.

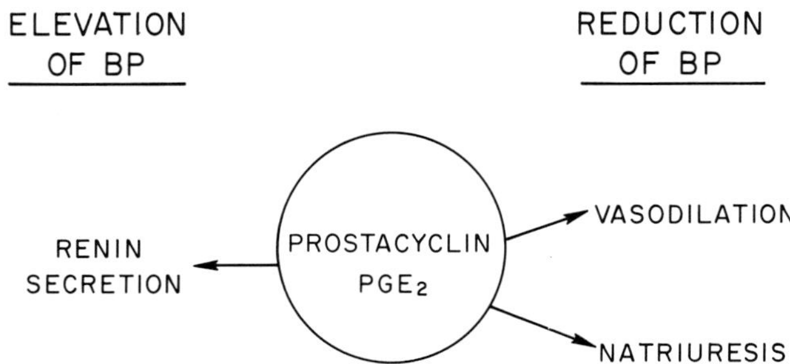

FIG. 2. Prostaglandin E_2 and prostacyclin act at several different sites to influence arterial pressure.

Thromboxane A_2 is formed largely by platelets (16) and is also formed by other cells, including macrophages. Thromboxane A_2 stimulates platelet aggregation, and, accordingly, inhibition of its formation by aspirin and the NSAIDs inhibits platelet aggregation. Thromboxane A_2 also is a vasoconstrictor. There is not convincing evidence that thromboxane A_2 participates in the regulation of arterial pressure under physiological circumstances. However, in experimental animal models of glomerular injury, there is evidence that thromboxane A_2 contributes to renal vasoconstriction (17,18). Also, following the resection of the majority of renal mass in the rat, thromboxane synthase inhibition lowers blood pressure (19). The relevance of thromboxane A_2 to human hypertension awaits elucidation.

Thus, it can be seen that vasodilator prostaglandins, such as PGE_2 and prostacyclin, have effects at some sites that reduce arterial pressure, whereas their stimulation of renin secretion exerts a pressor effect (Fig. 2). Given these opposing actions of the vasodilator prostaglandins on arterial pressure regulation, it would be predicted that the net effect of inhibiting the prostaglandin biosynthesis would be dependent upon which of the factors regulated by prostaglandins were dominant in determining a given patient's blood pressure.

THE CLINICAL EFFECTS OF NONSTEROIDAL ANTI-INFLAMMATORY DRUGS IN HYPERTENSIVE PATIENTS

In normal individuals not receiving any antihypertensive drugs, orally administered cyclo-oxygenase inhibitors either do not raise arterial pressure (10,20) or elevate it only slightly, up to 5 mmHg systolic (21,22). In hypertensive patients who are not on therapy, blood pressure following indomethacin administration was increased by a modest but significant extent in some studies (up to 12 mmHg mean blood pressure) or not significantly changed in others (23–27).

In hypertensive patients receiving antihypertensive drugs, some of the cyclo-oxygenase inhibitors will elevate arterial pressure. In treated patients, the rise in arterial pressure during cyclo-oxygenase inhibition generally exceeds that observed in hypertensive patients who are not receiving antihypertensive drugs. Indomethacin is the prototype NSAID, and its effects on treated hypertensive patients have been evaluated most extensively. Indomethacin has been shown to elevate arterial pressure in hypertensive patients treated with diuretics, beta-adrenoreceptor antagonists, and combinations of diuretics with a number of other antihypertensive agents (10,21–23,25,27–31). With regard to the antagonism of the antihypertensive effects of β-adrenoreceptor blockers by NSAIDs, it is of interest that excretion of the urinary metabolite of prostacyclin, 2,3-dinor-6-keto-$PGF_{1\alpha}$, is increased by propranolol (27).

The effect of indomethacin on arterial pressure in patients treated with converting-enzyme inhibitors has not been fully resolved. All studies have shown that indomethacin produces partial reversal of the acute antihypertensive effect of captopril (32–36). In addition, the hypotensive effect of chronic captopril treatment also is inhibited by indomethacin (37,38). One study has demonstrated that the hypotensive effect of continuing treatment with enalapril is reversed by indomethacin (39). However, a separate study did not show a significant effect of indomethacin on the hypotensive effect of chronically administered enalapril (40); whether the lack of effect of indomethacin in this study is related to the fact that most of the patients were black remains to be determined. Clearly, additional studies using captopril as a positive control will be required to determine whether enalapril differs from captopril with regard to reversal of its antihypertensive effect by indomethacin.

DIFFERENCES BETWEEN THE NONSTEROIDAL ANTI-INFLAMMATORY DRUGS

Other cyclo-oxygenase inhibitors have been studied less extensively than indomethacin. Piroxicam and ibuprofen have been shown to antagonize the effects of antihypertensive drugs (41,42). In contrast, sulindac does not interfere with the effect of antihypertensive drugs. For example, sulindac at a dose of 400 mg daily did not interfere with the effect of propranolol in the same group of patients who became hypertensive in response to piroxicam (41). Sulindac was also shown not to alter the antihypertensive effect of combination drug therapy (31,43). The lack of a hypertensive response to sulindac in patients on antihypertensive therapy is convincing because in each of these studies there were positive controls in which other NSAIDs caused an elevation of pressure in the same patients. Similarly, aspirin in doses of 1.95–3.5 g daily was without effect on combination antihypertensive therapy (21,31). More information is needed on naproxen, but the data currently available suggest that its effect on blood pressure is more like that of indomethacin than that of aspirin (31,43). It would be prudent to assume that, with the exception of aspirin and sulindac, all NSAIDs will antagonize antihypertensive agents until appropriately controlled studies prove otherwise.

Thus, all cyclo-oxygenase inhibitors do not appear to produce equivalent effects on hypertension in treated patients. The reasons for these qualitative differences are not known with certainty, but several possibilities deserve consideration. The disparate effects on blood pressure could reflect differences in the tissue-specific biotransformation of the cyclo-oxygenase inhibitors. For example, sulindac sulfide, the active metabolite of sulindac, is oxidized back to the inactive prodrug by the kidney, an inactivation mechanism that could protect portions of the nephron from cyclo-oxygenase inhibition by sulindac sulfide (44). Metabolism also is important in the pharmacology of aspirin, which is an irreversible inhibitor of the cyclo-oxygenase enzyme, whereas its metabolite, salicylic acid, is a weak competitive inhibitor. A further consideration is that tissue-selective distribution of drugs could occur. Finally, it is conceivable that the potent antagonists of antihypertensive drug action, such as indomethacin and piroxicam, exert these effects by actions other than cyclo-oxygenase inhibition.

INTERINDIVIDUAL VARIATION IN THE EFFECT OF NONSTEROIDAL ANTI-INFLAMMATORY DRUGS ON ARTERIAL PRESSURE

The magnitude of the hypertension evoked by indomethacin and related NSAIDs varies considerably between patients receiving the same antihypertensive drug (21,28). For example, the elevation in supine systolic pressure produced by indomethacin in patients receiving thiazide diuretics was found to range from no increase to an increase of 44 mmHg (28). The finding that major increases in blood pressure occur in a subset of the patients in the reported studies indicates that inferences drawn from the mean increases in blood pressure evoked by the NSAIDs greatly underestimate the risk to which this subset of susceptible patients is exposed when NSAIDs are added to their therapy. Furthermore, carefully monitored trials that also exclude patients with the most severe hypertension would underestimate the extent to which blood pressure

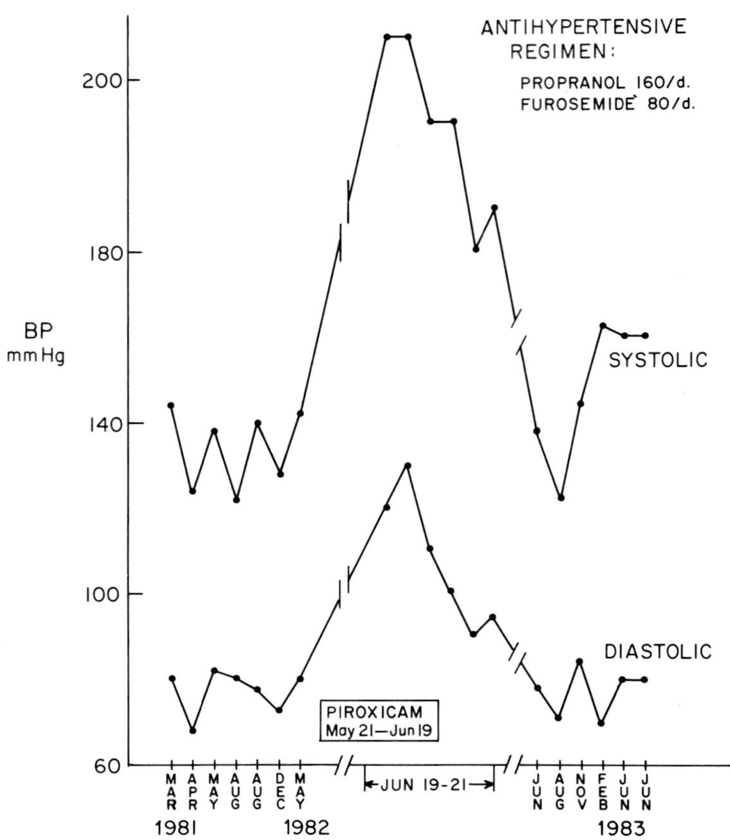

FIG. 3. Loss of blood pressure control following administration of piroxicam.

can rise in the subset of patients at greatest risk. For example, ethical considerations would limit the magnitude to which blood pressure could rise before intervention. In the less closely monitored circumstance of clinical practice, there is greater potential for an elevation in arterial pressure that is of major clinical importance, a conclusion that is illustrated by the severity of such interactions in individual patients. An example of the severity of such interactions is illustrated in Fig. 3, which depicts the problem of a 77-year-old Caucasian man. His hypertension had been characterized as being of the low-renin type; that is, following the administration of furosemide 80 mg and 3 hr in the upright posture, his plasma renin activity rose only to 1.05 ng/ml/hr. Good control of his blood pressure during treatment with propranolol (160 mg daily) and furosemide (80 mg daily) had been documented repeatedly. This patient had chronic osteoarthritis, which had been treated with a low dose of sulindac (200 mg daily). Because of incomplete relief of the osteoarthritis, a second physician initiated treatment with piroxicam (20 mg daily) as a substitute for sulindac. About 3 weeks after initiation of piroxicam, he developed a headache that became progressively worse. Fortunately, his wife had been trained to take his blood pressure, which she found to be 230/130 mmHg. He was immediately hospitalized, where the severe level of hypertension was confirmed. Only after the discontinuation of piroxicam did the blood pressure gradually return to the levels previously observed. It is clear that this remarkable hypertensive response to piroxicam pushed the patient to the brink of disaster. Not all patients have the benefit of such timely intervention. A 63-year-old Caucasian man, who also had documented low-renin hypertension, did not fare so well. His blood pressure also had been well controlled with a combination of propranolol and a diuretic. Because of cervical osteoarthritis, he was started on piroxicam. Three weeks later he suffered a massive intracerebral hemorrhage with hemiplegia and aphasia. Such an occurrence is tragic, considering the extreme rarity of cerebral hemorrhage in treated hypertensive patients.

To be able to predict which patients are at risk for marked elevations in blood pressure, it will be necessary to better understand the mechanisms that determine the wide variability in response of arterial pressure to the NSAIDs. Given the fact that prostaglandins can produce both pressor and depressor effects, it is not surprising that underlying baseline differences in the contributions of these opposing effects of prostaglandins to arterial pressure could yield differences in response to the inhibition of prostaglandin biosynthesis. For example, there is evidence suggesting that the effect of indomethacin on blood pressure is a function of baseline renin status. In a highly renin-dependent model of hypertension in the rat, indomethacin actually lowers the blood pressure (45). Furthermore, in rare instances in which hypertension in humans is unusually dependent upon renin secretion, indomethacin has produced a significant reduction in blood pressure (13,46)! In contrast to the effects in these exceptionally renin-dependent hypertensive patients, inhibition of prostaglandin synthesis with indomethacin or ibuprofen elevated arterial pressure in normal humans with a low-renin state produced by administration of fludrocortisone (47). Thus, opposite effects of indomethacin on arterial pressure are observed at the polar extremes of the renin spectrum; in drawing inferences from these observations it must be recognized that factors in addition to renin in these patients with high- and low-renin states could be influencing the response to inhibitors of prostaglandin biosynthesis.

Prior renin status also correlates with the extent to which indomethacin blocks the antihypertensive effect of captopril. Indomethacin has been shown to reverse the antihypertensive effect of maintenance captopril treatment in patients with low-renin hypertension, whereas indomethacin had no effect on the hypotensive response to captopril in patients who initially had normal plasma renin activity (38). Consistent with this observation are the results of a study in which the effect of indomethacin or ibuprofen on the acute hypotensive response to a single dose of captopril was evaluated in patients receiving, at different times, a high-salt or a low-salt diet. Full reversal of the acute antihypertensive effect of captopril was seen only when the patients were on a high-salt diet; when the same individuals were on a low-salt diet and the baseline renins were higher, indomethacin or ibuprofen produced only a slight and not significant reversal of captopril's hypotensive effects (32). Whereas these two studies are internally consistent regarding the effect of indomethacin on captopril's antihypertensive action, being greatest in patients with low renin, the results in untreated hypertensive patients demonstrated that indomethacin raised blood pressure only in the group with normal plasma renin levels but not in patients with low renin. These findings have led to a hypothesis that the effect of captopril in low-renin states could be exerted largely by stimulation of prostaglandin release, perhaps through an exaggeration of bradykinin's effect by converting-enzyme inhibition. The various studies attempting to evaluate the effect of converting-enzyme inhibitors on prostaglandin biosynthesis have yielded inconsistent results; thus, remaining unresolved is the extent to which the hypotensive action of converting-enzyme inhibitors is dependent on prostaglandin release. Increased urinary excretion of PGE_2 and 6-keto-$PGF_{1\alpha}$ (the hydration product of prostacyclin) has been seen with converting-enzyme inhibitors in some studies (38,40) but not in all (34). Changes in urinary excretion of primary prostaglandins could reflect changes in their renal biosynthesis but could also mirror changes in the distribution of prostaglandins into and out of the urine during its formation in the glomerulus and passage through the tubules. Elevation in the metabolite of PGE_2, 15-keto-dihydro-PGE_2, was measured in one study (33) but did not correlate temporally with the changes in blood pressure or the converting enzyme, and the extreme lability of that metabolite confounds analyses undertaken without internal standards added at the time of blood sampling. Perhaps most importantly, the acute effect of a converting-enzyme inhibitor may not necessarily be determined by the same mechanism that exerts the long-term hypotensive effects of converting-enzyme inhibition. No change in the urinary metabolite of prostacyclin, 2,3-dinor-6-keto-$PGF_{1\alpha}$, was found during continuing enalapril administration (48). Therefore, further studies need to be done to ascertain the extent to which prostaglandin release mediates a component of the hypotensive action of the converting-enzyme inhibitors, to determine whether NSAIDs antagonize the chronic antihypertensive effects of the structurally different converting-enzyme inhibitors to the same extent, and to explore interindividual differences in the reversal of the hypotensive action of converting-enzyme inhibitors by NSAIDs with regard to baseline renin status, sodium balance, race, and age.

The influence of renin status and other factors on the hypertensive effects of NSAIDs during treatment with other antihypertensive drugs also remains to be established; certainly the interaction with converting-enzyme inhibitors cannot be considered to predict the effects seen with other antihypertensive drugs. Research that enables identification of a subset of patients who will exhibit a hypertensive response to NSAIDs should also provide valuable insights into mechanisms of cardiovascular control.

CONCLUSION

In summary, some of the nonsteroidal anti-inflammatory drugs antagonize the hypotensive effects of antihypertensive agents. This antagonism is not observed with aspirin and sulindac, and these drugs may be used in conjunction with antihypertensive therapy. There is considerable interpatient variability in the extent of the elevation in blood pressure evoked by the NSAIDs, and, in some patients, dangerous levels of hypertension occur. The potential for cerebral hemorrhage clearly attends these drug interactions in which platelet function also is suppressed by cyclo-oxygenase inhibition.

REFERENCES

1. Moncado S, Higgs EA, Vane JR. Human arterial and venous tissues generate prostacyclin, a potent inhibitor of platelet aggregation. *Lancet* 1977;1:1–20.
2. Gerkens J, Faust T, Branch R. The effects of indomethacin and hemorrhage on splanchnic blood flow. *Eur J Pharmacol* 1982;78: 81–90.
3. Hedqvist P. Basic mechanisms of prostaglandin action on autonomic neurotransmission. *Annu Rev Pharmacol Toxicol* 1977; 17:259–279.
4. Wennmalm Å. Prostaglandin-mediated inhibition of noradrenaline release. A comparison of the neuroinhibitory effect of three prostaglandins: E_2, I_2, and 6-keto-$PGF_{1\alpha}$. *Prostaglandins Med* 1978;1:49–54.
5. Jackson EK, Campbell WB. A possible antihypertensive mechanism of propranolol: antagonism of angiotensin II enhancement of sympathetic nerve transmission through prostaglandins. *Hypertension* 1981;3:23–33.
6. Negus P, Tannen RL, Dunn MJ. Indomethacin potentiates the vasoconstrictor actions of angiotensin II in normal man. *Prostaglandins* 1976;12:175–180.
7. Vierhapper H, Waldhausl W, Nowotny I. Effect of indomethacin upon angiotensin-induced changes in blood pressure and plasma aldosterone in normal man. *Eur J Clin Invest* 1981;II:85–89.
8. Glänzer K, Prübing B, Düsing R, Kramer HJ. Hemodynamic hormonal responses to 8-arginine-vasopressin in healthy man: effects of indomethacin. *Klin Wochenschr* 1982;60:1234–1239.
9. Stokes JB, Kokko JP. Inhibition of sodium transport by prostaglandin E_2 across the isolated, perfused rabbit collecting tubule. *J Clin Invest* 1977;59:1099–1104.
10. Donker AJM, Arisz L, Brentjens JRH, van der Hem GK, Hollemans HJG. The effect of indomethacin on kidney function and plasma renin activity in man. *Nephron* 1976;17:288–296.
11. Larsson C, Weber P, Änggård E. Arachidonic acid increases and indomethacin decreases plasma renin activity in the rabbit. *Eur J Pharmacol* 1974;28:391–394.

12. Oates JA, Whorton RA, Gerkens JF, Branch RA, Hollifield JW, Frolich JC. The participation of prostaglandins in the control of renin release. *Fed Proc* 1979;38:72–74.
13. Frolich JC, Hollifield JW, Michelakis AM. Reduction of plasma renin activity by inhibition of the fatty acid cyclooxygenase in human subjects: independence of sodium retention. *Circ Res* 1979;44:781–787.
14. Gerber JG, Nies AS, Olsen RD. Control of canine renin release: macula densa requires prostaglandin synthesis. *J Physiol (Lond)* 1981;319:419–429.
15. Linas SL. Role of prostaglandins in renin secretion in the isolated kidney. *Am J Physiol* 1984;246:F811–F818.
16. Hamberg M, Svenson J, Samuelsson B. Thromboxanes: a new group of biologically active compounds derived from prostaglandin endoperoxides. *Proc Natl Acad Sci* 1975;72:2994–2998.
17. Saito H, Ideura T, Takeuchi J. Effects of a selective thromboxane A_2 synthetase inhibitor on immune complex glomerulonephritis. *Nephron* 1984;36:38–45.
18. Cadnapaphornchai P, Bondar NP, McDonald FD. Effect of imidazole on the recovery from bilateral ureteral obstruction in dogs. *Am J Physiol* 1982;243:F532–F536.
19. Purkerson ML, Joist JH, Yates J, Valdes A, Morrison A, Klahr S. Inhibition of thromboxane synthesis ameliorates the progressive kidney disease of rats with subtotal renal ablation. *Proc Natl Acad Sci USA* 1985;82:193–197.
20. Güllner, Hans-Georg, Gill JR, Bartter FC, Düsing R. The role of the prostaglandin system in the regulation of renal function in normal women. *Am J Med* 1980;69:718–724.
21. Mills EH, Whitworth JA, Andrews J, Kincaid-Smith P. Non-steroidal anti-inflammatory drugs and blood pressure. *Aust NZ J Med* 1982;12:478–482.
22. Patak RV, Mookerjee BK, Bentzel CJ, Hysert PE, Babej M, Lee JB. Antagonism of the effects of furosemide in normal and hypertensive man. *Prostaglandins* 1975;10:649–659.
23. Lopez-Ovejero JA, Weber MA, Drayer JIM, Sealey JE, Laragh JH. Effect of indomethacin alone and during diuretic or beta-adrenoreceptor-blockade therapy on blood pressure and the renin system in essential hypertension. *Clin Sci Mol Med* 1978;55:203S–206S.
24. Ylitalo P, Pitkäjärvi T, Metsä-Ketalä T, Vapaatalo H. The effect of inhibition of prostaglandin synthesis on plasma renin activity and blood pressure in essential hypertension. *Prostaglandins Med* 1978;1:479–488.
25. Ylitalo P, Pitkäjärvi T, Pyykönen ML, Nurmi A-K, Seppälä, E, Vapaatalo H. Inhibition of prostaglandin synthesis by indomethacin interacts with the antihypertensive effect of atenolol. *Clin Pharmacol Ther* 1985;38:443–449.
26. Ruilope L, Garcia Robles R, Barrientos A, Bermis C, Alcazar J, Tresquerres JAF, Mancheno E, Millet VG, Sancho J, Rodichicio, J-L. The role of PGE_2 and renin–angiotensin–aldosterone system in the pathogenesis of essential hypertension. *Clin Exp Hypertens* 1982;4:989–1000.
27. Beckmann ML, Gerber JG, Bynny RL, LoVerde M, Nies AS. Propranolol increases prostacyclin synthesis in patients with essential hypertension. *Hypertension* 1988;12:582–588.
28. Watkins J, Abbott EC, Hensby CN, Webster J, Dollery CT. Attenuation of hypotensive effect of propranolol and thiazide diuretics by indomethacin. *Br Med J* 1980;281:702–705.
29. Salvetti A, Arzilli F, Pedrinelli R, Beggi P, Motolese M. Interaction between oxprenolol and indomethacin on blood pressure in essential hypertensive patients. *Eur J Clin Pharmacol* 1982;22:197–201.
30. Wing LMH, Bune AJC, Chalmers JC, Graham JR, West MJ. The effects of indomethacin in treated hypertensive patients. *Clin Exp Pharmacol Physiol* 1981;8:537–541.
31. Chalmers JP, West MJ, Wing LM, Bune AJ, Graham JR. Effects of indomethacin, sulindac, naproxen, aspirin, and paracetamol in treated hypertensive patients. *Clin Exp Hypertens* 1984;A6:1077–1093.
32. Goldstone R, Martin K, Zipes R, Horton R. Evidence for a dual action of converting enzyme inhibition on blood pressure in normal man. *Prostaglandins* 1981;22:587–598.
33. Moore TJ, Crantz FR, Hollenberg NK. Contribution of prostaglandins to the antihypertensive action of captopril in essential hypertension. *Hypertension* 1981;3:168–173.
34. Witzgall H, Scherer B, Weber PC. Involvement of prostaglandins in the actions of captopril. *Clin Sci* 1982;63(Suppl):265S–267S.
35. Silberbauer K, Stanek B, Templ H. Acute hypotensive effect of captopril in man modified by prostaglandin synthesis inhibition. *Br J Clin Pharmacol* 1982;14:875–935.
36. Seto S, Aoi W, Iwami K, Yamaguebi T, Ashizana N, Kusauo S, Baba K, Doi Y, Kuramochi M, Hashiba K. Effects of propranolol and indomethacin on the depressor action of captopril in patients with essential hypertension. *Clin Exp Theory Practice* 1987;9A:623–627.
37. Salvetti A, Pedrinelli R, Magagna A, Ugenti P. Differential inhibition on the pharmacological responses to captopril in patients with essential hypertension. *Clin Sci* 1982;63:261S–263S.
38. Abe K, Itoh T, Imai Y. Implication of endogenous prostaglandin system on the antihypertensive effect of captopril SQ 14225, in low renin hypertension. *Jpn Circ J* 1980;44:422–425.
39. Salvetti A, Abdel Haq B, Magagna A, Pedrinelli R. Indomethacin reduces the antihypertensive action of enalapril. *Clin Exp Hypertens [A]* 1987;9A:559–567.
40. Oparil S, Horton R, Wilkins LH, Irwin J, Hammett DK. Antihypertensive effect of enalapril in essential hypertension: role of prostacyclin. *Am J Med Sci* 1987;294:395–402.
41. Pugliese F, Simonetti BM, Cinotti GA. Differential interaction of piroxicam and sulindac with the antihypertensive effect of propranolol [Abstract]. *Eur J Clin Invest* 1984;14:54.
42. Radack KL, Deck CC, Bloomfield SS. Ibuprofen interferes with the efficacy of antihypertensive drugs; a randomized, double-blind, placebo-controlled trial of ibuprofen compared with acetaminophen. *Ann Intern Med* 1987;107:628–635.
43. Wong DG, Spence JD, Lamki L, Freeman D, McDonald JWD. Effect of nonsteroidal and anti-inflammatory drugs on control of hypertension by beta-blockers and diuretics. *Lancet* 1986;1:997–1001.
44. Miller MJS, Bednar MM, McGiff JC. Renal metabolism of sulindac, a novel non-steroidal anti-inflammatory agent. *Adv Prostaglandin Thromboxane Leukotriene Res* 1983;11:487–491.
45. Jackson EK, Oates JA, Branch RA. Indomethacin decreases arterial blood pressure and plasma renin activity in rats with aortic ligation. *Circ Res* 1981;49:180–185.
46. de Jong PE, Donker AJ, van der Wall E, Erkelens DW, van der Hem GK, Doorenbos H. Effects of indomethacin in two siblings with a renin-dependent hypertension, hyperaldosteronism and hypokalemia. *Nephron* 1980;25:47–52.
47. Martin K, Zipser R, Horton R. Effect of prostaglandin inhibition on the hypertensive action of sodium-retaining steroids. *Hypertension* 1981;3:622–628.
48. Nadeau JH, FitzGerald GA, Oates JA, Wood AJJ. The effect of converting enzyme inhibition on sodium balance and systemic prostacyclin synthesis in man. *Clin Res* 1983;31:844A.

Hypertension: Pathophysiology, Diagnosis, and Management, edited by J. H. Laragh and B. M. Brenner. Raven Press, Ltd., New York © 1990.

CHAPTER 119

Phenylpropanolamine

Emmanuel L. Bravo

Biochemistry and Clinical Pharmacology of Phenylpropanolamine, 1911
Structure–Activity Relationship, 1911
Isomers of Phenylpropanolamine: Pharmacologic and Clinical Distinction, 1912
Pharmacology of Phenylpropanolamine, 1912
Proprietary Preparations Containing Phenylpropanolamine, 1913
Clinical Responses to Phenylpropanolamine, 1913
Effect of Phenylpropanolamine Alone on Systemic Arterial Pressure, 1913
Complications Attributed to Phenylpropanolamine, 1914
Drug–Drug Interactions, 1914
Population at Risk of Developing Hypertensive Complications, 1915
Summary and Recommendations, 1915
References, 1915

Phenylpropanolamine (PPA) is a sympathomimetic amine that is widely used as a constituent of over-the-counter nasal decongestants and appetite suppressants. It is estimated that about five billion dosage units of the compound are consumed annually. Ever since its introduction to clinical medicine, it has enjoyed a remarkable safety record; furthermore, evidence of its toxicity has been minimal (1–3). Nevertheless, PPA has recently become a center of controversy. Concern about its potential for adversely affecting health has been raised by reports of PPA causing hypertension (4–7), cardiac arrhythmias (8), stroke (9), and death in previously healthy individuals (10).

The precise effect of PPA on blood pressure has been an area of particular controversy. Although the medical literature abounds with articles addressing this issue, the question of whether PPA at currently recommended doses raises blood pressure remains unresolved. The difficulty of reaching some consensus is primarily because of the different drug preparations employed in these reports. The dextroisomer of PPA is much more potent than the racemic mixture of the drug, and the latter is the only form marketed in the United States. Furthermore, both immediate-release and slow-release preparations have been employed by different investigators. In addition, toxic reactions of the cardiovascular system to PPA may have been related to use of large doses, to concurrently used drugs, or to concomitant disease.

This review has the following objectives: (a) to give a brief survey of the biochemistry and clinical pharmacology of PPA, (b) to review the reported clinical responses to PPA, (c) to assess the prevalence and extent of complications attributed to PPA, (d) to determine the population at risk of developing complications to PPA, and (e) to offer some recommendations based on information gathered from a review of the literature on the subject.

BIOCHEMISTRY AND CLINICAL PHARMACOLOGY OF PHENYLPROPANOLAMINE

Structure–Activity Relationship (Fig. 1)

β-Phenylethylamine is considered to be the parent compound of the sympathomimetic amines. It consists of a benzene ring and an ethylamine side chain. Substitutions on the aromatic ring, on the α- and β-carbons, and on the terminal amino group yield various compounds with sympathomimetic activity. The greatest sympathomimetic activity occurs when two carbon atoms separate the benzene ring from the amino group.

In general, *substitution of the amino terminal group* increases β-receptor activity; furthermore, the less the substitution, the greater the selectivity for α-receptor activity. *N*-methylation increases the potency of primary amines. Phenylethylamine has little β-receptor activity because, unlike ephedrine, it lacks a methyl substitution at the amino terminal end.

Substitution at the third and fourth positions of the aromatic nucleus results in maximal α- and β-receptor activity. Absence of aromatic substitutions results in reduction of overall potency and some loss of direct peripheral sym-

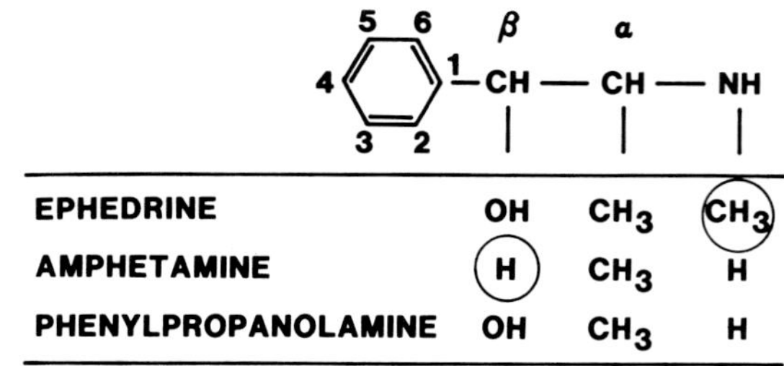

FIG. 1. Structure–activity relationship of phenylpropanolamine.

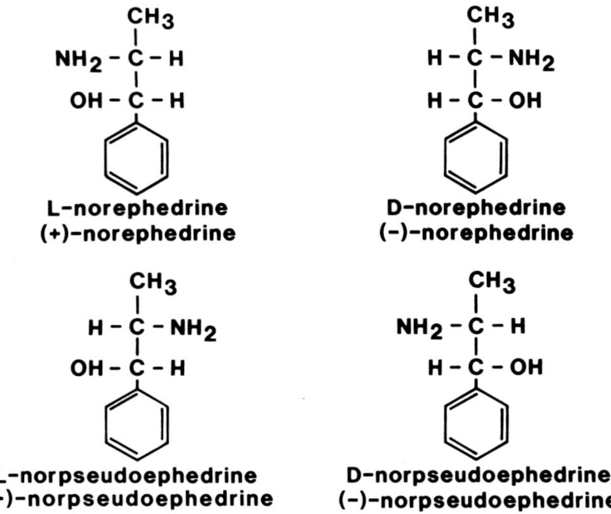

FIG. 2. Isomers of phenylpropanolamine.

pathomimetic activity. In addition, lack of polar hydroxyl (OH) groups on the phenylethylamine structure makes the resultant compound more lipophilic, makes it cross the blood–brain barrier more readily, and makes it have more central activity. Absence of the 3-OH group also increases the oral effectiveness and the duration of action of such compounds.

Substitution on the α-carbon atom blocks oxidation by monoamine oxidase (MAO), thereby greatly prolonging the duration of action of the compounds. Protection from rapid degradation by MAO allows these compounds to persist in nerve terminals and release norepinephrine from storage sites.

Substitution of an OH group on the β-carbon atom generally decreases central stimulant action, largely because of the lower lipid solubility. However, such substitutions greatly enhance agonistic activity of both α- and β-receptors.

In summary: (a) PPA has more marked α-activity than β-activity because of the absence of an alkyl substituent at the terminal amino group and the presence of a OH substituent at the β-carbon atom. (b) PPA has central nervous system activity that results from the absence of aromatic substitutions; however, it is less potent than amphetamine because of substitution at the β-carbon atom, which tends to lower lipid solubility, thereby decreasing the ability of the compound to enter cells. (c) PPA is likely to persist in nerve terminals and release norepinephrine from storage sites. This property results from substitution on the α-carbon atom, which blocks degradation by intraneuronal MAO. (d) PPA is orally active, with prolonged duration of action by virtue of the absence of the 3-OH group on the benzene ring, which blocks the MAO enzyme in liver and intestine.

Isomers of Phenylpropanolamine: Pharmacologic and Clinical Distinction

Norephedrine, the *N*-demethylated congener of ephedrine, is generally known by the more descriptive name *phenylpropanolamine* (PPA). The isomeric forms of PPA are shown in Fig. 2. Optically active forms that rotate a beam of polarized light clockwise are preceded by (+)-; those that rotate a beam of light counterclockwise are preceded by (−)-. Very often, the lowercase letters "*d*" (dextrorotatory) and "*l*" (levorotatory) are used for these distinctions. Equal mixtures of optically active isomers are called *racemic mixtures* and are labeled (±)- or *d,l*-. Isomers in which the major functional groups (NH_2, OH) are represented on different sides of the two-carbon skeleton are called "pseudo" forms; hence norpseudoephedrine.

The term PPA applies to all structures in Fig. 2. However, the material marketed in the United States is the racemic form, (±)-norephedrine. In contrast, the PPA sold in Europe and Australia is often the (+)-norpseudoephedrine isomer, a pharmacologically distinct agent that has central nervous system (CNS)-stimulating activity. There is evidence of human habituation and abuse of (+)-norpseudoephedrine.

Pharmacology of Phenylpropanolamine

As previously noted, PPA shares structural similarities with amphetamine. However, it has significantly less of the adverse CNS effects and abuse potential attributed to amphetamine. This property derives from substitution of an OH group on the β-carbon, which markedly lowers lipid solubility and increases water solubility, thereby decreasing the ability to penetrate cells. It is equal in potency to ephedrine but has less CNS-stimulating effects.

PPA is well absorbed after oral administration; about 80–90% of the administered dose is excreted unchanged in the urine within 24 hr, with a urinary elimination half-life of about 4 hr. Plasma level studies show a similar half-life.

The effects of PPA are largely the result of α-adrenergic agonist activity resulting from direct stimulation of adrenergic receptors and from release of norepinephrine from neuronal storage sites. PPA-induced elevations in arterial pressure are presumably due to these effects. The increase in arterial blood pressure is characterized by increases in cardiac output, peripheral vascular resistance, stroke volume, ejection fraction, and decreases in heart rate (11).

PROPRIETARY PREPARATIONS CONTAINING PHENYLPROPANOLAMINE

PPA is an ingredient in more than 70 over-the-counter preparations. Table 1 shows the products containing 25 mg or more per unit dose of PPA. Eleven have PPA as the only ingredient. These are usually sold as decongestants or as appetite suppressants. All others are combined with an antihistamine (chlorpheniramine), an antitussive (dextromethorphan), an expectorant (guaifenesin), or an analgesic (acetaminophen). These are usually sold as decongestants and cold remedies. The dose varies widely from preparation to preparation. It is as little as 3.125 mg in children's cold remedies and as much as 75 mg in adult diet pills. The highest recommended adult dosage of PPA for use as anorectics is 75 mg/day; for use as decongestants and cough remedies, 150 mg/day is recommended.

PPA is also an ingredient of pills made to look like amphetamine-containing drugs and like other prescription drugs. These preparations are called "look-alike" pills and are sold in the streets as "uppers"; they are also sold legally in "pick-me-up" shops and mail-order shops. They contain as much as 50 mg PPA combined with 25 mg ephedrine and/or 200 mg caffeine.

CLINICAL RESPONSES TO PHENYLPROPANOLAMINE

The numbers of patients exposed to significant doses of the drug are unknown, and the reporting scheme may only gather details of a proportion of these patients who develop significant signs and symptoms. The following summarizes clinically significant signs and symptoms from limited studies and case reports in the literature.

Effect of Phenylpropanolamine Alone on Systemic Arterial Pressure

Concerns regarding adverse hypertensive effects of PPA stem largely from reports by Horowitz et al. (5,6). In a prospective study in healthy normotensive subjects, they observed significant and potentially dangerous rises in blood pressure after ingestion of a single capsule of a preparation containing 85 mg of PPA. In this study, 12 of 37 subjects had a supine diastolic blood pressure rise to 100 mmHg or more, and one had a blood pressure rise to 190/142 mmHg. Some questions have been raised con-

TABLE 1. *Proprietary preparations containing 25 mg or more of phenylpropanolamine (PPA)*

Product	Formulation	PPA content (mg per unit dose)	Recommended adult dose (total, mg)
Tablet/capsule			
Acutrim[a]	Slow release	75	75
Acutrim II[a]	Slow release	75	75
Contac	Slow release	75	150
Dietac[a]	Slow release	75	75
Cold Factor 12	Slow release	75	150
Dexatrim (Caffeine free)[a]	Slow release	75	75
Dexatrim (Plus vitamins)[a]	Slow release	75	75
Headway	Slow release	75	75
Dexatrim (Extra strength)[a]	Immediate release	75	75
Triaminic 12	Immediate release	75	150
Allerest	Slow release	50	100
Dexatrim[a]	Slow release	50	50
Prolamine[a]	Slow release	37.5	75
Tussagesic	Slow release	25	75
Super Odrinex[a]	Slow release	25	75
A.R.M. Allergy Relief	Slow release	25	150
Sucrets[a]	Slow release	25	150
Coryban D	Slow release	25	100
Dristan	Slow release	25	100
Head and Chest	Slow release	25	150
Appedrine[a]	Slow release	25	75
Pyrroxate	Slow release	25	150
Triaminic	Immediate release	25	150
Triaminicin	Immediate release	25	100
Cold Factor	Liquid	75	150
Comtrex	Liquid	25	100
Formula 44D	Liquid	37.5	225
Cremacoat 3	Syrup	37.5	150
Cremacoat 4	Syrup	37.5	150

[a] Not combined with other drugs. All others are combined with an antihistamine (chlorpheniramine), an antitussive (dextromethorphan), an expectorant (guaifenesin), or an analgesic (acetaminophen).

From ref. 29, with permission.

cerning the chemical composition of the compound used in this report. There is reason to believe that the PPA preparation is not the racemic slow-release PPA but, rather, the related immediate-release stereoisomer, (+)-norpseudoephedrine, which is a CNS stimulant. This could explain the much lower incidence of toxicity reported in the United States, where the marketed PPA products contain the racemic form, *d,l*-norephedrine, which is devoid of CNS-stimulating activity.

More recently, however, Pentel et al. (11) demonstrated that single oral doses of 37.5 mg and 75 mg PPA (immediate-release formulation of the racemic isomer) produced dose-related increases in supine systolic blood pressure. In 10 subjects, the average rise in systolic blood pressure was 18.5 mmHg; one subject showed an increase of 43 mmHg in systolic blood pressure. This study has been loudly criticized (1,12) because (a) it involved a relatively small number of subjects, (b) no increases in diastolic blood pressure were noted, and (c) the overall magnitude of the pressor effect appeared to have been exaggerated by the response of one subject.

Similar doses of PPA in slow-release preparation have been shown to produce only modest or no increases in blood pressure. However, in some patients, significant increases in blood pressure have been observed with slow-release preparation, suggesting that some subjects may be more sensitive to PPA than others. Liebson et al. (12) recently reported their findings in two controlled studies that evaluated the effects of slow-release PPA on subjective and cardiovascular variables at recommended over-the-counter dose levels. In the first study, 159 subjects participated in a parallel group design that compared a 75-mg slow-release preparation with a 25-mg thrice-daily dosing regimen and placebo. In the second study, 59 subjects from the first study participated in a cross-over study that compared 75-mg slow-release PPA with placebo. These studies did not reveal clinically significant cardiovascular effects due to drug treatment.

Krakoff (13) reviewed results of five controlled (but four unpublished) studies using identical study designs. The subjects in these studies totaled 659 healthy normotensives and included 209 subjects from the study of Liebson et al. (12). He found no consistent pattern in arterial pressure responses. Although most normal subjects did not have detectable increases in arterial pressure, small increases occurred more consistently for the 75-mg slow-release preparation. In addition, a few subjects were found to exhibit idiosyncratic excessive elevations of blood pressure. Krakoff proposed that these studies may have failed to detect uniform findings of small differences because of (a) the inherent variability of arterial pressure and (b) the poor precision of traditional clinical methods for noninvasive measurement of arterial pressure.

In a recent study, using 24-hr ambulatory blood pressures to assess responses, Goodman et al. (14) reported that a 75-mg slow-release preparation given either acutely or chronically had no effect on the blood pressure of 18 normotensive males. Mitchell (15) also reported no pressor effect of PPA at daily doses of 100 mg after a 1-week chronic ingestion regimen.

Complications Attributed to Phenylpropanolamine

Reports of serious complications (4–7) (i.e., stroke, seizures, and cerebral hemorrhage) resulting from significant hypertension have generally been related to intake of PPA-containing drugs in more than the recommended doses or to self-medication with look-alike or fake amphetamine pills. Because these pills are not as potent as amphetamines, the user is more likely to take several at a time to obtain an effect equivalent to taking amphetamines. Because PPA and ephedrine have much more pronounced peripheral effects than do amphetamines, the hypertensive reactions from these stimulants are greater. Hypertensive crises and intracerebral hemorrhages culminating in death have been reported with use of these drugs. In contrast to these case reports, prospective clinical studies of PPA have generally been favorable. Silverman et al. (16) reported no adverse effects of a 25-mg dose of PPA either alone or in combination with 100 mg of caffeine.

In addition to hypertensive effects, arrhythmias have been reported by Weesner et al. (8). These authors postulate that the hypertension produced by PPA results in reflex bradycardia that may allow the ectopic pacemaker to assume control of the ventricles. Clinical evidence of acute myocardial injury following acute ingestion of PPA has also been substantiated (17).

Headaches, neuropsychiatric symptoms, and generalized convulsive seizures are common toxic reactions caused by large doses of PPA (18–20). Amphetamine-like reactions have also been described (21). These effects include (a) stimulation of the medullary respiratory center to tremor, (b) restlessness, (c) increased motor activity, (d) agitation, and (e) hallucinations.

Drug–Drug Interactions

An important question concerning any active and widely consumed agent is the effect of its use in the presence of other drugs. Interactions between PPA and MAO inhibitors (22), indomethacin (23), and antihypertensive drugs (24) (α-methyldopa and oxprenolol) have been described. MAO inhibitors potentiate the pressor effects of PPA by raising the concentration of catecholamines at nerve endings and making them available for release. By the same token, tyramine in foodstuff can act synergistically with PPA to enhance release of norepinephrine at nerve endings. Indomethacin, an inhibitor of prostaglandin synthesis, potentiates the direct and indirect effects of PPA. The mechanisms by which this interaction occurs are unclear. The widespread use of nonsteroidal anti-inflammatory drugs makes the use of PPA a greater risk to the public than is generally recognized. The mechanism by which PPA and methyldopa interact to produce a hypertensive crisis is not well understood. It is possible that PPA and α-methylnorepinephrine, a metabolite of methyldopa, act synergistically at vascular sites to cause severe peripheral vasoconstriction. Alternatively, patients receiving α-methyldopa could be supersensitive to the direct α-adrenergic agonist activity of PPA.

From these reports, it may be concluded that products containing PPA at currently marketed preparation and dosages do not pose a unique cardiovascular risk for normal, healthy adults. However, in some subjects, significant adverse reactions have occurred, suggesting that some individuals may be more sensitive to PPA than others.

The ability of PPA to induce toxic reactions depends, to a large extent, on the preparation and on the dose and rate of absorption. Those preparations in which PPA is present in the immediate-release form rather than in the slow-release form seem particularly apt to produce severe hypertensive reactions. Other factors such as concomitant medications may sensitize patients to the effects of PPA. In general, toxic reactions attributed to slow-release PPA-containing preparations have been related to intake of more than the recommended dosages.

POPULATION AT RISK OF DEVELOPING HYPERTENSIVE COMPLICATIONS

Since PPA acts by a direct α-agonist activity as well as by indirectly releasing norepinephrine (25), a major concern is that significant hypertensive reactions may occur in subjects who may be sensitized to the effects of catecholamines. There is little information in the literature about the incidence and severity of hypertensive reactions in the hypertensive population. Nonetheless, it seems prudent that patients with hypertension be made especially aware of a potential adverse reaction to PPA. Consideration should be given to small increases in blood pressure that may mislead physicians to a false impression of "resistant or refractory" hypertension.

Patients with impairment of autonomic function can develop an adverse hypertensive reaction to PPA. The number of such patients is not small. They include (a) the elderly (26), (b) patients with peripheral neuropathy from disorders such as diabetes mellitus or chronic uremia, and (c) the group of patients with overt autonomic dysfunction. Such patients have significant hypersensitivity to pressor stimuli (27); this is due, in part, to impairment of baroreflex functioning. Biaggioni et al. (28) have recently showed that extremely low doses of phenylpropanolamine (from 12.5 to 25 mg) in its immediate-release form produced marked increases in blood pressure in patients with overt autonomic insufficiency. Furthermore, the data showed that the more severely affected patients had the greater pressor responses to PPA. While no studies are available that assessed the effect of PPA in patients with milder degrees of autonomic impairment, it would be prudent to consider these patients at increased risk of developing a hypertensive reaction to the drug.

SUMMARY AND RECOMMENDATIONS

PPA is a potent sympathomimetic, and its hypertensive effect is dose-related. Hypertensive episodes are more likely to occur with preparations containing PPA in the immediate-release, as opposed to the slow-release, form. Most reported reactions result from either self-medication or intake of more than the recommended dosage (or both). However, reactions from single oral doses (50–75 mg) have been reported, and adverse interactions with commonly used drugs have been demonstrated.

Effects of PPA are the result of α-adrenergic agonist activity, largely from both direct stimulation of adrenergic receptors and release of neuronal norepinephrine. As such, PPA has the potential to interact with other drugs to produce toxic reactions, especially in treated hypertensive patients and in those with impairment of autonomic function. The occurrence of complications with single oral doses suggests that some normal subjects may be more sensitive to the drug than others. Although the incidence of serious complications in the general population is probably small, the availability of high-dose PPA-containing preparations without medical supervision is potentially dangerous. A possible safety measure against significant hypertensive reactions might be to limit PPA use to slow-release preparations or to single, small dosages not exceeding 50 mg.

REFERENCES

1. Morgan JP. *Phenylpropanolamine: a critical analysis of reported adverse reactions and overdosage.* Fort Lee, NJ: JK Burgess, 1986;13–25.
2. Lasagna L. Phenylpropanolamine and blood pressure. *JAMA* 1985;253:2491–2492.
3. Silverman HI, Lewis GP. Phenylpropanolamine. *JAMA* 1982;247:460.
4. Berstein E, Diskant B. Phenylpropanolamine: a potentially hazardous drug. *Ann Emerg Med* 1982;11:311–315.
5. Horowitz JD, Lang WJ, Howes LG, et al. Hypertensive response induced by phenylpropanolamine in anorectic and decongestant preparations. *Lancet* 1980;1:60–61.
6. Horowitz JD, McNiel JJ, Sweet B, Medelsohn FAO, Louis WJ. Hypertension and postural hypotension induced by phenylpropanolamine (trimolets). *Med J Aust* 1979;1:1975–1976.
7. McEwen J. Phenylpropanolamine-associated hypertension after the use of "over-the-counter" appetite suppressant products. *Med J Aust* 1983;2:71–73.
8. Weesner KM, Denison M, Roberts RJ. Cardiac arrhythmias in an adolescent following ingestion of an over-the-counter stimulant. *Clin Pediatr (Phila)* 1982;21:700–701.
9. Johnson DA, Etter HS, Reeves DM. Stroke and phenylpropanolamine [Letter]. *Lancet* 1983;2:970.
10. King J. Hypertension and cerebral hemorrhage after trimolets ingestion [Letter]. *Med J Aust* 1979;2:258.
11. Pentel PR, Asinger RW, Benowitz NL. Propanolol antagonism of phenylpropanolamine-induced hypertension. *Clin Pharmacol Ther* 1985;37:488–494.
12. Liebson I, Bigelow G, Griffiths RR, et al. Phenylpropanolamine: effects on subjective and cardiovascular variables at recommended over-the-counter dose levels. *J Clin Pharmacol* 1987;27:685–693.
13. Krakoff LR. Review of recent studies on the effect of phenylpropanolamine on systemic arterial blood pressure in human subjects. In: Morgan JP, Kagan DV, Brody JS, eds. *Phenylpropanolamine: risks, benefits, and controversies.* New York: Praeger, 1985;210–222.
14. Goodman RP, Wright JT, Barlascini CO, et al. The effect of phenylpropanolamine on ambulatory blood pressure. *Clin Pharmacol Ther* 1986;40:144–147.
15. Mitchell CA. Possible cardiovascular effects of phenylpropanolamine and belladonna alkaloids. *Curr Ther Res* 1968;10:47–53.

16. Silverman HI, Kreger BE, Lewis GP, et al. Lack of side effects from orally administered phenylpropanolamine with caffeine: a controlled three phase study. *Cur Ther Res* 1980;28:185–194.
17. Pentel PR, Mikell FL, Zavorol JH. Myocardial injury after phenylpropanolamine ingestion. *Br Heart J* 1982;47:51–54.
18. Mueller SM, Solow EB. Seizures associated with a new combination "pick-me-up" pill. *Ann Neurol* 1982;11:322.
19. Novenius G, Widerlov E, Lonnerholm G. Phenylpropanolamine and mental disturbance. *Lancet* 1979;2:1367–1368.
20. Schaffer CB, Pauli MW. Psychotic reaction caused by proprietary oral diet agents. *Am J Psychiatry* 1980;137:1256–1257.
21. Dietz AJ. Amphetamine-like reactions to phenylpropanolamine. *JAMA* 1983;245:601–602.
22. Cuthbert MF, Greenberg MP, Morley SW. Cough and cold remedies: a potential danger to patients on monoamine oxidase inhibitors. *Br Med J* 1969;1:404–406.
23. Lee KY, Bielin LJ, Vandongen R. Severe hypertension after ingestion of an appetite suppressant (phenylpropanolamine) with indomethacin. *Lancet* 1979;1:1110–1111.
24. McLaren EH. Severe hypertension produced by interaction of phenylpropanolamine with methyldopa and oxprenolol. *Br Med J* 1976;II:283–284.
25. Trendelenburg U, Muskus A, Fleming WW, et al. Effects of cocaine, denervation and decentralization on the response of the nictitating membrane to various sympathomimetic amines. *J Pharmacol Exp Ther* 1962;138:181–193.
26. Sachs C, Kaijser L. Autonomic cardiovascular responses in old age. *Clin Physiol* 1985;5:347–357.
27. Robertson D, Hollister AS, Carey EL, et al. Vascular β_2-adrenergic hypersensitivity in autonomic dysfunction. *J Am Coll Cardiol* 1984;3:850–856.
28. Biaggioni I, Onrot J, Stewart CK, Robertson D. The potent pressor effect of phenylpropanolamine in patients with autonomic impairment. *JAMA* 1987;258:236–239.
29. Bravo EL. Phenylproponolamine in other over the counter vasoactive compounds. *Hypertension* 1988;11:II-9.

Hypertension: Pathophysiology, Diagnosis, and Management, edited by J. H. Laragh and B. M. Brenner. Raven Press, Ltd., New York © 1990.

CHAPTER 120

Smoking and Cardiovascular Disease

Henry R. Black

Historical Perspective, 1917
Smoking as a Cardiovascular Risk Factor, 1918
The Interrelationships Among Cigarette Smoking and Other Cardiovascular Risk Factors, 1918
Blood Pressure, 1918
Prognosis, 1919
Choice of Therapy, 1920
Hypertension Syndromes in Smokers, 1920
Fibrinogen, 1921
Platelet Function, 1921
Leucocyte Counts, 1921
Other Hematologic Parameters, 1921
Cardiovascular Consequences of Cigarette Smoking, 1922
Effects on the Heart and Coronary Arteries, 1922
Effects of Smoking on Cerebrovascular Disease, 1923
Effects of Smoking on Peripheral Vascular Disease and the Aorta, 1923
Other Arterial Lesions Seen in Cigarette Smokers, 1924
The Pharmacology and Clinical Effects of Nicotine, 1924
The Pathologic and Clinical Effects of Carbon Monoxide, 1925
The Effects of Smoking Cessation, 1926
Techniques of Getting Patients to Stop Smoking, 1927
Conclusions, 1929
References, 1929

HISTORICAL PERSPECTIVE

Tobacco was introduced to Western society nearly 500 years ago, when Columbus and his crew saw Indians in San Salvador inhaling the smoke of burning leaves through a reed called *tabacum* (1). These and other Indians also smoked the leaves of this plant, which were rolled in a cigarette or cigar-like form, while others snorted fragments of unburned leaves. Columbus' sailors brought tobacco to Europe, where it received a mixed reception. Many, especially King James I of England, considered tobacco smoking a "loathsome," "harmful," and "dangerous" practice. But Jean Nicot, for whom nicotine is named, a physician to Queen Catherine de Medici of France, used extracts of the tobacco plant to treat a wide variety of ailments. John Rolfe brought tobacco seeds from Trinidad to the Jamestown, Virginia colony in 1613, giving the new colony the cash crop needed to survive where other British settlements had failed. In 1828, Posselt and Reiman isolated the alkaloid nicotine from tobacco leaves (2). By the early 19th century, tobacco was rolled in paper and smoked as cigarettes. After the Civil War, it became apparent that the land in the Confederacy, particularly in North Carolina, was well suited for growing a light tobacco, ideal for cigarettes. In 1881, the cigarette machine was invented and, largely through the efforts of James Buchanan Duke, inexpensive cigarettes were produced and widely marketed, especially in the United States. By World War I, the majority of American men were regular cigarette smokers, though women did not take up the habit until much later.

In 1938, Pearl (3) showed that heavy smokers up to the age of 70 had a shorter life span than did nonsmokers and that moderate smokers were also likely to die prematurely. In 1940, English et al. (4) pointed out that younger smokers, aged 40–59, were more likely to develop coronary artery disease (CAD). Both studies evaluated white men, the only citizens who smoked cigarettes to any degree.

In 1958, Hammond and Horn (5,6) analyzed the death rates of 187,783 men followed for an average of 44 months, and they showed a consistent increase in smokers as compared to nonsmokers. This increase was largest for cigarette smokers (68%) as compared to those who used other products (12% increase for pipes and 22% for cigars). Heavy smokers (more than two packs per day) had the largest relative risk (123%), but a dose–response relationship was evident. The majority of the increase in deaths was attributable to bronchogenic carcinoma, where the increase was nearly 10-fold, and to CAD, where the death rate was 70% higher in cigarette smokers than in nonsmokers (6). An increase in fatalities from cerebrovascular disease (46%) was also evident. These authors also noted a dose–response relationship for CAD mortality and pointed out that men who had quit smoking reduced this risk accordingly. Though there was a greater impact on the frequency of certain carcinomas, 52.1% of the excess deaths in smokers were attributable to cardiovascular disease (CVD) while 27% were due to carcinomas (13.5% to lung cancer and 13.5% to other cancers). Several years later, Hammond (7) reported on a similar survey of 442,094 men followed for an average of nearly 3 years. Again, death rates, especially from CAD and lung cancer, were significantly higher in smokers, particularly young and heavy smokers. These increases were evident even when other factors such as heredity, lifestyle, alcohol consumption, place of residence, and occupation were taken into account.

Doll and co-workers (8–11) surveyed 59,600 British physicians, of whom 40,637 (34,445 men and 6,192 women) replied. In their early reports and also at 20 years, there was a significant increase in CAD (52%) for all ages (35–84 years old) in men—with the largest effect occurring in younger smokers (15-fold increase in those aged 35–44), though still evident for the oldest age group (9,10). Strokes [cerebrovascular accident (CVA)] and "myocardial degeneration" were also attributable, in part, to cigarette smoking. Similar effects on CAD were seen in women, though the rate was only half that of men; furthermore, the effect of smoking was present only in those who smoked 15 cigarettes/day or more (11). These data were so compelling that, in 1964, the U.S. Surgeon General issued the first of several reports warning the public about the dangers of smoking (12). Though there have been some skeptics, numerous other studies have confirmed the detrimental effect of cigarette smoking in both sexes and all ages and suggest that differences in cigarette smoking habits of men and women are primarily responsible for the reduced life expectancy of men (13–23).

Smoking as a Cardiovascular Risk Factor

By the middle of the 20th century, it was clear that the United States, along with the rest of the industrialized world, was in the midst of a CVD epidemic. Death rates from CAD, in the United States particularly, increased progressively from 1910 to 1968, though the rate has been declining for the past 20 years (24). More than a million Americans have a myocardial infarction (MI) annually, and 20% of men develop CAD by the age of 60. Current estimates are that 640,000 lives are lost each year from CAD, with an additional 200,000 individuals dying from CVA (24).

The basis of this epidemic is multifactional. It has resulted primarily from atherosclerosis (AS). No single etiology for AS has been identified, and so the concept of "risk factors" has been developed. A risk factor is a condition or characteristic that increases the likelihood that an individual having that characteristic or condition will develop a particular disease. The presence of this factor, even to a large degree, does not guarantee that the disease will occur, nor does its absence ensure protection. As Kannel and Schatzkin (24) have emphasized, for a risk factor to be causally, not just statistically, related, the association should meet several criteria. The association must be consistent and robust and have biologic plausibility. It should precede the development of subclinical or clinical disease, and a dose–response gradient should be demonstrable. Lastly, for a risk factor to have real significance, interventions that reduce or eliminate it should result in less disease. Hopkins and Williams (25,26) have recently analyzed available data and have identified nearly 300 candidate risk factors for CVD. In their view and that of many others, high blood pressure (HBP), hypercholesterolemia, and cigarette smoking are the primary risk factors for CVD, particularly CAD, though this was not true in every population examined (26–29). Burch (30) has accepted the association between these three risk factors and CAD, but he feels that causality has not been demonstrated convincingly. Hopkins and Williams (25) have further considered how risk factors could lead to AS and have classified them into four categories: initiators, promoters, potentiators, and precipitators. Initiators are substances which injure arterial endothelium; promoters, on the other hand, enhance the deposition of lipids in the arterial wall, known as *atheromata.* Potentiators enhance thrombosis or platelet aggregation, while precipitators actually are responsible for triggering the clinical event. Cigarette smoking, because of the many direct and indirect effects which result, is the only risk factor listed which contributes to AS by all four mechanisms.

It is now well established that CVD risk factors interact with each other and that the presence of several of these factors will enhance the likelihood that a particular individual will develop CVD. In most, though not all, populations analyzed, cigarette smoking contributes significantly, and in an additive fashion, to the probability that an individual will develop or succumb to CVD (26). The relative impact of each of the major cardiovascular risk factors is difficult to judge for all related diseases and for each population subgroup. Hopkins and Williams (26) have calculated that 43% of CAD could be reduced if all tobacco product use, particularly cigarette smoking, were discontinued. Using the same calculations, 44% of CAD would be prevented if serum cholesterol was ≤160 mg% in everyone, as compared to 36% if diastolic blood pressure (DBP) was reduced to 80 mmHg or less in the population. While achieving ideal serum cholesterol levels and blood pressure (BP) requires major lifestyle adjustments or expensive and often poorly tolerated toxic medications in asymptomatic people, eliminating cigarette smoking is an essentially risk-free endeavor with an equivalent, if not greater, benefit.

THE INTERRELATIONSHIPS AMONG CIGARETTE SMOKING AND OTHER CARDIOVASCULAR RISK FACTORS

Cigarette smoking interacts with virtually all of the important and well-characterized CVD risk factors (see Table 1).

Blood Pressure

Numerous epidemiologic surveys, though not all, have shown that smokers tend to have lower BP than do non-

TABLE 1. *Effect of smoking on other cardiovascular risk factors*

I. Blood pressure
   A. *Rises* with smoking (acutely)
   B. Smokers have *lower* blood pressures
   C. Hypertensive smokers:
      1. are harder to control
      2. have a worse prognosis
      3. are more likely to have atherosclerotic renovascular hypertension (fibromuscular dysplasia?)
      4. are more likely to develop malignant and accelerated hypertension
      5. should not be given noncardioselective beta-blockers as monotherapy

II. Serum lipids

Increased	*Decreased*
Total cholesterol	HDL cholesterol
LDL cholesterol	
Free fatty acids	
Triglycerides?	

III. Obesity: Reduced body weight

IV. Hemorrheology

Increased	*Decreased*
Fibrinogen	Platelet survival
Blood viscosity	Bleeding time
Leucocyte count	Erythrocyte distensibility
Hematocrit	
Platelet aggregation	

V. Oral contraceptives: Further increases risk of myocardial infarction, stroke, and thromboembolic events

VI. Hormonal changes: Increased plasma estradiol (men) and vasopressin; worsens glucose tolerance

smokers (31–39). This finding has been noted in both sexes, adolescents, adults and in many different populations. These observations contrast sharply with the well-described acute increase in BP seen within minutes of smoking a cigarette (40–45). The reason for the lower levels of BP in smokers is not clear, though differences in body weight (BW) have been implicated. Smokers of 30 or fewer cigarettes per day usually weigh less than nonsmokers, and both BP and BW usually, but not always, rise when smokers quit (32,34,37,39,46–49). Though cigarette smoking is not associated with the development of essential hypertension, it has a significant impact on prognosis for hypertensives, on the appropriate choice of therapy, and on the development of several unusual, but important, consequences and of secondary forms of hypertension.

Prognosis

Isles et al. (50) reported mortality data from the Glasgow Blood Pressure Clinic on 3783 patients with nonmalignant hypertension seen during a 15-year period. The mortality rate in this population of primarily referred patients was significantly higher in smokers (50% of men and 36% of women). In several large clinical trials, the impact of smoking was equally clear. The Multiple Risk Factor Intervention Trial (MRFIT) discovered more than 100,000 hypertensive men in their screening program (51,52). At all levels of BP, the age-adjusted rate of CAD death was greater in smokers than in nonsmokers. The difference was more evident with increasing levels of serum cholesterol. In the Hypertension Detection and Follow-up Program (HDFP), where approximately 27% of the 10,940 participants smoked, cigarette smoking was a highly significant predictor of mortality for the cohort as well as for the subset with mild hypertension (DBP 90–104 mmHg) (53,54). Smoking ranked just behind renal failure, age, and evidence of prior CVA as a predictor of mortality and was more important than the level of DBP, prior MI, angina pectoris (AP), left ventricular hypertrophy (LVH), diabetes mellitus (DM), or the treatment group to which the patient was assigned (55). In mild hypertensives, similar data were obtained—with only age, LVH, prior MI, and renal dysfunction being more significant than cigarette use. The death rates for smokers were nearly twice those of nonsmokers regardless of the treatment assignment. The relative benefit of stepped-care therapy was less in smokers. These findings were also true in mild hypertensives with no other risk factors or end-organ damage. Thiazide diuretics were the primary treatment in this trial. The Australian National Blood Pressure Study also showed a greater rate of trial endpoints in smokers, regardless of whether the subject received active or placebo therapy (52,56). The relative reduction in trial endpoints was the same in smokers and nonsmokers when active therapy was compared to placebo (52). This trial, too, used thiazides as primary treatment.

In several other studies, the comparative benefit of thiazides and beta-blockers in smokers has been elucidated. In the Medical Research Council Trial, where 31% of the men and 26% of the women volunteers were smokers, those randomized to a nonselective beta-blocker (propranolol) or placebo had less of a BP response to treatment than did nonsmokers (57,58). Patients getting thiazides did equally well, regardless of their smoking status. In this large trial (17,354 patients), the benefit of treatment in preventing CVA and all CVD deaths, but not coronary events, was the same in the thiazide group, whether subjects smoked or not. In the propranolol group, however, smokers had no benefit from treatment, though nonsmokers showed a reduction in CVA, coronary events, and all CVD deaths (59). In the International Prospective Primary Prevention Study in Hypertension (IPPPSH), smokers (37% of men and 23% of women) had twice the rate of CVA and cardiac events as compared to nonsmokers (60). Those nonsmokers receiving oxprenolol, a noncardioselective beta-blocker with intrinsic sympathomimetic activity, had a reduction in cardiac events, a benefit absent in smokers (61). In this trial, smokers needed larger doses of both active drug and placebo but were as well controlled as nonsmokers and tended to have more symptoms than did nonsmokers.

The Heart Attack Primary Prevention in Hypertensives (HAPPHY) Trial had somewhat different results (62). In this study, men aged 40–64 with well-established diastolic hypertension (DBP 100–130 mmHg) received either a thiazide or a cardioselective beta-blocker (atenolol or metoprolol) as initial treatment with second and third drugs added if needed. Thirty-five percent of the 6569 patients smoked cigarettes. Mortality, as in other trials, was twice as high in smokers, but here the beta-blockers did afford protection to smokers. In a follow-up trial done with this population (MAPHY), those who received metoprolol were continued for another 4.2 years (63). Again, death rates were twice as high in smokers; however, those randomized to metoprolol did better than those given thiazides, with no difference in nonsmokers. The significance of this apparent advantage of one cardioselective beta-blocker (metoprolol) over another (atenolol) requires further confirmation.

The mechanism for the advantage of treating smokers with HBP with cardioselective beta-blockers rather than nonselective agents has been suggested by several authors. Trap-Jensen et al. (64) showed that atenolol reduced the rise in BP which occurs acutely after smoking, an effect not seen with propranolol. Freestone and Ramsay (65,66) showed that atenolol, but not propranolol or thiazides, blocked the combined pressor effect of cigarettes and caffeine. Tango et al. (67) and Houben et al. (68), however, did not find any difference in patients receiving propranolol and atenolol chronically.

Choice of Therapy

These data have significant implications, especially for initial treatment of hypertensives who smoke. Nonselective beta-blockers should probably not be used as monotherapy in these patients, though the cardioselective agents may be acceptable. Though thiazides do not block the acute effects of smoking as well as do selective beta-blockers, they have reduced the rate of CVA events—but not of CAD events—in smokers. Whether this failure to reduce CAD is due to adverse effects on lipids is still hotly debated, but addition of further lipid elevations to HBP and smoking may enhance the already-high likelihood that these individuals will develop CVD. Drugs that are effective and do not raise lipids—such as converting-enzyme inhibitors, calcium entry blockers, or peripheral alpha-1 blockers—may be attractive choices in smokers. No studies have as yet been done, however, that have confirmed the success of these classes of agents in smokers or that have compared them to each other or to thiazides in this population.

Hypertension Syndromes in Smokers

In addition to hypertensive smokers being perhaps somewhat more difficult to treat and having a worse prognosis, they are more likely to develop renovascular hypertension (RVHBP) and malignant hypertension (MHBP). Mackay et al. (69) reported on 85 inpatients with unilateral or bilateral renal artery stenosis (RAS). All had DBP $\geq$ 100 mmHg at presentation, and 22 had MHBP. The 63 patients without MHBP were compared to an age- and sex-matched group in the same outpatient clinic and to another matched group of inpatients with normal intravenous pyelograms and thus presumably normal renal arteries. In this study, 84% of the patients with RAS, including all those with bilateral involvement, were smokers, as compared to 45% of controls. Further analysis showed that the differences were significant only for those with atherosclerotic RAS but not for fibromuscular hyperplasia (FMD). Nicholson et al. (70) confirmed those findings in another retrospective study. They compared 71 patients with renovascular hypertension with 308 age-matched essential hypertensives seen only in the outpatient service. In their analysis, both atherosclerotic RAS and FMD were significantly more common in smokers than in controls (71% versus 41%). Black and Cooper (71) compared 21 patients with definite atherosclerotic RVHBP, who had been cured or improved by surgery or angioplasty, to 27 controls who had undergone arteriography looking for RAS, but in whom the disease was absent. Another 18 patients with typical RAS, but in whom no procedure was done (suspected cases), were also analyzed. In this series, 91% of the cases were smokers (usually heavy smokers) as compared to 59% of the controls ($p < 0.04$, odds ratio 6.53:1). All of the suspected cases were smokers. Though RVHBP is thought to be rare, it is particularly important to diagnose this disease when present. RVHBP may be curable, may require intervention to achieve any semblance of good BP control, and may dictate the choice of antihypertensives if medical therapy is selected or required. The clinician should have a higher index of suspicion that RVHBP may be present if the patient is a cigarette smoker.

Though the HDFP study did not find a higher prevalence of smokers in those with DBP > 115–129 mmHg, malignant or accelerated hypertension is more likely to occur in smokers (54,72–76). Isles et al. (72) calculated that hypertensives who smoked were five times more likely to develop MHBP than were nonsmokers, though only 82% of their patients [76% of those reported by Bloxham et al. (73)] were cigarette smokers. Tuomilehto et al. (75) pointed out that younger (15–44 years of age) and older (over 65) patients were more likely to show the association between smoking and MHBP. None of these investigators systematically evaluated these patients for RVHBP, so it is unclear whether MHBP might have developed as a consequence of this smoking-related complication.

Serum Lipids

Karvonen et al. (32) were among the first to report that smokers had higher total serum cholesterol levels than did nonsmokers. This observation has been repeatedly confirmed; and, more recently, others have shown not only that total serum cholesterol is higher in smokers but that high-density lipoprotein (HDL) serum cholesterol tends to be lower in smokers as well (37,38,77–87). But Haffner et al. (84) have questioned the relevance of this association. They found no correlation between the level of HDL_2 cholesterol (the lipoprotein subfraction inversely related to the risk of CAD) and cigarette consumption. A significant negative correlation existed, however, between smoking and HDL_3 cholesterol (a subfraction considered to be unrelated to CAD). But a more recent study by Mjos (77) did find reduced levels of HDL_2 cholesterol in smokers. Some authors have also observed elevations of triglycerides in smokers (85,86).

Obesity

Numerous studies have demonstrated that smokers are thinner than nonsmokers (32,87–89). Characteristically, smokers gain an average of 10 pounds when they quit smoking (90). Comstock and Stone (91) measured BW and subscapular and triceps skinfold thickness in men, aged 40–59, and repeated the measurements 5 years later. Nonsmokers and those who continued smoking gained a mean of 1.1 kg in that time, as compared to 5.1 kg for those who quit. The increase in both measurements was more than double when ex-smokers were compared to current smokers.

The mechanism for the lower BW in smokers is uncertain. It has been established that nicotine reduces the consumption of sweets in both animals and humans and that smokers expend approximately 10% more energy on days that they smoke as compared to days that they abstain (92–94). In general, most studies have shown that smokers actually consume more calories than nonsmokers but appear to use those calories less efficiently (90).

Abnormal Hematorrheology

The importance of abnormal coagulation in the pathogenesis of clinically significant atherosclerotic CVD has become increasingly obvious in the past several years (26,95). Though numerous factors contribute to the development of atherosclerotic lesions, atheromata alone, without total occlusion due to formation of clots, may not cause clinical disease. Cigarette smoking can accelerate coagulation in a variety of ways.

Fibrinogen

The fact that smokers have higher levels of fibrinogen was discovered in the 1970s and has been confirmed by numerous other investigators (96–100). Wilhelmsen et al. (97) reported on a 13.5-year follow-up of 794 middle-aged men. In their analysis, the level of serum fibrinogen was a significant risk factor for both MI and CVA, and a strong correlation was evident between fibrinogen level and cigarette smoking. More recent studies from Framingham and from the Northwick Park Heart Study also demonstrated a powerful relationship between fibrinogen levels and CVD, particularly MI. In both of these populations, fibrinogen levels were more closely related to CVD than was cigarette smoking per se (98,99). Kannel et al. (98) showed a progressive rise in age-adjusted fibrinogen levels in smokers compared to nonsmokers in both men and women, with ex-smokers having values similar to those of nonsmokers. The levels were closely correlated with the number of cigarettes smoked per day. Meade et al. (99) showed that fibrinogen levels fall in ex-smokers but don't return to normal for 5 years after smoking is stopped (101). Elevated fibrinogen levels will increase blood viscosity, a finding also noted in smokers and hypertensives (102,103). Levenson et al. (104) showed that both hypertension and increased blood viscosity independently increased arterial rigidity. Fibrinolytic activity is also reduced in smokers (105).

Platelet Function

Ross et al. (106) have suggested that platelets may be responsible for initiating the endothelial injury that results in intimal proliferation and atherosclerotic injury. Mustard and Murphy (107) were among the first to demonstrate shortened platelet survival and increased platelet turnover in smokers. This group, as well as others, later showed increased platelet aggregation in chronic smokers (108–111). Several investigators have found that cigarette smoking can acutely and chronically affect prostaglandin (PG) and prostacyclin (PGI_2) synthesis by platelets (112–114). This results in shortened bleeding times and evidence of increased synthesis of the proaggretory PGs (115,116). Others have shown direct effects of cigarette smoking on endothelial cell function, resulting in impaired PGI_2 production (114–119). Antiplatelet agents (such as aspirin and dipyridamole) or the cessation of smoking can correct these abnormalities (119–121).

Leucocyte Counts

Elevations of leucocyte (WBC) counts, though modest (800–1500 cells/mm^3) and usually well within the normal range, have been repeatedly demonstrated in cigarette smokers (122–127). This finding has occurred in both sexes and in adolescents and is related to the amount smoked and whether or not the smoker inhales. The increase is not due to pulmonary infection or industrial exposure (123,126). Friedman et al. (128) first suggested that the level of WBC count in the range seen in smokers, when measured on an earlier routine screening, was a strong predictor of a future MI. Cigarette smoking was highly correlated with the WBC count and explained most (two-thirds), but not all, of the association between CAD and the level of the WBC count. Zalokar et al. (129) confirmed these results, but only in those smokers who inhaled. In their study, WBC count rose from a mean of 6460/mm^3 for those inhaling one to nine cigarettes per day to 7670/mm^3 in those who inhaled 25 or more per day. The incidence of MI rose from 0.7/1000 patient-years in the light smokers to 5.2/1000 patient-years in the heavy smokers. In this study of 7206 Frenchmen, the mean WBC was 5740/mm^3 in nonsmokers and 7280/mm^3 in smokers who inhaled. Noninhalers had a mean WBC of 7040/mm^3.

Other Hematologic Parameters

In addition to the effect of cigarette smoking on platelets, WBCs, and fibrinogen, researchers have reported that smokers have higher red blood cell (RBC) counts, increased hematocrits, and abnormalities in RBC distensibility and size (102,124,127,130). These changes could also contribute to an increased likelihood of thrombosis and subsequent cardiovascular events.

Oral Contraceptives and Estrogen

Well into the sixth and seventh decades, CVD is less common in women than in men. Premenopausal women who smoke and also use estrogen-containing oral contraceptives, however, are at considerably greater risk of MI, stroke, and thromboembolic disease (131–133).

Other Hormonal Changes

Male cigarette smokers have been shown to have higher levels of plasma estradiol, a hormone which has been shown to be elevated in men with CAD (134,135). Smoking causes abnormal glucose metabolism in both animals and humans (136,137). There is no evidence, however, that smokers are more likely to develop DM.

Alcohol

Alcohol has not been considered to be a cardiovascular risk factor, but a recent Swedish study showed that smokers who used alcohol were considerably more likely to develop a nonfatal MI than were individuals who neither smoked nor drank alcohol (138). But others have shown that alcohol reduced the likelihood that smokers, even heavy smokers, would have abnormal coronary angiograms (139). Fried et al. (140) showed that smokers with angiographically normal coronary arteries had smaller coronary arteries than nonsmokers but that those who also drank had significantly larger vessels with greater cross-sectional areas than did nondrinkers.

CARDIOVASCULAR CONSEQUENCES OF CIGARETTE SMOKING

Though cigarette smoking is clearly a major contributor to a wide variety of cardiovascular diseases, smoking affects certain vascular beds and organs more than others. Thus smokers are especially prone to developing particular forms of CVD (Table 2).

TABLE 2. *Cardiovascular consequences of smoking*

- I. Cardiac effects
  - A. Coronary arteries
    - 1. Atherosclerosis in native circulation
      - a. Myocardial infarctions
      - b. Fatal infarctions
      - c. Recurrent infarctions
      - d. Silent ischemia
    - 2. Spasm
    - 3. Restenosis after angioplasty
    - 4. Atherosclerosis in bypass grafts
  - B. Sudden death
  - C. Unstable angina pectoris
  - D. Cardiomyopathy
  - E. Myocardial arteriolar hyperplasia
- II. Cerebral effects
  - A. Atheroembolic brain infarcts
  - B. Subarachnoid hemorrhage
  - C. Transient ischemic attack
  - D. Recurrent carotid artery stenosis after endarterectomy
- III. Other arterial pathologies
  - A. Aortic atherosclerosis
  - B. Iliofemoral atherosclerosis
  - C. Intermittent claudication
  - D. Lower-limb ischemia and amputations
  - E. Recurrent atherosclerosis of the bypass grafts
  - F. Abdominal aortic aneurysm
  - G. Renal arteriolar hyperplasia
  - H. Failure of skin grafts
  - I. Uteroplacental arterial hyperplasia
  - J. Diabetic microangiopathy—retinal and ? renal

Effects on the Heart and Coronary Arteries

The effects on the heart and coronary arteries are the most important factors attributable to cigarette smoking. The epidemiologic evidence cited above, in addition to numerous other studies, has unequivocally proven the relationship between smoking and CAD (5,7,8,21,25–29,141–154). Smokers are more likely to have a fatal MI and are at significantly greater risk of sudden death than are nonsmokers (155–157). The extent of coronary atherosclerosis correlates with the number of cigarettes smoked (144,149). In normotensive individuals, those with single-vessel disease had smoked an average of 38.3 pack-years, as compared to 44.9 pack-years in patients with double-vessel disease and 67.5 pack-years in patients with triple-vessel disease (144).

In otherwise low-risk individuals, such as younger people (especially women and normotensive or normocholesterolemic subjects), cigarette smoking has a particularly significant effect on increasing the risk of an MI. In a case-control study by Rosenberg et al. (150), women under 50 who smoked 15–24 cigarettes per day had a relative risk (RR) of 2.5 when compared to those who never smoked. In that population, the RR of developing an MI was sevenfold greater for very heavy smokers (≥35 cigarettes/day) than for nonsmokers. No other risk factor had anywhere near that impact, and the authors concluded that 65% of MI in younger women could be attributed to cigarette smoking. A recent Italian study found that the effect of smoking was even greater, up to 10-fold higher (152). In the Coronary Artery Surgery Study, the impact of smoking in men was especially significant for those under 35 (RR of 2.73) but not significant after age 50 (151). The interaction with other risk factors was also demonstrated. Young men (≤35 years) with elevated serum cholesterol who also smoked had a sevenfold increased likelihood of having CAD. The Framingham Heart Study has stated that an increase in cardiovascular mortality due to smoking is not present in those over 65 years of age (154). Others, however, have disagreed (158).

In addition to coronary atherosclerosis and MI, cigarette smokers are more likely to (a) have recurrent MI, (b) develop atherosclerotic lesions in bypass grafts, (c) re-stenose after percutaneous transluminal angioplasty, (d) have silent MI, and (e) develop coronary artery spasm and unstable AP (154,159–166). The MRFIT group found that ventricular premature beats were associated with cigarette smoking, though other investigators were unable to confirm the relationship (51,167–170). Davis et al. (168) and Myers et al. (169), who used ambulatory monitors, and McHenry et al. (170), who employed exercise testing, did not find that smoking increased significant ventricular arrhythmia, nor did smokers have more ventricular ectopy during exercise. In normal dogs and in those with experimental MI, ventricular fibrillation threshold was reduced after the animals inhaled the smoke from three cigarettes (2 mg of nicotine in 10 min) (171). In Framingham, typical AP was not more common in smokers (154). A recent cross-sectional analysis, the Primary Prevention Trial of middle-age men in Sweden, confirmed this finding for uncomplicated AP (typical ischemic chest pain unrelated to an MI) but did find that cigarette smoking was associated with AP following an MI (172). Aronow et al. (173) showed that smoking one cigarette reduced the time to the development of angina during standardized bicycle exercise. Martin et al. (174) showed that smoking reduced coronary sinus flow and increased coronary vascular resistance during atrial pacing, thus reducing myocardial O_2 delivery.

Hartz et al. (175) described a diffuse cardiomyopathy associated with cigarette smoking, independent of coronary artery atherosclerosis in a group of men under the age of 55. One hundred twenty-three individuals (62 under age 55 and 61 over age 55) were selected from a group of 6763 men without valvular heart disease who underwent coronary angiography. These patients all had diffuse hypokinesis of the left ventricle (LV), depressed LV ejection fraction (average 44%), and elevated LV end-diastolic pressures. Fifty-eight of the 62 younger subjects were smokers with a RR of 2.73 of developing this syndrome compared to nonsmokers, $p < 0.04$. This effect of smoking was not found in older patients. Black et al. (176) and others (177) have demonstrated intimal thickening in myocardial arterioles in subjects without clinical CAD, HBP, or DM, and Lough (178) was able to produce a cardiomyopathy in guinea pigs forced to smoke. Congestive heart failure (CHF) from all causes was more common in smokers in the Framingham Heart Study and the Coronary Drug Project (154,179).

Effects of Smoking on Cerebrovascular Disease

Though HBP is the cardiovascular risk factor most directly related to cerebrovascular disease, cigarette smoking has also been convincingly shown to be a significant independent contributor. In Framingham, a similar dose-related relationship between smoking and CVA was seen (RR of 1.8) when those who smoke more than 20 cigarettes/day were compared to nonsmokers (154). At the 26th year of follow-up, these earlier observations were confirmed (180). This study showed a significantly increased RR for all CVA and for atherothrombotic brain infarction, in both sexes, when the analysis was adjusted for HBP and age. The RR was dose-related, with that for light smokers (<10 cigarettes/day) being barely above that for nonsmokers. Heavy smokers (≥40 cigarettes/day) were nearly twice as likely to have a CVA as compared to nonsmokers. As with CAD, smokers who also had HBP had a much higher incidence of CVA as compared to normotensive smokers. Bonita et al. (181) found a similar interrelationship, with hypertensives who smoked having a nearly 20-fold increase in likelihood of developing a CVA as compared to normotensive nonsmokers. In this large case-control study, the CVAs attributed to smoking and HBP were equal (37% versus 36%). In HDFP, smoking status was a major factor in the development of CVA (182). A large population study done in eastern Finland showed an adjusted RR of 4.2 for cerebral infarctions and 2.2 for other CVA in men, a ratio slightly higher than that attributable to elevated DBP (183). In women, smoking was not shown to be a significant factor for either type of CVD. The Honolulu Heart Program, which studied 8006 men of Japanese origin, also showed a more than twofold increase in the risk of CVA, both of the thromboembolic and hemorrhagic types (184). Welin et al. (185) were not able to confirm the association between CVA and smoking, but their population was smaller. Colditz et al. (186) followed 121,700 female nurses and showed a definite dose-related increase for CVA, especially for subarachnoid hemorrhages (SAH) in smokers as compared to nonsmokers (186). Multivariate analysis in this predominantly young and middle-aged population showed that adjusting for BP, oral contraceptive use, and other cardiovascular risk factors did not significantly reduce the impact of cigarette smoking. Other investigators have also shown that SAH is more common in smokers in both men and women (186–188). Analogous to what has been observed in the coronary circulation, smoking may cause transient cerebral ischemia by reducing cerebral blood flow and is the major reason for the development of recurrent carotid artery stenosis after carotid endoarterectomy (189–191).

Effects of Smoking on Peripheral Vascular Disease and the Aorta

Though DM and Type III hyperlipidemia contribute to aortoiliac and more distal peripheral arterial disease (PVD) and intermittent claudication (IC), cigarette smoking is unquestionably the most important risk factor for this condition (154,179,192–200). In the Framingham Heart Study, the RR was 3.0, higher than that for any other cardiovascular syndrome (154,200). A dose–response relationship between the amount of smoking and symptoms was evident (154). IC is very rare in nonsmokers; and in one large surgical practice, 70% of the PVD seen was related to smoking (193). Smokers who don't quit are also more likely to require amputation or to have their grafts fail (196,199,201). Thomas (202) has suggested that arterial reconstructive surgery should not be offered to smokers with IC who will not stop smoking.

Several early pathologic studies showed that cigarette smokers had considerably more aortic atherosclerosis than did nonsmokers (141,203–205). Auerbach and Garfinkel (206) showed that aortic atherosclerosis is more common in smokers, and they also showed that abdominal aortic aneurysms (AAAs) occur eight times more often in smokers of one or more packs of cigarettes per day. Ribeiro et al. (207) have suggested that the collagen content of the aortas of smokers is abnormally high, and Cannon et al. (208) have found increased serum proteolytic activity in smokers with AAAs. The significance of these observations is unclear.

Other Arterial Lesions Seen in Cigarette Smokers

Other abnormalities of the arterial tree are also felt to be related to smoking. These include: changes in the uteroplacental circulation with an increase in the number of premature deliveries and small babies; the intrarenal circulation, though no clinical correlate has emerged except, perhaps, diabetic nephropathy; the skin, where smokers are much more likely to slough a graft than are nonsmokers; and possibly the retina, where the incidence of retinopathy in diabetics has been reported, by some, to be higher in smokers than in nonsmokers (176,177,209–217).

Richardson (218) demonstrated that young asymptomatic smokers have reduced reactive hyperemia in their hands after occlusion, suggesting reduced vasodilatory reserve and possibly small-vessel, rather than large-vessel, disease. Smoking has also been associated with impotence, both acutely after smoking two high nicotine cigarettes and chronically in patients with arterial disease (219,220).

The reasons for the development of AS lesions and the myriad clinical sequelae that result are exceedingly complex with a multitude of antecedents, the interrelations of which are poorly understood (221). Cigarette smoking contributes to CVD in a variety of ways, perhaps primarily because of the vascular, hematorrheologic, and metabolic effects of nicotine and carbon monoxide (CO), the two most important toxic products of cigarette smoking. Certainly, others of the 4000 or so substances identified as constituents of cigarettes are toxic as well, but the role of these compounds and ions is not as clear.

THE PHARMACOLOGY AND CLINICAL EFFECTS OF NICOTINE

The initially pleasurable effects of nicotine appear to be the primary reason why people who try tobacco products continue to use them. Addiction to nicotine is probably the reason why fewer than 25% of heavy smokers can limit or quit smoking as compared to 90% of regular users of alcohol (222,223).

Nicotine is an alkaloid composed of a pyridine and pyrrolidine ring with a methyl group attached and is about 10% of the particulate weight of cigarette smoke (224). It has a p*K* of 7.9 and is generally monoprotonated at physiologic pH (224,225). The pH of the cigarette smoke from most American brands is acidic (5.5), and little absorption occurs through the buccal mucosa. The pH of pipe and cigar smoke is 8.5, and that of chewing tobacco is adjusted to similar levels, so nicotine from these products is absorbed through the mouth (226). Nicotine is absorbed regardless of pH once tobacco smoke reaches the alveoli. Russell et al. (227) and McNabb et al. (228) have shown that hourly smoking of one cigarette will achieve peak serum levels of 30–40 ng/ml and trough levels of 10–20 ng/ml in regular cigarette smokers. The amount of nicotine delivered from one cigarette is approximately 1 mg; however, the plasma level achieved varies considerably, depending on smoking habits (how often the smoker inhales, how much the smoke is diluted by room air, and how much of the cigarette is smoked) (229–235). All currently marketed cigarettes contain similar amounts of nicotine, but the lower-yield varieties remove both nicotine and tar by filtration (225). Numerous recent studies have shown that the so-called "low-yield" cigarettes are probably not safer, since smokers will manipulate the smoking process to obtain the requisite amount of nicotine and may be at even greater risk from the non-nicotine components of cigarettes (222,224,232,236–238).

Nicotine has diverse pharmacologic actions, and it affects the cardiovascular system in a wide variety of ways. It stimulates autonomic ganglia and skeletal neuromuscular junctions by stimulating muscarinic receptors (225). It is a potent stimulator of the adrenergic nervous system and acutely increases heart rate (HR) and BP, presumably through stimulation of sympathetic ganglia and chromaffin tissue (40–43,45,238,239). Direct effects in the central nervous system (CNS)—perhaps at the ventrolateral medulla, nucleus tractus solitarius, and/or area postrema—may also contribute to nicotine's cardiovascular effects (239). Cryer et al. (40) showed significant increases in plasma norepinephrine and epinephrine in chronic cigarette smokers who smoked two cigarettes (40). These changes did not occur with sham cigarettes and were blocked by phenotalamine and propranolol. But Hill and Wynder (44) showed that smoking two nicotine-containing cigarettes increased plasma epinephrine, but not norepinephrine, within a short time after smoking. No changes in catecholamines were seen when these subjects smoked non-nicotine cigarettes. More recent work has shown that the primary effect of nicotine on adrenergic neurons is to directly release norepinephrine and to facilitate its release (41).

Smoking, presumably because of nicotine stimulation of the adrenergic nervous system, has a wide-ranging effect on the heart and peripheral and coronary vasculature. Acutely, cardiac output and myocardial contractility rise and peripheral vasoconstriction occurs (240,241). But in patients with AP, nicotine will reduce myocardial contractility and LV function (237,238). Coronary blood flow may fall as a result of increased coronary artery resistance, especially in those with CAD, though similar effects are seen in normal individuals (241–244). Coronary reserve, as assessed by the hyperemic response to coronary injection of contrast material, is depressed in smokers in a dose-related fashion (245). Winniford et al. (244) have shown that alpha-blockade increased coronary sinus blood flow after smoking, an effect not demonstrable with beta-blockade, suggesting that alpha-stimulation was responsible for the coronary vasoconstriction associated with smoking (244). Adrenergic stimulation also increases free fatty acids and cholesterol, probably as a result of direct effects of sympathetic stimulation (243,246–249). Elevations of free fatty acids increase myocardial oxygen requirements and may contribute to ischemic injury and arrhythmias (249). In addition, nicotine stimulates carotid and aortic body chemoreceptors, produces CNS arousal and relaxation, causes muscle relaxation, increases levels of growth hormone, beta-endorphins, cortisol, ACTH, and vasopressin but not plasma renin activity, and depresses prolactin secretion (225,250–254).

Nicotine is absorbed through the buccal mucosa or alveoli (225). It enters the circulation more rapidly through the lungs than by the systemic or portal routes and reaches the brain more quickly from the lungs than intravenously. It is metabolized primarily by the liver but is also excreted unchanged by the kidney, especially in an acid urine (227). Nicotine has a short half-life (approximately 2 hr) and a large volume of distribution (183 liters) (255). Cotinine, the major metabolite, is inactive, has a long half-life, and, hence, has been used as a measure of tobacco use (224). The plasma levels of nicotine and cotinine correlate reasonably well with the number of cigarettes smoked, and those who smoke low-yield cigarettes have only slightly lower levels (256). Interestingly, pipe and cigar smokers, who have a minimally increased risk of CVD, often have higher levels of plasma nicotine, cotinine, and thiocyanate than do cigarette smokers (257–261). But smokers of cheroots, small open-ended cigars which are usually inhaled, are at significant risk of MI (262).

In addition to the wide-ranging effects on the cardiovascular system, nicotine affects platelets and the endothelium and may be responsible for the wide variety of hematorrheologic abnormalities seen in smokers. Renaud et al. (263) showed that platelet aggregation in response to a variety of stimuli (such as thrombin, ADP, collagen, and epinephrine) was increased after smoking (263). The increase was directly related to inhaling high-nicotine cigarettes and was present for a short time (30–60 min); furthermore, it was not measurable in smokers who did not smoke for 24 hr (263). Folts and Bonebrake (264) showed that in dogs, cigarette smoke and intravenous nicotine reduced coronary blood flow distal to coronary artery stenoses as a result of the formation of platelet thrombi. Phentolamine prevented both the formation of platelet thrombi and the reduction in flow, supporting the hypothesis that the primary effect of smoking and nicotine was to stimulate platelet alpha-receptors, possibly resulting from an increase in catecholamines.

Others have felt that the effects of nicotine or smoking on clotting are best explained by actions on platelet and vessel-wall PG metabolism. Cigarette smoking (but not pipe smoking) raises urinary thromboxane B_2 (TxB_2), the stable metabolite of the proaggregatory thromboxane A_2 (TxA_2) (265). But *in vitro* studies showed inhibition of TxB_2 synthesis by nicotine, suggesting that some other constituent of smoking is responsible. Several groups have evaluated the effect of nicotine on vascular endothelium. Some, but not all, have shown nicotine-related inhibition of PGI_2 synthesis by blood vessels, including the aorta, umbilical artery, and veins (266–269). The reduced production of PGI_2 by blood vessel walls increases platelet aggregation and thrombus formation and may be the cause of the reduced reactive hyperemia in the forearm of humans seen after smoking (270).

Nicotine also inhibits PG synthesis in the heart (271). This effect may limit the ability of the coronary vasculature to hypertrophy appropriately and provide adequate flow and O_2 on demand (272). Nicotine has also been shown to damage endothelium and to reduce superoxide production by WBCs (273,274). The clinical relevance of these observations is unclear.

Nicotine has a wide variety of psychological and psychophysiologic effects which are largely responsible for an individual's continuing to smoke despite the well-known hazards. Smokers derive considerable pleasure from their habit, which they claim reduces stress, both calms and arouses them, increases work performance, and improves their concentration and information processing (222,275). Recent reviews and studies in humans and animals have supported many of these assertions (276–280). Schachter (222) feels that much of the data can be interpreted as showing decreased performance and increased dysphoria in smokers forced to abstain, who then feel and function better when they smoke. These observations support the contention that nicotine is a strongly addictive substance with a significant potential for abuse. Henningfield and Nemeth-Coslett (226) have reviewed this subject and point out that nicotine, either smoked as tobacco or given intravenously, has euphoriant effects very similar to cocaine and marijuana. Whether the stimulation of endorphin production by nicotine is related to this euphoria is unknown (226,281).

THE PATHOLOGIC AND CLINICAL EFFECTS OF CARBON MONOXIDE

The second major constituent of tobacco smoke implicated in the CVD associated with smoking is carbon monoxide (CO). CO is a naturally occurring gas released from combustion of organic matter, including petroleum products. CO is also released endogenously as a product of hemoglobin (Hb) catabolism (282). CO has a strong affinity for Hb, approximately 245 times that of O_2, and binds to it to form carboxyhemoglobin (COHb). Normal individuals have COHb levels of 0.5–1.0%, whereas the levels in smokers vary from 1% to 20%—depending on the number of cigarettes, pipes, or cigars smoked daily (283). Heavy smokers (two to three packs per day) generally have COHb levels of 7–9%, depending on (a) how much CO is present in the air as a result of pollution and (b) whether other sources of CO production are well-vented in a closed room (283). Fatal, acute CO poisoning occurs when blood levels are much higher (20–80%). Cigarette smoke contains 3–6% CO, whereas the concentration from cigar or pipe smoke, which burns at lower temperatures, is two- to threefold higher (284).

CO contributes to CVD in a variety of ways. The increased affinity of CO for Hb reduces the O_2 carrying capacity of the blood. CO, by binding so tightly to Hb, shifts the O_2 dissociation curve to the left, and Hb cannot release O_2 until pO_2 falls to low levels, thus impairing tissue oxygenation. This is especially critical in areas which normally function with low pO_2, such as the heart. CO also binds to myoglobin and other heme-containing compounds (285). Astrup and Kjeldsen (286) have shown that exposure to levels of CO somewhat higher than occur with smoking can cause necrosis of myofibrils, degeneration of mitochondria, and a variety of other subcellular abnormalities of muscle cells in laboratory animals, including lipid deposition (284,287). In addition, CO damages the arterial wall, thereby increasing the filtration and, hence, the accumulation of lipids from the plasma (287,288). Increased serum cholesterol feeding and hypercholesterolemia greatly accelerate this deposition, as does hypoxia (289). Hyperoxia retards the process (287).

Ayres et al. (290) studied the hemodynamic response to raising levels of COHb to 9% by inhalation, values seen in smokers (290). In their study, venous pO_2 dropped from 39 torr, at COHb levels of 0.95%, to 31 torr. Significant increases were noted in minute ventilation, cardiac output, O_2 extraction, O_2 consumption, and alveolar–arterial O_2 differences. Coronary blood flow increased in normal humans but not in those with CAD. Aronow and colleagues (291–293) have extensively studied the effects of carbon monoxide on the development of AP. They showed that smokers will develop AP sooner with supervised exercise when they smoke either nicotine or non-nicotine cigarettes. Though only nicotine-containing cigarettes had hemodynamic effects (increasing BP and HR), both increased CO levels in expired air to equivalent levels, raised COHb to nearly 8%, and reduced the time to development of AP from 110 sec to 84 sec. Further studies using inspired air with modestly increased levels of CO (50 ppm) compared to purified air showed similar results (294). COHb levels rose to 2.68%, as compared to 0.77% with purified air; and the time to AP fell from 224 sec to 188 sec. Other studies (295) using higher inhaled CO (150 ppm) achieved arterial CO concentration of just over 4% (the same achieved by smoking three cigarettes), corroborating many (but not all) of Ayres' findings. LV end-diastolic pressure rose, whereas stroke index, cardiac index, and coronary sinus, arterial, and venous pO_2 levels all fell. Changes in HR and BP were only seen when cigarettes were smoked but not when CO was inhaled, implying that those hemodynamic changes were due to nicotine or other products of smoking. All of these patients had documented CAD. Other investigators have found similar results (296). In animals, similar levels of inhaled CO have reduced the ventricular fibrillation threshold in some, but not all, studies (297–299). In the study that showed an effect, monkeys with an experimental MI were more sensitive than normal animals (298).

In 1973, Wald et al. (300) suggested that the level of COHb was a better predictor of CVD than was smoking history. In their study of 950 smokers aged 50–69, those with COHb levels greater than 5% had 21 times the risk of developing CAD, AP, or IC than did smokers with levels of less than 3%. Finnish investigators could not confirm the superiority of using COHb levels to predict atherosclerotic disease compared to other measures of smoking behavior (301). Smokers of low-yield cigarettes do not have lower COHb levels than do smokers of regular brands, but pipe and cigar smokers, who don't inhale, usually do (302,303).

The toxicity of even low doses of CO, due to both air pollution and passive smoking, is clear. Russell et al. (304) showed that nonsmokers exposed for less than an hour to ambient air with 38 ppm of CO had an increase in their COHb levels, from 1.6% to 2.6%. Aronow (305) demonstrated that, under similar conditions, subjects with AP had a reduction in exercise time to the development of symptoms when these subjects were in an unventilated room where three volunteers had smoked five cigarettes each within a 2-hr period. COHb levels in these patients were 2.28% in the unventilated, smoke-filled room, as compared to a level of 1.29% without smoking and 1.77% with good ventilation. Numerous studies have shown that nonsmokers have significant levels of nicotine or metabolites in urine, saliva, and amniotic fluid (306–308). The appreciation of the increased risks of passive smoking for CVD and noncardiovascular disease has changed the political climate in the United States (309–313). Many communities and industries have banned smoking in public places, and, in 1988, a nationwide ban on smoking on airline flights of 2 hr or less went into effect. Such a law would have been inconceivable a decade earlier.

THE EFFECTS OF SMOKING CESSATION

Shortly after the association between smoking and cardiovascular risk became evident, Doll and colleagues (8–10) reported that smoking cessation significantly reduced the excess risk attributed to smoking. Though there has been some disagreement about how substantial this reduction actually is, and whether the reduction extends to all individuals and all related problems, most investigators agree that physicians should try to get patients to stop smoking (154,314–329) (Table 3). Smoking cessation reduces mortality, reverses many of the changes noted in cardiovascular risk factors, and reverses the metabolic and hemodynamic variables affected by cigarette smoking.

Friedman and Siegelaub (320) studied a large subset of individuals who were members of the Kaiser–Permanente Medical Center and who had participated in multiphasic health checkups over a 10-year period. In their two groups [current smokers (n = 9392) and quitters (n = 3825)], those who quit had gained more weight (2–3 pounds), had a rise in mean systolic BP of 3.8 mmHg, a rise in serum uric acid (0.2–0.5 mg%), and a fall in serum glucose, hematocrit, and WBC count. No changes were noted in serum cholesterol.

TABLE 3. *Effects of smoking cessation*

Increased	Decreased
Blood pressure	Cardiovascular mortality
Body weight	Coronary artery disease
HDL cholesterol	Cerebrovascular disease
	Peripheral vascular disease
	Total serum cholesterol
	LDL cholesterol
	Glucose
	Hematocrit
	Leucocyte count
	Uric acid

Others have shown similar effects on BP. Green et al. (39) have shown that ex-smokers have higher BP than do smokers (134/80 mmHg for ex-smokers compared to 129/77 mmHg for those who smoked less than 20 cigarettes per day) but have the same BP as nonsmokers (133/80 mmHg). In Framingham, similar small changes in BP were noted (a 1.6-mmHg systolic increase over 20 years for quitters, as compared to a 0.7-mmHg increase in systolic BP for persistent smokers) (316). In Evans County, Georgia, no significant increase in BP was found in quitters versus those who continued to smoke over a 7-year period (330). In MRFIT, no significant independent effect on systolic or DBP was noted when appropriate adjustments were made for weight and the initiation of antihypertensives when needed (331). Quitters tended not to gain weight but lost less than the remainder of the subjects studied. Though both BP and BW tend to change in a direction that might increase, rather than decrease, cardiovascular risk, the changes in both are small and not important enough to recommend that smoking be continued.

Changes in serum cholesterol are more likely to be in a desirable direction. Though Friedman and Siegelaub (320) and the Framingham Study (316) did not find a consistent effect on cholesterol with smoking cessation, MRFIT did note a significant drop in total serum cholesterol in those who quit, even though they did not lose weight (331). HDL cholesterol may rise significantly in a short period of time when smoking is stopped (332,333).

Numerous observational studies have clearly delineated the benefits of smoking cessation on cardiovascular mortality and morbidity. Friedman et al. (321) showed that in the Kaiser–Permanente patients, persistent smokers had more than twice the risk of dying from CAD than did those who quit. The benefit of quitting was slightly larger in those who had overt CAD at baseline. Many other studies (314,315,326) have shown similar benefits for MI for both men and women, but Cook et al. (329) still found an increased risk of MI for ex-smokers, even after 20 years. This group reported that the cumulative effect of smoking is most important and that quitting is helpful, since it reduces the overall exposure to cigarettes. Most data, however, support the contention that reduction in risk occurs within 5 years and that the risk in ex-smokers is the same as that in nonsmokers within 10–20 years (154,323,324,326). Patients with unstable AP have a significantly reduced mortality if they stop smoking (325). Patients who quit smoking after an MI have significantly fewer fatal and nonfatal MIs and a delayed appearance of AP, even though those who stop smoking are usually the patients with more severe disease when initially hospitalized (316,319,327,334).

In addition to CAD, other complications of smoking are reduced in those who can quit. CVA rate, for example, is reduced within 2 years and is similar to that of nonsmokers in 5 years (180,328). Patients with IC also do much better if they can stop smoking, something that only 11% of patients studied by Jonason and Bergstrom (201) could manage. In this large series (n = 343), all of the patients who developed rest pain over a minimum of 3 years of observation were persistent smokers, whereas none of those who quit developed this complication. Survival and other vascular complications were also statistically and significantly more common in those who continued to smoke. In Juergens et al.'s series of 520 patients with PVD, the only patients who required amputation of the lower extremity (11.3%) were smokers (199).

Though the evidence favoring the benefit of smoking cessation is overwhelming, some have raised questions. Unfortunately, Rose and Hamilton (317) were unable to show significant benefit of aggressive intervention to get middle-aged men to stop smoking. But many of the subjects who did not get the special program stopped smoking anyway, thus reducing the power of the study to show benefit. Friedman et al. (335) have looked at the behavioral characteristics of subjects who quit as compared to those of persistent smokers. They tried to determine whether quitters were a lower risk group at the outset and whether the apparent benefit achieved from quitting was actually due to some baseline characteristic. Quitters tended to (a) smoke fewer cigarettes, (b) inhale less, and (c) have lower WBC counts, and they were less likely to have an abnormal electrocardiogram. BP and serum cholesterol were not different, and other differences were small. Lee (318) has questioned whether the reduction in CVD mortality seen in British doctors was replaced by an almost equal increase in death from other causes such as accidents and suicides, potentially stress-related causes that cigarette smoking might have prevented. In the Oslo trial, the investigators felt that the major reason for the reduction in CAD was the lowering of serum cholesterol, not smoking cessation (336).

TECHNIQUES OF GETTING PATIENTS TO STOP SMOKING

Physicians have consistently rated "advising patients to stop smoking" as being the most important facet of preventive medicine and health promotion worth teaching to patients (337–339). In 1987, only 9% of U.S. physicians currently smoked, considerably less than the nearly 30% of Americans who still use tobacco products (340). Yet doctors are not as likely as they should be to counsel patients against smoking. Anda et al. (341) showed that only 44% of smokers who had been to a doctor in the year prior to their survey had been told to stop smoking. The percentage was higher (73%) in patients who had a smoking-related cardiovascular event (MI or CVA)—consistent with Wells et al. (342), who found that specialists and generalists are more likely to counsel those with heart disease than discuss smoking cessation with patients who are as yet unaffected. The major reasons that physicians don't pursue these issues vigorously are the perception that such efforts will fail and that they are neither well prepared, skilled, nor appropriately reimbursed for the time it takes to advise patients adequately (337,343,344).

The best way to promote and implement smoking cessation is not certain (Table 4). Some have advocated community-based programs, taking advantage of the fact that 80–90% of smokers wish to quit and that 75% of successful quitters have done so on their own either because of economic, social, or medical reasons (345–348). Others have recommended work-site programs with strong physician support (349,350). Evans et al. (351), who reviewed avail-

TABLE 4. *Methods of smoking cessation*

I. Community approaches
II. Economic incentives
III. Work-site programs
IV. Behavior modification
V. Physician-based approaches
VI. Pharmacologic approaches
   1. Nicotine gum
   2. Centrally acting nicotine antagonists
   3. Clonidine

able data a decade ago, concluded that the results of the programs available were all disappointing and that an effort should be directed at education of teenagers, especially girls (the one demographic group in the U.S. where smoking rates are rising), so that they never start smoking. Wynder and Hoffman (352) do not feel that these programs help. Schwartz (353) and Thompson (354) are somewhat more hopeful that counseling and specialized smoking cessation clinics are promising methods which need more emphasis.

In the past 20 years, however, considerable work has been done on how physicians may play a greater role in getting their patients to quit smoking. The key to this effort is a better understanding of both the psychologic and biologic reasons why patients continue to smoke even though they understand the consequences of smoking and wish to stop.

Fisher et al. (348) reviewed the five stages of quitting. The first stage is *precontemplation,* during which time the smoker is not interested in stopping and not susceptible to any intervention. The second stage is *contemplation,* when a smoker seriously entertains the idea to quit. The third stage is *action,* when programs are tried. The fourth stage is *maintenance,* to keep the patient from returning to smoking. The fifth stage is *relapse,* which is quite common because most ultimately successful quitters have stopped several times before, an average of 2.6 times. This group suggests that advice be given in a nonthreatening way and that the physician try to move the patient from the precontemplation stage through to the stage of action. At that point, numerous well-validated techniques—providing written materials, setting a quit date, giving positive reinforcement, discovering the barriers to stopping, writing contracts with the patient, and emphasizing social support —can help (344). Follow-up is critical; and patients should be allowed to slip a little, given that minor transgressions are expected (355,356). In MRFIT, a similar intensive program got nearly 40% of the smokers to stop (51). In the Oslo study, results were not quite as good (25%), but the program was not as extensive (336). Ockene et al. (339) claim that the essence of these techniques can be successfully taught to house staff in a 3-hr program, easily incorporated into an ambulatory care experience. The actual impact on smoking reduction in the patients of these trainees is not known. Smoking cessation workshops claim to have long-term success rates of about 25% (357).

The value of a general physician's simply mentioning cessation during routine patient visits is debatable. Since well over 70% of smokers see a doctor annually, even a small increase in quit rates would significantly reduce the number of cigarette smokers. In the first large controlled trial of systematic physician advice, 5.1% of patients quit in conjunction with a warning that follow-up would be done —as compared to 3.3% of those given advice only, 1.6% of those who just asked about smoking, and 0.3% of those in the control group (358). Other programs have been somewhat more successful but rarely exceed 20% quit rates at 1 year (344,356,359–361). Kottke et al. (356) recently evaluated 39 controlled trials of smoking cessation. They concluded that unique approaches were not especially successful but that a personalized program with frequent reinforcement was the most successful method to get patients to stop smoking. The use of spirometry to measure vital capacity or level of exhaled CO, combined with measurements of blood levels of cotinine and COHb, enhanced the success of counseling (362,363).

An important advance in reducing smoking is the appreciation of the biologic impact of nicotine addiction and the development of pharmacologic tools, especially nicotine gum, which helps addicted smokers withdraw. In this gum, nicotine is bound to an ion-exchange resin and buffered so that it will be at pH 8.5 in the mouth, thus allowing buccal absorption. The gum is made in 1-, 2-, 4-, and 8-mg sizes which release increasing amounts of nicotine when chewed properly for approximately 30 min. The 2-mg size (the only one available in the United States) delivers 1.02 mg of nicotine and the 4-mg size delivers 2.39 mg, as compared to approximately 1.1 mg in the ordinary cigarette (364). The plasma nicotine levels obtained with the 2-mg size (11.8 ng/ml) are less than generally seen in regular smokers (15.7 ng/ml), but the 4-mg gum achieves comparable levels (227,228).

Nicotine gum allows addicted smokers to substitute the gum when they sense the need for a cigarette. Addicted smokers are more likely to (a) inhale, (b) smoke many high-nicotine cigarettes, (c) be unable to wait more than 30 min for their morning cigarette, (d) smoke more in the morning than later in the day, and (e) have trouble not smoking where it is prohibited (365). The Fagerstrom tolerance scale ratings, which take these factors into account, are high in those addicted to smoking. Nicotine gum is well-tolerated, but some patients will become dependent on it while others develop nausea, local mouth irritation, and hiccups which don't increase as the dose is raised (366–370). Cardiovascular side effects are very rare, though the gum should not be used in patients with recent MI, HBP, AP, or arrhythmias (369). The gum works best in addicted smokers (368,371,372).

Lam et al. (373) analyzed the available studies and concluded that the gum was superior to advice alone in a general practice, but not compared to placebo in that setting. The highest 1-year abstinence rate was achieved in smoking cessation clinics (27%), as compared to 18% with placebo gum in that milieu. Tonnesan et al. (368) suggested that the 4-mg dose was considerably more effective (44.4% abstinence at 1 year) compared to the 2-mg gum (12.1% at 1 year), the dose level used in most of the studies reported by Lam et al. (373). Oster et al. (374) feel that nicotine gum is cost-effective, but Kottke et al. (356) did not find it superior to other modalities. Different ways of giving nicotine (transcutaneously and intranasally) have been developed, but it is too early to tell whether they will add anything to treatment (375,376). Other approaches, such as centrally acting nicotine-receptor antagonists, mecamylamine, or the antihypertensive agent clonidine, have been proposed and warrant further investigation (377,378).

CONCLUSIONS

Cigarette smoking is the most important preventable cause of premature mortality and morbidity in America. The annual excess mortality attributable to smoking is more than 350,000 deaths, of which 170,000 are due to CAD and 125,000 to cancer (80% of which are in the lung). The average reduction in life expectancy of a smoker is 5–8 years, with current estimates being that $5\frac{1}{2}$ min of life are lost with each cigarette smoked (379).

The economic costs of smoking are enormous. The estimated annual health care bill associated with smoking exceeds $16 billion (1985 dollars), with an additional $37 billion yearly due to lost productivity, morbidity, and premature death (379). Kristein (380) has estimated that cigarette smoking costs employers $336 to $601 per year (1980 dollars) in health and life insurance costs, absenteeism, reduced productivity, and workmen's compensation. Smoking is the cause of a large percentage of fires, with significant loss of life and property. But, in spite of these data, 56,220,000 Americans (29.3%) were estimated in 1982 to still be smokers, including 14.7% of those 12–17 years of age (381). Though the annual consumption of cigarettes has fallen to the lowest level in 35 years (3494 cigarettes per person over age 18), the percentage of heavy smokers (>25 cigarettes/day) is increasing, as is the percentage of teenage girls and women who smoke (382). The same trend, a reduction in cigarette consumption, especially in men, is also evident in the United Kingdom—though not necessarily throughout Europe or in nonindustrialized countries, where smoking and smoking-related disease are increasing (383).

The health consequences of cigarette smoking were noted for the first time in the 1930s and have now become undeniable. Yet tobacco is the largest cash crop in America, providing $60 billion per year to the United States economy and accounting for 5% of all U.S. exports. Tobacco farmers still get government subsidies; and until 1988, when a New Jersey jury awarded Mr. Antonio Cipollone $400,000 in damages due to the impact of smoking on his wife's death, no liability has been legally assigned to tobacco use, in spite of the medical evidence. Tobacco has been credited with saving the Jamestown settlement in Virginia, with restoring the economic viability of the Confederacy, and, indirectly, with the flourishing of a great American university, Duke. I think that the debt is paid.

REFERENCES

1. McCusker K. Landmarks of tobacco use in the United States. *Chest* 1986;93:34S–36S.
2. Gilman AG, Goodman LS, Rall TW, Murad F. *The pharmacological basis of therapeutics,* 7th edition. New York: Macmillan, 1985.
3. Pearl R. Tobacco smoking and longevity. *Science* 1938;87:216–217.
4. English JP, Willius FA, Berkson J. Tobacco and coronary disease. *JAMA* 1940;115:1327–1329.
5. Hammond EC, Horn D. Smoking and death rates—report on forty-four months of follow-up of 187,783 men. I. Total mortality. *JAMA* 1958;166:1159–1172.
6. Hammond EC, Horn D. Smoking and death rates—report on forty-four months of follow-up of 187,783 men. II. Death rates by cause. *JAMA* 1958;166:1294–1308.
7. Hammond EC. Smoking in relation to mortality and morbidity. Findings in first thirty-four months of follow-up in a prospective study started in 1959. *J Natl Cancer Inst* 1964;32:1161–1188.
8. Doll R. The mortality of doctors in relation to their smoking habits. *Br Med J* 1954;1:1455–4877.
9. Doll R, Hill AB. Mortality in relation to smoking: ten years' observations of British doctors. *Br Med J* 1964;1:1399–1410.
10. Doll R, Peto R. Mortality in relation to smoking: 20 years' observations on male British doctors. *Br Med J* 1976;2:1525–1536.
11. Doll R, Gray R, Hafner B, Peto R. Mortality in relation to smoking: 22 years' observations on female British doctors. *Br Med J* 1980;280:967–971.
12. United States Department of Health, Education, and Welfare, Public Health Service. *Smoking and health: report of the Advisory Committee to the Surgeon General of the Public Health Service.* PHS Publication No. 1103. Washington, DC: Government Printing Office, 1964.
13. Kannel WB, McGee DL, Castelli WP. Latest perspectives on cigarette smoking and cardiovascular disease: the Framingham Study. *J Cardiac Rehabil* 1984;4:267–277.
14. Friedman GD, Dales LG, Ury HK. Mortality in middle-aged smokers and nonsmokers. *N Engl J Med* 1979;300:213–217.
15. Abramson JH. The hazard of persistent cigarette smoking in later life. *Am J Med Sci* 1977;274:35–43.
16. Wenger NK. Coronary disease in women. *Annu Rev Med* 1985;36:285–294.
17. Willett WC, Green A, Stampfer MJ, et al. Relative and absolute excess risks of coronary heart disease among women who smoke cigarettes. *N Engl J Med* 1987;317:1303–1309.
18. Criqui MH. Epidemiology of atherosclerosis: an updated overview. *Am J Cardiol* 1986;57:18C–23C.
19. Bain C, Rosner B, Hennekens CH, Speizer FE, Jesse MJ. Cigarette consumption and deaths from coronary heart-disease. *Lancet* 1978;1:1087–1088.
20. Seltzer CC. Smoking and coronary heart disease: what are we to believe? *Am Heart J* 1980;100:275–280.
21. Burch PRJ. Smoking and mortality in England and Wales, 1950 to 1976. *J Chronic Dis* 1981;34:87–103.
22. Waldron I. The contribution of smoking to sex differences in mortality. *Public Health Rep* 1986;101:163–173.
23. Miller GH, Gerstein DR. The life expectancy of nonsmoking men and women. *Public Health Rep* 1983;98:343–349.
24. Kannel WB, Schatzkin A. Risk factor analysis. *Progr Cardiovasc Dis* 1983;XXVI:309–332.
25. Hopkins PN, Williams RR. A survey of 246 suggested coronary risk factors. *Atherosclerosis* 1981;40:1–52.
26. Hopkins PN, Williams RR. Identification and relative weight of cardiovascular risk factors. *Cardiol Clin* 1986;4:3–31.
27. Gordon T, Garcia-Palmieri MR, Kagan A, et al. Differences in coronary heart disease in Framingham, Honolulu and Puerto Rico. *J Chronic Dis* 1974;27:329–344.
28. The Pooling Project Research Group. Relationship of blood pressure, serum cholesterol, smoking habit, relative weight and ECG abnormalities to incidence of major coronary events: final report of the Pooling Project. *J Chronic Dis* 1978;31:201–306.
29. Borhani NO. Prevention of coronary heart disease in practice—implications of the results of recent clinical trials. *JAMA* 1985;254:257–262.
30. Burch PRJ. Ischaemic heart disease: epidemiology, risk factors and cause. *Cardiovasc Res* 1980;14:307–338.
31. Gordon T, Kannel WB. Multiple risk functions for predicting coronary heart disease: the concept, accuracy, and application. *Am Heart J* 1982;103:1031–1039.
32. Karvonen M, Keys A, Orma E, Fidanza F, Brozek J. Cigarette

smoking, serum-cholesterol, blood-pressure, and body fatness. Observations in Finland. *Lancet* 1959;1:492–494.
33. Ballantyne D, Devine BL, Fife R. Interrelation of age, obesity, cigarette smoking, and blood pressure in hypertensive patients. *Br Med J* 1978;1:880–881.
34. Higgins MW, Kjelsberg M. Characteristics of smokers and nonsmokers in Tecumseh, Michigan. II. The distribution of selected physical measurements and physiologic variables and the prevalence of certain diseases in smokers and nonsmokers. *Am J Epidemiol* 1967;86:60–77.
35. Seltzer CC. Effect of smoking on blood pressure. *Am Heart J* 1974;87:558–564.
36. Arkwright PD, Beilin LJ, Rouse I, et al. Effects of alcohol use and other aspects of lifestyle on blood pressure levels and prevalence of hypertension in a working population. *Circulation* 1982; 66:60–66.
37. Goldbourt U, Medalie JH. Characteristics of smokers, nonsmokers and ex-smokers among 10,000 adult males in Israel. II. Physiologic, biochemical and genetic characteristics. *Am J Epidemiol* 1977;105:75–86.
38. Morrison JA, Kelly K, Mellies M, et al. Cigarette smoking, alcohol intake, and oral contraceptives: relationships to lipids and lipoproteins in adolescent school-children. *Metabolism* 1979;28:1166–1170.
39. Green MS, Jucha E, Luz Y. Blood pressure in smokers and nonsmokers: epidemiologic findings. *Am Heart J* 1986;111:932–940.
40. Cryer PE, Haymond MW, Santiago JV, et al. Norepinephrine and epinephrine release and adrenergic mediation of smoking-associated hemodynamic and metabolic events. *N Engl J Med* 1976;295:573–577.
41. Che S. Actions of nicotine and smoking on circulation. *Pharmacol Ther* 1982;17:129–141.
42. Aronow WS, Goldsmith JR, Kern JC, et al. Effect of smoking cigarettes on cardiovascular hemodynamics. *Arch Environ Health* 1974;28:330–332.
43. Trap-Jensen J. Effects of smoking on the heart and peripheral circulation. *Am Heart J* 1988;115:263–267.
44. Hill P, Wynder EL. Smoking and cardiovascular disease. Effect of nicotine on the serum epinephrine and corticoids. *Am Heart J* 1974;87:491–496.
45. Cellina GU, Honour AJ, Littler WA. Direct arterial pressure, heart rate, and electrocardiogram during cigarette smoking in unrestricted patients. *Am Heart J* 1975;89:18–25.
46. Lund-Larsen PG, Tretli S. Changes in smoking habits and body weight after a three-year period—the Cardiovascular Disease Study in Finnmark. *J Chronic Dis* 1982;35:773–780.
47. Hjermann I, Helgeland A, Holme I, et al. The intercorrelation of serum cholesterol, cigarette smoking and body weight. The Oslo Study. *Acta Med Scand* 1976;200:479–485.
48. Khosla R, Lowe CR. Obesity and smoking habits. *Br Med J* 1971;4:10–13.
49. Jacobs DR, Gottenborg S. Smoking and weight: the Minnesota Lipid Research Clinic. *Am J Public Health* 1981;71:391–396.
50. Isles CG, Walker LM, Beevers GD, et al. Mortality in patients of the Glasgow Blood Pressure Clinic. *J Hypertens* 1986;4:141–156.
51. Multiple Risk Factor Intervention Trial Research Group. Multiple risk factor intervention trial. Risk factor changes and mortality results. *JAMA* 1982;248:1465–1477.
52. Heyden S, Schneider KA, Fodon JG. Smoking habits and antihypertensive treatment. *Nephron* 1987;47:99–103.
53. Hypertension Detection and Follow-up Program Cooperative Group: Five-year findings of the Hypertension Detection and Follow-up Program. I. Reduction in mortality of persons with high blood pressure, including mild hypertension. *JAMA* 1979;242:2562–2571.
54. Davis BR, Ford CE, Remington RD, et al. The Hypertension Detection and Follow-up Program design, methods, and baseline characteristics and blood pressure response of the study population. *Prog Cardiovasc Dis* 1986;XXIX:11–28.
55. Langford HG, Stamler J, Wassertheil-Smoller S, et al. All-cause mortality in the Hypertension Detection and Follow-up Program: findings for the whole cohort and for persons with less severe hypertension, with and without other traits related to risk of mortality. *Prog Cardiovasc Dis* 1986;XXIX:29–54.
56. The Management Committee of the Australian National Blood Pressure Study. Prognostic factors in the treatment of mild hypertension. *Circulation* 1984;69:668–676.
57. Medical Research Council Working Party. MRC trial of treatment of mild hypertension: principal results. *Br Med J* 1985;291:97–104.
58. Greenberg G, Thompson SG, Brennan PJ. The relationship between smoking and the response to anti-hypertensive treatment in mild hypertensives in the Medical Research Council's trial of treatment. *Int J Epidemiol* 1987;16:25–30.
59. Medical Research Council Working Party on Mild Hypertension. Coronary heart disease in the Medical Research Council trial of treatment of mild hypertension. *Br Heart J* 1988;59:364–378.
60. The IPPPSH Collaborative Group. Cardiovascular risk and risk factors in a randomized trial of treatment based on the beta blocker oxprenolol: the International Prospective Primary Prevention Study in Hypertension (IPPPSH). *J Hypertens* 1985;3:379–391.
61. Buhler FR, Vasenen K, Watters JT, et al. Impact of smoking on heart attacks, strokes, blood pressure control, drug dose, and quality of life aspects in the International Prospective Primary Prevention Study in Hypertension. *Am Heart J* 1988;115:282–288.
62. Wilhelmsen L, Berglund G, Elmfeldt D, et al. Beta-blockers versus diuretics in hypertensive men: Main results from the HAPPHY trial. *J Hypertens* 1987;5:561–572.
63. Wikstrand J, Warnold I, Olsson G, et al. Primary prevention with metoprolol in patients with hypertension. Mortality results from the MAPHY Study. *JAMA* 1988;259:1976–1982.
64. Trap-Jensen J, Carlsen JE, Svendsen TL, et al. Cardiovascular and adrenergic effects of cigarette smoking during immediate non-selective and selective beta adrenoceptor blockade in humans. *Eur J Clin Invest* 1979;9:181–183.
65. Freestone S, Ramsay LE. Effect of coffee and cigarette smoking on the blood pressure of untreated and diuretic-treated hypertensive patients. *Am J Med* 1982;73:348–353.
66. Freestone S, Ramsay LE. Effect of beta-blockade on the pressor response to coffee plus smoking in patients with mild hypertension. *Drugs* 1983;25:141–145.
67. Tango M, Krogsgaard AR, Trap-Jensen J, et al. Haemodynamic effects of cigarette smoking before and during long-term non-selective and selective beta-adrenergic blockade in patients with arterial hypertension. *Acta Med Scand* 1985;693:111–114.
68. Houben H, Thien T, Van't Laar A. Haemodynamic effects of cigarette smoking during chronic selective and non-selective beta-adrenoceptor blockade in patients with hypertension. *Br J Clin Pharmacol* 1981;12:67–72.
69. Mackay A, Brown JJ, Cumming AMM, et al. Smoking and renal artery stenosis. *Br Med J* 1979;2:770–772.
70. Nicholson JP, Alderman MH, Pickering TG, et al. Cigarette smoking and renovascular hypertension. *Lancet* 1983;2:765–766.
71. Black HR, Cooper KA. Cigarette smoking and atherosclerotic renal artery stenosis. *J Clin Hypertens* 1986;4:322–330.
72. Isles C, Brown JJ, Cumming AMM, et al. Excess smoking in malignant-phase hypertension. *Br Med J* 1979;1:579–581.
73. Bloxham CA, Beevers DG, Walker JM. Malignant hypertension and cigarette smoking. *Br Med J* 1979;1:581–583.
74. Elliott JM, Simpson FO. Cigarettes and accelerated hypertension. *NZ Med J* 1980;91:447–449.
75. Tuomilehto J, Elo J, Nissinen A. Smoking among patients with malignant hypertension. *Br Med J* 1982;284:1086.
76. Petitti DB, Klatsky AL. Malignant hypertension in women aged 15 to 44 years and its relation to cigarette smoking and oral contraceptives. *Am J Cardiol* 1983;52:297–298.
77. Mjos OD. Lipid effects of smoking. *Am Heart J* 1988;115:272–275.
78. Heyden S, Heiss G, Manegold C, et al. The combined effect of smoking and coffee drinking on LDL and HDL cholesterol. *Circulation* 1979;60:22–25.
79. Phillips NR, Havel RJ, Kane JP. Levels and interrelationships of serum and lipoprotein cholesterol and triglycerides. Association with adiposity and the consumption of ethanol, tobacco, and beverages containing caffeine. *Arteriosclerosis* 1981;1:13–24.

80. Halfon S-T, Kark JD, Baras M, et al. Smoking, lipids and lipoproteins in Jerusalem 17-year-olds. *Isr J Med Sci* 1982;18:1150–1157.
81. Brischetto CS, Connor WE, Connor SL, et al. Plasma lipid and lipoprotein profiles of cigarette smokers from randomly selected families: enhancement of hyperlipidemia and depression of high-density lipoprotein. *Am J Cardiol* 1983;52:675–680.
82. Garrison RJ, Kannel WB, Feinleib M, et al. Cigarette smoking and HDL cholesterol. The Framingham Offspring Study. *Atherosclerosis* 1978;30:17–25.
83. Criqui MH, Wallace RB, Heiss G, et al. Cigarette smoking and plasma high-density lipoprotein cholesterol. The Lipid Research Clinics Program Prevalence Study. *Circulation* 1980;62:IV70–IV76.
84. Haffner SM, Applebaum-Bowden D, Wahl PW, et al. Epidemiological correlates of high density lipoprotein subfractions, apolipoproteins A-1, A-11, and D, and lecithin cholesterol acyltransferase. Effects of smoking, alcohol and adiposity. *Arteriosclerosis* 1985;5:169–177.
85. Eriksson J, Enger SC. The effect of smoking on selected coronary heart disease risk factors in middle-aged men. *Acta Med Scand* 1978;203:27–30.
86. Freedman DS, Srinivasan SR, Shear CL, et al. Cigarette smoking initiation and longitudinal changes in serum lipids and lipoproteins in early adulthood: the Bogalusa Heart Study. *Am J Epidemiol* 1986;124:207–219.
87. Khosla T, Lowe CR. Obesity and smoking habits. *Br Med J* 1971;4:10–13.
88. Lincoln JE. Relation of income to body weight in cigarette smokers and nonsmokers. *JAMA* 1970;214:1121.
89. Gordon T, Kannel WB, Dawber TR, et al. Changes associated with cigarette smoking: the Framingham study. *Am Heart J* 1975;90:322–328.
90. Wack JT, Rodin J. Smoking and its effects on body weight and the systems of caloric regulation. *Am J Clin Nutr* 1982;35:366–380.
91. Comstock GW, Stone RW. Changes in body weight and subcutaneous fatness related to smoking habits. *Arch Environ Health* 1972;24:271–276.
92. Grunberg NE. The effects of nicotine and cigarette smoking on food consumption and taste preferences. *Addict Behav* 1982;7:317–331.
93. Grunberg NE. Nicotine as a psychoactive drug: appetite regulation. *Psychopharmacol Bull* 1986;22:875–881.
94. Hofstetter A, Schutz Y, Jequier E, et al. Increased 24-hour energy expenditure in cigarette smokers. *N Engl J Med* 1986;314:79–82.
95. Ross R. The pathogenesis of atherosclerosis—an update. *N Engl J Med* 1986;314:488–500.
96. Korsan-Bengtsen K, Wilhelmsen L, Tibblin G. Blood coagulation and fibrinolysis in a random sample of 788 men 54 years old. II. Relations of the variables to "risk factors" for myocardial infarction. *Thromb Diathes Haemorrhol* 1972;28:99–108.
97. Wilhelmsen L, Svardsudd K, Korsan-Bengtsen K, et al. Fibrinogen as a risk factor for stroke and myocardial infarction. *N Engl J Med* 1984;311:501–505.
98. Kannel WB, D'Agostino RB, Belanger AJ. Fibrinogen, cigarette smoking, and risk of cardiovascular disease: insights from the Framingham Study. *Am Heart J* 1987;113:1006–1010.
99. Meade TW, Brozovic M, Chakrabarti RR, et al. Haemostatic function and ischaemic heart disease: principal results of the Northwick Park Heart Study. *Lancet* 1986;2:533–537.
100. Balleisen L, Bailey J, Epping PH, et al. Epidemiological study on factor VII, factor VIII and fibrinogen in an industrial population: 1 Baseline data on the relation to age, gender, body-weight, smoking, alcohol, pill-using, and menopause. *Thromb Haemost* 1985;54:475–479.
101. Meade TW, Imeson J, Stirling Y. Effects of changes in smoking and other characteristics on clotting factors and the risk of ischaemic heart disease. *Lancet* 1987;2:986–988.
102. Dintenfass L. Elevation of blood viscosity, aggregation of red cells, haematocrit values and fibrinogen levels in cigarette smokers. *Med J Aust* 1975;1:617–620.
103. Letcher RL, Chien S, Pickering TG, et al. Direct relationship between blood pressure and blood viscosity in normal and hypertensive subjects. Role of fibrinogen and concentration. *Am J Med* 1981;70:1195–1202.
104. Levenson J, Simon AC, Cambien FA, et al. Cigarette smoking and hypertension—factors independently associated with blood hyperviscosity and arterial rigidity. *Arteriosclerosis* 1987;7:572–577.
105. Meade TW, Chakrabarti R, Haines AP, et al. Characteristics affecting fibrinolytic activity and plasma fibrinogen concentrations. *Br Med J* 1979;1:153–156.
106. Ross R, Glomset J, Harker L. Response to injury and atherogenesis. *Am J Pathol* 1977;86:675–684.
107. Mustard JR, Murphy EA. Effect of smoking on blood coagulation and platelet survival in man. *Br Med J* 1963;1:846–849.
108. Glynn MF, Mustard JF, Buchanan MR, et al. Cigarette smoking and platelet aggregation. *Can Med Assoc J* 1966;95:549–553.
109. Levine PH. An acute effect of cigarette smoking on platelet function. A possible link between smoking and arterial thrombosis. *Circulation* 1973;XLVIII:619–623.
110. Davis JW, Davis RF. Acute effect of tobacco cigarette smoking on the platelet aggregate ratio. *Am J Med Sci* 1979;278:139–143.
111. Bierenbaum ML, Fleischman AI, Stier A, et al. Effect of cigarette smoking upon *in vivo* platelet function in man. *Thromb Res* 1978;12:1051–1057.
112. Hawkins R. Smoking, platelets and thrombosis. *Nature* 1972;236:450–452.
113. Fitzgerald GA, Oates JA, Nowak J. Cigarette smoking and hemostatic function. *Am Heart J* 1988;115:267–271.
114. Nadler JL, Velasco JS, Horton R. Cigarette smoking inhibits prostacyclin formation. *Lancet* 1983;1:1248–1250.
115. Mehta P, Mehta J. Effects of smoking on platelets and on plasma thromboxane-prostacyclin balance in man. *Prostaglandins Leukotrienes Med* 1982;9:141–150.
116. Nowak J, Murray JJ, Oates JA, et al. Biochemical evidence of a chronic abnormality in platelet and vascular function in healthy individuals who smoke cigarettes. *Circulation* 1987;76:6–14.
117. Reinders JH, Brinkman HM, Mourik JA, et al. Cigarette smoke impairs endothelial cell prostacyclin production. *Arteriosclerosis* 1986;6:15–23.
118. Pittilo RM, Mackie IJ, Rowles PM, et al. Effects of cigarette smoking on the ultrastructure of rat thoracic aorta and its ability to produce prostacyclin. *Thromb Haemost* 1982;48:173–176.
119. Madsen H, Dyerberg J. Cigarette smoking and its effects on the platelet–vessel wall interaction. *Scand J Clin Lab Invest* 1984;44:203–206.
120. Fuster V, Chesebro JH, Frye RI, et al. Platelet survival and the development of coronary artery disease in the young adult: effects of cigarette smoking, strong family history and medical therapy. *Circulation* 1981;63:546–551.
121. Davis JW, Davis RF. Prevention of cigarette smoking-induced platelet aggregate formation by aspirin. *Arch Intern Med* 1981;141:206–207.
122. Corre F, Lellouch J, Schwartz D. Smoking and leucocyte-counts. *Lancet* 1971;2:632–634.
123. Friedman GD, Siegelaub AB, Seltzer CC, et al. Smoking habits and the leukocyte count. *Arch Environ Health* 1973;26:137–143.
124. Helman N, Rubenstein LS. The effects of age, sex, and smoking on erythrocytes and leukocytes. *Am J Clin Pathol* 1975;63:35–44.
125. Billimoria JD, Pozner H, Metselaar B, et al. Effect of cigarette smoking on lipids, lipoproteins, blood coagulation, fibrinolysis and cellular components of human blood. *Atherosclerosis* 1975;21:61–76.
126. Yeung MC, Buncio AD. Leukocyte count, smoking, and lung function. *Am J Med* 1984;76:31–37.
127. Tell GS, Grimm RH, Vellar OD, et al. The relationship of white cell count, platelet count, and hematocrit to cigarette smoking in adolescents: the Oslo Youth Study. *Circulation* 1985;72:971–974.
128. Friedman GD, Klatsky A, Siegelaub AB. The leukocyte count as a predictor of myocardial infarction. *N Engl J Med* 1974;290:1275–1278.
129. Zalokar JB, Richard JL, Claude JR. Leukocyte count, smoking, and myocardial infarction. *N Engl J Med* 1981;304:465–468.
130. Isager H, Hagerup L. Relationship between cigarette smoking

and high packed cell volume and haemoglobin levels. *Scand J Haematol* 1971;8:241–244.
131. Petitti DB, Wingerd J, Pellegrin F, Ramcharan S. Risk of vascular disease in women. Smoking, oral contraceptives, noncontraceptive estrogens, and other factors. *JAMA* 1979;242:1150–1154.
132. Dalen JE, Hickler RB. Oral contraceptives and cardiovascular disease. *Am Heart J* 1981;101:626–639.
133. Wilson PWF, Garrison RJ, Castelli WP. Postmenopausal estrogen use, cigarette smoking, and cardiovascular morbidity in women over 50. The Framingham Study. *N Engl J Med* 1985;313:1038–1043.
134. Lindholm J, Winkel P, Brodthagen U, et al. Coronary risk factors and plasma sex hormones. *Am J Med* 1982;73:648–651.
135. Klaiber EL, Broverman DM, Dalen JE. Serum estradiol levels in male cigarette smokers. *Am J Med* 1984;77:858–862.
136. Janzon L, Berntorp K, Hanson M, et al. Glucose tolerance and smoking: A population study of oral and intravenous glucose tolerance tests in middle-aged men. *Diabetologia* 1983;25:86–88.
137. Rogers WR, Bass RL, Johnson DE, et al. Atherosclerosis-related responses to cigarette smoking in the baboon. *Circulation* 1980;61:1188–1193.
138. Rosengren A, Wilhelmsen L, Wedel H. Separate and combined effects of smoking and alcohol abuse in middle-aged men. *Acta Med Scand* 1988;223:111–118.
139. Barboriak JJ, Anderson AJ, Hoffmann RG. Smoking, alcohol and coronary artery occlusion. *Atherosclerosis* 1982;43:277–282.
140. Fried LP, Moore RD, Pearson TA. Long-term effects of cigarette smoking and moderate alcohol consumption on coronary artery diameter. *Am J Med* 1986;80:37–44.
141. Wilens SL, Plair CM. Cigarette smoking and arteriosclerosis. *Science* 1962;138:975–977.
142. Auerbach O, Hammond EC, Garfinkel L. Smoking in relation to atherosclerosis of the coronary arteries. *N Engl J Med* 1965;273:775–779.
143. Ball K, Turner R. Smoking and the heart. The basis for action. *Lancet* 1974;2:822–826.
144. Herbert WH. Cigarette smoking and arteriographically demonstrable coronary artery disease. *Chest* 1975;67:49–52.
145. Reid DD, McCartney P, Hamilton PJS, et al. Smoking and other risk factors for coronary heart-disease in British civil servants. *Lancet* 1976;2:979–984.
146. Miettinen OS, Neff RK, Jick H. Cigarette-smoking and nonfatal myocardial infarction: rate ratio in relation to age, sex and predisposing conditions. *Am J Epidemiol* 1976;103:30–36.
147. Uhl GS, Farrell PW. Myocardial infarction in young adults: risk factors and natural history. *Am Heart J* 1983;105:548–553.
148. Holmes DR, Elveback LR, Frye RL, et al. Association of risk factor variables and coronary artery disease documented with angiography. *Circulation* 981;63:293–299.
149. Ramsdale DR, Faragher EB, Bray CL, et al. Smoking and coronary artery disease assessed by routine coronary arteriography. *Br Med J* 1985;290:197–200.
150. Rosenberg L, Kaufman DW, Helmrich SP, et al. Myocardial infarction and cigarette smoking in women younger than 50 years of age. *JAMA* 1985;253:2965–2969.
151. Vlietstra RE, Frye RL, Kronmal RA, et al. Risk factors and angiographic coronary artery disease: a report from the Coronary Artery Surgery Study (CASS). *Circulation* 1980;62:254–261.
152. LaVecchia C, Franceschi S, DeCarli A, et al. Risk factors for myocardial infarction in young women. *Am J Epidemiol* 1987;125:832–843.
153. Wilhelmsen L. Coronary heart disease: epidemiology of smoking and intervention studies of smoking. *Am Heart J* 1988;115:242–249.
154. Kannel WB. Update on the role of cigarette smoking in coronary disease. *Am Heart J* 1981;101:319–328.
155. Spain DM, Bradess VA. Sudden death from coronary heart disease. Survival time, frequency of thrombi, and cigarette smoking. *Chest* 1970;58:107–110.
156. Kannel WB, Doyle JT, McNamara PM, et al. Precursors of sudden coronary death. Factors related to the incidence of sudden death. *Circulation* 1975;51:606–613.
157. Hallstrom AP, Cobb LA, Ray R. Smoking as a risk factor for recurrence of sudden cardiac arrest. *N Engl J Med* 1986; 314:271–275.
158. Jajich CL, Ostfeld AM, Freeman DH. Smoking and coronary heart disease mortality in the elderly. *JAMA* 1984;252:2831–2834.
159. Rechnitzer PA, Cunningham DA, Donner AP, et al. Characteristics that predicted recurrence of infarction within 3 years in the Ontario Exercise–Heart Collaborative Study. *Can Med Assoc J* 1983;128:1287–1290.
160. FitzGibbon GM, Leach AJ, Kafka HP. Atherosclerosis of coronary artery bypass grafts and smoking. *Can Med Assoc J* 1987;136:45–47.
161. Scholl J, Benacerraf A, Ducimetiere P, et al. Comparison of risk factors in vasospastic angina without significant fixed coronary narrowing to significant fixed coronary narrowing and no vasospastic angina. *Am J Cardiol* 1986;57:199–202.
162. Roubin GS, Spencer BK, Douglas JS. Restenosis after percutaneous transluminal coronary angioplasty: the Emory University Hospital experience. *Am J Cardiol* 1987;60:39B–43B.
163. Medalie JH, Goldbourt U. Unrecognized myocardial infarction: five-year incidence, mortality, and risk factors. *Ann Intern Med* 1976;84:526–531.
164. Maquad J, Fernandez F, Barrillon A, et al. Diffuse or segmental narrowing (spasm) of the coronary arteries during smoking demonstrated on angiography. *Am J Cardiol* 1984;53:354–355.
165. Jugdutt BI, Stevens GF, Zacks DJ, et al. Myocardial infarction, oral contraception, cigarette smoking, and coronary artery spasm in young women. *Am Heart J* 1983;106:757–761.
166. Heliovaara M, Karvonen MJ, Punsar S, et al. Importance of coronary risk factors in the presence or absence of myocardial ischemia. *Am J Cardiol* 1982;50:1248–1252.
167. Hennekens CH, Lown B, Rosner B, et al. Ventricular premature beats and coronary risk factors. *Am J Epidemiol* 1980;112:93–99.
168. Davis MJE, Hockings BEF, El Dessouky MAM, et al. Cigarette smoking and ventricular arrhythmia in coronary heart disease. *Am J Cardiol* 1984;54:282–285.
169. Myers MG, Benowitz NL, Dubbin JD, et al. Cardiovascular effects of smoking in patients with ischemic heart disease. *Chest* 1986;93:14–19.
170. McHenry PL, Faris JV, Jordan JW, et al. Comparative study of cardiovascular function and ventricular premature complexes in smokers and nonsmokers during maximal treadmill exercise. *Am J Cardiol* 1977;39:493–498.
171. Bellet S, DeGuzman NT, Kostis JB, et al. The effect of inhalation of cigarette smoke on ventricular fibrillation threshold in normal dogs and dogs with acute myocardial infarction. *Am Heart J* 1972;83:67–76.
172. Hagman M, Wilhelmsen L, Wedel H, et al. Risk factors for angina pectoris in a population study of Swedish men. *J Chronic Dis* 1987;40:265–275.
173. Aronow WS, Kaplan MA, Jacob D. Tobacco: a precipitating factor in angina pectoris. *Ann Intern Med* 1968;69:529–536.
174. Martin JL, Wilson JR, Ferraro N, et al. Acute coronary vasoconstrictive effects of cigarette smoking in coronary heart disease. *Am J Cardiol* 1984;54:56–60.
175. Hartz AJ, Anderson AJ, Brooks HL, et al. The association of smoking with cardiomyopathy. *N Engl J Med* 1984;311:1201–1206.
176. Black HR, Zeevi GR, Silten RM, et al. Effect of heavy cigarette smoking on renal and myocardial arterioles. *Nephron* 1983;34:173–179.
177. Oberai B, Adams CWM, High OB. Myocardial and renal arteriolar thickening in cigarette smokers. *Atherosclerosis* 1984; 52:185–190.
178. Lough J. Cardiomyopathy produced by cigarette smoke. Ultrastructural observations in guinea pigs. *Arch Pathol Lab Med* 1978;102:377–386.
179. The Coronary Drug Project Research Group. Cigarette smoking as a risk factor in men with a prior history of myocardial infarction. *J Chron Dis* 1979;32:415–425.
180. Wolf PA, D'Agostino RB, Kannel WB, et al. Cigarette smoking as a risk factor for stroke. The Framingham Study. *JAMA* 1988;259:1025–1029.
181. Bonita R, Scragg R, Stewart A, et al. Cigarette smoking and risk of premature stroke in men and women. *Br Med J* 1986;293:6–8.
182. Daugherty SA, Berman R, Entwisle G, et al. Cerebrovascular

events in the Hypertension Detection and Follow-up Program. *Prog Cardiovasc Dis* 1986;XXIX:63–72.

183. Salonen JT, Puska P, Tuomilehto J, et al. Relation of blood pressure, serum lipids and smoking to the risk of cerebral stroke. A longitudinal study in eastern Finland. *Stroke* 1982;13:327–333.
184. Abbott RD, Yin Y, Reed DM, et al. Risk of stroke in male cigarette smokers. *N Engl J Med* 1986;315:717–720.
185. Welin L, Svardsudd K, Wilhelmsen L, et al. Analysis of risk factors for stroke in a cohort of men born in 1913. *N Engl J Med* 1987;317:521–526.
186. Colditz GA, Bonita R, Stampfer MJ, et al. Cigarette smoking and risk of stroke in middle-aged women. *N Engl J Med* 1988;318:937–941.
187. Bonita R. Cigarette smoking, hypertension and the risk of subarachnoid hemorrhage: a population-based case-control study. *Stroke* 1986;17:831–835.
188. Fogelholm R, Murros K. Cigarette smoking and subarachnoid haemorrhage: a population-based case-control study. *J Neurol Neurosurg Psychiatry* 1987;50:78–80.
189. Grainger K, Mastaglia F. Smoking, transient ischaemic attacks and stroke. A temporal association. *Med J Aust* 1976;2:302–303.
190. Rogers RL, Meyer JS, Shaw TG, et al. Cigarette smoking decreases cerebral blood flow suggesting increased risk for stroke. *JAMA* 1983;250:2796–2800.
191. Clagett GP, Rich NM, McDonald PT, et al. Etiologic factors for recurrent carotid artery stenosis. *Surgery* 1983;93:313–318.
192. Tomatis LA, Fierens EE, Verbrugge GP. Evaluation of surgical risk in peripheral vascular disease by coronary arteriography: a series of 100 cases. *Surgery* 1972;71:429–435.
193. Weiss NS. Cigarette smoking and arteriosclerosis obliterans: an epidemiologic approach. *Am J Epidemiol* 1972;95:17–25.
194. Hughson WG, Mann JI, Garrod A. Intermittent claudication: prevalence and risk factors. *Br Med J* 1978;1:1379–1381.
195. Brooks SH, Blankenhorn DH, Chin HP, et al. Design of human atherosclerosis studies by serial angiography. *J Chronic Dis* 1980;33:347–357.
196. Greenhalgh RM, Laing SP, Cole PV, et al. Smoking and arterial reconstruction. *Br J Surg* 1981;68:605–607.
197. Puchmayer V. Smoking as a risk factor for the development of arterial occlusive disease. *Acta Univ Carol* [*Med Monogr*] *(Praha)* 1984;105:1–134.
198. Couch NP. On the arterial consequences of smoking. *J Vasc Surg* 1986;3:808–812.
199. Juergens JL, Barker NW, Hines EA. Arteriosclerosis obliterans: review of 520 cases with special reference to pathogenic and prognostic factors. *Circulation* 1960;XXI:188–195.
200. Kannel WB, Shurtleff D. The Framingham Study. Cigarettes and the development of intermittent claudication. *Geriatrics* 1973;1:61–68.
201. Jonason T, Bergstrom R. Cessation of smoking in patients with intermittent claudication. Effects on the risk of peripheral vascular complications, myocardial infarction and mortality. *Acta Med Scand* 1987;221:253–260.
202. Thomas M. Smoking and vascular surgery. *Br J Surg* 1981;68:601–604.
203. Hammond EC, Garfinkel L. Coronary heart disease, stroke, and aortic aneurysm. Factors in the etiology. *Arch Environ Health* 1969;19:167–182.
204. Sackett DL, Gibson RW, Bross IDJ, et al. Relation between aortic atherosclerosis and the use of cigarettes and alcohol. An autopsy study. *N Engl J Med* 1968;279:1413–1420.
205. Strong JP, Richards ML. Cigarette smoking and atherosclerosis in autopsied men. *Atherosclerosis* 1976;23:451–476.
206. Auerbach O, Garfinkel L. Atherosclerosis and aneurysm of aorta in relation to smoking habits and age. *Chest* 1980;78:805–809.
207. Ribeiro P, Walesby R, Edmondson S, et al. Collagen content of atherosclerotic arteries is higher in smokers than in non-smokers. *Lancet* 1983;1:1070–1072.
208. Cannon DJ, Casteel L, Read RC. Abdominal aortic aneurysm, Leriche's syndrome, inguinal herniation, and smoking. *Arch Surg* 1984;119:387–389.
209. Sexton M, Hebel JR. A clinical trial of change in maternal smoking and its effect on birth weight. *JAMA* 1984;251:911–915.
210. Mochizuki M, Maruo T, Masuko K, et al. Effects of smoking on fetoplacental–maternal system during pregnancy. *Am J Obstet Gynecol* 1984;149:413–420.
211. Armussen I, Kjeldsen K. Intimal ultrastructure of human umbilical arteries. Observations on arteries from newborn children of smoking and nonsmoking mothers. *Circ Res* 1975;36:579–589.
212. Riefkohl R, Wolfe JA, Cox EB, et al. Association between cutaneous occlusive vascular disease, cigarette smoking, and skin slough after rhytidectomy. *Plast Reconstr Surg* 1986;77:592–595.
213. Paetkau ME, Boyd TAS, Winship B, et al. Cigarette smoking and diabetic retinopathy. *Diabetes* 1977;26:46–49.
214. Klein R, Klein BEK, Davis MD. Is cigarette smoking associated with diabetic retinopathy? *Am J Epidemiol* 1983;118:228–238.
215. Telmer S, Christiansen JS, Andersen AR, et al. Smoking habits and prevalence of clinical diabetic microangiopathy in insulin-dependent diabetics. *Acta Med Scand* 1984;215:63–68.
216. Muhlhauser I, Sawicki P, Berger M. Cigarette-smoking as a risk factor for macroproteinuria and proliferative retinopathy in Type 1 (insulin-dependent) diabetes. *Diabetologia* 1986;29:500–502.
217. Stegmayr B, Lithner F. Tobacco and end stage diabetic nephropathy. *Br Med J* 1987;295:581–582.
218. Richardson DR. Effects of habitual tobacco smoking on reactive hyperemia in the human hand. *Arch Environ Health* 1985;40:114–119.
219. Hagen RL, D'Agostino JA. The effects of cigarette smoking on human sexual potency. *Addict Behav* 1986;11:431–434.
220. Virag R, Bouilly P, Frydman D. Is impotence an arterial disorder? A study of arterial risk factors in 440 impotent men. *Lancet* 1985;1:181–184.
221. McGill HC. The cardiovascular pathology of smoking. *Am Heart J* 1988;115:250–257.
222. Schachter S. Pharmacological and psychological determinants of smoking. *Ann Int Med* 1978;88:104–114.
223. Pollin W, Ravenholt RT. Tobacco addiction and tobacco mortality. Implications for death certification. *JAMA* 1984;252:2849–2854.
224. Darby TD, McNamee JE, van Rossum JM. Cigarette smoking pharmacokinetics and its relationship to smoking behaviour. *Clin Pharmacokinet* 1984;9:435–449.
225. Benowitz NL. Clinical pharmacology of nicotine. *Annu Rev Med* 1986;37:21–32.
226. Henningfield JE, Nemeth-Coslett R. Nicotine dependence. Interface between tobacco and tobacco-related disease. *Chest* 1988;93:37S–55S.
227. Russell MAH, Feyerabend C, Cole PV. Plasma nicotine levels after cigarette smoking and chewing nicotine gum. *Br Med J* 1976;1:1043–1046.
228. McNabb ME, Ebert RV, McCusker K. Plasma nicotine levels produced by chewing nicotine gum. *JAMA* 1982;248:865–868.
229. Ebert RV, McKendree EM, McCusker KT, et al. Amount of nicotine and carbon monoxide inhaled by smokers of low-tar, low-nicotine cigarettes. *JAMA* 1983;250:2840–2842.
230. Hill P, Marquardt H. Plasma and urine changes after smoking different brands of cigarettes. *Clin Pharmacol Ther* 1980;27:652–658.
231. Jaffe JH, Kanzler M, Friedman L, et al. Carbon monoxide and thiocyanate levels in low tar/nicotine smokers. *Addict Behav* 1981;6:337–343.
232. Russell MAH, Jarvis M, Iyer R, et al. Relation of nicotine yield of cigarettes to blood nicotine concentrations in smokers. *Br Med J* 1980;280:972–976.
233. Benowitz NL, Hall SM, Herning RI, et al. Smokers of low-yield cigarettes do not consume less nicotine. *N Engl J Med* 1983;309:139–142.
234. Herning RI, Jones RT, Benowitz NL, et al. How a cigarette is smoked determines blood nicotine levels. *Clin Pharmacol Ther* 1983;33:84–90.
235. Higenbottam T, Shipley MJ, Rose G. Cigarettes, lung cancer, and coronary heart disease: the effects of inhalation and tar yield. *J Epidemiol Community Health* 1982;36:113–117.
236. Castelli WP, Dawber TR, Feinleib M, et al. The filter cigarette and coronary heart disease: the Framingham Study. *Lancet* 1981;2:109–113.
237. Aronow WS, Swanson AJ. The effect of low-nicotine cigarettes on angina pectoris. *Ann Intern Med* 1969;71:599–601.
238. Aronow WS, Cassidy J, Vangrow JS, et al. Effect of cigarette

smoking and breathing carbon monoxide on cardiovascular hemodynamics in anginal patients. *Circulation* 1974;50:340–347.
239. Robertson D, Appalsamy M. Smoking and mechanisms of cardiovascular control. *Am Heart J* 1988;115:258–263.
240. Klein LW, Gorlin R. The systemic and coronary hemodynamic response to cigarette smoking. *NY State J Med* 1983;2:1264–1266.
241. Klein LW. Cigarette smoking, atherosclerosis and the coronary hemodynamic response: a unifying hypothesis. *J Am Coll Cardiol* 1984;4:972–974.
242. Klein LW, Ambrose J, Pichard A, et al. Acute coronary hemodynamic response to cigarette smoking in patients with coronary artery disease. *J Am Coll Cardiol* 1984;3:879–886.
243. Nicod P, Rehr R, Winniford MD, et al. Acute systemic and coronary hemodynamic and serologic responses to cigarette smoking in long-term smokers with atherosclerotic coronary artery disease. *J Am Coll Cardiol* 1984;4:964–971.
244. Winniford MD, Wheelan KR, Kremers MS, et al. Smoking-induced coronary vasoconstriction in patients with atherosclerotic coronary artery disease: evidence for adrenergically mediated alterations in coronary artery tone. *Circulation* 1986;73:662–667.
245. Klein LW, Pichard AD, Holt J, et al. Effects of chronic tobacco smoking on the coronary circulation. *J Am Coll Cardiol* 1983;1(2):421–426.
246. Kershbaum A, Bellet S, Dickstein ER, et al. Effect of cigarette smoking and nicotine on serum free fatty acids. Based on a study in the human subject and the experimental animal. *Circ Res* 1961;IX:631–638.
247. Spohr U, Hofmann K, Steck W, et al. Evaluation of smoking-induced effects on sympathetic, hemodynamic and metabolic variables with respect to plasma nicotine and COHb levels. *Atherosclerosis* 1979;33:271–283.
248. Kershbaum A, Bellet S, Khorsandian R. Elevation of serum cholesterol after administration of nicotine. *Am Heart J* 1965;69:206–210.
249. Mjos OD. Lipid effects of smoking. *Am Heart J* 1988;115:272–275.
250. Comroe JH. The pharmacological actions of nicotine. *Ann NY Acad Sci* 1960;90:49–51.
251. Pomerleau OF, Fertig JB, Seyler LE, et al. Neuroendocrine reactivity to nicotine in smokers. *Psychopharmacology* 1983;81:61–67.
252. Baer L, Radichevich I. Cigarette smoking in hypertensive patients—blood pressure and endocrine responses. *Am J Med* 1985;78:564–568.
253. Husain MK, Frantz AG, Ciarochi F, et al. Nicotine-stimulated release of neurophysin and vasopressin in humans. *J Clin Endocrinol Metab* 1975;41:1113–1117.
254. DeSouza EMC, Silva MRE. The release of vasopressin by nicotine: further studies on its site of action. *J Physiol* 1977;265:297–311.
255. Benowitz NL, Jacob P, Jones RT, et al. Interindividual variability in the metabolism and cardiovascular effects of nicotine in man. *J Pharmacol Exp Therapeut* 1982;221:368–372.
256. Hill P, Haley NJ, Wynder EL. Cigarette smoking: carboxyhemoglobin, plasma nicotine, cotinine and thiocyanate vs self-reported smoking data and cardiovascular disease. *J Chronic Dis* 1983;36:439–449.
257. McCusker K, McNabb E, Bone R. Plasma nicotine levels in pipe smokers. *JAMA* 1982;248:577–578.
258. Turner HM, Sillett RW, McNicol MW. Effect of cigar smoking on carboxyhaemoglobin and plasma nicotine concentrations in primary pipe and cigar smokers and ex-cigarette smokers. *Br Med J* 1977;2:1387–1389.
259. Wald NJ, Idle M, Boreham J, et al. Serum cotinine levels in pipe smokers: evidence against nicotine as cause of coronary heart disease. *Lancet* 1981;2:775–777.
260. Pechacek TF, Folsom AR, de Gaudermaris R, et al. Smoke exposure in pipe and cigar smokers—serum thiocyanate measures. *JAMA* 1985;254:3330–3332.
261. Hickey N, Mulcahy R, Daly L, et al. Cigar and pipe smoking related to four year survival of coronary patients. *Br Heart J* 1983;49:423–426.
262. Gyntelberg F, Pedersen PB, Lauridsen L, et al. Smoking and risk of myocardial infarction in Copenhagen men aged 40–59 with special reference to cheroot smoking. *Lancet* 1981;1:987–989.
263. Renaud S, Blache D, Cumont E, et al. Platelet function after cigarette smoking in relation to nicotine and carbon monoxide. *Clin Pharmacol Ther* 1984;36:389–395.
264. Folts JD, Bonebrake FC. The effects of cigarette smoke and nicotine on platelet thrombus formation in stenosed dog coronary arteries: inhibition with phentolamine. *Circulation* 1982;65:465–470.
265. Toivanen J, Ylikorkala O, Viinikka L. Effects of smoking and nicotine on human prostacyclin and thromboxane production *in vivo* and *in vitro*. *Toxicol Appl Pharmacol* 1986;82:301–306.
266. Wennmalm A, Alster P. Nicotine inhibits vascular prostacyclin but not platelet thromboxane formation. *Gen Pharmacol* 1983;14:189–191.
267. Istoel, Giessen WJ, Ezwolsman, et al. Effect of nicotine on production of prostacyclin in human umbilical artery. *Br Heart J* 1982;48:493–496.
268. Alster P, Wennmalm A. Effect of nicotine on the formation of prostacyclin-like activity and thromboxane in rabbit aorta and platelets. *Br J Pharmacol* 1984;81:55–60.
269. Jeremy JY, Mikhailidis DP, Dandona P. Cigarette smoke extracts, but not nicotine, inhibit prostacyclin (PGI_2) synthesis in human, rabbit and rat vascular tissue. *Prostaglandins Leukotrienes Med* 1985;19:261–270.
270. Wennmalm A. Cigarette smoking, prostaglandins and reactive hyperaemia. *Prostaglandins Med* 1979;3:321–326.
271. Wennmalm A. Nicotine inhibits hypoxia- and arachidonate-induced release of prostacyclin-like activity in rabbit hearts. *Br J Pharmacol* 1980;69:545–549.
272. Gorlin R. Dynamic vascular factors in the genesis of myocardial ischemia. *J Am Coll Cardiol* 1983;1:897–906.
273. Sasagawa S, Suzuke K, Sakatani T, et al. Effects of nicotine on the functions of human polymorphonuclear leukocytes *in vitro*. *J Leuk Biol* 1985;37:493–502.
274. Hladovec J. Endothelial injury by nicotine and its prevention. *Experientia* 1978;34:1585–1586.
275. Wesnes K, Warburton DM. Smoking, nicotine and human performance. *Pharmacol Ther* 1983;21:189–208.
276. Domino EF. Nicotine: a unique psychoactive drug—arousal with skeletal muscle relaxation. *Psychopharmacol Bull* 1986;22:870–874.
277. Fertig JB, Pomerleau OF, Sanders B. Nicotine-produced antinociception in minimally deprived smokers and ex-smokers. *Addict Behav* 1986;11:239–248.
278. Dunne MP, Macdonald D, Hartley LR. The effects of nicotine upon memory and problem solving performance. *Physiol Behav* 1986;37:849–854.
279. Edwards JA, Wesnes K, Warburton DM, et al. Evidence of more rapid stimulus evaluation following cigarette smoking. *Addict Behav* 1985;10:113–126.
280. Clarke PBS. Nicotine and smoking: a perspective from animal studies. *Psychopharmacology* 1987;92:135–143.
281. Chernick V. The brain's own morphine and cigarette smoking: the junkie in disguise? *Chest* 1983;83:2–4.
282. Astrup P, Kjeldsen K. Carbon monoxide, smoking, and atherosclerosis. *Med Clin North Am* 1973;58:323–350.
283. Stewart RD. The effect of carbon monoxide on humans. *Ann Rev Pharm* 1975;15:409–423.
284. Balleisen L, Bailey J, Epping PH, et al. Epidemiological study on factor VII, factor VIII and fibrinogen in an industrial population: 1. Baseline data on the relation to age, gender, body-weight, smoking, alcohol, pill-using, and menopause. *Thromb Haemost* 1985;54:475–479.
285. Coburn RF. Mechanisms of carbon monoxide toxicity. *Prev Med* 1979;8:310–322.
286. Astrup P, Kjeldsen K. Model studies linking carbon monoxide and/or nicotine to atherosclerosis and cardiovascular disease. *Prev Med* 1979;8:295–302.
287. Astrup P. Some physiological and pathological effects of moderate carbon monoxide exposure. *Br Med J* 1972;4:447–452.
288. Stender S, Astrup P, Kjeldsen K. The effect of carbon monoxide on cholesterol in the aortic wall of rabbits. *Atherosclerosis* 1977;28:357–367.

289. Turner DM. Carbon monoxide, tobacco smoking, and the pathogenesis of atherosclerosis. *Prev Med* 1979;8:303–309.
290. Ayres SM, Mueller HS, Gregory JJ, et al. Systemic and myocardial hemodynamic responses to relatively small concentrations of carboxyhemoglobin (COHb). *Arch Environ Health* 1969; 18:699–709.
291. Aronow WS, Dendinger J, Rokaw SN. Heart rate and carbon monoxide level after smoking high-, low-, and non-nicotine cigarettes. A study in male patients with angina pectoris. *Ann Intern Med* 1971;74:697–702.
292. Aronow WS, Rokaw SN. Carboxyhemoglobin caused by smoking nonnicotine cigarettes. Effects in angina pectoris. *Circulation* 1971;XLIV:782–788.
293. Aronow WS. Effect of carbon monoxide on cardiovascular disease. *Prev Med* 1979;8:271–278.
294. Aronow WS, Isbell MW. Carbon monoxide effect on exercise-induced angina pectoris. *Ann Intern Med* 1973;79:392–395.
295. Aronow WS, Cassidy J, Vangrow JS, et al. Effect of cigarette smoking and breathing carbon monoxide on cardiovascular hemodynamics in anginal patients. *Circulation* 1974;50:340–347.
296. Anderson EW, Andelman RJ, Strauch JM, et al. Effect of low-level carbon monoxide exposure on onset and duration of angina pectoris. A study in ten patients with ischemic heart disease. *Ann Intern Med* 1973;79:46–50.
297. Aronow WS, Stemmer EA, Wood B, et al. Carbon monoxide and ventricular fibrillation threshold in dogs with acute myocardial injury. *Am Heart J* 1978;95:754–756.
298. DeBias DA, Banerjee CM, Birkhead NC, et al. Effects of carbon monoxide inhalation on ventricular fibrillation. *Arch Environ Health* 1976;31:38–42.
299. Foster JR. Arrhythmogenic effects of carbon monoxide in experimental acute myocardial ischemia: lack of slowed conduction and ventricular tachycardia. *Am Heart J* 1981;102:876–882.
300. Wald N, Howard S, Smith PG, et al. Association between atherosclerotic diseases and carboxyhaemoglobin levels in tobacco smokers. *Br Med J* 1973;1:761–765.
301. Heliovaara M, Karvonen MJ, Vilhunen R, et al. Smoking, carbon monoxide, and atherosclerotic diseases. *Br Med J* 1978;1:268–270.
302. Russell MAH, Sutton SR, Iyer R, et al. Long-term switching to low-tar low-nicotine cigarettes. *Br J Addict* 1982;77:145–158.
303. Goldman AL. Carboxyhemoglobin levels in primary and secondary cigar and pipe smokers. *Chest* 1977;72:33–35.
304. Russell MAH, Cole PV, Brown E. Absorption by non-smokers of carbon monoxide from room air polluted by tobacco smoke. *Lancet* 1973;1:576–579.
305. Aronow WS. Effect of passive smoking on angina pectoris. *N Engl J Med* 1978;299:21–24.
306. Feyerabend C, Higenbottam T, Russell MAH. Nicotine concentrations in urine and saliva of smokers and non-smokers. *Br Med J* 1982;284:1002–1004.
307. Russell MAH, Feyerabend C. Blood and urinary nicotine in non-smokers. *Lancet* 1975;1:179–181.
308. Andresen BD, Ng KJ, Iams JD, et al. Cotinine in amniotic fluids from passive smokers. *Lancet* 1982;1:791–792.
309. Garland CM, Barrett-Connor E, Suarez L, et al. Effects of passive smoking on ischemic heart disease mortality of nonsmokers—a prospective study. *Am J Epidemiol* 1985;121:645–650.
310. Frishman WH. Involuntary smoking: cardiovascular effects of smoke on nonsmokers. *Cardiovasc Med* 1979;1:289–291.
311. Lefcoe NM, Ashley MJ, Pederson LL, et al. The health risks of passive smoking. The growing case for control measures in enclosed environments. *Chest* 1983;84:90–95.
312. White JR, Froeb HF. Small-airways dysfunction in nonsmokers chronically exposed to tobacco smoke. *N Engl J Med* 1980;302:720–723.
313. Glantz SA. Achieving a smokefree society. *Circulation* 1987;76:746–752.
314. Wilhelmsson C, Vedin JA, Elmfeldt D, et al. Smoking and myocardial infarction. *Lancet* 1975;1:415–419.
315. Gordon T, Kannel WB, McGee D. Death and coronary attacks in men after giving up cigarette smoking. A report from the Framingham Study. *Lancet* 1974;2:1345–1348.
316. Gordon T, Kannel WB, Dawber TR, et al. Changes associated with quitting cigarette smoking: the Framingham Study. *Am Heart J* 1975;90:322–328.
317. Rose G, Hamilton PJS. A randomised controlled trial of the effect on middle-aged men of advice to stop smoking. *J Epidemiol Community Health* 1978;32:275–281.
318. Lee PN. Has the mortality of male doctors improved with the reductions in their cigarette smoking? *Br Med J* 1979;2:1538–1540.
319. Salonen JT. Stopping smoking and long-term mortality after acute myocardial infarction. *Br Heart J* 1980;43:463–469.
320. Friedman GD, Siegelaub AB. Changes after quitting cigarette smoking. *Circulation* 1980;61:716–722.
321. Friedman GD, Petitti DB, Bawol RD, et al. Mortality in cigarette smokers and quitters. *N Engl J Med* 1981;304:1407–1410.
322. Kuller L, Meilahn E, Townsend M, et al. Control of cigarette smoking from a medical perspective. *Annu Rev Public Health* 1982;3:153–178.
323. Mulcahy R. Influence of cigarette smoking on morbidity and mortality after myocardial infarction. *Br Heart J* 1983;49:410–415.
324. Aberg A, Bergstrand R, Johansson S, et al. Cessation of smoking after myocardial infarction. *Br Heart J* 1983;49:416–422.
325. Daly LE, Mulcahy R, Graham IM, et al. Long term effect on mortality of stopping smoking after unstable angina and myocardial infarction. *Br Med J* 1983;287:324–326.
326. Johansson S, Bergstrand R, Pennert K, et al. Cessation of smoking after myocardial infarction in women. Effects on mortality and reinfarctions. *Am J Epidemiol* 1985;121:823–831.
327. Daly LE, Graham IM, Hickey N, et al. Does stopping smoking delay onset of angina after infarction? *Br Med J* 1985;291:935–937.
328. Abbott RD, Yin Y, Reed DM, Yano K. Risk of stroke in male cigarette smokers. *N Engl J Med* 1986;315:717–720.
329. Cook DG, Pocock SJ, Shaper AG, et al. Giving up smoking and the risk of heart attacks. *Lancet* 1986;2:1376–1379.
330. Greene SB, Aavedal MJ, Tryoler HA, et al. Smoking habits and blood pressure change: a seven year follow-up. *J Chronic Dis* 1977;30:401–413.
331. Schoenberger JC. Smoking change in relation to changes in blood pressure, weight, and cholesterol. *Prev Med* 1982;11:441–453.
332. Stubbe I, Eskilsson J, Nilsson-Ehle P. High-density lipoprotein concentrations increase after stopping smoking. *Br Med J* 1982;284:1511–1513.
333. Hulley SB, Cohen R, Widdowson G. Plasma high-density lipoprotein cholesterol level. Influence of risk factor intervention. *JAMA* 1977;238:2269–2271.
334. Baile WF, Bigelow GE, Gottlieb SH, et al. Rapid resumption of cigarette smoking following myocardial infarction: inverse relation to MI severity. *Addict Behav* 1982;7:373–380.
335. Friedman GD, Siegelaub AB, Dales LG, et al. Characteristics predictive of coronary heart disease in ex-smokers before they stopped smoking: comparison with persistent smokers and nonsmokers. *J Chronic Dis* 1979;32:175–190.
336. Hjermann I, Holme I, Velve Byre K, et al. Effect of diet and smoking intervention on the incidence of coronary heart disease. Report from the Oslo Study Group of a randomised trial in healthy men. *Lancet* 1981;2:1303–1310.
337. Wechsler H, Levine S, Idelson RK, et al. The physician's role in health promotion—a survey of primary-care practitioners. *N Engl J Med* 1983;308:97–100.
338. Sobal J, Valente CM, Muncie HL, et al. Physicians' beliefs about the importance of 25 health promoting behaviors. *Am J Public Health* 1985;75:1427–1428.
339. Ockene JK, Quirk ME, Goldberg RJ, et al. A residents' training program for the development of smoking intervention skills. *Arch Intern Med* 1988;148:1039–1045.
340. Harvey L, Shubat S. *AMA surveys of physician and public opinion on health care issues, 1987.* Chicago: American Medical Association, 1987.
341. Anda RF, Remington PL, Sienko DG, et al. Are physicians advising smokers to quit? *JAMA* 1987;257:1916–1919.
342. Wells KB, Lewis CE, Leake B, et al. The practices of general and

subspecialty internists in counseling about smoking and exercise. *Am J Public Health* 1986;76:1009–1013.
343. Wells KB, Lewis CE, Leake B, et al. Do physicians preach what they practice? A study of physicians' health habits and counseling practices. *JAMA* 1984;252:2846–2848.
344. Sachs DPL. Office strategies to help your patients stop smoking. *J Respir Dis* 1984;5(2):35–48.
345. Puska P, Salonen JT, Nissinen A, et al. Change in risk factors for coronary heart disease during years of a community intervention programme (North Karelia project). *Br Med J* 1983;287:1839–1844.
346. Kottke TE, Puska P, Salonen JT, et al. Projected effects of high-risk versus population-based prevention strategies in coronary heart disease. *Am J Epidemiol* 1985;121:697–704.
347. The Research Group ATS-RF2-OB43 of the Italian National Research Council. Time trends of some cardiovascular risk factors in Italy. Results from the Nine Communities Study. *Am J Epidemiol* 1987;126:95–103.
348. Fisher EB, Bishop DB, Goldmuntz J, et al. Implications for the practicing physician of the psychosocial dimensions of smoking. *Chest* 1988;93:69S–78S.
349. Andrews JL. Reducing smoking in the hospital. An effective model program. *Chest* 1983;84:206–209.
350. Fisher EB, Bishop DB, Mayer J, et al. The physician's contribution to smoking cessation in the workplace. *Chest* 1988;93:56S–65S.
351. Evans RI, Henderson AH, Hill PC, et al. Current psychological, social, and educational programs in control and prevention of smoking: a critical methodological review. *Atherosclerosis Rev* 1979;6:203–243.
352. Wynder EL, Hoffmann D. Tobacco and health—a societal challenge. *N Engl J Med* 1979;300:894–903.
353. Schwartz JL. Review and evaluation of methods of smoking cessation, 1969–77. Summary of a monograph. *Public Health Rep* 1979;94:558–563.
354. Thompson EL. Smoking education programs 1960–1976. *Am J Public Health* 1978;68:250–257.
355. Fagerstrom K-O. Effects of nicotine chewing gum and follow-up appointments in physician-based smoking cessation. *Prev Med* 1984;13:517–527.
356. Kottke TE, Battista RN, DeFriese GH, et al. Attributes of successful smoking cessation interventions in medical practice. A meta-analysis of 39 controlled trials. *JAMA* 1988;259:2883–2889.
357. Evans D, Lane DS. Long-term outcome of smoking cessation workshops. *Am J Public Health* 1980;70:725–727.
358. Russell MAH, Wilson C, Taylor C, et al. Effect of general practitioners' advice against smoking. *Br Med J* 1979;2:231–235.
359. Stewart PJ, Rosser WW. The impact of routine advice on smoking cessation from family physicians. *Can Med Assoc J* 1982;126:1051–1054.
360. Wilson D, Wood G, Johnston N, et al. Randomized clinical trial of supportive follow-up for cigarette smokers in a family practice. *Can Med Assoc J* 1982;126:127–129.
361. Richmond RL, Austin A, Webster IW. Three year evaluation of a programme by general practitioners to help patients to stop smoking. *Br Med J* 1986;292:803–806.
362. Richmond RL, Webster IW. A smoking cessation programme for use in general practice. *Med J Aust* 1985;142:190–194.
363. Jamrozik K, Vessey M, Fowler G, et al. Controlled trial of three different antismoking interventions in general practice. *Br Med J* 1984;288:1499–1503.
364. Nemeth-Coslett R, Henningfield JE, O'Keefe MK, et al. Nicotine gum: dose-related effects on cigarette smoking and subjective ratings. *Psychopharmacology* 1987;92:424–430.
365. Fagerstrom K-O. Measuring degree of physical dependence to tobacco smoking with reference to individualization of treatment. *Addict Behav* 1978;3:235–241.
366. Hjalmarson AIM. Effect of nicotine chewing gum in smoking cessation—a randomized, placebo-controlled, double-blind study. *JAMA* 1984;252:2835–2838.
367. Russell MAH, Raw M, Jarvis MJ. Clinical use of nicotine chewing-gum. *Br Med J* 1980;1:1599–1602.
368. Tonnesen P, Fryd V, Hansen M, et al. Effect of nicotine chewing gum in combination with group counseling on the cessation of smoking. *N Engl J Med* 1988;318:15–18.
369. Marvis MJ, Raw M, Russell MAH, et al. Randomised controlled trial of nicotine chewing-gum. *Br Med J* 1982;285:537–540.
370. Hughes JR, Miller SA. Nicotine gum to help stop smoking. *JAMA* 1984;252:2855–2858.
371. Fagerstrom K-O. A comparison of psychological and pharmacological treatment in smoking cessation. *J Behav Med* 1982;5:343–351.
372. Raw M, Jarvis MJ, Feyerabend C, et al. Comparison of nicotine chewing-gum and psychological treatments for dependent smokers. *Br Med J* 1980;2:481–482.
373. Lam W, Sacks HS, Sze PC, et al. Meta-analysis of randomised controlled trials of nicotine chewing-gum. *Lancet* 1987;2:27–29.
374. Oster G, Huse DM, Delea TE, et al. Cost-effectiveness of nicotine gum as an adjunct to physician's advice against cigarette smoking. *JAMA* 1986;256:1315–1318.
375. Rose JE, Herskovic JE, Trilling Y, et al. Transdermal nicotine reduces cigarette craving and nicotine preference. *Clin Pharmacol Ther* 1985;38:450–456.
376. Jarvis MJ, Hajek P, Russell MAH, et al. Nasal nicotine solution as an aid to cigarette withdrawal: a pilot clinical trial. *Br J Addict* 1987;82:983–988.
377. Stolerman IP. Could nicotine antagonists be used in smoking cessation? *Br J Addict* 1986;81:47–53.
378. Glassman AH, Stetner F, Walsh T, et al. Heavy smokers, smoking cessation, and clonidine. Results of a double-blind, randomized trial. *JAMA* 1988;259:2863–2866.
379. Fielding JE. Smoking: health effects and control. *N Engl J Med* 1985;313:491–498 and 555–561.
380. Kristein MM. How much can business expect to profit from smoking cessation? *Prev Med* 1983;12:358–381.
381. Warner KE. Smoking and health implications of a change in the federal cigarette excise tax. *JAMA* 1986;255:1028–1032.
382. Council on Scientific Affairs. Smoking and health. *JAMA* 1980;243:779–781.
383. Cooper R, Schatzkin A. Recent trends in coronary risk factors in the USSR. *Am J Public Health* 1982;72:431–440.

SECTION VIII

Management of the Hypertensive Patient

PART A

Application and Value of Nonpharmacologic Therapies

Hypertension: Pathophysiology, Diagnosis, and Management, edited by J. H. Laragh and B. M. Brenner. Raven Press, Ltd., New York © 1990.

CHAPTER 121

Clinical Trials as a Guide to Intervention

Michael H. Alderman and Paul R. Marantz

Potential Benefit of Treatment, 1942
Major Clinical Trials of Antihypertensive Therapy, 1943
The Veterans Administration Cooperative Study Group (VACSG) Trials, 1943
The U.S. Public Health Service (USPHS) Hospital Study, 1943
The Hypertension Detection and Follow-up Program (HDFP), 1944
The Australian National Blood Pressure Study, 1945
The Oslo Study, 1945
The Multiple Risk Factor Intervention Trial (MRFIT), 1945
The Medical Research Council (MRC) Treatment Trial for Mild Hypertension, 1946
The European Working Party on High Blood Pressure in the Elderly (EWPHE) Trial, 1946
The International Prospective Primary Prevention Study in Hypertension (IPPPSH), 1947
The Metoprolol Atherosclerosis Prevention in Hypertensives (MAPHY) Study, 1947
Summary of Clinical Trials, 1948
Potential Harm of Antihypertensive Therapy, 1948
Specific Side Effects, 1949
The Risk of Excessive Blood Pressure Reduction (How Low Is Too Low?), 1949
Labeling and Quality of Life, 1950
Individualization of Therapeutic Decisions, 1950
Race, 1950
Sex, 1950
Age, 1951
Preexisting End-Organ Damage, 1951
Multiple Risk Factors, 1951
Conclusions, 1951
References, 1952

A direct relationship between blood pressure and the incidence of cardiovascular disease has been widely believed for almost as long as we have been able to measure blood pressure. That belief was ultimately confirmed through the elegant epidemiologic study of the people of Framingham, Massachusetts (1). Not surprisingly, therefore, the introduction of orally effective hypotensive drugs in the mid-1950s was met with the hope that treatment of persons with high blood pressure would substantially reduce the incidence of stroke and heart disease.

That hope has been realized only in part. The fundamental problem has been that high blood pressure is not the cause of cardiovascular disease in the way that *Streptococcus pneumoniae* is the cause of pneumococcal pneumonia. Along with cigarette smoking and hyperlipidemia, elevated pressure is strongly correlated with cardiovascular disease events; however, this correlation is more accurately described as a "risk factor" than as a cause (2). Not everyone with hypertension will have a stroke or heart attack; in fact, during the foreseeable future, only a small minority experience a vascular calamity. Moreover, many persons with "normal" blood pressure (and therefore without the risk factor) will nevertheless suffer a cardiovascular event. Paradoxically, because those who lack the risk factor outnumber those with it, the majority of all cardiovascular events probably occurs in normotensive individuals, even if it is true that hypertension accounts for 35–45% of cardiovascular disease (3).

A strategy for management must reflect the nature of this relationship between hypertension and cardiovascular disease. Clearly, the goal in these circumstances cannot be to lower blood pressure, because that is not the cause of the disease, nor is it in itself a disease. Although the Framingham data suggest that reducing pressure will prevent —or at least delay—some cardiovascular events, some of those treated will nevertheless go on to have an event; and finally, the majority of those treated will not benefit, since they were never destined to have a premature stroke or heart attack. The mystery is to identify those who are carrying the risk factor and whose future event could be avoided by timely treatment. Because we do not have the key to that riddle, we need a strategy, based on the available evidence, to guide medical management until knowledge of cause makes specific preventive therapy possible. Great strides have been made in understanding how to manage hypertension since the introduction of effective oral hypotensive agents. Our task now is to assure that these modern tools are applied in the most efficient and effective way.

POTENTIAL BENEFIT OF TREATMENT

"Potential benefit" is the theoretical value that could be achieved by changing blood pressure from one level to another. This is calculated as the difference in probability of developing cardiovascular disease at the different levels of pressure.

Estimates of potential benefit derived from this calculation depend upon the validity of at least three assumptions: (i) that the blood pressure reductions postulated can be achieved and maintained for long periods of time; (ii) that antihypertensive drugs possess no inherent hazard which would diminish the efficacy of treatment; and (iii) that artificially lowering blood pressure produces for that individual the same life expectations as would be experienced by someone who was naturally at that lower point (4). In fact, however, probably none of these assumptions is entirely sound. First, there are insufficient data to show that long-term blood pressure reductions can be maintained, given the well-documented problem of compliance in antihypertensive treatment (5). The second assumption, that there is no inherent harm in antihypertensive drugs, has been shown not to be valid in a variety of clinical trials. Finally, the hope that artificial lowering of blood pressure will produce the full potential benefit associated with that lower blood pressure, while conceptually appealing, has not been proven. Indeed, available data suggest that only a fraction of that benefit has actually been observed, especially with regard to incidence of coronary artery disease (6).

Nevertheless, accepting these three assumptions permits estimation of the benefit that might accompany blood pressure reduction (4). To illustrate this point, the theoretical experience of persons grouped by age, gender, and associated other risk factors, at varying blood pressure, has been calculated (Table 1). Relative benefit (presented in parentheses) for each subgroup is the reduction in risk as a percentage of the original probability of having a cardiovascular disease event. Absolute potential benefit is the actual number of persons of each 100 treated who would benefit: It is this figure which is of greatest help in guiding individual decision making. The absolute potential benefit of blood pressure reduction decreases with age for men at high risk and increases with age for men at low risk. At all ages in the low-risk category, the potential benefit of blood pressure reduction is greater for men than for women.

Systolic blood pressure reduction from 195 to 135 mmHg, sustained for 15 years for 100 low-risk men, would benefit 9 at the cost of treating 91 who would not benefit. Expressed as a ratio (potential nonbenefit to potential benefit), as presented in Table 2, the value of 10:1 is calculated. This provides another way of evaluating the risk:benefit equation in contrast to the reduction in the original chance of developing cardiovascular disease, which in this case would be 60%. This ratio increases to 49:1 when a change in systolic blood pressure (SBP) from 165 to 135 mmHg

TABLE 1. *Probability (per 100) of cardiovascular disease (CVD) developing over a period of 15 years, according to sex, starting age, levels of risk, and the potential benefits from blood pressure (BP) reduction*[a]

Systolic BP (mmHg)	Low risk at age (years)			High risk at age (years)		
	35	45	55	35	45	55
Men						
195	15	32	47	86	95	97
180	12	27	41	81	93	96
165	10	22	35	76	90	94
135	6	15	24	63	82	88
Potential benefits[b]						
195→135	9 (60)	17 (53)	23 (49)	23 (27)	13 (14)	9 (9)
180→135	6 (50)	23 (44)	17 (41)	18 (22)	11 (12)	8 (8)
165→135	4 (40)	7 (32)	11 (31)	13 (17)	8 (9)	6 (6)
Women						
195	7	18	32	42	66	82
180	6	15	27	36	60	77
165	5	12	23	31	54	71
135	3	8	16	22	42	59
Potential benefits[b]						
195→135	4 (57)	10 (56)	16 (50)	20 (48)	24 (36)	23 (28)
180→135	3 (50)	7 (47)	11 (41)	14 (39)	18 (30)	18 (23)
165→135	2 (40)	4 (33)	7 (30)	9 (29)	12 (22)	12 (17)

[a] From ref. 4.

[b] Figures in parentheses are the relative benefit expressed as a percent of the original probability of having CVD; the arrows mean "reduced to."

TABLE 2. *Ratio of "nonbenefited to benefited" caused by blood pressure (BP) reduction*[a]

Reduction in systolic BP (mmHg)[b]	Men		Women	
	Low risk	High risk	Low risk	High risk
Fifteen years of follow-up				
195→135	10:1	3:1	24:1	4:1
180→135	16:1	5:1	32:1	6:1
165→135	24:1	7:1	49:1	10:1
Twenty-five years of follow-up				
195→135	5:1	7:1	10:1	3:1
180→135	7:1	9:1	16:1	5:1
165→135	12:1	12:1	32:1	7:1
Thirty years of follow-up				
195→135	3:1	19:1	6:1	3:1
180→135	5:1	24:1	9:1	4:1
165→135	8:1	32:1	16:1	7:1

[a] From ref. 4. The figures in the table are for 35-year-old men and women, years of follow-up, and levels of risk.
[b] The arrows mean "reduced to."

among low-risk young women is postulated; that is, for each low-risk woman who is helped by the reduction of systolic pressure from 165 to 135 mmHg, 49 others do not benefit from the experience. In their case, treatment at best does no harm but at worst produces unwanted side effects.

These data clearly predict that a benefit may result from blood pressure reduction at every level of raised pressure. But within each blood pressure stratum, the risk of cardiovascular disease, as well as the potential for benefit from blood pressure reduction, varies substantially, depending on a constellation of factors other than blood pressure (Fig. 1). Thus, while being a convenient tool to stratify groups with some relation to disease risk, blood pressure by itself is not a very precise predictor of individual outcome.

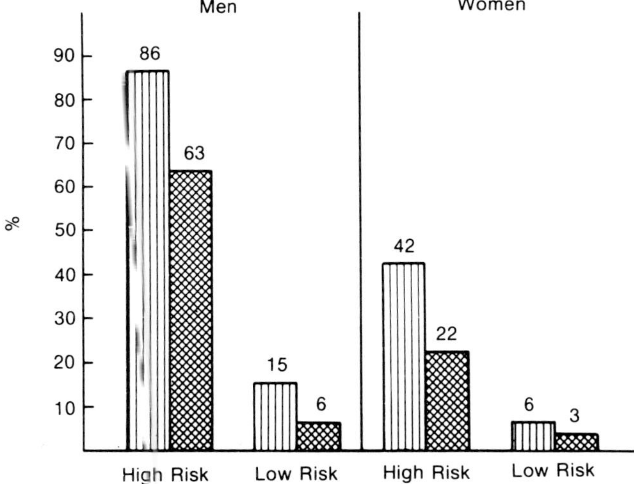

FIG. 1. Risk of cardiovascular disease developing over a period of 15 years for men and women aged 35 years, according to systolic blood pressure (BP) level and risk status. Striped bar indicates systolic BP of 195 mmHg; hatched bar indicates systolic BP of 135 mmHg. (From ref. 50.)

MAJOR CLINICAL TRIALS OF ANTIHYPERTENSIVE THERAPY

Empiric evidence from many clinical trials supports the theoretical postulation that blood pressure reduction in hypertensive patients would prevent cardiovascular morbidity and mortality. The practitioner must translate this aggregate information to guide the care of a single patient. Thus, studies must be carefully analyzed to see how they relate to the patient in question. This section reviews the randomized clinical trials in hypertension treatment (Table 3). In general, all trials have demonstrated benefit of blood pressure reduction but have varied substantially according to the group treated, the agents employed, and the outcome assessed.

The Veterans Administration Cooperative Study Group (VACSG) Trials

Completed about two decades ago, these trials were designed to determine whether application of active hypotensive agents could reduce cardiovascular disease morbidity and mortality (7,8). Participants, selected according to demanding criteria, were randomly allocated to either placebo or active treatment. Thereafter, except for drug therapy, all participants received the same follow-up care.

It turned out that among these veterans were a preponderance of high-risk patients, which may help explain the finding that the value of treating patients with diastolic pressures over 114 mmHg was so quickly demonstrated (7). At mild or moderate levels of diastolic hypertension, results were less dramatic, and, indeed, in the mild range (90–104 mmHg) (8), no statistically significant benefit of treatment was found. Subgroup analysis did suggest that subjects with mild hypertension who had evidence of cardiovascular abnormalities at entry were more likely than those without to benefit from treatment, as were older as compared to younger subjects.

Although the VACSG experience left important questions unanswered, its results demonstrated conclusively that blood pressure manipulation could save lives. These results naturally stimulated a desire to define more precisely the population for which chemotherapy could produce a benefit that would outweigh any risk.

The U.S. Public Health Service (USPHS) Hospital Study

A preliminary attempt to address some of the issues not resolved by the VACSG study was undertaken by the USPHS Hospital Study Group (9). Since it involved only 389 middle-aged subjects without prior evidence of end-organ disease, who had diastolic pressures below 104 mmHg, it is not surprising that few events occurred and that the outcome of this study was inconclusive. No significant difference in overall mortality emerged—although in the untreated control group, progression of blood pressure level and emergence of left ventricular hypertrophy were greater than among treated subjects. The greatest value of

TABLE 3. *Randomized clinical trials in hypertension*[a]

Trial	*N*	DBP Range	Blinded?	Females? (%)	Blacks? (%)	Age
VACSG (7)	143	115–129	Double	No	Yes (54%)	30–73
VACSG (8)	380	90–114	Double	No	Yes (41%)	N/S
USPHS (9)	389	90–114	Double	Yes (20%)	Yes (28%)	<55
HDFP (10)	10,940	>90	No	Yes (46%)	Yes (44%)	30–69
Australian (13)	3,427	95–110	Single	Yes (37%)	No	30–69
Oslo (14)	785	95–110	No	No	No	40–49
MRFIT (15)	12,866	>90 (62%)	No	No	Yes (7%)	35–57
MRC (19)	17,354	90–109	Single	Yes (40%)	No	35–64
EWPHE (20)	840	90–119	Double	Yes (70%)	N/S	>59
IPPPSH (21)	6,357	100–125	Double	Yes (50%)	N/S	40–64
MAPHY (22)	3,234	100–130	No	No	No	40–64

[a] DBP, diastolic blood pressure; N/S, not stated.

this study was to confirm that blood pressure control could be achieved in the general population.

The Hypertension Detection and Follow-up Program (HDFP)

The HDFP, the first large trial to test the value of antihypertensive therapy in mild hypertensives, has contributed as much to the development of controversy as it has to the resolution of the therapeutic issues (10). Unfortunately, its methodologic shortcomings make it difficult to confidently draw conclusions from its results. Study subjects were identified through community screening. They had mostly mild (90–104 mmHg diastolic) hypertension and were randomly allocated to either (a) a special care (SC) group for whom the therapeutic regimen involved incremental addition of drugs until goal pressure was achieved or (b) a referred care (RC) control group advised to seek care through conventional community sources. Since SC subjects were offered comprehensive free care through a program designed to enhance compliance, and RC subjects received varying treatment of unknown nature for a fee, both antihypertensive treatment and the organization of medical care were altered in the study design. It is not possible to decide whether the outcomes observed were due to differences in the care or to differences in hypotensive therapy.

At 14 centers, 158,000 persons were screened to yield more than 10,000 participants. In the study, blood pressure reduction was significantly greater, by about 5 mmHg, in the SC group. Coincident with this finding, there was a 16.9% lower cardiovascular mortality rate in the SC group when compared to the RC group. In addition, however, the noncardiovascular mortality improvement for the SC group was about 60% of that for cardiovascular mortality. This unanticipated benefit, appearing in such conditions as breast cancer, lends credence to the notion that aspects of care other than antihypertensive therapy may have contributed to the observed outcomes (10).

When the experience of the group with mild hypertension was subjected to more detailed scrutiny, the anticipated heterogeneity emerges. For example (Fig. 2), it can be seen that blacks had high event rates and substantial benefit, whereas white women experienced few deaths and did not seem to benefit from a lowered blood pressure (11).

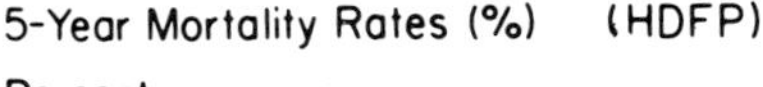

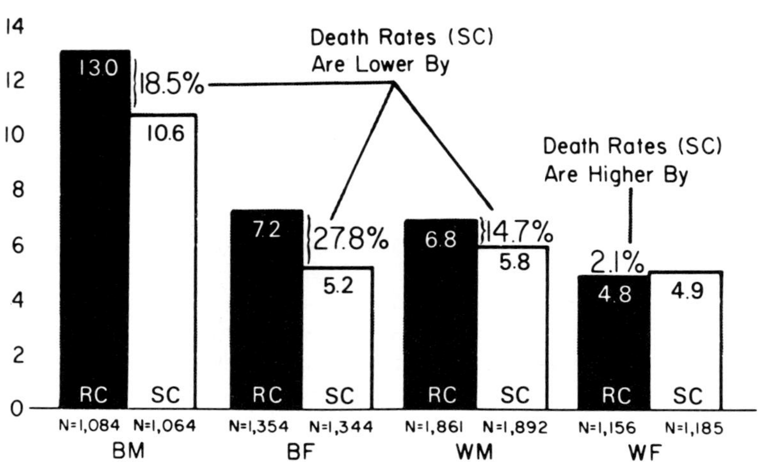

FIG. 2. Five-year mortality rates (in percent) for all causes, according to sex and race. BM, black male; BF, black female; WM, white male; WF, white female; RC, regular care; SC, special care; HDFP, Hypertension Detection and Follow-up Program. (From ref. 50.)

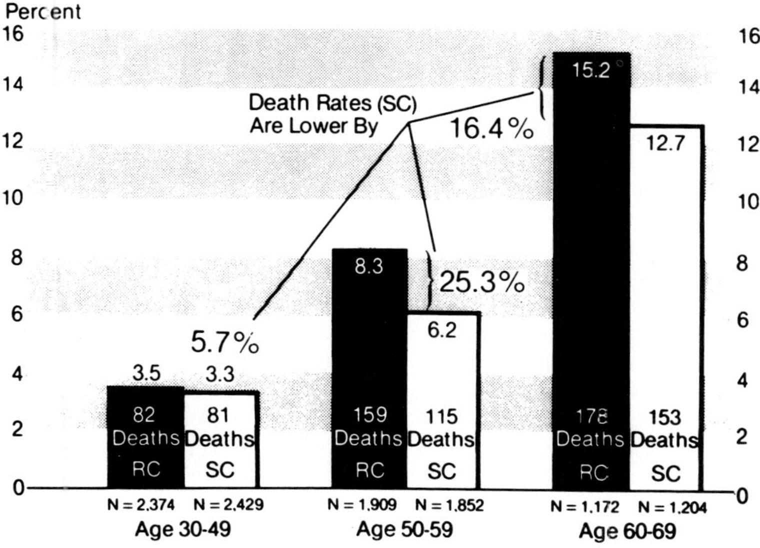

FIG. 3. Five-year mortality rates (in percent) for all causes, according to age at entry. RC, regular care; SC, special care. (From ref. 50.)

Furthermore, persons under 50 years of age had a low mortality rate which was not noticeably reduced by SC (Fig. 3), while older persons did show mortality reductions with SC (12).

Nevertheless, the main finding was that SC participants with mild hypertension experienced less cardiovascular disease mortality while having lower pressures than did their conventional care controls. Of note, however, was the low cardiovascular mortality rate in this mild group. More than 92% of both groups, including persons up to 69 years of age at entry, survived the 5-year experiment. The actual difference in total survival between the two groups was 1.5%. In absolute terms, this means that three fewer persons per 1000 died each year in the SC group than in the RC group.

The Australian National Blood Pressure Study

The Australian trial, like the HDFP, involved community recruited men and women volunteers (13). Participants had mild hypertension (diastolic pressure between 95 and 110 mmHg, along with systolic pressure less than 200 mmHg) and no evidence of end-organ disease at entry. Unlike the HDFP, however, patients were randomized to either drug or placebo treatment in the same setting. The treatment assignment was single-blind: That is, the physician was aware of whether the patient was taking an active drug or a placebo. All subjects, both experimental and control, were also counseled on weight, smoking, and diet.

According to both an "intention-to-treat" and an "on-treatment" analysis, the study revealed a significant reduction (following active treatment) in overall trial endpoints (which included death, cardiovascular and cerebrovascular complications, retinal changes, renal failure, or hypertensive encephalopathy) as well as in cardiovascular death rates (1.1 versus 2.6 per 1000 person-years, $p < 0.025$ by intention-to-treat analysis).

Of particular note in this trial was the observation that some placebo-treated patients with initially elevated pressure experienced a decline in pressure over the 4 years of the study. In fact, 78% of those whose initial diastolic blood pressure (DBP) was 100–104 mmHg had diastolic pressure below 100 mmHg at trial's end. Most importantly, these participants had the same risk of morbid and mortal endpoints as did those whose pressure had been reduced to that same level by drug. The great excess in morbidity was experienced by those untreated subjects whose pressure remained greater than 100 mmHg. The results suggest, therefore, that delayed drug therapy might be appropriate in mild hypertensives as long as pressure was declining and/or remained below 100 mmHg diastolic. A clue to when to start drugs would be provided by a clinical transformation (e.g., a rise in pressure). Adoption of this approach may delay the application of drugs in many, if not most, mild hypertensives.

The Oslo Study

The Oslo Study included only 785 men aged 40–49, without end-organ damage at entry, with mild hypertension (systolic 150–180 mmHg, diastolic 95–110 mmHg). The control group was untreated and was not given a placebo (14).

After 5 years, there was (a) no difference in mortality and (b) a statistically significant reduction in cerebrovascular events with treatment (0 versus 7 events, $p < 0.02$); however, there was a trend toward a greater number of coronary events in treated patients (20 versus 13 events, $p > 0.10$). The small sample size limited the power to detect a small positive result if it had been present. This study is consistent, however, with the general finding that stroke prevention is easier to demonstrate than heart attack prevention.

The Multiple Risk Factor Intervention Trial (MRFIT)

The MRFIT was not purely a trial of antihypertensive therapy (only 62% of the subjects had hypertension) but was of sufficient magnitude and importance to merit mention here. It was a randomized, primary prevention trial of 12,866 high-risk men (in the upper 15% of a risk score for blood pressure, cigarette smoking, and serum cholesterol), aged 35–57 years (15). Participants were assigned either to a special intervention (SI) program (consisting of stepped-care treatment for hypertension, counseling for cigarette smoking, and dietary advice for lowering blood cholesterol) or to their usual sources of care (UC) and followed for an average of 7 years. Despite successful reduction of all three risk factors in the SI group compared to the UC group, there was no statistically significant difference in cardiovascular or total mortality rates (overall 32.8/1,000 in SI and 34.0/1,000 in UC at 6 years). Subgroup analysis revealed that the SI subjects who had hypertension and an abnormal electrocardiogram (ECG) at baseline experienced a 65% increase in coronary heart disease (CHD) deaths when compared to the UC group. Also of concern was that SI subjects with the lowest initial DBP (90–94 mmHg) experienced greater mortality than did comparable UC subjects: 17 deaths in the SI group as compared to 12 in the UC group. This finding raises questions about the adverse effect of antihypertensive drug therapy (specifically diuretics) (16) and suggests that there may be some individuals with "mild hypertension" put at increased risk for cardiovascular morbidity and mortality by certain drug treatment.

The Medical Research Council (MRC) Treatment Trial for Mild Hypertension

The MRC Treatment Trial for Mild Hypertension was a population-based, placebo-controlled, single-blind, randomized therapeutic trial of generally healthy white men and women, aged 35–64, with DBPs of 90–109 mmHg, determined after multiple screenings by averaging six to eight measurements (17). This study excluded (a) individuals under prior treatment for hypertension, (b) those with recent myocardial infarction, or (c) those with secondary hypertension, angina, gout, or diabetes (18). Given the design parameters, which biased the group toward healthier subjects, the researchers calculated that 18,000 participants would have to be followed for up to 5 years (90,000 patient-years) to obtain statistically significant results. The actual study nearly met this goal, with 85,572 patient-years of observation at its conclusion (19).

The major positive finding of this study was a statistically significant reduction in the rate of strokes (1.4 versus 2.6 per 1000 patient-years, $p < 0.01$). Rates of coronary events (5.8 versus 5.9 per 1000 person-years) demonstrated neither clinically nor statistically significant differences between the treated and placebo groups (19).

Subgroup analysis suggested that: (a) women gained no demonstrable benefit overall and actually, with treatment, had a small increase in overall death rate (not statistically significant); (b) bendrofluazide seemed to be slightly more efficacious than propranolol at preventing strokes (Fig. 4); and (c) propranolol was less effective in cigarette smokers but demonstrated a trend toward prevention of coronary disease in nonsmoking men (Fig. 5).

The authors' final overall conclusion was that "if 850 mildly hypertensive patients are given active antihypertensive drugs for 1 year, about one stroke will be prevented. This is an important, but rare, benefit."

The European Working Party on High Blood Pressure in the Elderly (EWPHE) Trial

The EWPHE trial, begun in 1972, assessed the impact of antihypertensive drugs in patients 60 years of age or greater at entry (20). The study subjects were recruited from clinics, rather than by population screening. Entry criteria included the following: (a) age 60 or greater; (b) sitting blood pressure in the range of 160–239/90–119 mmHg; and (c) informed consent. Exclusion criteria included the following: (a) secondary, curable hypertension; (b) complications of hypertension such as congestive heart failure, history of cerebral or subarachnoid hemorrhage, or retinopathy (Grade III or IV); or (c) concurrent serious disease.

Subjects were randomized to receive either placebo or diuretics, followed in stepped fashion with further placebo or methyldopa. Specific study endpoints included death, nonfatal cerebral or subarachnoid hemorrhage, retinopathy (Grade III or IV), dissecting aneurysm, severe congestive heart failure, hypertensive encephalopathy, severe in-

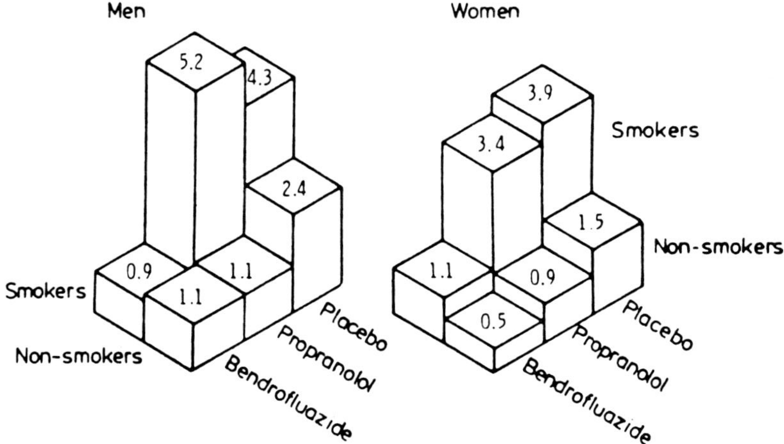

FIG. 4. Incidence of stroke per 1000 person-years of observation according to randomized treatment regimen and cigarette smoking status at entry to trial. (From ref. 19.)

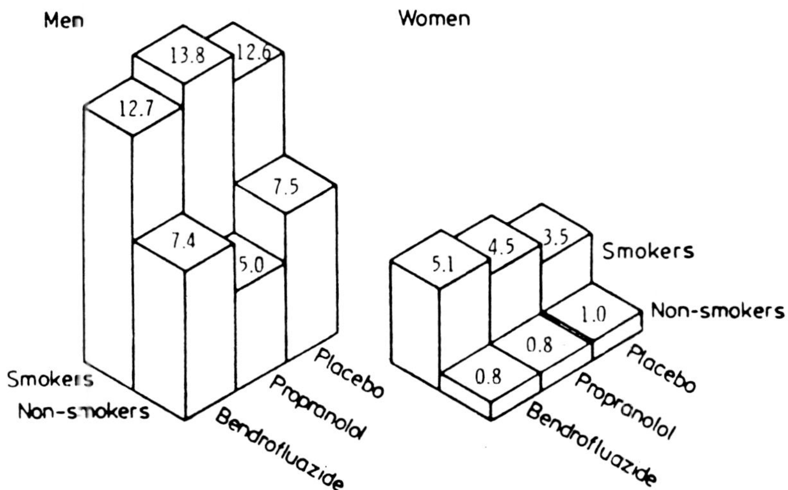

FIG. 5. Incidence of coronary events per 1000 person-years of observation according to randomized treatment regimen and cigarette smoking status at entry to trial. (From ref. 19.)

crease in left ventricular hypertrophy, or a rise in blood pressure beyond preset limits.

Treated subjects experienced a nonsignificant reduction in overall mortality (−9%, p = 0.41), but they did have a reduction in cardiovascular mortality which was both clinically and statistically significant (−27%, p = 0.037). Surprisingly, and in contrast to other clinical trials, the reduction in cerebrovascular deaths was not significant (−32%, p = 0.16), but decline in cardiac death did reach significance (−38%, p = 0.036). Morbid, nonfatal cardiovascular endpoints were also reduced by therapy (−60%, p = 0.0064). Overall, the study found that there were 29 fewer cardiovascular events, and 14 fewer cardiovascular deaths, per 1000 patient-years of observation.

Initially, these results appear to be at variance with some of the findings discussed above. For instance, the British MRC trial found only 1.2 strokes prevented per 1000 patient-years, in contrast to 6 per 1000 in this study. However, such apparent discrepancies may be resolved by reference to the earlier theoretical discussion of "potential benefit." As noted, greater benefit can be expected with a greater risk of disease. Perhaps subjects in the EWPHE trial were at greater risk, since they were both elderly and referred from clinics, as compared with the MRC trial participants, who were young and enrolled by population screening. This supposition is supported by the observed event rates. For cardiovascular mortality, the overall rates in the MRC trial were 3.1 and 3.3 per 1000 patient-years for active and placebo groups, respectively. In the EWPHE trial, comparable rates were 10-fold greater, i.e., 34 and 47 per 1000 patient-years.

The EWPHE trial then confirms earlier studies and, in addition, provides some evidence that antihypertensive therapy may prevent ischemic heart disease death.

The International Prospective Primary Prevention Study in Hypertension (IPPPSH)

The trials previously discussed had all shown some therapeutic benefit with respect to stroke, but the results with respect to ischemic heart disease had been generally disappointing. To determine whether the use of a beta-blocker as an initial therapy would improve the effect on cardiac events, the IPPPSH compared beta-blocker to placebo (21).

This study, begun in 1977, enrolled men and women aged 40–64 who had diastolic blood pressure between 100 and 125 mmHg. Exclusion criteria included history of angina, previous myocardial infarction or cerebrovascular accident, atrioventricular (AV) block, sick sinus syndrome, diabetes, and asthma. A total of 6357 subjects were randomized to receive either oxprenolol (a nonselective beta-blocker with intrinsic sympathomimetic activity) or placebo, plus other medications to achieve a goal of <95 mmHg diastolic blood pressure. Although the use of the beta-blocker was associated with greater antihypertensive effect and generally good patient tolerance, there was no overall protection against sudden death [relative risk (RR), 1.08; 95% confidence interval (CI), 0.68–1.72], myocardial infarction (RR, 0.83; 95% CI, 0.59–1.16), or stroke (RR, 0.97; 95% CI, 0.64–1.47).

However, in men, an interaction was noted between cigarette smoking and response to oxprenolol; such an interaction was not apparent in women. Rates for critical cardiac events among nonsmoking men were 5.4 versus 11.6/1000 patient-years, comparing beta-blocker with non-beta-blocker subjects. Comparable rates among male smokers were 18.1 and 14.5/1000 patient-years, respectively. This finding in moderate and severe hypertension is similar to the previously noted trend found among mild hypertensives in the MRC data (Fig. 6), suggesting that beta-blockers may have prevented cardiac disease in nonsmoking hypertensives. However, since both reflect trends dependent on subgroup analysis, they must be viewed cautiously.

The Metoprolol Atherosclerosis Prevention in Hypertensives (MAPHY) Study

A recent clinical trial compared metoprolol with thiazide diuretic in the initial treatment of 3234 newly detected hypertensive males aged 40–64 who had a diastolic blood pressure between 100 and 130 mmHg (i.e., not mild hy-

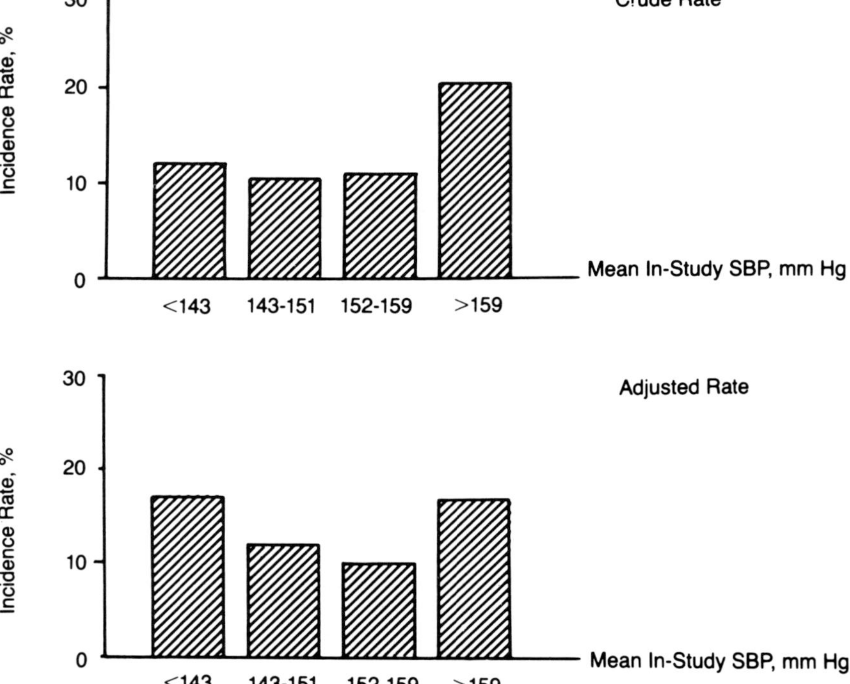

FIG. 6. Coronary heart disease incidence over 12 years of antihypertensive treatment by quartiles of mean in-study systolic blood pressure. The lower chart shows adjusted rates for coronary heart disease risk at entry. (From ref. 37.)

pertension) (22). Initially, these subjects were part of a multicenter international study called HAPPHY (Heart Attack Primary Prevention in Hypertensives), which also studied the beta-blockers propranolol, alprenolol, and atenolol; MAPHY represents an analysis of data from the centers studying metoprolol. Excluded were persons with past history of myocardial infarction or stroke, angina, diabetes, and certain other conditions. Participants were randomized to receive either metoprolol (200 mg/day) or a thiazide [hydrochlorothiazide (50 mg/day) or bendroflumethiazide (5 mg/day)]. These drugs were administered in an open, nonblinded fashion.

Overall mortality was less in the metoprolol group (8.0 versus 10.3 per 1000 patient-years at the conclusion of the study, $p = 0.028$). Cause-specific mortality rates were lower with metoprolol treatment for cardiovascular disease (42 versus 57 deaths, $p = 0.012$), including CHD (36 versus 43 deaths, $p = 0.048$) and stroke (2 versus 9 deaths, $p = 0.043$).

Interestingly, when the authors stratified the results to compare cigarette smokers with nonsmokers, they found that the significant reduction in mortality with metoprolol was confined to smokers ($p = 0.013$); nonsmokers showed only a nonsignificant trend toward reduced mortality in the group treated with the beta-blocker. This finding is at some variance with those of the MRC and IPPPSH trials. The authors point out that only the MAPHY study prospectively stratified subjects on the basis of smoking history and that the study employed a cardioselective beta-blocker instead of propranolol or oxprenolol, which may have led to unopposed alpha-adrenegic vasoconstriction in smokers. This possibly harmful effect would have been minimized by the use of metoprolol, a relatively beta-1-selective drug. This speculation is interesting, but it leaves somewhat confused the question of the interaction between beta-blockers and cigarette smoking. The MAPHY study, however, suggests strongly that patients with moderate or severe hypertension treated with a cardioselective beta-blocker are more likely to achieve coronary artery disease prevention than are those treated with a diuretic.

Summary of Clinical Trials

Taken together, the available evidence supports several conclusions:

1. Antihypertensive treatment reduces the risk of stroke, even among those with mild hypertension (diastolic pressure 90–105 mmHg).
2. The effect of antihypertensive treatment with diuretics on the incidence of coronary disease is minimal at best.
3. Cardioselective beta-blockade may offer an advantage over diuretics and may actually lead to coronary artery disease prevention, especially at higher levels of blood pressure. No data exist to describe the relative benefit of calcium-channel blockers or angiotensin-converting-enzyme inhibitors.
4. Benefits of therapy are greatest in those subgroups at highest risk: in particular, the elderly, blacks, those with diastolic blood pressure above 100 mmHg, those with other cardiovascular risk factors, and males.

POTENTIAL HARM OF ANTIHYPERTENSIVE THERAPY

Although treatment of mild hypertension, in the aggregate, reduces cardiovascular morbidity and mortality, this benefit is neither universally received nor evenly distributed. Virtually all drugs cause side effects. Those who enjoy the benefit of treatment are not necessarily the same as those who endure the side effects. Moreover, some side effects, though mild, may affect many more persons than the smaller number who benefit. Widespread drug treatment must therefore be based upon a clear understanding of its potential hazard, to ensure that the risk of harm is consistent with the benefit.

Specific Side Effects

Symptoms

In the treatment of mild hypertension, the MRC trial compared a diuretic (bendrofluazide), a beta-blocker (propranolol), and a placebo. About 30% of subjects were no longer taking their primary drug at 5 years (23). The specific reasons for drug withdrawal were noted (Table 4). Most commonly associated with the diuretic were gout, impotence, and lethargy. Beta-blockade produced impotence, lethargy, Raynaud's phenomenon, and dyspnea.

Chemical Changes

Some of the potentially important negative effects of antihypertensive drugs include changes in (a) blood lipids, (b) electrolytes, and (c) glucose metabolism.

Some studies have shown that antihypertensive medications can increase serum lipids. For example, in short-term studies, some beta-blocking drugs have been shown to raise serum triglycerides and to lower high-density lipoproteins (24,25). Diuretics raise total and low-density lipoprotein cholesterol (26). These effects may explain, at least partially, the observed lack of efficacy in antihypertensive therapy trials in reducing coronary heart disease.

Thiazide diuretics produce glucose intolerance (23). Whether such an effect would attenuate the benefits of blood pressure reduction is unclear but should be considered.

Another common effect of diuretic drugs is the reduction of serum potassium (27). While some have claimed that too much attention is paid to clinically insignificant reductions in serum potassium (28), others argue that such reductions may be important (29). For instance, in a subgroup analysis of the MRFIT, it was found that mortality rates were increased in diuretic treated subjects whose baseline ECGs were abnormal. It has been suggested that the arrhythmogenic effects of hypokalemia may have been partly responsible for this (30).

Diuretics also increase serum uric acid levels (31). While elevated urate levels had been previously implicated as a risk factor for coronary artery disease, such a relationship is not independent of other cardiovascular risk factors (1). Asymptomatic hyperuricemia does not require treatment (32). However, in the MRC trial, withdrawal of 13 patients per 1000 patient-years as a result of gout was noted in patients treated with diuretics (23). If serum levels are rising alarmingly in a patient receiving diuretic, it might be wise to substitute other therapy.

The Risk of Excessive Blood Pressure Reduction (How Low Is Too Low?)

Because the epidemiologic rationale for the treatment of hypertension is that a higher blood pressure, at any level, is linked to an increased risk of cardiovascular disease, it might seem logical to assume that the further the pressure was reduced, the greater the benefit received. In fact, it has been suggested that a goal for diastolic pressure should be the lowest diastolic pressure consistent with safety and tolerance (33). New knowledge suggests that this approach may no longer be prudent.

There has always been a conceptual basis for questioning this recommendation, because it rests on the flawed assumption that blood pressure reduction is cost-free. Patients with hypertension are rarely completely free of ath-

TABLE 4. *Withdrawals from randomized treatment: numbers and rates per 1000 patient-years*[a]

Condition	Bendrofluazide	Propranolol	Placebo
	Men		
Glucose intolerance	60 (7.7)	27 (3.4)	53 (3.3)
Gout	100 (12.8)	12 (1.5)	14 (0.9)
Impotence	98 (12.6)	50 (6.3)	20 (1.3)
Raynaud's phenomenon	0	41 (5.1)	3 (0.2)
Dyspnea	1 (0.1)	57 (7.1)	7 (0.4)
Lethargy	28 (3.6)	42 (5.3)	8 (0.5)
Nausea, dizziness, and headache	33 (4.2)	33 (4.1)	22 (1.4)
	Women		
Glucose intolerance	46 (5.9)	16 (2.1)	31 (2.0)
Gout	12 (1.5)	0	0
Raynaud's phenomenon	2 (0.3)	34 (4.5)	4 (0.3)
Dyspnea	2 (0.3)	53 (7.1)	3 (0.2)
Lethargy	13 (1.7)	62 (8.3)	4 (0.3)
Nausea, dizziness, and headache	58 (7.4)	70 (9.4)	27 (1.8)

[a] From ref. 51.

erosclerosis. Therefore, excessive lowering of the blood pressure might reduce tissue perfusion in areas served by a narrowed vessel. This may be particularly true in the heart, which is especially sensitive to decreased blood flow; in normal circumstances, its oxygen extraction is near-maximal. A greater autoregulatory reserve in cerebral vessels may explain why, in clinical trials, antihypertensive treatment has consistently reduced stroke in the face of less convincing results regarding heart attack (34). Since elderly hypertensives are most likely to have preexisting atherosclerosis, they may be at greatest risk from overzealous treatment (35). Now, recently reviewed older data (36), along with newer information from the study of a sample of men aged 47–54 in the Primary Prevention Trial in Göteborg, Sweden (37), provide empiric support for the view that lower may not always be better. In fact, a J-shaped curve appears to more accurately describe the relationship between attained blood pressure and coronary heart disease incidence (Fig. 6). These observations have been extended by an analysis of mortality data from the HDFP (38), which showed that the percentage fall, as well as the absolute final value of blood pressure achieved, may bear a J-shaped relationship to outcome. Thus, while "lower is better" in the natural state, it does not seem to be true for patients whose blood pressure is artificially manipulated by drugs.

Labeling and Quality of Life

Although often overlooked, many asymptomatic persons labeled hypertensive are instantly transformed from healthy persons into "patients." The impact of such labeling may be considerable. In a Canadian study (39), absenteeism was found to significantly increase among male steelworkers previously unaware of their elevated blood pressure after being informed of their condition (even if they were untreated). Such an effect was even more pronounced in those who were treated.

An analysis of data from the HDFP challenged some of these conclusions (40)—although the HDFP, too, noted an increase in disability days in previously unaware hypertensives who were diagnosed and referred to their usual sources of care (mean at baseline, 11.3 days versus 13.6 days at 1 year, $p = 0.017$). However, in another study, when a supportive, comprehensive, workplace-based treatment program was provided, it was found that while absenteeism for the newly diagnosed hypertensive did increase, it was still less than that of a control group (41).

The quality-of-life issue has received increased attention lately, because it has become clear that tangible benefits of treating asymptomatic hypertension are realized by only a minority of those treated. Although "quality of life" is difficult to measure, improved methodology is making its assessment more reproducible and quantifiable (42). It has been shown, for example, that captopril has a less unfavorable impact on quality of life, compared with methyldopa and propranolol (43). Perhaps most notable was that some worsening in "general well-being" was observed by (a) 51% of patients treated with methyldopa, (b) 45% of patients treated with propranolol, and (c) 31% of patients treated with captopril; that is, upwards of a third of patients on any of these antihypertensive drugs feel worse than they did without drugs. The point is that selection of therapy should be guided, in part, by these considerations as well as by the impact on blood pressure, since many agents are equally able to reduce blood pressure.

INDIVIDUALIZATION OF THERAPEUTIC DECISIONS

In sum, a wide body of clinical data supports the link between hypertension and cardiovascular disease, and data nearly as robust demonstrate that risk falls with successful antihypertensive therapy. This therapeutic benefit is, however, neither predictable nor equally distributed. In fact, some treated patients may actually be harmed. In these circumstances, data from subgroup analysis may be cautiously applied in view of the statistical vagaries associated with such *post hoc* analyses.

Race

The burden of cardiovascular disease falls disproportionately on blacks in the United States (44), very likely due to a greater prevalence of hypertension (45). Beyond the impact of increased prevalence, it has been speculated that the adverse consequences of hypertension, at a given level of blood pressure, are greater for blacks than for whites (46). Our own experience does not support this contention. On the contrary, when socioeconomic and access issues are controlled, blacks have an equal likelihood of success in treatment and, if anything, a greater degree of cerebrovascular disease protection (M. H. Alderman, *unpublished data*).

There are, however, observed racial differences in response to diuretics and beta-blockers (47), which may relate to a generally lower plasma renin activity among black hypertensives (48). It is problematic to make universal recommendations in terms of antihypertensive care on the basis of race alone. However, thiazides may be a good first-line agent in black patients. As previously noted, a stratified analysis of HDFP showed no survival benefit for white women (Fig. 2). The greatest observed benefit was for black women (27.8% mortality reduction), followed by black men (18.5%) and white men (14.7%) (10), suggesting that blacks may achieve a greater benefit from the stepped-care approach (beginning with thiazides) used in the HDFP.

Sex

It would be expected that women would have a lesser benefit from antihypertensive therapy, since they are, in general, at lesser risk for the adverse consequences of hypertension. As noted above, the HDFP found benefit for black women treated with antihypertensive drugs. The EWPHE trial did not provide a sex-specific analysis, but it did show benefit of therapy in a population including 70%

women (20). None of the other clinical trials has demonstrated a significant benefit from therapy for women.

In the HDFP, all sex and race subgroups showed some overall reduction in mortality with stepped-care treatment—except for white women, who had a slight (2.7%) increase in mortality (10). This difference was not statistically significant in the overall analysis. However, white women with initial diastolic blood pressure greater than 105 mmHg had a 5-year mortality increase of 168% in SC compared with RC ($p < 0.05$) (11).

The Australian trial, which also included women, failed to demonstrate a statistically significant reduction in trial endpoints for them (13), but this may have been due to inadequate power. In the British MRC trial, however, the all-cause mortality was lower among actively treated men (157 versus 181 deaths) but higher among actively treated women (91 versus 72 deaths). Although neither of these differences was significant, the difference between the sexes was statistically significant ($p < 0.05$) (19).

Thus, the observational data to suspect that hypertensive white women would be less likely than men to benefit from intervention have been borne out by clinical experience. Since all drugs do carry some risk, it is possible that the minimal intrinsic harm of antihypertensive therapy or the risk of excessive blood pressure fall may have exceeded the benefit derived by blood pressure reduction in this naturally favored group of white women. It should be kept in mind, however, that no study has been specifically designed to answer the question of treatment efficacy for women. Thus, the failure to demonstrate, unequivocally, that benefit does exist by *ex post facto* subgroup analysis cannot be taken to mean that drug therapy is not of benefit. Overall, it would suggest that drug therapy should be used even more sparingly than usual in this group.

Age

The theoretical basis for a relationship between age and antihypertensive therapy response is the same as that between sex and antihypertensive therapy response: If younger patients have fewer complications, they can be expected to realize a lesser benefit. If that benefit becomes small enough, it might, at least in the near term, be overshadowed by the adverse consequences of drug treatment. As indicated in Table 1, absolute potential benefit rises with increasing age for all groups except high-risk males.

Experimental data again support the expectation that older subjects will benefit more from treatment. In the HDFP, the reduction in mortality with stepped care was only 0.9% in subjects aged 30–49, whereas it was 23.6% and 16.8% in age groups 50–59 and 60–69, respectively (10). The Australian trial showed a significant reduction in trial endpoint for subjects 50–69 years old (69 versus 96, $p < 0.05$) but not for those 30–49 years old (22 versus 31, $p > 0.05$) (13); this, again, may be due to small numbers. In addition, the EWPHE trial (20) provided evidence that antihypertensive therapy could reduce the incidence of CHD in persons over the age of 60.

Preexisting End-Organ Damage

The impact of measurable end-organ disease as a predictor of response to hypotensive therapy is difficult to assess. Only the VACSG and HDFP studies included patients with preexisting end-organ damage. However, the greatest treatment benefit was realized in these trials, suggesting that patients with existing end-organ damage may experience greater benefit in the near term. Indeed, comparing patients with or without specific manifestations of existing end-organ damage (previous myocardial infarction, left ventricular hypertrophy, and/or cardiomegaly) showed that subjects with such damage experienced greater benefit from therapy. Of course, this still leaves open the possibility that even earlier treatment may have been preferable in the long term.

Not all end-organ abnormalities will predict greater benefit, and not all drugs will have the same effect. For example, there was the unexpected finding in the MRFIT that hypertensive men with baseline ECG abnormalities treated with diuretics had an increased CHD mortality (30). Furthermore, while a beta-blocker might be the drug of choice in a hypertensive patient 1 month after a myocardial infarction, it may not be appropriate in a patient with cardiomegaly and symptomatic heart failure.

Multiple Risk Factors

Theoretical extrapolation from Framingham (*supra vide*) suggests that persons with multiple risk factors should benefit more from antihypertensive therapy than those with fewer risk factors. However, the MRFIT study does not confirm this, since multifactorial intervention was, overall, not of value (15). This could have been because of the choice of drugs in some patients (i.e., diuretics in mild hypertensives with ECG abnormalities) or because of the tendency to reduce blood pressure too far (i.e., the J-shaped relation between attained blood pressure and ischemic heart disease incidence).

Still, hypertensives who smoke should stop, not because it will lower the blood pressure but because it is an absolutely safe way to reduce cardiovascular risk. Likewise, reduced dietary fat intake and increased exercise will safely reduce serum cholesterol; these measures will also, along with weight loss, reduce blood pressure (50).

CONCLUSIONS

Many, if not most, patients with hypertension should be treated. The great clinical challenge is to determine when, and by what means, to treat each individual patient. Since the cause of hypertension is usually unknown, and available therapy is generally imprecise, the clinician must craft, for each patient, a management strategy that is securely anchored in the experience of large-scale trials, yet tempered by the unique characteristics of that person. In these circumstances, the data justify only the most general recommendations.

1. Treatment of patients with moderate and severe hypertension produces greater benefit than does treatment of persons with mild hypertension.

2. In patients with mild hypertension of unknown etiology, watchful temporizing enhanced by efforts to control weight—and, when appropriate, by vigorous efforts to eliminate cigarettes—may be the best approach as long as diastolic blood pressure remains below 100 mmHg and shows no tendency to increase. Certain clinical transformations, such as an increase in blood pressure or the appearance of end-organ disease, would merit initiation of drug therapy.

3. Furthermore, among patients with otherwise uncomplicated mild hypertension, drug therapy is most likely to benefit males, blacks, older patients, and possibly smokers, hyperglycemics, and hyperlipidemics. By contrast, drug treatment of white women with mild hypertension has not been demonstrated to reduce cardiovascular morbidity and mortality.

4. Individualization of the drug regimen should be guided by an awareness of underlying end-organ disease.

5. In this silent "disease," the impact of therapy on quality of life must be carefully assessed and continuously reassessed. In a setting where the indication for treatment is borderline (perhaps most mild hypertensives), the inability to identify a drug which is well-tolerated by the patient may be an indication to withhold pharmacologic therapy.

6. Excessive reduction of blood pressure (<85 mmHg diastolic) may be counterproductive.

REFERENCES

1. Kannel WB. Some lessons in cardiovascular epidemiology from Framingham. *Am J Cardiol* 1976;37:269–282.
2. Rothman KJ. *Modern epidemiology*. Boston: Little, Brown & Co., 1986;7–21.
3. Kannel WB. Hypertension and other risk factors in coronary heart disease. *Am Heart J* 1987;114:918–925.
4. Madhavan S, Alderman MH. The potential effect of blood pressure reduction on cardiovascular disease: a cautionary note. *Arch Intern Med* 1981;141:1583–1586.
5. Sackett DL, Haynes RB, Gibson ES, et al. Randomized clinical trial of strategies for improving medication compliance in primary hypertension. *Lancet* 1975;1205–1207.
6. Rose G. Review of primary prevention trials. *Am Heart J* 1987;1013–1017.
7. Veterans Administration Cooperative Study Group on Antihypertensive Agents. Effects of treatment on morbidity in hypertension: results in patients with diastolic blood pressure averaging 115 through 129 mmHg. *JAMA* 1967;202:1028–1034.
8. Veterans Administration Cooperative Study Group on Antihypertensive Agents. Effects of treatment on morbidity in hypertension II. Results in patients with diastolic blood pressure averaging 90 through 114 mmHg. *JAMA* 1970;213:1143–1152.
9. Smith EW. Treatment of mild hypertension: results of a ten-year intervention trial. *Circ Res* 1977;40:I-98–I-105.
10. Hypertension Detection and Follow-up Program Cooperative Group. Five-year findings of the hypertension detection and follow-up program. I. Reduction of mortality in persons with high blood pressure, including mild hypertension. II. Mortality by race–sex and age. *JAMA* 1979;242:2562–2577.
11. Schnall PL, Alderman MH, Kern R. An analysis of the HDFP trial. Evidence of adverse effects of antihypertensive treatment on white women with moderate and severe hypertension. *NY State J Med* 1984;84:299–301.
12. Alderman MH. The epidemiology of hypertension: etiology, natural history, and the impact of therapy. *Cardiovasc Rev Rep* 1980;1:509–519.
13. The Management Committee. The Australian Therapeutic Trial in Mild Hypertension. *Lancet* 1980;1:1261–1267.
14. Helgeland A. Treatment of mild hypertension: a five-year controlled drug trial. The Oslo Study. *Am J Med* 1980;69:725–732.
15. Multiple Risk Factor Intervention Trial Research Group. Multiple Risk Factor Intervention Trial. Risk factor changes and mortality results. *JAMA* 1982;248:1465–1477.
16. Multiple Risk Factor Intervention Trial Research Group. Coronary heart disease death, nonfatal acute myocardial infarction and other clinical outcomes in the Multiple Risk Factor Intervention Trial. *Am J Cardiol* 1986;58:1–13.
17. MRC Working Party on Mild to Moderate Hypertension. Randomized controlled trial of treatment for mild hypertension: design and pilot trial. *Br Med J* 1977;2:1437–1440.
18. WHO/ISH Mild Hypertension Liaison Committee. Trials of treatment of mild hypertension. An interim analysis. *Lancet* 1982;1:149–156.
19. MRC Working Party. MRC trial of treatment of mild hypertension: principal results. *Br Med J* 1985;291:97–104.
20. Amery A, Birkenhager W, Brix P, et al. Mortality and morbidity results from the European Working Party on High Blood Pressure in the Elderly Trial. *Lancet* 1985;1:1349–1354.
21. The IPPPSH Collaborative Group. Cardiovascular risk and risk factors in a randomized trial of treatment based on the beta-blocker oxprenolol. *J Hypertens* 1985;3:379–392.
22. Wikstrand J, Warnold I, Olsson G, Tuomikhto J, Elmeldt D, Berghund G. Primary prevention with metoprolol in patients with hypertension. *JAMA* 1988;259:1976–1982.
23. MRC Working Party. Adverse reactions to bendrofluazide and propranolol for the treatment of mild hypertension. *Lancet* 1981;2:539–543.
24. Helgeland A, Hjermann I, Leren P, Enger SC, Holme I. High density lipoprotein cholesterol and antihypertensive drugs. The Oslo Study. *Br Med J* 1978;2:403.
25. Holtzman E, Rosenthal T, Goldbourt U, Segal P. Do beta-blockers alter lipids and what are the consequences? *J Cardiovasc Pharmacol* 1987;10(Suppl 2):S86–S92.
26. Ames RP. The influence of non-beta-blocking drugs on the lipid profile: Are diuretics outclassed as initial therapy for hypertension? *Am Heart J* 1987;114:998–1006.
27. Morgan DB, Davidson C. Hypokalemia and diuretics: an analysis of publications. *Br Med J* 1980;1:905.
28. Harrington JD, Isner JM, Kassirer JP. Our national obsession with potassium. *Am J Med* 1982;73:155.
29. Kaplan NM. Our appropriate concern about hypokalemia. *Am J Med* 1984;77:1.
30. Kuller LH, Hulley SB, Cohen JD, Neaton J. Unexpected effects of treating hypertension in men with electrocardiographic abnormalities: a critical analysis. *Circulation* 1986;73:114–123.
31. Breckenridge A. Hypertension and hyperuricemia *Lancet* 1966;1:15–18.
32. Fessel WJ. Renal outcomes of gout and hyperuricemia. *Am J Med* 1979;67:74–82.
33. Joint National Committee on Detection, Evaluation, and Treatment of High Blood Pressure. The 1980 Report of the Joint National Committee on Detection, Evaluation, and Treatment of High Blood Pressure. *Arch Intern Med* 1980;140:1280–1285.
34. Strandgaard S, Haunso S. Why does antihypertensive treatment prevent stroke but not myocardial infarction? *Lancet* 1987;2:658–661.
35. Fry J. National history of hypertension: a case for selective non-treatment. *Lancet* 1974;2:431–433.
36. Cruikshank JM, Penneret K, Sorman AE, et al. Low mortality from all causes including myocardial infarction, in well-controlled hypertensives treated with a beta-blocker plus other antihypertensives. *J Hypertens* 1987;5:489–498.
37. Samuelsson O, Wilehlmsen L, Andersson OK, Pennert K, Berglund G. Cardiovascular morbidity in relation to change in blood pressure and serum cholesterol levels in treated hypertension. *JAMA* 1987;258:1768–1776.

38. Cooper SP, Hardy RJ, La Barthe DR, et al. The relation between degree of blood pressure reduction and mortality among hypertensives in the Hypertension Detection and Follow-up Program. *Am J Epidemiol* 1988;127:387–403.
39. Haynes RB, Sackett DL, Tayler DW, Gibson ES, Johnson AL. Increased absenteeism from work after detection and labeling of hypertensive patients. *N Engl J Med* 1978;299:741–744.
40. Polk BF, Harlan LC, Cooper SP, et al. Disability days associated with detection and treatment in a hypertension control program. *Am J Epidemiol* 1984;119:44–53.
41. Alderman MH, Schoenbaum EE. Detection and treatment of hypertension at the worksite. *N Engl J Med* 1975;293:65–68.
42. Testa MA. Interpreting quality-of-life clinical trial data for use in the clinical practice of antihypertensive therapy. *J Hypertens* 1987;5(Suppl 1):S9–S13.
43. Croog SH, Levine S, Testa MA, et al. The effects of antihypertensive therapy on the quality of life. *N Engl J Med* 1986;314:1657–1664.
44. National Center for Health Statistics, Public Health Service. *Vital Statistics of the United States, Vol II. Mortality, Part A, 1950–84.* Washington, DC: US Government Printing Office, 1987.
45. Prineas R, Gillum R. *US epidemiology of hypertension in blacks: epidemiology, pathophysiology, and treatment.* Chicago: Year Book Medical, 1985;17–36.
46. Gillum RF. Pathophysiology of hypertension in blacks and whites: a review of the basis of racial blood pressure differences. *Hypertension* 1979;1:468–475.
47. Veterans Administration Cooperative Study Group on Antihypertensive Agents. Comparison of propranolol and hydrochlorothiazide for the initial treatment of hypertension. I. Results of short-term titration with emphasis on racial differences in response. *JAMA* 1982;248:1996–2003.
48. Brunner HR, Laragh JH, Barr L, et al. Essential hypertension: renin and aldosterone, heart attack, and stroke. *N Engl J Med* 1972;286:441–449.
49. Kaplan NM. Maximally reducing cardiovascular risk in the treatment of hypertension. *Ann Intern Med* 1988;109:36–40.
50. Alderman MH, Madhavan S. Management of the hypertensive patient: a continuing dilemma. *Hypertension* 1981;3:192–197.
51. Dollery CT. An update on the Medical Research Council Hypertension Trial. *J Hypertens* 1987;5:S75–S78.

Hypertension: Pathophysiology, Diagnosis, and Management, edited by J. H. Laragh and B. M. Brenner. Raven Press, Ltd., New York © 1990.

CHAPTER 122

The Meaning of Clinical Trials

Controversies in the Treatment of Hypertension

Göran Berglund

The Four Controversies, 1956
Above What Blood Pressure Limits Has Treatment Been Shown to Be Beneficial?, 1956
Can Coronary Heart Disease Be Prevented, and, If So, Do Beta-Blockers Have a Specific Cardioprotective Effect?, 1957
Is There a Blood Pressure Level in Treated Hypertensives Below Which Further Blood Pressure Reduction Precipitates Myocardial Infarction?, 1962
Clinical Implications, 1962
Recommendations, 1963
References, 1964

Few areas in clinical medicine have been so well documented as have the effects of antihypertensive drugs on mortality and morbidity. There have been an abundance of controlled clinical trials: The initial trial, in 1967, was the first Veterans Administration (VA) study, which included patients with diastolic blood pressures of 115–129 mmHg (1). Three years later, the results of the second VA study (2), concerning patients with initial diastolic blood pressures between 90 and 114 mmHg, were published. Additional reports from this study were presented in 1972 (3) and in 1974 (4).

The U.S. Public Health Service Study (5) was published in 1977. Three years later the results from the Oslo Study of mild hypertension (6) were presented. The first full report of the Australian National Blood Pressure Study (ANBP) (7) was presented the same year, although a short presentation of the main results had appeared the previous year (8). Later analyses of placebo effects (9) and of prognostic factors (10) were published in 1982 and 1984, respectively.

The main results of the large American study, the Hypertension Detection and Follow-up Program (HDFP), appeared as early as 1979 (11,12) and were later followed by a series of publications (13–16).

In 1982, the Multiple Risk Factor Intervention Trial (MRFIT) presented their findings for blood pressure intervention and also presented the main results with regard to multifactorial intervention (17).

In 1985, the results of a study concerning the effects of treatment of hypertension in the elderly, The European Working Party of Hypertension in the Elderly (EWPHE), appeared (18).

The design and pilot results of the British Medical Research Council (MRC) trial were published in 1977 (19), whereas results regarding side effects appeared in 1981 (20) —with the main results appearing as late as 1985 (21). A similar study, the International Prospective Primary Preventive Study in Hypertension (IPPPSH) (22), was presented the same year, with aims and methods having been described the year before (23).

The Heart Attack Primary Prevention in Hypertension (HAPPHY) trial—which, similar to the MRC trial and the IPPPSH, compared the ability of beta-blockers and thiazide diuretics to prevent hypertensive complications—was presented regarding aims and design in 1981 (24); the main results were presented during the autumn of 1986 (25).

Another study from Göteborg, the Primary Prevention Trial (GPPT), was presented the same year. While the main results (26) showed that specific intervention against the risk factors smoking, hypercholesterolemia, and hypertension did not prevent the appearance of coronary heart disease better than did usual care, an analysis of the management of hypertension revealed interesting findings which were presented as a dissertation in 1985 (27) and as separate publications (28–32).

In 1988, another major Göteborg-based study—the Metoprolol Arteriosclerosis Prevention in Hypertension (MAPHY) trial—was presented (33). In contrast to the MRC, IPPPSH, and HAPPHY trials, the MAPHY trial disclosed a significant reduction in total mortality and cardiovascular mortality in hypertensives treated with a selective beta-blocker, metoprolol, as compared to those treated with thiazide diuretics.

Thus, today's knowledge of the effects of antihypertensive treatment is based on a vast databank. What conclusions can be drawn from the studies presented here with respect to the daily care of hypertensive patients?

A general problem must first be addressed. In many fields of medicine it is known that patients participating in clinical tests are not always representative of the type of patient a physician would normally encounter in community health care. Often 50% or more of all subjects initially considered eligible for entry into a study are eliminated because of inclusion and exclusion criteria. These mechanisms of selection have probably resulted in the inclusion of a greater number of patients with milder hypertension into the major hypertension studies than was originally intended. This, in turn, could mean that the treatment gains have been underestimated. Other factors inherent to a clinical study might possibly have the opposite effect. Improved education for physicians, established treatment principles, more thorough follow-up, and greater information than what is currently prevalent could result in greater therapy benefits than what is now expected in ordinary community health care.

THE FOUR CONTROVERSIES

Four major controversies in the interpretation of the vast databank presented above will be addressed here:

1. a. Above what blood pressure limit has treatment been shown to be beneficial?
   b. In which age, sex, and race groups are these benefits proven?
2. Can coronary heart disease be prevented?
3. Do beta-blockers have a specific cardioprotective effect?
4. Is there a blood pressure level in treated hypertensives below which further blood pressure reduction precipitates myocardial infarction?

Above What Blood Pressure Limits Has Treatment Been Shown to Be Beneficial?

When combined, the studies mentioned in this chapter indicate that antihypertensive therapy reduces the complications of high blood pressure. This applies to mild hypertension as well (diastolic blood pressure of 90–105 mmHg). The effectiveness of treatment (i.e., the number of complications that can be prevented), however, decreases dramatically the milder the hypertension. This is evident in Table 1, which shows the efficacy of treatment in the studies having an untreated or placebo-treated control group.

In reviewing the results from the VA Study I concerning severe hypertension, the VA Study II and GPPT dealing with moderate hypertension, and the studies of mild hypertension, respectively, we see a gradual decrease in the ability of drug-based antihypertensive treatment to prevent (or postpone) complications, from 93% to 19%. Accordingly, almost all complications were prevented by treatment in the VA Study I, while only one of every five complications could be prevented in the MRC trial. What is the cause of this apparently paradoxical relationship between the severity of the hypertension and the effectiveness of the treatment? The relationship was paradoxical in the sense that if therapy was initiated at an early stage, early organ damage and accelerated blood pressure increases should be avoidable, and therefore the prognosis should be improved (compare, for example, the recommendations from the HDFP concerning early aggressive therapy). The most probable explanation is that the complications in severe hypertension are more directly caused by the pressure level per se, whereas in mild hypertension there are other risk factors that play an important role in the occurrence of the complications, which are primarily arteriosclerotic.

TABLE 1. *Effectiveness of antihypertensive treatment in the large hypertension studies*[a]

Study	Diastolic blood pressure	Effectiveness of treatment (%)
VA Study I	115–129 mmHg	93
VA Study II	105–114 mmHg	69
	90–104 mmHg	45
GPPT[b]	>100 mmHg	50
ANBP	90–104 mmHg	20
MRC	90–104 mmHg	19

[a] Effectiveness of treatment is defined as the number of cardiovascular events that were delayed.
[b] Screening diastolic blood pressure (DSP) limit of 115 mmHg is comparable to a DBP of 101 mmHg at the clinic.

As a result of the decreasing effectiveness of treatment in milder hypertension, we see that the milder the hypertension, the greater the number of patients that have to be treated in order for one patient to benefit from treatment (i.e., that a complication is prevented or postponed) (Table 2). Thus, an increasing number of patients have to be treated (six patients in the VA Study I; 16 in the VA Study II; 49 in the GPPT; 116 in the ANBP study; and 264 in the MRC trial), with the negative effects that this involves (worries about the diagnosis, time consumption, costs to patient and society, risk for side effects). This drastic increase in the number of treated patients necessary to postpone one cardiovascular complication must be taken into consideration when recommendations are given regarding blood pressure limits above which treatment should be instituted.

The current Swedish recommendations at the end of this chapter are based on (a) the integration of the evidence

TABLE 2. *Number of patients in the different hypertension studies who must be treated for 1 year in order to postpone one cardiovascular event for 1 year*

Study	*n*
VA Study I	6
VA Study II	16
GPPT	49
ANBP	116
MRC	264

from the major hypertension studies and (b) consideration of the above-mentioned factors with respect to the limits for pharmacological treatment.

In these recommendations it is emphasized that numerous blood pressures (a minimum of six) over an extended period of time (at least 4–6 months) are necessary prior to establishing the diagnosis of hypertension. This drastic sharpening of the diagnostic criteria is based on the findings from the ANBP study and the MRC trial that almost 50% of the patients with mild hypertension will become normotensive in the absence of active therapy and that the frequency of complications among these patients is lower than that among actively treated patients with the same blood pressure levels.

Our conclusion from the data given above is that antihypertensive drug treatment has been shown, beyond doubt, to decrease hypertensive complications in hypertensive subjects with *repeated* blood pressure ≥ 100 mmHg diastolic.

The space alotted to this review does not allow a detailed discussion on the benefit of treatment in various age, sex, and race groups. Strictly speaking, the proven benefits do only apply to middle-aged men. The great majority of men included in the above-cited trials have been white; however, in the trials where substantial numbers of black men have been included, the benefit of treatment has been of the same order for whites and blacks (12,13). In most trials, the benefit of treatment has been the least in white women, and so far no trial has been able to show a significant beneficial effect of antihypertensive treatment in white women (13,21). The EWPHE (18) addressed the benefit of treatment in hypertensive patients above 60 years of age and can be said to cover the age span from 60 to 70 years. The EWPHE results indicate that the benefit of treatment proven for middle-aged patients seems to extend also to the ages between 60 and 70 years. Above 70, however, there are no data available.

Can Coronary Heart Disease Be Prevented, and, If So, Do Beta-Blockers Have a Specific Cardioprotective Effect?

The VA study proved to be very effective in preventing direct hypertension-related complications (Fig. 1; Table 3). However, an effect on coronary heart disease could not be detected except for a tendency for a lower number of fatal cases, compensated, though, by a higher number of nonfatal infarctions, in the actively treated group.

In the MRC trial, active therapy, irrespective of type, had no discernible effect on coronary heart disease, and it saved no lives. In nonsmoking men a trend toward a lower incidence of coronary heart disease during treatment with propranolol was found. On the whole, however, the MRC study is a strong setback for those claiming that beta-blockers exhibit a cardioprotective effect.

The finding that smoking habits made a difference in the effect of treatment with propranolol was surprising. Blood pressure, however, was higher for smokers than for nonsmokers in the propranolol group, which could be a contributing factor to such a finding.

The IPPPSH is a study that paralleled, to a great extent, the MRC trial. The fact that there was no purely placebo-treated control group is understandable, when considering the blood pressure inclusion criteria (100–120 mmHg diastolic). The basic design of double-blind treatment is superior to that of the MRC trial, even if one questions the possibility of maintaining the "blindness" due to the known adverse reactions associated with beta-blockers and diuretics, namely, bradycardia and hypokalemia, respectively.

The main result was that beta-blockers did not appear to prevent the occurrence of coronary catastrophes any better than did the antihypertensive therapy based primarily on diuretics, nor was the incidence of stroke lower in the group treated with beta-blockers. These main findings agree with the results of the MRC trial, as does the finding that nonsmoking men seem to be the group, if any, in which beta-blockers might have a better preventive effect than would other antihypertensive treatment.

The HAPPHY was an open, randomized study that, similar to the MRC trial and the IPPPSH, compared the ability of beta-blockers in preventing coronary heart disease to treatment with thiazide diuretics. Inclusion of patients with diastolic blood pressures of 100–130 mmHg precluded a control group treated with placebo. A double-blind design was regarded as impossible to maintain, bearing in mind the known effects of the drugs on heart rate and serum potassium. Clearly, the open design entailed that the value of the analyses of side effects would be very limited; the

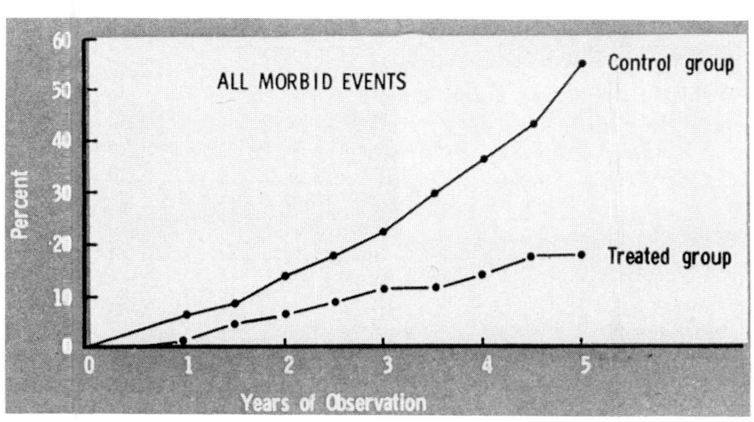

FIG. 1. Veterans Administration Study II. Estimated cumulative incidence of all fatal and nonfatal endpoints over a 5-year period.

TABLE 3. *Veterans Administration Study II: effectiveness of treatment with respect to diastolic blood pressure (DBP), age, and cardiovascular–renal (CVR) abnormalities during randomization*

Parameter	Effectiveness of treatment (%)
DBP	
90–104 mmHg	45
105–114 mmHg	69
Age	
<50 years	56
>50 years	58
CVR abnormalities	
Without abnormalities	50
With abnormalities	64
With CVR abnormalities	
DBP 90–104 mmHg	21
105–114 mmHg	73
With CVR abnormalities	
DBP 90–104 mmHg	52
105–114 mmHg	71
Age < 50 years	
DBP 90–104 mmHg	27
105–114 mmHg	74
Age > 50 years	
DBP 90–104 mmHg	50
105–114 mmHg	64

preconceived opinions of the physicians regarding the side effects of the drugs influenced these results.

Blood pressure was measured "blind," and endpoints were assessed by an independent committee; this improved the validity of the results.

The HAPPHY study verified the results of the MRC trial and of the IPPPSH; that is, it was not possible to demonstrate that beta-blockers had a greater cardioprotective effect than diuretics (Table 4). The results show that the findings in patients who have suffered a myocardial infarction could not be generalized to the large group of patients with mild uncomplicated hypertension.

The trial was designed in order to demonstrate a 30% difference between the drug groups. Such an effect could not be demonstrated, although even a smaller difference could be clinically relevant. The power to demonstrate a lesser difference, however, was weak in this study, as in the MRC trial and the IPPPSH. The results of these three studies do not exclude a slight cardioprotective effect of beta-blockers. The demonstration of such a weak effect, however, demands very large studies and is unlikely to be realized.

It has occasionally been asserted that negative metabolic effects such as increase in atherogenic lipid fractions might counteract the positive effects of beta-blockers. In the HAPPHY study, however, a reduction in total cholesterol during beta-blocker treatment was detected, which sheds new light on the value of short-term studies concerning the effects of the drug.

Consequently, a tendency toward lower stroke mortality was detected among the patients treated with beta-blockers in this trial. The difference was not significant, and the finding can be random. Among men in the IPPPSH, the same positive trend toward lower stroke mortality in the beta-blocker group was detected, whereas the opposite prevailed in the MRC trial. The finding (in the two latter studies) that smokers might benefit less from beta-blockers than from diuretics could not be verified in the HAPPHY study. The use, in this trial, of selective beta-blockers (which produce smaller increases in pressure during smoking than do nonselective beta-blockers) is a possible explanation. In the MRC trial, blood pressure was shown to be higher among smoking patients treated with propranolol than among nonsmokers treated with propranolol, implying that differences in blood pressure between smokers and nonsmokers could explain the differences between these studies.

The negative effects of diuretics on serum potassium and serum urate were verified. In spite of a 15–20% frequency of hypokalemia, the number of fatal myocardial infarctions was lower in the diuretic-treated group. The finding in the

TABLE 4. *Heart Attack Primary Prevention in Hypertension (HAPPHY) trial: total and cause-specific mortality, nonfatal myocardial infarction (MI), and nonfatal stroke*

Event	Diuretic (n = 3272)		Beta-blockers (n = 3297)	
	n	Rate/1000 patient-years	n	Rate/1000 patient-years
Coronary heart disease (CHD)				
Fatal CHD	50	4.09	54	4.35
Nonfatal MI	75	6.13	84	6.76
Fatal and/or nonfatal CHD	116	9.48	132	10.62
Stroke				
Fatal stroke	10	0.82	3	0.24
Nonfatal stroke	32	2.61	29	2.33
Fatal and/or nonfatal stroke	41	3.35	32	2.58
Deaths				
Fatal CHD	50	4.09	54	4.35
Fatal stroke	10	0.82	3	0.24
Other deaths	41	3.35	39	3.14
All deaths	101	8.25	96	7.73
Patients with an endpoint[a]	192	15.65	197	15.85
Total number of endpoints	224		225	

[a] Death, nonfatal MI, nonfatal stroke.

HAPPHY, VA, ANBP, HDFP, and EWPHE studies indicates that the marketing image vigorously presented by certain pharmaceutical companies—that thiazide diuretics, through their hypokalemia-producing effect, cause sudden cardiac death—is without scientific foundation. In all of these studies, the group that received treatment based on diuretics had a tendency toward a *lower* coronary mortality.

The Göteborg Primary Prevention Trial tested the "high-risk" philosophy for the prevention of coronary disease. The design was scientifically acceptable, although the effect of intervention on the multiple risk factors was less satisfactory, except for the effect on blood pressure. The absence of a preventive effect has to be attributed to a combination of (a) the contemporaneous reduction of the risk factors in the society in general (as reflected in the control groups) and (b) a rather unsatisfactory effect of the intervention on smoking and serum cholesterol.

The hypertension portion that has been reported in some detail, however, revealed some findings that raise expectations concerning the possibilities of intervention. Other findings raise doubts as to the beneficial effects of one-sided concentration on blood pressure reduction.

The fact that only two-thirds of the patients achieved the treatment goal has been criticized. The finding is, however, in accordance with other studies of mild to moderate hypertension. The fact that one out of every five patients took three drugs, combined with the fact that one out of every 20 patients took four drugs or more, also indicates that the patients had received intensive antihypertensive drug treatment. Yet, it is possible that an improved pressure reduction in patients with high pressures would have further reduced the number of cardiovascular complications.

The treatment was effective regarding the prevention of cardiovascular events (Fig. 2). As to coronary heart disease, the finding that fatal myocardial infarction is reduced while nonfatal myocardial infarction is not significantly affected recurs (compare VA, HDFP, ANBP, and EWPHE studies). Possible reasons for this recurrent finding are discussed above.

In spite of this positive effect on cardiovascular events, it is still these events that dominate the hypertensive's complication profile. During the 10 years of treatment, a very large number of patients suffered arteriosclerotic complications in the heart, brain, and peripheral vessels (Fig. 3). Previously known risk factors have been shown to be of

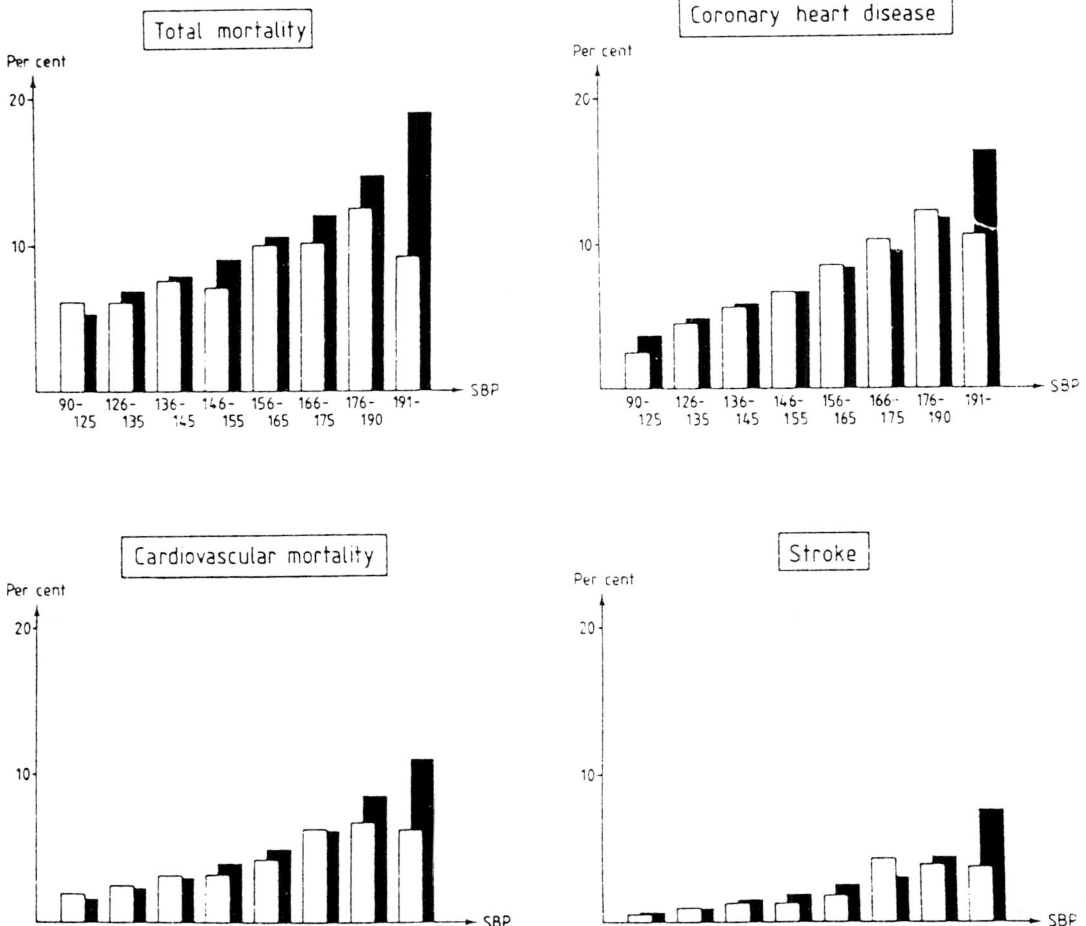

FIG. 2. Göteborg Primary Prevention Trial. Mortality and cardiovascular morbidity in relation to initial systolic blood pressure (SBP). Observed (*unshaded bars*) compared to predicted incidence (*shaded bars*) during 10 years of follow-up.

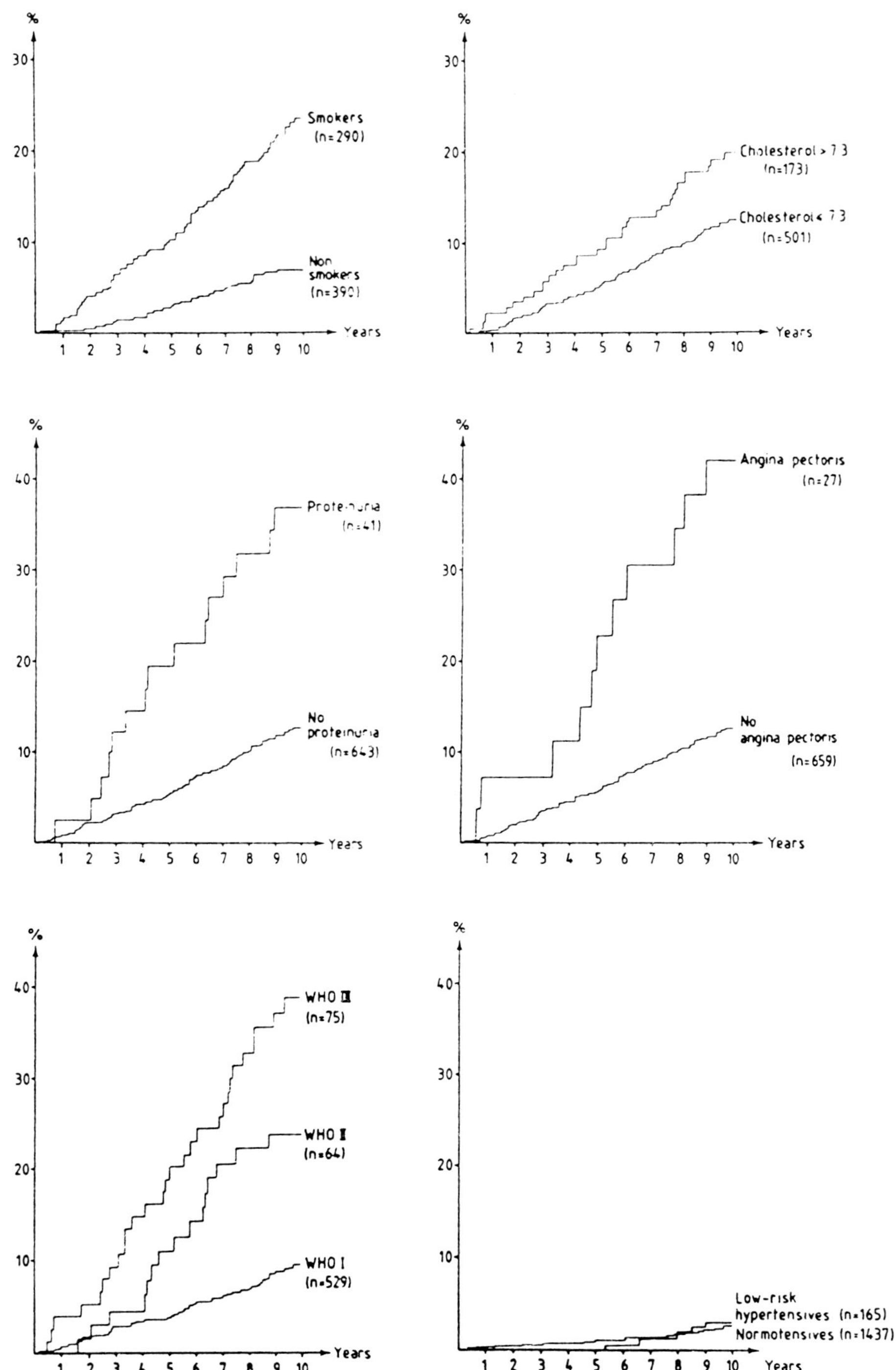

FIG. 3. Göteborg Primary Prevention Trial. Ten-year cumulative cardiovascular morbidity in relation to initial risk factor levels/categories.

importance in the occurrence of these complications, even in hypertensives. Smoking and serum cholesterol appear once again as important risk indicators that we, as doctors, *must* attempt to influence. The strong predictive ability of proteinuria provides incentive for future research concerning an easily identifiable indicator of vascular damage.

The great importance of serum cholesterol with respect to cardiovascular events is even more evident in the analysis of changes during the course of treatment. The finding that antihypertensive treatment lacked a preventive effect if the level of cholesterol was not reduced (Fig. 4) indicates once again that we must identify and influence all of the cardiovascular risk factors of the patient in order to prevent the occurrence of complications.

The recently published MAPHY trial (33), which compared the cardioselective beta-blocker metoprolol with

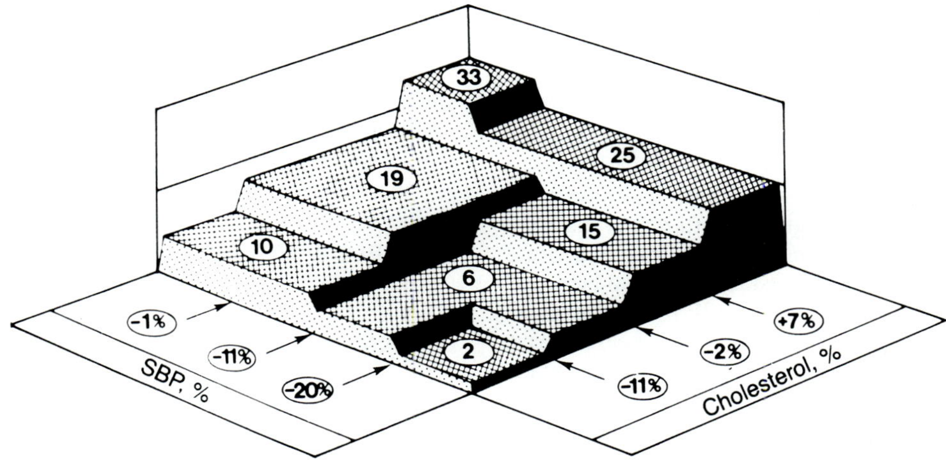

FIG. 4. Göteborg Primary Prevention Trial. Incidence of coronary heart disease during 10 years of follow-up in relation to the change in percentage of systolic blood pressure (SBP) and serum cholesterol during year 1.

thiazide diuretics, reported that the beta-blocker as initial therapy lowered both total mortality and coronary heart disease mortality better than the diuretics. Patients were randomly allocated to treatment with metoprolol (n = 1609, 1809 patient-years) or with a thiazide diuretic (bendroflumethiazide or hydrochlorothiazide, n = 1625; 8071 patient-years). The mean dose of metoprolol was 174 mg daily, and that of the thiazide diuretics was 46 mg for hydrochlorothiazide and 4.4 mg for bendroflumethiazide. Median follow-up time was 4.2 years.

Identical blood pressure control was achieved using a fixed therapeutic schedule. Total mortality was significantly lower (p = 0.028) for metoprolol than for thiazide diuretics (see Fig. 5), owing to fewer deaths from coronary heart disease and stroke. At the median follow-up time of 4.2 years, there were 28 deaths in the metoprolol group and 54 in the diuretic group—a 48% reduction in total mortality (95% confidence limits −68% to −17%). Total mortality was also significantly lower in smokers given metoprolol (p = 0.013). Long-term safety of the treatment was good, supported also by a somewhat lower number of deaths due to noncardiovascular disorders.

The results of the MAPHY trial are, thus, contrary to the results of the MRC, IPPPSH, and HAPPHY trials. The discrepancy is difficult to explain; perhaps it was the inclusion of a more homogeneous (only men) study population, combined with the use of a cardioselective beta-blocker, that led to the more beneficial effect of the beta-blockers in the MAPHY trial. Further trials and analyses of the existing databank are needed before it can be answered as to whether beta-blockers are superior to thiazide diuretics as the first-choice drug in hypertension.

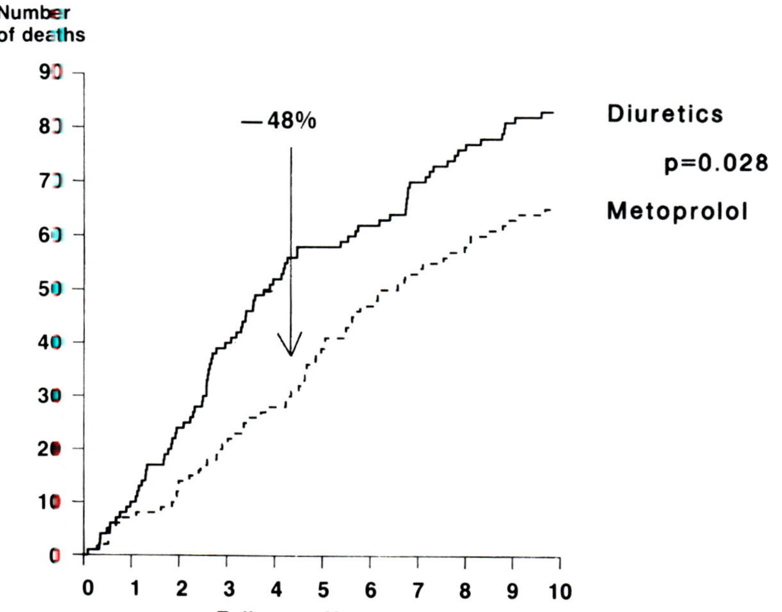

FIG. 5. Total cumulative mortality in two randomization groups. Solid line indicates diuretics (n = 1625); broken line indicates metoprolol (n = 1609) (p = 0.028).

Is There a Blood Pressure Level in Treated Hypertensives Below Which Further Blood Pressure Reduction Precipitates Myocardial Infarction?

Both in the HAPPHY trial and in the Göteborg Primary Prevention Trial (Fig. 6), a higher coronary morbidity was found in patients with mean in-study diastolic blood pressure below 86 mmHg than in patients with higher diastolic pressures. Studies by Cruickshank et al. (34,35) corroborate these findings. In-study blood pressures have also been analyzed in the ANBP study and in the IPPPSH. However, in the ANBP study the multiple risk of coronary heart disease at entry was not taken into account. It is obvious that a hypertensive subject who has a diastolic blood pressure of 120 mmHg, is a smoker, and has a serum cholesterol of 8.5 mmol/liter will have a drastically higher coronary risk than another subject who enters with a diastolic blood pressure of 100 mmHg, is a nonsmoker, and has a serum cholesterol of 5.5 mmol/liter. It is equally obvious that he will carry this risk with him into the trial irrespective of the type of treatment given to him. If then the impact of the in-study blood pressure, per se, should be analyzed, this difference in initial coronary risk must in some way be corrected for.

In the IPPPSH trial, mean in-study blood pressure and coronary heart disease incidence was related by means of an isotonic regression analysis. Because this method assumes a steadily increasing or decreasing relationship, it is obvious that this type of statistical analysis cannot be used to reveal a U- or J-shaped relationship.

The finding that there appears to be a blood pressure limit below which further reduction of pressure *increases* the risk for complications ought to prevent us from uncritically accepting recommendations that the lowest possible blood pressure level should always be sought. The underlying cause of this finding was not possible to clarify in these studies. One possible explanation might be that a drastic reduction of blood pressure could endanger the blood supply to vital organs, (e.g., if arteriosclerotic abnormalities exist in the supplying vessels). Additional analyses are necessary to clarify this point. Until such are at hand, the aim of the treatment ought to be a diastolic blood pressure below 90 mmHg; however, drastic decreases (e.g., to below 85 mmHg diastolic) should be avoided.

CLINICAL IMPLICATIONS

What conclusions as to clinical care are drawn by the authors of the publications concerning the large hypertension studies? If the studies are systematically perused, one will find that very few attempts have been made to interpret how the results might be transferred to practical, clinical treatment. The VA Study II concludes that even a partial normalization of blood pressure can be satisfactory, since such did not appear to have a lower preventive effect on complications. The ANBP study interprets its findings in the placebo group in such a way that a minimum of 4 months of follow-up with repeated blood pressure measurements is recommended prior to diagnosing hypertension. The HDFP recommends its systematical care model for all hypertensive patients and, further recommends initiating therapy at an early stage before organ complications arise. In the Oslo Study, the MRFIT, the EWPHE trial, the MRC trial, the IPPPSH, and the HAPPHY study, no interpretations are provided as to how the results are to be transferred to daily clinical practice. The recommendation from the GPPT was that smoking and hypercholesterolemia must

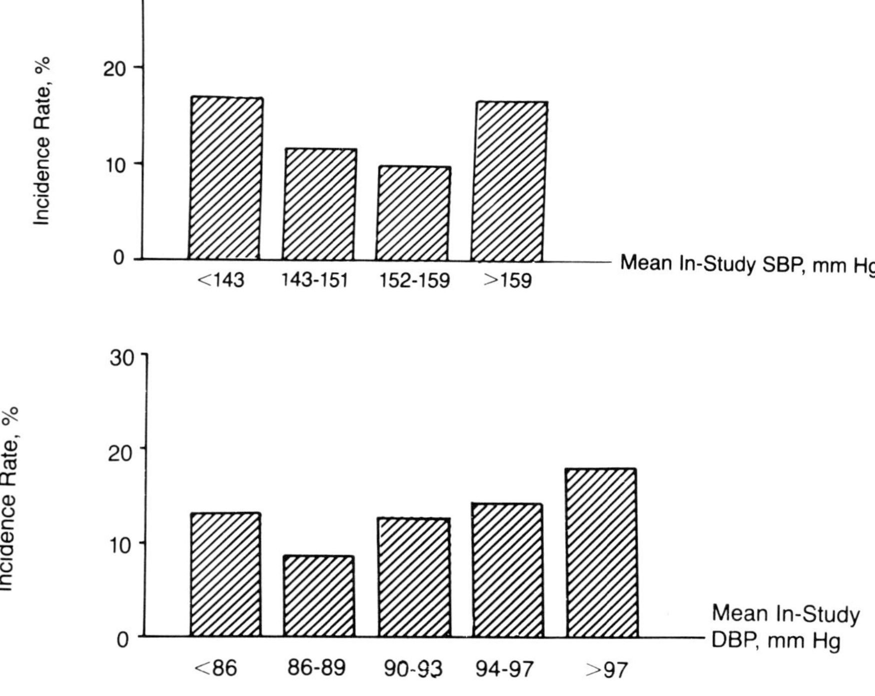

FIG. 6. Göteborg Primary Prevention Trial. Coronary heart disease (CHD) incidence in quartiles of mean in-study systolic blood pressure (SBP) (**upper panel**) and mean in-study diastolic blood pressure (DBP) (**lower panel**). Rates are corrected for CHD risk at entry.

also be acted upon if cardiovascular complications were to be prevented.

Thus, the publications from the major hypertension studies supply very little information regarding clinical problems. Why is this so? The causes are probably numerous. Manuscripts are produced under time constraints, and frequently many opinions are involved in the formulation of the text. Often only the main results have been analyzed, and analyses with more direct clinical value have had low priority in relation to the analysis of the main hypothesis. Furthermore, many researchers in the field of epidemiology fear that individuals who are involved in a major study will interpret the findings from a clinical point of view. Thus, it is left to the rest of the scientific community to interpret the results. This intellectual snobbishness has definite disadvantages. Researchers who have worked intensively with a major study over a period of years naturally have a better working knowledge, as well as a better overall understanding, of the results of the study than those who merely read the publication. They are, accordingly, better suited to translate the results into clinical recommendations. The results of clinical studies can obviously be interpreted in different ways. If one completely abstains from interpreting the findings into terms of clinical action, different interested parties are given free rein to render the interpretation best suited to their own aims. Everyone naturally has the right to interpret research results in partly different ways, yet an "official" interpretation by the group having performed the study makes it more difficult to interpret the findings completely according to one's own interests. Every research should endeavor to transform the research results into measures benefiting the patient. This is the ultimate reason for all clinical research.

The studies discussed in this chapter indicate that antihypertensive treatment with thiazide diuretics, as well as with beta-blockers, reduces the risk of cardiovascular complications in patients with repeated diastolic blood pressures above 100 mmHg. The documentation in support of this is greater for diuretics (VA Studies, ANBP, HDFP, EWPHE) than for beta-blockers (MRC trial). A direct comparison between the drug groups (MRC, IPPPSH, HAPPHY, and MAPHY), however, suggests a similar treatment effect with respect to cardiovascular complications. These three studies have documented that the effect of beta-blockers is comparable to the effect of thiazide diuretics in preventing cardiovascular complications in hypertensives. The question of whether beta-blockers prevent coronary heart disease more effectively than diuretics has been tested in the MRC, IPPPSH, HAPPHY, and MAPHY trials. The first three studies could not demonstrate such a cardioprotective effect with beta-blockers. However, as earlier mentioned, a lower total mortality and cardiovascular mortality was found in the metoprolol-treated group in the MAPHY trial, indicating that this beta-blocker has a better effect on cardiovascular complications than do thiazide diuretics. However, it should be observed that although the first three studies were large, they only had a limited power to demonstrate minor differences with regard to a cardioprotective effect between the drug groups. For example, in the HAPPHY study the power to demonstrate a 15% difference between the drugs was only 25%. None of the three studies had an acceptable power to demonstrate such a minor difference. The clinical relevance of such a minor difference is, however, difficult to evaluate.

Is there then any evidence to suggest that beta-blockers have a minor, but clinically relevant, cardioprotective effect? If the findings among men in the MRC trial, the IPPPSH, and the HAPPHY study (the latter contained only men) are pooled, a 15% lower total mortality rate for coronary heart disease and cardiovascular disease is found in the beta-blocker group (Table 5). Stroke mortality was 41% lower. However, none of these differences was statistically significant, in spite of the large number of patients. As to the corresponding nonfatal endpoints, the same tendency was not apparent, and for that reason the relevance of the findings must be questioned. The analysis is still justifiable, because it indicates the power problems that even these very large studies have.

RECOMMENDATIONS

Concluding this chapter are the recommendations drawn up by the Swedish National Association Against Heart and Lung Disease; these are very similar to the guidelines composed by a panel organized by the Social Board of Health.

1. The diagnosis of hypertension is to be established only after repeated blood pressure measurements; the milder the hypertension, the greater the number of blood pressure readings necessary. For mild hypertension, six blood pressure measurements (and the same number of visits) are recommended over a period of 4–6 months. Several of these blood pressure readings can be taken by a

TABLE 5. *Pooled results for men in the MRC trial, the IPPPSH, and the HAPPHY study*[a]

	Non-beta-blocker based (diuretic), *n* = 7099	Beta-blocker based, *n* = 7187	Percent difference
Entry blood pressure (mmHg):	165/104	165/104	
Blood pressure at last visit (mmHg):	144/90	144/89	
Fatal CHD:	4.47	3.81	−15%
Fatal stroke:	0.68	0.40	−41%
Fatal cardiovascular disease:	5.15	4.22	−18%
Fatal noncardiovascular disease:	3.82	3.51	−8%
Total mortality:	8.98	7.74	−14%

[a] Total patient-years = 59.633; *n* = 14.286.

nurse. For moderate/severe hypertension (diastolic blood pressure ≥ 105 mmHg), the diagnosis can be established after fewer blood pressure measurements.

2. An average diastolic blood pressure of 90 mmHg is required for diagnosing hypertension. This level applies regardless of age.

3. Systolic blood pressure is not to be used in diagnosing hypertension. Isolated increases in systolic blood pressure can, however, be treated in extreme cases (see below).

4. The diagnostic examination of younger and middle-aged patients with hypertension should include:

a. Patient history and physical examination
b. Serum potassium
c. Serum creatinine
d. Serum cholesterol
e. Blood glucose
f. Urine test for albuminuria and glucosuria
g. Electrocardiogram with precordial leads

The extent of the diagnostic investigation in elderly patients is to be based upon the clinical picture.

5. If mean blood pressure is ≥100 mmHg diastolic *and* the diagnostic examination indicates any of the following conditions, antihypertensive drugs should be instituted in combination with nonpharmacological treatment:

a. Previous myocardial infarction or stroke
b. Angina pectoris, heart decompensation, intermittent claudication, kidney disease
c. Diabetes mellitus
d. Hypertensive organ manifestations (left ventricular hypertrophy on electrocardiogram and/or albuminuria or elevated serum creatinine)
e. Other cardiovascular risk factors (smoking, hypercholesterolemia, and/or glucose intolerance)

If other cardiovascular risk factors are present, specific therapy against the same should be initiated.

6. Try nonpharmacological measures for approximately 6 months if mean blood pressure is ≥100 mmHg diastolic and none of the above conditions (point 5) are present. If the therapeutic goal (diastolic blood pressure below 90 mmHg) is not achieved, antihypertensive drugs may be added.

7. Antihypertensive treatment—pharmacological or nonpharmacological—*may* be instituted at diastolic blood pressure levels of 90–100 mmHg if any of the above conditions (point 5) are present. Pharmacological therapy should be the primary choice if previous myocardial infarction, stroke, heart decompensation, intermittent claudication, diabetes mellitus, or hypertensive organ manifestations are present, whereas nonpharmacological treatment can be attempted if other cardiovascular risk factors exist.

8. In elderly persons with isolated increases in systolic blood pressure (e.g., ≥220 mmHg), pharmacological treatment is initiated only if signs of vascular organ damage are present or if systolic blood pressure is extremely high. A preventive effect on hypertensive complications is not documented. The treatment is chiefly motivated by the expectation of preventing a stroke.

9. Response to therapy should be checked within 1–8 weeks, depending on entry blood pressure. If the drug initially given does not result in achievement of the treatment goal, the other primary drug (beta-blockers or diuretics) can be instituted instead. Combine beta-blockers and thiazide diuretics if the treatment goal is still not achieved. Addition of, or combination with, hydralazine, spironolactone, calcium antagonists, or angiotensin-converting-enzyme inhibitors can be tried if the treatment goal is not achieved through the combination of beta-blockers and thiazide diuretics. Chronic treatment should consist of the least number of drugs in the lowest doses possible, allowing for the treatment goal to be attained.

REFERENCES

1. Veterans Administration Cooperative Study Group on Antihypertensive Agents. Effects of treatment on morbidity in hypertension. Results in patients with diastolic blood pressures averaging 115 through 129 mmHg. *JAMA* 1967;202:116–122.
2. Veterans Administration Cooperative Study Group on Antihypertensive Agents. Effects of treatment on morbidity in hypertension. II. Results in patients with diastolic blood pressure averaging 90 through 114 mmHg. *JAMA* 1970;213:1143–1152.
3. Veterans Administration Cooperative Study Group on Antihypertensive Agents. Effects of treatment on morbidity in hypertension. III. Influence of age, diastolic pressure, and prior cardiovascular disease; further analysis of side effects. *Circulation* 1972;45:991–1004.
4. Taguchi J, Freis ED. Partial reduction of blood pressure and prevention of complications in hypertension. *N Engl J Med* 1974;291:329–331.
5. U.S. Public Health Service Hospitals Cooperative Group; McFate Smith W. Treatment of mild hypertension: results of a ten year intervention trial. *Circ Res* 1977;40:I-98–I-105.
6. Helgeland A. Treatment of mild hypertension: a five year controlled drug trial. The Oslo Study. *Am J Med* 1980;69:725–732.
7. Management Committee. The Australian Therapeutic Trial in Mild Hypertension. *Lancet* 1980;1:1261–1267.
8. Management Committee. Initial results of the Australian Therapeutic Trial in Mild Hypertension. *Clin Sci* 1979;57:449s–52s.
9. Management Committee of the Australian Therapeutic Trial in Mild Hypertension. Untreated mild hypertension. *Lancet* 1982;1:185–191.
10. Management Committee of the Australian National Blood Pressure Study. Prognostic factors in the treatment of mild hypertension. *Circulation* 1984;69:668–676.
11. Hypertension Detection and Follow-up Program Cooperative Group. Five-year findings of the Hypertension Detection and Follow-up Program. *JAMA* 1979;242:2562–2571.
12. Hypertension Detection and Follow-up Program Cooperative Group. Five-year findings of the Hypertension Detection and Follow-up Program. II. Mortality by race-sex and age. *JAMA* 1979;242:2572–2577.
13. Schnall PL, Alderman MH, Kern R. An analysis of the HDFP trial. Evidence of adverse effects of antihypertensive treatment on white women with moderate and severe hypertension. *NY State J Med* 1984;84:299–301.
14. Hypertension Detection and Follow-up Program Cooperative Group. Effect of stepped care treatment on the incidence of myocardial infarction and angina pectoris. 5-year findings of the Hypertension Detection and Follow-up Program. *Hypertension* 1984;6(Suppl 1):I-198–I-206.
15. Hypertension Detection and Follow-up Program Cooperative Research Group. The effect of antihypertensive drug treatment on mortality in the presence of resting electrocardiographic abnormalities at baseline: the HDFP experience. *Circulation* 1984;70:996–1003.
16. Hypertension Detection and Follow-up Program Cooperative Research Group. The effect of treatment on mortality in "mild"

hypertension. Results of the Hypertension Detection and Follow-up Program. *N Engl J Med* 1982;307:976–980.

17. Multiple Risk Factor Intervention Trial Research Group. Multiple Risk Factor Intervention Trial. Risk factor changes and mortality results. *JAMA* 1982;248:1465–1477.
18. Amery A, Brixko P, Clement D, et al. Mortality and morbidity results from the European Working Party on High Blood Pressure in the Elderly trial. *Lancet* 1985;2:1349–1354.
19. MRC Working Party on Mild to Moderate Hypertension. Randomised controlled trial of treatment for mild hypertension: design and pilot trial. *Br Med J* 1977;ii:1437–1440.
20. Medical research council working party on mild to moderate hypertension. Adverse reactions to bendrofluazide and propranolol for the treatment of mild hypertension. *Lancet* 1981;2:539–543.
21. Medical Research Council Working Party. MRC trial of treatment of mild hypertension: principal results. *Br Med J* 1985;291:97–104.
22. The IPPPSH Collaborative Group. Cardiovascular risk and risk factors in a randomized trial of treatment based on the beta-blocker oxprenolol: the International Prospective Primary Prevention Study in Hypertension (IPPPSH). *J Hypertens* 1985;3:379–392.
23. The IPPPSH Collaborative Group. The International Prospective Primary Prevention Study in Hypertension (IPPPSH): objectives and methods. *Eur J Clin Pharmacol* 1984;27:379–391.
24. Wilhelmsen L, Berglund G, Elmfeldt D, Wedel H. β-Blockers versus saluretics in hypertension. Comparison of total mortality, myocardial infarction, and sudden death: study design and early results on blood pressure reduction. *Prev Med* 1981;10:38–49.
25. Wilhelmsen L, Berglund G, Elmfeldt D, et al. Beta-blockers versus diuretics in hypertensive men. Main results from the HAPPHY trial. Presented at the Meeting of the International Society of Hypertension, Heidelberg, September 1986.
26. Wilhelmsen L, Berglund G, Elmfeldt D, et al. The multifactor primary prevention trial in Göteborg, Sweden. *Eur Heart J* 1986;7:279–288.
27. Samuelsson O. Hypertension in middle-aged men. Management, morbidity and prognostic factors during long-term hypertensive care. *Acta Med Scand* [*Suppl.*] 1985;219(Suppl 702).
28. Samuelsson O, Andersson O, Wilhelmsen L, Berglund G. Treatment of hypertension at an outpatient hypertension clinic. Blood pressure control, dropout rate, and side effects. *Prev Med* 1982;11:521–535.
29. Samuelsson O, Wilhelmsen L, Pennert K, Berglund G. Angina pectoris, intermittent claudication and congestive heart failure in middle-aged male hypertensives. Development and predictive factors during long-term antihypertensive care. The primary preventive trial, Göteborg, Sweden. *Acta Med Scand* 1987;221:23–32.
30. Samuelsson O, Wilhlemsen L, Elmfeldt D, Pennert K, Wedel H, Wikstrand J, Berglund G. Predictors of cardiovascular morbidity in treated hypertension. Results from the primary preventive trial in Göteborg, Sweden. *J Hypertens* 1985;3:167–176.
31. Samuelsson O, Wilhelmsen L, Svärdsudd K, Pennert K, Wedel H, Berglund G. Mortality and morbidity in relation to systolic blood pressure in two populations with different management of hypertension. Results from the study of men born in 1913 and the primary prevention trial, Göteborg, Sweden. *J Hypertens* 1987;5:57–66.
32. Samuelsson O, Wilhelmsen L, Andersson OK, Pennert K, Berglund G. Cardiovascular morbidity in relation to blood pressure control and changes in blood pressure and serum cholesterol during long-term treatment of hypertension. Results from the primary prevention trial in Göteborg, Sweden. *JAMA* 1987;258:1768–1776.
33. Wikstrand J, Warnold I, Olsson G, Tuomilehto J, Elmfeldt D, Berglund G. Primary prevention with metoprolol in patients with hypertension. Mortality results from the MAPHY study. *JAMA* 1988;259:1976–1982.
34. Cruickshank JM, Thorp JM, Zacharias FJ. Benefits and potential harm of lowering high blood pressure. *Lancet* 1987;i:581–584.
35. Cruickshank JM, Pennert K, Sörman AE, Thorp JM, Zacharias FM, Zacharias FJ. Low mortality from all causes, including myocardial infarction, in well-controlled hypertensives treated with a beta-blocker plus other antihypertensives. *J Hypertens* 1987;5:489–498.

Hypertension: Pathophysiology, Diagnosis, and Management, edited by J. H. Laragh and B. M. Brenner. Raven Press, Ltd., New York © 1990.

CHAPTER 123

What Blood Pressure Level Should Be Treated?

Alberto Zanchetti

Blood Pressure as a Guideline to Commence Treatment, 1967
Diastolic Blood Pressure, 1967
Systolic Blood Pressure, 1969
Blood Pressure as a Guideline to Conduct Treatment, 1972
Evidence from Controlled Trials, 1972
The Problem of the J-Shaped Curve, 1973
Conditions Under Which Blood Pressure Should Be Measured as a Guideline to Treatment, 1976
Casual and Office Blood Pressure, 1976
Ambulatory Blood Pressure Monitoring: Is 24-hr Blood Pressure Likely to Become a More Precise Guideline to Treatment?, 1977
Conclusions, 1980
References, 1982

It is apparently easy to answer the question, What blood pressure level should be treated? by paraphrasing the well-known definition by Geoffrey Rose (1) and saying, It is the level of blood pressure at which treatment does more good than harm. However, to translate this operational answer in more practical operative terms, it should be realized that the question implies two separate aspects and that the evidence relating to either of these aspects should be separately discussed.

The first aspect is that of the blood pressure level at which a decision to commence treatment should be taken. This is the more usual aspect, that which has been explored in many controlled therapeutic trials. The second, and equally important, aspect of the question is that of the level to which blood pressure should be brought by treatment.

There are further interrelated problems one has to consider when asking the general question about what blood pressure level should be treated. Which blood pressure should be taken as a guideline to start and maintain treatment: diastolic or systolic, or both (2)? And since it is well known that blood pressure is a highly variable parameter (3), at what time and under what conditions should blood pressure be measured to be used as a guide to treatment? This important aspect of the more general question has long been neglected or oversimplified, but it has received new attention because of the recent availability of 24-hr ambulatory blood pressure monitoring techniques (4); this subject deserves to be discussed separately.

BLOOD PRESSURE AS A GUIDELINE TO COMMENCE TREATMENT

Diastolic Blood Pressure

For the last 30 years or so, experts in hypertension—and, consequently, medical practitioners—have placed an almost exclusive emphasis on high diastolic blood pressure values as a risk factor and as a guideline for treatment (5). Undoubtedly, there is overwhelming evidence that increased diastolic blood pressure is a risk factor for cardiovascular disease—both cerebrovascular and coronary heart disease—in both males and females, with the most convincing traditional evidence coming from epidemiologic studies—first and foremost the one conducted in Framingham, Massachusetts.

There have been at least two major reasons for this predominant interest in diastolic blood pressure (2). The first reason has been the physiologic consideration that increased peripheral vascular resistance is the intrinsic hemodynamic disturbance in hypertension and that diastolic blood pressure is, though in an oversimplified way, a better indicator of peripheral resistance than is systolic pressure. The second reason is a historical one. When, at the beginning of the 1950s, hypertension first became treatable, attention was naturally directed to the most life-threatening forms [namely, malignant (or accelerated) and severe hypertension], which were associated with extreme elevations of diastolic blood pressure. The great success in treating these severe forms of hypertension led to the use of diastolic blood pressure as a guideline when the efficacy of antihypertensive therapy was also tested in more moderate forms of hypertension.

As a result of this attitude, all the controlled therapeutic trials upon which the management of hypertension is currently based have taken diastolic blood pressure values as the criteria for recruitment and for randomization of treatment. Figure 1 illustrates the diastolic blood pressure values used in each of the major trials planned to identify the diastolic blood pressure level above which treatment does more good than harm.

The results of these major trials have been presented and discussed in detail in previous chapters of this volume. To briefly illustrate the evidence relating to the decision-making process that is the main topic of this chapter, Table 1 [modified from a recent report by Strasser (6)] reports the therapeutic quotient (TQ) and the prevented event rate (PER) calculated for all large controlled trials of active versus placebo treatment (7–13). For each trial, the TQ gives the rate of morbid events (deaths, strokes, infarctions, etc.) in the placebo group, divided by those in the actively treated group, and is therefore a relative measure of benefit. The TQ figures in Table 1 show that within the range of mild hypertension, morbidity in the placebo groups exceeds that in the actively treated groups by 20–50% (TQ between 1.2 and 1.5).

It is equally important to consider the PERs (i.e., the difference between the rates of events in the placebo and actively treated groups), since it is an absolute measure of the rate of morbid events that have been prevented by active treatment of hypertension. Table 1 shows that while the PER values are very large in moderate to severe hypertension, the PER values are between 0.15 and 0.6 in most of the mild hypertension trials. A notable exception is the European Working Party on Hypertension in the Elderly (EWPHE), a trial on hypertensive patients aged 60 or more, in which the PER values are markedly higher (namely, 3.0), indicating that the higher mortality and morbidity of elderly subjects appear to make the results of hypertension treatment more rewarding at an older age than in middle-aged subjects.

One has to recognize that PER values as low as 0.15–0.6 do not make the results of mild hypertension treatment very exciting. The authors of the MRC trial, who have reported the lowest PER value of 0.15, have calculated from their data that 850 subjects with mild hypertension have to be actively treated for 1 year in order to prevent one stroke (13). However, another way of looking at these data is that of the public health expert. Strasser (6) has calculated that PER values of 0.15–0.6 indicate that in the seven to eight million population of a small country or of a large city, 800–3000 morbid events (predominantly strokes) might be prevented at the cost of treating half a million mild hypertensive subjects; and the authors of the Australian trial (10) have commented that "If the reduction in the rate of trial endpoints found in our volunteers were applied in the general population of Australia, we estimate that on average there would be 7000 fewer episodes of cardiovascular disease per year, including about 2000 fewer strokes and 2000 fewer deaths per year, at least over a 4-year period."

Furthermore, it has to be recognized that the conclusions of some controlled therapeutic trials may have been somewhat too pessimistic. For instance, before extrapolating to the general population the pessimistic conclusions of the Medical Research Council (MRC) trial that 850 patients

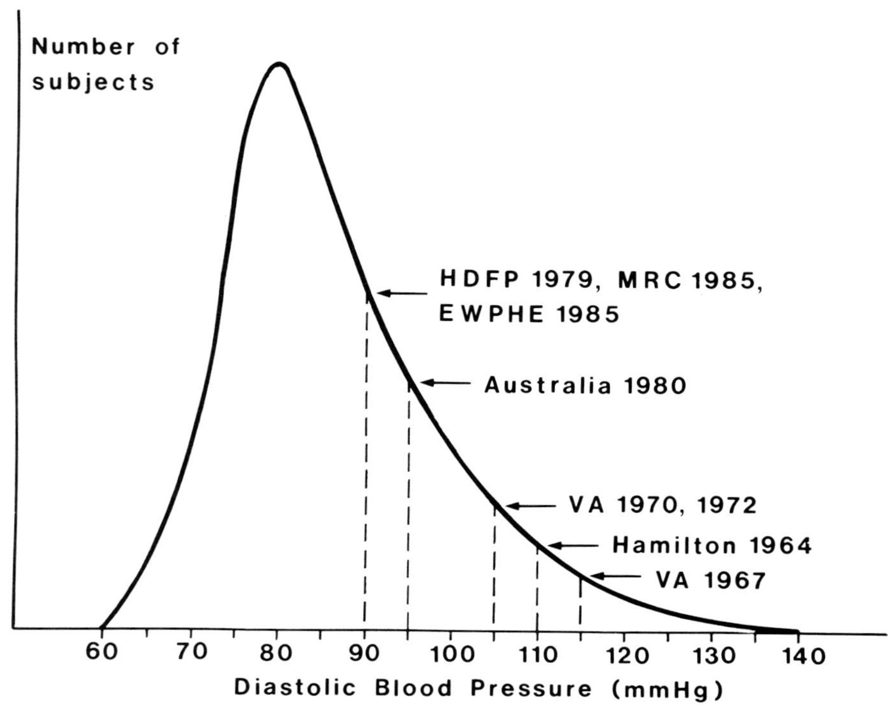

FIG. 1. Schematic diagram showing distribution of diastolic blood pressures in a community. The diagram indicates some of the major controlled therapeutic trials, and it also shows the levels of diastolic pressure above which a protective effect was demonstrated by active antihypertensive drug treatment. (From ref. 2.)

TABLE 1. *Results of controlled trials of placebo versus active treatment of hypertension*[a]

Study	Reference	DBP[b] (mmHg)	TQ[c]	PER[d]
VA 1967	7	115–129	14.3	23.9
VA 1970	8	105–114	4.0	7.3
VA 1970	8	90–104	1.5	2.7
USPHS	9	90–114	1.6	2.4
ANBPS	10	95–109	1.5	0.6
Oslo	11	90–109	1.4	0.5
EWPHE	12	90–119	1.25	3.0
MRC	13	90–109	1.2	0.15

[a] Modified from ref. 6.

[b] Diastolic blood pressure.

[c] Therapeutic quotient: the rates of events (deaths, strokes, infarctions, etc.) in the placebo groups, divided by these rates in the active-treatment groups.

[d] Prevented event rate: the absolute difference between the event rates in the placebo and active-treatment groups, expressed as per 100 patients per year.

with mild hypertension have to be treated for 1 year in order to prevent one stroke only, three aspects of the trial should be considered.

The first aspect is that in the MRC study, about 20% of the subjects with mild hypertension assigned to placebo had a diastolic blood pressure rising above 110 mmHg and were therefore given antihypertensive drugs. For statistical reasons, these subjects were analyzed in the placebo group, although they could be hardly considered untreated patients. It is clear that if progression to more severe hypertension (diastolic 110 mmHg or more) were to be classified as a morbid event, both the TQ and the PER in the MRC trial would have been higher.

A second aspect to be considered is that at least 18% of the subjects classified as mild hypertensives (diastolic 90–109 mmHg) at the entry into the MRC trial and assigned to placebo treatment were found not to be hypertensive according to the entry criteria in the following 3–5 years. This confirms what had previously been observed in the Australian trial on mild hypertension, where the proportion of mild hypertensives whose blood pressure became "normalized" under placebo treatment was even greater (14). It is likely that exclusion of these "false" hypertensives from the trial (e.g., by prolonging pretreatment observation to 3–4 months, as recommended below) would have increased the prevented event rate in the more restricted population of "true" mild hypertensives.

Finally, the problem of the patients withdrawn from treatment in the MRC trial has to be discussed. In the actively treated groups, as compared with the placebo group, there was an excess of over 15% of withdrawals because of adverse effects attributed to the drugs used. While this underscores the observation that treatment is not without disadvantages, this rather large proportion of withdrawals appears to depend on the nature of trials, in which patients obviously have to either (a) stick to the type of treatment and of drug to which they have been randomized or (b) withdraw. In common practice, doctors and patients have greater freedom in choosing and finding the most effective and least troublesome therapeutic regimen, and this is likely to increase effectiveness and reduce adverse effects of therapy, thus improving the TQ and the PER.

It should also be mentioned that a more recent analysis of the data of the MRC trial (15) has shown that the absolute benefit of treatment is much greater in the mild hypertensives who are classified as high risk by having other risk factors besides the mildly elevated diastolic pressure: About four high-risk patients would need to be treated (by a diuretic) for 5 years in order to avoid one stroke, whereas 242 low-risk patients would have to be treated for 5 years in order to avoid one stroke.

In summary, a precise indication of the level of diastolic blood pressure at which to commence treatment cannot be given. It is clear that at levels of 100 mmHg or above, the benefits of treatment are substantial; however, between 90 and 99 mmHg, the risk, albeit increased, is still relatively low, while the benefits, though significant, seem (on the whole) unimpressive, at least for the individual (but more consistent for public health goals). The 1989 guidelines provided by the Fifth Mild Hypertension Conference, jointly organized by the World Health Organization and the International Society of Hypertension (16), appear to be the wisest practical solution at this time (Fig. 2): Initiation of treatment should be considered when diastolic blood pressure is between 95 and 100 mmHg, but only after 3–6 months of observation with repeated measurements. As with all guidelines, these should be taken with some flexibility; furthermore, the limit for commencing treatment may be lowered to 90 mmHg if, for instance, there are other concomitant risk factors or if there is a strong family history of cardiovascular disease. As in all conditions, when the individual benefit is uncertain, the decision to start treatment at the 90–95 mmHg diastolic blood pressure level should be made by the physician together with the patient, and the conduct of treatment will be influenced by the occurrence (or nonoccurrence) of untoward effects of drugs, including symptoms.

Systolic Blood Pressure

For the reasons explained above, systolic blood pressure values have not been used as the recruitment criteria in controlled trials, and therefore no firm guidelines can be provided based on proven benefits of lowering systolic blood pressure. Even in the recent recommendations of the WHO/ISH (16), the authors had to be content with the vague statement, "At any level of diastolic blood pressure, increased levels of systolic blood pressure carry an additional risk."

This lack of solid information is particularly unfortunate in view of the observation that in moderate and mild hypertension, target organ damage is atherosclerotic rather than arteriolosclerotic or necrotic (17); moreover, for this type of damage, systolic values might represent a better predictive index than would diastolic values. This hypothesis is supported by three different sets of arguments: pathophysiologic, epidemiologic, and therapeutic.

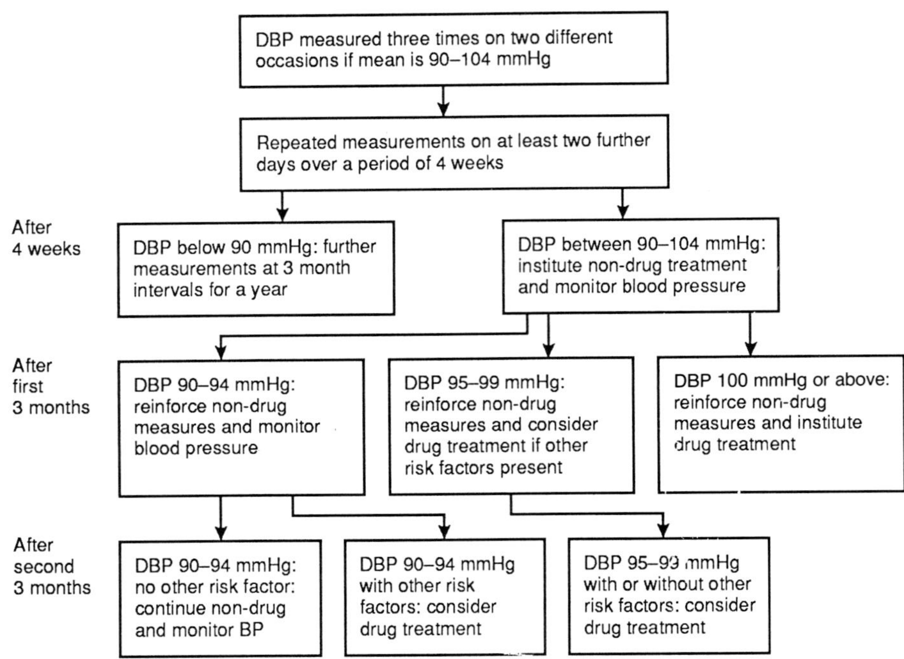

FIG. 2. Guidelines for treating mild hypertension, World Health Organization and International Society of Hypertension. (From ref. 16.)

Pathologic Considerations

Birkenhäger and de Leeuw (17) have pointed out that "Systolic pulse waves are known to create turbulence and reflected waves at sites of curving or branching arteries. It is possible that these disturbances of flow and pressure contribute to the disintegration of the endothelial lining and to plaque formation and its sequelae." Not only is loss of large-artery distensibility or compliance a characteristic of hypertension in the elderly, but it also appears to be an early phenomenon in essential hypertension, revealed by a concomitant increase in systolic blood pressure and in pulse-wave velocity (18). Furthermore, reduced aortic compliance with the consequent increase in systolic blood pressure is most important in the rise in parietal stress, is responsible for the development of left ventricular hypertrophy, and is, in the long term, a contributor to left ventricular failure (19).

Epidemiologic Considerations

Figure 3, from the Framingham Study (20), compares the impact of systolic blood pressures on the incidence of coronary heart disease. For both men and women aged 45 years and over, the slopes relating coronary heart disease incidence to systolic blood pressure were steeper than those relating it to diastolic pressure. Only in younger men did there appear to be a significant difference in the slopes favoring diastolic pressure. Calculation of coefficients for the regression of cardiovascular events of any type on systolic and diastolic pressures (Table 2) reveals that systolic blood pressure is the more potent contributor to all clinical sequelae of hypertension—not only coronary heart disease but also cerebrovascular accidents, congestive heart failure, cardiovascular death, and death by all causes (21).

Evidence from Controlled Clinical Trials

The recent trials of controlled therapeutic intervention also provide useful information on the importance of systolic blood pressure as a predictor of mortality and morbidity, although they have not been planned to explore the level of systolic pressure at which treatment should be started (2). In the MRC trial on mild hypertension (13), initial systolic blood pressure was found to correlate significantly with subsequent incidence of strokes, coronary events, cardiovascular events, and death by all causes, whereas initial diastolic blood pressure correlated less well with any type of event. Figure 4 illustrates the relation existing between pretreatment systolic blood pressure and stroke rates in the patients of the MRC trial treated by placebo; the figure also shows that stroke incidence is reduced by treatment with bendrofluazide and, in nonsmokers, with propranolol (15). Furthermore, we have already mentioned that a recent analysis of the MRC data (15) has shown that high-risk patients with mild hypertension have a greater absolute benefit from treatment. It should be stressed here that a high systolic blood pressure was included among the additional risks considered for the high-risk profile (15). This means that, for the same level of diastolic blood pressure, high systolic levels add to the risk of cardiovascular events and increase the benefits of treatment.

The recent EWPHE trial (12) has also provided useful information. The effects of active treatment and of placebo were analyzed according to systolic and diastolic blood pressures measured before randomization (22). As shown in Fig. 5, cardiovascular event rates rose in parallel with increasing initial systolic blood pressure levels in both the actively treated and the placebo-treated groups, but no relation was apparent with pretreatment diastolic values. Furthermore, at all systolic blood pressure levels above 160

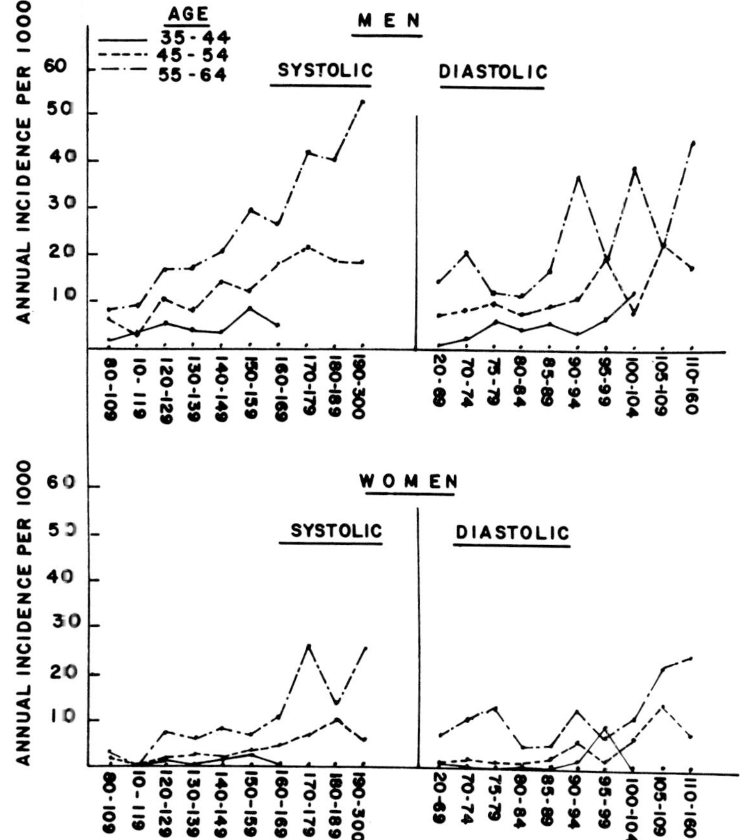

FIG. 3. Average annual incidence of coronary heart disease (14-year follow-up), according to systolic versus diastolic blood pressure, for men and women aged 35–64 years, Framingham Study. (From ref. 20.)

mmHg, active treatment was associated with lower morbidity rates than was placebo treatment (Fig. 5).

Evidence for Isolated Systolic Hypertension

Isolated systolic hypertension in both men and women appears to be associated with increased risk for cardiovascular disease. According to the Framingham Study (21), in men and women aged 55–74 years the incidence of cardiovascular disease is 3.5 times (men) and 3.8 times (women) greater among people with isolated systolic hypertension than among normotensives. However, no solid evidence is available from controlled trials as to whether treatment of isolated systolic hypertension carries benefits that outweigh its disadvantages. Although showing, as mentioned above, a net benefit of therapeutic lowering of systolic pressure levels of 160 mmHg or above, the data of the study performed by the EWPHE refer to patients whose diastolic pressure values were also elevated, and they cannot be extrapolated to patients with isolated systolic hypertension. Available evidence from two trials including isolated systolic hypertension patients is conflicting. A subanalysis of the trial on elderly patients in primary care (23) suggests that treatment of hypertension in the elderly is beneficial when diastolic pressure also is elevated, whereas the trend is reversed (i.e., greater morbidity in the actively treated than in the placebo group) when isolated systolic hypertension is considered. On the other hand, the pilot study of the Systolic Hypertension in the Elderly Program (24) has shown a trend, albeit nonsignificant, in favor of active treatment.

In summary, precise guidelines about commencement of antihypertensive treatment of systolic blood pressure levels are not available, but there is clear evidence not only that elevated systolic pressure is an important risk factor (probably even greater than diastolic pressure) but also that, when systolic blood pressure is 160 mmHg or above, active treatment is associated to reduced morbidity. This evidence is limited to hypertensive patients whose diastolic pressure also is elevated, and it cannot be extrapolated to patients with isolated systolic hypertension until results of current trials directed at this type of hypertension become avail-

TABLE 2. *Coefficients for regression of specific cardiovascular events with respect to systolic and diastolic blood pressure: Framingham Study 20-year follow-up, men and women 45–74 years old*[a]

	Men		Women	
Event	SBP	DBP	SBP	DBP
CHD	0.3299	0.2697	0.4630	0.3519
CHD death	0.4081	0.3424	0.5380	0.4091
CVA	0.5966	0.5324	0.6096	0.5924
CHF	0.5298	0.3264	0.5466	0.3563
Death	0.2770	0.1850	0.2662	0.1709
CV death	0.3672	0.2452	0.4859	0.2996

[a] From ref. 21. CHD, coronary heart disease; SBP, systolic blood pressure; DBP, diastolic blood pressure; CVA, cerebrovascular accident; CV, cardiovascular; CHF, congestive heart failure.

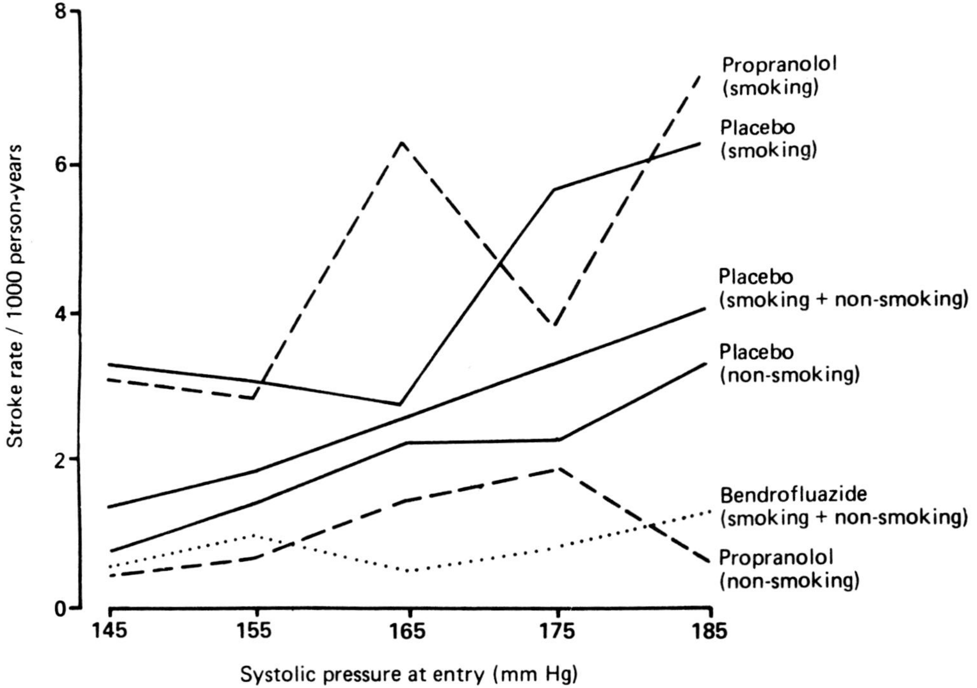

FIG. 4. Stroke rate per 1000 person-years versus systolic pressure at entry, with respect to treatment and smoking state. (From ref. 15.)

able. For the moment, it can be concluded that whenever diastolic blood pressure is 90 mmHg or above, systolic blood pressure values of 160 mmHg or greater carry an additional risk and should favor the doctor's decision toward active treatment.

BLOOD PRESSURE AS A GUIDELINE TO CONDUCT TREATMENT

In this section, we will discuss the following important problem: To what level should blood pressure be lowered in order to optimize the results of antihypertensive treatment?

Evidence from Controlled Trials

The Hypertension Detection and Follow-up Program (HDFP) (25) showed that the lower mortality of patients under stepped care (SC) as compared to that of patients under referred care (RC) was associated with an average reduction in diastolic blood pressure to 83.4 mmHg (SC) as compared to 87.8 mmHg (RC). It was therefore suggested that even a slightly more marked reduction of diastolic blood pressure induced by treatment carried significant benefits, and it was hinted that an even greater reduction of diastolic blood pressure to below 85 mmHg might have induced additional benefits. It has been remarked, how-

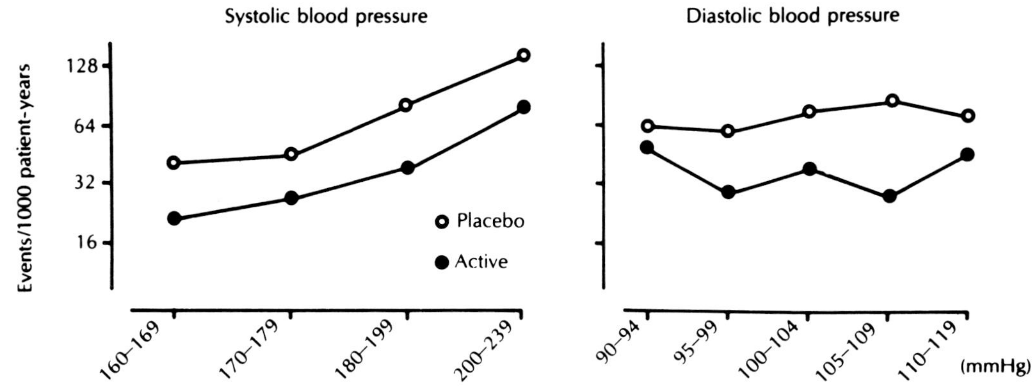

FIG. 5. Cardiovascular-study terminating events in four systolic blood pressure groups (obtained at randomization) show a steady increase in both placebo-treated and actively treated subjects. This trend is absent in five diastolic blood pressure groups, indicating that systolic pressure is more important than diastolic pressure as a risk factor in these patients aged 60 years and over. (Data from ref. 22.)

ever, that the lower diastolic blood pressure attained by SC treatment was the average result of a greater number of patients receiving antihypertensive therapy in the SC group than in the RC group (63.8% versus 43.0%) and that this is the most likely explanation of the lower mortality in SC patients (26). Therefore, no definite conclusion about the best level of diastolic blood pressure to be attained by antihypertensive therapy can be drawn from the HDFP study.

More definite information on this problem is provided by analysis of the MRC data (13,15,27,28). Systolic blood pressure achieved during treatment was found to correlate with morbid events better than diastolic blood pressure, therefore appearing to be a better guideline as to how to conduct treatment. Figure 6 shows the good relationship observed in the MRC trial between systolic blood pressure measured after 6 months of placebo and event rates for coronary disease, stroke, and all-cause mortality. Even in patients actively treated by either the beta-blocker propranolol or the diuretic bendrofluazide, stroke incidence was clearly related to the level of systolic blood pressure attained after 6 months of treatment and was less well related to diastolic blood pressure at the same time (Fig. 7). Figure 7 also shows that the curves relating systolic and diastolic pressure values during treatment of stroke flatten below systolic values of 135–144 mmHg and below diastolic values of 85–89 mmHg, suggesting little additional benefit from further blood pressure reduction.

The Problem of the J-Shaped Curve

It is obvious that blood pressure cannot be reduced to increasingly lower levels without reaching a point at which organ perfusion may be compromised and where morbidity and mortality increased rather than decreased. This phenomenon means that the curve relating morbidity to systolic or diastolic blood pressure values reached during treatment should be J- or U-shaped (i.e., the lowest morbidity rate would occur at intermediate pressure values, inflecting upwards not only at higher pressures but also at lower pressures). The real problem, however, is whether blood pressures that are commonly taken as goals of treatment or of controlled therapeutic trials may already be in the upwards inflecting part of the J-curve. The evidence is rather controversial, but the problem is of such a great practical importance as to deserve detailed discussion.

We have reported above that the data of the MRC trial show flattening of the incidence of cardiovascular events for systolic blood pressure levels below 135–144 mmHg and for diastolic blood pressure levels below 85–89 mmHg; however, from Figs. 6 and 7, no J-shaped curve is detectable, even for blood pressure levels below 125/85 mmHg. A specific search (by the MRC investigators) for a J-shaped relationship between blood pressure and the incidence of myocardial infarction in either the placebo or actively treated group has found no support for such a relationship (15). Likewise, the International Prospective Primary Prevention Study in Hypertension (IPPPSH), a prospective trial comparing beta-blocker treatment with non-beta-blocker-based treatment, did not observe any trend toward a J-shaped curve in either treatment group, even at diastolic pressures below 80 mmHg (Fig. 8) (29). On the other hand, the authors of another similar study (the Heart Attack Primary Prevention in Hypertension, or HAPPHY, trial) (30) have briefly reported to have calculated a J-shaped curve in their patients (31).

The issue of the J-shaped curve has been revived by another recent, albeit noncontrolled, study in which 939 patients with moderate to severe hypertension were treated with the $beta_1$-selective blocker atenolol over a 10-year period (32). This study confirmed that blood pressure achieved on treatment, particularly systolic blood pressure, is an excellent predictor of death from all causes and death from myocardial infarction, particularly for men. Good control of systolic blood pressure was associated with fewer deaths. These observations are in general agreement with

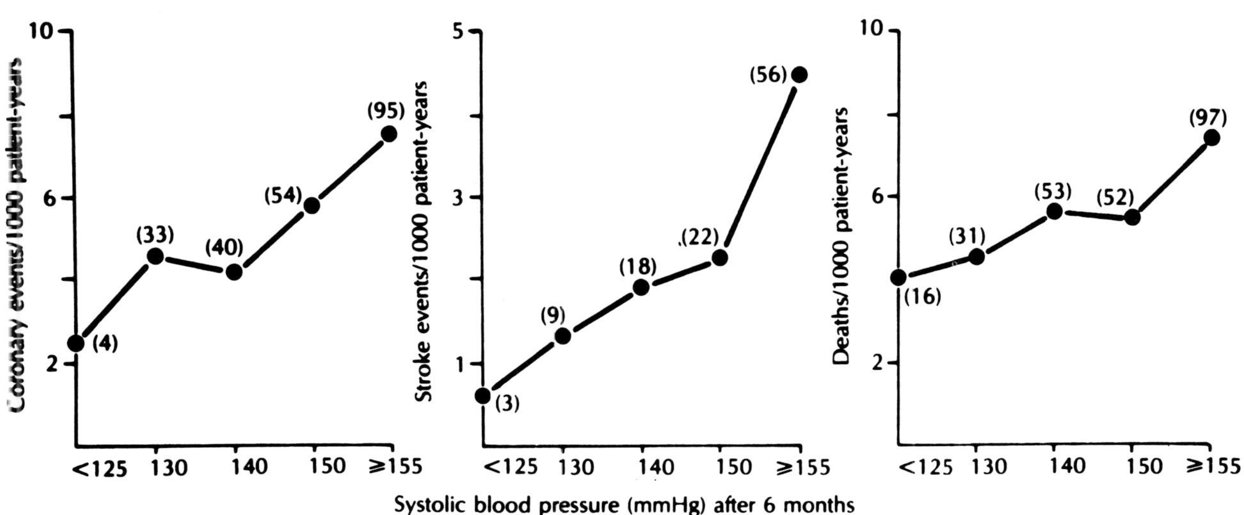

FIG. 6. Relationship between event rates and systolic blood pressure measured after 6 months of placebo. The three panels give event rates (fatal and nonfatal) for coronary disease, stroke, and all-cause mortality. Men and women and smokers and nonsmokers are analyzed together. Figures in parentheses give the number of events. (From ref. 27.)

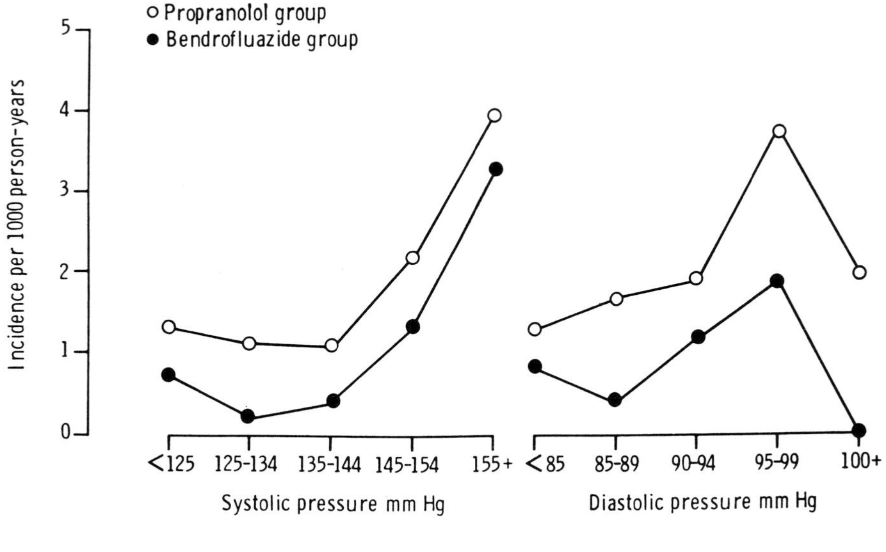

FIG. 7. Stroke incidence per 1000 person-years according to 6-month systolic and diastolic pressure and randomized active treatment (both sexes). (From ref. 28.)

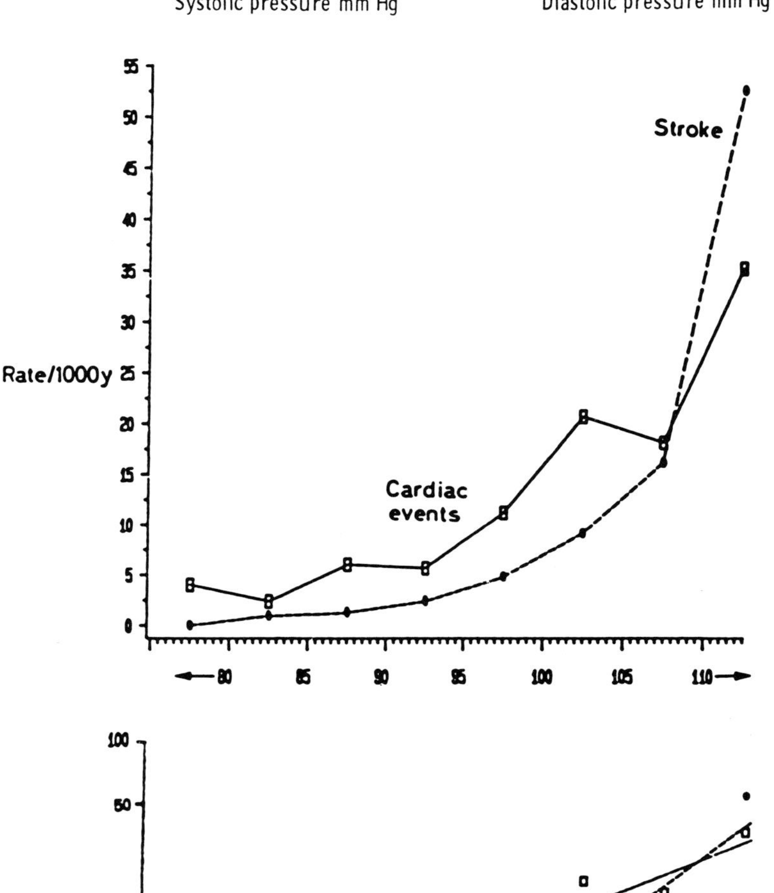

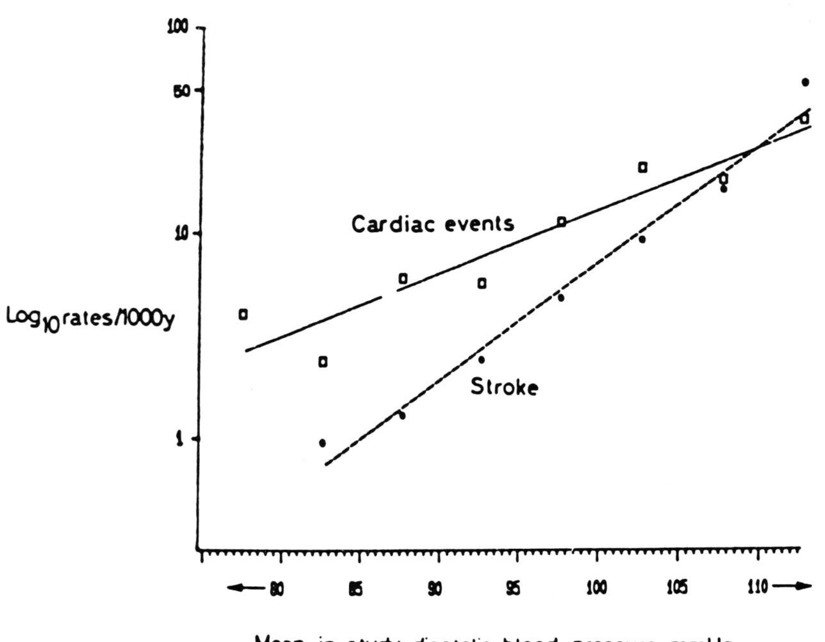

FIG. 8. Cardiac events and stroke rates related to diastolic blood pressure during antihypertensive treatment. (From ref. 29.)

the results of the MRC trial (13,15,27). More detailed analysis of the study by Cruickshank et al. (32) suggests some interesting implications. In Fig. 9 the patients are divided into tertiles according to mean systolic blood pressure achieved during treatment. Total mortality and deaths from myocardial infarction rose progressively and significantly from the lowest to the highest tertile of systolic blood pressure (from 129 to 163 mmHg). However, the data from Fig. 9 suggest that the relationship between systolic blood pressure and death from stroke may be J-shaped, with fewer deaths in the middle tertile but a somewhat greater incidence of fatal strokes in the tertile with lowest systolic pressures. This was particularly evident in older patients. There also appeared to be a J-shaped curve for deaths from myocardial infarction, when these were related to diastolic (rather than systolic) blood pressure; however, Fig. 10 shows that this was only found in patients with clinical signs of ischemic heart disease (33). Likewise, a recent analysis of the DHSS Hypertension Care Computing Project (DHCCP) (34) has also calculated a higher rate of ischemic heart disease deaths in hypertensive patients with treated diastolic pressures below 86 mmHg, but this relationship was found in patients with a positive history of ischemic heart disease as well as in patients with a negative history of the disease.

The study by Cruickshank et al. (32,33) is unfortunately a noncontrolled one; furthermore, in the absence of a control group, it is impossible to be certain that the greater mortality in the group of patients with lowest blood pressures was a real consequence of overtreatment, and it is difficult to exclude that low blood pressures were simply a sign, for instance, of a more severe impairment of left ventricular function and, hence, a predictor of death from myocardial infarction. The latter explanation is strengthened by reports—from surveys (35,36) and from a randomized trial (37)—that a J-curve relationship between diastolic pressure and coronary mortality may also be found among untreated hypertensive patients. Furthermore, the investigators of the Glasgow Blood Pressure Clinic, although calculating a nonlinear relationship between treated diastolic pressure and coronary death rate, did not find any relationship between (a) the change in diastolic blood pressure during treatment and (b) coronary death (38). Finally, if the really important question is not whether there is a J-shaped curve but, rather, how to determine the low level of blood pressure at which the mortality or morbidity curve inflects toward higher values, little help can be derived from calculations such as those provided by the authors stressing the J-shaped curve [e.g., Cruickshank et al. (33)], in which all values from 85 mmHg downward are lumped in a single group: Is the danger already in the 80–85 mmHg range, or does it result from much lower blood pressure values?

Despite these limitations, the strength of Cruickshank's general interpretation is in its correlation with physiologic considerations. Physiology of cerebral circulation makes it reasonable to expect that excessive reduction of systolic blood pressure in elderly hypertensives may blunt the benefits of antihypertensive therapy in preventing strokes; this is because cerebral perfusion is known to depend on systolic blood pressure—particularly in elderly patients, in whom occlusive carotid lesions are more likely to occur. It is equally reasonable to expect that excessive reduction of diastolic (rather than systolic) pressure in patients with ischemic heart disease may blunt the benefits of antihypertensive therapy in preventing myocardial infarction, since

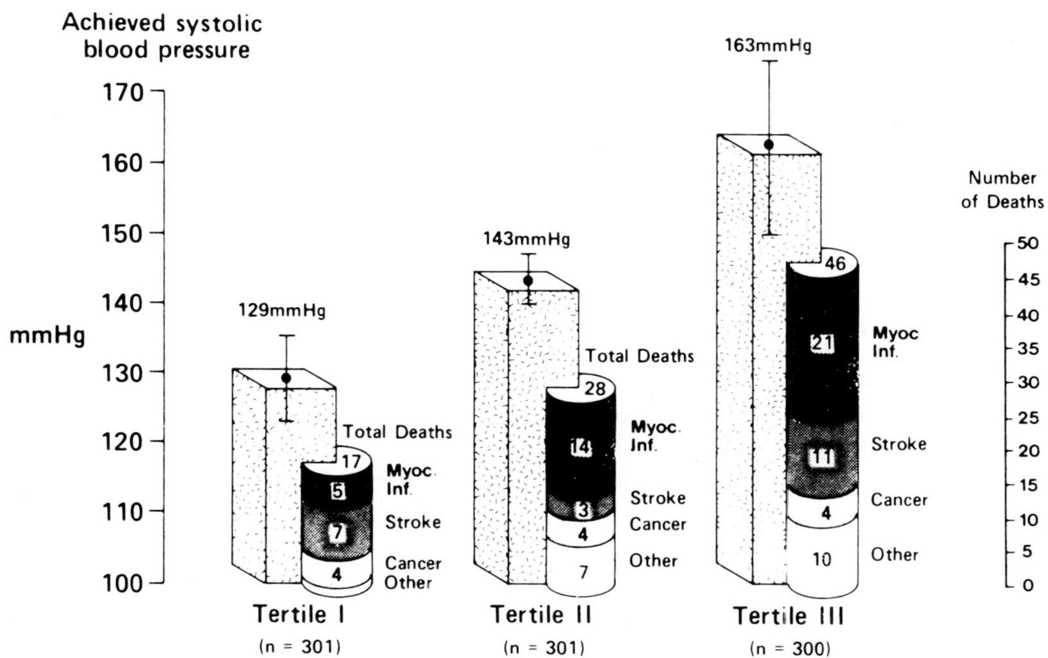

FIG. 9. Effect of controlling systolic blood pressure (SBP) upon mortality in a group of 939 hypertensive patients treated with atenolol for 10 years. Population of patients is divided into tertiles according to SBP level achieved by treatment. Myoc. Inf., myocardial infarction. (From ref. 32.)

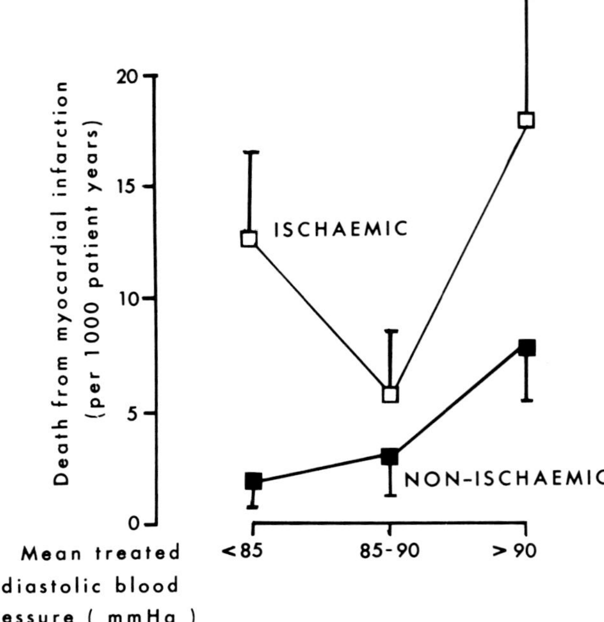

FIG. 10. Relationship between mortality rate (SEM shown) from myocardial infarction in ischemic and nonischemic patients, and treated diastolic blood pressure (age-adjusted). (From ref. 33.)

coronary perfusion is known to depend on diastolic (rather than systolic) blood pressure. On physiologic grounds, Strandgaard and Haunsø (39) have recently argued that a J-shaped curve should be more easily found when myocardial (rather than cerebral) ischemic events are considered, because autoregulation of myocardial blood flow (especially in the subendocardium) is seemingly more severely impaired by hypertension than is cerebral blood flow autoregulation and because oxygen delivery to the myocardium more critically depends on perfusion than does oxygen delivery to the brain, with myocardial (but not cerebral) oxygen extraction being already near-maximum in normal conditions.

In summary, both systolic and diastolic blood pressure values achieved during treatment (and particularly systolic values) are good guidelines to be followed in order to properly conduct antihypertensive therapy and to predict its outcome. The risk that excessive lowering of blood pressure may blunt the advantages of treatment is a reasonable concern, although there is no solid proof, for the time being, that, at least for the majority of hypertensive patients, the blood pressure values most commonly achieved by current treatment and established as goal of trials are of any substantial risk. However, the observation (in the MRC and in other controlled trials) that no additional benefits can be expected from lowering systolic blood pressure to below 135–144 mmHg and diastolic blood pressure to below 85–89 mmHg suggests that these levels should be taken as reasonable treatment goals, at least for most patients. The risk of excessively lowering blood pressure in complicated patients, especially those with occlusive arterial lesions, is a realistic one, however, but it can easily be avoided by carefully, slowly, and progressively lowering blood pressure and by looking at the global response of the patient, which also includes assessment of neurologic, cardiac, and renal changes accompanying blood pressure reduction (40,41).

CONDITIONS UNDER WHICH BLOOD PRESSURE SHOULD BE MEASURED AS A GUIDELINE TO TREATMENT

Casual and Office Blood Pressure

Posture

Posture, rest, and exercise are known to influence blood pressure; and since the beginning of the era of hypertension research and antihypertensive therapy, it has been clear that conditions of measurement had to be standardized in order to have common tools for description and risk prediction. The choice of the seated position has been determined less by physiologic considerations (systolic and diastolic values in the seated position are commonly intermediate between the slightly different values in the supine and upright positions) than by practical considerations—the seated position being the easiest to use in epidemiologic studies (*casual blood pressure*) and in medical practice (*office blood pressure*). All epidemiologic studies from which risk has been calculated, as well as all controlled therapeutic trials from which guidelines to treatment can be derived, have measured blood pressure in the seated position. Therefore, measurements in this position should commonly be used in the decision-making process of the doctor (16,42).

Measurements in the supine and upright positions have also been used in guiding antihypertensive therapy—especially in the early years, when several of the available drugs could easily induce postural hypotension. This is rarely necessary with current drugs, but measurement in the upright posture is still recommended—not only in clinical studies of new compounds but also in the treatment of elderly or of diabetic hypertensives, who may be particularly prone to falls in blood pressure on standing upright.

Rest and Exercise

The choice of the seated position obviously means that blood pressure is taken at rest, and current recommendations are that the subjects remain seated quietly for about 5 min before measurements are taken (16,42). It is also recommended (42) that the patients avoid smoking for at least half an hour before the visit (because smoking can raise blood pressure) (43) and also avoid a large meal during the few hours preceding measurement (because a large meal can considerably lower blood pressure) (44). Even at rest, blood pressure values can change from moment to moment (see below); therefore it is recommended that at least two or three measurements be taken at each occasion during a 2- to 3-min period and that the values be averaged (16,45). This average is the common guideline to treatment.

Exercise, both dynamic and static, is known to markedly influence blood pressure, and there is a periodically recurrent discussion as to whether the blood pressure peaks elicited by either type of exercise should also be considered for treatment (46). Unfortunately, no prospective study has explored whether exercise blood pressure is a better or an additional predictor of the risk of high blood pressure. In lack of this evidence, little use can be made of exercise blood pressure values as guidelines to treatment. However, the recently reported finding that echocardiographic indices of left ventricular hypertrophy are more closely related to blood pressure measured at the worksite, in a stressful condition, than to physician or home measurements on a non-working day (Fig. 11) (47) suggests that the issue of exercise or stress blood pressure as a predictor of risk deserves appropriate investigation.

Ambulatory Blood Pressure Monitoring: Is 24-hr Blood Pressure Likely to Become a More Precise Guideline to Treatment?

It has already been remarked in another section of this chapter that, although casual and office blood pressures, both systolic and diastolic values, are predictors of subsequent cardiovascular damage, the predictive power is strong only when blood pressure values are very high. Unfortunately, casual and office blood pressures are much less satisfactory predictors when blood pressure is in the so-called range of mild hypertension; as a consequence, a large number of mild hypertensives must receive treatment in order to prevent only few cardiovascular events. An important reason for that may be in the limitations by which the risk factor "hypertension" is quantitatively assessed. Indeed, blood pressure is highly variable (3); and it is something of a paradox that the diagnosis of a condition such as hypertension, which is defined in terms of blood pressure values, relies upon crude and occasional measurements such as casual or office blood pressures and that too often a decision to treat for life is based upon a single blood pressure measurement or upon a few blood pressure measurements, often taken over a period of less than a minute (2,4).

Invasive and noninvasive techniques for 24-hr ambulatory blood pressure monitoring in hypertensive patients are now available. Their use in research and in clinical practice has been extensively reviewed (48) and is also reviewed in other chapters of this volume. Only those aspects that have an impact on the decision-making process regarding what level of blood pressure should be treated are discussed below.

Blood Pressure Variability

Invasive ambulatory blood pressure techniques have allowed the marked variability of blood pressure throughout the 24-hr period to be quantified. The average 24-hr standard deviation of ± 10–12 mmHg that we have measured in both normotensives and hypertensives (3) indicates that in many subjects, blood pressure is above or below the conventional levels separating normotension from hypertension several times during the 24-hr period.

Pressor Effect of Blood Pressure Measurement

Ambulatory blood pressure monitoring has also allowed the recognition and quantification of the pressor effect resulting from the doctor or nurse taking the measurement. Although we have shown that the alarm pressor reaction induced by a nurse is smaller and shorter-lasting than that elicited by a doctor (Fig. 12) (49), these considerable and

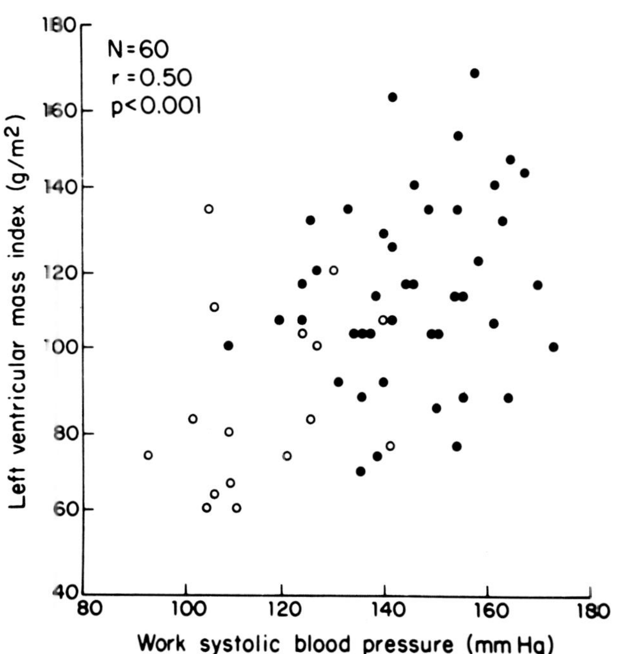

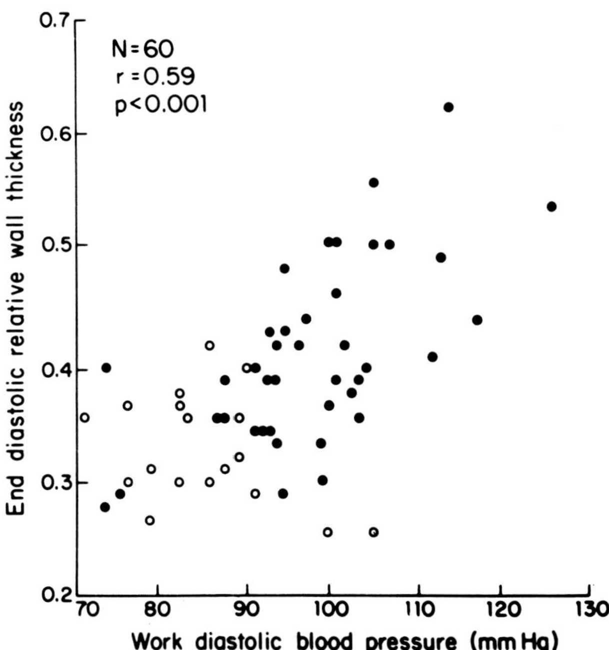

FIG. 11. Correlation between left ventricular mass index and worksite systolic blood pressure (**left**) and between relative wall thickness and worksite diastolic blood pressure (**right**). (From ref. 47.)

frequent pressor reactions may conceal the more limited number of true, permanent hypertensives in a large group of false occasional hypertensives, thus making the predictive value of office blood pressure often uncertain. This alarm pressor reaction to measurement is likely to account, at least in part, for the 18–50% of subjects who were classified as mild hypertensives at the entry into the MRC (13) and Australian (14) trials and who were found not to be hypertensive in the following 3–5 years, despite receiving no antihypertensive treatment.

Evaluation of Efficacy of Antihypertensive Therapy

Ambulatory blood pressure monitoring devices have been shown to be useful in assessing the efficacy of different antihypertensive agents in drug trials (50); in principle, these devices might become useful in clinical practice to provide a more faithful evaluation of the results of therapy.

Evaluation and Prediction of Risk Related to Blood Pressure

Ambulatory blood pressure monitoring has given some support to the common and reasonable (though unproven) hypothesis that the adverse cardiovascular effects of hypertension are related to both the height and the duration of the blood pressure elevation (51). In this context, ambulatory blood pressure monitoring may provide an important forecast of future damage. Blood pressure measurements thus provided are unspoiled by the alarm pressor reaction,

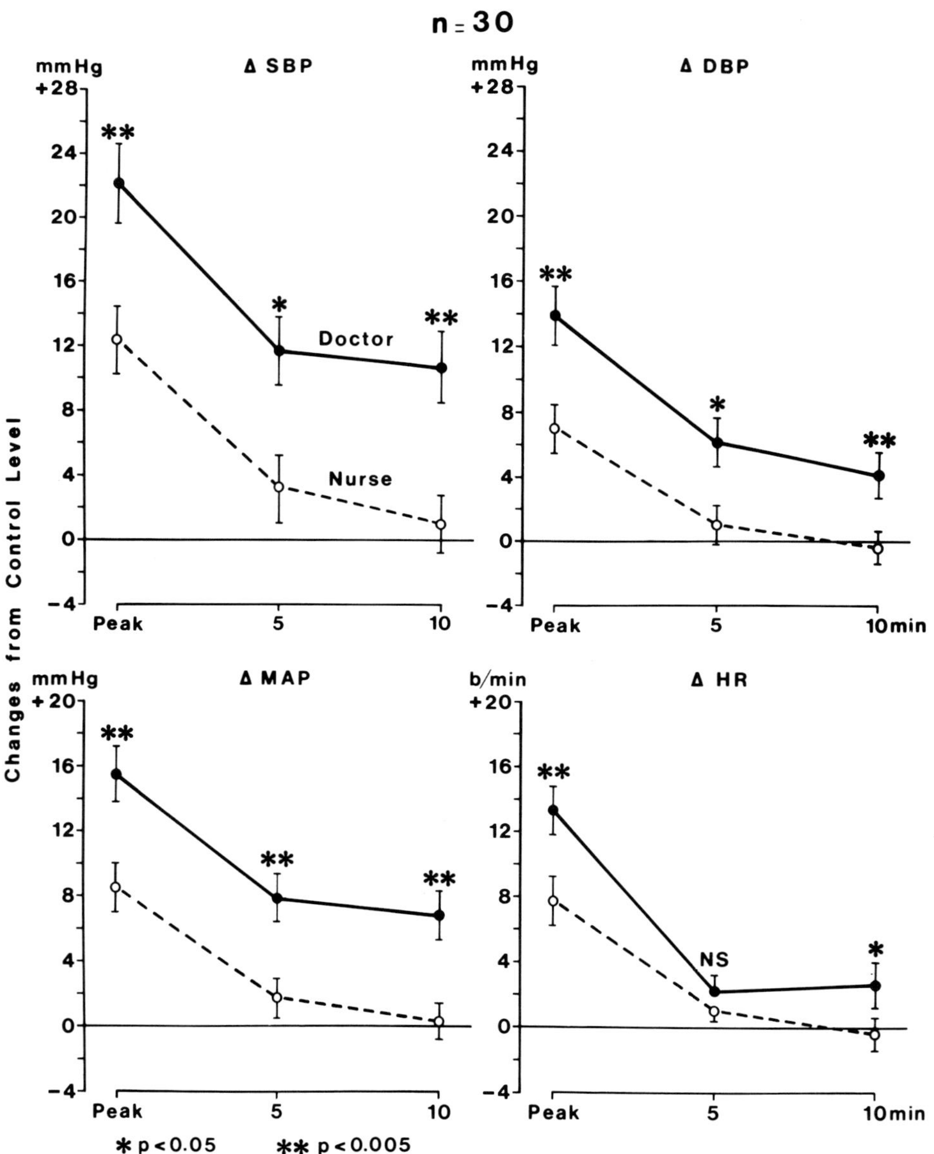

FIG. 12. Comparison of maximum (or peak) rises in systolic blood pressure (SBP), diastolic blood pressure (DBP), mean arterial pressure (MAP), and heart rate (HR) occurring in 30 subjects during a physician's and a nurse's visits. The rises occurring at the 5th and 10th minutes of the visits are also shown. Data are expressed as mean (±SEM) changes from a control value taken 4 min before each visit. (From ref. 49.)

even at the times when the cuff is inflated (52); furthermore, it is likely that frequently repeated measurements during the day and night, as well as during exertion and rest, provide a better time integral of the strain exerted upon the heart and blood vessels.

Several studies suggest that both daytime and 24-hr blood pressure means obtained by either invasive (53–55) or noninvasive (47,56–58) blood pressure monitoring correlate with target organ damage and cardiovascular complications better than do casual or office blood pressure measurements.

In a recent study by our group (51,59), 24-hr blood pressure was recorded intra-arterially by the Oxford method in 108 hospitalized subjects with essential hypertension ranging from mild to severe. The 24-hr means and standard deviations for systolic, mean, and diastolic blood pressures were related to the rate and severity of target organ damage, assessed by clinical examination and quantified according to a predetermined score. Twenty-four-hour blood pressure means were found to be variably different from blood pressure determined by cuff measurements: In most subjects, 24-hr blood pressure means were lower than cuff blood pressures.

The 108 patients were ranked in five groups according to whether the cuff mean blood pressure on admission to the hospital ward was (1) <110 mmHg, (2) between 111 and 124 mmHg, (3) between 125 and 140 mmHg, (4) between 141 and 155 mmHg, and (5) >155 mmHg. Each group was subdivided into two classes according to whether the 24-hr mean blood pressure of the patient was below or above the average 24-hr mean blood pressure of the respective group. Figure 13 shows that although cuff blood pressure was the same in both classes of each of the five groups, within each group the proportion of patients with target organ damage (as well as the overall severity of target organ damage) was always greater in the class with higher 24-hr pressure than in the class with lower 24-hr pressure, with the only exception being the group with the highest cuff blood pressures (group 5).

The 108 patients were also ranked in five groups according to whether their 24-hr mean arterial pressure was (1) <93 mmHg, (2) between 94 and 105 mmHg, (3) between 106 and 117 mmHg, (4) between 118 and 130 mmHg, and (5) >130 mmHg. Each group was subdivided into two classes according to whether the variability index of mean blood pressure was below or above the average value of the respective group. Figure 14 shows that although the mean 24-hr blood pressure was the same in both classes of each of the five groups, within each group the proportion of patients with target organ damage (as well as the overall severity of target organ damage) was always greater in the class with higher 24-hr variability than in the class with lower 24-hr variability. These findings demonstrate that the severity of hypertension is more closely related to 24-hr mean blood pressure than to cuff values. They also provide an unequivocal demonstration that hypertension-dependent target organ damage also relates to the extent of blood pressure variability.

Although this study (51,59), as well as the previous studies already mentioned (47,53–58), supports the superiority of ambulatory over more traditional blood pressure measurements in the diagnosis of hypertension and in the evaluation of the risk related to blood pressure, the limitation of this correlative approach should be recognized—the most important limitation being that a correlation cannot safely be translated into a cause–effect relationship and into a prediction without additional proof (2).

The only prospective investigation comparing the prognostic value of office and noninvasive ambulatory blood pressure measurements is that conducted by Perloff et al. (58), who have followed up a large cohort (1076) of hypertensive patients who were initially evaluated using both techniques. During the average 5-year follow-up, cardiovascular morbidity and mortality were significantly greater in those patients whose ambulatory blood pressure was higher than expected from office measurements, compared with the patients whose ambulatory blood pressure was lower than expected.

Problems Related to the Use of Ambulatory Blood Pressure Monitoring as a Guide to Treatment

These are certainly promising data. Various types of noninvasive ambulatory blood pressure machines are available now, either with nonautomatic or with automatic cuff inflation (48), and although all these machines are not without problems, there is no doubt that their noninvasive nature will spread the use of these machines and will be providing a lot of useful information in the near future.

However, the widespread introduction of ambulatory blood pressure monitoring in clinical practice should be observed with both hope and concern (4,60). The reasons for hope have been illustrated in the previous paragraphs. The reasons for concern are the following.

First, the present prognostic standards with regard to the level of blood pressure to be treated are based on (a) large population studies (such as that of Framingham, Massachusetts) performed over several decades and (b) the results of controlled therapeutic trials which include many thousands of patients. It would be unwise to substitute these admittedly inaccurate, yet well-tested, guidelines with the results of studies based on small numbers of subjects followed up for short periods of time, regardless of the sophistication of these studies.

Second, even if ambulatory blood pressure were to be proven as a more precise and reliable predictor of cardiovascular damage secondary to hypertension, new standards of prediction should be elaborated for ambulatory blood pressure. It would be unwarranted, and probably misleading, to use the same standard values originally used to calculate the risk of casual or office blood pressure and to decide about the level of blood pressure to be treated. Even a prospective study such as that by Perloff et al. (58) has not provided new guidelines to treatment besides the important (but generic) observation that, for the same level of office blood pressure, there is less risk when 24-hr blood pressure is lower than when it is higher.

Third, elaborate criteria and complicated devices are unlikely to help in screening, diagnosing, and treating such a widespread condition as arterial hypertension, where cost and time are important factors. However, it cannot be denied that the cost of an advanced diagnostic procedure,

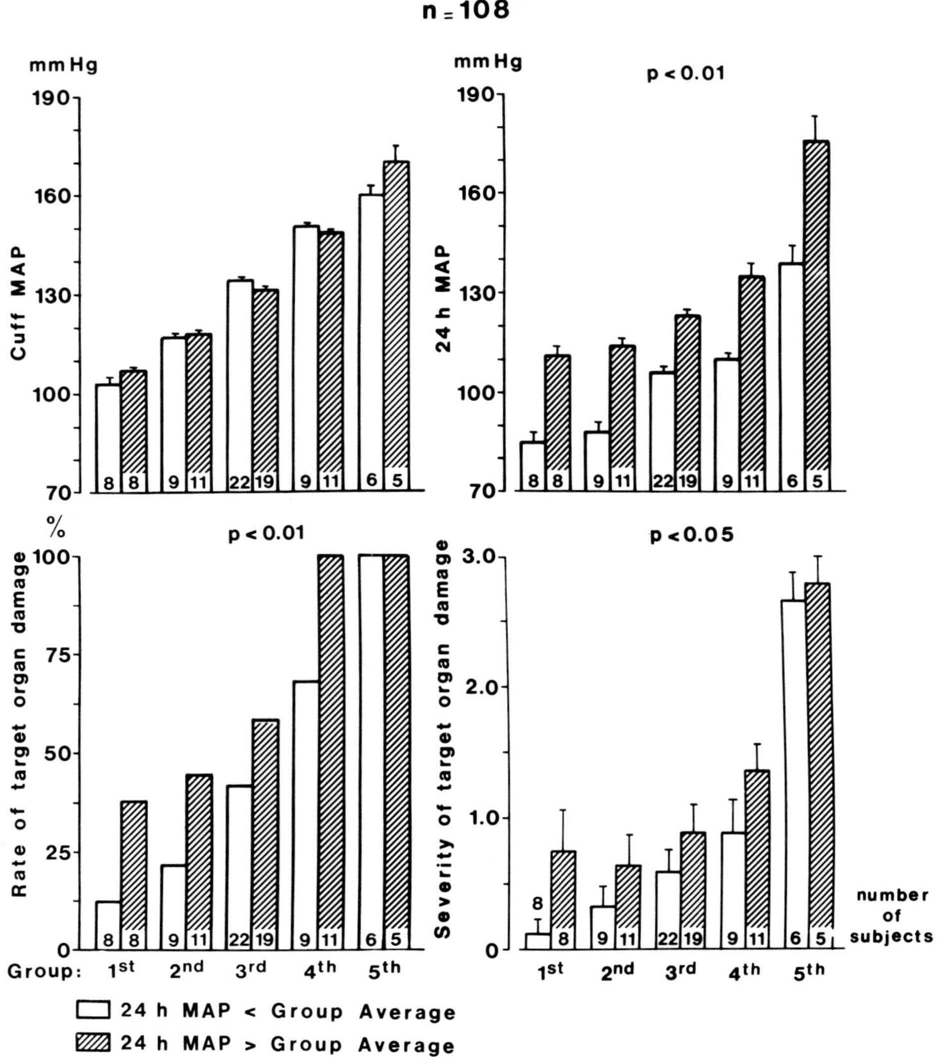

FIG. 13. Rate and severity in target organ damage in 108 subjects. The subjects were divided into five groups according to the increasing value of their mean arterial pressure (MAP) as measured by the cuff method on admission to a hospital ward. The patients of each group were subdivided into two classes according to whether their 24-hr MAP was below or above the 24-hr average MAP of the group. Note that within each group the two classes had a similar cuff blood pressure but that the rate and the severity of target organ damage were less in the classes in which 24-hr average MAP were lower. For each class, rate of target organ damage is expressed as the percentage of subjects exhibiting the damage, and severity of target organ damage is expressed as the subjects' average score; *p* refers to the difference between all couples of classes. (From ref. 59.)

such as ambulatory blood pressure monitoring, may be worthwhile in offsetting the greater cost and the longer time required for treating thousands of mild hypertensive subjects in order to save only a few lives. In this frame of mind, one should not disregard the possibility that other procedures, which might be simpler than ambulatory blood pressure monitoring but more meaningful than casual or office blood pressure, such as home blood pressure assessment, may also improve our present low power of predictability.

CONCLUSIONS

Information concerning the level of blood pressure at which treatment should be commenced, as well as the level which should be taken as the goal of treatment, is incomplete; moreover, current guidelines have to be considered as provisional suggestions about which consensus is large but not unanimous.

As to the issue of the blood pressure level at which treatment should start, solid information is only available concerning diastolic values, although it is known that elevated systolic pressure is at least as important a risk factor as is elevated diastolic pressure. There is general agreement on the need to administer antihypertensive therapy when diastolic pressure is 100 mmHg or above. At diastolic values between 90 and 99 mmHg the risk, albeit increased, is still relatively low; and the wisest practical solution, which coincides with suggestions from the World Health Organization and the International Society of Hypertension, is to com-

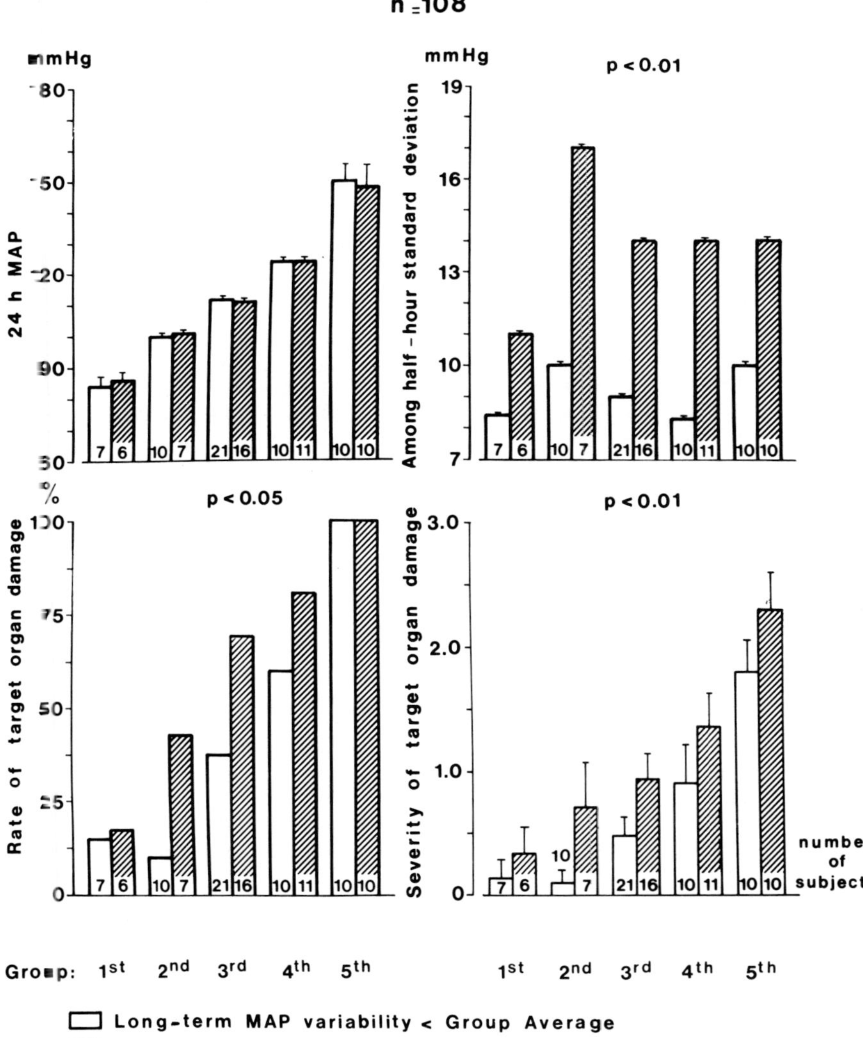

FIG. 14. Rate and severity of target organ damage in the 108 subjects of Fig. 13. The subjects were divided into five groups according to the increasing value of their 24-hr average MAP. The patients of each group were subdivided into two classes according to whether their standard deviation of 24-hr MAP (long-term variability) was below or above the average long-term variability of the group. Note that within each group the two classes had a similar 24-hr MAP but that the rate and the severity of target organ damage were less in the class in which long-term variability was lower. For other explanations see Fig. 13. (From ref. 59.)

mence treatment if diastolic pressure is between 95 and 100 mmHg, but only after 3–4 months of observation with repeated measurements. At values between 90 and 95 mmHg, decision in favor of treatment will be influenced by concomitant elevation of systolic values and by the occurrence of other risk factors or of a strong family history of cardiovascular disease. Because individual benefit is uncertain, the decision to start treatment at 90–95 mmHg diastolic pressure should be taken by the physician and the patient together. Although isolated systolic hypertension is known to carry an increased cardiovascular risk, no evidence is yet available that its treatment causes benefits that outweigh the disadvantages, and no firm general guidelines can be provided until the results of current trials become available.

As to the issue of the level to which blood pressure should be lowered by treatment, the dilemma whether levels currently suggested are low enough or too low can easily be solved by careful, slow, and progressive lowering of blood pressure, especially in the elderly hypertensive or whenever there are signs of occlusive arterial disease. Furthermore, the observation in recent trials that no additional benefits can be expected by lowering systolic pressure to below 135–144 mmHg and diastolic pressure to below 85–89 mmHg suggests that these levels should be taken as reasonable treatment goals, at least for most patients.

The limitations of casual and office blood pressures, the indices currently recommended for decision-making about antihypertensive therapy, should also be kept in mind, but before resorting to more complicated criteria and more sophisticated devices, such as ambulatory blood pressure monitoring, more solid evidence from prospective studies should be provided and new standards of risk should be elaborated.

Finally, it is likely that blood pressure, however measured, is not the only factor in cardiovascular damage and that, in deciding to commence treatment, attention should be paid not only to blood pressure values and other risk factors of cardiovascular disease but also to other markers, either of genetic predisposition or of physiologic activity (e.g., catecholamines, angiotensin, platelet activity, endothelial factors, etc.), which should be investigated to find out whether they might help us predict how the cardiovascular system would react to potentially damaging factors. The best therapeutic response is also likely to be achieved if not only blood pressure but all risk factors and mechanisms of cardiovascular damage, whenever altered, are suitably corrected.

REFERENCES

1. Evans JG, Rose G. Hypertension. *Br Med Bull* 1971;27:37.
2. Zanchetti A. Systolic, diastolic and 24-hour blood pressure: which should be treated? In: Hansson L, ed. *Hypertension annual.* London: Gower Academic Journals, 1988;3–19.
3. Mancia G, Zanchetti A. Blood pressure variability. In: Zanchetti A, Tarazi RC, eds. *Pathophysiology of hypertension: cardiovascular aspects, vol 7. Handbook of hypertension.* Amsterdam: Elsevier, 1986;125–152.
4. Zanchetti A. Blood pressure measurement and definition of hypertension. *Eur J Intern Med* 1989 (*in press.*)
5. Zanchetti A. Opening Remarks. *Curr Opin Cardiol* 1987;2(Suppl 1):S1.
6. Strasser T. Inferences from drug trials: risks, probabilities, ethics, and decision taking. In: Strasser T, Ganten D, eds. *Mild hypertension: from drug trials to practice.* New York: Raven Press, 1987:77–83.
7. Veterans Administration Cooperative Study Group on Antihypertensive Agents: Effects of treatment on morbidity in hypertension. Results in patients with diastolic blood pressure averaging 115 through 129 mmHg. *JAMA* 1967;202:1028–1034.
8. Veterans Administration Cooperative Study Group on Hypertension. Effects of treatment of morbidity in hypertension. II. Results in patients with diastolic blood pressure averaging 90 through 114 mmHg. *JAMA* 1970;213:1143–1152.
9. Smith WM. Treatment of mild hypertension: results of a ten-year intervention trial. US Public Health Service Hospitals Cooperative Study Group. *Circ Res* 1977;40(Suppl 1):98–105.
10. Report from the Management Committee. The Australian therapeutical trial in mild hypertension. *Lancet* 1980;1:1261–1267.
11. Helgeland A. Treatment of mild hypertension: a five-year controlled drug trial. The Oslo Study. *Am J Med* 1980;69:725–732.
12. Amery A, Birkenhäger W, Brixko P, et al. Mortality and morbidity results from the European Working Party on High Blood Pressure in the Elderly trial. *Lancet* 1985;1:1349–1354.
13. Medical Research Council Working Party. MRC trial of treatment of mild hypertension: principal results. *Br Med J* 1985;291:97–104.
14. Report by the Management Committee. The Australian Therapeutic Trial in Mild Hypertension: untreated mild hypertension. *Lancet* 1982;1:185–191.
15. Medical Research Council Working Party. Stroke and coronary heart disease in mild hypertension: risk factors and the value of treatment. *Br Med J* 1988;296:1565–1570.
16. World Health Organization. 1989 Guidelines for the management of mild hypertension: memorandum from a WHO/ISH meeting. (*in press*).
17. Birkenhäger WH, de Leeuw PW. Systolic blood pressure as a risk factor. *Curr Opin Cardiol* 1987;2(Suppl 1):S2–S5.
18. Tarazi RC, Magrini F, Dustan HP. The role of aortic distensibility in hypertension. In: Milliez P, Safar M, eds. *Recent advances in hypertension,* vol 2. Reims: Societé Alinea, 1975;133–142.
19. Safar ME, Simon AC. Hemodynamics in systolic hypertension. In: Zanchetti A, Tarazi RC, eds. *Pathophysiology of hypertension: cardiovascular aspects, vol 7. Handbook of hypertension.* Amsterdam: Elsevier, 1986;225–241.
20. Kannel WB, Gordon T, Schwartz MJ. Systolic versus diastolic blood pressure and risk of coronary heart disease. *Am J Cardiol* 1971;27:335–346.
21. Kannel WB, Dawber TR, McGee DL. Perspectives on systolic hypertension: the Framingham Study. *Circulation* 1986;61:1179–1182.
22. Amery A, Birkenhäger WH, Brixho P, et al. Efficacy of antihypertensive drug treatment according to age, sex, blood pressure and previous cardiovascular disease in patients over the age of 60. *Lancet* 1986;2:588–592.
23. Coope J, Warrander TS. Randomized trial of treatment of hypertension in elderly patients in primary care. *Br Med J* 1986; 293:1145–1148.
24. Furberg CD, Cutler JA, Probstfield JL, Page L, Hulley SP. The Systolic Hypertension in the Elderly program. In: Strasser T, Ganten D, eds. *Mild hypertension: from drug trials to practice.* New York: Raven Press, 1987;59–63.
25. Hypertension Detection and Follow-up Program Cooperative Group. Five-year findings of the Hypertension Detection and Follow-up Program. I. Reduction in mortality of persons with high blood pressure, including mild hypertension. *JAMA* 1979; 242:2562–2571.
26. Zanchetti A. Clinical trials on the treatment of hypertension. A critical appraisal. *J Clin Hypertens* 1986;2:179–182.
27. Lever AF on behalf of the Medical Research Council Working Party. Relationship between risk of stroke and systolic blood pressure in mild hypertension: observations from the Medical Research Council trial. *Curr Opin Cardiol* 1987;2(Suppl 1):S6–S14.
28. MRC Working Party on Mild to Moderate Hypertension. The MRC Mild Hypertension Trial: some subgroup results. In: Strasser T, Ganten D, eds. *Mild hypertension: from drug trials to practice.* New York: Raven Press, 1987;9–20.
29. The IPPPSH Collaborative Group. Cardiovascular risk and risk factors in a randomized trial of treatment based on the beta-blocker oxprenolol: the International Prospective Primary Prevention Study in Hypertension (IPPPSH). *J Hypertens* 1985;34:379–392.
30. Wilhelmsen L, Berglund G, Elmfeld D, et al. Beta-blockers versus diuretics in hypertensive men: main results from the HAPPHY trial. *J Hypertens* 1987;5:561–572.
31. Berlund G, Samuelsson O. Lowered blood pressure and the J-shaped curve. *Lancet* 1987;1:1154–1155.
32. Cruickshank JM, Pennert K, Sorman AE, et al. Low mortality from all causes, including myocardial infarction, in well-controlled hypertensives treated with a beta-blocker plus other antihypertensives. *J Hypertens* 1987;5:489–498.
33. Cruickshank JM, Thorp JM, Zacharias FJ. Benefits and potential harm of lowering high blood pressure. *Lancet* 1987;1:581–583.
34. Fletcher AE, Beevers DG, Bulpitt CJ, et al. The relation between a low treated blood pressure and IHD mortality: a report from the DHSS Hypertension Care Computing Project (DHCCP). *J Hum Hypertens* 1988;8:11–15.
35. Lindholm L, Lanke J, Bengtsson B, Ejlertsson G, Thulin T, Schersten B. Both high and low blood pressure risk indicators of death in middle-aged males. *Acta Med Scand* 1985;218:473–480.
36. Aromaa A. Blood pressure level, hypertension and five-year mortality in Finland. *Acta Med Scand* [*Suppl*] 1980;646:43–50.
37. Coope J, Warrender TS. Lowering blood pressure. *Lancet* 1987;1:1380.
38. Waller PC, Isles CG, Lever AF, Murray GD, McInnes GT. Does therapeutic reduction of diastolic blood pressure cause death from coronary heart disease? *J Hum Hypertens* 1988;2:7–10.
39. Strandgaard S, Haunsø S. Why does antihypertensive treatment prevent stroke but not myocardial infarction? *Lancet* 1987;2:658–661.
40. Zanchetti A. Which drug to which patients? *J Hypertens* 1985;3(Suppl 2):S57–S63.
41. Hansson L. Assessment of the patient's response. *J Hypertens* 1985;3(Suppl 2):S65–S69.
42. Gross F, Pisa Z, Strasser T, Zanchetti A. *Management of arterial hypertension. A practical guide for the physician and allied health workers.* Geneva: World Health Organization, 1984.
43. Trap-Jensen J. Effects of smoking on the heart and peripheral circulation. *Am Heart J* 1988;115(Suppl 1, part 2):263–267.
44. Lipsitz LA, Nyquist RP, Wei JY, Rowe JW. Postprandial reduction in blood pressure in the elderly. *N Engl J Med* 1983;309:81–83.
45. WHO Expert Committee. *Arterial hypertension.* Technical Report Series, No. 628. Geneva: World Health Organization, 1978.
46. Mancia G, Parati G. Reactivity to physical and behavioral stress and blood pressure variability in hypertension. In: Julius S, Bassett DR, eds. *Behavioral factors in hypertension, vol 9. Handbook of hypertension.* Amsterdam, Elsevier, 1987;104–122.
47. Devereux RB, Pickering TG, Harshfield GA, et al. Left ventricular hypertrophy in patients with hypertension: importance of blood pressure response to regularly recurring stress. *Circulation* 1983;68:470–476.
48. Mancia G. Ambulatory blood pressure monitoring in hyperten-

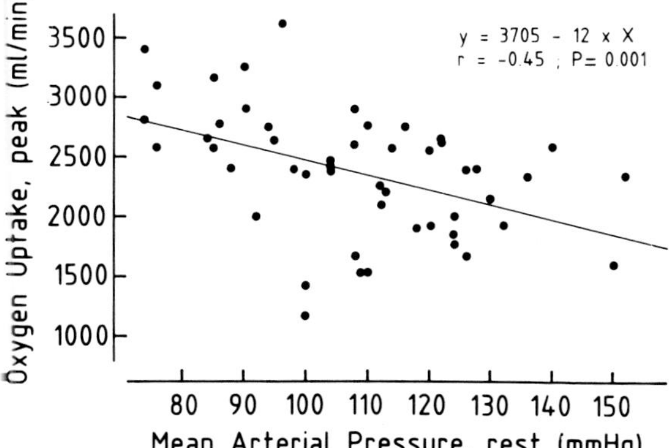

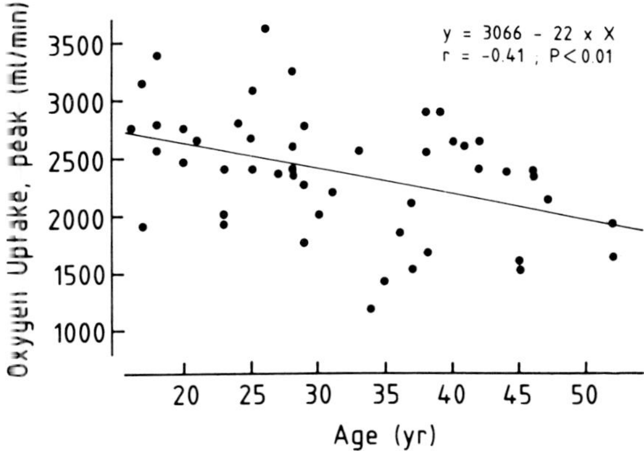

FIG. 3. Relationship between peak oxygen uptake (ml/min) and mean intra-arterial brachial artery pressure at supine rest (mmHg) (**upper panel**) and age (years) (**lower panel**).

of maximal aerobic power was associated with a pressure-related suppression of maximal stroke volume, together with a higher pulmonary wedge pressure at maximal exercise with increasing severity of hypertension. These findings suggest that the impairment of exercise capacity in hypertension could be the result of (a) the high-pressure load imposed on the heart at exhaustive exercise and/or (b) impaired left ventricular filling at high heart rates due to reduced left ventricular compliance. On the other hand, the age-related decline of oxygen uptake was associated with an age-related lowering of maximal heart rate, without evidence of impaired cardiac function.

Prognostic Significance of Exercise Blood Pressure

In the epidemiologic studies on the association between blood pressure, morbidity, and mortality, resting pressure was a major indicator for cardiovascular morbidity and mortality, and even for all-cause mortality. It is presently not known whether blood pressure during exercise is a better predictor of the patient's outcome than resting pressure. In the absence of such epidemiologic data, an analysis of the relationship between target organ damage and blood pressure at rest and during exercise could be useful. We analyzed this relationship in hypertensive patients, after exclusion of patients with WHO stage III complications because of the possible influence of these complications on exercise blood pressure. Table 1 summarizes the correlation coefficients of systolic intra-arterial pressure at supine rest, at sitting rest, at 50-watt exercise, and at maximal exercise, and also of age, with respect to (a) eye-fundus grade [stages 0 (normal), 1, and 2 according to Keith et al. (9)], (b) the Sokolow index on the electrocardiogram (SV1 + RV5), and (c) serum creatinine, which was ≤1.4 mg/dl in all 71 patients. In single regression analysis, the strongest association of eye-fundus grade was with age, but the relationship was also significant for blood pressure at all levels of activity. The Sokolow index was significantly related to blood pressure at rest but not with pressure during exercise. Serum creatinine was not related to blood pressure. In multiple regression analysis, in which age, weight, height, maximal oxygen uptake, and the blood pressures at the various levels of activity were introduced as independent variables, the following equations were obtained:

1. For eye-fundus grade (0–2): $-2.2 + 0.041$ age (years) ($t = 7.0$; $p < 0.001$) $+ 0.010$ supine-rest systolic blood pressure (mmHg) ($t = 3.6$; $p < 0.001$) ($R = 0.71$; $p < 0.001$).
2. For SV1 + RV5 (mm): $+11 - 0.25$ age (years) ($t = 2.1$; $p < 0.05$) $+ 0.20$ supine-rest systolic blood pressure (mmHg; $t = 3.4$; $p = 0.001$) ($R = 0.36$; $p < 0.01$).

Therefore, after allowing for age, systolic blood pressure at supine rest showed the strongest correlation with the eye-fundus grade and with the Sokolow index on the electrocardiogram. From these data there is no evidence that exercise blood pressure is a better determinant of target organ damage than blood pressure at rest.

TABLE 1. *Single correlation coefficients of eye-fundus grade, Sokolow index, and serum creatinine with age and systolic blood pressure at various levels of activity in 71 hypertensive patients*

			Systolic blood pressure			
			Rest		Exercise	
Parameter		Age	Supine	Sitting	50-watt	Maximal
Eye-fundus grade	*r:*	0.63	0.36	0.40	0.39	0.34
	p:	<0.001	<0.01	<0.001	<0.001	<0.01
SV1 − RV5	*r:*	−0.20	0.36	0.27	0.17	0.09
	p:	NS	<0.01	<0.05	NS	NS
Serum creatinine	*r:*	−0.02	0.03	0.05	0.15	0.12
	p:	NS	NS	NS	NS	NS

[a] NS, not significant.

Blood Pressure and Exercise-Related Sudden Death

Hypertension is undoubtedly a risk factor for sudden death (10). The question whether it is also a risk factor for exercise-related sudden death can be addressed by analyzing various studies on subjects who died during sport activity (11–17). Table 2 shows that exercise-related sudden death occurs almost exclusively in men (mostly in the fifth decade of life) which is not only due to greater sport participation (18); the table also shows that ischemic heart disease was found in approximately 80% of the subjects. Furthermore, an effort was made to obtain the risk factor profile of those who died. Hypertension was found in approximately one-third of the subjects in whom blood pressure could be traced. This is more than expected in men of similar age. Although such retrospective data are, of course, open to criticism, they suggest that patients with hypertension run a higher risk of sudden death during exercise, mainly due to coronary heart disease. This should be taken into consideration when counseling the hypertensive patient with regard to physical training. It is possible, however, that exercising men run a lower risk for sudden death in-between exercise sessions (19). Finally, hypertension has not been implicated in exercise-related death of young athletes (20).

PHYSICAL TRAINING AND BLOOD PRESSURE

Many studies have assessed the effect of physical training on blood pressure. Since it is well known that blood pressure decreases on repeated measurements, it is necessary to follow a control group during the same period of time. Ideally, the control group should be equal to the treatment group in all variables (particularly those with potential effect on blood pressure), except for the intervention itself. Several studies did include a control group, but usually the strictest criteria have not been followed; for example, the subjects were mostly not randomly allocated to experimental and control groups, and the controls have not been seen as often as the training subjects. Others followed the subjects in a detraining phase or randomly allocated them to periods with various levels of activity. Only controlled studies will be considered in this review. Most studies involve dynamic (predominantly isotonic) exercise, and few involve mainly isometric effort; the terms *endurance training* and *strength training* will be used to denote these forms of conditioning.

Endurance Training

Blood Pressure at Rest

Data obtained in studies in which the average control systolic blood pressure in the trained subjects was ≤140 mmHg (21–36) are summarized in Table 3, and data from studies in which this pressure was above this level (24,30,34,37–44) are summarized in Table 4. It should be noted that Table 3 includes studies on borderline hypertensives (31,34) and that Table 4 includes studies on individuals drawn from a normal elderly population (37,43).

Both male and female subjects have been studied, but most were male. The average age ranged from 16 to 70 years. Antihypertensive treatment was continued in few studies (38,39). The duration of the training period ranged from 1 to 8 months, with a frequency of mostly three sessions per week, each lasting 30–120 min. The training consisted mainly of bicycling, walking, jogging, running, and calisthenics. The training intensity was usually high, but this is difficult to compare between studies. In some studies, intensity was expressed as a percentage of maximal oxygen uptake; in others, it was expressed as a percentage of maximal heart rate or of heart rate reserve (difference between maximal and resting heart rates). In one study (44), training was performed at the lactate threshold, which was a rather low percentage of maximal oxygen uptake (47%). It can also be seen that the number of observations was sometimes less than the number of patients who entered the studies, usually due to drop-out or to low adherence rate.

The training programs resulted in average increases of exercise capacity (expressed as estimated or measured maximal oxygen uptake or as the workload at a certain submaximal heart rate) of 6–38%. The changes in working capacity were not significant in the control groups of the various studies. Weight usually remained unchanged, but small significant decreases were occasionally observed.

When all studies are considered together, the range of average blood pressures in the unfit state was wide, from 120 to 182 mmHg for systolic blood pressure and from 69 to 113 mmHg for diastolic blood pressure. In the parallel

TABLE 2. *Hypertension and exercise-related sudden death*

Authors (reference number)	Number of deaths	Age (years)	Gender (male/female)	IHD[a] (%)	Hypertension %	Hypertension n/n
Opie (11)	21	40 (17–58)	21/0	76	20	2/10
Thompson et al. (12)	18	? (42–59)	17/1	72	31	4/13
Walker and Roberts (13)	5	46 (40–53)	5/0	100	40	2/5
Thompson et al. (14)	12	47 (28–74)	12/0	92	0	0/8
Virmani et al. (15)	30	36 (18–57)	30/0	73	46	11/24
Jackson et al. (16)	9	47 (35–56)	9/0	100	33	3/9
Northcote et al. (17)	30	47 (22–66)	29/1	77	35	8/23

[a] IHD, ischemic heart disease; *n/n*, subjects with hypertension/subjects in whom blood pressure could be traced.

TABLE 3. *Effects of training on resting blood pressure*[a–c]

Authors (reference number)	Characteristics of subjects: Sex	Group	Number entered	Age	Training program: Dur (mo)	Weekly freq	Time (min)	Int	Methods	Blood pressure (mmHg): n	Pos	SBP (mean): Control	Intervention	DBP (mean): Control	Intervention	ΔPWC (%)	ΔWeight (%)
Gettman et al. (25)	M	TG	20	20–35	5	5×	30	85–90% of HRr	walk, run	13	sit	120	120 (NS)	74	75 (NS)	$\dot{V}O_2$ + 17%*	NS
	M	CG	30		5	2×	?	—	recreational	11	sit	118	115 (NS)	73	77 (NS)	NS	NS
Pollock et al. (23)	M	TG	16	49 (40–56)	5	4×	40	63–76% of HRm	walk	15	?	121	118 (NS)	78	76 (NS)	$\dot{V}O_2$ + 28%*	−1.7%*
	M	CG	8	?	5	—	—	—	—	8	?	117	118 (NS)	77	81 (NS)	?	NS
Seals et al. (32)	M + F	TG	14	62 ± 1 (SD)	6	⩾3×	30–45	80–90% of HRm	by, walk, jog	10	sup	121	111*	78	68*	$\dot{V}O_2$ + 18%*	NS
	M + F	CG	10	63 ± 3 (SD)	6	—	—	—	—	10	sup	121	124 (NS)	77	80 (NS)	NS	NS
Bonanno and Lies (24)	M	TG	8	30–58	3	3×	40–55	70–85% of HRm	walk, jog, cal	8	sit	123	126 (NS)	84	78*	$\dot{V}O_2$ + 6%*	NS
	M	CG	4		3	—	—	—	—	4	sit	135	132 (NS)	87	78*	NS	NS
Martin et al. (35)	M + F	TG	12	38 ± 7 (SD)	3	3×	60	Intense	swim, circuit weight	12	sup	123	118 (NS)	74	67 (NS)	$\dot{V}O_2$ + 16%*	NS
	M + F	CG	5	38 ± 8 (SD)	3	—	—	—	—	5	?	?	? (NS)	?	? (NS)	NS	?
Wolfe et al. (28)	M	TG	20	37 (29–48)	6	4×	30	60–80% of HRm	jog	12	?	126	121 (NS)	?	?	$\dot{V}O_2$est + 18%*	NS
	M	CG	13	35 (29–51)	6	—	—	—	—	10	?	119	118 (NS)	?	?	NS	NS
Van Hoof et al. (36)	M	TP	30	39 ± 10 (SD)	4	3×	60	70% of HRr	by, jog, cal	26	sit	—	122 (NS)	—	81*	$\dot{V}O_2$ + 14%*	−1.6%*
		NTP			4	—	—	—	—			126	—	86	—	—	—
Mann et al. (21)	M	TG	105	38 ± 0.9 (SE)	6	4–5×	60	HR = 160–190	walk, jog, run, cal	62	sup	129	124*	81	75*	ex time + 18%*	−?*
	M	CG	28	35 ± 1.8 (SE)	6	—	—	—	—	20	sup	132	125 (NS)	82	78 (NS)	?	?
Pollock et al. (26)	M	TG	22	55 (49–65)	5	3×	30	83–91% of HRm	walk, jog	20	sit	130	127 (NS)	84	79 (NS)	$\dot{V}O_2$ + 18%*	−1.5%*
	M	CG	8	?	5	—	—	—	—	6	sit	130	129 (NS)	86	84 (NS)	NS	NS
Myrtek and Villinger (27)	M	TG	20		1.2	3×	15	HR = 140	by	?	?	130	126 (NS)	80	78 (NS)	PWC_{140} + 25%*	?
	M	CG	20	23 ± 0.4 (SE)	1.2	—	—	—	—	?	?	132	133 (NS)	88	84 (NS)	?	?
Länsimies et al. (29)	M	TG	50	40–45	4	3–4×	50	40–66% of HRr	walk, jog, swim, ski, by	44	?	130	122*	84	83 (NS)	$\dot{V}O_2$est + 10%*	−1.1%*
													ns		ns	+	ns
	M	CG	50		4	—	—	—	—	46	?	128	123*	84	86 (NS)	NS	−0.9%* (NS)
Jennings et al. (33)	M + F	TP	12	22 (19–27)	1	3×	40	60–70% of $\dot{V}O_2$m	by	12	sup	—	122*	—	62*	$\dot{V}O_2$ + 10%*	NS
		TP			1	7×	40	60–70% of $\dot{V}O_2$m	by			—	120*	—	02*	$\dot{V}O_2$ + 20%*	NS
		NTP			1	—	—	—	—			132	—	69	—	—	—
Kukkonen et al. (30)	M	TG	17	35–50	4	3×	50	40–66% of HRr	walk, jog, by, ski	17	sit	133	127 (NS)	86	80*	$\dot{V}O_2$est + 9%*	NS
	M	CG	17		4	—	—	—	—	17	sit	129	124 (NS)	86	75*	NS	NS
Cléroux et al. (34)	M + F	TG	7	37 ± 4 (SE)	5	3×	20–45	60% of $\dot{V}O_2$m	by	7	sup	133	129 (NS)	83	80 (NS)	$\dot{V}O_2$est + 13%*	NS
	M + F	CG	7	33 ± 4 (SE)	5	—	—	—	—	7	sup	136	134 (NS)	81	83 (NS)	NS	NS
Hagberg et al. (31)	M + F	TP	25	16 ± 0.3 (SE)	6	3×	30–40	60–65% of $\dot{V}O_2$m	jog	25	sup	137	129*	80	75*	$\dot{V}O_2$ + 10%*	NS
		DP			9	—	—	—	—			139	—	78	—	NS	NS
deVries (22)	M	TG	112	70 (51–87)	1.5	3×	60	HR < 140	walk, run, cal, . . .	66	sit	140	136*	76	73*	PWC_{145} + 9%*	−1.1%*
	M	CG	32	?	1.5	—	—	—	—	32	sit	140	141 (NS)	76	75 (NS)	NS	NS

[a] Data are from controlled studies in which the average control systolic blood pressure in the trained group was ⩽140 mmHg. Studies are ranked according to this pressure.

[b] *Abbreviations:* by, bicycling; CG, control group; cal, calisthenics; condit, conditioning; DP, detraining phase; DBP, diastolic blood pressure; Dur, duration; ex, exercise; F, female; freq, frequency; HRm, maximal heart rate; HRr, heart rate reserve (max-rest); Int, intensity; jog, jogging; M, male; mo, month; *n*, number; NTP, nontraining phase; Pos, position; PWC, physical working capacity; run, running; SBP, systolic blood pressure; SD, standard deviation; SE, standard error; sit, sitting; ski, skiing; sup, supine; swim, swimming; TG, training group; TP, training phase; $\dot{V}O_2$m, maximal oxygen uptake; $\dot{V}O_2$est, estimated oxygen uptake; walk, walking.

[c] *Statistics:* comparison of trained versus control—NS, not significant; *, $p < 0.05$; ?, unknown. Comparison of change between exercise group and control group—ns, not significant; +, $p < 0.05$.

TABLE 4. *Effects of training on resting blood pressure*[a]

Authors (reference number)	Characteristics of patients				Training program					Blood pressure (mmHg)						ΔPWC (%)	ΔWeight (%)
												SBP (mean)		DBP (mean)			
	Sex	Group	Number entered	Age	Dur (mo)	Weekly freq	Time (min)	Int	Methods	*n*	Pos	Control	Intervention	Control	Intervention		
Cléroux et al. (34)	M + F	TG	5	32 ± 4 (SE)	5	3×	20–45	60% of $\dot{V}O_2$m	jog	5	sup	141	130*	71	75*	$\dot{V}O_2$est + 21%*	NS
	M + F	CG	7	33 ± 4 (SE)	5	—	—	—	—	7	sup	136	134 (NS)	81	83 (NS)	NS	NS
Cunningham et al. (43)	M	TG	113	63 (54–68)	12	3×	50	66–71% of HRr	walk, jog	106	?	141	135 (?) ns	86	82 (?) ns	$\dot{V}O_2$ + 10% (?) +	−0.5% (?) ns
	M	CG	111	63 (55–68)	12	—	—	—	—	106	?	142	136 (?)	86	82 (?)	NS	+1.3% (?)
Nelson et al. (42)	M + F	TP	17	44 (25–62)	1	3×	45	60–70% of $\dot{V}O_2$m	by	13	sup	—	132*	—	87*	$\dot{V}O_2$ + 17%*	NS
		TP			1	7×	45	60–70% of $\dot{V}O_2$m	by			—	127*	—	85*	$\dot{V}O_2$ + 19%*	NS
		NTP			1	—	—	—	—			143	—	96	—	—	—
Kukkonen et al. (30)	M	TG	13	35–50	4	3×	50	40–66% of HRr	walk, jog, by, ski	13	sit	145	136*	99	88*	$\dot{V}O_2$est + 10%*	−1.1 kg*
	M	CG	12		4	—	—	—	—	12	sit	140	140 (NS)	97	90*	NS	NS
Duncan et al. (41)	M	TG	44	30 (21–37)	4	3×	60	70–80% of HRm	walk, jog	44	sit	146	134 (?) ns	94	87 (?) +	$\dot{V}O_2$ + 12% (?) +	+0.5% (?) ns
	M	CG	12		4	—	—	—	—	12	sit	145	139 (?)	93	96 (?)	$\dot{V}O_2$ − 1% (?)	+1.2% (?)
Barry et al. (37)	M + F	TG	8	70 (55–78)	3	3×	40	HR > 130	by, condit, ex	8	sit	148	128*	88	82 (NS)	$\dot{V}O_2$ + 38%*	NS
	M + F	CG	5	72 (58–83)	3	—	—	—	—	5	sit	152	156 (NS)	94	91 (NS)	?	?
Bonanno and Lies (24)	M	TG	12	30–58	3	3×	40–55	70–85% of HRm	walk, jog, cal	12	sit	148	135*	97	83*	$\dot{V}O_2$ + 6%*	NS
	M	CG	15		3	—	—	—	—	15	sit	150	147 (NS)	101	90*	NS	NS
Schleusing et al. (38)	?	TG	10	35–45	8	3–4×	60–120	HR = 100–160	walk, jog, by, swim	8	?	153	145 (?)	106	99 (?)	$\dot{V}O_2$ + 21%*	?
	?	CG	11	?	8	—	—	—	—	11	?	159	157 (?)	105	108 (?)	NS	?
Urata et al. (44)	M + F	TG	10	51 ± 3 (SE)	2.5	3×	60	Lactate threshold	by	10	sit	156	144* +	103	98 (NS) ns	$\dot{V}O_2$est + 12%*	NS
	M + F	CG	10	51 ± 3 (SE)	2.5	—	—	—	—	10	sit	154	156	98	98 (NS)	?	NS
DePlaen and Detry (39)	F	TG	7	44	3	3×	60	>60% of $\dot{V}O_2$m	walk, jog, cal, by	5	sit	162	158 (NS)	104	104 (NS)	$\dot{V}O_2$ + 10%*	NS
	F	CG	8	47	3	—	—	—	—	4	sup	156	154 (NS)	110	107 (NS)	NS	NS
Roman et al. (40)	F	TP	30	55 (30–69)	3	3×	30	70% of HRm	walk, jog, cal, . . .	27	sit	182	161*	113	97*	$\dot{V}O_2$ + 24%*	?
		DP			3	—	—	—	—	24	sit	179	—	113	—	NS	?

[a] Data are from controlled studies in which the average control systolic blood pressure in the trained group was >140 mmHg. Studies are ranked according to this pressure. See Table 3 for abbreviations and statistics.

and how many would sustain the effort. There is no evidence up to now that low-level exercise results in a favorable effect on blood pressure, except perhaps for the study of Urata et al. (44) in which patients trained at the lactate threshold or at 47% of estimated maximal oxygen uptake; however, this effort was sustained during three sessions, 60 min per week. It is likely that only the highly motivated patient will be prepared to embark on such demanding exercise programs. Furthermore, several studies have shown that the antihypertensive effect of training disappears when the training program is stopped.

Physical training can be advocated together with other nonpharmacologic measures in the mild hypertensive, or as an adjunct to pharmacologic treatment in more severe hypertension. Whether the effect on blood pressure control of these various measures is additive or synergistic is not known. It is proposed that the usual guidelines for initiating drug therapy should be followed (124) and that blood pressure should be sufficiently controlled before starting the program.

Dynamic endurance exercise is usually advised. This consists of rhythmic movements of large muscle groups, as is the case in brisk walking, jogging, cycling, cross-country skiing, swimming, and calisthenics. Many authors feel that predominantly isometric exercise, as in strength training, wrestling, and weight-lifting, should be avoided because it may cause a considerable increase in blood pressure during the activity and because the benefits for the hypertensive patient are doubtful.

Since hypertension is a risk factor for cardiovascular disease, an exercise test prior to training is recommended in the hypertensive patient. The exercise test also helps to determine the training heart rate for the individual patient, particularly when he or she is taking drugs which interfere with the response of heart rate during exercise. One usually starts training at a heart rate equal to the resting heart rate plus 60% of the difference between maximal and resting heart rate. When no exercise test is performed and when the patient is not on antihypertensive treatment, exercise intensity can be set at a heart rate of 190 beats/min minus age. Training should be regular and progressive, avoiding exhaustion and sudden bursts of energy.

When there are no signs of ischemic heart disease, the patient can exercise without supervision; otherwise, more intense training should best be started in supervised training programs. Some complications of hypertension, such as cardiac failure, renal insufficiency, cerebrovascular accidents, and peripheral artery disease, will, of course, entail specific recommendations on physical activity and rehabilitation, which is beyond the scope of this chapter.

Finally, one should be careful in the choice of antihypertensive drugs for the exercising patient. Beta-blockers do have an unfavorable effect, particularly on sustained submaximal exercise; diuretics, particularly during acute or short-term treatment, seem to reduce exercise capacity, probably through the reduction of plasma volume.

The Athlete with Hypertension

Although rare in the young, hypertension could be a problem for the individual who wishes to excel in competitive sports. When there is no certainty with regard to the necessity of pharmacologic treatment, a waiting attitude could be justified because (a) hypertension has not been associated with sudden death in the young athlete (20) and (b) there is no evidence that sport activity affects the prognosis unfavorably.

Practically (125,126), one can propose that the diagnosis of hypertension in the athlete justifies a screening investigation including history, physical examination, electrocardiogram, chest x-ray, funduscopy, urine analysis, blood hemoglobin and glucose, renal function, and serum electrolytes and lipids. After three visits, if diastolic blood pressure is less than 95–100 mmHg and if neither target organ damage nor an obvious underlying disorder can be demonstrated, high-level sport activity can be allowed without pharmacologic treatment, provided that there be regular follow-up visits. When diastolic blood pressure remains higher than 95–100 mmHg at rest (124) or when there is target organ damage or a probable secondary cause of hypertension, further investigation is advised and treatment is indicated. High-level sport activity can possibly be allowed when blood pressure is controlled and when it is not precluded or rendered unwise by severe target organ damage or an underlying illness. Finally, when pharmacologic treatment is indicated in the athlete, the drug regimen should be such that exercise capacity is preserved. It is likely that a vasodilator-based treatment is most appropriate.

SUMMARY

Both dynamic predominantly isotonic and static or isometric exercise—two major forms of exercise—increase blood pressure, but pressure reaches higher levels during static effort. One should be aware, however, that blood pressure may rise considerably when hypertensive patients perform dynamic exercise. Blood pressure per se adversely affects maximal aerobic power, which is related to an impaired maximal stroke volume that can be ascribed to the high afterload or to impaired ventricular filling at high heart rate.

Dynamic, relatively intense physical training, performed at least 3 times 30 minutes per week for 1 to 8 months, has been shown to reduce blood pressure. The hypotensive effect was small in normotensive subjects, but averaged −11 and −6 mmHg for systolic and diastolic pressure, respectively, in the controlled studies on hypertensive patients. After training, blood pressure was also reduced when measured during exercise and during daytime ambulatory monitoring. Physical training can therefore be advocated in the management of the hypertensive patient in combination with other non-pharmacologic measures in mild hypertension or as an adjunct to pharmacologic treatment in more severe hypertension. Blood pressure should be controlled according to the usual guidelines before embarking in a training program. Further, an exercise test is recommended because: 1) hypertension is a risk factor for cardiovascular disease and 2) to establish the heart rate at which the individual patient should train. Finally, when prescribing antihypertensive medication to exercising patients, one should be aware that some drugs, particularly beta-blockers and diuretics, may reduce exercise performance or even impair the conditioning response.

REFERENCES

1. Staessen J, Cattaert A, Fagard R, Lijnen P, Vanhees L, Amery A. Epidemiology of treated, compared to untreated hypertension. In: Genest J, Kuchel O, Hamet P, Cantin M, eds. *Hypertension.* New York: McGraw-Hill, 1983;1069–1093.
2. Fagard R, M'Buyamba-Kabangu JR, Staessen J, Vanhees L, Amery A. Physical activity and blood pressure. In: Bulpitt CJ, ed. *Handbook of hypertension, vol 6: epidemiology of hypertension.* Amsterdam: Elsevier, 1985;104–130.
3. Fagard R. Habitual physical activity, training and blood pressure in normo- and hypertension. *Int J Sports Med* 1985;6:57–67.
4. Amery A, Julius S, Whitlock LS, Conway J. Influence of hypertension on the haemodynamic response to exercise. *Circulation* 1967;36:231–237.
5. Asmussen E. Similarities and dissimilarities between static and dynamic exercise. *Circ Res* 1981;48(Suppl I):I-3–I-10.
6. Wong HE, Kasser IS, Bruce RA. Impaired maximal exercise performance with hypertensive cardiovascular disease. *Circulation* 1969;39:633–638.
7. Bruce RA, Fisher LD, Cooper MN, Gey GO. Separation of effects of cardiovascular disease and age on ventricular function with maximal exercise. *Am J Cardiol* 1974;34:757–763.
8. Fagard R, Staessen J, Amery A. Maximal aerobic power in essential hypertension. *J Hypertens* 1988;6:859–865.
9. Keith NM, Wagener HP, Barker NW. Some different types of essential hypertension: their course and prognosis. *Am J Med Sci* 1939;197:332–343.
10. Kreger BE, Kannel WB. Influence of hypertension on mortality. In: Amery A, Fagard R, Lijnen P, Staessen J, eds. *Hypertensive cardiovascular disease: pathophysiology and treatment.* Dordrecht: Martinus Nijhoff, 1982;451–463.
11. Opie CH. Sudden death and sport. *Lancet* 1975;1:263–266.
12. Thompson PD, Stern MP, Williams P, Duncan K, Haskell WL, Wood PD. Death during jogging and running. *JAMA* 1979;242:1265–1267.
13. Waller BF, Roberts WC. Sudden death while running in conditioned runners aged 40 years or over. *Am J Cardiol* 1980;45:1292–1300.
14. Thompson PD, Funk ES, Carleton RA, Sturner WQ. Incidence of death during jogging in Rhode Island from 1975 through 1980. *JAMA* 1982;247:2535–2538.
15. Virmani R, Robinowitz M, McAllister HA. Non-traumatic death in joggers. *Am J Med* 1982;72:874–882.
16. Jackson RT, Beaglehole R, Sharpe N. Sudden death in runners. *NZ Med J* 1983;96:289–292.
17. Northcote RS, Evans ADB, Ballantyne D. Sudden death in squash players. *Lancet* 1984;1:148–151.
18. Pool J. Sudden death and sports. In: Fagard RH, Bekaert IE, eds. *Sports cardiology: exercise in health and cardiovascular disease.* Dordrecht: Martinus Nijhoff, 1986;223–227.
19. Siscovick DS, Weiss NS, Fletcher RH, et al. The incidence of primary cardiac arrest during vigorous exercise. *N Engl J Med* 1984;311:874–878.
20. Maron BJ, Roberts WC, McAllister HA, Rosing DR, Epstein SE. Sudden death in young athletes. *Circulation* 1980;62:218–229.
21. Mann GV, Garrett HL, Farhi A, Murray H, Billings FT. Exercise to prevent coronary heart disease. An experimental study of the effects of training on risk factors for coronary disease in men. *Am J Med* 1969;46:12–27.
22. deVries HA. Physiological effects of an exercise training regimen upon men aged 52–88. *J Gerontol* 1970;25:325–336.
23. Pollock ML, Miller HS Jr, Janeway R, Linnerud AC, Robertson B, Valentino R. Effects of walking on body composition and cardiovascular function of middle-aged men. *J Appl Physiol* 1971;30:126–130.
24. Bonanno JA, Lies JE. Effects of physical training on coronary risk factors. *Am J Cardiol* 1974;33:760–764.
25. Gettman LR, Pollock ML, Durstine JL, Ward A, Ayres J, Linnerud A. Physiological responses of men to 1, 3 and 5 day per week training programs. *Res Q* 1976;47:638–646.
26. Pollock ML, Dawson GA, Miller HS, et al. Physiologic responses of men 49 to 65 years of age to endurance training. *J Am Geriatr Soc* 1976;24:97–104.
27. Myrtek M, Villinger U. Psychologische und physiologische Wirkungen eines fünfwochigen Ergometertrainings bei Gesunden. *Med Klin* 1976;71:1623–1630.
28. Wolfe LA, Cunningham DA, Reichnitzer PA, Nichol PM. Effects of endurance training on left ventricular dimensions in healthy men. *J Appl Physiol* 1979;47:207–212.
29. Länsimies E, Hietanen E, Huttunen JK, Hanninen O, Kukkonen K, Raumaraa R, Voutilainen E. Metabolic and hemodynamic effects of physical training in middle-aged men. A controlled trial. In: Komi PV, Nelson RC, Morehouse CA, eds. *Exercise and sport biology.* Champaign, IL: Human Kinetics Publishers, 1979;199–206.
30. Kukkonen K, Raumaraa R, Voutilainen E, Länsimies E. Physical training of middle-aged men with borderline hypertension. *Ann Clin Res* 1982;14(Suppl 34):139–145.
31. Hagberg JM, Goldring D, Ehsani AA, Heath GW, Hernandez A, Schechtman K, Holloszy JO. Effect of exercise training on the blood pressure and hemodynamic features of hypertensive adolescents. *Am J Cardiol* 1983;52:763–768.
32. Seals DR, Hurley BF, Hagberg JM, Schultz J, Linder BJ, Natter L, Ehsani AA. Effects of training on systolic time intervals at rest and during isometric exercise in men and women 61 to 64 years old. *Am J Cardiol* 1985;55:797–800.
33. Jennings G, Nelson L, Nestel P, Esler M, Korner P, Burton D, Bazelmans J. The effects of changes in physical activity on major cardiovascular risk factors, hemodynamics, sympathetic function, and glucose utilization in man: a controlled study of four levels of activity. *Circulation* 1986;73:30–40.
34. Cléroux J, Péronnet F, de Champlain J. Effects of exercise training on plasma catecholamines and blood pressure in labile hypertensive subjects. *Eur J Appl Physiol* 1987;56:550–554.
35. Martin WD, Montgomery J, Snell PG, et al. Cardiovascular adaptations to intense swim training in sedentary middle-aged men and women. *Circulation* 1987;75:323–330.
36. Van Hoof R, Hespel P, Fagard R, Lijnen P, Staessen J, Amery A. Effect of endurance training on blood pressure at rest, during exercise and during 24 hours in normal men. *Am J Cardiol* 1989;in press.
37. Barry AJ, Daly JW, Pruett EDR, Steinmetz JR, Page HF, Birhead NC, Rodahl K. The effects of physical conditioning on older individuals. I. Work capacity, circulatory–respiratory function, and work electrocardiogram. *J Gerontol* 1966;21:182–191.
38. Schleusing G, Luther Th, Liebold F, Kunadt F. Einfluss des sportlichen Trainings auf Blutdruckverhalten und Leistungsvermögen bei Patienten mit Hypertonie. *Med Sport* 1969;9:197–201.
39. DePlaen JF, Detry JM. Hemodynamic effects of physical training in established arterial hypertension. *Acta Cardiol* 1980;35:179–188.
40. Roman O, Camuzzi AL, Villalon E, Klenner C. Physical training program in arterial hypertension. A long-term prospective follow-up. *Cardiology* 1981;67:230–243.
41. Duncan JJ, Farr JE, Upton SJ, Hagan RD, Oglesby ME, Blair SN. The effects of aerobic exercise on plasma catecholamines and blood pressure in patients with mild essential hypertension. *JAMA* 1985;254:2609–2613.
42. Nelson L, Jennings GL, Esler MD, Korner PI. Effect of changing levels of physical activity on blood pressure and haemodynamics in essential hypertension. *Lancet* 1986;2:473–476.
43. Cunningham DA, Rechnitzer PA, Howard JH, Donner AP. Exercise training of men at retirement: a clinical trial. *J Gerontol* 1987;42:17–23.
44. Urata H, Tanabe Y, Kiyonaga A, Ikeda M, Tanaka H, Shindo M, Arakawa K. Antihypertensive and volume-depleting effects of mild exercise on essential hypertension. *Hypertension* 1987;9:245–252.
45. Gill JS, Zezulka AV, Beevers DG, Davies P. Relation between

initial blood pressure and its fall with treatment. *Lancet* 1985;1:567–569.

46. Somers VK, Conway J, Sleight P. Physical training and ambulatory and sleep blood pressures in borderline hypertensive patients. In: *Abstract book of the 12th Scientific Meeting of the International Society of Hypertension,* 1988;1183.
47. Kinoshita A, Urata H, Tanabe Y, Ikeda M, Shindo M, Tanaka H, Arakawa K. What types of hypertensives respond better to mild exercise therapy? In: *Abstract book of the 12th Scientific Meeting of the International Society of Hypertension,* 1988;420.
48. Hartley LH, Mason JW, Hogen RP, et al. Multiple hormonal responses to prolonged exercise in relation to physical training. *J Appl Physiol* 1972;33:607–610.
49. Winder WW, Hagberg JM, Hickson RC, Ehsani AA, McLane JA. Time course of sympathoadrenal adaptation to endurance exercise training in man. *J Appl Physiol* 1978;45:370–374.
50. Péronnet F, Cléroux J, Perrault H, Cousineau D, de Champlain J, Nadeau R. Plasma norepinephrine response to exercise before and after training in humans. *J Appl Physiol* 1981;51:812–815.
51. Hickson RC, Hagberg JM, Conlee RK, Jones DA, Ehsani AA, Winder WW. Effect of training on hormonal responses to exercise in competitive swimmers. *Eur J Appl Physiol* 1979;41:211–219.
52. Winder WW, Hickson RC, Hagberg JM, Ehsani AA, McLane JA. Training-induced changes in hormonal and metabolic responses to submaximal exercise. *J Appl Physiol* 1979;46:766–771.
53. Ekblom B, Kilbom A, Soltysiak J. Physical training, bradycardia and autonomic nervous system. *Scand J Lab Invest* 1973;32: 251–254.
54. Pavlik G, Frenkl R. Sensitivity to catecholamines and histamine in the trained and in the untrained human organism and sensitivity changes during digestion. *Eur J Appl Physiol* 1975;34:199–204.
55. LeBlanc J, Boulay M, Dulac S, Jobin M, Labrie A, Rousseau-Migneron S. Metabolic and cardiovascular responses to norepinephrine in trained and non-trained human subjects. *J Appl Physiol* 1977;42:166–173.
56. Ostman I. Changed vascular sensitivity to noradrenaline in rats trained by physical exercise. *J Physiol (Lond)* 1975;252:38p–39p.
57. Krotkiewski M, Mandroukas K, Morgan L, et al. Effects of physical training on adrenergic sensitivity in obesity. *J Appl Physiol* 1983;55:1811–1817.
58. Lehmann M, Dickhuth HH, Schmid P, Porzig H, Keul J. Plasma catecholamines, beta-adrenergic receptors, and isoproterenol sensitivity in endurance trained and non-trained volunteers. *Eur J Appl Physiol* 1984;52:362–369.
59. Butler J, O'Brien M, O'Malley K, Kelly JG. Relationship of beta-adrenoceptor density to fitness in athletes. *Nature* 1982;298:60–62.
60. Öhman M, Kelly J. Beta-adrenoceptor changes in exercise and physical training. In: Fagard RH, Bekaert IE, eds. *Sports cardiology: exercise in health and cardiovascular disease.* Dordrecht: Martinus Nijhoff, 1986:136–142.
61. M'Buyamba-Kabangu JR, Fagard R, Lijnen P, Amery A. Relationship between plasma renin activity and physical fitness in normal subjects. *Eur J Appl Physiol* 1985;53:304–307.
62. Fagard R, Grauwels R, Groeseneken D, Lijnen P, Staessen J, Vanhees L, Amery A. Plasma levels of renin, angiotensin II and 6-keto-prostaglandin $F_{1\alpha}$ in endurance athletes. *J Appl Physiol* 1985;59:947–952.
63. Melin B, Eclache JP, Geelen G, et al. Plasma AVP, neurophysin, renin activity, and aldosterone during submaximal exercise performed until exhaustion in trained and untrained men. *Eur J Appl Physiol* 1980;44:141–151.
64. Skipka W, Böning D, Deck KA, Külpmann WR, Meurer KA. Reduced aldosterone and sodium excretion in endurance-trained athletes before and during immersion. *Eur J Appl Physiol* 1979;42:255–262.
65. Geyssant A, Geelen G, Denis Ch, et al. Plasma vasopressin, renin activity and aldosterone: effect of exercise and training. *Eur J Appl Physiol* 1981;46:21–30.
66. Hespel P, Lijnen P, Van Hoof R, et al. Effects of physical endurance training on the plasma renin–angiotensin–aldosterone system in normal man. *J Endocrinol* 1988;116:443–449.
67. Fagard R, Lijnen P, Amery A. Effects of angiotensin II on arterial pressure, renin and aldosterone during exercise. *Eur J Appl Physiol* 1985;54:254–261.
68. Viinika L, Vuori J, Ylikorkala O. Lipid peroxides, prostacyclins and thromboxane A_2 in runners during acute exercise. *Med Sci Sports Exerc* 1984;16:275–277.
69. Raumaraa R, Salonen JT, Kukkonen-Harjula K, Seppänen K, Seppälä E, Vapaatalo H, Huttinen JK. Effects of mild physical exercise on serum lipoproteins and metabolites of arachidonic acid: a controlled randomised trial in middle-aged men. *Br Med J* 1984;288:603–606.
70. Hespel P, Lijnen P, Fagard R, et al. Changes in erythrocyte sodium and plasma lipids associated with physical training. *J Hypertens* 1988;6:159–166.
71. Adragna NC, Chang JL, Morey MC, Williams RS. Effect of exercise on cation transport in human red cells. *Hypertension* 1985;7:132–139.
72. Hurley BF, Seals DR, Ehsani AA, Cartier LJ, Dalsky GP, Hagberg JM, Holloszy JO. Effects of high-intensity strength-training on cardiovascular function. *Med Sci Sports Exerc* 1984;16:483–488.
73. Hurley BF, Hagberg JM, Goldberg AP, Seals DR, Ehsani AA, Brennan RE, Holloszy JO. Resistive training can reduce coronary risk factors without altering $\dot{V}O_2$ max or percent body fat. *Med Sci Sports Exerc* 1988;20:150–154.
74. Fripp RR, Hodgson JL. Effect of resistive training on plasma lipid and lipoprotein levels in male adolescents. *J Pediatr* 1987;111:926–931.
75. Baechle TR. Effects of heavy resistance weight training on arterial blood pressure and other selected measures in normotensive and borderline hypertensive college men. In: Landry F, Orban W, eds. *Sports medicine.* 1978;169–175.
76. Pennock W, Fischer DE, Swanbom CD. Effect of chronic weight lifting on the blood pressure in hypertensive adolescents [Abstract]. *Prev Med* 1979;8:184.
77. Harris KA, Holly RG. Physiological response to circuit weight training in borderline hypertensive subjects. *Med Sci Sports Exerc* 1987;19:246–252.
78. Danzinger RG, Cumming SR. Effects of chlorothiazide on working capacity of normal subjects. *J Appl Physiol* 1964;19:636–638.
79. Caldwell JE, Ahonen E, Nousiainen U. Differential effects of sauna-, diuretic-, and exercise-induced hypohydration. *J Appl Physiol* 1984;57:1018–1023.
80. Nielsen B, Kubica R, Bonnesen A, Rasmussen IB, Stoklosa J, Wilk B. Physical work capacity after dehydration and hyperthermia. *Scand J Sports Sci* 1981;3:2–10.
81. Armstrong LE, Costill DI, Fink WJ. Influence of diuretic-induced dehydration on competitive running performance. *Med Sci Sports Exerc* 1985;17:456–461.
82. Kindermann W, Lehrmann S, Schmitt W. Körperliche Leistungsfähigkeit und Metabolismus. *Munch Med Wochenschr* 1986;128:53–56.
83. Andersen K, Vik-mo H. Role of the Frank–Starling mechanism during maximal semisupine exercise after oral atenolol. *Br Heart J* 1982;48:149–155.
84. Hespel P, Lijnen P, Vanhees L, Fagard R, Amery A. Beta-adrenoceptors and the regulation of blood pressure and plasma renin during exercise. *J Appl Physiol* 1986;60:108–113.
85. Vanhees L, Fagard R, Amery A. Effect of calcium channel blockade and beta-adrenoceptor blockade on short graded and single level endurance exercises in normal men. *Eur J Appl Physiol* 1988;58:87–91.
86. Epstein SE, Robinson BF, Kapler RL, Braunwald E. Effects of beta-adrenergic blockade on the cardiac response to maximal and submaximal exercise in man. *J Clin Invest* 1965;44:1745–1753.
87. Anderson SD, Bye PTP, Perry CP, Hamor GP, Theobald G, Nyberg G. Limitation of work performance in normal adult males in the presence of beta-adrenergic blockade. *Aust NZ J Med* 1979;9:515–520.
88. Petersen ES, Whipp BJ, Davis JA, Huntsman DJ, Brown HV, Wasserman K. Effects of beta-adrenergic blockade on ventilation

and gas exchange during exercise in humans. *J Appl Physiol* 1983;54:1306–1313.

89. Tesch PA, Kaiser P. Effects of beta-adrenergic blockade on O_2-uptake during submaximal and maximal exercise. *J Appl Physiol* 1983;54:901–905.
90. Wilmore JH, Ewy GA, Morton AR, et al. The effects of beta-adrenergic blockade on submaximal and maximal exercise performance. *J Cardiac Rehabil* 1983;3:30–36.
91. Galbo H, Holst JJ, Christensen NJ, Hilsted J. Glucagon and plasma catecholamines during beta-receptor blockade in exercising man. *J Appl Physiol* 1976;40:855–863.
92. Lundborg P, Åström H, Bengtsson C, et al. Effect of beta-adrenoceptor blockade on exercise performance and metabolism. *Clin Sci* 1981;61:299–305.
93. Hansson BG, Dymling JF, Hedeland H, Hulthen UL. Long-term treatment of moderate hypertension with the $beta_1$-receptor blocking agent metoprolol. *Eur J Clin Pharmacol* 1977;11:239–245.
94. Reybrouck T, Amery A, Billiet L. Hemodynamic response to graded exercise after chronic beta-adrenergic blockade. *J Appl Physiol* 1977;42:133–138.
95. Reybrouck T, Amery A, Fagard R, Billiet L. Haemodynamic response to graded exercise during chronic beta-adrenergic blockade with bunitrolol, an agent with intrinsic sympathomimetic activity. *Eur J Clin Pharmacol* 1977;12:333–339.
96. Ambrosio GB, Benussi P, Trevi GP, Pessina AC. Maximal exercise test in patients with essential hypertension treated with propranolol. *Eur J Cardiol* 1978;7:137–145.
97. Reybrouck T, Amery A, Fagard R, Jousten P, Lijnen P, Meulepas E. Beta-blockers: once or three times a day? *Br Med J* 1978;1:1386–1388.
98. Yamakado T, Oomishi N, Kondo S, Noziri A, Nakano T, Takezawa H. Effects of diltiazem on cardiovascular responses during exercise in systemic hypertension and comparison with propranolol. *Am J Cardiol* 1983;52:1023–1027.
99. Franciosa JA, Johnson SM, Tobian LJ. Exercise performance in mildly hypertensive patients. Impairment by propranolol but not oxprenolol. *Chest* 1980;78:291–299.
100. Myburgh DP, Gordon NF. Comparison of diltiazem and atenolol in young, physically active men with essential hypertension. *Am J Cardiol* 1987;60:1092–1095.
101. Szachcic J, Hirsch AT, Tuban JF, Vollmer C, Henderson S, Massie BM. Diltiazem versus propranolol in essential hypertension: responses of rest and exercise blood pressure and effects on exercise capacity. *Am J Cardiol* 1987;59:393–399.
102. Mooij J, Van Baak M, Boehm R, Does R, Petri H, Van Kemenade J, Rahn KH. The effects of verapamil and propranolol on exercise tolerance in hypertensive patients. *Clin Pharmacol Ther* 1987;41:490–495.
103. Sable DL, Brammell HL, Sheehan MW, Nies AS, Gerber J, Horwitz LD. Attenuation of exercise conditioning by beta-adrenergic blockade. *Circulation* 1982;65:679–684.
104. Marsh RC, Hiatt WR, Brammell HL, Horwitz LD. Attenuation of exercise conditioning by low dose beta-adrenergic receptor blockade. *J Am Coll Cardiol* 1983;2:551–556.
105. Ewy GA, Wilmore JH, Morton AR, et al. The effect of beta-adrenergic blockade on obtaining a trained exercise state. *J Cardiac Rehabil* 1983;3:25–29.
106. McLeod AA, Kraus WE, Williams RS. Effects of $beta_1$-selective and non-selective beta-adrenoceptor blockade during exercise conditioning in healthy adults. *Am J Cardiol* 1984;53:1656–1661.
107. Savin WC, Gordon EP, Kaplan SM, Hewitt BF, Harrison DC, Haskell WL. Exercise training during long-term beta-blockade treatment in healthy subjects. *Am J Cardiol* 1985;55:101D–109D.
108. Vanhees L, Fagard R, Amery A. Influence of beta-adrenergic blockade on effects of physical training in patients with ischaemic heart disease. *Br Heart J* 1982;48:33–38.
109. Froelicher V, Sullivan M, Myers J, Jensen D. Can patients with coronary artery disease receiving beta-blockers obtain a training effect? *Am J Cardiol* 1985;55:155D–161D.
110. Fagard R, Lijnen P, Vanhees L, Amery A. Hemodynamic response to converting enzyme inhibition at rest and exercise in humans. *J Appl Physiol* 1982;53:576–581.
111. Fagard R, Cattaert A, Lijnen P, et al. Response of the systemic circulation and of the renin–angiotensin–aldosterone system to ketanserin at rest and exercise in normal man. *Clin Sci* 1984;66:17–25.
112. Raffestin B, Denjean A, Legrand A, et al. Effects of nifedipine on responses to exercise in normal subjects. *J Appl Physiol* 1985;58:702–709.
113. Fagard R, Amery A, Reybrouck T, Lijnen P, Billiet L. Response of the systemic and pulmonary circulation to alpha- and beta-receptor blockade (labetalol) at rest and during exercise in hypertensive patients. *Circulation* 1979;60:1214–1219.
114. Fagard R, Fiocchi R, Lijnen P, et al. Haemodynamic and humoral responses to chronic ketanserin treatment in essential hypertension. *Br Heart J* 1984;51:149–156.
115. Cody RJ, Kubo SH, Covit AB, Müller FB, Lopez-Ovejero J, Laragh JH. Exercise hemodynamics and oxygen delivery in human hypertension. *Hypertension* 1986;8:3–10.
116. Pool PE, Seagren SC, Salel AF, Skalland ML. Effects of diltiazem on serum lipids, exercise performance and blood pressure: randomized, double-blind placebo-controlled evaluation of systemic hypertension. *Am J Cardiol* 1985;56:86H–91H.
117. Reybrouck T, Amery A, Billiet L, Fagard R. Triple antihypertensive therapy: a hemodynamic approach. In: Rorive G, Van Cauwenberghe H, eds. *The arterial hypertensive disease.* Paris: Masson, 1976;255–274.
118. Duffey DJ, Horwitz LD, Brammell HL. Nifedipine and the conditioning response. *Am J Cardiol* 1984;53:908–911.
119. Paffenbarger RS, Hyde RT, Wing AL, Hsieh CC. Physical activity, all-cause mortality, and longevity of college alumni. *N Engl J Med* 1986;314:605–613.
120. Leon AS, Connett J, Jacobs DR, Rauramaa R. Leisure-time physical activity levels and risk of coronary heart disease and death. *JAMA* 1987;258:2388–2395.
121. Pekkanen J, Martin B, Nissinen A, Tuomilehto J, Punsar S, Karvonen MJ. Reduction of premature mortality by high physical activity: a 20-year follow-up of middle-aged Finnish men. *Lancet* 1987;1:1473–1477.
122. Tran ZV, Weltman A, Glass GV, Mood DP. The effects of exercise on blood lipids and lipoproteins: a meta-analysis of studies. *Med Sci Sports Exerc* 1983;15:393–402.
123. Haskell WL. The influence of exercise training on plasma lipids and lipoproteins in health and disease. *Acta Med Scand* [*Suppl*] 1986;711:25–37.
124. Guideline for the treatment of mild hypertension: memorandum from a WHO/ISH meeting. *Lancet* 1983;1:457–458.
125. Strong WB. Hypertension and sports. *Pediatrics* 1979;64:693–695.
126. Langster JF. The sportsman with hypertension. *Aust Fam Physician* 1980;9:239–244.

Hypertension: Pathophysiology, Diagnosis, and Management, edited by J. H. Laragh and B. M. Brenner. Raven Press, Ltd., New York © 1990.

CHAPTER 125

Clinical Studies of the Role of Dietary Sodium in Blood Pressure

Myron H. Weinberger

Estimating Sodium Intake, 1999
Epidemiological Studies, 2000
Information from Studies on High Dietary Sodium Intake, 2000
The Relationship Between Sodium Intake and Added Potassium or Calcium, 2002
The Effects of Deliberate Dietary Sodium Loading on Blood Pressure in Humans, 2003
Observations with Extremely Low Dietary Sodium Intake, 2003
Physiological Rationale in Background for the Effects of Sodium on Blood Pressure, 2004
Observations of the Effect of Sodium Loading on Blood Pressure, 2005
Experimental Evidence Regarding Dietary Sodium Restriction, 2005
Sodium Sensitivity and Resistance of Blood Pressure, 2006
References, 2007

ESTIMATING SODIUM INTAKE

Before consideration of the observations stemming from epidemiological studies relating sodium intake to blood pressure, it is useful to review the current state of knowledge regarding the methods of estimating sodium intake. Sodium is a ubiquitous mineral found in abundant quantities in nature. The sodium content of foods is derived primarily from the sodium content of the soil and water in the areas where vegetables are grown and where animals are raised for human consumption. About 16% of average daily sodium intake occurs naturally in food. In industrialized societies, the majority of dietary sodium comes from the processing, preserving, and flavoring of foods, which contributes about 50% of the sodium ingested (1). In addition, approximately 33% of the sodium intake in industrialized societies results from the addition of sodium in cooking or at the table (1). Over 90% of ingested sodium is in the form of sodium chloride. Many techniques have been applied to estimate dietary sodium intake. None have proved ideal and each has advantages and limitations. Among the least reliable approaches for the estimation of sodium intake is personal recall of food consumption over a 24-hr period or longer (2). Dietary history records are slightly better than personal recall but are still not very accurate (3). Incomplete record-keeping, variability of sodium content of common foods, and inaccuracy in estimation of quantity plague personal food records. Records maintained at times of food ingestion covering 24 hrs, 72 hr, or even longer are slightly better than dietary histories but are still often incomplete (3). The most reliable single technique for estimation of dietary intake of nutrients is the preparation of duplicate meals in which the food ingested is replicated in a container which is saved for subsequent analysis (3). This is an expensive and inconvenient method of estimating nutrient intake. Furthermore, it is not widely applicable for long-term or population-based studies.

The urinary measurement of sodium excretion is very useful as an estimate of dietary intake of sodium, since, at steady-state conditions, 95% or more of ingested sodium is excreted in the urine over a 24-hr period. However, the estimates of sodium intake based on measurement of urinary sodium excretion are also fraught with variability. Incomplete urine collections can provide misleading data which can over- or underestimate the actual level of sodium intake. It is usually useful to measure urinary creatinine excretion as an index of completeness of the urine collection. While variability exists in creatinine excretion between individuals, based on activity, body weight, muscle mass, and renal function, the amount of creatinine excreted is quite consistent for a given individual. Barring marked variation in individual sodium intake, excessive dehydration, or treatment with agents affecting sodium and fluid balance, a complete 24-hr urine collection reflects sodium intake, as estimated by duplicate diets, with a high degree of accuracy. Therefore, most epidemiological and clinical studies have relied on this technique to estimate dietary sodium intake.

Some investigators have achieved success in estimating dietary sodium intake by examination of urinary excretion of sodium covering a period of less than 24 hr (4,5). The overnight timed urine collection is an example of such a technique which minimizes the variability due to incomplete collection of urine over a 24-hr period and which is unlikely to be influenced by marked alterations in dietary sodium intake in a given individual. The sodium excretion in a timed overnight urine sample has been found to correlate highly with that of the 24-hr urine collection in the same individual (4,5). The precision of estimation of dietary sodium intake by means of 24-hr urine collections is dependent on (a) the number of urine samples collected and (b) the variability of sodium intake for a given individual over a 24-hr period (6). Liu et al. (6) have reported that seven 24-hr urine collections are required in order to accurately estimate sodium intake in ambulatory subjects. Luft et al. (7) examined the accuracy of 24-hr and overnight urine collections in estimating sodium intake for subjects who received known amounts of sodium in their diet, ranging from normal to reduced and high. These observations indicated that timed overnight urine collections were reliably correlated with intake at the lower ranges of sodium consumption but were less reliable during a normal or high sodium intake. These investigators further examined the usefulness of a chloride-sensitive titrator strip in estimating urinary sodium content (8). Similarly, they observed a correlation between known dietary sodium intake and this semiquantitative measure of chloride excretion (8).

EPIDEMIOLOGICAL STUDIES

A variety of studies indicate that in Americans, average sodium intake for females ranges from 2 to 4 g/day, while that for males is approximately 50% higher, owing to their greater caloric intake, reaching 4–6 g/day (8–10). Potassium intake similarly varies on the base of sex and body size. American women generally consume 1–1.5 g/day of potassium, whereas men consume 2–6 g/day (11). Estimates of dietary sodium consumption in an English population, which was not separated on the basis of sex, indicated a range from 2.8 to 3.6 g/day (12). Thus, it would appear that these represent similar ranges of values for average sodium intake in industrialized societies. Epidemiologic studies have provided information regarding the extremes of sodium intake among populations examined throughout the world.

Evolutionary evidence indicates that the sodium content of the typical hunter–gatherer diet of our ancestors was very low in sodium and high in potassium (13). Indeed, recent population studies have demonstrated the ability of primitive people to survive quite adequately, even in a tropical environment, on levels of sodium intake of less than 250 mg/day (14). Low-sodium diets are not exclusively a feature of people living far from the sea where sodium is more abundant than in inland sites. Many islanders and coastal dwellers also follow low-sodium diets (15,16).

INFORMATION FROM STUDIES ON HIGH DIETARY SODIUM INTAKE

Factors such as age and genetic background may influence the response to dietary sodium intake. For example, studies of Dutch infants revealed that those given low-sodium formula had significantly lower blood pressures at the end of 6 months of feeding than did those given formulas high in sodium content (17). Similar observations were made by the same investigators, who demonstrated that infants and children drinking water in which the sodium content was high had higher blood pressures than did those in a similar community whose sodium content was lower (18). Furthermore, changing the water to bottled water low in sodium content lowered blood pressure in the children from the higher-sodium community (18). In the United States, a similar observation was made with respect to blood pressure in children from communities having markedly different sodium content of their drinking water (19). Calabrese and Tuthill (19) demonstrated that elementary school children from the community where the sodium content of drinking water was increased (because the reservoir for that community was located near the Massachusetts Turnpike, a site with extensive salting of the highway during the winter because of ice) had higher blood pressure levels than did children from an ethnically similar community nearby, whose water was supplied by a reservoir with lower sodium content. Thus, it would appear from these studies in Holland and America that even the content of sodium in drinking water can influence blood pressure.

Several investigators have reported on the relationship between apparent dietary sodium intake and the prevalence of hypertension in societies around the world. The original observations of Dahl (20) and Gleiberman (21) in this regard have been extended and complemented by the observations of MacGregor (22), who demonstrated a linear relationship between the prevalence of hypertension and increases in the levels of sodium intake in societies consuming above 50–100 mEq/day of sodium. These investigators demonstrated that hypertension and its cardiovascular sequelae, as well as the previously thought inexorable increase in blood pressure with age, were not seen below that level of sodium intake (22). This relationship was initially described by Gleiberman (21), who observed a linear correlation between systolic and diastolic blood pressure and levels of sodium intake in humans. However, that study was plagued by concerns regarding the confirmation of sodium intake, as well as the accuracy of blood pressure measurements, reported for differing societies.

It can be observed that in most industrialized cultures ingesting 8–15 g/day of sodium chloride (3.2–6 g/day of sodium), hypertension occurs with the frequency of about 10–15% among an unselected population (22). In addition, in these societies, approximately one-third of individuals will develop a rise in blood pressure with increasing age (22). Examples of extremes of sodium intake come from detailed studies of northern Japan, where intakes of 20–50 g/day of sodium chloride have been reported. This appears to be related to the dietary habits of using a great deal of soy paste, high-sodium miso soup, pickled vegetables, salt fish, and soy sauce (23). These eating habits may have been a cultural development dating to the time when sodium was used to preserve vegetables, fish, and meat over the winter period. It is also known that inhabitants of this region of Japan, in addition to having the highest incidence of hypertension (in excess of 60%), reported the major cause of death to be cerebral vascular disease, a sequelae of hypertension (23).

It is of interest to note that changes in dietary intake of sodium in this region occurred as a result of two government programs. The first one was mounted in the period from 1959 to 1971 and resulted in a modest decrease in average sodium chloride intake. The second one was conducted in the period from 1971 to 1981, was much more extensive, and reduced average sodium intake from 14.5 to 12.5 g/day. Both were associated with a decline in the incidence of stroke and hypertension (23). In Belgium, a similar campaign was conducted between 1968 and 1981, resulting in a decrease in average salt consumption from 15 to 9 g/day. This was accompanied by a decrease in stroke mortality (24).

Additional information regarding the effects of changes in sodium intake comes from studies of populations migrating from one area to another. One such study involves the inhabitants of the Tokelau Islands, who left their isolated environment and migrated to New Zealand (25). They adopted the increased sodium intake of the more acculturated New Zealanders and subsequently developed a greater prevalence of elevated blood pressure (25). Inhabitants of the Cook Islands can be separated into those who habitually consume an increased sodium intake (in whom the incidence of hypertension is 28%) and those subsisting on a low-sodium diet (in whom the incidence of hypertension is only approximately 3%) (15). Similar differences have been noted among the inhabitants of New Guinea. The coastal tribes of this locale have a high sodium intake and a substantial prevalence of hypertension that is not found among their highland compatriots, who have both a low sodium intake and a low incidence of hypertension (26) Additional relationships have been seen between sodium intake in blood pressure among inhabitants of the Solomon Islands (27). An African study examined changes in blood pressure in members of the Samburu Tribe recruited into the Kenyan Army (28). The native Samburu diet is very low in sodium and high in potassium. Similarly, the prevalence of hypertension is natively quite low in those individuals. When they were recruited into the Kenyan Army, however, the sodium intake increased markedly because of the high salt content of Army rations, and most of the Samburu demonstrated a significant rise of blood pressure (28). However, dietary changes were not the only one encountered by the Samburu recruited into the Kenyan Army. They were obviously subjected to many stressful environmental factors. When these individuals returned to their tribal environment and resumed their customary low-sodium–high-potassium intake, blood pressure also declined (28).

In America, one of the most extensive studies of cardiovascular disease and its associated risk factors has been mounted in Framingham, Massachusetts. Among the early observations in that study were measurements of urinary sodium excretion: 78% of the Framingham population was found to be excreting more than 8 g/day of salt (29). Furthermore, in comparing the range of sodium intake exhibited by the free-living inhabitants of Framingham, Massachusetts, it was found that in those who habitually ingested less than 8 g/day, as evidenced by decreased urinary sodium excretion, the incidence of hypertension was about 20%. However, in the individuals in whom salt intake was greater than 13 g/day, the incidence of hypertension almost doubled, to 36% (29). Thus, a relationship between sodium intake and blood pressure can be demonstrated in virtually any population in which it is examined, if care is taken to define the range of sodium intake and if that range is relatively wide.

Another component contributing to the inability to identify relationships between blood pressure and sodium intake in some societies is the issue of genetic susceptibility. Obviously, if a population with high susceptibility to the blood-pressure-raising effects of sodium is not exposed to a high-sodium diet for an extended period of time, hypertension may not be observed. On the other hand, if a population with inherent susceptibility to the pressure effects of sodium is exposed to an increased level of sodium intake, it is likely that all of the susceptible individuals will manifest an increase in blood pressure, whereas those who are not susceptible will not. Thus, individuals with both high and low blood pressure will be observed at the same level of increased sodium intake. Moreover, if there is a temporal component to blood pressure sensitivity to sodium, only those susceptible individuals with sufficient exposure to excess sodium will manifest the blood pressure rise.

Among populations where sodium intake is low, hypertension is virtually unknown, as are the cardiovascular complications thereof. In contemporary times, these societies have largely been primitive and isolated; thus it has been difficult to dissociate the effects of exercise and lean body mass, as well as relative absence of the confounding psychological accompaniments of societal stress, from the influence of a low dietary sodium intake in influencing their blood pressure level. These observations have, however, given us some insight into the minimal need for sodium of human beings. Studies of the Yanamamo Tribe in the Amazon Jungle have revealed average daily sodium excretion of less than 10 mEq/day (representing less than 250 mg/day of sodium intake) as well as no evidence of hypertension or its cardiovascular effects (14). The Eskimos in the Arctic Circle regularly ingest less than 80 mEq/day of sodium and have a low incidence of coronary disease, atherosclerosis, and stroke (20). Similarly, populations have been identified in various islands, in Central and South America, in Africa and Australia, at high altitudes, and in the Arctic, as well as in desert environments (where sodium intake is consistently less than 2 g/day). In those environments, hypertension is rare, as are its cardiovascular sequelae.

While extensive epidemiologic data are available linking sodium intake to blood pressure in a large number of human populations, there is less critically obtained information concerning the minimum requirements for sodium in human beings. The discovery of several isolated societies in whom average daily sodium intake is less than 10 mEq/day (less than 250 mg/day) suggests that even in arid or tropical environments, where losses of sodium and water from perspiration are considerable, the minimum need for sodium does not exceed that minute amount (14,22). The observation that average daily sodium intake of humans living in acculturated societies ranges from 2 to 4 g/day further suggests that the average consumption of sodium by free-living individuals in much of the civilized world is many orders of magnitude greater than is required for their biological needs.

Less precise information is available concerning the needs for subsets of a given population. Specific information regarding the sodium requirements of infants, growing children, young adults, pregnant women, and elderly individuals is not at hand. However, some scattered reports can shed some light on these issues. Studies in Holland indicate that newborn infants receiving a formula containing a normal amount of sodium have a significantly higher blood pressure after 6 months of feeding than do infants given a low-sodium formula from birth (17). As will be discussed subsequently, in consideration of the physiological relationships between sodium and blood pressure proposed by Guyton et al. (30), it may be that an increased level of blood pressure is required to enable the infant to excrete the additional, unneeded sodium provided by the higher-sodium-containing formula. Furthermore, the long-term impact of even subtle excesses of sodium, above that required for biological function, is not clearly defined. No specific information is available regarding the minimum sodium requirements of growing children or young adults. In normal pregnancy, alterations in the hormonal milieu favor sodium loss. This appears to be primarily due to the antimineralocorticoid, natriuretic effects of progesterone, which increase sodium excretion (31). In addition, the developing fetus and its uterine environment require sequestration of additional stores of sodium such that a normal pregnancy represents a non-steady-state condition, at least in part (32). For these reasons, progressive activation of the renin–aldosterone system is observed during the course of normal pregnancy which increases in parallel with the rise in levels of progesterone (33). Thus, in the normal pregnant woman, sodium restriction may not be advisable. In the pregnant individual with hypertension, these relationships may be altered. Nonetheless, extracellular fluid volume expansion is not considered to be a regular feature of pregnancy-induced hypertension, and thus diuretics and severe salt restriction are not usually advocated (34).

Little information is available regarding the sodium needs of aging individuals. Since renal function is a major determinant of the ability to excrete excess sodium, the general decline in renal function accompanying aging, thought to be due to a naturally occurring obsolescence of glomerular function, may impair the ability to excrete a salt load. This may account, in large part, for the increase in blood pressure, which generally accompanies aging in industrialized societies and which appears to be so strongly influenced by the level of sodium intake (22). An additional difference between acculturated and less acculturated societies in conjunction with their differences in levels of sodium intake is the observation that acculturated individuals have an extracellular fluid volume space which is approximately 15% greater than that of unacculturated individuals (35). This observation further suggests that the surfeit of sodium ingested in acculturated individuals produces an increase in extracellular fluid volume and blood pressure which is not biologically requisite.

THE RELATIONSHIP BETWEEN SODIUM INTAKE AND ADDED POTASSIUM OR CALCIUM

Several epidemiologic and interventional studies have provided evidence for an interactive role between sodium and potassium in influencing blood pressure (36–39). However, much less data are available concerning such an interaction between sodium and calcium (40). One of the earliest clinical descriptions, involving the blood-pressure-raising effects of sodium, came from the reports of observations in diabetic children given large amounts of sodium chloride (41). In those studies, an increase in potassium intake appeared to blunt the blood-pressure-raising effects of an increase in sodium intake. It has previously been noted that societies in whom sodium intake is habitually low are usually societies in whom potassium intake is higher than that of acculturated societies (22,25–28). A corollary to the observations relating high potassium and low sodium intake to a decreased blood pressure level are the observations that a low potassium intake may be associated with a rise in blood pressure (36,42). Furthermore, evidence exists that individuals consuming a high fruit and vegetable diet have a decreased incidence of stroke (43). Other epidemiologic data indicate a positive correlation between blood pressure and the urinary excretion of potassium observed from communities as disparate as Belgium (44) and Kenya (45). Watson et al. (37) studied adolescent black students on two occasions separated in time and found that the urinary sodium–potassium ratio was a good predictor of the future rise in blood pressure. It is also known that individuals who are traditionally thought to be at increased risk to the blood-pressure-raising effects of sodium, such as black subjects, have a dietary potassium intake which is significantly less than that of their white counterparts in comparative studies, although no differences in sodium intake could be detected (40). Thus, evaluation of the dietary intake of sodium in relation to that of potassium may be more important than consideration of the level of sodium intake alone. Watson and his colleagues also suggest that a similar relationship may exist between the urinary sodium–calcium ratio and blood pressure, with higher values being associated with higher pressures (40). Thus, the intake of these two minerals, potassium and calcium, may influence the responsiveness of blood pressure to sodium.

To examine the relationship between potassium and blood pressure further, several studies are informative. Lever et al. (46) investigated several components of total body electrolyte and fluid status and found a strong inverse correlation between total body potassium and blood pressure. Several studies which have utilized an increased sodium intake to examine the role of sodium on blood pressure have noted a net loss of potassium at sodium intake levels of 400 mEq/day or greater (47,48). Increases in sodium intake have thus been shown to increase potassium excretion. Other studies have demonstrated that an increase in potassium intake designed to prevent net potassium loss with sodium loading blunts or prevents the sodium-induced rise in blood pressure (49). Furthermore, in the course of such studies, documentation of a lesser increase in plasma volume and cardiac output and of a greater fall in plasma levels of norepinephrine were seen during the potassium-supplemented, sodium-loading phase (49). Potassium also has long been known to reduce blood pressure (50). More detailed studies indicate that potassium administration increases the excretion of sodium and lowers blood pressure (51–53). Several observations in both the acute and extended term have provided documentation of the antihypertensive effects of potassium. Furthermore, potassium has been shown to blunt the blood-pressure-raising effect of sodium loading (49,54).

THE EFFECTS OF DELIBERATE DIETARY SODIUM LOADING ON BLOOD PRESSURE IN HUMANS

Accidental and purposeful increases in sodium intake above the normal range have been reported to raise blood pressure in a variety of circumstances. McQuarrie et al. (41) observed a rise in blood pressure in diabetic children given large amounts of sodium salts. Furthermore, they observed that potassium administration caused a lesser increase in blood pressure. Ingestion of large amounts (1200 mEq/day) of sodium bicarbonate were observed to raise blood pressure in a single individual (55). Kirkendall et al. (47) administered 400 mEq/day of sodium for a period of 1 month to volunteer subjects without observing a significant increase in blood pressure. However, the precision of the blood pressure measurements was difficult to evaluate in that study, and the degree of compliance to the regimen was variable (47).

Our group conducted systematic studies of dietary sodium restriction and dietary sodium loading covering a range from 10 to 1200 or 1500 mEq/day in incremental steps (48,56). At the highest level of sodium intake, blood pressure and cardiac output increased. Eight of the subjects were black, and eight were white. This permitted comparison of the racial responses to the salt load. The black normotensives involved in this study had a lower threshold of blood pressure response to salt loading and a greater magnitude of increase in blood pressure than did the whites (48). In that study, as in the observations of Kirkendall et al. (47), levels of sodium intake greater than 300 mEq/day were associated with net potassium loss (48). The pressor effect of sodium loading was blunted when potassium was supplemented to prevent potassium depletion (48,49). In a more recent study, Roos et al. (57) administered 1100 mEq/day of sodium to normotensive white subjects and observed no change in blood pressure, further confirming the enormous capacity of white normotensives to excrete a massive sodium load.

OBSERVATIONS WITH EXTREMELY LOW DIETARY SODIUM INTAKE

A variety of investigators have made important contributions to the treatment of hypertension by the institution of diets that featured marked sodium restriction. The most famous of these was the "Rice Diet" instituted by Kempner (58). This diet, containing rice and fruit, was not only low in sodium but high in potassium and deficient in protein. Adherence to this diet proved lifesaving in many patients with accelerated or malignant hypertension before the advent of antihypertensive drugs. Other investigators also reported on their experience with diets structured to be markedly reduced in sodium content. However, most of these diets required rigid or severe dietary sodium restriction to a level of 30 mEq/day (0.7 g/day) or less (59,60). Although these diets were achievable in an institutionalized setting, they were often deemed to be unpalatable, and they frequently were not continued by free-living outpatients. Because of the notion that dietary sodium restriction had to be severe in order to be effective in reducing blood pressure and, more importantly, because of the advent of diuretic therapy in the late 1950s, about 30 years ago the interest in dietary sodium restriction as a therapeutic approach to hypertension waned. It has only been recently, when concern has been raised regarding the potential adverse effects of diuretic therapy, that a reevaluation of the role of modest dietary sodium restriction has been conducted.

There are a variety of studies which have compared the effects of sodium restriction with those of weight loss and have examined the issue of whether the two may confound each other in terms of their benefit on blood pressure. Although there are some inconsistencies between the results of these studies, the general agreement is that sodium restriction of a modest degree (50–80 mEq/day; 1–2 g/day) is of benefit in reducing blood pressure in many, but not all, hypertensive patients (61–69). Beard et al. (65) conducted a study among treated hypertensives in whom dietary sodium was reduced from a control value of 161 mEq/day to 37 mEq/day (65). They demonstrated the ability to maintain blood pressure control in their hypertensive subjects with fewer medications than were previously required. Morgan et al. (62) reduced sodium intake from 168 mEq/day to 85 mEq/day in hypertensives and achieved a significant decrease in blood pressure. Furthermore, they observed a correlation between the change in urinary sodium excretion and the change in blood pressure. They observed that the blood pressure fall was blunted by the responsiveness of the renin system. This provided an explanation for the greater efficacy of salt restriction and diuretic administration in patients in whom renin responsiveness is known to be diminished, such as black or elderly hypertensives. A variety of studies have demonstrated that modest dietary sodium restriction enhances the efficacy of a variety of antihypertensive agents (61,65,70). We have recently completed a study where free-living, treated hypertensives were taught to reduce their sodium intake by approximately half and to maintain that level of dietary sodium restriction for a period of 3 months (71). Among those who were successful in achieving this modest degree of dietary sodium restriction, the number and doses of medications required to maintain blood pressure control was significantly reduced

(71). Although an institutionalized setting was not required to achieve the reduction in sodium intake in these study subjects, individualized dietary counseling by a registered dietitian was employed. The dietitian reviewed the patients' personal food preferences in order to identify the major dietary sources of sodium (72). Substitutes and alternatives were then identified to enable the modest degree of dietary sodium restriction desired. Attention was paid to helping the individual while eating at restaurants, in fast-food sites, or outside of the home, as well as in reading labels while shopping (72). Granted that the subjects in this study were highly motivated and volunteered for participation, it is nonetheless likely that a similar level of success could be replicated in a less-selected population given proper resources and adequate motivation.

PHYSIOLOGICAL RATIONALE IN BACKGROUND FOR THE EFFECTS OF SODIUM ON BLOOD PRESSURE

Although the evidence that sodium is related to blood pressure, as previously cited, is substantial, the mechanisms by which an increased renal sodium intake or increased sodium reabsorption occurs and by which this may alter blood pressure is not as well defined. Guyton et al. (73) have developed an elegant model of the circulation and of blood pressure control which regards the kidney as the final common denominator in influencing blood pressure. In this conceptual framework, the physiological alterations which accompany sodium loading and volume expansion serve, by an intricate set of modulating mechanisms, to increase systemic blood pressure—and, thus, renal perfusion pressure—in an attempt to enhance the excretion of the excess sodium and water. This concept, termed the *renal function curve,* has its origins in older observations demonstrating that an increase in blood pressure produced an increase in sodium excretion in experimental animals (74). Human observations suggested that hypertensive patients, as a group, excreted more of an administered sodium load than did their normotensive counterparts (75). These observations were taken as confirmation of the pressure–natriuresis hypothesis. Subsequent studies in humans, which will be detailed below, indicate that there is marked heterogeneity in the renal response to sodium loading among hypertensive and normotensive humans. Among those with elevated pressures, the natriuretic response following an intravenous saline load was observed to be greatest in patients with primary aldosteronism (76). Low-renin essential hypertensive patients without evidence of hyperaldosteronism also had a significant natriuretic response to an intravenous salt load when compared to their hypertensive counterparts who had normal- or high-renin forms of essential hypertension or who had renal vascular hypertension (76). Even within the normotensive population, subsets of individuals can be identified who have an enhanced natriuretic response to the same intravenous saline load. These include black normotensives when compared to their white counterparts, as well as those over the age of 40 who were matched with younger individuals for gender and race (77). Furthermore, while these two subgroups of the normotensive population had an exaggerated immediate natriuretic response to intravenous saline loading, their total sodium excretion over the 24-hr period was observed to be less than that of their white or younger cohorts (77). The first-degree relatives of hypertensive subjects comprise another group in whom renal sodium handling has been observed to be abnormal despite the presence of a normal blood pressure (78). These individuals are less able to excrete an intravenous saline load than are their (age, gender, and race-matched) counterparts with no family history of hypertension. These three subsets of the normotensive population—black subjects, older individuals, and those with a family history of hypertension—are all known to be at greater risk for the development of hypertension later in life. Thus these abnormalities of sodium handling may serve to identify those at an increased risk for subsequent blood pressure elevation among normotensive subjects.

The renal handling of sodium and water is regulated by multiple and complex mechanisms. Many of these have been detailed in other chapters. We examined several components of renal function which are known to influence sodium and potassium handling for clues regarding the etiology of the aforementioned abnormalities. Plasma renin activity was found to be lower in those individuals in whom an exaggerated natriuretic response was seen, whereas aldosterone values were not significantly different (76). Furthermore, sympathetic nervous system components were also influenced by sodium loading, as will be detailed subsequently (79). Several other investigators have examined different aspects of the physiological rationale previously cited for the effects of sodium on blood pressure. Kokubu et al. (80) have also observed an exaggerated natriuretic response to sodium administration, as did several investigators who have reported abnormalities in the response of the renin–aldosterone system to alterations in sodium balance (81–87). Some investigators have hypothesized that these abnormalities may be related to sodium-sensitive blood pressure changes. Recent studies in humans (57) have confirmed the adaptation to sodium loading observed in our earlier studies (48,56,76–78). Roos et al. (57) further confirmed our previous observation (48) regarding the differential suppression of the renin–aldosterone and sympathetic nervous systems by sodium loading.

Investigators have sought evidence for sodium-related alterations in intrarenal hemodynamics and in factors which might influence differential renal blood flow. Several studies have provided evidence for participation of the kallikrein–kinin system in modulating renal sodium excretion (88–92). Other studies have shown differences in renal blood flow (93). The recent elucidation of a link between cardiac volume receptors and the kidney, coupled with the identification of atrial natriuretic factors, has provided an additional mechanism whereby the kidney may influence sodium excretion (94–96). Haddy et al. (97) have proposed that sodium-sensitive hypertension involved increased production of an endogenous inhibitor of Na-K-ATPase activity. Blaustein (98) has elaborated on this concept with a potential explanation for increased vascular responsiveness due to an increased intracellular sodium concentration in vascular smooth muscle. Extensive information has been generated regarding the participation of the sympathetic nervous system in sodium-related changes in blood pressure. There is substantial evidence that stimulation of proximal tubular alpha-adrenergic receptors enhances sodium reabsorption (99). Other investigators have reported a variety of alterations in sympathetic function with changes in sodium balance. These range from reports of alterations in baroreflex sensitivity (100) to increases in adrenergic activity (54,79,85,100–111). Finally, we have demonstrated that the vascular response to exogenous norepinephrine in humans is altered by the state of sodium balance (112).

A variety of studies have examined the role of genetic factors in influencing the blood pressure response to sodium. In experimental animals, some sodium-related forms of hypertension appear to be genetically determined and mediated by the kidney (113,114). Furthermore, studies have demonstrated heterogeneity in sodium handling in humans which appears to be genetically mediated. Whitfield and Martin (115) have demonstrated, by studies in monozygotic and dizygotic twin pairs, that basal renal tubular handling of both sodium and potassium, measured by the fractional excretion of sodium and potassium, are genetically influenced. These observations confirm earlier studies by our group regarding genetic influences on renal sodium handling following an intravenous saline load (116). In addition, those studies also demonstrated a genetic contribution to the responsiveness of the renin–angiotensin–aldosterone and sympathetic nervous systems as indicated by genetic influences on renin activity, aldosterone, and plasma norepinephrine levels (116,117). Furthermore, genetic influences on blood pressure responsiveness to alterations in dietary intake have been demonstrated by several groups, including our own (118–121). The importance of family history and of the activity of the sympathetic nervous system has also been emphasized by Skrabal et al. (104) as well as by other investigators.

Vascular responsiveness to pressor agents has been shown to be influenced by the state of sodium balance. This provides yet another mechanism by which sodium may influence blood pressure. In experimental animals, a variety of studies demonstrate that the dose–response curve to pressor agents, including angiotensin II and norepinephrine, can be modified by the state of sodium balance (122). Similarly, studies have been conducted in humans showing that angiotensin II responses (123), as well as responses to norepinephrine (112), can be influenced by dietary sodium intake or sodium balance. In addition, several studies have demonstrated vascular changes as a result of changes in sodium balance (124–126).

OBSERVATIONS OF THE EFFECT OF SODIUM LOADING ON BLOOD PRESSURE

Several of the early studies demonstrating the effects of an increase in sodium intake on blood pressure were largely anecdotal or accidental (41,42,55,59). Some of these have already been reviewed in this chapter and include (a) the observations of McQuarrie et al. (41) regarding excessive ingestion of sodium in diabetic children in 1936 and (b) the observations of McDonough and Wilhelmj in 1954 (127). An evaluation of the effects of sodium intake on blood pressure was initially performed by Kirkendall et al. (47), who studied four normal male prison volunteers following 4 weeks of low (10 mEq), moderate (210 mEq), and high (410 mEq) sodium intake in the presence of a potassium intake of 100 mEq/day. These investigators found no significant change in blood pressure between any of these diets. They did, however, note that there was a net loss of potassium when individuals were ingesting the highest level of sodium. It is possible that the disproportionately high potassium intake provided during this study, in comparison with the usual intake of free-living Americans, may have attenuated the effect of sodium on blood pressure. We systematically studied 16 normotensive, young male volunteers following equilibration on a 10-, 300-, 600- or 800-, and 1200- or 1500-mEq/day sodium intake, each given for 3-day periods with the exception of the 10-mEq/day sodium intake, which was given for 1 week (48,56). During this study, potassium intake was maintained constant at 80 mEq/day. A significant increase in mean arterial blood pressure was observed in these 16 normotensive subjects with sodium loading and was accompanied by a significant increase in cardiac output (48,56). Marked suppression of plasma renin activity and plasma aldosterone levels were noted at the 300-mEq/day sodium intake level, which was maintained at the higher levels of sodium ingestion (48). Plasma and urinary norepinephrine values also decreased with sodium loading, but suppression of these sympathetic nervous system markers was less complete than that of the renin–aldosterone system (48,128). As had been previously observed by Kirkendall et al. (47), a kaliuresis was observed at levels of sodium intake greater than 300 mEq/day, which led to net potassium loss (48). Among the study subjects, who were equally divided between black and white males, blacks were noted to have a lower threshold of blood pressure responsiveness and a greater magnitude of blood pressure increase with sodium loading than were whites (48,49). A subgroup of this study population participated in a second study following the same protocol, with the exception that potassium losses were prevented by ingestion of supplemental potassium on a daily basis, equivalent to urinary potassium losses, at levels of sodium intake above 300 mEq/day (49). The prevention of potassium depletion significantly attenuated the blood pressure response to sodium loading (49).

The role of the sympathetic nervous system in the responsiveness of blood pressure to sodium was investigated in another population of normotensive young men (112). In this study, an incremental intravenous infusion of norepinephrine was conducted following equilibration during a 10- or 800-mEq/day sodium diet period given in random order to all of the subjects. In this study, sodium restriction markedly attenuated the blood pressure to norepinephrine (112). Thus, the state of sodium balance modifies the blood pressure response to norepinephrine.

EXPERIMENTAL EVIDENCE REGARDING DIETARY SODIUM RESTRICTION

The evidence with respect to the effects of reduced dietary sodium intake on blood pressure in normotensive subjects is extremely sparse. We have recently studied normotensive, free-living adults (namely, parents of monozygotic twin children) who were willing to participate in a study designed to reduce dietary sodium intake to levels of less than 60 mEq/day for 3 months or more (129). These goals were accomplished by individualized dietary counseling by a registered dietitian in order to evaluate the specific food preferences of individual families (72). It was not difficult for these free-living, normotensive volunteers to achieve and maintain this level of dietary sodium restriction. Despite the fact that the subjects were normotensive, a significant reduction in blood pressure was observed (129). Furthermore, when the individual blood pressure responses were examined, marked heterogeneity was seen (130). These observations were utilized to develop one of our operative definitions of sodium sensitivity and resistance (131). Individuals who were found to be sodium-sensitive in this study were significantly older than their sodium-resistant counterparts, and they were more likely to have the haptoglobin 1–1 phenotype than other haptoglobin patterns (132). This suggests that haptoglobin may be a genetic marker for sodium sensitivity of blood pressure. Furthermore, when the individuals in this normotensive population were separated on the basis of haptoglobin phenotype, it was found that mean blood pressure among those individuals with haptoglobin 1–1 phenotype was significantly higher than that of the 2–2 phenotype group (132).

SODIUM SENSITIVITY AND RESISTANCE OF BLOOD PRESSURE

A variety of studies have been conducted to define sodium sensitivity and resistance of blood pressure, primarily in hypertensive subjects. Most of these studies have utilized dietary sodium restriction of a severe degree (10 mEq/day), usually followed by a period of dietary sodium loading ranging from 250 to 300 or more mEq/day (133–137). Blood pressure responses to the two periods of dietary sodium manipulation were then compared, and individuals showing marked differences were considered to be sodium-sensitive. Thus, most of these studies have begun with a period of dietary sodium restriction followed by that of dietary sodium loading. It is difficult to evaluate whether the blood pressure response used to define sodium sensitivity in these studies is related specifically to the response to sodium restriction or to the effects of sodium loading (133–137). In most of the studies for which data are given, the blood pressure at the end of the high dietary period is no different from that before dietary sodium restriction, suggesting that the sodium sensitivity defined in these situations is related to dietary sodium restriction alone. The interpretation of these observations is made even more difficult because of the heterogeneity of responsiveness of the humoral systems, such as the renin–angiotensin–aldosterone system, to sodium restriction. Thus, some individuals may begin the high dietary sodium period with a much higher or much lower level of renin and aldosterone than others. This variability may then determine the amount of sodium retained during the sodium loading period and may thus influence blood pressure responsiveness. Finally, in all of the previous studies, observations were confined to hypertensive subjects (133–137).

We have utilized a different protocol for the assessment of sodium sensitivity and resistance and have applied this not only to hypertensive subjects but to normotensives as well (131). Our protocol employed sodium and volume expansion by means of an intravenous saline load (2 liters over a 4-hr period) (138), followed the next day by sodium and volume depletion induced by a low sodium intake (10 mEq/day) and three 40-mg oral doses of the potent loop diuretic, furosemide (139). The blood pressure observed at the end of the saline infusion was compared to that following sodium and volume depletion. Individuals in either normotensive or hypertensive groups exhibiting a decrease in mean arterial pressure equal to or greater than 10 mmHg following sodium and volume depletion were considered to be sodium-sensitive, whereas those demonstrating a decrease in mean arterial pressure of less than 5 mmHg, and including those in whom blood pressure actually rose following sodium and volume depletion, were defined as sodium-resistant (131). Individuals whose blood pressure response fell between 5 and 9 mmHg were considered to be unclassifiable with respect to sodium responsivity. Among over 200 hypertensive subjects that we have studied in this fashion, 51% were found to be sodium-sensitive whereas 33% were sodium-resistant (131). Among the more than 400 normotensive subjects that we studied in a similar fashion, 58% were found to be sodium-resistant whereas 26% were sodium-sensitive (131). The sodium-sensitive individuals in both blood pressure populations were compared to their sodium-resistant cohorts in a variety of ways. The sodium-sensitive subjects were significantly older than the sodium-resistant subjects, in both the normotensive and hypertensive groups, despite the fact that the mean age for both populations was less than 45 years (131). Plasma renin activity was found to be significantly lower in sodium-sensitive subjects than in sodium-resistant individuals (131). Sodium-sensitive individuals had an enhanced natriuretic response to the saline infusion when compared to their resistant counterparts (131). However, the renin responsiveness was not accurately predictive of sodium responsivity. Thus, the observations could not be explained by low renin status alone. The sodium-resistant individuals were also found to have higher baseline or stimulated levels of plasma norepinephrine than those who were sodium-sensitive (131).

Finally, the haptoglobin 1–1 phenotype was more apt to be encountered among sodium-sensitive individuals of both hypertensive and normotensive groups than among the sodium-resistant cohorts in this independent study (132). These observations suggest that the blood pressure response to a low sodium diet and volume depletion may be determined by the responsiveness of the renin–angiotensin–aldosterone system to this maneuver. Individuals in whom the humoral responses are brisk are less apt to have a marked fall in blood pressure.

These observations corroborate similar observations using different protocols for the definition of sodium sensitivity and resistance reported by other investigators (133–137,140). Furthermore, Koolen and van Brummelen (141) have reported a similar blunted renin responsiveness in individuals that they characterized as being sodium-sensitive by means of a 2-week period of a high (300 mM) or low (50 mM) dietary sodium intake. They also observed that administration of intravenous furosemide was not helpful in predicting sodium sensitivity in their study (141). Further studies to define the mechanisms involved in establishing sodium responsivity of blood pressure are clearly needed. The observation that marked heterogeneity of sodium responsiveness exists not only among hypertensives but also among normotensives mandates clarification of the relationship between this phenomenon and the subsequent development of hypertension.

ACKNOWLEDGMENTS

The author wishes to express gratitude to Mrs. Cassandra Brown for her expertise in the preparation of this manuscript.

REFERENCES

1. Fregly MS, Fregly MJ. The estimates of sodium intake by man. In: Fregly MJ, Kare MR, eds. *The role of salt in cardiovascular hypertension.* New York: Academic Press, 1982;3–15.
2. Schacter J, Harper PH, Radin ME, et al. Comparison of sodium and potassium intake with excretion. *Hypertension* 1980;2:695–699.
3. Clark AJ, Mossholder S. Sodium and potassium intake measurements: dietary methodology problems. *Am J Clin Nutr* 1986;43:470–476.
4. Liu K, Dyer AR, Cooper RS, Stamler R, Stamler J. Can overnight urine replace 24-hour urine collections to assess salt intake? *Hypertension* 1979;1:529–534.
5. Luft FC, Fineberg NS, Sloan RS. Overnight urine collections to estimate sodium intake. *Hypertension* 1982;4:494–498.
6. Liu K, Cooper R, McKeever J, et al. Assessment of the association between habitual salt intake and blood pressure: methodological problems. *Am J Epidemiol* 1979;110:219.
7. Luft FC, Fineberg NS, Sloan RS. Estimating dietary sodium intake in individuals receiving a randomly fluctuating intake. *Hypertension* 1982;4:805–808.
8. Luft FC, Fineberg NS, Sloan RS. Overnight urine collections to estimate sodium intake. *Hypertension* 1982;4:494–498.
9. National Center for Health Statistics. *National Health Survey.* Washington, DC: US Government Printing Office, 1983.
10. Caggiula AW, Wing RR, Nowalk MP, Milas NC, Lee S, Langford H. The measurement of sodium and potassium intake. *Am J Clin Nutr* 1985;42:391–398.
11. Fischer DR, Morgan KJ, Zabik ME. Cholesterol, saturated fatty acids, polyunsaturated fatty acids, sodium and potassium intakes of the United States population. *J Am Coll Nutr* 1985;4:207–224.
12. Farleigh CA, Shepherd R, Land DG. Measurement of sodium intake and its relationship to blood pressure and salivary sodium concentration. *Nutr Res* 1985;5:815–826.
13. Eaton SB, Konner M. Paleolithic nutrition: a consideration of its nature and current implications. *N Engl J Med* 1985;312:283–289.
14. Oliver WJ, Cohen EL, Neel JV. Blood pressure, sodium intake and sodium-related hormones in the Yanomamo Indians, a "no-salt" culture. *Circulation* 1975;52:146–151.
15. Prior IAM, Grimley-Evans J, Harvey HPB, Davidson F, Lindsey M. Sodium intake and blood pressure in two Polynesian populations. *N Engl J Med* 1968;279:515–520.
16. Meneely GR, Dahl LK. Electrolytes in hypertension: the effects of sodium chloride. *Med Clin North Am* 1961;45:271–283.
17. Hofman A, Hazebroek A, Valkenburg HA. A randomized trial of sodium intake and blood pressure in newborn infants. *JAMA* 1983;250:370–373.
18. Calabrese EJ, Tuthill RW, Sieger TL, Klar JM. The role of elevated levels of sodium in diet and drinking water on the development of hypertension in animal models and humans. *Environ Pathol Toxicol* 1980;2:143–151.
19. Calabrese EJ, Tuthill RW. Elevated blood pressure levels and community drinking water characteristics. *J Environ Health Sci* 1978;A13:781–802.
20. Dahl LK. The possible role of chronic excess salt consumption in the pathogenesis of essential hypertension. *Am J Cardiol* 1961;8:571–575.
21. Gleiberman L. Blood pressure and dietary salt in human populations. *Ecol Food Nutr* 1973;2:143–155.
22. MacGregor GA. Sodium is more important than calcium in essential hypertension. *Hypertension* 1985;7:628–637.
23. Sasaki N. Epidemiological studies on hypertension in the northeastern part of Japan. *Jap Circ J* 1977;4:1139–1142.
24. Joosens JV, Geboers J. Salt and hypertension. *Prev Med* 1983;12:53–59.
25. Prior IAM, Stanhope JM. Blood pressure patterns, salt use and migration in the Pacific. In: Kesteloot H, Joosens JV, eds. *Epidemiology of arterial blood pressure.* The Hague: Martinus Nijhoff, 1980.
26. Maddocks I. Blood pressure in Melanesians. *Med J Aust* 1967;i:1123–1126.
27. Page LB, Damon A, Moellering RC. Antecedents of cardiovascular disease in six Solomon Island societies. *Circulation* 1974;29:1132–1146.
28. Shaper AG, Leonard PJ, Jones KW, Jones M. Environmental effects on the body build, blood pressure and blood chemistry of nomadic warriors serving in the army of Kenya. *East Afr Med J* 1969;46:282–289.
29. Dawber TR, Kannel WB, Kaga ANA, Donabedian RK, McNamara PM. Environmental factors in hypertension. In: Stamler J, et al, eds. *Epidemiology of hypertension.* New York: Grune and Stratton, 1967;255–288.
30. Guyton AC, Coleman TG, Cowley AW, Scheel KW, Manning RD, Norman RA. Arterial pressure regulation. *Am J Med* 1972;52:584–591.
31. Landau RL, Lugibihl K. The catabolic and natriuretic effects of progesterone in man. *Recent Prog Horm Res* 1961;17:249–255.
32. Weinberger MH, Kramer NJ, Grim CE, Petersen LP. The effect of posture and saline loading on plasma renin activity and aldosterone concentration in pregnant, non-pregnant and estrogen-treated women. *J Clin Endocrinol Metab* 1977;44:69–77.
33. Weinberger MH, Kramer NJ, Petersen LP, Cleary RE, Young PCM. Sequential changes in the renin-angiotensin-aldosterone systems and plasma progesterone concentration in normal and abnormal human pregnancy. In: Lindheimer MD, Katz AI, Zuspan FP, eds. *Hypertension in pregnancy.* New York: John Wiley & Sons, 1976;263–269.
34. Lindheimer MD, Katz AI. Sodium and diuretics in pregnancy. *N Engl J Med* 1973;288:891–895.
35. Freis ED. Salt volume and the prevention of hypertension. *Circulation* 1976;53:589–595.
36. Meneely GR, Battarbee HD. High sodium–low potassium environment and hypertension. *Am J Cardiol* 1976;38:768–785.
37. Watson RL, Langford HG, Abernethy J, Barnes TY, Watson MJ. Urinary electrolytes, body weight and blood pressure. *Hypertension* 1980;2(Suppl 1):I93–I98.
38. Pietinen PI, Wong O, Altschul AM. Electrolyte output, blood pressure and family history of hypertension. *Am J Clin Nutr* 1979;32:997–1003.
39. Liu LS, Tao SC, Lai SH. Relationship between salt excretion and blood pressure in various regions in China. *Bull WHO* 1984;62:255–260.
40. Langford HG, Watson RL. Electrolytes, environment and blood pressure. *Clin Sci Mol Med* 1973;45:1115–1119.
41. McQuarrie I, Thompson WH, Anderson JA. Effects of excessive ingestion of sodium and potassium salts on carbohydrate metabolism and blood pressure in diabetic children. *J Nutr* 1936;11:77–82.
42. Bulpitt CJ. Sodium excess or potassium lack as a cause of hypertension: a discussion paper. *J R Soc Med* 1981;74:896–900.
43. Khaw KT, Barrett-Connor E. Dietary potassium and stroke mortality. *N Engl J Med* 1987;316:235–240.
44. Staessen J, Bulpitt CJ, Fagard R, Joosens JV, Lunen P, Amery A.

Familial aggregation of blood pressure anthropometric characteristics and urinary excretion of sodium and potassium—a population study in two Belgian towns. *J Chron Dis* 1985;38:397–407.
45. Poulter N, Khaw KT, Hopwood BEC, Mugambi M, Peart WS, Rose G, Sever PS. Blood pressure and associated factors in a rural Kenyan community. *Hypertension* 1984;6:810–813.
46. Lever AF, Beretta-Piccoli C, Brown JJ, Davies DL, Fraser R, Robertson JIS. Sodium and potassium in essential hypertension. *Br Med J* 1981;283:463–468.
47. Kirkendall WM, Connor WE, Abbound F, Rasboggi SP, Anderson TA, Fry M. The effect of dietary sodium chloride on the blood pressure body fluids, electrolytes, renal function and serum lipids of normotensive man. *J Lab Clin Med* 1976;87:418–427.
48. Luft FC, Rankin LI, Bloch R, et al. Cardiovascular and humoral responses to extremes of sodium intake in normal black and white men. *Circulation* 1979;60:697–706.
49. Weinberger MH, Luft FC, Bloch R. The blood pressure-raising effects of high dietary sodium intake: racial differences and the role of potassium. *J Am Coll Nutr* 1982;1:139–148.
50. Addison W. The uses of sodium chloride, potassium chloride, sodium bromide and potassium bromide in cases of arterial hypertension which are amenable to potassium chloride. *Can Med Assoc J* 1928;18:281–285.
51. Young DB, McCaa RE, Pan YJ, Guyton AC. The natriuretic and hypotensive effects of potassium. *Circ Res* 1976;38(Suppl II):II-84–II-90.
52. Bauer JH, Gauntner WC. Effect of potassium chloride on plasma renin activity and plasma aldosterone during sodium restriction in normal man. *Kidney Int* 1979;15:286–291.
53. Morgan T, Creed R, Hopper J. Factors that determine the response of people with mild hypertension to a reduced sodium intake. *Clin Exp Hypertens* 1986;A8:941–962.
54. Fujita T, Noda H, Ando K. Sodium susceptibility and potassium effects in young patients with borderline hypertension. *Circulation* 1984;69:468–476.
55. Lowder SC, Brown RD. Hypertension corrected by discontinuing chronic sodium bicarbonate ingestion. *Am J Med* 1975;58:272–275.
56. Murray RH, Luft FC, Bloch R, Weyman AE. Blood pressure response to extremes of sodium intake in normal man. *Proc Soc Exp Biol Med* 1978;159:432–438.
57. Roos JC, Koomans HA, Dorhout Mees EJ, Delawi IMK. Renal sodium handling in normal humans subjected to low, normal and extremely high sodium supplies. *Am J Physiol* 1985;249: F941–F947.
58. Kempner W. Treatment of hypertensive vascular disease with rice diet. *Am J Med* 1948;4:545–577.
59. Ambard L, Beaujard E. Causes de l'hypertension arterielle. *Arch Gen Med* 1904;1:520–533.
60. Allen FW, Sherrill JW. The treatment of arterial hypertension. *J Metab Res* 1922;2:429–546.
61. Parijs J, Joosens JC, Van der Linden L, Virstreken G, Armery A. Moderate sodium restriction and diuretics in the treatment of hypertension. *Am Heart J* 1973;85:22–24.
62. Morgan T, Adams W, Gellies A, Wilson M, Morgan G, Carney S. Hypertension treated by salt restriction. *Lancet* 1978;i:227–230.
63. MacGregor GA, Markandu ND, Best FE, et al. Double-blind randomized cross-over trial of moderate sodium restriction in essential hypertension. *Lancet* 1982;i:352–354.
64. Skrabal F, Aubock J, Hortnagel H. Low sodium/high potassium diet for prevention of hypertension. *Lancet* 1981;ii:895–900.
65. Beard TC, Cooke HM, Gray WR, Barge R. Randomized controlled trial of a no-added sodium diet for mild hypertension. *Lancet* 1982;ii:455–458.
66. Watt GCM, Edwards C, Hart JT, Hart M, Walton P, Foy CJW. Dietary sodium restriction for mild hypertension in general practice. *Br Med J* 1983;286:432–436.
67. Silman AJ, Locke C, Mitchell P, Humpherson P. Evaluation of the effectiveness of a low sodium diet in the treatment of mild to moderate hypertension. *Lancet* 1983;i:1179–1182.
68. Richards AM, Nicholls MG, Espiner EA. Blood pressure response to moderate sodium restriction and to potassium supplementation in mild essential hypertension. *Lancet* 1984;i:757–760.
69. Longworth DL, Drayer JIM, Weber MA, Laragh JH. Divergent blood pressure responses during short-term sodium restriction in hypertension. *Clin Pharmacol Ther* 1980;27:544–546.
70. Erwteman TM, Nagelkerke N, Lubsen J, Koster M, Dunning AJ. β blockade, diuretics and salt restriction for the management of mild hypertension: a randomized double-blind trial. *Br Med J* 1984;289:406–409.
71. Weinberger MH, Cohen SJ, Miller JZ, Luft FC, Grim CE, Fineberg NS. Dietary sodium restriction as adjunctive treatment of hypertension. *JAMA* 1988;259:2561–2565.
72. Lang CL, Weinberger MH, Miller JZ. Dietary counseling results in effective dietary sodium restriction. *J Am Diet Assoc* 1985;85:477–479.
73. Guyton AC, Coleman TG, Cowley AW, Scheel KW, Manning RD, Norman RA. Arterial pressure regulation. *Am J Med* 1972;52:584–594.
74. Selkurt EE, Hall PW, Spencer MP. Influence of graded arterial pressure decrement in renal clearance of creatinine, *p*-aminohypurate and sodium *Am J Physiol* 1949;159:369–376.
75. Farnsworth EB, Barker MH. Tubular resorption of chloride in hypertensive and normal individuals. *Proc Soc Exp Biol Med* 1943;52:74–86.
76. Luft FC, Grim CE, Willis LR, Higgins JT, Weinberger MH. Natriuretic response to saline infusion in normotensive and hypertensive man. *Circulation* 1977;55:779–784.
77. Luft FC, Grim CE, Fineberg NS, Weinberger MH. Effects of volume expansion and contractions in normotensive whites, blacks and subjects of different ages. *Circulation* 1979;59:643–671.
78. Grim CE, Luft FC, Miller JZ, Brown PL, Gannon MH, Weinberger MH. Effects of sodium loading and depletion in normotensive first-degree relatives of essential hypertensives. *J Lab Clin Med* 1979;94:764–771.
79. Henry DP, Luft FC, Weinberger MH, Fineberg NS, Grim CE. Norepinephrine in urine and plasma following provocative maneuvers in normal and hypertensive subjects. *Hypertension* 1980;2:20–28.
80. Kokubu T, Hiwada K, Kobayashi T, Takada Y, Hashimoto H. An exaggerated natriuretic response to hypertonic saline infusion in the Stage II (WHO stage classification) essential hypertensive patients. *Clin Exp Hypertens* 1984;A6:731–742.
81. Taylor T, Moore TJ, Hollenberg NK, Williams GH. Converting enzyme inhibition corrects the altered adrenal response to angiotensin II in essential hypertension. *Hypertension* 1984;6:92–99.
82. Williams GH, Hollenberg NK, Brown C, Mersey JH. Adrenal responses to pharmacological interruption of the renin–angiotensin system in sodium restricted normal man. *J Clin Endocrinol Metab* 1978;47:725–731.
83. Hollenberg NK, Chemitz WR, Adams DF, Williams GH. Reciprocal influence of salt intake on adrenal glomerulosa and renal vascular responses to angiotensin II in normal man. *J Clin Invest* 1974;54:34–42.
84. Capuccio FP, Markandu ND, Sagnella GA, MacGregor GA. Sodium restriction lowers blood pressure through a decreased responsiveness of the renin system: direct evidence using saralasin. *J Hypertens* 1985;3:243–247.
85. Fagerberg B, Andersson OK, Isaksson B, Bjortorp P. Blood pressure control during weight reduction in obese hypertensive men: separate effects of sodium and energy restriction. *Br Med J* 1984;288:11–14.
86. Dawson-Hughes BF, Moore TJ, Dluhy RG, Hollenberg NK, Williams GH. Plasma angiotensin II concentration regulates vascular but not adrenal responsiveness to restriction of sodium intake in normal man. *Clin Sci* 1981;61:527–534.
87. Myers J, Morgan T, Waga S, Manley K. The effect of sodium intake related to the age of the patients. *Clin Exp Pharmacol Physiol* 1982;9:287–289.
88. Koolen MI, Daha MR, van Brummelen P. Is the renal kallikrein system relevant to sodium sensitivity in patients with essential hypertension? *Eur J Clin Invest* 1985;15:151–156.

89. Haddy FJ. Natriuretic hormone—the missing link in low renin hypertension? *Biochem Pharmacol* 1982;31:3159–3161.
90. Shimamoto K, Ura N, Nakao T, Nishimiya T, et al. Role of the kallikrein–kinin system in sodium metabolism in normotensives and essential hypertensives. *NZ Med J* 1983;96:905–907.
91. Ando K, Fujita T. Abnormal renal hemodynamics in salt-sensitive patients with essential hypertension. *Jpn Circ J* 1985;49:984–989.
92. Harris PJ, Navar G. Tubular transport responses to angiotensin I. *Am J Physiol* 1985;248:F621–F630.
93. Redgrave J, Rabinowe S, Hollenberg NK, Williams GH. Correction of abnormal renal blood flow response to angiotensin II by converting enzyme inhibition in essential hypertensives. *J Clin Invest* 1985;75:1285–1290.
94. Kokubu T, Hiwada K, Shishido M, Murakami E, Hashimoto H. Reduced responses of renin release to three different stimuli in essential hypertensives of stage II (WHO stage classification). *Clin Exp Hypertens* 1980;2:183–187.
95. Kohno M, Yasunari K, Murakawa K, Kanayama Y, Matsuura T, Takeda T. Effects of high-sodium and low-sodium intake on circulating atrial natriuretic peptides in salt-sensitive patients with systemic hypertension. *Am J Cardiol* 1987;59:1212–1213.
96. Morise T, Miyamori I, Hifumi S, et al. Effect of sodium intake on the excretion of urinary natriuretic factor in essential hypertensives. *Endocrinol Jpn* 1985;32:405–411.
97. Haddy F, Pamnani M, Clough D. The sodium–potassium pump in volume expanded hypertension. *Clin Exp Hypertens* 1978;1:295–336.
98. Blaustein M. Sodium ions, calcium ions, blood pressure regulation and hypertension: a reassessment and a hypothesis. *Am J Physiol* 1977;232:C165–C172.
99. Dibona GF. Neurogenic regulation of renal tubular sodium reabsorption. *Am J Physiol* 1977;233:F73–F81.
100. Weinstock M, Schorer-Apelbaum D. Impaired baroreflex sensitivity in the aetiology of salt hypertension in the rabbit. *Clin Sci* 1985;68:489–493.
101. de Champlain J, Krakoff L, Axelrod J. Interrelationships of sodium intake, hypertension and norepinephrine storage in the rat. *Circ Res* 1969;24(Suppl I):I75–I92.
102. Koolen MI, van Brummelen P. Adrenergic activity and peripheral hemodynamics in relation to sodium sensitivity in patients with essential hypertension. *Hypertension* 1984;6:820–825.
103. Vollmer RR. Effects of dietary sodium on sympathetic nervous system control of cardiovascular function. *J Auton Pharmacol* 1984;4:133–144.
104. Skrabal F, Herholz H, Neumayr M, Hamburger L, et al. Salt sensitivity in humans is linked to enhanced sympathetic responsiveness and to enhanced proximal tubular reabsorption. *Hypertension* 1984;6:152–158.
105. Haywood JR, Brennan TJ, Hinojosa C. Neurohumoral mechanisms of sodium-dependent hypertension. *Fed Proc* 1985;44:2393–2399.
106. Harvey JN, Casson IF, Clayden AD, Cope GF, Perkins CM, Lee MR. A paradoxical fall in urine dopamine output when patients with essential hypertension are given added dietary salt. *Clin Sci* 1984;67:83–88.
107. Masuo K, Ogihara T, Kumahara Y, Yamatodani A, Wada H. Plasma norepinephrine and dietary sodium intake in normal subjects and patients with essential hypertension. *Hypertension* 1983;5:767–771.
108. Watson RDS, Esler MD, Leonard P, Korner PI. Influence of variation in dietary sodium intake on biochemical indices of sympathetic activity in normal man. *Clin Exp Pharmacol Physiol* 1984;11:163–170.
109. Dustan HP. Physiologic regulation of arterial pressure: an overview. *Hypertension* 1982;4(Suppl 3):III-62–III-67.
110. Meldrum MJ, Badino L, Westfall TC. Role of dietary sodium on noradrenergic neurotransmission. *Fed Proc* 1982;41:1645–1649.
111. Campese VM, Rornoff MS, Levitan D, Saglikes Y, Friedler RM, Massry SG. Abnormal relationship between sodium intake and sympathetic nervous system activity in salt-sensitive patients with essential hypertension. *Kidney Int* 1982;21:371–378.
112. Rankin LI, Luft FC, Henry DP, Gibbs PS, Weinberger MH. Sodium intake alters the effects of norepinephrine on blood pressure. *Hypertension* 1981;3:650–656.
113. Dahl LK, Heine M, Thompson K. Genetic influence of the kidneys on blood pressure: evidence from chronic renal homografts in rats with opposite predisposition to hypertension. *Circ Res* 1974;34:94–101.
114. Bianchi G, Fox U, DiFrancesco GF, Boordi U, Radice M. The hypertensive role of the kidney in spontaneously hypertensive rats. *Clin Sci Mol Med* 1973;45:135–139.
115. Whitfield JB, Martin NG. Genetic and environmental causes of variation in renal tubular handling of sodium and potassium: a twin Study. *Gen Epidemiol* 1985;2:17–27.
116. Grim CE, Miller JZ, Luft FC, Christian JC, Weinberger MH. Genetic influences on renin, aldosterone and the renal excretion of sodium and potassium following volume expansion and contraction in normal man. *Hypertension* 1979;1:583–590.
117. Miller JZ, Luft FC, Grim CE, Henry DP, Christian JC, Weinberger MH. Genetic influences on plasma and urinary norepinephrine following volume expansion and contraction in normal man. *J Clin Endocrinol Metab* 1980;50:219–222.
118. Gudmundsson O, Cederblad A, Wikstrand J, Berglund G. Sodium elimination rate and blood pressure during normal and high salt intake in subjects with and without familial predisposition to hypertension. *Acta Med Scand* 1984;216:345–352.
119. Watt CCM, Foy CJW, Hart JT, et al. Dietary sodium and arterial blood pressure: evidence against genetic susceptibility. *Br Med J* 1985;291:1525–1528.
120. Nielsen JR, Pedersen KE, Klitgaard NA, et al. Genetic influence on sympathetic nervous activity and cellular sodium/potassium regulation in borderline and mild hypertension. Personal communication.
121. Miller JZ, Weinberger MH, Christian JC, Daugherty SA. Familial resemblance in the blood pressure response to sodium restriction. *Am J Epidemiol* 1987;126:822–830.
122. Weinberger MH, Ramsdell JW, Rosner DR, Geddes JJL. The effect of chlorothiazide and sodium on vascular responsiveness to angiotensin II in the rat. *Am J Physiol* 1972;223:1049–1052.
123. Gavras H, Brunner HR, Turini GA, et al. Antihypertensive effect of the oral angiotensin converting enzyme inhibitor SQ 14225 in man. *N Engl J Med* 1978;298:991–995.
124. London GM, Levenson JA, London AM, Simon AC, Safar ME. Systemic compliance, renal hemodynamics, and sodium excretion in hypertension. *Kidney Int* 1984;26:342–350.
125. London GM, Safar ME, Simon AC, Alexandre JM, Levenson JA, Weiss YA. Total effective compliance, cardiac output and fluid volumes in essential hypertension. *Circulation* 1978;57:995–1000.
126. Sullivan JM, Prewitt RL, Ratts TE, Josephs JA, Connor MJ. Hemodynamic characteristics of sodium-sensitive human subjects. *Hypertension* 1987;9:398–406.
127. McDonough J, Wilhelmj CM. The effect of excess salt intake on human blood pressure. *Am J Digest Dis* 1954;21:180–185.
128. Luft FC, Rankin LI, Henry DP, et al. Plasma and urinary norepinephrine values at extremes of sodium intake in normal man. *Hypertension* 1979;1:261–265.
129. Miller JZ, Daugherty SA, Weinberger MH, Grim CE, Christian JC, Lang CL. Blood pressure response to dietary sodium restriction in normotensive adults. *Hypertension* 1983;5:790–795.
130. Miller JZ, Weinberger MH, Daugherty SA, Fineberg NS, Christian JC, Grim CE. Heterogeneity of blood pressure response to dietary sodium restriction in normotensive adults. *J Chronic Dis* 1987;40:245–250.
131. Weinberger MH, Miller JZ, Luft FC, Grim CE, Fineberg NS. Definitions and characteristics of sodium sensitivity and blood pressure resistance. *Hypertension* 1986;8(Suppl II):II-127–II-134.
132. Weinberger MH, Miller JZ, Fineberg NS, Luft FC, Grim CE, Christian JC. Association of haptoglobin with sodium sensitivity and resistance of blood pressure. *Hypertension* 1987;10:443–446.
133. Kawasaki T, Delea CS, Bartter FC, Smith H. The effect of high sodium and low sodium intakes on blood pressure and other related variables in human subjects with idiopathic hypertension. *Am J Med* 1978;64:193–198.
134. Fujita T, Henry WL, Bartter FC, Lake CR, Delea CS. Factors

influencing blood pressure in salt-sensitive patients with hypertension. *Am J Med* 1980;69:334–344.

135. Fujita T, Noda H, Ando K. Sodium susceptibility and potassium effects in young patients with borderline hypertension. *Circulation* 1984;69:468–476.
136. Dustan HP, Tarazi RC, Bravo EL. Physiologic characteristics of hypertension. *Am J Med* 1972;52:610–622.
137. Sullivan JM, Ratts TE, Taylor JC, et al. Hemodynamic effects of dietary sodium in man: a preliminary report. *Hypertension* 1980;2:506–514.
138. Kem DC, Weinberger MH, Nugent CA. Saline suppression of plasma aldosterone in hypertension. *Arch Intern Med* 1971;128:380–386.
139. Grim CE, Weinberger MH, Higgins JT, Kramer NJ. A rapid and efficient protocol for the diagnosis of secondary forms of hypertension. *JAMA* 1977;237:1331–1335.
140. Falkner B, Onesti G, Angelakos E. Effect of salt loading on the cardiovascular response to stress in adolescents. *Hypertension* 1981;3(Suppl II):II-195–II-199.
141. Koolen MI, van Brummelen P. Sodium sensitivity in essential hypertension: role of the renin-angiotensin-aldosterone system and predictive value of an intravenous furosemide test. *J Hypertens* 1984;2:55–59.

Hypertension: Pathophysiology, Diagnosis, and Management, edited by J. H. Laragh and B. M. Brenner. Raven Press, Ltd., New York © 1990.

CHAPTER 126

Dietary Sodium Restriction in Hypertension

John D. Swales

Intervention Studies: Secondary Hypertension, 2011
Intervention Studies: Essential Hypertension, 2011
Design of Studies, 2012
Statistical Power, 2013
Differences in Initial Blood Pressure of Recruited Patients, 2013
Conclusions, 2013
Salt Sensitivity in Hypertension, 2014
Therapeutic Value of the Concept of Salt Sensitivity, 2015
Salt Restriction and Antihypertensive Medication, 2016
Diuretics, 2016
Other Antihypertensive Drugs, 2016
Adverse Effects of Salt Restriction, 2017
How Far Should Salt Intake Be Restricted?, 2018
References, 2018

Dietary salt has been implicated in the pathogenesis of hypertension on experimental, epidemiological, and clinical grounds. Others have argued that a high salt intake is a fairly recent aberration in the evolution of humans and that hypertension is therefore a consequence of this change in dietary habit (1). Such evolutionary arguments carry little weight in determining the advice to be given to individual hypertensive patients. Indeed the invocation of Darwinian natural selection would not seem relevant to the needs of Western man. Although correlations have been reported between salt intake and blood pressure in cross-cultural studies (2), such studies are equally tenuous as a basis for dietary advice. The present chapter will therefore be confined to analysis of the guidance provided by intervention studies which have examined the effect of changes in dietary salt upon blood pressure. The heavy reliance (particularly in public health campaigns) upon paleontology and anthropology perhaps underlines the controversial nature of much evidence in this field.

INTERVENTION STUDIES: SECONDARY HYPERTENSION

Sodium retention is demonstrably responsible for high blood pressure in the majority of patients with advanced renal failure managed by intermittent dialysis (3–5). Removal of sodium excess in such patients lowers blood pressure. Furthermore, it is possible to demonstrate a relationship between exchangeable sodium and blood pressure (4,5) On the other hand, blood pressure in some patients on chronic dialysis is not reduced by sodium depletion and requires bilateral nephrectomy for adequate control. In some patients with renovascular hypertension due to unilateral renal artery stenosis (6) and in severe malignant hypertension (7,8), high blood pressure levels may give rise to a negative sodium balance, presumably through perfusion pressure natriuresis. Isolated case reports suggest that saline infusion may produce clinical improvement in these cases (8,9).

Such secondary forms of hypertension are, however, unusual. Amongst patients with essential hypertension there is usually no evidence for sodium retention unless cardiac failure has supervened. Indeed, recent studies have demonstrated a slight reduction in exchangeable sodium and extracellular fluid in mildly hypertensive and young hypertensive subjects (10–12). In older subjects, one group has described a positive correlation between body sodium and blood pressure; this was interpreted as indicating secondary renal changes resulting in sodium retention (12). Excluding patients with advanced renal failure or with mineralocorticoid-induced hypertension—and, perhaps, some elderly individuals—dietary salt restriction cannot be advocated on the grounds that it corrects a pathophysiological abnormality. In such patients, its justification lies in claims that reducing salt intake lowers blood pressure.

INTERVENTION STUDIES: ESSENTIAL HYPERTENSION

The observation that sodium restriction lowers blood pressure dates from the early years of this century (13,14). Kempner's rice–fruit diet was shown to lower blood pressure effectively in severely hypertensive patients (15,17). This diet reduced sodium intake to approximately 5 mmol/day and also radically altered other dietary components. The Medical Research Council (MRC) study, however, provided evidence that the reduction in sodium was, at least partially, responsible for the fall in blood pressure, since the addition of only modest amounts of sodium chloride to the diet restored blood pressure to baseline levels (16). The unpleasantness of the Kempner rice–fruit diet, combined with the grave social disadvantages attendant upon it, led to poor compliance; as a result, relatively few clinicians were persuaded to incorporate it into routine clinical practice. In addition, the development of effective antihypertensive drugs shortly thereafter removed some of the clinical need for dietary methods of blood pressure lowering. In the 1970s, however, salt restriction began to be reassessed. This followed from the appreciation that lowering blood pressure, even in patients with mild to moderate hypertension, carried significant benefit. The need to treat increasingly large numbers of patients for the duration of their lives created new economic and social pressures to find alternatives to pharmacological therapy (18). The earliest studies, such as that conducted by the MRC (16), suggested that only severe salt restriction to 10 mmol/day (or less) of sodium had significant blood-pressure-lowering effect. This was clearly unacceptable to the majority of active hypertensive patients. However, more moderate degrees of salt restriction (i.e., reducing intake to 60–100 mmol/day) are feasible, although with some social difficulty. Accordingly, since the mid-1970s a series of dietary intervention maneuvers has been carried out to assess the effect of moderate salt restriction on blood pressure (Table 1). The interpretation of these studies has given rise to considerable debate. The apparent conflict of results recorded in Table 1 is attributable to at least three factors. These are: design of studies, number of patients included in each study (statistical power), and differences in initial blood pressure of patients recruited.

Design of Studies

The nature of the control group or period is critical in view of the need to detect a small effect upon blood pressure in the presence of a marked placebo effect when blood pressure is repeatedly measured. Thus in the trial reported by Silman et al. (24), blood pressures in the control group (whose members continued to attend for a year) fell from 159/98 to 139/87. In the intervention group, blood pressure fell from 167/99 to 139/81. The difference between the two was not statistically significant. The fall in blood pressure in the control group was, however, greater than that recorded in intervention groups in any of the other studies. A significant fall in blood pressure from baseline to intervention periods was also observed in both salt-restricted and control groups in another study (25), although there was no significant increase in blood pressure in either group during the final washout phase. The fall in blood pressure in the control group is also evident in the parallel group design trial reported by Morgan et al. (21). The most sensitive and specific design is undoubtedly a cross-over trial in which subjects are randomly allocated, in random sequence, to intervention and control periods (19,20, 23,26,28).

There is another difficulty in the design of trials of salt restriction. When patients are placed on a low-salt diet, other potentially relevant factors besides sodium are altered (19,21,22,24,25–27). The potential importance of such confounding effects became distressingly evident in the Australian National Health and Medical Research Council trial (29). This was, by far, the largest study to address the problem of sodium and potassium intake. Two hundred twelve subjects were randomized to normal diet, high-potassium diet, reduced-sodium diet, or high-potassium, low-sodium diet. Systolic and diastolic blood pressure fell by 3.8/1.6 in the normal diet group and by 8.9/5.8 in the low-sodium group. However, when patients were re-randomized to placebo or sodium chloride supplements, blood pressure was not elevated significantly by restoring sodium intake. The authors concluded that factors other than changes in sodium/potassium intake contributed to the fall in blood pressure during the diet phase of their study. In the most sophisticated cross-over design, all patients are stabilized on a low-salt diet and then, in random sequence, allocated (in a double-blind fashion) a placebo or salt sup-

TABLE 1. *Controlled trials on the efficacy of salt restriction in hypertension*

Study	n^a	Duration	Blood pressure (mmHg)		Sodium (mmol/day)		
			Baseline	Change	Initial	Final	Change
Parijs et al. (19)	17	4 weeks	147/98	−9.1/−5.8	191	93	−98
MacGregor et al. (20)	19	4 weeks	117^b	−7.1	191	83	−108
Morgan et al. (21)	31	2 years	160/97	−7.3	191	157	−34
Erwteman et al. (22)	44	4 weeks	143/94	−1.9/−0.5	130	72	−58
Watt et al. (23)	18	4 weeks	136/82	0.5/−0.3	143	87	−56
Silman et al. (24)	12	1 year	165/98	$-8.7^c/-6.3^c$	151	117	−34
Puska et al. (25)	34	6 weeks	138/86	$-0.7^d/+0.8$	192	77	−115
Richards et al. (26)	12	4–6 weeks	$137/86^e$	−4.0/−3.0	180	80	−100
Longworth et al. (27)	82	10 days	121^b	−1.7	197	70	−127
Grobbee et al. (28)	40	18 weeks	141/76	−0.8/−0.8	129	57	−72

[a] *n* represents the number of subjects who underwent salt restriction. In parallel group design studies, the overall number included is of course greater.
[b] Mean
[c] Taken as difference between salt restricted and non-salt-restricted groups.
[d] Change from baseline at end of study.
[e] Intra-arterial.

plement. This allows for discrimination between effects of sodium chloride and other dietary components (20,23,26). However, even these studies have yielded conflicting results.

Statistical Power

The statistical power of some studies has been severely constrained by their relatively small size, which makes the detection of a small change in blood pressure difficult. Thus, in some cases, apparently appreciable falls in blood pressure are documented which do not reach statistical significance (24,26). Duration of intervention is another feature of published studies which is open to criticism. The trials documented in Table 1 are of relatively short duration. In view of the fact that lifelong recommendations are being assessed, possible long-term changes in compliance and in physiological adaptation to a low-salt diet require evaluation. In diuretic-treated patients, for instance, progressive rises in plasma renin activity have been recorded over a 2-year period (30). Whether a similar phenomenon occurs with dietary salt restriction is unknown. Conversely, it is possible that reversal of long-standing vascular hypertrophy might result in amplification of any blood-pressure-lowering effect.

Differences in Initial Blood Pressure of Recruited Patients

Probably the most important explanation for the discordance in published reports lies in differences in initial blood pressure of the patients recruited. There is a necessary mathematical relationship between the degree of change in a variable and the initial value of that variable, since each shares a common component (31). The relationship shown in Fig. 1 is therefore predictable. However, the position of points indicates approximately zero benefit from moderate salt restriction when patients have an initial mean blood pressure in the range 100–105 mmHg. There is another physiological explanation for the lesser efficacity of salt restriction in the lower blood pressure ranges. One of the mechanisms by which the circulation is protected against volume depletion is the renin–angiotensin system. The activity of this system is inversely related to the height of blood pressure in unselected populations of normal subjects and patients with essential hypertension (32). Inhibition of the system may therefore be associated with a blood pressure response to salt depletion which is not observed in patients with a normally responding renin–angiotensin system. Two of the reported studies have thus shown a close relationship between the blood pressure response to salt restriction and initial renin (26,33).

This interpretation of published studies is supported by published data on the effects of moderate salt restriction in normotensive subjects (Table 2). Although these trials tend to be of shorter duration than those in hypertension, there is no indication of any blood-pressure-lowering effect. The suggestion of a pressor action in some reports (Fig. 1) may reflect small numbers and wide confidence limits, although severe salt restriction in some strains of laboratory rat has been found to result in blood pressure elevation (43–45).

Conclusions

The potential importance of long-term moderate salt restriction in the management of the major public health problem of mild hypertension has not been reflected in the

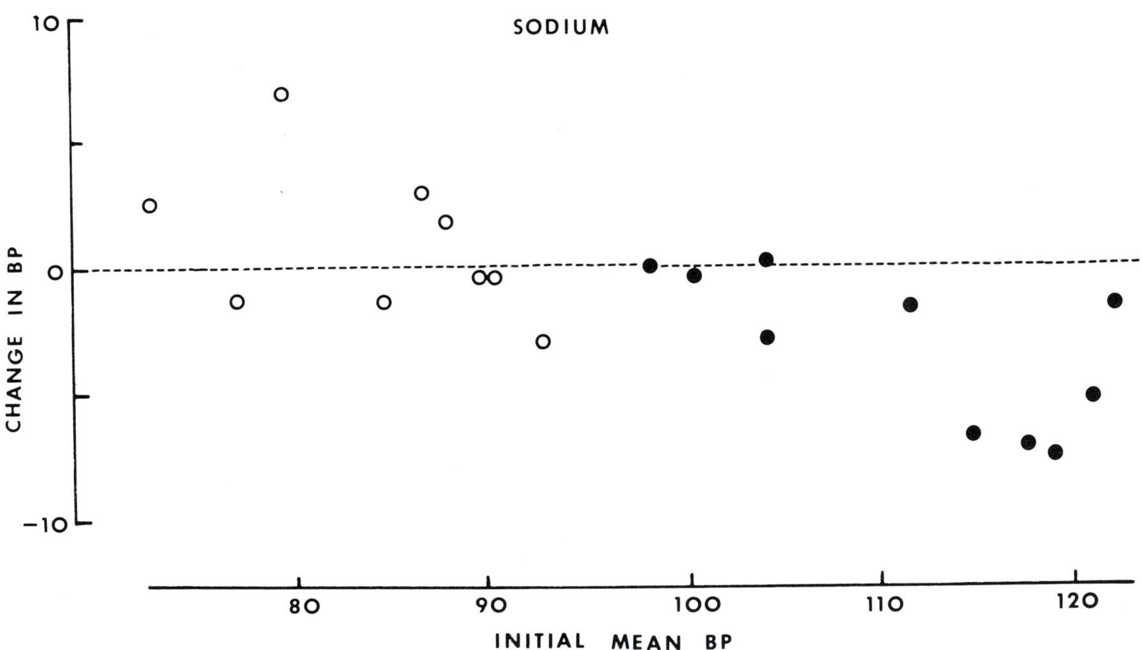

FIG. 1. Change in mean blood pressure produced in hypertensive patients (●) and normotensive subjects (○) by moderate salt restriction. Each point represents one reported trial (Tables 1 and 2).

TABLE 2. *Controlled trials of the effect of changes in salt intake on blood pressure of healthy volunteers*

Study	*n*	Duration	Blood pressure (mmHg)		Sodium (mmol/day)		
			Baseline	Change	Initial	Final	Change
Kirkendall et al. (34)	8	4 weeks	88[a]	+2	159	10	−149
				0	159	307	+148
Burstyn et al. (35)	7	8	120/79	−2.9/−3.1	143	414	+271
Murray et al. (36)	8	3–8 days	83.6[a]	−1.2	265	12	−253
				+5.7	265	702	+437
				+15.4	265	1442	+1177
Sullivan et al. (37)	27	5 days	75.4	+3.1	170	24	−146
Parfrey et al. (38)	28	5 days	119/75	−2.6/+0.9	168	15	−153
				+0.3/+0.4	168	310	+142
Cooper et al. (39)	124	24 days	109/61	−0.7/−1.3	110	45	−65
Heagerty et al. (40)	31	14 days	129/70	+0.5/−1.0	260	39	−221
Skrabal et al. (41)	20	2 weeks	125/76	−2.7/−3.1	210	40	−170
McNabb et al. (42)	8	5–6 days	108/70	Consistently higher up to +12.4/+12.9	300	10	−290

[a] Mean.

investment in scientific assessment of this therapy. So far, studies have been of short duration and small size. In addition, problems in design have led to uncertain results. On present evidence, however, it seems likely that moderate salt restriction down to a daily intake of 70–80 mmol sodium produces modest blood pressure reduction in patients with moderate to severe hypertension. The benefits in patients with borderline and mild hypertension are unproven. On present evidence, however, moderate salt restriction would seem to carry least benefit in those patients where dietary therapy is being considered as an alternative to single-drug therapy. Two additional problems require examination in this context: Are certain hypertensive patients likely to benefit from salt restriction, and does salt restriction have a role in combination with drug therapy?

SALT SENSITIVITY IN HYPERTENSION

The heterogeneity of essential hypertension has provided a tantalizing prospect to numerous research workers since the original debate between Platt and Pickering on the modality of blood pressure distribution curves (46). Although there is now agreement that the bi- or multimodality reported by Platt was an artefact of small numbers, unimodality does not exclude the presence of distinct subgroups within essential hypertension. As was pointed out by contributors to the debate (46), a unimodal distribution of, for instance, intelligence quotients or hemoglobin conceals discrete genetically determined disorders such as phenylketonuria or sickle cell anemia.

Dahl's development of an inbred strain of rats which developed sustained hypertension after being fed a high-salt diet (47) led logically to the search for analogous forms of hypertension in humans (Table 3). Kawasaki et al. (48) changed salt intake from 9 to 249 mmol sodium per day in 19 patients with essential hypertension, allowing a week for equilibration on each diet. Patients were classified into salt-sensitive and non-salt-sensitive groups, depending on whether they showed an increase in mean blood pressure of more than 10%. The salt-sensitive patients retained more sodium with sodium loading and showed less of a rise in renin (measured in the supine posture) with salt depletion. A later study from the same group (49) attributed a rise in blood pressure to a greater increase in cardiac output in salt-sensitive subjects who also showed higher plasma norepinephrines with salt loading and lesser decreases in plasma renin activity (PRA) and aldosterone. They concluded that salt sensitivity was associated with higher activity of the sympathetic nervous system, causing greater sodium retention and a greater increase in cardiac output on a high-sodium diet. In a later study, Fujita et al. (50) used 25 mg of mefruside daily, instead of a period of low-salt diet, and then supplemented subjects' salt intake to a level of approximately 390 mmol/day. A group of subjects with borderline hypertension were compared with matched normal controls. The hypertensive subjects showed some of the characteristics of salt-sensitive hypertensive patients (i.e., a rise in blood pressure with salt loading, associated with a rise in cardiac output and higher plasma norepinephrine). However, basal PRA and PRA after diuretics were also higher, and there was no difference in sodium excretion or in weight change between the two groups. The hemodynamic consequences of salt loading have been examined by other groups with different results. In other studies (51,52), hypertensive patients after moderate salt loading (345 ml/day) showed increased forearm vascular resistance at maximal vasodilatation and decreased forearm distensibility: The former was interpreted as indicating structural change. Skrabal et al. (41) reduced salt intake of 20 normotensive volunteers from a normal dietary level of 200 mmol/day to 50 mmol/day. Twelve of them showed a fall in systolic and diastolic blood pressure of at least 5 mmHg. These were classified as *responders.* They had a significantly higher baseline diastolic blood pressure, and a family history of hypertension was rather more common. There was no difference in plasma renin, aldosterone, vasopressin, or catecholamine levels in responders and nonresponders, nor did urinary electrolytes differ. The

TABLE 3. *Studies on salt sensitivity in hypertensive and normotensive subjects*

Study	Change in salt intake	Blood pressure criteria for salt sensitivity	Subjects studied	Associated characteristics in salt-sensitive subjects[a]
Kawasaki et al. (48)	9 → 249 mmol/day	10% increase in mean	19 untreated hypertensives	Greater retention of Na; lesser supine PRA on low-salt diet
Fujita et al. (49)			18 untreated hypertensives	Greater increase in cardiac output and plasma norepinephrine with salt loading; lower PRA and aldosterone on low-salt diet
Fujita et al. (50)	Diuretic → 390 mmol/day	—	21 borderline hypertensives, 12 normotensives	Rise in BP and cardiac output in hypertensives; higher aldosterone and plasma norepinephrine in hypertensives
Skrabal et al. (41)	50 → 200 mmol/day	Fall in systolic or diastolic pressure of at least 5 mmHg on low-salt diet	20 male normotensives	Higher diastolic pressure; family history of hypertension
Skrabal et al. (53)	50 → 200 mmol/day	Fall in systolic or diastolic pressure of at least 5 mmHg on low-salt diet	52 normotensives	Family history of hypertension; higher systolic and diastolic pressure; greater pressor response to norepinephrine; ?Enhanced proximal tubular Na reabsorption (but no net change); lower PRA on low-salt diet
Weinberger et al. (56)	2 liters saline, then 10 mmol Na^+ + 120 mg frusemide	Decrease of 10 mmHg or more on low-salt diet	378 normotensives, 198 hypertensives	Higher mean pressure; older; lower baseline PRA and lower PRA with salt depletion; higher basal norepinephrine; more common in blacks

[a] PRA, plasma renin activity; BP, blood pressure.

same group (53) later reported increased pressor response to infused norepinephrine in responders; this was associated with increased platelet alpha-2-adrenergic-receptor density (54). Although there was no difference in weight change or sodium excretion between responders and nonresponders, uric acid clearance fell more during sodium restriction in responding subjects. This was interpreted as indicating enhanced proximal tubular sodium reabsorption, not reflected in total sodium excretion. In addition, PRA was stimulated less by a low-salt diet. There was no difference in erythrocyte sodium fluxes between the two groups.

Luft et al. (55) used the opposite approach to the question of genetic predisposition to salt sensitivity and reached contrary findings. Forty-three first-degree relatives of patients with essential hypertension were given a 4-hr infusion of normal saline followed on the next day by a low-salt diet (10 mmol/day) and frusemide (120 mg). Compared with matched controls, blood pressure was consistently higher throughout these maneuvers in the relatives with no evidence for a differential response, although 24-hr sodium excretion was decreased and baseline PRA was increased. A larger series was later reported using the same regime in 378 normal volunteers and 198 patients with essential hypertension (56). The salt-sensitive normotensive and hypertensive subjects were older and had a lower baseline PRA and a lower PRA after stimulation with a low-salt diet as compared with salt-resistant subjects. Plasma norepinephrine was no different in salt-sensitive and salt-resistant normotensives and hypertensives—except with regard to baseline values, which were significantly higher in normotensive salt-sensitive subjects.

THERAPEUTIC VALUE OF THE CONCEPT OF SALT SENSITIVITY

In the above-mentioned reports, the hypothesis has been put forward that hypertension is the result of exposure of genetically salt-sensitive subjects to the high levels of salt contained in Western diet. In such individuals, dietary salt is therefore considered to be pathogenetic. Identification of salt-sensitive individuals could therefore theoretically enable blood pressure to be lowered in hypertensive patients, and hypertension could be prevented in genetically predisposed salt-sensitive normotensive subjects. The present evidence is not persuasive enough to support such a conclusion. The most important deficiency in all the cited reports is the absence of data on reproducibility. Blood pressure variability will inevitably lead to pressures which are higher or lower at the end of different interventions. Where individual changes in blood pressure are reported, they clearly represent a continuum with no evidence of two separate groups (48,56). Under these circumstances, many subjects stand to be misclassified. To provide meaningful therapeutic guidance, the clinician needs to know how consistent and how great a fall in blood pressure can be produced by dietary salt restriction carried out on several occasions. The specificity of the response also requires further study. Genetically predisposed subjects may show an abnormally great pressor response to several stressful stimuli. This is also the case with the Dahl sensitive rat (57). The presence, in some studies, of indices of sympathetic adrenergic activation emphasizes the need for studies of specificity.

In these studies, the fairly consistent presence of certain characteristics of salt-sensitive subjects would support the view, however, that the differences between salt-sensitive and salt-resistant subjects are, to some extent, real. Most notably, the baseline renin levels and renin responsiveness to salt depletion appear to be greater in salt-resistant normotensive and hypertensive subjects. This is consistent with the observation that salt sensitivity is more frequent in blacks and in the elderly (56). The relationship between salt sensitivity and essential hypertension is dubious, since PRA is slightly elevated in first-degree relatives of hypertensive patients (55). In addition, in some of the reports where age-matching has not been attempted, salt-sensitive hypertensive subjects were older, suggesting an acquired abnormality. Therefore, there is a strong possibility of secondary impairment of renin responsiveness—or, perhaps, biological variability in renin secretion—as a major factor in salt sensitivity. The renin–angiotensin system helps maintain blood pressure in the face of sodium depletion, and inhibition of the renin response would exacerbate the fall in blood pressure produced by salt depletion. In the articles published to date, there are no grounds to support the contention originally put forward by Kawasaki et al. (48) that there is a subgroup of hypertensive subjects with a genetically determined abnormality of sodium excretion. Although Luft et al. (55) reported reduced capacity to excrete a sodium load in first-degree relatives of hypertensives over a 24-hr period, after saline infusion, other protocols have suggested that in such individuals the immediate response to saline infusion was an accelerated sodium excretion (58). Recently one group has reported an association between the haptoglobin phenotype Hp1-1 and sodium sensitivity. However, there was considerable overlap between salt-sensitive and salt-resistant individuals in this respect (58a).

In summary, while it seems likely that certain hypertensive patients will respond preferentially to dietary salt restriction, apart from renin responsiveness there are no biochemical or physiological markers which are currently of value to the clinician in treating the individual patient. There is no justification for attempting to identify salt-sensitive normotensive subjects for prophylactic dietary advice on salt intake.

SALT RESTRICTION AND ANTIHYPERTENSIVE MEDICATION

Dietary advice in multifactorial intervention trials has been associated with a reduction in the amount of antihypertensive medication required to control blood pressure (59). A more specific study of the interaction between dietary salt restriction and antihypertensive medication was carried out by Beard et al. (60). Ninety patients receiving medication were randomly allocated to a fairly severe salt-restriction regime (37 mmols/day) or to a control group. Members of the salt-restricted group were able to halve their medication, and one patient in three was able to discontinue medication entirely. Two-thirds of the control group remained on the same dose of medication, and only 9% discontinued drugs. Initial medication included diuretics, beta-blockers, and other antihypertensives. The protocol selectively resulted in diuretics being withdrawn from the diet-treated group, since diuretics were discontinued (and other agents substituted) if urinary sodium fell below 50 mmol/24 hr. Despite this, however, the consumption of beta-blockers and other antihypertensives was reduced in the diet group, suggesting that the interaction between diet and therapy was indeed a real one. The duration of the trial was 12 weeks, and therefore it is uncertain how sustained the reduction in medication was.

These studies, while clinically important, do not help to define adjuvant effects of dietary salt restriction on specific forms of antihypertensive medication. Several investigations have addressed this problem.

Diuretics

The extent to which the natriuresis induced by diuretics accounts for their blood-pressure-lowering action is still controversial. There is, however, evidence that dietary salt intake influences the efficacy of diuretics as antihypertensive agents. Thus, in one study, ingestion of 20 g of sodium chloride daily for a week abolished the antihypertensive response to thiazide diuretics (61). In other investigations, raising salt intake from 50 to 100 mmol/day (62) and from 4.25 to 11.25 g/day (63) virtually inhibited the blood-pressure-lowering action of diuretics. Finnerty et al. (64) replaced urinary sodium losses induced by thiazides or frusemide with a saline infusion and found that blood pressure was restored to baseline levels. Interestingly, plasma volume expansion with dextran had no such effect. In another study, the blood pressure rise produced by the cessation of diuretic therapy was prevented by severe salt restriction (65). More recent controlled studies have been less encouraging. One cross-over trial reported a small additive effect when salt restriction was combined with diuretic therapy (19), whereas two other groups reported no effect (22,66). Although this may reflect inadequate power, it is notable that one of these studies was able to detect an additive effect of sodium restriction on beta-blocker treatment (22).

Sodium depletion increases salt appetite, and therefore it is possible that diuretic-treated patients may voluntarily increase sodium intake. It has been postulated that this phenomenon may explain "secondary escape" from the antihypertensive action of diuretics in some cases. Thus, Langford et al. (67) reported significantly higher urinary sodium excretion in women on antihypertensive therapy as compared with untreated women. However, these patients were known to be taking a variety of drugs. In the previously cited cross-over trial, Parijs et al. (19) reported increased urinary sodium excretion in diuretic-treated hypertensives. However, Bing et al. (30), in a longitudinal study, followed up 32 hypertensive patients treated with bendrofluazide (5 mg daily) as sole medication for 2 years. No change in mean 24-hr urinary sodium excretion occurred over this period, and individual patients showing an increase in urinary sodium showed no preferential tendency for blood pressure to increase. Interestingly, a progressive rise in PRA suggested that renin–angiotensin activation was a more likely mechanism for secondary escape.

Other Antihypertensive Drugs

Much less work has been carried out on the interaction between dietary salt restriction and other antihypertensive drugs. There is, however, good physiological and clinical support for the belief that the antihypertensive potency of converting-enzyme inhibitors is potentiated by sodium depletion (68). Ewrteman et al. (22) carried out a double-blind cross-over study of beta-blockade, diuretics, and moderate sodium restriction (sodium intake reduced from 130 to 72 mmol/day). They observed a useful additive effect when salt restriction was combined with a selective beta-blocker metoprolol.

There is no evidence for any useful interaction between sodium restriction and calcium-channel blockers. Thus, sodium restriction did not potentiate the antihypertensive action of either nitrendipine (69) or verapamil (70), while in another brief report there was a slight pressor effect when nifedipine-treated patients were salt-restricted (71).

In summary, it is probable that sodium restriction potentiates the action of angiotensin-converting-enzyme (ACE) inhibitors and perhaps also beta-blockers and diuretics. Except for the special case of ACE inhibitors where an effect occurs, the additive effect of moderate salt restriction (60–80 mmol/day) on antihypertensive agents is probably small and may be a useful alternative to adding another drug.

ADVERSE EFFECTS OF SALT RESTRICTION

In any assessment of drug treatment, both the risks and benefits of therapy require evaluation. There is much less published evidence on the adverse effects of dietary modifications in hypertension. There are no data on the incidence of adverse reactions to salt restriction, although this is of central importance when recommendations are to be made to large populations of patients with mild hypertension. Folkow and Ely (72) have emphasized the need for critical examination of the consequences of both low and high salt intake. Both low and high salt intakes can compromise the circulation in experimental studies. Thus, severe salt restriction impairs the cardiovascular response to such challenges as blood loss; furthermore, hypertensive animals are particularly susceptible in this regard—at least in the rat (72).

One of the important factors in this context seems to be reduced noradrenaline release per nerve impulse, causing the animal to maintain a higher level of sympathetic activity and higher renin secretion in order to maintain blood pressure. This, in turn, may reduce the potential neuroendocrine support which can be called upon in the face of an emergency (72). This impairment of a normal physiological response may account for the greater operative mortality when salt-depleted animals undergo surgical procedures (45). It seems likely that sodium depletion has similar adverse consequences when major surgery is carried out in humans (73). The predisposition of salt-depleted animals to acute renal tubular necrosis may reflect the same physiological effect (74,75).

Laboratory analysis of the harmful effects of salt depletion has not unnaturally concentrated upon severe dietary salt restriction. Lesser degrees of salt restriction have not been systematically studied from this viewpoint in the rat or in humans. Moderate salt restriction may be relatively free of these problems, or the incidence of adverse sequelae may be merely reduced, depending upon whether the degree of salt depletion is linearly related to the risk of adverse effects. Patients may not be homogeneous in this respect: The elderly, for instance, are particularly at risk from diuretic-induced sodium and water depletion and may also be exposed to greater risks when consuming a low-salt diet.

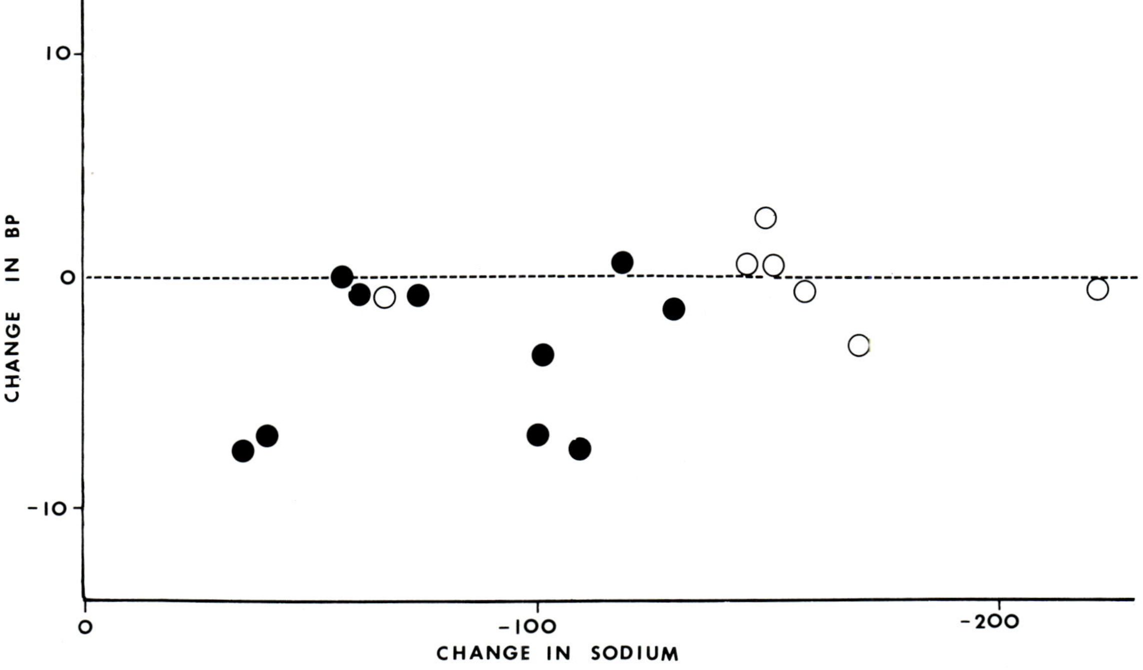

FIG. 2. Change in mean blood pressure in relation to degree of sodium restriction in trial reported in Tables 1 and 2.

Whether hypertensive patients (like hypertensive rats) are at increased risk is also unknown.

HOW FAR SHOULD SALT INTAKE BE RESTRICTED?

Earlier studies of salt restriction showed substantial blood pressure lowering in severely hypertensive patients when salt intake was reduced to levels below 10 mmol/day (15–17). The only significant attempt at detecting a dose–response relationship was carried out by Murray et al. (36), who exposed normal subjects to changes in salt intake ranging between 10 and 1500 mmol/day. Although the resultant graph showed a clear reduction in blood pressure at the extreme lower ends of salt intake (10 mmol/day), there was little relationship with blood pressure over the physiological range of sodium intake encountered in Western society. Freis (76) has postulated that efficacy of dietary salt restriction requires extracellular fluid and plasma volume contraction, which occurs only when salt intake is reduced to below 3 g (50 mmol of sodium per day). The available trial evidence (Fig. 2) does not support such a low cut-off point for benefit, although the heterogeneous nature of patients and protocols makes any attempt at detecting a dose–response relationship hazardous. However, as far as it goes, the available trial data (Table 1) would indicate that where blood pressure lowering has been demonstrated, it can be obtained with dietary intakes of sodium of 70–80 mmol/day. No adequate trial of untreated patients who reduce sodium intake significantly below these levels has been carried out, so that any recommendation to reduce intake below 70 mmol/day can only be based upon extrapolation. In view of the social difficulties and consequent problems with compliance, until more data is available it would seem unjustified to recommend a reduction in sodium intake below 70 mmol/day in hypertensive patients.

REFERENCES

1. Denton D. Hypertension a malady of civilisation? In: Sambhi MP, ed. *Systemic effects of antihypertensive agents.* New York: Grune & Stratton, 1976;577–583.
2. Glieberman L. Blood pressure and dietary salt in human populations. *Ecol Food Nutr* 1973;2:143–156.
3. Merrill JP, Schupak E. Mechanisms of hypertension in renoprival man. *Canad Med Assoc J* 1964;90:328.
4. Vertes V, Cangiano JL, Berman LB, Gould A. Hypertension in end-stage renal disease. *N Engl J Med* 1969;280:978–981.
5. Wilkinson R, Scott DF, Uldall PR, Kerr DNS. Plasma renin and exchangeable sodium in the hypertension of chronic renal failure. *Q J Med* 1970;39:377–394.
6. McAreavey D, Brown JJ, Cumming AMM, Davies DL, Fraser R, Lever AF, MacKay A, Morton JJ, Robertson JIS. Inverse relation of exchangeable sodium and blood pressure in hypertensive patients with renal artery stenosis. *J Hypertens* 1983;1:297–302.
7. Barraclough MA. Sodium and water depletion with acute malignant hypertension. *Amer J Med* 1966;40:265–272.
8. Kaneda H, Yamauchi T, Murata R, Matsumoto J, Haruyama T. Treatment of malignant hypertension with infusion of sodium chloride; a case report and a review. *Tohoku J Exp Med* 1980;132:179–186.
9. Thomas RD, Lee MR. Sodium repletion and beta-adrenergic blockade in treatment of salt depletion with accelerated hypertension. *Br Med J* 1976;2:1425–1426.
10. Bing RF, Smith AJ. Plasma and interstitial volumes in essential hypertension: relationship to blood pressure. *Clin Sci* 1981;61:287–293.
11. Bauer JH, Brooks CS. Body-fluid composition in normal and hypertensive man. *Clin Sci* 1982;62:43–49.
12. Beretta-Piccoli C, Davies DL, Boddy K, Brown JJ, Cumming AMM, East BW, Fraser R, Lever AF, Padfield PL, Semple PF, Robertson JIS, Weidmann P, Williams ED. Relation of arterial pressure with body sodium, body potassium and plasma potassium in essential hypertension. *Clin Sci* 1982;63:257–270.
13. Ambard L, Beaujard E. Causes de l'hypertension arterielle. *Arch Gen Med* 1904;1:520–533.
14. Allen FM, Sherrill JW. The treatment of arterial hypertension. *J Metab Res* 1922;2:429–545.
15. Dole VP, Dahl LK, Cotzias GC, Eder HA, Krebs ME. Dietary treatment of hypertension: clinical and metabolic studies of patients on the rice–fruit diet. *J Clin Invest* 1950;29:1189–1206.
16. Medical Research Council. The rice diet in the treatment of hypertension. *Lancet* 1950;2:509–513.
17. Corcoran AC, Taylor RD, Page IH. Controlled observations on the effect of low sodium dietotherapy in essential hypertension. *Circulation* 1951;3:1–16.
18. Joint National Committee on Detection, Evaluation and Treatment of High Blood Pressure. Non-pharmacological approaches to the control of high blood pressure. *Hypertension* 1986;8:444–467.
19. Parijs J, Joossens JV, Van der Linden L, Verstreken G, Amery AKPC. Moderate sodium restriction and diuretics in the treatment of hypertension. *Am Heart J* 1973;85:22–34.
20. MacGregor GA, Markandu N, Best F, Elder D, Cam J, Squires M. Double-blind randomised crossover trial of moderate sodium restriction in essential hypertension. *Lancet* 1982;1:351–354.
21. Morgan T, Gillies A, Morgan G, Adam W, Wilson M, Carney S. Hypertension treated by salt restriction. *Lancet* 1978;1:227–233.
22. Erwteman RM, Nagelkerke N, Lubsen J, Koster M, Dunning AJ. β-Blockage, diuretics and salt restriction for the management of mild hypertension: a randomised double blind trial. *Br Med J* 1984;289:406–409.
23. Watt GCM, Edwards C, Hart JJ, Hart M, Walton P, Foy CJW. Dietary sodium restriction for mild hypertension in general practice. *Br Med J* 1983;286:432–436.
24. Silman AJ, Locke C, Mitchell P, Humpherson P. Evaluation of the effectiveness of a low sodium diet in the treatment of mild to moderate hypertension. *Lancet* 1983;1:1179–1182.
25. Puska P, Iacono JM, Nissinen NA, Korhonen HJ, Vartianen E, Pietenen P, Dougherty R, Leino U, Mutanen M, Moisio S, Huttimen J. Controlled randomised trial of the effect of dietary fat on blood pressure. *Lancet* 1983;1:1–5.
26. Richards AM, Espiner EA, Mashowski AH, Nicholls MG, Ikram H, Hamilton EJ, Walls JE. Blood pressure response to moderate sodium restriction and to potassium supplementation in mild essential hypertension. *Lancet* 1984;1:757–761.
27. Longworth DK, Drayer JIM, Weber MA, Laragh JH. Divergent blood pressure responses during short term sodium restriction in hypertension. *Clin Pharmacol Ther* 1980;27:544–546.
28. Grobbee DE, Hofman A, Roelandt JT, Boomsma F, Schalekamp MA, Valkenburg HA. Sodium restriction and potassium supplementation in young people with mildly elevated blood pressure. *J Hypertens* 1987;5:115–119.
29. Chalmers J, Morgan T, Doyle A, Dickson B, Hopper J, Matthews J, Matthews G, Moulds R, Myers J, Nowson C, Scoggins B, Stebbing M. Australian National Health and Medical Research Council dietary salt study in mild hypertension. *J Hypertens* 1986;4(Suppl 6):S629–S637.
30. Bing RF, Thurston H, Swales JD. Salt intake and diuretic treatment of hypertension. *Lancet* 1979;ii:121–123.
31. Oldham PD. A note on the analysis of repeated measurements of the same subjects. *J Chronic Dis* 1962;15:967–977.
32. Meade TW, Imeson JD, Gordon D, Peart WS. The epidemiology of plasma renin. *Clin Sci* 1983;64:273–280.
33. Cappuccio FP, Markandu ND, Sagnella GA, MacGregor GA. Sodium restriction lowers high blood pressure through a decreased response of the renin system Direct evidence using saralasin. *J Hypertens* 1985;3:243–247.

34. Kirkendall WM, Connor WE, Arboud F, Rastogi SP, Anderson TA, Fry M. The effect of dietary sodium chloride on blood pressure, body fluids, electrolytes, renal function and serum lipids of normotensive man. *J Lab Clin Med* 1976;87:418–434.
35. Burstyn E, Hornall D, Watchorn C. Sodium and potassium intake and blood pressure. *Br Med J* 1980;281:537–539.
36. Murray RH, Luft FC, Bloch R, Weyman E. Blood pressure response to extremes of sodium intake in normal man. *Proc Soc Exp Biol Med* 1978;159:432–436.
37. Sullivan JM, Ratts TE, Taylor JC, Kraus DH, Barton BR, Patrick DR, Reeds SW. Hemodynamic effects of dietary sodium in man: a preliminary report. *Hypertension* 1980;2:506–514.
38. Parfrey PS, Markandu ND, Roulston JE, Jones BE, Jones JC, MacGregor GA. Relation between arterial pressure, dietary sodium intake and renin system in essential hypertension. *Br Med J* 1981;283:94–97.
39. Cooper R, Van Horn L, Liu K, Trevisan M, Nanas S, Ueshima H, Larbi E, Yu CS, Sempos C, Le Grady D, Stamler J. A randomised trial on the effect of decreased dietary sodium intake on blood pressure in adolescents. *J Hypertens* 1984;2:361–366.
40. Heagerty AM, Alton SM, El-Ashry A, Bing RF, Thurston H, Swales JD. Effect of changes in sodium balance on leucocyte sodium transport: qualitative differences in normotensive offspring of hypertensives and matched controls. *J Hypertens* 1986;4:333–338.
41. Skrabal F, Auback J, Hortnagl H. Low sodium/high potassium diet for prevention of hypertension: probable mechanism of action. *Lancet* 1981;2:895–900.
42. McNabb WR, Noormohamed FH, Lant AF. The effects of enalapril on blood pressure and the kidney in normotensive subjects under altered sodium balance. *J Hypertens* 1986;4:39–47.
43. Seymour AA, Davis JO, Freeman RH, DeForrest JM, Rowe BP, Stephens GA, Williams GM. Hypertension produced by sodium depletion and unilateral nephrectomy: a new experimental model. *Hypertension* 1980;2:125–129.
44. Munoz-Ramirez H, Chatelain RE, Bumpus FM, Khairallah PA. Development of two-kidney Goldblatt hypertension in rats under dietary sodium restriction. *Am J Physiol* 1980;238:H889–H894.
45. Webb DJ, Clark SA, Brown WB, Fraser R, Lever AF, Murray GD, Robertson JIS. Dietary sodium deprivation raises blood pressure in the rat but does not produce irreversible hyperaldosteronism. 1987;5:525–532.
46. Swales JD, ed. *Platt v Pickering.* London: Keynes Press, British Medical Association, 1985.
47. Dahl LK, Heine M, Tassinari L. Effects of chronic excess salt ingestion: evidence that genetic factors play an important role in susceptibility to experimental hypertension. *J Exp Med* 1962;115:1173–1190.
48. Kawasaki T, Delea CS, Bartter FC, Smith H. The effect of high-sodium and low-sodium intakes on blood pressure and other related variables in human subjects with idiopathic hypertension. *Am J Med* 1978;64:193–198.
49. Fujita T, Henry WL, Bartter FC, Lake CR. Factors influencing blood pressure in salt-sensitive patients with hypertension. *Am J Med* 1980;69:334–344.
50. Fujita T, Noda H, Ando K. Sodium susceptibility and potassium effects in young patients with borderline hypertension. *Circulation* 1984;69:468–476.
51. Takeshita A, Imaizumi T, Arhihora T, Nakamura M. Characteristics of responses to salt loading and deprivation in hypertensive subjects. *Circ Res* 1982;51:457–464.
52. Takeshita A, Ashihara T, Yamamoto K, Imaizumi T, Hoka S, Ito M, Nakamura M. Venous responses to salt loading in hypertensive subjects. *Circulation* 1984;69:50–56.
53. Skrabal F, Hergholz H, Neumayr M, Hamberger L, Ledochowski M, Sporer H, Hortnagl H, Schwarz, Schoritzer D. Salt sensitivity in humans is linked to enhanced sympathetic responsiveness and enhanced proximal tubular sodium reabsorption. *Hypertension* 1984;6:152–158.
54. Skrabal F, Gruber G, Meister B, Ledochowski M, Doll P, Lang F, Czerny E. Salt sensitivity in normotensives with family history of hypertension: Studies of membrane transport, intracellular electrolytes and alpha 2 adrenergic receptors. *J Hypertens* 1985;3(Suppl 3):S25–S28.
55. Luft FC, Weinberger MH, Grim CE. Sodium sensitivity and resistance in normotensive humans. *Am J Med* 1982;72:726–736.
56. Weinberger MH, Miller JZ, Luft FC, Grim CE, Fineberg NS. Definitions and characteristics of sodium sensitivity and blood pressure resistance. *Hypertension* 1986;8(Suppl II):II-127–II-134.
57. Dahl LK, Heine M, Thompson K. Genetic influence of the kidneys on blood pressure: evidence from chronic renal homografts in rats with opposite predispositions to hypertension. *Circ Res* 1974;34:94–101.
58. Wiggins RC, Basar I, Slater JDH. Effect of arterial pressure and inheritance on the sodium excretory capacity of normal young men. *Clin Sci Mol Med* 1978;54:639–647.
58a. Weinberger MH, Miller JZ, Fineberg NS, Luft FC, Grim CE, Christian JC. Association of haptoglobin with sodium sensitivity and resistance of blood pressure. *Hypertension* 1987;10:443–446.
59. Stamler R, Grimm R, Gisch FC, Elmer P, Dyer A, Berman R, Fishman J, Van Heel IV, Civinelli J, McDonald A, Stamler J. Control of high blood pressure by nutritional therapy: final report of a 4-year randomised controlled trial—the Hypertension Control Program. *JAMA* 1987;257:1484–1491.
60. Beard TC, Gray WR, Cooke HM, Barge R. Randomised controlled trial of a no-added-sodium diet for mild hypertension. *Lancet* 1982;ii:455–463.
61. Winer N. The antihypertensive mechanisms of salt depletion induced by hydrochlorothiazide. *Circulation* 1961;24:788–796.
62. Johnson OD, Ruchelman H, Ford RV. Diuretics and hypertension: effect of sodium balance. *N Engl J Med* 1962;267:336–338.
63. Fries ED, Wanko A, Wilson IM. Treatment of essential hypertension with chlorothiazide (Diuril). Its use and combined with other antihypertensive agents. *JAMA* 1958;166:137–139.
64. Finnerty FA, Davidov M, Kakaviatos IV. Relation of sodium balance to arterial pressure during drug-induced saluresis. *Circulation* 1968;37:175–183.
65. Hollander W, Chobanian AV, Wilkins RW. Relationship between diuretic and antihypertensive effects of chlorthiazide and mercurial diuretics. *Circulation* 1959;19:827–838.
66. Van Brummelen P, Schalekamp M, de Graeff J. Influence of sodium intake on hydrochlorothiazide-induced changes in blood pressure, serum electrolytes, renin and aldosterone in essential hypertension. *Acta Med Scand* 1978;204:151–157.
67. Langford HG, Watson RL, Gavras J. Increased salt appetite in the treated hypertensive. *Clin Res* 1975;23:55A.
68. MacGregor GA, Markandu ND, Smith SJ, Sagnella GA, Morton JJ. Angiotensin converting enzyme inhibition reveals an important role for the renin system in the control of normal and high blood pressure in man. *Clin Exp Hypertens* 1983;5:1367–1380.
69. Nicholson JP, Resnick LM, Di Fabio B, James HD, Jennis R, Laragh JH. Sodium restriction and the antihypertensive effect of nitrendipine. *Clin Res* (Abstrct.) 1986;34:404A.
70. Nicholson JP, Resnick LM, Laragh JH. The anti-hypertensive effect of verapamril at extremes of dietary sodium intake. *Ann Intern Med* 1987;107:329–334.
71. Morgan T, Anderson A, Wilson D, Myers J, Murphy J, Nowson C. Paradoxical effect of sodium restriction on blood pressure in people on slow channel calcium blocking drugs. *Lancet* 1986;i:793.
72. Folkow B, Ely DL. Dietary sodium effects on cardiovascular and sympathetic neuroeffector function as studied in various rat models. *J Hypertens* 1987;5:383–395.
73. Thompson JE, Vollman RW, Austin DJ, Kartchner MM. Prevention of hypotensive and renal complications of aortic surgery using balanced salt solutions. *Ann Surg* 1968;167:767–776.
74. McDonald FD, Thiel G, Wilson DR, Di Bona GF, Oken DE. The prevention of acute renal failure in the rat by long term saline loading: a possible role of the renin–angiotensin axis. *Proc Soc Exp Biol Med* 1969;131:610–614.
75. Di Bona GF, Sawin LL. The renin–angiotensin system in acute renal failure in the rat. *Lab Invest* 1971;25:528–532.
76. Freis ED. Does moderate salt restriction lower blood pressure? *Hypertension* 1986;8:265–266.

Hypertension: Pathophysiology, Diagnosis, and Management, edited by J. H. Laragh and B. M. Brenner. Raven Press, Ltd., New York © 1990.

CHAPTER 127

Role of Dietary Chloride in Hypertension

R. Curtis Morris, Jr., Hamoudi Al-Bander, and Theodore Kurtz

Salt-Sensitive Hypertension Studies, 2021
Conclusion, 2023
References, 2023

Although Ambard and Beaujard (1) suggested in 1904 that increased retention of chloride might be important in the pathogenesis of hypertension, Dahl (2) stated in 1954 the now prevalent view that "the sodium ion alone is important" (in the pathogenesis of hypertension). Indeed, chloride has been specifically dismissed as a pathogenetic determinant of hypertension (3,4). To a considerable extent, this view stems from three sets of observations made some 40 years ago in metabolic studies of humans and animals with hypertension: (i) Restriction of dietary sodium chloride decreased blood pressure, whereas subsequent supplementation of dietary sodium chloride increased blood pressure (5–7)—responses now said to characterize "salt sensitivity" (8,9). (ii) When restriction of dietary sodium chloride had decreased blood pressure, supplementation of dietary chloride without sodium (ammonium chloride) failed to increase blood pressure (5,7). (iii) When supplementation of dietary sodium chloride had increased blood pressure, the increase was abolished by restricting sodium alone (by substituting ammonium chloride or potassium chloride for the supplement of sodium chloride) (7).

According to the originally stated interpretation of these data (7), which was recently restated (10), "it was observed that sodium, but not chloride, restriction was *necessary*" to attenuate hypertension. The data, however, indicate only that restriction of dietary sodium alone is sufficient to attenuate NaCl-induced hypertension and that supplementing dietary chloride alone is not sufficient to induce hypertension. The data do not indicate that restriction of sodium is *necessary* to attenuate NaCl-induced hypertension, because they do not exclude the possibility that restriction of chloride alone is also sufficient to attenuate the hypertension. If, in fact, dietary restriction of either chloride or sodium were sufficient to attenuate NaCl-induced hypertension, this would suggest that both the Na and Cl components of dietary NaCl are necessary for its capacity to induce hypertension.

Positive tests of this hypothesis have recently been reported in two well-characterized rat models of salt-sensitive hypertension and in men with salt-sensitive essential hypertension.

SALT-SENSITIVE HYPERTENSION STUDIES

In uninephrectomized rats given NaCl and desoxycorticosterone, the so-called "DOC" model, Kurtz and Morris (11) asked the question, "Do non-chloride sodium salts induce hypertension in the DOC rat?" They found that the extent to which a given dietary intake of sodium induced an increase in blood pressure depended on whether or not the anionic component of the sodium salt was chloride. With normal and high dietary intakes of sodium, sodium chloride induced increases in blood pressure much greater than those induced by approximately equimolar amounts of either sodium bicarbonate or sodium ascorbate, or a combination of sodium bicarbonate and sodium ascorbate. A normal amount of dietary sodium chloride induced hypertension, whereas an equimolar amount of sodium bicarbonate did not increase blood pressure. Specifically, after 5 weeks of a normal dietary intake of sodium, the mean blood pressure in the rats given sodium bicarbonate was not different from that of rats given sodium chloride without DOC, but the mean blood pressure in both groups was substantially less than that of rats given sodium chloride and DOC. The difference observed in the relative capacities of NaCl and $NaHCO_3$/Na-ascorbate to increase blood pressure could not be attributed to differences in sodium or potassium balances, weight gain, or caloric intake. The failure of $NaHCO_3$ to induce hypertension appears to be independent of the hypokalemia that is characteristic of the DOC model, and it also appears to be independent of hypokalemia's predictable exaggeration by administration of $NaHCO_3$ (12).

In the Dahl salt-sensitive rat, Kotchen and co-workers

(13) compared the blood pressure response to sodium chloride loading and to equimolar sodium loading provided as a mixture of non-chloride-containing sodium salts. For 5 weeks the rats were fed a diet containing normal or high concentrations of sodium chloride or containing high concentrations of sodium provided as a mixture of sodium bicarbonate, sodium phosphate, and the sodium salts of amino acid. To prevent chloride depletion, both sodium chloride and the non-chloride-containing sodium salt mixture were added to a "normal" sodium chloride diet. At 1 week, the rats receiving high concentrations of sodium chloride had higher systolic blood pressures than did the rats in the other two groups. The investigators observed no statistically significant group differences in (a) plasma volume, (b) arterial pH, (c) plasma concentrations of Na^+, K^+, Cl^-, Ca^{2+}, or creatinine, or (d) renomedullary prostaglandin E_2 production. Compared to the animals receiving normal concentrations of sodium chloride, those receiving high concentrations of either sodium chloride or the sodium salts of amino acids had decreased plasma renin activity and plasma aldosterone concentrations. The investigators concluded that development of hypertension in the Dahl salt-sensitive rat is dependent on the provision of sodium as sodium chloride.

Recently, in a detailed metabolic study of five men with salt-sensitive essential hypertension, Kurtz et al. (14) asked two questions: (i) When blood pressure has decreased to normal values with restriction of dietary sodium chloride, does supplementation of dietary sodium without chloride (sodium citrate) increase blood pressure? (ii) When blood pressure has increased with supplemental dietary sodium chloride, does continued dietary supplementation of an equimolar amount of sodium without chloride (by replacing supplemental sodium chloride with sodium citrate) sustain the increase in blood pressure? After blood pressure had decreased to normal with restriction of dietary sodium chloride to 10 mmol/day (0.23 g of sodium per day), oral administration of sodium chloride for 7 days (240 mmol/day) induced significant increases in systolic and diastolic blood pressure of 16 ± 2 and 8 ± 2 mmHg (mean $\pm$ SEM), respectively. An equimolar amount of sodium given as sodium citrate induced no change in blood pressure. Replacing supplemental sodium chloride with an equimolar amount of sodium as sodium citrate abolished the increase in blood pressure induced by sodium chloride. Both salts induced substantial and comparable sodium retention, weight gain, and suppression of plasma renin activity and plasma aldosterone, but supplemental sodium chloride increased plasma volume and urinary excretion of calcium, whereas sodium citrate did not.

These findings, which demonstrate that the anionic component of an orally administered sodium salt can determine whether that salt can induce or maintain an increase in blood pressure, are not without precedent. In 1929, in a study of seven patients with hypertension in whom dietary salt was apparently unrestricted, Berghoff and Geraci (15) found that daily oral administration of 200 mmol of sodium chloride for 1 month induced increases in blood pressure, whereas oral administration of 278 mmol of sodium bicarbonate did not. In 1936, in a study of diabetic children, McQuarrie et al. (16) reported that the pressor effect of orally administered NaCl appeared to be greater than that of either sodium citrate or sodium bicarbonate. In recent preliminary observations in outpatients with essential hypertension, Morgan (17) found that oral loading with sodium bicarbonate (70 mmol/day for 2 weeks) induced a lesser increase in blood pressure as compared to that induced by oral loading with an equimolar amount of sodium chloride. The patients given sodium bicarbonate were not found to be different from those given sodium chloride with respect to urinary excretion of sodium. Detailed metabolic studies, however, were not performed to determine whether patients given sodium chloride ingested or retained more sodium than those given sodium bicarbonate; measurements of blood volume, plasma renin activity, or plasma aldosterone concentration were not reported. In patients with chronic renal failure, Husted et al. (18) found that orally administered sodium bicarbonate (200 mmol/day for 4 days) did not induce an increase in blood pressure, whereas an equimolar amount of sodium chloride did. Although the urinary excretion of sodium in patients given sodium bicarbonate was somewhat greater than that of patients given sodium chloride, substantial sodium retention occurred in both groups. In the single study in humans in which orally administered sodium bicarbonate is reported to have induced hypertension, blood pressure appeared to increase with administration of massive amounts of alkali (over 1000 mmol/day) only after supplementing the oral intake of chloride with potassium chloride, (80 mmol/day) (19).

Non-chloride-containing sodium salts might fail to increase blood pressure because of their inability to evoke substantial and sustained renal retention of sodium (20,21). But in the study of Kurtz et al. (14), both sodium chloride and sodium citrate induced substantial sodium retention, weight gain, and comparable suppressions of plasma renin activity and the plasma aldosterone concentration. Furthermore, replacing the dietary supplement of sodium chloride with an equimolar amount of sodium as sodium citrate not only corrected the hypertension induced by sodium chloride but did so despite continued retention of sodium, minimal changes in plasma aldosterone, and no decrease in body weight. Since only sodium chloride induced detectable increases in plasma volume and blood pressure, the differing effects of sodium chloride and sodium citrate on blood pressure may be a consequence of their differing effects on plasma volume, in keeping with the proposal of Hamlyn and Blaustein (21).

Administration of either sodium chloride or sodium citrate appeared to induce a striking retention of sodium (approximately 500 mmol) but a relatively small increase in weight (approximately 1 kg) and in plasma sodium concentration (2–4 mmol/liter). The finding is similar to the results of several studies in hypertensive subjects in whom supplementing a low-sodium diet with sodium chloride (approximately 250 mmol/day for 3–7 days) induced substantial sodium retention (260–450 mmol) but only a small gain in weight (less than 1 kg) (8,22,23). These observations suggest the possibility that some of the retained sodium may have become sequestered in tissue sites so that it became osmotically inactive.

It has recently been suggested that a disorder in calcium metabolism underlies salt-sensitive hypertension, both in experimental animal models (24,25) and in humans (26).

In a group of patients with essential hypertension, all of whom were on a low-calcium diet (200–350 mg/day), supplementation of dietary sodium with sodium chloride (200 mmol/day for 5 days) induced changes in blood pressure that correlated directly with changes in the serum level of $1,25(OH)_2D$ and correlated inversely with changes in the serum level of ionized calcium (26). These observations were interpreted as evidence that NaCl-induced changes in calcium metabolism mediated the changes in blood pressure. In the patients with essential hypertension studied by Kurtz et al. (14), their normal dietary intake of calcium (800 mg/day) may account for the observation that supplementation of dietary sodium with either sodium chloride or sodium citrate induced no detectable changes in circulating levels of ionized calcium or $1,25(OH)_2D$. The hypercalciuria induced by supplemental sodium chloride may have been an isolated consequence of the observed NaCl-induced increase in plasma volume (27), and the decrease in urinary excretion of calcium induced by sodium citrate may be an isolated consequence of increased delivery of bicarbonate to the distal renal tubule (28). The possibility that the chloride ion itself may contribute to NaCl-induced increases in blood pressure is raised by recent studies demonstrating important biologic effects of chloride in the brain (29), kidney (30–32), and smooth muscle (33). In erythrocytes of humans with essential hypertension, the recent finding that chloride concentrations and activity are decreased as compared with their levels in normotensive humans suggests the need for further research on the possible role of the chloride ion itself in hypertension (34).

Essential hypertension is presumably a heterogeneous disorder, and Kurtz et al. (14) studied only five affected men. In some patients with essential hypertension, nonchloride-containing sodium salts may induce increases in blood pressure as large as those induced by sodium chloride. Yet, in published studies in patients with essential hypertension and in animal models of salt-dependent hypertension, the anionic component of the sodium salt consumed has determined whether dietary intake of that salt increased blood pressure (11–15) and has also determined the extent of that increase (17).

It is of interest that dietary sodium bromide has been reported to be hypertensinogenic in patients with hypertension also found to be NaCl-sensitive (16). In the DOC model of salt-sensitive hypertension, both sodium bromide and sodium iodide appear to be hypertensinogenic (35). Bromide can effectively substitute for chloride in the Na^+–K^+–Cl^- cotransport system in the Madin–Darby canine kidney (MDCK) cell line (36). Thus, halide salts of sodium other than NaCl may have the hypertensinogenic capacity, possibly because they can be readily reclaimed by the kidney and distributed principally in the extracellular space, like sodium chloride (21).

CONCLUSION

It should be emphasized that the results of Kurtz et al. (14) provide no basis for making recommendations with respect to the dietary management of essential hypertension. Their results do suggest the need for further studies in humans with hypertension, to determine the relative capacities of different sodium salts to affect blood pressure. The results of such studies could be relevant to the dietary management of essential hypertension and to our understanding of the pathogenesis of NaCl-sensitive hypertension.

REFERENCES

1. Ambard L, Beaujard A. Causes de l'hypertension arterielle. *Arch Gen Med* 1904;I:520–533.
2. Dahl LK, Love RA. Evidence for relationship between sodium (chloride) intake and human essential hypertension. *Arch Intern Med* 1954;94:525–531.
3. Dahl LK. Possible role of salt intake in the development of essential hypertension. In: Bock KD, Cottier PI, eds. *Essential hypertension, an international symposium.* Berlin: Springer-Verlag, 1960;58–65.
4. Jacobson M, Liebman BF, Moyer G. *Salt: The brand name guide to sodium content.* New York: Workman Publishing, 1983.
5. Grollman A, Harrison TR, Mason MF, Baxter J, Crampton J, Reichsman F. Sodium restriction in the diet for hypertension. *JAMA* 1945;129:533–537.
6. Grollman A, Harrison TR. Effect of rigid sodium restriction on blood pressure and survival of hypertensive rats. *Proc Soc Exp Biol Med* 1945;60:52–55.
7. Dole VP, Dahl LK, Cotzias GC, Eder HA, Krebs ME. Dietary treatment of hypertension. Clinical and metabolic studies of patients on the rice–fruit diet. *J Clin Invest* 1950;29:1189–1206.
8. Kawasaki T, Delea C, Barrter F, Smith H. The effect of high-sodium and low-sodium intakes on blood pressure and other related variables in human subjects with idiopathic hypertension. *Am J Med* 1978;64:193–198.
9. Fujita T, Henry W, Barrter F, Lake C, Delea C. Factors influencing blood pressure in salt-sensitive patients with hypertension. *Am J Med* 1980;69:334–344.
10. Denton D. *The hunger for salt: an anthropological, physiological and medical analysis.* Berlin: Springer-Verlag, 1982.
11. Kurtz TW, Morris RC, Jr. Dietary chloride as a determinant of "sodium-dependent" hypertension. *Science* 1983;222:1139–1141.
12. Passmore JC, Whitescarver SA, Ott CE, Kotchen TA. Importance of chloride for deoxycorticosterone acetate-salt hypertension in the rat. *Hypertension* 1985;7(Suppl I):I-115–I-120.
13. Whitescarver SA, Ott CE, Jackson BA, Guthrie GP Jr, Kotchen TA. Salt-sensitive hypertension: contribution of chloride. *Science* 1984;223:1430–1432.
14. Kurtz TW, Al-Bander HA, Morris RC, Jr. "Salt-sensitive" essential hypertension in men: Is the sodium ion alone important? *N Engl J Med* 1987;317:1043–1048.
15. Berghoff RS, Geraci AS. The influence of sodium chloride on blood pressure. *IMJ* 1929;56:395–397.
16. McQuarrie I, Thompson WH, Anderson JA. Effects of excessive ingestion of sodium and potassium salts on carbohydrate metabolism and blood pressure in diabetic children. *J Nutr* 1936;11:77–101.
17. Morgan T. The effect of potassium and bicarbonate ions on the rise in blood pressure caused by sodium chloride. *Clin Sci* 1982;63:407s–409s.
18. Husted F, Nolph K, Maher J. $NaHCO_3$ and NaCl tolerance in chronic renal failure. *J Clin Invest* 1975;56:414–419.
19. Lowder SC, Brown RD. Hypertension corrected by discontinuing chronic sodium bicarbonate ingestion: subsequent transient hypoaldosteronism. *Am J Med* 1975;58:272–279.
20. Liebman BF, Langford HG. Hypertension and sodium salts. *Science* 1985;228:351–352.
21. Hamlyn JM, Blaustein MP. Sodium chloride, extracellular fluid volume, and blood pressure regulation. *Am J Physiol* 1986;251:F563–F575.
22. Ishii M, Atarashi K, Ikeda T, et al. Role of the aldosterone system in the salt-sensitivity of patients with benign essential hypertension. *Jpn Heart J* 1983;24:79–90.
23. Dustan HP, Valdes G, Bravo EL, Tarazi RC. Excessive sodium

retention as a characteristic of salt-sensitive hypertension. *Am J Med Sci* 1986;292:67–74.

24. Kageyama Y, Bravo EL. Neurohumoral and hemodynamic responses to dietary calcium supplementation in deoxycorticosterone–salt hypertensive dogs. *Hypertension* 1987;9:III-166–III-170.
25. Resnick LM, Sosa RE, Corbett ML, Gertner JM, Sealey JE, Laragh JH. Effects of dietary calcium on sodium volume vs. renin-dependent forms of experimental hypertension. *Trans Assoc Am Physicians* 1986;99:172–179.
26. Resnick LM, Nicholson JP, Laragh JH. Alterations in calcium metabolism mediate dietary salt sensitivity in essential hypertension. *Trans Assoc Am Physicians* 1985;98:313–321.
27. Massry SG, Coburn JW, Chapman LW, Kleeman CR. Effect of NaCl infusion on urinary Ca^{++} and Mg^{++} during reduction in their filtered loads. *Am J Physiol* 1967;213:1218–1224.
28. Peraino RA, Suki WN. Urine HCO_3^--augments renal Ca^{2+} absorption independent of systemic acid–base changes. *Am J Physiol* 1980;238:F394–F398.
29. Harris RA, Allan AM. Functional coupling of gamma-aminobutyric acid receptors to chloride channels in brain membranes. *Science* 1985;228:1108–1110.
30. Schnermann J, Ploth DW, Hermle M. Activation of tubulo-glomerular feedback by chloride transport. *Pflugers Arch* 1976;362: 229–240.
31. Kotchen TA, Galla JH, Luke RG. Failure of $NaHCO_3$ and $KHCO_3$ to inhibit renin in the rat. *Am J Physiol* 1976;231:1050–1056.
32. Wilcox CS. Regulation of renal blood flow by plasma chloride. *J Clin Invest* 1983;71:726–735.
33. Aickin CC, Brading AF. Intracellular chloride activity of guinea-pig vas deferens. *J Physiol* 1980;380:56p–57p.
34. Zidek W, Losse H, Lange-Asschenfeldt H, Vetter H. Intracellular chloride in essential hypertension. *Clin Sci* 1985;68:45–47.
35. Kurtz TW, Morris RC Jr. Halides as possible determinants of Na^+-dependent hypertension. *Kidney Int* 1986;29:250a.
36. McRoberts JA, Erlinger S, Rindler MJ, Saier MH. Furosemide sensitive salt transport in the Madin–Darby canine kidney cell line: evidence for the cotransport of Na, K, and Cl. *J Biol Chem* 1982;257:2260–2266.

Hypertension: Pathophysiology, Diagnosis, and Management, edited by J. H. Laragh and B. M. Brenner. Raven Press, Ltd., New York © 1990.

CHAPTER 128

Weight Reduction as a Therapeutic Modality in Hypertension

The Influence of Concurrent Sodium Deprivation

Efrain Reisin

Mechanisms Involved in Obesity–Hypertension Interaction, 2025
Changes in Fluid Volume Distribution and in Systemic Hemodynamics in Obesity Hypertension, 2026
Endocrinic–Adrenergic–Metabolic Changes in Obesity Hypertension, 2027
The Effect of Weight Loss in the Control of Blood Pressure: Clinical Experience—Short- and Long-Term Effect, 2028
Changes in Fluid Volume Distribution and in Systemic Hemodynamics Produced by Weight Reduction, 2030
Endocrinic–Adrenergic–Metabolic Changes Produced by Weight Reduction, 2031
Sodium Restriction Versus Weight Reduction, 2032
Feasibility of Weight-Reduction and/or Salt-Reduction Programs, 2033
References, 2033

"Excessive eating is like a deadly poison to the body of any man and it is the principle [cause] of all illnesses."
Maimonides, M. (1180): Mishneh Torah. Ch IV, No. 15.

Cross-sectional studies have shown that the association between obesity and hypertension is strong at any age, irrespective of the gender or race of the subject (2–7). Moreover, other investigators (8–10) have shown by longitudinal studies that with increase in weight and age, persons are at a greater risk of being hypertensives.

Earlier studies have explained that the identification of hypertension in obese subjects is not produced by a methodological inaccuracy (inappropriately sphygmomanometric cuff sizes) (11–16). Forsberg et al. (17) summarized studies that compared standard sphygmomanometric pressure measurements in the arm and intra-arterial pressures and concluded that the arm circumference probably is only a minor influential factor when a larger cuff is used. Consequently, the use of a bladder wider than the arm diameter (40% of arm circumference) and long enough to encircle 80% of the arm circumference is recommended to obtain more reliable measurements in obese hypertensives (18).

More recent studies (19–23) investigated the correlation between fat distribution and hypertension and found that obese individuals with high waist–hip ratio (upper-body obesity) have a higher incidence of hypertension than those with low waist–hip ratio (lower-body obesity) and that when the fat distribution is constant (intermediate type), obesity shows an uncertain correlation with high blood pressure (24). In consequence, apparently the role of fat distribution in the association is more important than the role of obesity; however, this theory deserves further investigation.

This chapter describes the pathophysiologic mechanisms that seem to be involved in obesity hypertension, together with the changes in those mechanisms produced by weight reduction independent of caloric or salt restriction. Other sections of this chapter include the existent clinical experience (short- and long-term-effect studies) regarding the effect of weight reduction on hypertension, the effect of the concurrent salt deprivation in hypertensive patients, and the feasibility of weight reduction and/or salt restriction programs.

MECHANISMS INVOLVED IN OBESITY–HYPERTENSION INTERACTION

Various mechanisms have been suggested by previous investigations to explain the association between obesity and hypertension. Only a few of those mechanisms, how-

TABLE 1. *Physiological mechanisms involved in obesity hypertension; effect of weight reduction*[a]

Endocrinic–metabolic mechanisms	Obesity hypertension	Weight reduction
Na^+ intake	↑	↓
Na^+-K^+-ATPase activity	↓	↓ or ↑
Adrenergic activity	↑	↓
Plasma renin activity	→ or ↓	↓ or →
Plasma aldosterone levels	→	↓ or →
Plasma insulin concentration	↑	↓
Fluid compartmental and hemodynamics		
Intravascular volume	↑	↓
Cardiopulmonary blood volume	↑	↓
Plasma volume/interstitial fluid volume ratio	→	↑
Intracellular fluid volume/total body water ratio	↑	↑
Cardiac output	↑ or →	↓ or →
Total vascular peripheral resistance	→	→
Left ventricular stroke work	↑	↓

[a] Adapted from ref. 115. ↑, increased; ↓, decreased; →, unchanged.

ever, were specifically studied in patients with upper- or lower-body obesity. Some authors studying the obese hypertensive population as a whole have described (a) alterations in the fluid volume distribution, (b) hemodynamic changes (19,25–29), and (c) cardiac morphologic alterations (30–32), and others have shown variations in the adrenergic, metabolic, and endocrinic factors as discussed below (Table 1).

Changes in Fluid Volume Distribution and in Systemic Hemodynamics in Obesity Hypertension

Plasma and Total Blood Volume

The plasma and total blood volume have been shown to be increased when absolute values in obese hypertensive patients are considered (26). Other investigators (27) have shown that the intravascular volume may be normal if it is calculated by deviation from desirable weight or from ideal weight. When one considers the lack of definition of appropriate indices to express changes in fluid volume distribution and in hemodynamics in patients with different body weight, however, the absolute values are considered an appropriate reference to relate to the absolute circulating volume in obese subjects (26).

In our laboratory, we measured plasma volume and total blood volume using radioisotope-tagged human serum albumin and hematocrit, respectively, and found a definitive increase in the absolute amount of circulating intravascular blood volume (26). Intravascular volume in obese subjects is non-uniformly distributed throughout the body because of the distribution of body fat. As total body fat increases, the ratio of intravascular volume to body weight falls from ±95 ml/kg to ±45 ml/kg. These data indicate that adipose tissue seems to be underperfused when compared with lean tissue (26).

Consequently, as earlier studies have noted (25,33), the absolute increase in blood volume for obese subjects reflects not only an increased size of the vascular bed but also an altered distribution of blood volume (26). We underscore the pathophysiologic importance of the increased absolute values because the absolute measured intravascular volume is the actual volume pumped by the heart and is generally redistributed centrally (cardiopulmonary area), thereby augmenting the venous return to the heart and increasing the cardiac output (29).

Extracellular and Intracellular Fluid Volumes

The extracellular fluid volume (28) was studied by only one group of investigators in the obese hypertensive subject, and they expressed the results by analyzing the indices of the partition of the plasma fluid volume (PV)/interstitial fluid volume (IF) and of the intracellular fluid volume/interstitial fluid volume. They have shown that the PV/IF ratio was within the normal range in obese hypertensive patients and correlated negatively with the mean arterial pressure and that the intracellular body water/interstitial fluid volume ratio was increased in obesity hypertension. They concluded that these findings might be caused either by an intracellular body water level that is too high for the level of interstitial fluid volume or by an interstitial fluid volume that is too low for the level of intracellular body water (28).

Systemic Hemodynamics

Earlier studies (25,33) and more recent investigations performed in our laboratory (26) have shown that the absolute cardiac output was elevated and that the total peripheral resistance was inappropriately normal in obese hypertensive patients compared with lean essential hypertensive patients. The increase in cardiac output is related to the expanded total blood volume. The increased arterial pressure, cardiac output, and blood volume were associated with an increased oxygen consumption, left ventricular stroke volume, and left ventricular stroke work (26). When the left ventricular structure was evaluated by echocardiographic techniques, we found an increase in the left arterial, left ventricular, and aortic root diameters as well as in post and septal well thicknesses and in left ventricular mass (31).

Based on those results, we summarized that arterial hypertension provides a concentric left ventricular hypertrophy, associated with the increased arterial pressure and its attendant increased afterload. In obesity, the increased plasma and cardiopulmonary volumes lead to ventricular dilatation and eccentric hypertrophy. Consequently, the obese hypertensive patient will have a dimorphic cardiac structural change, expressed by the concentric and eccentric left ventricular hypertrophy (30).

Peripheral Circulation

Previous studies in obese patients have shown a normal blood distribution to brain and kidneys but an increased blood flow distribution to the spleen (33). In a recent investigation we showed that obese hypertensive patients, compared with matched (by age, sex, and race) lean hypertensive subjects, had an increased renal blood flow and a decreased renal vascular resistance (32). Based on these results, we have suggested that the high output state and volume expansion that we observed in obese patients could maintain renal perfusion through lower total peripheral and renovascular resistance. This inappropriately lower total peripheral resistance in the obese hypertensive could counteract the opposing effect of vasoconstriction produced by hypertensive disease in the kidneys (32).

In summary, the hemodynamic characteristics of the obese hypertensive, studied in the whole obese hypertensive population without a specific differentiation between upper- and lower-body obesity, are the following: (a) increased absolute total blood volume and (b) a high redistribution to the cardiopulmonary area, thereby increasing the venous return. The increased intravascular volume and venous return increase cardiac output, stroke volume, and left ventricular work, with normal or inappropriately normal total peripheral resistance. These changes lead to ventricular dilatation and eccentric hypertrophy that, associated with the concentric hypertrophy produced by hypertension and the increased afterload, will induce a dimorphic structural change, expressed by concentric–eccentric left ventricular hypertrophy. Study of the peripheral circulation has shown an increased renal blood flow with a decreased renal vascular resistance.

Endocrinic–Adrenergic–Metabolic Changes in Obesity Hypertension

Insulin Resistance and Hyperinsulinemia

Previous studies have shown that obese subjects with upper-body obesity have hyperinsulinemia and insulin resistance that result from (a) a large accumulation of lipolytic hyperactive abdominal cells and (b) release of large amounts of free fatty acids into the portal vein. These changes caused (a) an excess hepatic synthesis of triglycerides, (b) inhibition of insulin intake, (c) hyperinsulinemia, and (d) insulin resistance (34,35).

The link between insulin alterations and the development of hypertension has been explained on the following basis: Insulin produces an increased absorption of sodium in the diluting segment of the distal nephron, with consequent water retention and increased cardiac output (36). The alteration of the sodium–potassium distribution causes increased vascular peripheral resistance. Insulin also increases adrenergic activity (36–39).

Thus, hyperinsulinemia and insulin resistance are considered to be the possible initial trigger of the endocrinic–adrenergic–metabolic changes described in obese patients with high blood pressure (34,36–39).

Sympathetic Nervous System

Previous investigations showing increased sympathetic activity (measured as norepinephrine turnover) during overfeeding (40,41) suggested that those changes produce an increased incidence of arrhythmias, angina pectoris, and hypertension in obese subjects (41). These changes were explained by some authors as being produced by an increased plasma insulin concentration, which may have a stimulatory effect on the sympathetic nervous system (42), or by an increased concentration of triiodothyronine, which increases the reactivity of the tissues to catecholamines (43,44). Clinical studies have shown that the increased triiodothyronine after overfeeding produced changes in thermogenesis induced by increased metabolism and caloric expenditure (40,44). This increase in caloric expenditure apparently reflects increased sympathetic activity (44). Based on these studies, it is believed today that chronic overfeeding may contribute to the presence of hypertension in obese subjects by adrenergic stimulation; however, most of the studies have not proved an increase in catecholamine levels or sympathetic activity in obese hypertensive subjects.

The Renin–Angiotensin–Aldosterone System

The importance of the renin–angiotensin–aldosterone system in obese hypertensive patients is controversial. Plasma renin activity has been shown to be unchanged (26) or reduced (45,46) in inverse proportion to weight. An inverse proportion has been explained on the basis of an increased total body sodium and water retention found in obese subjects (45).

The levels of aldosterone related to the low plasma renin activity levels are inappropriately increased in obese hypertensive patients (45). The aldosterone/plasma renin activity ratio was found to increase progressively with the increase in relative weight (45). More recent studies, however, have shown increased aldosterone levels in obese adolescents and adults (47), suggesting that hyperaldosteronism in obese subjects triggers the sodium and water retention that produces hypervolemia and increased cardiac output, previously described in the obese hypertensive subjects (45).

Sodium and Na^+-K^+-ATPase Activity

Previous investigations have suggested that increased sodium intake is one of the most important factors promoting hypertension in the obese subject (48). The hypertensive mechanisms produced by an excess of sodium are (a) an increased sensitivity to catecholamines, (b) an altered angiotensin II receptor sensitivity, (c) a passive waterlogging of the vessel wall, and (d) a reduced sodium–potassium exchange (49–51,57).

In obesity hypertension, the last mechanism is important, because researchers have shown a decreased Na^+-K^+-ATPase activity in the red blood cells of obese patients (52,53), which will produce an increase in intracellular concentration and a decrease in calcium efflux, with a concomitant increase in intracellular calcium concentration; these changes increase the smooth muscle tone and vascular resistance (54,55). All of these changes have been found in obese patients, particularly in those having upper-body obesity (56), who, according to previous studies, have a greater incidence of hypertension (19–23,52).

In summary, the importance of the endocrinic, adrenergic, and metabolic theory in obesity hypertension is controversial, but finding the link between some of these mechanisms should help in the understanding of obesity hypertension. These changes are probably initiated by (a) an increased insulin resistance, (b) hyperinsulinemia (which increases the adrenergic activity), and (c) reabsorption of sodium at renal tubular level. These changes are followed by: (a) an increased aldosterone level, which induces sodium and water retention, thereby producing hypervolemia; (b) an increased venous return and an increased cardiac output; and (c) an increased sodium intake with decreased Na^+-K^+-ATPase activity, which increases the intracellular sodium concentration. Only some of these mechanisms have been shown to be specifically altered in the upper-body obese subjects, who, as was previously emphasized, are more prone to the obesity–hypertension association.

THE EFFECT OF WEIGHT LOSS IN THE CONTROL OF BLOOD PRESSURE: CLINICAL EXPERIENCE—SHORT- AND LONG-TERM EFFECT

Although the positive role of weight control in the management of hypertension was once considered controversial (58), several publications during the last 10 years have shown the benefit of weight reduction in obese hypertensive patients (29,46,58–63). Some of these studies are summarized in Table 2.

To argue against the concept that weight loss has a causal role in reducing blood pressure, several associated factors were considered, including (a) a concomitant low sodium intake, (b) a reduced caloric intake when the patients are on a weight-reduction program, (c) the use of an inappropriate sphygmomanometer cuff, or (d) a familiarity with the procedure used to measure blood pressure (58).

Some recent experimental studies have shown that fasting animals demonstrated a suppressive adrenergic activity, suggesting a means for conservation of calories by diminishing metabolism and heat production (40,64–66); this finding was also confirmed by a clinical study (67), suggesting that a rapid decrease in arterial pressure, 48 hr after the initial hypocaloric consumption (low-carbohydrate diet), is responsible for a reduced plasma norepinephrine concentration level and is associated with an immediate decrease in blood pressure (68,69). All our clinical prospective studies, however, have shown a statistically significant reduction in blood pressure after an equilibration period in which the caloric intake was held normal for at least 10 days before the final blood determinations (29,62,63). Other investigators have shown a sustained late control of blood pressure by weight reduction when the patients have maintained their initial weight loss (or have slightly increased it) and were on an adequate diet or maybe a high-calorie diet (59,61). Earlier studies, as was previously discussed, have shown that the use of a cuff that is too narrow overestimates the blood pressure measurements, whereas a cuff that is too wide underestimates them (11–17). To avoid misinterpretations based on the accuracy of auscultatory measurements in obese subjects, however, some authors have also recorded the positive effect of weight reduction on blood pressure directly, by using intra-arterial pressure measurements (28,29).

Many of the studies that we discuss in this section have used control groups, some of them with a randomized design to evaluate the effect of weight reduction. Consequently, those studies ruled out the theory that familiarity with the procedure used to measure blood pressure could account for the positive effect of weight reduction on blood pressure (46,59–63).

In a study (62) in which salt intake was not restricted (intake of $\pm$165 mEq/24 hr), we showed that after a weight reduction of $\pm$10 kg the arterial pressure levels of 75% of the obese hypertensive patients treated only with this nonpharmacological approach returned to normal. In a long-term follow-up (8–12 months) with the patients on a regular diet and with the weight reduction maintained at similar levels, 52% of the patients maintained normal blood pressure ($\leq$140/90 mmHg) (63). A second group of 57 obese hypertensive patients were treated with hypocaloric diet and concomitant antihypertensive medications that previously had been inadequate to control blood pressure. Two months after the initiation of the diet, when the average weight reduction totaled $\pm$10 kg, the blood pressure of 61% of patients returned to normal levels (62). In the long-term follow-up, 8–12 months after the end of the dietary intervention, 86% of those who maintained their weight reduction had normal blood pressure (63). In the initial short-term follow-up, we included a group of 26 obese hypertensive patients, considered a control group, who did not receive dietetic advise. At the end of the follow-up period, they still had their initial overweight and high blood pressure (62).

Since those initial studies, other investigators have confirmed these results (46,59–61). One study used a low-calorie diet in obese hypertensive patients randomly divided into two groups according to their sodium intake, which was either 120 or 40 mEq/24 hr. The average weight reduction obtained (12 weeks after the initiation of the hypocaloric diet) was more than 20 kg. At the end of the follow-up, both groups of patients had statistically significant reductions in systolic and diastolic blood pressure regardless of their sodium consumption, and a positive correla-

TABLE 2. *Effects of weight loss on blood pressure: studies that mention sodium intake*

Study (reference number)	Total number of patients	Design	Duration in weeks	Weight reduction of treated patients (kg)	Conclusions
Dahl et al. (48)	12	Alternative caloric restriction with or without salt restriction	4 to 59	8 to 102	Fall of BP was closely correlated with decreased salt intake and not with decreased caloric intake
Reisin et al. (62)	107	Three study groups: weight reduction; weight reduction and antihypertensive treatment; and control	26	±7 to ±10	Weight reduction normalized BP in most of the patients
Tuck et al. (46)	25	Patients randomly assigned to 120-mEq/day or 40-mEq/day sodium intake; all in low caloric intake	12	±20	Positive correlation between reduction in body weight and BP
Reisin et al. (63)	66	Long-term study following weight reduction with patients on uncontrolled caloric intake; sodium intake 166 mEq/day	52 to 78	±7 to ±8	Weight loss induced a considerable fall in BP; pressure–weight reduction was maintained for at least 12–18 months
Gillum et al. (60)	87	Patients nonrandomly assigned to: baseline, weight reduction, sodium restriction, or baseline sodium restriction weight reduction; sodium intake 166 or 70 mEq/day	22	±6	Modest weight reduction is associated with a BP decrease independent of changes in sodium intake
Reisin et al. (29)	12	Intra-arterial pressure measured before and after weight reduction; sodium excretion ±167 to ±198 mEq/day	±26	±10	Reduction of mean BP is significantly correlated with the fall in body weigh[t]
Haynes et al. (73)	60	Patients randomized in weight reduction sodium intake ±167 to ±198 mEq/day	26	±4	Weight loss was not useful in lowering BP
Fagerberg et al. (72)	30	Patients randomized in hypocaloric diet; two different sodium intakes, 195 and 96 mEq/day; alcohol intake was ±133 to 232 g over a 14-week period	9 to 12	±8	Dietary-induced weight loss was associated with BP reduction only if there was a concomitant restriction of sodium intake
Dornfeld et al. (59)	256	Retrospective study; weight loss obtained with PSMF; BP was compared with that of patients on unrestricted caloric and sodium intake (±166 mEq/day)	28 to 90	±55 to ±64	Long-term changes in BP were correlated with changes in body weight
Langford et al. (61)	325	Patients treated with antihypertensive medications for at least 5 years were randomized with regard to the following instructions: continue taking medications, discontinue medications, discontinue medications with sodium restriction (±100 mEq/day), or discontinue medication and reduce weight (Na ± 150 mEq/day)	56	±4	Weight loss or sodium restriction more than doubles success in withdrawal of drug therapy

[a] BP, blood pressure; PSMF, low calorie protein supplemented fast diet.

tion was found between reduction in body weight and arterial pressure (46). The same group of investigators, with the same dietetic design as in the previous study, found, by calculating consecutive blood pressure measurements in two groups of obese hypertensives on hypocaloric diet, that after an initial blood pressure loss attributable to negative sodium and water balance, the further blood pressure reduction independent of sodium intake was produced by weight loss (±23 kg). They also showed that a long-term weight loss (6 months) was associated with a long-term blood pressure reduction in obese hypertensive subjects (59).

Using a careful design, another group of investigators (60) studied the different and independent effects of weight reduction and low salt (sodium) intake in obese hypertensives. In this study a randomized group of obese hypertensives were treated with caloric restriction and regular sodium intake for a period of 10 weeks and were also treated with sodium restriction and normal caloric intake for a similar period of time. The blood pressure reduction was statistically significant after weight reduction or after a sodium restriction, and the effect on blood pressure of the two dietetic approaches was additive.

In a study published by the Dietary Intervention Study in Hypertension (DISH) (61), a large number of obese patients (20% overweight) receiving antihypertensive therapy for at least 5 years were offered the following management: The therapy was withdrawn and was then replaced by either sodium restriction (101 patients) or weight reduction (87 patients). These two groups were compared with patients in whom the drug therapy was also withdrawn but without change in their diet (89 patients) or who continued on drug therapy (48 patients). The different groups studied included patients with a mean age of 56–59 years old; most of the patients were black (62–75%) and women (59–69%). The average weight loss of participants in the weight reduction program was 4.5 kg after a 1-year follow-up: 60% of them remained off medication and maintained normal blood pressure, whereas only 35% of the control subjects remained normotensives without medication. They also found that 46% of those patients who had reduced their sodium intake by 40 mEq remained off medication. The authors concluded that patients with mild hypertension whose blood pressure has been well controlled with medication for several years should be considered for withdrawal of their antihypertensive drug therapy if they are willing to enter a program of dietary changes, such as weight reduction or sodium restriction (61). Another group of investigators in Finland, however, showed that a weight reduction program with even modest success (±6 kg) reduced systolic (±11 mmHg) and diastolic (±7 mmHg) blood pressure in obese hypertensive patients, whereas salt restriction (±51 mEq) gives little benefit in the control of blood pressure (67).

In a more recent work, all the subjects (135 obese hypertensive patients) had significant weight loss accompanied by a decrease in blood pressure, and the correlation between changes in weight and blood pressure was significant. The investigators arrive at the conclusion, however, that the patients had shown a "floor effect"—that is, a degree of weight loss beyond which further reduction in blood pressure will not occur (70).

In another study involving a randomized control trial of 56 obese mild hypertensive patients, the effect of weight reduction (±7 kg) was compared with the effect of (a) drug intervention (metoprolol 200 mg daily) and (b) a placebo. The changes in the systolic blood pressure in patients who underwent weight reduction were greater than in those who were treated with metoprolol. The changes in diastolic blood pressure in patients who lost weight were also significantly greater than the changes obtained with either the metoprolol or placebo medication (71).

During the last decade, only two groups of investigators (72,73) contradicted the positive effect of weight loss on high blood pressure reduction. Those studies, however, were limited by (a) the small number of subjects studied, (b) the inclusion of only mild hypertensive patients, (c) diagnosis being made on only one clinic visit, and (d) inclusion of some patients who had a relatively high alcoholic consumption during the dietetic trial (72). Their conclusions were thus also limited to a small and specific group of patients studied, rather than being capable of refuting findings previously published by others, whose studies included patients of both sexes, two races (blacks and whites), and moderate-to-morbid obese subjects with mild to severe hypertension. Findings that are considered in a large review are not only statistically significant but also clinically significant (74).

In conclusion, it is believed today that weight loss reduces systolic and diastolic blood pressure, independently of changes in sodium intake, and that the blood pressure decrease can be maintained for long periods. Weight control could be not only an important tool in the treatment of blood pressure in the obese population but also an important approach in the prevention of hypertension. Data in the medical literature reject the concept that the decrease in arterial pressure with weight reduction results from the use of an inappropriate sphygmomanometer cuff, dietary sodium restriction, caloric restriction, or familiarity with the procedure used to determine blood pressure.

Existent data, however, have not included the effect of weight reduction in persons classified according to their fat distribution in upper- or lower-body obesity.

Changes in Fluid Volume Distribution and in Systemic Hemodynamics Produced by Weight Reduction

Previous studies have shown that after weight reduction, the intravascular fluid volume decreases significantly in normotensive and hypertensive patients (75,76). We have reported that in obese hypertensive patients a moderate weight reduction (±10 kg) resulted in a decrease in intravascular and cardiopulmonary blood volume (29). These differences, however, were abolished when the volumes were expressed with relation to body weight (29), a finding that, as we have explained earlier, might be related to the lack of definition of appropriate indices to express hemodynamic values for patients having different weights (26). Only one group of investigators studied the effect of weight reduction on the extracellular and intracellular fluid volume in a group of obese hypertensive patients. These studies showed a significant increase in the plasma volume/interstitial fluid volume ratio and in the intracellular fluid volume/total body water ratio, changes that they explained expressed a shift of fluid volume from the intracellular space to the interstitial space (28).

Studies on hemodynamic changes in obese normotensives and hypertensives following weight reduction have shown a reduced oxygen consumption, a reduced cardiac output, and a reduced left ventricular stroke work without changes in total peripheral resistance (29,75,76). We reported (a) only a moderate weight reduction in obese hypertensives on a controlled, regular-sodium-intake diet (±173 mEq/day), (b) a significant decrease in cardiac output directly related to a contracted blood volume, and (c) a decreased cardiopulmonary blood volume. The left ventricular stroke work was also reduced. These findings imply an improved cardiac function. The total peripheral resistance remained unchanged in our study group (29). All of these results have also been duplicated by later investigations that have also reported an improvement in arterial distensibility and compliance after weight reduction (77). Echocardiographic studies have shown that weight reduction decreased the interventricular, septal, and posterior wall thickness and the left ventricular mass, changes which suggest (according to the authors) that in the obese hypertensive patient, weight reduction should be considered not only for the control of blood pressure but also for the prevention of left ventricular hypertrophy (78).

In conclusion, the hemodynamic change produced by weight reduction in obese hypertensives is a decreased intravascular volume that induces both a reduced cardiac output and a reduced left ventricular stroke work, without changes in total peripheral resistance. These changes improve cardiac function (Table 1). Echocardiographic studies indicate a decrease in interventricular septal and posterior wall thickness and in the left ventricular mass.

Endocrinic–Adrenergic–Metabolic Changes Produced by Weight Reduction

Insulin Concentration Levels and Insulin Resistance

One previous study (79) examined the insulin secretion over a 3-year period in one obese, diabetic, normotensive woman during four consecutive phases: (i) when the patient was morbidly obese and diabetic, (ii) when she lost weight and was no longer diabetic, (iii) when she regained weight, and (iv) when she again became diabetic. In the baseline period, the patient had a resistance to insulin; this was manifested by high plasma levels, which reflect plasma insulin resistance. When the patient had reduced weight, fasting insulin levels were normal; moreover, the peak postprandial insulin levels were up to 10 times greater than fasting insulin concentrations. After an increase in weight, however, the patient again had high insulin levels and marked insulin resistance. This interesting and well-done metabolic study showed that weight loss clearly improved insulin resistance and improved the responsiveness of the beta cells as well.

The improvement of the diabetic status after weight loss was, according to some investigations, attributed to the fact that weight reduction permits the target cells to increase the number of their binding receptors, resulting in less insulin resistance and improved glucose utilization (80,81).

In studies on obese hypertension, caloric restriction reduces plasma insulin levels within a day, due to an increase in the number of insulin receptors and an increased affinity of the receptors for the insulin (82). Nevertheless, studies showing the effect of reduced insulin concentration on obese hypertensive patients remain to be done.

Sympathetic Nervous System

Earlier studies in rats have defined the role of the sympathetic system in the metabolic adaptation of fasting (64–66). After 48 hr of fasting in those animals, the norepinephrine turnover in the heart and other organs was found to be decreased by 40% (83).

In clinical studies, obese normotensive women on hypocaloric diet (low carbohydrate content) with a constant sodium intake had a significant fall in plasma norepinephrine levels with a concomitant decrease in blood pressure (68). More recent studies on obese hypertensive patients on various salt intakes have shown that weight loss reduces norepinephrine levels with a concomitant reduction in blood pressure, and the authors explained the fall in blood pressure on the basis of the diminished sympathetic nervous system activity, which probably will conserve calories by diminishing metabolism and heat production (84).

The Renin–Angiotensin–Aldosterone System

One group of investigators found, in a group of obese hypertensive patients, that weight reduction decreased the levels of plasma renin activity by 50%, with an also statistically significant decrease in plasma aldosterone levels; these changes were explained on the basis of a decrease in sympathetic activity (46). These results were confirmed by other studies (85–87). In our laboratory, however, we have shown that the initial low levels of plasma renin activity were only slightly, but not statistically significantly, decreased in a group of obese hypertensive patients who had lost an average of 10 kg of their body weight (29). Others showed that plasma renin activity and aldosterone secretion rate rose significantly after 10 days of starvation (88).

Sodium and Na^+-K^+-ATPase Activity

As has been previously shown, a moderate sodium intake reduces blood pressure of essential hypertensive patients (89). In earlier investigations, the changes in blood pressure of obese hypertensive patients, obtained after weight reduction, was attributed to a simultaneous decrease in sodium intake (48). As was previously explained, however, enough mechanistic and epidemiological data support the positive effect of weight reduction and blood pressure, independent of the also-positive effect of salt (sodium) restriction (90). During the initial first days of fasting, patients had a natriuretic phase, and, if fasting was prolonged, this phase was followed by a sodium conservation step. Also during this second phase, however, a continuous decrease in blood pressure is noticed and attributed to weight reduction (85).

A more recent study determined a change in the blood pressure sensitivity to sodium after weight loss in a group of adolescent normotensives. Blood pressure, plasma volume, and cardiac output were measured after 2 weeks on a high-sodium diet (250 mEq Na per day) and after 2 weeks on a low-sodium diet (<30 mEq Na per day), before and after a weight loss program. The authors found that weight loss altered blood pressure sensitivity to sodium through a concomitant reduction in plasma volume and cardiac output. These findings are useful in clarifying the combined effect of sodium restriction and weight reduction (91) but fail to rule out, to my understanding, the independent action of these two dietetic components in the control of blood pressure in obese hypertensive patients.

The effects of dieting on the Na^+-K^+-ATPase activity were reported by two previous studies (92,93). One group of investigators studied young, normotensive, obese subjects and found that after a 6-month hypocaloric diet with normal sodium intake, the sodium concentration of the erythrocytes significantly increased and the mean arterial pressure decreased (93). Others, however, studied obese hypertensive patients on a hypocaloric, low-sodium diet and found an increase in Na^+-K^+-ATPase uptake, with a considerable decrease in the intracellular sodium concentration (92).

In conclusion, after weight reduction, insulin levels are reduced, and an apparent increase in the number of binding receptors in the target cells results in less insulin resistance and improved glucose utilization. Weight reduction also diminishes the sympathetic nervous system activity; however, the effect of weight loss on the renin–angiotensin–aldosterone system is controversial. Changes in sodium intake decrease blood pressure, but apparently by different mechanisms than those attributed to the decrease in weight. More data are necessary in order to evaluate the changes in Na^+-K^+-ATPase and intracellular sodium concentration in obese hypertensive patients after weight reduction. Most of the studies that have studied the effect of weight reduction in the obese hypertensive population did not, however, specify the effects on those patients with upper- or lower-body obesity.

SODIUM RESTRICTION VERSUS WEIGHT REDUCTION

Previous epidemiological studies have shown that populations in primitive or industrialized societies with high sodium intake have a higher prevalence of hypertension than do those populations that have a low salt consumption (94–96). In controlled studies of normotensive subjects, sodium intake of up to 1500 mEq/day usually resulted in only small increases in blood pressure (97).

The use of rigid sodium restriction in an earlier study has proved the efficacy of salt reduction in hypertensive patients (98), findings that were later confirmed by other investigators (89,99–101,116).

Dahl et al. (48) found that during the concurrent effect of weight reduction and salt restriction, the decrease of blood pressure occurred during the first few weeks of caloric restriction before a significant weight loss had occurred. In a study by Paris et al. (99), a moderate reduction in salt intake decreased systolic and diastolic blood pressure, but not all the studies have been successful in demonstrating a statistically significant reduction in blood pressure with low-salt diet (69,102). This controversy can be explained on the basis of the existence of two different types of individuals—those with salt sensitivity and those with salt resistance (103). Salt sensitivity includes individuals with a dependency that apparently is associated with a reduced renal sodium excretory ability and/or a genetic predisposition for salt sensitivity (104).

Two other factors complicating the understanding of the effect of sodium restriction on hypertension are (a) the role of chloride reduction concomitant with sodium restriction and (b) the "protective" role of high potassium intake against the hypertensive effect of the sodium ion (100, 105–109).

Regarding the role of chloride versus sodium, some experimental studies have shown that sodium chloride raised the blood pressure but that sodium bicarbonate or bicarbonate-ascorbate did not increase blood pressure (107,109). A recent study (106) of a small group of patients with "salt-sensitive" hypertension found that oral administration of sodium chloride for 1 week significantly increased the systolic and diastolic blood pressure. An equimolar amount of sodium given as sodium citrate induced no change in blood pressure. The researchers concluded that these findings might be caused by the ability of the anionic component of the salt to increase plasma volume.

In a series of early and excellent experimental works, Meneely et al. (108) found that high-potassium feeding had a protective effect in the survival of rats loaded with high sodium intake, a finding that was associated with a decreased blood pressure. More recent studies showed that blood pressure levels were universally correlated with the intake and urinary excretion of potassium in black subjects studied in Evans County (105). However, other control studies that have studied the effect of additional potassium in the diet on blood pressure had contradictory results (100).

The concurrent effect of sodium restriction and weight control has been demonstrated by large clinical trials. Stamler et al. (110) reported that 30% of 189 patients treated with a caloric- and sodium-restricted diet had, after 4 years of dieting, lost at least 4–5 kg in weight and that 36% of the subjects had reduced their sodium intake. Following those changes in dietetic habits, 39% of the patients remained normotensive, as compared with only 5% who were normotensive in the control group without a nutritional or antihypertensive medication program. These results are consistent with those obtained by another group (111), in which a hypocaloric diet (1230 kcal/24 hr) and low sodium intake (95 mEq/24 hr) resulted in a decrease in systolic/diastolic blood pressure of 17/10 mmHg following an average weight reduction of 8 kg. Not all the investigators agree with this finding, and a study previously discussed in this chapter showed that the addition of salt reduction to weight control gave little benefit in the control of blood pressure (67).

In summary, the low-sodium, high-potassium diet is effective in reducing arterial pressure; however, this effect is apparently independent of the positive response produced by weight reduction, namely, the reduction in blood pressure that was previously explained on the basis of different and well-proved hemodynamic and endocrinic–adrenergic–metabolic changes induced by weight reduction. Not enough data are yet available to support the hypothesis that the chloride ion, rather than the sodium ion, is responsible for inducing hypertension in humans. There is enough laboratory evidence, however, to sustain the theory that salt-sensitive persons are probably better responders, or the only responders, to a decreased sodium intake diet; furthermore, the inclusion of salt restriction to the weight control approach offers an additive effect to the control of blood pressure in obese hypertensive patients.

FEASIBILITY OF WEIGHT-REDUCTION AND/OR SALT-REDUCTION PROGRAMS

Dietary compliance poses a significant problem, and some studies suggest that dropout rates in weight-loss programs range from 50% to 70% within 1–2 years (112). One study, however, reviewed the data from 36 publications on the long-term effect of behavior modification programs for weight control and from 12 studies that examined compliance with a sodium-restricted diet. In the weight-control studies, the mean post-treatment weight loss was 14 kg, with an average dropout rate of 15% (113). In studies of sodium restriction, the average decrease in post-treatment sodium intake (measured by urinary sodium excretion) from baseline values was 84 mEq/24 hr, with an average dropout rate of 8%. Many factors have been discussed as being responsible for affecting compliance; these include (a) interference from other prescribed antihypertensive regimen (diuretics), (b) diet–diet interactions (low sodium, low calorie, high potassium, etc.), (c) lifestyle, (d) skill, (e) perception of the disease, and (f) social support (112). Consequently, several recommendations have been given to improve dietary compliance: (a) Use an easy design, such as introducing a stepwise approach, with the easy component of the diet being introduced first. (b) Offer good information on the dietetic regimen and on how the regimen can be carried out. (c) Use a fear of the consequences of disease as a good motivator. (d) Tailor the regimen to the lifestyle of the individual patient. (e) Use goal-setting (short in term and easily obtained). (f) Encourage self-monitoring of blood pressure weight. (g) Use stimulus control (remove salt shaker, remove high-calorie food, etc.). (h) Encourage social support (inform wife or husband as to the importance of compliance to the regimen. (i) Apply the team approach (physician, dietitian, nurse, etc.) (114).

In conclusion, the nutritional approach in the treatment of hypertension should be advocated either alone or in combination with antihypertensive medications. Long-term compliance can be achieved and has been shown to be effective in large groups of hypertensive patients. To improve the compliance to the diastolic regimens, patients should be involved in a behavior-change program that should have at least a 6-month follow-up period.

ACKNOWLEDGMENT

To my wife, Ilana, and my children, Eyal and Thalia Alexis, for their love and support.

REFERENCES

1. Maimonides, M. *Mishneh Torah,* 1180;Chapter IV, No. 15.
2. Aullen JP, Hucher M. Hypertension artérielle-obésité: une étude épidémiologique sur 7002 sujets dans un département français. *Ann Cardiol Angeiol (Paris)* 1979;29:463–470.
3. Court JM, Hill GJ, Dunlop M, Boulton TJ. Hypertension in childhood obesity. *Aust Paediatr J* 1974;10:296–300.
4. Epstein FH. Prevalence of chronic disease and distribution of selected physiological variables in a total community of Tecumseh, Michigan. *Am J Epidemiol* 1965;81:307–322.
5. Kannel WB, Brand N, Skinner JJ, MacNamera P. The relation of adiposity to blood pressure and development of hypertension: the Framingham Study. *Ann Intern Med* 1976;67:48–49.
6. Stamler R, Stamler J, Riedlinger WF, Algera R, Roberts RH. Weight and blood pressure findings in hypertension screening of 1 million Americans. *JAMA* 1978;240:1607–1610.
7. Tyroler HA, Heyden S, Haines CG. Weight and hypertension: Evans County Study of Blacks and Whites. In: O'Glesby, P., ed. *Epidemiology and control of hypertension.* New York: Stratton Intercontinental, 1973:177–202.
8. Hsu PH, Mathewson FAL, Rabkin SW. Blood pressure and body mass index patterns: a longitudinal study. *J Chronic Dis* 1977;30:93–113.
9. Levi RL, White PD, Stroud WD. Overweight: a prognostic significancy in relation to hypertension and cardiovascular renal diseases. *JAMA* 1946;131:951–953.
10. Rabkin SW, Mathewson FAL, Hsu PH. Relation of body weight to development of ischemic heart disease in a cohort of young North American man after a 26-year observation period. The Manitoba Study. *Am J Cardiol* 1977;39:452–458.
11. Holland WW, Humerfelt S. Measurement of blood pressure: comparisons of intraarterial and cuff values. *Br Med J* 1964;2:1241–1249.
12. Karvonen MJ, Telivino LJ, Jarvin EKJ. Sphygmomanometer cuff size and the accuracy of indirect measurement of blood pressure. *Am J Cardiol* 1964;13:688–692.
13. King GE. Errors in clinical measurement of blood pressure in obesity. *Clin Sci* 1967;32:223–237.
14. Kvols LK, Rohlfing BM, Alexander JK. A comparison of intra-arterial and cuff blood pressure measurements in very obese subjects. *Cardiovasc Res Cent Bull* 1969;7:118–123.
15. Simpson JA, Jamieson G, Dickhaus DW, Grover RF. Effect of size of calf-bladder on accuracy of measurement of indirect blood pressure. *Am Heart J* 1965;70:208–215.
16. Trout KW, Bertrand CA, William MH. Measurement of blood pressure in obese persons. *JAMA* 1956;162:970–971.
17. Forsberg SA, Guzman MD, Berlund S. Validity of blood pressure measurement with cuff in the arm and forearm. *Acta Med Scand* 1970;188:389–396.
18. Kirkendall WM, Feinleib M, Freis ED, Mark AL. Recommendations for human blood pressure determination by sphygmomanometers. *Circulation* 1980;62:1146A–1155A.
19. Albrink MJ, Meigs JW. The relationship between serum triglycerides and skinfold thickness in obese subjects. *Ann NY Acad Sci* 1965;131:673–683.
20. Edwards DAW. Observations on the distribution of subcutaneous fat. *Clin Sci* 1950;9:259–270.
21. Garm SM. Relative fat patterning. An individual characteristic. *Hum Biol* 1967;26:75–89.
22. Seidell JC, Bokx JC, Deboer R, Deurerberg P, Heutwast JGAJ. Fat distribution of overweight persons in relation to morbidity and subjective health. *Int J Obesity* 1985;9:363–374.
23. Vogue J. The degree of masculine differentiation of obesities: a factor determining predisposition to diabetes, atherosclerosis, gout and uric calculus disease. *Am J Clin Nutr* 1956;4:20–34.

24. Robinson SC, Brucer M. Hypertension body build and obesity. *Am J Med Sci* 1940;199:819–829.
25. Backman L, Freyschuss V, Hallberg D, Melcher A. Cardiovascular function in extreme obesity. *Acta Med Scand* 1973;193:437–446.
26. Messerli FH, Christie B, DeCarvalho JGR, Aristimuno GS, Suarez DH, Dreslinski GR, Frohlich ED. Obesity and essential hypertension. Hemodynamics, intravascular volume and plasma renin activity. *Arch Intern Med* 1981;141:81–85.
27. Mujais SK, Tarazi RC, Dustan HP, Fouad FM, Bravo EL. Hypertension in obese patients, hemodynamic and volume studies. *Hypertension* 1982;4:84–92.
28. Raison J, Achimastos A, London G, Safar M. Intravascular volume, extracellular fluid volume and total body water in obese and nonobese hypertensive patients. *Am J Cardiol* 1983;51:165–170.
29. Reisin E, Frohlich ED, Messerli FH, Dreslinski GR, Dunn FG, Jones MM, Batson HM Jr. Cardiovascular change after weight reduction in obesity hypertension. *Ann Intern Med* 1983;98:315–319.
30. Messerli FH, Sundgaard-Riise K, Reisin E, Dreslinski GR, Dunn FG, Frohlich ED. Disparate cardiovascular effects of obesity and essential hypertension. *Am J Med* 1983;74:808–812.
31. Messerli FH, Sundgaard-Riise K, Reisin E, Dreslinski GR, Ventura HO, Oigman W, Frohlich ED. Dimorphic cardiac adaptation to obesity and arterial hypertension. *Ann Intern Med* 1983;99:757–761.
32. Reisin E, Messerli FH, Ventura HO, Frohlich ED. Renal hemodynamic studies in obesity-hypertension. *J Hypertens* 1987;5:397–400.
33. Alexander JK. Obesity and the circulation. *Mod Cardiovasc Dis* 1963;32:799–803.
34. Jarret RJ, Keen H, McCartney J, Fuller JH, Hamilton PJS, Reid DD, Rose G. Glucose tolerance and blood pressure in two populations sample their relation to diabetes mellitus and hypertension. *J Epidemiol* 1978;7:15–34.
35. KrotKiewski M, Bjorntorp P, Sjostrom L, Smith V. Impact of obesity on metabolism in men and women. Importance of regional adipose tissue distribution. *J Clin Invest* 1983;72:1150–1162.
36. DeFronzo RA, Cooke CR, Andres R, Faloona GR. The effect of insulin an renal handling of sodium, potassium, calcium and phosphate in man. *J Clin Invest* 1975;55:845–855.
37. Christensen NJ. Acute effects of insulin on cardiovascular function and noradrenaline uptake and release. *Diabetologia* 1983;25:377–381.
38. Voors AW, Webber LS, Frenchs RR, Berenson GS. Body height and body mass as determinants of basal blood pressure in children. The Bogalusa Heart Study. *Am J Epidemiol* 1981;106:101–108.
39. Winquist RJ, Webb RC, Bohr DF. Vascular smooth muscle in hypertension. *Fed Proc Am Soc Exp Biol* 1982;41:2386–2393.
40. Landsberg L, Young JB. Fasting, feeding and regulation of the sympathetic nervous system. *N Engl J Med* 1978;298:1295–1301.
41. Young JB, Landsberg L. Diet induced changes in sympathetic nervous system activity, possible implication for obesity and hypertension. *J Chronic Dis* 1982;35:879–886.
42. Evans DJ, Hoffman RG, KelKhoff R, Kissebah AH. Relationship of adrenergic activity to body fat topography, fat cell morphology and metabolic alterations in premenopausal women. *J Clin Endocrinol Metab* 1983;57:304–310.
43. Danforth JE, Horton ES, O'Connell M, Sims EAH, Banger AG, Ingbar SH, Braverman L, Vigenakis AG. Dietary induced alterations in thyroid hormone metabolism during over nutrition. *J Clin Invest* 1979;64:1346–1347.
44. Sims EAH. Mechanisms of hypertension in the overweight. *Hypertens* 1982;4:III43–III49.
45. Hiramatzu K, Yamada T, Ichekawa K, Izumiyama T, Nagata H. Changes in endocrine activity relative to obesity in patients with essential hypertension. *J A Geriatr Soc* 1981;29:25–30.
46. Tuck MJ, Sowers J, Dornfeld L, Kledzik G, Maxwell MH. The effect of weight reduction on blood pressure, plasma renin activity and plasma aldosterone levels in obese patients. *N Engl J Med* 1982;304:12–13.
47. Rochini AP, Katch VL, Grakin R, Moorehead C, Anderson J. Role for aldosterone in blood pressure regulation of obese adolescents. *Am J Cardiol* 1986;57:613–617.
48. Dahl KK, Silver L, Christie RW. Role of salt in the fall of blood pressure accompanying reduction of obesity. *N Engl J Med* 1958;258:1186–1192.
49. Cole FE, Frohlich ED, MacPhee AA. Angiotensin binding affinity and capacity in the midbrain area of spontaneously hypertensive and normotensive rats. *Brain Res* 1978;154:178–181.
50. Dechamplain J. The sympathetic system in hypertension. *J Clin Endocrinol Metab* 1977;6:633–655.
51. Tobian L. Salt and hypertension. *Ann NY Acad Sci* 1978;304:178–202.
52. DeLuise M, Blackburn GG, Ther JJ. Reduced activity in the red cell sodium potassium pump in human obesity. *N Engl J Med* 1980;303:1017–1022.
53. Klimes I, Nagulesparan M, Unger RH, Aronoph SL, Matt DM. Decreased Na^+-K^+-ATPase activity in erythrocyte membranes and intact erythrocytes from obese men. *J Clin Endocrinol* 1982;54:721–724.
54. Avenell A, Leeds AR. Sodium intake, inhibition of Na^+-K^+-ATPase and obesity (letter). *Lancet* 1981;1:836.
55. Blaunstein MP. Sodium ions, calcium ions, blood pressure regulation and hypertension. A reassessment and a hypothesis. *Am J Physiol* 1977;232:C165–C173.
56. Baungart AV, Zidek W, Losse H. Obesity, hypertension and intracellular electrolytes. *Klin Wochenschr* 1983;6:803–805.
57. Garsy RP, Meyer P. A new test showing abnormal net Na^+ and K^+ ATPase in erythrocytes of essential hypertensive patients. *Lancet* 1979;7:349–353.
58. Chiang BN, Perlman LV, Epstein FM. Overweight and hypertension: a review. *Circulation* 1969;39:403–410.
59. Dornfeld LP, Maxwell MH, Waks AV, Schnoth P, Tuck ML. Obesity and hypertension. Long term effect of weight reduction on arterial pressure. *Int J Obesity* 1985;9:381–389.
60. Gillum RF, Prineas RJ, Jeffery RW, Jacobs DR, Elmer PJ, Gomez O, Blackburn H. Nonpharmacological therapy of hypertension: the independent effect of weight reduction and sodium restriction in overweight borderline hypertensive patients. *Am Heart J* 1983;105:128–133.
61. Langford GH, Blaufox MD, Oberman A, Hawkins M, Curb JD, Cutter GR, Wassorteil-Smoller S, Pressel MS, Babcock C, Abenerthy MB, Tyler M. Dietary therapy slows the return of hypertension after stopping prolonged medication. *JAMA* 1985;253:657–669.
62. Reisin E, Abel R, Modan M, Silverberg DS, Eliahou HE, Modan B. Effects of weight loss without salt restriction on the reduction of blood pressure. *N Engl J Med* 1978;298:1–5.
63. Reisin E, Frohlich ED. Effects of weight reduction on arterial pressure. *J Chronic Dis* 1982;35:887–891.
64. Young JB, Landsberg L. Suppression of sympathetic nervous system during fasting. *Science* 1977;196:1473–1475.
65. Young JB, Landsberg L. Catecholamine and intermediary metabolism. *J Clin Endocrinol Metab* 1977;6:559–631.
66. Young JB, Landsberg L. Catecholamines and the regulation of hormone secretion. *J Clin Endocrinol Metab* 1977;6:657–695.
67. Rissanen A, Pietinen P, Siljamaki-Ojonsuu V, Piirainen H, Reissel P. Treatment of hypertension in obese patients: efficacy and feasibility of weight and salt reduction programs. *Acta Med Scand* 1985;218:149–156.
68. Jung RL, Shetty PS, Barroud M, Callingham BA, James WPT. Role of catecholamines in hypotensive response to dieting. *Br Med* 1979;1:12–13.
69. Kirkendall WH, Connor WE, Abboud F, Rastogi SP, Anderson TA, Fry M. The effect of sodium chloride on blood pressure, body fluids, electrolytes, renal function and serum lipids of normotensive man. *J Lab Clin Med* 1976;87:418–434.
70. Cohen W, Flamenbaum W. Obesity and hypertension: demonstration of a "floor effect." *Am J Med* 1985;80:177–181.
71. MacMahon SW, Bernstein L, MacDonald GS, Andrews G, Blocket RB. Comparison of weight reduction with metoprolol in treatment of hypertension in young overweight patients. *Lancet* 1985;I:1233–1250.
72. Fagerberg B, Anderson OK, Isaksson B, Bjorntorp P. Blood pressure control during weight reduction in obese hypertensive

men: Separate effects of sodium and energy restriction. *Br Med J* 1984;228:11–14.
73. Haynes AB, Harper AC, Costley SR. Failure of weight reduction to reduce mildly elevated blood pressure: a randomized trial. *J Hypertens* 1984;2:535–539.
74. Hovell MF. The experimental evidence for weight loss treatment of essential hypertension: a critical review. *Am J Public Health* 1982;72:359–368.
75. Alexander JK, Peterson KL. Cardiovascular effect of weight reduction. *Circulation* 1972;45:310–318.
76. Backman L, Freyschuss V, Hallberg D, Melcher A. Reversibility of cardiovascular changes in extreme obesity. *Acta Med Scand* 1979;205:367–373.
77. Toto-Moukouo JJ, Achimastos A, Asmar RG, Huges CJ, Safar M. Pulse wave velocity in patients with obesity and hypertension. *Am Heart J* 1986;21:136–140.
78. MacMahon SW, Wilcken DEL, MacDonald GJ. The effect of weight reduction on left ventricular mass. A randomized controlled trial in young overweight hypertensive patients. *N Engl J Med* 1986;314:334–339.
79. Genuth SM. Insulin secretion in obesity and diabetes. An illustrative case. *Ann Intern Med* 1977;87:714–716.
80. Olefsky JM, Kolterman OG. Mechanism of insulin resistance in obesity and non-insulin-dependent (Type II) diabetes. *Am J Med* 1981;70:151–168.
81. Roth J. Insulin binding to its receptor: Is the receptor more important than the hormone? *Diabetes Care* 1981;4:27–32.
82. Grey N, Kipinis DM. Effect of diet composition on the hyperinsulinemia of obesity. *N Engl J Med* 1971;385:827–831.
83. Young JB, Landsberg L. Stimulation of the sympathetic nervous system during sucrose feeding. *Nature* 1977;269:615–617.
84. Shetty PS, Jung RT, James WPT. Effect of catecholamine replacement with levodopa on the metabolic response to semistarvation. *Lancet* 1979;1:77–79.
85. Boulter PR, Spark RF, Arky RA. Dissociation of the renin aldosterone system and refractoriness to the sodium retaining action of mineralocorticoid during starvation in man. *J Clin Exp Metab* 1973;38:248–254.
86. Marks P, Wilson B, Delassale A. Aldosterone studies in obese patients with hypertension. *Am J Med Sci* 1985;289:224–228.
87. Sowers JA, Nyby M, Nafteli BE, Stern N, Beck F, Baron S, Catania R, Vlachis N. Blood pressure and hormone changes associated with weight reduction in the obese. *Hypertension* 1983;4:686–691.
88. Garnett ES, Cohen H, Nehmias C, Viol G. The roles of carbohydrate, renin and aldosterone in sodium retention during and after total starvation. *Metabolism* 1973;22:867–874.
89. MacGregor GA, Best FE, Conn JM, Markandu D, Elder M, Sagnella GA, Squires M. Double blind randomized crossover trial of moderate sodium restriction in essential hypertension. *Lancet* 1982;I:351–354.
90. Reisin E, Frohlich ED. Hemodynamics in obesity. In: Zanchetti A, Tarazi RC, eds. *Handbook of hypertension,* vol 7. New York: Elsevier; 1987;280–297.
91. Rochini A, Chico R, Kotach V, Bondie D. Weight loss alters pressure sensitivity to sodium. *Circulation* 1987;76:IV-8.
92. Sowers JR, Whitfield LA, Beck IWJ, Catania RA, Tuck MI, Dornfeld L, Maxwell M. Role of enhanced syurpathetic nervous system activity and reduced Na–K dependent adenosine triphosphatase activity in maintenance of elevated blood pressure in obesity: effect of weight loss. *Clin Sci* 1982;63:1215–1245.
93. Weder AB, Toneti BA, Skatch VL, Rochini AP. The antihypertensive effect of caloric restriction in obese adolescents: association of effect on erythrocyte countertransport and cotransport. *J Hypertens* 1984;2:507–514.
94. Lowenstein JW. Blood pressure in relation to age and sex in the tropics and subtropics. A review of the literature and an investigation in the tribes of Brasil Indians. *Lancet* 1961;1:389–392.
95. Page LB, Damon A, Moellering RC Jr. Antecedents of cardiovascular disease in six Solomon Island societies. *Circulation* 1974;49:1132–1140.
96. Sasaki N. High blood pressure and the salt intake of the Japanese. *Jpn Heart J* 1962;3:313–324.
97. Luft FC, Rankin LI, Bloch R, Weyman AE, Willis LR, Murray RM, Grim CE, Weinberger MH. Cardiovascular and humoral responses to extremes of sodium intake in normal black and white men. *Circulation* 1979;60:697–706.
98. Kempner W. Treatment of hypertensive vascular disease with rice diet. *Am J Med* 1948;4:545–549.
99. Paris J, Joossens JV, Vander Linder L, Verstreken G, Amery AK. Moderate sodium restriction and diuretics in the treatment of hypertension. *Am Heart J* 1973;85:22–25.
100. Richards AM, Nicholls MG, Espiner EA. Blood pressure response to moderate sodium restriction and to potassium supplementation in mild essential hypertension. *Lancet* 1984;1:757–761.
101. Watt GCM, Edwards C, Hart JT, Hart M, Welton P, Foy CJW. Dietary sodium restriction for mild hypertension in general practice. *Br Med J* 1983;286:432–436.
102. Corcoran AC, Taylor RP, Page I. Controlled observation on the effect of low sodium diet therapy in essential hypertension. *Circulation* 1951;3:1–10.
103. Kawasaki T, Delea CS, Bartter FC, Smith H. The effect of high sodium and low sodium intake on blood pressure and other related variables in human subjects with idiopathic hypertension. *Am J Med* 1978;64:193–198.
104. Dustan HP. Role of nutrition in hypertension and its control. *Experimental Aspects Prog Biochem Pharmacol* 1983;19:177–191.
105. Grim CE, Luft FC, Miller JZ, Meneely GR, Battarbee HD, Hames CG, Dahl LK. Racial differences in blood pressure in Evans County, Georgia. Relationship to sodium and potassium intake and plasma renin activity. *J Chronic Dis* 1980;33:87–94.
106. Kurtz TW, Al-Bander HA, Morris RC Jr. "Salt-sensitive" essential hypertension in men. Is the sodium ion alone important? *N Engl J Med* 1987;317:1043–1048.
107. Kurtz TW, Morris RCJ. Dietary chloride as a determinant of "sodium-dependent" hypertension. *Science* 1983;222:1139–1141.
108. Meneely GR, Battarbee HD. High-sodium low-potassium environment and hypertension. *Am J Cardiol* 1976;38:768–785.
109. Whitescarver SA, Ott CE, Jackson BA, Guthrie GR Jr, Kotchen TA. Salt sensitive hypertension. Contribution of chloride. *Science* 1984;223:1430–1432.
110. Stamler R, Stamler J, Grimm R, Gosch FC, Elmer P, Dyer A, Fishman J, VanHeel N, Civinelli J, McDonald A. Nutritional therapy for high blood pressure. Final report of a four-year randomized controlled trial. The hypertension control program. *JAMA* 1987;257:1484–1491.
111. Heyden S, Tyroler A, Hames CG, Bartel A, Thompson JW, Krishan J, Rosenthal T. Diet treatment of obese hypertensives. *Clin Sci Mol Med* 1973;45:2094–2125.
112. Dunbar J. Practical aspects of dietary management of hypertension: Compliance. *Can J Physiol Pharmacol* 1986;64:831–835.
113. Schlundt DG, Langford HG, McDonel EC. Compliance in dietary management of hypertension. *Compr Ther* 1985;11:59–66.
114. Schlundt DG. Compliance with dietary changes. *Bibl Cardiol* 1987;41:22–28.
115. Reisin E. Weight reduction in the management of hypertension: epidemiologic and mechanistic evidence. *Can J Physiol Pharmacol* 1987;64:818–824.
116. Beard TC, Cooke HM, Gray WR, Barge R. Randomized controlled trial of no-added-sodium diet for mild hypertension. *Lancet* 1982;II:455–458.

Hypertension: Pathophysiology, Diagnosis, and Management, edited by J. H. Laragh and B. M. Brenner. Raven Press, Ltd., New York © 1990.

CHAPTER 129

The Role of Dietary Calcium and Magnesium in the Therapy of Hypertension

Lawrence M. Resnick

Calcium, 2037
- Rationale for Calcium Therapy: Calcium Metabolism in Hypertension, 2039
- Calcium and the Renin–Aldosterone System, 2040
- Uniform Versus Heterogeneous Defects in Calcium Metabolism: A Cellular Hypothesis, 2042
- Interaction of Calcium and Sodium Metabolism, 2044
- Oral Calcium Supplementation in Hypertension: The Clinical Experience—Who Responds?, 2046
- Why Does Calcium Supplementation Lower Blood Pressure? 2049
- Summary and Overall Hypothesis, 2051

Magnesium, 2052
- Rationale for Magnesium Therapy: Magnesium Metabolism in Hypertension, 2052
- Cellular Effects, 2052
- Altered Magnesium Metabolism and Blood Pressure, 2053
- Therapy with Magnesium: Experience and Future Directions, 2055

References, 2056

CALCIUM

The ability of oral calcium supplementation to lower blood pressure in patients with essential hypertension was first reported in 1924 by W. L. T. Addison (1,2) (Fig. 1). This intriguing observation was largely ignored for over 50 years; however, in 1979, similar observations in experimental hypertensive rat models once again raised the issue of whether dietary calcium could be used as a primary form of antihypertensive therapy (3). Since that time, numerous epidemiologic studies have confirmed an inverse relationship between dietary calcium intake and blood pressure, a lower intake of calcium being associated with a higher blood pressure (4–7). At the same time, many research groups have now reported that oral calcium supplementation can lower blood pressure in at least some human hypertensive and normotensive populations. Yet, these now widespread findings have not been uniformly confirmed, and much resistance has yet to be overcome in accepting the notion that clinical aspects of calcium metabolism (such as the dietary intake, absorption, tissue distribution, and excretion of calcium) are indeed relevant to the pathophysiology and therapy of hypertension.

Some of the controversy appears unnecessary, and some criticism emphasizes a preferential role for other mineral ions (e.g., sodium, potassium, and/or magnesium, etc.) in the hypertensive process. However, the wide variety of interactions among all such "candidate" mineral elements makes such issues appear somewhat artificial. Nevertheless, the accumulated evidence abounds with apparently paradoxical, mutually exclusive observations, suggesting that calcium excess (or, alternatively, calcium deficiency) underlies the pathophysiology of hypertension (Table 1). For instance, much circumstantial evidence suggests that high blood pressure is a disease of calcium excess. Measuring intracellular cytosolic free calcium levels in platelets of normotensive and hypertensive subjects reveals a striking direct relationship between calcium and pressure (8). The higher the level of cytosolic free calcium, the higher the level of blood pressure. Similarly, in large normotensive populations, serum total calcium and blood pressure demonstrate a similar linear, positive association: The higher the serum calcium level, the higher the blood pressure (9). Furthermore, as has long been known, short-term elevations of serum calcium may acutely elevate blood pressure, whereas acute suppression of serum calcium is associated with an acute fall in pressure (10,11). Moreover, certain diseases that result in chronic hypercalcemia, such as primary hyperparathyroidism, are associated with a much higher incidence of hypertension than would otherwise be expected (12). These data suggest that higher blood pressures are associated with higher calcium levels and that

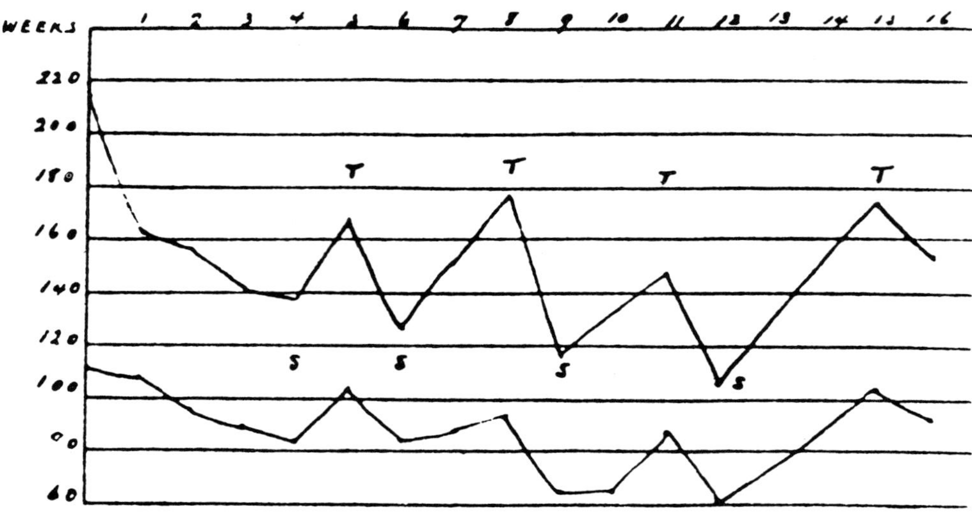

FIG. 1. Original description, by W. L. T. Addison, of the antihypertensive effect of oral calcium supplementation. A case showing marked susceptibility to $CaCl_2$ after a month's treatment. S, treatment discontinued; T, treatment restarted. The very low figures could be obtained in 24 hrs in warm weather. (From ref. 2.)

decreasing or blocking calcium might be an effective means of lowering pressure in hypertensive patients.

In apparent contradiction to this group of observations is other rapidly accumulating evidence that hypertension may be associated with a calcium deficiency. Many published studies utilizing a variety of sampling techniques describe the same phenomenon. A consistent inverse relationship is observed between dietary calcium intake and blood pressure (4–7); moreover, hypertensive patients may display a relative or absolute hypercalciuria (13). Thus, for the same level of urinary sodium excretion, patients with hypertension tend to have a higher excretion of calcium. As one might expect from these data, serum levels of ionized calcium may be lower in patients with essential hypertension (14). Lastly, in many rat strains and hypertensive humans, oral calcium supplementation may result in lower blood pressures (3,15–34). These observations would lend support to those who claim that higher blood pressure is a disease of calcium deficiency, which might be ameliorated if calcium could just be added to the system.

TABLE 1. *Calcium in hypertension: conflicting evidence*

High levels of calcium are associated with increased blood pressure:

1. Blood pressure is higher with higher levels of intracellular free calcium (8).
2. In large populations, higher blood pressures correlate with higher serum calcium levels (9).
3. Short-term elevation or depression of serum calcium levels raise and lower blood pressure, respectively (10, 11).
4. The chronic hypercalcemia of primary hyperparathyroidism and vitamin D intoxication is commonly associated with chronic hypertension (12).

Low levels of calcium may increase blood pressure:

1. Epidemiologic studies demonstrate an inverse relation between dietary calcium and blood pressure (4–7).
2. Hypertension is associated with an absolute or relative hypercalciuria (13).
3. Serum levels of ionized calcium may be lower than normal in some patients with essential hypertension (14).
4. Oral calcium supplementation may lower blood pressure in hypertensive rats and in normotensive and hypertensive humans (3,15–33).

How can these data be reconciled, and can a therapeutic role for dietary calcium supplementation be defined in clinical hypertension? It appears axiomatic that the utility of any nutritional recommendation in human disease implies an underlying connection between (a) the nutrient itself and/or its metabolism and (b) the pathophysiology of the disease process. Although hypertension is clinically and biochemically heterogeneous, much heated debate and many unfulfilled expectations have resulted from approaching this clinical syndrome as if it were one uniform process. One such example is the long-standing, still controversial role of dietary salt in hypertension, still an issue even though it has been more than 80 years since the first observations linking salt to blood pressure were made (35). Significant progress was finally made simply by observing that blood pressure in some hypertensive subjects was very sensitive to altered dietary salt intake, whereas in others, increased intake of salt either had no effect on blood pressure or even lowered blood pressure. We believe (36) that these same considerations apply to calcium in the pathophysiology and therapy of hypertensive disease. Furthermore, the proper role of dietary calcium in the treatment of hypertension can only be hinted at but cannot be resolved by epidemiologic analyses or even by a "clinical trials" approach in which all hypertensives are lumped together. Indeed, in using such an approach, large numbers of patients are often needed to show modest effects simply because different hypertensives, possibly with different underlying states of calcium metabolism, respond differently to the same dietary maneuver. This approach may thus obscure those clinical conditions and subgroups of hypertensives for whom increased dietary calcium intake would be particularly beneficial, and it may prevent a more routine use of increased calcium intake as a non-drug form of antihypertensive therapy.

Thus, the underlying heterogeneity of hypertension, both biochemically and clinically, needs to be emphasized, allowing for a more individualized approach to the choice of therapy. This heterogeneity has now been shown to extend to divalent cation metabolism as well and may help explain the diversity of blood pressure responses to the same environmental input, such as alterations of dietary salt, calcium, or magnesium intake.

Rationale for Calcium Therapy: Calcium Metabolism in Hypertension

Rapidly accumulating research data attests to an increasing focus on calcium in the pathophysiology of hypertension. This progress has largely proceeded along two parallel lines. At the more basic level, calcium is critical as part of a second messenger system in transducing cellular responses to a wide variety of stimuli. In at least four organ systems, this appears to be of special relevance to blood pressure homeostasis. First, since the time of Ringer (37), when calcium was shown to be important in cardiac contraction, it is now recognized that the generation and regulation of contractile force in all types of muscle is calcium dependent. This is especially true in smooth muscle, where, in the absence of fast, Na^+-linked channels, the slow, voltage-dependent calcium channels are of predominant importance. Second, calcium also participates in the final common pathway of stimulus–secretion coupling mechanisms and is thus central to endocrine function, including the renin–aldosterone system, calcium-regulating hormones, and other adrenal hormones. A special case of calcium-mediated endocrine function involves neurotransmitter release and postsynaptic responses, which, similarly, are calcium-dependent processes. It is understandable, therefore, that much research has also focused on how altered calcium-dependent processes might underlie an endocrine contribution to the pathogenesis of hypertension. Lastly, abnormalities of intrinsic renal endocrine and excretory function (in particular, of sodium handling and renin secretion) also seem to characterize the hypertensive process. Both renal tubular sodium reabsorption and renin secretion are influenced by altered cellular calcium handling; moreover, tubuloglomerular feedback, linking excretory signals to intrarenal vascular and renin responses, is also calcium dependent. Much attention has thus been appropriately focused on defining key renal abnormalities in hypertension, and a hypothesis to account for linked alterations of renin secretion and tubular sodium handling has recently been suggested (38). The challenge confronting calcium research at this basic, mechanistic level is to develop a more unified view in order to identify defects in cellular calcium handling which are common to all tissues and which manifest themselves as the wide variety of organ-defined abnormalities rapidly being catalogued in hypertensive syndromes.

A second, previously separate line of investigation has proceeded more slowly and empirically but has increasingly called attention to the involvement of calcium in hypertension at the epidemiological and clinical levels. The data often appear contradictory, since they support both (a) a positive, pathogenetic role for excess calcium in the hypertensive process and (b) an ameliorative role for calcium in hypertension, the latter implying that hypertension is somehow associated with a calcium deficiency (*vide supra,* Table 1). The challenge confronting this type of calcium-related research is first to resolve the apparent paradox regarding calcium—namely, that it contributes to, as well as protects from, hypertensive disease. Equally important, however, must be the challenge of how to integrate the knowledge obtained at these two different levels of investigation, namely, the clinical–environmental level and the molecular–cellular level. How do the cells know that environmental changes in dietary mineral intake have occurred? What determines their response to these signals? How do the molecular–cellular alterations characteristic of hypertension either contribute to, or result from (or both), clinically relevant alterations of calcium mineral balance?

Not only is the relevance of clinical calcium metabolism to hypertension still largely unexplained, but little attention has been focused on a possible role for those factors normally serving to regulate calcium homeostasis—the calcium-regulating hormones, namely, parathyroid hormone (PTH), calcitonin (CT), and 1,25-dihydroxyvitamin D (1,25D).

The vasoactive properties of PTH were first described in 1925 by Collip and Clark (39). PTH is a vasoactive molecule that has multiple postreceptor effects, and its action is associated with alteration of ion movements across cell membranes, involving sodium, hydrogen, potassium, and calcium (40–43). Circulating PTH levels appear to be abnormal in various hypertensive syndromes, both in experimental animal models and in human hypertension (44–47). When elevated, PTH appears to be appropriately responding to decreased circulating ionized calcium levels, as observed in spontaneously hypertensive rats (SHRs) and deoxycorticosterone acetate (DOCA)–saline rats and in primary hyperaldosteronism and low-renin essential hypertensive human subjects (*vide infra*). PTH has also been hypothesized to have either (a) a compensatory, offsetting effect on elevated blood pressure or (b) a primary pathogenetic role in syndromes of elevated blood pressure (44,48). This issue remains unresolved and perhaps should be best considered in the particular types of hypertensive disease in which it may serve either of these roles. Whatever its particular role in the pathogenesis of hypertensive disease, it now appears that PTH is linked to the function of the renin–aldosterone system (47), to sympathetic nerve activity (49), and, thus, to the control not only of blood pressure but of monovalent, as well as divalent, ion metabolism.

A physiological role for CT in human physiology has not yet been established, although in different tissues it alters the distribution of calcium between intracellular and extracellular spaces. In a given tissue, it may also stimulate or inhibit calcium influx according to the ambient membrane potential (50,51). CT is also a vasoactive peptide, either increasing or decreasing peripheral vascular resistance

(52,53). These effects on blood vessel tone seem to depend on the underlying state of calcium metabolism and salt balance and may also differ among differing renin subgroups of hypertensive individuals. It is unknown to what extent these alterations in circulating levels of CT found in human essential hypertensives and in experimental rat models of hypertension contribute to the elevation in pressure.

Lastly, both peripheral vascular and cardiac tissues appear to be target organs for the vitamin D steroid hormone, 1,25D (54–56). In these tissues, 1,25D mediates calcium influx, stimulates contraction, and potentiates contractile responses to other circulating agonists (56,57). A role for 1,25D (at least in some forms of human hypertension) seems likely, particularly in low-renin, salt-sensitive forms (58,59). As such, this vitamin D hormone species may mediate the hypertensive effects of dietary salt loading and help to explain the antihypertensive effects of dietary calcium loading (*vide infra*).

Calcium and the Renin–Aldosterone System

We have attempted to better define the role of calcium metabolism in hypertension, adopting an approach that attempts to bridge the basic, cellular–clinical gap and that emphasizes both the biochemical and clinical heterogeneity of the hypertensive process (36). Utilizing this approach, we have studied calcium metabolism in both experimental and clinical forms of hypertensive disease and have found broad-based deviations of ionic and hormonal circulating calcium indices. Indeed, divalent cation metabolism appears to be shifted (in both directions) away from average normotensive values among different types of hypertension, paralleling shifts in the activity of the hormonal system involved in regulating monovalent cation metabolism, namely, the renin–aldosterone system. Furthermore, these renin-linked shifts in calcium ionic and hormonal metabolism are clinically relevant in understanding the mechanism by which dietary intake of, for example, salt or calcium may affect blood pressure. Thus, assessment of calcium metabolism and of plasma renin activity may help target specific subgroups of hypertensive individuals for whom calcium supplementation may provide a nonpharmacologic alternative to dietary salt restriction, especially in elderly and black hypertensive populations.

We began by measuring circulating levels of ionized calcium and of the calcium-regulating hormones—namely, PTH, CT, and 1,25D—in subjects with primary, essential hypertension (60,61). Distinct pathophysiologic subgroups were identified by means of renin–sodium profiling. The renal pressor hormone, renin, released by the juxtaglomerular apparatus in response to a variety of ionic, neural, humoral, and direct-pressure–stretch stimuli, both reflects and contributes to pressure and volume homeostasis. Of interest, renin, like PTH, is unusual among hormones, increasing intracellular calcium levels associated with suppression of cellular hormone secretion. Approximately one-third of hypertensive individuals have renin levels inappropriately suppressed as compared to those of normotensive subjects at the same average level of urinary sodium excretion. These subjects are more commonly found in black and elderly hypertensive populations, in whom sodium-volume factors may predominate. On the other hand, inappropriately high levels of renin usually signify angiotensin II-dependent hypertension, in which sodium-volume mechanisms appear to be less clinically relevant. Thus, renin–sodium profiling may allow for a more pathophysiologically oriented way of categorizing hypertensive subjects and has allowed us to more logically fashion the appropriate antihypertensive treatment regimens (62).

When patients were categorized in this manner, serum ionized calcium levels in hypertensives were within the normal range but were distinguishably different among different renin subgroups (60) (Fig. 2). Low-renin hypertensives had lower average serum ionized calcium values, whereas high-renin subjects had values higher than other hypertensive or normotensive control subjects. With considerable overlap observed between individual subjects within renin subgroups, we sought to establish the pathophysiologic (rather than just the statistical) significance of the small ionized calcium changes within the normal range by measuring the calcium-regulating hormones PTH, CT, and 1,25D. What we found was that each of the calcium-regulating hormonal species measured was likewise shifted (61). Like serum ionized calcium values themselves, however, each hormone was deviated (in opposite directions) away from average normotensive values, appropriate for, and thus presumably secondary to, the altered circulating concentrations of calcium (Table 2). Thus, PTH values were consistently elevated in low-renin subjects, appropriate for the lower ionized calcium values found in these

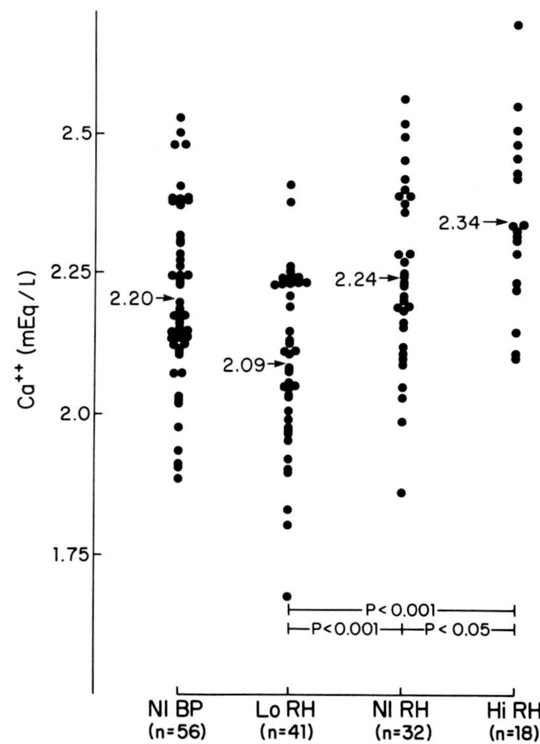

FIG. 2. Serum ionized calcium levels in normotensive and in different renin subgroups of essential hypertensive subjects. (From ref. 46.)

TABLE 2. *Calcium-regulating hormones in essential hypertension*[a]

Group	PTH	CT[b]	1,25D
Nl BF (n = 10)	244 ± 21 (254 ± 42)	68.0 ± 6.5	53.9 ± 5.3
Lo RH (n = 20)	433 ± 38** (398 ± 31)**	56.4 ± 1.8	75.4 ± 5.5***
Nl RH (n = 18)	318 ± 22* (307 ± 33)†	66.2 ± 4.0#	57.2 ± 4.3††
Hi RH (n = 13)	292 ± 37 (311 ± 39)	84.3 ± 3.9***,††††	43.1 ± 4.6†††

* $p < 0.05$; ** $p < 0.01$; *** $p < 0.008$ vs. Nl BP
† $p < 0.05$; †† $p < 0.008$; ††† $p < 0.0001$; †††† $p < 0.00001$ vs. Lo RH
\# $p < 0.005$ vs. Hi RH

[a] PTH, parathyroid hormone; CT, calcitonin; 1,25D, 1,25-dihydroxyvitamin D; Nl BP, normal blood pressure; Lo RH, low-renin hypertension; Nl RH, normal-renin hypertension; Hi RH, high-renin hypertension.
[b] The p-values for CT and 1,25D are for pooled variance T-statistics (Bonferroni).
[c] p for values in parentheses are means adjusted for covariance of urinary sodium excretion.

patients. Similarly, 1,25D values were elevated in these subjects whereas calcitonin levels were lower, again exactly what one would expect if calcium levels were physiologically sensed as being significantly lower in these individuals (Figs. 3 and 4). Conversely, high-renin subjects had elevated CT levels and suppressed values for both PTH and 1,25D as compared to the other hypertensive subjects, again consistent with the higher average circulating ionized calcium levels observed in these subjects. Low-renin essential hypertensive subjects are thus acting as if they have a "calcium deficit," whereas high-renin hypertensive subjects, as a group, act as if a calcium surfeit was present. It may be that apparently paradoxical calcium-related abnormalities of hypertensive subjects previously reported may, at least partly, reflect different hypertensive populations, with calcium metabolism shifted (in different directions) away from average normotensive values.

Further evidence linking calcium-regulating hormones to the renin–aldosterone system comes from studies of syndromes of mineralocorticoid excess. In essential hypertension, although alterations in calcium-regulating hormones may be relevant to the expression of the elevated blood pressure, they don't seem to be primary defects. Indeed, the hyperparathyroidism and the associated eleva-

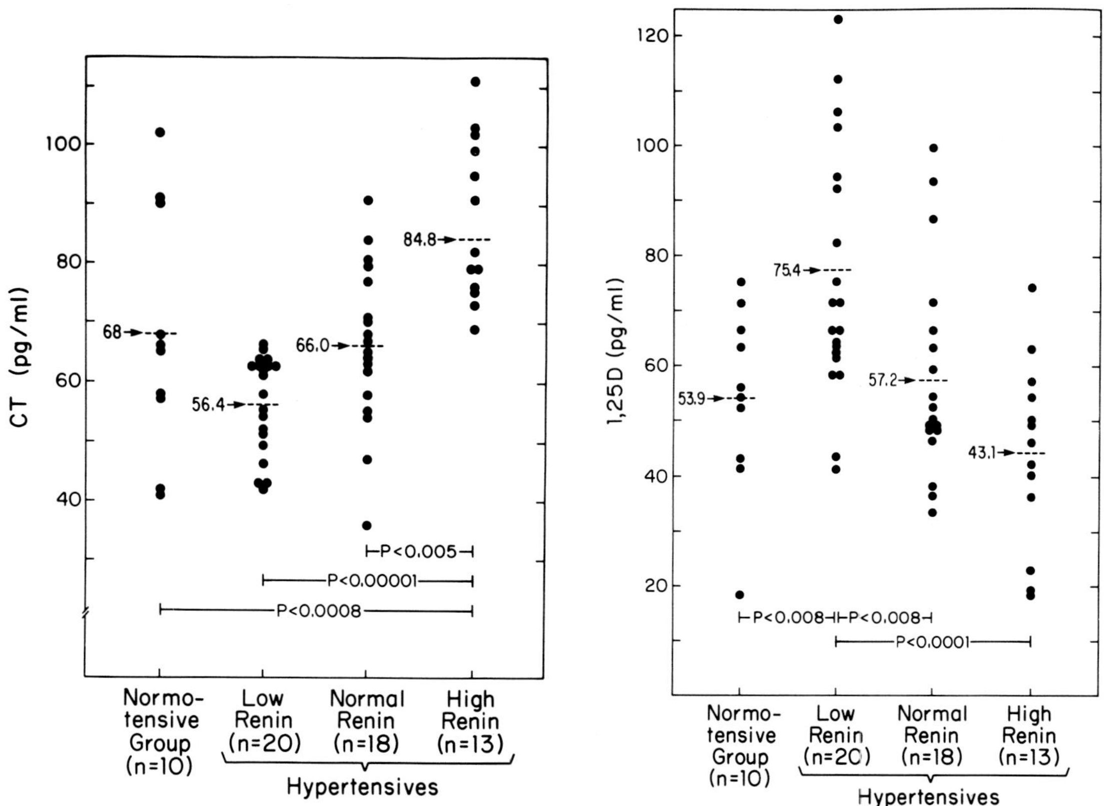

FIG. 3. Calciotropic hormones calcitonin (CT) and 1,25-dihydroxyvitamin D (1,25D) in normotensive and in different renin subgroups of essential hypertensive subjects. (From ref. 61.)

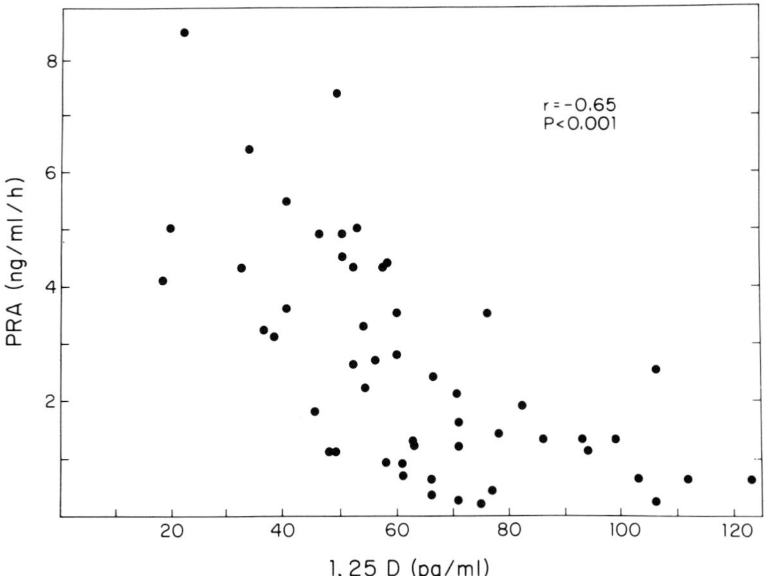

FIG. 4. Inverse relation between circulating levels of 1,25 dihydroxyvitamin D (1,25D) and plasma renin activity in normal and essential hypertensive subjects. (From ref. 61.)

tions of circulating 1,25D observed in low-renin and salt-sensitive forms of hypertension were appropriate for, and thus presumably secondary to, the lower serum ionized calcium levels measured in those hypertensive states. Conversely, the calcium hormonal patterns observed in high-renin, salt-insensitive hypertensives, suggestive of a calcium surfeit, are exactly what one would expect for the higher-than-average normotensive values for circulating ionized calcium measured in these subjects. These altered extracellular distributions of serum ionized calcium are themselves as yet unexplained, and we have hypothesized how they may reflect primary underlying abnormalities of cellular calcium handling (*vide infra*) (36).

In primary aldosteronism, unlike in essential hypertension, relationships between calcium hormones and circulating calcium levels are abnormal and suggest primary effects of mineralocorticoid excess on the renal production of 1,25D, independently of standard calcium signals. Although it had long been appreciated that mineralocorticoid excess causes renal calcium wasting and negative calcium balance (63,64), only recently has it been clinically recognized that the syndrome of primary aldosteronism is routinely associated with secondary hyperparathyroidism (65). As might be expected, serum ionized calcium levels in primary aldosteronism, a syndrome with the greatest degree of renin suppression, are even lower than in low-renin essential hypertension. Appropriately, PTH levels are even higher than in low-renin essential hypertension. At the same time, however, serum 1,25D levels are paradoxically suppressed in primary aldosteronism as compared with low-renin essential hypertension. This has also been found in deoxycorticosterone (DOC)–saline hypertensive rats as compared with NaCl-loaded control rats—lower calcium levels with concurrent paradoxically lower 1,25D levels (Fig. 5). Furthermore, the normal, direct, positive relationship between PTH and 1,25D is reversed in this syndrome. The higher the 1,25D, the lower the PTH, implying perhaps an intact feedback relationship between 1,25D and PTH but at the same time implying that neither calcium itself nor PTH is a primary influence on circulating 1,25D levels in primary aldosteronism. We hypothesize that mineralocorticoid hormones, here in opposition to physiologically "appropriate" calcium-related inputs, participate in the control of 1,25D synthesis (66).

Uniform Versus Heterogeneous Defects in Calcium Metabolism: A Cellular Hypothesis

If, as first demonstrated by Swiss workers, higher blood pressures are uniformly associated with higher levels of free cytosolic calcium in proportion to the elevation of the pressure (8), then how can one explain the diverse spectrum of extracellular ionized calcium values, some being lower, others higher, than average normotensive values? We have developed a hypothesis to reconcile this intracellular uniformity in the face of extracellular diversity (Fig. 6). This hypothesis also predicts clinical consequences that we have tested.

Analyzing hypertension with respect to calcium while disregarding magnesium (also the subject of recent investigation) (67), let us assume that there is an elevation of cytosolic free calcium in proportion to the elevation in blood pressure. At the same time, we have also observed that in low-renin hypertensive patients, serum ionized calcium levels are suppressed. Notice that the intracellular abnormality appears as the mirror image of the extracellular abnormality. The implied hypothesis would be a defect (call it Type I defect) in the plasma membrane separating intracellular from extracellular calcium pools. In the steady state, the plasma membrane incorrectly partitions calcium, with more calcium accumulating on the "inside," coming from the "outside." The result is the calcium metabolic pattern of the low-renin state, lower serum ionized calcium, and high cytosolic free calcium levels. This hypothesis is perfectly general, not dependent on any particular one of a variety of membrane defects already postulated in hypertension, including defects of Na-K-ATPase, sodium–

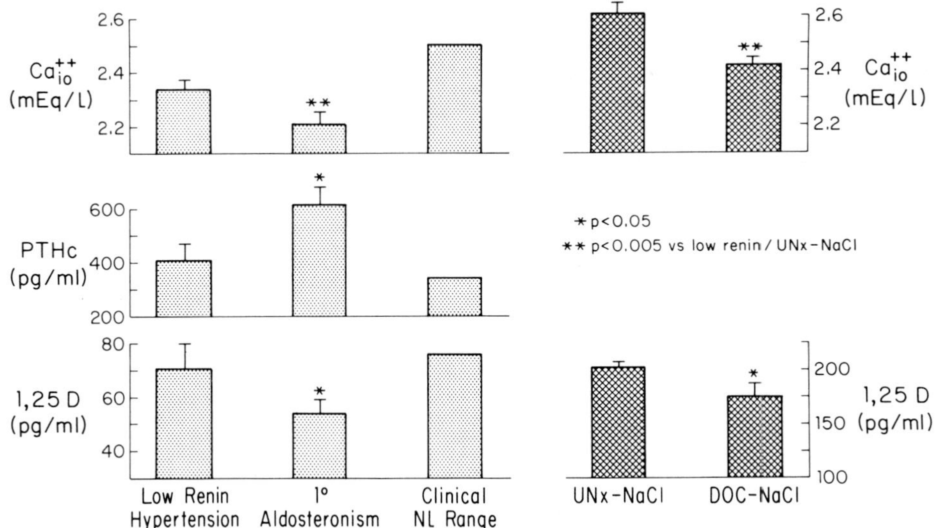

FIG. 5. Secondary hyperparathyroidism and inappropriately suppressed levels of 1,25 dihydroxyvitamin D (1,25D) in subjects with 1° aldosteronism (**left**) and in DOC–saline experimental hypertension in rats (**right**) compared with low-renin essential hypertension and salt-loaded control rats, respectively. (From ref. 66.)

potassium co-transport, sodium–sodium countertransport, sodium–calcium exchange, and Ca-ATPase, as well as humorally mediated calcium uptake (68–70). Furthermore, this Type I, plasma-membrane-dependent defect implies certain testable predictions. First, this kind of hypertension should be exquisitely sensitive to calcium-channel blockade, since the excess accumulated intracellular calcium must come from the extracellular calcium pool. Second, in accord with current molecular hypotheses regarding salt-sensitive hypertension, all of which link the ability of dietary salt to raise pressure with its ability to somehow increase the cellular uptake of calcium, we would predict that hypertensive patients with a low-renin, Type I defect should be more salt-sensitive than others, having a greater tendency to transport extracellular calcium intracellularly. These predictions have indeed been observed.

On the other hand, how can we reconcile the observations made in the high-renin hypertensive state? Once again, intracellular calcium levels are assumed to be increased, as demonstrated in all hypertensive patients (8). Yet, remember that in patients with high-renin hypertension, levels of ionized calcium outside the cell were also higher than in other people. Rather than the mirror-image picture of low-renin hypertension, the same distribution of free calcium seems to be going on inside and outside the cell. Here, we postulate that the problem is one of "domestic affairs"; let us call it a Type II defect. Most cells have organelles within which calcium is in steady-state equilibrium with cytoplasmic free calcium. The endoplasmic reticulum, the mitochondria, various cytoplasmic proteins, and calmodulin may all be involved. We hypothesize that an abnormal steady-state partitioning between stored and/

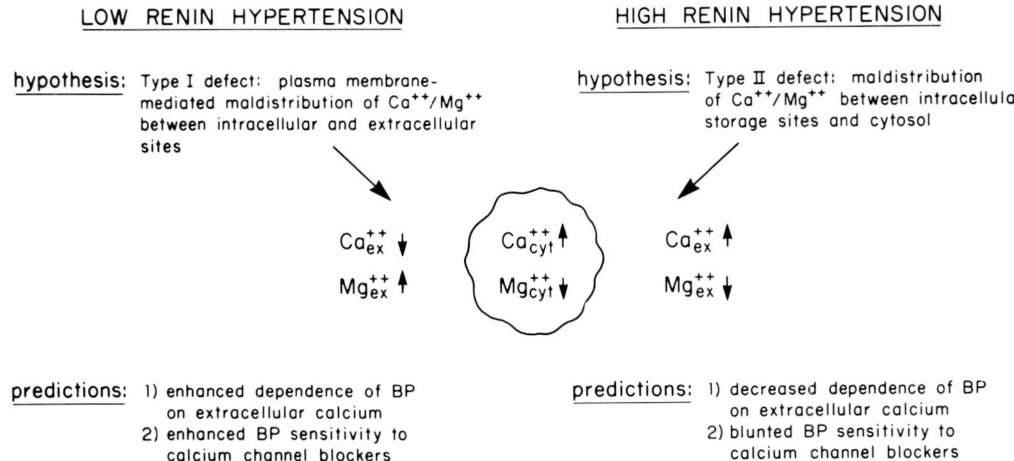

FIG. 6. Cellular hypothesis of hypertension to reconcile uniform intracellular deviation of divalent cations with heterogeneous extracellular distributions of calcium and magnesium among different renin subgroups of essential hypertension. (From ref. 36.)

or bound versus free intracellular calcium results in increased cytoplasmic free calcium. If indeed that is the primary abnormality, then one would expect an otherwise-normal outside plasma membrane to pump out the excess accumulated free cytoplasmic calcium, resulting in increased extracellular calcium levels. Indeed, angiotensin II recruits intracellular calcium stores, even to the extent of total cellular calcium depletion (71). Here, abnormal increases in intracellular calcium do not result from, but rather are the cause of, the increase in extracellular calcium. Once again, this hypothesis is independent of the various molecular mechanisms by which this might occur, such as endoplasmic reticulum or mitochondrial pump defects, abnormal calcium-binding protein interactions, or alterations of calcium–calmodulin binding. Regardless of how this "domestic affairs" Type II defect might arise, certain consequences can be predicted. First, since intracellular calcium is, in this model, less dependent on calcium entering from outside the cell, a patient with Type II, high-renin hypertension should be less sensitive to the blood-pressure-lowering effects of calcium-channel blockade. Second, since excess intracellular free cytoplasmic calcium can itself gate its own (calcium) channels, patients with high-renin hypertension would be predicted to be less sensitive to the hypertensive influences of dietary salt. These predictions are also consistent with published observations (*vide infra*).

Calcium-Channel Blockade in Essential Hypertension

To begin testing this cellular hypothesis, we studied the ability of a single dose of the calcium-channel antagonist nifedipine to lower blood pressure in relation to the ambient metabolic or hormonal circumstances. According to the pretreatment level of plasma renin activity, and in agreement with previous reports (72), low-renin patients exhibited the biggest decline in blood pressure after administration of nifedipine (Fig. 7) (73).

Similarly, elderly subjects have been reported to be more sensitive to calcium-channel blockers, which is consistent with the low-renin form of hypertension more prevalent among the elderly (72). Furthermore, in agreement with our earlier observations, we found that low-renin subjects had lower average ionized calcium values, which also predicted the blood pressure response to nifedipine: Patients with lower serum ionized calcium levels had a greater hypotensive response. The long-term blood pressure response to nifedipine after 1 month of therapy (10 mg, three times a day) was also predicted by pretreatment ionized calcium levels ($r = 0.71$, $p < 0.01$) (74). Moreover, longer-term nifedipine slightly but significantly raised both plasma renin activity and serum ionized calcium values, restoring them to levels indistinguishable from normotensive controls. In this way, a single measurement of serum ionized calcium or of plasma renin activity, as well as a single-dose nifedipine test, may be useful to predict the long-term efficacy of calcium-channel blockade in essential hypertension.

Interestingly, drug efficacy also depended on dietary salt sensitivity. If one does not measure renin activity or extracellular ionized calcium levels but merely distinguishes clinically between salt-sensitive and salt-insensitive people (i.e., those in whom elevations of dietary salt intake either did or did not significantly elevate blood pressure), then one will find that it is the salt-sensitive subgroup that exhibits an enhanced blood-pressure-lowering effect with calcium-channel blockade. Indeed, these salt-sensitive subjects had lower plasma renin activity, lower serum ionized calcium levels, and higher levels of 1,25D than did salt-insensitive subjects (75). Altogether, these results are in keeping with our hypothesis that a preferential response to calcium-channel blockade should be expected in a low-renin, Type I defect, plasma-membrane-dependent form of hypertension. Confirmatory evidence in experimental hypertensive models reveals a similar preferential response of salt-dependent, low-renin hypertension to calcium antagonists (76).

Interaction of Calcium and Sodium Metabolism

What additional clinical significance, if any, might there be of these subtle shifts in calcium metabolism among different renin-defined subgroups of essential hypertension? We reasoned that if these calcium metabolic shifts contributed to the pathogenesis of the hypertension itself, then maneuvers which were known to exacerbate hypertension

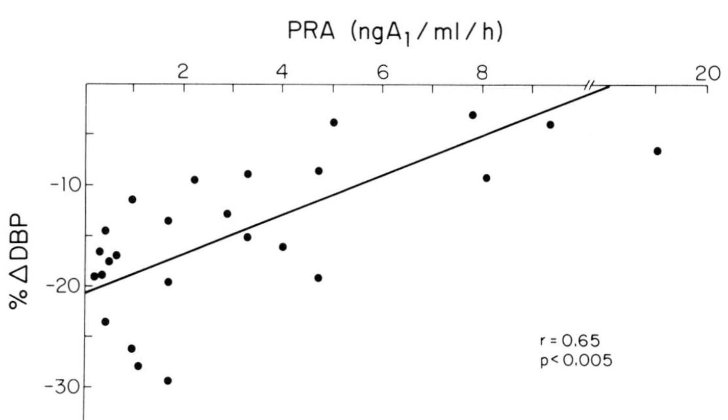

FIG. 7. The relation between the hypotensive response to a single dose of nifedipine and the pretreatment level of plasma renin activity (PRA). (From ref. 73.)

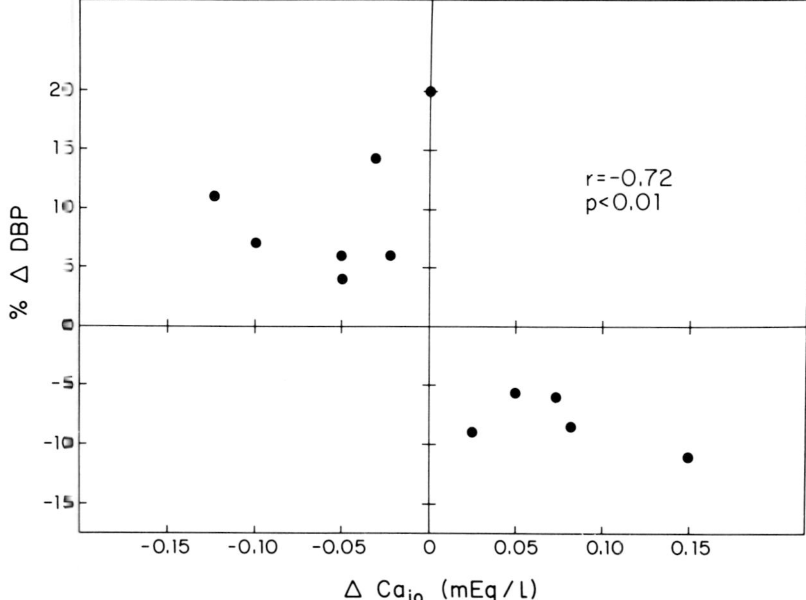

FIG. 8. Relation between salt-induced changes in diastolic blood pressure (%ΔDBP) and salt-induced alterations in serum ionized calcium (ΔCa_{io}) (From ref. 77.)

ought to necessarily provoke and/or exacerbate those same alterations in calcium metabolism. We therefore studied the short- and longer-term effects of dietary salt loading on blood pressure and calcium metabolism. Essential hypertensive subjects were randomly allocated to metabolic balance diets containing 10 and 200 mEq of sodium chloride for 5 days each. Longer-term studies among essential hypertensives provided for low-NaCl (<50 mEq/day) and high-NaCl (>200 mEq/day) diets for 1 month each under outpatient supervision (77,78).

In each group of studies, consistent relationships were observed between the ability of salt to raise blood pressure and its ability to alter calcium metabolism. Salt raised pressure significantly in approximately one-half of the hypertensive subjects in both short- and long-term studies, whereas pressure actually declined in some patients with salt loading. Regardless of the magnitude of the blood pressure change, however, continuous relationships were observed between (a) the changes in diastolic pressure on high versus low dietary salt and (b) salt-induced changes in both serum ionized calcium ($r = -0.72$, $p < 0.001$, short term; $r = -0.78$; $p < 0.001$, long term) and 1,25D ($r = 0.82$, $p < 0.001$, short term; $r = 0.71$, $p < 0.001$, long term) (Figs. 8 and 9). Salt raised pressure the most in those individuals in whom it most lowered ionized calcium levels and most elevated levels of 1,25D, provoking exactly those calcium metabolic changes characteristic of, and originally observed in, low-renin hypertension. This same linkage between the change in salt-induced blood pressure and in ionized calcium has also recently been observed by Cana-

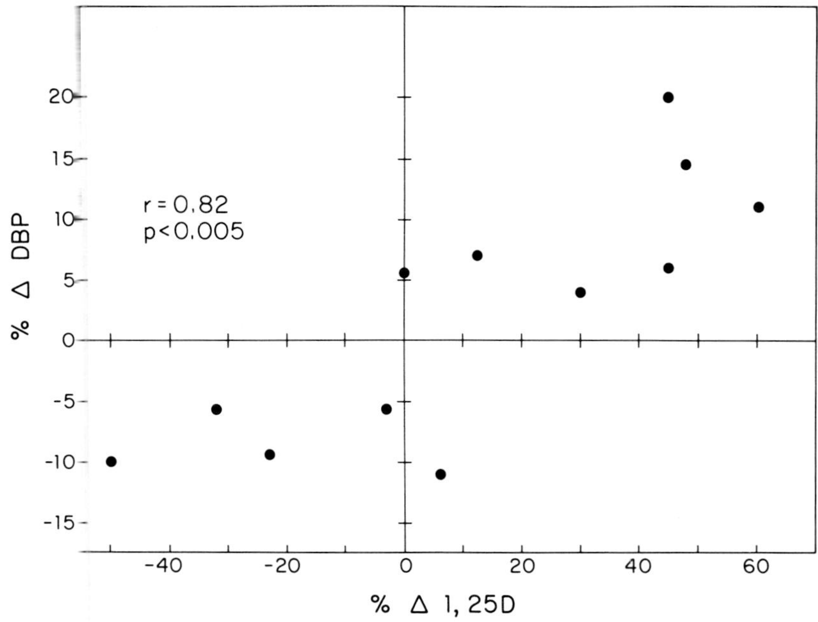

FIG. 9. Relation between salt-induced changes in diastolic blood pressure (%ΔDBP) and salt-induced stimulation of 1,25 dihydroxyvitamin D (%Δ1,25D). (From ref. 77.)

dian workers (79). Additionally, in hypertensive blacks, salt-induced changes in pressure were associated with increased circulating PTH levels (80).

It thus appears that the originally observed "calcium-deficient" ionic and hormonal pattern observed in low-renin patients is of pathophysiologic significance for hypertension, since it contributes to, and/or is reflective of, dietary salt sensitivity. Interestingly, preliminary studies by others also suggested that salt loading in normotensive subjects may elevate 1,25D and/or PTH levels, although pressure measurements were not reported in one of these studies (81,82). Conversely, when extremes of dietary salt intake did not result in significant changes in blood pressure, significant changes in serum ionized calcium were also not observed (83).

These data linking calcium metabolism to sodium-volume forms of hypertension are also supported by a variety of other observations in animal models (Table 3). The ability of increased dietary calcium intake to lower blood pressure in experimental hypertension is best documented in salt-dependent models such as DOC–saline and Dahl S rats (84,85). Similarly, in SHRs, high levels of dietary salt actually potentiates the hypotensive effects of calcium (86), and calcium feeding appears most therapeutically relevant in salt-sensitive strains of SHR (87). Furthermore, in the salt-independent, two-kidney, one-clip Goldblatt hypertensive rat, calcium may not be hypotensive (88).

TABLE 3. *Calcium–sodium interactions in hypertension*[a]

Experimental models

Calcium preferentially lowers blood pressure in salt-dependent models:
1. DOCA–NaCl hypertension (84)
2. Dahl S vs. Dahl R rats (85)
3. Salt-sensitive SHRs (87)
4. SHRs on high- vs. low-salt diets (86)

Calcium may raise blood pressure in salt-insensitive, renin-dependent, two-kidney, one-clip Goldblatt hypertension (88)

Clinical studies

Dietary salt loading alters calcium metabolism in:
1. Normotensives
   a. Increased PTH, increased 1,25D, ?ΔBP (81)
   b. No increased PTH but increased 1,25D and increased BP (82)
2. Hypertensives
   a. Salt-sensitive: decreased Ca^{2+}, increased 1,25D, increased BP (77,78)
   b. Salt-insensitive: No ΔCa^{2+}, Δ1,25D, or ΔBP (77,78)
   c. Increased PTH, increased BP, increased Ca_{int} (80)
   d. Decreased Ca^{2+}_{io}, increased BP (79)

Oral calcium supplementation blunts salt-induced hypertension in:
1. Black hypertensives (22)
2. White and black salt-sensitive subjects (19)

[a] Dahl S, Dahl salt-sensitive; Dahl R, Dahl salt-resistant; SHRs, spontaneously hypertensive rats; PTH, parathyroid hormone; 1,25D, 1,25-dihydroxyvitamin D; BP, blood pressure.

Oral Calcium Supplementation in Hypertension: The Clinical Experience—Who Responds?

These studies may provide a more rational basis on which to assess the potential antihypertensive effects of oral calcium supplementation. Specifically, while the above results indicated that the ability of salt to raise blood pressure was associated with its ability to alter calcium metabolism, the two phenomena need not have been causally linked, since the salt-induced blood pressure rise is perhaps only associated with, but not dependent on, the salt-induced shifts in calcium metabolism. If salt-induced hypertension depended on salt-induced effects on calcium metabolism, then preventing these calcium metabolic changes might at least partially prevent salt from raising blood pressure. Oral calcium supplementation was therefore utilized in attempting to suppress endogenous levels of PTH and of 1,25D and to reverse the elevated levels of those hormones measured in the low-renin, salt-sensitive patient. We thus proceeded to supplement hypertensive patients with calcium carbonate (2 g/day) in four divided doses under a variety of conditions: (a) in short-term studies of hypertensive patients on metabolic balance diets; (b) in longer-term outpatient studies; and (c) on high versus low dietary salt intakes. In each instance, calcium supplementation lowered blood pressure preferentially among those subjects with lower plasma renin activity (17) (Fig. 10, top), lower initial serum ionized calcium levels (89) (Fig. 10, bottom; Fig. 11), and among those who were salt-sensitive (19) (Fig. 12). Of note, while dietary calcium supplementation did not elevate circulating ionized calcium levels themselves, it always reversed the elevated PTH and 1,25D levels characteristic of the low-renin, salt-sensitive individual. Indeed, it was only among salt-sensitive subjects that calcium supplementation significantly lowered 1,25D levels, and only among salt-sensitive patients did calcium supplementation blunt salt-induced elevations in blood pressure. Interesting also were the pressor responses to oral calcium supplementation observed in subjects with high renin and higher initial ionized calcium levels and among those who were salt-insensitive. Once again, these results reflect the different, often opposite, clinical responses to the same dietary maneuver. These results also parallel the ameliorative effects of increased dietary calcium intake in salt-dependent, low-renin, lower ionized calcium, DOCA–saline rats versus the effects of calcium to exacerbate pressure in the renin-dependent, salt-sensitive, higher serum ionized calcium, Goldblatt hypertensive rat (Fig. 13) (88). These data thus emphasize the heterogeneity of hypertensive mechanisms among different hypertensive subjects and suggest the relevance of calcium metabolic indices in identifying and perhaps underlying this heterogeneity.

This divergent and often opposite pattern of blood pressure responses to oral calcium supplementation in different forms of hypertension may partly explain the heterogeneous responses observed in different published reports (Table 4). Different protocols employed different doses of calcium (600–2000 mg/day), administered for different lengths of time (4 days to 6 months) and on different schedules (q.H.S. to q.i.d.). Furthermore, with few exceptions (17–19,22,26), dietary salt intake was either not controlled

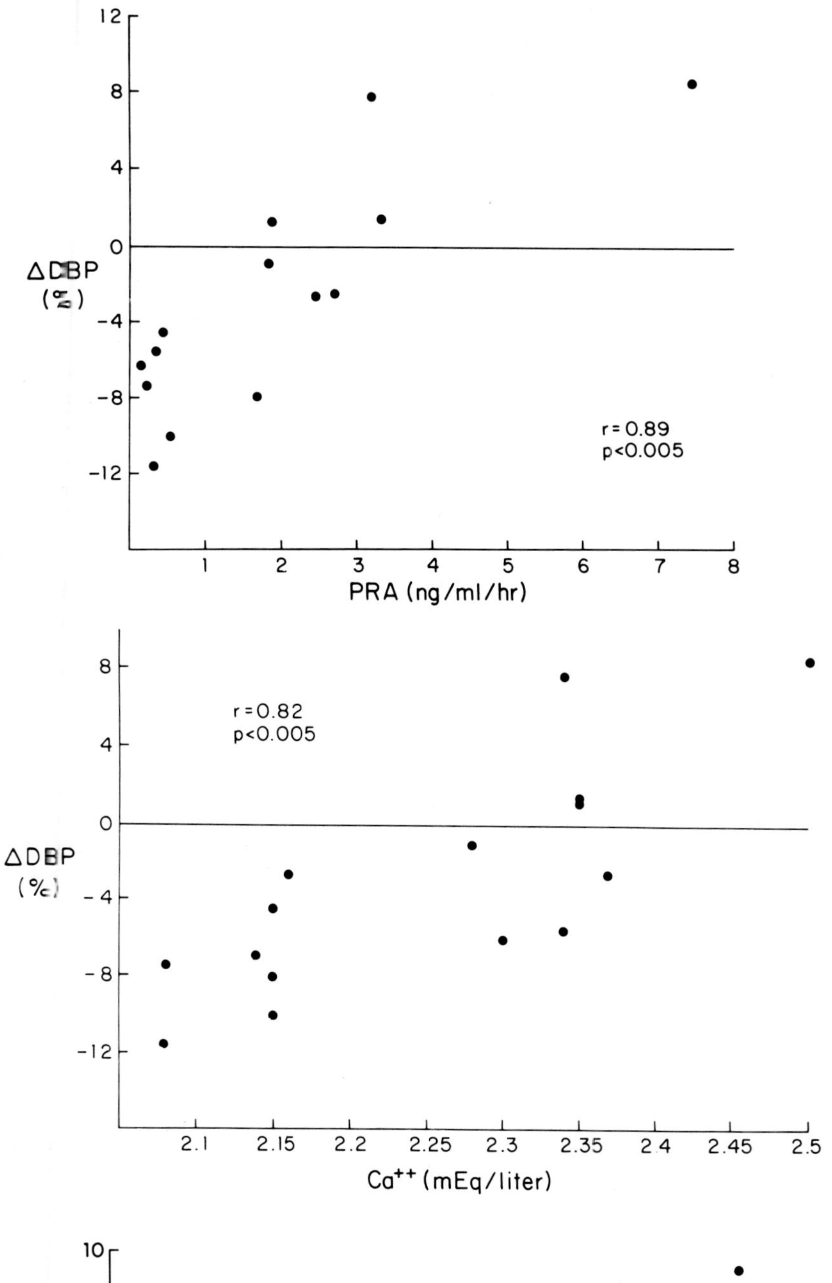

FIG. 10. The blood pressure effects of short-term oral calcium supplementation (2 g/day) in relation to pretreatment plasma renin activity (PRA) (**top**) and to the pretreatment level of fasting serum ionized calcium (Ca^{2+}) (**bottom**) (36).

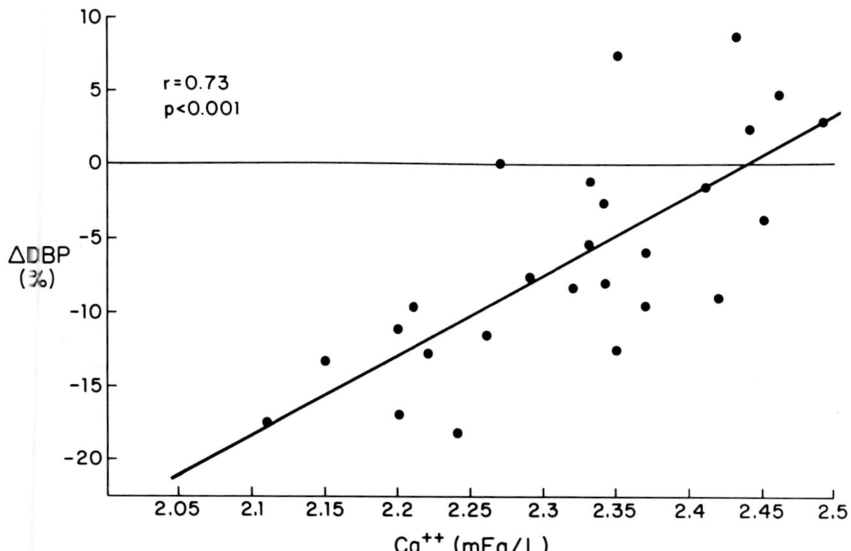

FIG. 11. Relation between the longer-term (6-month) blood pressure effects of oral calcium supplementation (2 g/day) and the pretreatment level of serum ionized calcium (Ca^{2+}). (From ref. 18.)

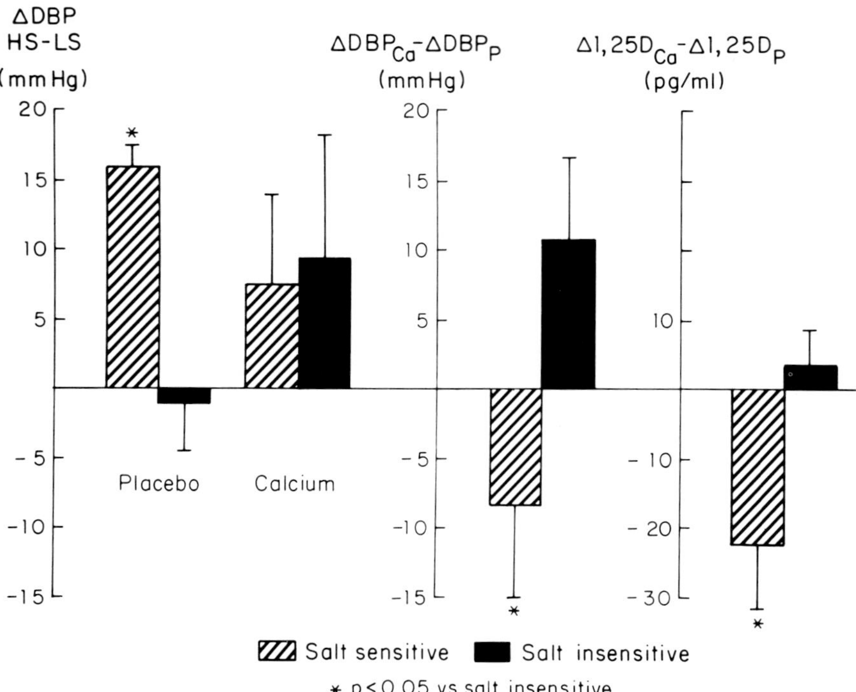

FIG. 12. Divergent blood pressure effects of oral calcium supplementation on salt-sensitive versus salt-insensitive essential hypertensive subjects. (From ref. 19.)

or not considered as a variable. Nevertheless, the major obstacle at present in accepting the ability of oral calcium supplementation to routinely and reproducibly affect blood pressure is a failure to recognize that this heterogeneous pattern of responses observed derives mainly from an underlying heterogeneity of pathophysiologies inherent in essential hypertension. This would help prevent the opposite interpretations of the utility of calcium in the therapy of hypertension arrived at by two different groups, using the same protocol and reporting almost identical data (21,29).

Hence, the subtle shifts in calcium metabolism initially observed among different renin subgroups of essential hypertensives and induced by dietary salt loading in salt-sensitive individuals are markers for, as well as indicators of, the selective utility of calcium, therapeutically, in hypertension. Specifically, sodium-volume-dependent hypertension is a "calcium-dependent" hypertension in which salt induces the "calcium metabolic deficit" that is characteristic of the low-renin state, namely, lower serum ionized calcium and elevated 1,25D levels. It is especially in this form of hypertension that calcium supplementation reverses and/or blunts both (a) the blood pressure and (b) the same calcium variables that sodium loading exacerbates. These conclusions are also supported by the work of Grobbee and Hofman (24), who reported that lower total serum calcium levels and/or higher initial PTH values predicted a fall in diastolic pressure following calcium supplementation. Similarly, these results were supported by Japanese workers who showed that among elderly hypertensives,

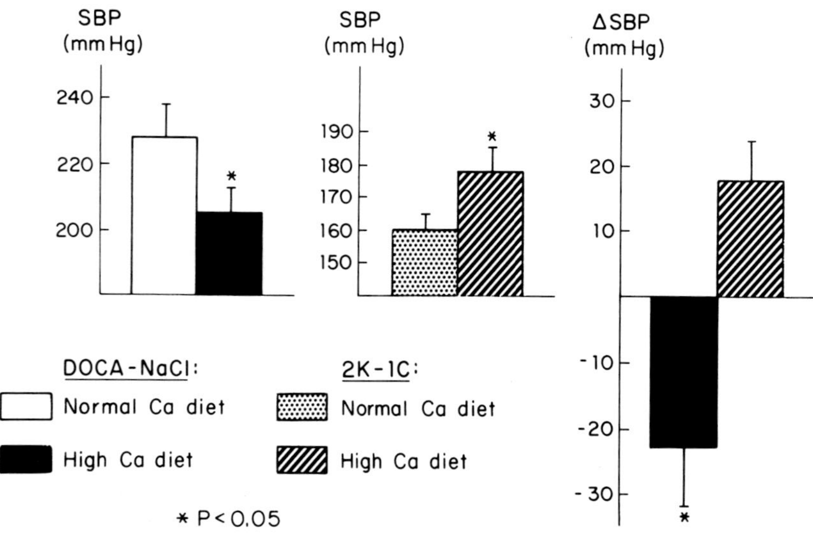

FIG. 13. Divergent effects of increased dietary calcium intake on pressure in salt-dependent, DOCA–saline rats versus salt-independent, renin-dependent, two-kidney, one-clip (2K–1C) Goldblatt rats. (From ref. 88.)

TABLE 4. *Does oral calcium supplementation lower blood pressure?*

Calcium lowers pressure in:	Calcium has no blood pressure effect in:
Normotensives	Normotensives
Belizan et al. (15)	Thomsen et al. (28)
Lyle et al. (16)	
Hypertensives	Hypertensives
Resnick et al. (17–19)	Meese et al. (29)
Johnson et al. (20)	Strazzullo (30)
McCarron et al. (21)	Nowson and Morgan (31)
Zemel et al. (22,23)	Zoccali et al. (32,33)
Grobbee and Hofman (24)	Cappucchio et al. (34)
Takeuchi et al. (25)	
Lasaridus et al. (26)	
Repke et al. (27)	

changes in 1,25D best predicted the long-term blood pressure response to calcium (Fig. 14, top) (25).

Why Does Calcium Supplementation Lower Blood Pressure?

Various explanations have been proposed to account for the observed hypotensive effects of calcium in hypertension. Addison initially observed a diuretic effect (1), and recent data by Zemel et al. (22,23) and by Lasaridis et al. (26) support this concept. The membrane-stabilizing effects of calcium have also been postulated to account for its clinical effects (90), but these effects are only observed at ambient calcium concentrations outside the physiologic range (91). If oral calcium supplementation does result in a stabilization of membrane potential or function, this effect would therefore be an indirect one, mediated by other effects of altered dietary calcium intake. Effects of increased dietary calcium intake on central and cardiac sympathetic tone have also been reported, and thus the hypotensive action of oral calcium supplementation may also involve central nervous system (CNS) mechanisms (87). The recent report that calcium supplementation elevates circulating levels of the potent vasodilating molecule, calcitonin-gene-related peptide (CGRP), supports a role for this molecule in blood pressure homeostasis and provides one more potential mechanism by which oral calcium supplementation may lower blood pressure (92,93) (Fig. 15).

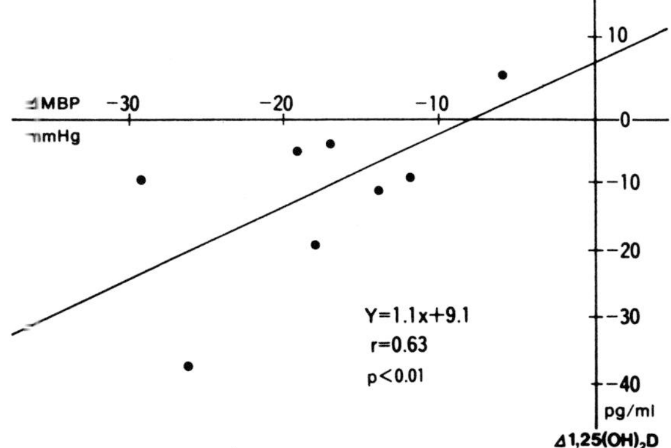

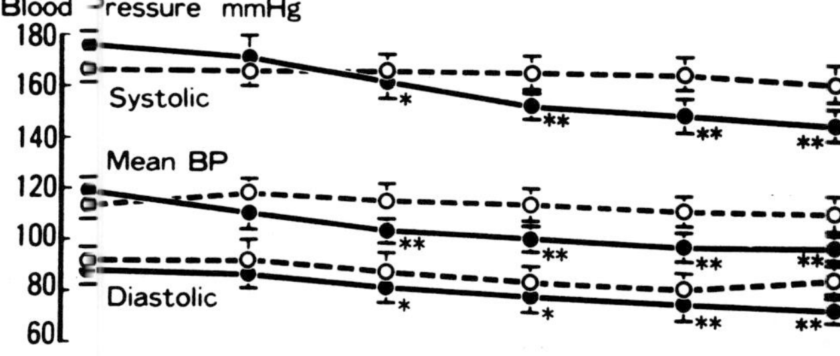

FIG. 14. Blood pressure effects of oral calcium supplementation in the elderly (*solid lines*): (**top**) in relation to the induced change in serum 1,25-dihydroxyvitamin D ($\Delta 1,25(OH_2)D$) (from ref. 25) and (**bottom**) in comparison with the effects of calcium with additional 1α-OH vitamin D (*dashed lines*) (From ref. 96)

Role of 1,25D Versus PTH

We wondered whether the observed "seesaw-like" opposing effects of dietary salt vis-à-vis dietary calcium on blood pressure were due to opposite salt- and calcium-induced effects on circulating calcium ion levels per se or due to induced alterations in calcium-regulating hormones, or both. We reasoned that adding 1,25D therapy to oral calcium supplementation would, by enhancing calcium absorption, provide a more positive calcium balance than would calcium supplementation alone. If total-body calcium balance and/or circulating calcium levels were themselves critical to the observed dietary mineral-induced blood pressure effects, then the addition of 1,25D to cal-

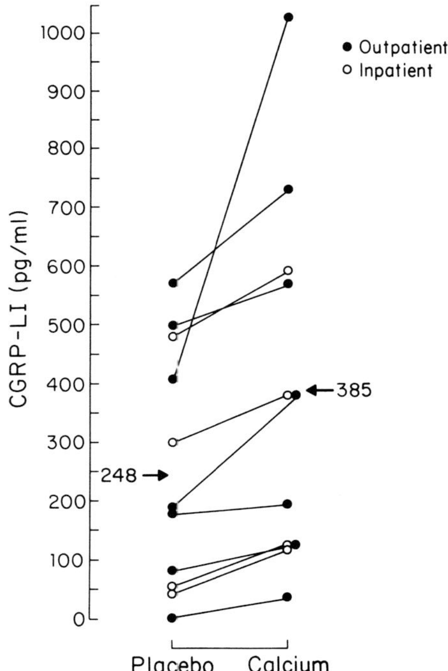

FIG. 15. Effect of oral calcium supplementation on serum circulating calcitonin-gene-related peptide-like immunoreactivity (CGRP-LI). (From ref. 93.)

cium itself would potentiate calcium effects on blood pressure. Interestingly, exactly the opposite was observed (94,95).

Essential hypertensive patients on metabolic balance diets, already receiving 2 g/day of supplemental calcium, were then given 1,25D (0.25 μg/day) for three additional days. Although calcium supplementation lowered blood pressure preferentially among low-renin hypertensives, who had lower initial levels of serum ionized calcium (Figs. 10 and 11), the addition of 1,25D to calcium reversed the calcium effects and elevated pressure in these same patients (Fig. 16). Conversely, blood pressure was ameliorated by calcium plus 1,25D in those high-renin, higher initial ionized calcium patients in whom calcium alone exerted a pressor effect. Similarly, Japanese workers demonstrated that compared to calcium alone, calcium given with a supplemental analogue of 1,25D, namely 1,α(OH)D_3, exacerbated blood pressure (Fig. 14, bottom) (25,96).

Comparing the effects of these two calcium maneuvers on circulating hormone levels was also revealing (Table 5). Calcium supplementation alone suppressed endogenous PTH and 1,25D levels, and it elevated plasma renin activity without significantly elevating serum ionized calcium levels. Calcium given with additional exogenous 1,25D also suppressed PTH levels while not significantly elevating serum ionized calcium. However, circulating 1,25D levels rose significantly with this regimen as compared to calcium supplementation alone, and plasma renin activity was suppressed. These opposite hormonal effects parallel their opposite blood pressure effects. Thus we arrive at the following conclusions: (a) PTH is probably of little significance in mediating the blood pressure effects of oral calcium supplementation, since it was suppressed by both calcium-related maneuvers, each having opposite blood pressure consequences. (b) At least part of the mechanism by which increased oral calcium intake influences blood pressure is

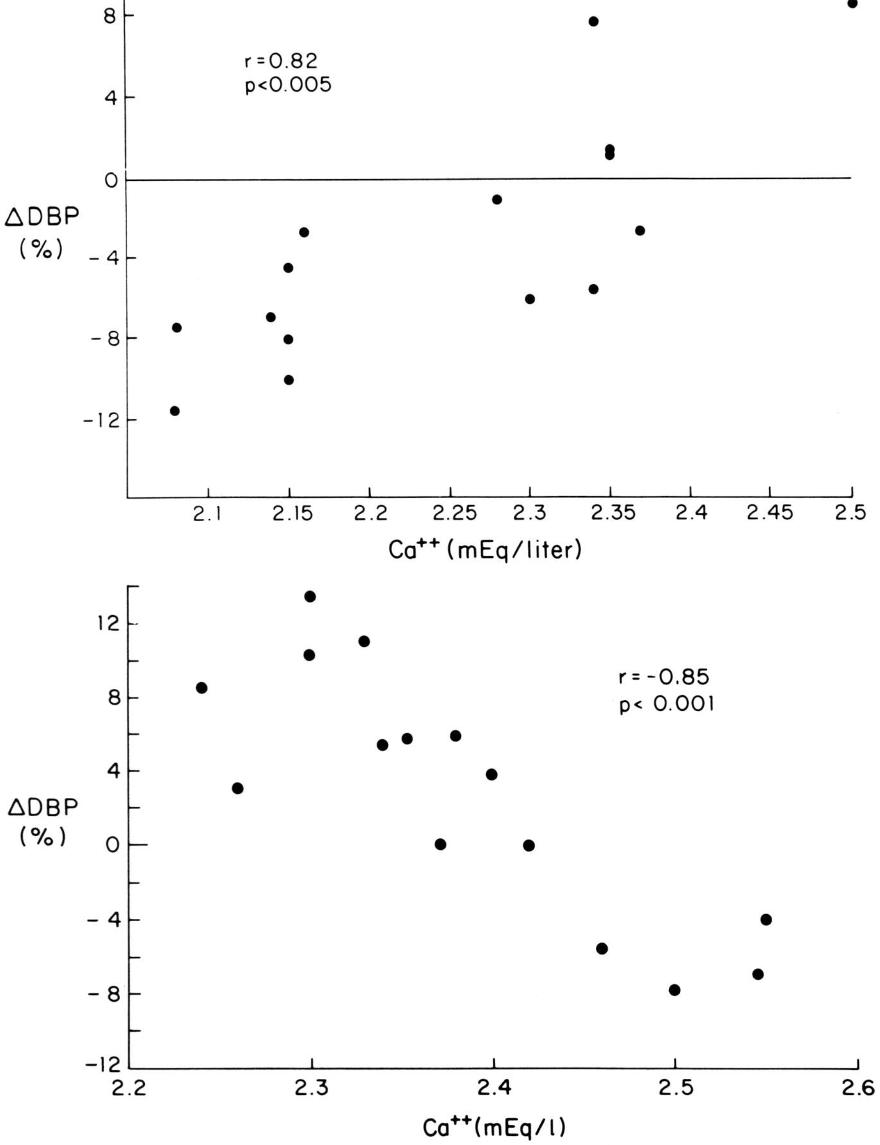

FIG. 16. Divergent blood pressure effects of oral calcium supplementation (**top**) versus calcium–1,25-dihydroxyvitamin D administration (**bottom**) in relation to pretreatment levels of ionized calcium (Ca^{2+}). (From ref. 95.)

TABLE 5. *Metabolic effects of calcium with and without 1,25-dihydroxyvitamin D*[a]

Treatment	ΔCa^{2+} (%)	ΔPTH (%)	Δ1,25D (%)	ΔPRA (%)
Ca^{2+}	3.2 ± 3.0	−35.7 ± 11.6	−53 ± 15	38 ± 8.3
Ca^{2+} − 1,25D	2.3 ± 1.1	−20 ± 7.7	63 ± 21[b]	−31 ± 9.5[b]

[a] PTH, parathyroid hormone; 1,25D, 1,25-dihydroxyvitamin D; PRA, plasma renin activity.
[b] $p < 0.001$ vs. Ca^{2+} alone.

by virtue of its ability to suppress circulating 1,25D levels. (c) The inverse relation of plasma renin activity to 1,25D observed in steady-state screening of hypertensive populations is also consistently observed dynamically. Calcium supplementation in suppressing endogenous 1,25D elevates plasma renin activity. This further strengthens the linkage between the renin–aldosterone system and calcium-regulating hormones. (d) The fact that calcium supplementation lowers blood pressure best among those subjects in whom it reverses the same renin and calcium hormonal deviations initially observed in low-renin, salt-sensitive hypertensive subjects emphasizes the clinical relevance of these hormonal deviations in the pathogenesis of the hypertensive process.

Summary and Overall Hypothesis

What emerges from these data is an appreciation of a critical role for calcium-regulating hormones, coordinately and reciprocally with the renin–aldosterone system, linking the humoral control of monovalent and divalent cation metabolism, in transducing dietary mineral signals at the cellular level. The resultant steady-state alterations in the distribution of calcium and magnesium, intracellularly and between intracellular and extracellular compartments in a variety of different tissues, directly influence (a) cardiac hemodynamic function, (b) central nervous and peripheral vasoactive hormone release, and (c) peripheral smooth muscle vasoconstrictor tone and, hence, the resultant blood pressure. This pattern of relationships is illustrated in Fig. 17. This scheme—in which the ability of an altered dietary mineral balance to affect blood pressure is necessarily mediated by, and thus affects, mono- and divalent cation-regulating hormones—provides a perspective for better understanding both the biochemical and clinical heterogeneity of hypertension. Specifically, this may help to resolve the bothersome observations that (a) a variety of genetically inherited ion transport defects found in hypertension are also found in normotensive family relatives and hence cannot by themselves explain elevated blood pressure and (b) chronic dietary sodium excess and/or calcium deficiency do not usually result in clinical hypertension. Therefore, in neither case can these factors be considered "causes" of hypertension, although they may each represent necessary, but not sufficient, conditions.

In essential hypertension, for instance, different primary genetically inherited or acquired alterations in cellular ion transport systems may result in the heterogeneous distribution of serum ionized calcium we have observed. These, in turn, create the metabolic setpoints of these two hormone systems (i.e., the renin–aldosterone system and calcium-regulating hormones), which would lead to hypertension only when access to dietary minerals such as sodium chloride, potassium, calcium, and magnesium is also shifted significantly, with each mineral either enhancing or suppressing these pathophysiologic hormone shifts. A high dietary salt intake in the setting of high endogenous 1,25D and secondary hyperparathyroidism would result in accelerated calcium transport intracellularly and would thus result in the vasoconstriction, enhanced cardiovascular function, and increased central neural hormonal release often observed in salt-sensitive hypertension. In the absence of this skewed metabolic profile, dietary salt loading would result in no elevation in blood pressure. Furthermore, by helping to offset the calcium metabolic profile characteriz-

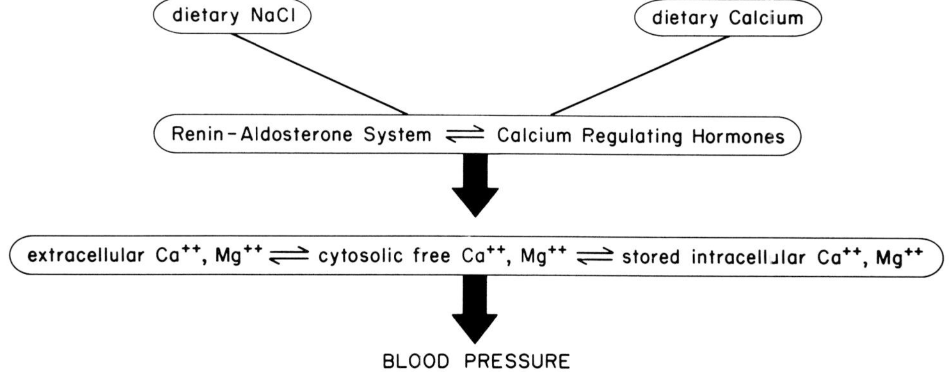

FIG. 17. General hypothesis in which the activities of the renin–aldosterone system and calcium-regulating hormones coordinately transduce environmental dietary mineral signals at the cellular level, thus determining the ultimate blood pressure effects of these minerals. (From ref. 36.)

ing the low-renin and salt-sensitive state, dietary calcium supplementation blunts the pressor effects of salt and, in already salt-loaded people, is significantly antihypertensive. These considerations also appear to help explain the heterogeneous blood pressure responses to a variety of different pharmacologic agents, including newer drug classes as calcium-channel antagonists and converting-enzyme inhibitors (62,73,75).

Knowing how these hormonal systems operate to preside coordinately over blood pressure homeostasis will not only afford additional meaningful insights into the pathophysiology of hypertension but will also allow us to diagnostically identify subgroups of hypertensives for whom more physiologic, individualized therapy can be constructed. Ultimately, long-term prophylactic strategies to prevent the onset of hypertensive disease might be developed.

MAGNESIUM

The therapeutic use of magnesium in human hypertensive disease dates back to the discovery (in the late 19th century) of its beneficial effect in the toxemia of pregnancy (97). At about the same time that Addison was reporting his experiences utilizing oral calcium supplementation, Blackfan and Hamilton (98), in 1925, reported the hypotensive effects of intravenous magnesium in malignant hypertension. However, interest in the routine use of magnesium in human hypertension declined in the face of inconsistent and heterogeneous blood pressure responses, as reported in 1942 by Winkler et al. (99). As is now documented for calcium (see above), magnesium supplementation lowered pressure in only some hypertensives. Consistent with our approach emphasizing the clinical and biochemical heterogeneity of calcium metabolism in the pathophysiology and treatment of hypertension, these early observations with magnesium therapy signal the need for careful subgroup analysis of human hypertension. It therefore seems reasonable to consider magnesium metabolism in hypertension in relation to (a) other pressor hormones systems such as the renin–aldosterone system and (b) the recent experience in the use of magnesium in the therapy of hypertension. This may allow for a more individualized approach to therapy, thereby making it possible to identify specific alterations that can serve as useful markers for individuals for whom magnesium supplementation would consistently lower blood pressure.

Rationale for Magnesium Therapy: Magnesium Metabolism in Hypertension

In a fashion parallel to calcium in the extracellular space, magnesium is the predominant intracellular divalent cation species. Yet, research in the cardiovascular role of magnesium metabolism has lagged behind that for calcium metabolism, at least partly because the accurate measurement of magnesium within various body compartments is still itself the focus of research. For example, in contrast to blood ionized calcium measurements (which utilize an ion-specific calcium electrode), circulating free or ionized magnesium levels cannot be routinely assessed. Similarly, despite the now wide use of fluorescent probes to analyze steady-state and acutely altered levels of intracellular cytosolic free calcium (100), the use of nuclear magnetic resonance (NMR) spectroscopy to assess intracellular levels of free magnesium has been restricted to few research groups, and only recently has it been applied to the clinical problem of hypertension (67). It also seems clear that those measurements of magnesium that are available reflect only poorly the total body magnesium stores, and thus the issue of a magnesium deficit or surfeit in any particular clinical situation is not easily assessed. Lastly, the control of magnesium metabolism, both in the extracellular space and intracellularly, is incompletely understood. Thus, although both calcium-regulating hormones (such as PTH, CT, and 1,25D) and aldosterone (101) affect magnesium (and, in turn, are influenced by magnesium), specific physiologically relevant feedback relationships have not been adequately established (102). Furthermore, the intracellular regulation of magnesium metabolism is still virtually unknown. Thus, despite its ability to modify and regulate a wide variety of transport processes involving calcium, potassium, and sodium, only one magnesium-specific plasma membrane pump has been defined that may have physiologic significance for magnesium transport (103,104). Hence, our ability to provide a physiologic basis for magnesium supplementation as a nonpharmacologic modality of antihypertensive therapy is limited.

Nevertheless, at least four considerations mandate further consideration of magnesium at this time: (i) presumed regulation of sodium-, potassium-, and calcium-dependent cardiac and smooth muscle contraction by magnesium, intracellularly, as well as endocrine and neurotransmitter secretion; (ii) the ability of abnormal magnesium metabolism to result in altered peripheral vascular reactivity and blood pressure; (iii) the presence of altered magnesium metabolism in clinical hypertension; and (iv) the ability of magnesium supplementation to change blood pressure.

Cellular Effects

The critical importance of ionic factors in controlling the integrity of intracellular metabolism, as well as the importance of triggering cellular responses to external stimuli, has become increasing recognized in the past decade. Magnesium can itself function as a calcium-channel blocker, modulating calcium-channel activity in heart cells (105) and causing vasodilatation comparable to pharmacologic calcium-channel blockade (106). Moreover, intracellular levels of magnesium at the free concentrations present in the cytoplasm serve to regulate a variety of the factors, including the following:

1. *Na-K-ATPase, which is critical for the establishment and maintenance of the resting cellular membrane potential, pumping sodium ions out and transporting potassium ions inward, both against their electrochemical potential gradients.* A decrease in the activity of this pump mechanism would lead to cellular depolarization and, in different tissues, would result in increased cardiac and smooth mus-

cle contractility, increased renal sodium excretion, and increased neurotransmitter release. The potential relevance of this enzyme in hypertensive disease has been emphasized by reports of decreased Na-K-ATPase activity present in hypertension, and the search for a humoral enzyme inhibitor is still intensely being pursued. Since magnesium stimulates Na-K-ATPase activity within the range of its concentrations found intracellularly (107), a deficit of intracellular free magnesium alone would lead to suppressed Na-K-ATPase activity, partial cellular depolarization, and the above-mentioned events that predispose to and/or cause increased blood pressure.

2. *Calcium-dependent potassium channels, which serve to offset the potential depolarizing influence of cellular calcium accumulation.* Increasing cytosolic free calcium triggers plasma-membrane potassium efflux, which has a hyperpolarizing influence. Excess activity of this pump mechanism may result in cellular hyporesponsiveness to external stimuli as has been documented in paramecia. Conversely, inhibiting this pump would tend to make cells hyperresponsive and, in excitable tissues, would result in the increased vascular reactivity and neural excitability reported in hypertension. Magnesium also regulates the activity of this pump activity and stimulates calcium-activated potassium efflux (108); magnesium deficiency at this site may also thus predispose to hypertension.

3. *Numerous other intracellular calcium-dependent processes.* Since calcium as a second messenger stimulates many events leading to cardiac and smooth muscle contraction, the ability of magnesium to antagonize these calcium-dependent processes suggests it would have an ameliorative effect on elevated blood pressure. Specifically, magnesium competes for calcium-binding sites on calmodulin (109), thus serving as a break on calcium–calmodulin stimulation of myosin light-chain kinase and other calmodulin-mediated, calcium-triggered kinases. Additionally, the steady-state equilibrium between free cytosolic calcium and intracellular calcium stores in endoplasmic (sarcoplasmic) reticulum, in calciosomes, and in mitochondria is also influenced by the ambient concentrations of magnesium (110). Thus, above and beyond its ability to individually modulate calcium-related biochemical processes, magnesium also regulates the intracellular sequestration and distribution of calcium itself.

Altered Magnesium Metabolism and Blood Pressure

A variety of studies, both *in vitro* and *in vivo,* have consistently reported that primary alterations in magnesium metabolism may lead to increased vascular reactivity and/or elevated blood pressure. These phenomena have been well documented by Altura and colleagues, as well as by others (111–113). Specifically, it was found that (i) extracellular magnesium concentrations directly influence basal smooth muscle vascular tone, (ii) hypomagnesemia enhances *in vitro* agonist-induced vascular contractility while attenuating relaxation, and (iii) hypermagnesemia blunts agonist-induced vascular contractions. These effects were associated with (a) altered vascular calcium handling and (b) greater levels of magnesium, thereby potentiating ^{45}Ca efflux in rat portal veins. Altura et al. (114) also studied the effects of dietary-induced magnesium deficiency in intact rats. These workers documented *in vivo* vasoconstriction and decreased lumen diameter of the mesenteric microcirculation, proportionate to the degree of magnesium deficiency. Furthermore, these changes were reflected in elevated blood pressures. Similarly, French workers showed an accelerated development of hypertension in magnesium-deficient SHRs (115). As a caveat, however, levels of serum magnesium achieved by these depletion protocols were significantly hypomagnesemic levels, which were not present in the vast majority of essential hypertensive clinical states. Nevertheless, these *in vitro* and animal studies provide a basis for understanding the possible relation between clinical magnesium depletion and hypertension.

Conversely, altered magnesium metabolism in already hypertensive subjects has long been recognized, although early observations were possibly affected by coexisting renal failure (116). In nonuremic subjects, levels of serum magnesium were lower in essential hypertensive subjects than in normotensive subjects (117). Similarly, one Scandinavian study reported age-related, gradually decreasing serum magnesium levels: The older subjects had lower average magnesium levels, which were, in turn, inversely related to the height of the blood pressure. These findings were interpreted as suggesting that a magnesium deficit might contribute to the gradually increasing incidence of hypertension with increasing age (118). These early suggestions were supported by broader epidemiologic studies in which estimated dietary magnesium intake was inversely elevated to levels of blood pressure. Individuals ingesting foods containing less magnesium had higher blood pressures (119–121).

The considerable overlap between serum magnesium levels among normotensive and hypertensive subjects led Iseri and co-workers (117) to suggest an underlying heterogeneity of magnesium metabolism in essential hypertension. Indeed, the biochemical and clinical heterogeneity of human hypertensive disease is now well established and does indeed extend to magnesium metabolism as well. When serum magnesium levels are measured in normotensive and essential hypertensive subjects, distinctly different results are obtained among different renin-defined subgroups of hypertension (Fig. 18) (46). In a manner parallel but opposite to serum ionized calcium levels (Fig. 2), serum magnesium levels were inversely related to (a) levels of plasma renin activity in subjects of equal age, (b) level of blood pressure, and (c) urinary sodium excretion. Within the same "normal" range found among normotensive control subjects, low-renin essential hypertensives had higher levels of serum magnesium, whereas high-renin subjects had magnesium levels significantly below average normotensive values. Thus, in a fashion parallel to calcium, but possibly relevant to a different hypertensive subgroup, the ability of dietary magnesium intake to influence blood pressure may differ according to the underlying state of magnesium metabolism and may only significantly benefit some, but not all, forms of clinical hypertension.

Intracellularly, however, a more unified disturbance of magnesium metabolism has been reported. Recently ^{31}P-NMR spectroscopy has been used to noninvasively assess

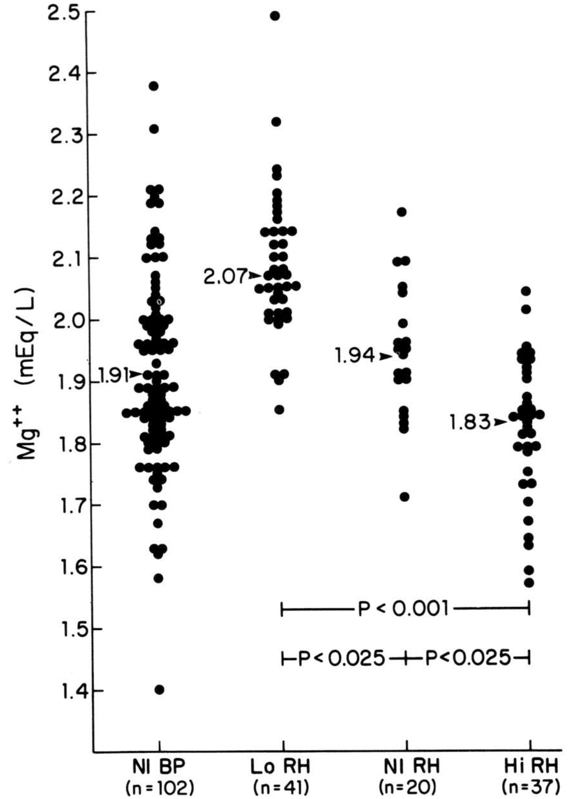

FIG. 18. Serum magnesium levels in a normotensive group and in different renin subgroups of essential hypertensive subjects. Nl BP, normal blood pressure; Lo RH, low-renin hypertension; Nl RH, normal-renin hypertension; Hi RH, high-renin hypertension. (From ref. 36.)

intracellular levels of free magnesium in erythrocytes of human and experimental models of hypertension. Fasting levels of intracellular free magnesium were significantly suppressed in hypertensive subjects as compared with normotensive subjects. These results have been subsequently confirmed in preeclampsia as compared to normotensive pregnancy (122), as well as in experimental SHR versus WKY rat models (123). Moreover, a continuous, inverse linear relationship was observed between the ambient intracellular free magnesium level and the height of the blood pressure (Fig. 19). In a fashion again parallel and opposite to the relation defined by Swiss workers for intracellular cytosolic free calcium and blood pressure (8), lower free magnesium levels were associated with higher systolic and diastolic blood pressures. This inverse relationship between intracellular free magnesium and blood pressure was not only observed in the steady state among human hypertensives but was also observed dynamically in sodium-volume dependent, DOC–saline rats and in renin-dependent, two-kidney, one-clip Goldblatt hypertensive rats (124). On different dietary calcium intakes, regardless of whether calcium lowered or elevated blood pressure, lower pressures were associated with higher intracellular free magnesium levels.

This apparent uniformity of altered magnesium levels intracellularly, despite the heterogeneous deviations (in both directions) in serum magnesium levels away from average normotensive values in different renin subgroups of hypertension, has been reconciled by the same cellular hypothesis suggested for altered calcium metabolism of hypertension (Fig. 6). In this scheme, different cellular defects result in different distributions of extracellular magnesium, despite a uniform deficit of intracellular cytosolic free magnesium. In the low-renin subject, plasma membrane defects of magnesium binding and/or transport result in increased circulating magnesium levels at the expense of, and directly reflecting, the depleted intracellular magnesium. Conversely, among high-renin subjects, similar decreased levels of intracellular free magnesium reflect altered intracellular compartmentalization of magnesium among storage sites vis-à-vis the cytoplasm. Hence, less cytosolic free calcium is available to exchange with the extracellular space, resulting in the lower serum magnesium levels observed in the high-renin hypertensive state. Whether this diverse, renin-linked pattern of magnesium metabolism in

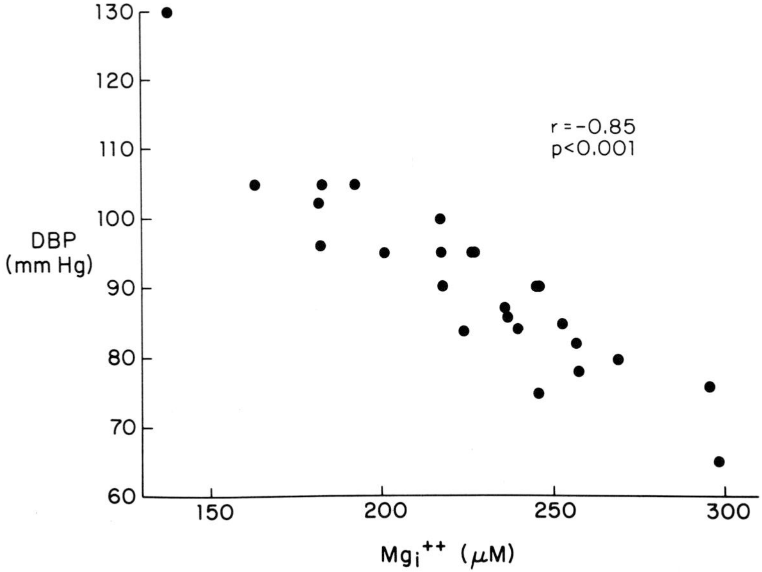

FIG. 19. Inverse relation between erythrocyte intracellular free magnesium (Mg_i^{2+}) and diastolic blood pressure (DBP) in normotensive and essential hypertensive subjects. (From ref. 67.)

hypertension provides a basis by which to select patients for whom magnesium supplementation may be significantly hypertensive is as yet unknown (*vide infra*).

Lastly, additional evidence suggests that these alterations of magnesium metabolism may be clinically relevant to the elevated blood pressure, providing an additional rationale for the therapeutic use of magnesium in at least some forms of hypertensive disease. First, as mentioned above, the ability of altered dietary calcium intake to lower blood pressure was associated with its ability to elevate intracellular free magnesium (124). Second, Zemel et al. (107) demonstrated that the ability of increased dietary salt intake to elevate blood pressure was associated with its ability to lower erythrocyte magnesium levels. Finally, the ability of the calcium-channel blocker nifedipine to lower blood pressure was also related to the pretreatment serum magnesium level: The lower the magnesium, the lesser the effectiveness of nifedipine; the higher the magnesium, the greater the hypotensive effect (73).

Therapy with Magnesium: Experience and Future Directions

Current experience utilizing oral magnesium supplementation as a nonpharmacologic means of antihypertensive therapy is severely limited. A variety of factors have contributed to this. Historically, emphasis was placed on short-term parenteral use, and this route is still commonly employed in the clinical setting of the pregnancy-induced hypertensive syndromes, preeclampsia and eclampsia. Indeed, even in pregnancy, the efficacy of parenteral magnesium as an antihypertensive is not what mandates its continued use; rather, it is used because of its action to suppress the increased neuromuscular irritability predisposing to, and sometimes resulting in, frank seizure activity (125). Furthermore, when magnesium did significantly lower blood pressure, it was found to do so best in situations of acute hypertension, with only sporadic success in cases of chronic "essential" hypertension (99). Lastly, the doses of magnesium used almost always resulted in significant hypermagnesemia, achieving levels which were grossly unphysiologic and which could not be reached by oral supplementation in patients having adequate renal function. In this regard, it is thus unclear to what extent the reported action of magnesium to stimulate prostacyclin formation is relevant to changes in magnesium within the physiologic range (126).

Recently, in a small series of essential hypertensive patients, hospitalized and in sodium balance for 5 days on a metabolic ward, magnesium sulfate was administered parenterally at low doses, 2 g/day (intramuscularly) for 4 days. Levels of serum magnesium rose, but not outside of the normal range. Similar to the experience of Winkler et al. (99) in essential hypertensives, using a high-dose protocol, a heterogeneous pattern of blood pressure responses was observed: Pressure in some patients worsened; in others, however, magnesium had significant hypotensive effects (62). As seen in Fig. 20, decreases in blood pressure occurred predominantly among the high-renin hypertensive patients having lower average circulating serum magnesium values. Interestingly, in the high-renin subjects, calcium supplementation was either ineffective or pressor (see Fig. 10). Perhaps the analysis of renin system activity also provides a clue to the efficacy of magnesium supplementation in hypertension. This important issue is still unexplored.

Similar to results of parenteral magnesium therapy, the clinical experience with oral magnesium supplementation is incomplete. Two early reports suggested that in diuretic-treated subjects, oral magnesium administration, either as the chloride or asparate hydrochloride salt, significantly lowered blood pressure (127,128). In one study, cellular magnesium depletion was documented on diuretic therapy alone, and repletion of these losses presumably contributed to its antihypertensive efficacy, as observed in magnesium-deficient animal preparations (115). However, in 17 un-

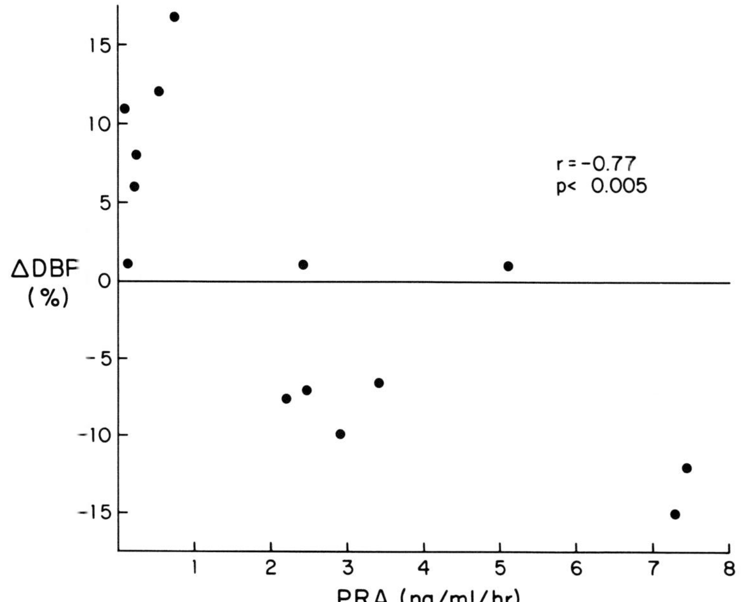

FIG. 20. The diastolic blood pressure effects (%ΔDBP) of short-term parenteral (intramuscular) magnesium sulfate in essential hypertension in relation to the pretreatment plasma renin activity (PRA). (From ref. 62.)

treated essential hypertensive subjects, no blood pressure effects were measured when magnesium was the sole form of therapy used (129). Furthermore, even in patients who were previously treated with diuretics, no hypotensive effects were reported by other Scandanavian workers (130).

Thus, progress has been made in magnesium research, and a role for decreased intracellular free magnesium levels in the pathophysiology of hypertension appears likely. Furthermore, the common clinical coincidence of hypertension, peripheral insulin resistance, glucose intolerance, and/or frank diabetes mellitus may have a common intracellular ionic basis, at least partially ascribable to the intracellular magnesium deficiency (131). However, a consistent, reproducible effect of magnesium supplementation on blood pressure has not yet been confirmed in hypertension, and therefore a definite role cannot yet be assigned to magnesium as a nonpharmacologic option in hypertension. Nevertheless, since (a) magnesium was first reported to lower blood pressure in both malignant hypertension and in pregnancy (both high-renin states as compared to nonpregnant, nonhypertensive states), (b) parenteral magnesium sulfate lowered pressure preferentially in high-renin essential hypertensives, and (c) oral magnesium supplementation may be effective in a setting of ongoing diuretic therapy (also a hyperreninemic state), it seems reasonable to hypothesize that the high-renin state and/or its attendant alterations in magnesium metabolism may provide a guide by which to further explore and identify those specific subgroups for whom magnesium itself may represent an effective form of antihypertensive therapy.

REFERENCES

1. Addison WLT. The use of calcium chloride in arterial hypertension. *Can Med Assoc J* 1924;14:1059–1061.
2. Addison WLT, Clark HG. Calcium and potassium chloride in the treatment of arterial hypertension. *Can Med Assoc J* 1925;15:913–915.
3. Ayachi S. Increased dietary calcium lowers blood pressure in the spontaneous hypertensive rats. *Metabolism* 1979;28:1234–1238.
4. McCarron D, Morris CD, Henry JH, Standon JL. Blood pressure and nutrient intake in the United States. *Science* 1984; 224:1392–1398.
5. Ackley S, Connor-Barrett E, Suarez L. Dairy products, calcium and blood pressure. *Am J Clin Nutr* 1983;38:457–461.
6. Gruchow HW, Sobocinski KA, Barbariak JJ. Threshold effects of dietary calcium on blood pressure. *J Hypertens* 1986;4(Suppl 5):S355–S357.
7. Reed D, McGee D, Yamo K, Hankin J. Diet, blood pressure and multicollinearality. *Hypertension* 1985;7:405–411.
8. Erne P, Bolli P, Burgissen E, Buhler FR. Correlation of platelet calcium with blood pressure; effect of antihypertensive therapy. *N Engl J Med* 1984;319:1084–1088.
9. Kesteloot H, Geboers J. Calcium and blood pressure. *Lancet* 1982;1:813–815.
10. Weidmann P, Massry SG, Coburn JW, Maxwell MH, Atelson J, Kleeman CR. Blood pressure effects of acute hypercalcemia: studies in patients with chronic renal failure. *Ann Intern Med* 1972;76:741–745.
11. Clowes GHA Jr, Simeone FA. Acute hypocalcemia in surgical patients. *Ann Surg* 1957;145:530–540.
12. Brinton GS, Jubiz W, Lagerquist LD. Hypertension in primary hyperparathyroidism: the role of the renin–angiotensin system. *J Clin Endocrinol Metab* 1975;41:1025–1029.
13. Strazzullo P, Nunziata V, Cirillo M, et al. Abnormalities of calcium metabolism in essential hypertension. *Clin Sci* 1983; 65:137–141.
14. McCarron DA. Low serum concentrations of ionized calcium in patients with hypertension. *N Engl J Med* 1982;307:226–228.
15. Belizan JM, Villar J, Pineda O, Gonzalez AE, Soing E, Garrera G, Sibrian R. Reduction of blood pressure with calcium supplementation in young adults. *JAMA* 1983;249:1161–1165.
16. Lyle RM, Melby CL, Hyner GC, Edmondson JW, Miller JZ, Weinberger MH. Blood pressure and metabolic effects of calcium supplementation in normotensive white and black men. *JAMA* 1987;257:1771–1776.
17. Resnick LM, Sealey JE, Laragh JH. Short and long-term oral calcium alters blood pressure (BP) in essential hypertension. *Fed Proc* 1983;42(3):300.
18. Resnick LM, Nicholson JP, Laragh JH. Calcium metabolism and essential hypertension—relationship to altered renin system activity. FASEB symposium on calcium and hypertension. *Fed Proc* 1986;34:2739–2745.
19. Resnick LM, DiFabio B, Marion RM, James GD, Laragh JH. Dietary calcium modifies the pressor effects of dietary salt intake in essential hypertension. *J Hypertens* 1986;4(Suppl 6):S679–S681.
20. Johnson NE, Smith EL, Freudenheim JL. Effects on blood pressure of calcium supplementation of women. *Am J Clin Nutr* 1985;42:12–17.
21. McCarron DA, Morris CD. Blood pressure response to oral calcium in persons with mild to moderate hypertension: a randomized, double-blind, placebo-controlled, crossover trial. *Ann Intern Med* 1985;103:825–831.
22. Zemel MB, Gualdoni SM, Sowers JR. Sodium excretion and plasma renin activity in normotensive and hypertensive black adults as affected by dietary calcium and sodium. *J Hypertens* 1986;4(Suppl 6):S343–S345.
23. Zemel MB, Gualdoni SM, Sowers JR. Reduction in total and extracellular water associated with calcium-induced natriuresis and the antihypertensive effect of calcium in blacks. *Am J Hypertens* 1988;1:70–72.
24. Grobbee DE, Hofman A. Effect of calcium supplementation on diastolic blood pressure in young people with mild hypertension. *Lancet* 1986;2:703–707.
25. Tabuchi Y, Ogihara T, Hashizume K, Sait H, Kumahara Y. Hypotensive effect of long-term oral calcium supplementation in elderly patients with essential hypertension. *J Clin Hypertens* 1986;3:254–262.
26. Lasaridis AN, Zanaieri KI, Kaisis CN, Syrgassis CD, Toukantonis AA. Oral calcium supplementation promotes renal sodium excretion in essential hypertension. *J Hypertens* 1987;5(Suppl 5):S307–S309.
27. Repke JT, Villar J, Anderson C, Pareja G, Dubin N, Beligan JM. Biochemical changes associated with blood pressure reduction induced by calcium supplementation during pregnancy. *Am J Obstet Gynecol* 1989;160:684–690.
28. Thomsen K, Nilas L, Christiansen C. Dietary calcium intake and blood pressure in normotensive subjects. *Acta Med Scand* 1987;222:51–56.
29. Meese RB, Gonzales DG, Casparian JM, Ram CVS, Peck CYC, Kaplan NM. The inconsistent effects of calcium supplements upon blood pressure in primary hypertension. *Am J Med Sci* 1987;254:219–224.
30. Strazzullo P, Siani A, Gugliemi S, DiCarlo A, Galletti F, Cirillo M, Mancini M. Controlled trial of long-term oral calcium supplementation in essential hypertension. *Hypertension* 1986; 8:1084–1088.
31. Nowson C, Morgan T. Effect of calcium carbonate on blood pressure. *J Hypertens* 1986;4(Suppl 6):S673–S675.
32. Zoccali C, Mallamaci F, Delfino D, Parlongo S, Iellamo D, Moscato D, Maggiore Q. Does calcium have a dual effect on arterial pressure? response to 1,25 dihydroxyvitamin D_3 and calcium supplements in essential hypertension. *J Hypertens* 1987;5(Suppl 5):S267–S269.

33. Zoccali C, Mallameci F, Delfino D, Ciccarelli M, Parlongo S, Iellamo D, Moscato D, Maggiore Q. Long-term oral calcium supplementation in essential hypertension: double-blind randomized, crossover study. *J Hypertens* 1986;4(Suppl 6):2676–2678.
34. Cappuccio FP, Markandu ND, Singer DRJ, Smith SJ, Shore AC, MacGregor GA. Does oral calcium supplementation lower high blood pressure? A double blind study. *J Hypertens* 1987;5:67–71.
35. Laragh JH, Pecker MS. Dietary sodium and essential hypertension: some myths, hopes and truths. *Ann Intern Med* 1983;98:735–743.
36. Resnick LM. Uniformity and diversity of calcium metabolism in hypertension: a conceptual framework. *Am J Med* 1987; 82(Suppl 1B):16–26.
37. Ringer S. A third contribution regarding the infusion of the inorganic constituents of the blood of the ventricular contraction. *J Physiol (Lond)* 1883;4:222–225.
38. Sealey JE, Blumenfeld JD, Bell GM, Pecker MS, Sommers SC, Laragh JH. On the renal basis for essential hypertension: nephron heterogeneity with discordant renin secretion and sodium excretion causing a hypertensive vasoconstriction–volume relationship. *J Hypertens* 1988;6:763–777.
39. Collip JB, Clark EP. Further studies on the physiological action for parathyroid hormone. *J Biol Chem* 1925;54:485–507.
40. DeLuise M, Harkner M. Parathyroid hormone stimulation of the Na^+/K^+ pump in rat clonal osteosarcoma cells. *J Endocrinol* 1986;111:61–66.
41. Kahn AM, Zimmer RA, Navran SS. Parathyroid hormone inhibits Na-H exchange in cultured vascular smooth muscle cells [Abstract]. *Kidney Int* 1988;33:298.
42. Sugarman A, Kahn T. Parathyroid hormone impairs extrarenal potassium tolerance in the rat. *Am J Physiol* 1988;254:F385–F390.
43. Bogin E, Massry SG, Harary I. Effect of parathyroid hormone on rat heart cells. *J Clin Invest* 1981;67:1215–1227.
44. Young EW, Bukowski RD, McCarron DA. Calcium metabolism in experimental hypertension. *Proc Soc Exp Biol Med* 1988;1987:123–141.
45. McCarron DA, Pingree PA, Rubin RJ, Goucher SM, Molitch M, Krutzik S. Enhanced parathyroid function in essential hypertension: a homeostatic response to a urinary calcium leak. *Hypertension* 1980;2:162–168.
46. Resnick LM, Laragh JH, Sealey JE, Alderman MA. Divalent cations in essential hypertension. Relations between serum ionized calcium, magnesium, and plasma renin activity. *N Engl J Med* 1983;309:888–891.
47. Resnick LM, Müller FB, Laragh JH. Calcium regulating hormones in essential hypertension: relation to plasma renin activity and sodium metabolism. *Ann Intern Med* 1986;105:649–654.
48. Hulter HN, Melby JC, Peterson JC, Cooke CR. Chronic continuous PTH infusion results in hypertension in normal subjects. *J Clin Hypertens* 1986;2:360–370.
49. Campese VM. Calcium, parathyroid hormone, and sympathoadrenal system. *Am J Nephrol* 1986;6(Suppl 1):29–32.
50. Resnick LM, Churchill MC, Churchill PC, Laragh JH, Orlowski R. The effects of calcitonin, calcitonin analogs and calcitonin-gene-related peptide on renin secretion: evidence for hormone-modulated calcium transport. *Fed Proc* 1986;45:1011.
51. Resnick LM, Churchill PC, Churchill M, Laragh JH, Orlowski R. The direct effect of calcitonin (CT), calcitonin analogues, and calcitonin gene-related peptide (CGRP) on renin secretion: evidence for calcium channel antagonism. *Clin Res* 1986;34:552A.
52. Resnick LM, Müller FB, Nicholson JP, Laragh JH. Calcitonin is a vasoactive hormone in hypertensive man. *Clin Res* 1984;32:523A.
53. Resnick LM, Müller FB, Nicholson JP, Laragh JH. Hormonal and hemodynamic effects of graded calcitonin infusion in hypertensive man. Presented at the Seventh International Congress of Endocrinology, Quebec City, June 1984.
54. Merks J, Hofmann W, Goldenschmidt D, Ritz E. Demonstration of 1,25 (OH_2) vitamin D_3 receptors and actions in vasular smooth muscle cells *in vitro. Calcif Tissue Int* 1987;41:112–114.
55. Kawashima, H. Receptor for 1-25-dihydroxyvitamin D in a vascular smooth muscle cell line derived from rat aorta. *Biochem Biophys Res Commun* 1987;146:1–6.
56. Walters MR, Wicki DC, Riggle PC. 1,25 Dihydroxy-vitamin D_3 receptors identified in the rat heart. *J Mol Cell Cardiol* 1986;18:67–72.
57. Bukoski RD, Xue H, McCarron DA. Effect of $1,25(OH)_2$ vitamin D_3 and ionized Ca^{2+} on ^{45}Ca uptake by primary cultures of aortic myocytes of spontaneously hypertensive and Wistar Kyoto normotensive rats. *Biochem Biophys Res Commun* 1987; 146(3):1330–1335.
58. Resnick LM, Laragh JH. Does dihydroxyvitamin D (1,25D) cause low renin hypertension? *Hypertension* 1984;6:792.
59. Resnick LM, Nicholson JP, Laragh JH. Alterations in calcium metabolism mediate dietary salt sensitivity in essential hypertension. *Trans Assoc Am Physicians* 1985;98:313–321.
60. Resnick LM, Laragh JH, Sealey JE, Alderman MH. Divalent cations in essential hypertension. Relations between serum ionized calcium, magnesium, and plasma renin activity. *N Engl J Med* 1983;308(15):888–891.
61. Resnick LM, Müller FB, Laragh JH. Calcium regulating hormones in essential hypertension: relation to plasma renin activity and sodium metabolism. *Ann Intern Med* 1986;108:649–654.
62. Resnick LM, Laragh JH. Renin, calcium metabolism and the pathophysiologic basis of antihypertensive therapy. *Am J Cardiol* 1985;56:68H–74H.
63. Luft R, Sjogren B. Some aspects of the metabolic effects of deoxycorticosterone acetate. *Metabolism* 1953;2:313–321.
64. Massry S, Coburn LW, Chapman LW, Kleeman CR. The effect of long-term deoxycorticosterone acetate administration on the renal excretion of calcium and magnesium. *J Lab Clin Med* 1968;71:212–219.
65. Resnick LM, Laragh JH. Calcium metabolism and parathyroid function in primary aldosteronism. *Am J Med* 1985;78:385–389.
66. Resnick LM, Gertner JM, Laragh JH. Abnormal vitamin D metabolism in primary aldosteronism and experimental mineralocorticoids excess. *J Hypertens* 1987;5(Suppl 5):S99–S101.
67. Resnick LM, Gupta RK, Laragh JH. Intracellular free magnesium in erythrocytes of essential hypertension: relation to blood pressure and serum divalent cations. *Proc Natl Acad Sci USA* 1984;81:6511–6516.
68. Kuriyama H, Uyshi I, Sueuk H, Kitamure A, Itoh T. Factors modifying contraction–relaxation cycle in vascular smooth muscles. *Am J Physiol* 1982;243:H641–H662.
69. Robertson BR. Altered calcium handling as a cause of primary hypertension. *Hypertension* 1984;2:453–460.
70. McCarron DA. Is calcium more important than sodium, in the pathogenesis of essential hypertension? *Hypertension* 1985;7: 607–627.
71. Smith JB, Smith L. Extracellular Na^+ dependence of changes in free G^{2+}, G^{2+} efflux, and total cell Ca^{2+} produced by angiotensin II in cultural arterial muscle cells. *J Biol Chem* 1987;262:17455–17460.
72. Erne P, Bolli P, Bertel O, et al. Factors influencing the hypertensive effects of calcium antagonists. *Hypertension* 1983;5(Suppl II):II-97–II-102.
73. Resnick LM, Nicholson JP, Laragh JH. Calcium, the renin–angiotensin system, and the hypertensive response to nifedipine. *Hypertension* 1987;10:254–258.
74. Resnick LM, Nicholson JP, Sealey JE, Laragh JH. Acute and long-term effects of calcium channel blockade on divalent ions, blood pressure, and plasma renin activity. *Clin Res* 1985;31(2): 253A.
75. Resnick LM, Nicholson JP, Laragh JH. The antihypertensive effects of calcium channel blockade: role of sodium and calcium metabolism. *J Cardiovasc Pharmacol* 1988;12(Suppl 6):S114–S115.
76. Hall CE, Hungerford S. Prevention of DOCA–salt hypertension with the calcium blocker nitrendipine. *Clin Exp Hypertens (A)* 1983;5:721–728.
77. Resnick LM, Nicholson JP, Laragh JH. Alterations in calcium metabolism mediate dietary salt sensitivity in essential hypertension. *Trans Assoc Am Physicians* 1985;98:313–321.
78. Resnick LM. Calcium as a mediated of salt sensitive hyperten-

sion. In: Massery SG, Omer M, Tirz E, eds. *Phosphate and mineral homeostatsis.* New York: Plenum Press, 1986;297–404.
79. Burgess ED, Keene PM, Watanabe M. Blood pressure and serum calcium responses to altered sodium intake in high renin hypertension. *Am J Hypertens* 1989;2:182–184.
80. Zemel MB, Gualdoni SM, Walsh MF, et al. Effects of sodium and calcium on calcium metabolism and blood pressure regulation in hypertensive black adults. *J Hypertens* 1986;4(Suppl 5):S364–S366.
81. Breslau NA, McCurie JL, Zerwith JE, Pak CYC. The role of dietary sodium on renal excretion and intestinal absorption of calcium and on vitamin D metabolism. *J Clin Endocrinol Metab* 1982;55:369–372.
82. Hughes GS, Oexmann MJ, Margolius HS, Epstein S, Bell NH. Normal vitamin D and mineral metabolism in essential hypertension. *Am J Med Sci* 1988;296:252–259.
83. McCarron DA, Rankin LI, Bennett MLU, Krutzik S, McClung MR, Luft FC. Urinary calcium excretion at extremes of sodium intake in normal man. *Am J Nephrol* 1981;1:84.
84. Kurtz TW, Morris RC. Attenuation of deoxycorticosterone-induced hypertension by supplemental dietary calcium. *J Hypertens* 1986;4(Suppl 5):S182–S131.
85. Peuler JD, Morgan DA, Mark AL. High calcium diet reduces blood pressure in Dahl salt-sensitive rats by neural mechanisms. *Hypertension* 1987;9(Suppl III):159–165.
86. McCarron DA, Lucas PA, Shneidman RS, Drüeke T. Blood pressure development of the spontaneously hypertensive rat following concurrent manipulation of the dietary Ca^{2+} and Na^{+}: relation to intestinal Ca^{2+} fluxes. *J Clin Invest* 1985;76:1147–1154.
87. Yang R-H, Jin H, Chen Y-F, Oparil S, Wyss JM. Dietary calcium supplementation prevents the exaggerated responsiveness of anterior hypothalamic α adrenoceptors in NaCl-loaded spontaneously hypertensive rats. *J Cardiovasc Pharmacol* 1989;13:162–167.
88. Resnick LM, Sosa RE, Corbett ML, Gertner JM, Sealey JE, Laragh JH. Effects of dietary calcium on sodium volume vs. renin-dependent forms of experimental hypertension. *Trans Assoc Am Physicians* 1986;99:172–179.
89. Resnick LM, Nicholson JP, Laragh JH. Outpatient therapy of essential hypertension with dietary calcium supplementation. *J Am Coll Cardiol* 1984;3:616.
90. Bukoski RD, McCarron DA. Altered aortic reactivity and lowered blood pressure associated with high Ca^{2+} intake in the SHR. *Am J Physiol* 1986;251(20):H976–H983.
91. Bohr DF. Vascular smooth muscle: dual effect of calcium. *Science* 1963;139:597–599.
92. Resnick LM. Calciotropic hormones in clinical and experimental hypertension. In: Laragh JH, Brenner BM, eds. *Perspectives in hypertension, vol. 2: endocrine mechanisms in hypertension.* New York: Raven Press, 1989;265–297.
93. Resnick LM, Preibisz JJ, Laragh JH. Calcitonin gene-related peptide-like immunoreactivity in hypertension: relation to blood pressure, sodium, and calcium metabolism. In: Ganten DS, Retteh R, eds. *Salt and hypertension.* New York: Springer-Verlag, 1989;190–199.
94. Resnick LM, Laragh JH. Does 1,25 dihydroxyvitamin D (1,25D) cause low renin hypertension? *Hypertension* 1984;6:792.
95. Resnick LM. Calcium and vitamin D metabolism in the pathophysiology of human hypertension. In: Levaner OA, ed. *Nutrition '87.* Washington, DC: American Institute of Nutrition, 1987;110–114.
96. Ogihara T, Saito H, Tabuchi Y, Hashizuma K, Kumahara Y. The hypotensive effect of long-term oral calcium loading in elderly hypertensive patients: the importance of endogenous vitamin D_3 suppression. *J Hypertens* 1986;4(Suppl 6):S685–S687.
97. Chesley LC. *Hypertensive disorders in pregnancy.* New York: Appleton-Century-Crofts, 1978;318–324.
98. Blackfan KD, Hamilton B. Uremia in acute glomerular nephritis: the cause and treatment in children. *Boston Med Surg J* 1925;193:617–628.
99. Winkler AW, Smith PK, Hoff HE. Intravenous magnesium sulfate in the treatment of nephritis convulsions in adults. *J Clin Invest* 1942;21:207–216.
100. Tsien RY. A nondisruptive technique for loading calcium buffers and indicators into cells. *Nature* 1981;290:527–528.
101. Horton R, Biglieri EG. Effects of aldosterone on the metabolism of magnesium. *J. Clin Endocrinol Metab* 1962;22:1187–1192.
102. Brautbar N, Massry S. Disorders of magnesium metabolism. In: Maxwell MH, Kleeman CR, Narins RG, eds. *Clinical disorders of fluid and electrolyte metabolism.* New York: McGraw-Hill, 1987;831–850.
103. Günthren T, Vormann J. Mg^{2+} efflux is accomplished by an amelioride sensitive Na^{+}/Mg^{2+} antiport. *Biochem Biophys Res Commun* 1985;130:540–545.
104. Feray JC, Garay R. An Na^{+}-stimulated Mg^{2+} transport system in human red blood cells. *Biochem Biophys Acta* 1986;856:76–84.
105. Agus ZA, Kalipourie E, Dukes I, Morad M. Cytosolic magnesium modulates calcium channel activity in mammalian ventricular cells. *Am J Physiol* 1989;256:C452–C455.
106. Ji BH, Erne P, Kiowski W, Bühler FR, Bolli P. Magnesium-induced vasodilation is comparable to that induced by calcium entry blockade, *J Hypertens* 1983;1(Suppl 2):368–371.
107. Zemel MB, Kraniak J, Standley PR, Sowers JR. Erythrocyte cation metabolism in salt-sensitive hypertensive blacks as affected by dietary sodium and calcium. *Am J Hypertens* 1988;1:386–392.
108. Bolowasch J, Kirkwood A, Miller C. Allosteric effects of Mg^{2+} on the gaiting of Ca^{2+}-activated K^{+} channels from mammalian skeletal muscle. *J Exp Biol* 1986;124:5–13.
109. Tsai MD, Drakenberg T, Thulin E, Foreen S. Is the binding of magnesium (II) to calmodilin significant? An investigation by magnesium-25 nuclear magnetic resonance. *Biochemistry* 1987;26:3635–3643.
110. Haselback W, Fassold E, Migola A, Rauch B. Magnesium dependence of sarcoplasmic reticulum calcium transport. *Fed Proc* 1981;40:2657–2661.
111. Altura BM, Altura BT. Magnesium ions and contraction of vascular smooth muscles: relationship to some vascular diseases. *Fed Proc* 1981;40:2672–2679.
112. Stephenson EW. Magnesium effects on activation of skinned fibers from striated muscle. *Fed Proc* 1981;40:2662–2666.
113. Somlyo AP, Somlyo AV. Effects and subcellular distribution of magnesium in smooth and striated muscle. *Fed Proc* 1981; 210:2667–2671.
114. Altura BM, Altura BT, Gebrewold A, Ising H, Güntter T. Magnesium deficiency and hypertension: correlation between magnesium deficient diets and microcirculatory changes *in situ. Science* 1984;223:1415–1317.
115. Berthelot A, Espisito J. Effects of dietary magnesium on the development of hypertension in the spontaneously hypertensive rat. *J Am Coll Nutr* 1983;4:343–353.
116. Walker BS, Walker DW. Normal magnesium metabolism and its significant disturbances. *J Lab Clin Med* 1936;21:713–720.
117. Albert DG, Morita Y, Iseri LT. Serum magnesium and plasma sodium levels in essential vascular hypertension. *Circulation* 1958;17:761–764.
118. Petersen B, Schroll M, Christiansen C, Tranavol I. Serum and erythrocyte magnesium in normal elderly Danish people. *Acta Med Scand* 1977;201:31–34.
119. McCarron DA, Morris CD, Cile C. Dietary calcium vs human hypertension. *Science* 1982;217:267–269.
120. Joffres MR, Reed DM, Yano K. Relationship of magnesium intake and dietary factors to blood pressure: the Honolulu Heart Study. *Am J Clin Nutr* 1987;45:459–475.
121. Witteman JCM, Willett WC, Stampfer MJ, Colditz GA, Sacks FM, Rosner B, Speizer FE, Hennekens CH. Dietary calcium and magnesium and hypertension: a prospective study [Abstract]. *Circulation* 1987;76(Suppl IV):35.
122. Dawson MJ, McFarlene DK, McFarlin GL, Nouszeski EA, Trupin SR. The biochemistry of female reproductive tissues studied by ^{31}phosphorus nuclear magnetic resonance spectroscopy: effects of pregnancy, hormonal manipulation, and disease. *Biol Reprod* 1988;38:31–38.
123. Maturra T, Kihno M, Kanayama Y, Yasunari K, Murahawa K,

Takeda T, Ischimiri K, Morihima I, Yongawa T. Decreased intracellular free magnesium in erythrocytes of spontaneously hypertensive rats. *Biochm Biophys Res Commun* 1987;143:1012–1017.

124. Resnick LM, Gupta RK, Sosa RE, Corbett ML, Seaby JE, Laragh JH. Effects of altered calcium intake in experimental hypertension: role of intracellular free magnesium. *J Hypertens* 1986;4(Suppl 5):S182–S185.

125. Lazard EM. Analysis of 575 cases of eclampsia and pre-eclampsia toxemias treated by intravenous injection of magnesium sulfate. *Am J Obstet Gynecol* 1933;25:647–656.

126. Nadler JL, Goodson S, Rude RK. Evidence that prostacyclin mediates the vascular action of magnesium in humans. *Hypertension* 1987;9:378–383.

127. Reyes AJ, Leary WP, Acosta-Barrios TN, Cavis WH. Magnesium supplementation in hypertension treated with hydrochlorothiazide. *Curr Ther Res* 1984;36:2.

128. Dyckner T, Wester PO. Effects of magnesium on blood pressure. *Br Med J* 1983;286:1847–1849.

129. Cappuccio FP, Markandu ND, Beynon GW, Shore AC, Sampson B, MacGregor GA. Lack of effect of oral magnesium on high blood pressure; a double-blind study. *Br Med J* 1985;291:235–238.

130. Henderson DG, Scherys J, Schott T. Effect of magnesium supplementation on blood pressure and electrolyte concentrations in hypertensive patients receiving long-term diuretic treatment. *Br Med J* 1986;293:664–665.

131. Resnick LM, Gupta RK, Gruenspan H, Laragh JH. Intracellular free magnesium in hypertension: relation to peripheral insulin resistance and obesity. *Clin Res* 1988;35:431A.

Hypertension: Pathophysiology, Diagnosis, and Management, edited by J. H. Laragh and B. M. Brenner. Raven Press, Ltd., New York © 1990.

CHAPTER 130

Nursing Management of the Hypertensive Patient

RoseMerie Marion and Carolyn Ryan

Captopril Test, 2061
Renal Vein Renins and Digital Intravenous Angiogram, 2062
Medication, 2063
Accurate Blood Pressure Measurement, 2064
Measurement in the Clinic, 2064
Home Blood Pressure Readings, 2065
Nonpharmacologic Therapies, 2066
Weight Reduction, 2066
Restriction of Alcohol Use, 2066
Smoking Cessation, 2066
Exercise, 2067
Other Techniques, 2067
Psychosocial Factors in Hypertension, 2068
Conclusions, 2069
References, 2069

The main objective of this chapter is to present a teaching tool that will assist nurses in the care and management of the hypertensive patient.

The earlier chapters in this book have described the physiological characteristics of hypertension and have also described its various types and causes, both primary and secondary. We wish to elaborate further by discussing the total care of the hypertensive patient, based on a common-sense approach. We will describe the proper techniques for performing various studies and will also describe the important role of the nurse as patient advocate in a field where various alternatives are ever present.

Establishing the type of hypertension the patient may have is the first step in managing the hypertensive patient. Eighty-five percent of all hypertensives have *essential hypertension;* the other 15% have what is referred to as *secondary hypertension* (1).

To distinguish the various types of hypertension that may be present it is best to begin with two simple diagnostic measures, the renin–sodium and aldosterone–sodium profile tests (2). These tests help to identify the several different biochemical disorders that may contribute to hypertension. They assess and compare the levels of plasma renin and urine aldosterone against the amount of sodium excreted in a 24-hr urine collection (2). Patients may then be categorized into low-renin, medium-renin, or high-renin subgroups (3). Knowledge of a patient's renin subgroup can help the physician to predict which type of medication will be most effective in controlling the patient's blood pressure (3).

Renin–sodium and aldosterone–sodium profiling may also determine whether or not further investigation is needed to diagnose secondary forms of hypertension such as primary aldosteronism or renovascular hypertension (4). It is extremely important to achieve an accurate diagnosis of a secondary cause for hypertension because a complete cure for such hypertension is now possible and may obviate the need for a lifetime of medication.

Some of the most important procedures used in properly diagnosing a secondary form of hypertension are the captopril test, renal vein renins, and digital angiograms (4). Because the nurse is directly involved in these three kinds of tests, they will be described in detail.

CAPTOPRIL TEST

The captopril test is used as a screening device to identify renovascular hypertension. Although only 5% of the total hypertensive population may have renovascular hypertension (5), it is a potentially curable form of the disorder.

With proper instructions to the patient, as well as strict adherence to the following methods, the captopril test can be done simply, safely, and accurately in either a clinic or a physician's office.

The captopril test is most useful when it is performed on an unmedicated patient whose plasma renin value is 2.6 ng/ml/hr or higher (5), whose hypertension is of recent onset or in whom an existing hypertension has accelerated, who is relatively young (i.e., 20–50 years old), and who has an abdominal bruit and a history of smoking (6). In the younger age groups, more women than men have renovascular disease, and it is rare among blacks (7).

Ideally, the patient should be off all medications, including vitamins, antihistamines, and any other over-the-counter medication, for at least 3 weeks prior to the test. This is because medications may influence the secretion of renin and thus affect the interpretation of the test results (2). It is particularly important that the patient be off diuretics prior to receiving the first dose of captopril. Precipitous falls in blood pressure have been noted in patients who are taking diuretics at the time captopril is administered (8).

The patient should not be salt depleted and is instructed to follow a normal salt diet (120–150 mEq/Na) in preparation for this procedure (5). This is necessary not only to avoid false-positive results but also to avoid an extremely hypotensive response to captopril in the presence of salt depletion (9). If a patient has renal impairment, such a response could conceivably compromise the kidney.

A 24-hr urine is collected preceding the captopril test. The patient is instructed to collect the urine in a clean plastic or glass bottle. No preservatives are added to this collection. The collection is begun after the patient has emptied her or his bladder into the toilet upon arising the day before the test. Then every drop of urine is saved and refrigerated, when possible, for the next 24 hr. The last sample is the first morning void on the day of the captopril test (2).

The captopril test takes 90 min. The following is a detailed description of how the test is performed:

1. The patient fasts for 2 hr.
2. The patient remains in a seated position and in a quiet setting. Conversation should be limited during the test, since this may influence blood pressure response.
3. Prior to receiving captopril and over a period of 30 min, several control blood pressures are taken.
4. Ideally, a 0.9% normal saline intravenous infusion with a stopcock is inserted both for the withdrawal of blood samples and for use if a precipitous blood pressure fall occurs (8). Renin samples may be drawn by venipuncture if intravenous equipment is not available.
5. Two renin samples are drawn in 10-ml tubes that contain EDTA and should remain at room temperature. Chilling the sample causes inadvertent activation to prorenin, which could lead to unpredictable variations in the plasma renin value (1). These samples are drawn 30 min after the patient has been seated quietly, just prior to the patient receiving captopril, and again 60 min after the captopril is given.
6. Captopril (25 mg) is given orally, crushed, and dissolved in 30 ml of water to facilitate absorption.
7. Blood pressure is measured every 5 min for the remainder of the test.
8. Closely observe the patient for an extreme fall in blood pressure. If the patient experiences symptoms such as lightheadedness or pallor, be prepared to place the patient supine and rapidly increase intravenous fluids (8). If intravenous fluids are not available, the patient can be fed salty foods such as crackers and bouillon.

A number of criteria have been established to determine if a captopril test is positive. First, the renin values appear to be more powerful discriminators of a positive captopril test than are the blood pressure responses to captopril (10). This is not to say that the blood pressure responses are not important, but they are not the most sensitive and specific criteria for determining the results of this procedure. Most renovascular patients do experience a fall in blood pressure, but many people with essential hypertension also exhibit such a blood pressure drop (5).

In distinguishing patients with renovascular hypertension from those with essential hypertension, Müller's group evolved three specific criteria. They are (a) stimulated plasma renin activity of 12 ng/ml/hr or more, (b) absolute increase in plasma renin activity of 10 ng/ml/hr or more, and (c) percentage increase in plasma renin activity of 150% or more, or 400% or more if baseline plasma renin activity is less than 3 ng/ml/hr (5).

If a patient has renal impairment, however, or is taking other antihypertensive medications, these criteria are not appropriate. A complete analysis of the significance of the captopril test may be found in the chapter by Müller, entitled "Clinical Evaluation and Differential Diagnosis of the Patient with Hypertension."

RENAL VEIN RENINS AND DIGITAL INTRAVENOUS ANGIOGRAM

Renal vein renins and the digital intravenous angiogram are performed consecutively and, usually, on an outpatient basis. These tests are invasive procedures, and it would be an understatement to say that they may be anxiety provoking. As with any test, it is important to discuss with the patient and family members the length and purpose of the test, what the procedure involves, the risks posed by the test, and the care following the test.

The purpose of the renal vein renins and digital angiogram is simply to determine whether a blockage in either one or both renal arteries may be contributing to the patient's hypertension.

Candidates for these procedures have had a positive captopril test and have been screened for allergic reactions to contrast medium and given prophylactic antihistamines or steroids if deemed necessary (11). Azotemia, when present, precludes use of the digital intravenous angiogram because there is a risk of dye-induced nephrotoxicity (12). The patient should be off all medications except those considered essential. Special emphasis is placed on withholding aspirin and other products that contain acetylsalicylic acid because of aspirin's inhibitory action on platelet aggregation (13). Nonsteroidal anti-inflammatory agents such as ibuprofen and naproxen should also be withheld because they prolong bleeding time. Because the catheter entry is usually at the femoral vein site, development of a hematoma is another risk of these procedures (14). In practice, we have diminished this risk considerably by having the patient withhold both aspirin and nonsteroidal anti-inflammatory agents for 5 days prior to the test.

During the renin sampling there is a risk of arterial puncture. This occurs very infrequently; however, when it does, the patient must remain supine for 12 hr and stay overnight in the hospital for observation (14).

Because patients receive captopril during these tests, the use of diuretics and salt depletion should be avoided preceding these examinations (8,9).

On the day of the renal vein renins and digital angiogram, solid foods are withheld 6 hr prior to the procedure. It is important to have patients empty their bladder immediately prior to the test.

The procedures are performed under local anesthesia, and sampling of blood for renin levels from the renal veins and inferior vena cava is carried out before and after captopril administration (15). The digital angiogram follows the renin sampling to complete the combined study. The entire procedure takes approximately 2.5 hr and is carried out in a radiology suite.

Recommendations for care following the renal vein renins and digital angiogram may be found in Table 1.

Upon discharge from the outpatient facility, the patient should be instructed to drink several glasses of fluid to facilitate excretion of the dye.

Bleeding from the catheter site is very rare after discharge but occasionally does occur. The patient should be discouraged from driving and lifting heavy objects for 6 hr following the procedure in order to avoid this possibility. Instructions advising the patient to lie flat and apply pressure over the catheterization site if this complication occurs are also included in the postprocedure teaching.

The results of the digital angiogram are usually obtained the same day the test is performed; the results of the renal vein renins are not available for 3 days. If these tests are suggestive of renovascular hypertension, the patient is advised to undergo an inpatient arteriogram in order to confirm the diagnosis of renovascular hypertension; sometimes it will be necessary to perform percutaneous transluminal renal angioplasty or balloon dilation at the same time in order to alleviate the stenosis.

MEDICATION

Medications are prescribed in 74% of all patient visits in the United States, and the majority of these medications are antihypertensive drug agents (16). A major question to ask about these statistics is, Are patients safely taking their medication?

When a group of 41 patients were asked what they did if they forgot to take medication, nine patients denied forgetting, 22 said they skipped the dose, and six said they made up the missed dose the next time (17). None of the respondents reported having received instructions for taking medications from any health professional (17). Many subjects in this same study were unaware that various over-the-counter medications decrease the effectiveness of prescription drugs, and they were also unaware that they might risk harmful drug interactions by combining these different medications (17).

TABLE 1. *Nursing care following renal vein renins and digital angiogram*

1. Apply sandbag over catheterization site and observe site for bleeding or hematoma every 20 min.
2. Check blood pressure every 10 min for first hour, and then every 20 min for next hour.
3. Check pedal pulses every 20 min.
4. Infuse 1000 ml normal saline over recovery period to compensate for a possible fall in blood pressure (8, 9).
5. Encourage patient to drink and eat, once stabilized.
6. Slowly dangle and ambulate patient 2 hr after completion of procedure.
7. Patient is able to resume normal activities 24 hr after the procedure.

Patients must be made aware that many readily available nonprescription drugs, such as antihistamines, vitamins, analgesics, health food additives, and cathartics, are just as powerful as their prescription drugs and may interfere with the actions of the latter. An example that may be brought to a patient's attention is that even aspirin interferes with the natriuretic effect of spironolactone (18). A patient on this drug who is also taking 600 mg of aspirin a day is effectively blocking the antihypertensive and natriuretic effect of spironolactone.

It is naive, of course, to think that patients will stop taking over-the-counter medications, but they should be urged to at least inform their health care providers when they take any nonprescribed drug.

In one survey, only two-thirds of hypertensive patients were found to be taking their prescribed medications (19). The other one-third had discontinued medication primarily, they said, because of side effects, inconvenience, or expense (19).

Obviously, then, many patients are *not* taking their medication safely. Many feel worse after they begin antihypertensive treatment. Some patients are asked to make drastic changes in their lifestyles in order to meet a medication schedule without any type of education or assistance, and many have misconceptions about taking medications that are never confronted or dispelled.

One of the responsibilities patients must take in their own health care is that of knowing what medication they are taking and communicating with health practitioners about their general well-being while taking these medications.

This is not an easy task for many patients, and they must be instructed and supported in this area. Some feel embarrassed that they continually forget to take their medications, and a few think (incorrectly) that there are no alternatives to feeling "miserable" on medications. There certainly are alternatives, and there are "helpful hints" for patients to remember in taking their medication, but they have to be pointed out, discussed, reinforced, and reviewed.

Considering that the average physician's visit is only 9 min in length (16), time for patient discussion and education is very short. Therefore, the role of medication educator is assumed by the nurse.

The best way to begin is to obtain as thorough a drug history as possible and to evaluate what the patient is able to comprehend and retain, to assist in setting up a teaching plan (20).

The nurse should encourage the patient to have other family members participate in this aspect of care so that at home the patient may have needed support and reinforcement.

The patient's lifestyle (including eating, sleeping, work, and recreational habits) should be reviewed, and a drug regimen tailored to suit the patient's needs should be planned.

It is important to point out to the patient that if a specific medication does not work, whether it be due to side effects or ineffectiveness in lowering blood pressure, there are other choices and alternatives.

It is useful to add written information to oral instructions. Patients can refer to printed materials if specific questions arise (21). Whenever a new medication is prescribed, an answer guide (such as that outlined in Table 2) may be completed in order to assist the patient in understanding his or her own medication. Common-sense facts for all patients taking any kind of medication can be found in Table 3.

The patient should also be aware that the pharmacist is another person who can assist and answer questions concerning medication therapy and drug interactions. The patient should be encouraged to choose a pharmacist who is not only knowledgeable and approachable but who also keeps thorough records of all the patient's prescribed medications. Literature available in the library, bookstores, and drug package inserts are other sources to include in the patient's education.

In the end, for compliance with any therapy, a medication regimen must be compatible with a patient's lifestyle. Education, patient involvement, reinforcement, and continuity of care will greatly enhance adherence to prescribed regimens.

Most nurses are quite familiar with older antihypertensive agents such as beta-blockers, diuretics, vasodilators, centrally acting adrenergic inhibitors, and alpha$_1$-adrenergic blockers.

Recently, the angiotensin-converting-enzyme (ACE) inhibitors and calcium-channel blockers have been introduced, providing good results for the hypertensive patient. These drugs appear to have fewer side effects and to provide a better quality of life. Table 4 should familiarize the reader with these relatively new drugs.

ACCURATE BLOOD PRESSURE MEASUREMENT

Because of the great importance of accurate blood pressure measurement in the management of the hypertensive patient, some points for nurses to consider when taking the blood pressure or when instructing the patient who will be taking his or her own readings at home are briefly reviewed, including sources of erroneous readings.

TABLE 2. *Guide to use of new medication*

1. Name of drug.
2. Type of drug (e.g., blood pressure pill, antibiotic, blood thinner, etc.)
3. Schedule for taking medication (e.g., before or after meals), and suggestions for the best way for the patient to remember to take medication.
4. Side effects and what to do if they are experienced (e.g., call physician if sore throat erupts after beginning angiotensin-converting-enzyme inhibitor).
5. Food and drinks to avoid (e.g., whether alcohol may be taken and, if so, in what quantity).
6. What to do if dose is missed (e.g., do not double-up on a blood thinner).
7. Length of time for which medication should be taken (e.g.: antibiotics—entire amount prescribed; beta-blockers—do not stop abruptly).
8. When to call the physician (e.g., prior to stopping any medication, if unacceptable side effects occur, or if lifestyle is changed for the worse).

TABLE 3. *Facts all patients should know about medications*

1. Know the names of all medications you take, both prescribed and over-the-counter; inform your health care team of these.
2. Know your allergies and inform your physician, nurse, and pharmacist when obtaining a new medication.
3. Do not keep outdated drugs.
4. Know how to store medications; some must be kept out of sunlight or must be refrigerated.
5. Know how to take your medication, and keep a daily record of what you take.
6. Do not take anyone else's medication.
7. Inform your physician if medications are too expensive for you to buy (22).
8. Know the significant side effects of your medications, and call your physician if problems arise.

Measurement in the Clinic

Use of the proper cuff size is essential. Too small a cuff results in artificially high readings. The width of the bladder inside the cuff should be 40% of the arm circumference, and the length of the bladder should be 80% of the arm circumference (28).

Center the bladder correctly over the brachial artery. Fold the bladder in half for exact measurement, and then place the midpoint of the bladder directly over the brachial artery to ensure accurate readings.

Apply the cuff smoothly and firmly. A cuff applied too loosely results in higher readings. Constricting clothing above the cuff also interferes with accuracy.

Position the arm properly. The arm is supported at approximately heart level regardless of patient position, that is, supine, sitting, standing. A raised arm produces lower readings, whereas a lowered or dangling arm results in higher readings. The arm should be relaxed and supported palm up.

Inflation of the cuff should be smooth and rapid. Prolonged venous stasis (i.e., when cuff is inflated and deflated too slowly, or when cuff pressure not completely returned to zero before reinflation) results in falsely high values. The cuff is deflated 2–3 mm/sec. For successive measurements, allow 1–2 min between readings.

Diastolic blood pressure is read at the disappearance of sound (Korotkoff Phase V). If sound is heard to zero, use muffling of sound (Korotkoff Phase IV) as the diastolic reading. Sound heard to zero may occur in conditions such as severe anemia or aortic regurgitation, or after vigorous exercise.

Check for auscultatory gap, that is, after initial onset of sound, the sound disappears and then recurs at a lower level. To avoid overlooking an auscultatory gap, inflate the cuff until the radial pulse can no longer be palpated.

Because of the variability of blood pressure, take three readings to ensure validity. Record the position of the patient and the arm used for readings.

TABLE 4. *ACE inhibition and calcium antagonist therapy: nursing implications*

Drug	Side effects	Nursing considerations
ACE inhibitors Captopril Enalapril Lisinopril	Loss of taste Rash Cough Decreased white blood count Proteinuria Hyperkalemia Dizziness Fall in blood pressure will be increased by diuretics and dehydration (23,24)	1. Medication best absorbed on empty stomach. 2. White blood count with differential should be checked prior to therapy, 1–2 weeks after beginning medication, and every 3 months thereafter. 3. Patient should be advised to report any signs of infection, such as fever or sore throat. 4. Instruct patient not to take potassium supplements and salt alternatives, unless prescribed by physicians. 5. Advise patient that aspirin and other nonsteroidal anti-inflammatory drugs may reduce effectiveness of medication. 6. Screen patient carefully for diuretic use prior to beginning ACE inhibitor. 7. Advise patient to call physician if loss of taste or rash occurs. Decreasing dosage usually alleviates these problems (25).
Calcium-channel blockers Nifedipine Verapamil Diltiazem hydrochloride Nitrendipine	Tachycardia Constipation Edema Headache Dizziness Hypotension (26,27)	1. Recent electrocardiogram should be checked. Calcium-channel blockers are contraindicated in patients with second- or third-degree heart block. 2. Liver enzymes should be checked frequently. Drugs may cause liver dysfunction. 3. Use cautiously with beta-blockers. 4. Advise patient drugs may cause constipation. Diet manipulation or approved laxatives may alleviate problem. 5. Advise patient to report any noted edema, especially of ankles and feet. 6. Plasma digoxin levels may be increased by calcium-channel blockers.

When assessing the patient's blood pressure for the first time, take readings in both arms and use the higher arm for monitoring.

When obtaining supine blood pressure, the patient should be reclining for 5 min; when obtaining standing blood pressure, he or she should be standing for 2 min.

A cold environment, urinary distention, talking, or tense muscles (uncomfortable position of arm, anxiety) may all cause higher readings.

Home Blood Pressure Readings

Frequently in the management of the hypertensive patient the physician will determine that home blood pressure readings are desirable.

It has been shown that blood pressure varies considerably over a 24-hr period, being higher at work than at home or during sleep (pressure is lowest during sleep) (29). Blood pressure readings have been found to be higher when taken by a physician than when recorded at home (30). In addition ambulatory blood pressure monitoring has been found to be a better predictor of target organ damage and of future morbid events than are clinic pressures (31). Certainly, then, home blood pressure readings are helpful adjuncts to clinic readings.

Before initiating drug therapy, with its attendant side effects, it is prudent to determine whether the patient's blood pressure is high enough during normal daily activities to warrant medications. Home readings are also very useful in evaluating the response of the patient to medication if drug therapy is indicated.

Home blood pressure levels can be monitored either by use of a 24-hr automatic recorder or by teaching the patient to take his or her own blood pressure.

When teaching patients to take their own blood pressure, we prefer that the patient use a sphygmomanometer and stethoscope rather than relying on digital recorders designed for home use. It has been suggested that these machines may not be accurate in recording blood pressure levels (32). In those circumstances where digital home recorders must be used (hearing impairment, arthritis, patient refusal to use manual equipment), the recorders should be carefully and frequently checked against sphygmomanometer readings for proper function.

Patients tend to be quite anxious about their ability to learn to take their own blood pressure. The initial blood pressure that the patient hears is almost always high. "Sweaty palms" are literally the norm. The patient should be reassured that this is a response to anxiety and that most patients react in the same manner. The patient should also be assured that manipulation of the valve and equipment becomes smoother and easier with practice.

We routinely instruct the patient to take the blood pressure twice a day for 2 weeks. If readings are stable, then two readings per week thereafter are recommended. The patient is advised to take three readings at each sitting and to record all three results. Pulse and activity are also recorded at the time of the readings. The patient is taught to notify the physician of untoward readings or symptoms, including significant reportable parameters for his or her individual blood pressure levels.

Only if necessary is a family member taught to take the patient's blood pressure, since patients themselves are primarily responsible for their own health care.

NONPHARMACOLOGIC THERAPIES

Therapies involving alterations in behavior patterns may be included in the nursing management of the hypertensive patient. When we assess the patient for an individualized optimal plan of care, we consider risk factors such as obesity, sedentary lifestyle, smoking, and alcohol.

Weight Reduction

Obesity is a problem that requires serious attention in patients with hypertension. Numerous studies have demonstrated that weight loss is associated with decreased levels of blood pressure (33), as well as with a reduction in left ventricular mass (34). It is thought that obese patients with left ventricular hypertrophy are prone to ventricular arrhythmias (35). In addition, the combination of hypertension and obesity places a double burden on the heart and may result in premature congestive heart failure (35). The Framingham Study has associated obesity with an increased incidence of stroke and coronary disease (36). Therefore, each patient is evaluated for the necessity of including weight loss in the treatment regimen.

If weight reduction is indicated, the patient is not simply told to "lose weight" nor merely handed a list of low-calorie foods. Most people who are overweight have developed poor eating habits that are difficult to change. Fundamental to an acceptable diet plan is a review of what these eating patterns are, including food preferences and dislikes. Healthier appropriate substitutions can be made, and reasonable guidelines acceptable to the patient can be established. The eating patterns and caloric requirements of a taxi driver working nights will vary considerably from those of a woman employed in an active day-care center or of a traveling businessman who frequently dines out.

Compliance with any diet program is a daunting task. Motivation may be high, as everyone wishes to be "rich and thin." Many patients lose excess weight initially but are less successful in maintaining an optimal weight. A nutritionist may be consulted to assist in planning a more flexible diet and to work with the patient in identifying and correcting detrimental eating patterns.

The patient is taught that a gradual one- or two-pound weight loss per week will ensure more permanent results than a "fad" or "crash" diet that may actually be quite dangerous. Electrolyte imbalance leading to life-threatening arrhythmias as well as other metabolic damage may occur. Patients are cautioned against the use of diuretics to induce weight loss. Over-the-counter appetite suppressants may contain substances such as phenylpropanolamine, which can increase blood pressure levels.

Depending on the amount of weight to be lost, selected professional or commercial weight reduction programs may be helpful, but these must be very carefully screened for legitimacy and medical supervision. Again, behavior patterns must be changed or the patient may regain weight once he or she leaves the program and group support is no longer available.

The dietary management of hypertension may include a low-salt diet. Sodium restriction is not recommended for every patient with hypertension. Only 30–50% of patients with hypertension are sodium sensitive (37). In some instances, severe salt restriction may not only be ineffective but may also cause untoward effects (37). The efficacy of sodium restriction is discussed in the chapter by Simpson, entitled "Hypertension and Sodium Intake", as well as in the chapter by Swales, entitled "Dietary Sodium Restriction in Hypertension."

The role of minerals such as calcium, magnesium, and potassium in lowering blood pressure is currently being investigated.

Restriction of Alcohol Use

Reduction of alcohol intake is another important consideration when planning a comprehensive treatment regimen for the hypertensive patient. Careful screening for each patient's daily alcohol consumption is required. Studies have documented significant increases in systolic and diastolic blood pressure in people consuming five or six drinks per day. Blood pressure has been shown to increase in proportion to the amount of alcohol consumed at levels greater than two drinks per day (38). Pressor effects of alcohol have been found in both untreated (39) and treated patients with hypertension. Regular intake of approximately six drinks per day reduces the effectiveness of antihypertensive medication (40).

Among men, the risk of stroke was found to be four times higher in heavy drinkers than in nondrinkers (41). Just as obesity and hypertension place a double burden on the heart, excessive alcohol intake combined with hypertension may conceivably increase the risk for stroke. Studies of the effects of alcohol on blood pressure and stroke relate more strongly to men than to women, for unknown reasons. A recent study has suggested that "among middle-aged women, moderate alcohol consumption decreases the risk of coronary heart disease and ischemic stroke but may increase the risk of subarachnoid hemorrhage" (42).

Thus, in guiding the hypertensive patient toward healthier dietary habits, the use of alcohol is discouraged. If such a restriction is unacceptable to the patient, limiting alcohol consumption to one to two drinks per day is advised.

Smoking Cessation

Yet another concern in establishing a treatment plan for the hypertensive patient is smoking. As is well known, hypertension itself greatly increases the risk of stroke; it is the major risk factor in 80% of all strokes (43). In addition, smoking is an independent risk factor for stroke, particularly brain infarction (44). The risk of stroke has been found to increase as the number of cigarettes smoked increases (44). Stopping smoking, or at least reducing the number of cigarettes smoked per day, is therefore strongly indicated for the patient with hypertension.

Other serious, even dire, cardiovascular consequences of smoking have been documented. Smoking doubles the risk for myocardial infarction as well as for stroke, possibly due to increased platelet aggregation (45). Smoking greatly increases the risk of sudden death at a young age in persons who smoke more than one pack of cigarettes per day (43). Smoking increases heart rate and the incidence of premature ventricular arrhythmias (45). Between 80% and 90% of patients with atherosclerotic renovascular hypertension have been found to be cigarette smokers (46).

Recent studies have shown that cigarette smoking reduces the efficacy of beta-blockers (particularly propranolol) in preventing strokes (47) and decreases the blood-pressure-lowering effects of some beta-blockers in patients on long-term therapy (48). Smoking may also interfere with the beneficial effects of beta-blockers in patients with angina (45).

The risks for stroke and coronary heart disease are reversible (43,44) in persons who stop smoking. Thus, counseling the patient to stop may be the most important treatment modality in the nursing care of the patient with hypertension. Patients who smoke find it extremely difficult to stop, possibly because of the addictive or psychosocial factors involved in smoking. The American Cancer Society pamphlet, *Quitter's Guide,* identifies some of these factors and offers self-help suggestions for stopping smoking. Hypnosis, self-help groups, use of nicotine gum in the appropriate dosage, and behavior modification programs may all be attempted. Smoking filter cigarettes does not lower the incidence of coronary heart disease when compared with smoking nonfilter cigarettes (49) and is therefore not a useful option. Unperforated filter cigarettes that produce lower levels of tar and nicotine may produce higher levels of carbon monoxide, severely reducing oxygen delivery to the myocardium (49).

When assisting patients to devise strategies for stopping smoking or for reducing the number of cigarettes smoked (by patients who cannot stop), it is important to include preventive aspects. Patients can be encouraged to teach their children about the many health hazards associated with cigarette smoking and about the difficulties encountered when attempting to stop smoking.

Exercise

Aerobic exercise had been found to be effective in lowering blood pressure in some individuals with hypertension. Studies have shown that in sedentary patients with mild to moderate hypertension, regular exercise has resulted in long-term lowering of blood pressure (50). Also, plasma catecholamine levels are reduced with regular moderate exercise (51). A reduction in sympathetic nervous system activity would be of special benefit to the anxious hypertensive patient with cardiovascular hyperreactivity. A further consideration in motivating patients to exercise is the finding that lower levels of physical fitness are associated with increased incidence of coronary disease as well as a somewhat higher risk of developing hypertension when compared with fit persons (52). Regular aerobic exercise increases lipid metabolism and may be a positive adjunct to weight loss in the hypertensive patient's treatment plan.

Any exercise regimen undertaken by the patient must be approved by the physician, who should determine a tolerable level of activity based on the patient's overall physical condition and blood pressure levels. Some hypertensive patients have expressed concern that they may have a stroke while exercising. In general, vigorous exercise has not been found to be a precipitating factor in cerebral vascular events (53,54). However, isometric or anaerobic exercises such as weight lifting, a favorite among young male hypertensives, may cause a rise in blood pressure and are not usually recommended.

Bicycling, jogging, swimming, and brisk walking are all acceptable forms of exercise, depending on patient inclination and tolerance. Some patients who exercise vigorously and are on concomitant drug therapy are cautioned to increase salt intake if lightheadedness occurs because of excessive perspiration. Also, patients must be cautioned to report to the physician any unusual symptoms that occur during any type of exercise program. Symptoms such as dyspnea, mild chest pressure, epigastric discomfort, headache, and excessive fatigue may be underestimated or denied, resulting in serious consequences (55).

All patients embarking on an exercise program at whatever level are advised to begin slowly and to work gradually up to maximal tolerated levels. As with most regimens involving behavioral changes, perseverance may be enhanced by joining a reputable health club or recruiting family or friends to participate.

Table 5 offers an example of a walking program published by the American Heart Association that can be undertaken by most patients. Patients can proceed at their own rates, repeating any week that is found to be more strenuous than anticipated. A specific written program may induce more compliance than simply being advised to "go out and walk more."

Other Techniques

Relaxation therapies involving biofeedback, meditation, and muscle or breathing exercises have been employed in the management of hypertensive patients. Some studies (56,57) have indicated that relaxation training results in systolic and diastolic blood pressure reductions in some patients with hypertension. Immediate effects of biofeedback training have been likened to the effects of beta-adrenoreceptor blockade, producing at least short-term reduction in arterial blood pressure in borderline hypertension (58). It has been demonstrated that relaxation techniques result in a reduction of sympathetic nervous system activity and may be useful in the alleviation of stress and anxiety (59).

Training periods for some of these therapies may be long, and compliance may be difficult; in addition, some controversy remains regarding long-term effects. However, enough evidence of positive results exists to warrant recommending these therapies for the treatment of mild hypertension to forestall the need for drug treatment. These techniques may also be useful as an adjunct to drug therapy for the hypertensive patient who is difficult to control (60). A reduction in the amount of drug required to maintain blood pressure at acceptable levels may be another positive outcome.

Practicing simple relaxation techniques for 15–20 min twice a day in a quiet comfortable setting has been advocated and may have preventive as well as therapeutic bene-

TABLE 5. *Sample walking program*[a]

	Warm up	Target-zone exercising	Cool down	Total time
Week 1				
Session A	Walk slowly for 5 min	Walk briskly for 5 min	Walk slowly for 5 min	15 min
Session B	Repeat above pattern			
Session C	Repeat above pattern			
Continue with at least three exercise sessions during each week of the program.				
Week 2	Walk slowly for 5 min	Walk briskly for 7 min	Walk slowly for 5 min	17 min
Week 3	Walk slowly for 5 min	Walk briskly for 9 min	Walk slowly for 5 min	19 min
Week 4	Walk slowly for 5 min	Walk briskly for 11 min	Walk slowly for 5 min	21 min
Week 5	Walk slowly for 5 min	Walk briskly for 13 min	Walk slowly for 5 min	23 min
Week 6	Walk slowly for 5 min	Walk briskly for 15 min	Walk slowly for 5 min	25 min
Week 7	Walk slowly for 5 min	Walk briskly for 18 min	Walk slowly for 5 min	28 min
Week 8	Walk slowly for 5 min	Walk briskly for 20 min	Walk slowly for 5 min	30 min
Week 9	Walk slowly for 5 min	Walk briskly for 23 min	Walk slowly for 5 min	33 min
Week 10	Walk slowly for 5 min	Walk briskly for 26 min	Walk slowly for 5 min	36 min
Week 11	Walk slowly for 5 min	Walk briskly for 28 min	Walk slowly for 5 min	38 min
Week 12	Walk slowly for 5 min	Walk briskly for 30 min	Walk slowly for 5 min	40 min
Week 13 and thereafter: Check your pulse periodically to see if you are exercising within your target zone. As you get more in shape, try exercising within the upper range of your heart zone. Remember that your goal is to continue getting the benefits you are seeking and to enjoy your activity.				

[a] From ref. 77. If you find a particular weeks' pattern tiring, repeat it before going on to the next pattern. You do not have to complete the walking program in 12 weeks.

fits (59). Such a regimen may be introduced with some degree of ease into the patient's normal daily routine.

All behavioral therapies are not suitable for all patients. Careful assessment of the patient's needs, attitudes, and response is required. Each patient is unique, with a variety of genetic, physiological, environmental, and psychological influences that affect his or her blood pressure. Identifying which therapies are appropriate and acceptable to the patient is essential. Many times it is a question of trial and error. Some very anxious patients have tried so hard to "relax" that blood pressure actually rises. Another consideration is the plethora of self-help books, self-interest groups, and media advice that are currently available. It is necessary to assist the patient to sift through these choices for validity and safety. A combination of therapies may work best for some patients.

When planning any treatment regimen, the patient must understand that there are no quick fixes—i.e., that optimal control of blood pressure requires a long-term commitment. Soliciting the support of family or friends is most important in motivating the patient to incorporate any treatment modalities into his or her way of life. Family members and associates may be of assistance in altering dietary habits or in undertaking exercise regimens. Or, they may simply cooperate with efforts by the patient to reduce the amount of stress at work or at home.

PSYCHOSOCIAL FACTORS IN HYPERTENSION

The psychosocial aspects of hypertension are the most difficult to manage and frequently tend to be overlooked in caring for the patient with elevated blood pressure. Because of the time and effort required to address these aspects of patient care they are often ignored. It is a great deal easier to dispense blood pressure medication than it is to explore or alter deeply rooted behavioral patterns, psychological make-up, or elements in the patient's environment that are stressful to him or her.

Although psychosocial factors are not the sole cause, they may certainly contribute to elevated blood pressures in a significant number of patients. Assisting the patient to deal with these factors may ensure better control of blood pressure levels and may contribute to a reduction in the amount of medication required.

Many studies have been conducted over the years in an effort to determine exactly what role psychosocial factors play in inducing and sustaining elevated levels of blood pressure. That these factors do have an effect should no longer be in doubt, although many elements, such as genetic predisposition and diet, may combine to contribute to elevated pressures. The data remain speculative because of the difficulty in measuring these factors.

Behavioral stressors are thought to affect the action of the kidneys in influencing blood pressure (61) and also to affect the central nervous system, thereby eliciting neurohormonal responses to raise blood pressure levels (62). Persons with a positive family history for hypertension have been shown to have greater cardiovascular hyperresponsivity to behavioral stressors than do normotensive individuals (63). Controlling these stressors would certainly be indicated in the preventive care of the patient with hypertension.

There seems to be no specific personality type among hypertensive patients. Very early writings associate irritability, tension, and worry (64), as well as passive–aggressive behavior, with hypertensive patients (65). Numerous, more recent studies have shown a significant relationship between borderline hypertension and suppressed anger or hostility (66–68), although the mechanism of this relationship is still not established. We have observed that a number of our patients exhibit behavioral tendencies of impatience, anxiety, and rigidity.

It has been suggested that there are subtle behavioral deficits in the untreated mild hypertensive patient, although these do not appear to interfere with normal activities of daily life. Some patients tend to be slower and less accurate in tests involving psychomotor, cognitive, and sensory-perceptual (69) tasks. These deficits may be restored with successful treatment of the elevated blood pressure (70).

Still other psychosocial influences have been implicated in the incidence of hypertension. These include (a) the effects of modernization or of material success or the lack of it and (b) media-induced, unattainable expectations (71). Job stressors and dissatisfactions have also been linked with sustained hypertension in susceptible people (72,73).

Because of health organization emphasis on hypertension and its alarming sequelae via television, magazine articles, and screening programs, the public has been exposed to a great deal of anxiety-producing information about high blood pressure. Each individual patient presents with preconceived ideas of what it means to have hypertension and how it will affect his or her life. It is mandatory in treating each patient to first explore what these notions are and then to correct frequently held false impressions by replacing them with accurate information about this very treatable health problem.

The concerns and fears of the patient can be explored concurrently by the nurse during the several visits to the physician that are necessary to establish (a) whether or not hypertension truly exists, (b) what type it is, and (c) what kind of therapy will be most effective.

Patients present with a wide variety of responses to the diagnosis of hypertension. Some patients express anger and frustration because they feel they have "done everything right"—that is, they are nonsmokers and they follow a salt-restricted diet, exercise, and maintain a reasonable weight yet they have still developed hypertension. Others concentrate on numbers, taking blood pressure readings several times a day at home. Still others are so frightened about dying, having a stroke, or a heart attack that they are reluctant to face their health problem. Some patients feel they are becoming "hypochondriacs," attaching undue significance to "every little symptom." Feelings that "it is my fault for having high blood pressure because I cannot control my stress" have been expressed, as well as feeling "shaky and out of control." These are but a few of the wide-ranging patient reactions to the diagnosis of high blood pressure.

In addition, several studies have been undertaken to examine the effects of being labeled as hypertensive. Increased absenteeism from work, less earning capacity (74), diminished feelings of health and well being (75), poorer self-image, and decreased marital adjustment have all been associated with patient reactions to the diagnosis of hypertension (76). Further investigation is necessary to verify some of these relationships, but each patient must be assessed for any untoward psychosocial effects. Identifying and assisting the patient to cope with these effects is basic to the care of patients with hypertension.

The primary objective of nursing care is a well-adjusted patient whose blood pressure levels are well controlled. Essential to the success of any treatment plan for the patient is an understanding and acceptance of the diagnosis. Patients should know what hypertension is and should understand that control of blood pressure requires a lifelong commitment. They must be aware that the consequence of neglect is target-organ damage. The kinds of information given will depend upon the patient's temperament, intellectual capacity, and level of anxiety.

In a quiet setting, the nurse provides the opportunity to discuss any concerns that the patient may have. Reasonable, attainable goals determined by the lifestyle and habits of the patient are planned. The channeling of stress into healthy outlets is discussed. Ways to reduce stressors in the work or home environment are explored. This process is effectuated over many visits. Explanations of any events related to therapy or diagnostic tests are provided. Some patients may benefit from participating in group therapy focusing on problems of patients with hypertension.

Because of our society's current emphasis on fitness and health, patients' self-esteem may plummet when they are confronted with a major health problem. Although hypertension is usually asymptomatic, much reassurance, re-explanation, and support are necessary in order to help the patient feel "well" again. It is imperative to restore the patient's confidence that he or she can lead a healthy, productive life.

CONCLUSIONS

The nurse's role in the management of the hypertensive patient is all-encompassing. We see the patient for the longest periods of time and act as coordinators of their care. As resource persons, we answer their questions and act as confidants. We perform diagnostic tests and identify problems. We educate, evaluate, and assess compliance with therapy as well as response to it.

The field of hypertension has been changing rapidly, from the introduction of new medications to the discovery of new diagnostic techniques and the increased awareness of the efficacy of behavioral therapies. Exciting new concepts concerning minerals and their effect on blood pressure are also evolving. Research continues into the role of vitamins, peptides, and hormones in regulating blood pressure.

The nurse is in a unique position to inform and instruct the public about the many therapeutic choices available in the constantly expanding field of hypertension.

REFERENCES

1. Laragh JH. Renovascular hypertension: a paradigm for all hypertension. *J Hypertens* 1986;Suppl 4:S79–S88.
2. Laragh JH, Sealey JE. Renin–sodium profiling: why, how, and when in clinical practice. *Cardiovasc Med* 1977;2(11):1058–1075.
3. Case DB, Wallace JM, Keim H, Weber M, Sealey JE, Laragh JH. Possible role of renin in hypertension as suggested by renin–sodium profiling and inhibition of converting enzyme. *N Engl J Med* 1977;296:641–646.
4. Laragh JH. Hypertension, the silent killer. *Health and medical horizons.* New York: Macmillan, 1988;144–151.
5. Müller FB, Sealey JE, Case DB, Atlas SA, Pickering TG. The

captopril test for identifying renovascular disease in hypertensive patients. *Am J Med* 1986;80:663–644.
6. Maxwell MH, Blufer KH, Franklin SS, Varady P. Cooperative study of renovascular hypertension. *JAMA* 1972;220:1195–1204.
7. Keith T. Renovascular hypertension in black patients. *Hypertension* 1982;4:438–443.
8. Case DB, Atlas SA, Laragh JH, Sullivan PA, McKinstry DN. Clinical experience with blockade of the renin–angiotensin–aldosterone system by an oral converting enzyme inhibitor (captopril) in hypertensive patients. *Prog Cardiovasc Dis* 1978;21:195–206.
9. Case DB, Laragh JH. Reactive hyper-reninemia in renovascular hypertension after angiotensin blockade with saralasin or converting enzyme inhibitor. *Ann Intern Med* 1979;91:153–160.
10. Case DB, Atlas SA, Laragh JH. Reactive hyperreninaemia to angiotensin blockade identifies renovascular hypertension. *Clin Sci* 1979;57:3135–3165.
11. Newton K. Cardiac catheterization. *Cardiac nursing.* Philadelphia: Lippincott, 1982.
12. Pickering T, Sos T. Overview: medical aspects of renal angioplasty. *Renovascular hypertension.* New York: Raven Press, 1987.
13. DeGaetano G, Cerlitti C, DeJana E, Latini R. Pharmacology of platelet inhibition in humans: implications of the salicylate–aspirin interaction. *Circulation* 1985;72(6):1185–1193.
14. Johnsrude I. *A practical approach to angiography.* Boston: Little, Brown, 1979.
15. Sos T, Vaughan D, Pickering T, Case D, Sneiderman T, Sealey J, Laragh J. Diagnosis of renovascular hypertension and evaluation of surgical curability. *Urol Radiol* 1982;3:199–203.
16. *The national ambulatory care in general and family practice: United States 1980–1981* (Vital and Health Statistics, Series 13). Hyattsville, MD: National Center for Health Statistics, September 1983.
17. Ellor J, Kurz D. Misuse and abuse of prescription and nonprescription drugs by the elderly. *Nurs Clin North Am* 1982;17(2):319–325.
18. Tweeddale M, O'Gilvie R. Antagonism of spironolactone-induced natriuresis by aspirin in man. *N Engl J Med* 1973;289(4):198–200.
19. Eraker SA, Kerscht JP, Becker MH. Understanding and improving patient compliance. *Ann Intern Med* 1984;100:258–268.
20. Grancio S. Opportunities for nurses in high blood pressure control. *Nurs Clin North Am* 1981;16(2):309–320.
21. Wiederholt J, Kotzan J. Effectiveness of the FDA-designed patient package insert for benzodiazepines. *Am J Hosp Pharm* 1983;40:828–834.
22. Schulman BN, Martinez B, Brogan D. Financial cost as an obstacle to hypertension therapy. *Am J Public Health* 1986;76(9): 1105–1108.
23. Irwin J, Viau J. Safety profiles of the angiotensin converting enzyme inhibitors: captopril and enalapril. *Am J Med* 1986;81(4C):45–50.
24. Morlin C. Comparative trial of lisinopril and nifedipine in mild to severe essential hypertension. *J Cardiovasc Pharmacol* 1987;9(3):S49–S52.
25. Case D, Atlas S, Marion R, Laragh J. Long term efficacy of captopril in renovascular and essential hypertension. *Am J Cardiol* 1982;49:1440–1445.
26. Schulte KL, Sabellek WA, Haertenberger A, Thiede H, Roecker L, Distler A, Gotzen R. Antihypertensive and metabolic effects of diltiazem and nifedipine. *Hypertension* 1986;8(10):859–865.
27. Hamilton H. *Nursing '87 drug handbook.* Springhouse, PA: Springhouse, 1987.
28. Frolich ED, Grim C, Labarthe DR, Maxwell MH, Perloff D, Weidman WH. *Recommendations for human blood pressure determinations by sphygmomanometers.* American Heart Association Pamphlet, 1987. New York: AHA.
29. Pickering TG, Harshfield GA, Kleinert HD, Blank S, Laragh JH. Blood pressure during normal daily activities, sleep, and exercise. *JAMA* 1982;247:992–996.
30. Kleinert HD, Harshfield GA, Pickering TG, et al. What is the value of home blood pressure measurement in patients with mild hypertension? *Hypertension* 1984;6:574–578.
31. Pickering TG, Harshfield GA, Devereux RB, Laragh JH. What is the role of ambulatory blood pressure monitoring in the management of hypertensive patients? *Hypertension* 1985;7:171–177.
32. Pickering TG, Cvetkovski B, James GD. An evaluation of electronic recorders for self-monitoring of blood pressure. *J Hypertens* 1986;4(Suppl 5):S328–S300.
33. Reisin E, Abel R, Modan M. Effect of weight loss without salt restriction on the reduction of blood pressure in overweight hypertensive patients. *N Engl J Med* 1978;298:1–6.
34. MacMahon SW, Wilcken DEL, MacDonald GJ. The effect of weight reduction on left ventricular mass: a randomized controlled trial in young overweight hypertensive patients. *N Engl J Med* 1986;314:334–339.
35. Messerli FH. Cardiopathy of obesity—a not-so-Victorian disease. *N Engl J Med* 1986;314:378–380.
36. Hubert HB, Feinleib N, McNamara PM, Castelli WP. Obesity as an independent risk factor for cardiovascular disease: a 26-year follow-up of participants in the Framingham Heart Study. *Circulation* 1983;67(5):968–977.
37. Laragh JH, Pecker MS. Dietary sodium and essential hypertension: some myths, hopes and truths. *Ann Intern Med* 1983;98(P2):735–743.
38. MacMahon SW, Norton RN. Alcohol and hypertension: implications for prevention and treatment. *Ann Intern Med* 1986;105: 124–126.
39. Potter JF, Beevers DG. Pressor effect of alcohol in hypertension. *Lancet* 1984;1:119–122.
40. Puddey IB, Beilin LJ, Vandongen R. Regular alcohol use raises blood pressure in treated hypertensive subjects. *Lancet* 1987;1:647–651.
41. Gill JS, Zezulka AV, Shipley MJ, Beevers DG. Stroke and alcohol consumption. *N Engl J Med* 1986;315:1041–1046.
42. Stampfer MJ, Colditz GA, Willett WC, Speizer FE, Hennekens CH. A prospective study of moderate alcohol consumption and the risk of coronary disease and stroke in women. *N Engl J Med* 1988;319:267–273.
43. Castelli WP. Cardiovascular disease and multifactorial risk: challenge of the 1980s. *Am Heart J* 1983;106:1191–1200.
44. Wolf PA, D'Agostino RB, Kannel WB, Bonita R, Belanger AJ. Cigarette smoking as a risk factor for stroke. The Framingham Study. *JAMA* 1988;259(7):1025–1029.
45. Buhler FR, Vesanen K, Watters JT, Bolli P. Impact of smoking on heart attacks, strokes, blood pressure control, drug dose, and quality of life aspects in the International Prospective Primary Prevention Study in Hypertension. *Am Heart J* 1988;115:282–286.
46. Working Group on Renovascular Hypertension, National Institutes of Health. Detection, evaluation, and treatment of renovascular hypertension. *Arch Intern Med* 1987;147:820–829.
47. Dollery C, Brennan PJ. The Medical Research Council hypertension trial: the smoking patient. *Am Heart J* 1988;115:276–281.
48. Trap-Jensen J. Effects of smoking on the heart and peripheral circulation. *Am Heart J* 1988;115:263–267.
49. Castelli BP, Dawber TR, Feinleib M, Garrison RJ, McNamara PM, Kannel WB. The filter cigarette and coronary heart disease: the Framingham Study. *Lancet* 1981;109–113.
50. Nelson L, Jennings GL, Esler MD, Korner PI. Effect of changing levels of physical activity on blood pressure and haemodynamics in essential hypertension. *Lancet* 1986;2:473–476.
51. Kiyonaga A, Arakawa K, Tanaka H, Shindo M. Blood pressure and hormonal responses to aerobic exercise. *Hypertension* 1985;7:125–131.
52. Blair SN, Goodyear NN, Gibbons LW, Cooper KH. Physical fitness and incidence of hypertension in healthy normotensive men and women. *JAMA* 1984;252:487–490.
53. Mutlu N, Berry RG, Alpers BJ. Massive cerebral hemorrhage. Clinical and pathological correlations. *Arch Neurol* 1963;8:649–661.
54. Gibbons LW, Cooper KH, Meyer BM, Ellison RC. The acute cardiac risk of strenuous exercise. *JAMA* 1980;224(16):1799–1801.
55. Thompson PD, Stern MP, Williams MS, Duncan K, Haskell WL, Wood PD. Death during jogging or running. *JAMA* 1979;242: 1265–1267.
56. Southam MA, Agras WS, Taylor CB, Kraemer HC. Relaxation training: Blood pressure reductions during the working day. *Arch Gen Psychiatry* 1982;39:715–717.
57. Engel BT, Glasgow MS, Gaarder KR. Behavioral treatment of high blood pressure. III. Follow-up results and recommendations. *Psychosom Med* 1983;45:23–29.

58. Messerli FH, Decarvalho JG, Christie B, Frolich ED. Systemic haemodynamic effects of biofeedback in borderline hypertension. *Clin Sci* 1979;57:437S–439S.
59. Benson H. *The relaxation response.* New York: Morrow, 1975.
60. Chesney MA, Black GW. Behavioral treatment of borderline hypertension: An overview of results. *J Cardiovasc Pharmacol* 1986;8(Suppl 5):S57–S63.
61. Light K. Psychosocial precursors of hypertension: experimental evidence. *Circulation* 1987;76(Suppl I):I-67–I-76.
62. Folkow B. Stress and blood pressure. In: *Adrenergic blood pressure regulation: proceedings of a symposium conference 22–25 May, 1984.* Princeton: Excerpta Medica, 1985.
63. Halstrup HL, Kraemer DL, Hotchkiss AP, Johnson CA. Cardiovascular responsivity to stress: family patterns and the effects of instructions. *J Psychsom Res* 1986;30(2):233–241.
64. Moschcowitz E. Hypertension: its significance, relation to arteriosclerosis and nephritis and etiology. *Am J Med Sci* 1919;158:668–684.
65. Alexander F. Emotional factors in essential hypertension. *Psychosom Med* 1939;1:173–179.
66. Perini C, Müller FB, Rauchfleisch U, Battegay R, Bühler F. Hyperadrenergic borderline hypertension is characterized by suppressed aggression. *J Cardiovasc Pharmacol* 1986;8(Suppl 5):S53–S56.
67. Dimsdale JE, Pierce C, Schoenfeld D, Brown A, Zusman R, Graham R. Suppressed anger and blood pressure: The effects of race, sex, social class, obesity, and age. *Psychosom Med* 1986;48(6): 430–436.
68. Schneider RH, Egan BM, John EH, Drobny H, Julius S. Anger and anxiety in borderline hypertension. *Psychosom Med* 1986;48(3–4):242–248.
69. Shapiro AP, Miller RE, King HE, Ginchereau EH, Fitzgibbon K. Behavioral consequences of mild hypertension. *Hypertension* 1982;4:355–360.
70. Miller RE, Shapiro AP, King HE, Ginchereau EH, Hosutt JA. Effect of antihypertensive treatment on behavioral consequences of elevated blood pressure. *Hypertension* 1984;6:202–208.
71. James SA. Psychosocial precursors of hypertension: A review of the epidemiologic evidence. *Circulation* 1987;76(Suppl I):I-60–I-66.
72. Krantz DS, deQuattro V, Blackburn HW, et al. Psychosocial factors in hypertension. *Circulation* 1987;76(Suppl I):I-84–I-88.
73. Cottington EM, Matthews KA, Talbott E, Kuller LH. Occupational stress, suppressed anger and hypertension. *Psychosom Med* 1986;48(3–4):249–260.
74. Johnson ME, Gibson ES, Terry CW, Haynes RB, Taylor DW, Gafne A, Sicurella JI, Sackett DL. Effects of labelling on income, work and social function among hypertensive employees. *J Chronic Dis* 1984;37(6):417–423.
75. Soghikian K, Fallick-Hunkeler EM, Ury HK, Fischer AA. The effect of high blood pressure treatment awareness on emotional well-being. *Clin Invest Med* 1981;4:191–196.
76. Mossey JM. Psychosocial consequences of labelling in hypertension. *Clin Invest Med* 1981;4:201–207.
77. American Heart Association. *Exercise and your heart.* New York: AHA, 1984.

Hypertension: Pathophysiology, Diagnosis, and Management, edited by J. H. Laragh and B. M. Brenner. Raven Press, Ltd., New York © 1990.

CHAPTER 131

Physician–Patient Interaction in the Treatment of Hypertension

Jay I. Meltzer

Formal Descriptions of Physician–Patient Interaction, 2073
Why Patients Obey Doctors, 2074
What Is Happening to Change the Traditional Role?, 2074
Uncertainty and Physician–Patient Interaction, 2074
Cognitive Dissonance and Physician–Patient Interaction, 2075
Clinical Studies of Physician–Patient Interaction in the Treatment of Hypertension, 2075
Influence of the Traditional Role, 2075
The Traditional Role and Compliance, 2075
What Do Patients Think Hypertension Means?, 2076
The Use and Significance of Quality-of-Life Assessment, 2076
Can Decision Analysis Have a Role in Physician–Patient Interaction?, 2076
Role of Self-Care in Physician–Patient Interaction, 2077
A Clinical Model of Physician–Patient Interaction in the Treatment of Essential Hypertension, 2077
Conclusions, 2080
References, 2081

When the drug treatment of hypertension was concentrated on severe and symptomatic disease, there was little stimulus to focus on physician–patient interaction as a factor in treatment outcome, apart from its significance for all medical care. When drugs were extended to mild disease, millions of asymptomatic individuals who felt well were sought, recruited, labeled, and referred for a lifetime of treatment as hypertensive patients. Studies show that this group has to remain in treatment for decades before benefit is clear and that there is considerable diminution in the quality of life of the unbenefited (1). Many patients drop out of treatment completely or fail to follow prescribed drug regimens. Consequently, the percentage of the population that is well controlled is low (2). Doctors, blaming the patient, label this behavior *noncompliance.* However, careful study of the causes of noncompliance suggests that apart from drug side effects and lowered quality of life, physician–patient interaction has important influence on the success of long-term treatment (3). A medical system characterized by emphasis on acute, symptomatic care and traditional physician–patient relationships may be ill prepared to deal with chronic asymptomatic disease in ambulatory, autonomous patients. Thus, clinical realities suggest attention to physician–patient interaction in the treatment of hypertension at a time when this question has been extensively treated in the general medical literature, stimulated by rapid and dramatic changes in societal and patient attitudes. In this chapter, I will discuss analyses of various aspects of the physician–patient relationship in general and will compare them to clinical observations specific for hypertension. Most of the time, the argument will apply principally to the case of mild hypertension, which, by the most recent census, comprises 83% of all hypertension (4).

FORMAL DESCRIPTIONS OF PHYSICIAN–PATIENT INTERACTION

The traditional concept of the physician–patient relationship, the *Parsonian theory,* regards sickness as social deviance (5). The physician, granted professional dominance, is placed in the powerful role of (a) defining illness, (b) providing treatment, (c) assuring treatment outcome, and (d) restoring normalcy. The patient is placed in a passive, dependent, "sick" role, charged only with the duty to trust, obey, and get well. The theory fails to account for the case of preventive health care or for chronic disease (6).

Another view considers the physician–patient relationship as an abstraction describing two interacting, yet independent, beings (7). In this fluid view, different treatment situations require different relationships. In medical emergencies such as diabetic coma, where the physician does everything and the patient nothing, a parent–child model based on such activity–passivity is appropriate. For acute medical care problems such as infection, where the patient cooperates by contributing data and by complying with the regimen, a parent–adolescent model based on guidance–cooperation is appropriate. For chronic conditions, the physician cannot cure patients but can only help them to help themselves—as in diabetes mellitus, for which the appropriate model is adult–adult or mutual participation. This model also applies to patients wishing to participate actively in their own care (7).

One model is not necessarily better than another. Each is appropriate in a certain context but inappropriate in others. Often the model must change over time. The patient with acute diabetic coma enters medical care in the first model, progresses to the second model with recovery (instruction in diet and insulin regulation), and later may enter a third phase, of chronic illness. If patient and physician cannot adapt to these changing conditions, the relationship may break down and the quality of care may suffer.

Each model has a different psychology. The first is one of complete physician control and a certain disidentification with the patient. The second model requires more identification with the patient, but as an adolescent molded in the parent's image. It assumes that only the physician knows what is right and then induces the patient to accept those aims as the patient's own, i.e., compliance. Only the third model, the mutual participation model, recognizes limitations on physician knowledge and power.

In treating disease for which there is no clear-cut agreement as to what constitutes a "cure" (where uncertainties exist and where patient evaluation of treatment outcome is required), the continuing, evolving search for what is the best treatment for each individual becomes the basis for physician–patient interaction. Here, physician gratification does not come from power or control over someone else, or from a mechanistic act such as lowering blood pressure, but from a phenomenon not well understood, possibly akin to the delayed rewards of teaching.

WHY PATIENTS OBEY DOCTORS

Aesculapian authority differs from other forms of authority because of a unique combination of three elements: wisdom, morality, and charisma (8). The first element, which is based on superior knowledge, does not of itself compel obedience. The second element, moral authority, deriving from the rightness and goodness of the physician's art, also cannot stand alone. Medical knowledge is limited and uncertain. Medical decisions are often made urgently, with life in the balance, and even the best moral intentions do not guarantee success. Therefore, physicians are also invested with charismatic authority, derived from a God-given grace.

Traditionalists believe a good doctor uses Aesculapian authority to dominate the patient for the beneficent purpose of removing doubt and uncertainty. This idea is strongly reinforced by those patients who want and need to believe in a physician and who therefore have a duty to find one from whom they will accept dominance (9). Traditionally, even highly informed physicians should, when they are sick, become "patients" and accept the "sick role." The concept of Aesculapian authority reveals a strong bias in our medical system toward authoritarian charismatic Parsonian care, fostering the use of models one and two by patients as well as by doctors.

WHAT IS HAPPENING TO CHANGE THE TRADITIONAL ROLE?

The principle of informed consent, as elegantly and thoroughly stated in the Report of the President's Commission for the Study of Ethical Problems in Medicine, now requires not only that patients be informed but also that they understand the information well enough to participate independently in medical decision-making (10). The report argues that the more Aesculapian authority is used to remove doubt and allay fear, the more patient autonomy is undermined by a subtle coercion, making informed consent an illusion. Authoritarian models and informed consent are mutually exclusive. There are many arguments advanced for maintaining authoritarian, paternalistic models. Some of these arguments are as follows: (a) Patients are too anxious or too irrational; (b) mutuality takes too much time or costs too much money; (c) only physicians know their patients' real needs; (d) relinquishing power and control to patients may be a threat to professional standing and competence; and (e) patients do not want to take a conscious role in decisions that may have unfavorable outcomes (11).

The alternative to paternalistic care—namely, mutual participation—poses a complex challenge for which there is no universal solution, since patients will vary in their capacity, and physicians in their competence, to manage this type of approach. However, all physicians should be encouraged to "experiment with varying degrees of patient participation in their daily practice," with particular attention to those situations involving uncertainty (12).

UNCERTAINTY AND PHYSICIAN–PATIENT INTERACTION

Assertion of Aesculapian authority may be the consequence of a failure or an unwillingness on the part of doctors to admit uncertainty (12). This failure to discuss uncertainty candidly and clearly in every encounter with patients (physicians, after all, discuss their uncertainties with colleagues) can lead to a "doctor knows best" attitude and to coercion of compliance. Only when doctor and patient together confront uncertainties—recognizing, for example, that doctors make mistakes or may not be completely objective—will patients begin to ask the right questions and help make the decisions that affect their lives. A down-to-earth conversation that frankly and candidly covers the important medical uncertainties enables doctors to decide with, and not for, their patients and enables patients to decide consciously and autonomously for themselves, not unconsciously by compliance (12). This kind of physician–patient interaction—which is not merely a matter of disclosing risks and benefits but involves a thorough give and take over time, keyed to how and why a decision is made—develops in a mutual participation model.

COGNITIVE DISSONANCE AND PHYSICIAN–PATIENT INTERACTION

Physicians are trained to analyze problems in terms of pathophysiology even though they realize that there is often a poor correlation between pathology and symptoms—that is, many patients feel sick without any diagnosable disease, whereas many others have a disease and are not sick. The difference between the way physicians think about disease and the way it is experienced by patients is the basis for cognitive dissonance (13,14).

Disease is felt as a loss, or a sense of disorder, or a shattering of the taken-for-grantedness of things (14). Since hypertension usually has no symptoms when first detected, the patient has nothing to experience except the shock of the diagnosis. "You have hypertension" are words that have powerful folk and social meanings, quite apart from their meaning for the doctor (15). Essential hypertension is a mistranslation of the French term, "hypertonie essentielle," referring to the tension on the blood vessel walls caused by elevated blood pressure. This misnomer causes patients, prisoners of words, to feel that tension, stress, and emotions cause the disease. One wonders how much less confusion there would be if we called it hyperpyesia.

Ideally, physicians should attempt to examine the disease as experienced by the patient; however, this kind of empathy may be hampered by authoritarian models, which emphasize that treatment should involve "doing something" to the patient (lowering the pressure) and that therapeutic success is something the physician determines. This cognitive dissonance can be bridged by the physician's ability to understand the patient's view of the disease and of the suffering it may cause, as well as by the patient's ability to understand the medical view, the rationale for treatment. In this way, both the sickness and the disease can be treated together.

CLINICAL STUDIES OF PHYSICIAN–PATIENT INTERACTION IN THE TREATMENT OF HYPERTENSION

Influence of the Traditional Role

Patients with hypertension tend to view their physician in the Parsonian mold (15). Consequently, unless otherwise informed, they may develop behavior patterns in concordance with Parson's concept of being sick, including increased job absenteeism and other forms of secondary gain (1,15–17).

The Traditional Role and Compliance

Compliance means conformity, obedience, and consent—in sum, submission to authority (18). The basic question of compliance goes to the heart of physician–patient interaction because it is a direct consequence of the traditional role as all-knowing parent getting the child to obey, highlighting the special type of professional authority (Aesculapian) that physicians have come to expect. The cause of noncompliance is the assumption that physicians, like all-knowing parents, are in charge of their patients (19). Philosophers have indicated that physicians have a right to expect compliance: "Departure from an expected standard without reasonable justification can appropriately involve blame" (20). But who is to define "departure" and "expected standards"? Is a patient who takes medication regularly for hypertension, even though advised against it by a doctor, noncompliant? Since compliance refers to a process (obeying doctors' orders) and not to an outcome, it is entirely possible, in situations involving uncertainty, that noncompliance might in fact be the road to recovery. Despite logical weaknesses in the concept of compliance, it has consumed enormous attention; as a matter of fact, a massive bureaucracy has developed just to deal with it (19).

Epidemiologic surveys show that treatment success as a percentage of newly discovered cases of hypertension is disappointing (21); half the patients drop out and half the remainder are poorly controlled (22). Both of these phenomena have been related to noncompliance (23). Noncompliance was recognized in 1975 as the critical missing element in the successful treatment of hypertension (24). With increased attention to noncompliance, the dropout rate has recently decreased in some series to 10–15% the first year and to 16–25% the second year (as yet, there are only spotty long-term statistics) (23). The special Veterans Administration hypertension clinics had a 37.8% dropout rate at 6 years (25). No data are available for treatment over 10–20 years. Of those remaining in treatment, 20–40% are noncompliant, although it is by no means assumed that all of these patients are suffering as a result (20). Assessments of noncompliance are said to require objectivity; thus, they emphasize pill counts, urine drug sampling, appointment keeping, and highly technical interviewing techniques, all requiring major investments in time, space, personnel, and money (26).

There are many studies designed to develop strategies for increasing compliance. To the extent that they all induce the patient to obey the doctor, they are coercive; thus, they require (but do not always employ) moral restraint. Physicians generally expect patient compliance and are often perplexed and angry when it is not forthcoming (27), to the point of using medical threats (28). In response to this coercion, noncompliant behavior may be a plea for patient control (29) or to get the doctor to listen or negotiate (30). Fear, a powerful influence on patient behavior, may be used to further compliance; the "fear" approach is specifically geared toward fear of strokes and heart attacks, even though these morbid events cannot be completely averted by treatment, only reduced. Hypertensives do not realize the probabilistic nature of their morbidity risks and usually feel they *will* eventually have a stroke or a heart attack. Exaggerating the threat protects the physician from chagrin and invites the patient to attribute the unexpected good outcome to good care (31). Thus the physician has other reasons to magnify the threat besides using it to coerce compliance. Curiously, some studies have shown fear to be an ineffective inducer of compliance (32,33). Thus, the use of fear rests on shaky empirical, as well as moral, grounds.

Studies show that almost any extra attention given the patient increases compliance, no doubt in direct relation to the poverty of the existing physician–patient interaction (34–36). In study after study, the following simple physician actions are shown to increase compliance: (a) increasing the quality of the instructions, ensuring that the patient understands what to do; (b) putting treatment regimens in writing; (c) being friendly, courteous, and compassionate; (d) increasing patient participation; (e) responding sensitively to complaints; and (f) sharing responsibility (37–41). Studies emphasizing patient participation show that the more the patient is autonomously committed to treatment, the greater the success of blood pressure reduction.

What if the enormous effort to solve the problem of compliance were directed toward achieving mutuality in the physician–patient relationship, giving patients choices and helping them to decide, autonomously, what they want to do about their hypertension? Not all patients at all times want to participate actively in their own care, nor should they be forced to, but what about those who do? Can we all honestly say we are fully prepared to identify and help them?

What Do Patients Think Hypertension Means?

Recent essays emphasize the impact of differences between the patient's view of sickness (illness) and the physician's view of disease on physician–patient interaction (13,14,42). Studies of blacks (43), Israelis (44), and urban Americans (15) all found considerable divergence between patient and physician beliefs concerning hypertension. In a study of mainstream urban males in a Veterans Administration clinic, 72% believed they had "hyper-tension," a folk illness with a medical name, (15) caused by chronic external stress due to psychopersonal factors augmented by fear, worry, anger, tension, overactivity, exhaustion, and excitement. The disease, patients think, causes symptoms such as dizziness, tiredness, headache, nosebleeds, flushing, and emotional lability, and, finally, bursting blood vessels. This view enables patients to assume various aspects of the sick role (15) in an effort to treat themselves quite apart from physician advice. Blacks have the idea that there are two diseases, hypertension and "high blood." Hypertension, in this view, is a very dangerous nervous disorder that is not in their power to control, nor amenable to drug treatment, thereby discouraging compliance (43). Cognitive dissonance leads to less effective care, apparently by fostering confusion and faulty communication.

The relevance to physician–patient interaction concerns the extent to which cognitive dissonance affects not only control of blood pressure but also patient suffering (45). Patients use the symbolic nature of their disease to link affective experience with physiologic events (15). They socialize their illness. Physicians need to understand this process of socialization in order to help patients avoid harmful negative interpretations of their disease that may damage health and happiness.

In conclusion, there are two processes to treat, the physiologic disease "hypertension" (the physician's health belief) and the affective disorder "hyper-tension" (the patient's health belief). Therefore, successful treatment not only would result in lowered blood pressure but also would lead to concordant beliefs that answer the basic patient questions: What causes it? Why me? Why now? What will happen? What can be done? To achieve this concordance takes time, conversation, supplementation by written material, and cross-questioning. It is a continuing process, leading to effective partnership in long-term treatment and better control.

The Use and Significance of Quality-of-Life Assessment

Looking back over decades of drug treatment, one finds discussions of side effects, but not until very recently have physicians considered the patient's assessment of therapeutic outcome. In one study, for example, when doctors felt that a set of hypertensives were 100% improved, only 48% of the patients felt improved, 8% felt worse, and 64% had no (or very weak) sexual activity (46). The rating by patients' relatives was even worse, with only 2% considered as being improved (46). This discordance is understandable because the physician looks at the problem mechanistically, in terms blood pressure reduction, and pronounces the patient cured, whereas the patient feels, and therefore is, worse. New physician interest in the patient's evaluation of treatment takes the form of a highly technical questionnaire, quality-of-life assessment (47).

This new dimension is used to help identify the best antihypertensive drug (48–53), but questions have been raised as to the significance of these interpretations (54); moreover, there are no data to prove that this "scientific" assessment (55) is any more accurate than a sensitive conversation between a mutually interactive physician and patient. The danger is in assuming that the results of a quality-of-life study automatically apply to a specific patient. A questionnaire will not solve the problem of physician–patient interaction; instead, this type of interaction requires personal assessment and reassessment over years of treatment as the dual conditions of disease and suffering change. Although attention to quality of life is welcomed, attempts to make it just another piece of scientific data in the determination of a specific drug regimen may have the undesirable effect of discouraging physicians from greater patient involvement.

Can Decision Analysis Have a Role in Physician–Patient Interaction?

Decision analysis can be applied to health policy, classes of problems, and individual patient decisions. Three steps are required. First, a clinical problem is defined and each decision option is described schematically as a branch of a tree. Second, probability is used to quantify the uncertainties in each option—the expected gains and risks. Step three, the most complex and controversial, assigns a relative value (utility) to each outcome. To elicit these values, patient and physician are required to understand each other's utility systems. This is where the patient expresses preferences, and there are various techniques for quantitation.

Formal decision analysis has rarely been used at the level of assessing individual patient utilities, and never for the treatment of essential hypertension from the individual's perspective (56). One early study suggests that decision analysis has value for physician–patient interaction in treatment of hypertension apart from the formal, mathematical process (57).

Each of the three steps in decision analysis can make substantial contributions to clinical thinking even if they cannot be integrated into a mathematical whole (58). For example, the probabilities of a decision tree should apply to a specific patient; thus, the personal physician needs to take average values from the literature on risks of morbid events and tailor them to that patient. How physicians combine many clinical findings into a single probability estimate is not known (59), but awareness of the need to do so may improve a physician's self-knowledge of the process. More important, when using decision analysis, physician and patient must work as a team (60). It is only a beginning to say that decisions should be shared or that doctors should decide with, and not for, their patients. One needs specific guidelines for the role and the responsibility of physician and patient in the shared decision act, yet one should do nothing to diminish the scientific value of the process. The physician's role is to lay out the medical facts. The patient's role is to understand the personal consequences (utility) of a potential outcome (60). This interaction is inhibited by authoritarian systems which neither admit uncertainty nor view the patient as fit for autonomous decision-making.

The search for the best probabilities to assign to each outcome forces the physician to face the very uncertainties upon which decisions are based. Consciousness of these uncertainties, as well as sharing decisions with patients, has the additional moral value of achieving informed consent.

There are many problems with decision analysis, but those physicians who try to use it to the extent possible have to get closer to their patients. To date, there are no studies to prove that using the informal decision analysis technique improves care in hypertension; however, to the extent that it contributes to the patient's feelings of control, there is a rational and clinical basis (from the studies on compliance) for believing that it will.

Role of Self-Care in Physician–Patient Interaction

Studies of self-care have generally been conducted in hypertension clinics and thus are shaped by the traditional models of physician–patient interaction available there. Therefore, patient compliance became the yardstick by which self-care was evaluated. In one study, physician–patient interaction and patient involvement in their own care were felt to be critical as compliance-enhancing factors (33). "Orienting medical services to patients as passive recipients is probably dysfunctional in the treatment of chronic ambulatory illness" (61). Assuming that active patient involvement would improve outcome, a measured scale of the degree of patient activity was developed by Schulman, based on four factors—patients being (i) addressed as partners, (ii) informed of treatment rationale, (iii) encouraged to report negative effects, and (iv) helped to make treatments operational (61). When patients with high APO scores were compared to those with low ones, the former showed better blood pressure control. These studies, conducted in hypertension clinics with traditional physician–patient relationships, led to the observation that "patients desiring to play an increased role . . . may experience difficulties . . . unless physicians are willing to change."

Greenfield et al. (62), in a study of peptic ulcer, tried to separate patient involvement from the context of compliance, attempting to direct it instead toward increased physician–patient interaction, thereby creating a forum for the development of the knowledge, skills, and confidence needed in the daily management of chronic disease. A tutorial intervention was designed to alter the traditional physician–patient relationship. Patients reviewed their medical records and were taught medical logic and information-seeking skills; they were also taught to recognize when and how decisions are made and to be assertive in asking relevant questions, getting answers, and negotiating disagreements. A matched control group received standard treatment. Results showed that tutorials increased physician–patient interaction and led to twice as much conversation, less functional disability, increased sense of control, and increased preference for more of the same in the future. The needs of hypertensives for confidence and sense of control over daily management are even greater than those of peptic ulcer patients and are of much longer duration. The authors planned to study hypertension next.

Barofsky (63) has analyzed the relationship between self-care and physician–patient interaction. Patients undertake the tasks of a therapeutic regimen by way of compliance, adherence, and therapeutic alliance. These involve, respectively, coercion, conformity, and negotiation in a continuum that varies directly with patients' active involvement and inversely with authoritarian physician dominance. Compliance is the necessary outcome of a process of coercion. Patient's enter the health care system socialized to expect control (Parsons), but only a few proceed to take advantage of what is inherently possible, namely, the development of full partnership involving self-care.

Since the knowledge base and the skills necessary for self-care are not complicated, anyone with a basic education and the right attitude can participate, given a helpful physician. It seems to work very well for patients with end-stage renal disease on home dialysis or for patients with insulin-dependent diabetes mellitus, and these conditions are hardly less complicated than hypertension.

A Clinical Model of Physician–Patient Interaction in the Treatment of Essential Hypertension

The Joint National Committee report of 1984, in its section on patient–professional interaction, states the follow-

TABLE 1. *Clinical model of physician–patient interaction in the treatment of hypertension*

Knowledge (patient needs to know)	Attitude (patient needs to believe)	Skill (patient needs to be able to)
Stage 1: Making the decision to control blood pressure		
Average blood pressure for age and sex; blood pressure varies considerably during the day; diagnosis of high blood pressure is problematic, defined in terms of excess risks	I can help determine whether my own blood pressure risk exceeds average risk	Measure own pressure accurately; keep good blood pressure records including pulse and weight; track blood pressure over the course of the day as needed
Hypertension can be asymptomatic	My blood pressure can be high without my feeling it	
Untreated hypertension can lead to stroke, heart disease, and kidney failure	Specific morbid events may not occur for years, or ever; nevertheless, the risk is always real and serious	Distinguish between average, goal, and high-risk levels of blood pressure
Goal blood pressure and patient's blood pressure		
Nonpharmacologic treatments should be tried first; high salt intake, overweight, sedentary life, alcohol, cigarettes can all raise blood pressure; if nonpharmacologic treatment does not lower blood pressure to goal, drugs may be needed	If blood pressure is lowered without drugs, so much the better for me	Maintain a low-salt diet; employ a proper exercise regimen; control associated risk factors, namely, alcohol, cigarettes, weight, cholesterol, stress
Although necessity for drugs may not be lifelong, necessity for maintaining control to goal blood pressure *is* lifelong	Potential problems can be solved by partnership with my doctor; benefits of control outweigh costs	Distinguish control from cure
Physician's *health belief model* in writing	Need for concordance in *health belief models*	Read physician material and discuss; question and get answers to questions; discuss own health beliefs concerning hypertension
Decision to treat with drugs is complex, subject to a modified decision analysis	Decision analysis is a good method for sharing decision-making between physician and patient	Distinguish probabilistic from mechanistic reasoning; cooperate in the evaluation of outcomes; evaluate quality of life; identify potential problems relating to control, i.e., demands of drug regimen, expense
Stage 2: Taking medication to control blood pressure		
Medical drug regimen, names of drugs, dose, and timing; what to do if dose is missed; side effects (see Stage 4, part B)	Antihypertensive therapy is a daily regulation—try to make it a habit	Tailor drug schedule to personal habits and blood pressure response
Drug control is a steady state of balance between patient's hypertensive mechanism and drug's antihypertensive action	Dose and regimen should not be changed by either doctor alone or patient alone	Develop cues that ensure regular therapy; make arrangements to have regular supply of needed medicines, i.e., renew prescription before supply runs out
Drug treatment requires understanding that medical physiology and physician expertise is valuable and necessary	Doctor is always available for telephone consultation regarding dosage adjustment, side effects, etc.	Become familiar with drug action in a general way
Stage 3: Monitoring progress toward blood pressure control		
Blood pressure goal	Goals may change with time and events	Monitor home blood pressure with sufficient frequency and accuracy so that *progress toward goal* is easily seen
Blood pressure may vary considerably during day and over time	Daily fluctuations within defined ranges are normal and should be of no undue concern	Track blood pressure and report results honestly and accurately
How often to check with physician by telephone, letter, and office visit	Appointments may be necessary to check on side effects, calibrate home blood pressure machine, and confirm blood pressure measurement skill	Know potential side effects and recognize them

TABLE 1. *Continued.*

Knowledge (patient needs to know)	Attitude (patient needs to believe)	Skill (patient needs to be able to)
Physician and patient need to consult and evaluate the results of experiments on drug treatment	Evaluation of therapeutic success is mutual	Effectively communicate results of patient data, home blood pressure response, side effects, and quality of life
Periodic physician–patient evaluation of new findings in drug treatment is advisable (necessary)		
Results of drug treatment experiments require review by physician and patient		
	Stage 4: Cooperation in long term BP control	
A. Communication: Blood pressure control is a combined effort of physician and patient	Physician is concerned for patient's long-term problem; physician acts as teacher/guide to transfer knowledge and skills to enable patient to control blood pressure through self-care	Evaluate own abilities and ask questions; get help when needed
Other health professionals can help solve problems	Others can be helpful	Select appropriate health care professional when indicated
Blood pressure control requires emotional support of family	Patient can ask family for help; as a partner, patient has responsibility to know what is expected and can freely state what is expected of physician	State when and how family members are or are not helping With physician, identify problems and work out solutions, evaluate progress
B. Medication: Side effects of drug(s) being taken	Side effects can occur at any time; physician will correct problems if they occur	Recognize side effects as possibly drug-induced Consult physician about side effects
Some side effects are symptoms, others involve asymptomatic metabolic changes	Physician will monitor me properly	Keep scheduled appointments
Other medications are available if side effects occur	Side effects can usually be eliminated or minimized	Balance certain inconveniences against value of blood pressure control achieved
New drugs are constantly being introduced	Physician will reevaluate drug regimen in light of new knowledge	Stimulate physician to reevaluate treatment program annually
Other drugs can interfere with blood pressure control: nonsteroidal anti-inflammatory agents, steroids, poor diabetic control, birth control pills, nose drops, appetite-control pills	Drug interactions can interfere with regulation	Consult with physician before taking other drugs; inform other physicians of current drug regimen
Intercurrent disease may affect steady state; i.e., acute gastroenteritis with dehydration and high fever requires dose adjustments	Doctor is always available for telephone consultation if needed regarding dosage adjustment; I don't necessarily like controlling my blood pressure, but I do it because I have found that it is effective	Know when to adjust treatment downward or upward using home blood pressure measurements or call for help

ing: "While diagnosis and treatment are the primary responsibility of the physician, making the decision to control blood pressure and adhering to the prescribed regimen are critical behaviors for the patient" (64). "Patient Behavior for Blood Pressure Control" (65) is a primer for physician–patient interaction, the vital factor in achievement and maintenance of long-term control. The patient is the decision-maker and problem solver; the physician is advisor, guide, and promoter.

Four critical steps are involved (Table 1): (i) making the decision to control blood pressure, (ii) taking medication, (iii) monitoring progress; and (iv) maintaining control over the years by problem solving. Each step requires specific knowledge, attitudes, and skills, which, over time, develop from, as well as modify, physician–patient interaction. Although no specific model of physician–patient interaction is discussed or even implicit in these guidelines, the general tone emphasizes the need to involve patients and keep them in control of the treatment process.

A clinical model emphasizing mutual participation is shown in Table 1. The first stage, making the decision to control blood pressure, involves establishing mutual participation, concordance in beliefs concerning hypertension, and involvement in self-care.

An important step is for patients to learn to take their own blood pressure. Written directions are required, and an appropriate blood pressure device is selected. The patient needs to be reassured that home blood pressures are scientifically valid data (66–69); these may, in fact, be even more accurate for evaluating blood pressure control as compared to doctor-elicited blood pressures, which may be overestimated (70) or may be biased by observer expectation (71). Page (72) has emphasized that blood pressure be measured by patients and that many readings over time are required because of different rhythms, patterns, and wide fluctuations. It is important to be sure that the patient obtains accurate measurements. The development of this skill is a cornerstone of one type of successful partnership. Medical sociologists feel that a physician's ability to preserve power over the patient depends largely on the ability to control the patient's uncertainty (37). The physician's willingness to transfer this power graciously, actively, and surely to the patient is an act of compassion and trust, fostering strong mutual bonding. Patient's home monitoring obtains data on the diurnal cycle and on the influence of the activities of daily living. Variations will be noted, but the patient should not be upset or confused by them.

Once the home blood pressure skill is developed, the effect of nonpharmacologic treatment can be observed for an appropriate period of time. Some claim that a placebo effect may occur (73,74).

If blood pressure reaches goal with nondrug treatment, the patient goes on a maintenance program (Table 1, Stage 4). The fact that the patient sees the success as partially self-managed is strong motivation for continuing maintenance and monitoring. If pressure does not come down to goal, the decision to use drugs will have to be made.

A modified form of decision analysis is used to help the patient conceptualize the steps in the decision, to see it as a principled gamble that treatment will do more good than harm. Framingham data, or any other similar data, may be used to show mean blood pressure for age and sex and to show the average risk for heart disease and stroke. The patient's risk can then be taken from the same tables and compared with the assumed risk at goal blood pressure.

In following out the steps of a decision analysis model, it becomes evident that patients really cannot make an informed decision based on drug studies, because they need to know what a specific drug does to *them,* not just in terms of their pressure response but also in terms of the cost in time, money, side effects, and quality of life. Thus, the initial exposure to drugs is an experiment in taking medication and in monitoring progress conducted in the home under physician guidance (Table 1, Stages 2 and 3). Nothing improves physician–patient interaction like success, so a wise choice of the first drug is important. The goal may be met with or without side effects, or it may not be met at all. If it is achieved with no ill effects, physician and patient proceed to Stage 4, namely, long-term control. If it is not, a second experiment is begun with another drug, and so on, until goal blood pressure, with a minimum of side effects, is achieved. At the end of the experiments, physician and patient can evaluate the costs, side effects, and quality of life against the gains in blood pressure control.

After a drug regimen is established, physician–patient interaction enters Stage 4, the long-term control. By this time, the patient should have acquired considerable knowledge and skill along with a positive attitude toward self-care. Schedules for follow-up treatment vary; however, for asymptomatic uncomplicated hypertension, no more than a yearly evaluation might be indicated. This annual examination, besides evaluating blood pressure control, organ damage, and quality of life, should also involve (a) a reexamination of the decision to treat with drugs and (b) a recommitment to the same regimen or to a new one if indicated by new information.

Table 1 features one type of physician–patient interaction. It is not the only possibility. Every physician can design one suited to his or her own practice. The more physician–patient interaction is thought out and made explicit, the more both parties will know how to communicate and cooperate.

CONCLUSIONS

Reasoned arguments from general medicine emphasize the importance of a mutual participation model of physician–patient interaction in dealing with autonomous ambulatory patients who are not feeling sick yet have a chronic disease, conditions which apply to essential hypertension. Uncertainty also favors mutual participation. The diagnosis itself is uncertain, more operational than scientific. According to Pickering (75), hypertension is that level of blood pressure at which the harm likely to ensue exceeds the nuisance value to the patient with regard to treatment. Even when there is agreement that diastolic pressures of 90–104 are to be diagnosed as hypertension, there is uncertainty concerning drug treatment. In a debate held at the first meeting of the American Society of Hypertension, "Should Mild Hypertension Be Treated?," 40% of the society thought yes and 60% thought no (76). Thus, medical uncertainty, the special needs of chronic care, and the increased desire of patients to participate all recommend that physicians treating hypertension give far more consideration to active patient participation than they have done in the past.

The decision to treat mild hypertension with drugs committed over 22 million healthy, autonomous Americans to becoming "patients" in the existing health care system (4). That system, with strong traditions favoring paternalism, authoritarianism, and scientism, made no concerted effort (despite the uncertainties) to relate to these healthy hypertensives as anything other than "sick." Thus, traditional medicine forced them into a "sick role," demanding compliance while at the same time failing in empathy, compassion, communication, and sometimes plain common courtesy.

Only a minority of referred patients remain in treatment or on medication, and only a minority remain well-controlled. Since the drugs are proven effective, physicians laid the blame for the failure on the patient and labeled it *noncompliance,* a nice term for not obeying doctor's orders. But studies consistently showed that patients and physicians were not talking about the same things: Physicians did not give clear instructions and did not bother to take time for detailed explanations, nor were they compassionate or even friendly. They did not, until recently, attempt to evaluate sickness, quality of life, or the effect of the disease on the person, nor did they allow patients to evaluate treatment outcome or participate in their own care to any significant extent. Not all patients want increased involvement in their own care, but those that do want to be involved have difficulty getting physicians to cooperate. When physicians are specifically oriented toward mutuality attitudes, change and care improves by means of a reallocation of physician time to patient teaching activities (77).

The present health care system allows for a wide range of physician–patient interaction. There is nothing to prevent patients moving from initial dependency to a partnership with considerable autonomy, self-motivation, self-regulation, and self-care. Construction of an explicit clinical model (Table 1) by each treating physician or clinic can focus attention on physician–patient interaction, the key to achieving the goal of improved blood pressure control.

In the course of years, patients come to know a great deal about their own blood pressure, having seen the raw data for themselves. Through development of their own skills and physician–patient interaction, a strong sense of partnership emerges. Since a significant number of patients, particularly those with mild hypertension, never experience a specific morbid event that is unquestionably linked to hypertension, it would be a blessing if, at the end of a lifetime of taking medication and monitoring blood pressure, physician and patient together could still say, "It was worth it." On the other hand, if there was a heart attack, a stroke, or kidney failure, it would be equally important to be able to say, "We did everything we could, and there are no regrets."

REFERENCES

1. Schoenberger JA. Antihypertensive drugs and the quality of life. *J Hypertens* 1986;4(Suppl 5):S390–S392.
2. Winnckoff RN, Murphy PK. The persistent problem of poor blood pressure control. *Arch Intern Med* 1987;147:1393–1396.
3. Stamler J. The mass treatment of hypertensive disease: defining the problem. *Ann NY Acad Sci* 1978;304:333–362.
4. Blood pressure levels in persons 18–74 years of age in 1976–80, and trends on blood pressure from 1960 to 1980 in the United States. National Health Survey Series 11, No. 234, July 1986.
5. Parsons T. *The social system.* Glencoe, IL: Free Press, 1951.
6. Gallagher EB. Lines of reconstruction and extension in the parsonian sociology of illness. *Soc Sci Med* 1976;10:207–218.
7. Szasz T, Hollander M. A contribution to the philosophy of medicine. *Arch Intern Med* 1956;585–592.
8. Osmond HG. God and the doctor. *N Engl J Med* 1980;302(10):555–558.
9. Inglefinger F. Arrogance. *N Engl J Med* 1980;303(26):1507–1511.
10. President's commission for the study of ethical problems in medicine. *Making health care decisions, vol 1: report of the ethical and legal implications of informed consent in the patient–practitioner relationship.* Washington, DC: US Government Printing Office, October 1982.
11. Brody DS. The patient's role in clinical decision-making. *Ann Intern Med* 1980;93:718–722.
12. Katz J. *The silent world of doctor and patient.* Glencoe, IL: Free Press, 1984.
13. Kleinman A, Eisenberg L, Good B. Culture, Illness, and care: clinical lessons from anthropologic and cross-culture research. *Ann Intern Med* 1978;88:251–258.
14. Baron RJ. An introduction to medical phenomenology: I can't hear you while I'm listening. *Ann Intern Med* 1985;103:606–611.
15. Blumhagen D. Hyper-tension: a folk illness with a medical name. *Cult Med Psychiatry* 1980;4:197–227.
16. Polk BF, Harlan LC, Cooper SP, Stromer M, Ignatius J, Mull H, Blaszkowski TP. Disability days associated with detection and treatment in hypertension control program. *Am J Epidemiol* 1984;119:44–53.
17. Macdonald LA, Sackett DL, Haynes RB, Taylow DW. Labelling in hypertension: a review of the behavioural and psychological consequences. *J Chronic Dis* 1984;37(12):933–942.
18. *Roget's thesaurus of words and phrases.* New York: Grosset & Dunlap, 1941.
19. Slack WV. The patient's right to decide. *Lancet* 1977:240.
20. Eraker SA, Kirscht JP, Becker MH. Understanding and improving patient compliance. *Ann Intern Med* 1984;100:258–268.
21. Stason WB, Weinstein MC. Allocation of resources to manage hypertension. *N Engl J Med* 1977;296(13):732–739.
22. Vetter H. Compliance-improving strategies in hypertension: introduction. *J Hypertens* 1985;3(Suppl 1):1.
23. Luscher TF, Vetter H, Siegenthaler W, Vetter W. Compliance in hypertension: facts and concepts. *J Hypertens* 1985;3(Suppl 1):3–9.
24. Greenfield S, Blumhagen D. Non-compliance comes to be reorganized as the cortical missing element in the successful treatment of hypertension. In: Poell RN, ed. *Physicians guide to compliance in hypertension.* Rahway, NJ: Merck & Co, 1975.
25. Perry HM Jr, Meyer G, Freis E, Neal W, Ramirez E, Schnaper H, Thomas JR, Carmody S. Six-year compliance with a treatment regimen and resultant control of blood pressure in special veterans administration hypertension clinics. *J Hypertens* 1986;4(Suppl 5):S393–S394.
26. Caron H. Compliance: the case for objective measurement. *J Hypertens* 1985;3(Suppl 1):11–17.
27. Gorlin R, Zucker HD. Physicians' reactions to patients. A key to teaching humanistic medicine. *N Engl J Med* 1983;308(18):1059–1062.
28. Heszen-Klemens I. Patients' noncompliance and how doctors manage this. *Sci Med* 1987;24(5):409–416.
29. Hayes-Bautista DE. Modifying the treatment: patient compliance, patient control and medical care. *Soc Sci Med* 1976;10:223–238.
30. Heaton PB. Negotiation as an integral part of the physician's clinical reasoning. *J Fam Pract* 1981;13(6):845–848.
31. Feinstein AR. The chagrin factor and qualitative decision analysis. *Arch Intern Med* 1985;145:1257–1259.
32. Garrity TF, Garrity AR. The nature and efficacy of intervention studies in the national high blood pressure education research program. *J Hypertens* 1985;3(Suppl 1):91–95.
33. Nelson EC, Stason WB, Neutra R, Solomon HS, McArdle PJ. Impact of patient perceptions on compliance with treatment for hypertension. *Med Care* 1978;16(11):893–906.
34. Binstock ML, Franklin KL, Formica EK. Therapeutic adherence programme improves compliance and lowers blood pressure. *J Hypertens* 1986;4(Suppl 5):S375–S377.
35. Ley P. Doctor–patient communication: Some quantitative estimates of the role of cognitive factors in noncompliance. *J Hypertens* 1985;3(Suppl 1):51–55.
36. Haehn K-D. Psychological approaches to improve patient compliance. *J Hypertens* 1985;3(Suppl 1):61–64.
37. Waitzkin H, Stoeckle JD. The communication of information about illness. Clinical, sociological, and methodological considerations. *Adv Psychosom Med* 1972;8:180–215.
38. Coleman VR. Physician behaviour and compliance. *J Hypertens* 1985;3(Suppl 1):69–71.
39. Becker MH, Maiman LA. Strategies for enhancing patient compliance. *J Community Health* 1980;6(2):113–135.
40. Haynes RB, Gibson ES, Hacket BC, Sackett DL, Taylor DW, Roberts RS, Johnson AL. Improvement of medication compliance in uncontrolled hypertension. *Lancet* 1976;June 12:1265–1268.
41. Svarstad BL. Physician–patient communication and patient conformity with medical advice. In: Mechanic D, ed. *The growth of bureaucratic medicine,* New York: John Wiley & Sons, 1976.
42. McWhinney IR. Are we on the brink of a major transformation of clinical method? *CMAJ* 1986;135:873–878.
43. Heurtin-Roberts S, Reisin E. Differences in patient and practitioner models of hypertension relate to compliance in black hypertensives. *J Hypertens* 1986;4(Suppl 5):S372–S376.
44. Greenfield SF, Barhan J, Yodfat Y. Health beliefs and hyperten-

sion: A control study in a Moroccan Jewish community in Israel. *Cult Med Psychiatry* 1987;11:79–95.
45. Cassel CJ. The nature of suffering and the goals of medicine. *N Engl J Med* 1982;306(11):639–645.
46. Jachuck SJ, Brierley H, Jachuck S, Willcox PM. The effect of hypotensive drugs on the quality of life. *J R Coll Gen Pract* 1982;32:103–105.
47. Williams GH. Quality of life and its impact on hypertensive patients. *Am J Med* 1987;82:98–105.
48. Callender JS. Quality of life in hypertension treatment: methods of assessment and results of recent trials. *Curr Opinion Cardiol* 1986;1:603–606.
49. Crogg SH, Levine S, Testa MA, Brown B, Bulpitt CJ, Jenkins CD, Klerman GL, Williams GH. The effects of antihypertensive therapy on the quality of life. *N Engl J Med* 1986;314(26):1657–1664.
50. Robertson JIS. The treatment of hypertension and quality of life. *J Hypertens* 1985;3(Suppl 2):S89–S90.
51. Williams GH, Croog SH, Levine S, Testa MA, Sudilovsky A. Impact of antihypertensive therapy on quality of life: effect of hydrochlorothiazide. *J Hypertens* 1987;5(Suppl 1):S29–S35.
52. Edmonds D, Vetter H, Vetter W. Angiotensin converting enzyme inhibitors in the clinic: quality of life. *J Hypertens* 1987;5(Suppl 3):S31–S35.
53. Hollenberg NK. Initial therapy in hypertension: quality-of-life considerations. *J Hypertens* 1987;5(Suppl 1):S3–S7.
54. Testa MA. Interpreting quality-of-life clinical trial data for use in the clinical practice of antihypertensive therapy. *J Hypertens* 1987;5(Suppl 1):S9–S13.
55. Siegrist J, Williams GW. Introduction. *J Hypertens* 1987;5(Suppl 1):S1–S2.
56. Kassirer JP, Moskowitz AJ, Lau J, Pauker SG. Decision analysis: a progress report. *Ann Intern Med* 1987;106:275–291.
57. Bursztaijn H, Feinbloom RI, Hann RN, Brodsky A. *Medical choices, medical chances.* New York: Delacorte Press/Seymour Laurence, 1981.
58. Ransohoff DF, Feinstein AR. Is decision analysis useful in clinical medicine? *Yale J Biol Med* 1976;49:165–168.
59. Sox HC Jr. Decision analysis: a basic clinical skill? *N Engl J Med* 1987;316(5):271–272.
60. Pauker SG, Kassirer JP. Decision analysis. *N Engl J Med* 1987;316(2):250–258.
61. Schulman BA. Active patient orientation and outcomes in hypertensive treatment. *Med Care* 1979;17(3):267–280.
62. Greenfield S, Kaplan S, Ware JE Jr. Expanding patient involvement in care. Effects on patient outcomes. *Ann Intern Med* 1985;102:520–528.
63. Barofsky I. Compliance, adherence and the therapeutic alliance: Steps in the development of self-care. *Soc Sci Med* 1978;12:369–376.
64. The 1984 report of the Joint National Committee on detection, evaluation, and treatment of high blood pressure. *Arch Intern Med* 1984;144:1045–1057.
65. Patient behavior for blood pressure control. Guidelines for professional. *JAMA* 1979;241(23):2534–2537.
66. Mancia G, Parati G, Pomidossi G, Di Rienzo M. Validity and usefulness of non-invasive ambulatory blood pressure monitoring. *J Hypertens* 1985;3(Suppl 2):S5–S11.
67. Brunner HR, Waeber B, Nussberger J. Clinical use of non-invasive ambulatory blood pressure recording. *J Hypertens* 1985;3(Suppl 2):S13–S17.
68. Sleight P. Differences between casual and 24-h blood pressures. *J Hypertens* 1985;3(Suppl 2):S19–S23.
69. Parati G, Pomidossi G, Albini F, Malaspina D, Mancia G. Relationship of 24-hour blood pressure mean and variability to severity of target-organ damage in hypertension. *J Hypertens* 1987;5:93–98.
70. Mancia G, Parati G, Pomidossi G, Casadei R, Groppelli A, Sposato E, Zanchetti A. *J Hypertens* 1985;3(Suppl 3):S421–S423.
71. Sassano P, Chatellier G, Corvol P, Menard J. Influence of observer's expectation on the placebo effect in blood pressure trials. *Curr Ther Res* 1987;41(3):305–312.
72. Page IH. The continuing failure to understand and treat hypertension. *JAMA* 1979;241(18):1897–1898.
73. Management committee of the Australian therapeutic trial in mild hypertension: the Australian therapeutic trial in mild hypertension. *Lancet* 1980;1:1261–1277.
74. Medical research council working party on need to moderate hypertension: randomized controlled trial of treatment for mild hypertension: design and pilot trial. *Br Med J* 1977;1:1437–1440.
75. Pickering G. *The nature of essential hypertension.* New York: Grune & Stratton, 1961.
76. American Society of Hypertension. Should mild hypertension be treated? Presented at the First Meeting of the American Society of Hypertension.
77. Inui TS, Yourtee EL, Williamson JW. Improved outcomes in hypertension after physician tutorials. A controlled trial. *Ann Intern Med* 1976;84:646–651.

Hypertension: Pathophysiology, Diagnosis, and Management, edited by J. H. Laragh and B. M. Brenner. Raven Press, Ltd., New York © 1990.

CHAPTER 132

Autonomic Nervous and Behavioral Factors in Hypertension

A Rationale for Treatment

Stevo Julius and Jurij Petrin

Behavioral and Neurogenic Factors in Early Phases of Hypertension, 2084
Neurogenic Early Hypertension as a Precursor of Later Established Hypertension, 2085
Mechanism of Transition from a Neurogenic to a Non-Neurogenic Form of Hypertension, 2087
Behavioral Treatment of Hypertension, 2088
References, 2089

Despite the prevailing popular belief that human hypertension is synonymous with nervous tension, the scientific evidence for the role of behavioral and neurogenic factors in the etiology of hypertension leaves much to be desired. Even when the evidence is reasonably good, it fails to gain general acceptance among the experts. Historical reasons for this scientific skepticism lay in the early demonstrations by Pickering (1) that after the forearm sympathetics are blocked with local anesthesia the vascular resistance in hypertensive patients remains elevated. In a similar vein were the findings by Conway (2) and Sivertsson (3), who utilized the maximal vasodilation after ischemic exercise to abolish the effects of autonomic tone on the forearm vasculature. Both authors found a residual "structural" increase of forearm vascular resistance in hypertensive patients and viewed this as evidence that the enhanced autonomic drive is not the major factor in the vascular abnormality of hypertension. Later, Korner et al. (4) demonstrated that the total systemic vascular resistance in hypertensive patients remains elevated even after a thorough cardiovascular autonomic blockade. Since the major hemodynamic abnormality in hypertension is an elevation of total peripheral resistance (5), and the elevation persisted in the absence of sympathetic drive, this suggested that the autonomic nervous system is not involved in the genesis of hypertension.

Such a negative attitude about the role of the autonomic nervous system in hypertension draws additional support from animal experimentation. Whereas it is reasonably easy to develop severe and self-sustaining forms of hypertension with a large number of experimental techniques, investigators using strictly neurogenic methods to elicit chronic hypertension were less successful. Removal of arterial baroreceptors (6), direct stimulation of the defense area in the brain (7), stimulation of the stellate ganglion (8), exposing rats to noise (9), and operant conditioning of primates (10) cause only temporary or labile elevations in blood pressure. Failure to show that the nervous system can induce a permanent state of accelerating hypertension, combined with strong evidence from their own laboratory, convinced Guyton and Coleman (11) and many others that the nervous system is a short-term blood pressure regulator of little importance with regard to the development of human hypertension. Closest to a self-sustaining behaviorally induced form of experimental hypertension are the socially stressed mice of Henry and Meehan (12). However, the renal pathology in these animals resembles pyelonephritis without classical vascular changes of hypertension.

The negative background notwithstanding, it will be shown in this chapter that autonomic nervous abnormalities and behavioral factors clearly play an important pathophysiologic role in some patients with hypertension. No claim will be made that these aberrations are present in the whole spectrum of essential hypertension. Nevertheless, inasmuch as behavioral treatment of hypertension is likely to be efficacious in patients with a strong neurogenic component, it is important to characterize and properly define this subgroup.

BEHAVIORAL AND NEUROGENIC FACTORS IN EARLY PHASES OF HYPERTENSION

In the early 1950s, investigators from Prague (13) observed that (in contradistinction to more severe forms of hypertension) in very mild hypertension a high cardiac output (and not a high total peripheral resistance) is the major hemodynamic feature. This observation was later confirmed by numerous investigators (14–18). Frequently, though not invariably, the high cardiac output is accompanied by a fast heart rate. Consequently, the condition is often referred to as the "hyperkinetic state" or "hyperkinetic borderline hypertension." Three independent studies showed that when oxygen consumption was measured, both the cardiac output and oxygen consumption values were elevated (15–17). Fast heart rates, high oxygen consumption, and elevated cardiac output are characteristic of hypermetabolic states (physical exercise, hyperthyroidism). However, in these states the vascular resistance is invariably low and the blood pressure remains close to normal. We pointed out that in hyperkinetic borderline hypertension the vascular resistance, while nominally normal, is inappropriately high for the observed levels of cardiac output (19). A high sympathetic tone could, theoretically, be responsible for this discrepancy between the cardiac output, the oxygen consumption, and the total peripheral resistance. More sympathetic drive to the heart may raise the cardiac output, and enhanced stimulation of peripheral metabolic receptors could increase the oxygen consumption, whereas a simultaneously enhanced alpha-adrenergic tone could cause vasoconstriction and thereby prevent the hypermetabolic vasodilation.

Based on such reasoning, the Ann Arbor group proceeded to investigate whether a generalized autonomic nervous abnormality may be the cause of the unusual hemodynamic constellation in hyperkinetic borderline hypertension. The hypothesis was tested with receptor-blocking agents, which, if properly used, can provide better information about the autonomic nervous tone than can the traditional measurement of catecholamine levels or even the assays of catecholamine turnover (20). An illustration of the type of information gained with acute pharmacologic intervention is given in Fig. 1. When large doses of propranolol (0.2 mg/kg, intravenously) are combined with a subsequent injection of 0.04 mg/kg of atropine, the response to propranolol symbolizes the amount of beta-adrenergic drive to the heart, whereas the response to atropine describes the degree of cardiac parasympathetic inhibition (21). First, Fig. 1 shows that the elevation of cardiac output in borderline hypertension is neurogenic, since a combined sympathetic and parasympathetic blockade abolishes the difference between patients and normotensive control subjects. The figure illustrates yet another important point: The elevation of the cardiac output is not due to an isolated sympathetic hyperactivity. Hypersensitivity of beta-receptors has been described in a group of patients

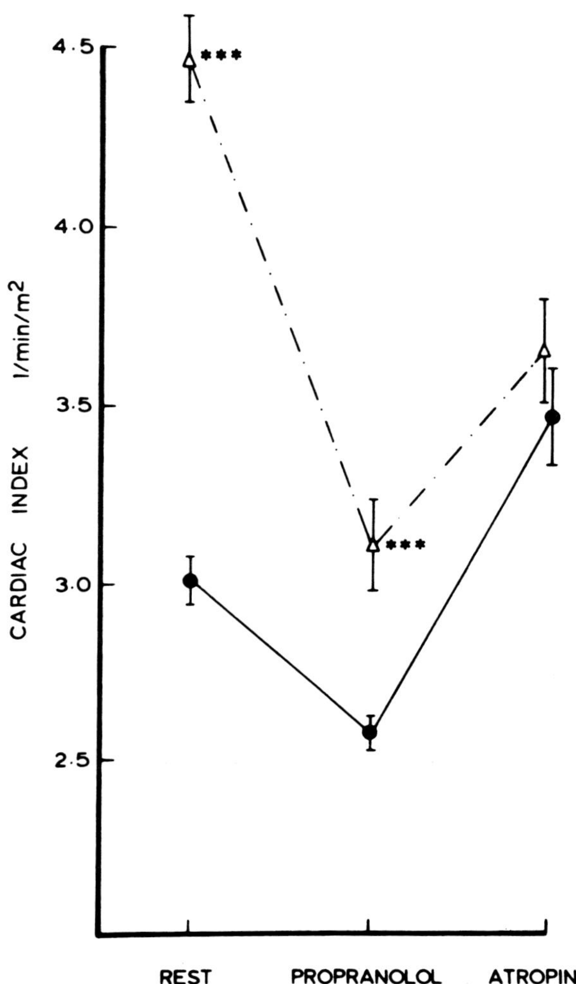

FIG. 1. Influence of the stepwise blockade of the autonomic system on cardiac index. First, propranolol (0.2 mg/kg, intravenously) was given, and the measurement was taken 7 min after completion of the injection. Another measurement was taken 7 min after atropine (0.04 mg/kg, intravenously). Patients were selected for an elevated cardiac index (1 SD above the mean of the controls). There were 16 such patients and 18 control subjects. (From ref. 21.)

(22) with hyperkinetic circulation, some of whom also had mild hypertension. However, in the patients in Fig. 1, after the beta-adrenergic blockade the cardiac output was still significantly higher than in normotensive control subjects and became normal only after the additional parasympathetic blockade with atropine. Thus both branches of the autonomic innervations of the heart were involved in the elevation of the cardiac output. This, in turn, suggests that the abnormality most likely originates in the central nervous system and is not due to an isolated hypersensitivity of beta-adrenergic receptors. A closer look at Fig. 1 brings to focus a third important point. Patients had a larger fall of cardiac output and heart rate than did control subjects, attesting to a higher-than-normal sympathetic drive. After atropine the situation is reversed; patients respond with lesser increase and therefore have less of a parasympathetic inhibitory tone. Such a reciprocal relationship in which a

higher sympathetic discharge is coupled with a lesser parasympathetic activity (or vice versa) is typical for the integrative function of the cardiovascular center in the medulla oblongata.

Numerous inputs descend upon the medulla, and many of them elicit the typical reciprocal change in the sympathetic and parasympathetic tone. Some of these lend themselves to experimental testing. Alteration of the stretch of arterial baroreceptors characteristically elicit a reciprocal sympathoparasympathetic response. Therefore, an abnormal baroreceptor function might be responsible for the hemodynamic constellation in neurogenic borderline hypertension, and a number of articles suggest that this, in fact, is the case (23–26). We were, however, not able to confirm these observations with regard to our patients (27). It is conceivable that the difference stems from variations in the patient population. For example, Eckberg (24) has shown that within the borderline blood pressure range, baroreceptor abnormality is related to the prevailing blood pressure; he also showed that the mildest patients had normal baroreceptor sensitivity. Nevertheless, a recent report that the arterial baroreceptors are less sensitive in children of hypertensive parents (26) casts doubt on our own contention of normal baroreceptor function in early borderline hypertension. Should it, in the future, be proven beyond doubt that baroreceptors are defective in very early phases of hypertension, this still will not establish the primacy of this defect. Baroreceptor function can be altered through changes of the afferent arc or as a result of a different central processing of an essentially normal input from the periphery. There is good evidence that influences from higher regions of the brain, such as activation of the defense reaction and sleep (28,29), can alter the function of arterial baroreceptors. Consequently, on theoretical grounds, psychosomatic factors may be responsible for the integrative abnormality of autonomic control in borderline hypertension.

Actual research data further support the theoretical notion that behavioral (psychosomatic) factors may be responsible for the abnormal autonomic control of the circulation in borderline hypertension. Patients with borderline hypertension are outward oriented, submissive to other people's opinions, and unable to express anger while harboring feelings of hostility and suspiciousness (30,31). Such personality profiles should render them vulnerable to stressful influences. It is therefore not surprising to find that patients with the mildest forms of hypertension (32–34), as well as normotensive children of hypertensive parents (35), show larger blood pressure responses to various mental stresses than do normal control subjects. Interestingly, the hyperreactivity is limited only to mental stress, whereas the blood pressure responses to other (physical) stressors tend to be normal (34). Thus the ability to regulate the blood pressure response to various stimuli is not diminished, and the observed hyperresponsiveness to mental stresses most likely reflects these subjects' behavioral styles (e.g., a tendency to readily perceive psychologic challenges). Unfortunately, this hyperreactivity has frequently been misconstrued and equated with the *mechanism* of the development of hypertension. The notion that hypertension develops through a summation of repeated emotionally induced pressor episodes is widely entrenched in the behavioral literature. Intellectually, the proponents of this concept draw support from Folkow et al.'s work on the role of the structural reinforcement in the course of hypertension (36). Whereas Folkow et al.'s results are factually indisputable and provide a clear framework to explain how hypertension accelerates, to our knowledge it has never been experimentally shown that repeated pressor episodes can lead to permanent, self-perpetuating hypertension. Clinical experience of acute cures of longstanding hypertension, after the cause has been surgically removed, suggests that hypertension cannot be maintained in the absence of a constant pressor stimulus. Psychosomatic or behavioral factors can cause hypertension only if they cause a permanent enhancement of the central nervous autonomic drive.

Those who, on theoretical grounds, accept the notion that repeated pressor episodes may elicit permanent hypertension must pass yet another hurdle. Most of their concepts are based on observations of hyperresponsiveness to mental stresses elicited in experimental laboratories. It is then assumed that the laboratory experience is representative of actual daily events and that emotional stress is the single most important cause of the overall variability of the blood pressure. However, the blood pressure variability observed under natural conditions shows no relationship to the magnitude of the pressor response in the laboratory. In fact, patients who are most hyperresponsive in the laboratory, the borderline hypertensives, do not show an abnormal blood pressure variability outside of the laboratory (37,38). Furthermore, as already pointed out in the introductory paragraphs of this chapter, it has been exceptionally difficult, if not impossible, to create sustained hypertension by repeated pressor episodes in animals.

NEUROGENIC EARLY HYPERTENSION AS A PRECURSOR OF LATER ESTABLISHED HYPERTENSION

Patients with borderline hypertension have a higher risk of developing future hypertension than do average normotensives, but that risk is not overwhelming. Review of the literature (39) suggests that after 10 years about 20% of borderline hypertensives will develop a more advanced form of hypertension. Even when the hypertension is considered to be established but mild (e.g., diastolic readings exceeding 95 mmHg on three separate occasions) (40), 3 years later about one-third will show improvement and revert to lower values. Since in this group of borderline and mild hypertensive patients one finds the largest proportion of subjects with a neurogenic component (but all patients will not necessarily develop a more severe form of hypertension), it is not clear whether those with neurogenic stigmata are less or more likely to progress to established hypertension. Does the behaviorally linked sympathetic overactivity in the "prehypertensive" phase carry a good or a bad prognosis?

Modern clinical practice is a historic extension of the tradition of differentiating between "organic" and "functional" conditions, and the present trend for objective laboratory work-up further reinforces this attitude. It is therefore frequently assumed that "anxiety" and "nervousness" are inherently benign conditions which may be bothersome to the patients but which are not likely to cause any permanent damage. This attitude certainly is not justified in the case of borderline hypertension. All the evidence points to the contrary; the subset of patients with a "neurogenic" mechanism is at the highest risk. As indicated earlier, the best case for a participation of the autonomic nervous system in the pathophysiology of the hypertension is in the subjects with hyperkinetic circulation. High cardiac output and resting tachycardia are the hallmarks of the hyperkinetic state. A number of studies have shown that fast resting heart rates, independent of the blood pressure elevation, are a predictor of future hypertension (41–43). This point is illustrated in Fig. 2, from the classical study of Levy et al. (41) on the 5-year incidence of hypertension among the U.S. military personnel. Normotensive subjects with normal heart rate had a very low incidence of hypertension. Subjects whose blood pressure readings were normal but whose resting heart rate was fast developed hypertension two to three times more frequently than did their counterparts with normal heart rate values. The incidence of hypertension in these hyperkinetic normotensive individuals was about the same as in individuals who had borderline hypertension but normal resting heart rate values. When these soldiers had both tachycardia and borderline hypertension, the risk for future hypertension substantially increased.

In a few hemodynamic studies, the cardiac output was measured and the measurement was repeated after periods of years. These studies offer yet another glimpse at the potential significance of the problem (44–47). The periods of observation were relatively short, but in all studies the

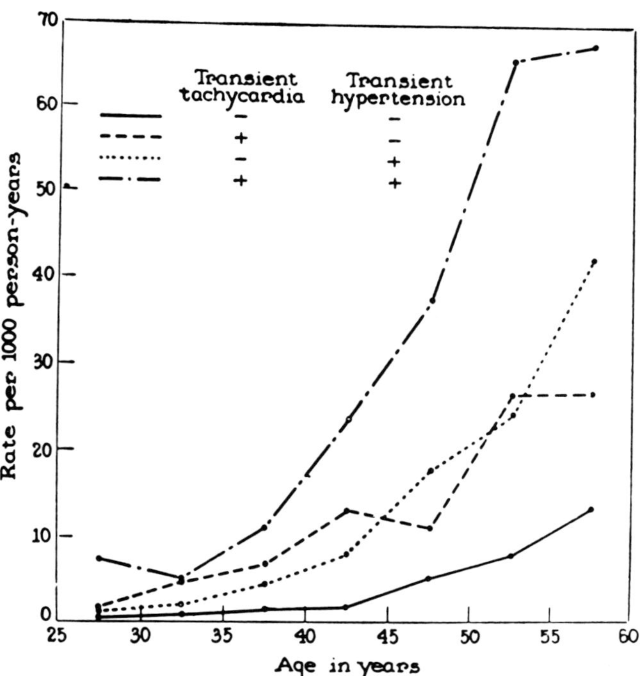

FIG. 2. Rates of development of sustained hypertension after a period of 5 years for specified age groups (From ref. 41.)

cardiac output decreased on the second exam, whereas the blood pressure tended to remain in the borderline range. Only one study reported an increase of the average blood pressure (45). The relatively short period of observation is the most likely reason why these studies failed to show progression toward hypertension. Thanks to the efforts of Lund-Johansen (16) in Norway, we now know that the time factor is very important. He investigated the hemodynamics in subjects who had Stage I hypertension (e.g., a minimal blood pressure elevation without target-organ damage). At the first exam, many of his subjects had hyperdynamic circulation (16). After 10 years there was no evidence of hyperdynamic circulation, but the blood pressure remained in the same range as at the outset. When the observations were extended to 15 years, the picture radically changed (48). At that point, many subjects developed high-resistance established hypertension, and the majority of them required antihypertensive treatment. Though the Lund-Johansen sample was small, when his observations are combined with the epidemiologic data on tachycardia as a predictor of hypertension a strong suggestion emerges. The hyperkinetic state and its neurogenic stigmata appear to be a precursor of future hypertension. However, the prevalence of the hyperkinetic state in the general population is not known. Is the neurogenic etiology of hypertension the rule or the exception? In our laboratory, about a third of the patients have hyperkinetic circulation, but our subjects were young male University students; whether they are representative of the population at large is a matter of conjecture. However, the data do provide a base to analyze whether patients with hyperkinetic circulation are a separate and qualitatively distinguishable subgroup. Over the years, we have accumulated invasive hemodynamic data on normotensive subjects and on patients with borderline hypertension. These individuals were selected by their blood pressure level, and we had no prior knowledge of their hemodynamic profile. Since both patients and control subjects were of the same age and sex, we combined the total population and first investigated whether the distributions of the heart rate and cardiac output were normal or skewed. This interim analysis indicated that for both variables the distribution curve was skewed toward the high values. In the next step, multiple models were fitted separately for the heart rate and cardiac output, to reject or accept the hypothesis that the distribution represents a single population. The single-population hypothesis was rejected, and, as seen in Figs. 3 and 4, there was a highly significant fit for two populations. Based on this, a secondary analysis was performed using the co-mingling technique developed by Schork and Schork (49). The data were adjusted for age, weight, and blood pressure; then, co-mingling analysis determined that when high heart rate and cardiac output are combined, two different populations are still present. In the final step, individuals belonging to the high-cardiac-output–high-heart-rate population were identified, and their original diagnostic classification was determined. Only 2% of the normotensive individuals were hyperkinetic, whereas 25% of the borderline hypertension group belonged to the hyperkinetic subset. This analysis confirms that amongst patients with borderline hypertension there exists a subgroup whose hemodynamic charac-

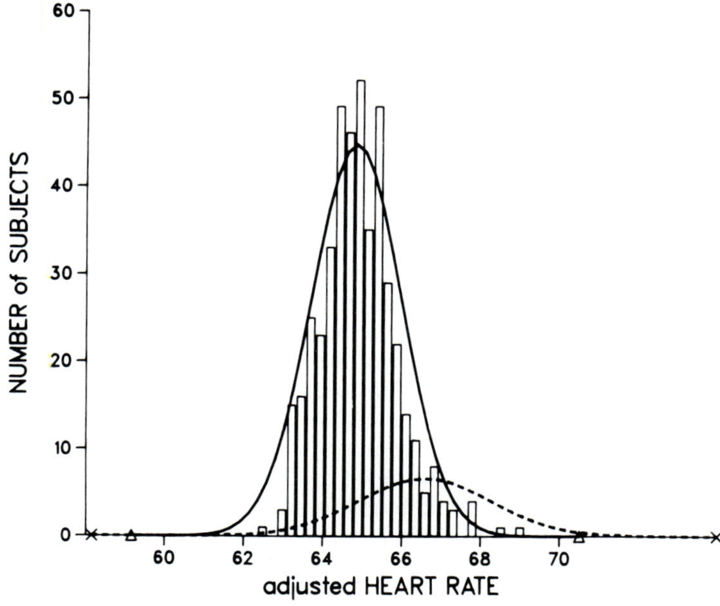

FIG. 3. Adjusted distribution of heart rate based on invasive hemodynamic data of 186 patients with borderline hypertension and 257 normal control subjects. Adjusted for age, sex, height, and weight. Solid line represents normokinetics; broken line represents hyperkinetics.

teristics are different from those of normotensive subjects and from those of the rest of patients with borderline hypertension. As it has been repeatedly stated, the blood pressure elevation in these hyperkinetic individuals is maintained through a neurogenic mechanism.

MECHANISM OF TRANSITION FROM A NEUROGENIC TO A NON-NEUROGENIC FORM OF HYPERTENSION

In the previous section, we suggested that hyperkinetic borderline hypertension eventually evolves into established hypertension. However, on the surface, a number of issues argue against such a chain of events. In early hypertension the cardiac output is elevated, but the hemodynamic hallmark of established hypertension is a normal cardiac output and a high vascular resistance. Regional and systemic vascular resistance in established hypertension remains elevated after a complete blockade of the autonomic nervous system (1,4). Furthermore, if plasma norepinephrine levels are used as the yardstick to evaluate the sympathetic nervous system in hypertension, high plasma catecholamine levels are found only in the early phases of hypertension; in established hypertension the catecholamine levels are normal (50). Consequently, if there is a transition from the hyperkinetic state to established hypertension, one ought to answer two important questions: (a) What is the mechanism whereby the cardiac output decreases and the vascular resistance increases? (b) How does the initial

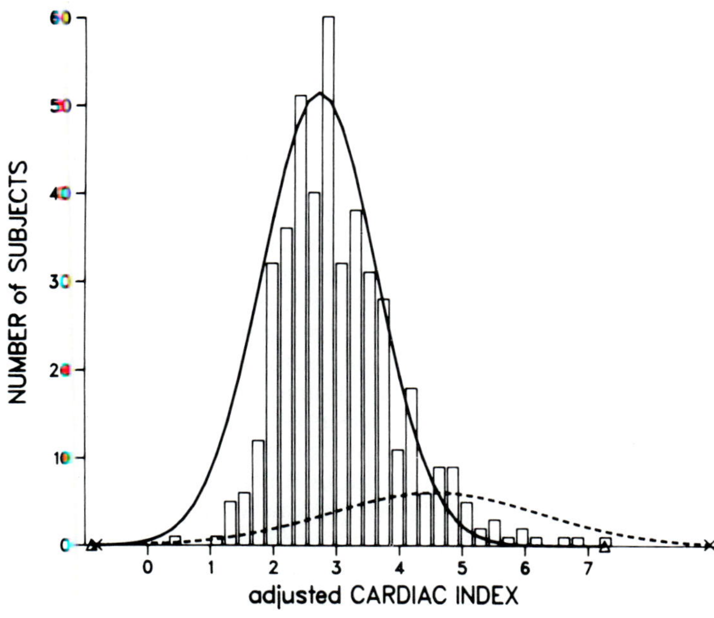

FIG. 4. Results for cardiac index (see legend for Fig. 3).

state of enhanced sympathetic drive revert to a more normal pattern?

The "total body autoregulation" has been invoked to explain the transition from a high to a normal cardiac output in the course of hypertension (11). Within the framework of this concept, an initial overperfusion (e.g., a flow exceeding the metabolic need of the tissues) triggers an increase of vascular resistance which, in turn, limits the flow. However, it is doubtful whether the mechanism is involved in the changing hemodynamic patterns in hypertension. The basic stimulus for autoregulation is overperfusion (e.g., a cardiac output that exceeds the oxygen demands of the body). However, patients with high cardiac output also have increased oxygen consumption (15–17). Such a hemodynamic constellation, where cardiac output is appropriately increased to match the higher oxygen consumption, provides no support for the autoregulatory concept. We believe that the decrease of cardiac output in the course of hypertension is a direct consequence of the combined effects of the elevated blood pressure and the enhanced sympathetic tone in patients with hyperkinetic circulation. An enhanced sympathetic tone may elicit a functional down-regulation of the beta-adrenergic receptors in the heart. Whereas there are no data on the actual number of cardiac beta-receptors in patients with borderline hypertension, pertinent observation of the cardiac responsiveness to beta-adrenergic stimulation supports the concept of a functional down-regulation. We (51), as well as others (52), have shown that patients with a normal cardiac output type of borderline hypertension respond to the same doses of isoproterenol with a lesser increase of heart rate and cardiac output than do control subjects. In addition, such patients also exhibit a limitation of the stroke volume. The decrease of stroke volume becomes particularly evident after a functional "denervation" of the heart with beta-adrenergic and a parasympathetic blockade (51) and is most likely due to a decrease of cardiac compliance. The decreased sympathetic responsiveness and the low stroke volume could account for the transition from hyperkinetic borderline hypertension to normal cardiac output established hypertension.

The increase of vascular resistance in the course of hypertension can be best explained by the structural reinforcement concept of Folkow (53). He postulated that elevated blood pressure leads to vascular hypertrophy and a thickening of the medial (muscular) layer of the resistance vessels. This change in wall-to-lumen ratio of the resistance vessels renders them hyperresponsive to all vasoconstrictive stimuli. Such early changes in vascular structure have been documented in hypertension (2,3), and we recently examined them in some detail (54). The clinical observations are in full agreement with Folkow's concept.

Whereas the transition from a high cardiac output to a high total peripheral resistance state can be explained by the secondary effects of the enhanced sympathetic drive and the elevated blood pressure on the heart and the blood vessels, this still leaves a major question unanswered. The sympathetic tone is enhanced in the early hyperkinetic phase, but it becomes normal in later phases of hypertension (50). What is the mechanism for this "resetting" of the sympathetic tone? We recently proposed a comprehensive conceptual framework to explain this transition (55). In short, the concept, supported by a substantial body of cross-sectional observations, suggests that the central nervous system exhibits a "blood-pressure-seeking behavior." It is postulated that in subserving the circulation, the central nervous system tightly regulates the blood pressure while allowing large variations in the flow. In order to achieve such a close regulation of the pressure, the central nervous system must sense the achieved and prevailing blood pressure. If the central nervous system is, in fact, organized in such a way and controls the circulation by regulating and sensing the blood pressure, it is easy to explain the disappearance of the enhanced sympathetic tone in the course of hypertension. As the structural reinforcement takes place, the blood vessels become hyperresponsive. If the central nervous system is responsible for the initial elevation of the blood pressure and has a mechanism to sense the achieved blood pressure, then with the advent of structural reinforcement a less sympathetic drive is needed to maintain the same blood pressure elevation. Within this context, the resetting of the sympathetic tone toward normal is an expected physiologic outcome. We wish to underscore the speculative nature of this concept and by no means consider it to be proven. Nevertheless, the concept provides a logical explanation for a chain of events known to occur in the course of hypertension. Further experimentation to prove or disprove this hypothesis is in order.

BEHAVIORAL TREATMENT OF HYPERTENSION

Observations quoted above about involvement of behavioral factors in hypertension suggest that such patients might benefit from behavioral methods for blood pressure reduction. The behavioral approach to treatment is particularly appealing in view of the high cost of medication, drug side effects, reports in literature about adverse effects of antihypertensive medication on blood lipids, and the tendency of patients not to comply with pharmacologic treatment.

In the last two decades a number of reports on behavioral treatment of hypertension became available (56–62). Three authoritative reviews (63–65) examine the results of such studies in some detail. Several methods of behavioral treatment have been used in an attempt to influence blood pressure; these include progressive muscular relaxation (PMR) (55,56,65,66), biofeedback (58–60), transcendental meditation (64), and some combinations of these. It is difficult to evaluate the influence of these methods on blood pressure levels and on the progression of the disease, mainly because of numerous methodological problems.

Usually a small number of subjects were studied, and the populations were highly selected. Often there were no control groups, blood pressure was measured mainly in the office, and compliance with treatment was usually not reported. In several studies, patients were kept on various regimens of antihypertensive medication, and the response to behavioral treatment was evaluated as a decrease in the amount of medication needed to control their blood pressure. The number of blood pressure readings before entry into the study and upon follow-up was frequently not standardized. In one of the reviews (63), only 29% of studies met all the criteria required for scientific evaluation of their results.

In spite of these shortcomings, some conclusions can be drawn. Some types of behavioral treatment are better for blood pressure control than others. PMR seems to have the most beneficial influence on hypertensive patients, whereas biofeedback is consistently showing inferior results (63). It is also apparent that the patient response to behavioral treatment is not uniform. For example, it has been shown that hyperkinetic borderline hypertensives who have a high level of sympathetic drive tend to be the best responders (56). In this study, more than 50% of mild hypertensives with fast heart rate, high norepinephrine plasma concentration, and high anxiety scores at rest responded to PMR, and 30% of them achieved normotension. Subjects reported improvement in their general well-being, with pleasant feelings of free floating and warm numbness in their arms and legs. Oxygen consumption, plasma norepinephrine concentration, and anxiety scores decreased at the end of the treatment.

Long-term results with behavioral treatment of hypertension are not very promising. In a review by Ward et al. (63), the follow-up data from several studies were evaluated across 12 months of follow-up. It was shown that the beneficial effects of behavioral treatment were stable up to 9 months following the initiation of treatment, but then faded to reach negative values at 12 months for both systolic and diastolic blood pressure. The reason for this is not clear, but the most logical explanation is that patients' compliance with regular treatment—which is time-consuming —decreases with months of training and that the small decline of both systolic and diastolic blood pressure discourages the patient from participating in regular treatment schedule.

At present, behavioral treatments of hypertension have serious limitations which preclude their routine use. PMR is the most promising method, but only a small percentage of hypertensive patients will benefit from this time-consuming procedure, with hyperkinetic borderline and mild hypertensive patients being the best responders. But even they will have favorable results only for several months and might become hypertensive again. Decreased patient compliance after several months of treatment probably explains the short-acting reduction of blood pressure. By no means can behavioral treatment replace drug treatment of arterial hypertension when this becomes indicated. It ought to be kept in mind that, while not necessarily improving the blood pressure, behavioral modalities very frequently positively affect the patients' general feeling of well-being, which in itself is a very desirable outcome.

Future research will have to elucidate whether behavioral treatment can ever play a major role in the treatment of arterial hypertension. A proper strategy would be to narrow the studies to "responders" and then to (a) evaluate the effect of treatment on the average blood pressure over 24 hr, (b) develop methods to improve patient compliance, and (c) investigate new and simplified methods for retention and practice of relaxation skills. It may then become possible to define the subset of patients in whom the behavioral treatment might have a long-term beneficial effect. Until these issues are resolved, behavioral treatment should be used as an adjunct to other, well-established methods of nonpharmacologic treatment of mild forms of arterial hypertension.

REFERENCES

1. Pickering GW. The peripheral resistance in persistent arterial hypertension. *Clin Sci* 1936;2:209.
2. Conway J. A vascular abnormality in hypertension. A study of blood flow in the forearm. *Circulation* 1963;27:520–529.
3. Sivertsson R. The hemodynamic importance of structural vascular changes in essential hypertension. *Acta Physiol Scand* 1970;79(Suppl 343):3–56.
4. Korner PI, Shaw J, Uther JB, West MJ, McRitchie RJ, Richards JG. Autonomic and non-autonomic circulatory components in essential hypertension in man. *Circulation* 1973;48:107–117.
5. Julius S, Egan B. Hemodynamics of hypertension. In: Zanchetti A, Tarazi RC, eds. *Handbook of hypertension, vol 7: pathophysiology of hypertension—Cardiovascular aspects.* Amsterdam: Elsevier, 1986;153–178.
6. Ferrario CM, McCubbin JW, Page IH. Hemodynamic characteristics of chronic experimental neurogenic hypertension in unanesthetized dogs. *Circ Res* 1969;29:911.
7. Folkow B, Rubinstein EH. Cardiovascular effects of acute and chronic stimulation of the hypothalamic defense area in the rat. *Acta Physiol Scand* 1966;68:48–57.
8. Liard JF, Tarazi RC, Ferrario CM, et al. Hemodynamic and humoral characteristics of hypertension induced by prolonged stellate ganglion stimulation in conscious dogs. *Circ Res* 1975;36:455.
9. Rothlin E, Cerletti A, Emmenegger H. Experimental psychoneurogenic hypertension and its treatment with hydrogenated ergot alkaloids (hydergine). *Acta Med Scand* 1956;154(Suppl 312):27–35.
10. Herd JA, Morse WH, Kelleher RT, Jones LG. Arterial hypertension in the squirrel monkey during behavioral experiments. *Am J Physiol* 1969;217:24–29.
11. Guyton AC, Coleman TG. Quantitative analysis of the pathophysiology of hypertension. *Circ Res* 1967;24–25(Suppl I):1–19.
12. Henry JP, Meehan JP. Psychosocial stimuli, physiologic specificity and cardiovascular disease. In: Weiner H, Hofer MA, eds. *Brain, behavior and bodily diseases.* New York: Raven Press, 1981;305–334.
13. Widimsky J, Fejfarova MH, Fejfar Z. Changes of cardiac output in hypertensive disease. *Cardiologia* 1957;31:381–389.
14. Eich RH, Peters RJ, Cuddy RP, Smulyan Y, Lyons RH. The hemodynamics in labile hypertension. *Am Heart J* 1962;63:188.
15. Sannerstedt R. Hemodynamic response to exercise in patients with arterial hypertension. *Acta Med Scand* 1966;458:1.
16. Lund-Johansen P. Hemodynamics in early essential hypertension. *Acta Med Scand* 1967;482(Suppl):1.
17. Julius S, Conway J. Hemodynamic studies in patients with borderline blood pressure elevation. *Circulation* 1968;38:282–288.
18. Frohlich ED, Kozul VJ, Tarazi RC, Dustan HP. Physiological comparison of labile and essential hypertension. *Circ Res* 1970;26 (Suppl I):55.
19. Julius S, Pascual A, Sannerstedt R, Mitchell C. Relationship between cardiac output and peripheral resistance in borderline hypertension. *Circulation* 1971;43:382–390.
20. Julius S, Ibsen H, Colfer HT. Hemodynamic and pharmacologic correlates of plasma norepinephrine in hypertension. In: Ziegler MG, Lake CR, eds. *Norepinephrine, vol 2: frontiers of clinical neuroscience.* Baltimore: Williams & Wilkins, 1984;401–409.
21. Julius S, Pascual AV, London R. Role of parasympathetic inhibition in the hyperkinetic type of borderline hypertension. *Circulation* 1971;44:413–418.
22. Frohlich ED, Tarazi RC, Dustan HP. Hyperdynamic beta-adrenergic circulatory state: Increased beta-receptor responsiveness. *Arch Intern Med* 1969;123:1–7.

23. Takeshita A, Tanaka S, Kuroiwa A, Nakamura M. Reduced baroreceptor sensitivity in borderline hypertension. *Circulation* 1975;51:738.
24. Eckberg DL. Carotid baroreflex function in young men with borderline blood pressure elevation. *Circulation* 1979;59:632.
25. Volpe M, Trimarco B, Ricciardelli B, Vigorito C, DeLuca N, Rengo F, Condorelli M. The autonomic nervous tone abnormalities in the genesis of the impaired baroreflex responsiveness in borderline hypertensive subjects. *Clin Sci* 1982;62:581–588.
26. Ookuwa H, Takata S, Ogawa J, Iwase N, Ikeda T, Hattori N. Abnormal cardiopulmonary baroreflexes in normotensive young subjects with a family history of essential hypertension. *J Clin Hypertens* 1987;3:596–604.
27. Julius S. Borderline hypertension: clinical and pathophysiologic significance. In: von Frick PH, von Harnack G-A, Martini GA, Prader A, Schoen R, Wolff HP, eds. *Advances in internal medicine and pediatrics.* Heidelberg: Springer-Verlag, 1978;52–84.
28. Hilton SM. Inhibition of baroreceptor reflexes on hypothalamic stimulation. *J Physiol* 1963;165:56–57.
29. Conway J, Boon N, Jones JV, Sleight P. Involvement of the baroreceptor reflexes in the changes in blood pressure with sleep and mental arousal. *Hypertension* 1983;5(5):746–748.
30. Harburg E, Julius S, McGinn NF, McLeod J, Hoobler SW. Personality traits and behavioral patterns associated with systolic blood pressure levels in college males. *J Chronic Dis* 1964;17:405–414.
31. Esler M, Julius S, Zweifler A, Randall O, Harburg E, Gardiner H, DeQuattro V. Mild high-renin essential hypertension: neurogenic human hypertension? *N Engl J Med* 1977;296:405–411.
32. Nestel PJ. Blood pressure and catecholamine excretion after mental stress in labile hypertension. *Lancet* 1969;1:692–694.
33. Light KC, Obrist PA. Cardiovascular reactivity to behavioral stress in young males with and without marginally elevated casual systolic pressures. Comparison of clinic, home, and laboratory measures. *Hypertension* 1980;2:802–808.
34. Eliasson K, Hjemdahl P, Kahan T. Circulatory and sympatho-adrenal responses to stress in borderline and established hypertension. *J Hypertens* 1983;1:131–139.
35. Falkner B, Onesti G, Angelakos ET, Fernandes M, Langman C. Cardiovascular response to mental stress in normal adolescents with hypertensive parents. Hemodynamics and mental stress in adolescents. *Hypertension* 1979;1:23–30.
36. Folkow B, Grimby G, Thulesius O. Adaptive structural changes of the vascular wall in hypertension and their relationship to control of the peripheral resistance. *Acta Physiol Scand* 1958;44:255.
37. Mancia G, Zanchetti A. Blood pressure variability. In: Zanchetti A, Tarazi RC, eds. *Handbook of hypertension, vol 7: pathophysiology of hypertension—cardiovascular aspects.* Amsterdam: Elsevier, 1986;125–152.
38. Horan MJ, Kennedy HL, Padgett NE. Do borderline hypertensive patients have labile blood pressure? *Ann Intern Med* 1981;94(1):466–468.
39. Julius S, Schork MA. Borderline hypertension—a critical review. *J Chronic Dis* 1971;23:723–754.
40. Australian National Blood Pressure Study Management Committee. The Australian therapeutic trial in mild hypertension. *Lancet* 1980;1:1261–1267.
41. Levy RL, White PD, Stroud WD, Hillman CC. Transient tachycardia: prognostic significance alone and in association with transient hypertension. *JAMA* 1945;129:585–588.
42. Paffenbarger RS, Jr., Thorne MC, Wing AL. Chronic disease in former college students—VIII. Characteristics in youth predisposing to hypertension in later years. *Am J Epidemiol* 1968;88:25–32.
43. Stamler J, Berkson DM, Dyer A, Lepper MH, Lindberg HA, Paul O, McKean H, Rhomberg P, Schoenberger JA, Shekelle RB, Stamler R. Relationship of multiple variables to blood pressure—findings from four Chicago epidemiologic studies. In: Paul O, ed. *Epidemiology and control of hypertension.* Miami: Symposia Specialists, 1975;307–352.
44. Eich RH, Cuddy RP, Smulyan H. Hemodynamics in labile hypertension: a follow-up study. *Circulation* 1966;34:299–307.
45. Safar ME, Weiss YA, Levenson JA, London GM, Milliez PL. Hemodynamic study of 85 patients with borderline hypertension. *Am J Cardiol* 1973;31:315–319.
46. Julius S, Quadir H, Gajendragadkar S. Hyperkinetic state: a precursor of hypertension? A longitudinal study of borderline hypertension. In: Gross F, Strasser T, eds. *Mild hypertension: natural history and management.* London: Pittman Medical Publishing Co., 1979;116–126.
47. Lund-Johansen P. Haemodynamic observations in mild hypertension. In: Gross F, Strasser T, eds. *Mild hypertension: natural history and management.* London: Pittman Medical Publishing Co., 1979;102–115.
48. Lund-Johansen P. Hemodynamic alterations in early essential hypertension: recent advances. In: Gross F, Strasser T, eds. *Mild hypertension: recent advances.* New York: Raven Press, 1983;237–249.
49. Schork NJ, Schork MA. Skewness and mixtures of normal distributions. *Commun Statist–Theory Meth* 1988;17:3951–3969.
50. Goldstein DS. Plasma catecholamines and essential hypertension. An analytical review. *Hypertension* 1983;5:86–99.
51. Julius S, Randall OS, Esler MD, Kashima T, Ellis CN, Bennett J. Altered cardiac responsiveness and regulation in the normal cardiac output type of borderline hypertension. *Circ Res* 1975;36–37(Suppl I):I-199–I-207.
52. Trimarco B, Volpe M, Ricciardelli B, Galva MA, Petracca R, Condorelli M. Studies of the mechanisms underlying impairment of beta-adrenoceptor mediated effects in human hypertension. *Hypertension* 1983;5:584–590.
53. Folkow B. Physiological aspects of primary hypertension. *Physiol Rev* 1982;62:347–503.
54. Egan B, Panis R, Hinderliter A, Schork N, Julius S. Mechanism of increased alpha-adrenergic vasoconstriction in human essential hypertension. *J Clin Invest* 1987;80:812–817.
55. Julius S. The blood pressure seeking properties of the central nervous system. *J Hypertension* 1988;6:177–185.
56. Cottier C, Shapiro K, Julius S. Treatment of mild hypertension with progressive muscle relaxation. *Arch Intern Med* 1984;144:1954–1958.
57. Bali LR. Long-term effect of relaxation on blood pressure and anxiety levels of essential hypertensive males: a controlled study. *Psychosom Med* 1979;41:637–646.
58. Bertilson HS. Treatment program for borderline hypertension among college students: relaxation, finger temperature, biofeedback, and generalization. *Psychol Rep* 1979;44:107–114.
59. Datey KK. Role of biofeedback training in hypertension and stress. *J Postgrad Med* 1980;26:68–73.
60. Frankel BL, Patel DJ, Horwitz D, Friedewald DT, Gaardner KR. Treatment of hypertension with biofeedback and relaxation techniques. *Psychosom Med* 1979;40:276–293.
61. Stone RA, DeLeo J. Psychotherapeutic control of hypertension. *N Engl J Med* 1976;294:80–84.
62. Blockwell B, Bloomfield S, Gartside P, Robinson A, Hanenson I, Magenheim H, Nidich S, Zigler R. Transcendental meditation in hypertension: individual response patterns. *Lancet* 1976;223–226.
63. Ward MM, Swan GE, Chesney MA. Arousal-reduction treatments for mild hypertension: a meta-analysis of recent studies. In: Julius S, Bassett DR, eds. *Handbook of hypertension, vol 9: behavioral factors in hypertension* Amsterdam: Elsevier, 1987;285–301.
64. Julius S, Cottier C. Behavior and hypertension. In: Dembroski TM, Schmidt TH, Blumchen, eds. *Biobehavioral bases of coronary heart disease.* Basel: Karger, 1983:271–289.
65. Shapiro AP, Schwartz GE, Ferguson DC. Behavioral methods in the treatment of hypertension: a review of their clinical status. *Ann Intern Med* 1977;86:626–636.
66. Brauer AP, Horlick L, Nelson E. Relaxation therapy for essential hypertension: a Veterans Administration outpatient study. *J Behav Med* 1979;2:21–29.

PART B

Drug Therapy

Hypertension: Pathophysiology, Diagnosis, and Management, edited by J. H. Laragh and B. M. Brenner. Raven Press, Ltd., New York © 1990.

CHAPTER 133

Origins and Development of Antihypertensive Treatment

Edward D. Freis

Ancient Beginnings, 2093
Growth of Knowledge in the Nineteenth Century, 2094
The Measurement of Blood Pressure, 2095
Forerunners of Modern Treatment, 2095
Low-Salt Diets, 2095
Surgical Sympathectomy, 2096
The Beginnings of Drug Treatment, 2096
Ganglion-Blocking Drugs, 2097
Veratrum viride, Hydralazine, and Reserpine, 2098
The Modern Era of Antihypertensive Drugs, 2099
Thiazide Diuretics, 2099
Guanethidine and Alpha-Methyldopa, 2100
Beta-Adrenergic Blocking Drugs, 2100
Converting-Enzyme Inhibitors, 2100
Calcium-Channel Blockers, 2100
Proving the Efficacy of Antihypertensive Drug Treatment, 2101
Summary and Conclusions, 2102
References, 2103

ANCIENT BEGINNINGS

Arterial blood pressure (BP) was not measured clinically until this century. However, the hardness of the arterial pulse has been the subject of great medical attention, including treatment, since ancient times. The early history related to hypertension has been collected by Ruskin in his masterful treatise, *Classics in Arterial Hypertension* (1), and I am indebted to him for most of the following discussion of that period.

As early as 2600 B.C., the *Yellow Emperor's Classic of Internal Medicine* (2) stated, "Nothing surpasses the examination of the pulse, for with it errors cannot be committed. In order to examine whether Yin or Yang predominates, one must distinguish a gentle pulse and one of low tension from a hard and bounding pulse. The heart influences the force and fills the pulse with blood." With remarkable insight the author states, "If too much salt is used in food, the pulse hardens." Also, he indicated the relationship between hypertension and congestive heart failure by stating that, "When the pulse is abundant but tense and hard like a cord there are dropsical swellings."

In the *Pulse Classic of Wang,* published in 280 A.D., some prognostic guidelines are given such as, "In cases of apoplexy, the pulse should be superficial and slow; if it is firm, rapid and large there is danger (1). Where there is pulmonary congestion a wiry and large pulse is favorable; but few can recover quickly if it is small and thready." The Ashurbanipal Library at Nineveh (669–626 B.C.) recommended venesection (which reduces BP) and cupping for the treatment of apoplexy. Leeches were used for apoplexy throughout the ancient world. Some ancient Chinese texts advised acupuncture or venesection when the pulse hardens (1).

The Romans also were much concerned with the pulse. The Roman patrician Cornelius Celsus (3) pointed out the increased rate and tenseness of the pulse with exercise, passion, and even the doctor's arrival! The latter is especially relevant today, when multiple visits are customary to allow the blood pressure to "settle down."

Lack of temperance in eating and in emotions was regarded as injurious by the ancient Chinese. The Arabic text *Al-Azkhora* (The Therapy) (1) was even more explicit in stating that "Nothing is more harmful to an aged person than to have a clever cook and a beautiful concubine." Hippocrates also said that sudden death is more common in the fat than in the lean (4).

Galen (131–201 A.D.) was greatly revered until the eighteenth century. Yet he probably held back medical progress by a combination of ignorance and authority. For example, he claimed that the pulse in apoplexy was weak and denied that the plethoric pulse syndrome described by Erasistrates was associated with stroke (5). By failing to associate increased arterial tension with apoplexy, Galen may have delayed the understanding of their relationship for many years.

On the other hand, Hippocrates (4) believed that paralysis was caused by apoplexy, which, in turn, resulted from plethora of the brain. From examining head wounds, he made the important observation that the paralysis occurs on the side opposite the lesion. Venesection, which could reduce the arterial blood pressure, was recommended by the Hippocratic School to relieve cerebral plethora. This method continued as the major treatment for stroke into the eighteenth century.

The ancient Greek and Romans treated apoplexy as an independent disease entity and did not realize its frequent connection with high blood pressure, then known as hardening of the pulse. For the treatment of the paralysis, Soravas of Ephesus (120 A.D.) recommended cupping of the spine to draw the animals spirits down and out (1). He also recommended bleeding and emetics to be followed by an enema if necessary. If any patient was strong enough to live through all this, he or she would probably make a good recovery.

For many centuries there had been bans on doing autopsies. These bans were lifted (at least in Basel, Switzerland) in the seventeenth century, when J. J. Wepfer reported four individuals who had died of apoplexy in 1658 (6). In each case he found a cerebral hemorrhage on the side opposite to the paralysis.

GROWTH OF KNOWLEDGE IN THE NINETEENTH CENTURY

Thomas Young is known for his 1808 Croonian Lecture on the functions of the heart and arteries (7). Young was a man of universal interests and accomplishments. He mastered seven languages; he developed theories of light (Young–Huygens wave theory) and accommodation (lens curvature, color vision, astigmatism) and even carried out a partial translation of the Rosetta stone! These were only a part of his many diverse accomplishments.

In his studies of the circulation, he proved "that the pressure which the blood possesses at the beginning of the great trunk of the aorta is kept up without noticeable loss down to the branches of the lower order." The statement is essentially correct. He claimed to have measured the percent fall in systolic and diastolic blood pressure in dogs from the aorta to mesenteric arteries of 200-μm diameter. The decrement averaged 16 mmHg. Approximately 150 years later, we remeasured the pressure drop using modern dynamic equipment (8) and found an average pressure drop of 17% systolic and 12% diastolic from aorta to mesenteric arteries of 200-μm diameter—a remarkable agreement, considering the methods used in Young's time. Young also affirmed the dependence of the quality of the arterial pulsation upon the force of the heart.

One of the best known contributors to the history of hypertension is Richard Bright (9), although there were others who preceded him in some aspects of his work. In the sixth century A.D., Aetios described sclerosis of the kidneys with possible manifestations of oliguria, hematuria, and dropsy in the absence of pain. Albuminuria was first noted by Cotugno in 1770 (1). In 1761, Morgagni found enlargement of the heart in autopsies exhibiting extensive hardening of the arteries (1).

Bright's principal contribution was to bring these various observations together, such as albuminuria, fullness and hardness of the pulse, and dropsy with hardening of the kidneys. These were presented in well-described case histories illustrated by superb color illustrations. By 1836 he expanded his observations to include apoplexy, serositis, hypertrophy of the left ventricle, and diminution of the specific gravity and urea content of the urine with increase in blood urea. He listed scarlatina or some other acute disease as the cause of this condition. Because of these accurate observations, Bright's disease and glomerulonephritis became synonymous. Bright provided a true pathological description of glomerulonephritis and probably of nephrosclerosis as well. With respect to the latter, he noted the thickening of the arterioles not only in the kidneys but also throughout the body.

In 1872, Gull and Sutton postulated that Bright's disease was due, in fact, to a primary generalized deposition of "hyaline fibrinoid" in arterioles and capillaries (10). This arteriolar change, in turn, resulted in both hypertrophy of the left ventricle and contracted kidneys. In 1874, Mahomed (11) was the first to state that hypertension could occur without primary renal disease, that arteriocapillary fibrosis represented generalized hypertensive (not nephrogenic) lesions, and that in most patients the increase of arterial pressure precedes any symptoms of renal disease, a remarkable insight considering how poor the BP measuring devices were at the time. Although the ophthalmoscope was developed by Helmholtz in 1851, a clear description of the constricted retinal vessels as related to hypertension was not described until 1876, by Gowers (12). He was unable to determine whether the constriction was functional or organic.

The physician principally responsible for popularizing the concept of hypertensive disease developing in the absence of Bright's disease was Sir Clifford Allbutt. In 1895 he presented his views on "senile plethora" and "hyperpiesia" as a generalized primary vascular disease separate from glomerulonephritis (13). However, this was not original, since he was using the concepts previously developed by Mahomed. Although he had little new to contribute, he wrote well and spoke well, which won him fame and a knighthood. Allbutt also separated hypertensive vascular disease from arteriosclerosis, stating that hypertension could occur without arteriosclerosis and vice versa.

The disease was finally named by Frank (14), in German: He called it "hypertonie essential," which might be freely translated as "primary hypertension." Unfortunately, many physicians interpreted the term to mean that hypertension was an essential adaptive reaction, a concept which discouraged any attempt to lower the blood pressure. This lead to the confusing term "essential hypertension." A more accurate term was given by Janeway (15), who, in 1913, described the varied course of hypertension and called the disorder "hypertensive cardiovascular disease"; however, it did not replace the former name.

THE MEASUREMENT OF BLOOD PRESSURE

Real progress in understanding hypertension and its treatment came with the measurement of BP quantitatively beginning with the studies of a small-town parson in eighteenth-century England. Stephen Hales performed his now-famous BP experiments in his backyard using horses. The animals were tied down to a wooden gate without anesthesia (16). A brass pipe was inserted into the carotid artery connected to a vertical glass tube by a flexible connection made from the windpipe of a goose. While a servant stood on a chair to hold up the tube, the blood rose 9 ft 6 in. in height initially and then gradually fell. The animals died when the blood in the tube fell to approximately 2 ft.

Fifty years after Hales measured BP directly, Poiseuille (17) introduced the mercury hydrodynometer thereby greatly reducing the height of the column needed for measuring the blood pressure. In 1846, Carl Ludwig (18), the great German physiologist from Leipsig, added a float to Poiseuille's mercury manometer with a connecting arm which inscribed the arterial pulse wave on a moving smoked drum, thereby making a permanent record.

Essential hypertension as a clinical entity was clearly defined, however, only after the development of noninvasive methods for measuring BP in humans, which occurred at the beginning of this century. Since hypertension is an asymptomatic disorder, its recognition in humans depended upon the development of a simple noninvasive instrument for recording the level of blood pressure in the doctor's office. The early indirect attempts proved to be impractical. They were mostly aimed at measuring the systolic BP only, by determining the force that was required to obliterate the pulse. For example, von Basch (19), in 1880, employed a mercury-filled manometer with a rubber bulb resting on the radial artery. He recorded the systolic blood pressure as the force required to obliterate the pulse. In 1889, von Helmholtz made important improvements in the von Basch instrument; this led him to find, for the first time, hypertension in the radial and temporal arteries but not in the dorsalis pedis artery in coarctation of the aorta, which he also correctly surmised caused the left ventricular hypertrophy found in this disorder.

The next important step was made by Riva-Rocci (20). It was he who, in 1896, thought of using a wrap-around inflatable rubber cuff to occlude the artery in the upper arm. Subsequently, von Recklinghausen (21) increased the width of the cuff from 5 to 13 cm to obtain better accuracy on the adult arm. Riva-Rocci recorded only the systolic blood pressure, which he determined by using the first pulse that he could palpate as the cuff was slowly deflated.

The landmark breakthrough which made blood pressure measurement a routine office procedure came from Nikolai Sergeyevich Korotkoff (22). In 1905 he described the sounds that he heard with a stethoscope placed over the brachial artery below the Riva-Rocci–von Recklinghausen inflatable cuff during its slow deflation. Korotkoff was a privat-dozent at the Imperial Military Medical Academy of St. Petersburg when Pavlov was a professor of physiology. Unlike the lengthy reporting style of his time, Korotkoff's communication was very succinct, covering less than two pages. In fact, it is suspected that it was dictated to a stenographer. In it he described the phases of the sounds and their probable origins based on his animal experiments. He also clearly defined the sounds which indicated systolic and diastolic blood pressure. Clinical recording of blood pressure then spread rapidly throughout the world.

FORERUNNERS OF MODERN TREATMENT

The invention of a clinically useful method for measuring BP opened the way for further progress in our understanding and management of hypertension. Another highly important development at that time was the discovery of renin by Tigerstedt and Bergman, the Scandinavian researchers who, in 1897, demonstrated a pressor principle in kidney extracts (23). Their pioneering effort led to the later discoveries by Goldblatt (24), Page (25), and Braun-Menendez (26). In addition to exerting a considerable influence on research on the pathogenesis of hypertension, the discovery of the renin–angiotensin system led to the recent development of a series of important antihypertensive drugs, the converting-enzyme inhibitors.

Low-Salt Diets

The importance of salt in the diet was discovered in 1904 by Ambard and Beaujard (27), who were then medical students in Paris. Their emphasis was on chloride; however, in reducing dietary chloride they also restricted sodium which is probably more important in hypertension control. Their observations preceded the use of diets extremely low in salt, which became popular in the 1940s. The success of these diets stimulated the development of the thiazide diuretics. Representing a major advance in treatment, thiazide diuretics revolutionized the management of hypertension.

Several investigators, such as Watkin (28) and Murphy (29), found that the rice diet of Kempner (30) depended on severe sodium restriction, to levels as low as 20–30 mEq/day. Moderate salt restriction (as is often prescribed today) was ineffective in these patients, possibly because they all had severe hypertension. Whether moderate restriction (approximately 80 mEq/day) is effective in milder forms of hypertension remains a controversial question: Some investigators claim that it is (31–33), whereas others claim that it is not (34–36).

Several investigators of the rice and fruit diet found that the marked sodium restriction leads to a reduction in plasma and extracellular fluid volume, which, in turn, is associated with the fall of BP (28,29). Extracellular fluid volume was reduced about 1–2 liters, and plasma volume was reduced by approximately 500 ml. Dustan (37) and ourselves (38) independently found a similar reduction of plasma and extracellular fluid volumes during treatment with thiazide diuretics. This suggests that the antihypertensive mechanism in both of these reductions is probably volume-dependent, and it also suggests that sodium deprivation will probably not be effective unless it is restrictive enough to cause some volume depletion (28,29,38,39).

Surgical Sympathectomy

The vasoconstrictor and cardioaccelerator properties of the sympathetic nervous system had long been known, but it was Kraus who urged the surgeon Fritz Bruening (40) to perform the first sympathectomy operation for hypertension in 1923. More extensive operations were developed by American surgeons in subsequent years, including Peet (41), Smithwick (42), and others. The experience with surgical sympathectomy led to the development of drugs producing chemical sympathectomy. These ganglion-blocking agents included tetraethylammonium chloride (43), hexamethonium (44), large doses of pentaquine (45), bretylium, quanethidine (46), and others.

THE BEGINNINGS OF DRUG TREATMENT

Prior to World War II there were no effective antihypertensive drugs. Sodium thiocyanate was first used by Treupel and Edinger in 1900 (47) and sporadically thereafter, including Hines at the Mayo Clinic (48). Its effectiveness was not demonstrated by controlled trials, and it was potentially toxic. Blood level measurements were required in order to keep the dosage within a safe range; even then, side effects were not infrequent. For these reasons the drug never became popular.

Drug treatment, however, was held back primarily by the prevailing attitude of therapeutic nihilism, popularized and given respectability by leading medical authorities. Well into the 1960s, some experts in the field believed that the arterial disease was the cause of the hypertension, rather than the result (49). The prevailing opinion scoffed at the use of drugs as "treatment of the manometer rather than of the patient." The frequent toxicity associated with the early drug treatment of hypertension only reinforced this opinion.

To my knowledge, the first effective drug treatment of malignant hypertension was in 1947 with the World War II antimalarial agent, pentaquine. At that time, the head of the Squibb Institute for Medical Research, which developed pentaquine, was James Shannon, who later became the first director of the National Institutes of Health. During the preclinical testing phase, it had been found that large oral doses of pentaquine led to a reduction of BP with severe orthostatic hypotension. Shannon was uninfluenced by the prevailing therapeutic nihilism and proposed that Squibb should initiate a program to develop drugs that would lower BP, of which pentaquine would be the first example. To carry out the clinical portion of the program he turned to Chester Keefer, Chairman of the Department of Medicine at Boston University, where I was a medical resident. Keefer asked me to test pentaquine and subsequent drugs, if any, in hypertensive patients.

In 1946, I gave pentaquine in antihypertensive doses to 17 patients with moderately severe to severe hypertension, including three with malignant hypertension (45). All patients were hospitalized for the therapeutic trial. After several days of treatment, supine blood pressure fell 10–40% below the baseline level (Fig. 1). Orthostatic hypotension was often severe at first but was usually moderated with continued administration of the drug. Side effects were, however, especially troublesome, consisting of abdominal pain and tenderness, back and chest pains, facial pallor, anorexia, nausea and vomiting, and constipation or diarrhea. Methemoglobinemia developed but was later successfully prevented by administering methylene blue orally with each dose of the drug. Agranulocytosis occurred in one patient and increased capillary fragility in another, both of which remitted after stopping the drug.

The three patients with malignant-phase hypertension showed (a) reversal of their neuroretinitis, (b) relief of headache, and (c) clearing of congestive heart failure; however, there was no improvement in renal failure, which was already far advanced. Hemodynamic studies disclosed a reduction of sympathetic vasopressor reflexes such as orthostatic hypotension, inhibition of the Valsalva overshoot following a forced expiration, and abolition of skin temperature gradients from foot to abdomen.

The side effects of pentaquine in large doses were too severe to recommend its use in treating hypertension. However, it was an important step on the road to effective treatment, because it demonstrated for the first time that some of the pathological manifestations of malignant hypertension were reversed by reducing BP with a drug and that amelioration of less severe forms of hypertension might occur with the same approach. Our results with pentaquine, therefore, were contrary to the prevailing opinion that reduction of BP, per se, was not beneficial; they also encouraged the development of new and more improved

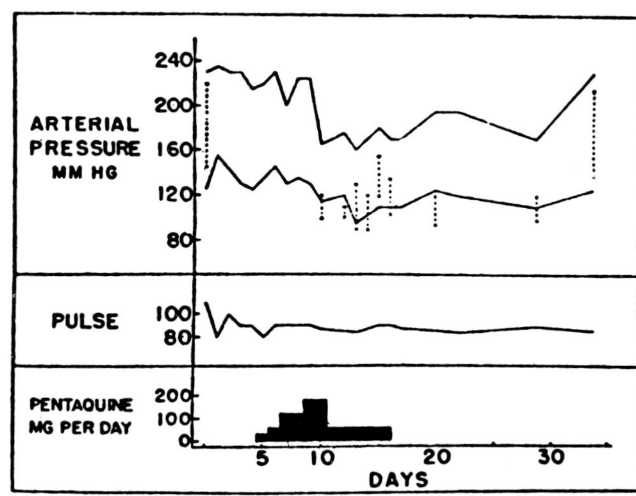

FIG. 1. Response to pentaquine in a patient with severe hypertension. The drug was increased, by daily increments, to a dose of 200 mg/day, at which point supine BP fell from approximately 230/130 to 170/105 mmHg. The dotted vertical lines represent BP in the orthostatic position. Following discontinuation of pentaquine the BP gradually rose, over a period of 2 weeks, to pretreatment levels. (From ref. 45.)

drugs for the treatment of hypertension. Two years later, Page and Taylor (50) reported on reversal of malignant hypertension using pyrogen therapy. However, side effects such as chills, fever, nausea, vomiting, and intense back and chest pains limited its use.

Ganglion-Blocking Drugs

Interest in the ganglion-blocking drugs began with the observations of Acheson and Moe (51), who demonstrated in animals that tetraethylammonium blocks transmission of autonomic nerve impulses. In 1947, Lyons et al. (43) reported on studies in humans (43). Because of the need for parenteral administration and especially because of its brief duration of action, it was not a practical drug for treating hypertension; Lyons et al. recommended it primarily for evaluation of sympathetic activity in selecting patients for surgical sympathectomy and for the treatment of causalgic states.

Hoobler et al. (52) described the hemodynamic effects of tetraethylammonium. Following intravenous administration of the drug, they found a marked increase in blood flow to the extremities, particularly to the foot. Digital skin temperature rose to equal that of the thigh. Vasodilatation was not found in the sympathectomized extremity, proving that the effect of the drug on limb blood flow was due to sympathetic blockade. The blockade was probably incomplete, however, because the vasodilatation in the foot was only about 56% as great as that achieved with lumbar paravertebral block, but it was greater than with any of the then-available vasodilators such as papaverine, nicotinic acid, and nitroglycerine.

More potent and longer-acting ganglion-blocking agents such as hexamethonium were developed later which completely blocked the sympathetic nerves as judged by increases in foot blood flow (53). Hexamethonium was introduced by Paton and Zaimis, who described its pharmacological properties in 1948 (54). Arnold and Rosenheim (55) used the drug in hypertensive patients that same year but used it only for brief periods of time and for studies on the peripheral circulation, not as a therapeutic agent in hypertension. Finnerty and Freis (56) were similarly intrigued with the effects of hexamethonium in patients with peripheral vascular disease. Our main objections to hexamethonium for long-term use in treating hypertension were that it required parenteral injections at least twice per day and that the side effects of both sympathetic and parasympathetic blockade were frequent and unpleasant.

To my knowledge, the first published report on the short-term effects of hexamethonium in hypertension was by Burt and Graham in 1950 (57). In the supine position in normotensive subjects, they found only a moderate fall in BP—which contrasted with the hypertensive patients, who exhibited a marked fall in BP, particularly in systolic BP. Orthostatic hypotension was often severe but could be reversed by tilting the foot of the bed up on blocks.

Horace Smirk first saw the possibilities of prolonged treatment of hypertension with hexamethonium despite its side effects. In 1950, Restall and Smirk (58) described the treatment of 15 patients with severe hypertension. BP was controlled by repeated subcutaneous injections two to three times per day. Effective dosage varied widely, from 5 to 500 mg per dose. Despite orthostatic hypotension, dry mouth, impotence, chilling in a cold environment due to failure of vasoconstriction, difficulty in urination, and a host of possible side effects that could result from both sympathetic and parasympathetic blockade, Restall and Smirk reported regression of the funduscopic signs of malignant hypertension, reduction in heart size, and dramatic clearing of the signs and symptoms of heart failure. This is the response we had seen previously with pentaquine (46).

Our group carried out a variety of hemodynamic studies with hexamethonium. It produced apparently complete sympathetic blockade, since the increase in blood flow to the foot following hexamethonium was equal to that produced by spinal or epidural anesthesia (53). In hypertensive patients with normal hearts the BP was reduced primarily by a fall in cardiac output (59). Pressures fell not only on the left side but also on the right side of the circulation; that is, there was venodilatation as well as arterial dilatation. By contrast, we found that in patients with congestive heart failure the cardiac output increased (59). The marked improvement in cardiac failure was not limited to hypertensive patients but also included those with other forms of heart disease except for patients with mitral stenosis, who not surprisingly did worse when filling pressure was lowered (60).

We interpreted our results (60) as follows: "It is suggested that hexamethonium may interrupt the congestive failure cycle at two points: (1) By decreasing the total peripheral resistance the work demand on the left ventricle is lessened." (Before that the entire emphasis was on reducing the overloaded right side of the heart with phlebotomy, venous tourniquets, and the like.) "(2) By reducing the filling pressure of the right heart the overloaded right ventricle is able to contract more effectively. These data supply additional evidence that the degree of constriction of the peripheral vessels both arterioles and veins may have an important influence on the function of the failing heart" (Fig. 2). These results, incidentally, were opposite to the prevailing opinion that blockade of the cardiac sympathetic drive is contraindicated in congestive heart failure. Our data suggested that decreased BP and afterload were more important while the sympathetic cardiac drive was less so. This concept passed unnoticed by the medical community until 20 years later, when it was rediscovered by Cohn (61) and others (62)—although similar findings and conclusions had been made by the Czech investigators, Brod and Fejfar (63).

Hexamethonium also provided us with a vivid picture of the critical importance of the sympathetic nervous system in stabilizing the BP in the face of minor degrees of blood loss. In supine subjects following hexamethonium blockade, we removed blood by venesection into a blood transfusion bottle. With each 50 ml of blood taken from the patient there was a definite fall in BP, and when only approximately 350 ml was removed the BP had fallen to collapse levels (Fig. 3). We then rapidly reinfused the blood;

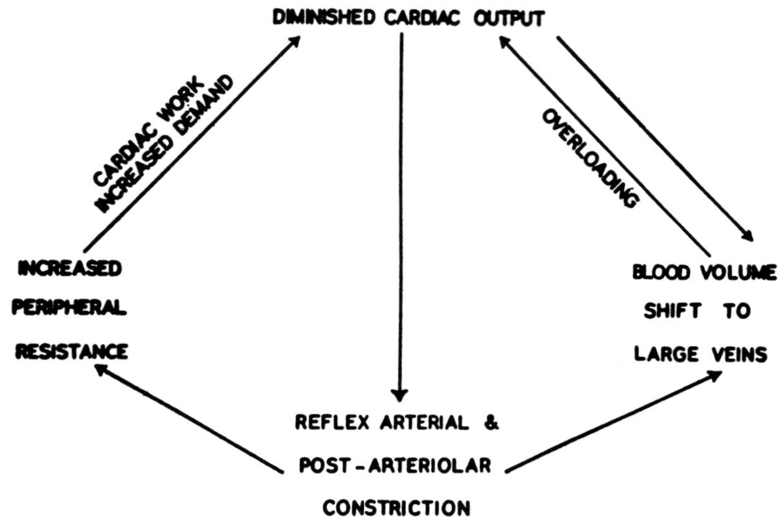

FIG. 2. Chart illustrating concept of combined effects of arteriolar resistance (increased afterload) and post-arteriolar constriction (increased preload) in establishing a "vicious cycle" in the failing heart, which was reversed by blocking the alpha-sympathetic system to both arterioles and veins with hexamethonium. (From ref. 60.)

and with each increment of blood returned, there was a corresponding rise of BP. When all the blood had been returned the BP was restored to the baseline level (64). Therefore, in the presence of sympathetic blockade, blood pressure rises or falls in direct proportion to even minor degrees of blood loss that would have no effect when the sympathetic nervous system is intact.

Veratrum viride, Hydralazine, and Reserpine

Veratrum viride is a shrub that grows wild in the foothills of the Allegheny mountains and elsewhere. It was used by the American Indians in initiation rites of puberty. When taken in sufficient amounts it causes violent retching, sweating, and collapse. In the nineteenth century, tincture of *Veratrum viride* was used by some American physicians to soften and slow the pulse (the former being due to a large fall in BP) in patients with febrile illnesses (65).

By studying the hemodynamic effects of veratrum and other drugs, we believed that we might provide information for the development of more effective and less toxic drugs (67). Almost every antihypertensive drug in use today was not found by indiscriminant screening but, instead, started with a knowledge of basic physiology and pharmacology. The two most recent examples are the converting-enzyme inhibitors and the calcium-channel blockers, both derived from knowledge of basic physiology.

Veratrum produced an initial decrease in BP, heart rate, and regional blood flows followed within a few minutes by a further decrease in arterial pressure and heart rate and a return of hepatic, renal, and muscle blood flows to essentially normal values. Unlike hexamethonium, cardiac out-

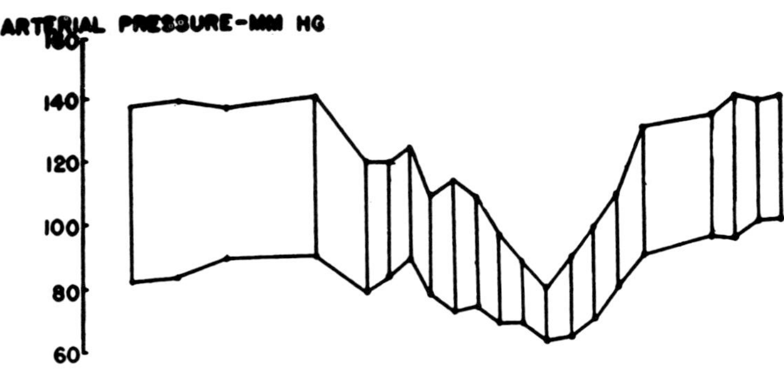

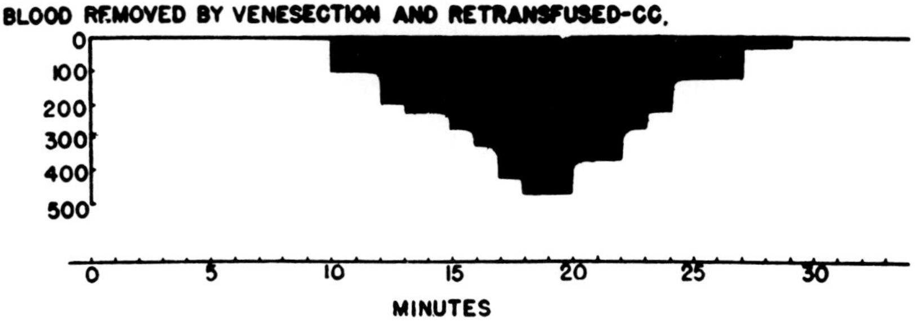

FIG. 3. Chart of arterial pressure and of the amount of blood removed by venesection and retransfused following administration of hexamethonium (50 mg, intravenously). With the sympathetic nervous system blocked, there was a stepwise decrease of BP—beginning with the first 50 ml removed. With reinfusion of blood, BP paralleled the volume of blood reinfused. There was no evidence of "compensation" as occurs with an unblocked sympathetic nervous system. (From ref. 64.)

put remained essentially unchanged after veratrum while total peripheral resistance fell (67).

The decrease in peripheral resistance appeared to occur in all areas under study, including the hepatic–portal circulation, the limbs, and the retinal arterioles. Sympathetic reflex responses remained intact, and there was no orthostatic hypotension with therapeutic doses of the drug. Vasopressor responses to the Valsalva maneuver, the erect posture test, and the cold pressor test also remained intact. Similar to hexamethonium, evidence of autonomous adjustment of the renal arterioles to the fall in blood pressure was also seen following the use of veratrum. Renal blood flow and glomerular filtration rate fell with the initial reduction in blood pressure but, after 30–60 min, returned to normal levels despite continued reduction in blood pressure (67). Like hexamethonium, veratrum produced oliguria which continued for several hours after changes in renal plasma flow and glomerular filtration rate had returned to normal. However, there was no rise in blood urea nitrogen or creatinine; in addition, the urine, though small in volume, was highly concentrated. The oliguria was a first-dose phenomenon; moreover, with continued oral administration of the drug, urine volume returned to normal. It was unfortunate that this drug, which had a favorable hemodynamic profile, should also induce severe and often intolerable side effects, especially nausea and vomiting.

Hydralazine was developed soon after the administration of the ganglion-blocking agents. It was first studied by Reubi (68), who pointed out that it was a vasodilator which increased renal blood flow. Our hemodynamic studies of this drug indicated that as blood pressure fell, cardiac output increased while central venous and right heart pressure rose (69). To explain these findings, we postulated that hydralazine dilates only the arterial side of the circulation and not the veins. In fact, the latter probably constrict through activation of the sympathetic nerves via the baroreceptors. This results in the unusual combination of (a) arteriolar dilatation due to direct drug action and (b) venoconstriction due to reflex action—resulting in a rise of venous pressure and, therefore, an increase in the preload of the heart.

Whereas some physicians abandoned hydralazine because of the toxicity observed with high doses, we and others found that severe toxicity need not occur if doses are restricted to less than 200 mg/day. Hydralazine is still used today, primarily as a Step 2 or 3 drug and for specific conditions such as toxemia of pregnancy.

Reserpine appears to be a much underrated drug. Although it can produce side effects such as stuffy nose, depression, and impotence, these appear to be uncommon with low doses (70). In combination with a diuretic, it is one of our most effective antihypertensive regimens (70). The effectiveness of this combination has been demonstrated in several Veterans Administration Cooperative Studies (70,71). Furthermore, its effectiveness remains unchanged if the dose is reduced from the usual 0.25 mg/day to a dose of 0.1 mg/day (70), thereby further minimizing side effects. One thiazide–reserpine combination tablet containing 0.1 mg reserpine and 25 or 50 mg hydrochlorothiazide should be an ideal treatment for Third-World countries because it is not only effective in a high percentage of patients but also is easy to administer, being given in a fixed dose only once daily. It is also by far the most affordable of all effective antihypertensive combinations.

THE MODERN ERA OF ANTIHYPERTENSIVE DRUGS

Thiazide Diuretics

The greatest breakthrough in the history of the drug treatment of hypertension came with the discovery of the orally effective diuretic, chlorothiazide (72). This development stimulated our interest because of prior successes with diets very low in sodium and with short-term treatment with mercurial diuretics. Chlorothiazide was effective in reducing BP and produced the same volume changes (37,38) as the strict low-salt diet (28,29). Furthermore, the drug was much more acceptable to the patients than a strict diet. We reported these results at the 19th annual meeting of the American Heart Association (72).

We not only emphasized the effectiveness of thiazide used alone but also emphasized its great advantage in enhancing the antihypertensive activity of other drugs. This permitted smaller and less toxic doses of the other drugs, thereby allowing effective BP control in most patients—with greatly reduced side effects. Because of these properties, more than any other development the drug treatment of hypertension came of age. Despite a number of excellent drugs that have been developed in subsequent years, the thiazides remain, perhaps, the most effective and generally useful of all agents, provided that they are given in adequate diuretic doses. Except for its use with digitalis, the current fear of hypokalemic effects of thiazides on the heart or of long-term elevation of cholesterol appears to be unfounded (74,78). Furthermore, the current trend to use very small doses or none at all may seriously compromise our ability to control hypertension effectively. The diuretics are the only drugs that reduce extracellular volume. This appears to be a most important mechanism for controlling BP over the long term.

An interesting feature of the hemodynamic effects of thiazide diuretics is that although the early reduction of BP is associated with a fall in cardiac output, this becomes converted (after approximately 1 month) to a fall in total peripheral resistance and a rise in cardiac output, back to pretreatment levels (73).

Ledingham and Cohen (75), Borst and Borst (76), and Guyton et al. (77) demonstrated the opposite effect during the development of salt-loading hypertension; that is, with the rise of BP during salt loading, cardiac output rose—resulting in a high-output, normal resistance type of hypertension. After 1–2 months, however, total peripheral vascular resistance increased and cardiac output fell, returning to normal—resulting in the high resistance type of chronic hypertension seen clinically.

Although occurring in opposite directions, the hemodynamic changes associated with sodium overloading on the one hand and sodium depletion on the other are remarkably similar. The BP change—either up (salt loading) or down (salt depletion)—is initiated by an appropriate change in cardiac output. However, the maintenance of the BP change is later taken over by a compensatory alteration in total peripheral resistance, thereby allowing the cardiac output to revert to normal. While the mechanism of these late changes is unknown, it has been called "delayed autoregulation" in the case of salt-loading hypertension and "reverse autoregulation" (79) in the case of reduced BP secondary to salt depletion.

Guanethidine and Alpha-Methyldopa

Following the thiazides, two new drugs appeared for clinical use. Guanethidine is a selective blocker of the peripheral sympathetic nervous system without blocking the parasympathetic system (80). This drug was never very successful because of difficulty in adjusting dosage to avoid orthostatic hypotension. Guanethidine had some unusual side effects, including (a) retrograde ejaculation into the urinary bladder and (b) urgency of defecation due apparently to unopposed parasympathetic activity. Because of side effects, guanethidine has gradually drifted into obsolescence.

The centrally acting alpha-methyldopa is a moderately effective Step 2 agent that was particularly useful in patients with renal impairment (81). Today, however, other, more recently developed agents appear to be more effective.

Beta-Adrenergic Blocking Drugs

Prichard and Gillam (82) were the first to demonstrate the effectiveness of the beta-blockers in hypertension. These drugs became very popular, and some physicians even preferred them to diuretics as primary therapy in certain types of patients. Some are more cardioselective than others, some have sympathomimetic effects, and others (such as labetolol) have additional alpha-adrenergic blocking effects. Each of these blockers with special effects may be preferred in certain types of hypertension. Several years ago the Veterans Administration Cooperative Study Group carried out a comparison between propranolol and hydrochlorothiazide, both titrated to rather high doses as needed as primary monotherapy (83). This was a double-blind, randomized trial involving over 600 patients.

The thiazide was more effective than propranolol after 1 year of treatment (84). It lowered BP more effectively over the long-term in whites and still further in blacks. There was less need to readjust dosage with the diuretic than with propranolol, and fewer patients were dropped from the trial because of side effects or cardiovascular complications. Also, the thiazide appeared to induce a greater carry-over effect when the drugs were discontinued. Substituting placebo for 2 weeks at the end of the 1-year trial resulted in a greater and more rapid return of BP with the beta-blocker than with the thiazide. Therefore, if the patient forgets his medication or runs out of it, his BP will remain in better control if he has been taking a diuretic rather than a beta-blocker.

One of the reasons some physicians prefer beta-blockers over diuretic drugs as initial monotherapy is the observation that beta-blockers are more effective than diuretics in patients with high renin hypertension (85). Renin profiles carried out in the Veterans Study (83) confirmed that patients with a low renin profile had a greater response to hydrochlorothiazide, whereas propranolol was more effective in patients with a high renin profile. The differences in diastolic BP were small, however, averaging 3 mmHg lower with hydrochlorothiazide than with propranolol in the low-renin group and 3 mmHg lower with propranolol in the high-renin patients. These differences were minor compared to the falls from pretreatment levels in both low- and high-renin hypertension produced by either drug and, in our judgment, did not warrant routine use of renin determinations as a guide to choice of treatment.

Converting-Enzyme Inhibitors

In 1980 the Veterans Administration Cooperative Study Group had contacted several clinical research directors of pharmaceutical companies concerning important new drugs. In reply, John Alexander, of Squibb, explained his need for a cooperative study on captopril. He was interested in demonstrating that small doses of captopril were effective in controlling BP. This was important because toxicity seemed to be dose-related—hence the desire to keep doses low.

Our Veterans Administration study demonstrated that captopril was as effective in small doses as in large doses (86). Doses of 25 mg b.i.d. or t.i.d. were as effective as 50 mg, and even doses of 12.5 mg were nearly as effective. Thus, at least in mild and moderate essential hypertension there was no need to use large and potentially toxic doses.

The study also demonstrated that when hydrochlorothiazide (25 mg, b.i.d.) was added to the captopril the fall in BP was significantly greater than with captopril alone and was without side effects of faintness, weakness, or impotence (87). Small doses of thiazide plus a converting-enzyme inhibitor were well tolerated, and this was generally a most effective antihypertensive regimen except in the rare patients with renovascular hypertension.

Calcium-Channel Blockers

Calcium ions play an important role in many biologic processes, including vascular smooth muscle contraction. A number of calcium-channel blockers are effective vasodilator antihypertensive agents such as nifedipine, verapamil, and diltiazem. They are also effective in treating angina pectoris; and verapamil, in particular, slows atrioventricular conduction, making it valuable in certain forms of arrhythmias. Other favorable features in the hypertensive heart include coronary vasodilatation, accelerated ventricular relaxation, and improvement in subendocardial perfusion.

Calcium-channel blockers are the most recent major drugs to become part of the antihypertensive armamentarium. Their initial major deficiency was a short duration of action, but this is being corrected by the development of sustained-release formulations. They have been used successfully both as Step 1 or Step 2 drugs. It is claimed that they reduce BP without causing fluid retention; therefore, diuretics may not be needed as frequently as with most other antihypertensive drugs.

PROVING THE EFFICACY OF ANTIHYPERTENSIVE DRUG TREATMENT

In the late 1960s and early 1970s the Veterans Administration Cooperative Study Group reported on the effects of treatment on morbidity and mortality in hypertension. In 1962 a group of physicians in Veterans Administration Hospitals organized a cooperative study group to evaluate antihypertensive agents under well-controlled conditions (88). Patients were randomly assigned, in a double-blind manner, to a treatment group or a placebo group. Treatment consisted of a combination of diuretic, reserpine, and hydralazine, which we knew from prior studies to be quite effective in lowering BP (89).

Principal results in the group of patients with initial diastolic BP between 90 and 114 mmHg were as follows: There were 19 cardiovascular deaths in the placebo group as compared to eight in the treated patients. The most frequent cause of death was myocardial infarction or sudden death, of which 11 occurred in the control patients and six occurred in the treated group. When nonfatal myocardial infarction was included, the incidence of coronary heart disease events was essentially equal between the control and treated groups. Stroke was the next most common fatal event, with eight occurring in the placebo group versus only one in the treated group.

For the combined fatal and major nonfatal cardiovascular complications, the life-table method of analysis (Fig. 4) indicated that the risk of developing a major cardiovascular complication over a 5-year period was reduced from 55% to 18% with treatment, a significant difference. The difference was highly significant in those entering with diastolic levels

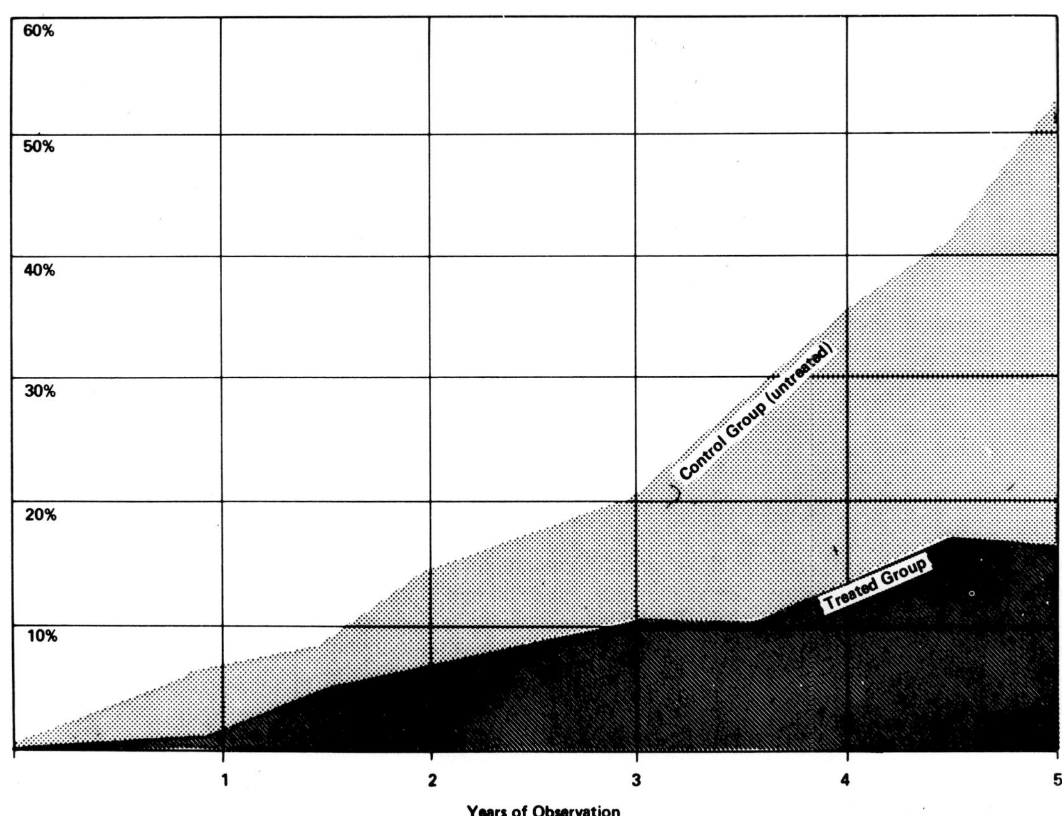

FIG. 4. Estimated cumulative incidence of major cardiovascular morbidity over a 5-year period as calculated by the life-table method. There is an increasing difference in morbidity–mortality over 5 years (55% minus 18%) between the control and treated groups, representing a 67% effectiveness of treatment (37/55). (From ref. 87.)

of 105–114 mmHg. Between 90 and 104 mmHg diastolic pressure, results were favorable toward treatment, but to much lesser degree; moreover, the difference was not statistically significant. However, the number of patients entered was too small to provide a definitive answer concerning the value of treating mild hypertension, despite the rigorous design of the trial (87).

The importance of this study was that it represented the first randomized, placebo-controlled, multiclinic trial to demonstrate that treatment of moderate to moderately severe hypertension is effective in preventing major complications such as stroke, renal damage, congestive heart failure, and dissecting aortic aneurysm. It also demonstrated that progression to a more severe degree of hypertension in patients with mild or moderate hypertension was prevented. This evidence led Mary Lasker, who has been a driving force in American medicine, to visit Elliot Richardson, who was then the head of Health, Education and Welfare. Mrs. Lasker presented the reprints of the Veterans study and asked that a special fund be allocated to educate the public and the physicians concerning the results. Thus was born the National High Blood Pressure Education Program, which soon became a successful and vigorous educational program that used the media and other modalities to popularize the treatment of hypertension.

How well have the results of the Veterans Administration trial stood the test of time compared with the results derived from subsequent controlled trials? In the Veterans Administration trial, treatment was only marginally effective in mild hypertension, perhaps because the number of patients with mild, uncomplicated hypertension was too small to allow for reliable conclusions. However, the results in mild hypertension were similar to those in the large MRC trial (89), which found the benefit to be so small in mild hypertension that the justification of treating many millions of mild hypertensives becomes questionable. The VA trial also reported a significant benefit of treatment against stroke but not against heart attack. This difference in effectiveness is in agreement with most controlled studies, including the MRC trial and the Australian trial (90).

The VA trial results differed from the Hypertension Detection and Follow-up Program in several respects (91). The latter found that antihypertensive treatment afforded considerable protection against myocardial infarction. Furthermore, the latter observed that treatment was more effective in mild than in more severe hypertension, whereas the Veteran's Administration trial found the opposite. Whereas the recent trials reported only on coronary disease and stroke, our study—probably because it also included moderately severe patients—demonstrated that other complications also were prevented. These included congestive heart failure, progressive renal disease, and dissecting aortic aneurysm (88); that is, most of the major complications of hypertension were preventable with antihypertensive drug treatment. The degree of protection seems to depend on the extent of damage already present at the time of initiating treatment and on the adequacy of BP control. Equally important, the drugs prevent progression of hypertension, which leads to early complications.

Why are myocardial infarction and sudden death not prevented by reduction of BP with antihypertensive agents? Probably lifestyle changes are also required, particularly stopping cigarette smoking and adapting a diet restricted in saturated fats and cholesterol. Reduction of BP alone is not enough.

SUMMARY AND CONCLUSIONS

A method for measuring BP clinically was discovered less than 100 years ago. Prior to this, the disorder that we now call hypertension could be suspected only by the quality of the pulse. In ancient times a hard pulse—that is, one that was difficult to compress—was often treated with bleeding and leeches, which resulted in at least some reduction of BP. Progress was made when autopsies were permitted and particularly in the latter half of the nineteenth century, when histology provided microscopic examination of the small vessels. In 1827, Bright recognized an inflammatory disease of the kidney which caused a generalized cardiovascular disease leading to dropsy, apoplexy, and uremia. Later, Mahomed and Allbutt described a primary, generalized, fibrosis of the arterioles that did not originate in the kidney—a condition that we now recognize as severe essential hypertension.

In 1905, Korotkoff developed a clinically applicable method for measuring BP. This landmark discovery permitted epidemiological studies of BP in relation to cardiovascular mortality. It was primarily the Society of Actuaries who, in the 1920s, recognized the great prevalence of the disorder (92). Although it was clear to the Insurance Companies that a diastolic BP of 95 mmHg or higher of BP shortened life because of cardiovascular complications, their data relative to mild and moderate hypertension was dismissed by most physicians of the time as being of no great consequence. However, definitive proof was eventually provided by Kannel and co-workers in the classical Framingham Study, which demonstrated beyond any doubt the importance of hypertension as a cardiovascular risk factor (93).

Except for rest and sedatives (which had no real antihypertensive effect), hypertension remained an untreated disease until the late 1930s and the 1940s, when sympathectomy and the rice diet were advised for patients with severe hypertension. The first successful use of antihypertensive drugs in causing remission of malignant hypertension occurred in the late 1940s—initially with pentaquine and a few years later with hexamethonium.

The early drugs had many side effects; and it was not until the 1950s that the great breakthrough occurred in antihypertensive drug treatment, with the development of chlorothiazide. This drug was highly effective orally, it was well tolerated, and it enhanced the antihypertensive effectiveness of other drugs when given in combination with them. It permitted, in fact, the birth of effective step-therapy. The beta-blockers represented the leading advance of the 1960s, followed in recent years by the converting-enzyme blockers and the calcium-channel blockers as major therapeutic agents.

As recently as 20 years ago the effectiveness of antihypertensive drug treatment of moderate essential hypertension was still disputed. The issue was finally settled by a controlled clinical trial, the Veterans Administration Cooperative Study, which demonstrated beyond any reasonable doubt that drug treatment was effective in preventing the complications of moderate hypertension (diastolic BP of 105 mmHg and above). Larger-scale trials followed to determine whether treatment was also effective in mild asymptomatic hypertension (diastolic BP of 90–104 mmHg). The results of these studies have been conflicting, and the cost/benefit ratio of treatment—particularly for the large group of patients with diastolic levels in the range of 90–94 mmHg—remains in doubt. Whether such patients should be actively treated or carefully monitored for early detection of progression still remains an undecided question. Patients with persistent BP levels above 95 mmHg diastolic or 160 mmHg systolic, as well as patients with evidence of cardiovascular damage associated with hypertension (such as left ventricular hypertrophy by electrocardiogram or echocardiography), generally are treated.

It is remarkable that it has taken less than 90 years from the time high blood pressure was first recognized clinically to the present period of effective control. Coronary heart disease remains as the most common cause of death in hypertensive patients. Reduction of BP has been least successful in preventing myocardial infarction and sudden death. However, it is now realized that control of BP alone is not enough. It seems probable that with simultaneous reduction of other leading risk factors for coronary heart disease (such as normalization of blood lipids and elimination of cigarette smoking), we may look forward to the conquest of this last and most important cause of death in hypertension.

Hypertension is a public health problem. The prevention of stroke is less expensive than the care of those incapacitated by its effects. The prevention of other complications, especially in wage earners and heads of households, has a payoff not only in the quality of life but also in economic gain. I have had the good fortune to have been engaged in antihypertensive drug research at a time when it was making great progress. The advances were made possible by the collaboration of many individuals, both in industry and in clinical pharmacology.

REFERENCES

1. Ruskin A. *Classics in arterial hypertension.* Springfield IL: Charles C Thomas, 1956.
2. Nei Ching. *Yellow emperor's classic of internal medicine.* Books 2–9, published between 2698 and 2598 BC.
3. Celsus AAC. *De Re Medicina,* translated by W Spencer. London: Heinemann, 1935–1938, 3 vols.
4. Hippocrates. *Genuine works of Hippocrates,* translated by F Adams. London: Sydenham Society, 1849, 2 vols.
5. Galen C. *Introductio in Pulsus ad Teuthram,* interpreted by M Gregory. London: Guliel Rovillius, 1959.
6. Wepfer JJ. *Observationes Anatomicae ex Cadaveribus eorum quos sustulit Apoplexia. Cum Exercitatione de ejus Loco Affecto.* Shaffhausen: Johann Casper Suterus, 1958.
7. Young TI. The Croonian Lecture. On the functions of the heart and arteries. *Philos Trans R Soc Lond* 1809;1:1–31.
8. Sugiura T, Freis ED. Pressure pulse in small arteries. *Circ Res* 1962;11:838–843.
9. Bright R. Cases and observations illustrative of renal disease accompanied with the secretion of albuminous urine. *Guy's Hosp Rep* 1836;1:338–379.
10. Gull WW, Sutton HG. On the pathology of the morbid state commonly called chronic Bright's disease with contracted kidneys ("arteriocapillary fibrosis") *Med Chir Trans Lond* 1872;65:273–326.
11. Mahomed FA. Chronic Bright's disease without albuminuria. *Guy's Hosp Rep* 1881;25:295–416.
12. Gowers W. The state of the arteries in Bright's disease. *Br Med J* 1876;2:743–745.
13. Allbutt TC. Senile plethora or high arterial pressure in elderly persons. *Abstracts, Transactions of the Hunter Society 1895–1896. 77th Session.* London: Headley Bros, 1896;38–57.
14. Frank O. Ein neues optisches Federmanometer. *Z Biol* 1925;82:49–80.
15. Janeway TC. Clinical study of blood pressure. *Guide to the use of the sphygmomanometer.* New York: D Appleton 1904.
16. Hales S. Statistical essays containing haemostaticks; or an account of some hydraulick and hydrostattical experiments made on the blood and blood pressure of animals. London: Innys and Manby, 1933.
17. Poiseuille JLM. Recherches sur le force du coeur aortique. *Arch Gen Med* 1828:550–554.
18. Ludwig C. Zur Kenntniss des einglusses der respirations—bewegungen auf den Blutlauff in aortensysteme. *Arch Anat Physiol Wissensch Med (Mueller's Arch)* 1847:242–302.
19. von Basch S. Ueber die Messung des blutdrucks am menschen. *Z Klin Med* 1880;2:79–96.
20. Riva-Rocci S. Un sfigmomanometro nuovo. *Gaz Med Torino* 1896;47:981–1001.
21. von Recklinghausen H. Ueber Blutdruck Messung beim Menschon. *Arch Exp Pathol Pharmacol* 1901;46:78–96.
22. Korotkoff NS. A contribution to the problem of methods for the determination of the blood pressure. *Izvestiya Imperatorskoi Voenno-Meditsinskoy Akademii (Rep Imper Mil-Med Acad St Petersburg)* 1905;11:365–367.
23. Tigerstedt R, Bergman PG. Niere und kreislauf. *Scand Arch Physiol* 1897–1898;7–8:223–271.
24. Goldblatt H, Lynch T, Hanzal RF, Summerville WW. Studies on experimental hypertension. I. The production of persistent elevation of systolic blood pressure by means of renal ischemia. *J Exp Med* 1934;59:347–379.
25. Page IH, Helmer OM. A crystalline pressor substance (angiotonin) resulting from the reaction between renin and renin activator. *J Exp Med* 1940;71:495–520.
26. Braun-Menendez EJ, Fasciolo C, Le Loir F, Munoz M. The substance causing renal hypertension. *J Physiol Lond* 1940;98:283–298.
27. Ambard L, Beaujard E. Causes de l'hypertension arterielle. *Arch Gen Med (NS)* 1904;1:520–523.
28. Watkin DM, Fraeb HF, Hatch FT, Gutman AB. Effects of diet in essential hypertension. II. Results with unmodified Kempner rice diet in fifty hospitalized patients. *Am J Med* 1950;9:441–448.
29. Murphy RJF. The effects of "rice diet" on plasma volume and extracellular fluid space in hypertensive subject. *J Clin Invest* 1950;29:912–920.
30. Kempner W. Treatment of kidney disease and hypertensive vascular disease with rice diet. *N Carolina Med J* 1944;5:125 and 273.
31. MacGregor GA, Best FE, Cam JM, et al. Double-blind randomized crossover trial of moderate sodium restriction in essential hypertension. *Lancet* 1982;1:351–355.
32. Parijs J, Joosens JV, Van der Linden L, Verstrecken G, Amery AKPC. Moderate sodium restriction and diuretics in the treatment of hypertension. *Am Heart J* 1973;85:22–34.
33. Morgan T, Gillies A, Morgan G, Adam W, Wilson M, Carney S. Hypertension treated by salt restriction. *Lancet* 1978;1:227–230.
34. Richards AM, Espiner EA, Maslowski AH, et al. Blood pressure

response to moderate sodium restriction and to potassium supplementation in mild essential hypertension. *Lancet* 1984;1:757–761.
35. Watt GCM, Edward C, Hart JT, Walton P, Fay CJW. Dietary sodium restriction for mild hypertension in general practice. *Br Med J* 1983;286:432–435.
36. Silman AJ, Mitchell P, Locke C, Humpherson P. Evaluation of the effectiveness of a low sodium diet in the treatment of mild to moderate hypertension. *Lancet* 1983;1:1179–1182.
37. Dustan HP, Cumming GR, Corcoran AC, Page IH. A mechanism of chlorothiazide enhanced effectiveness of antihypertensive ganglioplegic drugs. *Circulation* 1959;19:360.
38. Wilson IM, Freis ED. Relationship between plasma and extracellular fluid volume depletion and the antihypertensive effects of chlorothiazide. *Circulation* 1959;20:1028.
39. Beard T, Gray WR, Cooke HM, Barge R. Randomized controlled trial of a no-add-sodium diet for mild hypertension. *Lancet* 1982;2:455–458.
40. Bruening F. Die operative Behandlung der Angina Pectoris durch Extirpation des Halsbrustsympathetics und Bemerkungen ueber die operative Behandlung der abnormen Blutdrucksteigerung. *Klin Wochnschr* 1923;2:777–780.
41. Peet MM. Results of subdiaphragmatic splanchnicectomy for arterial hypertension. *N Engl J Med* 1947;236:270–276.
42. Smithwick RH, Thompson JE. Splanchnicectomy for essential hypertension: results in 1266 cases. *JAMA* 1953;152:1501–1504.
43. Lyons RH, Moe GK, Neligh RM, Hoobler SW, Campbell KN, Berry RL, Rennick BR. The effects of blockade of the autonomic ganglia in man with tetraethylammonium. *Am J Med Sci* 1947;213:315–323.
44. Smirk FH. Practical details of the methonium treatment of high blood pressure. *NZ Med J* 1950;49:637–643.
45. Freis ED, Wilkins RW. Effect of pentaquine in patients with hypertension. *Proc Soc Exp Biol Med* 1947;64:731–736.
46. Freis ED. Bretylium and guanethidine: two new drugs producing specific blockade of the sympathetic nervous system. *Heart Bull* 1960;9:88.
47. Treupel G, Edinger A. Untersuchungen uber Rhoden-Verbindungen. *Munch Med Wochenschr* 1900;47:717–720.
48. Hines EA. The thiocyanates in the treatment of hypertensive disease. *Med Clin N Am* 1946;30:869–877.
49. Goldring W, Chasis H. Antihypertensive drug therapy. In: Ingelfinger FJ, ed. *Controversies in internal medicine.* Philadelphia: WB Saunders, 1966;83–91.
50. Page IH, Taylor RD. Pyrogens in the treatment of malignant hypertension. *Mod Concepts Cardiovascular Dis* 1949;18:51–52.
51. Acheson GH, Moe GK. The action of tetraethylammonium ion on the mammalian circulation. *J Pharmacol Exp Ther* 1946;87:220–226.
52. Hoobler SW, Malton SD, Ballantine TH Jr, Cohen SW, Neligh RB, Peet MM, Lyons RH. Studies on vasomotor tone. I. The effect of the tetraethylammonium ion on the peripheral blood flow of normal subjects. *J Clin Invest* 1949;28:638–647.
53. Schnaper HW, Johnson RL, Touhy EB, Freis ED. The effect of hexamethonium as compared to procaine or metycaine block on the blood flow to the foot of normal subjects. *J Clin Invest* 1951;30:786–791.
54. Paton WDM, Zaimis EJ. Clinical potentialities of certain bisquaternary salts causing neuromuscular and ganglionic block. *Nature* 1948;162:810.
55. Arnold P, Rosenheim ML. Effect of pentamethonium iodide on normal and hypertensive persons. *Lancet* 1949;2:321–323.
56. Finnerty FA Jr, Freis ED. Experimental and clinical evaluation in man of hexamethonium (C6) a new ganglionic blocking agent. *Circulation* 1950;2:828–836.
57. Burt CC, Graham AJP. Pentamethonium and hexamethonium iodide in investigation of peripheral vascular disease and hypertension. *Br Med J* 1950;1:455–460.
58. Restall PA, Smirk FH. The treatment of high blood pressure with hexamethonium iodide. *NZ Med J* 1950;49:206–209.
59. Freis ED, Rose JC, Partenope A, Higgins TF, Kelley RT, Schnaper HW, Johnson RL. The hemodynamic effect of hypotensive drugs in man. III. Hexamethonium. *J Clin Invest* 1953;32:1285–1298.
60. Kelley RT, Freis ED, Higgins TF. The effects of hexamethonium on certain manifestations of congestive heart failure. *Circulation* 1953;7:169–174.
61. Cohn JN. Vasodilator therapy for heart failure. *Circulation* 1973;48:5–8.
62. Miller RR, Vismara LA, Williams DO, Amsterdam EA, Mason DT. Pharmacological mechanisms for left ventricular unloading in clinical congestive heart failure. *Circ Res* 1976;39:127.
63. Brod J, Fejfar Z. Mechanism of transient increase of the cardiac output in adrenergic blockade with dibenamine. *Sb Lek* 1951;53:154–163.
64. Freis ED, Stanton JR, Finnerty FA Jr, Schnaper HW, Johnson RL, Rath CE, Wilkins RW. The collapse produced by venous congestion of the extremities or by venesection following certain antihypertensive agents. *J Clin Invest* 1951;30:435–442.
65. Krayer O, Acheson GH. The pharmacology of the veratrum alkaloids. *Physiol Rev* 1946;26:383–446.
66. Freis ED, Stanton JR. A clinical evaluation of veratrum viride in the treatment of essential hypertension. *Am Heart J* 1948;36: 723–738.
67. Freis ED, Stanton JR, Culbertson JW, Litter J, Halperin MH, Burnett CH, Wilkins RW. The hemodynamic effects of hypotensive drugs in man. I. Veratrum viride. *J Clin Invest* 1949;28:353–368.
68. Reubi F. Influence of some peripheral vasodilators on the renal circulation. *Helvet Med Acta* 1949;16:297.
69. Freis ED, Rose JC, Higgins TF, Finnerty FA Jr, Kelley RT, Partenope EA. The hemodynamic effects of hypotensive drugs in man. IV. Hydrozinophthalazine. *Circulation* 1953;8:199–203.
70. Veterans Administration Cooperative Study Group on Antihypertensive Agents. Low doses vs standard dose of reserpine, a randomizing double-blind multiclinic trial in patients taking chlorothalidone. *JAMA* 1982;248:2471–2477.
71. Veterans Administration Cooperative Study on Antihypertensive Agents. A double-blind control study of antihypertensive agents. I. Comparative effectiveness of reserpine and hydralazine, and three ganglion blocking agents. *Arch Intern Med* 1960;106:96–101.
72. Freis ED, Wilson IM, Parrish AE. Enhancement of antihypertensive activity with chlorothiazide. Presented at the 19th annual meeting of the American Heart Association, Chicago, Illinois, Oct 28, 1957.
73. Shah S, Khatri I, Freis ED. Mechanism of antihypertensive effect of thiazide diuretics. *Am Heart J* 1978;95:611–618.
74. Freis ED. The cardiovascular risks of thiazide diuretics. *Clin Pharmacol Exp Ther* 1986;39:224–239.
75. Ledingham JM, Cohen RD. The role of the heart in the pathogensis of renal hypertension. *Lancet* 1963;2:979–981.
76. Borst JGG, Borst De G. Hypertension explained by Starling's theory of circulatory homeostatis. *Lancet* 1963;1:677–682.
77. Guyton AC, Coleman TG, Cawley AW, Manning RD Jr, Norman RA, Ferguson JD. A systems analysis approach to understanding long range arterial blood pressure control and hypertension. *Circ Res* 1974;35:159–164.
78. Freis ED, Papademetriou V. How dangerous are diuretics? *Drugs* 1985;30:469–474.
79. Tobian L. Hypertension and the kidney. *Arch Intern Med* 1974;133:959–967.
80. Cohn JN, Liptak TE, Freis ED. Hemodynamic effects of guanethidine in man. *Circ Res* 1963;12:298–307.
81. Oates JA, Gillespie L Jr, Udenfriend S, Sjoerdsma A. Decarboxylase inhibition and blood pressure reduction by alpha-methyl-3,4-dehydroxy-DL-phenylalamine. *Science* 1960;131:1890–1891.
82. Prichard BNC, Gillam PMS. Use of propranolol (Inderal) in treatment of hypertension. *Br Med J* 1964;2:725–732.
83. Veterans Administration Cooperative Study Group on Antihypertensive Agents. Comparison of propranolol and hydrochlorothiazide for the initial treatment of hypertension. I. Results of short-term titration with emphasis on racial difference in response. *JAMA* 1982;248:1996–2003.
84. Veterans Administration Cooperative Study Group on Antihypertensive Agents. Captopril: evaluation of low doses, twice daily

patients: They quiet the heart rate and reduce cardiac work. These properties are also shared by a subclass of calcium antagonists (i.e., verapamil and diltiazem).

Altogether then, the availability of the above five major drug types, given either as monotherapy or in creative combination when necessary, makes individualized therapy an achievable goal.

It is appropriate here to comment on the results to date of clinical trials evaluating the effects of these newer agents on cardiac and vascular sequelae of hypertension. For both financial and ethical reasons, large-scale controlled trials on the scale conducted in the past are no longer likely to occur. Moreover, until recently, clinical trials employing crossover monotherapy designs were not considered feasible or conceptually desirable.

Notwithstanding, it has been shown convincingly that long-term beta-blocker therapy can protect from a subsequent myocardial infarction in either normotensive or hypertensive subjects (10). Weaker evidence suggests that beta-blockers can also provide protection from a subsequent coronary event in hypertension. Two studies showed primary cardioprotection in nonsmoking men (11,12), and one (13) showed no effect. Another, the MAPHY (Metoprolol Atherosclerosis Prevention in Hypertension) trial (14), concluded that metoprolol was significantly more effective than a sulfonamide diuretic in preventing coronary events. However, overall event rates were small, and there were differing effects of smoking in the two groups being compared. Also, this study, a subgroup of a larger trial (13) (HAPPY—Heart Attack Primary Prevention in Hypertension), produced results conflicting with those of the parent study. Nevertheless, a comprehensive review of all trials using beta-blockers for secondary cardioprotection revealed an impressive 25% reduction in cardiac mortality, a 33% reduction in sudden death, and a 35% reduction in reinfarction rate (10). Thus, beta-blockers can now be recognized as extremely effective agents for protecting from further coronary disease.

The calcium antagonists can convincingly prevent atherosclerosis and vascular injury in animal models (see Chapters 32 and 33) but the evidence that they can provide cardioprotection in humans is, so far, either negative or only suggestive (15,16). ACE inhibitors also protect from vascular damage in Dahl salt-sensitive (Dahl-S) and stroke-prone, spontaneously hypertensive models, but less rapidly than calcium antagonists. ACE inhibitors have been shown to improve both exercise tolerance and longevity in patients with congestive heart failure (17), but there are no similar data in other hypertensive patients. Alpha-blocker therapy has not been critically evaluated for its impact on cardiac and vascular consequences of hypertension.

In summary, the results so far are promising for the newer agents, which reduce cardiac work either directly or indirectly. (Cardiac work is reduced indirectly by vasodilation, which also increases flow to vital organs.)

The Heterogeneity of Human Essential Hypertension

Clinical and epidemiological observations made over the past 25 years provide compelling evidence for the heterogeneity of essential hypertension. From clinical studies and observation, it is abundantly evident that individual patients with comparable degrees of hypertension may differ significantly in their endocrinologic profiles, in their response or lack of response to particular drugs, and in their prognosis and outcome. Confirming this evidence—indeed, making some of it possible—is a battery of new, exciting antihypertensive drugs targeted against specific hypertensive mechanisms.

Today we know a great deal more about the pathophysiology of human hypertension, too. As indicated above, the range of drugs available for treatment is much broader not only in number but in mechanisms of action, covering biologic pathways not even suspected of being implicated when the concept of stepped care was promulgated. It is now clear that just as there is no single cause of hypertension, there is also no single universally effective treatment. However, that realization does not leave us as helpless as it might have done years ago: With today's advanced techniques of serum assay for measuring plasma renin activity, along with the availability of highly specific pharmacologic probes, we are increasingly able to differentiate in diagnosis and in treatment.

Recognizing Two Vasoconstrictor Mechanisms

Sustained arteriolar vasoconstriction is the basis for all diastolic hypertension. Two long-term mechanisms have been identified that account for major portions of this vasoconstriction (18) (see Chapter 82). One occurs because of an excess of the vasoconstrictive hormone angiotensin II, generated by plasma renin as a consequence of excessive renal secretion of renin. Its presence is generally quantifiable by the height of the plasma renin in untreated patients, and it can be addressed therapeutically by anti-renin-system agents. The other long-term mechanism is marked by a low plasma renin value. Because a lowered plasma renin is a uniform response to sodium administration in both normal and hypertensive people, and because the blood pressure of such hypertensive people is often normalized by diuretic or dietary sodium depletion, it is likely that this form of arteriolar vasoconstriction is induced by antecedent excessive renal sodium retention. The physiologic pathways for this sodium-related vasoconstrictor mechanism are still not entirely clear but may be associated with an imbalance between intracellular and extracellular calcium (19) (see Chapter 82). Accordingly, this form of vasoconstriction is correctable either by diuretics or by treatment with calcium-channel antagonists or alpha-adrenergic blockers. The meaning of all this is that we are at last able to mount a rational diagnostic and management strategy for hypertensive patients that is several important steps removed from the blind empiricism of the past.

THE MODERN PATIENT WORK-UP

The modern evaluation of each new patient (see Chapter 85) provides the fullest possible definition of the two forms of long-term vasoconstriction described in detail in Chapters 69 and 82. The biochemical package of the initial work-up includes the measurement of serum K^+, urea and creatinine, 24-hr urinary electrolytes and microalbumin excretion rate, and the plasma renin profile. Target organ appraisal and risk assessment are further sharpened by a fasting sugar and a lipid profile and by a baseline electrocardiogram and echocardiogram to assess left ventricular status.

The ambulatory renin profile is the basic screen in searching for curable forms of hypertension because it is markedly suppressed in primary aldosteronism and is usually elevated and never below 2.5 ng/ml/hr in curable renovascular disease. Accordingly, patients in the latter subgroup, in order to rule curable renovascular disease in or out, are next ones who are given the powerful captopril screening test (20) or, alternatively, a trial of an ACE inhibitor. The renin profile and the plasma renin response to captopril also provide information about renin involvement and nephron status, which, together with the baseline laboratory data, is useful for defining pathophysiology, pace, and prognosis and for planning specifically targeted, simpler, long-term drug therapy (see Chapter 85).

CHOOSING DRUGS FOR THE INDIVIDUAL PATIENT

In selecting drugs, the physician should keep in mind the major goal of long-term drug therapy. With the initial work-up in hand, the physician is in position to achieve a primary pharmacotherapeutic goal of long-term antihypertensive therapy (21) (see Table 1). This is to prescribe the fewest number of drugs in the smallest effective amount and lowest frequency. Such a goal is particularly important in hypertension, considering that every antihypertensive drug presents a toxic problem of one degree or another and that the commitment to it is sure to be long-term, possibly lifelong. Effective monotherapy of hypertension is now more possible than ever before, and all five drug types described above qualify as candidates for monotherapy in appropriately studied individual patients. This opportunity represents a great advance in a field characterized in the past by additive, multiple drug therapy.

Renin System Patterns to Guide Drug Choice

Patients with very high renin and without renovascular disease are most certainly candidates for monotherapy with an ACE inhibitor or beta-blocker. Conversely, those with very low plasma renin values or no blood pressure or plasma renin response to captopril (22) are definitely candidates for monotherapy with calcium antagonists, diuretics, or alpha-blockers. It should be kept in mind, however, that while the renin system patterns revealed by the work-up provide valuable guidelines for making appropriate selections among antihypertensive agents, the predictive power of the renin profile is strongest at the extremities of the range. At the middle ranges, renin-mediated and sodium-related mechanisms may overlap or may express an inappropriate interaction between the two, and here the physician must lean more heavily on the pragmatic clinical arts, using the specific drug types now available as pharmacologic probes, with the patient serving as his own control. The right drug for each patient thus can be validated individually [the "*n* of 1" concept (23)].

TABLE 1. *Overall goals for evaluating and treating hypertensive patients*

Goals of evaluation
To identify all curable and definable forms of hypertension
To stratify all other forms of hypertension based on their underlying pathophysiologic mechanisms
Goals of long-term drug therapy
To give the minimum number of drugs, in the minimum effective amounts, with the minimum frequency possible, thus minimizing both short- and long-term side effects.

Using Drug Response to Validate Optimal Efficacy and to Confirm Mechanisms

This approach is especially relevant for patients in the medium range of renin values, where the renin profile has its least predictive value. It is also applicable to all patients whenever renin profiling is not available. The strategy of informed empiricism involves the single-file testing of the five major, mechanism-specific drug types: The optimum response points to mechanisms involved. Such a clinical approach, known as *diagnosis ex juvantibus,* has a long tradition (24). Used with renin profiling, it addresses the basic heterogeneity of essential hypertension in order to achieve a drug response tailored to the individual, thereby treating the patient as well as the disease. Indeed, as will be discussed below, this general strategy is gaining increased support from recent clinical studies demonstrating the advantages of single-file testing in a double cross-over design, which tests every drug in question in every patient.

DRUG THERAPY FOR HIGH-RENIN PATIENTS

Renin dependency can be assessed with a single oral test dose of captopril. This simple and inexpensive captopril test, as described in Chapter 85, has been successfully used for the screening of renovascular hypertension (20). In applying the test for the screening of renovascular hypertension, it must be emphasized that the reactive rise in renin, rather than the blood pressure response, is the main discriminator of renovascular hypertension. Nevertheless, a dramatic decrease in blood pressure confirms renin dependency, just as a total lack of response generally indicates a nonrenin vasoconstrictor mechanism (also see the chapter by Spence, entitled "Pseudohypertension").

For those patients with a medium- to high-renin profile (plasma renin activity greater than 2.5 ng/ml/hr) in whom the captopril test confirms renin dependency but who turn out not to have curable renovascular disease, the modern choice for first-line therapy is an ACE inhibitor, chosen because of the specificity of these drugs: There is no longer any doubt that the overwhelming portion of their depressor effect is the result of their inhibition of angiotensin II formation (25–27). The effectiveness of converting-enzyme inhibition is well illustrated in Chapter 69. The higher the baseline renin, the more dramatic the blood pressure correction. An additional long-term effect is attained by the accompanying blockade of aldosterone's sodium retention.

In the medium- to high-renin group, a reasonable alternative first choice is a beta-blocker. Although not as potent as ACE inhibitors, beta-blockers are extremely effective in lowering renin secretion (28,29); moreover, in certain subgroups (e.g., those with tachycardia or coronary disease) they have the added value of reducing cardiac work and perhaps protecting from future coronary events. Furthermore, unlike therapy with diuretics, monotherapy with beta-blockers has been shown in controlled trials to protect from coronary events, the major sequelae of hypertension (10) (see above).

DRUG THERAPY FOR LOW-RENIN PATIENTS

A low-renin profile suggests a nonrenin, sodium-related factor in the diastolic hypertension. Here the choice of first-line therapy is somewhat broader. Historically, the first choice for this group was a diuretic (30), the cornerstone of the old-fashioned stepped-care empirical approach to treating all essential hypertension. In the past, all other drugs were then added on in "steps." The diuretic was needed because all of the other older drugs caused reactive fluid retention. However, with modern agents, reactive fluid retention generally is not a problem. Now, even in low-renin patients, the ground occupied by diuretics is under sharp challenge by the newer calcium antagonists and by $alpha_1$-adrenergic blockers (31–33). Calcium antagonists are especially effective in low-renin patients (34–36), many of whom have the sodium-dependent type of vasoconstriction.

The specificity of calcium antagonists for this group is by no means absolute; these drugs often can produce significant depressor responses in medium- and even high-renin patients, possibly because increased cytosolic calcium may be a final pathway for sustaining all forms of vasoconstriction. However, the finding of their selective effectiveness in low-renin hypertension is also supported by work showing that a calcium antagonist fails to block the pressor action of angiotensin II while readily blocking norepinephrine action (37).

The calcium blockers' greater effectiveness against low-renin hypertension may be exploited in an interesting way. We have shown that concurrent sodium administration does not oppose, and even might enhance, the antihypertensive action of these agents (38). Allowing salt in the diet reduces renin and shifts the patient to the sodium-dependent type of vasoconstriction, against which calcium antagonists are most effective. On the other hand, verifying the same principle, sodium depletion and high-renin secretion induced by diet or diuretic therapy may rob these agents of their depressor power while enhancing the antihypertensive effect of converting-enzyme inhibitors. These relationships are in keeping with (a) a number of reports that indicate greater effectiveness of calcium antagonists in low-renin forms of hypertension (31,32,34) and (b) other reports indicating little or no added benefit from combining these agents with a diuretic (39–41). The results are of practical interest because patients given calcium antagonists can liberalize their sodium intake and thereby improve volume and flow and—it is to be hoped—well being, without adverse effect on blood pressure.

Calcium-channel blockers are theoretically more attractive agents than diuretics because, like ACE inhibitors, they actually *improve* blood flow to the heart, brain, and kidneys as they reduce blood pressure. They are not associated, as the diuretics are, with dehydration, hemoconcentration, impotence, abnormal lipid profiles, hyperuricemia, and azotemia. Indeed, the fact that long-term clinical trials utilizing a diuretic-based regimen have failed to show protection against coronary artery disease may be attributable to some of these problems (30). Quite possibly, as preliminary evidence suggests, converting-enzyme inhibitors (17) and calcium-channel blockers (16) might demonstrate cardioprotection in long-term controlled trials.

Another class of agents that maintain tissue flow as they lower pressure are the alpha-blockers such as prazosin. The best responders to alpha-blockers, as well as the best responders to calcium antagonists, are those patients with low-renin hypertension (33,42). These $alpha_1$-receptor blockers are less potent than the calcium-channel blockers but appear to address the same vasoconstrictor mechanism, perhaps because of the close proximity of alpha- and calcium receptors on the cell wall (43). Combination of the two drug types can produce additive effects (43,44).

SEEKING MONOTHERAPY FOR THE MEDIUM-RENIN PATIENT OR FOR THE UNPROFILED PATIENT

As can be seen from an inspection of Fig. 1, plasma renin activity values above 8–10 ng/ml/hr or under 1.0 point reliably to selective and effective monotherapy, but intermediate-range values show far less accurate marksmanship. Possibly, in this range, renin-mediated and sodium-related mechanisms of vasoconstriction overlap or function reciprocally. Unfortunately, this is where the majority of patients with essential hypertension are to be found, and the clinician is left to draw on the empiric process described above. Five major drug types (see Fig. 1) are now available for this exercise.

The empiric process need not be as blind as it was formerly, however, and it most surely is not as limited in its alternatives. For one thing, the renin profile may be available to add its weight to other tests in the baseline evaluation: As already discussed, values on the high side (as opposed to the low side) suggest which type of drug should be tried first.

The rationale for this choice is that the converting-enzyme inhibitor, of all the medications available, is the most specific, so that a negative result is as informative as a positive one. The strongest immediate effect of converting-enzyme inhibition is against angiotensin's direct vasoconstriction. Over the longer term (2–3 weeks), however, the impact of converting-enzyme inhibitors in blocking aldosterone secretion is also expressed; thus these agents work

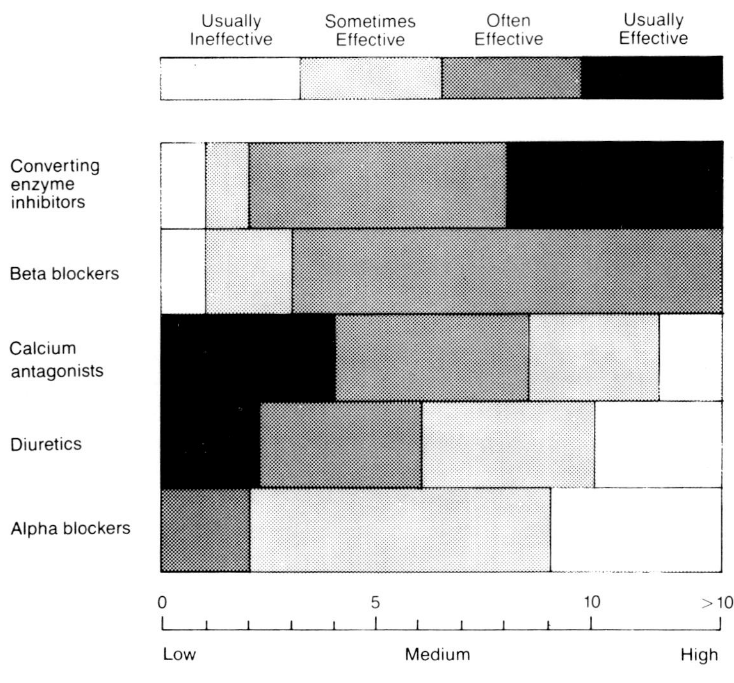

FIG. 1. A schematized representation of the selective action of major types of antihypertensive drugs. Research that has defined two fundamentally different mechanisms of long-term vasoconstriction—one renin-dependent, the other mediated by sodium and volume factors—is supported by assessments of the level of activity of renin in the blood. Some 30% of people with essential hypertension have low levels of renin activity, about 50% have medium levels, and about 20% have high levels. The plasma renin activity measurement is an aid in predicting the potential effectiveness of antihypertensive drug treatment. Converting-enzyme inhibitors and beta-receptor blockers are most useful in people whose hypertension is renin-mediated. Converting-enzyme inhibitors also lower blood pressure in many patients with intermediate or even somewhat low levels of plasma renin. They are ineffective when plasma renin is near zero. Beta-blockers resemble converting-enzyme inhibitors in their spectrum of effectiveness but are less useful when high renin levels are brought about by sodium depletion. Calcium antagonists, diuretics, and alpha-receptor blockers are most useful in people with the renin-independent, sodium–volume-mediated type of vasoconstriction. Alpha-blockers may be effective in low-renin patients, but, more often than calcium antagonists or diuretics, they fail to fully control blood pressure in such patients.

on the sodium-related side as well. If after a few weeks they still fail, the next alternative is to stop the antirenin drug and pursue a purely sodium-related solution. The choices are, in sequence, calcium-channel blockers, alpha$_1$-adrenergic blockers, and, lastly, diuretics. The reason for this ranking is that the first two of the three agents, when they bring about a successful depressor result, do so without reducing the blood flow that could be so vital to cardiovascular health and that may be compromised by diuretics. There are, of course, exceptions to this sequence. Diuretics may be the first choice in patients with overt hemodilution or fluid retention, phenomena that are often present in obese and low-renin hypertensive subjects.

Two important caveats should be observed in applying the empirical evaluation–treatment process to patients with medium renin values. First, the clinician should resist the temptation to begin adding other drugs when converting-enzyme monotherapy seems inadequate at first. Converting-enzyme inhibitors also suppress aldosterone secretion, but because the effect of this action only reaches its full expression slowly [endogenous aldosterone activity accounts for 1–2% (at most) of daily renal sodium reabsorption], several weeks may pass before the full benefits of converting-enzyme inhibitors are seen in patients in whom sodium dependency shares culpability with renin dependency. This component of the converting-enzyme inhibitor's antihypertensive action resembles that of spironolactone in the delayed onset of what eventually can be a considerable depressor effect, an effect often greater than that of full-dose thiazide diuretic agents (9).

Second, the clinician must be willing to pursue monotherapy and try only one drug at a time. Unless a rigorous, systematic trial of monotherapies makes additive therapy the last resort, it is no trial at all. Additive therapy provides (a) few clues to the nature of the basic hypertensive lesion, (b) little advance in understanding the pathophysiology of hypertension, and (c) less-than-optimal service to the patient. Superimposing one drug on another, as in the stepped-care regimen, makes the entire pursuit impossible to analyze and allows many patients to take nontherapeutic (and possibly detrimental) drug agents for life. A recent review of 1486 clinical trials showing that many patients whose blood pressures were controlled by combination therapy rather than by monotherapy most likely represents a summing of patients rather than a demonstration of drug effectiveness (24). These patients, responding separately and specifically to the effective components in their antihypertensive recipe, would have been better served had there been an orderly effort to discover to which component of the combination they were responding. Therefore, one must be wary of these older reports, which focus primarily on the *mean* responses for groups. Often hidden by this analysis is the fact that, within such a group, very good responders may be averaged with nonresponders and with those who actually exhibit pressor response (24). This point is well illustrated by some recent reports (45,46).

Recently, strong new support has been provided for the treatment algorithm developed herein, which seeks to fully explore monotherapy before considering combination therapy. One such study (47) has evaluated separately in each subject the effectiveness of a beta-blocker, an ACE inhibitor, and a diuretic in randomized, 4-month, changeover sequence. All three drugs had equal mean effectiveness; however, each agent was effective in different, particular groups of patients, and this selective effectiveness, or lack of it, was predictable by renin profiling. This study verifies an earlier cross-over design study (32). Moreover, there is statistical validity and considerable potential for

cardiodepression, vascular resistance rose and blood pressure did not change. A gradual fall in blood pressure was observed in all patients between 2 and 5 hr after receiving any beta-blocker. The fall in blood pressure was caused in all cases by a reduction of vascular resistance. The antihypertensive and vasodilator effect of the drugs was associated with the return of cardiac output, heart rate, and stroke volume to baseline values (for pindolol to a point above baseline values). After 24 hr the antihypertensive effect of all beta-blockers was associated with a reduction of vascular resistance below pretreatment level. However, at any level of blood pressure, cardiac output was higher and vascular resistance was lower with pindolol treatment as compared with other drug treatment. Thus, all beta-blockers exert their antihypertensive effect through vasodilatation. Their degree of vasodilation depends on cardiac sympathetic drive and ISA as determinants of the magnitude of their effect on cardiac output.

Hemodynamic Interrelationships and Adaptations During Beta-Blockade

For all five beta-blockers, highly significant correlations emerged over the 24-hr period between arterial pressure on the one hand and vascular resistance and cardiac output on the other (Fig. 5). Thus, the lower pressure, the lower vascular resistance, and the higher cardiac output are consistent with one another. Apparently, a low cardiac output during beta-blockade prevents, rather than causes, a reduction in blood pressure. The regression lines were not different for the beta-blockers—with the exception of pindolol, which, for any value of blood pressure, showed higher values of cardiac output and lower values of vascular resistance.

How does one explain the increments in cardiac output, heart rate, and stroke volume when blood pressure and vascular resistance start to fall after starting beta-blockade? It has been demonstrated that changes in heart rate, cardiac output, and stroke volume after vasodilatation during beta-blockade depend on vagal withdrawal and on an increase in venous return (34). Thus, during the vasodilator phase of the beta-blockers, the initial hemodynamic changes are offset by interference of the arterial baroreflex. This sequence of events is further elaborated and clarified in Fig. 6. Also in our previously mentioned literature review (28), changes in stroke volume and changes in vascular resistance after using the various beta-blockers were inversely correlated both acutely after (Fig. 7) and during long-term beta-blockade (Fig. 8). Furthermore, the uniform "vasodilator" response to long-term beta-blockade, which is underlying the beta-blockers' antihypertensive effect, was always associated with an increase in stroke volume. Moreover, in the acute 24-hr study of five beta-blockers we found that the changes in stroke volume, as well as the changes in heart rate, were inversely correlated with the changes in vascular resistance (33).

Effects of "Direct" Vasodilators on Cardiovascular Hemodynamics

Provided that baroreceptor reflexes are intact, the response to a fall in systemic blood pressure will be enhanced sympathetic and reduced parasympathetic nervous activity. The increase in heart rate, cardiac contractility, and cardiac output, which often accompany treatment with vasodilators, reflect counterregulatory activity. The higher levels of plasma catecholamine and plasma renin activity

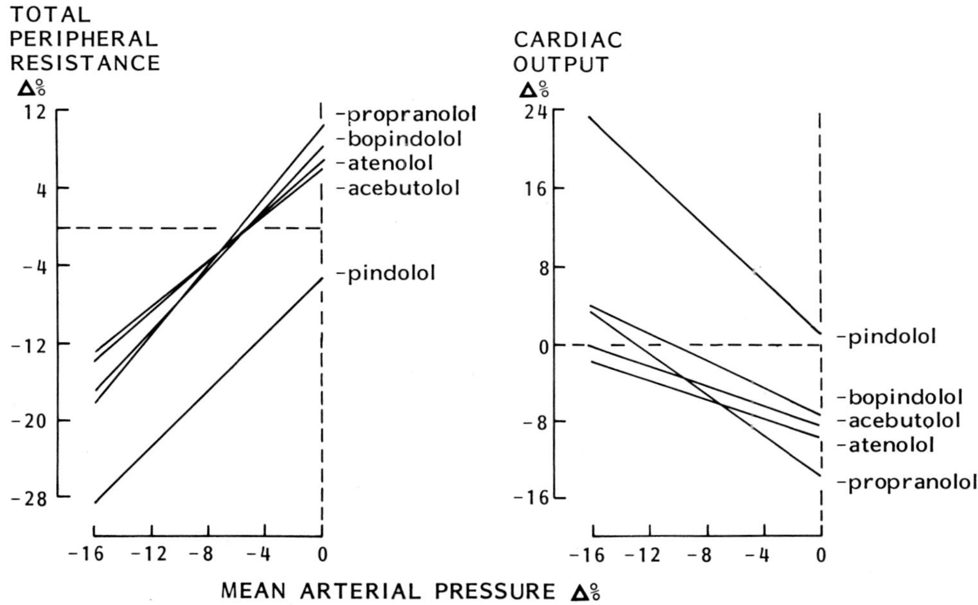

FIG. 5. Relationship between changes in mean arterial pressure and changes in peripheral resistance or cardiac output during the gradual onset of the antihypertensive effect of five beta-adrenoceptor antagonists over a 24-hr period. Every regression line represents 160 points, with $p < 0.001$ for every regression equation. (From refs. 4 and 33.)

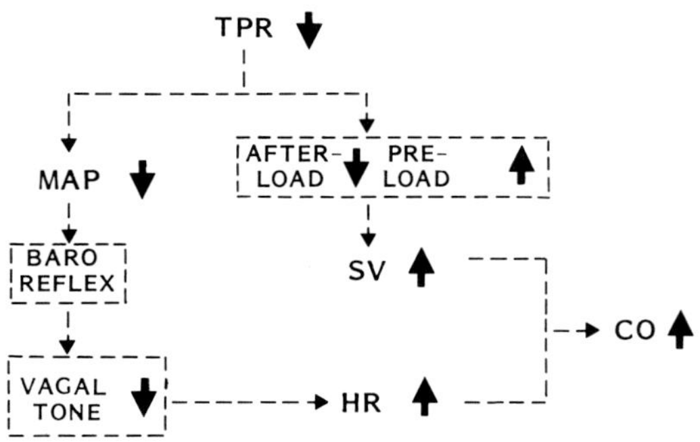

FIG. 6. Hemodynamic adaptations after the onset of the antihypertensive effect of beta-adrenoceptor antagonists. TPR, total peripheral resistance; MAP, mean arterial pressure; SV, stroke volume; HR, heart rate; CO, cardiac output.

that follow administration of various vasodilators (35) are an additional indication of increased sympathetic drive. Intravenous administration of vasodilators that cause an immediate and pronounced reduction in blood pressure are the most likely to cause marked reflex increases in heart rate and cardiac conduction.

"Vasodilating" drugs, whatever the underlying mechanism, may be classified according to their primary site of action on blood vessels (Table 2). The relative effects of vasodilator drugs on arteriolar resistance and venous capacitance are controversial (36). Organic nitrates, which act primarily on the venous capacitance vessels but also on the large conductive arteries, are of historical interest only in the treatment of essential hypertension and are not discussed further.

Hydralazine

Hydralazine has a direct relaxing effect on the smooth muscle of arterial resistance vessels. As a result, diastolic pressure is usually reduced to a greater extent than systolic pressure (37). Similarly, left ventricular systolic and end-diastolic pressure are decreased as a result of the reduction in afterload, which leads to an improvement in left ventricular pump function and an increase in heart rate and cardiac output. Increases in the pressure of the small circulation sometimes occur because of a lack of action on the venous circulation. However, these increases may be more prominent under the acute influence of other vasodilators in this category, such as minoxidil or diazoxide (34).

Minoxidil

The magnitude of the antihypertensive response to minoxidil is related to the baseline level of hypertension; the response to initial or incremental doses declines with reduced blood pressure, so that there is little or no response at a pretreatment diastolic pressure of 85 mmHg. Minoxidil, therefore, has minimal blood-pressure-lowering activity in normotensive subjects (38). Like the other vasodilators with little effect on venous capacitance, minoxidil does not produce orthostatic hypotension and does not affect the function of carotid and aortic baroreceptors (39). In common with other agents in this class, minoxidil also decreases arteriolar resistance, reduces cardiac afterload, and increases blood flow. The absence of venous vasodilator activity leads to increased venous return by reducing venous pooling and also leads to a consequent increase in heart rate, cardiac output, cardiopulmonary blood volume, and pulmonary artery pressure (40).

Pinacidil

Pinacidil is a newer, potent arterial vasodilator (41,42). The acute hemodynamic effects of intravenous pinacidil

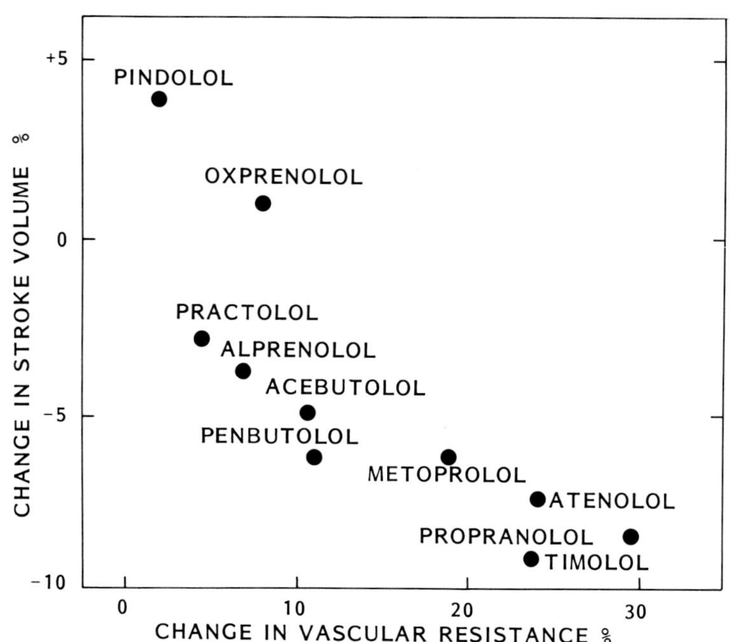

FIG. 7. Relationship between changes in total peripheral resistance and changes in stroke volume acutely after intervenous beta-adrenoceptor blockade. Note that the degree of ISA decreases from left to right in this graph. (See also Table 1 and Figs. 2 and 3.)

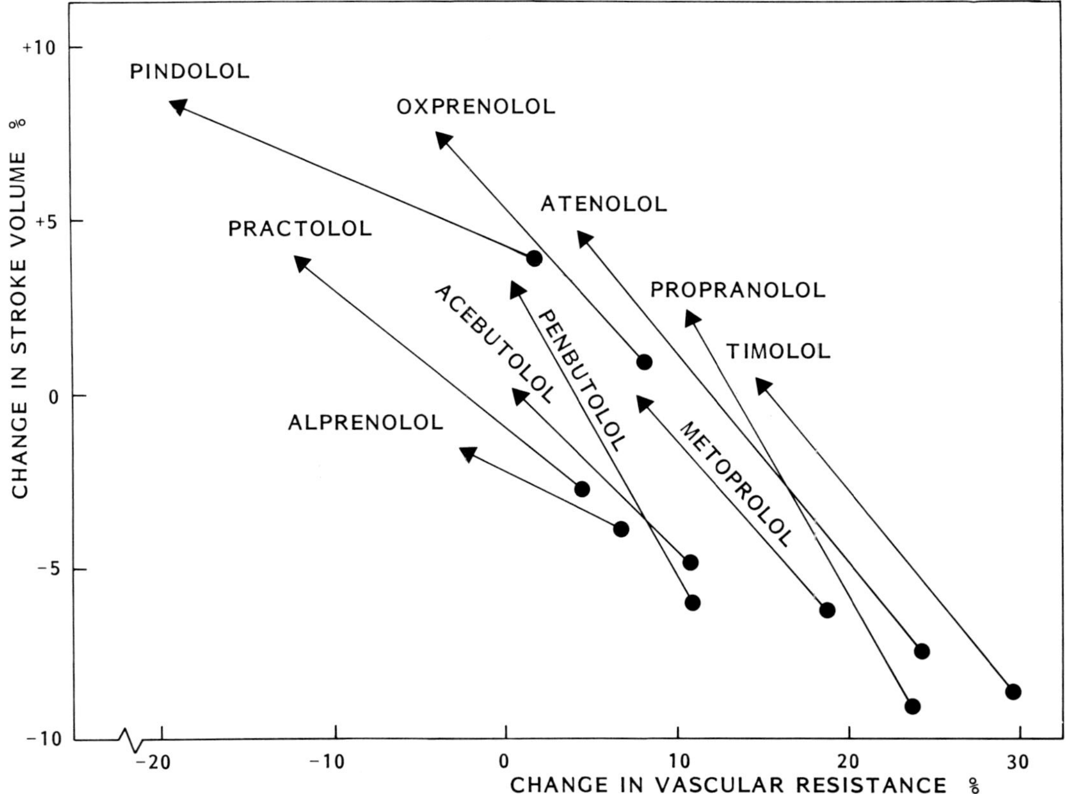

FIG. 8. Relationship between changes in total peripheral resistance and changes in stroke volume after acute intravenous beta-blockade (●) and during long-term beta-blocker therapy for hypertension (▲). Note that the reduction in vascular resistance, which is always underlying the antihypertensive action of beta-blockers, is associated with an increase in stroke volume.

(0.2 mg/kg) infused over 8 min reduced mean arterial blood pressure from 94 to 74 mmHg in normotensive subjects. Ten minutes after beginning drug administration, heart rate had increased from 75 to 106 beats/min and remained significantly elevated after 70 min; cardiac index had increased by 25%, and systemic vascular resistance had decreased by more than 37%. Other studies have shown similar effects in hypertensive patients (43,44). As with hydralazine and minoxidil, the reflex tachycardia produced by pinacidil can be greatly reduced by concomitant administration of a beta-blocker (42,45).

TABLE 2. *Classification of "vasodilating" drugs according to their predominant hemodynamic effect*

Resistance vessels	Capacitance vessels	Capacitance and resistance vessels
Endralazine	Organic nitrates	Sodium nitroprusside
Hydralazine		Guanabenz
Diazoxide		Guanfacine
Minoxidil		Clonidine
Pinacidil		Alpha-methyldopa
Nifedipine		Prazosin
Nitrendipine		Terazosin
Nicardipine		Phentolamine
Nisoldipine		Urapidil
Felodipine		Captopril
Isradipine		Ramipril
Verapamil		Enalapril
Diltiazem		Lisinopril

Effects of Centrally Acting Antihypertensive Agents on Cardiovascular Hemodynamics

This group of drugs includes alpha-methyldopa, clonidine, and guanfacine. These drugs cause a global reduction in central sympathetic outflow through stimulation of central alpha-2-adrenoceptors. As a consequence, a reduced sympathetic activity on both the venous and arterial site of the circulation, as well as a reduced cardiac sympathetic drive, is the result. In general, blood pressure is reduced by vasodilatation, with a small decrease in cardiac output (3,46,47). Orthostatic hypotension is a predictable feature, with vasodilators acting on both the capacitance and the resistance vessels, so that minimal postural changes may have profound hemodynamic effects.

Effects of Alpha-Adrenoceptor Antagonists on Cardiovascular Hemodynamics

Prazosin, terazosin, and urapidil are selective alpha-1-adrenoceptor antagonists. Both drugs have a combined effect on the venous and arteriolar site of the circulation, like sodium nitroprusside and the centrally acting drugs. The fall in blood pressure is associated with no change in cardiac output and a decrease in cardiac filling pressures (40). Terazosin has a longer duration of action than does prazosin, but otherwise has a similar hemodynamic action (48). Urapidil also reduces total peripheral resistance (and, hence, blood pressure) with both acute and long-term administration (49). In contrast to hydralazine, which loses its antihypertensive potency with prolonged treatment (due to activation of reflex mechanisms), no tachyphylaxis is observed with urapidil in hypertensive patients (50). A degree of preload reduction, caused by intravenous urapidil in normotensive volunteers, suggests that in addition to affecting arteriolar dilatation, the drug has some effects on the venous system (49). As a rule, vasodilatation and the lowering of blood pressure with urapidil are not accompanied by reflex tachycardia. Indeed, bradycardia has been reported in several studies (49,50).

Angiotensin-Converting-Enzyme (ACE) Inhibitors

In general, the hemodynamic responses to individual ACE inhibitors are similar, despite their structural differences. Captopril, the first orally active ACE inhibitor, reduces blood pressure in patients with essential or renovascular hypertension via arteriolar and venous dilatation (51,52). Total peripheral resistance and mean arterial pressure are reduced with acute administration, and in the longer term there is no significant increase in heart rate or cardiac output. Enalapril lacks the sulfhydryl group of captopril and differs only in the onset and duration of antihypertensive effects, since it is a prodrug requiring *in vivo* de-esterification to its active form, enalaprilat. Lisinopril, the lysine analogue of enalapril, appears to have a longer duration of antihypertensive effect than does enalapril. In mild to moderate hypertension there is no alteration in cardiac output with short-term ACE inhibition, although there may be a slight increase in cardiac output toward normal values if hypertension is severe. A degree of venous pooling may account for the absence of augmentation of cardiac output observed in general, but any such increase in venous capacitance is not sufficient to promote orthostatic hypotension. In general, dilatation of arteriolar resistance vessels would be expected to result in a baroreceptor-mediated increase in heart rate. However, studies with ACE inhibitors indicate a notable absence of reflex tachycardia subsequent to blood pressure reduction by arteriolar vasodilatation (53–55). The mechanism of this effect remains uncertain. Baroreceptor and cardiovascular hemodynamic reflexes in response to posture and exercise appear to be maintained despite ACE inhibition (54). The venodilator action of ACE inhibitors appears not to be predominant, and whereas modification of vagally mediated responses may occur with ACE inhibitors (53), it is unlikely to be a significant mechanism for their antihypertensive effect. The most probable mechanism is reduced sympathetic activity after withdrawal of the synergistic action of angiotensin II on norepinephrine release from sympathetic nerves.

Effects of Calcium Antagonists on Cardiovascular Hemodynamics

The net hemodynamic effects of the calcium antagonistic drugs (also called slow-channel inhibitors, calcium-channel inhibitors, or calcium-entry blockers) are a consequence of a complex interplay of (a) their direct actions on the myocardium and the coronary and peripheral circulations and (b) their indirect effects on the autonomic nervous system (56,57). Despite widely varying chemical structures, all calcium antagonists act as vasodilators, lowering vascular resistance (afterload) and blood pressure through interference with calcium metabolism primarily in vascular smooth muscle cells. The effects of the various agents on heart rate and atrioventricular conduction differ (27). Clinically, the hemodynamic effects induced by different calcium antagonists will be influenced by the reactivity of the patient's cardiovascular homeostatic reflex mechanisms and ventricular function. Here, the most important indirect hemodynamic effect is the baroreceptor-mediated reflex increase in beta-adrenergic tone (especially with the dihydroxypyridine group), which is a response to widespread systemic vasodilatation (58). The increase in tone consists of a positive inotropic and chronotropic response, which tends to counteract any direct associated negative chronotropic/inotropic effects of the drug (59).

The various calcium antagonists differ in their effects on the cardiovascular system (60) (Table 3). The dihydropyridine group (nifedipine and its congeners) are the most potent vasodilators. These agents have minimal negative inotropic activity *in vivo* and are more likely to produce reflex stimulation of the sympathetic nervous system. Diltiazem and verapamil have a lesser vasodilating effect; verapamil has significant direct negative inotropic and chronotropic effects as compared with diltiazem and nifedipine.

Verapamil and Congeners

In addition to causing marked vasodilatation in most peripheral beds, verapamil is an extremely potent coronary vasodilator (61,62); this latter effect is more powerful than that elicited by papaverine or glyceryl trinitrate (63,64). In patients in sinus rhythm, the mean arterial pressure is reduced, with a slight increase in cardiac output. No signifi-

TABLE 3. *Differential cardiovascular effects of the calcium antagonists nifedipine, verapamil, and diltiazem*[a]

Effect	Nifedipine	Verapamil	Diltiazem
Peripheral vasodilator effect	+++	++	++
Reflex sympathetic stimulation	++	+	+
Negative inotropic effect	+	++	+
Negative chronotropic effect (sinus node)	0	++	+
Slowing of AV conduction	0	+	+
Prolongation of refractory period in AV node	0	+	+

[a] AV, atrioventricular; 0, absence; +, ++, and +++, increasing degree of presence.

cant reduction in stroke volume occurs. Very similar results were found by others (65). In healthy adults, a slight negative inotropic action was found, but this was easily abolished by exercise (66). No increase in heart rate or cardiac output was observed after acute administration or treatment for 1–6 weeks with verapamil (67–70).

Diltiazem

Although it is chemically dissimilar to verapamil, diltiazem possesses many similarities to the verapamil group in terms of action; however, diltiazem differs in having less of a negative inotropic and chronotropic effect. Generally, single intravenous doses of diltiazem decrease systemic vascular resistance and blood pressure by 20–30% and increase cardiac output because of the arterial dilatory effect of the drug. Usually, heart rate decreases (71–74) or does not change, although increases have been reported (75). Single intravenous doses of diltiazem have also produced beneficial hemodynamic changes (decreased blood pressure, and unchanged or increased cardiac output/index) in patients with congestive heart failure and hypertensive or coronary artery disease (76,77) and in those with primary or secondary pulmonary hypertension (78,79). Hemodynamic effects following oral administration have been less consistent.

Nifedipine and Newer Dihydropyridines

The newer dihydropyridine calcium antagonists are structurally related to nifedipine. They have been developed to provide greater vascular selectivity, less myocardial depression, more flexible dosing regimens, and an improved side-effect profile, while sharing the fundamental hemodynamic profile of the parent drug. The pharmacology of several important new dihydropyridines has been recently reviewed (80). Significant reductions in blood pressure occur within 30 min of oral nifedipine administration (81). Intravenous nifedipine (1–4 mg) reduces blood pressure by up to 34% in patients with hypertension (82). The antihypertensive effect is due to a marked decrease in systemic vascular resistance, with cardiac output increased because of baroreceptor-mediated increases in beta-adrenergic tone (81,83–85). After treatment with nifedipine for 6–8 weeks, heart rate and cardiac output were no longer increased above baseline values, despite unchanged or increased baroreflex sensitivity (86,87). Similar effects have been reported with the dihydropyridines nitrendipine, nicardipine, and nisoldipine (80). The hemodynamic effects of a single dose of verapamil, diltiazem, and nifedipine have been compared in patients with recent myocardial infarctions (88). The drugs differ in their effects on heart rate and cardiac index, with nifedipine significantly increasing these parameters and both diltiazem and verapamil either decreasing them or having no effect on them (Fig. 9). All drugs decreased mean arterial pressure, and none affected either pulmonary wedge pressure or cardiac index. In further comparisons, nifedipine again increased heart rate (by 12–16%), whereas verapamil had no statistically significant effect on this parameter and diltiazem caused a reduction of 7%. The three agents had similar significant hypotensive effects, with the more rapid blood pressure reductions after nifedipine administration producing the reflex increases in heart rate (89,90).

HEMODYNAMIC PROFILES OF ANTIHYPERTENSIVE AGENTS DURING PHYSICAL EXERCISE

With only few exceptions, the effect of most antihypertensive agents on blood pressure is maintained during ex-

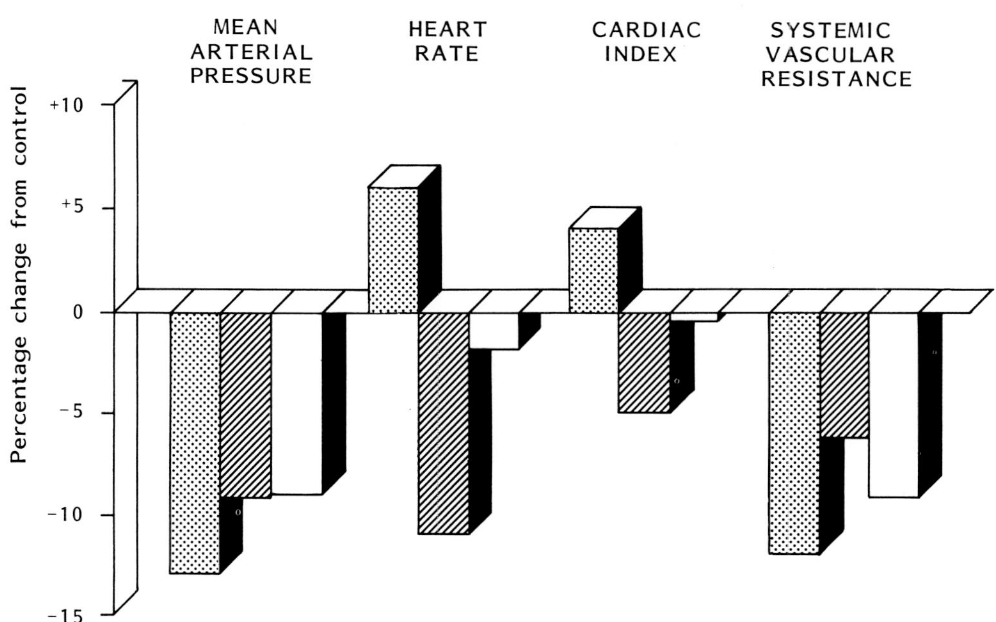

FIG. 9. Comparative hemodynamic effects of single doses of orally administered nifedipine (20 mg) (*stippled columns; n* = 12), diltiazem (120 mg) (*unshaded columns; n* = 12) and verapamil (160 mg) (*hatched columns; n* = 10) in patients with recent myocardial infarctions. (Based on data from ref. 88.)

ercise (3). The antihypertensive effect of the centrally acting drugs alpha-methyldopa and clonidine gradually wears off during increasing levels of exercise. The mechanism of this phenomenon is not clear. During treatment with diuretics, the beta-blockers, the alpha-blocker prazosin, labetalol, the calcium antagonists, and the ACE inhibitors, the blood-pressure-lowering effect is fully maintained at all levels of exercise. It is interesting to note that during treatment with the beta-adrenoceptor antagonists the vasodilator response to exercise is enhanced (3), which once again stresses the importance of vasodilatation for their antihypertensive action, not only at rest but also during sympathetic stimulation.

COMPARISON OF HEMODYNAMIC PROFILES OF THE VARIOUS ANTIHYPERTENSIVE AGENTS

The hemodynamic profile of an antihypertensive drug during prolonged treatment of hypertension is the net result of a number of processes:

1. the primary hemodynamic effect of pharmacological interference with cardiovascular and hormonal homeostasis,
2. secondary hemodynamic adaptations as a consequence of the reflex control of the circulation, and
3. tertiary changes such as regression of left ventricular hypertrophy and structural vascular changes in response to long-term resetting of blood pressure control.

The net result of at least the first two processes can be demonstrated in a pressure–flow–resistance diagram as based on the described acute and subacute intermediate long-term effects of the various antihypertensive drugs (Fig. 10). The classical direct vasodilators have a profound effect on vascular resistance, but part of their antihypertensive effect is offset by reflex cardiostimulation and renal retention of sodium and water. In the long run the diuretics, most calcium antagonists, the alpha-1-adrenoceptor blockers, and the ACE inhibitors lower blood pressure, with little or no effect on cardiac output. Apparently the drugs act at different levels of cardiovascular control in order to prevent reflex responses to the vasodilatation. The centrally acting drugs reduce both cardiac output and vascular resistance to some extent as a consequence of reduced central sympathetic outflow. Thus, apparently all antihypertensive agents lower blood pressure through interference with some vasoconstriction mechanism. The only exception to this rule seems to be the beta-blockers devoid of ISA, of which propranolol has been the prototype for more than 20 years. Showing a similar effect on blood pressure when compared with the other classes of antihypertensive agents, these drugs seem to reduce cardiac output and to maintain, or even further increase, vascular resistance. In other words, the hemodynamic profile of this type of beta-blockers exactly mirrors the profile of the classical vasodilators. It has been, however, extensively argued above that these hemodynamic profiles are the consequences of hemodynamic adaptations in response to the primary pharmacological intervention. Whereas the antihypertensive and vasodilator action of most antihypertensive agents is independent of sympathetic drive, the cardiac effects of beta-blockers are augmented by increased sympathetic activity (3). As a consequence, the reflex adaptations will be amplified as well under these conditions, and the primary antihypertensive (i.e., vasodilator) mechanism of beta-blockers will be completely masked (4). A way to unmask this vasodilator activity of beta-adrenoceptor antagonists is either to minimize cardiac sympathetic drive by absolute bedrest or by studying beta-blockers with ISA which can substitute for the loss of cardiac sympathetic tone caused by blockade of cardiac beta-receptors in order to prevent cardiodepression and reflex-vasoconstriction (33).

A UNIFYING CONCEPT: THE VASODILATOR RULE OF ANTIHYPERTENSIVE TREATMENT

All classes of antihypertensive agents lower blood pressure by causing vasodilatation through whatever mechanism. This vasodilatation may be produced by either reduced vasoconstrictor mechanisms or enhanced vasodilator factors. The principal ways to interfere with vasoconstrictor mechanisms are:

1. reduction of sympathetic vasoconstrictor nerve activity, (beta-blockers, alpha-1-antagonists, centrally acting alpha-2-agonists),
2. interference with humorally mediated vasoconstriction (ACE inhibitors, beta-blockers), or

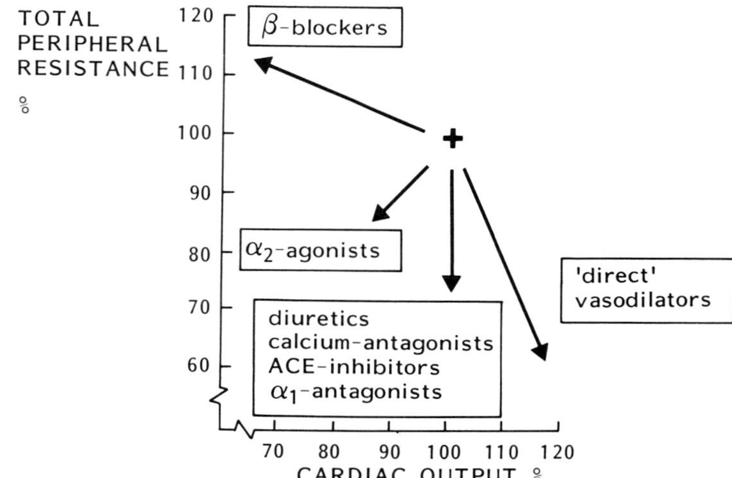

FIG. 10. Relative effects of the different categories of antihypertensive agents on cardiac output and total peripheral resistance in hypertension. The black cross indicates the hemodynamic situation in the untreated condition. The position of beta-blockers refers to those representatives of this group who are devoid of intrinsic sympathomimetic activity. (See also Table 1 and Figs. 2 and 3.) ACE, angiotensin-converting enzyme.

3. inhibition of excitation–contraction coupling in vascular smooth muscle cells (saliuretics, "direct" vasodilators, calcium-entry blockers).

The active interplay between these three main mechanisms at different sites of the circulation, in combination with the multiple effects of most antihypertensive drugs at different levels of hierarchy in circulatory homeostasis, may explain why antihypertensive agents lower blood pressure. Whenever they do so, it is always the reversal of the underlying hemodynamic abnormality (i.e., vasodilatation) which is initiating the return of blood pressure toward a lower value.

REFERENCES

1. Bohr D. What makes the pressure go up? *Hypertension* 1981;3(Suppl II):II-160–II-172.
2. Lund-Johansen P. State of the art review; haemodynamics in essential hypertension. *Clin Sci* 1980;59:343S–354S.
3. Lund-Johansen P. In: Birkenhäger WH, Reid JL, eds. *Handbook of hypertension, vol 5: clinical pharmacology of antihypertensive drugs.* New York: Elsevier, 1984; 39–66.
4. Man in't Veld AJ, Van den Meiracker AH, Schalekamp MADH. Do beta-blockers really increase peripheral vascular resistance? Review of the literature and new observations under basal conditions. *Am J Hypertens* 1988;1:91–96.
5. Gabriel R. Comparison of the hypotensive effects of bendrofluazide, bumetanide and xipamide. *Curr Med Res Opin* 1983;8:645–648.
6. Holland OB, Gomez-Sanchez CE, Kuhnert LV, et al. Antihypertensive comparison of furosemide with hydrochlorothiazide for black patients. *Arch Intern Med* 1979;139:1015–1021.
7. Andersson O. The use of diuretics in modern antihypertensive therapy. *Acta Pharmacol Toxicol (Copen)* 1984;54(Suppl I):79–87.
8. Conway J, Lauwers P. Hemodynamic and hypotensive effects of long-term therapy with chlorothiazide. *Circulation* 1960;21:21–26.
9. Dustan HP, Cumming CR, Corcoran AC, Page IH. A mechanism of chlorothiazide enhanced effectiveness of antihypertensive ganglioplegic drugs. *Circulation* 1959;19:360–365.
10. Frohlich ED, Schnaper HW, Wilson IM, Freis ED. Hemodynamic alterations in hypertensive patients due to chlorothiazide. *Engl J Med* 1960;262:1261–1263.
11. Lant A. Diuretics: clinical pharmacology and therapeutic use (part II). *Drugs* 1985;29:162–188.
12. Rudd P, Blaschke TF. Antihypertensive agents and the drug therapy of hypertension. In: Goodman X, Gilman Y, eds. *The pharmacological basis of therapeutics,* 7th edition. New York: Macmillan, 1985;784–805.
13. Bennett WM, McDonald WJ, Kuehnel E, Hartnett MN, Porter GA. Do diuretics have antihypertensive properties independent of natriuresis? *Clin Pharmacol Ther* 1977;22:499–504.
14. Shah S, Khatri I, Freis ED. Mechanism of antihypertensive effect of thiazide diuretics. *Am Heart J* 1978;95:611–618.
15. Van Brummelen P, Woerlee M, Schalekamp MADH. Long-term versus short-term effects of hydrochlorothiazide on renal haemodynamics in essential hypertension. *Clin Sci* 1979;56:463.
16. Kumar EB, Nelson GK, Silke B, Ahuja RC, Okoli RC, Taylor SH. Circulatory dose–response effects of HCT at rest and during dynamic exercise in essential hypertension. *J R Coll Physicians Lond* 1982:16.
17. Freis ED. Salt in hypertension and the effect of diuretics. *Annu Rev Pharmacol Toxicol* 1979;19:13–23.
18. Tobian L. How sodium and the kidney relate to the hypertensive arteriole. *Fed Proc* 1974;33:138–142.
19. Struyker-Boudier HAJ, Smits JFM, Kleinjans JCS, Van Essen H. Hemodynamic actions of diuretic agents. *Clin Exp Hypertens* 1983;5(Suppl 2):209–233.
20. Kelly DA, Hamilton S. A placebo-controlled trial to evaluate the antihypertensive efficacy and acceptability of indapamide. *Curr Med Res Opin* 1977;5:137–144.
21. Biddle TL, Yu PN. Effect of furosemide on hemodynamics and lung water in acute pulmonary edema secondary to myocardial infarction. *Am J Cardiol* 1979;43:86–90.
22. Al-Sadir J, Zimmet L, Zahavi I, Watanachai K, Resnekov L. The hemodynamic effect of intravenous furosemide on the treatment of cardiac failure following acute myocardial infarction. *Clin Res* 1974;22:256A–256A.
23. Davidson RM, Goldman J Jr, Whalen RE, Wallace AG. Hemodynamic effects of furosemide in acute myocardial infarction. *Circulation* 1971;(Suppl II):156.
24. Dikshit K, Vyden JK, Forrester JS, Chatterjee K, Prakash R, Swan HJC. Renal and extrarenal hemodynamic effects of furosemide in congestive heart failure after acute myocardial infarction. *N Engl J Med* 1973;288:1087.
25. Kiely J, Kelly DT, Taylor DR, Pitt B. The role of furosemide in the treatment of left ventricular dysfunction associated with acute myocardial infarction. *Circulation* 1973;48:581.
26. Aroaye MA, Chang MY, Khatri IM, et al. Furosemide compared with hydrochlorothiazide. *JAMA* 1978;240:1863–1866.
27. Lund-Johansen P. The role of drugs in countering adverse pathophysiological profiles: influence on hemodynamics. *Am Heart J* 1987;114:958–964.
28. Man in't Veld AJ, Schalekamp MADH. Effects of 10 different beta-adrenoceptor antagonists on hemodynamics, plasma renin activity, and plasma norepinephrine in hypertension: the key role of vascular resistance changes in relation to partial agonist activity. *J Cardiovasc Pharmacol* 1983;5:S30–S45.
29. Johnsson G, De Gusman M, Bergman H, Sannerstedt R. The hemodynamic effects of alprenolol and propranolol at rest and during exercise in hypertensive patients. *Pharmacol Clin* 1969;2:34–39.
30. Svendsen TL, Carlsen JE, Hartling O, McNair A, Trap-Jensen J. A comparison of the acute haemodynamic effects of propranolol and pindolol at rest and during supine exercise in man. *Clin Sci* 1980;59:465–468.
31. Brogden RN, Heel RC, Speight TM, Avery GS. Labetalol: a review of its pharmacology and therapeutic use in hypertension. *Drugs* 1978;15:251–278.
32. Lund-Johansen P. Pharmacology of combined alpha-beta-blockade II. Haemodynamic effects of labetalol. *Drugs* 1984;28(Suppl 2):35–50.
33. Meiracker van den AH, Man in't Veld AJ, Ritsema van Eck HJ, Boomsma F, Schalekamp MADH. Hemodynamic and hormonal adaptations to beta-adrenoceptor blockade: a 24-hour study of acebutolol, atenolol, pindolol and propranolol in hypertensive patients. *Circulation* 1988;78:957–968.
34. Man in't Veld AJ, Wenting GJ, Boomsma F et al. Sympathetic and parasympathetic components of reflex-cardiostimulation during vasodilator treatment of hypertension. *Br J Clin Pharmacol* 1980;8:547–551.
35. Cottrell JE, Illner P, Kittay MJ, Steele JM Jr, Lowenstein J, et al. Rebound hypertension after sodium nitroprusside-induced hypotension. *Clin Pharmacol Ther* 1980;27:32–46.
36. Brown MJ. Vasodilator drugs: systemic and regional considerations. *Anaesth Intensive Care* 1980;8:310–317.
37. Levenson J, Simon A, Achiwiastos A, Temmar M, Safar M. Effets hémodynamiques compares de deux vasodilateurs: la dihydralazine et le diltiazem dans l'hypertension artèrielle permanente essentielle. *Archives Mal Coeur* 1982;75(Suppl):167.
38. Lowenthal DT, Affrime MB. Pharmacology and pharmacokinetics of minoxidil. *J Cardiovasc Pharmacol* 1980;2(Suppl 2):93–106.
39. Bryan AK, Hoobler SW, Rosenweig J, Weller JM, Purdy JM. Effect of minoxidil on blood pressure and hemodynamics in severe hypertension. *Am J Cardiol* 1977;39:796–801.
40. Tarazi RC, Dustan HP, Bravo EL, Niarchos AP. Vasodilating drugs: contrasting haemodynamic effects. *Clin Sci Mol* 1976;51(Suppl 3):575S–578S.
41. Nicholls DP, McNeill J, Harron DWG, Shanks RG. Cardiovascular effects of pinacidil and propranolol alone and in combination in normal humans. *J Cardiovasc Pharmacol* 1986;8a:51–54.
42. Nicholls DP, Murtagh JG, Scott ME, Morton P, Shank RG. Acute haemodynamic effects of pinacidil in man. *Br J Clin Pharmacol* 1986;22b:287–292.
43. Carlsen JE, Kardel T, Hilden T, Tango M, Trap-Jensen J. Immediate central and peripheral haemodynamic effects of a new vasodilating agent pinacidil (P1134) in hypertensive man. *Clin Physiol* 1981;1:375–384.
44. Kardel T, Hilden T, Carlsen J, Trap-Jensen J. *N″*-cyano-*N*-4-pyridyl-*N′*-1,2,2-trimethylpropylguanidine, a new vasodilating agent: acute effects on blood pressure and pharmacokinetics in

hypertensive patients. *J Cardiovasc Pharmacol* 1981;3:1002–1007.
45. Carlsen JE, Kardel T, Lund JO, McNair A, Trap-Jensen J. Acute hemodynamic effects of pinacidil and hydralazine in essential hypertension. *Clin Pharmacol Ther* 1985;37:253–259.
46. Frohlich ED, Messerli FH, Pegram BL, Kardon MB. Hemodynamic and cardiac effects of centrally acting antihypertensive drugs. *Hypertension* 1984;6(Suppl II):76–81.
47. Feldstein CA, Cohen AA, Sabaris RP, Burucia JE. Hemodynamic effects of guanfacine in essential hypertension. *Clin Ther* 1984;6:325–334.
48. Titmarsh S, Monk JP. Terazosin. A review of its pharmacodynamic and pharmacokinetic properties, and therapeutic efficacy in essential hypertension. *Drugs* 1987;33:461–477.
49. Van Zwieten PA. Pharmacological and haemodynamic profile of urapidil. In: Amery A, ed. *Treatment of hypertension with urapidil: preclinical and clinical update* 1986; International Congress and Symposium Series No. 101. London: Royal Society of Medicine Services; 1–9.
50. Schoetensack W, Bruckschen EG, Zech K. Urapidil. In: Scriabine A, ed. *New drugs annual: cardiovascular drugs.* New York: Raven Press, 1983;19–48.
51. Tarazi RC, Bravo EL, Fouad FM, Omvik P, Cody RJ. Hemodynamic and volume changes associated with captopril. *Hypertension* 1980;2:576–585.
52. De Bruyn JHB, Man in't Veld AJ, Wenting GJ, Derkx FHM, Schalekamp MADH. Haemodynamic profile of captopril in various forms of hypertension. *Eur J Clin Pharmacol* 1981;20:163–168.
53. Ajayi AA, Campbell BC, Howie CA, Reid JL. Acute and chronic effects of the converting enzyme inhibitors enalapril and lisinopril on reflex control of heart rate in normotensive man. *J Hypertens* 1985;3:47–53.
54. Fitzpatrick MA, Julius S. Hemodynamic effects of angiotensin-converting enzyme inhibitors in essential hypertension: a review. *J Cardiovasc Pharmacol* 1985;7:S35–S39.
55. Thuillez C, Richer C, Guidicelli JF. Pharmacokinetics, converting enzyme inhibition and peripheral arterial hemodynamics of ramipril in healthy volunteers. *Am J Cardiol* 1987;59:380–440.
56. Block PJ, Winkle RA. Hemodynamic effects of anti-arrhythmic drugs. *Am J Cardiol* 1983;52:14C–23C.
57. Singh BN, Ellrodt G, Nademanee K. Calcium antagonists: cardiocirculatory effects and therapeutic applications. In: Hurst JW, ed. *Clinical essays on the heart,* vol 2. New York: McGraw-Hill, 1984;65–97.
58. Low RI, Takeda P, Mason DT, DeMaria AN. The effects of calcium channel blocking agents on cardiovascular function. *Am J Cardiol* 1982;49:547–553.
59. Henderson AH. Calcium antagonists in the treatment of ischaemic heart disease I. *Postgrad Med J* 1983;59(Suppl 2):7–10.
60. Henry PD. Comparative pharmacology of calcium antagonists: nifedipine, verapamil and diltiazem. *Am J Cardiol* 1980;46:047–1058.
61. Melville KI, Shister HE, Huq S. Iproveratril: experimental data on coronary-dilation and anti-arrhythmic action. *Can Med Assoc J* 1964;90:761–770.
62. Winbury MM, Howe BB, Hefner MA. Effects of nitrates and other coronary dilators on large and small coronary vessels: an hypothesis for the mechanism of action of nitrates. *J Pharmacol Exp Ther* 1969;168:70–95.
63. Fleckenstein A. Specific pharmacology of calcium in myocardium, cardiac pace-makers and vascular smooth muscle. *Annu Rev Pharmacol Toxicol* 1977;17:149–166.
64. Haas H, Hartfelder G. Alpha-isopropyl-alpha-[*N*-methyl-*N*-homoveratryl-alpha-amino propyl]-3-4-dimethoxyphenylacetonitril, eine Aulstanz mit coronasgefassen Eigenschaften. *Arzneimittelforschung* 1962;12:549–558.
65. Seabra-Gomes R, Richards A, Sutton R. Hemodynamic effects of verapamil and practolol in man. *Eur J Cardiol* 1976;4:79–85.
66. Ätterhog JH, Ekelund LG. Haemodynamic effects of intravenous verapamil at rest and during exercise in subjectively healthy middle aged males. *Eur J Clin Pharmacol* 1975;8:317–322.
67. De Leeuw PW, Smit AJPM, Willemse PJ, Birkenhäger WH. Effects of verapamil in hypertensive patients. In: Zanchetti A, Krikler Dm, eds. *Calcium antagonism in cardiovascular therapy—experience with verapamil.* Amsterdam: Excerpta Medica, 1981;233.
68. Doyle AE, Anavekar SN, Oliver LE. A clinical trial of verapamil in the treatment of hypertension. In: Zanchetti A, Krikler DM, eds. *Calcium antagonism in cardiovascular therapy—experience with verapamil.* Amsterdam: Excerpta Medica, 1981;252.
69. Lewis GRJ. Verapamil in the treatment of chronic hypertension. *Clin Invest Med* 1980;3:175.
70. Muiesan G, Agabiti-Rosei E, Alicandri C, Beschi M, Castellano M, et al. Influence of verapamil on catecholamines, renin and aldosterone in essential hypertensive patients. In: Zanchetti A, Krikler DM, eds. *Calcium antagonism in cardiovascular therapy—experience with verapamil.* Amsterdam: Excerpta Medica, 1981;238.
71. Bertrand ME, Dupuis BA, Lablanche JM, Tilmant PY, Thieuleux FA. Coronary haemodynamics following intravenous or intracoronary injection of diltiazem in man. *J Cardiovasc Pharmacol* 1982;4:695–699.
72. Dash H, Copenhaver G, Ensminger SM, Toggart EJ. Diltiazem improves left ventricular relaxation in coronary artery disease. *Clin Res* 1983;31:660A.
73. Nishimura N, Mori Y, Kusumoto H, Kamekawa R, Iino A, et al. Clinical evaluation of adjuvants for anaesthesia. II. effects f CRD-401 on circulatory function. *Jpn J Anesthesiol* 1972; 1:1147.
74. Walsh RA, Porter CB, Starling MR, O'Rourke RA. Beneficial haemodynamic effects of intravenous and oral diltiazem in severe congestive heart failure. *J Am Coll Cardiol* 1984;3:1044–1050.
75. Safar ME, Simon ACh, Levenson JA, Cazor JL. Hemodynamic effects of diltiazem in hypertension. *Circ Res* 1983;52:I169–I173.
76. Materne P, Legrand V, Vandormael M, Collignon P, Kulbertus HE. Hemodynamic effects of intravenous diltiazem with impaired left ventricular function. *Am J Cardiol* 1984;54:733–737.
77. Walsh RA, Porter CB, Starling MR, O'Rourke RA. Salutary hemodynamic effects of intravenous and oral diltiazem in severe congestive heart failure. *Circulation* 1982;66(Suppl II, Pt 2):II-138.
78. Bates ER, Crevey BJ, Dantzker DR, D'Alonzo G, Popat KD, et al. Acute haemodynamic effects of intravenous diltiazem in primary and secondary pulmonary hypertension. *J Am Coll Cardiol* 1984;3:579.
79. Gassner A. Günstige Beeinflussung der pulmonalen Hypertonie bei Patienten mit Chronischer obstruktiver Atemwegerkrankung durch Diltiazem. *Schweiz Med Wochenschr* 1984;114:332–337.
80. Freedman DD, Waters DD. "Second generation" dihydropyridine calcium-antagonists. Greater vascular selectivity and some unique applications. *Drugs* 1987;34:578–598.
81. Bonaduce D, Ferrara N, Petretta M, Romano E, Postiglione M, et al. Hemodynamic study of nifedipine administration in hypertensive patients. *Am Heart J* 1983;105:865–867.
82. Murphy MB, Scriven AJ, Brown MJ, Causen R, Dollery CT. The effects of nifedipine and hydralazine induced hypotension on sympathetic activity. *Eur J Clin Pharmacol* 1982;23:479–482.
83. Guazzi M, Olivari MT, Polese A, Fiorentini C, Magrini F, et al. Nifedipine, a new antihypertensive with rapid action. *Clin Pharmacol Therap* 1977;22:528.
84. Lederballe-Pederson O, Mikkelsen E. Acute and chronic effects of nifedipine in arterial hypertension. *Eur J Clin Pharmacol* 1978;14:375–381.
85. Olivari MT, Bartorelli C, Polese A, Fiorentini C, Moruzzi P, et al. Treatment of hypertension with nifedipine, a calcium antagonist agent. *Circulation* 1979;59:1056.
86. Kiowski W, Erne P, Bertel O, Hulthen UL, Ritz R, et al. Unchanged baroreflex sensitivity during acute and chronic antihypertensive therapy with nifedipine. *J Hypertens* 1983(1 Suppl 2):365.
87. McLeay RAB, Stallard TJ, Watson RDS, Littler WA. The effect of nifedipine on arterial pressure and reflex control. *Circulation* 1983;67:1084.
88. Theroux P, Waters DD, Debaisieux JC, Szlachcic J, Micgala HF, et al. Hemodynamic effects of calcium ion antagonists after acute myocardial infarction. *Clin Invest Med* 1980;3:81–85.
89. Chaitman BR, Wagniart P, Pasternac A, et al. Improved exercise tolerance after propranolol, diltiazem or nifedipine in angina pectoris. *Am J Cardiol* 1984;53:1–9.
90. Silke B, Verma SP, Nelson GIC, Ahuga RC, Hussain M, et al. The effects on left ventricular performance of nifedipine and verapamil on exercise-induced angina pectoris. *Br J Clin Pharmacol* 1984;17:735–743.

Hypertension: Pathophysiology, Diagnosis, and Management, edited by J. H. Laragh and B. M. Brenner. Raven Press, Ltd., New York © 1990.

CHAPTER 136

What Are We Really Achieving with Long-Term Antihypertensive Drug Therapy?

Lennart Hansson and Björn Dahlöf

What Can Be Expected from Antihypertensive Drug Therapy?, 2131
Reduction of Cardiocerebrovascular Complications (Normalization of Hypertension-Induced Mortality and Morbidity), 2131
Regression of Structural Cardiovascular Changes, 2132
Metabolic Side Effects, 2132
Compliance and Quality of Life, 2132
Benefits of Antihypertensive Treatment: The Controlled Trials, 2133
Malignant Hypertension, 2133
Nonmalignant Hypertension, 2133
Suboptimal Effects of Therapy, 2137
The Dalby Study, 2137
The Glasgow Blood Pressure Clinic Study, 2137
The Göteborg Study, 2137
Other Studies, 2138
Risk of Lowering Blood Pressure Too Far, 2138
Discussion, 2139
References, 2140

The question "What are we really achieving with long-term drug treatment in hypertension?" appears justified in view of the extensive treatment of patients with arterial hypertension that takes place in all industrialized countries of the world today. It is well known that the development in the field of antihypertensive treatment has been remarkably rapid during the last few decades. This can be attributed to several factors. Perhaps the most important of these is that numerous intervention trials have demonstrated clear benefits when patients with hypertension are treated with blood-pressure-lowering drugs. Some of the important studies in this area will be reviewed briefly here. Another important factor is that antihypertensive drugs, which are effective and generally well tolerated, have been developed and made available for general use.

The widespread use, and sometimes uncritical application, of antihypertensive drugs does not always produce the benefits expected. In fact, some recent studies, which will be reviewed briefly here, clearly indicate that results in treated hypertensive patients have been suboptimal; that is, treated hypertensive patients still have significant overmorbidity and overmortality as compared to matched normotensive subjects. These are, to some extent, unexpected and certainly disappointing findings, and an attempt will be made to explain the less-than-optimal results presented in these trials.

Finally, some recent intervention trials have suggested that lowering of arterial pressure in hypertensive patients below a certain point may be associated with an increasing rate of complications, particularly death from coronary artery disease. Other equally well conducted intervention studies have not shown this J-shaped relationship between blood pressure and risk in the hypertensive range; this is another issue that needs clarification when the achievements obtained with long-term drug treatment in hypertension are to be assessed.

WHAT CAN BE EXPECTED FROM ANTIHYPERTENSIVE DRUG THERAPY?

Reduction of Cardiocerebrovascular Complications (Normalization of Hypertension-Induced Mortality and Morbidity)

Hypertension (systolic or diastolic, labile or fixed) at any age, in either sex, has been shown to be a powerful contributor to each of the clinical manifestations of atherosclerosis (e.g., coronary artery disease, stroke, cardiac failure, and intermittent claudication) (1–5).

The association between blood pressure and all cardiovascular complications has been shown to be continuous throughout the range of systolic and diastolic blood pressure studied, and no definitive cut-off point can be defined (1–5). Thus, in the 1959 Build and Blood Pressure study, the blood pressure that appeared optimal for longevity was less than 110 mmHg systolic and 70 mmHg diastolic (4).

More than 50% of all deaths occurring during the second part of life are known to be due to a cardiovascular cause (6). Most of the blood-pressure-related cardiovascular events appear to result from the large number of individuals exposed to only a slight increase in risk rather than from a smaller number of individuals with high blood pressure who, of course, individually are exposed to a much greater risk. According to Whelton (8), based on Framingham data (1–3) and U.S. Health Statistics (7), more than 60% of the cardiovascular complications that are attributable to elevated diastolic blood pressure result from exposure to diastolic blood pressure below 95 mmHg, and 45% of such complications occur at diastolic blood pressures below 90 mmHg.

Against this background it is obvious that with today's "high-risk strategy," depending on the cut-off point for initiating treatment, only 10–20% of the general population would qualify for treatment. With this approach, the expected reduction in blood-pressure-induced cardiovascular events will not be 100% (8).

In 1981, Rose (9) estimated that even a 2- to 3-mmHg shift in the entire blood pressure distribution in Great Britain might produce life-saving benefits equal to those being achieved by the concurrent traditional approach to antihypertensive therapy there.

On the assumption that the treatment of hypertension would totally reverse hypertension-induced risk, it might be said that the lower the blood pressure on treatment without side effects or symptomatic hypotension, the better the prognosis.

Regression of Structural Cardiovascular Changes

Both heart and vessels show complex structural adaptations (left ventricular hypertrophy, vascular hypertrophy) in response to elevated blood pressure and metabolic demands. These structural changes of the cardiovascular system are (in most circumstances and, at least, temporarily) highly appropriate, especially on the local level (10). However, when all systemic resistance vessels in the chronic high-pressure state are involved, this gives a positive feedback interaction between structural and functional influences with unfortunate consequences (11–13).

Media hypertrophy of the precapillary resistance vessels causes a structurally based hyperreactivity, meaning that systemic resistance is kept increased also when smooth muscle tone of the vessels is normal or low (14,15). The vascular hypertrophy can be considered as the ultimate structural factor behind the progression of hypertension, independent of the initiating factor (16).

Hypertrophy of the heart is an adaptive process, initially well tolerated and clinically silent. With time, failing heart function may supervene, but even more important is the strong risk (independent of blood pressure elevation per se) for all kinds of cardiovascular complications associated with left ventricular hypertrophy (17–22).

Hypertrophy of both the large and small arterial vessels has been shown to follow the same general pattern of development and regression as in the heart (10). Regression of both the left ventricular hypertrophy and vascular hypertrophy has been shown to occur with several antihypertensive agents, especially drugs which interfere with both the sympathetic nervous system and the renin–angiotensin–aldosterone system (10,22).

Metabolic Side Effects

Several antihypertensive agents have negative influences on metabolic parameters. A summary of the best documented effects is shown in Table 1.

Diuretic drugs (first-line therapy in a majority of hypertension treatment trials), although highly effective in reducing blood pressure, have shown a detrimental effect on other risk factors for coronary heart disease (CHD) and may offset the positive effect of hypertension control. These metabolic disturbances induced by diuretics appear clinically unimpressive; however, risk-table analysis reveals that they could reverse the benefits of blood pressure control completely (23), although this was not the case in, for example, the large Medical Research Council (MRC) trial (24).

Compliance and Quality of Life

One major problem in treating mild to moderate hypertension is that treatment does not provide relief of symptoms, since this condition is usually free of symptoms.

TABLE 1. *Comparison between different antihypertensive drugs concerning metabolic side effects*[a]

	Beta-blockers	Diuretics	Alpha-blockers	ACE inhibitors	Ca antagonists
Blood glucose	↑?	↑	0	0	0?
Lipids					
HDL	↓ [b]	0	↑		
LDL	↑ [b]	↑	↓	0	0
TG	↑ [b]	↑	↓		
Serum urate	0	↑	0	0	0
Serum potassium		↓	0	↑	0?

[a] HDL, high-density lipoprotein; LDL, low-density lipoprotein; TG, triglycerides; ↑, increase; ↓, decrease; 0, no effect (effect uncertain or of no clinical significance).

[b] Less pronounced for selective beta-blockers, and vice versa for beta-blockers with marked intrinsic sympathomimetic activity.

Rather, the goal is to change the natural history, which is fundamentally more difficult, in part, because of the problem of compliance (25). Today, low patient compliance is one of the most important therapy-limiting factors in hypertension (26). It is estimated that 10–15% of hypertensives are lost from follow-up in the first year of therapy and that 20–40% of patients comply insufficiently with prescribed antihypertensive drugs (26).

Monk (27) investigated the general well-being of hypertensives. After diagnosis and starting of antihypertensive therapy, scores in the general well-being questionnaire were reduced (27). This may be due to the paradox seen in the management of hypertension—that the patient is more likely to feel worse than to feel better after diagnosis and initiation of treatment.

Data from the MRC trial confirms that subjective side effects are a major problem with today's first-line therapy. Eleven percent of the subjects in the diuretic group and 12% of the subjects in the beta-blocker group were withdrawn from randomized treatment because of side effects (such as impotence, gout, Raynaud's phenomenon, lethargy, nausea, dizziness, etc.). In the placebo group, only 2% were withdrawn for these reasons (28).

Newer drugs such as angiotensin-converting-enzyme (ACE) inhibitors have shown fewer or no negative effects on quality of life—probably because of more favorable side-effect profiles (29), which also may improve compliance.

BENEFITS OF ANTIHYPERTENSIVE TREATMENT: THE CONTROLLED TRIALS

Malignant Hypertension

The most severe form of hypertension, malignant phase hypertension, is associated with remarkably high mortality in the untreated state. Thus, a review of six series of patients with untreated malignant hypertension by Pickering et al. (30) in 1961 showed an average mortality of approximately 50% within 6 months after diagnosis of malignant hypertension had been made, and 5-year mortality approached 100% (Fig. 1). However, with the introduction of antihypertensive treatment, 5-year survival in malignant hypertension improved from 0% to about 75% (Table 2) (30–40).

It should be noted that the treated series of patients listed in Table 2 refers, in some instances, only to patients with grade IV retinopathy; however, in other series, patients with both grade III and grade IV have been included. Moreover, in some instances the 5-year survival rate has been estimated from survival curves. Therefore the 5-year survival data should not be regarded as fully comparable or absolutely exact, but the information provided still indicates a gradual improvement of 5-year survival in this serious condition.

It could also be added that the World Health Organization has recommended that both patients with grade III and IV retinopathy should be classified as having malignant hypertension (41). It should further be noted that in

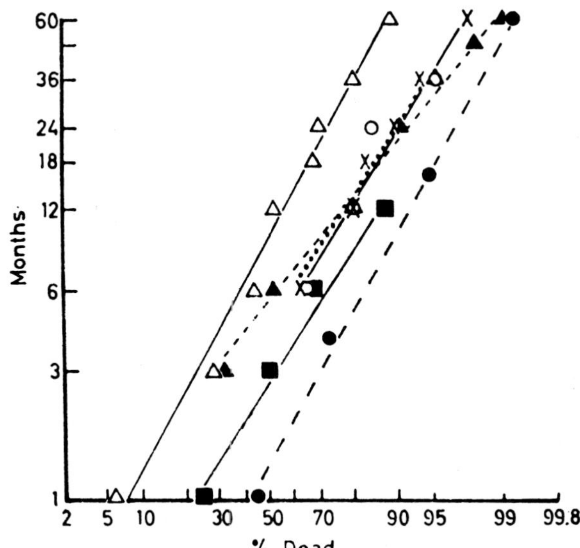

FIG. 1. Mortality in six series of patients with untreated malignant hypertension. (From ref. 30.)

most series of patients, some of the improved 5-year survival may be attributable to hemodialysis or renal transplantation (40).

Against the background of the evidence presented above, there can be no doubt that antihypertensive treatment in patients with malignant-phase hypertension is associated with a marked improvement in prognosis, although there is still room for further improvement. A potential further benefit of antihypertensive treatment in general is that this may prevent the development of the malignant phase, thereby making malignant hypertension more rare, as indicated by the findings in our series (40).

Nonmalignant Hypertension

The overwhelming majority of all hypertensive patients who receive antihypertensive medication today suffers from nonmalignant hypertension. Based on early clinical observations it soon became apparent that similar benefits of antihypertensive therapy were to be expected in nonmalignant hypertension as compared to those which had already been reported in malignant hypertension. One example of this is the analysis of survival rates in 381 patients on combined treatment with various antihypertensive drugs as reported by Björk et al. (42) in 1961. Benefits of treatment were more clearly established in controlled intervention series, sometimes conducted under double-blind conditions and with placebo control (Table 3) (24,43–49).

In the early study by Hamilton et al. (43), conducted in the United Kingdom, half of the patients in their series were left untreated, whereas the other half received active antihypertensive therapy, which reduced hypertension-induced complications in patients with diastolic blood pressures (phase IV) at 110 mmHg or above. All the other trials in Table 3 were placebo-controlled—with the exception of the Hypertension Detection and Follow-up Program study

TABLE 2. *Five-year survival in malignant hypertension*

Author(s)	Number of patients	Year	Five-year survival (%)	Reference
		Untreated		
Pickering et al.	407	1961	0	30
		Treated		
Dustan et al.	84	1958	33	31
Harington et al.	94	1959	22	32
Björk et al.	93	1960	50	33
Sokolow and Perloff	26	1960	15	34
Mohler and Freis	64	1960	22	35
Hodge et al.	497	1961	36	36
North et al.	106	1961	44	37
Farmer et al.	161	1963	29	38
Hood et al.	335	1970	50	39
Gudbrandsson et al.	69	1979	75	40

(49), which compared referred care (i.e., commonly available medical care) with stepped care (i.e., standardized and intensified treatment at special centers). As shown in Table 3, benefits obtained through antihypertensive therapy have been demonstrable in patients with ever milder degrees of hypertension during the 20-year period surveyed. However, it is also obvious from these trials that the number of patients required to show benefits at the milder degrees of blood pressure elevation has increased dramatically. However, overall the data do not provide consistent evidence of a differential relative effect of treatment at differing levels of blood pressure in the mild to moderately hypertensive range.

In deciding to treat or not to treat patients with mildly elevated blood pressures (where the absolute benefit for the individual in reduced hypertension related morbidity and mortality is hard to estimate), factors such as subjective or metabolic side effects of treatment (as well as effects on structural cardiovascular changes) become increasingly important. These circumstances have triggered a sometimes intense discussion on whether or not to treat mild hypertension. A perspective on treatment of malignant and mild hypertension is shown in Table 4. To throw some additional light on this question, the effect of pharmacological antihypertensive treatment on major endpoints in major controlled studies will be discussed in some detail.

Analysis of Major Endpoints in Mild to Moderate Hypertension

A majority of the trials in mild to moderate hypertension were designed to detect an effect of treatment on an aggregate of cardiovascular disease endpoints. The frequency of individual fatal and nonfatal events in these studies was sufficient to detect only a large effect of treatment, such as that commonly observed for cerebrovascular disease.

In order to provide a more stable estimate of the effect of treatment than provided by any single study, as well as to increase the power to detect moderate reductions in total mortality and fatal and nonfatal CHD, MacMahon et al. (50) pooled data from nine studies in mild to moderate hypertension. Data were pooled using the technique developed by Peto and colleagues (51), ensuring that treated subjects in one trial were compared only with control subjects in the same trial. Although there is a certainty of the comparability of total mortality data among the trials, the comparability of cause-specific mortality and morbidity is less certain.

The characteristics of the nine studies pooled are given in Table 5 (24,46,48,49,52–56). Only randomized, primary prevention trials in which the objective was to test the effect of blood pressure reduction were included. It may raise some concern to include studies such as the Hypertension

TABLE 3. *Improvement of prognosis by antihypertensive therapy in non-malignant hypertension*

Author(s)	Number of patients	Year	Benefits shown at diastolic blood pressure ≥ (mmHg)	Reference
Hamilton et al.	64	1964	110 (phase IV)	43
Wolff and Lindeman	87	1966	110	44
Veterans Administration	515	1967 and 1970	105	45 and 46
Australian National Study	3,943	1979	100	47
Australian National Study	3,427	1980	95	48
Hypertension Detection and Follow-up Program Study	10,940	1979	90	49
Medical Research Council Study	17,354	1985	90	24

TABLE 4. *Results of hypertension treatment—a perspective (5-year survival, in percent)[a]*

Untreated	Treated	Blood pressure level
Malignant hypertension (minority)		
0% "Symptomatic"	75% "Asymptomatic"	Very high
Mild hypertension (majority)		↓
95% "Asymptomatic"	96% "Symptomatic"	Normotension

[a] The numbers are approximate and should only be seen as measures of the treatment effects.

Detection and Follow-up Program (HDFP) (49) and the Multiple Risk Factor Intervention Trial (MRFIT) (56) in the analysis, since they both used referred-care controls. Taking into consideration the large proportion of placebo or "untreated" controls in the other studies who were known to be on active treatment (MRC study 13%, Oslo study 17%) or whose treatment status was unknown, as well as taking into account the number of control patients becoming normotensive, the distinction between the placebo or untreated control trials and the referred-care control trials is not sharp. In general, the active treatment of control patients in the trials can be expected to have led to an underestimation of the treatment effect.

The pooled analysis by MacMahon et al. (50) addressed the question as to what benefit you may get for a certain difference in blood pressure achieved by systematic drug treatment (intervention groups) versus lesser degree of blood pressure control (control groups). Together the studies in mild to moderate hypertension comprised 43,000 patients with an average follow-up of 5.6 years (240,800 patient-years). Treatment in all studies were diuretic-based (plus beta-blockers in some cases), and the difference in diastolic blood pressure between intervention groups and the control groups was 5.7 mmHg.

Effect on Total Mortality

The pooled difference in mortality between intervention groups and control groups was statistically significant, with a reduction in total mortality of 11% in subjects from the intervention groups (95% confidence interval: −19% to −2%) (Fig. 2).

Reduction in stroke mortality accounted for 50% of the total reduction in deaths (50).

If these pooled data are used for calculating survival instead, the 5-year survival in the intervention groups will be 96.1% compared to 95.6% in the control groups—in other words, an increase in 5-year survival of 0.5% for a difference in diastolic blood pressure of 5.7 mmHg in mild to moderate hypertension.

Effect on Stroke

In the intervention groups, stroke mortality was significantly reduced by 38% (95% confidence interval: −53% to −19%); furthermore, the incidence of nonfatal stroke was significantly reduced by 43% (95% confidence interval: −54% to −29%) (50).

The overall reduction in stroke was 39% (95% confidence interval: −48% to −28%). Exclusion of MRFIT data (56) (effort to reduce other risk factors) did not substantially alter the results.

Benefits of drug-induced blood pressure reduction on stroke were evident for both sexes and in both younger and older individuals and for all blood pressure levels included (50).

Effect on Coronary Heart Disease

The CHD event rate was considerably higher in the HDFP study (50); this was probably because data on nonfatal myocardial infarction which were derived from self-reports were included. Therefore, in the pooled analysis, it

TABLE 5. *Randomized treatment trials in mild to moderate hypertension—some characteristics*

Study	Age	Included BP diastolic	Excluded end-organic damage	*n*	Net change in DBP (placebo minus control)	Reference
Placebo or untreated controls						
VA 1970	Mean 52	90–114	Severe	380	−19	46
PHS 1977	21–55	90–114	+	389	−10	52
VA-NHLBI 1978	21–50	85–105	+	1,012	−7	53
Oslo 1980	40–49	<110 and DBP ≥ 95 or SBP ≥ 150	+	785	−10	54
ANBP 1980	30–69	95–109	+	3,427	−6	48
EWPHE 1985	≥60 (mean 72)	90–119	Severe	840	−10	55
MRC 1985	35–64	90–109	Severe	17,354	−6	24
Referred-care control						
HDFP 1979	30–69	90–114	−	10,940	−5	49
MRFIT 1982	35–57	90–114	+	12,866	−4	56

[a] BP, blood pressure; DBP, diastolic blood pressure; SBP, systolic blood pressure.

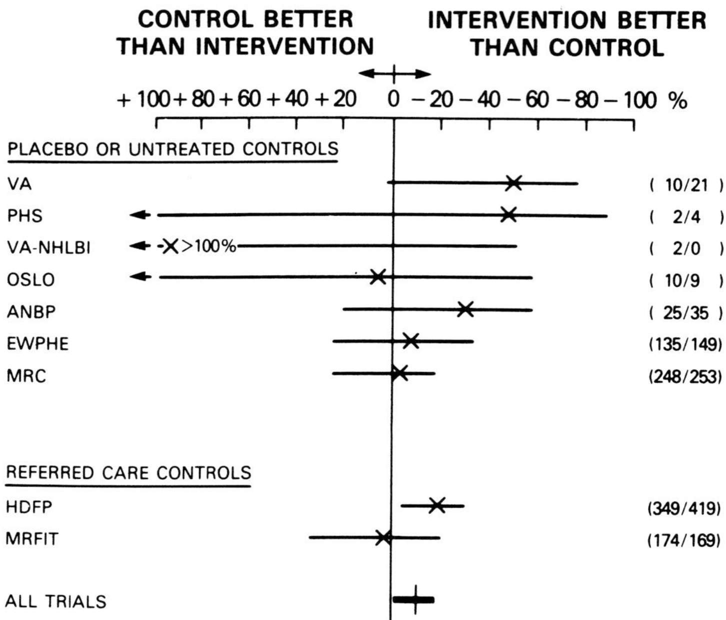

FIG. 2. Estimates (approximately 95% confidence intervals) of the relative difference in total mortality between study intervention and control groups. Number of events (intervention/control) are given in parentheses. (From ref. 50.)

was decided to include only those events from the HDFP study that were documented by serial electrocardiogram (ECG) changes (50).

The incidence of nonfatal myocardial infarction was 6% lower (95% confidence interval: −22% to +14%) and mortality from CHD was 8% lower (95% confidence interval: −26% to +6%) in patients from the intervention groups than in those from control groups (50). Exclusion of data from the MRFIT trial (56) did not alter the results, but inclusion of self-reported nonfatal events from the HDFP study (49) gave a significant reduction of CHD events by 12% (95% confidence interval: −20% to −3%) (50).

However, not even the pooled results from these studies give convincing evidence of reduced fatal and nonfatal CHD with drug-induced (diuretics and beta-blockers) reduction of diastolic blood pressure of about 5 mmHg for over 5 years. It should once again be stressed that active treatment among control subjects (as much as 58% of patients in the referred-care group of HDFP study) in these trials is likely to have reduced the ability to detect a significant effect of study treatments on CHD.

Post hoc analyses from the HDFP (49) and MRFIT (56) studies indicate that treatment (diuretic-based stepped care) was more favorable for CHD in those without borderline ECG abnormality than in those with such abnormalities, but of course these data must be interpreted with caution.

In the MRC trial (24), fatal CHD events were 15% fewer in the group with beta-blocker based therapy (103 versus 129), but this difference was not significant. Nonsmoking men seemed to have more benefit from beta-blockade in both the MRC (24) and the International Prospective Primary Prevention Study in Hypertension (IPPPSH) (57) studies, whereas benefits were similar for smoking and nonsmoking men in the Heart Attack Primary Preventive Study in Hypertension (HAPPHY) trial (58). In the IPPPSH study, which involved 6307 men and women, the primary aim was to determine if a beta-blocker based antihypertensive treatment was better than a non-beta-blocker-based treatment in reducing major cerebrovascular events. Overall there was no additional benefit of using a beta-blocker, but the trial showed that the frequency of both CHD (myocardial infarction and sudden death) and strokes was correlated with the diastolic blood pressure achieved in the course of the study. The slope of the correlation showing relative risk was steeper for stroke than for cardiac events (Fig. 3).

In the HAPPHY trial, which was an open comparison of antihypertensive therapy with diuretics or $beta_1$-selective blockers (atenolol and metoprolol) in more than 6000 men with untreated diastolic blood pressures in the range 100–130 mmHg, there was no difference between the two

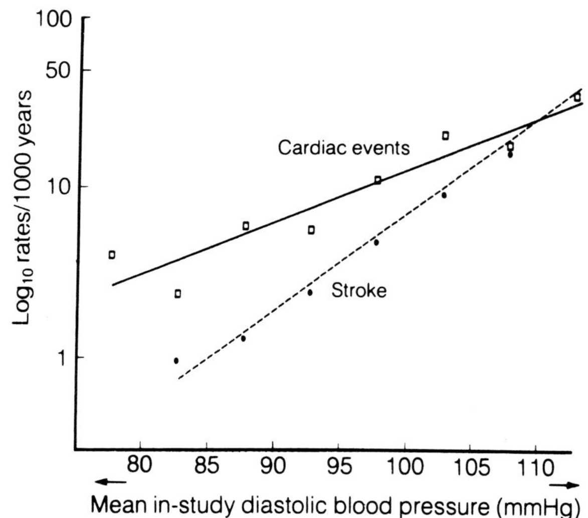

FIG. 3. Cardiac events and strokes in relation to treated diastolic blood pressure in the IPPPSH study. (From ref. 57.)

therapeutic modalities as regards the prevention of CHD or other cardiovascular complications (58).

There are several factors that may have contributed to the failure of the major intervention trials in hypertension to document a significant reduction of the incidence of CHD:

1. The trials are too small, even in combination, to detect important effects of 15% or less.
2. The trials are too short (mean follow-up time of 5.6 years).
3. Widespread use of antihypertensive therapy among control patients.
4. Other factors related to therapy itself or the underlying disease (see discussion).

SUBOPTIMAL EFFECTS OF THERAPY

As already noted, the positive experience obtained from treatment of malignant and nonmalignant hypertension, as briefly reviewed above, has contributed to the widespread use and general acceptance of antihypertensive therapy today. Against this background it was perhaps somewhat surprising and certainly disappointing when a number of recent studies showed that the results of treatment in hypertension appeared to be less favorable than expected. Only three such studies will be briefly reviewed here.

Furthermore, a comparison between the pooled data on mild to moderate hypertension mentioned above and on prospective mortality and morbidity associated with the same diastolic blood pressure difference will be made.

The Dalby Study

In southern Sweden, Lindholm (59) conducted a retrospective analysis of the morbidity in all treated hypertensive patients in the small community of Dalby and made comparisons to sex- and age-matched normotensive subjects living in the same community. As examplified in Table 6, cardiovascular morbidity was significantly more prevalent in several age groups of treated hypertensive patients than in the matched normotensive subjects (59). However, although highly significant reductions in arterial blood pressure had been obtained in the treated patients, the blood pressure in the patients was still markedly and significantly higher than in the matched normotensive subjects (59).

The Glasgow Blood Pressure Clinic Study

In Glasgow, Scotland, mortality in the treated hypertensive patients in the Glasgow Blood Pressure Clinic during an average of 6.5 years was compared to the mortality in two control populations near Glasgow (60). In the different patients groups, mortality was found to be two to five times higher than in the control populations, with benefits of treatment being most pronounced in the patients in whom blood pressure was reduced the most. However, even in the patients in whom the diastolic blood pressure on treatment had been reduced to ≤90 mmHg, there was still a certain overmortality as compared to the control populations of the same age and sex (60).

The Göteborg Study

Ten-year data from the Göteborg Primary Preventive Trial were reported by Samuelsson (61) in 1985 (Table 7). Of the 686 patients initially included in this study and who all were given pharmacological antihypertensive therapy, 80 died (mainly from cardiovascular causes) during the 10-year observation period (60). Data were not presented regarding 81 further patients, but cardiovascular morbidity and blood pressure control was reported for 525 patients at the end of 10 years of treatment. Although data on a normotensive control population were not presented, it is obvious that the cardiovascular morbidity in these middle-aged male hypertensives was considerable during the 10-year period of study. Moreover, it should be noted that more than one-third of all reported patients did not obtain the goal blood pressure ($<\frac{160}{95}$ mmHg) at the end of 10 years of treatment, and 10% had diastolic blood pressure >105 mmHg or systolic blood pressure > 170 mmHg (60).

These three recent studies all clearly demonstrate that treated hypertensive patients have a greater cardiovascular morbidity and/or mortality than expected. It is also clear

TABLE 6. *Morbidity in treated male hypertensive patients aged 40–59 in comparison to age- and sex-matched normotensive subjects in Dalby*[a]

Morbidity	Treated patients (n = 66)	Normotensives (n = 75)	Statistics
Cerebrocardiovascular disease	21%	1%	$p < 0.001$
Stroke	2%	0%	NS[b]
Coronary disease	20%	1%	$p < 0.001$
Intermittent claudication	2%	0%	NS
Diabetes mellitus	8%	5%	NS
Blood pressure (mmHg)			
Untreated	183/114		
	$p < 0.001/0.001$		
Treated	149/91	133/80	$p < 0.001/0.001$

[a] Data were taken from one of the age groups studied by Lindholm (59).
[b] NS, not significant.

TABLE 7. *Ten-year data on the hypertensive patients in the Göteborg Primary Preventive Study*[a]

At entry, *n* = 686, males aged 47–54 years, based on a random sample of 9,996 men born between 1915 and 1925.
Initial blood pressure 169/106 mmHg (*n* = 686); all were then treated with antihypertensive drugs.
Blood pressure after 10 years of treatment: 149/89 mmHg (*n* = 525)
Ten-year mortality (*n* = 80)
Cardiovascular disease: 58.8%
Diabetes mellitus: 22.5%
Malignant disease: 11.3%
Discontinued follow-up (*n* = 81)
Of the remaining 525 patients, 161 (30.7%) developed one or more cardiovascular complication (stroke, myocardial infarction, intermittent claudication, angina pectoris) or diabetes mellitus.
Thirty-four percent had blood pressure ≥ 160 mmHg systolic and/or ≥95 mmHg diastolic.
Ten percent had blood pressure > 170 mmHg systolic or >105 mmHg diastolic.

[a] Data were taken from ref. 61.

that treated patients quite frequently do not obtain the goal blood pressure. Similar difficulties in achieving the intended goal blood pressure have been reported in several other series of patients (Table 8).

Other Studies

The pooled mortality and morbidity from the nine randomized trials of antihypertensive treatment mentioned before (Table 5) has been used for comparison with data from two large prospective trials (63).

For the same diastolic blood pressure difference between intervention and control (change in diastolic blood pressure: ~6 mmHg) observed in the pooled analysis (50), the maximum predicted incidence of stroke and CHD, adjusted for other risk factors, over 6 years of follow-up, was estimated from the follow-up study of individuals screened for the MRFIT and Framingham studies (63).

The size of the observed effect of blood pressure reduction on stroke was 80% of the maximum predicted, suggesting that the effects of long-term blood pressure elevation on the cerebral vasculature are mostly reversible over 5–6 years of blood pressure reduction (63).

Regarding CHD, the nonsignificant observed reduction in incidence of 8–9% was approximately one-third of the maximum predicted (63).

In the open so-called Clatterbridge study, where 939 moderate to severe hypertensives were followed for approximately 6 years (on average) on a beta-blocker-based treatment, blood pressure was lowered from 183/109 mmHg to 145/87 mmHg (64). Total mortality and morbidity due to myocardial infarction were lowered to about 40% of the predicted levels expected in untreated patients, both being similar to levels in an age- and sex-matched reference control population. In contrast to the surprisingly good result in CHD, death rate from stroke was reduced by 50% but was still twice that of the reference population (64).

RISK OF LOWERING BLOOD PRESSURE TOO FAR

Although there is a direct relationship between the level of blood pressure and the risk for cardiovascular complications both in untreated and treated hypertension, it is obvious that if blood pressure is lowered too extensively, risk will not continue to decrease but will instead increase again (Fig. 4). In other words, the relationship between blood pressure and risk is J-shaped.

Based on a recent retrospective analysis of patients treated with a beta-1-selective agent (the Clatterbridge study), it has been proposed that the risk of coronary artery disease mortality would again increase if diastolic blood pressure were reduced to below 85 mmHg in patients with preexisting ischemic heart disease (65). In 1979, Stewart (66) claimed that lowering of diastolic blood pressure (phase IV) to below 105 mmHg was associated with an increase in myocardial infarction. A reanalysis of the Framingham data by Anderson (67) also supported this claim in a way; that is, when statistical "data smoothing" was "unsmoothed," diastolic blood pressures below 90 mmHg were associated with no further lowering of cardiovascular events (67). In fact, the interpretation of the "unsmoothed" Framingham data may also be that the lowest part of a J-shaped curve seen in an untreated population is observed at a somewhat higher blood pressure level than expected.

TABLE 8. *Goal blood pressures and percentage of patients at goal after 2–10 years of antihypertensive therapy in some large series of patients*

Authors	Goal diastolic blood pressure (mmHg)	Duration of therapy (months)	Results	Reference
Australian National Study	<80[a]	44	>90 mmHg in 24.5%	48
Hypertension Detection and Follow-up, stepped care	<90	60	≥90 mmHg in 29.9%	49
Hypertension Detection and Follow-up, referred care	<90	60	≥90 mmHg in 47.5%	49
Ménard et al.	<95	24	>95 mmHg in 21.1% ≥90 mmHg in 43.1%	62
Samuelsson	<95	120	≥95 mmHg in 34%	61

[a] Goal was reduced from 90 to 80 mmHg after 2 years.

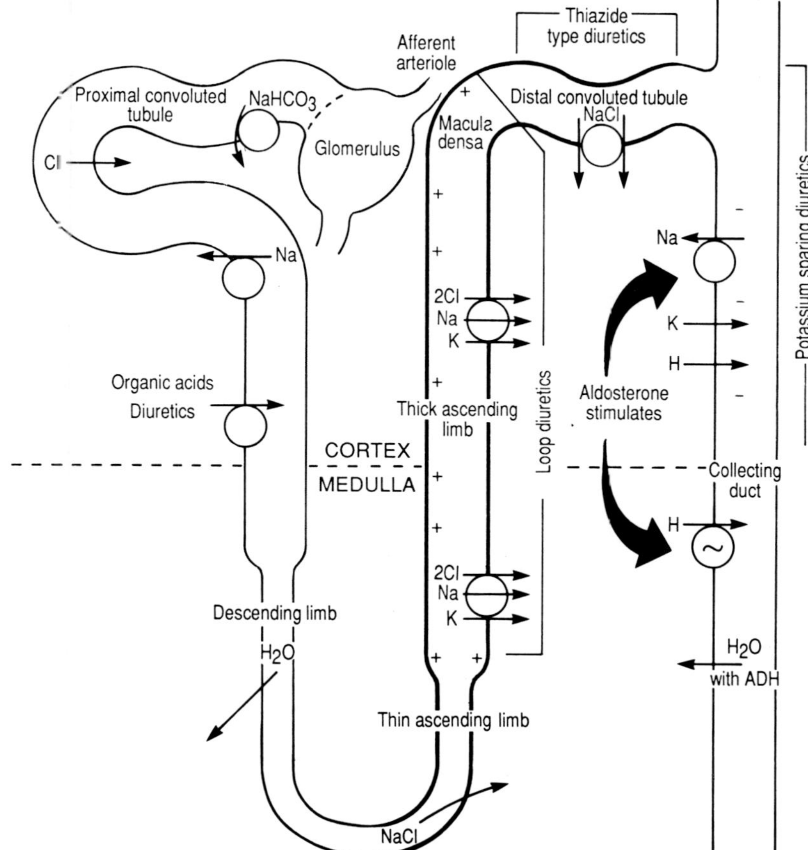

FIG. 2. Overall scheme of major transport processes in the nephron, with sites of diuretic action.

proves most useful (Figs. 1 and 2). The mechanism and site(s) of action within the nephron largely determine the maximum natriuretic effect possible with a given diuretic and also determine the other physiologic responses associated with its administration. The mechanisms of renal sodium reabsorption and the action of diuretics have been extensively reviewed (see refs. 14 and 16–18). Four primary sites of diuretic action within the nephron have been identified: the proximal tubule; the thick ascending limb of Henle's loop (the "high-ceiling" diuretics); the distal convoluted tubule (thiazides and related agents); and the connecting tubule and cortical collecting duct—the aldosterone-sensitive part of the nephron (aldosterone antagonists and sodium-channel blockers).

Proximal Tubule

Carbonic anhydrase inhibitors exert their principal diuretic effects on the proximal tubule. Their inability to sustain a diuretic effect makes them ineffective as antihypertensive agents. They are, however, of historical interest in that these sulfonamides were the progenitors of the development of most other diuretics. Although none of the diuretics used to treat hypertension act primarily on the proximal tubule, many of them are sulfonamide derivatives, and this structural feature generally is associated with their variable capacity to inhibit carbonic anhydrase (19). Other effects of these drugs on the proximal tubule may exist. In particular, metolazone, a relative of the thiazides, inhibits proximal tubular sodium reabsorption but does not inhibit carbonic anhydrase (20). This compound inhibits sodium-coupled phosphate transport in brush border vesicles of the proximal tubule (21).

The natriuresis caused by the use of thiazides or loop diuretics results in a reduction of extracellular volume. This, in turn, leads to an increase in proximal tubule sodium and water reabsorption which supersedes the direct natriuretic effect of carbonic anhydrase inhibition. As a consequence, proximal tubule reabsorption actually increases during diuretic therapy (22). In addition, the more distal segments of the nephron, especially the loop of Henle, can increase sodium reabsorption and further compensate for any reduction in proximal reabsorption (23–26). Despite these considerations, proximal actions may influence some of the effects of diuretics on acid–base balance and kaliuresis by increasing distal delivery of bicarbonate and may moderate the increase in proximal tubule reabsorption in response to volume depletion.

Thick Ascending Limb of Henle's Loop

This segment of the nephron has a major role in sodium and water homeostasis and is the site of action of the "loop" or "high-ceiling" diuretics. Sodium reabsorption is accomplished in this segment by an electroneutral Na–K–2Cl cotransport carrier located in the luminal membrane (Fig. 3). This cotransport is driven by the low intracellular sodium concentration which, in turn, is due to the activity of the Na^+,K^+ ATPase on the basolateral membrane (27). The segment has a high reabsorptive capacity for sodium chloride; furthermore, under most conditions, over 20% of the filtered sodium load is reabsorbed here. Since the water permeability of the thick ascending limb is low, urinary dilution takes place in this segment (28). Additionally, while actively separating solute from water, the medullary thick ascending limb provides the energy source for the countercurrent system that renders the medulla hypertonic (28). Therefore, sodium chloride reabsorption in this nephron segment is essential to both the dilution and concentration of urine.

The sulfonamide "high-ceiling" diuretics—furosemide and bumetanide—act on the thick ascending limb to inhibit the Na–K–2Cl cotransporter from the luminal side (27). Ethacrynic acid, a phenoxyacetic acid derivative, may act on this segment in a different manner (29,30). This latter drug also has effects when applied to the basolateral membrane of isolated thick ascending limb tubules (30). As expected from the characteristics of the thick ascending limb, these are powerful natriuretic–diuretic agents and impair the abilities both to concentrate and to dilute urine (14).

The thick ascending limb is also a major site of calcium and magnesium reabsorption (31). The mechanism(s) of reabsorption of divalent cations in this segment is unknown but may be linked to the lumen positive potential (31), which is a characteristic of the ion transport properties of this nephron segment (27). Reabsorption of both calcium and magnesium is disrupted by loop diuretics, resulting in increased calcium and magnesium excretion (31).

Loop diuretics have important vascular effects. Administration of furosemide promptly increases renin secretion, even when volume depletion is prevented (32,33). This effect has several potential mediators. Loop diuretics presumably inhibit transport of sodium chloride transport at the macula densa, which would increase renin secretion despite increased sodium chloride delivery (34) (as discussed elsewhere in this volume). Although the mechanism of sodium transport at the macula densa has not been directly studied, this segment of the nephron is flanked on either side by the thick ascending limb (35). It is likely, therefore, that transport at the macula densa is also sensitive to loop diuretics and that this is one mechanism by which they stimulate renin secretion. In addition, loop diuretics stimulate prostaglandin production, which, in turn, stimulates renin secretion (34–36). In keeping with this possibility, indomethacin administration diminishes the acute rise in renin seen after furosemide administration (37–39).

The increase in renal prostaglandin production following furosemide administration also decreases renal vascular resistance and increases renal blood flow (34,40). These effects are enhanced by volume depletion. Systemic vascular effects of furosemide, of which an increase in venous capacitance is especially prominent, are also mediated by renal prostaglandin production (41).

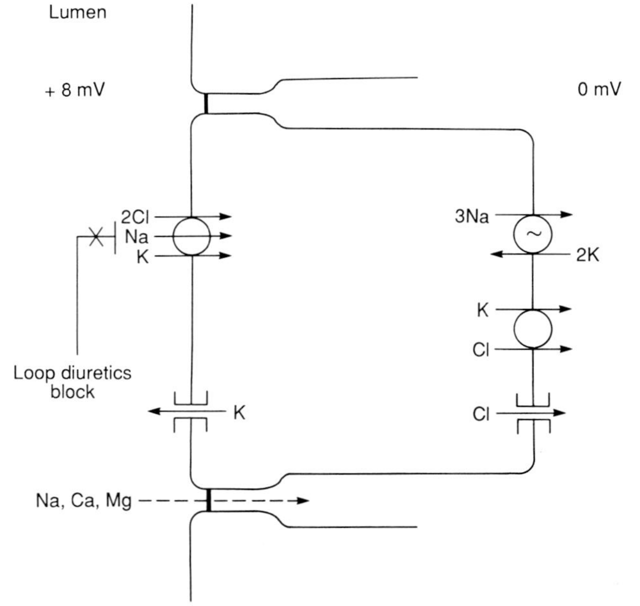

FIG. 3. Scheme of transport in the thick ascending limb of Henle's loop. The lumen-positive transepithelial electrical potential drives the reabsorption of cations, including sodium, calcium and magnesium, via a paracellular pathway. The Na-K-2Cl cotransporter in the luminal membrane is blocked, and the lumen positive potential abolished by "loop diuretics." "O" represents a carrier protein, "⊝" represents an ATP dependent transporter and "⊢⊣" represents a membrane channel. Adapted from references 27 and 30.

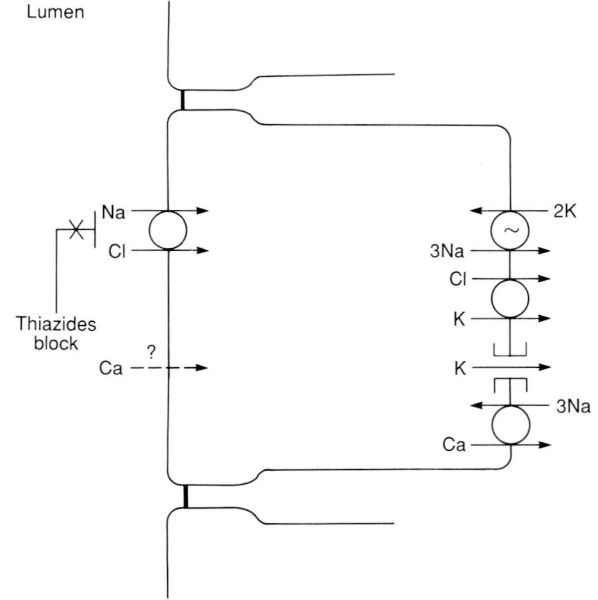

FIG. 4. Scheme of transport in the distal convoluted tubule. Thiazides and related diuretics block the Na-Cl cotransporter in the luminal membrane. The mechanism of calcium entry from the lumen is uncertain. Net reabsorption of calcium is governed by the activity of the Na-Ca exchanger in the basolateral membrane, which in turn depends on the level of intracellular sodium and hence sodium-chloride uptake from the lumen. "O" represents a carrier protein, "⊝" represents an ATP dependent transporter, and "⊢⊣" represents a membrane channel. Adapted from references 44, 53, and 54.

Distal Convoluted Tubule

An electroneutral cotransport mechanism in the luminal membrane in this segment serves to reabsorb sodium chloride. This transporter is blocked by thiazides and related diuretics (Fig. 4) (42–45).

The distal convoluted tubule is relatively water impermeable and is responsible for maintaining the dilute filtrate delivered from the cortical thick ascending limb and, perhaps, for further dilution of tubular fluid (46). Early on, it was recognized that thiazides impaired free water clearance without decreasing urine concentration and, at times, actually increased it (47). Thus, thiazides and their derivatives limit the capacity to dilute urine without impairing concentrating ability (48,49).

Although there is a direct relationship between urinary excretion of sodium and calcium in most situations, calcium excretion is diminished during thiazide administration (50). Increases in proximal tubular reabsorption of calcium and sodium which occur with volume depletion contribute to this effect (51,52). However, micropuncture studies showed that these agents also increase calcium reabsorption in the distal convoluted tubule (53). This most likely reflects the thiazide-induced inhibition of sodium influx into the tubular cells from the lumen which decreases intracellular sodium levels and which, in turn, increases sodium entry into the tubular cells via a Na–Ca exchanger located on the basolateral membrane. This entry is coupled to enhanced calcium extrusion from the cell into the peritubular space and, hence, to increased calcium reabsorption (53,54).

In contrast to their effects on calcium, thiazides tend to increase renal magnesium excretion, both acutely and chronically (55,56). The site within the nephron responsible for this effect is not known. The chronic effect may be localized to the cortical collecting duct, since magnesium loss can be prevented or corrected with diuretics active at that site (*vide infra*).

Aldosterone-Sensitive Part of the Nephron (Connecting Tubule and Cortical Collecting Duct)

This nephron segment is an important site of sodium, potassium, and acid transport. In addition, this site has a major role in the compensatory response to diuretics, with actions occurring at the more proximal sites in the nephron. Because of its location, it plays a key role in determining the final electrolyte composition of the urine.

This segment is composed of two types of epithelial cells: principal and intercalated cells. Sodium ions enter the principal cells from the tubular fluid via selective sodium channels in the luminal membrane and are pumped out of the cells into the interstitial space by the Na,K ATPase in the basolateral membrane (Fig. 5). The movement of sodium ions in this manner generates a lumen-negative transepithelial electrical potential, which, in turn, is largely responsible for potassium secretion (57) and chloride reabsorption (58). This part of the nephron has a low capacity for sodium reabsorption relative to more proximal segments, but it can establish very high transepithelial sodium gradients and remove virtually all of the remaining sodium from the urine. The amount of sodium reabsorbed by this segment depends on the interplay of two major factors—the plasma aldosterone level and the luminal sodium delivery.

Aldosterone increases both the luminal membrane sodium permeability and the capacity to extrude sodium across the basolateral membrane (59). This is accomplished by an increase in the number of sodium channels and sodium pumps inserted into the luminal and basolateral membrane, respectively. Neither conductance of the sodium channel nor activity of the sodium pump is changed directly by aldosterone (60–63).

This part of the nephron is also the major location for the related processes of urinary acidification and bicarbonate regeneration (64). Hydrogen ion secretion is accomplished by the intercalated cells of the collecting duct. Two transport processes have been identified in their luminal membrane—an ATP-dependent proton pump and a sodium–hydrogen ion exchanger. Although the mechanisms are not entirely clear, mineralocorticoids play an important role in promoting hydrogen ion secretion. This is an expected consequence of the mineralocorticoid-related increase in sodium transport and resulting increased luminal electronegativity which facilitates hydrogen ion secretion. However, there are also major effects that are independent of sodium transport (65). In addition to effects on hydrogen

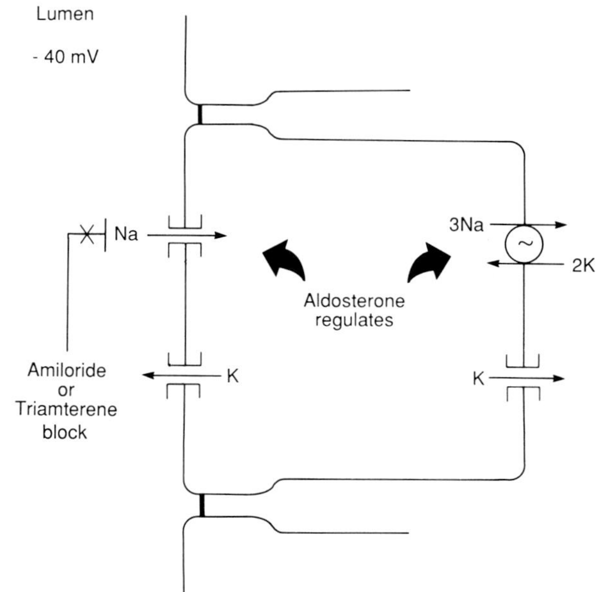

FIG. 5. Scheme of sodium and potassium transport in the aldosterone-sensitive nephron segment. Potassium secretion is a consequence of the lumen negative electrical potential generated by sodium transport. Aldosterone's effects to increase the capacity for sodium transport by increasing the number of luminal membrane sodium channels and sodium pumps in the basolateral membrane are antagonized by spironolactone. Amiloride and triamterene block the sodium channel from the luminal side. "○" represents a carrier protein, "⊝" represents an ATP dependent transporter, and "⊔⊓" represents a membrane channel.

ion secretion per se, mineralocorticoids also increase acid excretion by enhancing ammoniagenesis. Although this is an expected consequence of potassium wasting (66), the potassium loss does not seem to account for the entire effect (67,68).

Two types of diuretics are active in this segment—direct aldosterone antagonists, of which spironolactone is the only commercially available example, and direct inhibitors of sodium transport, including amiloride and triamterene. The discovery that cortisone could antagonize the action of aldosterone in the rat (69) and that progesterone could act similarly in an Addisonian patient treated with a mineralocorticoid (70) spurred the search for aldosterone antagonists and led to the development of spironolactone (71). Spironolactone is a competitive antagonist of the binding of aldosterone to its cytoplasmic receptor (72), which is the major basis of its natriuretic activity. In addition to this action, spironolactone also inhibits aldosterone biosynthesis (73, 74), but only at concentrations far in excess of those that inhibit the binding of aldosterone to its receptor (75). Although inhibition of biosynthesis is unlikely to be a major mechanism of action of spironolactone, it may play a role in the drug's effectiveness by blunting the rise in aldosterone levels that occur in reaction to spironolactone therapy. As an aldosterone antagonist, spironolactone causes natriuresis and antikaluresis. Spironolactone does not cause magnesium wasting and can be used to replete magnesium deficits (55).

Two drugs that block sodium transport in the collecting duct are currently available for clinical use. Of the two, amiloride has been the more intensively studied and has been widely used as a pharmacologic probe to study sodium transport in a variety of tissues (76). Triamterene, although less well studied, seems (in general) to act by the same mechanism as amiloride but is less potent. Triamterene may have additional activities independent of effects on the luminal membrane (77,78).

At submicromolar concentrations, amiloride acts from the luminal side of the tubule to block sodium channels in the collecting duct (76–78). This results in natriuresis and also prevents the development of a lumen negative potential, thereby reducing the driving force for potassium and hydrogen ion secretion. In addition, in higher concentrations, amiloride blocks Na–H exchange (76–78) and thus diminishes proton secretion. Concentrations of amiloride required for the latter effect are higher than those seen in the urine under clinical circumstances, suggesting that this mechanism is not operative with clinical use of the drug (78). Both amiloride and triamterene could impair urinary acidification by inducing potassium retention, which would impair ammoniagenesis as noted above. Both the sodium-channel blockers and direct aldosterone antagonists therefore tend to produce a systemic metabolic acidosis. This is usually mild or inapparent, except in special circumstances such as cirrhosis, diabetes, renal insufficiency, or concomitant nonsteroidal anti-inflammatory drug use (79–81).

Amiloride is also hypocalciuric, possibly owing to its reduction of the lumen negative potential or perhaps by a mechanism consequent to decreased sodium entry analogous to that described above for thiazides (54, 82). The hypocalciuric effects of thiazides and amiloride, acting as they do at different sites, are additive (83, 84). Amiloride reduces urinary magnesium excretion and is useful to help restore magnesium deficits (55, 56, 85, 86). Triamterene has been less well studied in this regard but may also reduce magnesium losses.

Thus, spironolactone, amiloride, and triamterene produce qualitatively similar effects on the composition of urine. It should be noted that the presence of mineralocorticoid, which is obligatory for the activity of spironolactone, is not required in order for amiloride or triamterene to exert their actions (87, 88). These latter drugs will, however, be more effective in the presence of mineralocorticoid activity. The effects of spironolactone and the sodium-channel blockers are additive, since they act by distinct mechanisms. A broad clinical experience indicates that, at clinical doses, spironolactone is the most powerful of the three in producing potassium retention and natriuresis; probably as a consequence, it has much more antihypertensive activity than the other two (89–91).

RENAL–METABOLIC EFFECTS OF CHRONIC DIURETIC THERAPY

After an initial period of natriuresis, patients on diuretic therapy come into a new steady state with maintained volume contraction. This new steady state is unlike most forms of volume depletion which are associated with decreased sodium excretion. Since external sodium balance is maintained, the homeostatic response to volume contraction is combined with a level of renal sodium excretion commensurate with intake, rather than being combined with a level that is appropriate for extracellular fluid volume status. The development of a new steady state has several bases that vary to some extent, depending on the type of diuretic involved.

Sodium-Volume Homeostasis

The attenuation of the natriuretic effect of diuretics with continued use has been termed the "braking phenomenon" (15). This renal response involves hemodynamic, humoral, and neural mediators. The volume depletion that follows diuretic therapy can lead to diminished renal blood flow and glomerular filtration rate, even with loop diuretics (which, as noted above, can acutely increase renal blood flow). In general, these changes are small; often, no changes in renal hemodynamics are found with chronic therapy, although small changes might remain of great importance and may be difficult to detect. The presence or absence of altered renal hemodynamics may depend on the degree of salt intake and of volume depletion.

A major consequence of volume depletion is enhancement of proximal tubular reabsorption of sodium and water (15), and this increase occurs even with those agents that have a proximal site of action (22). The increase in proximal reabsorption is mediated, in part, by peritubular Starling forces or "physical factors" (92) and results, in part, from a decrease in "backleak" of solutes and water into the tubular lumen. The backleak is relatively nonspecific, involving all solutes reabsorbed in this segment. The increase in proximal reabsorption reduces the flow rate of tubular fluid, thereby enhancing fractional sodium reabsorption in the distal nephron segments, especially the thick ascending limb (93).

During thiazide therapy, sodium reabsorption in Henle's loop is enhanced as a consequence of the steep medullary concentration gradient that accompanies volume depletion (15). Under this condition, water is passively extracted from the thin descending limb, which has a high permeability to water and low permeability to sodium, thereby increasing the luminal sodium concentration and decreasing the tubular flow rate. These factors, in turn, lead to passive sodium reabsorption in the thin ascending limb, which is highly permeable to sodium and relatively impermeable to water, and further enhance sodium reabsorption in the thick ascending limb (92). Thus, volume depletion leads to major adaptations in sodium reabsorption in the proximal nephron and loop of Henle.

Sodium reabsorption is also increased in the cortical collecting tubule by diuretics acting proximal to this segment. This occurs as a consequence of increased distal sodium supply (because of the shunting of sodium that normally would be reabsorbed at the diuretic's site of action to the distal nephron) and the increased capacity for sodium reabsorption (because of the elevations of aldosterone levels secondary to stimulation of plasma renin levels during diuretic therapy).

Potassium Homeostasis

Distal sodium supply inappropriately elevated for the level of aldosterone also promotes the potassium-wasting effects (and is the major mechanism underlying these effects) of those diuretics acting proximal to the cortical collecting duct, the "potassium-wasting diuretics." The aldosterone levels are stimulated with chronic diuretic therapy because of the stimulation of the renin–angiotensin system with volume depletion. In support of this are the findings that diuretics do not cause potassium wasting in Addisonian patients (94) or in adrenalectomized animals (95). Furthermore, aldosterone antagonists (96) or converting-enzyme inhibitors (97) not only block the diuretic-induced increase in aldosterone but also block the potassium loss. Several other mechanisms may also contribute to potassium wasting, such as an increase in distal tubular fluid flow rates (98), stimulation of potassium recycling in the kidney (99), carbonic anhydrase inhibition, and alkalosis (*vide infra*).

The loss of potassium is limited by several factors, the most important of which are (a) the increase in proximal tubule sodium reabsorption with consequent damping of the increase in sodium supply and distal flow rates and (b) the effects of decreased plasma potassium levels to diminish both potassium excretion (100) and aldosterone secretion (101, 102).

Acid–Base Homeostasis: Metabolic Alkalosis

A tendency toward metabolic alkalosis accompanies the use of "potassium-wasting" diuretics. This phenomenon was initially related to sodium chloride depletion without commensurate bicarbonate excretion, since in edematous patients on low-salt diets who are undergoing massive diuresis with ethacrynic acid, the elevation of serum bicarbonate was not entirely accounted for by the increase in urinary acid excretion. This situation was termed "contraction" alkalosis (103). With more modest diuresis, the magnitude of the induced alkalosis cannot be explained by volume contraction around a stable level of total body bicarbonate, and it is now clear that an increase in acid secretion (or bicarbonate regeneration) by the kidney must underlie diuretic-induced alkalosis (64, 104).

Several factors contribute to the generation and maintenance of the alkalosis with loop or thiazide diuretics (64, 105). Among these are (a) the stimulation of aldosterone (106), (b) sodium depletion (106), (c) maintained volume contraction (106), (d) enhanced proximal tubule bicarbonate reabsorption (107), (e) diminished glomerular filtration rate (108), (f) chloride depletion per se (103), (g) increased tubular fluid flow rates in the cortical collecting duct (109), and (h) potassium loss with resulting stimulation of ammoniagenesis and hydrogen ion secretion in the cortical collecting ducts (66). In addition, loop diuretics may increase acid secretion in the thick ascending limb (109).

Water Homeostasis: Hyponatremia

Diuretics also have important effects on water metabolism. As discussed above, both loop diuretics and thiazide derivatives directly impair free water clearance. This effect to lower sodium concentrations is amplified by diuretic-induced volume depletion, which provides a nonosmotic stimulus to antidiuretic hormone (ADH) secretion. In addition, as noted above, loop diuretics impair the urinating concentrating mechanism and prevent the kidney from responding to ADH levels with a concentrated urine. Thus, hyponatremia is relatively uncommon with the use of loop diuretics, except in the presence of marked volume depletion. Thiazide-type drugs, however, are active only in the cortex, thereby impairing urinary dilution without impairing the ability of ADH to concentrate urine, and are a common cause of hyponatremia (110–113).

Hyperuricemia

Currently available diuretics elevate uric acid levels by decreasing its excretion. Most diuretics, including the thiazides, are organic acids that may interfere with the secretion of uric acid into the proximal tubule. However, this is not the sole, or even major, mechanism of their effect on serum uric acid levels. The major effect seems to be mediated by volume depletion per se, with accompanying increased proximal tubule reabsorption of uric acid (15).

Consistent with this mechanism, the phenoxyacetic acid derivatives—ethacrynic acid, indacrinone, and tycrinafen (tienilic acid)—exert their uricosuric effect by blocking proximal tubule reabsorption of uric acid. Of the first two of these, ethacrynic acid is only acutely uricosuric (114). Indacrinone, a loop diuretic, can also lead to hyperuricemia with chronic use (115). Apparently, its natriuretic activity can cause enough volume depletion to elevate uric acid levels despite its direct inhibitory effects on urate reabsorption. Evidence of the independence (and opposition) of the natriuretic and uricosuric activities is provided by the observations that the uricosuric dose of ticrynafen is about one-fifth the natriuretic dose (116) and that indacrinone has two enantiomers, one with both uricosuric and natriuretic activity and one with predominantly uricosuric activity (117).

Divalent Cation Homeostasis

As discussed above, the thiazide-type diuretics increase calcium reabsorption. This property alone is not sufficient to account for their hypocalciuric effect, which requires volume contraction to be fully expressed (118).

Magnesium wasting by potassium-wasting diuretics is of relevance not only in its own right but also because of its effects on potassium (and, less commonly, calcium) homeostasis (119) (see below).

PHARMACOLOGY OF DIURETICS

The chemistry and pharmacology of diuretic agents has been the subject of extensive reviews (17, 120, 121) and will be discussed briefly and selectively here. It is important to bear in mind that, in general, all diuretics acting at a given site will have similar maximal effects.

With the exception of the direct aldosterone antagonists, the major mode of action of all diuretics used to treat hypertension involves inhibiting ion transporters in the luminal membrane of the renal tubule. Most are extensively protein bound and are therefore filtered minimally at the glomerulus. They arrive at their site of action by secretion into the tubular fluid. As organic acids, many share the probenecid-sensitive secretory pathway in the pars recta of the proximal tubule (122).

The response to loop diuretics has been clearly shown to depend on the concentration of drug in the urine and is therefore a function of both the amount (dose) and the time course of the delivery of the diuretic at its site of action (123). Loop diuretics vary in their bioavailability, with absorption being rapid and complete for bumetanide but with bioavailability of only 50–60% of the administered dose for furosemide. Absorption of furosemide seems to be delayed by intake with food (124). The duration of action of loop diuretics is short (usually substantially less than 2 hr) for all available compounds (114). Because of this short duration of action, their generation of negative sodium balance can be overcome readily by ingestion of sodium chloride (125, 126).

The thiazides diuretics are all sulfonamide derivatives. They differ mainly in their half-life, which is a function of their lipophilicity: The more lipophilic agents have larger volumes of distribution and longer half-lives. Half-lives vary from as little as 3 hr for bendroflumethazide to about 26 hr for polythiazide and to 40–60 hr for chlorthalidone, a member of the phthalimidine group (114, 120). Bioavailability of an oral dose is highly variable, based mainly on their absorption. For reasons that are not entirely clear, administration with food doubles the availability of chlorothiazide, a poorly absorbed agent and also increases that of hydrochlorothiazide to a lesser extent (120, 127). These effects are probably related to delayed gastric emptying, since propantheline, an anticholinergic agent that slows gastric emptying, also increases absorption of hydrochlorothiazide (128). The effect is not universal for all these agents, since food intake has no effect on absorption of bendroflumethiazide (129).

Although there is significant variability in absorption of chlorothiazide among patients, the degree of absorption for any given individual is highly reproducible (118). Different preparations of a given thiazide are usually of similar bioavailability (120).

The potassium-sparing agents, amiloride and triamterene, are generally well absorbed. In contrast to the thiazides, the absorption of amiloride seems to be reduced when it is given with food (130). Spironolactone is lipophilic and is absorbed best when given with food (131). Spironolactone undergoes extensive first-pass uptake and metabolism by the liver and is excreted in the bile, so that absorption and bioavailability may correlate poorly (120). Its major metabolite, canrenone, accounts for most of its biologic activity in clinical use. Original formulations of spironolactone were poorly absorbed compared to the currently available preparations. Therefore, current therapeutic doses may be substantially lower than those reported in earlier reports (132).

These observations imply that for uniform bioavailability of a given dose in a specific subject, many diuretics should be taken at a fixed time interval with respect to food.

HOW DO DIURETICS LOWER BLOOD PRESSURE?

The basis for the antihypertensive action of diuretic therapy is not completely understood. Relatively little progress has been made since Tobian's review of this subject over 20 years ago (133). Most of the data concerning the hypotensive action of diuretics derive from experiments with thiazide-type diuretics, which act on the distal convoluted tubule. Two possible mechanisms of action must be considered—that the hypotensive effect is a direct or indirect consequence of sodium (chloride) depletion or that diuretics act by direct or indirect vascular effects independent of natriuresis.

The Importance of Salt Depletion

Multiple lines of evidence support the view that salt and extracellular volume depletion underlies the hypotensive effect. The hemodynamic correlates of the hypotensive response to diuretics have been the focus of many studies. A reduction of plasma volume by 10–15% accompanies the initial diuresis during the first week of therapy with thiazides at doses approximately half those producing maximal natriuretic effects (134–138). Over this short-term period, cardiac output falls and peripheral vascular resistance rises (136–139). With chronic administration, blood volume returns toward normal (*vide infra*), cardiac output usually returns toward or to normal, and peripheral resistance falls to below pretreatment values (Fig. 6) (137, 138, 140–143).

A critical degree of blood volume deficit is sustained. Direct measurements of blood volume reveal such a sustained decrease in most (135, 137–138, 142, 144–148), but not all (135, 137, 140–143), studies. This inconsistency may be based on several methodologic difficulties. Among these is the variability of blood volume measurements (133, 149). In keeping with this, many of the negative studies show small, but statistically insignificant, decreases. In addition, studies have not been performed under balance conditions. Several investigators have found that salt intake increased in their subjects during chronic diuretic therapy (141, 150, 151), a finding that could obscure the detection of a small degree of volume depletion relative to intake. From a physiologic standpoint, the degree of sustained volume depletion needed may be quite small and within the variability of these measurements. The volume deficit must be evaluated with regard to the vascular capacitance. The reduction of peripheral resistance means that a "near-normal" absolute level of blood volume is inappropriately low for the state of the vascular tree. Using weight as an indirect measure of extracellular fluid volume in subjects on *ad libitum* diets who are presumed to be in a caloric steady state, chronic diuretic therapy is often associated with average weight losses in the range of 1–2 kg (137, 144, 152).

The role of sustained volume depletion in the antihypertensive action of thiazides is emphasized by the demonstration that upon cessation of diuretics, both body weight and plasma volume increase (135, 147). Body weight initially increases above baseline values, and patients often complain of swelling and puffiness during this period. Weight then declines, so that by 4 weeks after stopping the diuretic, body weight is above levels on chronic diuretic therapy by 1–2 kg (147).

The role of sustained volume depletion in maintaining the antihypertensive effect of diuretics is also supported by results from experiments with salt repletion during ongoing therapy. Ingestion of large amounts of salt can prevent or reverse the hypotensive actions of diuretics (153, 154). Thus, sodium chloride intake of 20 g for 1 week was found to reverse the antihypertensive effect of 150 mg/day of hydrochlorothiazide (144). This response to salt intake is dose-dependent, since addition of 6–12 g of salt to the diet had little or no effect (144). The amount of salt needed to affect the antihypertensive action of diuretics may vary with the diuretic dosage and duration of action. In other studies, utilizing lower doses of diuretics, smaller changes in sodium intake have been shown to alter the blood pressure response (155–157). The amount of salt needed to overcome the antihypertensive effect seems to vary directly with the dose and duration of action of the diuretic.

Additional, albeit indirect, evidence for sustained volume depletion with chronic diuretic therapy are (a) the responses to volume-sensitive hormone renin and (b) other biochemical parameters. Plasma renin levels during chronic diuretic therapy are elevated with respect to both pre- and post-treatment values (138, 147, 148, 158). A variety of routine blood chemistries of patients on chronic diuretic therapy are also consistent with volume depletion: Blood urea, serum creatinine, total protein, and hematocrit often tend to rise (137, 140, 158).

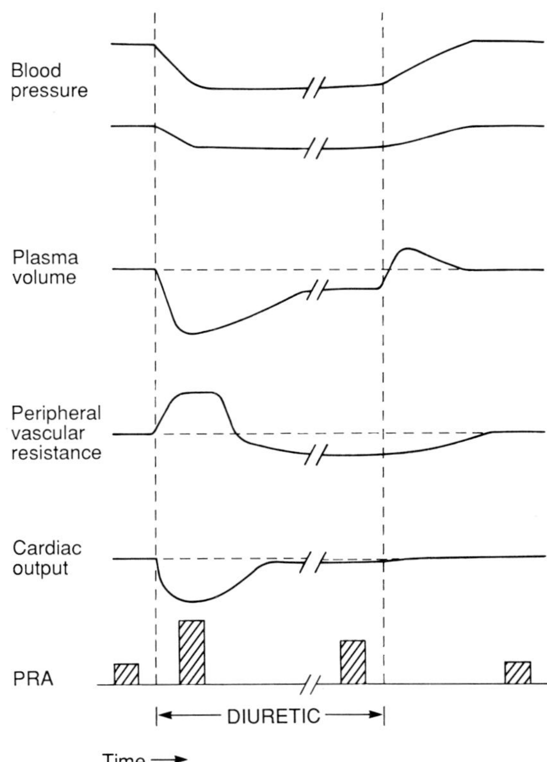

FIG. 6. Diagram of hemodynamic correlates of the antihypertensive effects of diuretic therapy.

The hemodynamic and extracellular volume effects of 150 mg chlorothiazide daily are quite similar to those of draconian salt restriction (less than 10 mEq/day) with the rice–fruit diet (133, 159). More recently, the blood pressure effects of smaller, now more commonly used doses of thiazide-type diuretics have been found to produce blood pressure effects similar to those of a diet with about 40 mEq/day of sodium (Fig. 7) (157, 160). Biochemical and hormonal profiles are also similar in patients who are on low-salt diets or who are taking diuretics (161). The antihypertensive effects of diuretics and dietary salt restriction would therefore appear to have the same basis.

Direct Vasodilator Effects of Diuretics

The observation that peripheral vascular resistance falls with diuretic therapy, coupled with the discovery of diazoxide (a benzothiadiazene that is a direct vasodilator without diuretic activity), led to the concept that thiazides are direct vasodilators. In fact, several diuretics do affect ion transport in vascular smooth muscle and other nonrenal cells. For example, thiazides and their derivatives, particularly the chlorobenzamide indapamide, diminish calcium influx in portal vein (and other smooth muscle) preparations (162). The mechanism of this effect is not clear. Loop diuretics and amiloride have been shown to inhibit ion

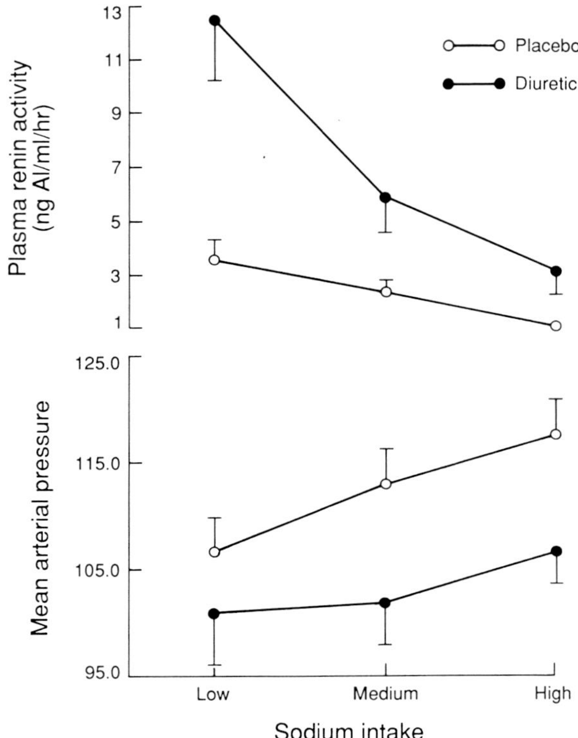

FIG. 7. Effect of diuretic therapy (chlorthalidone 25 mg daily or indapamide 2.5 mg daily) compared with placebo in 12 patients studied after 3 weeks of low (about 40 mEq per day), medium (about 100 mEq per day), and high (about 250 mEq per day) sodium intake. For each level of sodium intake, plasma renin activity was lower during diuretic therapy. The low sodium diet with placebo and the high sodium diet with diuretic resulted in similar levels of both blood pressure and plasma renin activity.

transporters that cause sodium entry into vascular smooth muscle cell (163, 164). The resulting decrease in intracellular sodium concentration would be expected to reduce smooth muscle contractility (165). This has been observed in experimental situations (163, 164). The concentrations at which these effects occur, however, are usually above those found with clinical use of these drugs.

With the possible exception of indapamide (166), it is clear that diuretics have minimal activity as direct vasodilators at plasma concentrations present during clinical use. Accordingly, peripheral resistance rises acutely with thiazide administration (*vide supra*). In addition, diuretics do not lower blood pressure in hypertensive patients on chronic hemodialysis (167) or in nephrectomized animals (168), supporting a key role for the kidney in their action.

HETEROGENEITY OF THE RESPONSE TO DIURETICS

Volume Depletion in Diuretic Responders and Nonresponders

The hypotensive response to diuretic therapy is not uniform (*vide infra*). If volume depletion is a necessary condition for the hypotensive response, is it also a sufficient one? That is, do patients with a hypotensive response to diuretics ("responders") differ from nonresponders as a function of their absolute reduction in blood volume?

Of course, it is possible to fail to respond to a diuretic because no net negative sodium balance is achieved. This could occur in several ways. In the presence of renal failure, the diuretic may not reach its site of action in the tubule in sufficient concentration. Alternatively, the dose may be too low to be effective; or the duration of action of the diuretic may be too short, and the dosing too infrequent, to achieve sustained negative sodium balance. This latter situation is a common reason for the ineffectiveness of loop diuretics (123, 125). As noted above, excessive salt intake may also obviate diuretic-induced volume depletion.

Barring the above considerations, the hypotensive response to monotherapy with diuretics does not seem to be solely related to the degree of negative sodium balance per se. In most studies, diuretic responders, usually defined as those patients with a decrease in mean arterial pressure of more than 10%, have similar (or occasionally even greater) decreases in plasma volume when compared to nonresponders (138, 148, 169). In one study, however, diuretic responders had falls in blood volume, whereas nonresponders did not (143). Low-renin patients with essential hypertension, predominantly diuretic responders, have been reported to have greater weight loss on diuretics than do normal or high-renin patients (170); usually, however, similar weight losses are found in nonresponders and responders (148, 152, 158). Analysis of 305 patients in the Veteran's Administration Cooperative Study, who underwent titration of hydrochlorothiazide at doses ranging from 50 to 200 mg daily, revealed that the degree of weight loss did not correlate with the response to a given dose of diuretic. However, those whose blood pressure responded only to the highest dose had greater weight loss than did either (a) nonresponders to that same dose or (b) responders to lower doses (152). In addition, the response to severely sodium-restricted diets was found to be extremely variable and to correlate poorly with the degree of negative sodium balance (171, 172). In keeping with this variability, normal subjects usually do not have a hypotensive response to diuretics (153, 173).

These results suggest that an individual's adaptation (or abnormal adaptation, since normal subjects do not respond) to extracellular volume depletion is the major determinant of the long-term blood pressure response. The finding that acute volume expansion with saline or dextran partially (at most) reverses the fall in blood pressure induced by chronic thiazide monotherapy (144, 154) is also consistent with a chronic adaptation underlying the blood pressure response.

Role of the Renin–Angiotensin–Aldosterone System

A key difference between diuretic responders and nonresponders appears to lie in the heterogeneity of the adaptive responses of peripheral vascular resistance, which is governed predominantly by the renin–angiotensin–aldosterone system.

An increase in the activity of the renin–angiotensin–aldosterone system plays a major role in conserving sodium and maintaining blood pressure in the face of short-term and long-term extracellular volume depletion (as discussed elsewhere in this volume) and is therefore a limiting factor in the blood pressure response to diuretics (174). Several investigators have found that hypertensive patients who fail to respond to diuretic therapy have a greater rise in renin or greater angiotensin II responsiveness than do those who respond (138, 148, 158, 175, 176). These data suggest that diuretic-induced volume depletion stimulates the renin–angiotensin system and thereby blunts their antihypertensive efficacy. This interpretation is supported by the demonstration that in patients whose blood pressure is refractory to volume depletion, addition of a converting-enzyme inhibitor to block the renin system promptly lowers blood pressure (177). This finding is further supported by the long-term efficacy of antirenin therapy (i.e., converting-enzyme inhibition or beta-blockade) in combination with diuretic therapy in resistant hypertension (*vide infra*).

Even in those subjects whose renin rises appropriately in response to diuretics, the renin–aldosterone axis may not be entirely normal. In one study, in 28 patients with normal renin essential hypertension, renin levels before and after 6 weeks of chlorthalidone (100 mg daily) were similar in responders and nonresponders, whereas nonresponders had greater increases in aldosterone with therapy (158). Hollenberg, Williams, and colleagues have defined an abnormality in the aldosterone response to angiotensin II in a large subset of essential hypertensives with overtly normal renin systems; they have termed this *nonmodulating hypertension* (178) (as discussed elsewhere in this volume).

In addition, the renin–aldosterone axis is abnormally suppressed in about 30% of hypertensive patients (179). In these patients with low-renin essential hypertension, the levels of plasma renin activity remain low in the face of stimuli to renin secretion, such as low salt intake, acute furosemide administration, or upright posture, either alone or in combination. These subjects would be expected to respond particularly well to diuretic therapy, and that is often found to be the case (158, 170, 180–188).

The pathophysiologic basis for the heterogeneity of the renin system is unknown. Sealey et al. (189) have suggested a renal basis for essential hypertension in which there are two subpopulations of nephrons: One ("ischemic") subpopulation has afferent arteriolar lesions, reduced perfusion pressure, and elevated renin secretion, whereas the other subpopulation has increased perfusion pressure, hyperfiltration, hypernatriuresis, and suppressed renin secretion. This discordance of nephron function may be aggravated further by volume contraction resulting from diuretic therapy, with additional stimulation of renin by the ischemic nephrons and a reduction of pressure-related natriuresis by the adapting, hyperfiltering nephrons. According to this hypothesis, the function of the ischemic nephrons would define the reactive rise in renin. Low-renin subjects might be expected to have a reduction in nephron number (189, 190). This hypothesis is discussed in Chapter 69.

Consistent with this hypothesis, animals with two-kidney one-clip Goldblatt hypertension (a renin-dependent model) (191), as well as patients with unilateral renal artery stenosis (192, 193), most often do not respond to diuretics. In contrast, models of hypertension such as mineralocorticoid excess, which depend on volume expansion or have suppressed renin levels, respond well to diuretics or to salt restriction.

Although the failure of renin to rise in reaction to volume depletion is a key element of the blood pressure response, it does not completely explain diuretic sensitivity, however. Many hypertensive diuretic responders have normal renin values that appear to rise appropriately in response to diuretics or volume depletion (158). As noted above, these patients may nonetheless have abnormalities in the renin–angiotensin–aldosterone axis. In addition, some of this discrepancy may be methodologic, a result of utilizing assays of renin activity which do not measure low values of renin accurately (194). Furthermore, the short half-life of plasma renin makes the detection of subtle changes in activity difficult and complicates the assessment of the integrated activity of the renin–angiotensin system.

Beyond these considerations, the lack of a rise in renin levels with diuretic therapy does not by itself explain the fall in peripheral vascular resistance seen with chronic diuretic therapy. The decrease in vascular responsiveness to angiotensin II which occurs with salt depletion may be an additional factor influencing the response to diuretic therapy (195).

Sympathetic Nervous System Activity During Diuretic Therapy

Decreased pressor responsiveness to norepinephrine infusion has been demonstrated in hypertensive subjects on acute or chronic diuretic therapy (154, 196, 197). Norepinephrine sensitivity can be restored by sodium loading (154). Such a decrease in pressor sensitivity may be specific to catecholamines, since, in dogs, angiotensin II sensitivity is unimpaired (198). In patients, however, pressor sensitivity to angiotensin II is also reduced during diuretic therapy (199) or while on a low-salt diet (195), so that the changes seen with norepinephrine may be nonspecific (200).

Supine plasma norepinephrine levels are elevated acutely and chronically during the course of diuretic therapy (148, 201). This may reflect increased sympathetic nerve activity, which is also elevated in hypertensive rats given diuretics (202). Any increase in nerve traffic appears to be relatively ineffective (198), perhaps owing to decreased release of norepinephrine or to postsynaptic impairment of norepinephrine's effect. Postural changes in norepinephrine, pulse, and blood pressure, as well as the response to the Valsalva maneuver, are not changed by chronic diuretic therapy in hypertensive patients as a group (143, 201) or in responders compared with nonresponders (143). Thus, reflex function of the sympathetic nervous system is unimpaired during chronic diuretic therapy.

Sympathetic nervous system blockade does, however, enhance diuretic sensitivity, in part, by decreasing renin secretion (*vide supra*). The hypotensive effect of diuretics during adrenergic blockade is markedly sensitive to intravascular volume (134, 203, 204). Baroreceptor sensitivity may play a role in determining the rate at which blood pressure returns to pretreatment levels after stopping diuretics (205).

Other Vasoactive Systems

Other vasoactive mediators are also affected by diuretic therapy. Prostacyclin production has been found to be increased during diuretic therapy (150). The increase of this vasodilator may be greater in diuretic responders as compared to nonresponders (206), implicating the prostaglandins in diuretic effectiveness. The loop diuretics are particularly powerful stimulators of prostaglandin synthesis, and their venodilating activity is mediated by these agents (40, 41). Additionally, most nonsteroidal anti-inflammatory agents, which inhibit cyclo-oxygenase, often blunt the hypotensive effect of diuretics (*vide infra*). Thus, the prostaglandin system clearly modulates the response to diuretics.

Kinins have also been reported to be affected by diuretic therapy. Urinary kallikrein excretion has been reported to be elevated in diuretic responders as compared with nonresponders (151).

Intracellular calcium levels in platelets are reported to be decreased in patients whose blood pressure is controlled on diuretics; and if these levels reflect those in vascular smooth muscle, vasodilation would be an expected result (207). This finding seems more likely to reflect a common final pathway for all vasodilatation and does not shed light on the specific mechanism of diminished vasoconstriction by diuretics.

Several other theories have also been invoked to explain the fall in peripheral resistance in diuretic responders. It has been proposed that the fall in extracellular volume and cardiac output leads to "reverse autoregulation" and thereby decreases arteriolar tone (208,209). A putative natriuretic hormone with vasoconstrictor properties, perhaps a Na,K-ATPase inhibitor, has been proposed as a mediator of volume-dependent hypertension (210–212). Such a hormone would presumably be suppressed by volume contraction resulting from diuretics. Pending further identification of such a hormone, this also remains an interesting speculation.

CLINICAL EFFICACY OF DIURETICS

Antihypertensive Efficacy

Thiazide-type diuretics have been used as first-line therapy in all major randomized clinical trials of the long-term treatment of hypertension (213–220) (as discussed elsewhere in this volume). As such, they are the most intensively evaluated of all antihypertensive therapies. As primary therapy of hypertension, diuretics lower blood pressure in slightly less than half of patients with essential hypertension—a success rate that is similar to, or better than, that found with other monotherapy. The variability in this fraction of responders depends, in all likelihood, on several factors, including the demographics of the patient population studied, the diet, the severity of the hypertension, and the dose of diuretic administered. The vast majority of patients can be successfully treated with combination regimens that include diuretics, a finding that further enhances their clinical value.

The large prospective trials of the treatment of hypertension assigned their treatment regimens randomly. As with other agents, it would be optimal to target diuretic therapy so that responders were the only ones receiving this therapy. To this end, several criteria can be used in an attempt to select diuretic responders from among all essential hypertensives. The simplest are demographic criteria. On average, elderly, black, and/or obese patients are found to respond especially well to diuretics as primary therapy (221–224). Because there is broad overlap between responders and nonresponders in these categories, they are of minor utility in selecting therapy for an individual.

Criteria for diuretic treatment based on the mechanisms underlying the blood pressure elevation in a specific individual would, of course, be ideal. Unfortunately, for most patients, no such criteria are available. Perhaps the most specific marker is the presence of suppressed renin activity, since over 80% of low-renin hypertensives respond to volume depletion therapy, with either diuretics or salt restriction (*vide supra*). However, a large number of patients with normal renin values also respond to diuretics, and selecting these patients often requires therapeutic trials. Unfortunately, no adequate marker exists for salt- or diuretic-sensitive hypertension.

Protection from Cardiovascular Disease

The goal of hypertensive therapy is not merely to lower blood pressure, but to do so in a manner that will prevent the cardiovascular and renal disease for which hypertension is a risk factor. The results of lowering blood pressure with diuretics have been intensively scrutinized over a wide range of severity of hypertension. As used in the prospective trials, diuretic therapy affords protection against stroke and the development of congestive heart failure, while, in general, it does not protect against mortality from ischemic heart disease (as discussed elsewhere in this volume). This failure is particularly important in the treatment of mild hypertension, where ischemic heart disease substantially outweighs stroke as a cause of morbidity and mortality. In the Multiple Risk Factor Intervention Trial (MRFIT), patients with abnormal electrocardiograms had an increased risk for sudden death with diuretic therapy (219,225). In this study, hydrochlorothiazide therapy was accompanied by the increased risk, while therapy with chlorthalidone was not. The Framingham study also found that therapy of hypertension, mostly diuretic-based, increased the risk of sudden death (226).

Left ventricular hypertrophy is a consequence of hypertension which is also a risk factor for cardiovascular morbidity that is independent of blood pressure (227) (see the chapter by Devereux, entitled "Hypertensive Cardiac Hypertrophy: Pathophysiologic and Clinical Characteristics," this volume). Diuretics do not seem to reverse left ventricular hypertrophy as successfully as do sympathetic antagonists, converting-enzyme inhibitors, or calcium-channel blockers (228,229) (see the chapter by Devereux, cited in this paragraph), although regression of left ventricular hypertrophy has been demonstrated in a population consisting predominantly of diuretic responders, perhaps with low plasma renin activity (230).

In addition, in rats, lowering blood pressure with diuretic-based regimens does not halt progression of renal disease (231), whereas treatment with a converting-enzyme inhibitor or calcium-channel blocker may do so (231,232).

The failure of diuretics to protect patients from many hypertensive sequelae may be universal to all agents, since none have been as carefully evaluated. Thus, despite its utility in the secondary prevention of heart attacks (233), nonselective beta-blockade with propranolol also failed to protect against heart attacks or to do as well as bendroflumethiazide against stroke in the one trial where it was compared as primary therapy (220). Only recently has evidence been gathered from a hybrid clinical trial to suggest that an agent, the beta-1-selective blocker metoprolol, can afford cardioprotection during the treatment of hypertension (234) (discussed elsewhere in this volume).

Although the disappointing results in regard to cardiovascular protection might be attributed to diuretics by default, several consequences of diuretic use might contribute to this failure by counteracting their beneficial effects on blood pressure. Among these are the decrease in cardiac output discussed above, potassium and magnesium losses, and disturbances of glucose and lipid metabolism.

METABOLIC SIDE EFFECTS OF DIURETIC THERAPY

The homeostatic responses to the renal actions of diuretics bring water and solute excretion back into balance over the course of several weeks. Although sodium intake equals output, the diuretic remains effective, since the new steady state is attained at the cost of sustained deficits of sodium and volume, potassium, and magnesium. Agents with a short duration of action induce alternating periods of (a) natriuresis immediately following administration and (b) sodium retention after the diuretic effect has abated (125). The implication of the development of a new steady state is that as long as dietary, metabolic, and circulatory parameters are unchanged, the deficits caused by diuretics should appear relatively early in the course of therapy and remain relatively stable (111,222,235–240).

The mechanisms by which diuretics produce alterations in fluid and electrolyte homeostasis are discussed above (see also Fig. 8). The focus in this section is on the clinical aspects of these disturbances (see Table 2).

Volume Depletion and Hyponatremia

The mild degree of volume depletion usually induced by diuretics is generally well tolerated by those with intact cardiac reflexes. With more severe volume depletion, symptoms of fatigue, weakness, and cramps may occur. Postural hypotension is also a problem with more severe volume depletion, especially in the setting of impaired cardiovascular reflexes; elderly patients appear to be particularly vulnerable (241).

TABLE 2. *Adverse effects of chronic diuretic therapy*

1. Direct consequences of diuretic action
   - Sodium-volume depletion
   - Orthostatic symptoms
   - Hyponatremia
   - Hypokalemia
   - Hypomagnesemia
   - Hyperuricemia
2. Secondary effects
   - Cardiac arrhythmias
   - Glucose intolerance
   - Increased cholesterol
   - Failure of cardioprotection
3. Idiosyncratic drug reactions

As discussed above, the combination of volume depletion and the direct effects of diuretics can result in hyponatremia, which can be severe (110–113). Excessive water drinking, which may not be immediately apparent, is a predisposing factor (240,242). Potassium depletion may also predispose to hyponatremia (110). The elderly are also particularly vulnerable to hyponatremia, perhaps because of the decrease in the ability to clear free water that often accompanies aging (243).

Potassium Wasting

The kaliuresis resulting from the use of diuretics acting proximal to the cortical collecting duct results in a decrease in total body potassium which is ameliorated with chronic therapy (144,244–246). Serum potassium also decreases, usually by about 0.5 mEq/liter (144,235,247,248). While levels may remain within the normal range, they are depressed below 3.5 mEq/liter, often severely so, in 10–50% of patients (222,235,238,249,250). The variability may reflect differences in sodium intake (*vide infra*) or potassium intake (251), among other factors. The incidence of hyperaldosteronism is extremely low among patients with diuretic-induced hypokalemia (252), so it is not a useful diagnostic finding in this regard.

The overall significance of these decreases, as well as whether the risks of repletion outweigh the benefits, has been hotly debated (253). The major hazards of hypokalemia with diuretics are ventricular irritability and glucose intolerance.

Diuretic therapy with associated hypokalemia has been reported to induce ventricular ectopy (254–257), but this is not a universal finding (258). Furthermore, potassium replacement may not reverse the ectopy (257), suggesting that another factor, perhaps magnesium depletion, is operative in diuretic-induced ectopy (see below). Adequate potassium replacement is difficult to gauge, however, so the failure of ectopy to decrease may reflect inadequate potassium repletion.

In addition to baseline lowering of serum potassium levels, the deficit in total body potassium without frank hypokalemia may make patients more vulnerable to stress-induced hypokalemia (259). This effect is mediated by beta-2-adrenergic stimulation (260) and involves the shift of potassium from the extracellular fluid into the cell, prob-

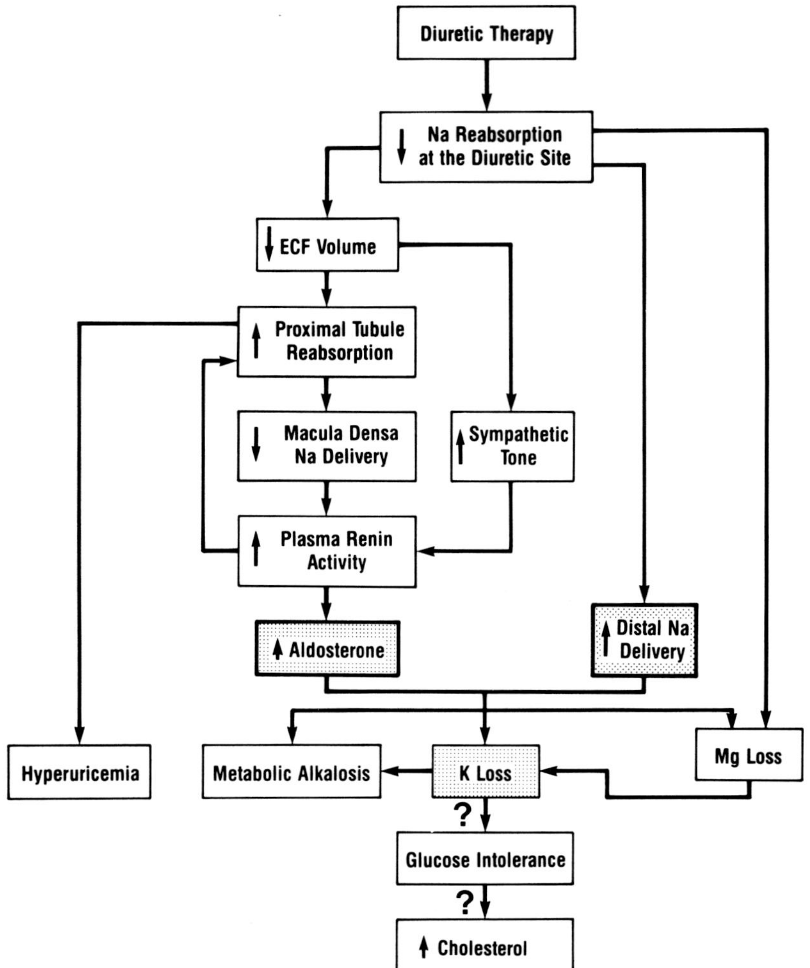

FIG. 8. Overview of major metabolic consequences of diuretics. The relationship of glucose intolerance to diuretic-induced increases in cholesterol is speculative.

ably by stimulation of the Na,K ATPase (261). This is particularly important in the context of acute myocardial ischemia, since it is associated with increased frequency of malignant ventricular arrhythmias (256,262).

The frequency of diuretic-induced hypokalemia depends, to some extent, on the type of diuretic used. Loop diuretics, despite their greater potency, seem to cause less hypokalemia (156,235,263,264). This is probably related to the duration of action of the agents in question. For example, a long-acting thiazide-type agent, such as chlorthalidone, causes greater potassium loss than do equivalent doses of shorter-acting agents, such as hydrochlorothiazide (156). The hypokalemia is dose-related over a wide range, from 25 to 200 mg for either hydrochlorothiazide or chlorthalidone (235,255). Since the antihypertensive dose often occurs at low doses, without much greater blood pressure responses at higher doses (221,255,265,266), the dose of diuretic should be kept at a minimum when these agents are used.

A related issue is the dietary sodium intake which best complements diuretic therapy, with respect to optimizing their antihypertensive efficacy and minimizing hypokalemia. Conflicting reports are present in the literature. Moderate sodium restriction, to about 60–80 mEq/day, has been reported to markedly decrease potassium loss to about half that seen with an intake of 180–200 mEq/day, while slightly enhancing the hypotensive effect of diuretics (156), in keeping with the finding that the addition of 20 g of salt to the diet increases potassium losses (144). In contrast, more severe sodium restriction has been shown to lower potassium levels in comparison to higher sodium intakes in acute (267,268) and 3-week (157) studies. The diuretic dose was lower in the latter study, but the discrepancy may also reflect differences in the activation of the renin–angiotensin system by the different levels of sodium restriction. Potassium secretion reflects levels of aldosterone and of distal sodium supply. The curvilinear relationship between aldosterone (or renin) and sodium intake is gradual at sodium intakes greater than 80 mEq, whereas levels of these hormones rise steeply at lower levels of dietary sodium (269). Thus, with more stringent sodium restriction the reactive increases in renin and aldosterone may limit the fall in blood pressure and accelerate potassium loss. The secretion of aldosterone in response to angiotensin II is also enhanced by sodium depletion (195,270); some hypertensives do not show this enhancement (178), which might modify the potassium wasting caused by diuretics.

Hyperkalemia

As discussed above, potassium-sparing diuretics predispose to hyperkalemic, hyperchloremic acidosis. This becomes of clinical importance, primarily in diabetes or renal insufficiency or with use of nonsteroidal anti-inflammatory drug therapy.

Magnesium Wasting

As noted above, thiazide-type and loop diuretics cause renal magnesium loss. As with potassium, serum levels may stay within the normal range. Magnesium loss can be an independent stimulus to cardiac arrhythmias, most often related to digitalis therapy (271,272). Importantly, magnesium depletion can also cause renal potassium wasting, which is refractory to potassium supplementation (273,274), and can contribute to the decrease in intracellular potassium present with diuretic use (55). Magnesium wasting is not a feature of potassium-sparing diuretics (55, 275,276) (*vide supra*).

Hypercalcemia

Despite producing hypocalciuria, thiazide-type diuretics rarely causes frank hypercalcemia. Hypercalcemia, when present, is usually related to an underlying disorder of calcium metabolism, most commonly hyperparathyroidism (277,278). In addition to hypocalciuria, thiazides can elevate serum calcium levels by enhancing the peripheral effects of parathyroid hormone (279). This view is supported by the finding that thiazides can induce an elevation of serum calcium levels in patients on chronic maintenance hemodialysis (280).

The hypercalciuria caused by loop diuretics is rarely of overt long-term significance. This is probably because the increase in proximal tubular calcium reabsorption with chronic use (*vide supra*) overrides the direct effect of these drugs on calcium reabsorption by the thick ascending limb.

Glucose Intolerance

This subject has been reviewed recently (278). Glucose intolerance or frank noninsulin-dependent diabetes may develop or worsen during diuretic therapy (281). In prospective trials, the average level of fasting glucose, as well as the number of subjects who develop glucose intolerance, is higher in those on diuretics (248,282). The abnormality is often partially reversible upon cessation of diuretic therapy (248,281,283). Concomitant use of beta-blockers increases the incidence of hyperglycemia (282,284).

Although the benzothiadiazine diazoxide is directly toxic to the pancreas, the mechanism of diuretic-induced glucose intolerance is most likely related to the hypokalemia (278, 285). Both impaired insulin release and impaired peripheral glucose uptake have been suggested as bases for the effect. Glucose-clamp experiments suggest that the primary mechanism involves impairment of insulin secretion (285). In keeping with this observation, the effect on glucose metabolism can be corrected by potassium repletion (286, 287) Impaired glucose metabolism is not seen with potassium-sparing diuretics, which actually may improve glucose tolerance (278).

Nonketotic hyperglycemic hyperosmolar coma, a catastrophic complication of non-insulin-dependent diabetes, occurs with increased frequency, albeit still rarely, in patients on loop diuretics or thiazides, with or without amiloride (288). This condition, which carries a high mortality, occurred on a background of diuretic therapy in 17 of 20 patients in one series (289).

Elevation of Cholesterol Levels

Serum cholesterol levels increase during the first 12 weeks of therapy with potassium-wasting diuretics, with low-density lipoprotein cholesterol levels increasing by about 5–15% (290–294) in men and postmenopausal women but not in premenopausal women (295). At 1 year of therapy, the levels decrease to pretreatment values (248, 296,297). This apparent normalization of cholesterol with prolonged therapy may reflect falling baseline levels. In placebo-controlled studies, both diuretic and placebo groups exhibited falling cholesterol levels, with levels in the diuretic group remaining elevated as compared to the group on placebo (248,298). The magnitude of this difference is 2–3% (248). Cessation of diuretic therapy is also associated with lowering of cholesterol levels (283, 299–301).

The precise significance of this elevation of cholesterol is unknown, although both epidemiologic and clinical trial data suggest that elevations of this magnitude can significantly increase the incidence of ischemic heart disease (302,303). The cause remains speculative. It may be related to impaired glucose tolerance (304) and, hence, potassium losses. In this regard, spironolactone does not adversely affect lipids (305,306). Additionally, therapy with thiazide-type diuretics and potassium-sparing agents such as amiloride, triamterene, or the converting-enzyme inhibitor captopril is usually not associated with adverse effects on serum lipids (306).

Hyperuricemia

As discussed above, serum uric acid levels are elevated by chronic diuretics, especially thiazide-type and loop diuretics. Renal excretion is not increased, so uric acid stones are not more common with these agents. In those who are predisposed to gout, the elevation of uric acid may lead to acute attacks of gout. In the Medical Research Council trial, gout led to withdrawal of diuretic therapy at a rate of 12.8 per 1000 patient-years of treatment (220). In general, asymptomatic hyperuricemia need not be treated (278).

TOXICITY AND DRUG INTERACTIONS OF DIURETICS

The treatment of hypertension is a strategy of prevention and therefore requires agents with minimal toxicity. Fortunately, diuretics have very little toxicity apart from the renal–metabolic effects discussed above. Nevertheless, they are frequently discontinued because of side effects. In the HDFP trial, chlorthalidone was discontinued in 20.6% of subjects taking these medicines, whereas spironolactone was discontinued in 16.9% (307).

As with all antihypertensive therapies, impotence is an all-too-common result of thiazide therapy, approximating 20% in some studies and often higher than seen with beta-blockers (248). The incidence is higher with spironolactone, particularly in high doses. Spironolactone is an androgen antagonist (308), an effect also responsible for the frequent gynecomastia the drug induces. Spironolactone can also cause amenorrhea. The endocrine side-effects are dose-related and are relatively infrequent at doses of 25–50 mg daily. Gastrointestinal discomfort is also a common side effect of this agent.

Acute interstitial nephritis, often accompanied by eosinophiluria, eosinophilia, a maculopapular rash, adenopathy, and fever, has been observed infrequently in patients on sulfonamide diuretics, including thiazides, chlorthalidone, furosemide, and triamterene (309, 310). This likely represents a hypersensitivity reaction. Oliguria is usually not part of the presentation (310). It is not dose-related and may occur after weeks or months of therapy (310). A facilitating role for concomitant triamterene or amiloride therapy may be present. Perhaps underdiagnosed, this syndrome cannot be very common.

Hypokalemic nephropathy, a result of long-standing severe hypokalemia, is also a possible consequence of diuretic use but is more commonly seen with diuretic abuse. Triamterene has been found in kidney stones and may form a nidus for stone formation (311). However, it does not appear that patients on triamterene have an unusually high incidence of kidney stones (312).

Idiopathic toxicities also include a possible doubling of the relative risk for acute cholecystitis in patients on thiazides, found in two case-control studies (313, 314) but not in the Boston Collaborative Drug Surveillance Program (315). Rashes occur in less than 0.5% of all patients on thiazides (316). Blood dyscrasias and pancreatitis are also seen on rare occasion. Ototoxicity can occur with use of loop diuretics, usually with intravenous administration and/or in the presence of renal insufficiency (310).

The most important drug interaction of diuretics is with nonsteroidal anti-inflammatory agents. A dramatic hyperkalemic nephropathy has been seen with triamterene (and less commonly with amiloride) and with nonsteroidal anti-inflammatory agents. This could be induced in normal volunteers by administering triamterene and indomethacin (317). Inhibitors of renal prostaglandin synthesis, which include all nonsteroidal anti-inflammatory agents except sulindac, also interfere with natriuresis and blood pressure control during diuretic therapy (318–320).

A second important interaction is with lithium. Any volume depletion can enhance proximal tubule reabsorption of lithium nonspecifically, which has been used as a marker of proximal tubule sodium reabsorption. Thiazide-type diuretics, in particular, can cause elevations of lithium levels, predisposing to toxicity (321). Loop diuretics tend to increase lithium excretion, which offsets the effects of volume contraction on lithium levels (322).

USE OF DIURETICS IN HYPERTENSION

For years after their introduction, diuretics were the foundation of antihypertensive therapy. This was institutionalized in the formulation of "stepped-care" therapy. As we have seen, diuretics are useful as primary therapy in many patients.

Additionally, a rationale existed for continuing diuretic therapy in nonresponders because agents such as the direct vasodilators hydralazine or minoxidil, the centrally acting sympatholytic agents methyldopa or clonidine, and sympatholytics such as reserpine or guanethidine all produce sodium retention, which decreases their antihypertensive effectiveness. Thus, diuretics are a necessary adjunct to their use. The introduction of beta-blockers, converting-enzyme inhibitors, calcium-channel blockers, and alpha-blockers, agents that do not produce fluid retention, has undermined this rationale. Diuretics are now one of several possible choices for initial therapy (323), and the decision to use them should be individualized to the extent possible (*vide supra*). Several studies have also shown that newer agents, such as converting-enzyme inhibitors, are better tolerated than diuretics, providing less interference with "quality of life" (324, 325). Nonetheless, diuretics are well tolerated, inexpensive, and effective in many patients.

Although newer antihypertensive agents do not require salt depletion to be effective, combining diuretics with beta-blockers or converting-enzyme inhibitors is often useful in hypertension refractory to monotherapy (282, 326, 327). Interestingly, diuretics often are found to not add to the hypotensive effects of calcium-channel blockers (328–330).

Diuretics may have particular value in hypertension associated with congestive heart failure; however, here too, other agents that reduce pre- and afterload are being found to be beneficial in supplementing (and, in some cases, supplanting) diuretic use.

Hypertension associated with renal disease is often accompanied by sodium retention. In this circumstance, the more powerful loop diuretics are particularly valuable. Metolazone may also be useful in the presence of renal insufficiency, perhaps because of its proximal tubule effects (331, 332). The other thiazide-type diuretics are not effective when the glomerular filtration rate (GFR) is less than 20 ml/min (47, 333). When the GFR is severely depressed, combinations of diuretics that act at different sites in the nephron may be useful (334).

Potassium-sparing agents are relatively contraindicated in these patients, who often have difficulty in disposing potassium. Kidney function in patients with renal disease is often very sensitive to volume depletion, so that diuretics must be used cautiously in this setting to avoid severe worsening of renal function due to oversaluresis.

Diuretics should be avoided in patients with glucose intolerance or non-insulin-dependent diabetes (335, 336). In addition to the concerns noted above, diabetics often have difficulty in handling potassium loads, so that potassium-sparing agents should also be avoided.

Choice and Dosage of Diuretic

In general, thiazide diuretics with intermediate or long duration of action are the preferred agents. They provide once-daily therapy. The longer-acting agents, perhaps with greater antihypertensive potency, also produce greater kaliuresis. Loop diuretics are short-acting and are perhaps less effective because of this (125). Although furosemide can be effective when taken once daily (337), even when taken twice daily it is less effective than thiazide derivatives in treating uncomplicated essential hypertension (263, 264, 338).

Spironolactone is the sole potassium-sparing agent with significant antihypertensive effects when used as a sole agent. In every study where it has been compared to potassium-wasting diuretics, it has been found to be of equal antihypertensive efficacy (89, 91, 183, 184, 186, 327, 339, 340), although the onset of its action is, in most cases, more gradual. Formerly used at doses of at least 100 mg/day, doses of 50 mg daily are often effective (340, 341). Spironolactone, at high doses, is particularly valuable in the treatment of primary hyperaldosteronism (91).

In most patients with otherwise uncomplicated essential hypertension, the blood pressure response to diuretics shows a relatively flat dose–response curve. Increasing the dose will, however, increase the number of responders as well as the frequency of side effects (152, 341, 342). Since the bioavailability of these agents shows large interindividual variability, rigid dosage recommendations are not very useful. Every effort should be made to find the minimum effective dose in a given patient. Often, this can be as low as 12.5–25 mg of hydrochlorothiazide daily, or its equivalent (96, 343–345). Although alternate-day treatment is often unsuccessful, less-than-daily treatment may be highly successful in individual patients (96, 342). The success of this therapy may depend on the level of dietary salt intake, with greater success found in patients on low-sodium diets.

Withdrawal of long-term diuretic therapy often results in prolonged periods of normotension (299, 346, 347). This finding may relate to the success of alternate-day therapy in subjects who were formerly on daily therapy. It also suggests that drug holidays might be incorporated in the routine long-term care of patients on chronic diuretic therapy.

The optimal sodium intake required to enhance diuretic effectiveness and reduce toxicity is not clear. Severe sodium restriction is best used to substitute for, rather than complement, diuretic therapy. Very high sodium intake should be avoided as well in the setting of diuretic therapy. Barring these extremes, relatively consistent dietary sodium intake should be followed in order to obtain a consistent response.

Approach to Hypokalemia

As with other agents, diuretics should be discontinued, and appropriate substitutes should be used, if significant side effects occur. The most common problems of diuretic therapy are a consequence of their potassium wasting (see above). The balance of the evidence suggests that if diuretic therapy must be continued, hypokalemia should be treated if it is symptomatic or severe, or if patients are at high risk for cardiovascular disease.

Adequate repletion may be difficult to gauge, since serum potassium levels may not reflect total body stores (348). There are four approaches to potassium repletion. First, the diuretic dose should be lowered to the minimum effective dose. Second, spironolactone may be substituted for the potassium-wasting diuretic. This has the attractions of providing equivalent antihypertensive treatment and of the parsimony of avoiding the treatment of a complication of a medication with a second medication. Third, electrolyte replacement therapy can be undertaken. Lastly, a potassium-sparing agent can be added to the regimen.

Administering enough potassium to replete body stores is often difficult. The potassium becomes an added stimulus to aldosterone secretion, which accelerates further potassium loss (100–102). Thus, complete repletion is usually difficult. As noted, potassium-wasting diuretics also waste magnesium, and magnesium deficits may result in hypokalemia refractory to potassium supplementation. At times, magnesium supplementation has had to be combined with potassium supplementation in order to replete potassium in patients with diuretic-induced hypokalemia (274).

Potassium supplementation can be attempted with intake of potassium-rich foods. This has the drawback of increased caloric intake in order to add enough potassium-rich foods to the diet to supply more than 40 mEq/day of extra potassium, an amount that is often required in order to normalize serum potassium levels (349, 350). In addition, if severe chloride depletion and metabolic alkalosis coexists with potassium depletion, chloride repletion will be necessary in order to effectively replace the potassium, and potassium-rich foods are generally low in chloride. Although generally safe, potassium chloride preparations are a cause of gastrointestinal irritation or ulceration (351). Newer microencapsulated preparations have excellent bioavailability and may decrease the incidence of this complication (96, 352). Oral potassium in any form can cause diarrhea.

Potassium-sparing diuretics have often been found to be more effective than potassium supplementation in repleting serum levels and body stores (353–355). This would be expected, since these agents either directly or indirectly antagonize aldosterone. The potassium-sparing agents also decrease magnesium excretion, allowing the correction of any magnesium deficits that might underlie the hypokalemia. The effectiveness of a given dose of any of the potassium-sparing diuretics in relation to the potassium loss caused by a given dose of thiazide varies greatly among individuals. Therefore, these agents should be titrated. Fixed dose combination should only be used when appropriate doses are established.

In addition to the potential benefits outlined above, potassium repletion with oral potassium supplementation (356) or with potassium-sparing diuretics may improve blood pressure control. This may be due to the natriuresis caused by either potassium supplementation or the potassium-sparing diuretics, or it may be related to other mechanisms involving potassium effects on the sympathetic nervous system, or vascular smooth muscle may be operative (357). Epidemiologic and animal studies suggest that high potassium intake protects both humans (358) and stroke-prone spontaneously hypertensive rats (359) from stroke, a potential added benefit of potassium repletion.

SUMMARY AND FUTURE PROSPECTS

Diuretics are effective antihypertensive agents in a substantial proportion of hypertensive patients. They are convenient, inexpensive, and generally well tolerated. While protecting patients from stroke, they fail to afford protection from ischemic heart disease and, possibly, from other hypertensive sequelae. This limitation, coupled with the increasing availability of agents that do not require adjunctive diuretic therapy to be successful, is reducing their role, even in those patients who respond to them.

When used, they should be used at lowest effective doses, an amount that can be found in an individual patient only by careful titration. It is possible that potassium wasting underlies the failure of diuretics to protect against ischemic heart disease; furthermore, in high-risk patients, potassium-wasting diuretics should be avoided, or potassium should be aggressively replaced. This is best accomplished by the addition of a potassium-sparing diuretic to the regimen.

Future developments in several aspects of diuretic therapy are awaited. Tests to predict diuretic sensitivity in individual patients are an important need. The possibility of producing a uricosuric diuretic has been realized, and it is hoped that agents with acceptable toxicity could be developed and made available. Spironolactone, the only potassium-sparing agent that is an effective antihypertensive agent in its own right, has endocrinological side effects that sharply limit its utility. The development of a direct aldosterone antagonist without these side effects would seem to be a realizable goal with great potential. Lastly, the discovery of atrial natriuretic factor raises the possibility of classes of diuretics with mechanisms of action unlike those of currently available diuretics (see the chapter by Atlas and Laragh, entitled "Atrial Natriuretic Factor and Its Involvement in Hypertensive Disorders," this volume). Such a diuretic, whose principal effects are on renal hemodynamics or the medullary collecting duct, may have significant advantages over current agents.

Diuretics are the oldest widely used antihypertensive therapy. Although their use is being increasingly limited, they remain valuable as antihypertensive agents. Despite their venerable status, much remains to be learned about the mechanism by which they lower blood pressure. It is unlikely that the optimal way to utilize them has yet been determined or that the optimal diuretic agents have yet been discovered.

ACKNOWLEDGMENTS

The author is grateful to Drs. Jon Blumenfeld, Gary James, and John Laragh for their helpful comments in reviewing this manuscript; he also would like to thank Margaret Blake and Elizabeth Held for their assistance. This manuscript was written while the author was supported by U.S. Public Health Service grants HL35886 and HL18323.

REFERENCES

1. Kempner W. Treatment of kidney disease and hypertensive vascular disease with rice diet. *NC Med J* 1944;5:125–133.
2. Kempner W. Treatment of hypertensive vascular disease with rice diet. *Am J Med* 1948;4:545–577.
3. Chapman CB, Gibbons TB. The diet and hypertension. *Medicine* 1950;29:29–69.
4. Megibow RS, Pollak H, Stollerman GH, Roston EH, Bookman JJ. The treatment of hypertension by accelerated sodium depletion. *J Mt Sinai Hosp NY* 1948;15:233–239.
5. Novello FC, Sprague J. Benzothiazine dioxides as novel diuretics. *J Am Chem Soc* 1957;79:2028–2029.
6. Beyer KH, Baer JE, Russo HF, Haimbach AS. Chlorothiazide (6-chloro-7-sulfamyl-1,2,4-benzothiadiazine-1,1-dioxide): enhancement of sodium chloride excretion. *Fed Proc* 1957;16:282.
7. Hollander W, Wilkins RW. Chlorothiazide: A new type of drug for the treatment of arterial hypertension. *Boston Med Q* 1957;8:69–75.
8. Wilkins RW. New drugs for hypertension with special reference to chlorothiazide. *N Engl J Med* 1957;257:1026–1030.
9. Freis ED, Wilson IM. *Med Ann District Columbia* 1957;26:468, 516.
10. Freis ED, Wanko A, Wilson IM, Parrish AE. Treatment of essential hypertension with chlorothiazide (Diuril). *JAMA* 1958;166:137–140.
11. Baum C, Kennedy DL, Knapp DE, Juergens JP, Faich GA. Prescription drug use in 1984 and changes over time. *Med Care* 1988;26:105–114.
12. Ray WA, Schaffner W, Oates JA. Therapeutic choice in the treatment of hypertension. Initial treatment of newly diagnosed hypertension and secular trends in the prescribing of antihypertensive medications for Medicaid patients. *Am J Med* 1986;81(6C):9–16.
13. Laragh JH. The proper use of the newer diuretics. *Ann Intern Med* 1967;67:606–613.
14. Goldberg M. The renal physiology of diuretics. In: Orloff J, Berliner R, eds. *Handbook of physiology, section 8: renal physiology.* Bethesda, MD: American Physiological Society, 1973;1003–1031.
15. Grantham JJ, Chonko AM. The physiological basis and clinical use of diuretics. In: Brenner BM, Stein JH, eds. *Sodium and water homeostasis.* New York: Churchill Livingstone, 1978;178–211.
16. Seldin DW, Giebisch G, eds. *The kidney: physiology and pathophysiology,* vols 1 and 2. New York: Raven Press, 1985.
17. Dirks JH, Sutton RAL, eds. *Diuretics: physiology, pharmacology and clinical use.* Philadelphia: WB Saunders, 1986.
18. Lang F, ed. Physiology of diuretic action. *Renal Physiol* 1987;10:135–220.
19. Peters G, Roch-Ramel F. Thiazide diuretics and related drugs. *Handbuch exp pharmakol* 1969;24:257–405.
20. Seely JF, Dirks JH. Site of action of diuretic drugs. *Kidney Int* 1977;11:1–8.
21. Kempson SA, Kowalski JC, Puschett JB. Direct effect of metalozone on sodium-dependent transport across the renal brush border membrane. *J Lab Clin Med* 1983;101:308–316.
22. Dirks JH, Cirksena WJ, Berliner RW. Micropuncture study of the effect of various diuretics on sodium reabsorption by the proximal tubules of the dog. *J Clin Invest* 1966;45:1875–1885.
23. Bernstein BA, Clapp JR. Micropuncture study of bicarbonate reabsorption by the dog nephron. *Am J Physiol* 1968;214:251–257.
24. Diezi J, Michoud P, Aceves J, Giebisch G. Micropuncture study of electrolyte transport across papillary collecting duct of the rat. *Am J Physiol* 1973;224:623–634.
25. Stein JH, Reineck HJ. Effect of alterations in extracellular fluid volume on segmental sodium transport. *Physiol Rev* 1975;55:124–141.
26. Stein JH, Lamiere NH, Earley LE. Renal hemodynamic factors and the regulation of sodium excretion. In: Andreoli TE, Hoffman JF, Fanestil DD, eds. *Physiology of membrane disorders.* New York: Plenum Press, 1978;739–772.
27. Greger R. Ion transport mechanisms in thick ascending limb of Henle's loop of mammalian nephron. *Physiol Rev* 1985;65:760–797.
28. Roy DR, Jamison RL. Countercurrent system and its regulation. In: Seldin DW, Giebisch G, eds. *The kidney: physiology and pathophysiology,* vol 2. New York: Raven Press, 1985;903–932.
29. Burg M, Green N. Effect of ethacrynic acid on the thick ascending limb of Henle's loop. *Kidney Int* 1973;4:301–308.

30. Greger R, Wangemann P. Loop diuretics. *Renal Physiol* 1987; 10:174–183.
31. Burg MB. Thick ascending limb of Henle's loop. *Kidney Int* 1982;22:454–464.
32. Vander AJ, Carlson J. Mechanism of the effects of furosemide on renin secretion in anesthetized dogs. *Circ Res* 1969;25:145–152.
33. Imbs JL, Schmidt M, Velly J, Schwartz J. Comparison of the effects of two groups of diuretics on renin secretion in the anesthetized dog. *Clin Sci Mol Med* 1977;52:171–182.
34. Keeton TK, Campbell WB. The pharmacologic alteration of renin release. *Pharmacol Rev* 1981;31:81–227.
35. Tisher CC, Madsen KM. Anatomy of the kidney. In: Brenner BM, Rector FC, eds. *The kidney,* vol 1. Philadelphia: WB Saunders, 1986;3–60.
36. Ratak RV, Fadem SZ, Rosenblatt SG, Lifschitz MD, Stein JH. Diuretic-induced changes in renal blood flow and prostaglandin E excretion in the dog. *Am J Physiol* 1979;236:F494–F500.
37. Rumpf KW, Frenzel S, Lowitz HD, Scheler F. The effect of indomethacin on plasma renin activity in man under normal conditions and after stimulation of the renin angiotensin system. *Prostaglandins* 1975;10:641–648.
38. Baille MD, Crosslan K, Hook JB. Natriuretic effect of furosemide after inhibition of prostaglandin synthetase. *J Pharmacol Exp Ther* 1976;199:469–476.
39. Donker AJM, Arisz L, Brentjens JRH, Van der Hem GK, Hollemans HJG. The effect of indomethacin on kidney function and plasma renin activity in man. *Nephron* 1976;17:288–296.
40. Gerber JG. Role of prostaglandins in the hemodynamic and tubular effects of furosemide. *Fed Proc* 1983;42:1707–1710.
41. Johnston GD, Hiatt WR, Nies AS, Payne NA, Murphy RC, Gerber JG. Factors modifying the early nondiuretic vascular effects of furosemide in man: the possible role of prostaglandins. *Circ Res* 1983;53:630–635.
42. Stokes JB. Sodium chloride absorption by the urinary bladder of the winter flounder: a thiazide-sensitive, electrically neutral transport system. *J Clin Invest* 1984;74:7–16.
43. Ellison DH, Velasquez H, Wright FS. Thiazide-sensitive sodium chloride cotransport in early distal tubule. *Am J Physiol* 1987; 253:F546–F554.
44. Velasquez H. Thiazide diuretics. *Renal Physiol* 1987;10:184–197.
45. Shimizu T, Yoshitori K, Nakamura M, Imai M. Site and mechanism of action of trichlormethiazide in rabbit distal nephron segments perfused *in vitro. J Clin Invest* 1988;82:721–730.
46. Jamison RL. Urine concentration and dilution. In: Brenner BM, Rector FC, eds. *The kidney,* vol 1. New York: WB Saunders, 1981;495–550.
47. Heinemann HO, Demartini FE, Laragh JH. The effect of chlorothiazide on renal excretion of electrolytes and free water. *Am J Med* 1959;26:853–861.
48. Earley LE, Kahn M, Orloff J. The effects of infusion of chlorothiazide on urinary dilution and concentration in the dog. *J Clin Invest* 1961;40:857–866.
49 Suki WN, Rector FC Jr, Seldin DW. The site of action of furosemide and other sulfonamide diuretics in the dog. *J Clin Invest* 1965;44:1458–1469.
50. Lamberg BA, Kuhlback B. Effect of chlorothiazide and hydrochlorothiazide on the excretion of calcium in the urine. *Scand J Clin Lab Invest* 1959;11:351–357.
51. Agus ZS, Chiu PJS, Goldberg M. Regulation of urinary calcium excretion in the rat. *Am J Physiol* 1977;232:F545–549.
52. Brickman AS, Massry SG, Coburn JW. Changes in serum and urinary calcium during treatment with hydrochlorothiazide: studies on mechanisms. *J Clin Invest* 1972;51:945–954.
53. Costanzo LS, Windhager EE. Calcium and sodium transport by the distal convoluted tubule of the rat. *Am J Physiol* 1978;235: F492–F506.
54. Costanzo LS. Mechanism of action of thiazide diuretics. *Semin Nephrol* 1988;8:234–241.
55. Wester PO, Dyckner T. Diuretic treatment and magnesium losses. *Acta Med Scand* 1981; Suppl 647:145–152.
56. Leary WP, Reyes AJ. Diuretic-induced magnesium losses. *Drugs* 1984;28(Suppl 1):182–187.
57. Wright FS, Giebisch G. Regulation of potassium excretion. In: Seldin DW, Giebisch G, eds. *The kidney: physiology and pathophysiology,* vol 2. New York: Raven Press, 1985;1223–1249.
58. Kokko JP, Jacobson HR. Renal chloride transport. In: Seldin DW, Giebisch G, eds. *The kidney: physiology and pathophysiology,* vol 2. New York: Raven Press, 1985;1097–1117.
59. Hierholzer K. Sodium reabsorption in the distal tubular system. In: Seldin DW, Giebisch G, eds. *The kidney: physiology and pathophysiology,* vol 2. New York: Raven Press, 1985;1063–1096.
60. Edelman IS, Marver D. Mediating events in the action of aldosterone. *J Steroid Biochem* 1979;12:219–224.
61. Edelman IS. Mechanism of action of aldosterone: energetic and permeability factors. *J Endocrinol* 1979;81:49P–53P.
62. Palmer LG, Li JH, Lindemann B, Edelman IS. Aldosterone control of the density of sodium channels in the toad urinary bladder. *J Membr Biol* 1982;64:91–102.
63. Geering K, Girardet M, Bron C, Kraehenbuhl JP, Rossier BC. Hormonal regulation of (Na^+,K^+)-ATPase biosynthesis in the toad bladder. Effect of aldosterone and 3,5,3′-triiodo-L-thyronine. *J Biol Chem* 1982;257:10338–10343.
64. Seldin DW, Rector FC Jr. The generation and maintenance of metabolic alkalosis. *Kidney Int* 1972;1:306–321.
65. Koeppen B, Giebisch G, Malnic G. Mechanism and regulation of renal tubular acidification. In: Seldin DW, Giebisch G, eds. *The kidney: physiology and pathophysiology,* vol 2. New York: Raven Press, 1985;1491–1525.
66. Tannen RL, McGill J. Influence of potassium on renal ammonia production. *Am J Physiol* 1976;231:1178–1184.
67. Welbourne TC, Francoeur D. Influence of aldosterone on renal ammonia production. *Am J Physiol* 1977;233:E56–E60.
68. DuBose TD Jr, Caflisch CR. Effect of selective aldosterone deficiency on acidification in nephron segments of the rat inner medulla. *J Clin Invest* 1988;82:1624–1632.
69. Sala G, Luetscher JA. Effect of sodium-retaining corticoid, electrocortin, desoxycorticosterone and cortisone on renal function and excretion of sodium and water in adrenalectomized rats. *Endocrinology* 1954;55:516–518.
70. Landau RL, Bergenstal DM, Lugibihe K, Kascht ME. The metabolic effect of progesterone in man. *J Clin Endocrinol* 1955;15: 1194–1215.
71. Kagawa CM, Cella JA, Van Arman CG. Action of new steroids in blocking effects of aldosterone and deoxycorticosterone on salt. *Science* 1957;126:1015–1016.
72. Fanestil DD. Mode of spironolactone action: competitive inhibition of aldosterone binding to kidney mineralocorticoid receptors. *Biochem Pharmacol* 1968;17:2240–2242.
73. Erbler HC. Stimulation of aldosterone production *in vitro* and its inhibition by spironolactone. *Arch Pharmacol* 1972;273:366–372.
74. Erbler HC. Inhibition of aldosterone production in diuretic-induced hyperaldosteronism by aldosterone antagonist canrenone in man. *Arch Pharmacol* 1974;285:395–401.
75. Corvol P, Claire M, Oblin ME, Geering K, Rossier B. Mechanism of the antimineralocorticoid effects of spironolactones. *Kidney Int* 1981;20:1–6.
76. Benos DJ. Amiloride: a molecular probe of sodium transport in tissues and cell. *Am J Physiol* 1982;242:C131–C145.
77. Shackleton CR, Wong NLM, Sutton RAL. Distal (potassium-sparing) diuretics. In: Dirks JH, Sutton RAL, eds. *Diuretics: physiology, pharmacology and clinical use.* Philadelphia: WB Saunders, 1986;117–134.
78. Horisberger J-D, Giebisch G. Potassium-sparing diuretics. *Renal Physiol* 1987;10:198–220.
79. Gabow PA, Moore S, Schrier RW. Spironolactone-induced hyperchloremic acidosis in cirrhosis. *Ann Intern Med* 1979;90: 338–340.
80. Greenblatt DJ, Koch-Weser J. Adverse reactions to spironolactone. *JAMA* 1973;225:40–43.
81. Levine DZ, Page D. Diuretic-induced acid–base disturbances. In: Dirks JH, Sutton RAL, eds. *Diuretics: physiology, pharmacology and clinical use.* Philadelphia: WB Saunders, 1986;320–340.
82. Costanzo LS. Comparison of calcium and sodium transport in early and late rat distal tubules: effect of amiloride. *Am J Physiol* 1984;246:F937–F945.
83. Costanzo LS, Weiner IM. Relationship between clearances of Ca

and Na: effect of distal diuretics and PTH. *Am J Physiol* 1976; 230:67–73.

84. Costanzo LS. Localization of diuretic action in the microperfused rat distal tubules: Ca and Na transport. *Am J Physiol* 1985;248:F527–F535.
85. Ryan MP, Ryan MF, Counihan TB. The effect of diuretics on lymphocyte magnesium and potassium. *Acta Med Scand* 1981; Suppl 647:153–161.
86. Devane J, Ryan MP. The effects of amiloride and triamterene on urinary magnesium excretion in conscious saline-loaded rats. *Br J Pharmacol* 1981;72:285–289.
87. Baba WL, Tudhope GR, Wilson GM. Triamterene, a new diuretic drug. *Br Med J* 1962;2:756–764.
88. Bull M, Laragh JH. Amiloride, a potassium sparing natriuretic agent. *Circulation* 1968;37:45–53.
89. Brooks CS, Johnson CA, Kotchen JM, Kotchen TA. Diuretic therapies in low renin and normal renin essential hypertension. *Clin Pharmacol Ther* 1978;22:14–20.
90. DeCarvalho JGR, Emery AC, Frohlich ED. Spironolactone and triamterene in volume-dependent essential hypertension. *Clin Pharmacol Ther* 1980;27:53–56.
91. Laragh JH. *Spironolactone for the treatment of hypertension or congestive heart failure: a review.* Princeton, NJ: Excerpta Medica, 1987.
92. Reineck HJ, Stein JH, Seldin DW. Integrated responses of the kidney to alterations in extracellular fluid volume. In: Seldin DW, Giebisch G, eds. *The Kidney: physiology and pathophysiology,* vol 2. New York: Raven Press, 1985;1137–1161.
93. Hebert SC, Andreoli TE. Control of NaCl transport in the thick ascending limb. *Am J Physiol* 1984;246:F745–F756.
94. Cannon PJ, Heinemann HO, Stason WB, Laragh JH. Ethacrynic acid: Effectiveness and mode of diuretic action. *Circulation* 1965;31:5–18.
95. Gantt CL, Synex JH. Observations on the mechanism of potassium excretion due to the administration of hydrochlorothiazide. *Proc Soc Exp Biol Med* 1961;106:27–28.
96. McMahon FG. *Management of essential hypertension. The new low-dose era,* 2nd edition. Mt. Kisco, NY: Futura Publishing, 1984.
97. Weinberger MH. Influence of an angiotensin converting-enzyme inhibitor on diuretic induced metabolic effects in hypertension. *Hypertension* 1983;5(Suppl III):132–138.
98. Good DW, Wright FS. Luminal influences on potassium secretion: sodium concentration and flow rate. *Am J Physiol* 1979; 236:F192–F205.
99. Bargman JM, Jamison RL. Disorders of potassium homeostasis. In: Dirks JH, Sutton RAL, eds. *Diuretics: physiology, Pharmacology and clinical use.* Philadelphia: WB Saunders, 1986;296–319.
100. Young DB. Qualitative analysis of aldosterone's role in potassium regulation. *Am J Physiol* 1988;255:F811–F822.
101. Davis JO, Urquhart J, Higgins JT. The effects of alterations of plasma sodium and potassium concentration on aldosterone secretion. *J Clin Invest* 1963;42:597–609.
102. Laragh JH, Sealey JE. The renin angiotensin aldosterone hormonal system and regulation of sodium, potassium and blood pressure homeostasis. In: Orloff J, Berliner R, eds. *Handbook of physiology, section 8: renal physiology.* Bethesda, MD: American Physiological Society, 1973;831–908.
103. Cannon PJ, Heinemann HO, Albert MS, Laragh JH, Winters RW. "Contraction" alkalosis after diuresis of edematous patients with ethacrynic acid. *Ann Intern Med* 1965;62:979–990.
104. Garella S, Chang BS, Kahn SI. Dilution acidosis and contraction alkalosis: review of a concept. *Kidney Int* 1975;8:279–283.
105. Emmett M, Seldin DW. Clinical syndromes of metabolic acidosis and metabolic alkalosis. In: Seldin DW, Giebisch G, eds. *The kidney: physiology and pathophysiology,* vol 2. New York: Raven Press, 1985;1567–1639.
106. Cohen JJ. Correction of metabolic alkalosis by the kidney after isometric expansion of extracellular fluid. *J Clin Invest* 1968;47: 1181–1192.
107. Bichara M, Paillard M, Carman B, DeRouffignac C, Leviel F. Volume expansion modulates $NaHCO_3$ and NaCl transport in the proximal tubule and Henle's loop. *Am J Physiol* 1984;247: F140–F150.
108. Cogan MG, Liv F-Y. Metabolic alkalosis in the rat. *J Clin Invest* 1983;71:1941–1960.
109. Hropot M, Fowler N, Karlmark B, Geibisch G. Tubular action of diuretics: Distal effects on electrolyte transport and acidification. *Kidney Int* 1985;28:477–489.
110. Fichman MP, Vorherr H, Kleeman CR, Telfer N. Diuretic-induced hyponatremia. *Ann Intern Med* 1971;75:853–863.
111. Ashraf N, Locksley R, Arieff AI. Thiazide-induced hyponatremia associated with death or neurologic damage in outpatients. *Am J Med* 1981;70:1163–1168.
112. Szatalowicz VL, Miller PD, Lacher JW, Gordon JA, Schrier RW. Comparative effect of diuretics on renal water excretion in hyponatremic edematous disorders. *Clin Sci* 1982;62:235–238.
113. Ashouri OS. Severe diuretic-induced hyponatremia in the elderly. A series of eight patients. *Arch Intern Med* 1986;146: 1355–1357.
114. Lant A. Diuretic drugs. *Drugs* 1986;31(Suppl 4):40–55.
115. Wilhelmson CE, Vedin JA, Moerlin C, Lund-Johansen P, Vorburger C, Enenkel W, Lutterbeck PM, Bolognese J, Cirillo VJ, Tempero KF. A double-blind comparison of a novel indanone diuretic (MK-196) with hydrochlorothiazide in the treatment of essential hypertension. *Br J Clin Pharmacol* 1979;8:261–266.
116. Stote RM, Dubb JW, Familiar RG, Alexander F. Ticrynafen: a uricosuric antihypertensive diuretic. *Clin Pharmacol Ther* 1978; 23:456–460.
117. Blaine EH, Fanelli GM, Irvin JD, Tobert JA, Davies RO. Enantiomers of indacrinone: a new approach to producing an isouricemic diuretic. *Clin Exp Hypertens [A]* 1982;4:161–176.
118. Breslau N, Moses AM, Weiner IM. The role of volume contraction in the hypocalciuric action of chlorothiazide. *Kidney Int* 1976;10:164–170.
119. Alfrey AC. Disorders of magnesium metabolism. In: Seldin DW, Giebisch G, eds. *The kidney: physiology and pathophysiology,* vol 2. New York: Raven Press, 1985;1281–1295.
120. Beermann B, Groschinsky-Grind M. Clinical pharmacokinetics of diuretics. *Clin Pharmacokinet* 1980;5:221–245.
121. Lant A. Diuretics: clinical pharmacology and therapeutic use. *Drugs* 1985;29:57–87,162–188.
122. Brater DC. Pharmacodynamic considerations in the use of diuretics. *Annu Rev Pharmacol Toxicol* 1983;23:45–62.
123. Brater DC. Resistance to loop diuretics: why it happens and what to do about it. *Drugs* 1985;30:427–443.
124. Kelly MR, Cutler CE, Forrey AW, Kimpel BM. Pharmacokinetics of orally administered furosemide. *Clin Pharmacol Ther* 1974;15:178–186.
125. Wilcox CS, Mitch WE, Kelly RA, Skorecki K, Meyer TW, Friedman PA, Souney PF. Response of the kidney to furosemide. I. Effects of salt intake and renal compensation. *J Lab Clin Med* 1983;102:450–458.
126. Kelly RA, Wilcox CS, Mitch WE, Meyer TW, Souney PF, Rayment CM, Friedman PA, Swartz SL. Response of the kidney to furosemide. II. Effect of captopril on sodium balance. *Kidney Int* 1983;24:233–239.
127. Welling PG, Barbhaiya RH. Influence of food and fluid volume on chlorothiazide bioavailability: comparison of plasma and urinary excretion methods. *J Pharm Sci* 1982;71:32–35.
128. Beermann B, Groschinsky-Grind M. Enhancement of the gastrointestinal absorption of hydrochlorothiazide by propantheline. *Eur J Clin Pharmacol* 1978;13:385–387.
129. Beermann B, Groschinsky-Grind M, Lindstrom B. Effect of food on the bioavailability of bendroflumethiazide. *Acta Med Scand* 1978;204:291–293.
130. Schmid E, Fricke G. Studies on urinary excretion of the potassium-retaining diuretic amiloride (desmethyl-pipazuroyl-guanidine, MK 870) in man. *Pharmacol Clin* 1969;1:110–113.
131. Melander A, Danielson K, Schersten B, Thulin T, Wahlin E. Enhancement by food of canrenone bioavailability from spironolactone. *Clin Pharmacol Ther* 1977;22:100–103.
132. Karim A. Spironolactone: Disposition, metabolism, pharmacodynamics, and bioavailability. *Drug Metab Rev* 1978;8:151–188.
133. Tobian L. Why do diuretics lower blood pressure in essential hypertension? *Annu Rev Pharmacol* 1967;7:399–408.
134. Dollery CT, Harington M, Kaufmann G. The mode of action of chlorothiazide in hypertension: with special reference to potentiation of ganglion-blocking drugs. *Lancet* 1959;1:1215–1218.

135. Wilson IM, Freis IM. Relationship between plasma and extracellular fluid volume depletion and the antihypertensive effect of chlorothiazide. *Circulation* 1959;20:1028–1036.
136. Frohlich ED, Schnaper HW, Wilson IM, Freis ED. Hemodynamic alterations in hypertensive patients due to chlorothiazide. *N Engl J Med* 1960;262:1261–1263.
137. Shah S, Khatri I, Freis ED. Mechanism of antihypertensive effect of thiazide diuretics. *Am Heart J* 1978;95:611–618.
138. van Brummelen P, Man in't Veld AJ, Schalekamp MADH. Hemodynamic changes during long-term thiazide treatment of essential hypertension in responders and nonresponders. *Clin Pharmacol Ther* 1980;27:328–336.
139. Villarreal H, Exaire JE, Revollo A, Soni J. Effects of chlorothiazide on systemic hemodynamics in essential hypertension. *Circulation* 1962;26:405–408.
140. Conway J, Lauwers P. Hemodynamic and hypotensive effects of long-term therapy with chlorothiazide. *Circulation* 1960;21:21–27
141. Gifford RW, Mattox VR, Orvis AL, Stones DA, Rosevear JW. Effect of thiazide diuretics on plasma volume, body electrolytes, and excretion of aldosterone in hypertension. *Circulation* 1961; 24 1197–1205.
142. Lund-Johansen P. Hemodynamic changes in long-term diuretic therapy of essential hypertension. *Acta Med Scand* 1970;187: 509–518.
143. de Carvalho JGR, Dunn FG, Lohmoller G, Frohlich ED. Hemodynamic correlates of prolonged thiazide therapy: comparison of responders and nonresponders. *Clin Pharmacol Ther* 1978;22: 875–880.
144. Winer BM. The antihypertensive actions of benzothiadizenes. *Circulation* 1961;23:211–218.
145. Hansen J. Hydrochlorothiazide in the treatment of hypertension. *Acta Med Scand* 1968;183:317–321.
146. Leth A. Changes in plasma and extracellular fluid volumes in patients with essential hypertension during long-term treatment with hydrochlorothiazide. *Circulation* 1970;42:479–485.
147. Tarazi RC, Dustan HP, Frohlich ED. Long-term thiazide therapy in essential hypertension. *Circulation* 1970;709–717.
148. Ibsen H, Leth A, Hollnagel H, Kappelgaard AM, Damkjaer Nielsen M, Christensen NJ, Giese J. Renin–angiotensin system in mild hypertension: the functional significance of angiotensin II in untreated and thiazide-treated hypertensive patients. *Acta Med Scand* 1979;205:547–555.
149. Feldschuh J, Enson Y. Prediction of the normal blood volume: relation of blood volume to body habitus. *Circulation* 1976;56: 605–612.
150. Webster J, Dollery CT, Hensby CN, Friedman LA. Antihypertensive action of bendroflumethiazide: increased prostacyclin production? *Clin Pharmacol Ther* 1980;28:751–758.
151. O'Connor DT, Preston RA, Mitas JA II, Frigon RP, Stone RA. Urinary kallikrein activity and renal vascular resistance in the antihypertensive response to thiazide diuretics. *Hypertension* 1981;3:139–147.
152. Freis ED, Reda DJ, Materson BJ. Volume (weight) loss and blood pressure response following thiazide diuretics. *Hypertension* 1988;12:244–250.
153. Freis ED, Wanko A, Wilson IM, Parish AE. Chlorothiazide in hypertensive and normotensive patients. *Ann NY Acad Sci* 1958;71:450–455.
154. Winer BM. The antihypertensive mechanism of salt depletion induced by hydrochlorothiazide. *Circulation* 1961;24:788–796.
155. Parijs J, Joosens JV, Van der Linden L, Verstrecken G, Amery AK. Moderate sodium restriction and diuretics in the treatment of hypertension. *Am Heart J* 1973;85:22–34.
156. Ram CVS, Garrett BN, Kaplan NM. Moderate sodium restriction and various diuretics in the treatment of hypertension: effects of potassium wastage and blood pressure control. *Arch Intern Med* 1981;141:1015–1019.
157. Case DB, Pickering TG, Laragh JH. High sodium intake prevents adverse metabolic effects of diuretic treatment without reversing antihypertensive effect. *Clin Res* 1984;32:329A.
158. Weber MA, Drayer JI, Rev A, Laragh JH. Disparate patterns of aldosterone response during diuretic treatment of hypertension. *Ann Intern Med* 1977;87:558–563.
159. Murphy RJF. The effect of "rice diet" on plasma volume and extracellular fluid space in hypertensive subjects. *J Clin Invest* 1950;29:912–917.
160. Beard TC, Cooke HM, Gray WR, Barge R. Randomized trial of a no-added sodium diet for mild hypertension. *Lancet* 1982;2: 455–458.
161. Laragh JH, Pecker MS. Dietary sodium and hypertension. *Ann Intern Med* 1983;77:1297–1305.
162. Mironneau J, Savineau J-P, Mironneau C. Compared effects of indapamide, hydrochlorothiazide and chlorthalidone on electrical and mechanical activities in vascular smooth muscle. *Eur J Pharmacol* 1981;75:109–113.
163. Cantiello H, Copello J, Muller A, Mikulic L, Villami MF. Effect of bumetanide on potassium transport and ionic composition of the arterial wall. *Am J Physiol* 1986;251:F537–F546.
164. Haddy FJ, Pamnani MB, Swindall BT, Johnston J, Cragoe EJ. Sodium channel blockers are vasodilators as well as natriuretic and diuretic agents. *Hypertension* 1985;7(Suppl I):I-121–I-126.
165. van Breemen C, Aaronson P, Loutzenhiser R. Sodium–calcium interactions in mammalian smooth muscle. *Pharmacol Rev* 1979;30:167–208.
166. Chaffman M, Heel RC, Brogden RN, Speight TM, Avery GS. Indapamide: a review of its pharmacodynamic properties and therapeutic efficacy in hypertension. *Drugs* 1984;28:189–235.
167. Bennett WM, McDonald WJ, Kuehnel E, Hartnett MN, Porter GA. Do diuretics have antihypertensive properties independent of natriuresis? *Clin Pharmacol Ther* 1977;22:499–504.
168. Orgison JL. Failure of chlorothiazide to influence tissue electrolytes in hypertensive and non-hypertensive nephrectomized dogs. *Proc Soc Exp Biol Med* 1962;110:161–164.
169. Leth A, Ibsen H. Changes in the ratio of plasma to interstitial fluid volume during long-term antihypertensive therapy. *J Lab Clin Med* 1976;87:781–791.
170. Dunn MJ, Tannen RL. Low renin hypertension. *Kidney Int* 1974;5:317–325.
171. Dole VP, Dahl LK, Cotzias GC, Elder HA, Krebs ME. Dietary treatment of hypertension. Clinical and metabolic studies of patients on the rice–fruit diet. *J Clin Invest* 1950;1189–1206.
172. Dahl LK, Stahl BG, Cotzias GC. Metabolic effects of marked sodium restriction in hypertensive patients: changes in total exchangeable sodium and potassium. *J Clin Invest* 1954;33:1397–1406.
173. Wilkins RW, Hollander W, Chobanian AV. Chlorothiazide in hypertension. Studies on its mode of action. *Ann NY Acad Sci* 1958;71:465–472.
174. Vaughan ED Jr, Carey RM, Peach MJ, Ackerley JA, Ayers CR. The renin response to diuretic therapy: a limitation of antihypertensive potential. *Circ Res* 1978;42:376–381.
175. Anderson GH, Dalakos TG, Elias A, Tomycz N, Streeten DHP. Diuretic therapy and response of essential hypertension to saralasin. *Ann Intern Med* 1977;87:183–187.
176. Leonetti G, Terzoli L, Sala C, Bianchetti C, Sernesi L, Zanchetti A. Relationship between the hypotensive and renin-stimulating actions of diuretic therapy in hypertensive patients. *Clin Sci Mol Med* 1978;55:307s–309s.
177. Gavras H, Brunner HR, Laragh JH, Sealey JE, Gavras I, Vukovitch RA. A converting enzyme inhibitor to identify and treat vasoconstrictor and volume factors in hypertension. *N Engl J Med* 1974;291:817–821.
178. Redgrave J, Rabinowe S, Hollenberg NK, Williams GH. Correction of abnormal renal blood flow response to angiotensin II by converting enzyme inhibition in essential hypertensives. *J Clin Invest* 1985;75:1285–1290.
179. Kaplan NM. *Clinical hypertension,* 3rd edition. Baltimore: Williams and Wilkins, 1982;318.
180. Spark RF, Melby JC. Hypertension and low plasma renin activity: evidence for mineralocorticoid excess. *Ann Intern Med* 1971;75:831–836.
181. Crane MG, Harris JJ, Johns VJ Jr. Hyporeninemic hypertension. *Am J Med* 1972;52:457–466.
182. Carey RM, Douglas JG, Schweikert JR, Liddle GW. The syndrome of essential hypertension and suppressed plasma renin activity: normalization of blood pressure with spironolactone. *Arch Intern Med* 1972;130:849–854.
183. Adlin EV, Marks AD, Channick BJ. Spironolactone and hydro-

chlorothiazide in essential hypertension: blood pressure response and plasma renin activity. *Arch Intern Med* 1972; 130:855–858.
184. Vaughan ED, Laragh JH, Gavras I, Buhler FR, Gavras H, Brunner HR, Baer L. Volume factors in low and normal renin essential hypertension. *Am J Cardiol* 1973;32:523–532.
185. Castenfors J, Johnsson H, Oro L. Effect of alprenolol on blood pressure and plasma renin activity in hypertensive patients. *Acta Med Scand* 1973;193:189–195.
186. Douglas JG, Hollifield JW, Liddle GW. Treatment of low-renin essential hypertension: comparison of spironolactone and a hydrochlorothiazide–triamterene combination. *JAMA* 1974;227: 518–521.
187. Karlberg BE, Kagedal B, Tegler L, Tolagen K, Bergman B. Controlled treatment of primary hypertension with propranolol and spironolactone: a crossover study with special reference to initial plasma renin activity. *Am J Cardiol* 1973;37:642–649.
188. MacGregor GA, Dawes P. Antihypertensive effect of propranolol and spironolactone in relation to plasma angiotensin II. *Clin Sci Mol Med* 1976;51:193s–196s.
189. Sealey JE, Blumenfeld JD, Bell GM, Pecker MS, Sommers SC, Laragh JH. On the renal basis for essential hypertension: nephron heterogeneity with discordant renin secretion causing a hypertensive vasoconstriction–volume relationship. *J Hypertens* 1988;6:763–777.
190. Brenner BM, Garcia DL, Anderson S. Glomeruli and blood pressure: less of one, more the other? *Am J Hypertens* 1988;1: 335–347.
191. Tobian L, Coffee K. Effect of thiazide drugs on renovascular hypertension in contrast to their effect on essential hypertension. *Proc Soc Exp Biol Med* 1964;115:196–198.
192. Baer L, Parra-Carrillo JZ, Radichevich I, Williams GS. Detection of renovascular hypertension with angiotensin II blockade. *Ann Intern Med* 1977;86:257–260.
193. Hollenberg NK. Medical therapy for renovascular hypertension: a review. *Am J Hypertens* 1988;1:338s–343s.
194. Sealey JE. Measurement of the hormones of the renin system in hypertensive patients. *Clin Biochem* 1981;14:273–281.
195. Williams GH, Hollenberg NK, Braley LM. Influence of sodium intake on vascular and adrenal angiotensin II receptors. *Endocrinology* 1976;98:1343–1350.
196. Aleksandrow D, Wysnacka W, Gajewski J. Influence of chlorothiazide upon arterial responsiveness to nor-epinephrine In hypertensive subjects. *N Engl J Med* 1959;261:1052–1055.
197. Freis ED, Wanko A, Schnaper HW, Frohlich ED. Mechanism of the altered blood pressure responsiveness produced by chlorothiazide. *J Clin Invest* 1960;39:1277–1281.
198. Zsoter TT, Hart F, Radde IC. Mechanism of antihypertensive action of prolonged administration of hydrochlorothiazide in rabbit and dog. *Circ Res* 1970;27:717–725.
199. Weidmann P, Beretta-Piccoli C, Meier A, Keusch G, Gluck Z, Ziegler WH. Antihypertensive mechanism of diuretic treatment with chlorthalidone: complementary roles of sympathetic axis and sodium. *Kidney Int* 1983;23:320–326.
200. Preziosi P, De Schaepdryver AF, Marmo E, Miele E. On the mechanism of the antihypertensive effect of hydrochlorothiazide. *Arch Int Pharmacodyn* 1961;131:209–229.
201. Lake CR, Ziegler MG, Coleman MD, Kopin IJ. Hydrochlorothiazide-induced sympathetic hyperactivity in hypertensive patients. *Clin Pharmacol Ther* 1979;26:428–432.
202. Aoki VS, Brody MJ. The effect of thiazide on the sympathetic nervous system of hypertensive rats. *Arch Int Pharmacodyn* 1969;177:423–434.
203. Dustan HP, Cumming GR, Corcoran AC, Page IH. A mechanism of chlorothiazide enhanced effectiveness of antihypertensive ganglioplegic drugs. *Circulation* 1959;19:360–365.
204. Dustan HP, Tarazi RC, Bravo EL. Dependence of arterial pressure on intravascular volume in treated hypertensive patients. *N Engl J Med* 1972;286:861–866.
205. Carreta R, Fabris B, Bellini G, Tonutti L, Battilana G, Bianchetti A, Campanacci L. Baroreflex function after therapy withdrawal in patients with essential hypertension. *Clin Sci* 1983;64:259–263.
206. Webster J, Dollery CT, Hensby CN, Friedman LA. Antihypertensive action of bendroflumethiazide: increased prostacyclin production? *Clin Pharmacol Ther* 1980;28:751–758.
207. Erne P, Bolli P, Burgisser E, Buhler FR. Correlation of platelet calcium with blood pressure—effect of antihypertensive therapy. *N Engl J Med* 1984;310:1084–1088.
208. Tobian L. Hypertension and the kidney. *Arch Intern Med* 1974; 133:959–967.
209. Guyton AC, Coleman TG, Cowley AW, Manning RD Jr, Norman RA, Ferguson JD. A systems analysis approach to understanding long-range arterial blood pressure control and hypertension. *Circ Res* 1974;35:159–176.
210. Haddy FJ, Overbeck JW. The role of humoral factors in volume expanded hypertension. *Life Sci* 1976;19:935–948.
211. Blaustein M. Sodium ions, calcium ions, blood pressure regulation, and hypertension: a reassessment and a hypothesis. *Am J Physiol* 1977;232:C165–C173.
212. MacGregor GA, de Wardener HE. Is a circulating sodium transport inhibitor involved in the pathogenesis of essential hypertension? *Clin Exp Hypertens* 1981;3:815–830.
213. Veteran's Administration Cooperative Study Group on Antihypertensive Agents. Effects of treatment on morbidity in hypertension: results in patients with diastolic blood pressures averaging 115 through 129 mmHg. *JAMA* 1967;202:1028–1034.
214. Veteran's Administration Cooperative Study Group on Antihypertensive Agents. Effects of treatment on morbidity in hypertension. II. Results in patients with diastolic blood pressures averaging 90 through 114 mmHg. *JAMA* 1970;213:1143–1152.
215. Smith WM. Treatment of mild hypertension: results of a ten-year intervention trial—U.S. Public Health Service Hospitals Cooperative Study Group. *Circ Res* 1977;40(Suppl I):I-98–I-105.
216. Hypertension Detection and Follow-up Program Cooperative Group. The effect of treatment on mortality in "mild" hypertension. *N Engl J Med* 1982;307:976–980.
217. The Management Committee. The Australian therapeutic trial in mild hypertension. *Lancet* 1980;1:1261–1269.
218. Helgeland A. Treatment of mild hypertension: a five-year controlled drug trial: the Oslo study. *Am J Med* 1980;69:725–732.
219. Multiple Risk Factor Intervention Trial Research Group. Multiple Risk Factor Intervention Trial: risk factor changes and mortality results. *JAMA* 1982;248:1465–1477.
220. Medical Research Council Working Party. MRC trial of treatment of mild hypertension: principal results. *Br Med J* 1985; 291:97–104.
221. Veterans Administration Cooperative Study Group on Antihypertensive Agents. Efficacy of nadolol alone and combined with bendroflumethiazide and hydralazine for systemic hypertension. *Am J Cardiol* 1983;52:1230–1237.
222. Veterans Administration Cooperative Study Group on Antihypertensive Agents. Comparison of propranolol and hydrochlorothiazide for the initial treatment of hypertension. I. Results of short-term titration with emphasis on racial differences in response. *JAMA* 1982;248:1996–2003.
223. Moser M, Lunn J. Responses to captopril and hydrochlorothiazide in black patients with hypertension. *Clin Pharmacol Ther* 1982;32:302–307.
224. Meserli FH, Sundgaard-Riise K, Reisin E, Dreslinski G, Dunn FG, Frohlich ED. Disparate cardiovascular effects of obesity and cardiovascular hypertension. *Am J Med* 1983;74:808–812.
225. Multiple Risk Factor Intervention Trial Research Group. Baseline resting electrocardiographic abnormalities, antihypertensive treatment, and mortality in the Multiple Risk Factor Intervention Trial. *Am J Cardiol* 1985;55:1–15.
226. Kannel WB, Cupples LA, D'Agostino RB, Stokes J III. Hypertension, antihypertensive treatment, and sudden coronary death: the Framingham study. *Hypertension* 1988;11(Suppl II):II-45–II-50.
227. Kannel WB. Prevalence and natural history of electrocardiographic left ventricular hypertrophy. *Am J Med* 1983;75(Suppl 3A):4–11.
228. Tarazi RC. Regression of left ventricular hypertrophy by medical treatment: present status and possible implications. *Am J Med* 1983;75(Suppl 3A):80–86.
229. Drayer JIM. Does left ventricular mass decrease during antihypertensive therapy? *Arch Intern Med* 1985;145:1583–1584.
230. Reichek N, Franklin BB, Chandler T, Muhammed A, Plappert T, St. John Sutton M. Reversal of left ventricular hypertrophy by

antihypertensive therapy. *Eur Heart J* 1982;3(Suppl A):165–169.
231. Anderson S, Rennke HG, Brenner BM. Therapeutic advantage of converting enzyme inhibitors in arresting progressive renal disease associated with systemic hypertension in the rat. *J Clin Invest* 1986;77:1993–2000.
232. Yoshiola T, Shiraga H, Yoshida Y, Fogo A, Glick AD, Deen WM, Hoyer JR, Ichikawa I. "Intact nephrons" as the primary origin of proteinuria in chronic renal disease: study in the rat model of subtotal nephrectomy. *J Clin Invest* 1988;1614–1623.
233. Frishman WH, Furberg CD, Friedewald WT. Beta-adrenergic blockade for survivors of acute myocardial infarction. *N Engl J Med* 1984;310:830–837.
234. Wikstrand J, Warnold I, Olsson G, Tuomilehto J, Elmfeldt D, Berglund G. Primary prevention with metoprolol in patients with hypertension: mortality results from the MAPHY study. *JAMA* 1988;259:1976–1982.
235. Morgan DB, Davidson C. Hypokalemia and diuretics: an analysis of publications. *Br Med J* 1980;280:905–908.
236. Wilkinson PR, Issler H, Hesp R, Raftery RE. Total body and serum potassium during prolonged thiazide therapy for essential hypertension. *Lancet* 1975;1:759–762.
237. Maronde RF, Milgrom M, Vlachakis ND, Chan L. Response of hydrochlorothiazide-induced hypokalemia to amiloride. *JAMA* 1983;249:237–241.
238. Ridgeway NA, Ginn DR, Alley K. Outpatient conversion of treatment to potassium-sparing diuretics. *Am J Med* 1986;80:785–788.
239. Rose BD, Turka LA. Diuretics. In: Kaplan NM, Brenner BM, Laragh JH, eds. *The kidney in hypertension.* New York: Raven Press, 1987;179–196.
240. Friedman E, Shadel M, Halkin H, Farfel Z. Thiazide-induced hyponatremia: reproducibility by single dose rechallenge and an analysis of pathogenesis. *Ann Intern Med* 1989;110:24–30.
241. Shannon RP, Wei JY, Rosa RM, Epstein F, Rowe JW. The effect of age and sodium depletion on cardiovascular response to orthostasis. *Hypertension* 1986;8:438–443.
242. Kennedy RM, Earley LE. Profound hyponatremia resulting from a thiazide-induced decrease in urinary diluting capacity in a patient with polydipsia. *N Engl J Med* 1970;282:1185–1186.
243. Ledingham JG, Crowe MS, Forsling ML, Phillips ML, Phillips PA, Rolls BJ. Effects of aging on vasopressin secretion, water excretion and thirst in man. *Kidney Int* 1987;Suppl:S90–S92.
244. Talso PJ, Carabello AJ. Effects of benzothiadiazines on serum and total body electrolytes. *Ann NY Acad Sci* 1960;88:822–840.
245. Edmonds CJ, Jasani B. Total body potassium in hypertensive patients during prolonged diuretic therapy. *Lancet* 1972;2:8–12.
246. Leemhuis MP, van Damme KJ, Struyvenberg A. Effects of chlorthalidone on serum and total body potassium in hypertensive patients. *Acta Med Scand* 1976;200:37–45.
247. Beevers DG, Hamilton M, Harpur JE. The long-term treatment of hypertension with thiazide diuretics. *Postgrad Med J* 1971;539–643.
248. Medical Research Council Working Party on Mild to Moderate Hypertension. Adverse reactions to bendrofluazide and propranolol for the treatment of mild hypertension. *Lancet* 1981;2:539–542.
249. Veterans Administration Cooperative Study on Antihypertensive Agents. Double blind control study of antihypertensive agents. III. Chlorothiazide alone and in combination with other agents; preliminary results. *Arch Intern Med* 1962;110:230–236.
250. Sandor FF, Pickens PT, Crallan J. Variations of plasma potassium concentrations during long-term treatment of hypertension with diuretics without potassium supplements. *Br Med J* 1982;284:711–715.
251. Abdulla M, Norden A, Jagerstad M. Dietary intake of potassium in the elderly. *Lancet* 1975;2:562.
252. Kaplan NM. Hypokalemia in the hypertensive patient: with observations on the incidence of primary aldosteronism. *Ann Intern Med* 1967;66:1079–1090.
253. Harrington JT, Isner JM, Kassirer JP. Our national obsession with potassium. *Am J Med* 1982;73:155–159.
254. Holland OB, Nixon JV, Kuhnert L. Diuretic-induced ventricular ectopic activity. *Am J Med* 1981;70:762–768.
255. Hollifield JW, Slaton PE. Thiazide diuretics, hypokalemia, and cardiac arrhythmia. *Acta Med Scand* 1981; Suppl 647:67–73.
256. Nordrehaug JE. Malignant arrhythmias in relation to serum potassium values in patients with acute myocardial infarction. *Acta Med Scand* 1981; Suppl 647:101–108.
257. Medical Research Council Working Party on Mild to Moderate Hypertension. Ventricular extra-systoles during thiazide treatment: substudy of MRC mild hypertension trial. *Br Med J* 1983;287:1249–1253.
258. Madias JE, Madias NE, Gavras HP. Nonarrhythmogenicity of diuretic-induced hypokalemia. Its evidence in patients with uncomplicated hypertension. *Arch Intern Med* 1984;144:2171–2176.
259. Struthers AD, Whitesmith R, Reid JL. Prior thiazide diuretic treatment increases adrenaline-induced hypokalemia. *Lancet* 1983;1:1358–1360.
260. Brown MJ, Brown DC, Murphy MB. Hypokalemia from beta-receptor stimulation of circulating epinephrine. *N Engl J Med* 1983;309:1414–1419.
261. Clausen T, Flatman JA. $Beta_2$-adrenoceptors mediate the stimulating effect of adrenaline on active electrogenic Na–K transport in rat soleus muscle. *Br J Pharmacol* 1980;68:749–755.
262. Nordrehaug JE, Johannessen KA, von der Lippe G. Serum potassium concentration as a risk factor of ventricular arrhythmias early in acute myocardial infarction. *Circulation* 1985;71:645–649.
263. Araoye MA, Chang MY, Khatri IM, Freis ED. Furosemide compared with hydrochlorothiazide. Long-term treatment of hypertension. *JAMA* 1978;240:1863–1866.
264. Holland OB, Gomez-Sanchez CE, Kuhnert L, Poindexter C, Pak CY. Antihypertensive comparison of furosemide with hydrochlorothiazide for black patients. *Arch Intern Med* 1979;139:1015–1021.
265. Magee PFA, Freis ED. Is low-dose hydrochlorothiazide effective? *Hypertension* 1986;8(Suppl II):II-135–II-139.
266. Materson BJ, Oster JR, Michael UF, Bolton SM, Burton ZC, Stambaugh JE, Morledge J. Dose response to chlorthalidone in patients with mild hypertension: efficacy of a lower dose. *Clin Pharmacol Ther* 1978;24:192–198.
267. Edmonds CJ, Wilson GM. The action of hydroflumethiazide in relation to adrenal steroids and potassium loss. *Lancet* 1960;1:505–509.
268. Landmann-Suter R, Struyvenberg A. Initial potassium loss and hypokalemia during chlorthalidone administration in patients with essential hypertension. *Eur J Clin Invest* 1978;8:155–164.
269. Brunner HR, Laragh JH, Baer L, Newton MA, Goodwin FT, Krakoff LR, Bard RH, Buhler FR. Essential hypertension: renin and aldosterone, heart attack and stroke. *N Engl J Med* 1972;286:441–449.
270. Delkers W, Brown JJ, Fraser R, Lever AF, Morton JJ, Robertson JIS. Sensitization of the adrenal cortex to angiotensin II in sodium deplete man. *Circ Res* 1974;34:69–77.
271. Dyckner T, Wester PO. *Diuretic treatment and magnesium losses in electrolytes and cardiac arrhythmias.* Royal Society of Medicine International Symposium Series, 1981;145–152.
272. Cohen L, Kitzes R. Magnesium sulfate and digitalis—toxic arrhythmias. *JAMA* 1983;249:2808–2810.
273. Shils MF. Experimental human magnesium depletion. *Medicine* 1969;48:61–85.
274. Dyckner T, Wester PO. Ventricular extrasystoles and intracellular electrolytes before and after potassium and magnesium infusions in patients on diuretic treatment. *Am Heart J* 1979;97:12–28.
275. Heidenreich O. Mode of action of conventional and potassium-sparing diuretics—aspects with relevance to Mg-sparing effects. *Magnesium* 1984;3:248–256.
276. Ryan MP. Magnesium and potassium-sparing diuretics. *Magnesium* 1986;5:282–292.
277. Christensson T, Hellstrom K, Wengle B. Hypercalcemia and primary hyperparathyroidism: prevalence in patients receiving thiazides as detected in a health screen. *Arch Intern Med* 1977;137:1138–1142.
278. Dawson KG, Sutton RAL. Metabolic disorders. In: Dirks JH, Sutton RAL, eds. *Diuretics: physiology, pharmacology and clinical use.* Philadelphia: WB Saunders, 1986;341–361.

279. Popovtzer MM, Subryan VL, Alfrey AC, Reeve EB, Schrier RW. The acute effect of chlorothiazide on serum ionized calcium. Evidence for a parathyroid hormone-dependent mechanism. *J Clin Invest* 1975;55:1295–1302.
280. Koppel MH, Massry SG, Shinaberger JH, Hartenbower DL, Coburn JW. Thiazide-induced rise in serum calcium and magnesium in patients on maintenance hemodialysis. *Ann Intern Med* 1970;72:895–901.
281. Murphy MB, Lewis PJ, Kohner E, Schumer B, Dollery CT. Glucose intolerance in hypertensive patients treated with diuretics; a 14-year follow-up. *Lancet* 1982;2:1293–1295.
282. Bengtsson C, Blohme G, Lapidus L, Lindquist O, Lundgren H, Nystrom E, Petersen K, Sigurdsson JA. Do antihypertensive drugs precipitate diabetes? *Br Med J* 1984;289:1495–1497.
283. Ames RP, Hill P. Improvement of glucose tolerance and lowering of glycohemoglobin and serum lipid concentrations after discontinuation of diuretic therapy. *Circulation* 1982;65:899–904.
284. Dornhorst A, Powell SH, Pensky J. Aggravation by propranolol of hyperglycemic effect of hydrochlorothiazide in type II diabetics without alteration of insulin secretion. *Lancet* 1985;1:123–126.
285. Helderman JH, Elahi D, Andersen DK, Raizes GS, Tobin JD, Shocken D, Andres R. Prevention of the glucose intolerance of thiazide diuretics by maintenance of body potassium. *Diabetes* 1983;32:106–111.
286. Rapaport MI, Hurd HF. Thiazide-induced glucose intolerance treated with potassium. *Arch Intern Med* 1964;113:405–408.
287. Gorden P. Glucose intolerance with hypokalemia. *Diabetes* 1973;22:544–551.
288. Fonseca V, Phear DN. Hyperosmolar non-ketotic diabetic syndrome precipitated by treatment with diuretics. *Br Med J* 1982;284:36–37.
289. Gerich JE, Martin MM, Recant L. Clinical and metabolic characteristics of hyperosmolar non-ketotic coma. *Diabetes* 1971;20:228–238.
290. Schoenfield MF, Goldberger E. Hypercholesterolemia induced by thiazides: a pilot study. *Br Thr Res* 1964;6:180–184.
291. Ames RP, Hill P. Elevation of serum lipid levels during diuretic therapy of hypertension. *Am J Med* 1976;61:748–757.
292. Grimm RH, Leon AS, Hunninghake DB, Lenz K, Hannan P, Blackburn H. Effects of thiazide diuretics on plasma lipids and lipoproteins in mildly hypertensive men. A double-blind controlled trial. *Ann Intern Med* 1981;94:7–11.
293. Weidmann P, Gerber A, Mordasini R. Effects of antihypertensive therapy on serum lipoproteins. *Hypertension* 1983;5(Suppl III):III-120–III-131.
294. Weinberger MH. Antihypertensive therapy and lipids: paradoxical influences on cardiovascular risk. *Am J Med* 1986;80(Suppl 2A):64–70.
295. Boehringer K, Weidmann P, Mordasini R, Schiff H, Bachman C, Riesen W. Menopause-dependent plasma lipoprotein alterations in diuretic treated women. *Ann Intern Med* 1982;97:206–209.
296. Berglund G, Andersson O. Beta-blockers or diuretics in hypertension? A six-year follow-up of blood pressure and metabolic side effects. *Lancet* 1981;1:744–747.
297. Veterans Administration Cooperative Study Group on Antihypertensive Agents. Efficacy of propranolol and hydrochlorothiazide for the initial treatment of hypertension. II. Results of long-term therapy. *JAMA* 1982;248:2004–2011.
298. Veterans Administration Cooperative Study Group on Antihypertensive Agents. Serum lipoprotein levels during chlorthalidone therapy. *JAMA* 1980;244:1691–1695.
299. Finnerty FA Jr. Step-down treatment of mild systemic hypertension. *Am J Cardiol* 1984;53:1304–1307.
300. Stamler R, Stamler J, Grimm R, Gosch F, Elmer P, Dyer A, Berman R, Fishman J, Van Heel N, Civinelli J, McDonald A. Nutritional therapy for high blood pressure. *JAMA* 1987;257:1484–1487.
301. Lasser NL, Grandits G, Caggiula AW, Cutler JA, Grimm RH, Kuller LH, Sherwin RW, Stamler J. Effects of antihypertensive therapy on plasma lipids and lipoproteins in the Multiple Risk Factor Intervention Trial. *Am J Med* 1984;76(Suppl 2A):52–66.
302. Kannel WB, Castelli WP, Gordon T. Cholesterol in the prediction of atherosclerotic disease. *Ann Intern Med* 1979;90:85–91.
303. Lipid Research Clinics Primary Prevention Trial Results. II. Relationship of reduction in incidence of coronary heart disease to cholesterol lowering. *JAMA* 1984;144:1947–1953.
304. Ames RP. Negative effects of diuretic drugs on metabolic risk factors for coronary heart disease: possible alternative therapies. *Am J Cardiol* 1983;51:632–638.
305. Ames RP, Peacock PB. Serum cholesterol during treatment of hypertension with diuretic drugs. *Arch Intern Med* 1984;144:710–714.
306. Lardinois CK, Neuman SL. The effect of antihypertensive agents on serum lipids and lipoproteins. *Arch Intern Med* 1988;148:1280–1288.
307. Curb JD, Borhani NO, Blaszkowski TP, Zimbaldi N, Fotiu S, Williams W. Long-term surveillance for adverse effects of antihypertensive drugs. *JAMA* 1985;253:3263–3268.
308. Loriaux DL, Menard R, Taylor A, Pita JC, Santen R. Spironolactone and endocrine dysfunction. *Ann Intern Med* 1976;85:630–636.
309. Magil AB, Ballon HS, Cameron EC, Rae A. Acute interstitial nephritis associated with thiazide diuretics: clinical and pathologic observations in three cases. *Am J Med* 1980;69:939–943.
310. Bennett WM. Diuretic toxicity and drug interactions. In: Dirks JH, Sutton RAL, eds. *Diuretics: physiology, pharmacology and clinical use.* Philadelphia: WB Saunders; 1986;362–373.
311. Ettinger B, Oldroyd NO, Sorgel F. Triamterene nephrolithiasis. *JAMA* 1980;244:2443–2445.
312. Jick H, Dinan BJ, Hunter JR. Triamterene and renal stones. *J Urol* 1982;127:224–225.
313. Rosenberg L, Shapiro S, Slone D, Kaufman DW, Miettinen OS, Stolley PD. Thiazides and acute cholecystitis. *N Engl J Med* 1980;303:546–548.
314. van der Linden W, Ritter B, Edlund G. Acute cholecystitis and thiazides. *Br Med J* 1984;654–655.
315. Porter JB, Jick H, Dinan BJ. Acute cholecystitis and thiazides. *N Engl J Med* 1981;304:954–955.
316. Arndt KA, Jick H. Rates of cutaneous reactions to drugs: a report from the Boston Collaborative Drug Surveillance Program. *JAMA* 1976;235:918–923.
317. Favre L, Glasson P, Vallotton MB. Reversible acute renal failure from combined triamterene and indomethacin: a study in healthy subjects. *Ann Intern Med* 1982;96:317–320.
318. Tweedale MG, Ogilvie RI. Antagonism of spironolactone-induced natriuresis by aspirin in man. *N Engl J Med* 1973;289:198–200.
319. Steiness E, Waldorff S. Different interactions of indomethacin and sulindac with thiazides in hypertension. *Br Med J* 1982;285:1702–1703.
320. Koopmans PP, Thien TT, Gribnau FWJ. Influence of non-steroidal anti-inflammatory drugs on diuretic treatment of mild to moderate essential hypertension. *Br Med J* 1984;289:1492–1494.
321. Himmelhoch JM, Poust RI, Mallinger AG, Hanin I, Neil JF. Adjustment of lithium dose during lithium–chlorothiazide therapy. *Clin Pharmacol Ther* 1977;22:225–227.
322. Jefferson JW, Kalin NH. Serum lithium levels and long-term diuretic use. *JAMA* 1979;241:1134–1136.
323. 1988 Joint National Committee. The 1988 report of the Joint National Committee on Detection, Evaluation, and Treatment of High Blood Pressure. *Arch Intern Med* 1988;148:1023–1038.
324. Croog SH, Levine S, Testa MA, Brown B, Bulpitt CJ, Jenkins CD, Klerman GL, Williams GH. The effects of antihypertensive agents on the quality of life. *N Engl J Med* 1986;314:1657–1664.
325. Helgeland A, Strommen R, Hagelund CH, Tretli S. Enalapril, atenolol, and hydrochlorothiazide in mild to moderate hypertension. A comparative multicentre study in general practice in Norway. *Lancet* 1986;1:872–875.
326. Zanchetti A. A re-examination of stepped-care: a retrospective and a prospective. *J Cardiovasc Pharmacol* 1985;7:S126–S131.
327. Lavenius B, Hansson L. A double-blind comparison of spironolactone and hydrochlorothiazide in hypertensive patients treated with metoprolol. *Int J Clin Pharmacol* 1982;20:291–295.
328. Hallin L, Anorzin L, Hansson L. Controlled trial of nifedipine and bendroflumethiazide in hypertension. *J Cardiovasc Pharmacol* 1983;5:1083–1095.

329. Massie B, McCarthy P, Ramanathan KB, Weiss RJ, Anderson M, Eidelson BA, Labreche DG, Tubau JF, Ulep D, Bartels D. Diltiazem and propranolol in mild to moderate essential hypertension as monotherapy or in combination with hydrochlorothiazide. *Ann Intern Med* 1987;107:150–157.
330. Nicholson JP, Resnick LM, Laragh JH. Hydrochlorothiazide is not additive to verapamil in treating essential hypertension. *Arch Intern Med* 1989;149:125–128.
331. Steinmuller SR, Puschett JP. Effects of metolazone in man: comparison with chlorothiazide. *Kidney Int* 1972;1:169–181.
332. Dargie HJ, Allison MEM, Kennedy AC, Gray MJB. High dosage metolazone in chronic renal failure. *Br Med J* 1972;4:196–198.
333. Swartz CD, Kim KE. Management of hypertension in the patient with chronic renal disease. *Cardiovasc Clin* 1978;9:263–272.
334. Wollam GL, Tarazi RC, Bravo EL, Dustan HP. Diuretic potency of combined hydrochlorothiazide and furosemide therapy in patients with azotemia. *Am J Med* 1982;72:929–938.
335. Prince MJ, Stuart CA, Padia M, Bandi Z, Holland OB. Metabolic effects of hydrochlorothiazide and enalapril during treatment of the hypertensive diabetic patient. *Arch Intern Med* 1988;148: 2363–2368.
336. Bloomgarden ZT, Ginsberg-Fellner F, Rayfield EJ, Bookman J, Brown WV. Elevated hemoglobin A_{1c} and low-density lipoprotein cholesterol levels in thiazide-treated diabetic patients. *Am J Med* 1984;77:823–827.
337. Mroczek WJ, Martin CH, Hattwick MAW, Kennedy M. Once-daily furosemide therapy in diuretic-treated hypertensive patients. *Curr Ther Res* 1978;24:824–830.
338. Healy JJ, McKenna TJ, Canning B St J, Brien TG, Duffy GJ, Muldowney FP. Body composition changes in hypertensive subjects on long-term diuretic therapy. *Br Med J* 1970;1:716–719.
339. Winer BM, Lubbe WF, Colton T. Antihypertensive actions of diuretics: comparative study of an aldosterone antagonist and a thiazide, alone and together. *JAMA* 1968;204:117–121.
340. Berglund G, Andersson O. Hydrochlorothiazide and spironolactone alone and in fixed combination in hypertension. *Curr Ther Res* 1980;27:360–364.
341. Schersten B, Thulin T, Kuylenstierna J, Engstrom M, Karlberg BE, Tolagen K, Nordlander S, Nilsson G. Clinical and biochemical effects of spironolactone administered once daily in primary hypertension: Multicenter Sweden study. *Hypertension* 1980;2: 672–679.
342. Bengtsson C, Johnsson G, Sannerstedt R, Werko L. Effect of different doses of chlorthalidone on blood pressure, serum potassium, and serum urate. *Br Med J* 1975;1:197–199.
343. Korduner I, Kabin I, Hagbarth G. Low-dose chlorthalidone treatment in previously untreated hypertension. *Curr Ther Res* 1981;29:208–215.
344. MacGregor GA, Banks RA, Markandu ND, Bayliss J, Roulston JE. Lack of effect of beta-blocker on flat dose response to thiazide in hypertension: efficacy of low dose thiazide combined with beta-blocker. *Br Med J* 1983;286:1535–1538.
345. Materson BJ, Oster JR, Michael UF, Bolton SM, Burton ZC, Stambaugh JE, Morledge J. Dose response to chlorthalidone in patients with mild hypertension: efficacy of a lower dose. *Clin Pharmacol Ther* 1978;24:192–198.
346. Levinson PD, Khatri IM, Freis ED. Persistence of normal BP after withdrawal of drug treatment in mild essential hypertension. *Arch Intern Med* 1982;142:2265–2268.
347. Maland LJ, Lutz LJ, Castle CH. Effects of withdrawing diuretic therapy on blood pressure in mild hypertension. *Hypertension* 1983;5:509–517.
348. Dyckner T, Wester PO. The relationship between extra- and intracellular electrolytes with hypokalemia and/or diuretic treatment. *Acta Med Scand* 1978;204:269–282.
349. Maronde RF, Barr J, Vlachakis ND, Spencer CA, Chan L. Oral potassium chloride and amiloride in hydrochlorothiazide-induced potassium loss. *Clin Pharmacol Ther* 1984;36:431–435.
350. Schwartz AB, Swartz CD. Dosage of potassium chloride to correct thiazide-induced hypokalemia. *JAMA* 1974;230:702–704.
351. Alsop WR, Moore JG, Rollins DE, Tolman KG. The effects of five potassium chloride preparations on the upper gastrointestinal mucosa in healthy subjects receiving glycopyrrolate. *J Clin Pharmacol* 1984;24:235–239.
352. McMahon FG, Ryan JR, Akdamar K, Ertan A. Effect of potassium chloride supplements on upper gastrointestinal mucosa. *Clin Pharmacol Ther* 1984;35:852–855.
353. Licht JH, Haley RJ, Pugh B, Lewis SB. Diuretic regimens in essential hypertension: a comparison of hypokalemic effects, BP control, and cost. *Arch Intern Med* 1983;143:1694–1699.
354. Ibsen H. The effect of potassium chloride and spironolactone on thiazide-induced potassium depletion in patients with essential hypertension. *Acta Med Scand* 1974;196:21–26.
355. Jackson PR, Ramsay LE, Wakefield V. Relative potency of spironolactone, triamterene, and potassium chloride in thiazide-induced hypokalemia. *Br J Clin Pharmacol* 1982;14:257–263.
356. Kaplan NM, Carnegie A, Raskin P, Heller JA, Simmons M. Potassium supplementation in patients with diuretic-induced hypokalemia. *N Engl J Med* 1985;312:746–749.
357. Tannen RL. Effects of potassium on blood pressure control. *Ann Intern Med* 1983;98:773–780.
358. Khaw KT, Barrett-Connor E. Dietary potassium and stroke-associated mortality: A 12-year prospective population study. *N Engl J Med* 1987;316:235–240.
359. Tobian L, Lange JM, Johnson MA, MacNeill DA, Wilke TJ, Ulm KM, Wold LJ. High-K diets reduce brain haemorrhage and infarcts, death rate and mesenteric arteriolar hypertrophy in stroke-prone spontaneously hypertensive rats. *J Hypertens* 1986;4(Suppl):S205–S207.

Hypertension: Pathophysiology, Diagnosis, and Management, edited by J. H. Laragh and B. M. Brenner. Raven Press, Ltd., New York © 1990.

CHAPTER 138

Calcium Antagonists

Fritz R. Bühler

Cardiovascular and Renal Adaptation in Essential Hypertension, 2169
Cardiovascular Action of Calcium Antagonists, 2171
Cardiovascular Counterregulation, 2172
Renal Effects of Calcium Antagonists, 2173
Renin, Age, and Race as Indicators of Antihypertensive Response, 2173
Effective Drug Combination for Severe and Renal Hypertension, 2174
Renal Tissue Protection with Calcium Antagonist Therapy?, 2175
References, 2176

In 1962, the calcium antagonist verapamil was shown by the nephrologist Heidland (1) to lower blood pressure acutely in patients with hypertension and renal disease, while no effect was seen in either normotensive patients with renal parenchymal disease or normal individuals following the intravenous administration of the drug. In all three groups, a comparable increase in renal blood flow was observed. This improved renal flow was the focus of that report, and the observed antihypertensive response was not appreciated at all at that time. In the late 1960s and early 1970s the antihypertensive effectiveness of both verapamil (2,3) and nifedipine (4,5) was documented, and it was found that the fall in blood pressure was greater in patients with higher pretreatment pressures (3). In 1979, one study detected better antihypertensive efficacy of calcium antagonists in black patients (6), a high proportion of whom also have a low plasma renin activity (7). It was only in the late 1970s that long-term administration of calcium antagonists in hypertension was studied (8–10). Widespread use of calcium antagonists in hypertension has developed. In the last 5–7 years only, studies that have provided convincing evidence for the usefulness of calcium antagonists in long-term antihypertensive therapy (11–13) have coincided with the development of new pathophysiological concepts linking derangements in transmembrane sodium and calcium transport to the pathophysiology of essential hypertension (14,15).

CARDIOVASCULAR AND RENAL ADAPTATION IN ESSENTIAL HYPERTENSION

Essential hypertension is characterized by different developmental phases. In an early phase, beta-adrenoceptor-mediated cardiovascular responses [i.e., heart rate (16,17), exercise tachycardia (16) (and hence cardiac output), plasma renin activity (18), and renin responsiveness (19–21)] are augmented; renovascular resistance is practically normal (22).

In a later phase of hypertension or with older age, beta-adrenoceptor-mediated effects tend to be blunted (Fig. 1). Accordingly, exercise-induced tachycardia and heart rate responses to isoproterenol are reduced (16,23,24), plasma renin activity is normal or low (7,18) and hyperresponsive to sympathetic stimuli (19,25), and peripheral vasodilator responses to beta-adrenoceptor stimulation are diminished (26,27). Similarly, isoproterenol causes a lesser increase in renal blood flow of older individuals or patients with low-renin hypertension (28). With blunting of beta-adrenoceptor-mediated functions, relative alpha-adrenoceptor-mediated vasoconstriction prevails. Hence, the established phase of essential hypertension is characterized by an elevated peripheral vascular resistance to which enhanced postjunctional alpha-1- and alpha-2-adrenoceptor-mediated (29,30) and calcium-influx-dependent (31) vasoconstriction contribute. Enhanced calcium-influx-dependent vasoconstriction may be operated to a great extent through postjunctional alpha-1- and alpha-2-adrenoceptors, and this eventually leads to increased intracellular free calcium concentration in vascular smooth muscle cells. This appears to be reflected by an increased calcium concentration in platelets of patients with essential hypertension and by its correlation with the height of blood pressure (32) (Fig. 2, left). Decreased beta-adrenoceptor-mediated function in the later phase of essential hypertension appears not to be the result of a change in receptor number or their affinity (33,34) and therefore is more likely due to alterations distal to the receptor site (e.g., at the level of the G-protein coupling).

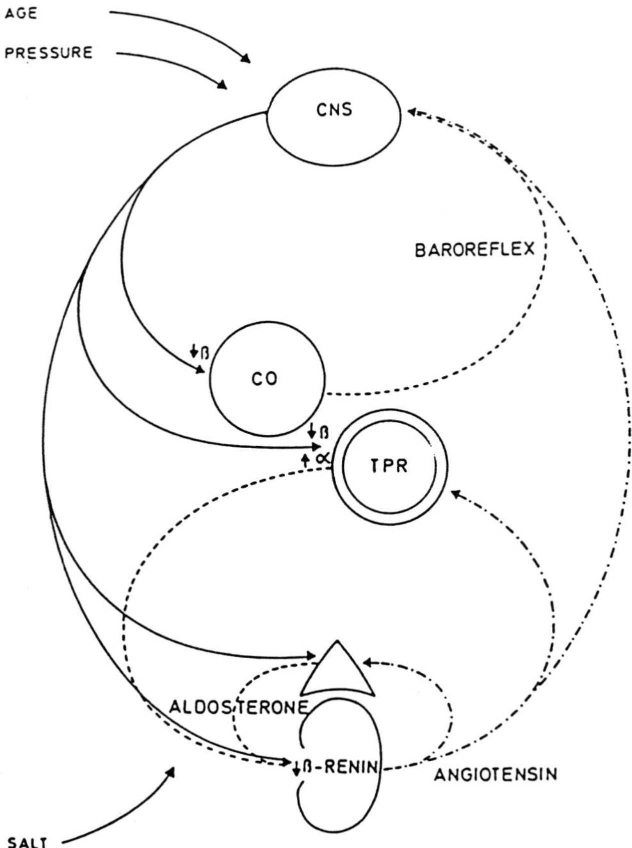

FIG. 1. Adrenergic and angiotensinergic regulation of the circulation. Age, salt, and blood pressure per se contribute to the transition from a predominantly hyper-beta-adrenoceptor-mediated cardiovascular regulation in younger patients to a later maintenance phase (older patients) where beta effects and renin are blunted and where alpha-adrenoceptor-mediated vasoconstriction prevails.

Such a transition from an early phase of essential hypertension where beta-adrenoceptor-mediated functions prevail to a later one where alpha-adrenoceptor-mediated and calcium-influx-dependent vasoconstriction dominates is exemplified by low-renin essential hypertension and by our patient reported above. These derangements tally with several other known features of low-renin essential hypertension, particularly in the kidney; some of them can be considered an enhanced aging process.

With increasing age, renal blood flow and glomerular filtration rate (GFR) tend to decrease; furthermore, the associated increase in filtration fraction (35,36) (i.e., the lower ratio of pre- and postglomerular resistances) eventually leads to a rise in hydraulic pressure in the glomerular capillary. Owing to increased glomerular ultrafiltration and the reduction in peritubular flow, the proximal tubular sodium reabsorption increases; this effect may be enhanced by alpha-2-adrenoceptor-mediated proximal tubular sodium reabsorption (37). If essential hypertension is characterized by a systemic plasma membrane defect (38), it is conceivable that mechanisms which lead to enhanced alpha-2-adrenoceptor-mediated slow calcium-channel influx, increased cytosolic calcium, and blunted calmodulin-dependent Ca^{2+}-ATPase-fueled calcium extrusion in platelets (39) may also be operative in renal tubular cells and accessible to calcium-entry blockade (40).

The disproportionate increase in aldosterone relative to the low renin occurring with aging and in low-renin essential hypertensive patients (41) may contribute further to sodium retention via enhanced sodium reabsorption in the distal and collecting tubule. Overt sodium volume retention (42)—other than the slightly elevated cardiopulmonary volume and elevated atrial natriuretic peptide (43)—is difficult to show in low-renin essential hypertension; this may be explained by the resulting pressure natriuresis. Cardiovascular, renal regulatory, and counterregulatory mech-

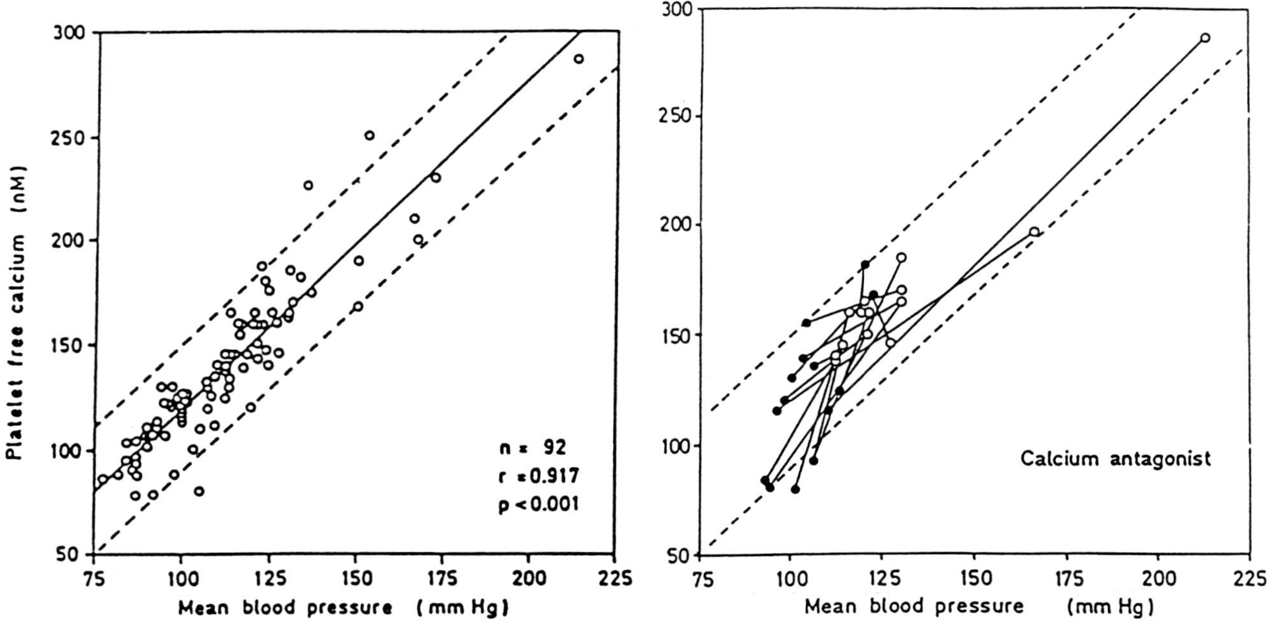

FIG. 2. Intracellular free calcium concentration in platelets from normotensive and hypertensive subjects as measured by the Quin-2 method (**left**) and in parallel reduction with blood pressure during calcium antagonist therapy (**right**).

anisms have to be borne in mind when discussing the mode of action and place of calcium antagonists in treating patients with different forms of hypertension.

CARDIOVASCULAR ACTION OF CALCIUM ANTAGONISTS

Increased systemic vascular resistance in essential hypertension depends on increased calcium influx (31,44). Calcium antagonists lower cytosolic free-calcium concentrations (Fig. 2, right), mainly through a reduction of transmembranous calcium influx, and are potent arteriolar vasodilators. Infusion of verapamil into the brachial artery produces vasodilation as assessed by venous occlusion plethysmography. The maximal vasodilator responses of the forearm circulation were inversely related to the patients' plasma renin activity and angiotensin II concentration (Fig. 3). This suggests greater calcium-influx-dependent vasoconstriction when the renin–angiotensin pressor system is suppressed.

Acute and chronic antihypertensive drug effects differ with respect to the underlying pathophysiological mechanisms, and they may also vary between the various types of calcium antagonists. Thus, when nifedipine was given sublingually to patients with essential hypertension there was a modest, yet significant, acute reduction of systolic and diastolic blood pressure (45). This decrease was associated with increases in heart rate, cardiac index, plasma norepinephrine concentrations, and plasma renin activity, whereas calculated systemic vascular resistance decreased. These findings suggest reflexly mediated sympathoneural activation due to arterial vasodilation. For a given stimulus, sympathetic stimulation will be greater in subjects with normally functioning baroreflexes.

Hypertension leads to blunting of the sensitivity of the arterial baroreflexes (46), as does old age (47). These effects of age and high blood pressure seem to be independent of each other (48). If this is so, then elderly hypertensive patients will have less counterregulatory reflex activation and sympathetically mediated vasoconstriction as compared to younger and high-renin patients, and the latter will have more than normotensive controls. Indirect evidence is derived from the observation that normotensive subjects have no change, or only a small decrease, in pressure after administration of calcium antagonists (31,49). More direct

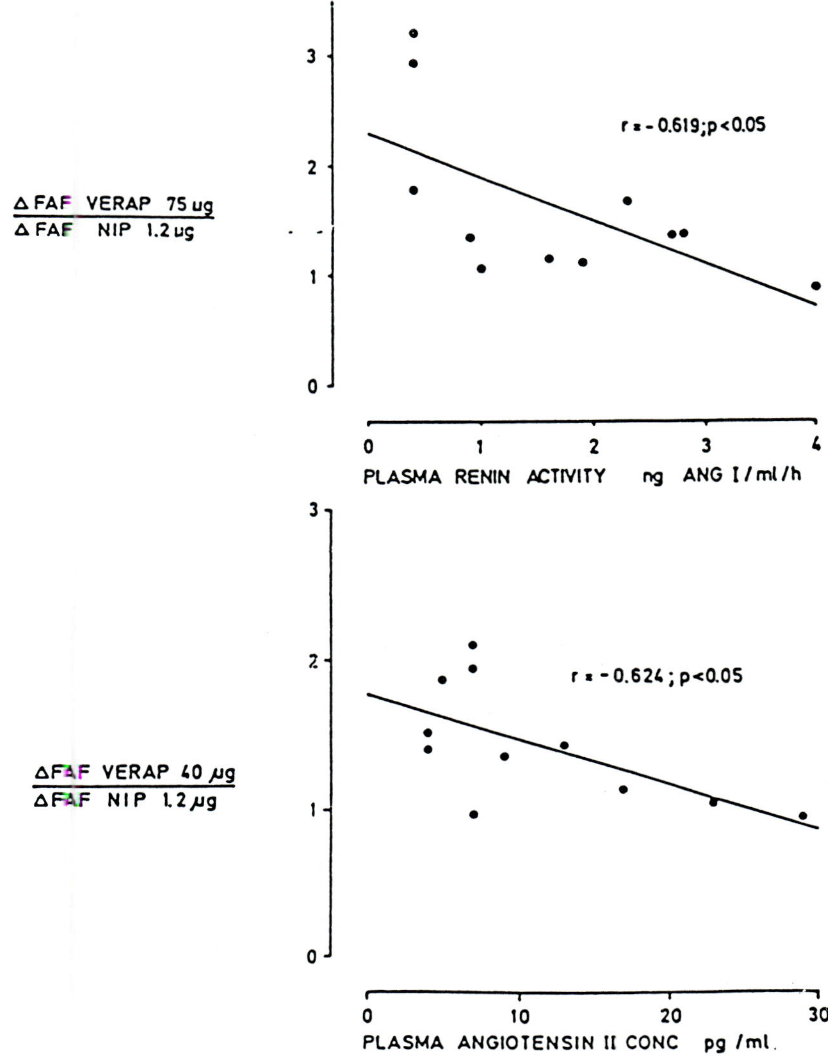

FIG. 3. Data showing that vasodilator response to interarterially infused verapamil (forearm venous occlusion plethysmography) relates inversely to plasma renin activity and angiotensin II concentration. FAF, forearm blood flow.

evidence comes from a study in which arterial baroreflex sensitivity was related to the acute fall in blood pressure after nifedipine given sublingually (50). Baroreflex sensitivity was inversely related to age, and subjects with low sensitivities had the greatest acute falls in blood pressure (Fig. 4). Also, subjects with the greatest increase in plasma norepinephrine levels as a marker of changes of sympathetic activity had the greatest increases in cardiac output, a hemodynamic response pattern that would tend to counteract the decrease of pressure the most.

Similar responses suggestive of mild chronic sympathetic stimulation have also been observed with another dihydropyridine, namely, nitrendipine (51). In contrast, verapamil and diltiazem do not seem to cause either acute or chronic reflex stimulation as judged by plasma norepinephrine measurements (52,53). Although plasma norepinephrine concentrations may not accurately reflect sympathetic nervous system activity under all circumstances (54,55), and changes of heart rate cannot be taken as indices of sympathetic activity because of these drugs' direct negative chronotropic effects, these findings raise the possibility that counterregulatory mechanisms may differ between the dihydropyridines and verapamil and diltiazem.

Other mechanisms probably also contribute to the antihypertensive effects of calcium antagonists, but their quantitative importance remains to be precisely defined. Vasoconstriction due to adrenergic stimulation is markedly reduced during therapy, but it has been debated whether this inhibition applies to both alpha-1- and alpha-2-adrenoceptor-mediated vasoconstriction (56–58); the latter system is effectively blocked by calcium antagonists (59). However, some interference with alpha-1-adrenoceptor-mediated vasoconstriction also seems likely, since nifedipine reduced the blood pressure increases produced by the alpha-1-adrenoceptor agonist phenylephrine in patients with hypertension. Although phenylephrine is not absolutely specific for the alpha-1-type adrenoceptor, this and other (60) findings suggest an interference of calcium antagonists with both alpha-1- and alpha-2-adrenoceptor-mediated vasoconstriction, although the latter effect may be more pronounced. Calcium antagonists also interfere with angiotensin-II-mediated vasoconstriction (61) and normalize blood pressure in an animal model in which hypertension was induced by continuous angiotensin II infusion (62). Equally important, calcium antagonists reduce angiotensin's stimulatory effect on aldosterone biosynthesis and secretion (63), an effect which may be particularly pertinent in a state where aldosterone is inappropriately high (e.g., low-renin essential hypertension) (41).

CARDIOVASCULAR COUNTERREGULATION

The experience with calcium antagonists in clinical investigation of hypertension has taught us a principal lesson on antihypertensive drug action. On the one hand, calcium antagonists eliminate excess calcium-influx-dependent vasoconstriction and thereby tend to normalize elevated peripheral vascular resistance. On the other hand, peripheral vasodilation is countered by baroreflex-induced sympathetic nervous system activation that results in alpha-1-adrenoceptor-, alpha-2-adrenoceptor-, and angiotensin-mediated vasoconstriction (as well as cardiac and renal stimulation). The more blunted the baroreflex, beta-adrenoceptor, and renin compensatory baroreflex, the greater the fall in blood pressure (see Fig. 1). At the level of the vascular smooth muscle cell, calcium antagonists block slow channel-calcium entry, but, for example, alpha-1-adrenoceptor- or angiotensin-receptor-activated and inositol-trisphosphate-mediated superficial sarcoplasmic calcium release may sustain vascular contraction (64). This logic helps in understanding the efficacious combination of a calcium-entry blocker with a renin-suppression beta-blocker or angiotensin-converting-enzyme inhibitor.

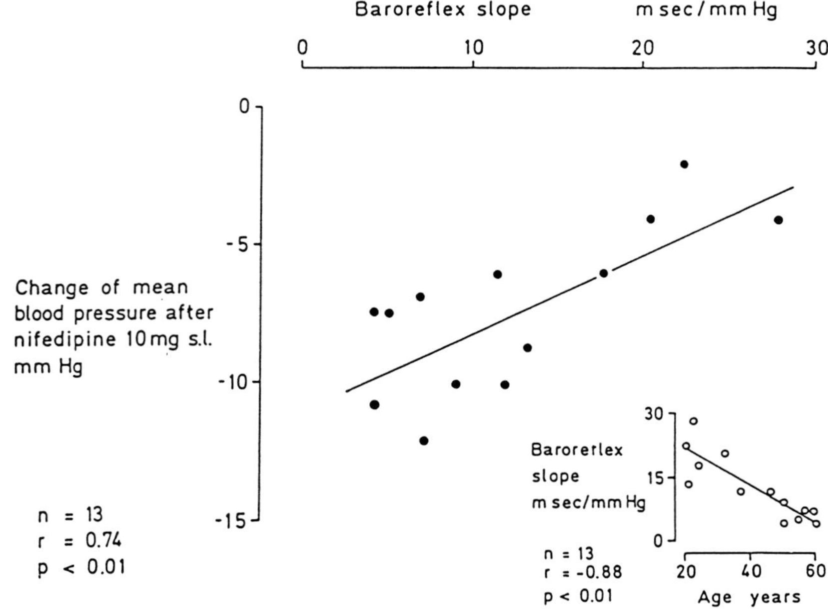

FIG. 4. Data showing that baroreflex sensitivity decreases with the patient's age **(inset)**; the more the baroreflex sensitivity is reduced, the greater the acute (and chronic) fall in blood pressure in response to nifedipine.

Unlike other vasodilating agents, calcium antagonists do not cause sodium-volume retention; moreover, no changes in blood volume have been observed in our (13,45) and other studies with nifedipine and verapamil (65,66). Accordingly, the mechanism by which calcium antagonists lower blood pressure without causing sodium retention awaits clarification.

RENAL EFFECTS OF CALCIUM ANTAGONISTS

Renal vascular dilating effects of calcium antagonists have been known since the early days (1,67), but their natriuretic effect of 6–10 g salt in the first few days of treatment only recently has been appreciated for nifedipine and nitrendipine (52,68–70). The case for verapamil is less clear, since natriuresis or diuresis was not found in some experiments (52,71) whereas decreased tubular sodium reabsorption was seen in others (72).

Renal hemodynamic responses to calcium antagonists greatly depend on the neural and hormonal determinants of renal vascular tone which are differently sensitive to calcium antagonists (73). Their common, and perhaps prominent, renal effect is to reduce (elevated) preglomerular resistance and to maintain or increase GFR (74–76). This also implies differential effects on pre- and postglomerular resistance which may lead to a greater GFR.

There are nonvascular sites of calcium antagonist action which seem to contribute to natriuresis. Diminished tubular sodium reabsorption was found in the isolated perfused kidney (74–76), even when renal plasma flow and GFR were kept constant (77). A proximal tubular action is inferred by increased phosphate and urate excretion after acute administration of calcium antagonists (78).

In humans, nitrendipine increased fractional sodium excretion and free water clearance during maximal water diuresis; this effect occurred without change in renal plasma flow or GFR, suggesting direct tubular action at a level proximal to the diluting segment (79). Reduction of distal tubular sodium reabsorption was shown in stop-flow studies (40,77). Although most of these studies represent acute effects, the changes observed were the opposite of those found with other vasodilating agents (i.e., hydralazine and minoxidil), which acutely decreased sodium and water excretion (72). A repetitive natriuretic effect was shown with the new dihydropyridine, namely, isradipine; moreover, the sodium excretion rate (or absolute proximal reabsorption) correlated with the fall in blood pressure (80).

Interference with aldosterone secretion (51,61,63), and thus reduced sodium reabsorption in the collecting tubule, is yet another factor by which calcium antagonists promote natriuresis. It is conceivable that the slightly elevated aldosterone in low-renin essential hypertension, in addition to the elevated preglomerular resistance, may form the renal substrate for calcium antagonist action.

The concept of sodium-volume filling is supported further by controlled studies showing that calcium antagonists intraindividually lower blood pressure more on a high sodium intake, both acutely (81,86) and chronically (87).

RENIN, AGE, AND RACE AS INDICATORS OF ANTIHYPERTENSIVE RESPONSE

The above (reno-) pathophysiological view of essential hypertension and the mechanisms of action have been tested in several pharmacotherapeutic studies. In the early phase of high blood pressure development, in younger patients or those with a high or normal renin ("normal" being too high for the elevated pressure), beta-blockers and converting-enzyme inhibitors were found to be more effective than in older or low-renin patients (88). About 80% of the patients under the age of 40 years normalize their diastolic blood pressure to below 95 mmHg with a beta-blocker (89) or converting-enzyme inhibitor (90). The response rates in the age group between 40 and 60 years are about 50%, and an age relationship with beta-blocker monotherapy was found in this subgroup as well (91). Over the age of 60 years, beta-blockers and converting-enzyme inhibitors normalize blood pressure in about 20% of the patients, and a combination therapy is required for pressure control more often. A similar picture emerges for the renin subgroups, with a response rate to beta-blockers of about 80% in high-, 50% in normal-, and 20% in low-renin essential hypertension (Fig. 5). These response rates are comparable to those found with converting-enzyme inhibitors (92). Although such an age- and renin-related response pattern has not been found in every beta-blocker or converting-enzyme inhibitor study, there is a substantial body of supportive information from investigators around the world (93).

Diuretic drugs were shown to be more effective than beta-blockers in older patients, who often exhibit low renin levels. Blood pressure normalization with diuretics has been interpreted as normalization of pretreatment volume overfilling (94,95). In addition to some elevation of cardiopulmonary volume (42), there are two other important cardiovascular characteristics in old and low-renin patients: enhanced calcium-influx-dependent vasoconstriction and blunted cardiovascular reflex regulation. Calcium antagonists were found to have a response pattern similar to that seen with diuretics (13). Calcium antagonists normalize blood pressure in about 80% of patients older than 60 years or having a low renin (Fig. 6), in 50% of those between the age 40 and 60 years or having a normal renin, and in only about 20% of patients under the age of 40 years or having a high renin (13,96–98). Some of the more recent studies are in keeping with this view (99–109) (Table 1). Using calcium antagonists in a retarded formulation (110) or using the newer longer-acting dihydropyridine types [e.g., nitrendipine (97) or amlodipine (111)], antihypertensive care may be equally simple as that with diuretic drugs.

Black hypertensive patients have a great prevalence of low renin, and diuretics were considered as drugs of first choice (112,113). Beta-blockers (114) and converting-enzyme inhibitors (115) were both less effective in black patients than in white patients. As a new alternative to diuretics, calcium antagonists have proven most efficacious in black hypertensives; moreover, in a recent double-blind, randomized comparison with atenolol, age dependency was also observed (102).

Why is it that a renin–, age–, or race–response relationship is not found in all the trials? There seem to be some

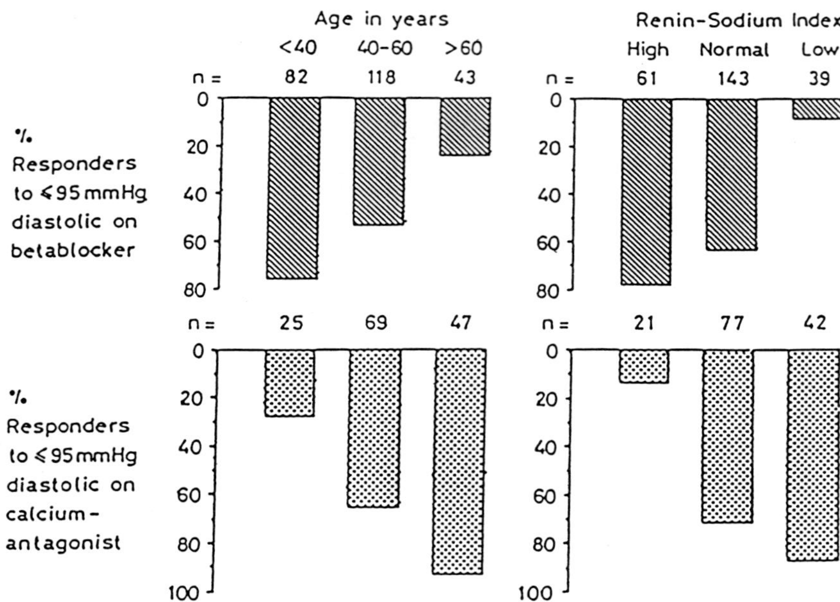

FIG. 5. Histogram showing that blood pressure normalization (≤95 mmHg diastolic) in response to beta-blockers (**upper panel**) occurs more often in younger (**left**) and high-renin (**right**) patients than with calcium antagonists (**lower panel**) and occurs more often with calcium antagonists in older patients and in those with lower plasma renin activity.

common problems with drug testing with regard to possible predictors. The impacts of these predictors, although highly significant, are not overwhelmingly strong. Analyses of these predictors have helped in the degree of treatment strategies, but they are not mandatory criteria for drug selection in an individual patient. Correlations are usually found only with relatively sizable study populations and in studies with a high degree of standardization (Table 2). Daytime variation, quality of blood pressure recording, renin assay variability, and recognition of drug kinetics and dose adjustment may be of importance here. For these reasons, and because of the background noise, multicenter trials in data collection often fail to show these relationships in spite of a large study population.

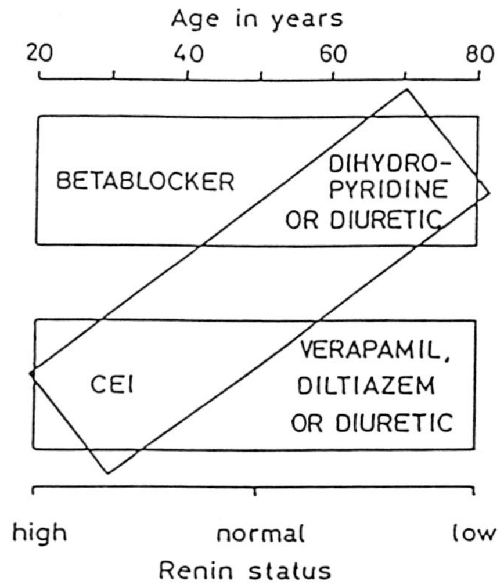

FIG. 6. The patient's age and plasma renin activity as used for designing pathophysiologically oriented and individualized antihypertensive treatment: Antihypertensive monotherapy (with beta-blockers and angiotensin-converting enzyme inhibitors) is used for younger and high-renin patients, whereas calcium antagonists are used for older and low-renin patients; there is preferential use of the combination of the beta-blocker dihydropyridine and the angiotensin-converting enzyme inhibitor verapamil.

EFFECTIVE DRUG COMBINATION FOR SEVERE AND RENAL HYPERTENSION

Even though age, renin, and race help in drug selection, about 20% of the patients require drug combinations to achieve a diastolic target pressure of 95 mmHg or below; about 30% if the new WHL/WHO/ISH recommendation of 90 mmHg (116) is applied. The quality of blood pressure control is the first aim of antihypertensive therapy. There are, however, more reasonable, effective, and usually better-tolerated drug combination approaches; the above-mentioned pathophysiological considerations help in this regard (Fig. 6). While it is of little benefit to combine a beta-blocker with a converting-enzyme inhibitor or to combine a calcium antagonist with a diuretic (117), crosswise combinations (Fig. 6) have been shown to be highly effective, particularly in patients with severe hypertension (118,119). Thus, calcium antagonists of the dihydropyridine type can be safely combined with beta-blockers (113,119), while both verapamil and diltiazem should only be added after great caution and consideration of contraindications such as sick sinus syndrome, AV-conduction defects, or impaired cardiac contractility (118). All calcium antagonists can be most effectively and safely combined with converting-enzyme inhibitors; this drug combination is preferred in those patients who are otherwise difficult to treat (119). It may well be that deterioration of renal function seen with converting-enzyme inhibitors in bilateral renovascular hypertension is prevented by the combination with calcium antagonists. Combination of different calcium antagonists may have additive effects; but similarly to this combination with a diuretic drug, there is little antihy-

TABLE 1. *Greater antihypertensive effectiveness of calcium antagonists in older, low-renin, and black patients*

Drug	Authors	Older	Low renin	Black
Verapamil	Leary et al. (6)			+
	Bühler et al. (13)	+	+	
	Müller et al. (110)	+		
Nifedipine	Erne et al. (96)	+	+	
	Kiowski et al. (98)	+	+	+
	Landmark	+		
	Resnick et al. (99)		+	
	Ribstein et al. (100)	+		
	Ueda	+		
Nitrendipine	Müller et al. (97)	+	+	
	Moser et al. (101)			+
	Dustan (103)		+	+
	Pedrinelli et al. (105)	+	+	
	Fritschka (107)	+		
	Zachariah et al. (106)		+	
	Weinberger (104)	+		
	M'Buyamba-Kabangu et al. (102)	+	+	+
Nicardipine	Cluzel	+		
Diltiazem	Moser et al. (108)			+
	Amodeo et al. (109)		+	
	Pool	+		
	Zachariah et al. (106)	+		

pertensive gain. In patients with essential hypertension, blood pressure control may rarely necessitate the use of a diuretic; however, there is no strong argument (other than the patient's well-being) against the addition of diuretics (provided that they have a potassium-sparing component and are administered a low dose), since the notion that diuretics may cause excessive cardiovascular morbidity or mortality (120) has been contradicted by recent large-scale trials (e.g., the IPPPSH (121), the MRC trial in mild hypertension (122), the EWPHE (123), the HAPPHY (124), and the MAPHY (125)]; there may be some beta-blocker benefit (121,122,125), particularly in men who do not smoke (121,122).

In patients with renal parenchymal hypertension, calcium antagonists were shown to be most efficacious (85); this may again be linked to their relative volume overfilling and often low renin status. However, as more renal function is reduced, calcium antagonists seem to benefit more from the addition of a diuretic agent (126). As to whether long-term effects of calcium antagonist therapy improve renal function under certain circumstances is still open to debate.

TABLE 2. *Linear correlations between factors influencing the antihypertensive response to calcium antagonists*[a]

Factor	Age	MBP	PRA	ΔMBP
Age	1.00 } NS	—	—	—
MBP	0.13 } NS	1.00	—	—
PRA	−0.44**	−0.25*	1.00	—
ΔMBP	−0.36**	−0.55**	0.49**	1.00

[a] Total number of patients, 138 (verapamil, 43; nifedipine, 66; nitrendipine, 29); MBP, pretreatment mean blood pressure; PRA, pretreatment plasma renin activity; ΔMBP, change of mean blood pressure during therapy; NS, not significant; *$p < 0.01$; **$p < 0.001$.

RENAL TISSUE PROTECTION WITH CALCIUM ANTAGONIST THERAPY?

Experimental evidence strongly suggests that calcium antagonists, combined with enhanced tissue perfusion, provide a protective effect on different tissues [i.e., myocardium (127) and vasculature], including a delaying effect on the development of arteriosclerosis (128). In the clinical setting, however, these potentials have not been proven. Several efforts using calcium antagonist therapy to show a reduction of cardiac death or reinfarction following a myocardial infarction (secondary prevention) have failed (129) except for recent studies with diltiazem (130,131). This points to a possible difference between the three major types of calcium antagonists in which the balance between the potential tissue protection and the drug-induced fall in coronary (or perhaps also cerebrovascular) perfusion pressure may be crucial.

Similarly, efforts were made in the maintenance of GFR and in the prevention of renal damage, and the renal inflammatory response to injury (e.g., in experimental glomerulonephritis) can be reduced with different calcium antagonists (132,133). Prostaglandin-induced reduction in glomerular filtration consequent to preglomerular vasoconstriction has been reversed by diltiazem (134). Radiocontrast-induced renal insufficiency has been attenuated with simultaneous administration of a calcium antagonist (135). More recently, calcium antagonists have been claimed to reduce or prevent the development of hypertension in renal transplant patients treated with the immunosuppressant cyclosporin A (136). The better understanding of low-dose cyclosporin-induced renal damage and hypertension in which the endothelium-related relaxing factor appears to play an important role (137), as well as of the mode of calcium antagonist action, may help to elucidate new pathophysiological mechanisms in hypertension.

REFERENCES

1. Heidland A, Klütsch K, Oebeck A. Myogenbedingte Vasodilatation bei Niereníschämie. *Münch Med Wochenschr* 1962;35:1636.
2. Hagino D. Application of ipoveratril in the pharmacotherapy of hypertension. *Jpn J Clin Exp Med* 1968;45:208–242.
3. Brittinger WD, Schwarzbeck A, Wittenmeier KW, Twittenhoff WD, Stegaru B, Huber W, Ewald RW, von Henning GE, Fabricius M, Stauch M. Klinisch-experimentelle Untersuchungen über die blutdrucksenkende Wirkung von Verapamil. *Dtsch Med Wochenschr* 1970;37:1837–1871.
4. Murakami M, Murakami E, Takekoshi N, Tsuchiya M, Kin T, Onoe T, Takeuchi N, Funatsu T, Hars S, Ishise S, Mifune J, Maede M. Antihypertensive effect of 4-(2′-nitrophenyl)-2,6-dimethyl-4-dihydropyridine-3,5-dicarbonic acid dimethylester (nifedipine, Bay-a 1040), a new coronary dilator. *Jpn Heart J* 1972;13:128–133.
5. Aoki K, Kondo S, Mochizuki A. Antihypertensive effects of cardiovascular Ca^{2+}-antagonists in hypertensive patients in the absence and presence of beta-adrenergic blockade. *Am Heart J* 1978;96:218–227.
6. Leary WP, Phil D, Asmal AC. Treatment of hypertension with verapamil. *Curr Ther Res* 1979;25:747–752.
7. Brunner HR, Sealey JE, Laragh JH. Renin subgroups in essential hypertension. *Circ Res* 1973;32(Suppl I):99–104.
8. Lederballe-Pederson O, Mikkelsen E, Christensen NJ, Kornerup HJ, Pedersen EB. Effect of nifedipine on plasma renin, aldosterone and catecholamines in arterial hypertension. *Eur J Clin Pharmacol* 1979;15:235–240.
9. Midtbø K, Hals O. Verapamil in the treatment of hypertension. *Curr Ther Res* 1980;27:830–835.
10. Lewis GRJ, Morley KD, Lewis BM, Bones PJ. The treatment of hypertension with verapamil. *NZ Med J* 1978;84:351–354.
11. Guazzi MD, Fiorentini C, Olivari MT, Bartorelli A, Necchi G, Polese A. Short and long-term efficacy of a calcium antagonist agent (nifedipine) combined with methyldopa in the treatment of severe hypertension. *Circulation* 1980;61:913–919.
12. Anavekar SN, Christophidis N, Louis WJ, Doyle AE. Verapamil in the treatment of hypertension. *J Cardiovasc Pharmacol* 1981;3:287–291.
13. Bühler FR, Hulthén UL, Kiowski W, Bolli P. Greater antihypertensive efficacy of the calcium channel inhibitor verapamil in older and low renin patients. *Clin Sci* 1982;63:439–442.
14. Blaustein MP. Sodium ions, calcium ions, blood pressure regulation and hypertension: a reassessment and a hypothesis. *Am J Physiol* 1977;232:C165–173.
15. Garay RP, Meyer Ph. A new test showing abnormal net Na^+ and K^+ fluxes in erythrocytes of essential hypertensive patients. *Lancet* 1979;17:349–353.
16. Bertel O, Bühler FR, Kiowski W, Lütold BE. Decreased beta-adrenoreceptor responsiveness as related to age, blood pressure and plasma catecholamines in patients with essential hypertension. *Hypertension* 1980;2:130–138.
17. Bühler FR, Kiowski W, van Brummelen P, Amann FW, Bertel O, Landmann R, Lütold BE, Bolli P. Plasma adrenoceptor-mediated and cardiac, renal and peripheral vascular adrenoceptor-mediated responses in different age groups of normal and hypertensive subjects. *Clin Exp Hypertens* 1980;2:409–426.
18. Bühler FR, Burkart F, Lütold BE, Küng M, Marbet G, Pfisterer M. Antihypertensive betablocking action as related to renin and age: a pharmacological tool to identify pathogenic mechanisms in essential hypertension. *Am J Cardiol* 1975;36:653–669.
19. Burkart F, Bühler FR, Pfisterer M, Lütold BE, Küng M. Hemodynamic responses to exercise and acute betablockade in renin subtypes of essential hypertension. *Clin Sci* 1976;51:70.
20. Perini C, Müller FB, Rauchfleisch U, Battegay R, Bühler FR. Hyperadrenergic borderline hypertension is characterized by suppressed aggression. *J Cardiovasc Pharmacol* 1986;8(Suppl 5):S53–S56.
21. Esler M, Julius S, Zweifler A, Randall O, Harburg E, Gardiner H, de Quattro V. Mild high renin essential hypertension: a neurogenic human hypertension? *N Engl J Med* 1977;296:405–411.
22. Hollenberg NK, Borucki LJ, Adams DF. The renal vasculature in early essential hypertension: evidence for a pathogenic role. *Medicine* 1978;37:167–178.
23. London GM, Safar ME, Weiss YA, Milliez PL. Isoproterenol sensitivity and total body clearance of propranolol in hypertensive patients. *J Clin Pharmacol* 1976;16:174–178.
24. Astrand PO, Rodahl K. *Textbook of work physiology*. New York: McGraw-Hill, 1970.
25. Lowder SC, Hamet P, Liddle GW. Contrasting effects of hypoglycemia on plasma renin activity and cyclic adenosine 3′,5′-monophosphate (cyclic AMP) in low renin and normal renin essential hypertension. *Circ Res* 1976;38:105–109.
26. Fleisch JH. Age-related changes in the sensitivity of blood vessels to drugs. *Pharmacol Ther* 1980;8:477–487.
27. van Brummelen P, Bühler FR, Kiowski W, Amann FW. Age-related decrease in cardiac and peripheral vascular responsiveness to isoproterenol. *Clin Sci* 1981;60:571–577.
28. Bauer JH, Brooks CS, Burch RN. Renal function and hemodynamic studies in low and normal renin hypertension. *Arch Intern Med* 1982;142:1317–1325.
29. Amann FW, Bolli P, Kiowski W, Bühler FR. Enhanced alpha-adrenoceptor-mediated vasoconstriction in essential hypertension. *Hypertension* 1981;3(Suppl I):119–123.
30. Bolli P, Erne P, Ji BH, Block LH, Kiowski W, Bühler FR. Adrenaline induces vasoconstriction through postjunctional alpha-2-adrenoceptors and this response is enhanced in patients with essential hypertension. *J Hypertens* 1983;1(Suppl 2):257–259.
31. Hulthén UL, Bolli P, Amann FW, Kiowski W, Bühler FR. Enhanced vasodilatation in essential hypertension by calcium channel blockade with verapamil. *Hypertension* 1982;4(Suppl II):26–31.
32. Erne P, Bolli P, Bürgisser E, Bühler FR. Correlation of platelet calcium with blood pressure. Effect of antihypertensive therapy. *N Engl J Med* 1984;310:1084–1088.
33. Feldman RD, Limbird LE, Nadean J, Robertson D, Wood AJS. Alterations in leucocyte beta-receptor affinity with ageing. *N Engl J Med* 1984;310:815–818.
34. Landmann RMA, van Brummelen P, Amann FW, Bühler FR. Increased beta-adrenoceptor binding capacity is associated with blunted beta-adrenoceptor-mediated cardiovascular responses in essential hypertension. *J Cardiovasc Pharmacol* 1985;7(Suppl 6):S168–S171.
35. Schalekamp MADH, Schalekamp-Kuyken MPA, Birkenhäger WH. Abnormal renal hemodynamics and renin suppression in hypertensive patients. *Clin Sci* 1970;38:101–107.
36. London GM, Safar ME, Sassard JE, Levenson JA, Simon AC. Renal and systemic hemodynamics in sustained essential hypertension. *Hypertension* 1984;6:743–754.
37. De Leeuw P, Birkenhäger WH. Sodium and adrenergic mechanisms. In: Birkenhäger WH, Reid JL, eds. *Handbook of hypertension,* vol 8. New York: Raven Press, 1987;203–216.
38. Postnov YV, Orlov SN. Cell membrane alteration as a source of primary hypertension. *J Hypertens* 1984;2:1–6.
39. Resink TJ, Dimitrov D, Zschauer A, Erne P, Tkachuk VA, Bühler FR. Platelet calcium-linked abnormalities in essential hypertension. *Ann NY Acad Sci* 1987;488:252–265.
40. Di Bona GF, Sawin LL. Renal tubular site of action of felodipine. *J Pharmacol Exp Ther* 1984;228:420–424.
41. Bühler FR, Laragh JH, Sealey JE, Brunner HR. Plasma aldosterone–renin interrelationships in various forms of essential hypertension: studies using a rapid assay of plasma aldosterone. *Am J Cardiol* 1973;32:554–561.
42. Kiowski W, Julius S. Renin response to stimulation of cardiopulmonary mechanoreceptors in man. *J Clin Invest* 1978;62:656–663.
43. Müller FB, Bolli P, Kiowski W, Erne P, Resink TJ, Raine AEG, Bühler FR. Atrial natriuretic peptide is elevated in low renin essential hypertension. *J Hypertens* 1986;4(Suppl 6):S489–S491.

44. Robinson BF, Dobbs BJ, Bayley S. Response of forearm resistance vessels to verapamil and sodium nitroprusside in normotensive and hypertensive men: evidence for a functional abnormality of vascular smooth muscle in primary hypertension. *Clin Sci* 1982;63:33–37.
45. Kiowski W, Bertel O, Erne P, Hulthén UL, Bolli P, Ritz R, Bühler FR. Haemodynamic and reflex mechanisms of acute and chronic antihypertensive therapy with the calcium channel blocker nifedipine. *Hypertension* 1983;5(Suppl 1):170–174.
46. Bristow JD, Honour AJ, Pickering GW, Sleight P, Peti R. Diminished baroreflex sensitivity in high blood pressure. *Circulation* 1969;39:48–55.
47. Gribbin B, Pickering TG, Sleight P, Peti R. Effect of age and high blood pressure on baroreflex sensitivity in man. *Circ Res* 1971;29:424–431.
48. Randall OS, Esler M, Culp B, Julius S, Zweifler A. Determinants of baroreflex sensitivity in man. *J Lab Clin Med* 1978;91:514–519.
49. MacGregor GA, Rotellar C, Markander ND, Sagnella GA. Contrasting effects of nifedipine, captopril and propranolol in normotensive and hypertensive subjects. *J Cardiovasc Pharmacol* 1982;4(Suppl 3):358–361.
50. Kiowski W, Erne P, Bertel O, Bolli P, Bühler FR. Acute and chronic sympathetic reflex activation and antihypertensive response to nifedipine. *J Am Coll Cardiol* 1986;7:344–348.
51. Fouad FM, Pedrinelli R, Bravo EL, Abi-Samra F, Textor SC, Tarazi RC. Clinical and systemic hemodynamic effects of nitrendipine. *Clin Pharmacol Ther* 1984;35:768–775.
52. Leonetti G, Cuspidi C, Sampieri L, Terzoli L, Zanchetti A. Comparison of cardiovascular, renal and humoral effects of acute administration of two calcium channel blockers in normotensive and hypertensive subjects. *J Cardiovasc Pharmacol* 1982;4(Suppl 3):S319–S324.
53. Muiesan G, Agabiti-Rosei E, Castellano M, et al. Antihypertensive and humoral effects of verapamil and nifedipine in essential hypertension. *J Cardiovasc Pharmacol* 1982;4(Suppl 3):S325–S329.
54. Floras J, Vann Jones J, Hassan O, Osikowska BA, Sever PS, Sleight P. Failure of plasma norepinephrine to consistently reflect sympathetic activity in humans. *Hypertension* 1986;8:641–649.
55. Folkow B, Di Bona GF, Hjemdahl P, Thorn P, Wollni PE. Measurements of plasma norepinephrine concentrations in human primary hypertension. A word of caution on their applicability for assessing neurogenic contributions. *Hypertension* 1983;5:399–404.
56. De Mey J, Vanhoutte P. Uneven distribution of postjunctional alpha-1- and alpha-2-like adrenoceptors in canine arterial and venous smooth muscle. *Circ Res* 1981;48:875–884.
57. Van Meel KA, DeJonge A, Kalkmann HO, Wilffert B, Timmermans PBMWM, van Zwieten PA. Vascular smooth muscle contraction initiated by postsynaptic-adrenoceptor activation is induced by an influx of extracellular calcium. *Eur J Pharmacol* 1981;69:205–208.
58. Cavero I, Shepperson NB, Lefevre-Borg F, Langer SZ. Differential inhibition of vascular smooth muscle responses to alpha-1- and alpha-2-adrenoceptor agonists by diltiazem and verapamil. *Circ Res* 1983;52:169–176.
59. Timmermans PBMWM, Mathy MJ, Thoolen MJMC, DeJonge A, Wilffert B, van Zwieten PA. Invariable susceptibility to blockade by nifedipine of vasoconstriction to various alpha-2 adrenoceptor agonists in pithed rats. *J Pharm Pharmacol* 1984;36:772–775.
60. Timmermans PBMWM, Mathy MJ, Wilffert B, et al. Differential effect of calcium entry blockers on alpha-1-adrenoceptor-mediated vasoconstriction *in vivo. Naunyn Schmiedebergs Arch Pharmacol* 1983;324:239–245.
61. Millar JA, McLean KA, Reid JL. The effects of the calcium antagonist nifedipine on pressor and aldosterone responses to angiotensin II in normal man. *Eur J Clin Pharmacol* 1983;24:315–321.
62. Sterzel RB, Huelsemann JL, McKenzie DE, Wilcox CS. Nitrendipine reverses vasoconstriction and renal hemodynamic changes in experimental hypertension. *J Cardiovasc Pharmacol* 1984;6(Suppl 7):S1032–S1035.
63. Millar JA, McLean K, Reid JL. Calcium antagonists decrease adrenal and vascular responsiveness to angiotensin II in normal man. *Clin Sci* 1981;61:65s–69s.
64. van Breemen C, Bühler FR. Vascular smooth muscle superficial calcium barrier and its role in antihypertensive drug therapy. *J Cardiovasc Pharmacol* 1988.
65. Bayley S, Dobbs RJ, Robinson BF. Nifedipine in the treatment of hypertension: report of a double blind controlled trial. *Br J Clin Pharmacol* 1982;14:509–514.
66. Bruun NE, Ibsen H, Nielsen F, Nielsen MD, Moelbak AG, Hartling OJ. Lack of effect of nifendipine on counterregulatory mechanisms in essential hypertension. *Hypertension* 1986; 8:655–661.
67. Kluetsch K, Schmidt P, Grosswendt J. Der Einfluss von Bay a 1040 auf die Nierenfunktion des Hypertonikers. *Arzneimittelforschung* 1972;22:377–380.
68. Thananoparvan C, Golub MS, Eggena P, Barrett JD, Sambhi MP. Renal effects of nitrendipine monotherapy in essential hypertension. *J Cardiovasc Pharmacol* 1985;6(Suppl 7):S1040–S1044.
69. Garthoff B, Kazda S, Knorr A, Thomas G. Factors involved in the antihypertensive action of calcium antagonists. *Hypertension* 1982;225:263–270.
70. Luft FC, Aronoff G, Sloan R, Fineberg N, Weinberger M. Calcium channel blockade with nitrendipine. *Hypertension* 1985;7:438–443.
71. Leonetti G, Sala C, Bianchini C, Terzoli L, Zanchetti A. Antihypertensive and renal effects of orally administered verapamil. *Eur J Clin Pharmacol* 1980;18:375–382.
72. Dietz JR, Davies JO, Freeman RH, Villareal D, Echtenlcamp SR. Effects of intrarenal infusions of calcium entry blockers in anesthetized dogs. *Hypertension* 1983;5:482–488.
73. Loutzenhiser R, Epstein M. Effects of calcium antagonists on renal hemodynamics. *Am J Physiol* 1985;249:F619–F629.
74. Loutzenhiser R, Horton C, Epstein M. Effects of diltiazem and manganese renal hemodynamics: studies in the isolated perfused rat kidney. *Nephron* 1985;39:382–388.
75. Marre M, Misumi J, Raensch KD, Corvol P, Ménard J. Diuretic and natriuretic effects of nifedipine on isolated perfused rat kidneys. *J Pharmacol Exp Ther* 1982;223:263–267.
76. Loutzenhiser R, Epstein M, Horton C, Sonke P. Reversal by the calcium antagonist nisoldipine of norepinephrine-induced reduction of GFR: evidence for preferential antagonism of preglomerular vasoconstriction. *J Pharmacol Exp Ther* 1984;232:382–387.
77. Yamaguchi I. Studies in a new 1,5-benzodiazepine derivative. *Jpn J Pharmacol* 1974;24:511–516.
78. Zanchetti A, Leonetti G. Natriuretic effect of calcium antagonists. *J Cardiovasc Pharmacol* 1985;7(Suppl 4):S33–S37.
79. Wallia R, Greenberg A, Puschett JB. Renal hemodynamic and tubular transport effects of nitrendipine. *J Lab Clin Med* 1985;105:498–503.
80. Krusell LR, Jespersen LT, Schmitz A, Thomsen K, Lederballe Pedersen O. Repetitive natriuresis and blood pressure. Long-term calcium entry blockade with isradipine. *Hypertension* 1987;10:577–581.
81. Nicholson JP, Resnick LM, Laragh JH. The antihypertensive effect of verapamil at extremes of dietary sodium intake. *Ann Intern Med* 1987;107:329–334.
82. Luque-Otero M, Fernandez-Pinilla C, Catalan P, Martell-Claros N, Fernandez-Cruz A, Martinez-Gomez ME. Acute antihypertensive effect of nifedipine on high and low salt diet. *J Cardiovasc Pharmacol* 1987;10(Suppl 10):S147–S148.
83. Leonetti G, Rupoli L, Sangiorgio P, Gradnik R, Cuspidi C, Bolla G, Zanchetti A. Effects of different sodium intakes on the antihypertensive and renal effects of single oral doses of nifedipine in hypertensive patients. *J Cardiovasc Pharmacol* 1987;10(Suppl 10):S138–S139.
84. MacGregor GA, Pevahouse JB, Cappuccio FP, Markandu ND. Nifedipine, sodium intake, diuretics and sodium balance. *Am J Nephrol* 1987;7(Suppl 1):44–48.
85. Salvetti A, Bozzo MV, Graziola M, Abdel-Haq B. Acute hemodynamic effect of nifedipine in hypertensives with chronic renal failure: the influence of volume status. *J Cardiovasc Pharmacol* 1987;10(Suppl 10):S143–S146.
86. MacGregor GA, Pevahouse JB, Cappuccio FP, Markandu ND.

Nifedipine, diuretics and sodium balance. *J Hypertens* 1987;5(Suppl 4):S127–S131.
87. Cappuccio FP, Markandu ND, MacGregor GA. Calcium antagonists and sodium balance: effect of changes in sodium intake and of the addition of a thiazide diuretic on the blood pressure lowering effect of nifedipine. *J Cardiovasc Pharmacol* 1987;10(Suppl 10):S57–S60.
88. Bühler FR, Bolli P, Kiowski W, Erne P, Hulthén UL, Block LH. Renin profiling to select antihypertensive baseline drugs. *Am J Med* 1984;20:36–42.
89. Bühler FR, Bertel O, Lütold BE. Simplified and age-stratified antihypertensive therapy based on betablockers. *Cardiovasc Med* 1978;3:135–148.
90. Lijnen P, M'Buyamba JR, Fagard R, Staessen J, Amery A. Age-related hypotensive response to captopril in hypertensive patients. *Methods Find Exp Clin Pharmacol* 1983;5(9):655–660.
91. Bühler FR, Laragh JH, Vaughan ED Jr, Brunner HR, Gavras H, Baer L. The antihypertensive action of propranolol: specific antirenin response in high and normal renin essential, renal, renovascular and malignant hypertension. *Am J Cardiol* 1973; 32:511–522.
92. Müller FB, Sealey JE, Case DB, Atlas SA, Pickering TG, Pecker M, Preibisz JJ, Laragh JH. The captopril-test for identifying renovascular disease in hypertensive patients. *Am J Med* 1986;80:633–644.
93. Bühler FR. Antihypertensive action of beta-blockers. In: Laragh JH, Bühler FR, Seldin DW, eds. *Frontiers in hypertension research.* New York: Springer, 1981;423–436.
94. Crane MG, Harris JJ, Johus VJ. Hyporeninemic hypertension. 1972;52:457–466.
95. Vaughan ED Jr, Laragh JH, Gavras I, Bühler FR, Gavras H, Brunner HR. The volume factor in low and normal renin essential hypertension: its treatment with either spironolactone or chlorthalidone. *Am J Cardiol* 1973;32:523–532.
96. Erne P, Bolli P, Bertel O, Hulthén UL, Kiowski W, Müller F, Bühler FR. Factors influencing the hypotensive effects of calcium antagonists. *Hypertension* 1983;5(Suppl II):97–102.
97. Müller FB, Bolli P, Erne P, Block LH, Kiowski W, Bühler FR. Antihypertensive therapy with the long-acting calcium-antagonist nitrendipine. *Pharmacology* 1984;6:S1073–S1076.
98. Kiowski W, Bühler FR, Fadayomi MO, Erne P, Müller FB, Hulthén UL, Bolli P. Age, race, blood pressure and renin: predictors for antihypertensive treatment with calcium antagonists. *Am J Cardiol* 1985;56:81H–85H.
99. Resnick LM, Nicholson JP, Laragh JH. Calcium metabolism and the renin–aldosterone system in essential hypertension. *J Cardiovasc Pharmacol* 1985;7(Suppl 6):S187–S193.
100. Ribstein J, de Treglode D, Mimran A. Acute effect of nifedipine on arterial pressure in healthy subjects and hypertensives. *Arch Mal Coeur* 1985;78:29–32.
101. Moser M, Cunn J, Nash DT, Burris JF, Winer N, Simon G, Vlachakis ND. Nitrendipine in the treatment of mild to moderate hypertension. *J Cardiovasc Pharmacol* 1984;6(Suppl 7):S1085–S1089.
102. M'Buyamba-Kabangu JR, Lepira B, Lijnen P, Tshiani K, Fagard R, Amery A. Intracellular sodium and the response to nitrendipine and acebutolol in African blacks. *Hypertension* 1988; 11:100–105.
103. Dustan HP. Nitrendipine in black U.S. patients. *J Cardiovasc Pharmacol* 1987;9(Suppl 4):267–271.
104. Weinberger MH. The role of age, race and plasma renin activity in influencing the blood pressure response to nitrendipine or hydrochlorothiazide. *J Cardiovasc Pharmacol* 1987;9(Suppl 4):272–275.
105. Pedrinelli R, Fonad FM, Tarazi RC, Bravo EL, Textor SC. Nitrendipine, a calcium-entry blocker: renal and humoral effects in human arterial hypertension. *Arch Intern Med* 1986;146:62–65.
106. Zachariah PK, Schwartz GL, Ritter SG, Strong CG. Plasma predictors of calcium channel blocker efficacy in hypertension. *J Cardiovasc Pharmacol* 1986.
107. Fritschka E. Crossover comparison of nitrendipine with propranolol in patients with essential hypertension. *J Cardiovasc Pharmacol* 1984;6(Suppl 7):1100–1108.
108. Moser M, Cunn J, Materson BJ. Comparative effects of diltiazem and hydrochlorothiazide in blacks with systemic hypertension. *Am J Cardiol* 1985;56:101H–104H.
109. Amodeo C, Kobrin I, Ventura HO, Messerli FH, Fröhlich ED. Immediate and short-term hemodynamic effects of diltiazem in patients with hypertension. *Circulation* 1986;73:108–113.
110. Müller FB, Ha HR, Hotz H, Schmidlin O, Follath F, Bühler FR. Once a day verapamil in essential hypertension. *Br J Clin Pharmacol* 1986.
111. Burger RA, Carter DG, Gardiner DG, Higgins AJ. Amlodipine, a new dihydropyridine calcium channel blocker with slow onset and long duration of action. *Br J Pharmacol* 1985;85:281P.
112. Veterans Administration Cooperative Study Group on Antihypertensive Agents. Comparison of propranolol and hydrochlorothiazide for the initial treatment of hypertension. I. Results of short-term titration with emphasis on racial differences in response. II. Results of long-term therapy. *JAMA* 1982;248:1996–2003 and 2003–2011.
113. Hall WD. Pharmacologic therapy of hypertension in blacks. In: Hall WD, Saunders E, Shulman NB, eds. *Epidemiology, pathophysiology and treatment.* Chicago: Year Book Medical Publishers, 1985.
114. Moser M, Cunn J. Comparative effects of pindolol and hydrochlorothiazide in black hypertensive patients. *Angiology* 1981;32:561.
115. Moser M, Cunn J. Responses to captopril and hydrochlorothiazide in black patients with hypertension. *Clin Pharmacol Ther* 1982;32:307.
116. 1986 Guidelines for the Treatment of Mild Hypertension. Memorandum from a WHO/ISH meeting. *J Hypertens* 1986;4:383–386.
117. Brouwer RML, Bolli P, Erne P, Conen D, Kiowski W, Bühler FR. Antihypertensive treatment using calcium antagonists in combination with captopril rather than diuretics. *J Cardiovasc Pharmacol* 1985;7(Suppl 4):S88–S91.
118. Brouwer RML, Follath F, Bühler FR. Review of the cardiovascular adversity of the calcium antagonist betablocker combination: implications for antihypertensive therapy. *J Cardiovasc Pharmacol* 1985;7(Suppl 4):S38–S44.
119. Müller FB, Bolli P, Linder L, Kiowski W, Erne P, Bühler FR. Calcium antagonists and the second drug for antihypertensive therapy. *Am J Med* 1986;81(Suppl 6A):25–29.
120. The Multiple Risk Factor Intervention Trial Research Group. Multiple risk factor intervention trial, risk factor changes and mortality results. *JAMA* 1982;248:1465–1477.
121. The IPPPSH Collaborative Group. Cardiovascular risks and risk factors in a randomized trial of treatment based on the betablocker oxprenolol. The International Prospective Primary Prevention Study in Hypertension (IPPPSH). *J Hypertens* 1985;3:379–392.
122. MRC trial of mild hypertension: principal results. *Br Med J* 1985;291:89–90.
123. European Working Party on High Blood Pressure in the Elderly. Mortality and morbidity results from the European Working Party on High Blood Pressure in the Elderly. *Lancet* 1985;1:1349–1354.
124. Wilhelmsen L, Berglund G, Elenfeldt D. Betablockers versus diuretics in hypertensive men: main results from the HAPPHY trial. *J Hypertens* 1987;5:561–572.
125. Wikstrand J, Warnold I, Olsson G, Tuomilehto J, Elenfeldt D, Berglund G. Primary prevention with metoprolol in patients with hypertension. *JAMA* 1988;259:1975–1982.
126. Sterzel RB. Renal actions of calcium antagonists. *J Cardiovasc Pharmacol* 1987;10(Suppl 10):S17–S21.
127. Fleckenstein A. *Calcium antagonism in heart and smooth muscle.* New York: Wiley, 1983;314–318.
128. Fleckenstein A, Frey M, Zora J, Fleckenstein-Grün G. Experimental basis for long-term therapy of arterial hypertension with calcium antagonists. *Am J Cardiol* 1985;56:3H–14H.
129. Furberg C. Calcium antagonists and secondary cardiac prevention. Submitted for publication.
130. Gibson RS, Boden WE, Therous P, Strauss HD, Pratt CM, Gheorghiade M, Capone RJ, Crawford MH, Schlant RC, Kleiger RE, Young PM, Schechtman K, Perryman BM, Roterts R, and the Diltiazem Reinfarction Study Group. Diltiazem and rein-

farction in patients with non-Q-wave myocardial infarction. Results of a double-blind, randomized, multicenter trial. *N Engl J Med* 1986;315:423–429.

131. Moss AJ, and the Multicenter Diltiazem Post-Infarction Research Group. Long-term effect of diltiazem on mortality and reinfarction after myocardial infarction (MI)—the MDPIT study [Abstract]. *J Am Coll Cardiol* 1988;11(2):27A.

132. Atkins RC, Holsworth SR, Hancock WW, Thomson NM, Glasgow EF. Cellular immune mechanisms in human glomerulonephritis: the role of mononuclear leukocytes. *Springer Sem Immunopathol* 1982;5:269–296.

133. Sterzel RB, McKenzie DE. Effects of nitrendipine on the course of experimental immunologic glomerulonephritis. *J Cardiovasc Pharmacol* 1987;9(Suppl I):S60–S64.

134. Loutzenhiser R, Epstein M, Horton C, Sonke P. Reversal of renal and smooth muscle actions of the thromboxane mimetic U-44069 by diltiazem. *Am J Physiol* 1986;250:F619–F626.

135. Bakris GL, Burnett JC Jr. A role for calcium in radiocontrast-induced reductions in renal hemodynamics. *Kidney Int* 1985;27:465–468.

136. Neumayer H-H, Wagner K. Prevention of delayed graft function in cadaver kidney transplants by diltiazem: outcome of two prospective, randomized clinical trials. *J Cardiovasc Pharmacol* 1987;10(Suppl 10):S170–S177.

137. Lüscher TF, Weber E, Bühler FR. Effects of cyclosporin A on endothelium-dependent relaxations in the rat renal artery [Abstract]. *Kidney Int* 1988.

Hypertension: Pathophysiology, Diagnosis, and Management, edited by J. H. Laragh and B. M. Brenner. Raven Press, Ltd., New York © 1990.

CHAPTER 139

Beta-Blockers in the Treatment of Hypertension

Peter Bolli, Peter G. Fernandez, and Fritz R. Bühler

Pharmacology and Clinical Pharmacology of Beta-Blockers, 2182
Pharmacology, 2182
Classification of Beta-Blockers, 2183
Clinical Pharmacology, 2184
Antihypertensive Mode of Action of Beta-Blockers, 2185
Reduction in Cardiac Output and Hemodynamic Effects of Beta-Blockers, 2186
Suppression of Renin Release, 2186
Resetting of Arterial Baroreceptors, 2186
Central Nervous System Mechanisms, 2187
Blockade of Prejunctional Beta-Adrenoceptors, 2188
Stimulation of Vasodilator Prostaglandins, 2188
Effect on Plasma Volume, 2188
Antihypertensive Beta-Blockade, 2188
Cardioselective or Nonselective Antihypertensive Beta-Blockade: Does It Matter?, 2189
Is Intrinsic Sympathomimetic (Partial Agonist) Activity Clinically Relevant?, 2190
Beta-Blockers with Additional Vasodilator Properties, 2191
Combination Therapy with Beta-Blockers, 2191
Beta-Blockers and Diuretics, 2191
Beta-Blockers and Vasodilators, 2191
Beta-Blockers and Prazosin, 2192
Beta-Blockers and Other Sympatholytic Drugs, 2192
Beta-Blockers and Calcium Antagonists, 2192
Beta-Blockers and Angiotensin-Converting-Enzyme Inhibitors, 2193
Age and Renin: Indicators for Antihypertensive Response to Beta-Blocker Treatment?, 2193
Beta-Blocker Treatment in the Elderly Hypertensive Patient, 2195
Renovascular Hypertension, 2195
Pheochromocytoma, 2195
Beta-Blocker Treatment in Complicated Hypertension, 2195
Antihypertensive Beta-Blockade in Ischemic Heart Disease and Postmyocardial Infarction Patients, 2195
Antihypertensive Beta-Blockade in Patients with Cardiac Arrhythmias, 2196
Beta-Blocker Treatment in Patients with Renal Impairment, 2196
Beta-Blocker Treatment in Patients with Diabetes Mellitus, 2196
Beta-Blockers in Patients with Lipid Disorders, 2196
Beta-Blocker Treatment and Anesthesia, 2197
Antihypertensive Beta-Blockade in Pregnancy, 2197
Antihypertensive Beta-Blockade in Patients with Migraine, 2197
Primary Prevention for Sudden Death and Myocardial Infarction with Antihypertensive Beta-Blockade, 2197
Tolerability, 2199
Heart Failure and Asthma, 2199
Raynaud's Phenomenon, 2200
Impotence, 2200
Insulin-Dependent Diabetes Mellitus, 2201
Gastrointestinal Side Effects, 2201
Peripheral Vascular Disease, 2201
Central Nervous System Side Effects, 2201
Skin, Mucous Membranes, and Eye Manifestations, 2201
Muscle Cramps, 2201
Drug Interactions with Beta-Blockers, 2201
Abrupt Withdrawal of Beta-Blocker Therapy, 2201
Treatment of Beta-Blocker Overdose, 2203
Summary, 2203
References, 2203

The concept of alpha- and beta-adrenoceptors as applied to current cardiovascular pharmacotherapy was first described by Ahlquist in 1948 (1). Specific to the cardiovascular system, alpha-adrenoceptors mediate vascular smooth muscle contraction and therefore mediate vasoconstriction; beta-adrenoceptors cause smooth muscle relaxation and therefore cause vasodilation, bronchodilation, and cardiac stimulation.

Although alpha-adrenoceptor-blocking agents were known at the time of Ahlquist's communication, it was 10 years later that the first beta-blocking compound, dichlorisoprenaline, was discovered (2). This was soon followed by pronethalol, the first clinically used beta-blocker (3). However, because of its carcinogenicity in mice, pronethalol was replaced by propranolol, which presently represents the standard to assess all subsequent beta-blocking agents. Pronethalol and propranolol were used initially to treat patients with angina pectoris and cardiac arrhythmias (4). Their antihypertensive efficacy was first described by Prichard (5), Prichard and Gillam (6), and Schroder and Werko (7). Although first met with some skepticism because of difficulties in understanding the antihypertensive mode of action of beta-blockers, these reports opened up a revolutionary era in the treatment of hypertension. Further developments of beta-blockers included the synthesis of compounds which preferentially block cardiac beta-1-adrenoceptors ("cardioselective" beta-blockers) and those which, besides their beta-blocking properties, possess partial intrinsic beta-adrenoceptor agonist properties as well as additional (e.g., vasodilating, alpha-blocking) properties. This line of development subsequently led to numerous beta-blocking drugs which are presently being evaluated for clinical use, and it also led to the novel compounds currently under investigation.

PHARMACOLOGY AND CLINICAL PHARMACOLOGY OF BETA-BLOCKERS

Pharmacology

Beta-blockers are structurally similar to catecholamines and isoprenaline, with which they have in common a ring structure and an aliphatic side chain (Fig. 1). Various alterations of the ring and side-chain structure determine changes in their pharmacological properties. The position of the hydroxyl group at the asymmetrical carbon atom in the side chain greatly influences the affinity of the beta-receptor, whereas substitution on the ring structure determines partial (intrinsic) agonist and membrane-stabilizing properties in addition to preferential selectivity for beta-1- or beta-2-receptor subtypes (8). The beta-blocking activity

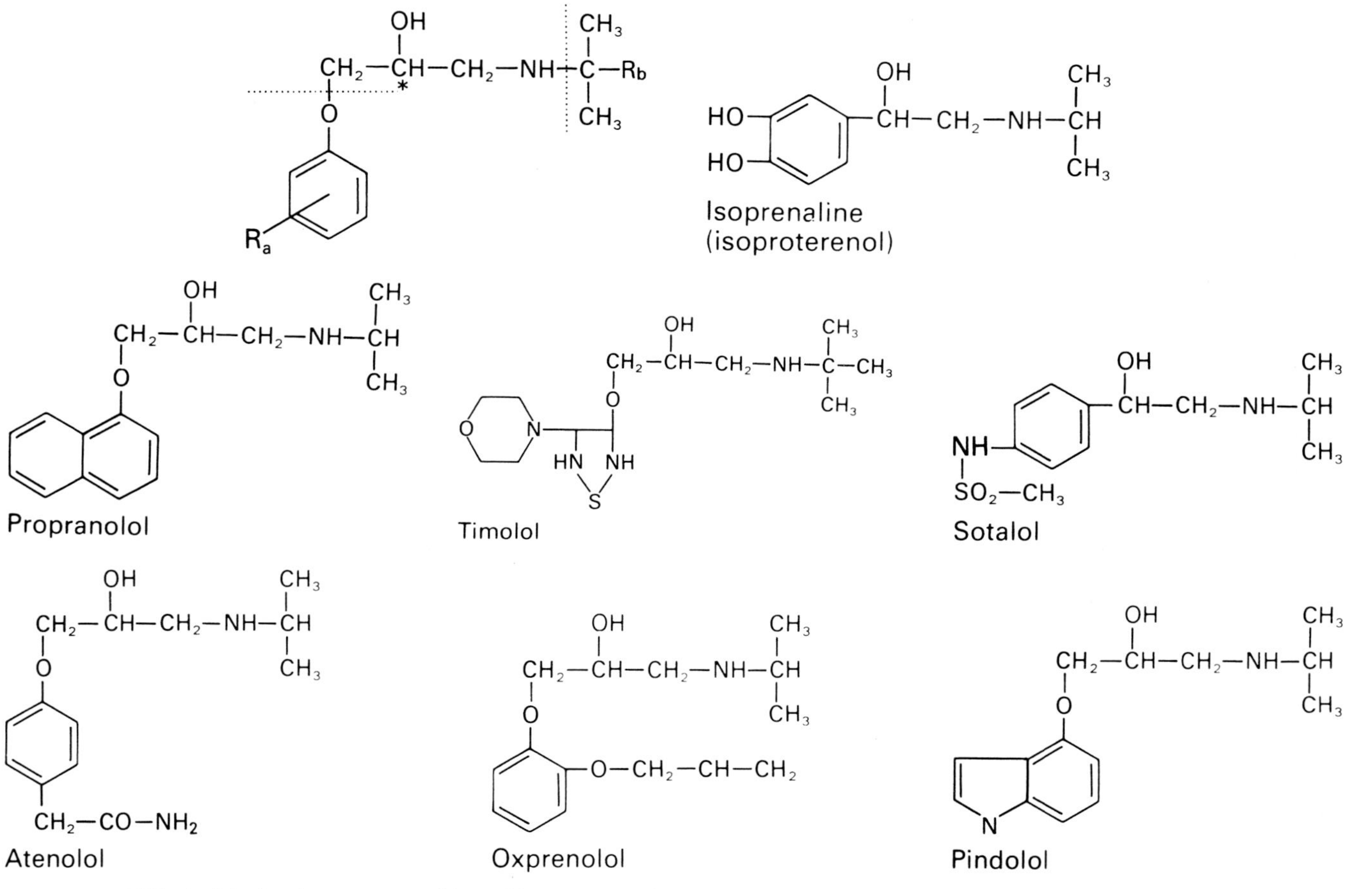

Isoprenaline (isoproterenol)

Propranolol

Timolol

Sotalol

Atenolol

Oxprenolol

Pindolol

FIG. 1. The basic structure of beta-blockers consists of an aliphatic side chain and a ring structure (**top left**). Shown also is the similarity to isoprenaline, the beta-agonist compound. Differences in the structure of the radical (R_a) determine the potency of the beta-blocking effect, the extent to which the drug exhibits intrinsic sympathomimetic activity, and whether or not it exerts an unspecific action on the cell membrane ("membrane-stabilizing effect"). The central portion of the molecule features an asymmetrical carbon atom (C). Substitution of R_b by hydrogen results in an isopropyl group, and its substitution by CH_3 in a tertiary butyl group determines the affinity of the beta-blocker for the beta-adrenoceptor. The lower part of the figure shows examples of the structural formula of some beta-blockers to demonstrate the aliphatic side chain and ring structure as the base of their molecule. (From ref. 8.)

TABLE 1. *Pharmacological characteristics of commonly used beta-blockers*

Beta-blocker	Beta-1-selectivity (cardioselectivity)	ISA[a]	Membrane-stabilizing effect	Beta-blocking metabolites
Acebutolol	+	+	+	+
Alprenolol	−	++	+	+
Atenolol	+	−	−	?
Bevantolol	+	−	−	?
Bisoprolol	+	+	−	−
Bopindolol[b]	−	+	?	+
Metoprolol	+	−	±	−
Nadolol	−	−	−	−
Oxprenolol	−	++	+	?
Penbutolol	−	+	+	+
Pindolol	−	+++	+	−
Propranolol	−	−	+	+
Sotalol	−	−	−	?
Timolol	−	−	+	−

[a] ISA, intrinsic sympathomimetic activity.
[b] Bopindolol is a prodrug whose pharmacological activity is exerted by its metabolite.

is limited to the levorotatory isomer of the compound; however, for clinical purposes, racemic preparations are used.

Classification of Beta-Blockers

For the treatment of hypertension, beta-blockers usually are classified into nonselective (beta-1 and beta-2) and cardioselective (beta-1) adrenoceptor-blocking compounds and, furthermore, into those which possess intrinsic sympathomimetic activity (ISA) and/or membrane-stabilizing pharmacologic effects (9). Table 1 shows such a classification of beta-blockers in current use. Differentiation of beta-blockers according to hydro- and lipophilicity (Table 2), as well as according to their renal and hepatic excretory pathways, may be important for the adverse reaction profile and for certain clinical conditions (e.g., impairment of renal or hepatic function) (10).

Cardioselectivity

In 1967, Lands et al. (11) provided evidence for two subtypes of beta-adrenoceptors as defined by their relative affinities for epinephrine and norepinephrine. Beta-1-adrenoceptor blockade lowers heart rate and reduces cardiac contractility and therefore reduces cardiac output and myocardial oxygen consumption. In humans, the neural component of renal renin release is mediated by beta-1-adrenoceptors. Beta-2-adrenoceptor blockade antagonizes catecholamine-induced relaxation of vascular and bronchial smooth muscle leading to broncho- and vasoconstriction. Prejunctional beta-receptors which mediate catecholamine-induced facilitation of neuronal norepinephrine release into the synaptic cleft are considered to be of beta-1 or beta-2 (12) subtype, though this is still debated.

Because beta-2-adrenoceptor blockade does not contribute to the antihypertensive effect (13), the logical step to take was the development of beta-1-selective drugs. How-

TABLE 2. *Lipophilicity (expressed as partition coefficient n-octanol/water at 37°C and pH = 7.4), plasma protein binding (%), oral bioavailability (approximate percent of dose), and beta-blocking plasma concentrations of commonly used beta-blockers*

Beta-blocker	Partition coefficient[a]	Protein binding	Bioavailability	Beta-blocking plasma concentration
Acebutolol	0.68	84	50	0.2–2 μg/ml
Alprenolol	3.27[b]	85	10	50–100 ng/ml
Atenolol	0.015	<5	50	0.2–0.5 μg/ml
Bevantolol	13.0[b]	98	50	0.2–0.6 μg/ml
Bisoprolol	4.8	30	90	10–40 ng/ml
Bopindolol	—	—	70	—
Nadolol	0.066	30	30	30–70 ng/ml
Metoprolol	0.93	12	40	50–100 ng/ml
Oxprenolol	2.28	79	40	80–100 ng/ml
Pindolol	0.82	57	85	50–150 ng/ml
Propranolol	20.2	93	30	50–100 ng/ml
Sotalol	0.039	54	100	0.5–4 μg/ml
Timolol	1.16	10	55	5–10 ng/ml

[a] The higher the partition coefficient, the greater the lipophilicity of the compound.
[b] At pH = 7.0.

ever, selectivity to beta-1-adrenoceptors is dose-dependent; with increasing doses, blockade of beta-2-adrenoceptors is inevitable and therefore the degree of "cardioselectivity" decreases (14). When expressed as the ratio between the blocking actions of beta-1- and of beta-2-mediated responses and taking the ratio obtained with propranolol as equal to 1, the relative beta-1-selectivity was found to be six orders of magnitude greater for metoprolol, nine for atenolol, and 12 for bisoprolol, a new beta-1-selective agent (15).

Intrinsic Sympathomimetic (Partial Agonist) Activity

The partial agonist effect causes mild activation of the beta-receptors and, at the same time, blocks access of endogenous catecholamines to the receptor site (16). ISA has an agonist effect on both beta-2- and beta-1-adrenoceptors; this effect may vary according to the type of beta-blocker (17). This explains both the vascular and the cardiac effects of ISA. However, the effect of ISA is limited by its flat dose–response curve; hence, with increasing doses of ISA-containing beta-blockers, the increase in agonist effect is relatively small compared to the beta-blocking action (18). The partial agonist activity is competitive and can be blocked with high doses of non-ISA-containing beta-blockers.

Membrane-Stabilizing (Local Anesthetic) Effect

This "quinidine-like" effect is unrelated to the competitive inhibition of catecholamines and therefore does not contribute to the antihypertensive efficacy of beta-blockers (19). The membrane-stabilizing effect on the cardiac action potential is seen only with drug concentrations of about 50–100 times greater than those inhibiting exercise-induced tachycardia (20). Therefore, this ancillary property is unlikely to be clinically relevant (21).

Clinical Pharmacology

Beta-blockers are rapidly absorbed, and most of them (except acebutolol, atenolol, and nadolol) are completely absorbed; moreover, the ingestion of food does not interfere with their absorption to any clinically relevant extent (22). They undergo a variable first-pass effect in the liver, resulting in differences with regard to their bioavailability. The distribution time for these drugs varies from 5 to 30 min (22).

Beta-blockers, which are metabolized mainly by the liver, are predominantly lipophilic (e.g., propranolol); predominantly hydrophilic compounds (e.g., atenolol) are excreted by the kidneys (Table 2). Impairment of renal function thus can result in higher plasma half-life of water-soluble beta-blockers (22). The more lipophilic a beta-blocker, the easier it equilibrates between the plasma compartment and brain tissue. Therefore, hydro- and lipophilicity may be important in determining the side-effect profile of beta-blockers (10). There is indeed a wide range of plasma protein binding with beta-blockers, with a range of no binding with atenolol to near complete binding (100%) with propranolol. In general, protein binding correlates with the degree of lipophilicity of the drug.

The plasma half-life of beta-blockers varies from 2 to 24 hr (Table 3), which, to some extent, dictates the dosage frequency per day (see section entitled "Antihypertensive Beta-Blockade"). Some beta-blockers form metabolites which, by themselves, exert beta-blocking effects (Table 2).

The dose of beta-blockers to achieve a satisfactory antihypertensive response is usually larger than the one required for beta-blockade (23), and the great individual variability of pharmacokinetics may explain the differences in individual doses required to achieve a similar antihypertensive effect. For some lipophilic beta-blockers (bufuralol, metoprolol, and timolol), the patients' debrisoquine/sparteine type of oxidation polymorphism may influence plasma drug concentration, thereby leading to higher

TABLE 3. *Plasma half-life, usual therapeutic daily dose range (for the majority of patients either as monotherapy or in combination with other antihypertensive drugs), dosage frequency, and equipotent single doses of commonly used beta-blockers*

Beta-blocker	Mean plasma half-life (hr)	Usual therapeutic daily dose range (mg/day)	Dosage frequency[c]	Equipotent single doses (mg)
Acebutolol	3–4	400–800	b.i.d.	200
Alprenolol[a]	2–3	200–800	b.i.d.	200
Atenolol	6–9	50–100	o.d.	100
Bevantolol	1.5–2.0	200–400	o.d./b.i.d.	200
Bisoprolol	10–11	5–10	o.d.	10
Bopindolol	4–7[b]	1–2	o.d.	1
Nadolol	14–24	80–240	o.d.	120
Metoprolol[a]	3–4	100–200	b.i.d.	100
Oxprenolol[a]	2–3	80–320	t.i.d./b.i.d.	100
Penbutolol	2–4	60–80	o.d./b.i.d.	—
Pindolol	3–6	5–30	b.i.d./o.d.	5
Propranolol[a]	3–6	80–320	b.i.d.	100
Sotalol	7–18	160–320	b.i.d./o.d.	200
Timolol	4–5	10–40	b.i.d./o.d.	10

[a] Long-acting or slow-release formulations with lower dosage frequency available.
[b] Half-life of the prodrug.
[c] Abbreviations: b.i.d., twice daily; o.d., once daily; t.i.d., thrice daily.

plasma drug levels and, hence, greater beta-blockade in those patients who are of poor metabolizer phenotype (3–10% of the European and North American population) as compared to "extensive metabolizers" (24). However, the large safety margin of beta-blocker usually allows for variation caused by such genetic differences. Although there is a close correlation between the degree of beta-blockade (e.g., isoproterenol antagonism) and the plasma levels of drugs, the latter usually do not relate to the degree of the antihypertensive action; this reflects the complexity of the beta-blockers' antihypertensive mode of action. However, the ratio of the dosage needed for different beta-blockers to produce comparable antihypertensive effects is similar to the relative beta-blocking potency of these drugs (23).

ANTIHYPERTENSIVE MODE OF ACTION OF BETA-BLOCKERS

Although the mechanisms by which beta-blockers lower blood pressure are not fully understood, their antihypertensive effect is the result of beta-adrenoceptor blockade; this is because the *d*-isomers, which have no beta-blocking properties, do not lower blood pressure (25). Accordingly, the antihypertensive pharmacologic action takes place at sites of beta-receptors; these beta-receptors competitively antagonize the actions of catecholamines, which include (a) postjunctional beta-adrenoceptors of the heart, of the blood vessels, and of the juxtaglomerular apparatus of the kidney, (b) prejunctional beta-adrenoceptors of the sympathetic nerve terminals, (c) beta-adrenoceptors related to baroreceptors of the carotid sinus and of the aortic arch, and (d) beta-adrenoceptors related to the autonomic pathways of the central nervous system (Fig. 2). Although lacking an integrated explanation of the mode of action of beta-blockers, the following mechanisms have been found to be most likely operative in the antihypertensive pharmacologic responses of beta-blockers: (a) reduction in cardiac output; (b) suppression of renin release; (c) resetting of baroreceptors; (d) direct action on the central nervous system; (e) release of vasodilator prostaglandins; and (f) blockade of prejunctional beta-receptors.

However, it has not been possible—with the exception of the renin classification (26,27)—to identify hypertensive patients as to their preferential response to one of these mechanisms. Furthermore, any of these mechanisms fall short of explaining the observation that there is a delay

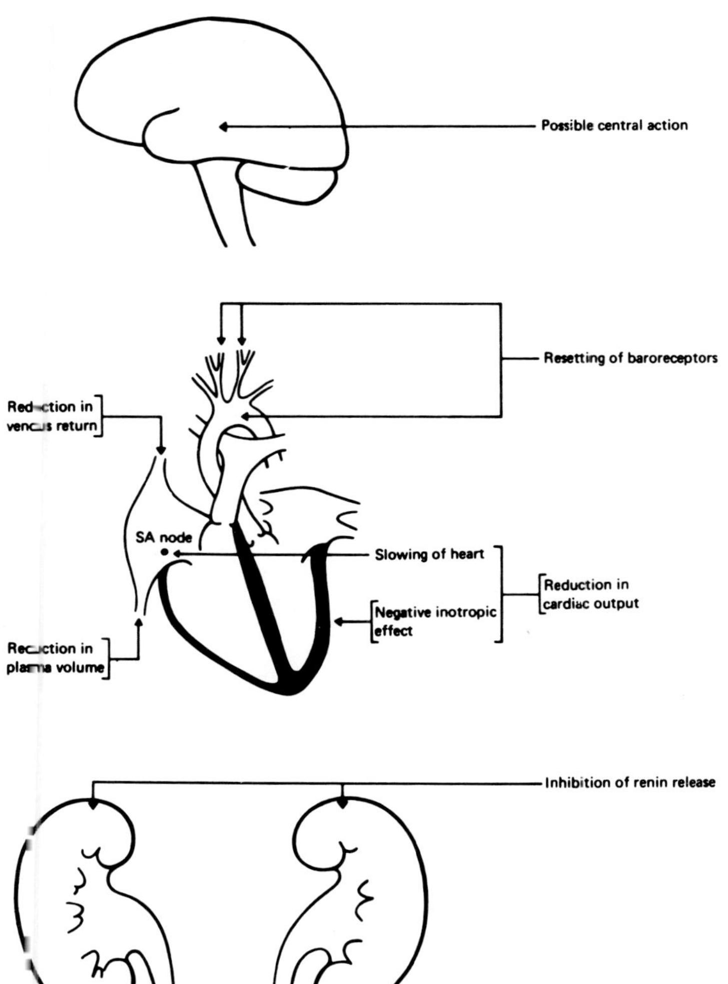

FIG. 2. Proposed antihypertensive modes of action of beta-blockers. (From ref. 71.)

between (a) the changes in the indices for the beta-blockers' effectiveness on the above mechanisms and (b) the fall in blood pressure (28–30).

Reduction in Cardiac Output and Hemodynamic Effects of Beta-Blockers

Acute administration of beta-blockers lowers cardiac output; this is a result of the beta-blockers' negative inotropic action consequent to the competitive inhibition of the catecholamines acting on beta-receptors in the myocardium, the sino-atrial node, and possibly the capacitance vessels (21), which result in slowing of heart rate and a decrease in myocardial contractility. Because of reflex sympathetic activation (31) mediated by vascular alpha-1- and alpha-2-adrenoceptors (32), vascular resistance increases while mean arterial pressure remains unchanged (33–36). Beta-blockers with ISA lower cardiac output and increase vascular resistance to a lesser extent (and may even induce slight vasodilation), as compared to non-ISA-containing beta-blockers (16,35,37,38) (Fig. 3).

During chronic treatment, the initial elevated vascular resistance falls to below the pretreatment levels within a variable time (days to weeks), and this inadvertently leads to a fall of blood pressure (33,34,39). Cardiac output remains reduced with non-ISA-containing blockers (33–35,39,40), representing the main factor for their antihypertensive beta-blockade; in contrast, ISA-containing blockers lower cardiac output to a lesser extent but lower peripheral resistance to a greater extent (Fig. 3). However, the lowered cardiac output does not entirely explain the primary antihypertensive mode of action of beta-blockers, since in the face of a reduced cardiac output during chronic therapy, peripheral vascular resistance may remain elevated, resulting in nonresponse to antihypertensive beta-blockade (32,33,36).

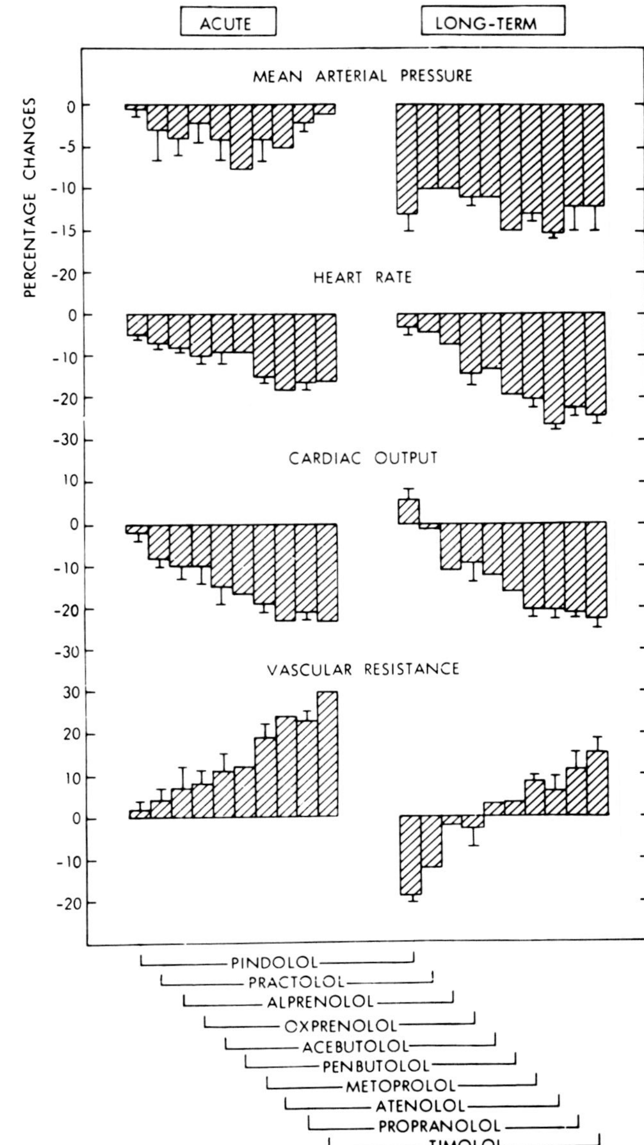

FIG. 3. Acute and long-term hemodynamic effects of 10 beta-receptor blockers in supine resting patients with hypertension. Indicated are mean percentage changes and standard errors of the mean in those cases where at least four studies for a given beta-blocker were available. The beta-blockers are presented according to a decreasing quantity of intrinsic sympathomimetic activity (ISA) or partial agonist activity (PAA) from left to right. (From ref. 35.)

Suppression of Renin Release

Renin release is suppressed at often small doses by all beta-blockers (26,27,41–46), though some investigators found a lesser renin suppressibility with ISA-containing beta-blockers (47,48). The fall in blood pressure in response to beta-blocker therapy has been found to relate directly to changes in plasma renin activity (26,42,44,46) (Fig. 4) in some studies; in others, however, although suppression of plasma renin was found, it was not possible to demonstrate a relationship between (a) the decrease in blood pressure and (b) the level of pretreatment renin or the treatment-induced fall in plasma renin activity (48–51). However, some of these discrepancies may be explained by differences in methodology (42). Beta-blockers also reduce aldosterone excretion rate (Fig. 5), but, relative to the renin-suppressing effect of beta-blockers, the reduction of plasma aldosterone is smaller; this may be due to the increased plasma potassium concentrations (consequent to renin suppression), independently stimulating aldosterone production and release while, at the same time, further suppressing renin release (52). In patients with high plasma renin activity, renin suppression appears to be the prevailing antihypertensive mode of action of beta-blockers (see section entitled "Combination Therapy with Beta-Blockers"); however, in patients with normal and low renin concentrations, the lowering of renin would have to operate in concert with other antihypertensive mechanisms (42).

Resetting of Arterial Baroreceptors

The baroreflexes are less sensitive to an increase in blood pressure in patients with established hypertension than in

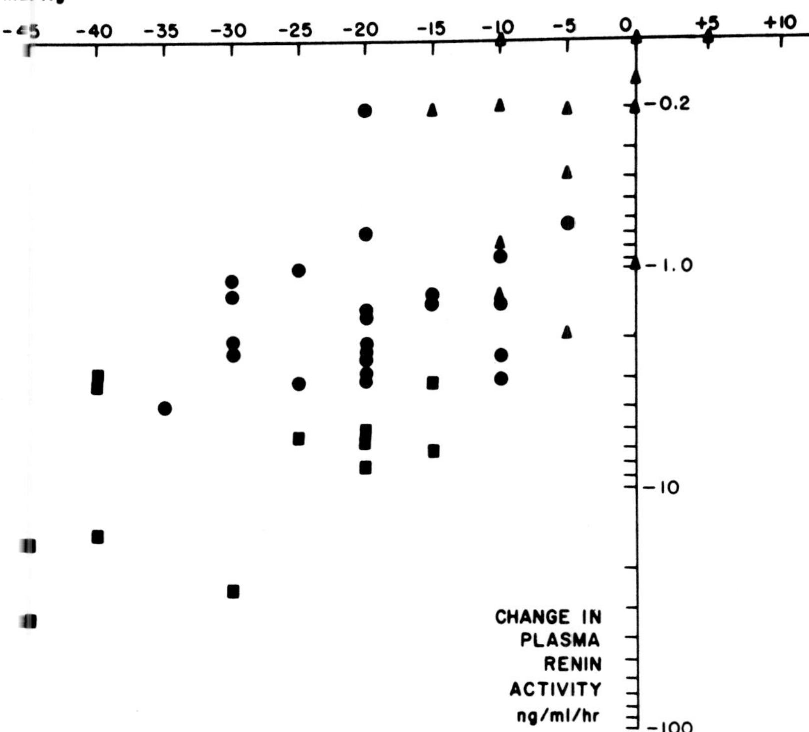

FIG. 4. Direct relationship of propranolol-induced changes in diastolic pressure plotted against the absolute decrements in plasma renin activity in patients with low (▲), normal (●), and high (■) renin. (From ref. 26.)

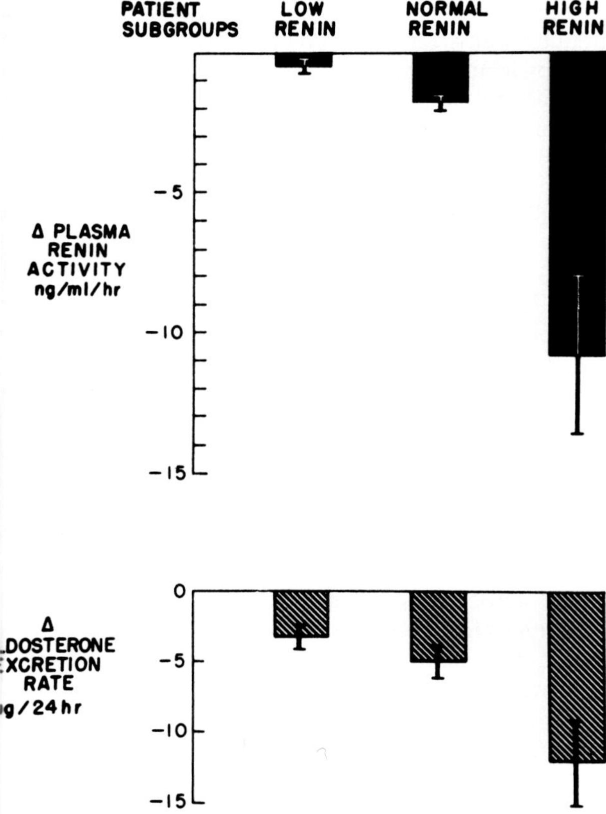

FIG. 5. Propranolol-induced concurrent reduction in plasma renin activity and aldosterone excretion rates in low-, normal-, and high-renin subgroups. (From ref. 26.)

normotensive subjects (53). Chronic beta-blocker treatment has been reported to restore this abnormality (53,54) and could serve as an explanation for the delayed fall in blood pressure during chronic beta-blocker administration (21,39). However, this finding has not been consistent (55), presumably owing to methodological problems associated with quantitative measurement of baroreflex sensitivity in humans.

Central Nervous System Mechanisms

The presence of beta-adrenoceptors in the brain (56) provided the basis for investigations into a possible central nervous system effect of beta-blockers. Reduction of central sympathetic outflow could be a mechanism whereby beta-blockers may lower the initially elevated peripheral vascular resistance (57). However, this notion is complicated by the following observations: (a) In animal experiments, high concentrations of intracerebrally injected beta-blockers are required in order to lower blood pressure; these high concentrations, through leakage from the brain, subsequently lead to therapeutic levels of the drug in the circulating blood, thereby confounding a centrally mediated effect (58). (b) A "nonspecific" effect contributes to the centrally mediated fall in blood pressure; this decrease can be achieved also by *d*-propranolol (59). (c) The degree of lipophilicity (and, therefore, the rapidness and degree of penetration into the cerebrospinal fluid) differs between various betablockers, yet the onset and magnitude of the antihypertensive efficacy is similar (60). (d) Finally, the reduction in sympathetic activity could be mediated through changes in afferent impulses arising from arterial baroreceptors; thus, strictly speaking, this reduction does not originate in the central nervous system (57).

Blockade of Prejunctional Beta-Adrenoceptors

Blockade of prejunctional beta-adrenoceptors (and, hence, attenuation of their facilitatory effect on norepinephrine release) seems an attractive (61), though as yet largely unproven, hypothesis. It has been shown that bevantolol lowered circulating levels of norepinephrine and exhibited a significant vascular sparing effect when compared with propranolol (62). However, in combination with a diuretic, plasma norepinephrine concentrations remained elevated until the diuretic was withdrawn (63) although the reflex elevation of plasma renin activity was lowered—suggesting that bevantolol, when administered alone, may reduce neuronal norepinephrine release, but not under circumstances of adrenergic stimulation. Also, an effect on prejunctional beta-receptors might explain why beta-blockers appear to interfere with alpha-adrenoceptor-mediated vasoconstriction (32) in patients with enhanced alpha-adrenoceptor-mediated vasoconstriction (64,65).

Stimulation of Vasodilator Prostaglandins

The possibility that prostaglandins may be invoked in the antihypertensive mode of action of beta-blockers (66) stems from the observation that indomethacin, a potent inhibitor of prostaglandin synthesis, attenuates the antihypertensive effect of beta-blockers (67). However, this effect is not specific for beta-blockers, since it is also documented with diuretics (67).

Effect on Plasma Volume

In early studies (68) it was found that propranolol reduced plasma volume, but this did not correlate with the fall in blood pressure. Furthermore, later studies showed that reduction of plasma volume during beta-blockade was not a constant feature and is unlikely to contribute to the antihypertensive mode of action of beta-blockers (69).

ANTIHYPERTENSIVE BETA-BLOCKADE

Beta-blockers, given either alone or in combination with other antihypertensive drugs (39,70–72), lower blood pressure of all grades of essential and renal hypertension (39,43,73,74). Overall, 40–60% of patients with mild to severe hypertension respond satisfactorily to beta-blocker monotherapy, and the antihypertensive effect of the various beta-blockers has been shown to be comparable and appears not to depend on ancillary pharmacologic properties (e.g., cardioselectivity, ISA, etc.) (23,41,75,76). Beta-blockers also lower exercise-induced increases in blood pressure (77,78) but do not induce postural or exercise hypotension (39), since increased adrenergic activity on assumption to upright posture induces vasoconstriction via intact alpha-adrenoceptor-mediated vasoconstriction. However, when combined with other antihypertensive drugs (e.g., bethanidine, methyldopa, or prazosin), postural and exercise hypotension may become apparent (70). In unselected patients, the antihypertensive response to beta-blockers is similar to that of methyldopa, adrenergic neuron-blocking agents (39), diuretics (71,79), calcium antagonists (80), and angiotensin-converting-enzyme inhibitors (81). In most patients, particularly in those with mild and moderate hypertension, the antihypertensive action is seen within the first few days after initiation of treatment, though the maximum attainable effect is usually reached within one to several weeks (33,34,39); this is usually preceded by other evidence of beta-blockade.

The commonly used beta-blockers, along with their usual doses, are shown in Table 3. Although high doses were prescribed at the beginning of the beta-blocker era (39,82), long-term experience has shown that the dose response to antihypertensive beta-blockade is flat and that in most patients whose blood pressure does not respond satisfactorily to beta-blocker monotherapy, combination treatment should be considered. On the other hand, low doses may give good blood pressure control; furthermore, in patients who initially required higher doses, an attempt to reduce them may be justified so as to reduce the potential of side effects. Tolerance to the antihypertensive action of beta-blockers is rare, and fluid retention does not occur except when given to patients with heart failure. The most frequent cause for blood pressure rise during beta-blocker therapy is noncompliance, which can easily be ascertained by a faster-than-usual rise in exercise heart rate. If a patient responds well or is resistant to a given beta-blocker he or she is likely to respond in the same way to another one (23).

The beta-1 ("cardioselective") type of blockers are atenolol (83), bevantolol (84), metoprolol (69,85), the newer, highly beta-1-selective compound bisoprolol (86) (all without ISA), and the ISA-containing beta-blocker acebutolol (87) (Table 3). Nonselective ISA-containing beta-blockers are bopindolol (88), pindolol (37), oxprenolol (89), penbutolol (90), and alprenolol (23), with pindolol having the most pronounced partial agonist effect (18). Nonselective non-ISA-containing beta-blockers are propranolol (39), sotalol (which has class III antiarrhythmic properties) (91), nadolol (14), and timolol (83). Owing to their longer plasma half-life (Table 3), atenolol, bisoprolol, nadolol, and sotalol provide blood pressure reduction for 24 hr when given once daily. However, it has been shown that drugs with a shorter plasma half-life can be given once daily with adequate blood pressure control (84,87). Bopindolol, a newer compound, is a prodrug; during its liver passage (plasma half-life 4–7 hr) it is rapidly metabolized to its active metabolite, thereby providing a 20- to 27-hr half-life of the pharmacological effects (92). Currently, bopindolol is the beta-blocker with the longest duration of action, allowing even a once-weekly administration (88). For those beta-blockers which have a shorter plasma half-life, a prolonged action has been achieved by providing slow-release or long-acting formulations (e.g., acebutolol, metoprolol, oxprenolol, or propranolol, which can be given once or twice daily) (14,75,93,94). Beta-blockers with additional vasodilating properties are discussed in the section entitled "Beta-Blockers with Additional Vasodilator Properties." This large number of available beta-blockers makes the selection of the most appropriate compound for a given condition difficult. However, although the antihypertensive and antianginal effect of beta-blockers are comparable, ancillary pharmacological properties, and differences in clinical pharmacological characteristics, as well as differences in side-effect patterns, may determine the use of a particular beta-blocker in the individual patient.

The following sections should provide some directional help, and Table 4 summarizes clinical situations that would influence the choice of beta-blocking drugs.

CARDIOSELECTIVE OR NONSELECTIVE ANTIHYPERTENSIVE BETA-BLOCKADE: DOES IT MATTER?

The main advantage of cardioselective beta-blockers probably lies in their sparing effects on airway resistance (95–97); however, this has remained controversial, presumably owing to differences in methodology applied in various studies (98). The risk of developing a bronchoconstriction increases considerably with higher doses and in susceptible patients (99). However, it is clear that bronchoconstriction can more readily be overcome by beta-2-agonistic (bronchodilator) drugs in the presence of cardioselective blockers than in the presence of nonselective blockers (22,95). The sparing effect on vascular beta-2-adrenoceptors by cardioselective beta-blockers results in a smaller blood pressure rise to stress and exercise (100).

Since pancreatic insulin release and catecholamine-stimulated glycogenolysis are predominantly beta-2-adrenoceptor-mediated (101), beta-1-selective and ISA-containing blockers should induce less impairment of glucose tolerance in diabetic patients (77,102,103) and should interfere less with the recovery from hypoglycemia (21,103–105) (see also section entitled "Beta-Blocker Treatment in Patients with Diabetes Mellitus").

Beta-1-selective blockers are less likely to alter plasma cholesterol concentrations and plasma lipoprotein fractions (106); however, similar to nonselective beta-blockers, beta-1-selective blockers increase plasma triglyceride con-

TABLE 4. *Clinical situations that would influence the choice of a beta-blocking drug*[a]

Condition	Choice of beta-blocker
Asthma, chronic bronchitis with bronchospasm	Avoid all beta-blockers if possible; however, if beta-blockade is necessary, small doses of beta-1-selective blockers (e.g., acebutolol, atenolol, metoprolol, bisoprolol) or drugs with ISA (e.g., pindolol, oxprenolol), as well as labetalol with alpha-adrenergic-blocking properties, can be used.
Congestive heart failure	Beta-blockers are contraindicated; if necessary, drugs with ISA and vasodilator properties might have an advantage.
Angina	In vasospastic angina, labetalol may be useful; other beta-blockers should be used with caution. In patients with angina at already low heart rates, drugs without ISA may be preferable. Patients who have angina at high heart rates but who have resting bradycardia might benefit from a drug with ISA.
Atrioventricular conduction defects	Beta-blockers are generally contraindicated; however, drugs with partial agonist activity, as well as labetalol, may be tried with caution.
Bradycardia	Beta-blockers with ISA, as well as labetalol, have less pulse-slowing effect and are preferable.
Raynaud's phenomenon, intermittent claudication, cold extremities	Beta-1-selective blocking agents, labetalol, and drugs with ISA or additional alpha-blocking (labetalol) or vasodilator properties might have an advantage.
Depression	Avoid propranolol. Substitute a beta-blocker with ISA or low lipid solubility.
Diabetes mellitus	Beta-1-selective agents and ISA drugs are preferable.
Thyrotoxicosis	All agents will control symptoms, but drugs without ISA are preferred.
Pheochromocytoma	Avoid all beta-blockers unless an alpha-blocker is given. Labetalol may be used as a treatment of choice.
Renal failure	Use reduced doses of compounds largely eliminated by renal mechanisms (nadolol, sotalol, atenolol) and those drugs whose bioavailability is increased in uremia (propranolol, alprenolol). Also consider possible accumulation of active metabolites (alprenolol, propranolol).
Use of insulin and sulfonylurea	Danger of hypoglycemia but is possibly reduced using drugs with beta-1-selectivity.
Clonidine	Avoid nonselective beta-blockers, and use labetalol for rebound effect with clonidine withdrawal.
Oculomucocutaneous syndrome	Stop drug.
Hyperlipidemia	Avoid nonselective beta-blockers; use agents with ISA or beta-1-selectivity, or use labetalol.
Migraine	Drugs with ISA may be less effective.

[a] Adapted from ref. 242. ISA, intrinsic sympathomimetic (partial agonist) activity.

centrations, though this may be less pronounced (with greater cardioselectivity) at equipotent antihypertensive doses (107,108). The increase in plasma triglyceride concentrations could be due to unopposed alpha-adrenoceptor stimulation counteracting lipoprotein lipase activity (106).

On the other hand, cardioselective beta-blockers block epinephrine-induced hypokalemia less effectively than do nonselective blockers (109); this is because epinephrine stimulates, via beta-2-adrenoceptors, a membrane-bound ATPase in skeletal muscle (109) which promotes the shift of potassium from the extracellular to the intracellular compartment. Increases in plasma concentrations of epinephrine, which can lead to clinically relevant falls in plasma potassium concentration (109), can occur in the event of a myocardial infarction (110). Epinephrine-induced hypokalemia is enhanced in diuretic-treated patients (111) and can be attenuated by the combination of the diuretic with a beta-blocker.

IS INTRINSIC SYMPATHOMIMETIC (PARTIAL AGONIST) ACTIVITY CLINICALLY RELEVANT?

The clinical manifestations of ISA and cardioselectivity are often very similar even though they are achieved through different mechanisms: Cardioselective beta-blockers leave beta-2-adrenoceptors accessible to stimulation by endogenous (or exogenous, therapeutic) catecholamines, whereas ISA stimulates mainly beta-2- and beta-1-adrenoceptors. With increasing doses of cardioselective beta-blockers, beta-1-selectivity decreases relative to the degree of beta-2-blockade; however, with ISA-containing beta-blockers, beta-2- and beta-1-adrenoceptor stimulation increases, but, owing to the flat dose–response curve of ISA, this stimulation decreases relative to the increase in the beta-receptor-blocking effect (18). ISA is most effective when endogenous catecholamine levels are low, but it is least effective when endogenous sympathetic nervous system activity is high (18,77,78). Under resting conditions (77,112) and during sleep (93), beta-blockers endowed with ISA reduce heart rate to a lesser extent than do those without ISA; during exercise, however, there was no difference between the two types of beta-blocker in terms of heart rate reduction (77,78) (Fig. 6). Therefore, beta-blockers with ISA are suitable for patients with low resting heart rates. In elderly patients, low resting heart rates can induce tiredness as cardiac output is reduced, and a change to an ISA-containing beta-blocker may result in subjective improvement (77). Furthermore, in some patients with orthostatic hypotension secondary to the loss of peripheral receptor stimulation, pindolol has been used to increase heart rate and thus maintain upright blood pressure (113).

Beta-blockers with ISA are less likely to reduce resting cardiac output (35,114) and peripheral blood flow (115) (Fig. 3); pindolol, as a result of its stimulating effect on beta-2-receptors (116), was shown to possess a vasodilator effect (35,47). Hence, it has been suggested that beta-blockers with ISA may be better tolerated in patients with cold extremities (115,117,118).

In acute studies (114,119), the lesser fall in cardiac output, the slight vasodilator effect, and the lower pulmonary wedge pressure of pindolol led to the notion that ISA-containing blockers may be less likely to precipitate heart failure. However, the beta-adrenergic-stimulatory effect of the ISA component cannot be relied on as being a sufficient safeguard to avert beta-blocker-induced heart failure, but if beta-blockers are absolutely necessary in patients with compromised cardiac function, ISA-containing drugs should be used (37,77).

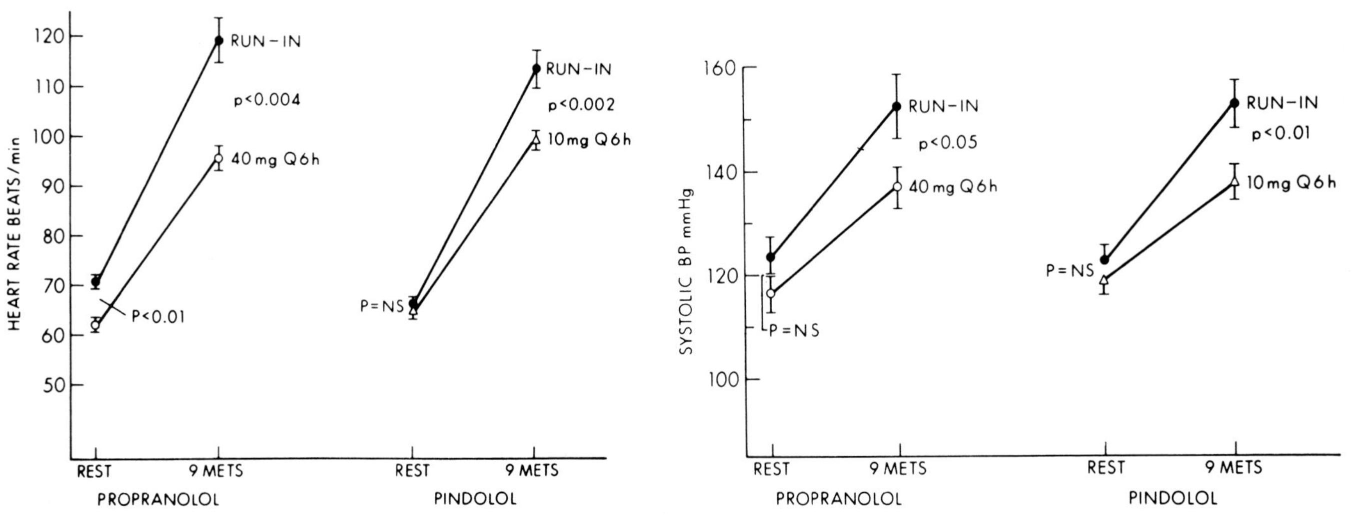

FIG. 6. Effects of pindolol and propranolol on the heart rate (**A**) and systolic blood pressure (**B**) at rest and during exercise [9 METS (3.0 miles per hr at 15% grade for 3 min)]. A significant decrease in resting heart rate and systolic pressure, as well as a significant decrease in heart rate and systolic pressure increments with exercise, is seen with propranolol (160 mg/day; *open symbols*) compared with the run-in (pretreatment) period (*filled symbols*). There is no significant change in the resting heart rate and systolic pressure in patients treated with pindolol (40 mg/day). However, the heart rate and systolic pressure increments with exercise are significantly blunted. (From ref. 77.)

The literature has shown that ISA-containing beta-blockers may have less of a bronchoconstrictor effect than do non-ISA-containing beta-blockers (77,120), and patients who developed such symptoms on non-ISA-containing compounds did not develop these symptoms on ISA-containing blockers (23). At low doses, cardioselective beta-blockers may cause less bronchoconstriction than do ISA-containing compounds. However, the clinical benefit of this pharmacological advantage is still being debated (98); moreover, as in patients with compromised cardiac function, ISA may not be regarded as a safeguard against beta-blocker-induced bronchoconstriction and should thus be avoided in asthmatic patients, since alternative antihypertensive drugs are available.

ISA-containing beta-blockers do not seem to alter plasma lipids unfavorably (121). This has been demonstrated for oxprenolol (122), bopindolol (123), and pindolol (124), the latter having been observed to possibly raise the HDL cholesterol fraction (125) while the non-ISA-containing compounds caused a decrease (124,126). The global results, however, are still inconsistent (127).

BETA-BLOCKERS WITH ADDITIONAL VASODILATOR PROPERTIES

Beta-blockers with additional vasodilating properties reduce vascular resistance and, at the same time, attenuate the vasodilator-induced reflex tachycardia (31), thereby tending to restore the central and peripheral hemodynamic abnormalities in the established hypertensive state (34). Vasodilation can be achieved with (a) high pharmacologic action of ISA (e.g., pindolol), (b) an additional postjunctional alpha-1- and/or alpha-2-adrenoceptor blockade, and (c) an additional direct vasodilator effect (Table 5). Labetolol vasodilates by additional postjunctional alpha-1-blockade and can be used in severe hypertension and hypertensive emergencies (given orally or intravenously) with rapid onset of the fall in blood pressure (128). For the same reasons, labetolol is used in patients with pheochromocytoma (129) and is also used for treating hypertensive crises during clonidine withdrawal (129). Medroxolol (130) also has alpha- and beta-blocking actions as well as beta-2-adrenoceptor-stimulating actions. Celiprolol (131) combines beta-1-selective blockade with beta-2-adrenoceptor stimulation and a direct vasodilator effect and has broncho-sparing properties which may provide a better safety margin (132). Carvedilol, a more recent compound, combines a well-balanced noncardioselective beta-blockade with a direct precapillary vasodilator effect and has shown good long-term antihypertensive efficacy (133) as has bucindolol, a beta-blocker with (a) a stimulating effect on beta-2-receptors and (b) a direct vasodilator action (134).

Beta-blockers with additional vasodilator properties are also effective antianginal agents, since besides the beta-blocker-related decrease in myocardial oxygen consumption the vasodilator-induced afterload reduction alleviates left ventricular work (131,135). Whether the newer beta-blocking, vasodilating drugs are associated with a greater response rate among older patients remains to be assessed; these drugs also need to be assessed in terms of their possible beneficial effect on plasma lipids owing to their alpha-blocking properties and ISA (106).

COMBINATION THERAPY WITH BETA-BLOCKERS

Beta-blockers can be combined with practically all other antihypertensive agents, the combination usually providing an antihypertensive response that is superior to that achieved with the single components; unwanted adverse reactions of the single components can, to a certain extent, be negated by the combination (31,79,136).

Beta-Blockers and Diuretics

Diuretics and beta-blockers are the most frequently used combination (39,71,79). They have a synergistic effect on cardiac output (137), and their antihypertensive effect is additive (49,79). While diuretics lower plasma volume, beta-blockers do not (49). Therefore they counter, to some extent, the diuretic-induced increase in plasma renin activity and, by reducing aldosterone secretion (Fig. 5), counter the diuretic-induced fall in plasma potassium (Fig. 7).

Beta-Blockers and Vasodilators

Beta-blockers counter the vasodilator-induced increase in heart rate, cardiac output, and plasma renin activity (31); conversely, the vasodilator drug attenuates the beta-blocker-induced, unopposed, alpha-adrenoceptor-mediated, enhanced vasoconstrictor effect, thereby adding to the antihypertensive effect (136,138). The combination of a

TABLE 5. *The vasodilating beta-blockers*[a]

	Receptor blockade					
	Alpha-1	Alpha-2	Beta-1	Beta-2	ISA beta	Direct vasodilation
Pindolol			+	+	+++	
Labetalol	+		+	+	±	
Celiprolol		±	+		+	+
Prizidilol			+	+		+
Carvedilol			+	+		+
Medroxalol	±		+	+	+	±
Bucindolol	±	±	+	+	+	+

[a] Adapted from ref. 47.

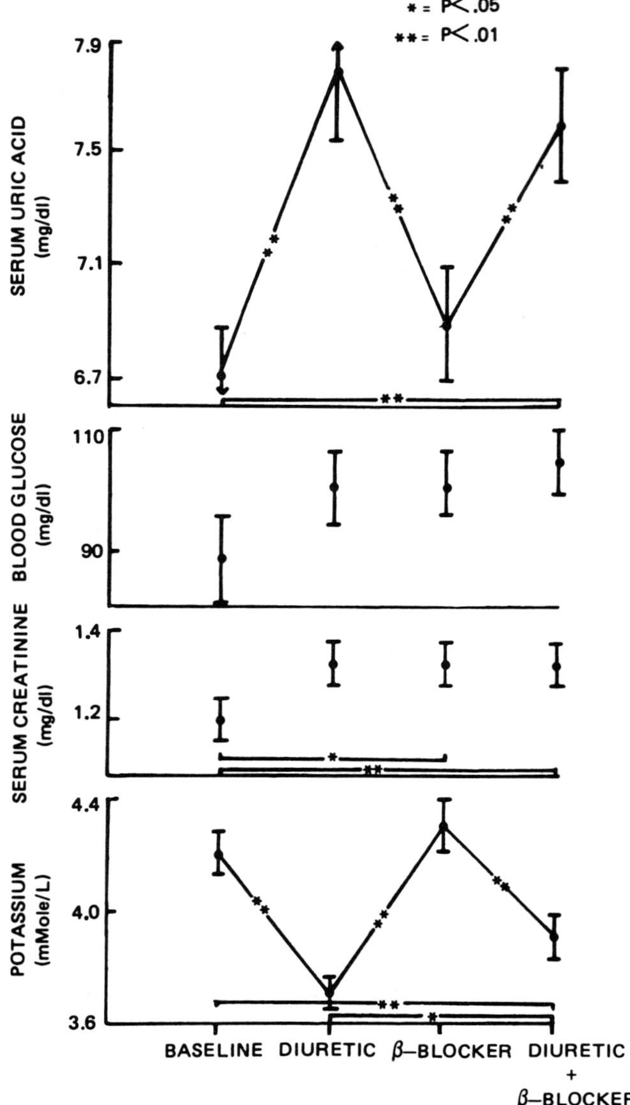

FIG. 7. Effects on clinical chemistry measurements of diuretics and beta-blockers (propranolol or metoprolol) given separately, or in combination, in 36 patients with essential hypertension. (From ref. 72.)

beta-blocker and a diuretic with the vasodilator is often essential for the treatment with the potent vasodilator minoxidil (136).

Beta-Blockers and Prazosin

Beta-blockade combined with prazosin enhances the antihypertensive effect (139); however, since the orthostatic blood pressure rise is blunted as a result of prazosin's alpha-blockade, postural hypotension may occur, particularly with the first dose of prazosin (140).

Beta-Blockers and Other Sympatholytic Drugs

The combination of a beta-blocker with sympatholytic drugs (methyldopa, guanethidine, reserpine, clonidine) has less of a logical pharmacologic basis because they all, by reducing sympathetic activity, ultimately lower heart rate and cardiac output even though they act on the sympathetic nervous system via different mechanisms. Usually, patients who respond well to methyldopa also do so to beta-blockers (39). When beta-blockers are combined with clonidine, they may expose the blood vessels to unopposed alpha-adrenoceptor-mediated vasoconstriction in case of a hypertensive crisis following acute discontinuation of clonidine (141). Treatment of such a condition consists of combined alpha- and beta-blockade with labetolol (129).

Beta-Blockers and Calcium Antagonists

More recently, the combination of a beta-blocker with calcium antagonists has been shown to be very effective and well tolerated, and beta-blockade counters the effects of reflex sympathetic stimulation evoked by the calcium antagonist (142,143) (Fig. 8). There is some concern as to the combination of verapamil with a beta-blocker because of their common prolonging action on atrioventricular conduction (144), though this seems to be less of a problem when the drugs are given orally (145).

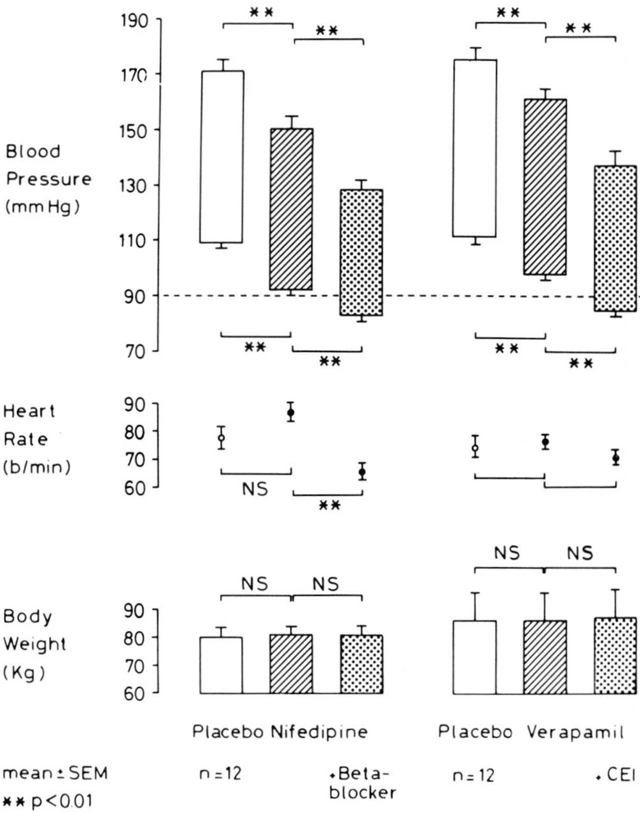

FIG. 8. Blood pressure response to combination treatment of a beta-blocker with nifedipine (**left panel**). The addition of the beta-blocker blunts the slight increase in heart rate on nifedipine alone. The antihypertensive response to the beta-blocker–calcium-antagonist combination is comparable to that of an angiotensin-converting-enzyme inhibition (CEI) and a calcium antagonist (**right panel**). (From ref. 143.)

atenolol, and hydrochlorothiazide in mild to moderate hypertension. *Lancet* 1986;1:872–875.

160. Yusuf S, Peto R, Lewis J, Collins R, Sleight P. Beta blockade during and after myocardial infarction: an overview of the randomized trials. *Prog Cardiovasc Dis* 1985;17:335–371.

161. Cove-Smith JR, Kirk CA. CNS-related side effects with metoprolol and atenolol. *Eur J Clin Pharmacol* 1985;28(Suppl):69–72.

162. Fodor JG, Chockalingam A, Drover A, Fifield F, Pauls CJ. A comparison of the side effects of atenolol and propranolol in the treatment of patients with hypertension. *J Clin Pharmacol* 1987;27:892–901.

163. Tarazi RC, Frohlich ED, Dustan HP. Contribution of cardiac output to renovascular hypertension. *Am J Cardiol* 1973;31:600–605.

164. Case DB, Atlas SA, Marion RM, Laragh JH. Long-term efficacy of captopril in renovascular and essential hypertension. *Am J Cardiol* 1982;49:1440–1446.

165. Berne RM. Regulation of coronary blood flow. *Physiol Rev* 1964;44:1–29.

166. Berdeaux A, Giudicelli JF. Intrinsic sympathomimetic activity and coronary blood flow. *Br J Clin Pharmacol* 1982;13:175S–180S.

167. Parratt JR, Wadsworth RM. The effect of 'selective' beta-adrenoceptor blocking drugs on the myocardial circulation. *Br J Pharmacol* 1970;39:296–308.

168. Olsson G, Oden A, Johansson L, Sjogren A, Rehnqvist N. Prognosis after withdrawal of chronic postinfarction metoprolol treatment: a 2–7 year follow-up. *Eur Heart J* 1988;9:365–372.

169. Frishman WH, Silverman R. Clinical pharmacology of the new beta-adrenergic blocking drugs. III. Comparative clinical experience and new therapeutic applications. *Am Heart J* 1979;98:119–131.

170. Burckhardt D, Raeder E. The effect of acebutolol on cardiac arrhythmias in patients with chronic coronary artery disease. *Am Heart J* 1980;99:443–445.

171. Burckhardt D, Pfisterer M, Hoffmann A, Burkart F, Emmenegger H, Jost M, Bolli P, Buhler FR. Effects of the beta-adrenoceptor blocking agent sotalol on ventricular arrhythmias in patients with chronic ischemic heart disease. *Cardiology* 1983;70(Suppl 1):114–121.

172. Echt DS, Berte LE, Clusin WT, Samuelsson RG, Harrison DC, Mason JW. Prolongation of the human cardiac monophasic action potential by sotalol. *Am J Cardiol* 1982;50:1082–1086.

173. Neuvonen PJ, Elonen E, Vuorenmaa T, Laakso M. Prolonged Q-T interval and ventricular tachyarrhythmias, common features of sotalol intoxication. *Eur J Clin Pharmacol* 1981;20:85–89.

174. McKibbin JK, Pocock WA, Barlow JB, Miller RNS, Obel IWP. Sotalol hypokalaemia, syncope and torsade de pointes. *Br Heart J* 1984;51:157–162.

175. Rasmussen S, Rasmussen K. Influence of metoprolol, alone and in combination with a thiazide diuretic on blood pressure, plasma volume, extracellular volume and glomerular filtration rate in essential hypertension. *Eur J Clin Pharmacol* 1979; 15:305–310.

176. Textor SC, Fouad FM, Bravo EL, Tarazi RC, Vidt DG, Gifford RW. Redistribution of cardiac output to the kidneys during oral nadolol administration. *N Engl J Med* 1982;307:601–605.

177. Waal-Manning HJ, Bolli P. Atenolol vs. placebo in mild hypertension: renal, metabolic and stress antipressor effects. *Br J Clin Pharmacol* 1980;9:553–560.

178. Bauer JH, Brooks CS. The long-term effect of propranolol therapy on renal function. *Am J Med* 1979;66:405–410.

179. Ibsen H, Sederberg-Ohlsen P. Changes in glomerular filtration rate during long-term treatment with propranolol in patients with arterial hypertension. *Clin Sci* 1973;44:128–134.

180. Warren DJ, Swainson CP, Wright N. Deterioration in renal function after betablockade in patients with chronic renal failure and hypertension. *Br Med J* 1974;2:193–194.

181. Rosenfeld J, Boner G, Wainer E. Renal function during acute and long-term pindolol treatment in hypertensive patients with normal and decreased glomerular filtration. *Br J Clin Pharmacol* 1982;13:237S–240S.

182. Herrera J, Vukovich RA, Griffith DL. Elimination of nadolol by patients with renal impairment. *Br J Clin Pharmacol* 1979;7(Suppl 2):227S–231S.

183. Moore SB, Goodwin FJ. Effect of beta-adrenergic blockade on plasma-renin activity and intractable hypertension in patients receiving regular dialysis treatment. *Lancet* 1976;2:67–70.

184. Janka HU, Ziegler AG, Disselhoff G, Mehnert H. Influence of bisoprolol on blood glucose, glucosuria, and haemoglobin A_1 in noninsulin-dependent diabetics. *J Cardiovasc Pharmacol* 1986;8(Suppl 11):S96–S99.

185. Lager I. Adrenergic blockade and hypoglycaemia. *Acta Med Scand [Suppl]* 1983;672:63–67.

186. Wilhelmsen L, Wedel H, Tibblin G. Multivariate analysis of risk factors for coronary heart disease. *Circulation* 1973;48:950–958.

187. Kannel WB, Castelli WP, Gordon T. Cholesterol in the prediction of atherosclerotic disease. *Ann Intern Med* 1979;90:85–91.

188. Oka Y, Frishman W, Becker RM, Kadish A, Strom J, Matsumoto M, Orkin L, Frater R. Clinical pharmacology of the new beta adrenergic blocking drugs. Part 10. Beta adrenoceptor blockade and coronary artery surgery. *Am Heart J* 1980;99:255–269.

189. Boudoulas H, Snyder GL, Lewis RP, Kates RE, Karayannacos PE, Vasko JS. Safety and rationale for continuation of propranolol therapy during coronary bypass operation. *Ann Thorac Surg* 1978;26:222–227.

190. Williams JB, Stephenson LW, Holford FD, Langer T, Dunkman WB, Josephson ME. Arrhythmia prophylaxis using propranolol after coronary artery surgery. *Ann Thorac Surg* 1982;34:435–438.

191. Leather HM, Humphrey SDM, Baker P. A controlled trial of hypotensive agents in hypertension in pregnancy. *Lancet* 1968;2:488–490.

192. Gallery EDM, Saunders DM, Hunyor SN, Gyory AZ. Randomized comparison of methyldopa and oxprenolol for the treatment of hypertension in pregnancy. *Br Med J* 1979;1:1591–1594.

193. Sandstrom B. Antihypertensive treatment with adrenergic betareceptor blocker metoprolol during pregnancy. *Gynecol Obstet Invest* 1978;9:195–204.

194. O'Hare MF, Murnaghan GA, Russell CJ, Leahey WJ, Verma MP, McDevitt DG. Sotalol as a hypotensive agent in pregnancy. *Br J Obstet Gynaecol* 1980;87:814–820.

195. Lunell N-O, Persson B, Aragon G, Friedholm BB, Astrom H. Circulatory and metabolic effects of acute beta-1 blockade in severe pre-eclampsia. *Acta Obstet Gynecol Scand* 1979;58:443–445.

196. Diamond S, Kudrow L, Stevens J. Long-term study of propranolol in the treatment of migraine. *Headache* 1982;22:268–271.

197. Ljung O. Treatment of migraine with metoprolol. *N Engl J Med* 1980;303:156–157.

198. Forssman B, Linslad CJ, et al. Atenolol for migraine prophylaxis. *Headache* 1983;23:188–190.

199. Markley HG, Cheronis JCD, Piepho RW. Verapamil in prophylactic therapy of migraine. *Neurology* 1984;34:973–976.

200. Veterans Administration Cooperative Study Group on antihypertensive agents. Effects of treatment on morbidity in hypertension. I. Results in patients with diastolic blood pressures averaging 115 through 129 mmHg. *JAMA* 1967;202:1028–1034.

201. The Multiple Risk Factor Intervention Trial Research Group. Multiple risk factor intervention trial, risk factor changes, and mortality results. *JAMA* 1982;248:1465–1477.

202. Medical Research Council Working Party: MRC trial of treatment of mild hypertension: principal results. *Br Med J* 1985;291:97–104.

203. Wilhelmsen L, Berglund G, Elmfeldt D, Fitzsimons T, Holzgreve H, Hosie J, Hornkvist PE, Pennert K, Tuomilehto J, Wedel H. Betablockers versus diuretics in hypertensive men: main results from the HAPPHY trial. *J Hypertens* 1987;5:561–572.

204. The IPPPSH Collaborative Group. Cardiovascular risks and risk factors in a randomized trial of treatment based on the betablocker oxprenolol: the International Prospective Primary Prevention Study in Hypertension (IPPPSH). *J Hypertens* 1985;3:379–392.

205. Buhler FR, Vesanen K, Watters JT, Bolli P. Impact of smoking on heart attacks, strokes, blood pressure control, drug dose, and

quality of life aspects in the International Prospective Primary Prevention Study in Hypertension. *Am Heart J* 1988;115:282–288.

206. European Working Party on High Blood Pressure in the Elderly: mortality and morbidity results from the European Working Party on High Blood Pressure in the Elderly Trial. *Lancet* 1985;1:1349–1354.
207. Wikstrand J, Warnold I, Olsson G, Tuomilehto J, Elmfeldt D, Berglund G. Primary prevention with metoprolol in patients with hypertension. Mortality results from the MAPHY Study. *JAMA* 1988;259:1976–1982.
208. Greenblatt DJ, Koch-Weser J. Adverse reactions to beta-adrenergic receptor blocking drugs. A report from the Boston Collaborative Drug Surveillance Program. *Drugs* 1974;7:118–129.
209. Kellaway GSM. Adverse drug reactions during treatment of hypertension. *Drugs* 1976;11(Suppl 1):91–99.
210. The Medical Research Council Working Party on Mild to Moderate Hypertension. Adverse reactions to bendrofluazide and propranolol for the treatment of mild hypertension. *Lancet* 1981;2:539–543.
211. Raine JM, Palazzo MG, Kerr JH, Sleight P. Near-fatal bronchospasm after oral nadolol in a young asthmatic and response to ventilation with halothane. *Br Med J* 1981;282:548–549.
212. Gokal R, Dornan TL, Ledingham JGG. Peripheral skin necrosis complicating betablockage. *Br Med J* 1979;i:721–722.
213. McSorley PD, Warren DJ. Effects of propranolol and metoprolol on the peripheral circulation. *Br Med J* 1978;2:1598–1600.
214. White C de B, Udwadis BP. Beta-adrenoceptors in the human dorsal hand vein, and the effects of propranolol and practolol on venous sensitivity to noradrenaline. *Br J Clin Pharmacol* 1975;2:99–105.
215. Bolli P, Erne P, Ji BH, Block LH, Kiowski W, Buhler FR. Adrenaline induces vasoconstriction through postjunctional alpha-2 adrenoceptors and this response is enhanced in patients with essential hypertension. *J Hypertens* 1984;2(Suppl 3):115–118.
216. Abramson EA, Arky RA, Woeber KA. Effects of propranolol on the hormonal and metabolic responses to insulin hypoglycemia. *Lancet* 1966;2:1386–1388.
217. Reveno WS, Rosenbaum H. Propranolol hypoglycaemia. *Lancet* 1968;1:920.
218. Roberts DH, Tsao Y, McLoughlin GA, Breckenridge A. Placebo-controlled comparison of captopril, atenolol, labetalol, and pindolol in hypertension complicated by intermittent claudication. *Lancet* 1987;3:650–653.
219. Reichert N, Shibolet S, Adar R, Gafni J. Controlled trial of propranolol in intermittent claudication. *Clin Pharmacol Ther* 1975;17:612–615.
220. Bayliss PFC, Duncan SM. The effects of atenolol (Tenormin) and methyldopa on simple tests of central nervous function. *Br J Clin Pharmacol* 1975;2:527–531.
221. Wright P. Untoward effect associated with practolol administration. Oculomucocutaneous syndrome. *Br Med J* 1975;1:595–598.
222. Greenblatt DJ, Koch-Weser J. Clinical toxicity of propranolol and practolol. A report from the Boston Collaborative Drug Surveillance Program. In: Avery G, ed. *Cardiovascular drugs,* vol 2. Baltimore: University Park Press, 1978;176–195.
223. Frishman WH, Christodoulou J, Weksler B, Smithen C, Killip T, Scheidt S. Abrupt propranolol withdrawal in angina pectoris: effects on platelet aggregation and exercise tolerance. *Am Heart J* 1978;95:169–179.
224. Miller RR, Olson HG, Amsterdam EA, Mason DT. Propranolol-withdrawal rebound phenomenon. Exacerbation of coronary events after abrupt cessation of antianginal therapy. *N Engl J Med* 1975;293:416–418.
225. Nattel S, Rangno RE, Van Loon G. Mechanism of propranolol withdrawal phenomena. *Circulation* 1979;59:1158–1164.
226. Lederballe Pederson O, Mikkelson E, Nielsen JL, Christensen NJ. Abrupt withdrawal of beta blocking agents in patients with arterial hypertension. Effects on blood pressure, heart rate and plasma catecholamines and prolactin. *Eur J Clin Pharmacol* 1979;15:215–217.
227. Rangno RE, Langlois S, Lutterodt A. Metoprolol withdrawal phenomena: mechanism and prevention. *Clin Pharmacol Ther* 1982;31:5–18.
228. Ross PJ, Lewis MJ, Sheridan DJ, Henderson AH. Adrenergic hypersensitivity after beta blocker withdrawal. *Br Heart J* 1981;45:637–642.
229. Walden RJ, Hernandez J, Yu Y, Al-Khader A, Prichard BNC. Withdrawal of betablocking drugs. *Am Heart J* 1982;104:515–520.
230. Hedberg A, Gerber JG, Nies AS, Wolfe BB, Molinoff PB. Effects of pindolol and propranolol on beta adrenergic receptors on human lymphocytes. *J Pharmacol Exp Ther* 1986;239:117–123.
231. Bolli P, Buhler FR, Raeder EA, Amann FW, Meier M, Rogg H, Burckhardt D. Lack of beta-adrenoceptor hypersensitivity after abrupt withdrawal of long-term therapy with oxprenolol. *Circulation* 1981;64:1130–1134.
232. Rangno RE, Langlois S, Stewart J. Cardiac hyper- and hyporesponsiveness after pindolol withdrawal. *Clin Pharmacol Ther* 1982;31:564–571.
233. Szecsi E, Kohlschutter S, Schiess W, Lang E. Abrupt withdrawal of pindolol or metoprolol after chronic therapy. *Br J Clin Pharmacol* 1982;13:353S–357S.
234. Walden RJ, Bhattacharjee P, Tomlinson B, Cashin J, Graham BR, Prichard BNC. The effect of intrinsic sympathomimetic activity on beta-receptor responsiveness after beta-adrenoceptor blockade withdrawal. *Br J Clin Pharmacol* 1982;13(Suppl 2):359s–364s.
235. Buhler FR, Erne P, Dimitrov D, Zschauer A, Resink TJ, Bolli P. Withdrawal of the long-acting betablocker bopindolol is not associated with beta-adrenoceptor supersensitivity. *J Cardiovasc Pharmacol* 1986;8(Suppl 6):64–69.
236. Lindenfeld J, Crawford MH, O'Rourke RA, Levine SP, Montiel MM, Horwitz LD. Adrenergic responsiveness after abrupt propranolol withdrawal in normal subjects and in patients with angina pectoris. *Circulation* 1980;62:704–711.
237. Skrabal F, Kotanko P, Gruber G, Meister B, Doll P. Alpha$_2$- and beta$_2$-adrenoceptors and haemodynamic parameters during beta-blockade with and without intrinsic activity and/or beta$_1$ selectivity. *J Hypertens* 1987;5(Suppl 5):S181–S183.
238. Kirsten R, Neff J, Heintz B, Nemeth N, Rahlfs VW, Nelson K. Influence of different bisoprolol doses on hemodynamics, plasma catecholamines, platelet aggregation, and alpha-2 and beta-receptors in hypertensive patients. *J Cardiovasc Pharmacol* 1986;8(Suppl 11):S113–S121.
239. Rangno RE, Nattel S, Lutterodt A. Prevention of propranolol withdrawal mechanism by prolonged low dose propranolol schedule. *Am J Cardiol* 1982;49:828–833.
240. Frishman W, Jacob H, Eisenberg E, Ribner H. Clinical pharmacology of the new beta-adrenergic blocking drugs. Part 8. Self-poisoning with beta-adrenoceptor blocking agents: recognition and management. *Am Heart J* 1979;98:798–811.
241. Buhler FR. Antihypertensive actions of betablockers. In: Laragh JH, Buhler FR, Seldin DW, eds. *Frontiers in hypertension research.* New York: Springer, 1981;423–435.
242. Frishman WH. Beta-adrenergic receptor blockers. Adverse effects and drug interactions. *Hypertension* 1988;11(Suppl II):II-21–II-29.

Hypertension: Pathophysiology, Diagnosis, and Management, edited by J. H. Laragh and B. M. Brenner. Raven Press, Ltd., New York © 1990.

CHAPTER 140

Angiotensin-Converting-Enzyme Inhibitors in Hypertension

Bernard Waeber, Jürg Nussberger, and Hans R. Brunner

The Renin–Angiotensin System, 2210
ACE Inhibitors, 2210
Effects of ACE Inhibition on Various Neurohumoral Pressor and Depressor Systems, 2210
ACE Inhibition and Angiotensin II, 2211
ACE Inhibition and Aldosterone Secretion, 2211
ACE Inhibition and Vasopressin Release, 2212
ACE Inhibition and Atrial Natriuretic Factor, 2212
ACE Inhibition and Prostaglandins, 2212
ACE Inhibition and the Kallikrein–Kinin System, 2213
ACE Inhibition and the Sympathetic Nervous System, 2214
ACE Inhibition and the Parasympathetic Nervous System, 2215
ACE Response to Chronic Inhibition, 2215
Response of Renin Secretion to ACE Inhibition, 2216
Hemodynamic Effects of ACE Inhibitors During Rest and Exercise, 2216
ACE Inhibition and Blood Flow Distribution, 2216
Renal Circulation, 2216
Coronary Circulation, 2216
Cerebral Circulation, 2217
ACE Inhibition in Different Types of Hypertension, 2217
Essential Hypertension, 2217
Renovascular Hypertension, 2217
Mineralocorticoid-Induced Hypertension, 2218
Hypertension Due to Renin-Producing Tumors, 2218
Hypertension Due to Pheochromocytoma, 2218
Hypertension and Pregnancy, 2218
ACE Inhibition in Hypertension Associated with Other Disorders, 2219
ACE Inhibition and Renal Disorders, 2219
ACE Inhibition and Cardiac Hypertrophy, 2219
ACE Inhibition and Congestive Heart Failure, 2219
ACE Inhibition and Coronary Heart Disease, 2220
ACE Inhibition and Peripheral Vascular Disease, 2220
ACE Inhibition in Diabetic Patients, 2220
ACE Inhibition in Patients with Respiratory Problems, 2220
ACE Inhibitors as a First-Step Treatment of Hypertension, 2220
Interactions of ACE Inhibitors with Other Antihypertensive Drugs, 2221
ACE Inhibitors and Diuretics, 2221
ACE Inhibitors and β-Adrenoceptor Blocking Agents, 2221
ACE Inhibitors and Calcium Antagonists, 2221
ACE Inhibitors in Patients with Treatment-Resistant or Malignant Hypertension, 2221
ACE Inhibitors in the Treatment of Hypertensive Crises, 2221
Metabolic Effects of ACE Inhibition, 2221
Effect of ACE Inhibition on Quality of Life, 2222
Dosage, 2222
Side Effects of ACE Inhibitors, 2222
Side Effects Related to the Blockade of the Renin–Angiotensin System, 2222
Side Effects Possibly Related to Inhibition of ACE Activity Per Se, 2223
Compound Related Side Effects, 2223
Conclusions, 2223
References, 2223

Angiotensin-converting-enzyme (ACE) inhibitors are now widely used in the treatment of patients with hypertensive disorders. These agents inhibit the generation of angiotensin II and thereby make it possible to block the renin–angiotensin system (RAS) chronically. Given alone or in combination with other antihypertensive drugs, these compounds are very effective in lowering blood pressure of most hypertensive patients. They have a favorable hemodynamic and metabolic profile, can be used safely even in the presence of associated diseases, elicit few side effects, and have an excellent subjective tolerability.

The aim of this chapter is to review the clinical experience accumulated with ACE inhibitors in the management of hypertensive patients.

THE RENIN–ANGIOTENSIN SYSTEM

Activation of the enzyme chain culminating in the formation of angiotensin II in the circulation starts with renin secretion from the kidney (Fig. 1). This proteolytic enzyme cleaves off the decapeptide angiotensin I from angiotensinogen, a protein substrate produced by the liver and circulating in the blood. Angiotensin I is devoid of any vasoactive effect; a converting enzyme splits it into two fragments. The larger fragment, an octapeptide, represents the final hormone angiotensin II (1). The ACE is also one of the enzymes physiologically involved in breaking down bradykinin, a vasodilating hormone (2). Most of the angiotensin I is converted to angiotensin II during its passage through the pulmonary circulation (3). Endothelial cells of the pulmonary vascular bed are known to be particularly rich in ACE (4), but this enzyme is also present in extrapulmonary blood vessel walls (2). ACE has been demonstrated within the endothelial cells as well as on their luminal surface (4,5). The vascular endothelial tissue is capable of synthesizing ACE (6).

During recent years, the concept of a vascular RAS has emerged (7–10). Indeed, there seem to exist in the vascular wall all the components required for the generation of angiotensin II. Some of the renin contained in the arterial wall is probably originating from the circulation (11). Additionally, renin may be produced directly by vascular smooth muscle cells (12). Compatible with an extrarenal synthesis of renin is the observation that the renin gene is expressed in a number of organs other than the kidney (13). Evidence for the presence of renin substrate in the vascular wall has also been provided (14). Angiotensinogen gene is, like that of renin, expressed in various tissues (15). Whether the vascular RAS leads to significant local angiotensin II formation and plays a role in cardiovascular control independently of circulating angiotensin II, however, remains to be clarified (7–10).

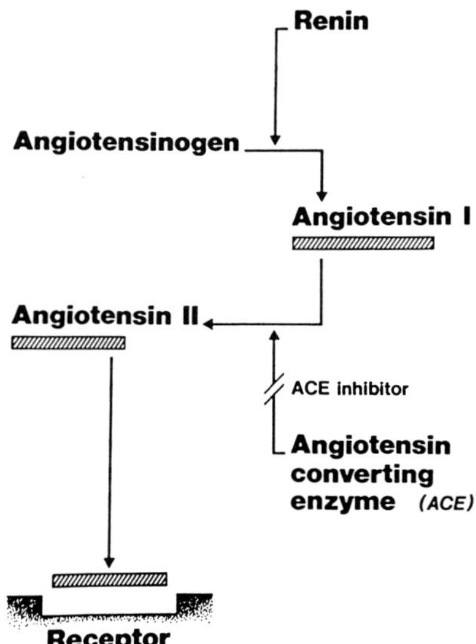

FIG. 1. Components of the renin–angiotensin system.

ACE INHIBITORS

The first ACE inhibitor to be used in humans was teprotide (16,17). This compound is a nonapeptide and had the shortcoming of being effective only when administered parenterally. Numerous orally active inhibitors were subsequently developed (18). The largest experience so far has been accumulated with captopril and enalapril, the two agents currently marketed in most countries. Captopril has a fast onset of action and can block ACE activity maximally within 15–30 min after oral administration but has a short plasma half-life (2 hr). Unlike captopril, enalapril has a delayed onset of action. With this agent, complete inhibition of ACE activity is achieved within only 2–4 hr. This is because enalapril maleate, the form used for the oral route, has to be hydrolyzed following intestinal absorption to its active diacid form called *enalaprilat.* The plasma half-life of enalaprilat (11 hr) is much longer than that of captopril.

There exist different approaches to evaluate in humans the potential of drugs to inhibit ACE activity (19). One possibility is to demonstrate blockade of the pressor response to exogenous angiotensin I. This method provides direct evidence of the efficacy of any ACE inhibitor but has the disadvantage that pharmacologic doses of angiotensin I have to be injected. A more convenient way is to measure plasma ACE activity (20). The degree of suppression of this enzyme activity in plasma generally reflects quite well the reduction of angiotensin II generation from angiotensin I (21). In the case of captopril, the enzyme activity has to be determined immediately following blood drawing; this is because *in vitro* the captopril–ACE complex tends to dissociate and could lead to an underestimation of the extent to which ACE is inhibited (22). Since plasma ACE is not responsible for the bulk of the conversion of angiotensin I to angiotensin II, its activity should be corroborated by simultaneous determinations of plasma angiotensin II. Unfortunately, although plasma angiotensin II can now be determined reliably, this assay remains laborious, partially because cross-reacting precursors and metabolites interfere with the measurement; furthermore, *in vitro* production of angiotensin II has to be taken into account (23–25).

EFFECTS OF ACE INHIBITION ON VARIOUS NEUROHUMORAL PRESSOR AND DEPRESSOR SYSTEMS

The regulation of blood pressure is permanently under the control of pressor (Fig. 2A) and depressor (Fig. 2B) systems and hormones. The contribution of the RAS to cardiovascular homeostasis is particularly complex. Angiotensin II influences vascular tone not only directly through its constrictor properties but also because it enhances the release and/or the action of a variety of vasoactive substances. ACE inhibitors may therefore lower blood pressure by altering the balance of various vasoconstrictor and vasodilator stimuli. Nevertheless, this still represents mainly the consequence of reduced angiotensin II levels.

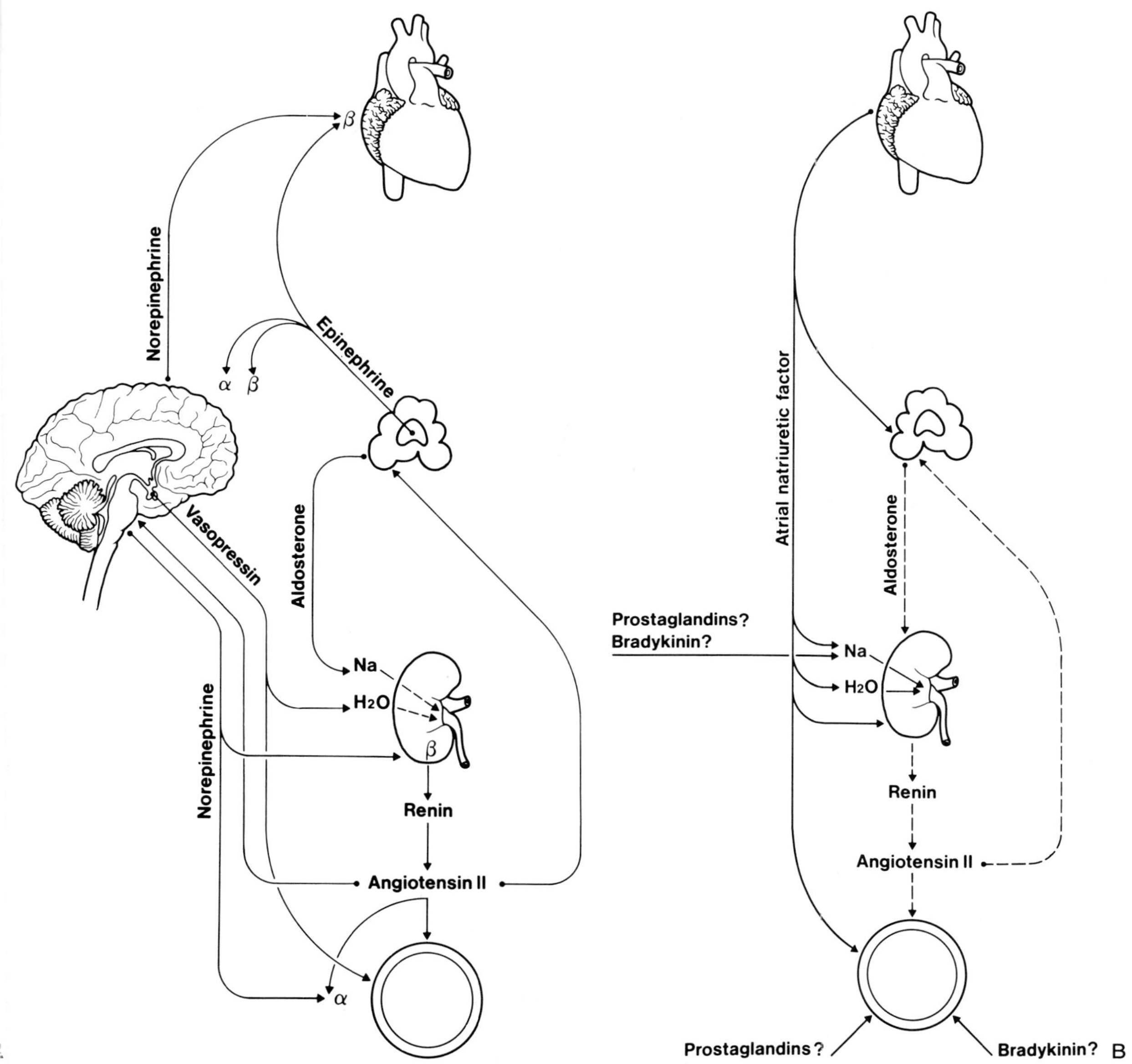

FIG. 2. Pressor (**A**) and depressor (**B**) systems and hormones involved in blood pressure regulation.

ACE Inhibition and Angiotensin II

It is very difficult to assess in the individual hypertensive patient the precise role of angiotensin II in maintaining his or her high blood pressure by stimulating receptors of vascular smooth muscle cells. A given level of circulating angiotensin II may indeed cause different degrees of contraction of blood vessels. For example, increasing total body sodium is known to enhance blood pressure responsiveness to this peptide (26). Vascular hyperreactivity to angiotensin II can also be anticipated in hypertensive patients exhibiting structural changes of blood vessels (27). On the other hand, it is possible that a vasodilating prostaglandin such as prostacyclin (28,29) synthesized in the vascular wall blunts the pressor effect of angiotensin II (30). A similar modulating action might be exerted by circulating bradykinin (31,32).

In response to ACE inhibition one would expect a fall in blood pressure proportional to the activity of the RAS. In fact, the magnitude of the initial blood pressure reduction induced by ACE inhibitors is related to pretreatment plasma renin activity and plasma angiotensin II levels (33–37). However, with long-term therapy the relationship between the blood pressure fall and the pretreatment renin and angiotensin II status becomes very weak (37–39). In many patients, sustained ACE inhibition for several weeks lowers blood pressure gradually to levels beyond those achieved at the beginning of treatment. Renin profiling appears therefore of relatively little practical value in predicting whether an ACE inhibitor is likely to normalize blood pressure of a particular patient. Nevertheless, good responders to acute ACE inhibition tend to remain well controlled during chronic therapy.

ACE Inhibition and Aldosterone Secretion

Angiotensin II is a well-established stimulus of aldosterone secretion (40,41). Not surprisingly, therefore, the rate of aldosterone production is decreased during ACE inhibition (34,35,42). This effect may be of great benefit to the hypertensive patient. It favors natriuresis and consequently helps to prevent the development of sodium retention when blood pressure is lowered. Indeed, in hypertensive patients, total body sodium content was found reduced after prolonged ACE inhibition (43,44). There has been some question as to whether aldosterone secretion is still angiotensin II dependent (and thus reduced) during chronic treatment (45,46). After having studied closely the plasma aldosterone and angiotensin II levels after long-term ACE inhibition (2 years), we found that both these parameters were still markedly reduced and that their changes were closely correlated (47).

ACE Inhibition and Vasopressin Release

Elevated plasma vasopressin levels have been reported in malignant and severe hypertension (48,49). In these patients, vasopressin secretion may be reduced during treatment with an ACE inhibitor (50,51). Whether this effect contributes to the antihypertensive action of ACE inhibition in these patients remains unclear. Furthermore, in the majority of hypertensive patients who have apparently normal vasopressin levels, there is no evidence that ACE inhibition affects vasopressin release.

ACE Inhibition and Atrial Natriuretic Factor

Atrial natriuretic peptides released into the circulation by atrial cardiocytes are thought to be involved in blood pressure regulation and sodium-volume homeostasis (52). It is noteworthy that these peptides have vasodilating, diuretic, and natriuretic properties but that they also oppose the action of the renin–angiotensin–aldosterone axis in different ways. They suppress renin and aldosterone secretion. Moreover, they inhibit the angiotensin-II-induced vasoconstriction (53). The plasma concentration of atrial natriuretic peptides is increased in a fraction of hypertensive patients (54,55). Synthetic atrial natriuretic peptides have recently been infused during ACE inhibition in hypertensive patients (56). ACE inhibition seemed to enhance the natriuretic and diuretic effect, but not the blood-pressure-lowering effect, of the investigational peptide. In contrast, in normotensive volunteers, ACE inhibition attenuated the natriuresis induced by the atrial natriuretic peptide (57).

ACE Inhibition and Prostaglandins

Prostaglandins represent a group of 20-carbon fatty acids that are synthesized from arachidonic acid, a component of the phospholipids contained in cell membranes (58) (Fig. 3). There exist complex interactions between prostaglandins and the RAS. Angiotensin II enhances the release of arachidonic acid, thereby triggering the production of prostaglandins (59). Arachidonic acid is converted to prostaglandin G_2 (PGG_2) by cyclo-oxygenase. PGG_2 is then transformed to either prostaglandin E_2 (PGE_2, a vasodilator), prostaglandin $F_{2\alpha}$ ($PGF_{2\alpha}$, a vasoconstrictor), thromboxane A_2 (TxA_2, a proaggregatory vasoconstrictor), or prostacyclin (PGI_2, an antiaggregatory vasodilator). Prostacyclin, unlike PGE_2, is not destroyed during its passage through the pulmonary vascular bed (60). For this reason it may play a role as a circulating vasoactive substance, whereas PGE_2 is more likely implicated in the local regulation of the tone of blood vessels. As already pointed out above, prostaglandins not only possess direct relaxant properties but also attenuate the vasoconstrictor effect of angiotensin II (30). Another important connection between the renin axis and prostaglandins deals with the secretion of renin. Both PGE_2 and PGI_2 have, indeed, been recognized to stimulate the release of renin (61,62). In the hypertensive patient, infusion of PGI_2 or of a PGE_2 analogue elicits a fall in blood pressure (63,64). Chronic transdermal administration of the prostaglandin analogue antagonizes the angiotensin-II-mediated vasoconstriction (64). On the contrary, inhibitors of cyclo-oxygenase (such as nonsteroidal anti-inflammatory drugs) tend to increase blood pressure of hypertensive patients (65).

Acute ACE inhibition with teprotide has been reported to increase prostaglandin levels in arterial blood of hypertensive patients (66). Subsequent studies have provided similar findings, such as significant increases in the plasma

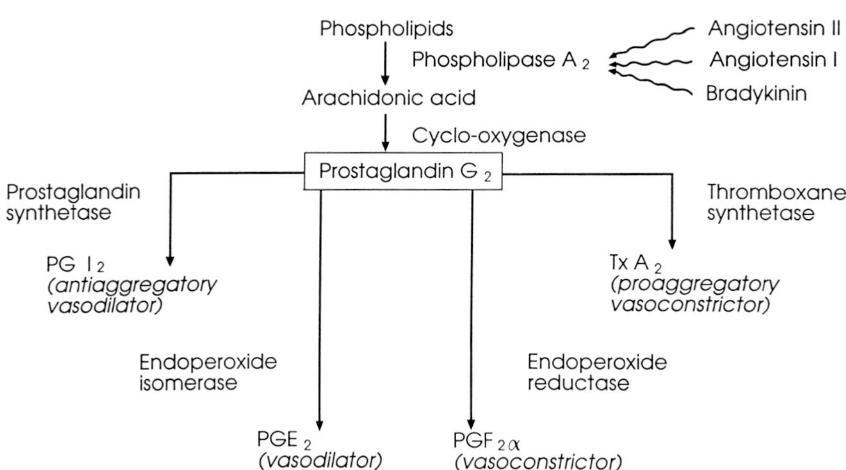

FIG. 3. Steps in prostaglandin synthesis.

levels of PGE_2 metabolites following treatment with a single oral dose of captopril. However, plasma levels of 6-keto-prostaglandin $F_{1\alpha}$, a stable metabolite of PGI_2, were not influenced by captopril (67,68). In normotensive subjects, the peak blood-pressure-lowering effect of captopril correlated well with the changes in plasma PGE_2 metabolites but not with the changes in plasma angiotensin II, which surprisingly were not found reduced by the ACE inhibitor (67). With regard to hypertensive patients, only those with elevated plasma concentrations of PGE_2 metabolites during chronic captopril treatment lowered their blood pressure (69). In another study performed in hypertensive patients, however, no change in plasma prostaglandins could be detected during chronic treatment with captopril (70).

Administration of the cyclo-oxygenase inhibitor indomethacin was shown to reduce the antihypertensive effect of captopril (68,70–72). When captopril and indomethacin are given together, the order of administration appears to be critical to the antihypertensive effect of the ACE inhibitor (71). The blood-pressure-lowering effect of captopril is attenuated in hypertensive patients pretreated with the cyclo-oxygenase inhibitor, whereas it is unaffected when captopril treatment precedes the administration of indomethacin. The results obtained with enalapril are less conclusive. The administration of a cyclo-oxygenase inhibitor was found by some (73), but not by others (74), to blunt the antihypertensive effect of this agent. In normal subjects, acute ACE inhibition with enalapril does not modify plasma levels of PGE_2 metabolites (69). These observations therefore raise the question of the similarity of ACE inhibitors in terms of their action on prostaglandin metabolism. For instance, captopril, but not enalapril, has been shown to stimulate PGE_2 biosynthesis in a culture of renomedullary interstitial cells (75). In this *in vitro* experiment, the tissues were exposed to drug concentrations comparable to those achieved in the plasma of humans. Captopril, unlike enalapril, contains a sulfhydryl group in its chemical structure. Whether this sulfhydryl group is responsible for the activation of phospholipase A_2 needs to be clarified. It should be stressed, however, that even enalapril may affect *in vivo* prostaglandin production, since an increased urinary excretion in 6-keto-prostaglandin $F_{1\alpha}$ has been detected in hypertensives treated for several weeks with this compound (74). Recently, a TxA_2 synthetase inhibitor was administered together with captopril (76). This enhanced the blood pressure drop, but the final blood pressure reached was not different whether captopril was administered with the TxA_2 synthetase inhibitor or with a placebo.

Prostaglandins are presumably involved in the regulation of extracellular fluid volume. There is indeed strong evidence that renal prostaglandins promote water and sodium excretion (77). Prostaglandin-related mechanisms seem to participate in the regulation of renal perfusion as well as of the intrarenal blood flow distribution (78). Renal prostaglandins are also known to antagonize the glomerular actions of angiotensin II (79) as well as the tubular effects of antidiuretic hormone (80). Theoretically, prostaglandins might therefore be involved in the renal response to ACE inhibition. In hypertensive patients, cyclo-oxygenase inhibition with indomethacin administration for several days decreased urinary sodium together with prostaglandin excretion (72). This response was observed both when ACE activity was intact and when it was suppressed by captopril, a finding that does not support a particular role of renal prostaglandins during ACE inhibition. Some investigators were unable to demonstrate any effect of captopril or enalapril (given for several weeks) on urinary excretion of 6-keto-$PGF_{2\alpha}$ (81). On the other hand, a selective increase in urinary PGE_2 has been observed in hypertensives treated for a few days with captopril (82). In the latter patients, the increases in urinary PGE_2 and sodium excretion were significantly and positively correlated. This is interesting, considering the fact that PGE_2 is believed to be the main prostaglandin synthesized in the kidney (83).

The contribution of prostaglandins to the antihypertensive effect of ACE inhibitors still needs to be clarified. It has to be remembered in this context that prostaglandins seem to be involved in the mechanism of the blood-pressure-lowering effect of various drugs other than ACE inhibitors (69).

ACE Inhibition and the Kallikrein–Kinin System

The basic elements of the kallikrein–kinin system are illustrated in Fig. 4. They consist of proteases (kallikreins) which release kinins from precursor proteins (kininogen) (84–86). There exist two kinds of kallikreins, namely, plasma and glandular kallikrein. The active plasma kallikrein is derived from the inactive prekallikrein when the latter is exposed, for instance, to the active fragment of factor XII (87). Plasma kallikrein produces bradykinin, a potent vasodilator nonapeptide, from a high-molecular-weight substrate. Kallikrein present in the renal tissue and in the urine is of the glandular subtype. Renal prekallikrein may be activated by phospholipase A_2 and arachidonic acid, thus suggesting a role for prostaglandins in the regulation of the renal kallikrein–kinin system (88). Renal kallikrein cleaves both low- and high-molecular-weight kininogen to produce kallidin, a decapeptide. Kallidin is then processed to bradykinin by an aminopeptidase. Kallidin and bradykinin are rapidly metabolized by kininases, one of them (kininase II) being identical with ACE (2).

There are important interrelations between the renin–angiotensin–aldosterone and the kallikrein–kinin systems. A key one is related to the common pathway of angiotensin II and bradykinin inactivation. Mineralocorticoids represent another link between the two hormonal systems. These salt-retaining steroids are indeed known to increase the release of renal kallikrein (89,90). Also to be considered is the fact that the vasoconstrictor effect of angiotensin II may be opposed by bradykinin (32) and that both angiotensin II and bradykinin stimulate prostaglandin synthesis (59,91,92). Finally, it is possible that kallikrein is involved in the activation of prorenin (93,94).

The question as to whether ACE inhibition results in accumulation of bradykinin and whether such an accumulation might substantially contribute to the antihypertensive effect of ACE inhibitors is still debated. Some investigators have reported increases in circulating bradykinin during acute ACE inhibition with teprotide and captopril (67,95). In most studies, however, no consistent changes in

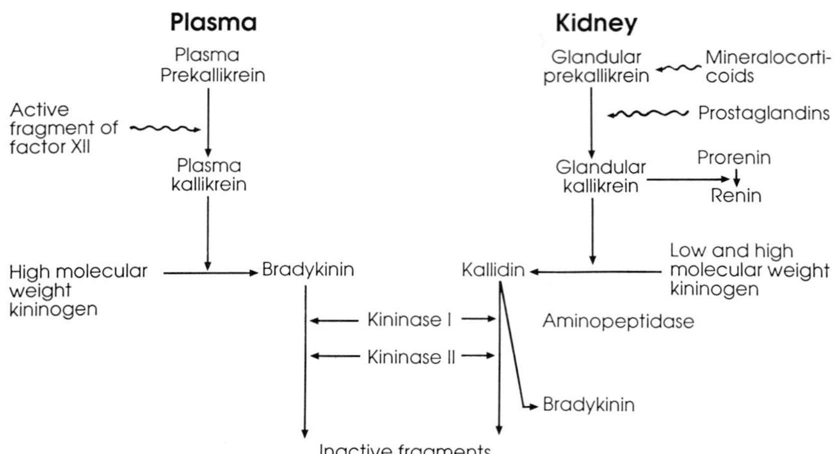

FIG. 4. Components of the kallikrein–kinin system.

circulating bradykinin could be detected, both during short- and long-term inhibition of the bradykinin-processing enzyme kininase II (70,96–98). Interestingly, a decrease in the number of bradykinin tissue receptors has been observed following prolonged captopril administration (97). The same investigators also demonstrated a down-regulation of these receptors by exogenous bradykinin. Based on these results, it was speculated that bradykinin may have accumulated in tissues. Acute and chronic ACE inhibition does enhance the vascular response to exogenous bradykinin (99,100). In this respect, the recent finding of an increased thickness of weals caused by intradermal injection of bradykinin during ACE inhibition is interesting, because it is at least compatible with the concept that bradykinin accumulates in tissues (101,102).

Different approaches other than the measurement of circulating kinins have been used to explore the cardiovascular role of the kallikrein–kinin system during ACE inhibition. In hypertensive animals, specific antikinin antibodies acutely attenuated the antihypertensive effect of captopril (103), whereas the use of competitive antagonists of bradykinin gave conflicting results (104,105). There are other experiments that do not substantiate a contribution of kinins to the blood-pressure-lowering effect of ACE inhibition. For instance, rats rendered hypertensive by an infusion of angiotensin II for more than 1 week failed to lower their blood pressure in response to ACE inhibition (106). Conversely, the concept that an accumulation of bradykinin might modulate the antihypertensive effect of ACE inhibitors was suggested by a study in which aprotinin, an inhibitor of serine proteases, was administered to patients treated with captopril and was found to reverse part of the antihypertensive effect of the ACE inhibitor (107).

The renal kallikrein–kinin system is presumably implicated in renal sodium handling (84–86). In sodium-loaded animals, treatment with aprotinin reduced sodium excretion (108). Urinary kallikrein is reduced by ACE inhibition (71,109), probably as a result of the decreased levels of aldosterone. During acute ACE inhibition, urinary kinin excretion was reported to increase in the absence of a concomitant change in circulating bradykinin (66). Indeed, these authors observed a correlation between the blood pressure response to acute ACE inhibition and the simultaneous rise in urinary kinin excretion, whereas no significant relationship emerged between the blood pressure and the plasma bradykinin changes. However, captopril administered by other investigators for several days did not change urinary kinin levels (71). Whether the renal kallikrein–kinin system facilitates the natriuresis while ACE activity is inhibited remains therefore speculative.

ACE Inhibition and the Sympathetic Nervous System

The sympathetic nervous system (SNS) participates in the regulation of human cardiovascular function already in the basal state (110). It is thought to be hyperactive in patients with high blood pressure (111–113). Much has been learned over the past few years on the connections between the SNS and the RAS (114). There exists a mutual influence between the two systems, with the activation of one amplifying the activity of the other.

This interplay between the SNS and the RAS occurs in the brain. Angiotensin II increases sympathetic efferent nerve activity when administered centrally (115,116). At present, it is uncertain whether circulating angiotensin II gains access to the brain through some areas (such as the circumventricular organs, the area postrema, or the subfornical organ) that lack a tight blood–brain barrier (117,118). Therefore, the capacity of ACE inhibitors to lower blood pressure by reducing the passage of angiotensin II into the central nervous system remains to be further explored. Also to be considered is the possible impact of ACE inhibitors on the brain–renin–angiotensin system (119). In this respect, still relatively little is known. There is some evidence that captopril penetrates the blood–brain barrier in humans in sufficient amounts to inhibit the ACE in cerebrospinal fluid (120). Hence, at least theoretically, captopril might block ACE activity in brain areas involved in blood pressure regulation.

At the periphery, angiotensin II seems to interact with the SNS both at pre- and postjunctional receptors. Angiotensin II has been suggested to inhibit the re-uptake of catecholamines (121). A probably important action of angiotensin II is the facilitation of norepinephrine release by terminal nerve endings (122) (Fig. 5). Angiotensin II also

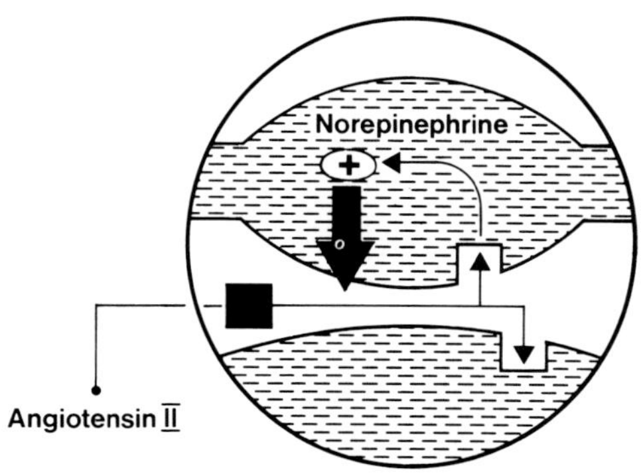

FIG. 5. Pre- and postsynaptic effects of angiotensin II (see text for detailed explanations).

potentiates the effect of norepinephrine postjunctionally (123). In humans, a postsynaptic interaction between norepinephrine and angiotensin II has been demonstrated recently with regard to systolic, but not diastolic, blood pressure (124). Finally, angiotensin II is a well-established mediator of epinephrine release from the adrenal medulla (125).

The influence of ACE inhibitors on cardiovascular responses to sympathetic activation has been studied in animals and in humans. Captopril has been shown experimentally to blunt the pressor effect of both sympathetic nerve stimulation (126–128) and α-adrenoceptor stimulation with exogenous norepinephrine (129–131). That captopril attenuates the blood pressure effect of norepinephrine has also been found in normal subjects (132), but others were unable to confirm this observation (133). It is worth noting that the captopril-induced attenuation of the pressor responses was not abolished by cyclo-oxygenase inhibition, which suggests a mechanism not related to prostaglandins. A reduced pressor effect of norepinephrine during captopril treatment was also demonstrated in hypertensive patients (134,135). This observation is of particular interest because hypertensive patients are expected to have an enhanced cardiovascular pressor reactivity when compared to normotensive subjects (136).

ACE inhibitors interfere minimally with circulatory reflexes in normotensive subjects as well as in hypertensive subjects (137–143). With respect to the baroreceptor reflex function, the observations are not unanimous. No change, a resetting, and a potentiation, as well as an increased sensitivity of the baroreflex, have been described with ACE inhibition (140–143). In most hypertensive patients, the blood pressure and heart rate response to changes in posture are not impaired (35,139,144–147). The risk of suffering postural hypotension, however, exists in excessively sodium-depleted patients. The same is true in normotensive subjects (148). In hypertensive patients, a normal adaptive response of blood pressure to changes in body position seems to be better maintained during chronic (35,144,145) than during acute (149) ACE inhibition. A possible explanation is the development, during long-term ACE inhibition, of an enhanced reflex sympathetic response to standing. The postural increase in plasma norepinephrine appears indeed to be greater during chronic than during acute treatment with captopril (144,145,149). This corresponds to the observation that patients chronically treated with an ACE inhibitor given either alone or in combination with a diuretic seem to rarely complain of orthostatic symptoms (150–153).

A hallmark of ACE inhibitors is that they lower blood pressure without inducing a cardioacceleration (33,35, 139,140,144,154). These agents usually induce no consistent change in circulating catecholamines (139,155,156). The various interactions between the SNS and the RAS probably account for a significant part of these properties. The fact that the elimination of the RAS does not lead to a functionally enhanced cardiovascular role of the SNS is certainly advantageous for the antihypertensive action of ACE inhibitors.

ACE Inhibition and the Parasympathetic Nervous System

It has been suggested that the heart rate acceleration which accompanies arteriolar dilatation is, to some extent, the consequence of a reflex withdrawal of vagal tone (157). A clear increase in the activity of the parasympathetic system could be demonstrated in normotensive subjects during both acute and chronic ACE inhibition (143,158–160). This action of ACE inhibitors cannot be explained by an inhibition of acetylcholinesterase. *In vitro,* neither captopril nor enalapril has a suppressing effect on bovine erythrocyte acetylcholinesterase activity (160). The parasympathomimetic effect of ACE inhibitors is probably a direct consequence of the disappearance of angiotensin II. It can indeed be reversed by infusion of subpressor doses of angiotensin II (160). It is relevant in this context that angiotensin II has been shown experimentally to inhibit vagal responses both centrally and peripherally (161,162). The stimulation of vagal activity by captopril has been observed not only in normotensive subjects but also in hypertensive patients (137). It is therefore possible that the hemodynamic response to ACE inhibitors is partly due to an increase in vagal tone.

ACE: RESPONSE TO CHRONIC INHIBITION

Prolonged treatment of animals with captopril or enalapril has been reported to increase the concentration of ACE in the serum and in the lungs (163–165). Induction of ACE biosynthesis by captopril has been demonstrated in cultured human endothelial cells (166). Induction of ACE production during chronic administration of captopril or enalapril appears to occur also in hypertensive patients (167,168). This adaptive increment in plasma ACE concentration passes completely unnoticed when ACE activity is assayed in the presence of an ACE inhibitor. ACE activity indeed remains inhibited during chronic treatment with captopril and enalapril (47,167,168). Since ACE induction occurs mainly with repeat administration of an ACE inhibitor, evidence of an increased ACE concentration provides proof that the drug has been taken not only on the day of the office visit. After withdrawal of therapy with an

ACE inhibitor, ACE concentration in plasma returns to normal over a period of weeks (167). There is no indication for a harmful effect of the induction of ACE by its inhibitors.

RESPONSE OF RENIN SECRETION TO ACE INHIBITION

The concentration of enzymatically active renin rises during short- and long-term ACE inhibition (33–35). This is thought to be due to the interruption of the feedback inhibition of renin release by angiotensin II (169). The active form of renin represents only one part of the total amount of renin found in the circulation. There exists indeed an inactive form of renin (often called *prorenin*) which is considered to be the precursor of active renin (170). Until recently, the plasma concentration of total renin has been assessed by measuring plasma renin activity after *in vitro* activation of prorenin. Inactive renin was calculated as the difference between total and active renin. Using this approach, it has been possible to show that both active and inactive renin increase during ACE inhibition (171–173). It became apparent, however, that the pattern of the changes in the two types of renin differed with time: The active renin tends to increase during the acute phase at the expense of inactive renin; during the chronic phase, however, active and inactive renin are both increased in parallel. These observations could be confirmed by the direct quantitation of active and total renin using monoclonal antibodies specific for different sites of the renin molecule (174). The rise in angiotensin I resulting from ACE inhibition appears to be due to an enhanced release of active renin rather than to an accumulation of angiotensin I (175). The renin response to ACE inhibition is blunted by β-adrenoceptor blockade (176) as well as by cyclo-oxygenase inhibition (71,73).

HEMODYNAMIC EFFECTS OF ACE INHIBITORS DURING REST AND EXERCISE

Like heart rate, cardiac output essentially does not change when blood pressure is lowered by an ACE inhibitor (144,154,177–180). During prolonged treatment, cardiac output may increase in some patients (177). This is most likely to occur in patients who have malignant hypertension and who are already exhibiting a reduced cardiac output (181). The fall in systemic vascular resistance resulting from ACE inhibition can be associated with a decrease in cardiac filling pressures (177,180). This observation reflects possibly a relaxant effect of ACE inhibitors on capacitance blood vessels or an improved cardiac performance. Pulmonary vascular resistance is not affected by ACE inhibitors (177,178). Adding a diuretic to an ACE inhibitor does not cause any major alteration in the profile of the hemodynamic response to ACE inhibition (182). In hypertensive patients subjected to moderate or strenuous physical exercise, both captopril and enalapril reduce the peak blood pressure increase but have no effect on the heart rate response (183,184). ACE inhibition does not alter the increase in cardiac output in response to dynamic exercise (184). When an ACE inhibitor is administered together with a diuretic, however, a fall in cardiac output may be observed during exercise (182).

ACE INHIBITION AND BLOOD FLOW DISTRIBUTION

Renal Circulation

In the kidney, angiotensin II exerts multiple regulatory functions, including modulation of renal blood flow, glomerular filtration rate, tubular reabsorption of sodium, and inhibition of renin release (169,185–190). With respect to the regulation of renal hemodynamics, angiotensin II acts on both the afferent and the efferent arterioles (191). Angiotensin II is not required to maintain normal renal function in subjects with a normal perfusion pressure (192). An increase in renal blood flow can, however, be demonstrated in normotensives receiving an ACE inhibitor (193). This rise in renal blood flow is more pronounced in salt-deplete subjects than in salt-replete subjects. This is not surprising, since the former are known to have a more active renin–angiotensin system than the latter.

Renal vascular tone is abnormally elevated in a substantial fraction of hypertensive patients (194,195). In these patients also, renal plasma flow is increased by blockade of angiotensin II generation. This has been shown during acute, as well as during chronic, ACE inhibition (43,44,193,196–200). The rises in renal blood flow resulting from ACE inhibition are, as anticipated, accentuated in patients with an activated renin–angiotensin system (193,197). Also, when combined with a diuretic, long-term ACE inhibition enhances renal blood flow (201). This is of great importance because the hyperreninemia induced by a diuretic given as monotherapy would be expected to have no, or even an opposite, renal hemodynamic effect. The rise in renal plasma flow evoked by ACE inhibitors is thought to be mediated by a preferential vasodilatation of the efferent arterioles of the glomeruli (197,200).

In a subset of hypertensive patients, renal plasma flow and renal vascular responsiveness to angiotensin II seem not to increase as expected in response to a dietary sodium load. ACE inhibition may correct these abnormalities while decreasing blood pressure (202). The significance of this observation, however, remains to be clarified.

Coronary Circulation

The coronary vasoconstrictor action of angiotensin II is well established (203). In the hypertensive patient as in the normotensive subject, coronary blood flow depends to a large extent on autoregulatory mechanisms that adjust oxygen supply to the myocardial needs. Under certain circumstances, angiotensin II may modulate the tone of the coronary tree of hypertensive patients and, consequently, impair coronary perfusion. Confirmation for such an influence of angiotensin II has been provided recently (204). In this study, diuretic therapy reduced coronary blood flow.

This effect could be reversed by acute ACE inhibition despite the concurrent blood pressure fall, thus confirming similar earlier observations made in dogs using teprotide (205). This suggests that angiotensin II actively participates in the control of coronary vascular tone, at least if the renin–angiotensin axis is activated.

Cerebral Circulation

A major concern when lowering blood pressure is the maintenance of an adequate cerebral perfusion. Over a wide range of blood pressure, cerebral blood flow is kept constant via autoregulation (206). There is a risk of causing a potentially harmful drop in cerebral blood flow when reducing blood pressure acutely below the lower limit of autoregulation. This is most likely to occur in hypertensive patients, since they exhibit an autoregulation curve which is shifted to higher blood pressure levels than that of normotensive subjects. These patients appear to be particularly prone to having their cerebral perfusion impaired when a very high blood pressure is reduced rapidly. With respect to ACE inhibitors, they lower blood pressure of hypertensives without diminishing cerebral blood flow (207,208). In one study (208), an increase in cerebral blood flow was observed after a few days. It appeared to be most pronounced in those patients who responded to ACE inhibition with the biggest blood pressure reduction. In another study of hypertensive patients with unilateral cerebrovascular disease, captopril actually enhanced cerebral blood flow to the affected hemisphere despite a 10% fall in blood pressure (209). Interestingly, in an experimental model of hypertension, acute ACE inhibition has been shown to acutely shift their lower limit of cerebral autoregulation by 20–30 mmHg (210).

ACE INHIBITION IN DIFFERENT TYPES OF HYPERTENSION

Essential Hypertension

Essential hypertension is by far the most common form of clinical hypertension. During the last decade, a considerable number of reports dealing with the effect of ACE inhibitors in patients with essential hypertension have been published (211–215). These agents effectively lower blood pressure as monotherapy in more than 50% of patients with mild to moderate hypertension (216–219). In general, white hypertensives tend to respond better than black patients (218). Some attenuation of the clinical efficacy of ACE inhibition has been reported during chronic treatment with captopril as well as with enalapril (219–221). Adding a diuretic restored the maximal response (221). A major advantage of ACE inhibitors, however, is their capability to maintain a satisfactory blood control for years.

With aging, renin secretion tends to fall (222). Based on this finding, it has been implied that therapy with an ACE inhibitor is less likely to be efficacious in the elderly than in the younger hypertensive patients (223). In fact, this assumption has not been confirmed by large-scale studies carried out by practitioners (224–226). The blood pressure reductions obtained with captopril as well as with enalapril turned out to be equal in the different classes of age. Like in the younger hypertensive patient, the blood-pressure-lowering effect of ACE inhibition in the elderly is influenced by race, with the white patients being the best responders (227).

Renovascular Hypertension

In patients with renovascular hypertension due to a unilateral renal artery stenosis, plasma renin levels are frequently increased (228). Renovascular hypertension is usually a condition difficult to treat by conventional antihypertensive agents. In these patients, acute and chronic ACE inhibition is often very effective in reducing blood pressure (37,229–232). ACE inhibitors generally achieve a good blood pressure control without requiring the association of multiple drugs.

The fact that circulating angiotensin II is markedly diminished following ACE inhibition can have an adverse effect on kidney function behind the stenosis (Fig. 6). When perfusion pressure to the glomeruli is considerably reduced, angiotensin II may become vital for maintaining adequate filtration pressure. This is because angiotensin II exerts its vasoconstrictor action predominantly on the efferent arterioles. That renal problems may occur during

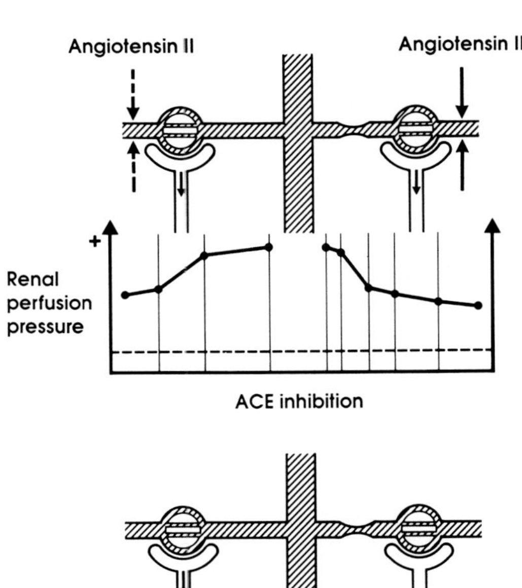

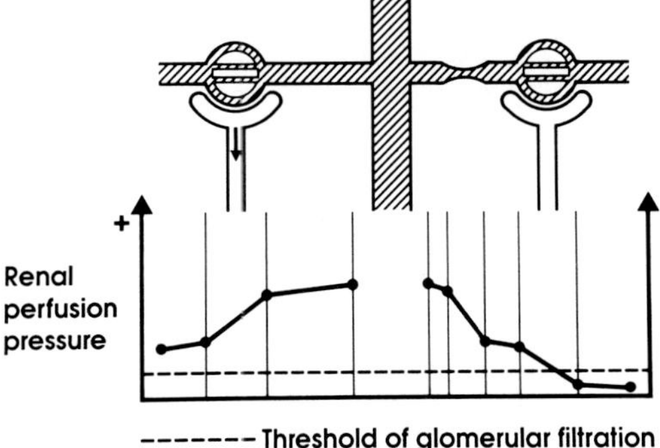

FIG. 6. Influence of angiotensin-II-mediated postglomerular vasoconstriction on renal perfusion pressure in the absence or presence of a renal artery stenosis (see text for detailed explanations).

ACE inhibition was first demonstrated in patients with bilateral renal artery stenosis and in patients with renal artery stenosis in a single kidney. Azotemia developed in these patients when blood pressure was lowered by captopril (233–236). The experience available so far suggests that the impairment of renal function caused by such a mechanism is reversible after withdrawal of the ACE inhibitor. Ironically, patients with bilateral renal artery stenosis or renal artery stenosis in a single kidney often exhibit a hypertension which is poorly responsive to ACE inhibition alone. Frequently in these patients, other antihypertensive drugs have to be combined with an ACE inhibitor in order to normalize blood pressure. In general, the risk of developing azotemia is most eminent when blood pressure is successfully reduced.

Cessation of glomerular filtration rate may also occur in case of unilateral renal artery stenosis; however, renal failure does not develop, because the intact contralateral kidney compensates for the decreased glomerular filtration (237). The function of the two kidneys can be assessed separately using radionuclide techniques. Using this approach, it became apparent that the glomerular filtration rate of the stenotic kidney is not always severely compromised by ACE inhibitors (237,238). Among the main determinants of the response of a stenotic kidney to ACE inhibition are such factors as the level of systemic pressure, the severity of the renal artery stenosis, the functional state of the contralateral kidney, and the degree of activation of the renin–angiotensin system. The risk of a persistent damage to the stenotic kidney—for instance, by facilitating renal artery thrombosis—seems to exist only when renal blood flow is markedly diminished as a result of ACE inhibition (239). Nevertheless, the presence of a unilateral renal artery stenosis does not totally preclude the use of ACE inhibitors. These agents may indeed be very helpful in patients who for different reasons cannot undergo reconstructive surgery or angioplasty. From a practical point of view, it is recommended to check renal function a few days after initiation of therapy with an ACE inhibitor in those patients presenting a hypertension difficult to control by conventional pharmacologic tools. The probability that these patients present a renovascular hypertension is indeed not negligible (240).

In searching in a given patient for a renal artery stenosis, it would seem more appropriate to evaluate the renin secretory response to ACE inhibition rather than the basic renin profile. The increments in plasma renin activity induced acutely by ACE inhibitors seem indeed more pronounced in patients with renovascular than in those with essential hypertension (241). The degree of hyperreninemia observed during long-term inhibition of ACE does not, however, seem to predict the blood pressure achieved subsequently by the surgical cure of the renal artery stenosis (230). ACE inhibitors, because of their stimulating effect on renin secretion, raise the sensitivity of the renal vein renin sampling test, making it more likely to uncover an asymmetry of renal renin secretion (242).

The extent to which blood pressure is reduced by acute ACE inhibition cannot serve as a reliable indicator of the outcome of renal artery repair or nephrectomy in the individual patient (229,230). In contrast, the blood pressure response to long-term ACE inhibition has some prognostic value. Thus, successful blood pressure control is likely to be obtained with surgery or angioplasty in a patient with proven renal artery stenosis in whom blood pressure could be normalized with an ACE inhibitor given as sole therapy for several weeks (37,230). It seems reasonable, however, not to prolong treatment with an ACE inhibitor for many weeks before correcting the stenosis.

Mineralocorticoid-Induced Hypertension

Renin secretion is typically suppressed in hypertensive patients with primary aldosteronism. No wonder, therefore, that acute ACE inhibition fails to lower blood pressure in most patients (243–245). Nevertheless, blood pressure can decrease slightly in some of these patients during both acute and prolonged ACE inhibition. Since blood pressure of some patients with essential hypertension may also not fall in response to ACE inhibition, the lack of a drop in blood pressure cannot be used to identify patients with primary aldosteronism. Acute ACE inhibition with captopril may, however, be useful for the differentiation of patients with an aldosterone-producing adenoma from those exhibiting bilateral micronodular hyperplasia. In the former, aldosterone production is supposed to be completely autonomous; for this reason, blockade of angiotensin II generation does not reduce the abnormally elevated plasma aldosterone levels. In the latter, it is known that aldosterone secretion can still be stimulated by angiotensin II. Not surprisingly, therefore, these patients tend to respond to captopril with a certain decrease in circulating aldosterone concentration (244,245). Whether this simple test ought to be performed systematically in patients with primary aldosteronism remains to be further explored.

Hypertension Due to Renin-Producing Tumors

Juxtaglomerular cell tumors with a hypersecretion of renin represent a rare cause of hypertension. In this prototype of angiotensin-II-dependent hypertension, ACE inhibitors usually reduce blood pressure to normal levels (246). However, the failure to normalize blood pressure in response to ACE inhibition does not necessarily rule out the presence of a renin-secreting tumor.

Hypertension Due to Pheochromocytoma

Plasma renin activity tends to be elevated in patients with pheochromocytoma (247). ACE inhibition has occasionally been shown to lower blood pressure substantially in these patients (248,249).

Hypertension and Pregnancy

At the present time, the use of ACE inhibitors in hypertensive pregnant women should be avoided. In the pregnant rabbits and ewes, captopril has been shown to enhance the rate of stillbirths (250). In the pregnant rabbit, placental perfusion is reduced by ACE inhibition (251). Captopril administered during human pregnancy seems to affect both the maternal and the fetal renin–angiotensin system (252). Neonatal anuria has been described after treatment with captopril (253) or enalapril (254) during pregnancy. In the latter case, peritoneal dialysis has proved to be lifesaving. ACE inhibition during pregnancy may impair closing of the ductus arteriosus (255). It should be said, however, that a number of pregnancies had a favorable outcome despite the administration of an ACE inhibitor (255).

ACE INHIBITION IN HYPERTENSION ASSOCIATED WITH OTHER DISORDERS

ACE Inhibition and Renal Disorders

Although renal disease undoubtedly represents a major cause of hypertension, it is also true that abnormally high blood pressure levels have a deleterious effect on renal function. In some patients with chronic renal failure, the renin–angiotensin system may contribute importantly to the development of their hypertension (256). In a majority of patients, however, it is the impaired sodium-handling capacity of the kidney which plays the predominant role in the pathogenesis of their hypertension (257). Plasma renin activity is often normal or even low in these patients (258–260). There is some suggestion, however, that the renin secretion, although seemingly not elevated, is inappropriately high in relation to the associated sodium retention (259,260). Moreover, it is possible that plasma renin activity measured in a vein does not closely reflect the amount of angiotensin II formed locally within the kidney (261). ACE inhibitors given as monotherapy in the presence of an underlying renal disease normalize blood pressure less frequently than do those given in the presence of an intact renal function (200,262).

Theoretically, ACE inhibitors might improve the natural history of renal disease not only because of their antihypertensive effect but also because of their effects on intrarenal hemodynamics and on the glomerular cells (187, 188, 190, 191). Thus, these agents are expected to prevent the development of glomerular hyperperfusion and hyperfiltration (i.e., of alterations which occur together with the loss of functional nephrons and which presumably contribute to injuring further the remnant glomeruli) (263). In hypertensive patients with a normal renal function, a rise in the glomerular filtration rate in response to ACE inhibition has been observed by some investigators (44,264). In a long-term survey, however, no such effect could be demonstrated (200). As assessed by plasma creatinine levels, a slight deterioration of glomerular filtration rate may also be observed (262). The potential of ACE inhibitors to stabilize or to improve renal function in hypertensive patients with chronic renal failure is difficult to investigate. This is because in some patients the progression of renal disease may, to a large extent, be unrelated either to the quality of blood pressure control or to the drugs used to achieve blood pressure normalization. In patients who already have impaired renal function, chronic ACE inhibition does not seem to alter glomerular filtration rate (265). On the other hand, a favorable effect on renal function cannot be ruled out, since the follow-up of a large number of hypertensive patients with impaired renal function has provided evidence for a decrease in the plasma concentration of creatinine (262). In patients who have essential hypertension and who exhibit a modest degree of renal failure, strict blood pressure control with an ACE inhibitor is followed by either a stabilization or an improvement in renal function (266). In hypertensive patients with no sign of renal failure, the long-term blood pressure reduction resulting from ACE inhibition is accompanied by a decrease in urinary protein excretion (200,267). Similar results have been obtained in patients with hypertension complicated by a renal parenchymal disease (200).

When arterial hypertension is associated with terminal renal failure, it usually can be corrected by hemodialysis and ultrafiltration of extracellular fluid. Patients who do not respond to such sodium depletion have a tendency to exhibit inappropriately high plasma renin activity (268). In such patients, chronic ACE inhibition offers an effective alternative to bilateral nephrectomy (269,270). ACE inhibitors are potentially useful in some patients who develop hypertension following renal transplantation (271,272). In such cases, however, hypertension may be due to a stenotic artery of the graft, and blood pressure reduction induced by an ACE inhibitor can therefore lead to the development of renal failure, for reasons that have been discussed (272).

ACE Inhibition and Cardiac Hypertrophy

Ventricular hypertrophy may be regarded as a compensatory process which, for some time, maintains the cardiac function and performance in spite of the increased ventricular afterload caused by sustained high blood pressure levels. Factors other than arterial pressure per se influence probably the development of ventricular hypertrophy (273). For instance, the presence of renin- and angiotensin-II-binding sites has been demonstrated in the cardiac myocytes (274,275). Angiotensin II has a positive inotropic effect on the myocardium (276) and possibly exerts a mitogenic action (277). Whether circulating or locally generated angiotensin II is involved in the development of cardiac hypertrophy, however, remains uncertain. Thus, there is no obvious difference in left ventricular muscle mass between hypertensive patients with high renin levels and those with low renin levels (278). Like most antihypertensive agents, ACE inhibitors induce a regression of left ventricular hypertrophy in the presence of prolonged blood pressure reduction (154,199,273,278).

ACE Inhibition and Congestive Heart Failure

Undoubtedly, ACE inhibitors have markedly improved the treatment of patients with severe congestive heart failure (279,280). These patients most often have a rather low blood pressure before initiation of treatment and respond to ACE inhibition with an additional drop in blood pressure. Typically, hemodynamic changes induced by blockade of the renin–angiotensin system consist of a decline in total peripheral resistance, in left ventricular filling pressure, and in right pressures, together with an increase in cardiac output and no heart rate modification (281,282). In hypertensive patients presenting with congestive heart failure, any reduction of blood pressure would be expected to be of great benefit to the cardiac function. Whether in this particular context there is some real advantage to decreasing blood pressure with an ACE inhibitor rather than with some other antihypertensive drug has not yet been established.

ACE Inhibition and Coronary Heart Disease

ACE inhibitors have been administered to hypertensive patients with coronary heart disease (283–285). Coronary blood flow and myocardial oxygen consumption decreased during acute ACE inhibition, but these changes occurred in parallel with a reduction of the double product (i.e., systolic blood pressure multiplied by heart rate), which means that the metabolic balance of the heart was not altered (283,285). In one study, chronic ACE inhibition appeared even to attenuate the ST segment depression observed at the maximal double product during ergometry (284). In normotensive patients with coronary artery disease treated for a few days with captopril, an overall improvement in myocardial perfusion has been demonstrated during exercise, but evidence for a coronary steal effect has been detected simultaneously in some cardiac areas (286). A main advantage of ACE inhibition in patients with angina may be the lack of a reflex increase in myocardial sympathetic tone (287).

ACE Inhibition and Peripheral Vascular Disease

ACE inhibitors dilate both small and large arteries when lowering blood pressure (288). Systemic arterial compliance is increased by these agents (288), but it is still unclear whether chronic ACE inhibition has any influence on the development of structural alterations in the vascular wall. Interestingly, chronic therapy with captopril in hypertension associated with claudication may increase blood flow to the limbs, as reflected by an improvement in both the pain-free interval and the maximum walking distance (289,290).

ACE Inhibition in Diabetic Patients

It is essential to normalize blood pressure of hypertensive patients with diabetes mellitus in order to preserve renal function as long as possible (291). Hypertensive patients with uncomplicated diabetes seem to respond to ACE inhibition as well as do patients with essential hypertension (292). Lowering blood pressure of hypertensive diabetics reduces urine protein excretion without modifying renal function (293,294). Such a favorable effect on proteinuria has been demonstrated even in normotensive diabetics with azotemia (295). Particularly relevant is the fact that ACE inhibition for 2 years did slow the rate of renal deterioration in patients with diabetic nephropathy (296). These beneficial effects have been attributed to a decrease in glomerular capillary pressure, a pressure which presumably is abnormally increased in diabetics, as suggested by micropuncture studies in diabetic rats (263). Captopril may also enhance insulin responsiveness in muscle tissue of patients with non-insulin-dependent diabetes mellitus (297). This phenomenon could be explained by a captopril-induced accumulation of local bradykinin (298).

ACE Inhibition in Patients with Respiratory Problems

ACE inhibitors have been used successfully to treat hypertensive patients suffering from chronic obstructive pulmonary disease (299). In this study, no deleterious effect of ACE inhibition on respiratory function tests was observed. Most important, antihypertensive therapy with ACE inhibitors was revealed to be safe also in asthmatic patients (300–302). Bronchial provocation testing was performed in asthmatics treated with an ACE inhibitor. The bronchial reactivity to metacholine (301) and bradykinin (302) was not enhanced by kininase II inhibition.

ACE INHIBITORS AS A FIRST-STEP TREATMENT OF HYPERTENSION

Diuretics and β-blockers are well established as drugs of first choice in the treatment of hypertension. It is now becoming more acceptable for ACE inhibitors and calcium-entry blockers to be used as an alternative for initiating antihypertensive therapy (303). A key point to be taken into account when considering the use of ACE inhibitors as a first-step treatment is their clinical efficacy as compared to other classes of antihypertensive agents.

A number of studies have shown that captopril and enalapril given in monotherapy have an antihypertensive effect practically similar to that of thiazide diuretics (153,304,305). Both types of agents are also equally potent in the elderly (306,307). Furthermore, the blood-pressure-lowering effect of ACE inhibitors appears to be quite similar to that of β-blockers, although there is a clear trend showing that ACE inhibitors decrease resting systolic pressure to a greater extent than do β-adrenoceptor blocking agents (308–313). During exercise, however, systolic blood pressure seems to be lower with β-adrenoceptor blockade than with ACE inhibition (314). The blood pressure reduction obtained in hypertensives with ACE inhibitors is, on the average, also very close to that achieved during calcium-entry blockade (315–319). Based on the results of all these trials, ACE inhibitors administered alone are effective antihypertensive drugs and can be proposed as first-line antihypertensive agents.

Starting the treatment with an ACE inhibitor may have the advantage of simplifying the therapeutic approach to the hypertensive patient. This is based on the findings of a study in which ACE inhibition as the first-step treatment of mild to moderate uncomplicated essential hypertension has been evaluated in double-blind fashion (168). Patients were randomly allocated to either enalapril or a placebo as the first step, followed (when necessary) by the successive addition of a thiazide diuretic, a β-blocker, and the vasodilator hydralazine. During the 6-month follow-up, enalapril given as the first drug in the stepped-care approach to the treatment of hypertension provided a better degree of blood pressure control than did the standard treatment. This result was achieved with a smaller number of tablets than those used in conventional therapy.

INTERACTIONS OF ACE INHIBITORS WITH OTHER ANTIHYPERTENSIVE DRUGS

ACE Inhibitors and Diuretics

The antihypertensive activity of ACE inhibitors is greatly enhanced by coadministration of a diuretic (17,153,218, 260,304–306,320). When ACE inhibition alone fails to normalize blood pressure, reduction of total body sodium (e.g., by a diuretic) triggers the release of renin and, consequently, causes the maintenance of high blood pressure to become angiotensin II dependent. Very low doses of diuretics may suffice to reduce blood pressure when combined with an ACE inhibitor (321). In fact, the hypertensive patient who has his or her angiotensin II generation blocked by ACE inhibition is unable to avoid hypotension if a critical level of sodium depletion is exceeded (36,260). To minimize the risk of hypotension when introducing an ACE inhibitor in a patient already on diuretic therapy, it is strongly recommended that the diuretic be withdrawn (or at least decreased in dosage) for a few days prior to the administration of the first dose. In hypertensive patients with ongoing diuretic therapy, it seems also possible to avoid the occurrence of hypotension by starting with small oral doses of ACE inhibitors (6.25 or 12.5 mg captopril or 5 mg enalapril) (322,323). As expected, a sodium-restricted diet also potentiates the blood pressure response to ACE inhibition (324). In this study, enalapril treatment caused a net natriuresis in salt-deplete, as well as in salt-replete, hypertensive patients.

ACE Inhibitors and β-Adrenoceptor Blocking Agents

The addition of a β-blocker to an ACE inhibitor is often thought not to provide a very rational combination. There exists evidence, however, that some individual hypertensive patients may benefit from such an association (176,304,313,314,325). Blockade of renal β-adrenoceptors blunts the hyperreninemia in response to ACE inhibition (176). It is perhaps partly by this mechanism that β-blockers sometimes induce a supplementary blood pressure reduction. The addition of a β-blocker seems to prolong the blood-pressure-lowering effect of the short-lasting inhibitor captopril (325).

ACE Inhibitors and Calcium Antagonists

The antihypertensive effect of ACE inhibitors is consistently enhanced by calcium antagonists (315,316,325–329). It has actually been proposed that calcium-entry blockers may be able to replace diuretics in the combination with an ACE inhibitor (326), but clear evidence of equal antihypertensive efficacy of these two combinations has not been provided so far. Interestingly, ACE inhibition buffers the counterregulation induced by acute calcium-entry blockade (330). ACE inhibition might attenuate the reflex increase in the tone of the sympathetic nervous system during chronic treatment with a calcium antagonist. This is suggested by the observation that the incidence of adverse effects of the calcium-entry blocker nifedipine tends to be diminished by the concomitant administration of captopril (316).

ACE INHIBITORS IN PATIENTS WITH TREATMENT-RESISTANT OR MALIGNANT HYPERTENSION

A number of studies have demonstrated the usefulness of ACE inhibitors in the management of hypertensive patients unresponsive to multiple drug combinations (260,331–334). In these patients, addition of a thiazide (or even a loop diuretic) is often necessary to control blood pressure. ACE inhibitors can also be successfully administered to patients with malignant hypertension (181,332).

ACE INHIBITORS IN THE TREATMENT OF HYPERTENSIVE CRISES

ACE inhibition represents a rational approach to the treatment of patients who need to have their blood pressure reduced within a few hours. In this indication, the rapidly acting captopril is preferable to enalapril. Captopril may be given either by the usual oral route (335) or sublingually (336). Substantial blood pressure reductions can be obtained within 15 min after oral captopril administration. In the patients unresponsive to acute ACE inhibition alone, usually the addition of a loop diuretic with quick onset of action allows blood pressure control to be achieved in a fast, but progressive, manner (335). Parenterally administered ACE inhibitors have also been utilized with good results in the management of hypertensive emergencies (337–339). Caution is necessary in patients suspected of having a markedly activated renin–angiotensin system (e.g., by previous excessive diuretic administration), since sudden hypotension may develop in these patients (335).

METABOLIC EFFECTS OF ACE INHIBITION

There is currently a growing concern about the potential adverse impact of antihypertensive drugs on lipid and glucose metabolism as well as on circulating levels of potassium and uric acid (340). Increases in plasma lipids, glucose, and uric acid levels are all linked with an increased risk of ischemic heart disease (341). Potassium depletion seems to enhance the risk of developing cardiac arrhythmias (342).

ACE inhibitors have no effect on serum levels of total cholesterol (218,343,344), very low-density and low-density lipoprotein cholesterol (344), triglyceride (343,344), and glucose (218,343), whereas there is some indication that serum apolipoproteins A-I and A-II, which are major apolipoproteins of the high-density lipoprotein fraction, are raised by ACE inhibition (344). In contrast, thiazide diuretics have untoward effects on lipid and glucose metabolism (218,345). In particular, they do cause increases in total serum cholesterol while reducing the concentration of high-density lipoproteins. It is of interest that ACE inhibitors may actually prevent the diuretic-induced hyperlipidemia and hyperglycemia (218,343).

ACE inhibitors seem to exert a uricosuric action (346). They reduce serum uric acid concentrations in patients with hyperuricemia. Interestingly, diuretic-induced hyperuricemia is attenuated by ACE inhibition (218,343).

ACE inhibitors, by blocking the generation of angiotensin II, reduce aldosterone secretion (34,35,42). This mineralocorticoid hormone leads to a urinary loss of potassium. Generally, the suppression of aldosterone synthesis mediated by ACE inhibition does not lead to a clinically relevant increase in serum potassium in patients with a normal renal function (218,347,348). The risk of developing a severe hyperkalemia during ACE inhibition seems to exist mainly in patients with terminal renal failure (347,348). ACE inhibitors have a clear potassium-sparing effect when combined with a diuretic (218,343). Intracellular potassium, as assessed by the determination of intralymphocytic potassium content, increases when an ACE inhibitor is coadministered with a diuretic (349), whereas it falls when a diuretic is given alone (350). This seems to indicate that the pool of intracellular potassium is preserved during ACE inhibition despite concomitant diuretic therapy. In a few patients, the addition of a potassium-sparing diuretic to an ACE inhibitor may be desirable in order to correct the hypokalemia induced by a diuretic (most often by a loop diuretic). This can often be done safely in patients with a normal renal function (351). However, such a combination should be avoided as soon as there is any evidence of renal failure. Caution should also be used when supplementing with potassium a patient treated with an ACE inhibitor (352). From a physiological point of view, it is interesting that the stimulation of aldosterone secretion by potassium is not abolished in hypertensive patients treated with an ACE inhibitor (353). The fact that these homeostatic mechanisms of potassium metabolism are still functioning in the face of ACE inhibition is probably the reason why serious hyperkalemia is rarely observed in hypertensive patients.

EFFECT OF ACE INHIBITION ON QUALITY OF LIFE

The goal of modern antihypertensive therapy should be to lower blood pressure without impairing the patient's enjoyment of life (354). Very early in the evaluation of ACE inhibitors, it became apparent that these drugs have a high acceptability because of a minimal interference with the well-being of patients. It has even been suspected that ACE inhibitors could produce euphoria. However, this turned out not to be true in hypertensive patients treated with captopril (355). In normal subjects, evidence for a modest increase in alertness has been found after a 2-week treatment with enalapril (356). In hypertensive patients, ACE inhibition by enalapril did not alter memory function; however, memory function was slightly, but consistently, impaired by atenolol (357). Recently, utilizing elaborate standardized questionnaires, it has been demonstrated that, in hypertensive patients, captopril improves the sense of well-being, the work performance, and the cognitive function, whereas it has no influence on other indices of quality of life such as physical symptoms, sexual function, sleep function, life satisfaction, and social participation (358). This was well in agreement with the results obtained earlier with less sophisticated methods in captopril-treated patients (359).

DOSAGE

During the early developmental phase of captopril, investigators used daily doses ranging from 600 to 1000 mg even though the first study of captopril in humans had shown clearly that maximal converting-enzyme blockade could be obtained with 20 mg taken orally (360). It was then realized that it is not necessary to suppress ACE activity throughout the day to achieve a satisfactory blood pressure control (167,361), and subsequently much lower doses of captopril were tested (362–368). In one study, 25 mg of captopril taken twice a day lowered blood pressure to the same extent as did 50 mg taken three times a day (362). In another trial, 50 mg of captopril taken twice a day appeared more efficacious than did 25 mg taken twice a day, but it provided results equivalent to those found in the group taking 100 mg twice a day (363). Hypertensive patients were found to decrease their blood pressure equally whether they received 50 mg of captopril once a day or 50 mg of captopril twice a day (367). As single morning doses, 50 mg of captopril produced blood pressure reductions comparable to those produced by 10 mg of enalapril (366,368).

With respect to enalapril, there is a dose–blood-pressure-response relationship in hypertensive patients for daily doses ranging from 2.5 to 20 (and maybe 40) mg (369). However, doses smaller than 10 mg/day may be insufficient to achieve satisfactory blood pressure control. Administration of a given amount of this compound once a day appears to be as effective as giving half that dose twice a day (217,370). Both captopril and enalapril are excreted by the kidney (371,372). Accordingly, the doses of these agents should be reduced in patients with impaired renal function.

SIDE EFFECTS OF ACE INHIBITORS

Side Effects Related to the Blockade of the Renin–Angiotensin System

Hypotension, hyperkalemia, and renal impairment represent typical side effects that are caused by blockade of angiotensin II production. They have all been discussed in detail in different sections of this chapter. Most often they are seen when ACE inhibitors are misused. On one occasion, the hypotensive episode caused by ACE inhibition has led to ischemic cardiovascular complications (373). As expected, dehydration favors the occurrence of hypotension in patients treated with an ACE inhibitor (374,375). Infusion of either saline or angiotensin II can restore a normal blood pressure, but the handling of a saline infusion is much easier; therefore, a saline infusion should preferably be used. A risk of inducing renal impairment by ACE inhibition exists mainly in patients with bilateral renal artery stenosis or with a stenosis of the artery to a solitary kidney. In the absence of renal artery stenosis, the development of renal insufficiency is very unlikely to be observed unless there are severe and widespread vascular lesions in the kidneys (376).

Side Effects Possibly Related to Inhibition of ACE Activity Per Se

Dry, nonproductive cough has been recognized as a class side effect of ACE inhibitors. Post-marketing surveillance of enalapril in a large number of patients has suggested a prevalence of cough of 1% (377). For captopril, post-marketing surveillance showed that 0.2% of the patients had to interrupt therapy because of the occurrence of irritable throat or cough (378). This figure may be somewhat too optimistic. The experience with lisinopril has shown cough to be a problem in 3.4% of hypertensive patients, as compared with 1.2% in placebo-treated patients (379). The mechanisms responsible for this adverse effect are under investigation. A recent report has stated that normal subjects acutely treated with an ACE inhibitor become hypersensitive to inhalation of a cough-inducing substance (380). One possibility is that the cough inducer releases kinins or substance P (i.e., peptides known to be degradated by ACE) (2,381). These peptides might accumulate and play the role of a second messenger in triggering the cough reflex. This is compatible with the observation that bradykinin inhalation produces cough in humans (382). Bradykinin is a well-established activator of prostaglandin synthesis (59,91,92). This renders particularly interesting the finding that cyclooxygenase inhibition reduces cough of hypertensive patients receiving an ACE inhibitor (383).

Compound Related Side Effects

During the course of the development of captopril, excessively high doses were used. This was associated with a rather high incidence of unwanted effects (151,347). The risk of suffering a serious adverse effect turned out to be particularly important in patients with some degree of renal failure and in those with associated connective tissue disease. The most troublesome was leucopenia, which was fatal in a few patients (384,385). There was also some worry about the renal effects of captopril. Some patients developed proteinuria while on captopril treatment (386,387), and the occurrence of immune complex glomerulopathy was feared (388). Taste disturbance and a variety of skin eruptions were observed not infrequently when using excessive doses of captopril. The incidence of all these adverse effects has declined drastically with the reduction of the total daily dose of captopril administered (151,225,378). In particular, leucopenias were not a problem anymore (225,378). Based on a broad survey, it appears that the occurrence of a cutaneous rash or of a dysgeusia necessitates withdrawal of captopril in around 0.80% and 0.35% of the patients, respectively (378). Captopril may cause very rarely a cholestatic jaundice (389) or an angioneurotic edema (390). At the doses recommended today, captopril is believed not to have any direct nephrotoxic effect (391).

The safety profile of enalapril is, in many aspects, very similar to that of captopril (152,217,224,377). However, the incidence of rash and taste disturbance tends to be lower with enalapril than with captopril (392,393). Interestingly, a number of patients having experienced a skin rash while on captopril could be maintained on long-term enalapril therapy with no recurrence of the adverse effect (394,395). However, whether this is because enalapril, unlike captopril, is free of a sulfhydryl group remains speculative. Of note is that enalapril may also cause angioneurotic edema (377,396). However, even extremely large doses of this agent are well tolerated (397).

Elderly hypertensive patients are particularly prone to having side effects during antihypertensive therapy. This seems not to be true for ACE inhibitors. Indeed, in two large field studies, the overall incidence of unwanted effects was found not to be influenced by age (224,225).

CONCLUSIONS

It has been proven that the pharmacological inhibition of ACE provides a highly effective means for the treatment of hypertensive patients. Increasing interest in ACE inhibitors is not only because of their efficacy but also because of their favorable hemodynamic and metabolic effects. These agents are generally very well tolerated, and their major advantage is that they do not interfere with the quality of life of patients.

REFERENCES

1. Oparil S, Haber E. The renin–angiotensin system. *N Engl J Med* 1974;291:389–401.
2. Erdös EG. Angiotensin I converting enzyme. *Circ Res* 1975;36:247–255.
3. Ng KKF, Vane JR. Conversion of angiotensin I to angiotensin II. *Nature* 1967;216:762–766.
4. Ryan JW, Ryan US, Schultz DR. Subcellular localization of pulmonary angiotensin converting enzyme (kininase II). *Biochem J* 1975;146:497–499.
5. Smith U, Ryan JW, Smith DS. Freeze-etch studies of the plasma membrane of pulmonary endothelial cells. *J Cell Biol* 1973;56:492–495.
6. Hial V, Gimbrone MA, Peyton MP, Wilcox GM, Pisano JJ. Angiotensin metabolism by cultured human vascular endothelial and smooth muscle cells. *Microvasc Res* 1979;17:314–329.
7. Swales JD. Arterial wall or plasma renin in hypertension? *Clin Sci* 1979;56:293–298.
8. Dzau VJ. Vascular angiotensin pathways: a new therapeutic target. *J Cardiovasc Pharmacol* 1987;10(Suppl 7):9–16.
9. Campbell DJ. Tissue renin-angiotensin system: sites of angiotensin formation. *J Cardiovasc Pharmacol* 1987;10(Suppl 7):1–8.
10. Swales JD, Heagerty AM. Vascular renin-angiotensin system: the unanswered questions. *J Hypertens* 1987;5(Suppl 2):1–5.
11. London M, Bing RF, Thurston H, Swales JD. Arterial wall up-

take of the renal renin and blood pressure control. *Hypertension* 1983;5:629–634.
12. Re RN, Fallon JT, Dzau VJ, Ouay S, Haber E. Renin synthesis by canine aortic smooth muscle cells in culture. *Life Sci* 1982;30:99–106.
13. Field LJ, McGowan RA, Dickinson DP, Gross KW. Tissue and gene specificity of mouse renin expression. *Hypertension* 1984;6:597–603.
14. Desjardins-Giasson S, Gutkowska J, Garcia R, Genest J. Renin substrate in rat mesenteric artery. *Can J Physiol Pharmacol* 1981;59:528–532.
15. Dzau VJ. Significance of the vascular renin-angiotensin pathway. *Hypertension* 1986;8:553–559.
16. Ondetti MA, Williams NJ, Sabo EF, Pluscec J, Cleaver ER, Kocy O. Angiotensin converting enzyme inhibitors from the venom of *Bothrops jararaca:* isolation, elucidation of structure and synthesis. *Biochemistry* 1971;10:4033–4039.
17. Gavras H, Brunner HR, Laragh JH, Sealey JE, Gavras I, Vukovich RA. An angiotensin converting enzyme inhibitor to identify and treat vasoconstrictor and volume factors in hypertensive patients. *N Engl J Med* 1974;291:817–821.
18. Brunner HR, Nussberger J, Waeber B. The present molecules of converting enzyme inhibitors. *J Cardiovasc Pharmacol* 1985;7(Suppl 1):2–11.
19. Brunner HR, Waeber B, Nussberger J. Does pharmacological profiling of a new drug in normotensive volunteers provide a useful guideline to antihypertensive therapy? *Hypertension* 1983;5(Suppl III):101–107.
20. Cushman DW, Cheung HS. Spectrophotometric assay and properties of the angiotensin converting enzyme in the rabbit lung. *Biochem Pharmacol* 1971;20:1637–1648.
21. Biollaz J, Burnier M, Turini GA, Brunner DB, Porchet M, Gomez HJ, Jones KH, Ferber F, Abrams WB, Gavras H, Brunner HR. Three new long-acting converting enzyme inhibitors: relationship between plasma converting enzyme activity and response to angiotensin I. *Clin Pharmacol Ther* 1981;29:665–670.
22. Roulston JE, McGregor GA, Bind R. The measurement of angiotensin-converting enzyme in subjects receiving captopril. *N Engl J Med* 1980;303:397.
23. Nussberger J, Brunner DB, Waeber B, Brunner HR. True versus immunoreactive angiotensin II in human plasma. *Hypertension* 1985;7(Suppl I):I-1–I-7.
24. Nussberger J, Brunner DB, Waeber B, Brunner HR. Specific measurement of angiotensin metabolites and *in vitro* generated angiotensin II in plasma. *Hypertension* 1986;8:476–482.
25. Nussberger J, Brunner DB, Waeber B, Brunner HR. In-vitro renin inhibition to prevent generation of angiotensins during determination of angiotensin I and II. *Life Sci* 1988;42:1683–1688.
26. Brunner HR, Chang P, Wallach R, Sealey JE, Laragh JH. Angiotensin II vascular receptors: their activity in relationship to sodium balance, the autonomic nervous system and hypertension. *J Clin Invest* 1972;51:58–67.
27. Folkow B. The haemodynamic consequence of adaptative structural changes of the resistance vessels in hypertension. *Clin Sci* 1971;41:1–12.
28. Terragno DA, Crowshaw K, Terragno NA, McGiff JC. Prostaglandin synthesis by bovine mesenteric arteries and veins. *Circ Res* 1975;36 & 37(Suppl I):76–80.
29. Dusting GJ, Moncada S, Vane JR. Prostacyclin (PGX) is the endogenous metabolite responsible for relaxation of coronary arteries induced by arachidonic acid. *Prostaglandins* 1977;13:3–15.
30. Lonigro AJ, Itskovitz HD, Crowshaw K, McGiff JC. Dependency of renal blood flow on prostaglandin synthesis in the dog. *Circ Res* 1973;32:712–717.
31. Vinci JM, Zusman RM, Izzo JL, Bowden RE, Horowitz D, Pisano JJ, Keiser HR. Human urinary and plasma kinins. Relationship to sodium-retaining steroids and plasma renin activity. *Circ Res* 1979;44:1228–1237.
32. Aubert JF, Waeber B, Nussberger J, Vavrek RJ, Stewart JM, Brunner HR. Influence of endogenous bradykinin on blood pressure response to vasopressors in normotensive rats assessed with a bradykinin-antagonist. *J Cardiovasc Pharmacol* 1988;11:51–55.
33. Gavras H, Brunner HR, Turini GA, Kershaw GR, Tifft CP, Cuttelod S, Gavras I, Vukovich RA, McKinstry DN. Antihypertensive effect of oral angiotensin converting enzyme inhibitor SQ 14225 in man. *N Engl J Med* 1978;298:991–995.
34. Case DB, Atlas SA, Laragh JH, Sealey JE, Sullivan PA, McKinstry DN. Clinical experience with blockade of the renin-angiotensin-aldosterone system by an oral converting-enzyme inhibitor (SQ 14,225 or captopril) in hypertensive patients. *Progr Cardiovasc Dis* 1978;21:195–206.
35. Brunner HR, Gavras H, Waeber B, Kershaw GR, Turini GA, Vukovich RA, McKinstry DN, Gavras I. Oral angiotensin-converting enzyme inhibitor in long term treatment of hypertensive patients. *Ann Intern Med* 1979;90:19–23.
36. Hodsman GP, Isles CG, Murray GD, Usherwood TP, Webb DJ, Robertson JIS. Factors related to first dose hypotensive effect of captopril: prediction and treatment. *Br Med J* 1983;286:832–834.
37. Atkinson AB, Brown JJ, Cumming AMM, Fraser R, Lever AF, Leckie BJ, Morton JJ, Robertson JIS. Captopril in renovascular hypertension: long-term use in predicting surgical outcome. *Br Med J* 1982;284:689–692.
38. Case DB, Atlas SA, Laragh JH, Sullivan PA, Sealey JE. Use of first dose response or plasma renin activity to predict the long-term effect of captopril: identification of triphasic pattern of blood pressure response. *J Cardiovasc Pharmacol* 1980;2:339–346.
39. Waeber B, Gavras I, Brunner HR, Cook CA, Charocopos F, Gavras H. Prediction of sustained antihypertensive efficacy of chronic captopril therapy: relationships to immediate blood pressure response and control plasma renin activity. *Am Heart J* 1982;103:384–390.
40. Laragh JH, Angers M, Kelly WG, Lieberman S. Hypotensive agents and pressor substances. The effect of epinephrine, norepinephrine, angiotensin II and others on the secretory rate of aldosterone in man. *JAMA* 1960;174:234–240.
41. Biron P, Koiw E, Nowaczynski W, Brouillet J, Genest J. The effects of intravenous infusion of saline-5-angiotensin II and other pressor agents on urinary electrolytes and corticosteroids, including aldosterone. *J Clin Invest* 1961;40:338–347.
42. Atlas SA, Case DB, Sealey JE, Laragh JH, McKinstry DN. Interruption of the renin-angiotensin system in hypertensive patients by captopril induces sustained reduction in aldosterone secretion, potassium retention and natriuresis. *Hypertension* 1979;1:274–280.
43. Sanchez RA, Marco E, Gilbert HB, Raffaele GP, Brito M, Gimenez M, Moledo LI. Natriuretic effect and changes in renal hemodynamics induced by enalapril in essential hypertension. *Drugs* 1985;30(Suppl I):49–58.
44. De Zeeuw D, Navis GJ, Donker AJM, De Jong PE. The angiotensin converting enzyme inhibitor enalapril and its effects on renal function. *J Hypertens* 1983;1(Suppl I):93–97.
45. Biollaz J, Brunner HR, Gavras I, Waeber B, Gavras H. Antihypertensive therapy with MK 421: angiotensin II–renin relationships to evaluate efficacy of converting enzyme blockade. *J Cardiovasc Pharmacol* 1982;4:966–972.
46. Griffing GT, Sindler BH, Aurecchia SA, Melby JC. Temporal enhancement of renin–aldosterone blockade by enalapril, an angiotensin-converting enzyme inhibitor. *J Clin Pharmacol Ther* 1982;32:592–598.
47. Brunner HR, Waeber B, Nussberger J, Schaller MD, Gomez JH. Long-term clinical experience with enalapril in essential hypertension. *J Hypertens* 1983;1(Suppl 1):103–107.
48. Padfield PL, Brown JJ, Lever AF, Morton JJ, Robertson JIS. Blood pressure in acute and chronic vasopressin excess. Studies of malignant hypertension and the syndrome of inappropriate antidiuretic hormone secretion. *N Engl J Med* 1981;304:1067–1070.
49. Thibonnier M, Aldigier JC, Soto ME, Sassano P, Ménard J, Corvol P. Abnormalities and drug-induced alterations of vasopressin in human hypertension. *Clin Sci* 1981;61:149–152.
50. Thibonnier M, Soto ME, Ménard J, Aldiger JC, Corvol P, Milliez P. Reduction of plasma and urinary vasopressin during treatment of severe hypertension by captopril. *Eur J Clin Invest* 1981;11:449–453.
51. Santucci A, Luparini RL, Ferri C, Ficara C, Giarrizzo C, Balsano

226. Cooper WD, Glover DR, Kimber GR. Influence of age on blood pressure response to enalapril. *Gerontology* 1987;33(Suppl 1):48–54.
227. Schnaper HW, Stein G, Schoenberger JA, Leon AS, Tuck ML, Taylor AA, Liss CL, Shapiro DA. Comparison of enalapril with thiazide diuretics in the elderly hypertensive patient. *Gerontology* 1987;33(Suppl 1):24–35.
228. Vaughan ED Jr, Bühler FR, Laragh JH, Sealey JE, Baer L, Bard RH. Renovascular hypertension: renin measurements to indicate hypersecretion and contralateral suppression, estimate renal plasma flow, and score for surgical curability. *Am J Med* 1973;55:402–414.
229. McGrath BP, Matthews PG, Johnston CI. Use of captopril in the diagnosis of renal hypertension. *Austral NZ J Med* 1981; 11:359–363.
230. Staessen J, Bulpitt C, Fagard R, Lijnen P, Amery A. Long-term converting enzyme inhibition as a guide to surgical curability of hypertension associated with renovascular disease. *Am J Cardiol* 1983;51:1317–1322.
231. Hollenberg NK. Medical therapy of renovascular hypertension: efficacy and safety of captopril in 269 patients. *Cardiovasc Rev Rep* 1983;4:854–879.
232. Smith RD, Franklin SS. Comparison of effects of enalapril plus hydrochlorothiazide versus standard triple therapy on renal function in renovascular hypertension. *Am J Med* 1985;79(Suppl 3C):14–23.
233. Hricik DE, Browning PJ, Kopelman RI, Goorno WE, Madias NE, Dzau VJ. Captopril-induced functional renal insufficiency in patients with bilateral renal artery stenoses or renal artery stenosis in a solitary kidney. *N Engl J Med* 1983;308:373–376.
234. Chrysant SG, Dunn M, Marples D, De Masters K. Severe reversible azotemia from captopril therapy. *Arch Intern Med* 1983;143:437–441.
235. Jackson B, Matthews PG, McGrath BP, Johnston CI. Angiotensin converting enzyme inhibition in renovascular hypertension: frequency of reversible renal failure. *Lancet* 1984;i:225–226.
236. Bussien JP, Schaller MD, Nussberger J, Waeber B, Brunner HR. Insuffisance rénale aiguë après inhibition de l'enzyme de conversion de l'angiotensine par différents agents. *Schweiz Med Wochenschr* 1984;114:236–239.
237 Wenting GJ, Derkx FHM, Tan-Tjiong LH, Van Seyen AJ, Man in't Veld AJ, Schalekamp MADH. Risks of angiotensin converting enzyme inhibition in renal artery stenosis. *Kidney Int* 1987;31(Suppl 20):S180–S183.
238 Reams GP, Singh A, Logan KW, Holmes RA, Bauer JH. Total and split renal function in patients with renovascular hypertension: effects of angiotensin converting enzyme inhibition. *J Clin Hypertens* 1987;3:153–163.
239 Williams PS, Hendy MS, Krill A. Captopril-induced renal artery thrombosis and persistent anuria in a patient with documented pre-existing renal artery stenosis and renal failure. *Postgrad Med J* 1984;60:561–563.
240 Davis BA, Crook JE, Vestal RE, Oates JA. Prevalence of renovascular hypertension in patients with grade III or IV hypertensive retinopathy. *N Engl J Med* 1979;301:1273–1276.
241 Case DB, Laragh JH. Reactive hyperreninemia following angiotensin blockade with either saralasin or converting enzyme inhibitor: a new approach to screen for renovascular hypertension. *Ann Intern Med* 1979;91:153–160.
242. Re RN, Novelline R, Escourron MT, Athanasoulis C, Burton J, Haber E. Inhibition of angiotensin converting enzyme for diagnosis of renal artery stenosis. *N Engl J Med* 1978;298:582–586.
243. Brunner HR, Gavras H, Waeber B, Textor SC, Turini GA. Clinical use of an orally acting converting enzyme inhibitor: captopril. *Hypertension* 1980;2:558–565.
244. Thibonnier M, Sassano P, Joseph A, Plouin PF, Corvol P, Ménard J. Diagnostic value of a single dose of captopril in renin- and aldosterone-dependent surgically curable hypertension. *Cardiovasc Rev Rep* 1982;3:1659–1664.
245. Lyons DF, Kern DC, Brown RD, Hanson CS, Carollo ML. Single dose captopril as a diagnostic test for primary aldosteronism. *J Clin Endocrinol Metab* 1983;57:892–896.
246. Baruch D, Corvol P, Alhenc-Gelas F, Dufloux MA, Guyenne TT, Gaux JC, Raynaud A, Brisset JM, Duclos JM, Ménard J. Diagnosis and treatment of renin-secreting tumors. Report of three cases. *Hypertension* 1984;6:760–766.
247. Harrison TS, Birbari A, Seaton JR. Malignant hypertension in pheochromocytoma: correlation with plasma renin activity. *Johns Hopkins Med J* 1972;130:329–332.
248. Lonte G, Guffens P, Waucquez JL, Firre E, Legrand JL, Klels E, Adam J. Effect of captopril on hypertension due to pheochromocytoma. *Lancet* 1984;ii:175.
249. Plouin PF, Rougeot MA, Chatellier G, Comoy E, Ménard J. Système rénine–angiotensine–aldostérone au cours du phéochromocytome: un rôle dans l'élévation tensionnelle? *Arch Mal Coeur* 1985;78:1734–1736.
250. Broughton-Pipkin F, Symonds EM, Turner SR. The effect of SQ 14,225 (captopril) upon mother and fetus in the chronically cannulated ewe and in the pregnant rabbit. *J Physiol* 1986;87:533–542.
251. Ferris TF, Wein EK. Effect of captopril on uterine blood flow and prostaglandin E synthesis in the pregnant rabbit. *J Clin Invest* 1983;71:809–815.
252. Bontroy MJ, Vert P, Hurault De Ligny B, Miton A. Captopril administration in pregnancy impairs fetal angiotensin converting enzyme activity and neonatal adaptation. *Lancet* 1984;ii:935–936.
253. Rothberg AD, Lorenz R. Can captopril cause fetal and neonatal renal failure? *Pediatr Pharmacol* 1984;4:189–192.
254. Schubiger G, Flury G, Nussberger J. Enalapril for pregnancy-induced hypertension: acute renal failure in a neonate. *Ann Intern Med* 1988;108:215–216.
255. Kreft-Joris C, Plouin PF, Tchobroutsky C. Angiotensin converting enzyme inhibitors during pregnancy. *J Hypertens* 1987;5(Suppl 5):553–554.
256. Ledingham JGG. Effects of angiotensin II and angiotensin converting enzyme inhibition in chronic renal failure. *Kidney Int* 1987;31(Suppl 20):112–116.
257. Weidmann P. Pathogenesis of hypertension associated with chronic renal failure. *Contrib Nephrol* 1984;41:47–65.
258. Wilkinson R, Scott DF, Udall PR, Kerr DNS, Swinney J. Plasma renin and exchangeable sodium in the hypertension of chronic renal failure. *Q J Med* 1970;39:377–394.
259. Davies DL, Beevers DG, Briggs JD, Medina AM, Robertson JIS, Schalekamp MADH, Brown JJ, Lever AF, Morton JJ, Tree M. Abnormal relationship between exchangeable sodium and the renin–angiotensin system in malignant hypertension and in hypertension with chronic renal failure. *Lancet* 1973;i:683–686.
260. Brunner HR, Waeber B, Wauters JP, Turini GA, McKinstry DN, Gavras H. Inappropriate renin secretion unmasked by captopril (SQ 14,225) in hypertension of chronic renal failure. *Lancet* 1978;ii:704–707.
261. Mendelsohn FAO. Angiotensin II: evidence for its role as an intrarenal hormone. *Kidney Int* 1982;22(Suppl 12):78–81.
262. Jenkins AC, Dreslinski GR, Tadros SS, Groel JT, Fand R, Herczeg SA. Captopril in hypertension: seven years later. *J Cardiovasc Pharmacol* 1985;7(Suppl 1):96–101.
263. Hostetter TH, Rennke HG, Brenner BM. The case for intrarenal hypertension in the initiation and progression of diabetic and other glomerulopathies. *Am J Med* 1982;72:375–380.
264. Hollenberg NK, Swartz SL, Passan DR, Williams GH. Increased glomerular filtration rate after converting enzyme inhibition in essential hypertension. *N Engl J Med* 1979;301:9–12.
265. Cooper WD, Doyle GD, Donohoe J, Laher M, Ledingham JGG, Raine AEG, Melinck C, Unsworth J, Raman GV, Van den Burg MJ, Woollard ML, Currie WJC. Enalapril in the treatment of hypertension associated with impaired renal function. *J Hypertens* 1985;3(Suppl 3):471–474.
266. Bauer JH, Reams GP, Lal SM. Renal protective effect of strict blood pressure control with enalapril therapy. *Arch Intern Med* 1987;147:1397–1400.
267. De Venuto G, Andreotti C, Mattarei M, Pegoretti G. Long-term captopril therapy at low doses reduces albumin excretion in patients with essential hypertension and no sign of renal impairment. *J Hypertens* 1985;3(Suppl 2):143–146.
268. Lifschitz MD, Kirschenbaum MA, Rosenblatt SG, Gibney R. Effect of saralasin in hypertensive patients on chronic dialysis. *Ann Intern Med* 1977;88:23–27.
269. Vaughan ED Jr, Carey RM, Ayers CR, Peach MJ. Hemodialy-

sis-resistant hypertension: control with an orally active inhibitor of angiotensin converting enzyme. *J Clin Endocrinol* 1979;48:869–871.

270. Wauters JP, Waeber B, Brunner HR, Guignard JP, Turini GA, Gavras H. Uncontrollable hypertension in patients on hemodialysis: long-term treatment with captopril and salt subtraction. *Clin Nephrol* 1981;16:86–92.
271. Hamilton DV, Evans DB, Maidment G, Pryor JS. Captopril in refractory hypertension in patients with chronic renal failure and renal transplantation. *J R Soc Med* 1981;74:357–362.
272. Curtiss JJ, Luke RG, Whelchel JD, Diethelm AG, Jones P, Dustan HP. Inhibition of angiotensin-converting enzyme in renal transplant recipients with hypertension. *N Engl J Med* 1983;308:377–381.
273. Frohlich ED. Pathophysiological considerations in left ventricular hypertrophy. *J Clin Hypertens* 1987;3:54–65.
274. Wright GB, Alexander RW, Eckstein LS, Gimbrone MA Jr. Characterization of rabbit ventricular myocardial receptors for angiotensin II: evidence for two sites with different affinities and specificities. *Mol Pharmacol* 1984;24:213–221.
275. Dzau VJ, Re RN. Evidence for the existence of renin in the heart. *Circulation* 1987;75(Suppl I):134–136.
276. Koch-Weser J. Nature of the inotropic action of angiotensin on ventricular myocardium. *Circ Res* 1965;16:230–237.
277. Re RN, La Biche RA, Bryan SE. Nuclear-hormone mediated changes in chromatin solubility. *Biochem Biophys Res Commun* 1983;110:61–68.
278. Devereux RB, Pickering TG, Cody RJ, Laragh JH. Relation of renin–angiotensin system activity to left ventricular hypertrophy and function in experimental and human hypertension. *J Clin Hypertens* 1987;3:87–103.
279. Captopril Multicenter Research Group. A placebo-controlled trial of captopril in refractory chronic congestive heart failure. *J Am Coll Cardiol* 1983;2:755–763.
280. The Consensus Trial Study Group. Effects of enalapril on mortality in severe congestive heart failure. *N Engl J Med* 1987;23:1429–1435.
281. Turini GA, Brunner HR, Ferguson RK, Rivier JL, Gavras H. Congestive heart failure in normotensive man: haemodynamics, renin, and angiotensin II blockade. *Br Heart J* 1978;40:1134–1142.
282. Turini GA, Brunner HR, Gribic M, Waeber B, Gavras H. Improvement of chronic congestive heart failure by oral captopril. *Lancet* 1979;1:1213–1215.
283. Daly P, Rouleau JL, Cousineau D, Burgess JH. Acute effects of captopril on the coronary circulation of patients with hypertension and angina. *Am J Med* 1984;76(5B):111–115.
284. Strozzi C, Cocco G, Portaluppi F, Padula A, Urso L, Alfiero R, Rizzo A, Tasini MT. Ergometric evaluation of the effects of captopril in hypertensive patients with stable angina. *J Hypertens* 1985;3(Suppl 2):147–148.
285. Mettauer B, Rouleau JL, Daly P. The effect of captopril on the coronary circulation and myocardial metabolism of patients with coronary artery disease. *Postgrad Med J* 1986;62(Suppl 1):54–58.
286. Tardieu A, Virot P, Vandroux JC, Vergnoux H, Pinaud D, Chabanier A, Bensaid J. Effects of captopril on myocardial perfusion in patients with coronary insufficiency: evaluation by the exercise test and quantitative myocardial tomoscintigraphy using thallium-201. *Postgrad Med J* 1986;62(Suppl 1):38–41.
287. Daly P, Mettauer B, Rouleau JL, Cousineau D, Burgess JH. Lack of reflex increase in myocardial sympathetic tone after captopril: potential antianginal effect. *Circulation* 1985;71:317–325.
288. Safar ME, Bouthier JA, Levenson JA, Simon AC. Peripheral large arteries and the response to antihypertensive treatment. *Hypertension* 1983;5(Suppl III):63–68.
289. Libretti A, Catalano M. Captopril in the treatment of hypertension associated with claudication. *Postgrad Med J* 1986;62(Suppl I):34–37.
290. Roberts DH, Tsao Y, McLoughlin GA, Breckenridge AM. Placebo-controlled comparison of captopril, atenolol, labetolol, and pindolol in hypertension complicated by intermittent claudication. *Lancet* 1987;ii:650–653.
291. Christlieb AR, Warram JH, Krowleski AS, Busick EJ, Gauda OP, Asmal AC, Soldnier JS, Bradley RF. Hypertension: the major risk factor in juvenile onset insulin-dependent diabetics. *Diabetes* 1981;30(Suppl 2):90–96.
292. Sullivan PA, Kelleher M, Twomey M, Dineen M. Effects of converting enzyme inhibition on blood pressure, plasma renin activity (PRA) and plasma aldosterone in hypertensive diabetics compared to patients with essential hypertension. *J Hypertens* 1985;3:359–363.
293. Gambaro G, Morbiato F, Cicerello E, Del Turco M, Sartori L, D'Angelo A, Grepaldi G. Captopril in the treatment of hypertension in type I and type II diabetic patients. *J Hypertens* 1985;3(Suppl 2):153–154.
294. Matthews DM, Wathen CG, Bell D, Collier A, Muir AL, Clarke BF. The effect of captopril on blood pressure and glucose tolerance in hypertensive non-insulin dependent diabetics. *Postgrad Med J* 1986;62(Suppl 1):73–75.
295. Taguma Y, Kitamoto Y, Futaki G, Ueda H, Monma H, Ishizaki M, Takanashi H, Sekino H, Sasaki Y. Effect of captopril on heavy proteinuria in azotemic diabetics. *N Engl J Med* 1985;313:1617–1620.
296. Björck S, Nyberg G, Mulec H, Granerus G, Herlitz H, Aurell M. Beneficial effects of angiotensin converting enzyme inhibition on renal function in patients with diabetic nephropathy. *Br Med J* 1986;293:471–474.
297. Jauch KW, Hartl W, Guenther B, Wicklmayr M, Rett K, Dietze G. Captopril enhances insulin responsiveness of forearm muscle tissue in non-insulin-dependent diabetes mellitus. *Eur J Clin Invest* 1987;17:448–454.
298. Dietze GJ, Rett K, Jauch KW, Wicklmayr M, Fink E, Hartl W, Guenther B, Fritz H, Mehnert H. Captopril bei Hypertonikern mit Diabetes mellitus Typ II. *Herz* 1987;12(Suppl I):16–21.
299. Bertoli L, Fusco M, Micallef RE, Busnardo I. Treatment of essential hypertension with captopril in patients with chronic obstructive pulmonary disease. *J Hypertens* 1985;3(Suppl 2):153–154.
300. Riska H, Stenius-Aarniala B, Sovijärvi ARA. Comparison of the efficacy of an ACE inhibitor and a calcium channel blocker in hypertensive asthmatics. A preliminary report. *Postgrad Med J* 1986;62(Suppl I):52–53.
301. Sala H, Abad J, Juanmiguel L, Plans C, Ruiz J, Roig J, Moura J. Captopril and bronchial reactivity. *Postgrad Med J* 1986;62 (Suppl I):76–77.
302. Dixon CMS, Fuller RW, Barnes PJ. The effect of an angiotensin converting enzyme inhibitor, ramipril, on bronchial responses in asthmatic subjects. *Br J Clin Pharmacol* 1987;23:91–93.
303. Zanchetti A. A re-examination of stepped-care: a restrospective and a prospective. *J Cardiovasc Pharmacol* 1985;7(Suppl 1):126–131.
304. Wing LMH, Chalmers JP, West MJ, Bune AJC, Russel AE, Elliott JM, Morris MJ. Treatment of hypertension with enalapril and hydrochlorothiazide or enalapril and atenolol: contrasts in hypotensive interactions. *J Hypertens* 1987;5(Suppl 5):603–606.
305. Pool JL, Gennari J, Goldstein R, Kochar MS, Lewin AJ, Maxwell MH, McChesney JA, Mehta J, Nash DT, Nelson EB, Rastogi S, Rofman B, Weinberger M. Controlled multicenter study of the antihypertensive effects of lisinopril, hydrochlorothiazide, and lisinopril plus hydrochlorothiazide in the treatment of 394 patients with mild to moderate essential hypertension. *J Cardiovasc Pharmacol* 1987;9(Suppl 1):36–42.
306. Muisan G, Agabiti-Rosei E, Buoninconti R, Cagli V, Carotti A, Corea L, Innocenti P, Malerba M, Paciaroni E, Pirrelli A, Toso M, Botta G. Antihypertensive efficacy and tolerability of captopril in the elderly: comparison with hydrochlorothiazide and placebo in a multicenter, double-blind study. *J Hypertens* 1987;5(Suppl 5):599–602.
307. Shapiro DA, Liss CL, Walker JF, Lewis JL, Lengerich RA, Irvin JD. Enalapril and hydrochlorothiazide as antihypertensive agents in the elderly. *J Cardiovasc Pharmacol* 1987;10(Suppl 7):S160–S162.
308. O'Connor DT, Mosley CA, Cervenka J, Bernstein KN. Contrasting renal haemodynamic responses to the angiotensin converting enzyme inhibitor enalapril and the β-adrenergic antagonist metoprolol in essential hypertension. *J Hypertens* 1984;2(Suppl 2):89–92.
309. Andren L, Karlberg BE, Svensson A, Ohman KP, Nilsson OR,

Hansson L. Long-term effects of captopril and atenolol in essential hypertension. *Acta Med Scand* 1985;217:155–160.

310. Edmonds D, Knorr M, Greminger P, Walger P, Frielingsdorf J, Vetter H, Vetter W. ACE inhibitor versus β-blocker in the treatment of essential hypertension. *Nephron* 1987;47(Suppl 1):90–93.

311. Bolzano K, Arriaga J, Bernal R, Bernardes H, Calderon JL, Debruyn J, Dienstl F, Drayer JIM, Goodfriend TL, Gross W, Guthrie GP, Holwerda N, Klein W, Krakoff L, Liebau H, Oparil S, Reams GP, Reed WG, Safar ME, Schubotz R, Seedat YK, Thind GS, Veriava Y, Wollam G, Wods JW, Zusman RM. The antihypertensive effect of lisinopril compared to atenolol in patients with mild to moderate hypertension. *J Cardiovasc Pharmacol* 1987;9(Suppl 3):43–47.

312. Zachariah PK, Bonnet G, Chrysant SG, De Backer G, Goldstein R, Herrera J, Lindner A, Materson BJ, Maxwell MH, McMahon FG, Merrill RH, Paton RR, Rapp AD, Roginsky MS, Seedat YK, Sime F, Vaicaitis JS, Weinberg MS, Zusman RM. Evaluation of antihypertensive efficacy of lisinopril compared to metoprolol in moderate to severe hypertension. *J Cardiovasc Pharmacol* 1987;9(Suppl 3):53–58.

313. Wing LMH, Chalmers JP, West MJ, Russel AE, Morris MJ, Cain MD, Bune AJC, Southgate DO. Enalapril and atenolol in essential hypertension: attenuation of hypotensive effects in combination. *Clin Exp Hypertens* 1988;10:119–133.

314. Franz IW, Behr U, Ketelhut R. Resting and exercise blood pressure with atenolol, enalapril and a low-dose combination. *J Hypertens* 1987;5(Suppl 3):37–41.

315. Stornello M, Di Rao G, Iachello M, Pisani R, Scapellato L, Pedrinelli R, Salvetti A. Hemodynamic and humoral interactions between captopril and nifedipine. *Hypertension* 1983;5 (Suppl III):154–156.

316. Salvetti A, Innocenti PF, Iardella M, Pambianco F, Saba GC, Rossetti M, Botta GF. Captopril and nifedipine interactions in the treatment of essential hypertensives: a crossover study. *J Hypertens* 1987;5(Suppl 4):139–142.

317. Mörlin C, Baglivo H, Boeijinga JK, Breckenridge AM, Clement D, Johnston GD, Klein W, Kramer R, Luccioni R, Meurer KA, Richardson PJ, Rosenthal J, Six R, Witzgall H. Comparative trial of lisinopril and nifedipine in mild to severe essential hypertension. *J Cardiovasc Pharmacol* 1987;9(Suppl 3):48–52.

318. Gennari C, Nami R, Bianchini C, Pavese G. Nitrendipine and the angiotensin converting enzyme inhibitors in the treatment of hypertension. *J Cardiovasc Pharmacol* 1987;9(Suppl 4):245–251.

319. Bidiville J, Nussberger J, Waeber G, Porchet M, Waeber B, Brunner HR. Are good antihypertensive responses to converting enzyme inhibitors or calcium antagonists mutually exclusive? *Hypertension* 1988;11:166–173.

320. Brunner HR, Gavras H, Waeber B. Enhancement by diuretics of the antihypertensive action of long-term angiotensin converting enzyme blockade. *Clin Exp Hypertens* 1980;2:639–657.

321. Andren L, Weiner L, Svensson A, Hansson L. Enalapril with either a "very low" or "low" dose of hydrochlorothiazide is equally effective in essential hypertension. A double-blind trial in 100 hypertensive patients. *J Hypertens* 1983;1(Suppl 2):384–386.

322. Thind GS, Mahapatra RK, Johnson A, Coleman RD. Low-dose captopril administration in patients with moderate-to-severe hypertension treated with diuretics. *Circulation* 1983;67:1340–1345.

323. Webster J, Robb OJ, Witte K, Petrie JC. Single doses of enalapril and atenolol in hypertensive patients treated with bendrofluazide. *J Hypertens* 1987;5:457–460.

324. Navis GJ, De Jong PE, Donker AJM, Van der Hem GK, De Zeeuw D. Diuretic effects of angiotensin-converting enzyme inhibition: comparison of low and liberal sodium diet in hypertensive patients. *J Cardiovasc Pharmacol* 1987;9:743–748.

325. McGregor GA, Markandu ND, Smith SJ, Sagnella GA. Captopril: contrasting effects of adding hydrochlorothiazide, propranolol, or nifedipine. *J Cardiovasc Pharmacol* 1985;7(Suppl 1):82–87.

326. Brouwer RML, Bolli P, Erne P, Conen D, Kiowski W, Bühler FR. Antihypertensive treatment using calcium antagonists in combination with captopril rather than diuretics. *J Cardiovasc Pharmacol* 1985;7(Suppl 1):88–91.

327. Donnelly R, Elliott HL, Reid JL. Nicardipine combined with enalapril in patients with essential hypertension. *Br J Clin Pharmacol* 1986;22:283s–287s.

328. Lang R, Degenhardt S, Ollenschläger G, Barth A. Effect of a low-dose combination nitrendipine/enalapril in less-severe degrees of hypertension. *J Cardiovasc Pharmacol* 1987;9(Suppl 4):254–255.

329. Singer DRJ, Markandu ND, Shore AC, McGregor GA. Captopril and nifedipine in combination for moderate to severe essential hypertension. *Hypertension* 1987;9:629–633.

330. Bellet M, Sassano P, Guyenne TT, Corvol P, Ménard J. Sympatho-inhibitory effect of angiotensin converting enzyme inhibition during counterregulation induced by dihydropyridine. *J Hypertens* 1987;5(Suppl 5):583–585.

331. Atkinson AB, Lever AF, Brown JJ, Robertson JIS. Combined treatment of severe intractable hypertension with captopril and diuretic. *Lancet* 1980;ii:105–107.

332. Case DB, Atlas SA, Sullivan PA, Laragh JH. Acute and chronic treatment of severe and malignant hypertension with the angiotensin converting enzyme inhibitor captopril. *Circulation* 1981;64:765–771.

333. Raine AEG, Ledingham JGG. Clinical experience with captopril in the treatment of severe drug-resistant hypertension. *Am J Cardiol* 1982;49:1475–1479.

334. Havelka J, Vetter H, Studer A, Greminger P, Lüscher T, Wollnik S, Siegenthaler W, Vetter W. Acute and chronic effects of the angiotensin converting enzyme inhibitor captopril in severe hypertension. *Am J Cardiol* 1982;49:1467–1474.

335. Biollaz J, Waeber B, Brunner HR. Hypertensive crisis treated with orally administered captopril. *Eur J Clin Pharmacol* 1983;25:145–149.

336. Tschollar W, Belz GG. Sublingual captopril in hypertensive crisis. *Lancet* 1985;ii:34.

337. Tifft CP, Gavras H, Kershaw GR, Gavras I, Brunner HR, Liang CS, Chobanian AV. Converting enzyme inhibition in hypertensive emergencies. *Ann Intern Med* 1979;90:43–47.

338. Di Pette DJ, Ferraro JC, Evans RR, Martin M. Enalaprilat, an intravenous angiotensin-converting enzyme inhibitor, in hypertensive crises. *Clin Pharmacol Ther* 1985;38:199–204.

339. Strauss R, Gavras I, Vlahakos D, Gavras H. Enalaprilat in hypertensive emergencies. *J Clin Pharmacol* 1986;26:39–43.

340. Ames RP, Hill P. Antihypertensive therapy and the risk of coronary heart disease. *J Cardiovasc Pharmacol* 1982;4(Suppl 2):206–212.

341. Castelli WP, Anderson K. A population at risk: prevalence of high cholesterol levels in hypertensive patients in the Framingham study. *Am J Med* 1986;80(2A):23–32.

342. Hollifield JW. Thiazide treatment of hypertension. Effects of thiazide diuretics on serum potassium, magnesium, and ventricular ectopy. *Am J Med* 1986;80(Suppl 4A):8–14.

343. Malini PL, Strochi E, Ambrosioni E, Magnani B. Long-term antihypertensive, metabolic and cellular effects of enalapril. *J Hypertens* 1984;2(Suppl 2):101–105.

344. Sasaki J, Arakawa K. Effect of captopril on serum lipids, lipoproteins, and apolipoproteins in patients with mild essential hypertension. *Curr Ther Res* 1986;40:898–902.

345. Weinberger MH. Antihypertensive therapy and lipids: evidence, mechanisms and implications. *Arch Intern Med* 1985;145:1102–1105.

346. Leary WP, Reyes AJ. Angiotensin I converting enzyme inhibitors and the renal excretion of urate. *Cardiovasc Drugs Ther* 1987;1:29–38.

347. Waeber B, Gavras I, Brunner HR, Gavras H. Safety and efficacy of chronic therapy with captopril in hypertensive patients: an update. *J Clin Pharmacol* 1981;21:508–516.

348. Textor SC, Bravo EL, Fouad FM, Tarazi RC. Hyperkalemia in azotemic patients during angiotensin converting enzyme inhibition and aldosterone reduction with captopril. *Am J Med* 1982;73:719–725.

349. Costa FV, Borghi C, Boshi S, Ambrosioni E. Differing dosages of captopril and hydrochlorothiazide in the treatment of hyperten-

sion: Long-term effects on metabolic values and intracellular electrolytes. *J Cardiovasc Pharmacol* 1985;7(Suppl 1):70–76.
350. Ryan MP, Ryan MF, Counihan TB. The effect of diuretics on lymphocyte magnesium and potassium. *Acta Med Scand* 1981;209:153–161.
351. Mooser V, Waeber G, Bidiville J, Waeber B, Nussberger J, Brunner HR. Kalemia during combined therapy with an angiotensin converting enzyme inhibitor and a potassium-sparing diuretic. *J Clin Hypertens* 1987;3:510–513.
352. Burnakis TG, Mioduch HJ. Combined therapy with captopril and potassium supplementation. A potential for hyperkalemia. *Arch Intern Med* 1984;144:2371–2372.
353. Barnes JN, Drew PJT, Furniss SS, Holly JMP, Knight AR, Skehan JD, Goodwin FY. Effect of angiotensin converting enzyme inhibition on potassium-mediated aldosterone secretion in essential hypertension. *Clin Sci* 1985;68:625–630.
354. Hollenberg NK. Initial therapy in hypertension: quality-of-life considerations. *J Hypertens* 1987;5(Suppl 1):3–7.
355. Callender JS, Hodsman GP, Hutcheson MJ, Lever AF, Robertson JIS. Mood changes during captopril therapy for hypertension: a double-blind pilot study. *Hypertension* 1983;5(Suppl III):90–93.
356. Olajide D, Lader M. Psychotropic effects of enalapril maleate in normal volunteers. *Psychopharmacology* 1985;86:374–376.
357. Lichter I, Richardson PJ, Wyke MA. Differential effects of atenolol and enalapril on memory during treatment for essential hypertension. *Br J Clin Pharmacol* 1986;21:641–645.
358. Croog SH, Levine S, Testa MA, Brown B, Bulpitt CJ, Jenkins CD, Klerman GL, Williams GH. The effects of antihypertensive therapy on the quality of life. *N Engl J Med* 1986;314:1657–1664.
359. Hill JF, Bulpitt CJ, Fletcher AE. Angiotensin converting enzyme inhibitors and quality of life: the European trial. *J Hypertens* 1985;3(Suppl 2):91–94.
360. Ferguson RK, Brunner HR, Turini GA, Gavras H, McKinstry DN. A specific orally active inhibitor of angiotensin converting enzyme in man. *Lancet* 1977;i:775–778.
361. Waeber B, Brunner HR, Brunner DB, Curtet AL, Turini GA, Gavras H. Discrepancy between antihypertensive effect and angiotensin converting enzyme inhibition by captopril. *Hypertension* 1980;2:236–242.
362. Veterans Administration Cooperative Study Group on Antihypertensive Agents. Low-dose captopril for the treatment of mild to moderate hypertension. *Arch Intern Med* 1984;144:1947–1953.
363. Drayer JIM, Weber MA. Monotherapy of essential hypertension with a converting-enzyme inhibitor. *Hypertension* 1983;5(Suppl 3):108–113.
364. De Gaudemaris R, Battistella P, Siche JP, Debru JL, Blatier JF, Mallian JM. Comparative study of the efficacy of captopril at a single daily dose of 100 mg and at a twice daily dose of 50 mg by measuring ambulatory pressure over 24 hours. *Postgrad Med J* 1986;62(Suppl 1):97–100.
365. Fogari R, Zoppi A, Corradi L, Poletti L, Tettamanti F, Botta GF. Hypotensive effect of once-daily administration of captopril. *Curr Ther Res* 1986;40:500–508.
366. Garanin G. A comparison of once-daily antihypertensive therapy with captopril and enalapril. *Curr Ther Res* 1986;40:567–575.
367. Schoenberger JA, Wilson DJ. Once-daily treatment of essential hypertension with captopril. *J Clin Hypertens* 1986;4:379–387.
368. De Cesaris R, Ranieri G, Salzano EV, Liberatore SM. Once daily therapy with angiotensin converting enzyme inhibitors in mild hypertension: a comparison of captopril and enalapril. *J Hypertens* 1987;5(Suppl 5):595–597.
369. Bergstrand R, Herlitz H, Johansson S, Berglund G, Vedin A, Wilhelmsson C, Gomez HJ, Cirillo VJ, Bolognese JA. Effective dose range of enalapril in mild to moderate essential hypertension. *Br J Clin Pharmacol* 1985;19:605–611.
370. Bergstrand R, Johansson S, Vedin A, Wilhelmsson C. Comparison of once-a-day and twice-a-day dosage regimens of enalapril (MK-421) in patients with mild hypertension. *Br J Clin Pharmacol* 1982;14:136P–137P.
371. Kripalani KJ, McKinstry DN, Singhvi SM, Willard DA, Vukovich RA, Migdalof BH. Disposition of captopril in normal subjects. *Clin Pharmacol Ther* 1980;27:636–641.
372. Fruncillo RJ, Rocci ML, Vlasses PH, Mojaverian P, Shepley K, Clementi RA, Oren A, Smith RD, Till AE, Riley LJ, Krishna G, Narins RG, Ferguson RK. Disposition of enalapril and enalaprilat in renal insufficiency. *Kidney Int* 1987;31(Suppl 20):117–122.
373. Baker KM, Johns DW, Ayers CR, Carey RM. Ischemic cardiovascular complications concurrent with administration of captopril. *Hypertension* 1980;2:73–74.
374. Benett PR, Cairns SA. Captopril, diarrhoea, and hypotension. *Lancet* 1985;i:1105.
375. Coulshed DJ, Davies SJ, Turney JH. Prolonged hypotension after fever during enalapril treatment. *Lancet* 1985;ii:222.
376. Thind GS. Renal insufficiency during angiotensin-converting enzyme inhibitor therapy in hypertensive patients with no renal artery stenosis. *J Clin Hypertens* 1985;4:337–343.
377. Cooper WD, Sheldon D, Brown D, Kimber GR, Isitt VL, Currie WJC. Post-marketing surveillance of enalapril: experience in 11710 hypertensive patients in general practice. *J R Coll Gen Pract* 1987;37:346–349.
378. Chalmers D, Dombey SL, Lawson DH. Post-marketing surveillance of captopril (for hypertension): a preliminary report. *Br J Clin Pharmacol* 1987;24:343–349.
379. Rush JE, Merrill DD. The safety and tolerability of lisinopril in clinical trials. *J Cardiovasc Pharmacol* 1987;9(Suppl 3):99–107.
380. Morice AH, Lowry R, Brown MJ, Higenbottam T. Angiotensin-converting enzyme and the cough reflex. *Lancet* 1987;ii:1116–1118.
381. Thiele EA, Strittmatter SM, Snyder SH. Substance K and substance P as possible endogenous substrates of angiotensin converting enzyme in the brain. *Biochem Biophys Res Commun* 1985;128:317–324.
382. Fuller RW, Dixon CMS, Cuss FMC, Barnes PJ. Bradykinin-induced bronchoconstriction in humans. *Annu Rev Respir Dis* 1987;135:176–180.
383. Nicholls MG, Gilchrist NL. Sulindac and cough induced by converting enzyme inhibitors. *Lancet* 1987;i:872.
384. Cooper RA. Captopril-associated neutropenia. Who is at risk? *Arch Intern Med* 1983;143:659–660.
385. Ersley AJ, Alexander JC, Caro J, Boyd RL. Hematologic side effects of captopril and associated risk factors. *Cardiovasc Rev Rep* 1982;3:660–671.
386. Prins EJL, Hoorntje SJ, Weening JJ, Donker AJM. Nephrotic syndrome in a patient on captopril. *Lancet* 1979;ii:306.
387. Case DB, Atlas SA, Mouradian JA, Fishman RA, Sherman RL, Laragh JH. Proteinuria during long-term captopril therapy. *JAMA* 1980;244:346–349.
388. Hoorntje SJ, Kallenberg CGM, Weening JJ, Donker AJM, The TH, Hoedemaeker PJ. Immune-complex glomerulopathy in patients treated with captopril. *Lancet* 1980;ii:1212–1214.
389. Rahmat J, Gelfand RL, Gelfand MC, Winchester JF, Schreiner GE, Zimmerman HJ. Captopril-associated cholestatic jaundice. *Ann Intern Med* 1985;102:56–58.
390. Jett GK. Captopril-induced angioedema. *Ann Emerg Med* 1984;13:489–490.
391. Donker AJM. Nephrotoxicity of angiotensin converting enzyme inhibitors. *Kidney Int* 1987;31(Suppl 20):132–137.
392. Irvin JD, Viau JM. Safety profiles of the angiotensin converting enzyme inhibitors captopril and enalapril. *Am J Med* 1986;8(Suppl 4C):46–50.
393. Case DB. Angiotensin-converting enzyme inhibitors: Are they all alike? *J Clin Hypertens* 1987;3:243–256.
394. Gavras I, Gavras H. Captopril and enalapril. *Ann Intern Med* 1983;88:556–557.
395. Rotmensch HH, Vlasses PH, Ferguson RK. Resolution of captopril-induced rash after substitution of enalapril. *Pharmacotherapy* 1983;3:131–133.
396. Singer DRJ, McGregor GA. Angioneurotic oedema associated with two angiotensin converting enzyme inhibitors. *Br Med J* 1986;293:1243.
397. Waeber B, Nussberger J, Brunner HR. Self poisoning with enalapril. *Br Med J* 1984;288:287–288.

Hypertension: Pathophysiology, Diagnosis, and Management, edited by J. H. Laragh and B. M. Brenner. Raven Press, Ltd., New York © 1990.

CHAPTER 141

Alpha-Adrenoceptor-Blocking Agents in the Treatment of Hypertension

Peter A. van Zwieten

Chemical Structures, 2233
Mode of Action and Pharmacodynamic Properties, 2235
Classification and Function of α-Adrenoceptors, 2235
Role of α-Adrenoceptors in Hypertensive Disease, 2237
Vasodilator and Hypotensive Activity of α-Adrenoceptor Blockers, 2237
α-Adrenoceptor-Blocking Agents with Additional Pharmacological Properties, 2239
Hemodynamic Properties of α-Adrenoceptor-Blocking Agents, 2240
Pharmacokinetics and Biotransformation, 2241
Therapeutic Application of α-Adrenoceptor Antagonists in Hypertension, 2242
Efficacy and Dosage, 2242
Side Effects and Toxicity, 2244
Contraindications, 2245
Drug Interactions and Combinations with Other Drugs, 2245
Interactions, 2245
Combinations with Other Drugs, 2245
Treatment of Elderly Hypertensives with α-Adrenoceptor Antagonists, 2246
References, 2247

Because elevated total peripheral resistance is the most consistent hemodynamic change observed in established hypertension, the application of arterial vasodilators seems to be a logical approach to treat this disorder. Moreover, since α-adrenoceptor antagonists are potent arterial (in particular, arteriolar) vasodilators, it is not surprising that these drugs have been investigated as potential antihypertensives.

However, classical α-adrenoceptor antagonists, such as phentolamine, phenoxybenzamine, tolazoline, and hydrogenated ergot alkaloids, have not proved to be useful in the long-term control of blood pressure in hypertensive patients. Reflex tachycardia, fluid and sodium retention, and difficulties in dosage adjustment have limited the occasional use of these agents, particularly phentolamine, to the preoperative preparation of patients with pheochromocytoma.

More recently, phentolamine has been studied as an experimental "unloading drug" in patients with congestive heart failure (1,2).

Indoramin has been studied as a potential antihypertensive drug and shown to be effective, although its adverse reactions proved to be considerable (3,4). At present, it cannot be judged whether or not indoramin is likely to become a currently applied antihypertensive drug.

A key development in the history of α-adrenoceptor blockers was the discovery of prazosin, the first selective α_1-adrenoceptor-blocking agent. Apart from being an interesting pharmacological tool, this compound was the first α-adrenoceptor blocker that could successfully be applied in the treatment of hypertension. One of the major advantages of prazosin over the classical nonselective α-blockers is the virtual absence of reflex tachycardia. The same appears to hold for the various successor drugs to prazosin, which are also selective α_1-adrenoceptor-blocking agents. For these reasons, the emphasis in this chapter shall be placed upon prazosin and closely related drugs. Some attention shall also be paid to drugs that display additional pharmacological activities besides their α_1-blocking potency, such as urapidil, labetalol, and ketanserin.

CHEMICAL STRUCTURES

Figures 1 and 2 show the chemical structures of those α-adrenoceptor-blocking agents which are clinically relevant or of some historical interest. Phentolamine is an imidazoline derivative, and attempts have been made to relate its activity to clonidine, a centrally acting hypotensive drug with an imidazolidine structure. Indoramine, a compound

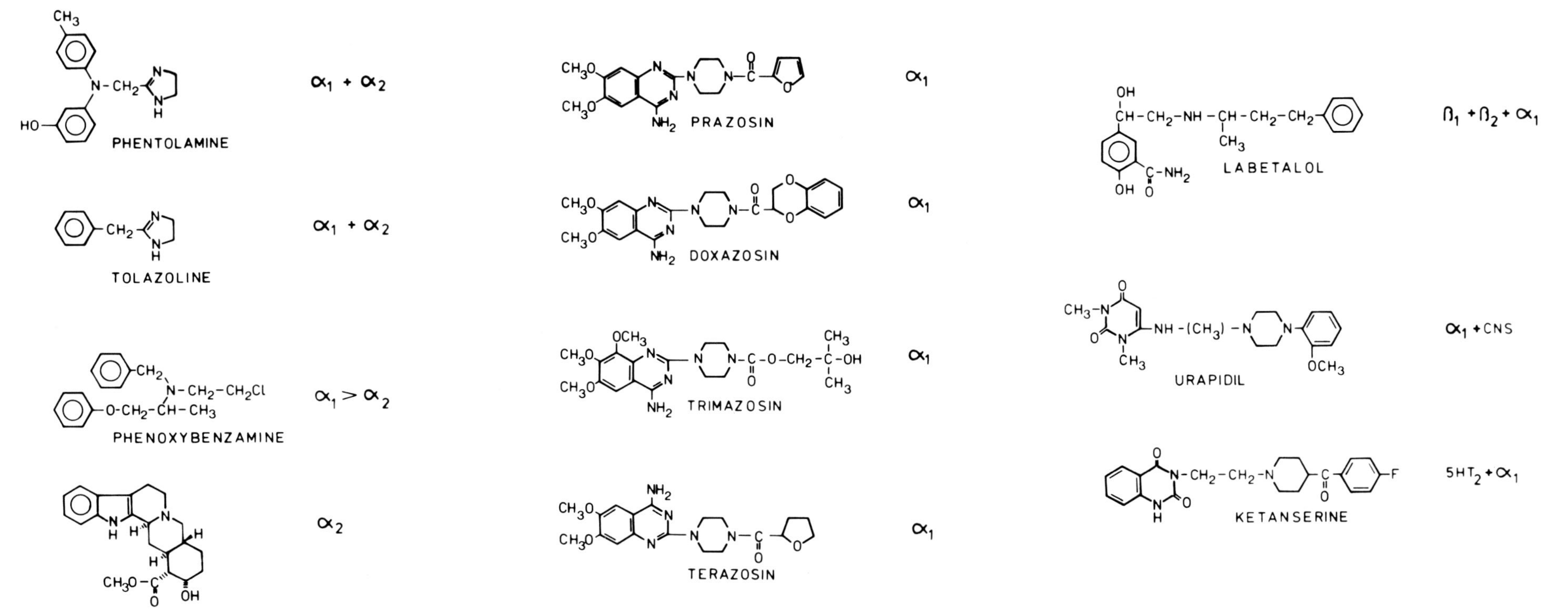

FIG. 1. Chemical structures of nonselective ($\alpha_1 + \alpha_2$)-adrenoceptor antagonists (**left**) and selective α_1-blockers (**center**). Urapidil, ketanserin, and labetalol (**right**) are selective blockers of α_1-adrenoceptors, but they possess additional pharmacological activities not related to α-adrenoceptors.

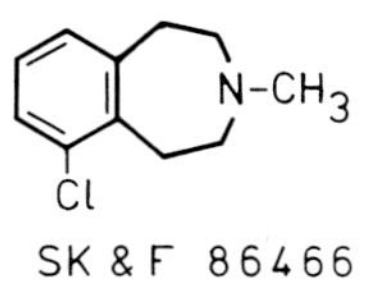

FIG. 2. Chemical structure of 6-chloro-*N*-methyl-2,3,4,5-tetrahydro-1*H*-3-benzazepine (SK&F 86466), a selective α_2-adrenoceptor antagonist with hypotensive potency in animal experiments. (From ref. 6.)

with miscellaneous activities, contains an indole moiety. Phenoxybenzamine is a phenylethylamine derivative and is thus chemically somehow related to the endogenous catecholamines noradrenaline and adrenaline. The prazosin molecule was deliberately designed as a compound with some resemblance to papaverine and to the aminopyrimidine moiety of cyclic AMP and cyclic GMP, with the intention to obtain a molecule with direct dilator activity on vascular smooth muscle. However, prazosin causes direct vasodilatation only at dosage levels which are well beyond those currently used in the treatment of hypertension (5).

Furthermore, the inhibition of phosphodiesterase by prazosin, an activity which can be well imagined for such a chemical structure, also occurs only at much higher doses than those applied therapeutically.

It should be realized, as will be discussed in more detail in the section entitled "Vasodilator and Hypotensive Activity of α-Adrenoceptor Blockers," that the vasodilator activity of prazosin which underlies its application as an antihypertensive is fully and satisfactorily explained by the blockade of postsynaptic α_1-adrenoceptors in the arterioles.

Doxazosin, trimazosin, and terazosin are the successor drugs to prazosin and, as such, are also selective antagonists of postsynaptic α_1-adrenoceptors. They show a close chemical resemblance to prazosin. Piperazino substitution at position 2 and 6,7-dimethoxy substitution in the aromatic ring proved to be requirements for optimal antihypertensive activity. As obvious from the structures of the successor drugs doxazosin, trimazosin, and terazosin, further substitution at the piperazino moiety can be largely varied without losing antihypertensive activity. In prazosin, this substituent is a furan moiety; in the closely related terazosin, however, this is a tetrahydrofuran nucleus. In the doxazosin molecule, this substituent consists of a benzdioxan moiety; in trimazosin, however, it is an ester with a hydroxy-substituent tertiary $-CH_2-C(CH_3)_2$ moiety. Concerning the α_1-adrenoceptor drugs with ancillary activities, to be discussed in more detail in the section entitled "α-Adrenoceptor-Blocking Agents with Additional Pharmacological Properties," urapidil appears to be chemically derived from uracil. It should be emphasized here that this molecule does not contain any stereoisomers, since no asymmetric carbon atoms are available. Labetalol, a combined α- and β-adrenoceptor blocker, is a derivative of salicylamide. The molecule contains a phenylalkyl moiety and also resembles the classical β-blocker structures found in propranolol and related drugs. As a result of having two asymmetric carbon atoms, the labetalol molecule contains four stereoisomers, with different pharmacological properties.

Ketanserin is a selective antagonist of $5HT_2$-receptors with additional, modest affinity for α_1-adrenoceptors. Its chemical structure is largely different from that of the various α-adrenoceptor blockers discussed in this chapter.

α_2-Adrenoceptor blocking agents have been of use as tools in pharmacological studies only. Yohimbine, rauwolscine, and idazoxan are the prototypes of more or less selective α_2-adrenoceptor antagonists. Yohimbine and rauwolscine are diasteromeric Rauwolfia alkaloids. The experimental compound SK&F 86466, which is also a selective α_2-adrenoceptor blocking agent, has been shown to lower blood pressure in some animal models of hypertension (6) and may be studied in humans as well. The structures of the α_2-adrenoceptor-blocking agents are shown in Figs. 1 and 2.

In general, it should be noted that a relationship between chemical structure and pharmacological activity can hardly be recognized for the α-adrenoceptor blocking agents so far developed; however, within certain subgroups (e.g., the prazosin-related drugs), such relationships appear to exist. This lack of structure–activity relationship (SAR) in α-adrenoceptor blockers clearly contrasts with that for the β-adrenoceptor-blocking drugs, where a SAR is easily detectable and adheres to quantitative criteria.

MODE OF ACTION AND PHARMACODYNAMIC PROPERTIES

The majority of mechanistic studies has been performed with the selective α_1-adrenoceptor antagonist prazosin. There is no doubt that the vasodilator and hypotensive activity of this compound and its successor drugs is predominantly based upon the blockade of α_1-adrenoceptors at postjunctional sites in the precapillary arterioles (resistance vessels) of the peripheral circulation. For those reasons, the discussion of the mode of action of α-blockers shall be focused upon α-adrenoceptors in general and upon prazosin as the best known example of an α-adrenoceptor-blocking agent.

Classification and Function of α-Adrenoceptors

α-Adrenoceptors are generally recognized to be a vital component of the transmission process in the synapses of the sympathetic nervous system. Their molecular, physiological, pathophysiological, and pharmacological aspects have been studied extensively over the past decade. The classification of α-adrenoceptors has been a matter of confusion and debate for several years. Fortunately, the availability of selective agonists and antagonists for the various α-adrenoceptor subtypes has led to a widely accepted and logical classification, which shall be briefly summarized here.

α-Adrenoceptors can be divided into the α_1- and α_2-subtypes (7–9). This subclassification is based on the affinity of selective agonists and antagonists for these two subtypes, whereas the subdivision into presynaptic and postsynaptic (prejunctional and postjunctional) α-adrenoceptors defines the localization with respect to the synapse (Fig. 3). Pre-

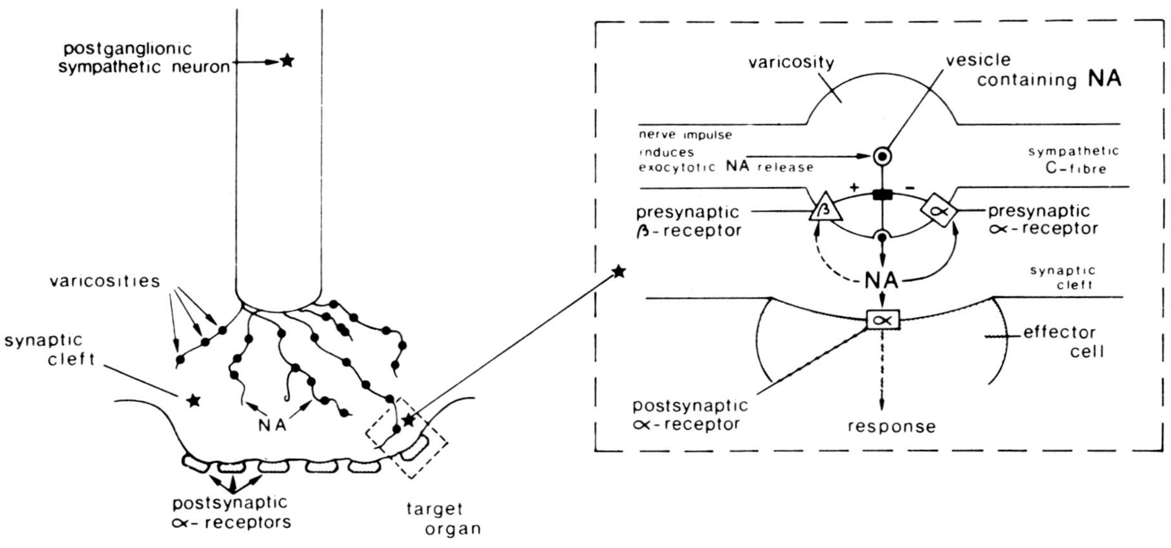

FIG. 3. Adrenergic synapse. Nerve activity releases the endogenous neurotransmitter noradrenaline (NA) and adrenaline from the varicosities. Noradrenaline and adrenaline reach the postsynaptic α- or β-adrenoceptors on the cell membrane of the target organ by diffusion. Upon receptor stimulation, a physiologic or pharmacologic effect is initiated. At postsynaptic sites, both α_1- and α_2-adrenoceptors are present. Their stimulation in blood vessels causes vasoconstriction. At presynaptic sites, predominantly α_2-adrenoceptors occur. Their stimulation causes a reduction of the noradrenaline release from the nerve ending. Noradrenaline release from presynaptic sites is enhanced when prejunctional α_2-adrenoceptors are blocked by selective α_2-adrenoceptor-blocking agents or by nonselective (α_1 + α_2)-adrenoceptor antagonists.

synaptic receptors are located on the sympathetic nerve ending and postsynaptic receptors on the target organ, such as a blood vessel (10–12). Noradrenaline and adrenaline are nonselective agonists; that is, they stimulate α_1- and α_2-adrenoceptors equally well. Similarly, classic α-adrenoceptor blockers, such as phentolamine and phenoxybenzamine, are nonselective compounds that antagonize both α_1- and α_2-adrenoceptors. At present we have a variety of agonists and antagonists at our disposal that are selective for either of the two receptor subtypes (Table 1). These

TABLE 1. *α-Adrenoceptor agonists and antagonists; characterization with respect to their selectivity for α_1- and α_2-adrenoceptors; possible therapeutic applications*

Agents	Receptor stimulated or blocked	Application
Agonists		
Noradrenaline (neurotransmitter)	$\alpha_1 + \alpha_2 + \beta_1$	Vasoconstrictor ($\alpha_1 + \alpha_2$)
Adrenaline	$\alpha_1 + \alpha_2 + \beta_1 + \beta_2$	Vasoconstrictor ($\alpha_1 + \alpha_2$)
Phenylephrine	$\alpha_1 > \alpha_2$	Vasoconstrictor (α_1), decongestant (α_1)
Cirazoline	α_1	Vasoconstrictor
Methoxamine	α_1	Vasoconstrictor
Clonidine	$\alpha_2 + \alpha_1$	Antihypertensive (central α_2)
Guanfacine	$\alpha_2 > \alpha_1$	Antihypertensive (central α_2)
Azepexole (B-HT 933)	α_2	Experimental antihypertensive (central α_2)
B-HT 920	α_2 + DA	Experimental
UK-14,304	α_2	Experimental
Antagonists		
Phentolamine (Regitine)	$\alpha_1 + \alpha_2$	Pheochromocytoma preoperative phase ($\alpha_1 + \alpha_2$)
Tolazoline	$\alpha_2 > \alpha_1$	Vasodilator ($\alpha_1 + \alpha_2$)
Prazosin (Minipress)	α_1	Antihypertensive (peripheral α_1)
Doxazosin	α_1	Antihypertensive (peripheral α_1)
Terazosin	α_1	Antihypertensive (peripheral α_1)
Trimazosin	α_1	Antihypertensive (peripheral α_1)
Corynanthine } Diastereoisomers	α_1	Experimental
Rauwolscine } Diastereoisomers	α_1	Experimental
Yohimbine } Diastereoisomers	α_2	Experimental
Idazoxan	α_2	Experimental
SK&F 86466	α_2	Experimental

selective compounds are useful tools in experimental pharmacology, but some of them (e.g., the selective blocker of the α_1-adrenoceptor prazosin) have become valuable drugs in the treatment of hypertension and, more recently, of congestive heart failure.

Presynaptic α-adrenoceptors are almost exclusively of the α_2-subtype, judged by their affinity for selective α_2-receptor agonists and antagonists. However, both α_1- and α_2-adrenoceptors occur in comparable numbers at postsynaptic sites. Stimulation of presynaptic α_2-adrenoceptors reduces the release of endogenous noradrenaline from the nerve ending. Stimulation of vascular postsynaptic α_1- and α_2-adrenoceptors by their respective agonists causes vasoconstriction (11–13).

α-Adrenoceptors of both subtypes are found in a variety of organs and tissues. We shall limit the discussion to those tissues in which the α-adrenoceptors are targets for antihypertensive drugs. Peripheral α_1- and α_2-adrenoceptors at postsynaptic sites are involved functionally in the constriction of precapillary arterioles (resistance vessels), which is brought about by the endogenous neurotransmitters noradrenaline and adrenaline. It seems likely that the postsynaptic α_2-adrenoceptors are not innervated; in other words, their location is extrasynaptic rather than intrasynaptic space. Accordingly, they may be considered as hormone receptors, reacting to circulating catecholamines rather than to the neurotransmitter (noradrenaline) that is released from presynaptic structures (13,14). The stimulation of both α_1- and α_2-adrenoceptors at postsynaptic sites by appropriate agonists causes vasoconstriction and a rise in blood pressure. Accordingly, the vasoconstriction caused by noradrenaline and adrenaline is an effect based upon both α_1- and α_2-adrenoceptor stimulation. The concept of the postsynaptic α_2-adrenoceptor is rather new, and it has considerably changed our views of the distribution and functional role of α-adrenoceptors. Recent experiments by our own group have demonstrated that postsynaptic α_2-adrenoceptors probably play an important role in maintaining vascular tone in human resistance vessels (15,16).

The modulation of noradrenaline release from presynaptic sites by presynaptic α_2-adrenoceptors may be involved in physiologic regulation, particularly blood pressure and heart rate. α_2-Adrenoceptors have been found in the heart, both at presynaptic and postsynaptic sites. Their functional role in regulating the circulation has remained unclear; however, presynaptic α_2-receptors may play a part in bradycardia induced by clonidine and related drugs (17,18). Accordingly, the role of these receptors in physiologic processes that regulate heart rate by the sympathetic nervous system is speculative.

In the central nervous system, α-adrenoceptors are located in the brain stem—more specifically, the nucleus tractus solitarii, the vasomotor center, and the nucleus of the vagal nerve. The region of the nucleus tractus solitarii contains a particularly high density of (nor)adrenergic synapses, suggesting a functional role of α-adrenoceptors. These receptors are mainly of the α_2-subtype, although the presence of α_1-adrenoceptors has been demonstrated by receptor-binding techniques.

The stimulation of central α_2-adrenoceptors by appropriate agonists induces a reduction of peripheral sympathetic tone. Arterial blood pressure and heart rate fall via the stimulation of an inhibitory neuron—probably the bulbospinal neuron. The stimulation of central α_2-adrenoceptors also induces an enhanced vagal tone, thus contributing to bradycardia. It seems likely that the central α_2-adrenoceptors are functionally involved in regulating blood pressure and heart rate. For reviews on central α-adrenoceptors and their involvement in blood pressure regulation and as targets of centrally acting antihypertensive drugs, see refs. 19–22.

Role of α-Adrenoceptors in Hypertensive Disease

To date, a clear and consistent picture regarding the characteristics and density of α-adrenoceptors in human hypertensive disease has not emerged. This limitation is explained so far by methodological shortcomings, which hardly allows investigation of α-adrenoceptors in vascular smooth muscle, with virtually all studies being limited to α_2-adrenoceptors on *ex vivo* thrombocytes.

Conflicting results have been reported with respect to the α_2-receptor density in thrombocytes of hypertensives.

Brodde et al. (23,24) have repeatedly found significantly increased densities of α_2-adrenoceptors in thrombocytes of hypertensives, as compared with those obtained from age- and sex-matched normotensive subjects. Jones et al. (25), however, found a lower α_2-adrenoceptor density in platelets from hypertensives, whereas Motulsky et al. (26) found no difference at all. A hyperreactivity to pressor stimuli has been reported repeatedly in hypertensive patients (27–29). In hypertensive subjects the hyperreactivity already described for the systemic circulation was also found in the vascular bed of the human forearm (15,30,31). Again, the hyperreactivity was a general phenomenon for both α_1- and α_2-adrenoceptor-mediated vasoconstriction, as well as for both adrenaline and noradrenaline. These findings cast doubt upon the specificity of the hyperreactivity phenomenon encountered in hypertensive subjects. For a review of this subject, see ref. 32.

Whether highly specific or not, the hyperreactivity to vasoconstrictor stimuli in hypertensives appears to be a logical basis for drug treatment with α-adrenoceptor antagonists and other vasodilators that will lower total peripheral resistance, which is consistently elevated in established hypertensive disease.

Vasodilator and Hypotensive Activity of α-Adrenoceptor Blockers

The vasodilator and hypotensive activity of α-adrenoceptor-blocking agents is fully explained on the basis of competitive interaction at the level of postsynaptic α-adrenoceptors in the resistance vessels of the peripheral circulation. The occupation of these receptors by the α-adrenoceptors antagonists prevents the access to, and the stimulation of, the receptors by the endogenous agonists noradrenaline and adrenaline. Nonselective α_1- and α_2-adrenoceptor antagonists such as phentolamine cause vasodilatation that is based upon blockade of both α_1- and

α_2-adrenoceptors. The application of such drugs is accompanied by marked reflex tachycardia, which is triggered by the baroreceptor reflex system and the autonomic nervous system. Owing to presynaptic α_2-receptor blockade, treatment with phentolamine is accompanied by enhanced release of catecholamines from the nerve endings. Probably as a result of reflex sympathetic activation, phentolamine treatment induces the stimulation of the renin–angiotensin–aldosterone system, accompanied by an increase in plasma renin activity, thereby causing the retention of sodium and water. The reflex tachycardia is a serious drawback in the use of nonselective (α_1 + α_2)-adrenoceptor-blocking agents as antihypertensives.

The introduction of the selective α_1-adrenoceptor-blocking agent prazosin as an antihypertensive offered much better possibilities for antihypertensive treatment, since reflex tachycardia was virtually absent. According to Constantine et al. (33), prazosin does not cause reflex tachycardia in conscious dogs, although weak reflex tachycardia in rats has been described (34,35). Several authors have reported that in hypertensive patients continuously treated with prazosin, no substantial reflex tachycardia is observed in the steady state (for reviews, see refs. 34,36, and 37).

The absence of a marked reflex stimulation of the heart cannot be explained in detail. A partial explanation is offered by the absence of noradrenaline release via a presynaptic (α_2) mechanism. α_1-Adrenoceptors are found almost exclusively at postjunctional sites; prejunctional α-receptors are predominantly of the α_2-subtype. For this reason, it would be expected that prazosin should not significantly interfere with the release of endogenous noradrenaline mediated by presynaptic α_2-adrenoceptors. It has indeed been observed by various investigators that prazosin does not enhance the release of noradrenaline from sympathetic nerve endings, whereas classical, nonselective blockers of α_1- and α_2-adrenoceptors do stimulate the liberation of noradrenaline via a presynaptic mechanism.

The lack of a pronounced reflex tachycardia following prazosin treatment may be the result of reduced baroreceptor modulation, since it has been found that prazosin depresses baroreflex function in cats (38), dogs (39), and man (40). However, such an effect could not be established for prazosin in rabbits (41). On the other hand, prazosin (and indoramin) reduced the number of sympathetic nerve discharges in cats (42) and rats (43). Furthermore, no increase in plasma dopamine-β-hydroxylase activity accompanied the fall in blood pressure caused by prazosin in humans, nor is an increase in plasma noradrenaline levels found following administration of prazosin in conscious dogs (44). Finally, prazosin has very little influence on plasma renin, the levels of which are usually unchanged or occasionally somewhat reduced (36,37,45). Nevertheless, some retention of sodium and water may occur, although less than that observed after treatment with directly acting vasodilators or phentolamine.

A second mechanism which may help to explain the lack of reflex tachycardia during prazosin treatment is the blockade of central α_1-adrenoceptors. It has been demonstrated by Huchet et al. (46) that the blockade of central α_1-adrenoceptors (e.g., by prazosin) modulates the baroreceptor reflex mechanism and thus counteracts the reflex tachycardia evoked by prazosin-induced vasodilatation. For a schematic presentation of this mechanism, see Fig. 4. At present, there is general agreement that the reversible blockade of vascular postsynaptic α_1-adrenoceptors is the underlying cause of the vasodilator and hypotensive effects of prazosin.

Various other mechanisms involved in the hypotensive effect can be excluded. Prazosin does not interfere with transmission in peripheral sympathetic ganglia or neurons (47). It does not clearly display acute central hypotensive activity (47–49), although blockade of central α_1-adrenoceptors in rat brain has been demonstrated by studies of radioligand binding. It has been reported by only one group that α_1-adrenoceptor antagonists such as prazosin can reduce blood pressure (and heart rate) in animals, not only via blockade of vascular α_1-adrenoceptors but also as a result of a centrally mediated decrease in sympathetic tone (43).

Central α_2-adrenoceptor stimulation decreases sympathetic nervous activity and increases vagal tone. Conversely, it has recently been suggested that activation of central α_1-adrenoceptors increases sympathetic tone and reduces vagal activity (46).

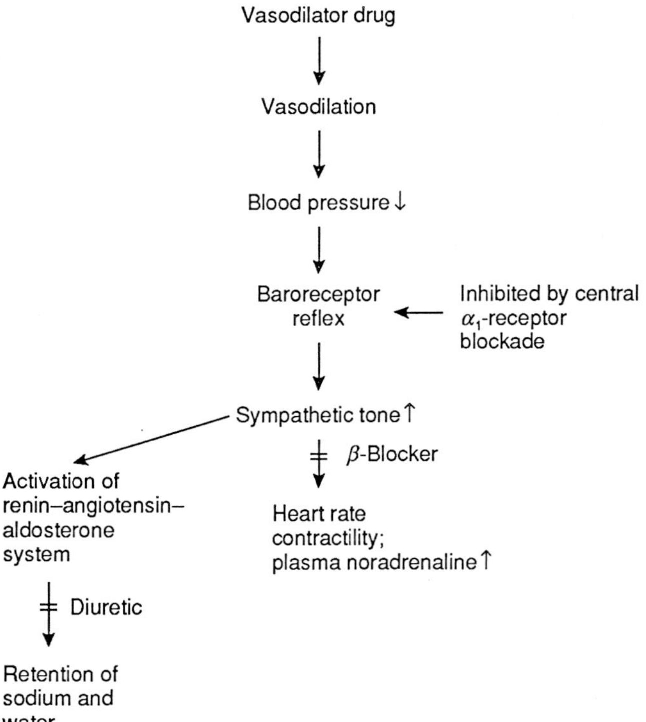

FIG. 4. Reflex activity, elicited by vasodilator drugs and mediated by the baroreceptor mechanism and the sympathetic nervous system. Enhanced sympathetic activity caused elevated plasma noradrenaline levels, a rise in heart rate and contractility, and also the activation of the renin–angiotensin–aldosterone system, thus giving rise to the retention of sodium and water. The rise in heart rate can be counteracted with a β-blocker; the retention of sodium and water can be counteracted by a diuretic. Blockade of central α_1-adrenoceptors by selective α_1-adrenoceptor antagonists modulates the baroreceptor reflex mechanism and hence suppresses reflex tachycardia.

Inhibition of phosphodiesterase by prazosin, as well as a direct vasodilator action, has been ruled out to play a role in therapeutic doses of the drug (36). Prazosin does not decrease cardiac output (47). The hypotensive effect of prazosin is due solely to a decrease in total peripheral resistance, reflecting dilatation of the precapillary arterioles as a result of the blockade of vascular α_1-adrenoceptors.

The selectivity of prazosin for α_1-adrenoceptors has been demonstrated in isolated perfused rabbit pulmonary artery (38), in the perfused cat spleen, and in rat brain slices, as well as in other *in vivo* and *in vitro* preparations (50,51). Studies on receptor binding using prazosin as the displacing drug (52) or as a tritiated ligand (53–56) have confirmed its marked affinity and selectivity for α_1-adrenoceptors.

The successor drugs to prazosin—namely, trimazosin, doxazosin, and terazosin—appear to have the same mode of action as prazosin, as far as can be judged at present.

Trimazosin is somewhat less selective for α_1-adrenoceptors than is prazosin (57,58); in contrast to prazosin, trimazosin shows weak direct vasodilator activity (59). It seems very likely that trimazosin, like prazosin, induces a hypotensive/antihypertensive effect and causes a reduction in total peripheral resistance, predominantly as a result of vascular postsynaptic α_1-adrenoceptor blockade. Since α_1-blockade by trimazosin is somewhat weaker than that caused by prazosin, it has been suggested that other mechanisms, possibly direct vasodilator activity, may contribute to the drugs' hypotensive effect (60). The possibility should also be considered that trimazosin's active metabolite (CP 23445) displays hypotensive activity as a result of direct vasodilator potency. Trimazosin does not significantly influence heart rate, probably for the same reason as discussed for prazosin (see above). Like prazosin, trimazosin causes the dilatation of both resistance and capacitance vessels (61).

Doxazosin is also a selective α_1-adrenoceptor-blocking agent in animal preparations (51,62) and in humans (63–65). Doxazosin has a somewhat lower potency as an α_1-antagonist than does prazosin (66), Doxazosin, probably for similar reasons as discussed for prazosin, does not cause relevant reflex tachycardia. Concomitantly, the mode of action of doxazosin appears to be the same as that of prazosin, but doxazosin has a longer duration of action.

Terazosin displays the same degree of selectivity for α_1-adrenoceptors as does prazosin; however, on a molar basis, terazosin's potency is threefold lower (67,68). It should be assumed, therefore, that terazosin's mode of hypotensive action is the same as that of prazosin. Terazosin has a longer duration of action than does prazosin and is more hydrophilic. As for prazosin, doxazosin, and trimazosin, virtually no reflex tachycardia is observed during treatment with terazosin (69).

α-ADRENOCEPTOR-BLOCKING AGENTS WITH ADDITIONAL PHARMACOLOGICAL PROPERTIES

Urapidil is a selective α_1-adrenoceptor antagonist with an additional central hypotensive action, which is not fully understood. On a molar basis, urapidil is less potent as an α_1-blocker than is prazosin, and urapidil is also somewhat less selective. A modest affinity of urapidil for β_1-adrenoceptors was found in both radioligand-binding and functional studies with isolated organs. However, this β_1-adrenoceptor-blocking activity does not play a role in the antihypertensive activity of urapidil in humans. In older studies, urapidil had been claimed to possess a presynaptic α_2-adrenoceptor-agonistic effect, but this could not be confirmed by several authors. Since urapidil has very little affinity for α_2-adrenoceptors, as concluded from radioligand-binding studies, a relevant presynaptic α_2-effect can hardly be expected.

Apart from its manifest α_1-adrenoceptor-blocking activity, urapidil shows central hypotensive activity in several animal models—for instance, after injection into cerebral ventricles or into the vertebral artery (Fig. 5). Although difficult to demonstrate in patients, the central mechanism can be expected to contribute to the drug's blood-pressure-lowering effect. In contrast to classical centrally acting drugs such as clonidine, guanfacine, and α-methyldopa, the central effect of urapidil is not mediated by central α_2-adrenoceptors. It has been speculated recently that the central hypotensive activity of urapidil might be mediated by $5HT_{1A}$-receptors in the central nervous system. This view, which is only based upon a certain affinity of urapidil for $5HT_{1A}$-receptors in radioligand-binding studies, has hardly been substantiated by conclusive pharmacological experiments so far. For reviews, see refs. 70–72.

In conclusion, urapidil should be considered a moderately selective α_1-adrenoceptor antagonist with an additional central hypotensive mechanism, which, unlike clonidine, does not involve central α_2-adrenoceptors. Urapidil's various pharmacological activities are shown schematically in Fig. 6.

Labetalol is a nonselective ($\beta_1 + \beta_2$)-adrenoceptor-blocking agent with rather modest α_1-adrenoceptor-antagonistic activity, which usually weakens after a few months of continuous antihypertensive treatment. As such, labetalol should be considered as a β-blocker rather than as an α-adrenoceptor-blocking agent—in particular, upon prolonged application. During the initial period of treatment, the vasodilatation, caused by labetalol's α_1-adrenoceptor-blocking activity, gradually wanes and fully disappears after a few months. Furthermore, it should be realized that labetalol is not a uniform compound but, instead, a mixture of four stereoisomers. Two of these isomers are biologically inactive, whereas the α_1- and ($\beta_1 + \beta_2$)-adrenoceptor-antagonistic activity is contained separately in the two other isomers. As such, labetalol is not a true hybrid compound, since its various properties are not concentrated in one and the same molecule. For reviews on labetalol, see refs. 73 and 74.

Ketanserin, a novel antihypertensive agent, is a selective and potent antagonist of serotonergic receptors of the $5HT_2$-type and is simultaneously a moderately active α_1-adrenoceptor-blocking agent (75). Ketanserin's antihypertensive potency, associated with vasodilatation and a reduction of total peripheral resistance, is not fully understood at the mechanistic/receptor level. It is difficult to explain its vasodilator activity solely on the basis of $5HT_2$-receptor blockade in the peripheral circulation, since

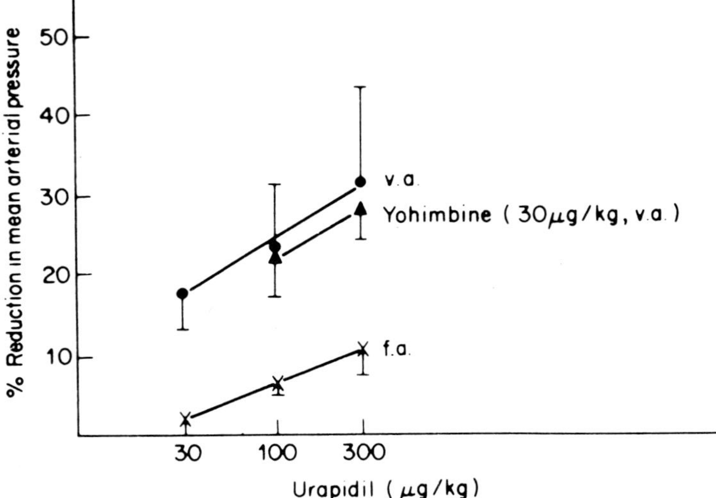

FIG. 5. Demonstration of the central hypotensive activity of urapidil. After infusion into the left vertebral artery, thereby inducing perfusion of the brain stem with the drug, the hypotensive effect is much stronger than after systemic administration via a femoral artery. The central hypotensive effect of urapidil is not reduced by prior treatment with the α_2-adrenoceptor antagonist yohimbine. Shown are the dose–response curves for the reduction in mean arterial pressure of chloralose-anesthetized cats by urapidil after infusion via the vertebral artery (v.a.) or via the femoral artery (f.a.) and after infusion via the vertebral artery 15 min after v.a. infusion of yohimbine (30 μg/kg). Symbols represent mean values $\pm$ SEM (n = 4–5). $p < 0.05$. (Data from ref. 72.)

a few other $5HT_2$-antagonists, which are devoid of α_1-adrenoceptor-antagonistic activity (e.g., ritanserin and LY 53857), do not lower blood pressure (76). On the other hand, the α_1-adrenoceptor-antagonistic activity of ketanserin is probably too weak to adequately explain its vasodilator potency, especially when compared with the pharmacodynamic profile of the standard α_1-blocker prazosin. It

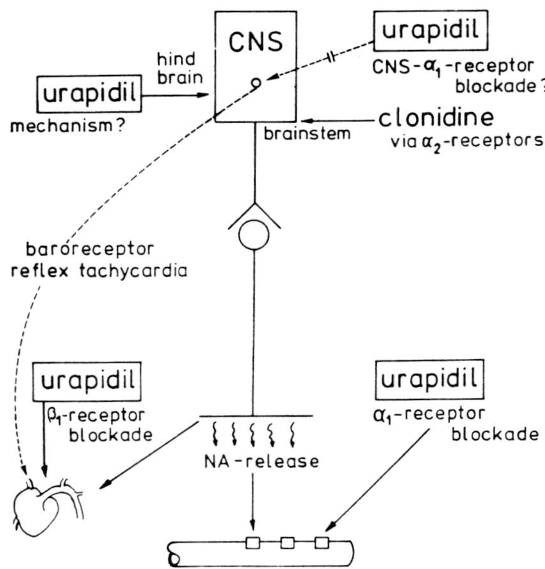

FIG. 6. Schematic representation of the mechanisms underlying the hemodynamic changes induced by urapidil. First, blockade of vascular postsynaptic α_1-adrenoceptors causes dilatation of the precapillary arterioles, a reduction in total peripheral resistance, and hence a fall in blood pressure. Second, a central hypotensive effect with a presently unknown mechanism is initiated, probably at the level of the hindbrain. Accordingly, peripheral sympathetic tone is reduced, causing vasodilatation. Third, the baroreflex-receptor-mediated tachycardia is blunted, probably at a central level, possibly involving blockade of central α_1-adrenoceptors. Fourth, urapidil shows modest antagonistic activity on cardiac β_1-adrenoceptors. This mechanism may offer a moderate contribution to hypotensive activity and to the impairment of reflex tachycardia.

has been speculated that there might be a mutual interaction between $5HT_2$- and α_1-receptors, in the sense of an amplification upon stimulation; conversely, there might be an enhanced vasodilatation as a result of simultaneous blockade by the combined antagonist ketanserin ($5HT_2$ + α_1) (77). So far, this issue remains unsettled, with insufficient experimental data being available to either support or discard it.

More recently, a central hypotensive effect of ketanserin has been reported, but this activity is probably insufficient to explain all of the antihypertensive potency of the drug (78).

In conclusion, the mode of action of ketanserin as a vasodilator and antihypertensive drug remains unclear. It has become more and more likely that the selective blockade of $5HT_2$-receptors in the peripheral circulation is not a general mechanism or principle causing vasodilatation and hypotension. For a recent review on ketanserin, see ref. 79.

HEMODYNAMIC PROPERTIES OF α-ADRENOCEPTOR-BLOCKING AGENTS

α-Adrenoceptor of both subtypes (α_1 and α_2) are known to be present in relevant densities in both arteries and veins. Accordingly, α-adrenoceptor-blocking agents should be expected to cause α-adrenoceptor blockade in both vascular beds. Indeed, dilatation is observed in both the resistance and the capacitance vessels upon systemic application of either nonselective blockers or α-selective adrenoceptor antagonistic drugs. The pronounced venous dilatation is understandable in view of the particular dependence of the veins on sympathetic stimulation (80,81). The dilatation of resistance vessels explains the hypotensive/antihypertensive effect of these drugs, whereas venodilatation is probably the reason for the well-known side effect known as *postural hypotension.* As already discussed in the section entitled "Mode of Action and Pharmacodynamic Properties," the nonselective (α_1 + α_2)-blockers (e.g., phentolamine) cause severe reflex tachycardia, mediated by the baroreceptor reflex mechanism and the autonomic nervous system. Fluid retention, a common adverse reaction to virtually all vasodilator drugs, is also a common observation during treatment with nonselective ($\alpha_1 + \alpha_2$)- and selective α_1-adrenoceptor blockers. Reflex tachycardia and fluid retention are satisfactorily explained by the activation of the sympathetic nervous system and the renin–angiotensin–aldosterone system, although this activation appears to be much less pronounced upon application of the selective α_1-blockers. The hemodynamic profile of the selective α_1-adrenoceptor blockers, of which prazosin and its successor drugs are the current examples, may be summarized as follows:

1. Prazosin and related drugs cause a reduction in total peripheral resistance and a fall in blood pressure as a result of dilatation of the precapillary arterioles (resistance vessels). Simultaneously, venodilatation occurs, owing to the blockade of α_1-adrenoceptors in the venous vascular bed. This effect is probably the background of the well-known side effect known as *orthostatic hypotension,* as reflected by the "first-dose" effect of prazosin.
2. A dilator effect of prazosin on renal resistance vessels which is not associated with impairment of renal function has been described in hypertensive patients (82).
3. As discussed previously (see section entitled "Mode of Action and Pharmacodynamic Properties"), prazosin and related drugs cause little or no reflex tachycardia, although some fluid retention is indeed observed upon prolonged treatment and usually requires the combined application of a natriuretic drug.
4. The newer α_1-adrenoceptor-blocking drugs, such as doxazosin, trimasozin, and terazosin, display a hemodynamic profile which is very similar to that of prazosin.
5. It should be realized that the hemodynamic profile of α_1-blockers in hypertensive patients closely resembles that in normotensive volunteers. However, when used in patients with congestive heart failure, the hemodynamic changes induced by α_1-adrenoceptor-blocking agents are clearly different. For instance, it was shown that in patients with congestive heart failure, the α_1-adrenoceptor antagonist terazosin (83) significantly reduced left ventricular filling pressure and systemic vascular resistance while increasing both heart rate and cardiac index.

For review literature on the hemodynamic profile of the selective α_1-adrenoceptor-blocking agents, see refs. 36, 37, and 45.

Urapidil, when administered intravenously to hypertensives, displayed a hemodynamic profile very similar to that of prazosin and related drugs (84). Accordingly, the acute fall in arterial blood pressure was accompanied by an increase in systemic, renal, and splanchnic blood flow, as well as transient reflex tachycardia, as a result of sympathetic activation. In several patients treated with urapidil, orthostatic hypotension was observed, reflecting venous dilatation. This hemodynamic profile is virtually the same as that observed for intravenously administered prazosin (37,85). As in the case of prazosin, reflex tachycardia does not occur during prolonged treatment with urapidil. A detailed hemodynamic analysis of the long-term effects of urapidil has not yet been performed.

Since the α-adrenoceptor-antagonistic activity of both ketanserin and labetalol is rather weak and probably hardly relevant to their hypotensive effects in long-term treatment of hypertension, we shall not discuss their hemodynamic profile here.

PHARMACOKINETICS AND BIOTRANSFORMATION

We wish to emphasize the pharmacokinetics and metabolism of prazosin and its successor drugs, because these drugs are the most clinically relevant α-adrenoceptor-blocking agents.

The kinetic behavior of phenoxybenzamine and phentolamine will also be summarized briefly in the following sections.

Phenoxybenzamine

After oral administration, approximately 30% of the administered phenoxybenzamine is absorbed (86). Inactivation occurs both through biotransformation in the liver and by renal excretion. Phenoxybenzamine has a long duration of action, thus requiring a once-daily dosage schedule (86). It is known from clinical experience that a patient should be maintained on one particular dose for at least 3 days before this dose is increased.

Phentolamine

Phentolamine is characterized by rapid oral absorption and rapid development of its hypotensive action. The drug is predominantly and rapidly inactivated by biotransformation in the kidney; hence its duration of action is short, requiring a new dose every 4 hr when applied orally (87).

Prazosin

Approximately 60% of prazosin is readily absorbed following oral administration (34). The drug is subject to a substantial first-pass effect in the liver. Maximal plasma concentrations are achieved 1–2 hr after oral ingestion of the drug. Both in animals and in humans, prazosin is subject to extensive biotransformation in the liver. Mainly *O*-dealkylation and conjugation with glucuronic acid occur in humans, whereas 6-*O*-demethylprazosin is the main metabolite in dogs (88). Less than 1% of the unchanged drug is excreted via the kidney. As shown with ^{14}C-labeled prazosin, the drug and its metabolites are rapidly taken up by various tissues. The highest concentrations were found in the lungs, various blood vessels, and the heart, whereas the brain level remained rather low in spite of the lipophilic character of prazosin (88,89). The plasma half-life was found to be 1–2 hr in dogs (89), whereas a $t_{\frac{1}{2}}$ of almost 3 hr was found in humans (90). Following intravenous injection there is a correlation between plasma levels and hypotensive effect, but only in the early phase of treatment (90).

However, after oral ingestion the plasma half-life (3–4 hr) (91) is shorter than that of the therapeutic, hypotensive effect. In the steady state, approximately 97% of the drug is bound to plasma proteins, predominantly albumin.

Trimazosin

The bioavailability for oral trimazosin has been reported to be approximately 60%. The drug is extensively metabolized in the liver (57), and its major metabolite (CP 23445) in humans is an alkyl-hydroxylated derivative of the parent drug. According to Reid et al. (57), the pharmacokinetic profile of trimazosin is best described by a two-compartment model. The terminal half-life of trimazosin was found to be 2.73 ± 0.90 hr, and that of the metabolite (CP 23445) was found to be 1.47 ± 0.65 hr. After oral and intravenous administration, a similar plasma elimination half-life was found (57).

Doxazosin

Relatively few detailed pharmacokinetic data on doxazosin are available at present. In healthy normotensive subjects, the major pharmacokinetic difference between prazosin and doxazosin has been found in the elimination half-life, which for doxazosin was significantly longer (11 hr) (64) than for prazosin (2.5 hr) (92).

Terazosin

Upon oral administration, 90% of terazosin is reported to be absorbed (68,93), which is higher than that observed for prazosin (60%). Food appeared to have no significant influence on oral absorption. The maximal plasma concentration was achieved 1–2 hr after oral administration. A good correlation appeared to exist between administered dose and plasma concentration. Protein binding in plasma was found to be 90–94%. Terazosin is extensively metabolized in the liver, according to the following pathways (93):

1. Hydrolysis of the amide bond occurs, thereby yielding the free piperazine derivative.
2. Smaller portions of the drug are subject to *O*-demethylation and *N*-dealkylation, respectively, as well as to cleavage of the piperazine ring.

The biliary tract is a major route of excretion, as concluded from the observation that approximately 60% of the radioactive material is recovered from the feces of healthy volunteers who had received [^{14}C]terazosin by mouth. Approximately one-third of the drug was recovered in the unchanged form from both the feces and the urine after oral administration.

After either oral or intravenous administration, the half-life of plasma elimination has been reported in the range of 10–18 hr, with an average of 12 hr (93,94). Accordingly, the drug is eliminated more slowly than prazosin, thus allowing a once-daily dosage in the treatment of hypertension. Sonders et al. (93) demonstrated that the half-life of elimination of terazosin was significantly prolonged in subjects over 70 years of age as compared with subjects 39 years old. Hypertensive disease and congestive heart failure appear not to cause relevant changes in the kinetic behavior of the drug.

Urapidil

After oral administration to healthy volunteers, urapidil was reported to have an average bioavailability of 78%. A first-pass effect is assumed to occur. Peak concentrations in plasma were achieved 4–6 hr after ingestion of the currently used slow-release preparation (standard capsule) (95). The time course of the plasma concentration following an intravenous bolus injection could be described by means of a two-compartment model, with half-lives of 35 min and 2.7 hr, reflecting distribution and elimination, respectively. Approximately 80% of the drug appears to be protein bound. The half-life of elimination following oral administration was found to be 3.1 hr. Approximately 50–70% of the drug was eliminated via the renal route, consisting of 15% parent compound and 85% metabolites (for review, see ref. 95). In humans, *p*-hydroxylated urapidil appears to be the major metabolite (M_1). *O*-methylated (M_2) and *N*-demethylated (M_3) urapidil are also demonstrable but are quantitatively of less importance. M_1 appears to be biologically inactive, whereas M_2 may contribute to the drug's blood-pressure-lowering effect. M_2 has a longer half-life than does urapidil and may therefore become more important upon prolonged treatment. In the elderly, the enteral absorption was not different from that in younger adults. However, the half-life of elimination was clearly prolonged in older hypertensives, and it would seem useful to apply lower doses of urapidil in the treatment of the elderly.

THERAPEUTIC APPLICATION OF α-ADRENOCEPTOR ANTAGONISTS IN HYPERTENSION

Efficacy and Dosage

As stated previously, the older α-blockers such as *phentolamine* and *phenoxybenzamine* are only used in the preoperative phase of pheochromocytoma and during surgery. Reflex tachycardia is the main drawback in the use of these compounds in the prolonged treatment of essential hypertension. If reflex tachycardia is problematic when these older α-adrenoceptor antagonists are applied in the preoperative treatment of pheochromocytoma, this adverse reaction can be readily suppressed by the simultaneous application of a β-adrenoceptor-blocking agent. Phentolamine is given orally every 4 hr in 20-mg doses, depending on the effect achieved. Intravenous doses of 5–10 mg are given preoperatively, to be repeated if necessary during surgery.

Phenoxybenzamine treatment is started with 10-mg doses, which can be raised up to a maximum of 20–60 mg daily, in three doses. As an intravenous infusion, a dose of 0.5–1 mg/kg body weight is given over a 2-hr interval, 36 and 12 hr prior to the surgical intervention. *Prazosin's* efficacy in mild to severe hypertension has been demonstrated in numerous therapeutic trials, against placebo and in comparison with other drugs. Follow-up studies have shown continued efficacy after 2–5 years of treatment. Its efficacy as monotherapy has been shown, but prazosin is frequently combined with a diuretic or a β-blocker, or both.

Among the various studies described in the literature, we shall briefly discuss the following examples:

1. The study by Inouye et al. (96), where, in 14 patients with mild to moderate essential hypertension, it was demonstrated that prazosin (monotherapy) was as effective as hydrochlorothiazide or propranolol when given twice daily (1–10 mg) for 2 months.
2. The study by Scharf et al. (97) in 10 hypertensive patients without end-organ damage, where prazosin was given in titrated doses (1–20 mg).
3. The study by Neusy and Lowenstein (98), where the antihypertensive effect of prazosin was shown to persist after 12 months of treatment.
4. The two-center randomized trial by Stamler et al. (99), where prazosin and hydrochlorothiazide were shown to cause the same degree of blood pressure reduction (97 mmHg diastolic at baseline was reduced by 10.3 mmHg in the prazosin group and by 8.6 mmHg in the hydrochlorothiazide group).

The various trials where prazosin's efficacy was demonstrated have been reviewed (100,101). Comparative studies discussed in these reviews have shown prazosin to be as effective as α-methyldopa, clonidine, hydralazine, atenolol, indoramin, propranolol, labetalol, and captopril. Prazosin does not significantly change renal function and does not cause adverse effects on renal function in hypertensives with renal impairment. The virtual absence of reflex tachycardia was already discussed (see section entitled "Mode of Action and Pharmacodynamic Properties"). Orthostatic hypotension, probably caused by dilatation of the venous vascular bed, is the basis of the so-called first-dose effect. It can be largely avoided by starting the therapy with a very low dose of 0.5 mg, to be ingested at bed time and to be followed by a gradual build-up of the dosage schedule. The following dosage schedule is therefore recommended: The first dose should be 0.5 mg in the evening; subsequently, two to three 0.5-mg doses should be given in the daytime during the following 3 days. If necessary, depending upon the effect, the dosage can be elevated up to three 1-mg portions. A maintenance dose should subsequently be given, up to a maximum of 20 mg daily (thrice daily).

A certain efficacy of prazosin as an unloading drug in the treatment of congestive heart failure has been described, usually in trials with a rather small number of patients. Most of the trials are rather short, and one would like to see more prolonged periods of observation to be convinced of the drug's long-term efficacy in cardiac failure. For a survey of the results with prazosin in clinical trials in congestive heart failure, see refs. 36, 37, and 45. A few reports in the literature suggest that prazosin can be useful in the preoperative treatment of pheochromocytoma, but it seems advisable to combine it with a β-blocker in those particular cases (102).

Trimazosin

The dose-related antihypertensive effect of trimazosin has been demonstrated both in double-blind, placebo-controlled studies and in open studies. Initially a thrice-daily regimen was applied, but in a later stage it was shown that a twice-daily schedule of treatment gave rise to an 80% responder rate. Similarly, after an initial maximal dose range of 900 mg daily it is now recognized that in most cases a satisfactory response is obtained at a daily dose of 300 mg. The duration of action of trimazosin is thus obviously longer than that of prazosin, although pharmacokinetic data would suggest that trimazosin should preferably be administered thrice daily.

Since both trimazosin and its most important metabolite are pharmacologically active, the onset of action is slower than that of prazosin; moreover, the first-dose effect may also be expected to be milder than that of prazosin. Nevertheless, it would seem wise to titrate the dosage schedule of trimazosin as carefully as that of prazosin, until more clinical experience has been obtained with this newer drug.

No consensus has yet been reached concerning the dosage regimen of trimazosin. In mild to moderate essential hypertension the following schedule could be submitted: Begin with 50 mg two times daily, to be increased up to a maximum dosage of 300 mg daily, divided into two 150-mg portions each day. Further clinical studies are required to establish such a schedule more firmly. For reviews on the clinical application of trimazosin, see refs. 103 and 104.

Doxazosin

The selective α_1-adrenoceptor antagonist doxazosin has been demonstrated to be effective in antihypertensive treatment in several studies, both in double-blind and in open, multicenter trials (105–112). Hemodynamic and other relevant data of five studies have been pooled (112) and may be summarized as follows: Doxazosin treatment maintains blood pressure control in mild to moderate hypertensive patients, both at rest and during exercise, for a period of treatment up to 1 year. Doxazosin treatment lowers blood pressure more so than does placebo, and its efficacy appears to be comparable to that of β-blockers such as metoprolol or nadolol, although somewhat less than the effect caused by atenolol or the diuretic hydrochlorothiazide. Doxazosin's onset of action is slower than that of prazosin, and its duration of action is clearly longer, thus allowing a once-daily dosage schedule. As observed for prazosin, little or no change in heart rate occurs; however, data so far obtained suggest that doxazosin, in contrast to prazosin, does not cause postural hypotension. A limited number of data suggest that doxazosin may be effective as monotherapy. As far as can be judged at present, the most currently applied dosage schedule for doxazosin may be summarized as follows: The initial dosage should be 1 mg daily; if necessary, the dosage can be increased to 2 mg after 1 or 2 weeks. Thereafter, the dosage can be changed, at similar intervals, to 4 or possibly 8 mg daily. Most patients so far studied appear to respond adequately to a daily dose of 4 mg. The manufacturer proposes a maximum daily dose of 16 mg, but this is a rather high dose which is hardly substantiated by clinical data.

For recent review literature on doxazosin, see refs. 113 and 114.

Terazosin

Terazosin has been studied in double-blind trials against placebo or against prazosin in periods of 4–13 weeks, in doses of 1–40 mg daily given orally to patients with mild to moderate essential hypertension. Terazosin was significantly more effective than placebo in lowering blood pressure. In most cases, no increase in heart rate was observed. As monotherapy, administered at a dosage of up to 20 mg once daily, terazosin displayed an antihypertensive efficacy similar to that of prazosin administered in doses of up to 10 mg twice daily. Both drugs reduced supine mean systolic and diastolic blood pressures by 5–10 mmHg. In doses of up to 10 mg once daily, however, terazosin proved to be less effective than hydrochlorothiazide administered in doses of 25–50 mg twice daily. Drayer et al. (115) observed that terazosin produced a downward shift in the circadian pattern of blood pressure, confirming persistent antihypertensive effects for 24 hr.

The available data suggest that terazosin can be applied as monotherapy in doses of 10–20 mg once daily, although a twice-daily dose of terazosin appears to be well tolerated.

More clinical experience is required in order to establish terazosin's optimal dosage schedule and its final position in the management of essential hypertension. Terazosin might be anticipated to be of potential use in congestive heart failure. So far, beneficial effects were seen in small numbers of patients only. For extensive reviews of the therapeutic efficacy of terazosin in hypertension, see refs. 68 and 69.

Urapidil

Urapidil's efficacy has been demonstrated in several smaller and larger clinical trials, against placebo or against other drugs. Clinical trials, including multicenter studies, have been performed for periods up to 2 years and led to the conclusion that efficacy is maintained upon prolonged treatment. In most cases, sustained-release capsules of 30 mg have been used, which were usually given twice daily. The possibility to apply this capsule once daily is subject to investigation at present.

In smaller studies, it has been shown that urapidil given intravenously as a bolus injection may be used to manage a hypertensive emergency. In a few small studies, the impression has been obtained that urapidil may be beneficial as an unloading drug in the treatment of congestive heart failure.

For reviews on the clinical efficacy of urapidil, see refs. 70–72.

A discussion of the therapeutic efficacy of labetalol and ketanserin, which are not primarily α-blockers, lies beyond the scope of this chapter.

SIDE EFFECTS AND TOXICITY

Most adverse reactions to α-adrenoceptor antagonists can be extrapolated from their vasodilator and α-blocking potency. Hypotension, dizziness, headache, reflex tachycardia, congestion of the nasal mucosa, and impaired ejaculation are logical side effects of the α-blockers—in particular, of the nonselective α_1- and α_2-blockers.

The virtual absence of reflex tachycardia during treatment with *prazosin* and related α_1-selective drugs was already discussed in the section entitled "Mode of Action and Pharmacodynamic Properties." Postural hypotension, known as the *first-dose effect of prazosin,* is probably reflecting venous dilatation. This phenomenon can be prevented, in large part, by careful titration of the dosage.

Experience so far available suggests that the successor drugs to prazosin—in particular, doxazosin and terazosin—cause less postural hypotension than does prazosin, and it has been claimed that doxazosin would not display this problem at all (103,104,112,114). This difference with prazosin may be explained by the slower onset of the hypotensive effects of doxazosin and terazosin.

Another explanation, although speculative, might be that prazosin would have a relatively stronger influence on venous tone than would the newer drugs, but this presumption remains to be substantiated.

Apart from the difference with respect to orthostatic hypotension, it seems very likely that trimazosin, doxazosin, and terazosin display a pattern of side effects related to α_1-receptor blockade which is very similar to that of prazosin. For reviews, see refs. 36,45,68,69,103,104, and 112–114.

Sexual dysfunction owing to prazosin treatment is very rare, and the association with the drug is not convincingly established. For the newer drugs, no relevant data in this respect are available.

Renal and respiratory functions remain uninfluenced by prazosin and other selective α_1-adrenoceptor antagonists.

Prazosin has been reported to favorably influence the profile of plasma lipids during long-term treatment of hypertension, with a tendency to improve the ratio HDL/LDL + VLDL-cholesterol, in the sense of increasing HDL and reducing LDL + VLDL-cholesterol. In some (but not all) studies, prazosin was found to decrease plasma triglyceride levels. Most of the studies on the influence of prazosin on lipid levels have included a smaller number of patients and have not adequately controlled other factors influencing plasma lipids, such as diet and smoking habits. Studies with larger numbers of patients under carefully controlled conditions will be required in order to definitely establish the influence of prazosin on the lipid profile. The influence of prazosin on plasma lipids—which is complex and, in many ways, insufficiently established—has been advocated as a potentially favorable factor in the cardiovascular risk profile of hypertensives treated with this and similar drugs, but this issue is so far not substantiated by data. With respect to the mechanism involved, it has been shown *in vitro* that α_1-adrenoceptor stimulation via lowering of adenyl cyclase activity activates hormone-sensitive lipoproteinlipase. However, it has never been demonstrated unequivocally that α_1-adrenoceptor antagonism is the only mechanism underlying the favorable changes of the plasma lipid profile by prazosin. Nevertheless, α_1-adrenoceptor antagonism is likely to be an important factor, since similar effects have been described for doxazosin and trimazosin. For reviews on this subject, see refs. 115–117.

Prazosin and its successor drugs doxazosin and terazosin do not influence blood glucose levels and are therefore considered safe drugs in the treatment of hypertensive diabetic patients (37,118,119).

Urapidil shows the usual side effects of a selective α_1-blocking agent as discussed above for prazosin, but a first-dose effect has not been clearly recognized and described. Mild sedation is sometimes observed in the beginning of the treatment period, but it usually is transient. There are virtually no reports on sexual dysfunction caused by urapidil treatment. As a whole, urapidil appears to be well tolerated. For reviews on its side effects, see refs. 70 and 71 and the literature quoted therein.

A discussion of the side effects of labetalol and ketanserin lies beyond the scope of this section.

CONTRAINDICATIONS

Although caution appears to be advisable in a few clinical conditions, specific contraindications for α-adrenoceptor-blocking agents are hardly known.

Orthostatic hypotension, with the risk of falling and trauma especially in old patients, is a potential risk of all α-blockers. This danger might be reduced for doxazosin and trimazosin, which are claimed to cause little or no postural hypotension in therapeutic doses (see section entitled "Side Effects and Toxicity").

An abrupt fall in blood pressure, as caused by intravenously administered α-adrenoceptor blockers (in particular, phentolamine or phenoxybenzamine), is potentially deleterious in patients (in particular, the elderly) with relevant cerebral or coronary ischemia. Hypersensitivity to prazosin is a rare contraindication.

α_1-Adrenoceptor-blocking agents may be safely used in patients with obstructive airways disorders, diabetes mellitus (119), or peripheral vascular disease. This appears to be an advantage over β-adrenoceptor blockers, which should be avoided in these conditions or at least applied most cautiously; only β_1-selective drugs should be used, if β-adrenoceptor blockers are to be used at all.

DRUG INTERACTIONS AND COMBINATIONS WITH OTHER DRUGS

Interactions

Very few relevant interactions between α_1-adrenoceptor antagonists and other drugs have been reported, and systematic investigations on this subject have rarely been carried out.

It was reported by Elliott et al. (120) that the postural hypotensive response to prazosin was aggravated by simultaneously applied propranolol, but this interaction did not occur in the experiments by Stokes et al. (121). In contrast to data obtained in animal experiments (122), an inhibitory effect of prazosin on the hypotensive action of clonidine could not be established under clinical conditions.

Indomethacin has been reported to significantly reduce the hypotensive effect of prazosin in four of nine patients (39). Simultaneously, the rise in plasma renin activity induced by prazosin treatment in these patients was prevented by indomethacin.

Combination with Other Drugs

The antihypertensive activity of α-adrenoceptor-blocking agents is enhanced by a variety of current antihypertensive drugs. As a whole, this should be considered as an additive, nonspecific effect which does not involve interaction at the receptor level. Potentiation does not occur. With respect to *prazosin,* a variety of different antihypertensive drugs can be combined with this α_1-adrenoceptor blocker (37) but are most frequently combined with a β-blocker and/or a diuretic. As such, prazosin is usually added to a combined therapy involving a β-blocker and a diuretic. The diuretic in this triple therapy counteracts potential fluid retention induced by prazosin. In all studies reported, prazosin appeared to cause an additive decrease in blood pressure. The pharmacological and therapeutic implications of the combination of prazosin with a diuretic and/or a β-blocker may be considered as follows:

α_1-Adrenoceptor Antagonists Plus Diuretics

Potentially, this combination of antihypertensives seems a logical and favorable one for the following reasons:

1. α_1-Adrenoceptor antagonists tend to induce the retention of sodium and water as a result of their vasodilator activity. This effect is counteracted by natriuretic agents.
2. The potentially unfavorable effect of the diuretics on the lipid profile is counteracted by α_1-adrenoceptor agents, which tend to improve this profile.
3. At a lower level of extracellular sodium, as induced by treatment with natriuretic agents, the vasoconstrictor response to endogenous noradrenaline is blunted. This may be an explanation for the antihypertensive activity of the diuretics. This mechanism is additive to the reduction of noradrenaline-induced vasoconstriction caused by the blockade of α_1-adrenoceptors.
4. α_1-Adrenoceptor antagonists and diuretics are both blood-pressure-lowering drugs, thus causing an additional antihypertensive effect.

Thiazides are the diuretic agents used most frequently in the treatment of hypertension; for this reason, they are the most obvious combination partners with α_1-adrenoceptor antagonists. The usefulness of this combination is well-documented (37). In addition, there is no fundamental objection against the simultaneous administration of α_1-adrenoceptor antagonists with potassium-sparing diuretics such as triamterene or amiloride, nor is there a basic pharmacological argument against the simultaneous application of an

α_1-adrenoceptor antagonist and a combination of a thiazide and a potassium-sparing diuretic.

α_1-Adrenoceptor Antagonists Plus β-Blockers

The combination of α_1- and β-adrenoceptor antagonists is potentially useful for the following reasons:

1. To a modest degree, the α_1-adrenoceptor-blocking agents may cause some reflex tachycardia. This adverse reaction is suppressed by the simultaneous application of β-adrenoceptor-blocking agents.
2. As was similarly discussed for the diuretics (see above), the potentially unfavorable influence of β-blockers on the lipid profile is counteracted by simultaneously applied α_1-adrenoceptor-blocking agents. It should be realized that the negative influence on the lipid spectrum appears to be the most pronounced for nonselective β_1- and β_2-blockers without intrinsic sympathomimetic activity (ISA) and much less obvious for β-blockers with strong ISA (e.g., pindolol or oxprenolol) or for β_1-selective drugs (atenolol, metoprolol, etc.).
3. Both α_1- and β-adrenoceptor antagonists are antihypertensives, although they act via clearly different mechanisms. Their combined application may be anticipated to cause an additive antihypertensive effect.

α_1-Adrenoceptor Antagonists Plus β-Blocker Plus Diuretic

The classical triple therapy in stepped-care treatment of hypertension implicates the combined application of a vasodilator, added to a regimen of β-blocker plus diuretic. Vasodilatation in the arteriolar vascular bed appears to be a logical approach to antihypertensive treatment, since in established hypertension the increased total peripheral resistance is the most consistent hemodynamic change in comparison to normotensive subjects. It is well-documented that monotherapy with a direct vasodilator such as hydralazine or minoxidil is unsatisfactory as a result of compensatory mechanisms caused by vasodilatation, such as reflex tachycardia and fluid retention. The addition of a β-blocker suppresses reflex tachycardia, whereas a simultaneously applied diuretic will counteract fluid retention.

It has been demonstrated in clinical studies (37) that α_1-adrenoceptor antagonists can be used as the vasodilator component in triple therapy, instead of a more classical vasodilator with a direct relaxing action on vascular smooth muscle. The basic mechanism of vasodilatation caused by α_1-adrenoceptor blockade is fundamentally different from that of the directly acting vasodilators. Nevertheless, the principle of triple therapy with an α_1-adrenoceptor blocker, a β-blocker, and a diuretic is basically the same as that of a combination of a directly acting vasodilator with a β-blocker and a diuretic.

Trimazosin, doxazosin, and terazosin can also be potentially combined with various other antihypertensives. As was similarly described for prazosin, these newer α_1-blockers can potentially be added to a diuretic, to a β-blocker, or to a combination of both, to yield an additive antihypertensive action. However, such combinations have rarely been studied systematically. There are only a few incidental reports on combined application of urapidil with other antihypertensives. At least on theoretical grounds, an outcome similar to the one described for prazosin and its successor drugs may be anticipated, but further studies are required.

TREATMENT OF ELDERLY HYPERTENSIVES WITH α-ADRENOCEPTOR ANTAGONISTS

Old age as such does not appear to be associated with obvious and significant changes in the density and sensitivity of α-adrenoceptors, but it should be realized that the present methodology does not allow the determination of adrenoceptors that would really matter (i.e., those located in blood vessels) (123). In a limited number of patients, the impression has been obtained that old age is accompanied by a reduced responsiveness of vascular α_1-adrenoceptors (124) to agonists. Irrespective of inconclusive changes in α-adrenoceptors in old age, it has been demonstrated that hypertensives show an enhanced reactivity to various vasoconstrictor stimuli, such as stimuli from both α_1- and α_2-adrenoceptor agonists (30–32).

So far, no consistent experimental findings have been published which suggest that prazosin would be more or less active in elderly hypertensives when compared with younger adult hypertensive patients.

In conclusion, prazosin and related drugs are probably at least as effective in the elderly as in younger hypertensive adults, and there are no studies available which suggest the contrary. Since prazosin is mainly inactivated by hepatic biotransformation, no important *kinetic* changes may be anticipated for this drug in the elderly, since impaired kidney function is the most obvious and relevant change in drug-handling processes associated with old age. Neither theoretical arguments nor clinical observations suggest that prazosin would display a different kinetic behavior in the elderly hypertensive.

Bronchial asthma, diabetes mellitus, and renal failure occur more frequently in the elderly. These conditions, however, are no clear contraindications for prazosin. Congestive heart failure, a condition also more frequently occurring in the elderly, may even be influenced favorably by prazosin treatment. *Orthostatic hypotension,* a common adverse reaction to prazosin, may be anticipated to cause more problems in the elderly, for the following two reasons: (i) the blunted baroreceptor reflex function in old age and (ii) the greater incidence of vertigo of the elderly. Other side effects to prazosin are probably not more frequent or severe in old patients than in younger adults. Finally, it should be realized that prazosin may cause or enhance urinary incontinence as a result of its relaxing effect on the sphincter of the bladder (125,126). It can be imagined that this adverse reaction may occur more frequently and cause more problems in old patients than in younger adults treated with prazosin. On the other hand, prazosin has also been used successfully in the treatment of benign prostatic obstruction (127). In conclusion, present knowledge and experience suggest that prazosin can be safely used in elderly hypertensives, even in presence of several concomitant diseases. Orthostatic hypotension is probably the most relevant adverse reaction, particularly in the elderly.

The use of the successor drugs to prazosin has not been studied systematically in elderly hypertensives, but a few incidental data on this subject have been published recently. The disposition of *doxazosin* was studied in two groups of normotensive volunteers who were 62–89 and 23–39 years of age. The volume of distribution increased significantly with age, but bioavailability and clearance were not significantly altered (128). It was concluded that old age, per se, is unlikely to influence the disposition of doxazosin to a significant degree.

Terazosin was studied in a small number of normotensives who were 54–62 and 19–30 years of age (129). In the older group, the mean plasma concentrations of terazosin were higher and the drug's half-life was longer. There were no indications that terazosin caused a stronger hypotensive effect in the older group.

REFERENCES

1. Georgopoulos AJ, Valasidis A, Siourthas D. Treatment of chronic heart failure with slow release phentolamine. *Eur J Clin Pharmacol* 1978;13:325.
2. Gould L, Becker WH, Macklin EE. Effects of intravenous phentolamine on hemodynamics and resting pulmonary gas exchange in man. *Angiology* 1980;31:120.
3. Stokes GS, Frost GW, Graham RM, MacCarthy EP. Indoramin and prazosin as adjuncts to beta-adrenoceptor blockade in hypertension. *Clin Pharmacol Ther* 1979;25:783–785.
4. Marshall AJ, Kettle MA, Barrit DW. Evaluation of indoramin added to oxprenolol and bendrofluazide as a third agent in severe hypertension. *Br J Clin Pharmacol* 1980;10:217.
5. Constantine JW. Analysis of the hypotensive action of prazosin. In: Cotton J, ed. *Prazosin—evaluation of a new antihypertensive agent.* Amsterdam: Excerpta Medica, 1974. Quoted in ref. 36.
6. Roesler JM, McCafferty JP, DeMarinis RM, Matthews WD, Hieble JP. Characterization of the antihypertensive activity of SK&F 86466, a selective α_2-antagonist in the rat. *J Pharmacol Exp Ther* 1986;236:1–7.
7. Berthelsen S, Pettinger WA. A functional basis for classification of α-adrenergic receptors. *Life Sci* 1977;21:595–606.
8. Starke K. α-Adrenoceptor subclassification. *Rev Physiol Biochem Pharmacol* 1981;88:199–236.
9. Timmermans PBMWM, van Zwieten PA. The postsynaptic α_2-adrenoceptor. *J Auton Pharmacol* 1981;1:171–183.
10. Langer SZ. Presynaptic regulation of the release of catecholamines. *Pharmacol Rev* 1981;32:337–362.
11. van Zwieten PA, Timmermans PBMWM. Cardiovascular α_2-adrenoceptors. *J Mol Cell Cardiol* 1983;15:717–733.
12. van Zwieten PA. Role of α-adrenoceptors in hypertension and antihypertensive drug treatment. *Am J Med* 1984;77:17–25.
13. Langer SZ, Massingham R, Shepperson NB. Presence of postsynaptic α_2-adrenoceptors of predominantly extrasynaptic location in the vascular smooth muscle of the dog hind limb. *Clin Sci* 1980;59(Suppl 6):225S–228S.
14. Wilffert B, Timmermans PBMWM, van Zwieten PA. Extrasynaptic location of α_2- and non-innervated β_2-adrenoceptors in the vascular system of the pithed normotensive rat. *J Pharmacol Exp Ther* 1982;221:762–768.
15. Jie K, van Brummelen P, Vermey P, Timmermans PBMWM, van Zwieten PA. Identification of vascular postsynaptic α_1- and α_2-adrenoceptors in man. *Circ Res* 1984;54:447–452.
16. van Brummelen P, Jie K, Timmermans PBMWM, van Zwieten PA. Postjunctional α-adrenoceptors and the regulation of arteriolar tone in humans. *J Cardiovasc Pharmacol* 1985;7:S149–S152.
17. De Jonge A, Timmermans PBMWM, van Zwieten PA. Participation of cardiac presynaptic α_2-adrenoceptors in the bradycardiac effects of clonidine and analogues. *Naunyn-Schmiedeberg's Arch Pharmacol* 1981;317:8–12.
18. Timmermans PBMWM, van Zwieten PA. α_2-Adrenoceptors: classification, localization, mechanisms and targets for drugs. *J Med Chem* 1982;25:1389–1401.
19. Schmitt H. Action des α-sympathomimétiques sur les structures nerveuses. *Actual Pharmacol* 1971;24:93–113.
20. Kobinger W. Central α-adrenergic systems as targets for hypotensive drugs. *Rev Physiol Biochem Pharmacol* 1978;81:40–100.
21. van Zwieten PA. Antihypertensive drugs with a central action. *Prog Pharmacol* 1975;1:1–63.
22. van Zwieten PA, Timmermans PBMWM. Pharmacological basis for the hypotensive activity and side-effects of α-methyl-DOPA, clonidine and guanfacine. *Hypertension* 1984;Suppl 6:28–33.
23. Brodde OE, Daul AE, O'Hara N, Bock KD. Increased density and responsiveness of α- and β-adrenoceptors in circulating blood cells of essential hypertensive patients. *J Hypertens* 1984;2(Suppl 3):111–113.
24. Brodde OE, Daul AE, O'Hara N, Khalifa AM. Properties of α- and β-adrenoceptors in circulating blood cells of patients with essential hypertension. *J Cardiovasc Pharmacol* 1985;7:S162–S167.
25. Jones CR, Hamilton CA, Whyte KF, Elliott HL, Reid JL. Acute and chronic regulation of alpha(2)-adrenoceptor number and function in man. *Clin Sci* 1985;68(Suppl 10):129S–132S.
26. Motulsky HJ, O'Connor DT, Insel PA. Platelet α_2-adrenergic receptors in treated and untreated essential hypertension. *Clin Sci* 1983;64:265–272.
27. Philipp T, Distler A, Cordes U. Sympathetic nervous system and blood pressure control in essential hypertension. *Lancet* 1978;2:959–963.
28. Amann FW, Bolli P, Kiowski W, et al. Enhanced α-adrenoceptor-mediated vasoconstriction in essential hypertension. *Hypertension* 1981;3(Suppl I):119–123.
29. Buehler FR, Bolli P, Erne P, Kiowski W, Mueller FB, Hulthén UL, Ji BH. Adrenoceptors, calcium and vasoconstriction in normal and hypertensive humans. *J Cardiovasc Pharmacol* 1985;7:S130–S136.
30. Jie K, van Brummelen P, Vermey P, Timmermans PBMWM, van Zwieten PA. α_1- and α_2-adrenoceptor mediated vasoconstriction in the forearm of normotensive and hypertensive subjects. *J Cardiovasc Pharmacol* 1986;8:190–196.
31. Kiowski W, Hulthén UL, Ritz R, Buehler FR. Alpha-2-adrenoceptor mediated vasoconstriction in human arterial vessels. *J Clin Pharmacol Ther* 1983;34:565–569.
32. van Zwieten PA, Jie K, van Brummelen P. Postsynaptic α_1- and α_2-adrenoceptor changes in hypertension. *J Cardiovasc Pharmacol* 1987;10(Suppl 4):S68–S75.
33. Constantine JW, Weeks RA, McShane WK. Prazosin and presynaptic α-receptors in the cardio-accelerator nerve of the dog. *Eur J Pharmacol* 1978;50:51.
34. Graham RM, Pettinger WA. Prazosin. *N Engl J Med* 1979;300:232–236.
35. Lefèvre-Borg F, Roach AG, Gomeni R, Cavero I. Mechanism of antihypertensive activity of orally administered prazosin in spontaneously hypertensive rats. *J Cardiovasc Pharmacol* 1979;1:31.
36. Brogden RN, Heel RC, Speight TM, Avery GS. Prazosin: a review of its pharmacological properties and therapeutic efficacy in hypertension. *Drugs* 1977;14:163–197.
37. Stanaszek WF, Kellerman D, Brogden RN, Romankiewicz J. Prazosin update. A review of its pharmacological properties and therapeutic use in hypertension and congestive heart failure. *Drugs* 1983;25:339–384.
38. Cambridge D, Davey MJ, Massingham R. The pharmacology of antihypertensive drugs with special reference to vasodilators, α-adrenergic blocking agents and prazosin. *Med J Aust* 1977;Special suppl 2:2.
39. Hardey DW, Lokhandwala MF. Influence of prazosin on cardiac reflex function. *Eur J Pharmacol* 1979;57:251.
40. Sasso EH, O'Connor DT. Prazosin depression of baroreflex function in hypertensive man. *Eur J Clin Pharmacol* 1982;22:7–9.

41. Cavero I. Effects of prazosin on reflex changes in heart rate evoked by vasopressor and vasodepressor stimuli in conscious rabbits. *J Cardiovasc Pharmacol* 1982;4(Suppl):S108.
42. Ramage AG. Why do α_1-adrenoceptor antagonists fail to cause reflex tachycardia? *Br J Pharmacol* 1982;77(Suppl):323P.
43. Persson B, Yao T, Thoren P. Correlation between decreased heart rate and central inhibition of sympathetic discharges after prazosin administration in the spontaneously hypertensive rat. *Clin Exp Hypertens* 1981;3:245–250.
44. Saeed M, Sommer O, Holtz J, Bassenge E. α-Adrenoceptor blockade by phentolamine causes β-adrenergic vasodilatation by increased catecholamine release due to presynaptic α-blockade. *J Cardiovasc Pharmacol* 1982;4:44–48.
45. Cavero I, Roach AG. The pharmacology of prazosin, a novel antihypertensive agent. *Life Sci* 1980;27:1525–1533.
46. Huchet AM, Velly J, Schmitt H. Role of α_1- and α_2-adrenoceptors in the modulation of the baroreflex vagal bradycardia. *Eur J Pharmacol* 1981;71:455–461.
47. Constantine JW, McShane WK, Scriabine A, Hess HJ. Analysis of the hypotensive action of prazosin. In: Onesti G, Kim KE, Moyer JH, eds. *Hypertension: mechanisms and management.* New York: Grune & Stratton, 1973;429.
48. Roach AG, Gomeni R, Mitchard M, et al. The blood pressure lowering effects of intravenous versus intracerebroventricular prazosin in anesthetized cats. *Eur J Pharmacol* 1978;49:271–274.
49. Timmermans PBMWM, Lam E, van Zwieten PA. The interaction between prazosin and clonidine at α-adrenoceptors in rats and cats. *Eur J Pharmacol* 1979;49:271–276.
50. Doxey JC, Smith CFC, Walker JM. Selectivity of blocking agents for pre- and postsynaptic α-adrenoceptors. *Br J Pharmacol* 1977;60:91.
51. Timmermans PBMWM, Kwa HY, Karamat Ali F, van Zwieten PA. Prazosin and its analogues UK-18,596 and UK-33,274: a comparative study on cardiovascular effects and α-adrenoceptor blocking activities. *Arch Int Pharmacodyn* 1980;245:218.
52. U'Prichard DC, Charness ME, Robertson D, Snyder S. Prazosin: differential affinities for two populations of α-adrenergic receptor binding sites. *Eur J Pharmacol* 1978;50:87.
53. Greengrass PM, Bremner R. Binding characteristics of ^{3}H-prazosin to rat brain α-adrenergic receptors. *Eur J Pharmacol* 1979;55:323.
54. Cambridge D, Davey MJ, Greengrass PM. The pharmacology of antihypertensive drugs with special reference to vasodilators, α-adrenergic blocking agents and prazosin. *Prog Pharmacol* 1980;3:107.
55. Hornung R, Presek P, Glossman H. Alpha-adrenoceptors in rat brain: direct identification with prazosin. *Naunyn Schmiedeberg's Arch Pharmacol* 1979;308:223.
56. Miach PJ, Dausse JP, Cardot A, Meyer P. ^{3}H-prazosin binds specifically to α_1-adrenoceptors in rat brain. *Naunyn Schmiedeberg's Arch Pharmacol* 1980;312:23.
57. Reid JL, Meredith PA, Elliott H. Pharmacokinetics and pharmacodynamics of trimazosin in man. *Am Heart J* 1983;106:1222–1228.
58. Singleton W, Sexton CAPD, Hernandez J, Prichard BN. Postjunctional selectivity of α-blockade with prazosin, trimazosin and UK-33,274 in man. *J Cardiovasc Pharmacol* 1982;4:S145–S155.
59. Constantine JW, Hess HJ. The cardiovascular effects of trimazosin. *Eur J Pharmacol* 1981;74:227.
60. Sands H, Jorgensen R. Effects of prazosin on cyclic nucleotide content and blood pressure of the spontaneously hypertensive rat. *Biochem Pharmacol* 1979;28:685–687.
61. Awan N, Hermanovich J, Vera Z, et al. Cardiocirculatory actions of trimazosin and sodium nitroprusside in ischemic heart disease. *Clin Pharmacol Ther* 1982;31:290.
62. Vincent J, Hamilton CA, Sumner DJ, Reid JL. A comparison of the hypotensive activity and *in vitro* and *in vivo* α_1-adrenoceptor antagonist properties of prazosin, trimazosin and doxazosin in the rabbit. *Br J Pharmacol* 1983;79(Suppl):388P.
63. Singleton W, Saxton CAPD, Hernandez R, Ferrer RS, Prichard BNC. Alpha blocking effect of prazosin, trimazosin and UK-33,274 in man. In: Turner P, ed. *World conference on clinical pharmacological therapy, abstracts.* London: Macmillan, 1980.
64. Elliott HL, Meredith PA, Sumner DJ, et al. A pharmacodynamic and pharmacokinetic assessment of a new α-adrenoceptor antagonist, doxazosin (UK 33274) in normotensive subjects. *Br J Clin Pharmacol* 1982;13:699.
65. Vincent J, Elliott HL, Meredith PA, Reid JL. Doxazosin, an α_1-adrenoceptor antagonist: pharmacokinetics and concentration effect relationships in man. *Br J Clin Pharmacol* 1983;15:719–725.
66. Hamilton CA, Reid JL, Vincent J. Pharmacokinetic and pharmacodynamic studies with two α-adrenoceptor antagonists, doxazosin and prazosin in the rabbit. *Br J Pharmacol* 1985;86:79–87.
67. Kyncl JJ. The pharmacology of terazosin. *Am J Med* 1986;80(Suppl 5B):12–19.
68. Titmarsch S, Monk JP. Terazosin. A review of its pharmacodynamic and pharmacokinetic properties and therapeutic efficacy in essential hypertension. *Drugs* 1987;33:461–477.
69. Moser M (Ed). Advances in the management of hypertension: focus on terazosin, a new alpha-1-adrenergic antagonist. *Am J Med* 1986;80(5B):1–105.
70. Schoetensack W, Bruckschen EG, Zech K. Urapidil. In: Scriabine W, ed. *New drugs annual: cardiovascular drugs.* New York: Raven Press, 1983;19–48.
71. Amery A, ed. Treatment of hypertension with urapidil. Preclinical and clinical update. *R Soc Med Serv* 1986;101:1–186.
72. van Zwieten PA, De Jonge A, Wilffert B, Timmermans PBMWM, Beckeringh JJ, Thoolen MJMC. Cardiovascular effects and interaction with adrenoceptors of urapidil. *Arch Int Pharmacodyn* 1985;276:180–201.
73. Richards DA, Prichard BNA. Proceedings of the second symposium on labetalol. *Br J Clin Pharmacol* 1979;8(Suppl 2):89S–239S.
74. Lund-Johansen P. Pharmacology of combined α-β-blockade. Hemodynamic effects of labetolol. *Drugs* 1984;28(Suppl 2):35–50.
75. Kalkman HO, Timmermans PBMWM, van Zwieten PA. Characterization of the antihypertensive properties of ketanserin (R 41468) in rats. *J Pharmacol Exp Ther* 1982;222:227–231.
76. Vanhoutte PM, Ball SG, Berdeaux A, et al. Mechanism of action of ketanserin in hypertension. *Trends Pharmacol Sci* 1986;7:58–59.
77. Medgett IC. Effect of neuronal uptake blockade on the amplifying effect of serotonin on sympathetic vasoconstriction in rat autoperfused hind limb. *J Cardiovasc Pharmacol* 1987;10(Suppl 3):S65–S68.
78. van Zwieten PA, Mathy MJ, Boddeke HWGM, Doods HN. Central hypotensive activity of ketanserin in cats. *J Cardiovasc Pharmacol* 1987;10(Suppl 3):S54–S58.
79. Frohlich ED, van Zwieten PA, eds. Serotonin in cardiovascular regulation. *J Cardiovasc Pharmacol* 1987;10(Suppl 3):S1–S137.
80. Lund-Johansen P. Hemodynamic changes at rest and during exercise in long-term prazosin therapy of essential hypertension. In: Cotton DKW, ed. *Prazosin—evaluation of a new antihypertensive agent.* Amsterdam: Excerpta Medica, 1974;43.
81. Robinson BF. Drugs acting directly on vascular smooth muscle: circulatory and secondary effects. *Br J Pharmacol* 1981;12:5S.
82. Preston RA, O'Connor DT, Stone RA. Prazosin and renal hemodynamics: arteriolar vasodilatation during therapy of essential hypertension in man. *J Cardiovasc Pharmacol* 1979;1:277.
83. Lui HK, Awan NA, Needham K, Mason DT. Comparative evaluation of the new oral systemic vasodilator terazosin and nitroprusside in severe chronic heart failure. *Clin Res* 1985;33:207A.
84. Messerli FH, Kobrin I, Amodeo C, Ventura HO, Forhlich ED. Immediate cardiovascular effects of urapidil in essential hypertension. In: Amery A, ed. Treatment of hypertension with urapidil. *R Soc Med Serv* 1986;101:87–91.
85. Kobrin I, Gallo A, Kumar A, Pegram BL, Frohlich ED. Immediate hemodynamic changes produced by urapidil in normotensive and spontaneously hypertensive rats. *Clin Exp Hypertens* 1984;A6:685–697.
86. Ball SG. Phaeochromocytoma. In: Robertson JIS, ed. *Handbook of hypertension, vol 2: Clinical aspects of secondary hypertension.* Amsterdam: Elsevier, 1984;238–275.

87. Imhoff PR, Garnier B, Brunner L, Keller G, Rohrer T. Human pharmacology of orally administered phentolamine. In: Taylor SH, ed. *Phentolamine in heart failure and other cardiac disorders.* Bern: H Huber, 1976;11–22.
88. Taylor LA, Twomey TM, Schuch von Wintenau M. The metabolic fate of prazosin. *Xenobiotica* 1977;7:357–364.
89. Hess HJ. Biochemistry and structure–activity studies with prazosin. In: Cotton DKW, ed. *Prazosin—evaluation of a new antihypertensive agent.* Amsterdam: Excerpta Medica, 1974;5.
90. Bateman DN, Hobbs DC, Twomey TM, et al. Prazosin, pharmacokinetics and concentration effect. *Eur J Clin Pharmacol* 1979;16:177–181.
91. Wood AJ, Bolli P, Simpson FO. Prazosin in normal subjects: plasma levels, blood pressure and heart rate. *Br J Pharmacol* 1976;3:199–202.
92. Elliott HL, McLean K, Sumner DJ, et al. Immediate cardiovascular responses to oral prazosin—effects on current β-blockers. *Clin Pharmacol Ther* 1981;29:303.
93. Sonders RC. The pharmacokinetics of terazosin. *Am J Med* 1986;80(Suppl 5B):77–81.
94. Kondo K, Ohashi K, Ebiwara A. Pharmacokinetics and pharmacological effects of terazosin, a new alpha-blocker. *Jpn J Clin Pharmacol Ther* 1982;13:137–138.
95. Zech K, Steinijans VW, Radtke HW. Pharmacokinetics of urapidil in normal subjects. In: Amery A, ed. Treatment of hypertension with urapidil. *R Soc Med Serv* 1986;101:29–38.
96. Inouye I, Massie B, Benowitz N, Simpson P, Lofe D, Topic N. Monotherapy in mild to moderate hypertension: comparison of hydrochlorothiazide, propranolol and prazosin. *Am J Cardiol* 1984;53:24A–28A.
97. Scharf SC, Lee HB, Wexler JP, Blaufox MD. Cardiovascular consequences of primary antihypertensive therapy with prazosin hydrochloride. *Am J Cardiol* 1984;53:32A–36A.
98. Neusy AJ, Lowenstein J. Effects of prazosin, atenolol and thiazide diuretics on plasma lipids in patients with essential hypertension. *Am J Med* 1986;80(Suppl 2A):94–99.
99. Stamler R, Stamler J, Gosch FC, Berkson DM, Dyer A, Hershinow P. Initial antihypertensive drug therapy: alpha-blocker or diuretic. Interim report of a randomized trial. *Am J Med* 1986;80(Suppl 2A):90–93.
100. Okun R. Effectiveness of prazosin as initial antihypertensive therapy. *Am J Cardiol* 1983;51:644–650.
101. Kincaid-Smith PC. Alpha blockade: an overview of efficacy data. *Am J Med* 1987;82(Suppl 1A):21–25.
102. Cubeddu LX, Zarate NA, Rosales CB, Zschaek W. Prazosin and propranolol in preoperative management of phaeochromocytoma. *Clin Pharmacol Ther* 1982;32:156–160.
103. Taylor CR, Leader JP, Singleton MB, Munster EW, Falkner FC. Profile of trimazosin: an effective and safe antihypertensive agent. *Am Heart J* 1983;106:1269–1285.
104. Perry RS. Trimazosin. *Drugs Today* 1985;21:243–252.
105. Hayduk K. Efficacy and safety of doxazosin in hypertension therapy. *Am J Cardiol* 1987;59:35G–39G.
106. Rosenthal J. A multicenter trial of doxazosin in West Germany. *Am J Cardiol* 1987;59:40G–45G.
107. Torvik D, Madsbu HP. An open one-year comparison of doxazosin and prazosin in mild to moderate essential hypertension. *Am J Cardiol* 1987;59:68G–72G.
108. Ott P, Storm T, Krusell LR, Jensen H, Badskjaer J, Faergeman O. Multicenter, double-blind comparison of doxazosin and atenolol in patients with mild to moderate hypertension. *Am J Cardiol* 1987;59:73G–77G.
109. Nash DT, Schonfeld G, Reeves RL, Black H, Wiedler DJ. A double-blind parallel trial to assess the efficacy of doxazosin, atenolol and placebo in patients with mild to moderate systemic hypertension. *Am J Cardiol* 1987;59:87G–90G.
110. Halttunen P, Himanen P, Frick MH, et al. A long-term double-blind comparison of doxazosin and atenolol in patients with mild to moderate essential hypertension. *Br J Clin Pharmacol* 1986;21(Suppl 1):55S–62S.
111. Baez MA, Garg DC, Jallad NS, Wiedler DJ. Antihypertensive effect of doxazosin in hypertensive patients: comparison with atenolol. *Br J Clin Pharmacol* 1986;21(Suppl 1):63S–68S.
112. Cox DA, Leader P, Milson JA, Singleton W. The antihypertensive effect of doxazosin: a clinical overview. *Br J Clin Pharmacol* 1986;21(Suppl 1):83S–90S.
113. Starke K, ed. Doxazosin: coronary artery disease; risk factor management. *Am J Cardiol* 1987;59:1G–104G.
114. Reid JL, Davies HC, eds. α_1-Adrenoceptor blockade in hypertension: pharmacological and clinical profile of doxazosin. *Br J Clin Pharmacol* 1986;21(Suppl 1):1S–92S.
115. Drayer JIM, Weber MA, De Young JL, Brewer DD. Long-term blood pressure monitoring in the evaluation of antihypertensive therapy. *Arch Int Med* 1983;143:898–901.
116. Ames RP. The effects of antihypertensive drugs on serum lipids and lipoproteins. Part II: non-diuretic drugs. *Drugs* 1986; 32:335–337.
117. Ferrier C, Beretta-Piccoli C, Wiedmann P, Mordasini R. Alpha-1-adrenergic blockade and lipoprotein metabolism in essential hypertension. *Clin Pharmacol Ther* 1986;40:525–530.
118. Weidmann P, Uchlinger DE, Gerber A. Antihypertensive treatment and serum lipoproteins. *J Hypertens* 1985;3:297–306.
119. Konigstein BP. Treatment with prazosin in patients suffering from a maturity onset diabetes. *Wiener Med Wochenschr* 1978;128:27–29.
120. Elliott HL, McLean K, Sumner DJ. Immediate cardiovascular responses to oral prazosin—effects on current β-blockers. *Clin Pharmacol Ther* 1981;29:303.
121. Stokes GS, Gain JM, Mahony JF, Raftos J, Stewart JH. Long-term use of prazosin in combination or alone for treating hypertension. *Med J Aust* 1977;Special suppl:13–16.
122. Timmermans PBMWM, Lam E, van Zwieten PA. The interaction between prazosin and clonidine at α-adrenoceptors in rats and cats. *Eur J Pharmacol* 1979;49:271–276.
123. Docherty JR. Aging and the cardiovascular system. *J Auton Pharmacol* 1984;6:77–84.
124. Kirkendall WM. Treatment of hypertension in the elderly. *Am J Cardiol* 1986;57:63C–68C.
125. Thien Th. Urinary incontinence caused by prazosin. *Br Med J* 1978;11:622–624.
126. Kiruluta GH, et al. Prazosin as cause of urinary incontinence. *Urology* 1981;XVIII:618–619.
127. Hedlund H, Andersson KE, Ek AK. Effects of prazosin in patients with benign prostatic obstruction. *J Urol* 1983;130:275–278.
128. Vincent J, Meredith PA, Elliott HL, Reid JL. The pharmacokinetics of doxazosin in elderly normotensives. *Br J Clin Pharmacol* 1986;21:521–524.
129. McNeil JJ, Drummer HE, Conway EL, Workman BS, Louis WJ. Effect of age on pharmacokinetics of and blood pressure responses to prazosin and terazosin. *J Cardiovasc Pharmacol* 1987;10:168–175.

Hypertension: Pathophysiology, Diagnosis, and Management, edited by J. H. Laragh and B. M. Brenner. Raven Press, Ltd., New York © 1990.

CHAPTER 142

Centrally Acting Sympathetic Inhibitors

Michael A. Weber, William F. Graettinger, and Deanna G. Cheung

Features of Individual Agents, 2251
Clonidine, 2252
Guanabenz, 2253
Guanfacine, 2254
Methyldopa, 2255
Reserpine, 2256
Clinical Characteristics, 2256
A Transdermal Form of Clonidine, 2257
Considerations in the Elderly, 2258
Centrally Acting Agents and Left Ventricular Hypertrophy, 2258
Summary, 2259
References, 2259

The best known of the centrally acting sympathetic nervous system inhibitors, methyldopa and clonidine, have been available for several years. Recently, most attention in the area of antihypertensive therapeutics has focused on newer classes of agents such as angiotensin-converting-enzyme inhibitors and calcium-channel blockers. But the centrally acting drugs, including the newer compounds guanabenz and guanfacine, continue to have an important role in the management of hypertension. This class of drugs is effective in reducing blood pressure and can be administered to patients with complex clinical forms of hypertension as well as to those with straightforward or mild hypertension. Patients with renal insufficiency, diabetes mellitus, ischemic heart disease, or chronic obstructive airway disease are suitable candidates for antihypertensive treatment with these drugs. Similarly, elderly patients and those with severe or treatment-resistant forms of hypertension can respond well to the centrally acting agents.

Contemporary issues in hypertension management include not only the reduction of blood pressure but also the effect of drugs on left ventricular structure and function, metabolic factors, and the avoidance of symptomatic side effects. There is growing evidence that centrally acting antihypertensive agents can produce regression of left ventricular hypertrophy, which may be especially important in older hypertensive patients. There appear to be only minimal effects of these drugs on glucose metabolism, and they may exhibit slightly beneficial actions on the plasma lipid profile. A concern with these drugs, however, has been their propensity to cause symptomatic side effects, especially dry mouth and drowsiness. These problems now appear to occur less commonly, and with less severity, as investigators and clinicians have become skilled in the use of these agents in far lower doses than were previously used. This chapter will describe the centrally acting agents in more detail and will demonstrate how they can be used as monotherapy or in combination therapy in ways that allow the overall goals of antihypertensive therapy to be satisfactorily accomplished.

FEATURES OF INDIVIDUAL AGENTS

The available agents comprising this group are methyldopa, clonidine, guanabenz, guanfacine, and reserpine. Although there are differences between these agents in their mechanisms of action, they work primarily by decreasing sympathetic outflow from the central nervous system.

The growing evidence for a role of the sympathetic nervous system in mediating hypertension has been recently reviewed in detail (1). It has been claimed, for example, that plasma norepinephrine concentrations are higher in hypertensives than in normals and that in such individuals there is a correlation between the plasma catecholamine concentration and the blood pressure (2,3). It has also been postulated that hypertensive patients, as well as individuals prone to hypertension, have exaggerated sympathetic responses to stressful stimuli (4,5). Beyond its direct effects, the sympathetic nervous system may also influence blood pressure through its interactions with other mechanisms such as the renin–angiotensin system and through its effects on sodium and water balance (6,7). The centrally acting agents themselves have helped to provide further evidence supporting a role for sympathetic activity in hypertension; thus, it has been shown that there is a close correlation between (a) the decreases in blood pressure produced by agents such as clonidine and (b) the inhibitory effects of these agents on central and peripheral nerve tone (8).

Although these agents all influence central sympathetic outflow, there are differences between them in their actions on the peripheral components of the sympathetic nervous system and in their effects on the heart and on endocrine function. For this reason, it is of value to consider these agents separately.

Clonidine

Although it was introduced more recently than reserpine or methyldopa, clonidine has received more detailed study than the other agents and has become the model upon which central nervous system mechanisms of action have been best defined (9). As with the other drugs in this group, as well as with some of the beta-blocking agents, clonidine can produce side effects (such as drowsiness or dry mouth) that tend to indicate an action in the central nervous system. But more specifically, when clonidine is injected directly into the intracerebral ventricles (10) or the cisterns (11), it produces decreases in blood pressure and in heart rate.

A major concept in the regulation of blood pressure by the central nervous system is that alpha-adrenergic receptors within specific neurons mediate cardiovascular events when stimulated by naturally occurring sympathomimetic substances or by exogenously administered drugs. Specifically, when these alpha-receptors (which are situated in the lower brain stem in the nucleus tractus solitarii of the medulla oblongata) are activated, there is a decrease in sympathetic outflow to the cardiovascular system (12). Thus, it has been concluded that the antihypertensive action of clonidine is probably dependent upon its alpha-receptor agonist properties within the central nervous system which produce inhibitory effects on peripheral sympathetic activity. In confirmation of this idea, it has been shown that pretreatment with the alpha-receptor-blocking agent phentolamine will agonize clonidine's blood-pressure-lowering action (13).

The alpha-adrenergic-stimulating properties of clonidine might produce an interesting effect in the peripheral circulation, but it might be opposite to that accomplished by its actions in the central nervous system. Within minutes of administering clonidine to hypertensive human subjects there is a small but definite increase in blood pressure. This phenomenon usually is short-lived, because it is soon overwhelmed by the antihypertensive effect of clonidine's action in the central nervous system. But it has been suggested that the pressor dose–response relationship in the periphery sometimes may exist for clonidine concentrations over a wider range than for clonidine's effect in the central nervous system; that is, the centrally mediated hypotensive action of clonidine might reach plateau stage while the peripheral blood-pressure-raising action may continue to parallel with the increasing doses. If this concept is true, it suggests that high doses of clonidine could be counterproductive and may even have a lesser overall antihypertensive effect than do lower doses.

In addition to its action at the postsynaptic alpha-receptor, clonidine also has an agonist effect at the presynaptic receptor, which, by activating mechanisms that inhibit neurotransmittor release, might thereby contribute to the decrease in plasma norepinephrine concentrations found during treatment. The importance of this effect in the overall antihypertensive action of clonidine is not yet clear. However, a recent report (8) showing close correlations between both cerebrospinal and plasma norepinephrine concentrations and clonidine-induced decrements in blood pressure indicate that the primary effect of clonidine on plasma norepinephrine levels originates from its actions in the central nervous system.

As suggested earlier, it is possible that sympathetic mechanisms might raise blood pressure through impairing the sensitivity of baroreflex function. Thus, it is possible that the action of clonidine in the nucleus tractus solitarii of the vasomotor center may restore sensitivity to baroreflex mechanisms. Indeed, such an action of clonidine in reversing baroreceptor impairment has been shown in hypertensive animals (14) as well as in patients with essential hypertension (15). The modest decrease in heart rate often observed with clonidine is at least partly due to direct stimulatory effects on vagal mechanisms (16,17).

Clonidine has actions on the renin–angiotensin–aldosterone system that potentially could also contribute to its antihypertensive properties. It is likely that the inhibition of renin release produced by clonidine is secondary to its inhibition of sympathetic activity, although it is also possible that a direct drug action within the kidney might contribute to the renin-lowering effect (18). It has been shown that there may be separate renin-dependent and renin-independent components to the antihypertensive action of clonidine. In one study using repeated measurement (13), the following observation was made: On the first day of treatment with a low dose of clonidine in hypertensive patients, a close correlation was found between decreases in plasma renin activity and decreases in blood pressure. Thereafter, blood pressure continued to fall during a period of several days by a mechanism that clearly was unrelated to the effect of clonidine on renin release. Even in low-renin patients, in whom clonidine did not cause any change in plasma renin activity, there was an appreciable fall in blood pressure. Of interest, clonidine can cause a suppressive effect on aldosterone production that also might contribute to its antihypertensive action. This effect might be independent of changes in the renin–angiotensin system and might result directly from clonidine's central action, perhaps mediated by changes in adrenocorticotropic hormone (ACTH) release (19).

The hemodynamic properties of clonidine are summarized in Table 1. During chronic administration, blood pressure and heart rate remain decreased in both the supine and erect postures (20). Despite the inhibition of sympathetic mechanisms, there is an appropriate cardiac output response during exercise in patients receiving clonidine (21). It has been speculated that the preservation of cardiovascular reflexes during clonidine treatment is due to the predominance of the central nervous system action, which allows peripheral effector mechanisms to remain virtually intact. This characteristic may help explain the particularly

TABLE 1. *Hemodynamic effects of centrally acting antihypertensive agents*

Drug	Cardiac output	Total peripheral vascular resistance	Orthostasis	Glomerular filtration rate	Plasma volume	Plasma renin activity
Reserpine	↓	↓	+	↓	↑	↓
Methyldopa	↓	↓	+	↔	↑	↓
Clonidine	↓	↓	−	↔	↔	↓ or ↔
Guanabenz	↓	↓	−	↔	↔	↓ or ↔
Guanfacine	↓	↓	−	↔	↔	↓ or ↔

low incidence of orthostatic symptoms with clonidine (13,22). Renal blood flow and glomerular filtration rate are well preserved during treatment with clonidine; the decrease in renovascular resistance produced by the drug appears to compensate for any fall in renal perfusion pressure (23). Clonidine may be particularly valuable in patients with renal insufficiency; it is effective in lowering blood pressure in both severe and milder forms of hypertension associated with renal failure and does not appear to cause deterioration in the level of renal function (24,25). Because renal clearance is important in the elimination of clonidine, its dosage should be modified in accordance with glomerular filtration rate.

Clinical experience has shown clonidine to be a highly effective antihypertensive agent (26,27). The addition of a diuretic potentiates its antihypertensive effect in many patients; it has been estimated that the clonidine–diuretic combination will adequately control blood pressure in well over 70% of patients with mild to moderate hypertension (28,29). In many instances, the antihypertensive effects of clonidine can be achieved with dosages of 0.4 mg daily or less; adherence to lower dosage regimens not only minimizes side effects but also virtually eliminates the possibility of rebound problems if the treatment is precipitously discontinued. Comparative studies have shown that clonidine is at least as effective as agents such as methyldopa (22,30). It has been suggested that clonidine may be less likely than methyldopa to produce orthostatic symptoms. In other studies, clonidine has been shown to be at least as effective as propranolol (31) or prazosin (32) in lowering blood pressure. The use of clonidine in combination with other antihypertensive agents is discussed below.

Adverse effects that may occur during treatment with clonidine are listed in Table 2. The most common side effects are drowsiness or sedation as well as dry mouth. These effects are seen soon after the institution of therapy but tend to decrease in severity during the first few weeks of treatment (33). Approximately 7% of patients will discontinue treatment because they consider the side effects to be intolerable (34). As discussed later, the use of clonidine in its transdermal preparation may markedly reduce the frequency and severity of unwanted symptomatic side effects.

Guanabenz

The central actions of guanabenz have been demonstrated in studies in which this agent was found to penetrate the central nervous system, decrease sympathetic discharge, and thereby decrease blood pressure (35). These studies have also indicated that the action of guanabenz is mediated by stimulation of alpha-receptors, because the effects of guanabenz can be blocked by concurrent alpha-adrenergic blockade. Competitive binding studies using brain homogenates have indicated that guanabenz has a strong affinity for the alpha-2 subtype; this selectivity may be even greater than that observed for clonidine (36). The same studies have indicated that the affinity of guanabenz for the alpha-2-receptor is approximately 1300-fold greater than that for the alpha-1-receptor. In hypertensive patients, the decrease in blood pressure produced by guanabenz is predictably associated with decreases in peripheral resistance. At the same time, there are only minimal changes in heart rate, myocardial contractility, or cardiac output (37). Moreover, the response of the heart to exercise does not appear to be affected by this agent.

The effects of guanabenz on renal function have been studied closely in the dog (38). In this species, guanabenz has been found to increase glomerular filtration rate and sodium excretion. There is no change in renal blood flow, but urine osmolality is decreased. The apparent increase in water excretion seems to be related to an alpha-2-specific

TABLE 2. *Relative frequencies of clinical adverse effects of centrally acting antihypertensive agents*[a]

Effect	Reserpine	Methyldopa	Clonidine	Guanabenz	Guanfacine
Depression	++	±	−	−	−
Drowsiness	±	++	++	++	+
Dry mouth	−	+	++	++	++
Headache	+	+	+	+	+
Nightmares	++	+	±	−	−
Nasal congestion	++	±	−	−	−
Sexual dysfunction	+	++	+	+	+
Fluid retention	++	++	−	−	−
Weight gain	+	+	−	−	−

[a] −, does not occur; ±, rare; +, infrequent; ++, common.

inhibitor effect of guanabenz on the release of antidiuretic hormone. The mechanism of the increase in sodium excretion is not as well understood but may be partly dependent on an increase in glomerular filtration rate. It is also possible that guanabenz has a direct effect on renal tubular alpha-receptors that mediate sodium excretion. Experience with other centrally acting agents indicates that an inhibitory action on aldosterone production could contribute to this effect (19), although this mechanism has not yet been studied directly with guanabenz. Experience with guanabenz in human subjects has indicated that it has relatively little effect on renal function. Importantly, long-term treatment with this agent does not cause retention of sodium or water and does not appear to produce changes in plasma or blood volume (39,40). Clinically, weight gain and edema do not occur. This characteristic of guanabenz enables it to be considered for single-agent therapy in mild to moderate hypertension.

As would be predicted with an agent that inhibits sympathetic outflow, it has been established that guanabenz decreases plasma concentrations of catecholamines and dopamine β-hydroxylase activity (41,42). It has also been shown that the greatest decreases in catecholamines occur in those patients whose resting catecholamines levels are highest, suggesting that hypertension characterized by increased sympathetic activity is particularly responsive to this form of treatment (43). This study has also shown that guanabenz attenuates the increases in plasma concentrations of both norepinephrine and epinephrine during exercise, whereas clonidine seems to diminish only the concentrations of norepinephrine. Thus, it is possible that these two agents might have differing effects on adrenomedullary responsiveness to sympathetic stimuli. Guanabenz also has a modest inhibitory effect on plasma renin activity. Although there is little change in renin values in low-renin hypertensive patients during guanabenz treatment, most patients with normal or high renin values tend to have decreases in plasma renin activity during treatment.

The metabolic effects of guanabenz may be of clinical relevance. Guanabenz has been shown to reduce serum concentrations of total cholesterol (44,45), sometimes by as much as 10%. The decrease appears to be due primarily to a reduction in the low-density lipoprotein fraction (46), and it has also been reported that triglyceride concentrations may be reduced. These effects may be related, at least in part, to direct actions of the drug on hepatic synthesis and on fatty acid oxidation (47). Guanabenz does not appear to influence glucose metabolism (45,48). Measurements of insulin, glucogen, and growth hormone remain unchanged during chronic treatment with this agent (48). Moreover, in a multicenter study in diabetic hypertensive patients, we found that no changes in diabetic therapy were necessitated by concurrent antihypertensive therapy with guanabenz (49).

Guanfacine

Guanfacine has recently become available for clinical use in the United States. Its essential characteristics resemble those of clonidine and guanabenz, but its once-daily efficacy may add to its acceptance in the clinical setting. Preliminary studies in animal models have documented that guanfacine is an alpha-adrenergic agonist in both the central nervous system and the peripheral arterial circulation. Low-dose infusions in the dog have shown that whereas intravenous guanfacine produced no consistent hemodynamic effect, administration directly into the vertebral artery produced marked blood-pressure-lowering responses. Moreover, these effects could be prevented by pretreatment with phentolamine (50). Guanfacine also has been shown to decrease sympathetic outflow from the central nervous system as measured directly in studies of sympathetic nerve flow (51). This agent slightly slows the heart rate, presumably through its facilitation of reflex bradycardia (52). It produces the expected transitory pressor responses when given to the pithed rat (50); these effects can be blocked by phentolamine, yohimbine, and prazosin (53,54). However, guanfacine has a far greater selectivity for the alpha-2-adrenergic receptor than for the alpha-1-receptor (55).

Guanfacine produces strong antihypertensive effects (56) in hypertensive patients. There are concomitant decreases in plasma concentrations of catecholamines and renin activity, but the relationship between these changes and those in blood pressure have not been directly established (56). Other metabolic changes include decreases in serum prolactin but not in growth hormone (57). The plasma lipid concentrations, including total cholesterol and triglycerides, are also slightly decreased; there appears to be no change in glucose metabolism as judged by glucose tolerance tests (57). Hemodynamically, guanfacine works primarily by decreasing peripheral resistance. Interestingly, it also appears to reduce right atrial pressure, suggesting that it may be a useful agent in patients with ventricular dysfunction in whom a reduction in preload may be of value (56).

Studies with guanfacine as antihypertensive monotherapy have established its efficacy when used once daily, most typically in doses of 1 mg (58–60). It has been found to be significantly more effective than placebo in decreasing blood pressure and has been observed to have efficacy similar to that of guanabenz. In these studies, guanfacine did not alter measurements of plasma volume, emphasizing its potential suitability as a single agent for the treatment of hypertension. However, it also has been shown to be highly effective when used as a second-line agent in addition to pretreatment with a diuretic. When added to chlorthalidone (61), it has been shown to produce significant further decrements in blood pressure. Interestingly, this effect of guanfacine occurs in a very narrow dosage range: 0.5 mg daily was found not to be more effective than placebo, and doses of 2 or 3 mg daily were no more effective than just 1 mg daily. This study, as well as a further wide-scale multicenter experience (62), emphasized that the incidence of significant symptomatic adverse effects was low and that only a very small percentage of patients voluntarily discontinued treatment. As with all drugs of this type, sudden discontinuation of treatment with guanfacine results in an increase in blood pressure, but the rate of rise is less than that observed with clonidine (62). A large multinational study, conducted primarily in Europe, has confirmed the efficacy and good side-effect profile of guanfacine when administered in low doses. This experience has documented the use of this agent, either alone or in combination with a variety of other drugs for up to 7 years, and has reported that antihypertensive efficacy and patient acceptance of guanfacine appears to be sustained during chronic administration (63).

Methyldopa

The antihypertensive efficacy of this agent was established in 1960, and it was made available for general use in 1963. As with clonidine, methyldopa appears to produce its antihypertensive action through its effects in the central nervous system. Injections of small doses of methyldopa directly into the vertebral artery or into the cerebral ventricle produce reductions in arterial blood pressure. It is likely that the antihypertensive action of methyldopa is dependent on stimulation of alpha-adrenergic receptors that are probably located in the nucleus tractus solitarii of the medulla. In confirmation of this idea that an alpha-agonist mechanism is involved, the antihypertensive action of methyldopa can be blocked by pretreatment with the alpha-blocking agent phentolamine (64). The activation of these receptors is not directly by methyldopa itself but, instead, by its metabolite α-methylnorepinephrine, which is formed within the brain. Indeed, inhibition of dopamine-β-hydroxylase, which is an essential factor in the formation of α-methylnorepinephrine, decreases the antihypertensive efficacy of methyldopa (65). Injection of the metabolite directly into the cerebral ventricle produces decreases in blood pressure that actually are greater than those produced by methyldopa itself (66).

Actions of methyldopa in the periphery may also contribute to its antihypertensive effect. The false neurotransmitter theory was long considered the best explanation for methyldopa's antihypertensive action. It has been shown that methyldopa and its metabolite, α-methylnorepinephrine, like norepinephrine, are taken up by the adrenergic nerve endings. At neuronal discharge, α-methylnorepinephrine is released together with the native norepinephrine and competes with it at the postsynaptic alpha-adrenergic receptor. It is likely that α-methylnorepinephrine is less potent than norepinephrine in producing vasoconstrictor effects when interacting with the alpha-receptor and thus causes an overall reduction in vascular tone and blood pressure. In animal studies, however, this mechanism has not been consistently verified (67), and it has not been possible to be totally certain that the antihypertensive action of methyldopa is due directly to the generation of α-methylnorepinephrine (68).

A further theory has postulated that methyldopa might interfere with the biosynthesis of norepinephrine. Thus, it was suggested that methyldopa might inhibit the enzyme dopa decarboxylase, which is responsible for the formation of dopamine from dopa and is a necessary part of the production of the final neurotransmittor, norepinephrine. Although inhibition of norepinephrine appears to be an effective way to reduce blood pressure, it now seems less likely that methyldopa works through this mechanism, because while the racemic (D, L) preparation of methyldopa is required for the full antihypertensive action (69), only the L-isomer poses decarboxylation properties (70). As with clonidine, methyldopa also has an inhibitory effect on renin release. Although this mechanism has not been highly studied, it has been shown that the antirenin action of methyldopa can potentially play a part during its use as single-agent therapy (71) or in combination with a diuretic (72).

The hemodynamic effects of methyldopa are summarized in Table 1. During chronic treatment there is a decrease in total peripheral resistance, with a maintenance of cardiac output at baseline levels (73). Although there is a tendency for blood pressure to be decreased to a greater extent in the standing posture than in the supine posture, this orthostatic effect is less than that seen with peripheral adrenergic blockers such as guanethidine (74). Like clonidine, the antihypertensive action of methyldopa is not associated with decreases in glomerular filtration rate or renal blood flow, factors that enhance the usefulness of this agent in patients with renal insufficiency (75).

The maximum antihypertensive effect of methyldopa occurs approximately 6 hr after an oral dose, and some antihypertensive effectiveness may persist for up to 48 hr. As single-agent therapy, methyldopa controls blood pressure in up to 70% of patients with mild hypertension and is also effective in patients with more severe forms of hypertension (76). The addition of a diuretic to methyldopa adds considerable antihypertensive effect: Approximately two-thirds of patients with mild, moderate, or severe hypertension can have their blood pressure normalized with this combination. Since methyldopa given alone frequently causes compensatory retention of salt and water, which then decreases its long-term antihypertensive effectiveness, it has become customary for this agent to be given in combination with a diuretic. Moreover, the addition of the diuretic often enables blood pressure control to be obtained with relatively modest doses of each drug.

The most common adverse effect with methyldopa, as shown in Table 2, is drowsiness or excessive sedation; this is troublesome in approximately one-quarter of all patients. The drowsiness will usually diminish with continued use of the drug. Less well defined problems with mentation—including difficulty in concentrating and amnesia-like episodes, as well as difficulties in calculation or the retention of newly obtained information—also may occur (77). Postural dizziness is seen in about 15% of patients taking methyldopa. Sexual dysfunction and fluid retention are not uncommon. Dry mouth and gastrointestinal upsets are also seen occasionally. Approximately 5–10% of patients will be forced to discontinue treatment with methyldopa because of adverse effects.

Methyldopa also may sometimes induce a positive direct Coomb's test, hemolytic anemia, hepatitis, or drug fever. The positive direct Coombs' reaction occurs in approximately 25% of patients taking methyldopa; the antibody is directed against the Rh locus, not against the drug (78). However, only about 5% of patients with a Coombs' reaction (i.e., less than 1% of all patients given methyldopa) will actually develop hemolytic anemia. A form of hepatitis indistinguishable from viral hepatitis occurs in approximately 2% of patients receiving methyldopa. This phenomenon is manifested by elevated liver enzymes and requires termination of the methyldopa treatment. Usually the liver function chemistries will return to normal after the drug has been stopped (79). Drug fever, either with or without associated liver findings, occurs in approximately 1% of patients receiving this drug (80). It is advised that methyldopa not be given to patients with a history of liver disease or hypersensitivity to the drug.

Despite these rare adverse effects, methyldopa has for a long time represented a palatable and effective form of antihypertensive therapy. Its future role will become clearer as it is compared with newer types of antihypertensive agents. Recently, this agent was a principal form of treatment in a major clinical trial of the benefits of antihypertensive therapy in the elderly (81); the positive findings of this study, as discussed elsewhere in this volume, have again emphasized that this long available agent may still have an important role to play in the management of clinical hypertension.

Reserpine

This agent is considered briefly in this chapter because it clearly has important central mechanisms of action despite the effects it exerts at other sites. It depletes norepinephrine and serotonin stores in the brain and in peripheral adrenergic nerve endings. In animal studies, tissue catecholamine concentrations begin to fall 1 hr after administration of reserpine and reach their nadir by 24 hr. There are two mechanisms postulated by which this effect could be achieved. First, it has been suggested that reserpine enhances the degradation of norepinephrine by blocking its incorporation into protective chromaffin granules. Second, it is possible that reserpine blocks the uptake of dopamine into the storage granules in which dopamine would be converted to norepinephrine (82). Within the central nervous system, these actions of reserpine presumably occur in the vasomotor center in the medulla oblongata and also in the hypothalamus (83).

Despite the importance of its action in the central nervous system, reserpine works in a fashion different from that postulated for clonidine, guanabenz, or methyldopa; it appears to have an inhibitory effect on adrenergic mechanisms rather than the agonist action suggested for the other agents. However, centrally determined side effects such as drowsiness and sedation occur as frequently with reserpine as with the other agents. There also appears to be an increase in vagal tone similar to that produced by clonidine, a factor which may explain the decrease in heart rate seen with reserpine (84). There is an increase in gastric acid secretion during reserpine treatment that also may be mediated through an increase in vagal tone. The cardiovascular effects of reserpine are summarized in Table 1, and its adverse effects are listed in Table 2. Reserpine remains an effective antihypertensive drug, is inexpensive, and has the convenience of once-daily dosage. Concern about some of its adverse effects has resulted, however, in a gradual decrease in its use during the last few years.

CLINICAL CHARACTERISTICS

There are many differing types of antihypertensive agents now available, and the selection of a particular drug is often a matter of the personal preference or experience of the prescribing physician. The most commonly used doses of the drugs described in this article are given in Table 3. The centrally acting agents continue to play an important role in antihypertensive therapy because of their generally safe profile and their effectiveness. They tend to have slightly more symptomatic side effects than are found with newer types of agents such as the converting-enzyme inhibitors or the calcium-channel blockers; however, a growing experience with the centrally acting drugs has indicated that their use in low dosages will minimize unwanted side effects without causing substantial decreases in efficacy. A comparison of these agents with diuretics and beta-blockers, which are probably the most commonly prescribed antihypertensive drugs, is given in Table 4. This comparison suggests that there are circumstances in which the centrally acting drugs might be preferable. Moreover, a major clinical trial recently completed in the United Kingdom by the Medical Research Council, using a diuretic and a beta-blocker, suggested that the incidence of adverse effects with these types of drugs was comparatively high (85).

The overall strategy of using antihypertensive drugs is not a focus of this chapter, but as a generalization, it can be stated that the centrally acting agents can be used at virtually any stage of a stepped-care approach to the treatment of hypertension. As already indicated, these agents all work well in combination with diuretics, often allowing good results to be achieved with comparatively low doses of the agents employed. These agents also work well in combination with vasodilators such as hydralazine or minoxidil. For example, it has been shown that clonidine is at least as effective as propranolol when given together with hydralazine and a diuretic in patients with more severe forms of hypertension (86). In patients with treatment-resistant hypertension, it also has been found that the superimposition of clonidine on complex multidrug antihypertensive regimens can be highly effective in inducing blood pressure control (24).

When clonidine or other centrally acting agents are combined with the beta-blocking agent propranolol (Table 5) there is an additive effect, and blood pressure falls more than with either agent given alone (31). This suggests that these two types of agents have differing antihypertensive mechanisms: The antirenin action of propranolol (together with its other mechanisms of action, which are poorly understood) contributes importantly to its blood-pressure-

TABLE 3. *Dosages of centrally acting antihypertensive agents*[a]

Drug	Starting dose	Recommended range	Maximum dose
Clonidine	0.1	0.1–0.4	1.2
Guanabenz	4	4–16	32
Guanfacine	1.0	1.0–3.0	3.0
Methyldopa	250	250–1000	1500
Reserpine	0.1	0.1–0.25	0.25

[a] All doses are in milligrams; each dose is usually given twice daily except for reserpine, which is usually given once daily. Lower starting doses can be employed, especially in elderly patients or when used in combination therapy.

TABLE 4. *Clinical effects of three types of antihypertensive therapy*

	Centrally acting agents	Beta-blockers	Diuretics
Young patients	Effective	Effective	Less effective
Elderly patients	Effective	Less effective	Effective
Black patients	Effective	Less effective	Effective
White patients	Effective	Effective	Less effective
Concurrent diabetes mellitus	Safe and effective	Caution with insulin-taking patients	May influence concurrent diabetes therapy
Cholesterol	Decrease	Possible HDL decrease	Possible increase
Adverse metabolic changes	None or rare	None or rare	Potassium and other factors influenced
Exercise tolerance	No change	Decrease	Decrease
Left ventricular abnormalities	Potential improvement	Inconsistent or no change	No change

lowering activity (87), whereas clonidine, while also exhibiting part of its antihypertensive action through its renin-lowering effect, works largely through inhibition of sympathetic activity. Of interest, the heart-rate-lowering effects of these two agents also are additive. Propranolol works presumably through its direct inhibitory action on the heart, whereas clonidine lowers heart rate through its enhancement of vagal tone.

It is also of interest to consider the interaction of clonidine with the alpha-adrenergic-blocking agent prazosin (Table 5). The sites of the principal antihypertensive actions of these two agents are different: Clonidine works chiefly within the central nervous system, whereas prazosin works at the peripheral postsynaptic alpha-adrenergic receptor. Despite this difference, both agents ultimately have the same effect—namely, blocking the vasoconstriction produced when the sympathetic nervous system, through its neurotransmittor norepinephrine, stimulates the postsynaptic alpha-adrenergic receptor. Thus, it is not surprising that it has been found that the addition of prazosin in patients already being treated with clonidine fails to bring about further antihypertensive effects (88). It is likely that the central action of clonidine (and presumably of guanabenz or methyldopa) in suppressing sympathetic outflow is so effective that there is virtually no peripheral sympathetic vascular drive remaining to be blocked by the prazosin

TABLE 5. *Blood pressure values (mean ± SEM) in crossover studies utilizing clonidine (0.3 mg/day) and propranolol (120 mg/day) (n = 8), or clonidine (0.3 mg/day) and prazosin (15 mg/day) (n = 13)*[a]

Treatment	Systolic blood pressure (mmHg)	Diastolic blood pressure (mmHg)
Control	166 ± 5	109 ± 2
Clonidine alone	149 ± 3[b]	96 ± 3[b]
Propranolol alone	149 ± 5[b]	100 ± 3[b]
Clonidine + propranolol	146 ± 7[b]	93 ± 3[b]
Control	158 ± 7	100 ± 3
Clonidine alone	142 ± 5[b]	92 ± 3[b]
Prazosin alone	144 ± 5	94 ± 1[b]
Clonidine + prazosin	143 ± 8[b]	93 ± 6[b]

[a] All measurements were in the seated position.
[b] $p < 0.05$ or better when compared with control value.

action. A further unproductive combination is that between reserpine and guanethidine; however, because each of these agents are now used infrequently, the likelihood of this combination being used is small.

Occasionally, the sudden cessation of treatment with the centrally acting agents can provoke a rapid rise in blood pressure to its pretreatment values, or to even higher levels. This effect, sometimes described as a discontinuation syndrome, has been described in detail elsewhere (89).

A TRANSDERMAL FORM OF CLONIDINE

Transdermal clonidine is administered in a small skin-colored patch that contains sufficient drug to provide treatment for 7 days at a time. Three differing sizes of this device provide, respectively, 0.1 mg, 0.2 mg, or 0.3 mg of clonidine per day. The skin patches are water resistant and adhere well to the skin, allowing patients to undertake a full range of physical activities while wearing them.

The pharmokinetic characteristics of the transdermal clonidine provide some of its main potential advantages as an antihypertensive therapy. After the skin patch is first applied it takes 2–3 days for the clonidine to reach its stable plasma concentration, owing to an initial period of skin sequestration of the drug. Once the clonidine has reached its plateau level, it remains constant on a relatively permanent basis. When one patch is removed (after approximately 1 week), the clonidine disappears slowly from the plasma, owing to the accumulated drug in the skin reservoir. Thus, when a new patch is administered (typically at another site), it starts providing sufficient clonidine so that, together with the residual drug from the previous patch, the plasma drug concentration remains constant. The actual amount of clonidine able to pass through the skin varies slightly according to the location used; the most practical and effective areas appear to be the chest or the upper outer arm.

The evenness of the plasma clonidine concentrations during transdermal therapy is a key to the attractiveness of this method of administration. When conventional oral medications are used, their plasma concentrations tend to reach high peak concentrations soon after the tablets are ingested; thereafter, there is a steady decline in plasma concentration to the trough level that immediately precedes administration of the next tablet. It is likely that symptomatic side effects associated with drug administration are associated with the peak plasma concentrations. Thus, it is not surprising that when transdermal clonidine has been substituted for the oral form of the agent, there has been a marked reduction in the incidence of symptomatic side effects (90).

The most common complaint with the transdermal clonidine preparation has been with skin reactions which occur most commonly between 3 weeks and 9 months after the start of treatment. Up to 20% of patients treated with this device complain of a localized reaction that occurs typically under the patch itself. This reaction can vary from a mild, nonspecific, superficial irritation to a localized allergic response. Occasionally, this latter reaction can be associated with formation of small vesicles or superficial ulcerations. Regardless of the type of reaction, cessation of treatment is associated with disappearance of the skin lesion. If the skin reaction is not severe, patients may elect to continue treatment; there have been no reports of systemic or generalized reactions to this form of treatment that are of clinical concern. Moreover, subsequent challenging of patients who have experienced allergic reactions to the skin patch with large oral doses of clonidine have reactivated the skin responses in only one or two instances; again, cessation of the treatment resulted in rapid disappearance of these manifestations. Patients most likely to incur a skin reaction are those with very fair skin. It is also possible that women are slightly more susceptible than men.

Multiple clinical trials with transdermal clonidine have shown its efficacy across the full demographic spectrum of hypertensive patients (91). It has been found to work well in elderly patients as well as in the young, and it has also been found to be equally effective in black and white patients. Moreover, it works well in patients with renal insufficiency and in those with diabetes mellitus. As with other forms of antihypertensive therapy, it is effective as monotherapy in approximately 60% of patients with mild to moderate essential hypertension.

Its greatest attribute, however, is its convenience and avoidance of generalized side effects. Table 6 summarizes physician and patient evaluations of this form of treatment as compared with previous forms of antihypertensive therapy. In this surveillance of over 3000 patients (92) there is clearly a strong acceptance of this newer form of treatment. The attraction of taking medication on a once-weekly basis appears to be strong, allowing patients to go for long periods of time without being reminded of their requirements for medical support. It is also of practical value in some older or infirm patients who are unable (for physical or emotional reasons) to be responsible for taking their own medications. The administration of this treatment in such individuals can be easily undertaken by relatives or other personnel. Overall, the interesting characteristics of this innovative form of therapy should make it attractive in a substantial proportion of hypertensive patients. Where unwanted side effects, poor compliance, or inadequate results have occurred with conventional forms of treatment, the transdermal clonidine preparation might offer a good alternative for achieving satisfactory and well-tolerated control of blood pressure.

TABLE 6. *Acceptability of transdermal clonidine therapy in patients switched from treatment with oral antihypertensive agents*[a]

	Patients (%)	Physicians (%)
Highly satisfied	46	43
Satisfied	32	36
Indifferent or dissatisfied	20	20
Highly dissatisfied	2	1

[a] Results were obtained in 3059 patients and 451 physicians responding to questionnaires concerning transdermal clonidine therapy (92).

CONSIDERATIONS IN THE ELDERLY

The centrally acting antihypertensive agents, with their ability to inhibit sympathetic mechanisms, would be appropriate forms of therapy for older hypertensive patients. There has been a strong experience with clonidine in treating elderly patients. It has been found that both the oral and the transdermal form of this agent are effective in decreasing the predominantly systolic hypertension found in this age group; moreover, this antihypertensive effect has been shown to occur without producing unwanted changes in cerebral blood flow (93). In an earlier study in patients with predominantly systolic hypertension, it was found that effective antihypertensive effects could be produced by low doses of clonidine administered in combination with the diuretic chlorthalidone (94). Moreover, these results could be achieved in a majority of patients with a single nighttime dosage, thereby adding to the convenience of the treatment and minimizing its potential symptomatic side effects.

A large-scale analysis of treatment with guanabenz in the elderly has also been carried out (95). Approximately 50% of these patients, aged 61–76 years, had decreases of at least 20 mmHg in systolic blood pressure when treated with guanabenz alone; similar results were found in patients receiving a combination of guanabenz and hydrochlorothiazide. As with clonidine, this agent was found to be generally well tolerated by the patients. Recently, methyldopa was used in a large-scale European study of the long-term benefits of treating hypertension in the elderly. In these subjects, whose age averaged 72 years and who were followed for up to 7 years, the combination of a diuretic with methyldopa produced sustained antihypertensive effects (81). Of even greater importance, major cardiovascular events and cardiovascular mortality were decreased by approximately 40% in patients receiving these active medications as compared with those receiving only placebo. These various studies, therefore, tend to indicate that the centrally acting antihypertensive agents might be particularly appropriate as antihypertensive therapy in elderly subjects.

CENTRALLY ACTING AGENTS AND LEFT VENTRICULAR HYPERTROPHY

Left ventricular hypertrophy, which is a common finding in hypertension, may be a risk factor that is independent of

65. Day MD, Roach AG, Whiting RL. The mechanisms of the antihypertensive action of alpha-methyldopa in hypertensive rats. *Eur J Pharmacol* 1973;21:271.
66. Heise A, Kroneberg G. Alpha-sympathetic receptor stimulation in the brain and hypotensive activity of alpha-methyldopa. *Eur J Pharmacol* 1972;17:315.
67. Haefely W, Hurlimann A, Thoeneu H. The effect of stimulation of sympathetic nerves in the cat treated with reserpine, alpha-methyldopa, and alpha-methylmetatyrosine. *Br J Pharmacol* 1966;26:172.
68. Van Zwieten PA. Centrally mediated action of alpha-methyldopa. In: Onesti G, Fernandes M, Kim KE, eds. *Regulation of blood pressure by the central nervous system.* New York: Grune & Stratton, 1976;293.
69. Gillespie L Jr, Oates JA, Crout JR, et al. Clinical and chemical studies with alpha-methyldopa in patients with hypertension. *Circulation* 1962;25:281.
70. Porter CC, Totaro JA, Leiby CM. Some biochemical effects of alpha-methyl-3,4-dihydroxyphenylalanine and related compounds in mice. *J Pharmacol Exp Ther* 1961;134:139.
71. Weidmann P, Hirsch D, Maxwell MH, et al. Plasma renin and blood pressure during treatment with methyldopa. *Am J Cardiol* 1974;34:671.
72. Kaplan NM. Antihypertensive drugs in combination. *Arch Int Med* 1975;135:660.
73. Onesti G, et al. Pharmacodynamic effects and clinical use of alpha-methyldopa at rest and during exercise in patients with arterial hypertension. *Acta Medica Scand* 1962;171:75.
74. Oates JA, et al. The relative efficacy of guanethidine, methyldopa and pargyline as antihypertensive agents. *N Engl J Med* 1965;273:729.
75. Brodwall EK, Myrhe E, Stenbaek O, et al. The effect of methyldopa on renal function in patients with renal insufficiency. *Acta Med Scand* 1966;191:339.
76 Johnson P, Kitching AA, et al. Treatment of hypertension with methyldopa. *Br Med J* 1972;1:133.
77 Adler S. Methyldopa-induced decrease in mental activity. *JAMA* 1974;230:1428.
78. Lo Buglio AF, Jandl JH. The nature of the alpha-methyldopa red-cell antibody. *N Engl J Med* 1967;176:658.
79. Elkington SG, Schreiber WM, Conn HO. Hepatic injury caused by L-alphamethyldopa. *Circulation* 1969;40:589.
80. Glontz GE, Saslow S. Methyldopa fever. *Arch Int Med* 1968;122:445.
81. Amery A, Birkenhager W, Brixko P, et al. Mortality and morbidity results from the European Working Party on high blood pressure in the elderly trial. *Lancet* 1985;1(8442):1349.
82. Rutledge CO, Weiner N. The effect of reserpine upon the synthesis of norepinephrine in the isolated rabbit heart. *J Pharmacol Exp Ther* 1967;157:290.
83. Molzbauer M, Vogt M. Depression by reserpine of the noradrenaline concentration in the hypothalamus of the cat. *J Neurochem* 1956;1:8.
84. Cohen SJ, et al. Effects of reserpine therapy on cardiac output and atrioventricular conduction during rest and controlled heart rates in patients with essential hypertension. *Circulation* 1968;37:738.
85. Medical Research Council Working Party. MRC trial of treatment of mild hypertension: principal results. *Br Med J* 1985;291(6488):97.
86. Mroczek WJ, Davidov ME. A randomized clinical trial of clonidine and propranolol in hypertensive patients receiving a diuretic and a vasodilator. *Curr Ther Res* 1978;23:294.
87. Buhler FR, Laragh JH, Baer L, et al. Propranolol inhibition or renin secretion. *N Engl J Med* 1972;287:1209.
88. Hubbell FA, Weber MA, Drayer JIM. Neutralization of prazosin's antihypertensive effect in the presence of clonidine [Abstract]. *Clin Res* 1981;29:272A.
89. Weber MA. Discontinuation syndrome following cessation of treatment with clonidine and other antihypertensive agents. *J Cardiovasc Pharmacol* 1980;2(Suppl 1):S73.
90. Weber MA, Drayer JIM. Clinical experience with rate-controlled delivery of antihypertensive therapy by a transdermal system. *Am Heart J* 1984;108:231.
91. Weber MA, Drayer JIM, McMahon FG, et al. Transdermal administration of clonidine for treatment of high BP. *Arch Int Med* 1984;144:1211.
92. Hollifield J. Clinical acceptability of transdermal clonidine: a large-scale evaluation by practitioners. *Am Heart J* 1986; 112:900–906.
93. Reed WG, Devous M, Kirk LM, et al. Effects of catapres-TTS on cerebral blood flow in elderly hypertensive patients. New York: Springer-Verlag, 1985;22.
94. Gray DR, Weber MA, Drayer JIM. Effects of low-dose antihypertensive therapy in elderly patients with predominant systolic hypertension. *J Gerontol* 1983;38:302.
95. Weber MA, Drayer JIM. Treatment of hypertension in the elderly. *South Med J* 1986;79:323.
96. Kannel WB. The Framingham study. *Am J Med* 1983;75:4.
97. Tarazi RC, Sen S, Saracoga M, et al. The multifactorial role of catecholamines in hypertensive cardiac hypertrophy. *Eur Heart J* 1982;3(Suppl A):103.
98. Reichek N, Franklin BB, Chandler T, et al. Reversal of left ventricular hypertrophy by antihypertensive therapy. *Eur Heart J* 1982;3(Suppl A):165.
99. Fouad FM, Nahashima Y, Tarazi RC, et al. Differential binding of guanabenz and its metabolites to cerebral alpha-2 receptors. *Drug Dev Res* 1983;3:91.
100. Drayer JIM, Gardin JM, Weber MA. Changes in cardiac anatomy and function during therapy with alpha-methyldopa: an echocardiographic study. *Curr Ther Res* 1982;32:856.
101. Drayer JIM, Weber MA, Gardin JM. Mediators of changes in left ventricular mass during antihypertensive therapy. In: Keurs HEDJ, Schipperheyn JJ, eds. *Cardiac LVH.* Boston: Martinus Nijhoff, 1984;224.
102. Walson PD, Graver P, Rath A, et al. Effects of guanabenz in adolescent hypertension. *J Cardiovasc Pharmacol* 1984;6:S814.
103. McMahon FG, Ryan MR Jr, et al. Regression of left ventricular hypertrophy in nineteen hypertensive patients treated with clonidine for eighteen months: a prospective study. In: Weber MA, Drayer JIM, Kolloch R, eds. *Low dose oral and transdermal therapy of hypertension.* Darmstadt: Steinkopff-Verlag, 1985;81.
104. Arevalo JV. Clonidine and left ventricular function in patients with arterial hypertension. *Trib Med* 1983;68:29.
105. Weber MA, Graettinger WF, Drayer JIM. The adrenergic inhibitors. *Med Clin North Am* 1987;71(5):959–977.
106. Dreslinski GR, Frolich ED, Dunn FG, et al. Echocardiographic diastolic ventricular abnormality in hypertensive heart disease: atrial emptying index. *Am J Cardiol* 1981;47:1087.

Hypertension: Pathophysiology, Diagnosis, and Management, edited by J. H. Laragh and B. M. Brenner. Raven Press, Ltd., New York © 1990.

CHAPTER 143

Vasodilators

Brian F. Robinson and N. Benjamin

Mechanisms of Vasodilatation, 2263
Classification of Vasodilators, 2264
Differential Effects of Dilators on Blood Vessels of Different Types, 2265
Hemodynamic Effects, 2265
Vasodilators Used in Hypertension, 2266
Factors Determining the Effectiveness of a Vasodilator in Hypertension, 2266
Nitro Vasodilators, 2266
Hydralazine, 2268
Diazoxide, 2270
Minoxidil, 2271
Antihypertensive Dilators: Similarities and Differences, 2272
References, 2273

Among the earliest drugs to be found effective in reducing severely elevated arterial pressure were arteriolar dilators such as thiocyanate and magnesium sulfate. Such agents were, however, potentially toxic and had to be given by intravenous infusion. Consequently, they could be used only for short periods in circumstances such as hypertensive encephalopathy or eclampsia. It was not until the early 1950s, with the introduction of hydralazine, that a dilator agent became available that could be given orally in long-term therapy. Since that time, many new vasodilators have been developed, and some (but by no means all) have proved effective in the treatment of systemic hypertension. It is still unclear, however, why one substance that is found to be a potent arteriolar dilator in acute experiments turns out to be highly effective in the treatment of hypertension, whereas another with a pattern of action that is superficially similar but which works in a different way is of no value at all.

The slow growth of our understanding of the mechanisms by which dilator substances exert their effects reflects, in part, the complexity of the processes governing contraction and relaxation in vascular smooth muscle, which are themselves only just beginning to be unraveled. It is now possible, however, to define some of the basic mechanisms by which drugs induce vasodilatation and to attempt a general classification of the various agents in this group.

MECHANISMS OF VASODILATATION

The contraction of vascular smooth muscle depends on an increase in the concentration of free calcium in the cytosol. It is now widely accepted that the effect of calcium is mediated through the formation of a calcium–calmodulin complex which leads to activation of myosin light-chain kinase with consequent phosphorylation of the myosin light chains (1). This, in turn, permits interaction of myosin and actin with the development of tension. The relation between ionic calcium concentration and tension development appears not to be constant, however, partly because of the influence of various modulators on the activity of the calcium–calmodulin complex. The trigger for the increase in cytosolic calcium may be either (a) an extrinsic constrictor such as norepinephrine or angiotensin II acting through receptors on the cell surface or (b) an intrinsic cellular mechanism acting in ways that are as yet incompletely defined. Either of these activating systems may give rise to (a) an influx of calcium through specific membrane channels (of which there are more than one type) and/or (b) the release of calcium from intracellular stores. Relaxation is effected by a reversal of this process, with a removal of calcium from the cytosol either by sequestration in the intracellular stores or by extrusion across the cell membrane.

The ion channels and transport systems that form the primary calcium-handling mechanisms are themselves subject to regulation by higher-level executive systems that coordinate the ionic fluxes, thereby exerting a modulating influence on the concentration of free calcium in the cytosol. Examples of such systems are provided by the various "second messenger" systems that mediate the action of certain constrictor and dilator agents. Thus the action of α_1-adrenoceptor agonists and many other constrictor substances that act through receptors is thought to result from the hydrolysis of phosphoinositides, leading to the liberation of inositol triphosphate and diacylglycerol, which have multiple actions on the calcium-handling mechanisms resulting in a controlled increase in cytosolic calcium (2). Many dilator agents, both physiological and pharmacological, act by increasing the intracellular concentration of one or other of the cyclic nucleotides, namely, cyclic adenosine monophosphate and cyclic guanosine monophosphate. These substances also have multiple actions within the cell, some of which will influence the calcium-handling processes.

From consideration of the processes known to be involved in the mediation of contraction and relaxation, it is clear that there are a limited number of basic mechanisms through which substances may act to produce vasodilatation:

1. They may inhibit the tonic effect of a constrictor system or may act to prevent depolarization of the cell membrane.
2. They may directly inhibit the entry of calcium through the cell membrane or may interfere with its release from the intracellular stores.
3. They may enhance the sequestration of calcium from the cytosol or may enhance the extrusion of calcium across the cell membrane.
4. They may interfere directly with activation of the contractile machinery.

Some drugs appear to act directly by one of these basic mechanisms (e.g., inhibition of calcium entry by a dihydropyridine), but many act by modulation of the higher-level systems through which the basic processes are regulated. In attempting a classification of dilator agents, it is therefore necessary to adopt a pragmatic approach which includes not only primary mechanisms but also the "second messenger" systems through which many agents act.

CLASSIFICATION OF VASODILATORS

Table 1 shows a functional classification of vasodilators according to the various known or putative modes of action.

Substances that decrease the local concentration of endogenous constrictors or increase the concentration of dilators. Examples include (a) converting-enzyme inhibitors, which reduce the concentration of angiotensin II, (b) agents such as reserpine, which deplete the adrenergic neuron terminals of transmitter, and (c) dipyridamole, which increases the local concentration of the dilator mediator adenosine by preventing uptake.

Dilators acting by blocking receptors for constrictor agonists. These include α-adrenoreceptor-blocking agents (phentolamine, prazosin, indoramin) and angiotensin-receptor blockers (saralasin). The magnitude of the dilatation induced by such drugs, as well as that induced by those drugs which decrease the availability of constrictors, will, of course, be entirely dependent on the extent to which vascular tone is being maintained by the action of the system they inhibit at the time they are given. The apparent effectiveness of these drugs can thus vary greatly according to the circumstances.

TABLE 1. *A classification of dilator substances*

Class	Action
0	Alter concentration of humoral mediators
	Reduce availability of endogenous constrictors
	Increase availability of endogenous dilators
1	Block receptors for constrictor agonists
2	Prevent membrane depolarization
	K^+-channel agonists
	Cl^--channel blockers
	Na^+,K^+-ATPase stimulators
3	Block membrane calcium channels
4	Increase concentration of cyclic GMP
	Endothelium-dependent dilators
	Nitrovasodilators
	Phosphodiesterase inhibitors
5	Increase concentration of cyclic AMP
	Activators of adenyl cyclase
	Phophodiesterase inhibitors
6	Act directly on contractile machinery
	Prevent phosphorylation of myosin

Dilators acting by inhibition of membrane depolarization. Several mechanisms are known (or have been suggested) by which membrane depolarization may be prevented, but it is not clear whether any existing pharmacological agents actually work in this way. Possible mechanisms include enhancement of potassium efflux (suggested as the mode of action of minoxidil), blockade of chloride efflux (suggested as a possible action of the nitroprusside ion), and stimulation of the electrogenic sodium pump (which is the basis of the dilator action of small increases in extracellular potassium concentration).

Dilators acting by inhibition of calcium influx through specific membrane channels. Examples include verapamil, diltiazem, and the dihydropyridines, of which nifedipine is the prototype. In those types of vascular smooth muscle exhibiting spontaneous electrical activity, the spike potentials are believed to depend on a calcium current; thus, calcium-channel blockers may also act to prevent certain types of membrane depolarization.

Dilators acting by increasing intracellular concentrations of cyclic guanosine monophosphate (cGMP). Cyclic GMP is now known to be an important regulator of intracellular calcium handling and of contractile tension (3). It causes activation of a cGMP-dependent protein kinase, with consequent phosphorylation of numerous smooth muscle proteins such as myosin light-chain kinase. The phosphorylation of the myosin light chains is decreased, but it is not yet known whether this results from (a) a reduced sensitivity of the myosin light-chain kinase to the calcium–calmodulin complex, (b) an increased activity of the phosphatase, or (c) a combination of the two. Whatever the mechanism, the reduced level of phosphorylation of myosin will be expected to cause reduced interaction with actin at any given concentration of cytosolic calcium, thereby inducing relaxation. In addition to this direct effect on the contractile machinery, the phosphorylation of calcium-handling proteins may lead to a fall in cytosolic calcium (4) by enhancing uptake into the sarcoplasmic reticulum or increasing net extrusion across the plasma membrane.

Four general mechanisms are known by which the concentration of cGMP may be elevated and by which relaxation may be induced. Dilators such as acetylcholine, histamine, bradykinin, thrombin, and ATP act on the endothelium to cause release of a mediator (endothelium-derived relaxing factor, EDRF) which diffuses to the adjacent smooth muscle, where it stimulates the soluble guanylate cyclase within the cell—thereby enhancing the synthesis of cGMP. The nitrovasodilators (nitroprusside, organic nitrates) act directly on the smooth muscle, again through activation of soluble guanylate cyclase; their detailed mechanism of action is discussed later. Atriopeptins act directly on the membrane-bound guanylate cyclase to increase the synthesis of cGMP. The concentration of cGMP may also be increased by drugs that inhibit breakdown, and experimental agents exist that selectively inhibit the cGMP phosphodiesterase.

Dilators acting by increasing intracellular concentrations of cyclic adenosine monophosphate (cAMP). Cyclic AMP is also an important regulator of the contractile process (5). It is thought to act through the activation of a cAMP-dependent protein kinase, with consequent phosphorylation of a variety of smooth muscle proteins. The final mechanism of action on the contractile system and on calcium handling may thus be very similar to that of cGMP, but cAMP may differ from cGMP in that it does not reduce the concentration of ionized calcium in the cytosol (4).

At least three mechanisms exist through which the concentration of cAMP within the cell may be increased. The β-adrenoceptor agonists increase production of cAMP by activating a membrane-bound adenylate cyclase that is linked to the β-adrenoceptor. Forskolin, a diterpene, is believed to activate the enzyme by acting directly on the catalytic subunit. Drugs such as theophylline and papaverine, which are selective inhibitors of the cAMP phosphodiesterase, increase concentrations of the cyclic nucleotide by reducing breakdown, and they also potentiate the action of drugs that increase synthesis.

Drugs acting directly on the contractile machinery. Both cGMP and cAMP may act, in part, by reducing activation of the contractile machinery, and drugs such as trifluoperazine and prenylamine have also been shown to have such an effect *in vitro.* There is no evidence, however, that any substance used clinically as a dilator works primarily through this mechanism, although it has been postulated that some such as diazoxide might act in this way.

DIFFERENTIAL EFFECTS OF DILATORS ON BLOOD VESSELS OF DIFFERENT TYPES

The mechanisms by which smooth muscle tone is maintained vary between blood vessels of different types. In cutaneous veins, for example, maintained constriction normally depends on the constrictor effect of the sympathetic nerves, and there is little or no intrinsic tone. In the resistance vessels of the forearm, on the other hand, the contribution of the sympathetic nerves is less important whereas intrinsic tone is much more important. With a diversity of activation mechanisms operating, it is not surprising that dilators acting in different ways show different patterns of action on (a) resistance vessels on the one hand and (b) capacitance vessels or larger arteries on the other. Of drugs in clinical usage, α-adrenoreceptor antagonists have a selective effect on veins when given acutely, reflecting the dependence of capacitance vessels on sympathetically mediated constriction. The magnitude of the effect, however, varies greatly in different patients and at different times, depending on the level of sympathetic constrictor tone. Organic nitrates are also highly venoselective in their action.

Calcium-entry blockers are selective for resistance vessels, reflecting the dependence of arteriolar tone on calcium influx through potential-operated membrane channels, a mechanism that is of little or no importance in the veins. Hydralazine, diazoxide, and minoxidil are also, in varying degrees, selective for resistance vessels; the reasons for the selective action of these drugs are not known and may well differ between them.

HEMODYNAMIC EFFECTS

The circulatory response to systemic administration of a dilator depends on the balance between (a) the primary effect of the drug on resistance and capacitance vessels and (b) the effect of the various compensatory mechanisms that are evoked (Fig. 1); the latter may be either short-term or long-term.

The immediate effect of a drug acting mainly on the capacitance system will be to reduce ventricular filling pressures and stroke volume; this will lead to a fall in cardiac output, with a consequent fall in arterial pressure. Because pooling of blood in the dilated venous bed is increased in the upright position, the circulatory changes will be much affected by posture. There will be a reflex increase in heart rate and an increase in sympathetic outflow to the peripheral vasculature. With all existing agents, there is almost always some effect on the resistance vessels which tends to reduce arterial pressure further and limit the fall in cardiac output; the final pattern of response is very variable, depending on the dose of the drug, the subject's posture, and whether the subject is at rest or exercising.

The immediate effect of drugs acting mainly on the arterioles is to reduce arterial pressure as a result of the fall in peripheral resistance. There is again a reflex activation of the sympathetic nerves which, in the presence of maintained ventricular filling pressures, leads to an increase in cardiac output. The circulatory changes are not usually much influenced by posture.

The sympathetic activation that follows administration of a dilator agent tends to wane with time, but it is usually accompanied by increased activity of the renin–angiotensin system which may or may not be maintained. The extent to which renin secretion is stimulated varies greatly, and the factors determining the response have not been clearly defined. A further compensatory mechanism is retention of salt and water by the kidney; this develops over days or weeks, is maintained indefinitely, and may be progressive. The scale of the retention varies greatly with different agents, even though their effect on arterial pressure appears similar.

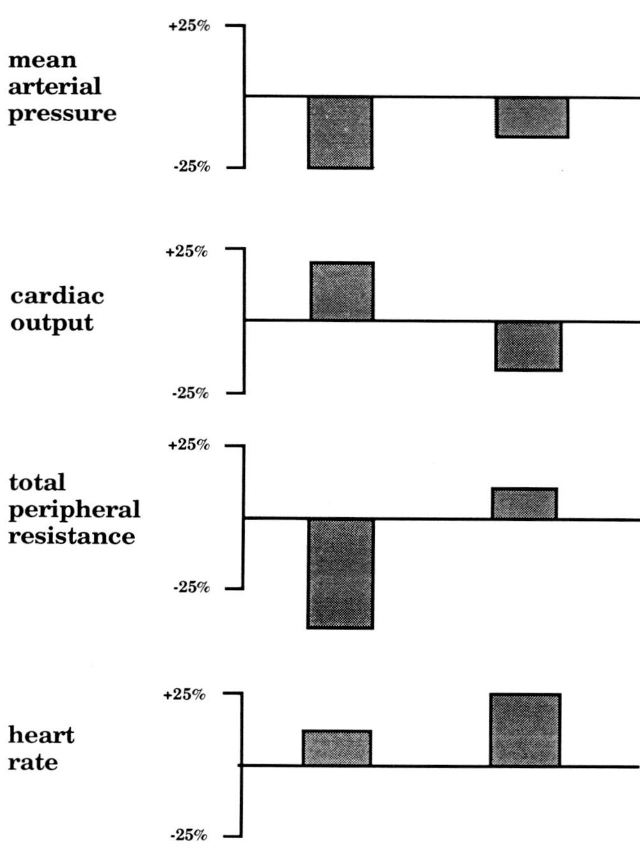

FIG. 1. Circulatory effects of drugs having predominant action on arterioles (diazoxide) and veins (nitroglycerin). Diazoxide reduces peripheral resistance, thereby causing a fall in arterial pressure; this is associated with a rise in heart rate and cardiac output (data from ref. 58). Nitroglycerin has a selective venodilator effect that is most clearly manifest when it is given during exercise. It then reduces cardiac output as a consequence of reduced filling pressure, thereby causing a fall in arterial pressure; this is associated with a rise in heart rate, and peripheral resistance may rise slightly (data from ref. 59). A dominant effect on the venous bed may also be observed in left ventricular failure. In other circumstances, however, the veins are usually less constricted and hence less susceptible to dilatation; nitroglycerin then appears to have a more balanced effect on resistance vessels and veins.

The overall effect of the compensatory mechanisms that have been described is to (a) provide a constrictor stimulus to the blood vessels which opposes the primary dilator action of the drug and (b) restore or increase cardiac output as a result of increased sympathetic stimulation of the heart and expansion of blood volume. All of these actions will tend to diminish the hypotensive effect of the drug.

VASODILATORS USED IN HYPERTENSION

Factors Determining the Effectiveness of a Vasodilator in Hypertension

The most important factors determining the effectiveness of a dilator as an antihypertensive appear to be (a) selectivity for resistance vessels and (b) maintenance of pharmacological action during long-term treatment. The blood-pressure-lowering action of drugs that have little effect on the resistance vessels and act mainly on the veins is essentially short-term, since it depends on the reduction of central venous pressure; with prolonged therapy, this change is quickly reversed by expansion of blood volume, and the effect on arterial pressure is lost.

In general, the arteriolar dilators that have been found to be useful in hypertension include those that inhibit the effect of extrinsic constrictors in some way, those that block calcium channels, and a miscellaneous group of drugs that act directly on the vascular smooth muscle but whose mode of action is uncertain.

Those "direct acting" dilators that work through the cyclic nucleotide control systems have, without exception, proved ineffective in the long-term treatment of raised blood pressure.

Nitro Vasodilators

Nitroglycerin (or glyceryl trinitrate as it is known in the United Kingdom) was first synthesized in 1846 by Ascania Sobrero, and in 1849 its use in the treatment of angina pectoris was suggested by Constantin Hering. In 1867, Lauder Brunton found that isoamyl nitrite has properties similar to those of nitroglycerin and proposed that the nitro group was important for their pharmacological effect. Isosorbide mono- and dinitrate were the product of research into sugar alcohols for use in diabetic diets in the 1930s (6). Clinical studies in the 1960s demonstrated the more prolonged action of these nitrodilators in preventing angina.

Sodium nitroprusside was first synthesized over 100 years ago, and its pharmacological properties were reported by Johnson in 1929, but it was not until its rapid hypotensive action was shown in 1955 (7) that clinical interest was aroused.

Mode of Action and Circulatory Effects

The relaxant effect of the nitrodilators is mediated through an increase in the concentration of cGMP within the cell (8). Their action is thus mediated through the same final mechanism as that of agonists such as acetylcholine, which work through the endothelium. The relaxing factor produced by the endothelium (EDRF) is now thought to be nitric oxide (9), and it is believed that this is the agent that diffuses to the smooth muscle and stimulates the soluble guanylate cyclase to increase production of cGMP. The nitrodilators appear to act directly on the smooth muscle rather than the endothelium, either by serving as a substrate for the generation of nitric oxide or perhaps by stimulating the guanylate cyclase directly. Sodium nitroprusside will spontaneously form nitric oxide in solution (10), whereas the organic nitrates such as isosorbide dinitrate and nitroglycerin must undergo an enzymatic or nonenzymatic reaction. The generation of nitric oxide from organic nitrates has been shown to be accelerated by sulfhydryl compounds, especially cysteine (11); thiols may also be required for subsequent steps in the activation of guanylate cyclase (8,12).

In addition to their effect on cGMP, nitrodilators may also affect cell membrane function. Reduction in membrane potential has been reported (13), although the effect is small and occurs at doses higher than those required to produce relaxation. Changes in membrane permeability to potassium (13) and chloride (10) have been suggested as the mechanism of relaxation in response to nitroprusside, although it is possible that these are secondary to intracellular changes in cGMP or calcium.

Organic nitrates show selectivity toward large arteries and veins and are relatively less potent arteriolar dilators (14). This selectivity may be accounted for by the observation that they are more potent elevators of cGMP in venous tissue than in arterial tissue (15).

At low doses the venodilator effects of organic nitrates predominate, reducing left and right ventricular filling pressure and end-diastolic ventricular volume (16). At higher doses the effects on resistance vessels become apparent, with a greater reduction in systemic arterial pressure. Skeletal muscle blood flow consistently increases, with a less marked effect on renal and mesenteric blood flow (17). Reflex responses to reduced arterial and venous pressure result in an increase in heart rate acutely, although long-term therapy is not associated with alterations in either blood pressure or heart rate in normotensive subjects. There appears to be little effect on renal sodium excretion from long-term use of nitrates.

Sodium nitroprusside shows a pattern of venoselectivity that is similar to that of the nitrates when given locally (14), but it appears to produce approximately equal effects on resistance and capacitance vessels when given systemically (18). This may be due to its rapid clearance on passage through capillary beds (10).

Nitroprusside infusion is rapidly effective in reducing systemic arterial pressure and both systemic and pulmonary venous pressure. Although there is no direct effect on cardiac muscle, cardiac output may be variably affected by the changes in filling pressure and arterial pressure and is also influenced by a reflex-induced increase in heart rate (19). In the anesthetized dog, nitroprusside has been shown to increase coronary, femoral, renal, and mesenteric blood flow (20).

Pharmacokinetics and Metabolism

Extensive reviews on the pharmacokinetics and metabolism of nitroglycerin (21) and isosorbide nitrates (22) show this to be a complex issue. Investigation has been hampered by the difficulty in measuring the extremely small concentrations of nitrate necessary to produce a therapeutic effect.

The organic nitrates are very lipid soluble and are easily absorbed following sublingual, oral, or dermal therapy. Nitroglycerin has a large volume of distribution and a plasma half-life of approximately 3 min following intravenous administration of a bolus in humans. The molecule is rapidly "denitrated" in the liver to produce the less active glyceryl dinitrate or mononitrate. Oral administration is less effective, probably because of extensive first-pass hepatic metabolism.

Isosorbide dinitrate is usually administered orally and also undergoes significant first-pass metabolism, but the resulting isosorbide mononitrate is also active and has a half-life of 4–6 hr.

The detailed pharmacokinetics of sodium nitroprusside have been reviewed by Kreye (10). Nitroprusside has a short biological half-life of less than 1 min as a result of its rapid destruction in the peripheral tissues. The most important metabolite is cyanide, which is rendered less toxic by conversion to thiocyanate and is then slowly excreted by the kidney.

Toxicity and Side Effects

Organic Nitrates

Organic nitrates commonly give rise to a throbbing headache, which is probably secondary to cerebral vasodilatation. The headache often abates within a few days of continued therapy, presumably reflecting tolerance to the drug. First-dose syncope is also common with sublingual nitroglycerin and is thought to result from orthostatic venous pooling. Methemoglobinemia may result from overdosage with organic nitrates, and contact dermatitis occurs occasionally following dermal application.

Sodium Nitroprusside

High-dose infusion may result in accumulation of cyanide, with evidence of poisoning manifested by metabolic acidosis, hypoxemia, tetanic spasms, and death. Thiocyanate poisoning is a hazard with prolonged (greater than 72 hr) infusions, particularly in patients with impaired renal function. A thiocyanate concentration of greater than 120 mg/liter in plasma is considered potentially toxic. Symptoms of thiocyanate poisoning include headache, nausea, vomiting, coma, and death. There is also a theoretical risk of formation of carcinogenic nitrosamines when nitroprusside is administered concurrently with drugs that possess a secondary amine structure (23).

Mode of Use

Organic Nitrates

Nitroglycerin and isosorbide di- and mononitrate produce a reduction of arterial pressure when given acutely. In long-term therapy, however, they are generally considered to be ineffective in reducing blood pressure in hypertensive patients. Recently, a small effect of sustained-release isosorbide dinitrate on systolic blood pressure has been reported in elderly patients with isolated systolic hypertension (24). It is possible that this results from an increased compliance of large vessels rather than from a sustained effect on vascular resistance.

Sodium Nitroprusside

Because of the rapid onset and offset of action, infusion of sodium nitroprusside at doses from 0.5 to 8 μg/kg/min has proved a safe and effective means of producing a controlled reduction of arterial pressure in patients with malignant hypertension, whatever the underlying cause. The wide range of effective doses makes it essential to monitor blood pressure intra-arterially. Nitroprusside has also been used to produce perioperative hypotension in surgical operations where avoidance of blood loss is important.

Tolerance

There is considerable controversy surrounding the subject of tolerance to organic nitrates. Reduction in their antianginal effect with chronic administration, as well as a reduction in therapeutic effect in heart failure, has been shown by most (but not all) studies (for review see ref. 25). The mechanism by which tolerance occurs is not clear. When exposed to high concentrations of organic nitrates *in vitro,* vascular smooth muscle rapidly becomes insensitive to further applications. Pharmacological tolerance also occurs in munitions workers who are subject to high levels of absorption, as evidenced by the coronary and digital vasospasm that may occur 2–3 days after exposure has ceased (26). There are several biochemical steps at which the changes leading to tolerance might occur. Stimulation of guanylate cyclase by nitrates requires the presence of sulfhydryl groups, and it has been suggested that depletion of sulfhydryl-containing cysteine may underlie the development of tolerance (27). It has also been suggested that cytosolic guanylate cyclase becomes less sensitive to nitric oxide with continued stimulation (28); a further possibility would be an increase in phosphodiesterase activity. The development of tolerance in clinical use of the organic nitrates is probably caused only in part, or in some cases not at all, by the induction of pharmacological tolerance. The most important cause of the waning of the circulatory effects is probably an expansion of blood volume in response to sustained dilatation of the capacitance vessels.

Pharmacological tolerance to the relaxant effect of nitroprusside has not been described when this drug is used in a clinical setting.

Hydralazine

Hydralazine was first introduced into clinical practice in the early 1950s. It was used in what are now regarded as very high doses, and initial enthusiasm quickly gave way to disillusion when the high incidence of side effects came to be recognized. There was a renaissance of interest in the 1970s, when it was realized that the drug could usefully be given in much lower doses if used in combination with a β-adrenoceptor antagonist and a diuretic. Since then it has been used widely as the third agent in the "stepped-care" approach, but it is now being replaced by newer drugs such as the calcium-entry blockers.

Analogues of hydralazine with similar, if not identical, pharmacological effects include dihydralazine and endralazine.

Mode of Action and Circulatory Effects

Despite much investigation, the mode of action of hydralazine remains unknown. In contrast to most other dilators, its relaxant effect is restricted to certain blood vessels; moreover, it has no action on other types of smooth muscle. It is a highly effective dilator of resistance vessels but is less effective in causing relaxation of conduit arteries, with variable effects depending on the species, vessel, and type of contraction; it has little or no effect on the veins. Hydralazine is, in general, more active in antagonizing norepinephrine-induced contractions than in antagonizing those induced by high concentrations of potassium (29,30). In rabbit aortic rings, there is evidence of an endothelium-mediated component to the relaxant effect that is important at low concentrations of the drug (30). Other suggested mechanisms of action include interaction with purinergic receptors and an effect on sympathetic constrictor function (see ref. 29 for review); direct inhibition of phosphorylation of myosin light chains has been observed in isolated myofibrils (31). The drug differs from all other dilator agents in the slow onset and prolonged duration of its effect. Following local infusion into the brachial artery over a period of 2 min, no effect can be discerned until shortly after the infusion, when blood flow gradually increases to reach a maximum after 30–60 min; the effect gradually wanes over the next 30–60 min (14). A slow onset of dilatation may also be observed *in vitro* (30).

In accordance with its delayed dilator action when given locally, the blood-pressure-lowering effect of hydralazine is slow to develop (even when the drug is given intravenously) and takes 15–30 min to become apparent. When hydralazine is given by itself, the fall in peripheral resistance is accompanied by tachycardia and an increase in cardiac output, so that the fall in arterial pressure may be relatively small (32).

Within the arterial circulation, hydralazine preferentially affects the coronary, cerebral, splanchnic, and renal circulations, with a lesser effect in skin and muscle (32). Chronic administration usually gives rise to sodium retention, but this is not so severe as with diazoxide or minoxidil; plasma renin activity increases. The reduction in arterial pressure produced by hydralazine correlates with the log plasma concentration when patients are studied as a group (33), but clearly there is much individual variation.

Pharmacokinetics and Metabolism

The drug is well absorbed when given orally, and bioavailability is increased when it is given with food (34). Hydralazine undergoes extensive first-pass metabolism involving acetylation, and fractional availability has been estimated at 0.10–0.15 in subjects with the fast acetylator phenotype and 0.30–0.35 in the slow; it is also subject to oxidative metabolism, and this step may either precede or follow acetylation (35). Free hydralazine in plasma condenses with ketones and keto-acids to form hydrazones, and from some of these at least it may be possible to regenerate hydralazine; there is also evidence that some of the

sion (hydralazine, diazoxide, and minoxidil) are all powerful arteriolar dilators. It is curious that the mode of action should be uncertain for all three, and one wonders if there is some common factor that accounts for their effectiveness.

Sodium retention is a prominent feature of therapy with minoxidil, diazoxide, and, to a lesser extent, hydralazine. It has been thought that sodium retention results from a direct effect of the drug on the renal tubule or that it is secondary to the effect of the drug on the renal vasculature. It is therefore surprising to find that direct infusion of both minoxidil (55) and diazoxide (56) into the renal artery cause an increase in the excretion of salt and water by the kidney. We must conclude that the sodium retention results from the systemic effects of the drugs. Reduction in blood pressure, and hence renal perfusion pressure, is presumably an important factor, but there is almost certainly a contribution from activation of hormonal or neural reflex mechanisms that inhibit sodium excretion. It remains unexplained why other dilators such as calcium-channel-blocking drugs do not promote sodium retention.

Stimulation of renin secretion is another frequent result of dilator therapy, and, as with sodium retention, which it frequently parallels, there is much variation with different drugs. The mechanisms are uncertain but almost certainly include increased sympathetic drive to the juxtaglomerular apparatus, since β-adrenoceptor blockers are effective in preventing the increase.

The development of tolerance is an important problem with all antihypertensive dilators. Physiological tolerance arising as a result of retention of salt and water, with activation of the sympathetic and renin–angiotensin systems, is widely recognized. Pharmacological tolerance (i.e., a reduced responsiveness of the vessels to the agent) has received much less attention. Tolerance to the organic nitrates is well documented, but other factors are probably more important in determining their lack of effectiveness in the treatment of hypertension. Evidence indicating that some patients develop a high degree of tolerance to hydralazine has been presented, and the magnitude of the changes observed makes it likely that pharmacological tolerance is one cause of a poor clinical response to this drug. No comparable studies have been performed on other dilator agents whether they be direct-acting, agonist-inhibiting, or calcium-entry-blocking. This is a surprising omission, since complex physiological systems such as that controlling the contraction and relaxation of vascular smooth muscle tend to be self-stabilizing and frequently respond to simple interventions with compensatory changes that seek to restore their former equilibrium. If, as is probable, a degree of tolerance does occur with some or all dilators, it would signal caution in interpreting the results of acute experiments with hypotensive agents. An encouraging initial response may not always be maintained, and formal studies to assess the occurrence and extent of pharmacological tolerance would seem appropriate at an early stage in the evaluation of all new drugs.

The possibility of using dilator agents in combination has rarely been considered. For such an approach to be successful, it would clearly be necessary for the drugs to have modes of action that were different and in some way complementary; prazosin and hydralazine provide one example of dilators that have a greater effect in combination than when given separately (57). Further exploration of the effect of such combinations would seem justified.

Dilator agents such as diazoxide and minoxidil offer a powerful means by which peripheral resistance can be lowered, and arterial pressure reduced, in patients with severe and resistant hypertension. They are crude instruments, however, acting in an unselective way and are not able to restore the pattern of vascular resistance, and hence of blood flow, to normal. It is, perhaps, not surprising that their use is associated with a high incidence of side effects. The effectiveness of such drugs however, offers the hope that it will be possible to develop dilators that are equally powerful but that have a more physiological pattern of action and that will consequently be more acceptable to patients.

REFERENCES

1. Van Breemen C, Leijten P, Yamamoto H, Aaronson P, Cauvin C. Calcium activation of vascular smooth muscle. *Hypertension* 1986;8(Suppl II):II-89–II-95.
2. Heagerty AM, Ollerenshaw JD. The phosphoinositide signalling system and hypertension. *J Hypertens* 1987;5:515–524.
3. Murad F. Cyclic guanosine monophosphate as a mediator of vasodilation. *J Clin Invest* 1986;78:1–5.
4. Morgan JP, Morgan KG. Alteration of cytoplasmic ionised calcium levels in smooth muscle by vasodilators in the ferret. *J Physiol (Lond)* 1984;357:539–551.
5. Kukovetz WR, Pöch G, Holzmann S. Cyclic nucleotides and relaxation of vascular smooth muscle. In: Vanhoutte PM, Leusen I, eds. *Vasodilatation.* New York: Raven Press, 1981;339–353.
6. Carr CJ. History of the synthesis and pharmacology of isosorbide dinitrate. *Am Heart J* 1985;110:197–201.
7. Page IH, Corcoran AC, Dustan HP, Koppanyi T. Cardiovascular actions of sodium nitroprusside in animals and hypertensive patients. *Circulation* 1955;11:188–198.
8. Ignarro LJ, Lippton H, Edwards JC, et al. Mechanism of vascular smooth muscle relaxation by organic nitrates, nitrites, nitroprusside and nitric oxide: evidence for the involvement of *S*-nitrothiols as active intermediates. *J Pharmacol Exp Ther* 1981;218:739–749.
9. Palmer RMJ, Ferrige AC, Moncada S. Nitric oxide accounts for the biological activity of endothelium-derived relaxing factor. *Nature* 1987;327:524–526.
10. Kreye VAW. Sodium nitroprusside. In: Scriabine A, ed. *Pharmacology of antihypertensive drugs,* New York: Raven Press, 1980;373–396.
11. Yeates RA, Laufen H, Leitold M. The reaction between organic nitrates and sulfhydryl compounds. *Mol Pharmacol* 1985; 28:555–559.
12. Schroder H, Noack E, Muller R. Evidence for a correlation between nitric oxide formation by cleavage of organic nitrates and activation of guanylate cyclase. *J Mol Cell Cardiol* 1985;17:931–934.
13. Cheung DW, MacKay MJ. The effects of sodium nitroprusside and 8-bromo-cyclic GMP on electrical and mechanical activities of the rat tail artery. *Br J Pharmacol* 1985;86:117–124.
14. Collier JG, Lorge RE, Robinson BF. Comparison of effects of tolmesoxide (RX 71107), diazoxide, hydrallazine, prazosin, glyceryl trinitrate and sodium nitroprusside on forearm arteries and dorsal hand veins of man. *Br J Clin Pharmacol* 1978;5:35–44.
15. Edwards JC, Ignarro LJ, Hyman AL, Kadowitz PJ. Relaxation of intrapulmonary artery and vein by nitrogen oxide-containing vasodilators and cyclic GMP. *J Pharmacol Exp Ther* 1984;228:33–42.
16. Bayley S, Valentine H, Bennett ED. The haemodynamic responses to incremental doses of intravenous nitroglycerin in left ventricular failure. *Intensive Care Med* 1984;10:139–145.
17. Abrahams J. Hemodynamic effects of nitroglycerin and long-acting nitrates. *Am Heart J* 1985;110:216–224.

18. Miller RR, Vismara LA, Williams DO, Amsterdam EA, Mason DT. Pharmacological mechanisms for left ventricular unloading in clinical congestive heart failure. Differential effects of nitroprusside, phentolamine and nitroglycerin on cardiac function and peripheral circulation. *Circ Res* 1976;39:127–133.
19. Palmer RF, Lasseter KC. Drug therapy: sodium nitroprusside. *N Engl J Med* 1975;292:294–297.
20. Pagani M, Vatner SF, Braunwald E. Hemodynamic effects of intravenous sodium nitroprusside in the conscious dog. *Circulation* 1978;57:144–151.
21. DiCarlo FJ. Nitroglycerin revisited: chemistry, biochemistry, interactions. *Drug Metab Rev* 1975;4:1–38.
22. Fung HL, Sutton SC, Kamiya A. Blood vessel uptake and metabolism of organic nitrates in the rat. *J Pharmacol Exp Ther* 1984;228:334–341.
23. Woo Park J, Means GE. Formation of *N*-nitrosamines from sodium nitroprusside and secondary amines. *N Engl J Med* 1985;313:1547–1548.
24. Duchier J, Iannascoli F, Safar M. Antihypertensive effect of sustained-release isosorbide dinitrate for isolated systolic systemic hypertension in the elderly. *Am J Cardiol* 1987;60:99–102.
25. Leier CV. Nitrate tolerance. *Am Heart J* 1985;110:224–232.
26. Lange RL, Reid MS, Tresch DD, Keelan MH, Bernhard VM, Coolidge G. Nonatheromatous ischemic heart disease following withdrawal from chronic industrial nitroglycerin exposure. *Circulation* 1972;46:666–678.
27. Needleman P, Johnson EM Jr. Mechanism of tolerance development to organic nitrates. *J Pharmacol Exp Ther* 1973;184:709–715.
28. Waldman SA, Rapoport RM, Ginsburg R, Murad F. Desensitization to nitroglycerin in vascular smooth muscle from rat and human. *J Pharmacol* 1986;35:3525–3531.
29. Kreye VAW. Direct vasodilators with unknown modes of action: the nitro-compounds and hydralazine. *J Cardiovasc Pharmacol* 1984;6(Suppl 4):S646–S654.
30. Spokas EG, Folco G, Quilley J, Chander P, McGiff JC. Endothelial mechanism in the vascular action of hydralazine. *Hypertension* 1983;5(Suppl I):I-107–I-111.
31. Jacobs M. Mechanism of action of hydralazine on vascular smooth muscle. *Biochem Pharmacol* 1984;33:2915–2919.
32. Koch-Weser J. Hydralazine. *N Engl J Med* 1976;295:320–323.
33. Zacest R, Koch-Weser J. Relation of hydralazine plasma concentration to dosage and hypotensive action. *J Clin Pharmacol Ther* 1972;13:420–428.
34. Melander A, Danielson K, Hanson A, et al. Enhancement of hydralazine bioavailability by food. *J Clin Pharmacol Ther* 1977;22:104–107.
35. Ludden TM, McNay JL Jr, Shepherd AMM, Lin MS. Clinical pharmacokinetics of hydralazine. *Clin Pharmacokinetics* 1982;7:185–205.
36. Raskin NH, Fishman RA. Pyridoxine-deficiency neuropathy due to hydralazine. *N Engl J Med* 1965;273:1182–1185.
37. Cameron HA, Ramsay LE. The lupus syndrome induced by hydralazine: a common complication with low dose treatment. *Br Med J* 1984;289:410–412.
38. Björck S, Svalander C, Westberg G. Hydralazine-associated glomerulonephritis. *Acta Med Scand* 1985;218:261–269.
39. Robinson BF, Collier JG, Dobbs RJ. Acquired tolerance to dilator action of hydrallazine during oral administration. *Br J Clin Pharmacol* 1980;9:407–412.
40. Takenaka T, Asano M, Shiono K, Shibasaki M, Inagaki O. Cardiovascular pharmacology of nicardipine in animals. *Br J Clin Pharmacol* 1985;20:7S–22S.
41. Robinson BF, Dobbs RJ, Phillips RJW. Effect of treatment with chlorthalidone and atenolol on response to dilator agents in the forearm resistance vessels of men with primary hypertension. *Br J Clin Pharmacol* 1983;16:327–332.
42. Rubin AA, Roth FE, Taylor RM, Rosenkilde H. Pharmacology of diazoxide, an antihypertensive, nondiuretic benzothiadiazine. *J Pharmacol Exp Ther* 1962;136:344–352.
43. Wilson WR, Okun R. The acute hemodynamic effects of diazoxide in man. *Circulation* 1963;28:89–93.
44. Sellers EM, Koch-Weser J. Protein binding and vascular activity of diazoxide. *N Engl J Med* 1969;281:1141–1145.
45. Gilmore E, Weil J, Chidsey C. Treatment of essential hypertension with a new vasodilator in combination with beta-adrenergic blockade. *N Engl J Med* 1970;282:521–527.
46. Johnson GA, Barsuhn KJ, McCall JM. Sulfation of minoxidil by liver sulfotransferase. *Biochem Pharmacol* 1982;31:2949–2954.
47. Meisheri KD, Cipkus LA. Minoxidil sulfate acts as a K^+-channel agonist to produce vasodilation [Abstract]. *Fed Proc* 1987;46:1383.
48. Hamilton TC, Weir SW, Weston AH. Comparison of the effects of BRL 34915 and verapamil on electrical and mechanical activity of rat portal vein. *Br J Pharmacol* 1986;88:103–111.
49. DuCharme DW, Freyburger WA, Graham BE, Carlson RG. Pharmacologic properties of minoxidil: a new hypotensive agent. *J Pharmacol Exp Ther* 1973;184:662–670.
50. Hall D, Truer KL, Loracher C. Treatment of severe hypertension with minoxidil and its effects on systemic and pulmonary hemodynamics. *Clin Sci Mol Med* 1976;51:587s–589s.
51. Ruskoaho H. Regression of cardiac hypertrophy with drug treatment in spontaneously hypertensive rats. *Med Biol* 1984;62:263–276.
52. Hall D, Froer K-L, Rudolph W. Serial electrocardiographic changes during long-term treatment of severe hypertension with minoxidil. *J Cardiovasc Pharmacol* 1980;2(Suppl 2):s200–s205.
53. Martin WB, Spodick DH, Zins GR. Pericardial disorders occurring during open-label study of 1,869 severely hypertensive patients treated with minoxidil. *J Cardiovasc Pharmacol* 1980;2(Suppl 2):s217–s227.
54. Krehlik JM, Hindson DA, Crowley JJ, Knight LL. Minoxidil-associated pericarditis and fatal cardiac tamponade. *West J Med* 1985;143:527–529.
55. Zins GR. Alterations in renal function during vasodilator therapy. In: Wesson LG, Fanelli GM, eds. *Recent advances in renal physiology and pharmacology.* Baltimore: University Park Press, 1974;165–186.
56. Allen WR, Brouhard BH, Lynch RE. Sodium reabsorption during intrarenal diazoxide infusion in the dog. *Pharmacology* 1983;27:336–342.
57. Vandenburg MJ, Sharman VL, Wright P, Drew PJ, Barnes JN. Hydralazine and prazosin in the treatment of hypertension. *Br J Clin Pharmacol* 1983;16:537–542.
58. Man in 't Veld AJ, Wenting GJ, Boomsma F, Verhoeven RP, Schalekamp MADH. Sympathetic and parasympathetic components of reflex cardiostimulation during vasodilator treatment of hypertension. *Br J Clin Pharmacol* 1980;9:547–551.
59. Christensson B, Katlefors T, Westling H. Haemodynamic effects of nitroglycerin in patients with coronary heart disease. *Br Heart J* 1965;27:511–519.

Hypertension: Pathophysiology, Diagnosis, and Management, edited by J. H. Laragh and B. M. Brenner. Raven Press, Ltd., New York © 1990.

CHAPTER 144

Hypertensive Emergencies

Samuel J. Mann and Steven A. Atlas

The Nature of Hypertensive Crises, 2275
Medical Emergencies and Urgencies, 2275
The Role of Blood Pressure Elevation, 2275
Hypertensive Encephalopathy, 2276
Accelerated or Malignant Hypertension, 2276
Etiology, 2276
Pathophysiology, 2276
Acute Hypertensive Crisis, 2277
Treatment of Hypertensive Emergencies and Urgencies, 2278
General Considerations, 2278
Drugs for Hypertensive Emergencies, 2279
Drugs for Hypertensive Urgencies, 2281
Management of Specific Conditions, 2283
Conclusions, 2286
References, 2286

Advances in pharmacotherapy have enabled acute lowering of blood pressure in essentially all patients presenting with a hypertensive emergency. However, reports of adverse outcomes are numerous; in many instances, the risk of rapid blood pressure lowering can exceed the benefit. The purpose of this chapter is to review (a) the current understanding of hypertensive emergencies and (b) the approaches to their management.

THE NATURE OF HYPERTENSIVE CRISES

The term "hypertensive emergency" covers an array of clinical situations, with differing severity of blood pressure elevation and differing degrees of urgency of treatment. In some emergencies, the severity or rapidity of blood pressure elevation is the determinant of urgency. In others, the underlying medical condition is more relevant to urgency of treatment than is the severity of blood pressure elevation.

Medical Emergencies and Urgencies

A true "emergency" requires blood pressure lowering as quickly as possible (i.e., within minutes) in order to protect life or vital organ function. The drug employed should have an onset of action that is nearly instantaneous and should be nearly universally effective, regardless of the underlying etiology of the blood pressure elevation. In these circumstances, monitoring in an intensive care unit is generally advisable. Table 1 lists the conditions that are considered to be true hypertensive emergencies. (Eclampsia and preeclampsia are considered further in another chapter).

The degree of blood pressure elevation per se does not define the need for immediate treatment. Factors such as the chronicity of blood pressure elevation, the nature of target organ damage, and the presence of underlying medical conditions may be more important than the blood pressure level in making this assessment.

There are many medical conditions, listed in Table 2, in which blood pressure lowering is needed urgently but not instantaneously. In such medical "urgencies," 30 min or longer can safely be allowed for blood pressure monitoring. In these circumstances, rapidly acting drugs requiring intra-arterial monitoring in an intensive care unit are not necessary.

Finally, it should be emphasized that most instances of severe blood pressure elevation do not constitute a hypertensive crisis. In situations where the risk of imminent major organ damage is considered minimal, rapid lowering of blood pressure can be associated with more risk than benefit. Clinical examples include the following: chronic but asymptomatic, severe hypertension (with Grade 0, I, or II fundi); acute blood pressure elevation associated with anxiety; pseudohypertension; and systolic hypertension in the elderly.

The Role of Blood Pressure Elevation

The manifestations of certain hypertensive crises are due to an extreme or rapid blood pressure elevation. Such crises may present either as a worsening of chronic hypertension, as represented by the syndrome of accelerated or malignant hypertension, or as an acute blood pressure rise in a previously normotensive patient, as seen in acute glomerulo-

TABLE 1. *Hypertensive emergencies*

Hypertensive encephalopathy
Hypertension associated with intracranial hemorrhage
Hypertension associated with stroke
Hypertension associated with pulmonary edema
Hypertension associated with acute myocardial infarction
Adrenergic crisis
Dissecting aortic aneurysm
Eclampsia

nephritis, preeclampsia, scleroderma renal crisis, and other conditions. The risk to vital organ function results from vascular damage or circulatory disturbances caused by extreme blood pressure elevation. The pathophysiology and clinical features of the "classical" hypertensive crises—hypertensive encephalopathy and malignant hypertension—will be considered in subsequent sections.

Perhaps more commonly, a hypertensive crisis may arise when coexisting blood pressure elevation aggravates an underlying medical condition such as acute myocardial infarction or acute aortic dissection. Such conditions may require immediate antihypertensive treatment in the absence of vascular changes and even at relatively modest degrees of blood pressure elevation. Selection of therapy is usually guided by the underlying condition, as will be discussed later in this chapter.

HYPERTENSIVE ENCEPHALOPATHY

Hypertensive encephalopathy is characterized by an alteration in neurological function in the setting of severe hypertension (1,2). Although encephalopathy is frequently a complication of malignant hypertension, it may occur without evidence of prior vascular damage, particularly following an abrupt blood pressure rise (3,4). Manifestations can include headache, alteration of mental status (confusion, somnolence, delirium, coma), visual impairment, and seizures (1,2). Focal neurological findings can also occur (1,2), in which case the possibility of a localized lesion (e.g., stroke or intracranial hemorrhage) must also be considered.

Pathological findings include microinfarctions and petechial hemorrhages (1,2,5). Areas of microinfarction are associated with arteriolar fibrinoid necrosis and luminal narrowing (1). Although cerebrospinal fluid pressure may or may not be elevated (1,6), cerebral edema is a constant finding (6–8).

The pathophysiology of hypertensive encephalopathy remains controversial. One theory ascribes encephalopathy to cerebral ischemia resulting from luminal narrowing and spasm (9,10) and possibly vascular occlusion (1). In another theory, it is postulated that breakdown (or failure) of autoregulation at very high systemic pressures leads to localized hyperperfusion and, eventually, edema (1,4,10).

ACCELERATED OR MALIGNANT HYPERTENSION

Malignant hypertension constitutes a syndrome of severe elevation of mean arterial pressure (usually, but not always, with a diastolic blood pressure exceeding 140 mmHg) associated with vascular damage which is manifest on physical examination by retinal hemorrhages, exudates, and papilledema (11). The term "accelerated hypertension" is often used when the syndrome appears without papilledema. Complications due to vascular damage may be evident at the time of presentation and include encephalopathy, renal impairment, and microangiopathic hemolytic anemia.

The distinction between accelerated and malignant hypertension has been de-emphasized recently for several reasons. First, although the presence or absence of retinal hemorrhages and exudates is clear to most observers, the presence of papilledema, unless severe, is more difficult to ascertain on funduscopic examination and is more subject to observer interpretation (12). Second, both the short- and long-term prognoses are independent of the presence or absence of papilledema (12–14), possibly as a result of improvements in pharmacotherapy. And finally, both the pathogenesis and clinical management of accelerated and malignant hypertension are the same. The degree of urgency is based on the risk to vital organ function, rather than on the presence or absence of papilledema.

Etiology

The process of vascular damage in malignant hypertension is generally thought to be initiated by chronically elevated arterial pressure (15), although contributions by other factors (discussed below) have also been proposed. In the past, severe and inadequately treated essential hypertension was the most prevalent antecedent of malignant hypertension (6). With more widespread and improved treatment of essential hypertension, progression to the malignant phase is seen less commonly (6) but still does occur, perhaps with increased frequency among smokers (16,17).

Other etiologies of hypertension are now more prevalent among patients who progress to the malignant phase (6). Renovascular (18) and renal parenchymal disorders (11) are the most common, but many other causes have been documented, including pheochromocytoma (19), renal vasculitis (20), and oral contraceptive use (21). Even patients with primary aldosteronism have rarely been reported to enter the malignant phase (22), presumably when hypertension has been long neglected.

Pathophysiology

The vascular lesions of accelerated hypertension consist predominantly of myointimal profileration and fibrinoid necrosis (6). *Myointimal profileration* is a pathological feature commonly seen in sustained, benign hypertension (23), and its severity parallels the severity and duration of

TABLE 2. *Hypertensive urgencies*

Malignant hypertension
Hypertension associated with left ventricular failure
Hypertension associated with unstable angina
Perioperative hypertension
Preeclampsia

the hypertension. Vascular smooth muscle hypertrophy and collagen deposition contribute to medial thickening, and this can be accompanied by cellular intimal profileration, which results in the "onion-skin" appearance of small vessels in patients with more severe hypertension (15,24). Medial and intimal thickening result in reduced lumen diameter and lumen-to-wall ratio (6,11). Although medial thickening is, to a variable extent, reversible after weeks to months of blood pressure control, intimal changes contribute to irreversible luminal narrowing, particularly in patients with more severe hypertension (24).

The accelerated phase of hypertension is characterized by the appearance of changes of *fibrinoid necrosis* (6,25). These changes can develop acutely and further compromise the lumen of small vessels (15), and they can be responsible for the rapid development of renal insufficiency. In contrast to medial and intimal thickening, these changes are more rapidly reversible with blood pressure control and can resolve within days of treatment (25,26).

In the early stages of fibrinoid necrosis, a critical level of blood pressure elevation causes spasm in some segments of small blood vessels while causing overdilatation in other segments (27). Spasm probably occurs as an autoregulatory phenomenon, whereas localized vasodilatation is believed to result from overstretching. Variations in the thickness of vascular smooth muscle along the course of the vessel walls may explain differences in vessel wall responses: Spasm occurs in thicker segments, whereas stretching occurs in segments with a thinner smooth muscle layer (27). Damage to endothelium has been documented, particularly in the overstretched regions (28). Endothelial damage is followed by entry of fibrin and other plasma components into the intercellular space, accompanied by swelling, fibrin deposition, edema, and thrombus formation (11,15,24,29). The resultant luminal narrowing contributes to target-organ ischemia. These changes, which are mirrored on funduscopic examination by the appearance of retinal hemorrhages and exudates, have been noted in arterioles of many organ systems but are more prominent in the renal vascular bed (2,25,30).

Why some patients proceed from benign hypertension to an accelerated phase and others do not is not entirely clear. Some believe that the extreme blood pressure elevation is responsible for initiating the vascular damage (29), whereas others postulate an interaction of blood pressure with hormonal changes (31). Certainly the latter contributes to sustaining and aggravating the process. An elevation of plasma renin activity (32–34) and of aldosterone secretion (35,36) is seen in a large proportion of patients with accelerated hypertension, and angiotensin-converting-enzyme inhibitors effectively lower blood pressure in many patients (37,38), consistent with the role of the renin–angiotensin–aldosterone axis in the malignant process. Preexisting hyperreninemia (e.g., in patients with renovascular hypertension) may contribute to the increased risk of developing the malignant phase in some patients. In others, hypersecretion of renin is probably secondary to the renal vascular changes produced by severe blood pressure elevation (36). Once initiated, hypersecretion of renin is thought to set into motion a vicious cycle in which increased angiotensin levels enhance vasoconstriction and worsen renal ischemia, leading to further increases in renin secretion (39,40). At this stage, a concomitant pressure natriuresis has been observed and can result in intravascular volume depletion and further elevation of renin secretion and sympathetic nervous system activity (40). In this regard, saline repletion, with accompanying reductions in plasma renin activity and in aldosterone secretion, has at least temporarily reversed the malignant process in some studies (41–43).

Although these demonstrated hormonal changes are commonly present, they are not absolute requirements for development of the malignant phase. Malignant hypertension has been reported in patients with normal renin levels (36,44) or even in patients with suppressed renin levels, as seen in those with aldosterone-producing adenoma (22). In experimental models, necrotizing vascular lesions can be seen in anephric animals in the absence of renin (30). Experimental malignant hypertension has also been produced by injection of various other vasopressors, including deoxycorticosterone–saline (29,45,46), vasopressin (27,47), and norepinephrine (28,48).

The most common target-organ complications include encephalopathy (discussed above), renal impairment, and microangiopathic hemolytic anemia. The vascular changes of malignant hypertension occur in other organs as well; uncommonly, hypertensive crises have presented with unexpected target-organ damage such as pancreatitis (49) or bowel necrosis (50).

Renal Failure

Myointimal profileration, associated with "onion-skin" lesions, develops slowly and may be associated with progressive renal insufficiency in its late stages (6,24). These changes lead to loss of nephron number and do not improve greatly with treatment of accelerated hypertension, thus being largely responsible for the irreversible component of renal failure (24).

The vascular changes of fibrinoid necrosis develop more acutely and resolve more quickly and completely, being inapparent on renal biopsies performed within 3 weeks following initiation of treatment (25,26). It is likely that the acute deterioration in renal function seen shortly before presentation with hypertensive crisis, as well as the improvement seen within weeks of treatment, may be largely explained by the development and subsequent resolution of fibrinoid necrosis.

Microangiopathic hemolytic anemia is manifested by hemolysis, red blood cell fragmentation, evidence of intravascular coagulation, and fibrin deposition (51). Platelet count is reduced, with increased amounts of fibrin degradation products (51). The occurrence of hemolytic anemia is associated with an elevated serum creatinine (51), suggesting that this process may potentiate renal damage.

ACUTE HYPERTENSIVE CRISIS

Whereas malignant hypertension usually represents an accelerated phase of a sustained blood pressure elevation, it can also occur in the absence of a prior history of hypertension. In such acute hypertensive crises, the vessel walls lack the protective structural thickening seen in chronic hypertensives (52). In this setting, the upper limit of autoregulation of blood flow has not yet increased, as it does in chronic hypertension (53), so that risk of encephalopathy or hemorrhage exists at much lower blood pressures than in the malignant phase of sustained hypertension. In patients with preeclampsia or acute glomerulonephritis, for example, and particularly in young patients, encephalopathy can be seen at diastolic blood pressures far below 140 mmHg, and immediate treatment may be required despite only "modest" blood pressure elevation.

TREATMENT OF HYPERTENSIVE EMERGENCIES AND URGENCIES

General Considerations

The task of acutely lowering severely elevated blood pressure has been facilitated by the availability of potent and rapidly acting drugs. However, complications arising from rapid lowering of blood pressure in hypertensive crisis have been reported widely (54–61); therefore, assessment of the risks and benefits of pharmacologic intervention is essential in management decisions. Aside from avoiding inappropriate use of these agents, careful attention to the clinical status of the patient during treatment can also help to minimize adverse outcomes.

Two important considerations in the early management of hypertensive emergencies are *how quickly* and *how much* to lower blood pressure. Many available pharmacologic agents can instantaneously normalize blood pressure in most crises. However, reversible and irreversible complications have been seen even at "normal" blood pressure levels (54,55,61). Furthermore, exaggerated and unintended falls in blood pressure, down to hypotensive levels, are not infrequent. Thus a margin of safety is warranted, and more gradual blood pressure reduction is preferable. In most clinical circumstances, complete normalization of blood pressure is not necessary and, with certain exceptions, should not be the goal of therapy. The specific target blood pressure to be achieved during initial treatment cannot be generalized. The target blood pressure will depend on the underlying medical condition, and its selection must take into consideration other clinical factors that vary from patient to patient.

The principal factors that need to be considered in selecting a particular drug, route of administration, dosage, and target blood pressure are listed in Table 3 and are discussed below.

TABLE 3. *Clinical factors relevant to the management of hypertensive emergencies*

Age
Volume status
Concurrent antihypertensive treatment
Duration of hypertension
Underlying medical conditions
Oral versus parenteral agents

Age

Elderly patients are at greater risk of adverse effects when blood pressure is lowered acutely (56). Because the incidence of known or occult coronary and cerebrovascular disease is greater than in younger patients, acute blood pressure lowering can often result in ischemic symptoms. Autoregulatory capacity is also reduced in the elderly, contributing further to hypoperfusion at lower blood pressures (62). In addition, increased sensitivity to the pharmacologic effect of drugs is often seen. Finally, the possibility that elevated systolic blood pressure represents "pseudohypertension" resulting from stiff, calcified vessels must also be borne in mind before deciding to acutely lower blood pressure. In general, the use of lower drug doses, the selection of a higher target blood pressure, and more careful attention to blood pressure monitoring are indicated in elderly patients.

Volume Status

Administration of potent loop diuretics has often been advocated as primary or adjunctive treatment of hypertensive crisis. In the setting of volume overload, such as hypertension due to renal parenchymal disease, acute glomerulonephritis, primary aldosteronism, or hypertension associated with left ventricular failure, the use of diuretics may be recommended. Their use consequent to the administration of sodium-retaining vasodilators is also commonly indicated.

In the absence of evident volume overload, however, the early use of diuretics in the treatment of hypertensive crisis must be questioned. A reduced intravascular volume has been demonstrated in many patients with sustained hypertension (63–66) and is particularly prominent in those who have entered the malignant phase (6). Prior use of diuretics, or reduced fluid intake due to anorexia, can further contribute to reduced intravascular volume. The administration of potent vasodilators in these patients can cause a precipitous blood pressure fall.

Hypotension, when it occurs, is best treated by halting or reducing infusion rates, as well as by the aggressive infusion of crystalloid to expand the dilated intravascular space. In the acutely dilated state, particularly in the presence of volume depletion, 1–2 liters or more may be necessary in order to restore blood pressure.

Concurrent Antihypertensive Treatment

Antihypertensive medications taken prior to presentation, while failing to lower blood pressure, may have blocked the compensatory reflexes or may have reduced the intravascular volume. In this setting, addition of the acutely administered drug may drastically lower blood pressure. Therefore, in such situations, the use of continuous, rather than bolus, administration of rapidly acting drugs may be preferable.

Duration of Hypertension

In patients with chronic hypertension, autoregulation of blood flow is altered (53), and rapid blood pressure lower-

coronary artery bypass graft hypertension (114), pheochromocytoma (115), and clonidine withdrawal (115,116). However, in patients with known or suspected pheochromocytoma, it is considered generally advisable to first establish alpha-blockade (e.g., with phentolamine or prazosin) before adding a beta-blocker, unless concurrent administration of the latter is clearly indicated by severe tachycardia or ectopy.

Oral labetolol has been shown to lower blood pressure within 1–3 hr when given in doses of 100–400 mg (117–119) and may be useful in some urgent situations. It has recently gained some popularity in the treatment of preeclampsia (120).

Other Beta-Receptor Blockers

Intravenous administration of propranolol or metoprolol generally has little acute blood-pressure-lowering effect but is often used as adjunctive therapy to minimize reflex cardiac stimulation. These agents are useful in combination with vasodilators such as sodium nitroprusside, in patients with acute aortic dissection, myocardial infarction, or coronary disease, and, when indicated, in combination with phentolamine in patients with pheochromocytoma.

Sympatholytic Agents

Oral administration of *clonidine* has been shown to effectively and smoothly lower blood pressure (121–124), with an onset of action of 30–60 min (124), a maximal response within a 2- to 4-hr period (124), and little risk of a precipitous fall. Beneficial effects on coronary blood flow have been reported (125). In this category of drugs, clonidine has largely replaced the use of intravenous *methyldopa* or intramuscular *reserpine* for urgent treatment of hypertension.

Drowsiness caused by this class of agents may interfere with clinical assessment of patients with hypertensive encephalopathy or stroke. Therefore, in patients with neurological deficit, selection of alternate drugs is probably advisable.

Treatment with clonidine or methyldopa can be continued for long-term blood pressure control, although the acute responses and dosage requirements do not necessarily predict the long-term situation. Furthermore, the high incidence of bothersome side effects (drowsiness, dry mouth, impotence) may contribute to noncompliance, with possible rebound hypertension if the drug is stopped abruptly.

Management of Specific Conditions

Table 5 lists the agents that are either recommended or contraindicated in specific hypertensive emergencies and urgencies. Current areas of controversy regarding the management of these conditions are considered here.

Accelerated or Malignant Hypertension

The syndrome of malignant hypertension constitutes a medical urgency, except in the presence of encephalopathy, symptomatic coronary insufficiency, severe congestive heart failure, or other conditions which require emergency treatment. In the absence of these complications, the use of oral or intravenous agents with an onset of action exceeding 15–30 min is acceptable and may even be preferable to instantaneously acting intravenous drugs requiring intraarterial monitoring in an intensive care unit. Acute normalization of blood pressure is not indicated. A target diastolic blood pressure of 100–110 mmHg, to be achieved over the first 24–48 hr of treatment, has been recom-

TABLE 5. *Drugs of choice for hypertensive emergencies or urgencies*

Condition	Drugs of choice	Contraindicated
Hypertensive encephalopathy	Nitroprusside; diazoxide + diuretic ± beta-blocker	Centrally acting sympatholytic agents
Malignant hypertension	Nifedipine ± beta-blocker; captopril; labetolol (infusion or bolus); clonidine	
Hypertension associated with:		
Intracranial hemorrhage	Nitroprusside; labetolol (infusion)	Diazoxide; ? nifedipine
Stroke	Nitroprusside; labetolol (infusion)	Diazoxide; ? nifedipine
Left ventricular failure		
Pulmonary edema	Nitroprusside ± loop diuretic; nitroglycerin ± loop diuretic	Beta-blockers; verapamil
Congestive heart failure	Nifedipine ± loop diuretic; captopril ± loop diuretic	Beta-blockers; verapamil
Coronary insufficiency		
Acute myocardial infarction	Nitroglycerin ± beta-blocker; nitroprusside ± beta-blocker	Diazoxide; hydralazine
Unstable angina	The above, or nitrates (S.L., P.O., or transdermal) ± beta-blocker or calcium blocker	Diazoxide; hydralazine
Adrenergic crisis	Nitroprusside ± beta-blocker; phentolamine ± beta-blocker; ? labetolol	Beta-blocker monotherapy
Dissecting aortic aneurysm	Nitroprusside ± beta-blocker; trimethaphan	Diazoxide; hydralazine; nifedipine
Perioperative hypertension	Nitroprusside; nitroglycerin; labetolol; nifedipine	

[a] S.L., sublingually; P.O., orally.

mended, and even higher target blood pressures may be appropriate in some clinical circumstances.

Although the major goal of acute intervention is lowering of blood pressure, observation of the acute response to specific agents can be useful for purposes of diagnosis and chronic management. Where time allows, observation of the response to agents that attack a specific pathophysiologic mechanism, such as an angiotensin-converting-enzyme inhibitor or an alpha-blocker, can be helpful, particularly before institution of other antihypertensive medications that can alter the acute response. Although, as already noted, positive responses to these agents in malignant hypertension are not necessarily diagnostic of correctable renovascular lesions or of pheochromocytoma, a failure to respond may be useful in identifying patients in whom further work-up is unnecessary.

Hypertensive Encephalopathy

In contrast to uncomplicated accelerated hypertension, hypertensive encephalopathy requires rapid blood pressure lowering because there is risk of imminent brain damage. The signs and symptoms of encephalopathy are generally rapidly ameliorated by blood pressure reduction (1). However, acute blood pressure reduction can, in some cases, worsen cerebral ischemia (126,127); therefore, use of rapidly acting parenteral drugs, such as sodium nitroprusside, whose effects are easily titrated and rapidly reversible, is generally recommended. In addition, deterioration of neurological status should prompt consideration of other diagnoses, such as cerebrovascular accident, head injury, or other cerebral pathology which can be accompanied by severe blood pressure elevation.

The effect of various antihypertensive agents on cerebral blood flow may be of relevance in the management of accelerated hypertension, and even more so in the management of hypertensive encephalopathy. If acute blood pressure lowering is accompanied by reduction of cerebral blood flow, cerebral ischemia can occur—particularly if large vessel narrowing from arteriosclerosis, or small vessel narrowing from malignant vasculitis, is present.

Maintenance of cerebral blood flow has been demonstrated with captopril (128,129), nifedipine (130), and labetolol (131). In one study, cerebral blood flow increased with nifedipine, despite blood pressure lowering (102). On the other hand, decreases in cerebral blood flow have been demonstrated with propranolol (132), sodium nitroprusside (133), diazoxide (134), and clonidine (102,135). The results of these studies must, however, be interpreted cautiously. Among these reports, study conditions varied considerably; in some cases, results for patients with chronic hypertension, acute hypertension, and normal blood pressure were included in analyses. Thus the observed effects on cerebral blood flow may not accurately predict the effect in patients with the vascular changes of malignant hypertension and encephalopathy, where cerebral blood flow may be nonhomogeneous. Additionally, microinfarctions, which have been documented in the territory of small-vessel disease (2), could result from aggravation of localized ischemia, regardless of the effect of a drug on overall cerebral blood flow. And finally, in the presence of diagnosed or undiagnosed cerebrovascular disease, cerebral blood flow may fall with blood pressure lowering, regardless of the antihypertensive agent employed.

The choice of a target blood pressure remains controversial. In general, the risk of extreme blood pressure lowering is likely to exceed the risk of moderate blood pressure lowering, with little loss of benefit. In chronically hypertensive patients, in whom there has been an upward shift in the limits of autoregulation (136), cerebral hypoperfusion may occur at normal or even mildly elevated blood pressures (54,61). In addition, reduction of mean arterial pressure by 40% has been associated with neurological symptoms (126,127). It is generally recommended that mean blood pressure be reduced initially (over the course of 1 hr) by a maximum of 20%, or to a diastolic blood pressure of 100–110 mmHg; however, in selected patients, even higher target blood pressures may be advisable.

Intracranial Hemorrhage

Acute management of blood pressure elevation, in the setting of intracranial bleeds, remains controversial. In some uncontrolled studies of patients with subarachnoid hemorrhage and with intraparenchymal hemorrhage or hematoma (137–139), but not in others (140), treated patients had a lower mortality than untreated patients. In one study of patients with subarachnoid hemorrhage, the mortality and incidence of re-bleeding were higher in patients with a systolic blood pressure exceeding 160 mmHg (141). However, the effect of acute lowering of blood pressure was not assessed.

The potential benefits of acute antihypertensive therapy include reduction of the incidence of re-bleeding and reduction of edema formation. However, blood pressure lowering can promote border zone ischemia by reducing cerebral perfusion, particularly in chronically hypertensive patients or in patients with increased intracranial pressure.

Thus, the role of blood pressure reduction in the acute management of subarachnoid hemorrhage and of intraparenchymal hemorrhage is not clear. It seems reasonable to treat acutely and severely elevated blood pressure levels with rapidly acting and easily titratable drugs. In patients with mildly elevated blood pressure, particularly in patients with chronic hypertension, benefits of blood pressure reduction are unproven.

Cerebrovascular Accidents

Blood pressure elevation commonly accompanies thrombotic stroke, in both previously hypertensive and normotensive patients (142). Although the cause is not fully understood, sympathetic tone is known to be increased, as documented by increased plasma catecholamine levels (143). Increased intracranial pressure may contribute (144).

The effect of elevated blood pressure on the clinical outcome of thrombotic stroke is not clear. Blood pressure elevation might increase blood flow through a stenotic vessel or through collateral vessels, but it might also aggravate edema formation in the region of the infarct.

Acute blood pressure lowering has been associated with reduction of cerebral blood flow (145) and with exacerbation of the neurological deficit (57,127,146). Therefore, considerable attention has been given to the question of whether or not to treat acute or preexisting hypertension. There is general agreement that *mild* blood pressure elevation should not be treated—particularly in patients with chronic hypertension, in whom reduction of blood pressure to "normal" levels can cause cerebral hypoperfusion as a result of changes in cerebral autoregulation (136). Cerebral autoregulation has also been shown to be impaired in the setting of stroke (145,147) and in the elderly (62). The treatment of *acute* and *severe* blood pressure elevations is more controversial. Currently, a consensus viewpoint would recommend treating hypertension associated with acute stroke if diastolic blood pressure is above 130 mmHg (88,136). The target diastolic blood pressure should be no lower than 100 mmHg, and blood pressure should probably be reduced gradually over the course of several hours. Nonetheless, many prefer to use rapidly acting drugs whose effects can be easily titrated should neurological signs worsen as pressure is lowered.

Hypertension Associated with Left Ventricular Failure

In the nonhypertensive patient, left ventricular failure is associated with physiologic increases in vasoconstrictor hormones, including catecholamines (148) and angiotensin II (149). The vasoconstrictor-mediated increase in peripheral resistance contributes greatly to left ventricular dysfunction. Treatment with nitrates, diuretics, and vasodilators (including angiotensin-converting-enzyme inhibitors) have been widely demonstrated to be effective.

In the hypertensive patient, acute hormonal changes may combine with the baseline elevation of peripheral vascular resistance to severely impair left ventricular performance. In this setting, vasodilators can have a dramatic beneficial effect on cardiac output. Intravenous nitroglycerin and sodium nitroprusside are each effective in treating pulmonary edema (86), although sodium nitroprusside may provide more effective blood pressure control (89). Many experts still recommend concurrent administration of a rapidly acting diuretic, although this is probably not necessary for acute benefit in the severely hypertensive patient given a vasodilator.

In situations that are not as urgent, converting-enzyme inhibitors (e.g., oral captopril or intravenous enalaprilat) can be combined with diuretics to provide effective vasodilation and rapid improvement in heart failure (150,151). Nifedipine (152,153) and alpha-adrenergic-blocking agents (e.g., prazosin) (154,155) have also been effective in this setting.

Hypertension Associated with Myocardial Infarction or Ischemia

The goal of acute antihypertensive therapy is to reduce myocardial oxygen consumption and to increase myocardial blood supply. Intravenous nitroglycerin, which induces a greater reduction of myocardial oxygen consumption than does sodium nitroprusside (87) and may better sustain regional blood flow distal to a stenosis (156,157), may be the preferred drug of the two. Nifedipine will lower blood pressure effectively, but the fall in blood pressure is not titratable; moreover, provocation of angina has occasionally been observed with its acute use (69).

Beta-blockade generally has little acute antihypertensive effect but can be helpful in reducing heart rate and oxygen consumption (at the expense, however, of reduced cardiac output). The combined effects of beta-blockade with nitrates are, of course, advantageous.

Dissecting Aortic Aneurysm

Acute blood pressure reduction is needed to reduce shear forces on the damaged aorta. Reflex sympathetic activation, which accompanies administration of most vasodilators, can increase both the rate and velocity of left ventricular ejection, thereby increasing shear forces in the aorta. Therefore, agents such as hydralazine and diazoxide are contraindicated. In the past, trimethaphan, which blocks such reflex effects while reducing both preload and afterload, was considered the only drug of choice. In recent years, however, sodium nitroprusside has been gaining wider acceptance because it is easier and safer to use. Reflex effects are minimized by its venodilator action and can be completely obviated by addition of a beta-blocker (e.g., intravenous propranolol or metoprolol, followed by conversion to an oral form). Such combinations are now considered the treatment of choice. In converting to chronic oral therapy, beta-blockers and/or sympatholytic agents are considered a mainstay of treatment.

Adrenergic Crises

These are characterized by an abrupt increase in adrenergic tone. Plasma catecholamine levels are elevated in rebound hypertension following clonidine (and, possibly, methyldopa) withdrawal (158), in hypertension associated with ingestion of alpha-agonists such as phenylpropanolamine (159), in the drug interaction of monoamine oxidase inhibitors with tyramine-rich foods (160), and in pheochromocytoma (161). Blood pressure elevation is due, principally, to increased alpha-adrenergic vasoconstriction, although beta-adrenergic overactivity may also occur (e.g., in epinephrine-secreting pheochromocytoma).

Although phentolamine, the nonselective alpha-blocker, is the ideal physiologic agent for blood pressure lowering, sodium nitroprusside has been shown to be equally effective, and greater familiarity with sodium nitroprusside's use commends it as a drug of choice in true emergencies. In cases where adjunctive therapy with beta-blockers is indicated (e.g., because of severe tachycardia or ventricular ectopy), establishment of alpha-blockade (with phentolamine, phenoxybenzamine, or prazosin) should probably be accomplished first. Intravenous administration of the combined alpha- and beta-blocker labetolol appears to be effective in many such situations (115,116), although further experience with its use in pheochromocytoma is needed.

Postoperative Hypertension

Postoperative hypertension is characterized by an increase in sympathetic tone and in total vascular resistance (162). Vasodilators are generally quite effective and have the advantage of not compromising cardiac output. Nitroglycerin and sodium nitroprusside have been compared and, in two studies, are of nearly equal efficacy (87,89). Nitroglycerin has been associated with lower myocardial oxygen consumption and with a greater increase in cardiac output when used in patients with post-coronary artery bypass graft hypertension (87). Intravenous nitroglycerin may therefore be preferable in trying to maximize cardiac output in the setting of possible myocardial ischemia.

CONCLUSIONS

In summary, the pathophysiologic basis and pharmacologic management of hypertensive emergencies have been reviewed. Short-acting intravenous agents remain the drugs of choice for true emergencies, with sodium nitroprusside generally providing the best combination of effectiveness and titratability. In urgent situations, it is possible to use the more convenient oral agents and, in particular, agents which may help to identify pathogenetic mechanisms or to direct the course of subsequent treatment. Several newer agents are effective, and their use has been reviewed. Finally, the need for restraint has also been emphasized, to avoid complications from unnecessary and overzealous lowering of blood pressure.

REFERENCES

1. Chester EM, Agamanolis DP, Banker BQ. Hypertensive encephalopathy: a clinicopathologic study of 20 cases. *Neurology* 1978;28:928–939.
2. Healton EB, Brust JC, Feinfeld DA, Thompson GE. Hypertensive encephalopathy and the neurological manifestations of malignant hypertension. *Neurology* 1982;32:127–132.
3. Kontos HA, Wei E, Dietrich WD, et al. Mechanism of cerebral arteriolar abnormalities after acute hypertension. *Am J Physiol* 1981;240:H511–H527.
4. Johansson B, Strandgaard S, Lassen NA. On the pathogenesis of hypertensive encephalopathy. The hypertensive "breakthrough" of autoregulation of cerebral blood flow with forced vasodilatation, flow increase, and blood–brain-barrier damage. *Circ Res* 1974;34 & 35(Suppl 1):I-167–I-171.
5. Finnerty FA. Hypertensive encephalopathy. *Am J Med* 1972;52:672–678.
6. Kincaid-Smith P, McMichael J, Murphy EA. The clinical course and pathology of hypertension with papilledema. *Q J Med* 1958;27:117–154.
7. Kwong YL, Yu YL, Lam KSL, Woo E, Ma JTC, Huang CY. CT appearance in hypertensive encephalopathy. *Neuroradiology* 1987;29:215.
8. Weingarten KL, Zimmerman RD, Pinto RS, Whelan MA. Computed tomographic changes of hypertensive encephalopathy. *Am J Neuroradiol* 1985;6:395–398.
9. Byrom FB. Pathogenesis of hypertensive encephalopathy and its relation to malignant phase of hypertension; experimental evidence in the hypertensive rat. *Lancet* 1954;2:201–211.
10. Dinsdale HB, Robertson DM, Haas RA. Cerebral blood flow in acute hypertension. *Arch Neurol* 1974;31:80–87.
11. Kincaid-Smith P. Malignant hypertension: mechanisms and management. *Pharmacol Ther* 1980;9:245–269.
12. McGregor E, Isles CG, Jay JL, Lever AR, Murray GD. Retinal changes in malignant hypertension. *Br Med J* 1986;292:233–234.
13. Ahmed MEK, Walker JM, Beevers DG. Lack of differentiation between malignant and accelerated hypertension. *Br Med J* 1986;292:235–237.
14. Yu SH, Whitworth JA, Kincaid-Smith P. Malignant hypertension: Aetiology and outcome in 83 patients. *Clin Exp Hypertens [A]* 1986;A8:1211–1230.
15. Susin M, Mailloux LU. Essential malignant hypertension. Clinicopathologic correlations. *NY State J Med* 1978;78:54–58.
16. Bloxham CA, Beevers DG, Walker JM. Malignant hypertension and cigarette smoking. *Br Med J* 1979;1:581–583.
17. Isles C, Brown JJ, Cumming AMM, et al. Excess smoking in malignant-phase hypertension. *Br Med J* 1979;1:579–581.
18. Davis BA, Crook JE, Vestal RE, Oates JA. Prevalence of renovascular hypertension in patients with grade III or IV hypertensive retinopathy. *N Engl J Med* 1978;301:1273–1276.
19. Gifford RW Jr, Kvale WF, Maher FT, Roth GM, Preistly JT. Clinical features, diagnosis and treatment of pheochromocytoma: a review of 76 cases. *Mayo Clin Proc* 1964;39:281–302.
20. O'Connell MT, Kubrusly DB, Fournier AM. Systemic necrotizing vasculitis seen initially as hypertensive crisis. *Arch Intern Med* 1985;145:265–267.
21. Hodsman GP, Robertson JIS, Semple PF, Mackay A. Malignant hypertension and oral contraceptives: four cases, with two due to the 30 μg oestrogen pill. *Eur Heart J* 1982;3:255–259.
22. Murphy BE, Whitworth JA, Kincaid-Smith P. Malignant hypertension due to an aldosterone producing adrenal adenoma. *Clin Exp Hypertens [A]* 1985(A7):939–950.
23. Schwartz GI, Strong CG. Renal parenchymal involvement in essential hypertension. *Med Clin North Am* 1987;71:843–858.
24. McCormack LJ, Beland JE, Schneckloth RE, Corcoran AC. Effects of antihypertensive treatment on the evolution of the renal lesions in malignant nephrosclerosis. *Am J Pathol* 1958; 34:1011–1022.
25. Pickering G. *High blood pressure,* 2nd ed. London: J & A Churchill, 1968;312.
26. Pitcock JA, Johnson JH, Hatch FE. Malignant hypertension in blacks. Malignant intrarenal arterial disease as observed by light and electron microscopy. *Hum Pathol* 1976;7:333–346.
27. Byron FB. The evolution of acute hypertensive arterial disease. *Program Cardiovasc Dis* 1974;17:31–37.
28. Giese J. Acute hypertensive vascular disease. 2. Studies on vascular reaction patterns and permeability changes by means of vital microscopy and colloidal tracer techniques. *Acta Pathol Microbiol Scand* 1964;62:497–515.
29. Beilin LJ, Goldby FS. High arterial pressure versus humoral factors in the pathogenesis versus humoral factors in the pathogenesis of malignant hypertension. The case for pressure alone. *Clin Sci* 1977;52:111–113.
30. Muirhead EE, Turner LB, Grollman A. Hypertensive cardiovascular disease. Vascular lesions of dogs maintained for extended periods following bilateral nephrectomy or ureteral ligation. *Arch Pathol* 1951;51:575–592.
31. Möhring J. High arterial pressure versus humoral factors in the pathogenesis of malignant hypertension. The case for humoral factors as well as pressure. *Clin Sci* 1977;52:113–117.
32. Davies DL, Beevers DG, Briggs JD, et al. Abnormal relation between exchangeable sodium and the renin–angiotensin system in malignant hypertension with chronic renal failure. *Lancet* 1973;1:683–686.
33. Bühler FR, Laragh JH, Vaughan ED. Anti-hypertensive action of propranolol. Specific anti-renin responses in high and normal renin forms of essential, renal, renovascular and malignant hypertension. *Am J Cardiol* 1973;32:511–522.

34. Brown JJ, Davies DL, Lever AF, Robertson JIS. Plasma renin concentration in human hypertension III: renin in relation to complications of hypertension. *Br Med J* 1966;1:505–508.
35. Laragh JH, Ulick S, Januszewicz V, Deming QB, Kelly WG, Lieberman S. Aldosterone secretion and primary and malignant hypertension. *J Clin Invest* 1960;39:1091–1106.
36. McAllister RG, Van Way CW III, Dayani K, et al. Malignant hypertension: effect of therapy on renin and aldosterone. *Circ Res* 1971;28(Suppl II):II-160–II-174.
37. Case DB, Atlas SA, Sullivan PA, Laragh JH. Acute and chronic treatment of severe and malignant hypertension with the oral angiotensin-converting enzyme inhibitor captopril. *Circulation* 1981;64:711–765.
38. Biollaz J, Waeber B, Brunner HR. Hypertensive crisis treated with orally administered captopril. *Eur J Clin Pharmacol* 1983;25:145–149.
39. Dauda G, Möhring J, Hofbauer, et al. The vicious circle in acute malignant hypertension of rats. *Clin Sci*(Suppl) 1973; 45(S1):251–255.
40. Kincaid-Smith P. Understanding malignant hypertension. *Aust NZ J Med* 1981;11(Suppl 1):64–68.
41. Gross F, Dietz R, Mast GJ, Szokol M. Salt loss as a possible mechanism eliciting an acute malignant phase in renal hypertensive rats. *Clin Exp Pharmacol Physiol* 1975;2:323–333.
42. Möhring J, Petri M, Szokol M, Haack D, Möhring B. Effects of saline drinking on malignant course of renal hypertension in rats. *Am J Physiol* 1976;230:849–857.
43. Baer L, Carrillo SZ, Radichevich I, Williams GS. Detection of renovascular hypertension with angiotensin II blockade. *Ann Intern Med* 1977;86:257–260.
44. Kawazoe N, Eto T, Abe I. Pathophysiology in malignant hypertension: With special reference to the renin–angiotensin system. *Clin Cardiol* 1987;10:513–518.
45. Gavras H, Brunner HR, Laragh JH, Vaughan ED Jr, Koss M, Cote LJ, Gavras I. Malignant hypertension resulting from deoxycorticosterone–acetate and salt excess. Role of renin and sodium in vascular changes. *Circ Res* 1975;36:300–309.
46. Reid JL, Zivin JA, Kopin IJ. Central and peripheral adrenergic mechanisms in the development of deoxycorticosterone–saline hypertension in rats. *Circ Res* 1975;37:569–579.
47. Möhring J, Möhring B, Petri M, Haack D. Vasopressor role of ADH in the pathogenesis of malignant DOC hypertension. *Am J Physiol* 1977;232:F260–F269.
48. Kincaid-Smith P, Hobbs JB, Friedman A, Mathews DC. Structural and ultrastructural alterations in mesenteric and renal arterioles following infusion of vasoactive agents. In: Genest J, Koiw E, eds. *Hypertension.* New York: Springer-Verlag, 1972;97–108.
49. Bercenas CG, Gonzalez-Molina M, Hull AR. Association between acute pancreatitis and malignant hypertension with renal failure. *Arch Intern Med* 1978;138:1254–1256.
50. Padfield PL. Malignant hypertension presenting as an acute abdomen. *Br Med J* 1975;3:353–354.
51. Gavras H, Oliver N, Aitchison J, et al. Abnormalities of coagulation and the development of malignant phase hypertension. *Kidney Int* 1975;8:S252–S261.
52. Folkow B. The haemodynamic consequences of adaptive structural changes of the resistance vessels in hypertension. *Clin Sci* 1971;41:1–12.
53. Strandgaard S, Olesen J, Skinhoj E, Lassen NA. Autoregulation of brain circulation in severe arterial hypertension. *Br Med J* 1973;1:507–510.
54. Ledingham JGG, Rajagopalan B. Cerebral complications in the treatment of accelerated hypertension. *Q J Med* 1979;48:25–41.
55. Nobile-Orazio E, Sterzl R. Cerebral ischemia after nifedipine treatment. *Br Med J* 1981;283:948.
56. Jackson G, Pierscianowski TA, Mahon W, Condon J. Inappropriate anti-hypertensive therapy in the elderly. *Lancet* 1976;2:1317–1318.
57. Graham DI. Ischaemic brain damage following emergency blood pressure lowering in hypertensive patients. *Acta Med Scand [Suppl]* 1983;678:61–69.
58. Hayreh SS, Sernais GE, Virdi PS. Fundus lesion in malignant hypertension. *Ophthalmology* 1986;93:74–87.
59. Kumar GK, Dastoor FC, Robayo JR, Razzaque MA. Side effects of diazoxide. *JAMA* 1976;235:275–276.
60. Cove DH, Sedden M, Fletcher RF, Dukes DC. Blindness after treatment for malignant hypertension. *Br Med J* 1979;2:246.
61. Haas DC, Streeten DHP, Kim RC, Naalbandian AN, Obeid AL. Death from cerebral hypoperfusion during nitroprusside treatment of acute angiotensin-dependent hypertension. *Am J Med* 1983;75:1071–1076.
62. Wollner L, McCarthy ST, Super ND, Macy DJ. Failure of cerebral autoregulation as a cause of brain dysfunction in the elderly. *Br Med J* 1979;1:1117–1118.
63. Messerli RH, DeCarvalho GR, Christie B, Frohlich ED. Essential hypertension in black and white subjects. Hemodynamic findings and fluid volume state. *Am J Med* 1979;67:27–31.
64. Tarazi RC, Frohlich ED, Dustan HP. Plasma volume in men with essential hypertension. *N Engl J Med* 1968;278:762–765.
65. Julius S, Pascual AV, Reilly K. Abnormalities of plasma volume in borderline hypertension. *Arch Intern Med* 1971;127:116–119.
66. Bauer J, Brooks CS. Body-fluid composition in normal and hypertensive man. *Clin Sci* 1982;62:43–49.
67. Brown P, Gross M, Harrison MJ. Paraplegia following oral hypotensive treatment of malignant hypertension. *J Neurol Neurosurg Psychiatry* 1987;50:104.
68. Frishman WH, Weinberg P, Peled HB, Kimmel B, Charlap S, Beer N. Calcium entry blockers for the treatment of severe hypertension and hypertensive crisis. *Am J Med* 1984;77(2B):35–45.
69. Yagil Y, Kobrin I, Leibel B. Ischemic ECG change with initial nifedipine therapy of severe hypertension. *Am Heart J* 1982;103:49–50.
70. Cohn JN, Burke LP. Nitroprusside. *Ann Intern Med* 1979;91:752–757.
71. Palmer RF, Lasseter KJ. Sodium nitroprusside. *N Engl J Med* 1975;292:294–297.
72. Bhatia SK, Frohlich ED. Hemodynamic comparison of agents useful in hypertensive emergencies. *Am Heart J* 1973;85:367–373.
73. Guiha NJ, Cohn JN, Mikulic E, Franciosa JA, Limas CJ. Treatment of refractory heart failure with infusion of nitroprusside. *N Engl J Med* 1974;291:587–592.
74. Meline LJ, Westenkow DR, Pace NL, Bodily MN. Computer-controlled regulation of sodium nitroprusside infusion. *Anesth Analg* 1985;64:38–42.
75. Merrifield AJ, Blundell MD. Toxicity of sodium nitroprusside. *Br J Anaesth* 1974;46:324.
76. Kanada SA, Kanada DJ, Hutchinson RA. Angina-like syndrome with diazoxide therapy for hypertensive crises. *Ann Intern Med* 1976;84:696–699.
77. Sellers EM, Koch-Weser J. Protein binding and vascular activity of diazoxide. *N Engl J Med* 1969;281:1141–1145.
78. Koch-Weser J. Diazoxide. *N Engl J Med* 1976;294:1271–1274.
79. Jeller LB, Dye MS, Michelakis AM. Individual titration of intravenous diazoxide therapy in patients with severe hypertension. *Clin Exp Pharmacol Physiol* 1975;2:423.
80. Garrett BN, Kaplan NM. Efficacy of slow infusion of diazoxide in the treatment of severe hypertension without organ hypoperfusion. *Am Heart J* 1982;103:390–394.
81. Lee WR, Mroczek WJ, Davidov ME, Finnerty FA. Non-emergency use of slow infusion of diazoxide. *Clin Pharmacol Ther* 1975;18:154–157.
82. Thien T, Koene RA. Acute treatment of hypertension with slow infusion of diazoxide. *Arch Intern Med* 1983;143:882–884.
83. Miller WE, Gifford RW, Humphrey DC, Vidt DG. Management of severe hypertension with intravenous injections of diazoxide. *Am J Cardiol* 1969;24:870–875.
84. Fajans SS, Floyd JC Jr, Thiffault CA, Knopf RF, Harrison TS, Conn JW. Further studies on diazoxide suppression of insulin release from abnormal and normal islet cell tissue in man. *Ann NY Acad Sci* 1968;150:261–280.
85. Dale RC, Schroeder ET. Respiratory paralysis during treatment of hypertension with trimethaphan camsylate. *Arch Intern Med* 1976;136:816–818.
86. Cottrell JE, Turndorf H. Intravenous nitroglycerin. *Am Heart J* 1978;96:550–553.
87. Fremes SE, Weisel RD, Mickle DAG. A comparison of nitroglyc-

erin and nitroprusside. I. Treatment of post-operative hypertension. *Ann Thorac Surg* 1985;39:53–60.

88. Garcia JY, Vidt DG. Current management of hypertensive emergencies. *Drugs* 1987;34:263–278.
89. Flaherty JT, Magee PA, Gardner TL, Potter A, MacAllister NP. Comparison of intravenous nitroglycerin and sodium nitroprusside for treatment of acute hypertension developing after coronary artery bypass surgery. *Circulation* 1982;65:1072–1077.
90. Saragoca MA, Homsi E, Ribeiro AB, Filho SRF, Ramos OL. Hemodynamic mechanism of blood pressure response to captopril in human malignant hypertension. *Hypertension* [*Suppl*] 1983;5:I-53–I-58.
91. Tschollar W, Belz GG. Sublingual captopril in hypertensive crises. *Lancet* 1985;2:34–35.
92. Ferguson RK, Turini GA, Brunner HR, Gavras H. A specific orally active inhibitor of angiotensin-converting enzyme in man. *Lancet* 1977;1:775–778.
93. Brunner HR, Gavras H, Waeber B. Oral angiotensin-converting inhibitor in long-term treatment of hypertensive patients. *Ann Intern Med* 1979;90:19–23.
94. Lopez-Ovejero JA, Saal SD, D'Angelo W, Cheigh JS, Stenzel KH, Laragh JH. Reversal of vascular and renal crises of scleroderma by oral angiotensin-converting-enzyme blockade. *N Engl J Med* 1979;300:1417–1419.
95. Zawada ET, Clements PJ, Furst DA. Clinical course of patients with scleroderma renal crisis treated with captopril. *Nephron* 1981;27:74–78.
96. Millar JA, McGrath BP, Matthews PG, Johnson CI. Acute effects of captopril on blood pressure and circulating hormonal levels in salt-replete and depleted normal subjects and essential hypertensive patients. *Clin Sci* 1981;61:75–83.
97. Müller FB, Sealey JE, Case DB, et al. The captopril test for identifying renovascular disease in hypertensive patients. *Am J Med* 1986;80:633–644.
98. Dipette DJ, Ferraro JC, Evans RR, Martin M. Enalaprilat, an intravenous angiotensin-converting enzyme inhibitor in hypertensive crises. *Clin Pharmacol Ther* 1985;38:199–204.
99. Alpert MA, Bauer JH. Rapid control of severe hypertension with monoxidil. *Arch Intern Med* 1982;142:2099–2104.
100. Wood BC, Sharma JN, Crouch TT. Oral minoxidil in treatment of hypertensive crisis. *JAMA* 1979;241:163.
101. Stone PH, Antman EM, Muller JE, Braunwald E. Calcium channel blocking agents in the treatment of cardiovascular disorders. Part II: hemodynamic effects and clinical applications. *Ann Intern Med* 1980;93:886–904.
102. Bertel O, Conen D, Radu EW, Müller J, Lang C, Dubach UC. Nifedipine in hypertensive emergencies. *Br Med J* 1983;286:19–21.
103. Schillinger DS. Nifedipine in hypertensive emergencies: a prospective study. *J Emerg Med* 1987;5:463–473.
104. Ellrodt AG, Ault MJ, Riedinger M, Sandmurata GH. Efficacy and safety of sublingual nifedipine in hypertensive emergencies. *Am J Med* 1985;79(4A):19–25.
105. Abraham G, Shukkur A, Van der Meulen J, Johny KV. Sublingual nifedipine—a safe and simple therapy for hypertensive emergencies. *Br J Clin Pract* 1986;40:478–481.
106. Beer N, Gallegos I, Cohen A, Klein N, Sonnenblick E, Frishman W. Efficacy of sublingual nifedipine in the acute treatment of systemic hypertension. *Chest* 1981;79:571–574.
107. Haft JI, Litterer WE. Chewing nifedipine to rapidly treat hypertension. *Arch Intern Med* 1984;144:2357–2359.
108. Takekoshi N, Murakami E, Murakami H, et al. Treatment of severe hypertension and hypertensive emergency with nifedipine, a calcium antagonist agent. *Jpn Circ J* 1981;45:582–860.
109. Wilson DJ, Wallin JD, Vlachachis N, et al. Intravenous labetolol in the treatment of severe hypertensive emergencies. *Am J Med* 1983;75(Suppl)(4A):94–102.
110. Lebel M, Langlois S, Belleau LJ. Labetolol infusion in hypertensive emergencies. *Clin Pharmacol Ther* 1985;37:615–618.
111. Vlachakis ND, Maronde RF, Maly JW, Medakovic M, Kassem N. Pharmacodynamics of intravenous labetolol and follow-up therapy with oral labetolol. *Clin Pharmacol Ther* 1985;38:503–508.
112. Wright JT Jr, Wilson JD, Goodman RP, Minisi AJ. Labetolol by continuous intravenous infusion in severe hypertension. *J Clin Hypertens* 1986;1:39–43.
113. Chauvin M, Deriaz H, Hiars P. Continuous I.V. infusion of labetolol for postoperative hypertension. *Br J Anaesth* 1987;59:1250–1256.
114. Meretoja OA, Allonen H, Arola M, Laaksonin VO. Combined alpha- and beta-blockade with labetolol in post-open heart surgery hypertension. *Chest* 1980;78:810–815.
115. Agabiti Rosei E, Brown JJ, Lever AF, Robertson AS, Robertson JIS, Trust PM. Treatment of phaeochromocytoma and of clonidine withdrawal hypertension with labetolol. *Br J Clin Pharmacol* 1978;3(S3):809–815.
116. Rosenthal T, Rabinowitz B, Boichis H, Elazar E, Brauner A, Neufeld HN. Use of labetolol in hypertensive patients during discontinuation of clonidine therapy. *Eur J Clin Pharmacol* 1981;21:237–240.
117. Davies AB, Subramanian VB, Gould B, Raftery EB. Rapid reduction of blood pressure with acute oral labetolol. *Br J Clin Pharmacol* 1982;13:705–710.
118. Ghose RR, Mathur YB, Upadhyay M, Morgan WD, Khan S. Treatment of hypertensive emergencies with oral labetolol. *Br Med J* 1978;2:96.
119. Serlin MJ, Maciuer M, Green GJ, Macnee CM, Breckenridge AM. Rate of onset of hypotensive effect of oral labetolol. *Br J Clin Pharmacol* 1979;7:165–168
120. Michael CA. Use of labetolol in the treatment of severe hypertension during pregnancy. *Br J Clin Pharmacol* 1979;8(Suppl 2):211S–215S.
121. Anderson RJ, Hart GR, Crumpler BP, Reed WG, Matthews CA. Oral clonidine loading in hypertensive urgencies. *JAMA* 1981;246:848–851.
122. Marks AD, Adlin EV, Channick BJ. Oral clonidine for rapid control of accelerated hypertension. *J Clin Pharmacol* 1987;27:193–198.
123. Cohen IM, Katz MA. Oral clonidine loading for rapid control of hypertension. *Clin Pharmacol Ther* 1978;24:11–15.
124. Spitalewitz S, Porush JG, Oguagha C. Use of oral clonidine for rapid titration of blood pressure in severe hypertension. *Chest* 1983;83(Suppl):404–407.
125. Houston MC. Clonidine hydrochloride: review of pharmacology and clinical aspects. *Prog Cardiovasc Dis* 1981;23:337–350.
126. Harden R, Russell R. Iatrogenically induced hypertensive encephalopathy. *Johns Hopkins Med J* 1979;145:44–48.
127. Strandgaard S, Paulson OB. Cerebral autoregulation. *Stroke* 1984;15:413–415.
128. Paulson OB, Vorstrup S, Andersen AR, Smith J, Godtfredsen J. Converting enzyme inhibition resets cerebral autoregulation at lower blood pressure. *J Hypertens* 1985;3(Suppl 3):487–496.
129. Tajagopalan B, Baine AEG, Cooper R, Ledingham JGG. Changes in cerebral blood flow in patients with severe congestive heart failure before and after captopril treatment. *Am J Med* 1984;76:86–90.
130. Sorkin EM, Clissold SP, Brogden RN. Nifedipine. A review of its pharmacodynamic, pharmacokinetic properties and therapeutic efficacy in ischaemic heart disease, hypertension and related cardiovascular disorders. *Drugs* 1985;30:182–274.
131. Pearson RM, Griffith DNW, Woollard M, James IM, Havard CWH. Comparison of effects on cerebral blood flow of rapid reduction in systemic arterial pressure by diazoxide and labetolol in hypertensive patients: preliminary findings. *Br J Clin Pharmacol* 1979;8(S2):195S–198S.
132. Aoyagi M, Deshmukh VD, Meyer JS, Kawamura Y, Tagashira Y. Effect of beta adrenergic blockade with propranolol on cerebral blood flow, autoregulation and CO_2 responsiveness. *Stroke* 1976;7:291–295.
133. Henriksen L, Paulson OB, Lauritzen M. The effects of sodium nitroprusside on cerebral blood flow and cerebral venous blood gases. I. Observations in awake man during and following moderate blood pressure reduction. *Eur J Clin Invest* 1982;12:383–397.
134. Goldberg HI, Codario RA, Banka RA, Reivich M. Patterns of cerebral dysautoregulation in severe hypertension to blood pressure reduction with diazoxide. *Acta Neurol Scand* [*Suppl*] 1977;64:64–65.
135. Lowenstein J. Clonidine. *Ann Intern Med* 1980;92:74–77.

136. Strandgaard S. Cerebral blood flow in hypertension. *Acta Med Scand [Suppl]* 1983;678:11–25.
137. Meyer JS, Bauer RB. Medical treatment of spontaneous intracranial hemorrhage by the use of hypotensive drugs. *Neurology* 1962;12:36–47.
138. Slosberg PS. Treatment of ruptured intracranial aneurysm by induced hypotension. *Mt Sinai J Med* 1973;40:82–90.
139. Nibbelink DW, Torner JC, Henderson WG. Randomized treatment study. Drug-induced hypotension. In: Sahs AL, Nibbelink DW, Torner JC, eds. *Aneurysmal subarachnoid hemorrhage: report of the cooperative study.* Baltimore: Urban and Schwartzenberg, 1981;77–106.
140. Mullan S. Conservative management of the recently ruptured aneurysm. *Surg Neurol* 1975;3:27–32.
141. Nibbelink DW. Antihypertensive and antifibrinolytic therapy following subarachnoid hemorrhage from ruptured intracranial aneurysm. In: Sahs AL, Nibbelink DW, Torner JC, eds. *Aneurysmal subarachnoid hemorrhage: report of the cooperative study.* Baltimore: Urban and Schwartzenberg, 1981;287–296.
142. Wallace JD, Levy LL. Blood pressure after stroke. *JAMA* 1981;246:2177–2180.
143. Myers GM, Norris JW, Hachinski VC, Sole MJ. Plasma norepinephrine in stroke. *Stroke* 1981;12:200–204.
144. Roozekrans NTP, Porsius AJ, Van Zwieten PA. Comparison between the pressor response and the rise in plasma catecholamines induced by acutely elevated intracranial pressure. *Arch Int Pharmacodyn* 1979;240:143–157.
145. Meyers JS, Shimazu K, Fukuuchi Y, Oghuchi T, Okamoto S, Koto A, Ericsson AD. Impaired neurogenic cerebrovasular control and dysautoregulation after stroke. *Stroke* 1973;4:169–186.
146. Lavin P. Management of hypertension in patients with acute stroke. *Arch Intern Med* 1986;145:66–68.
147. Meyer JS, Teraura T, Marx P, Hashi K, Sakamoto K. Brain swelling due to experimental cerebral infarction. Changes in vasomotor capacitance and effects of intravenous glycerol. *Brain* 1972;95:833–852.
148. Thomas JA, Marks BH. Plasma norepinephrine in congestive heart failure. *Am J Cardiol* 1978;41:233–243.
149. Dzau VH, Colucci WS, Hollenberg NK, Williams GH. Relation of the renin–angiotensin–aldosterone system to clinical state in congestive heart failure. *Circulation* 1981;63:645–651.
150. Ader R, Chatterjee K, Ports T, Brundage B, Hiramatsu B, Parmley W. Immediate and sustained hemodynamic and clinical improvement in chronic heart failure by an oral angiotensin-converting enzyme inhibitor. *Circulation* 1980;61:931–937.
151. Levine TB, Franciosa JA, Cohn JN. Acute and long-term response to an oral converting-enzyme inhibitor, captopril, in congestive heart failure. *Circulation* 1980;62:35–41.
152. Polese A, Fiorentini C, Olivari MT, Guazzi MD. Clinical use of a calcium antagonistic agent (nifedipine) in acute pulmonary edema. *Am J Med* 1979;66:825–830.
153. Bartorelli C, Magrini F, Moruzzi P, Olivari MT, Polese A, Fiorentini C, Guazzi M. Hemodynamic effects of a calcium antagonistic agent (nifedipine) in hypertension: therapeutic implications. *Clin Sci [Suppl]* 1978;55:291S–292S.
154. Mehta J, Iacono M, Feldman RL, Pepine CJ, Conti CR. Comparative hemodynamic effects of intravenous nitroprusside and oral prazosin in refractory heart failure. *Am J Cardiol* 1978;41:925–930.
155. Awan NA, Miller RR, Mason DT. Comparison of effects of nitroprusside and prazosin on left ventricular function and the peripheral circulation in chronic refractory congestive heart failure. *Circulation* 1978;57:152–159.
156. Flaherty JT. Comparison of intravenous nitroglycerin and sodium nitroprusside in acute myocardial infarction. *Am J Med* 1983;74(Suppl):53–60.
157. Mann T, Cohn PF, Holman BL, Green LH, Markis JE, Phillips DA. Effect of nitroprusside on regional myocardial blood flow in coronary artery disease. Results in 25 patients and comparison with nitroglycerin. *Circulation* 1978;57:732–758.
158. Hansson L, Hunyur SH. Blood pressure over-shoot due to acute clonidine (capatres) withdrawal: studies on arterial and urinary catecholamines and suggestions for management of the crisis. *Clin Sci [Suppl]* 1973;43:181S–183S.
159. Pentel P. Toxicity of over-the-counter stimulants. *JAMA* 1984;252:1898–1903.
160. Hollister LE. Psychiatric disorders. In: Melmon KL, Morelli HF, eds: *Clinical pharmacology. Basic principles in therapeutics.* New York: Macmillan, 1978;850–856.
161. Manger WM, Gifford RW Jr. *Pheochromocytoma.* New York: Springer-Verlag, 1977.
162. Fouad FM, Estafanous FG, Tarazi RC. Hemodynamics of postmyocardial revascularization hypertension. *Am J Cardiol* 1978;41:564–569.

Hypertension: Pathophysiology, Diagnosis, and Management, edited by J. H. Laragh and B. M. Brenner. Raven Press, Ltd., New York © 1990.

CHAPTER 145

The Pharmacology of Antihypertensive Drugs and Drug–Drug Interactions

K. R. Lees and J. L. Reid

Beta-Adrenoceptor Antagonists, 2292
Mode of Action and Clinical Features, 2292
Interactions, 2292
Diuretics, 2293
Mode of Action and Clinical Features, 2293
Interactions, 2293
ACE Inhibitors, 2294
Mode of Action and Clinical Features, 2295
Interactions, 2295
Calcium Antagonists, 2295
Mode of Action and Clinical Features, 2295
Interactions, 2295
Vasodilators, 2297
Mode of Action and Clinical Features, 2297
Interactions, 2297
Centrally Acting Drugs, 2297
Mode of Action and Clinical Features, 2297
Interactions, 2297
Summary and Conclusions, 2298
References, 2298

Modern regimens for the treatment of hypertension usually involve one or more drugs selected from the following classes: beta-adrenoceptor antagonists, diuretics, vasodilators, and centrally acting drugs. Since it is now well recognized that side effects of antihypertensive treatment are commonly dose-related, there has been an increasing tendency to use monotherapy only for mild hypertensives and to progress early to combination therapy using low doses of drugs having contrasting mechanisms of action. This is the basis of stepped-care approaches and standard triple therapy.

There is thus potential for additive effects and for synergism between the different classes of antihypertensive drugs; there is also potential for interactions between drugs within these classes.

Since antihypertensive drugs are widely used in long-term therapy, in middle-aged and elderly patients they may often be used in association with drug therapy for other common concomitant conditions. There is thus considerable scope for drug interactions in hypertensive patients either (a) between two antihypertensive drugs or (b) between an antihypertensive drug and another class of agent.

It is important to recognize that drug interactions may have adverse consequences or may be a useful combination. In the case of antihypertensive therapy, the consequences of a drug interaction may be as follows:

1. Synergism or additional blood-pressure-lowering effect, which, depending on the individual patient, may be beneficial (to achieve control of the poorly controlled patient) or adverse (if symptoms result from an excessive fall in blood pressure).
2. Antagonism of the antihypertensive effect either directly (when the effects of an antagonist are overcome by an agonist) or indirectly (e.g., when fluid retention occurs in response to sympathetic inhibitors).
3. Modification of the side effect profile, which makes therapy with the two drugs more or less acceptable to the patient—for example, the use of beta-adrenoceptor antagonists together with dihydropyridine calcium antagonists: the reflex sympathetic activation seen with calcium antagonists is blocked and blood-pressure-lowering effects are enhanced.

Drug interactions have been characterized into those depending on a pharmacokinetic interaction where the plasma level of the drug increases or decreases. This may be a consequence of (a) changes in bioavailability or protein binding of one or another drug or (b) influences on clearance by the liver or kidney. Alternatively, interactions may be pharmacodynamic. In this case the plasma level may be unchanged, but the effect is modified by an interaction at the level of the specific receptor or via other compensatory effector mechanisms. As discussed below, in practice, as in the case of the interaction between verapamil and prazosin, there may be both pharmacokinetic and pharmacodynamic contributions to the interaction. In addition, effects of disease (cardiac, hepatic, or renal) or age may lead to drug–disease interactions which may modify drug–drug interactions.

As a generalization, relevant drug interactions are most likely to occur when one or another drug has a steep dose (or plasma level)–response relationship *and* has an action on a vital body function. Most significant drug interactions thus involve cardioactive drugs, anticoagulants, and drugs influencing hemostasis as well as hypoglycaemic agents. Where there is a flat dose–response relationship and a broad therapeutic index, there is much less likelihood of life-threatening interactions.

A number of classical antihypertensive drug interactions of sympathomimetic amines with monoamine oxidase inhibitors, as well as of tricyclic antidepressants with sympatholytics such as guanethidine or bethanidine, are now largely of historical interest. These drugs are not now widely used in the treatment of hypertension. The interactions are predictable from the known pharmacological properties of the drugs concerned. They are also useful as examples, respectively, of interactions characterized by dangerous and excessive rises in blood pressure or by antagonism of the antihypertensive effect.

In this review, some of the more important drug interactions, both adverse and beneficial, will be described, especially those that are relevant to clinical practice in the late 1980s and/or early 1990s.

BETA-ADRENOCEPTOR ANTAGONISTS

Propranolol was identified as a useful antihypertensive agent in the 1960s. Many related compounds, which are all competitive antagonists of beta-blockers, have since become available, and these are now amongst the most widely used cardiovascular drugs.

Mode of Action and Clinical Features

There are two types of beta-receptor. Beta-1-receptors are found mainly in cardiac muscle (where they mediate the positive inotropic and chronotropic effects of the catecholamines) and in adipose tissue. Beta-2-receptors are found in bronchi, pancreas, and peripheral vasculature; in this site they produce vasodilatation. The consequences of administration of beta-blockers can be predicted from (a) the distribution of these receptors, (b) their function, and (c) the spectrum of pharmacological activity of the individual beta-blocker.

The beta-adrenoceptor antagonists are not a homogeneous group. Partial agonism is an additional feature of some beta-blockers. Other features include (a) relative selectivity for the beta-1-receptor, which may influence the spectrum of side effects, (b) hydrophilicity, and (c) hepatic metabolism. Membrane-stabilizing activity is unlikely to be of clinical relevance.

Interactions (Table 1)

Interactions with Antihypertensive Drugs

Interactions between beta-adrenoceptor antagonists and other antihypertensive drugs are usually predictable and beneficial. Most striking is the pharmacodynamic interaction with vasodilator drugs, particularly the direct vasodilators (1) and dihydropyridine calcium antagonists. Reflex sympathetic activation resulting from vasodilatation is inhibited by beta-blockade. This may make the addition of a vasodilator more tolerable to the patient and may also prevent homeostatic reversal of these drugs' antihypertensive effect.

A general interaction between beta-adrenoceptor antagonists and diuretics is well documented but of questionable clinical importance. Whereas diuretics invariably cause a rise in plasma renin activity, the beta-blockers generally depress renin activity. Overall, renin activity in the presence of the two drugs can be variable and correlates poorly with antihypertensive effect. Nevertheless, the combination of beta-blocker and diuretic is a logical and useful antihypertensive regimen.

Although beta-adrenoceptor antagonists and dihydropyridine calcium antagonists demonstrate a beneficial and possibly synergistic interaction, this cannot be applied to the papaverine-based calcium antagonists such as verapamil. Both verapamil and the beta-blockers have a nega-

TABLE 1. *Interactions of beta-adrenoceptor antagonists*

Interaction	Effect
With antihypertensive drugs	
Vasodilator	Synergistic antihypertensive effect; reduced reflex tachycardia
Diuretic	Opposing effects on plasma renin activity
Papaverine calcium antagonist	Negative inotropic and chronotropic effect; increased antianginal effect
With other drugs	
Beta-sympathomimetic agent	Competitive antagonism
Alpha-sympathomimetic agent	Profound vasoconstriction
Nonsteroidal anti-inflammatory drugs	Loss of antihypertensive effect
Antacids	Reduced absorption of beta-blockers
Oral contraceptive agent	Increased levels of metoprolol
Cimetidine	Increased levels of lipid-soluble beta-blockers
Rifampicin	Increased metabolism of lipid-soluble beta-blockers

tive inotropic and a negative chronotropic action. Their use in combination parenterally has been associated with heart block and with acute hypotension. Use of the combination for chronic oral treatment is, however, not absolutely contraindicated and may be advantageous in selected patients (2–5), but great caution should certainly be exercised when using these two drugs together.

Interactions with Other Drugs

Predictable interactions occur with sympathomimetic agents. All beta-adrenoceptor antagonists will antagonize the effects of isoprenaline (6). The bronchodilator action of salbutamol is inhibited by the beta-blockers, especially those that are not "cardioselective." The antagonism is competitive and therefore, cardioselective antagonists such as atenolol, when given in low dosage, can be overcome by higher doses of salbutamol. This has clinical relevance in that a patient with mild asthma and moderate or severe hypertension and/or angina could be treated with a cardioselective beta-blocker under appropriate supervision.

Also predictable is the interaction between beta-adrenoceptor antagonists and sympathomimetic drugs with combined alpha and beta or pure alpha properties: Unopposed alpha stimulation results in powerful vasoconstriction and reflex bradycardia. Such an interaction has been observed between adrenaline and propranolol (6–8) or timolol (9,10) but is not a striking feature if a cardioselective beta-adrenoceptor antagonist such as metoprolol is involved (6–8). With the pure alpha-agonist phenylephrine, fatal consequences have occurred in the presence of nonselective beta-blockade (11).

As with other antihypertensive agents such as diuretics, it has been found that indomethacin and possibly other nonsteroidal anti-inflammatory drugs can reduce the hypotensive effects of the beta-adrenoceptor antagonists. This is best documented with propranolol (12–14) and pindolol (12), but there is no evidence that the other beta-adrenoceptor antagonists are not similarly affected (15). Likewise, clinical experience would suggest that other nonsteroidal agents will have an equivalent interaction with antihypertensive drugs, though it has been claimed that sulindac is devoid of such effects (16).

Antacids have been reported to affect absorption of beta-blockers. Calcium carbonate has been shown to reduce significantly the peak plasma concentration, as well as the area under the curve, of atenolol following acute dosing; however, it has not been found to affect the chronic response of blood pressure (17). Aluminum hydroxide gel decreases the bioavailability of propranolol (18) and atenolol (17). These studies were small, however, and there are conflicting results for metoprolol in the literature (19). The dose–response relationship for beta-adrenoceptor antagonists is relatively flat; thus, despite the likely frequency of concomitant use of antacids and beta-adrenoceptor antagonists, any such interaction is not likely to be of major clinical significance.

The area under the curve for the lipid-soluble beta-adrenoceptor antagonist metoprolol, which undergoes first-pass metabolism, is increased in women taking oral contraceptive agents (20). It is possible that propranolol and other lipid-soluble beta-blockers would show a similar effect. Again, however, the clinical importance of such an interaction is not potentially great. The interaction between propranolol and cimetidine is more likely to be of significance. Propranolol concentrations may increase twofold in the presence of cimetidine (21–24). Evidence so far suggests that only beta-adrenoceptor antagonists metabolized by the liver are affected by cimetidine, and thus atenolol (24) and pindolol (25) are free from this interaction. Ranitidine does not interfere with the metabolism of beta-adrenoceptor antagonists (26–28).

The broad-spectrum antibiotic, rifampicin, which induces the production of hepatic microsomal enzymes, is reported to reduce the area under the curve for metoprolol by about one-third (29) and had a similar effect on propranolol (30). Loss of beta-blockade in hypertension is unlikely to be of clinical significance, though this may be more important in patients with angina.

In summary, there are a number of pharmacokinetic and pharmacodynamic interactions between beta-blockers and other drugs. Most are of doubtful clinical significance, however.

DIURETICS

There are three groups of diuretics in common use: the thiazides, the loop diuretics, and the potassium-sparing drugs. Those which are most widely used in hypertension are the thiazides.

Mode of Action and Clinical Features

Prolonged diuretic exposure results in (a) resetting of the renal threshold for salt and water retention and (b) a reduction in intravascular and (probably) intracellular volume. This certainly contributes to the hypotensive action but does not entirely explain it, since restitution of plasma volume will not completely restore the blood pressure (31) and since the dose–response relationships for diuresis and antihypertensive effect are not comparable (32). A combination of the following is probably responsible for the antihypertensive effect: (a) effects on vascular smooth muscle contractility; (b) structural changes in resistance vessels due to alterations in intracellular salt and water; and (c) the changes in extracellular volume (33).

Interactions (Table 2)

Interactions with Antihypertensive Drugs

The combination of diuretics and beta-adrenoceptor antagonists has already been mentioned. This is a very useful combination, and clinical experience with it is now extensive. Triple therapy, using a vasodilator, a beta-adrenoceptor antagonist, and a diuretic, is also common. Adequate blood pressure control is not always achieved with a beta-blocker–vasodilator combination, partly because of fluid

TABLE 2. *Interactions of diuretics*

Interaction	Effect
With antihypertensive drugs	
Beta-adrenoceptor antagonist	Opposing effects on renin release
Vasodilator	Synergistic antihypertensive effect and reduced fluid retention
Potassium-sparing diuretic	Opposing effects on potassium balance
ACE inhibitor	Synergistic antihypertensive effect and reduced potassium loss
With other drugs	
Potassium salts	Opposing effects on potassium balance
Digoxin	Increased toxicity in presence of diuretic-induced hypokalemia
Nonsteroidal anti-inflammatory drugs	Opposing effects on fluid balance and blood pressure
Indomethacin	Reversible renal impairment with triamterene
Colestipol	Reduced excretion of chlorothiazide
Probenecid	Enhanced diuresis; reduced uricosuric effect
Lithium	Enhanced toxicity

retention in an attempt to maintain blood pressure. A diuretic can reverse this response and exerts synergistic effects on blood pressure control. With very powerful vasodilators such as minoxidil, concomitant use of a diuretic is almost mandatory in order to prevent clinically evident fluid retention (34).

It is not uncommon in clinical practice to see two or more diuretics used together. The combination of a potassium-sparing diuretic and a thiazide is theoretically advantageous because it may not have any overall effect on plasma potassium. In practice, however, fixed dose combinations are not universally successful, since patients respond differently and either hypokalemia or hyperkalemia may still be observed under such circumstances.

One striking synergistic interaction of the diuretics is with the angiotensin-converting-enzyme (ACE) inhibitors. To some extent, the salt- and fluid-depleting effects of the diuretics are countered by reflex stimulation of the renin–angiotensin–aldosterone system. This is prevented by the use of an ACE inhibitor along with a diuretic. However, addition of an ACE inhibitor after diuretic "priming" may result in severe hypotension (35).

Interactions with Other Drugs

The effect of other drugs on plasma potassium levels is the subject of several further interactions. Oral potassium chloride supplements are frequently given in combination with thiazide diuretics, although such supplements are not universally required; moreover, the doses frequently given are not adequate if supplementation is required. Hypokalemia induced by thiazide diuretics may potentiate digoxin toxicity.

As with beta-adrenoceptor antagonists, there is evidence that indomethacin (and possibly other nonsteroidal anti-inflammatory drugs) can inhibit the antihypertensive effects of the diuretics (14). This is best documented with bendroflumethiazide (14) and chlorthalidone (13). There are conflicting results with hydrochlorothiazide (36–38). Once again, it has been suggested that sulindac does not impair the antihypertensive effect of thiazides and may indeed enhance this (39). Inhibition of prostaglandin synthesis (prostaglandin mediates both vasodilatation and renal sodium retention) is suggested to be the mechanism by which nonsteroidal drugs may increase blood pressure. Sulindac is reported to inhibit (exclusively) extrarenal prostaglandin synthesis and, thus, not to cause fluid retention. In general terms, the effect of nonsteroidal drugs on blood pressure control can be very striking in individual cases, and the frequency with which antihypertensive drugs and anti-inflammatory drugs are used together is such that this is an interaction of major significance.

One variant on the above involves the concurrent use of triamterine and indomethacin. In a limited number of healthy subjects, renal function has been significantly but reversibly impaired by the combination of triamterine and indomethacin but not by the individual drugs (40,41). Once again this appears to have been related to effects on prostaglandin synthesis.

A number of other less important interactions have been reported with the diuretics. These include (a) reduced excretion of chlorothiazide following colestipol (42) and (b) a two-way interaction between chlorothiazide and probenecid. Probenecid enhances the diuresis seen with chlorothiazide, but the uricosuric effect of probenecid may be inhibited by the diuretic (43,44). The combination of hydrochlorothiazide and triamterene with amantadine may produce toxic levels of amantadine (45) and diuretics may precipitate lithium toxicity.

In summary, the combination of diuretics with vasodilators and with beta adrenoceptor antagonists is a useful one. A number of diuretic interactions involve potassium. Some of these are useful, i.e. the combination of a thiazide with a potassium sparing agent, but there is also the potential for adverse interactions either between diuretics or with other groups. The diuretics may have a significant potentiating effect on the ACE inhibitors and the ACE inhibitors may protect against adverse metabolic effects with diuretics.

ACE INHIBITORS

This is a recently developed class of drugs that are finding increasing favor in the treatment of hypertension and heart failure. Compared with the beta-adrenoceptor antagonists or diuretics, experience with the ACE inhibitors is limited; thus, new interactions may still be identified.

Mode of Action and Clinical Features

ACE inhibitors such as captopril and enalapril interrupt the renin–angiotensin–aldosterone system at the level of conversion of angiotensin I to angiotensin II. They may therefore be associated with a reduction in fluid retention and a potassium-sparing effect. The main mechanism by which they lower blood pressure, however, appears to be associated with a vasodilator action through a combination of (a) withdrawal of the direct vasoconstrictor role of angiotensin II, (b) removal of angiotensin II facilitatory actions on the sympathetic nervous system, and (c) possibly also central actions. The possibility that some of their action depends on accumulation of bradykinin, for which ACE is one of the pathways for degradation, has been proposed but not established.

Interactions (Table 3)

Interactions with Antihypertensive Drugs

Since they act upon the renin–angiotensin system, the ACE inhibitors will potentiate the actions of diuretics or will be potentiated by the addition of a diuretic (46). The combination can be particularly useful in the treatment of hypertension but may be equally hazardous if the ACE inhibitor is added to a regimen including high-dose diuretics because severe first-dose hypotension may result (35). The combination of an ACE inhibitor and a diuretic is also attractive because hypokalemia is less likely to be encountered (47,48). However, if a potassium-sparing agent is used with an ACE inhibitor, then dangerous hyperkalemia may result (49) and thus this combination should be avoided.

Since the ACE inhibitors appear to lower blood pressure by vasodilatation, it might not appear logical to combine these drugs with other vasodilators. There is evidence from both volunteer and patient studies, however, that the combination of ACE inhibitor and calcium antagonist shows either no interaction (50) (i.e., simply additive effects) or a beneficial interaction (51–54).

Interactions with Other Drugs

For reasons already mentioned, the combination of ACE inhibitors and potassium salts may result in hyperkalemia. The potassium-sparing effect of the ACE inhibitors is not as powerful as that of the potassium-sparing diuretics, and it may therefore be appropriate to continue with some potassium supplements in certain cases; close supervision is clearly required.

As with other antihypertensive drugs, there is evidence that indomethacin may prevent the hypotensive action of captopril (55). Once again it seems reasonable to suggest that this may be a general interaction between the drug groups. High-dose naloxone inhibits the hypotensive action of captopril acutely (56) but not with chronic treatment (57). The absorption of captopril is reduced by antacids and food (58).

CALCIUM ANTAGONISTS

There are two main classes of drugs in this group: (i) the pyridine derivatives, such as nifedipine, and (ii) the papaverine derivatives, such as verapamil.

Mode of Action and Clinical Features

Smooth muscle contraction is initiated by membrane depolarization that is sodium dependent, followed by calcium influx through specific channels; the calcium antagonists restrict this influx, and thus they cause relaxation of vascular smooth muscle. Verapamil also inhibits atrioventricular conduction in the heart and inhibits the smooth muscle of the gut, whereas nifedipine appears more specific to vascular muscle. Diltiazem lies somewhere between these two.

Interactions (Table 4)

Interactions with Antihypertensive Drugs

All of the calcium antagonists show some pharmacodynamic interaction with beta-adrenoceptor antagonists (2–5). The dihydropyridine drugs show improved antihypertensive activity and antianginal effect when given in conjunction with a beta-adrenoceptor antagonist. This is due to reversal of the reflex sympathetic activation which would normally be encountered. A similar pharmacodynamic interaction with alpha-adrenoceptor antagonists has also been reported with nifedipine (59). Verapamil also

TABLE 3. *Interactions of the ACE inhibitors*

Interaction	Effect
With antihypertensive drugs	
Diuretic	Synergistic antihypertensive effect and reduced potassium loss
Potassium-sparing diuretic	Hyperkalemia
Calcium antagonists	Increased antihypertensive effect
With other drugs	
Potassium salt	Hyperkalemia
Nonsteroidal anti-inflammatory drugs	Opposing effects on blood pressure
Naloxone	Inhibits antihypertensive effect acutely
Antacids	Reduced absorption of captopril

TABLE 4. *Interactions of the calcium antagonists*

Interaction	Effect
With antihypertensive drugs	
Beta-adrenoceptor antagonist	Dihydropyridines: synergistic antihypertensive and antianginal effect; reduced tachycardia Papaverines: negative inotropic and chronotropic effect; increased levels of lipid soluble agents
Alpha-adrenoceptor antagonist	Increased antihypertensive effect
Prazosin	Verapamil causes increased levels of prazosin
ACE inhibitors	Increased antihypertensive effect
With other drugs	
Digoxin	Increased levels, especially with papaverines
Cimetidine	Increased levels of calcium antagonists
Carbamazepine	Verapamil increases levels
Cyclosporin	Diltiazem increases levels
Cytotoxic drug	Verapamil enhances effect
Quinidine	Verapamil increases levels; nifedipine reduces levels
Lithium	Increased lithium toxicity

shows a pharmacokinetic interaction with prazosin: Increased systemic bioavailability and higher peak levels of prazosin have been reported (60), possibly due to alterations either in hepatic blood flow (61) or enzyme activity (62). The combined alpha–beta-adrenoceptor antagonist, labetalol, enhances blood pressure fall with nifedipine, though this does not appear to be a synergistic interaction (63). While in normal volunteers there appears to be no pharmacokinetic or pharmacodynamic interaction between nifedipine and lisinopril (a new ACE inhibitor) (50), there have been some reports that the combination of calcium antagonist and ACE inhibitor is beneficial both in terms of antihypertensive efficacy and in reducing the biochemical effects, as well as the side effects, of both drugs (51–54). Although nifedipine does not appear to have any pharmacokinetic interaction with either atenolol or metoprolol (64), verapamil has been reported to increase the area under the curve for metoprolol by 30% (65). Diltiazem may also increase propranolol levels, perhaps by competing for protein-binding sites (66), though there is contrary evidence (67).

Interactions with Other Drugs

A number of interactions with other drugs has been reported. The most significant of these are effects on digoxin and effects caused by cimetidine. Verapamil, nifedipine, and diltiazem have each been reported to increase digoxin levels. In the case of nifedipine, this increase is around 15% (68,69); diltiazem increases digoxin levels by between 20% and 60% (70,71); and verapamil has been reported to cause a 60–70% increase in digoxin levels, probably by reducing renal clearance (72–74).

Cimetidine inhibits the metabolism of nifedipine (75) and has been reported to cause a 70% increase in the area under the curve for nifedipine (76). Cimetidine also inhibits the metabolism of verapamil (77). There is no evidence that ranitidine has an effect on either drug (76).

There is evidence that all of the calcium antagonists can affect liver metabolism. Both diltiazem and verapamil reduce antipyrine clearance (78,79); both nifedipine and verapamil increase indocyanine green clearance (79); and both verapamil and nifedipine may cause an increase in liver blood flow (79). It would therefore appear that nifedipine can be responsible for an increase in liver blood flow, that diltiazem can cause a reduction in oxidative drug metabolism, and that verapamil may produce both of these effects (78,79). There is some evidence that verapamil may thus increase carbamazepine levels significantly (80), and diltiazem has been reported to reduce the first-pass metabolism of propranolol (81). Cyclosporin metabolism is reduced by diltiazem, with resulting higher levels and increased risk of toxicity (82,83). Verapamil leads to enhanced toxicity of cytotoxic drugs *in vitro* and *in vivo* (84,85).

Verapamil and nifedipine appear to have conflicting effects on quinidine concentrations. Verapamil may increase quinidine concentrations through a reduction in clearance of approximately 50% (86) and may be associated with hypotension (87). Nifedipine, however, lowers quinidine levels (88). Other antiarrhythmic drugs that may interact with the calcium antagonists include disopyramide, whose effect may be increased by verapamil, and amiodarone, for which there is a solitary report of possible synergy with diltiazem resulting in sinus arrest (89).

There is a report of a possible interaction between diltiazem and lithium, resulting in lithium toxicity at "therapeutic" levels (90). A similar pharmacodynamic interaction has been reported in a larger number of subjects with verapamil and lithium, such that nausea, vomiting, muscular weakness, ataxia, and tinnitus were encountered when verapamil was added to lithium despite no significant change in plasma lithium concentrations (91).

In summary, the important interactions with the calcium antagonists are dependent on drug type. The agents with nifedipine-like effects show improved antihypertensive and antianginal efficacy in the presence of beta-blockade. The verapamil-like drugs may show increased toxicity in the presence of beta-blockade as a result of negative chronotropic, dromotropic, and inotropic actions. Similarly, although all calcium antagonists appear to increase digoxin levels and, to a much lesser extent, digitoxin levels, it is the verapamil-like drugs which are responsible for the greater effect. Despite the similar mechanisms of action, there appear to be useful improvements in antihypertensive efficacy when the calcium antagonists are added to other vasodilator regimens.

VASODILATORS

This heading includes the remaining vasodilators (such as hydralazine, minoxidil, and diazoxide) as well as the alpha-1-adrenoceptor antagonists (such as prazosin).

Mode of Action and Clinical Features

These drugs all have a direct relaxing effect on vascular smooth muscle. Apart from the known alpha-adrenoceptor antagonists, the effect does not appear to be mediated by actions on identified specific receptors or mechanisms. The result of vasodilatation of the precapillary arterioles is a fall in vascular resistance. This may be compensated for by an increase in sympathetic activity, which increases cardiac output (92); in addition, stimulation of the renin–angiotensin system may occur, leading to fluid retention (93).

Interactions (Table 5)

Interactions with Other Antihypertensive Drugs

The combination of vasodilators (which have a propensity to cause reflex sympathetic activation) and beta-adrenoceptor antagonists is, in general, beneficial. A useful increase in antihypertensive effect, along with a reduction in unpleasant subjective side effects, would be expected. However, the combination of prazosin and the beta-adrenoceptor antagonist propranolol has been reported to show increased intensity and duration of the orthostatic hypotension during introduction of prazosin treatment (94,95). The interaction does not appear to work in reverse, in that the addition of beta-blockade to long-term prazosin treatment is not associated with acute hypotension (96). Although the beta-adrenoceptor antagonists such as propranolol will enhance the antihypertensive activity of hydralazine (1), there is also evidence that hydralazine may significantly increase the bioavailability of propranolol (97) or metoprolol (98) but not of the remainder of the beta-adrenoceptor antagonists (98), which do not undergo significant first-pass metabolism.

Interactions with Other Drugs

The concurrent use of indomethacin with prazosin may reduce the hypotensive effect of prazosin (99). There is an interaction with sympathomimetic agents such that the alpha-adrenergic antagonists will inhibit the effects of these drugs. There do not, however, appear to be major interactions with other drug groups.

CENTRALLY ACTING DRUGS

Reserpine, clonidine, and alpha-methyldopa comprise this group. The first of these is undoubtedly an effective antihypertensive agent (100), but it causes sedation or depression and is now seldom used. Clonidine and related alpha-2-adrenoceptor agonists are used in low doses in the United States. Alpha-methyldopa has been in use for a quarter of a century and remains a widely prescribed drug.

Mode of Action and Clinical Features

After crossing the blood–brain barrier, alpha-methyldopa is decarboxylated to alpha-methylnoradrenaline, which is a relatively selective alpha-2-agonist (101). Clonidine also acts in the brain stem to stimulate alpha-2-receptors. Central control of blood pressure is modified, and the hemodynamic result is a fall in both peripheral vascular resistance and cardiac output (102).

Interactions (Table 6)

Interactions with Other Antihypertensive Drugs

A rapid blood pressure elevation may be encountered during clonidine withdrawal. This is exacerbated in the presence of beta-blockade (103–106) but not with labetalol (107). The combination of propranolol and methyldopa has been reported to result in a hypertensive reaction (108). This may occur more often with nonselective beta-adrenoceptor antagonists and is due to unopposed alpha-pressor activity.

Interactions with Other Drugs

There is some evidence that amitriptyline (109), but not all tricyclic antidepressants (110), may interact with methyldopa to antagonize the antihypertensive effects. This may

TABLE 5. *Interactions of vasodilators*

Interaction	Effect
With antihypertensive drugs	
Beta-adrenoceptor antagonists	Increased antihypertensive effect and reduced reflex tachycardia; hydralazine reduces the first-pass metabolism of lipid-soluble agents
With other drugs	
Nonsteroidal anti-inflammatory drugs	Opposing effects on blood pressure

TABLE 6. *Interactions of centrally acting drugs*

Interaction	Effect
With antihypertensive drugs	
Beta-adrenoceptor antagonists	Exacerbation of rebound hypertension during clonidine withdrawal; hypertensive reaction to combination of propranolol and methyldopa in some cases
With antihypertensive drugs	
Amitriptyline	Antagonizes antihypertensive effect of methyldopa and clonidine
L-Dopa	Methyldopa may increase or reduce the effect
Haloperidol	Reversible dementia with methyldopa
Noradrenaline	Enhanced pressor effect in presence of methyldopa

be due to central alpha-adrenoceptor-antagonist properties of the tricyclic antidepressants. The tricyclics antagonize the antihypertensive effect of both clonidine and methyldopa in animals (111). Other centrally acting drugs that may interact with methyldopa include L-dopa and haloperidol. Methyldopa may cause either an increase or a decrease in effect of L-dopa (112–116). There are reports of reversible dementia occurring after haloperidol was introduced on a background of methyldopa treatment (117–119). It has not been established whether this is due to synergistic inhibition of dopamine in the central nervous system. Finally, in view of the effects of methyldopa at adrenergic receptors, there is a potential for methyldopa to enhance the pressor effect of exogenous noradrenaline (120).

SUMMARY AND CONCLUSIONS

The major groups of drugs used in the treatment of hypertension have the potential for many drug interactions with each other and with other therapeutic agents. Fortunately, the vast majority of potential interactions do not result in any clinically significant effect; moreover, most of the identifiable drug reactions can be viewed as beneficial, since they either enhance antihypertensive effect or reduce adverse symptoms or side effects. Only a small number of therapeutically relevant adverse drug interactions have been characterized in spite of extensive world-wide use of antihypertensive drugs for more than 30 years. In general, these drug interactions, whether adverse or beneficial, can be predicted from the pharmacology or pharmacokinetics and metabolic features of the drugs concerned.

ACKNOWLEDGMENTS

The authors wish to thank Miss L. M. Gilbert and Mrs. R. Reid for invaluable help with research, as well as Miss N. Scott and Mrs. J. Hamilton for excellent secretarial assistance.

REFERENCES

1. Moses C. Drug treatment of mild hypertension: adverse consequences. *Ann NY Acad Sci* 1978;304:84–98.
2. Krikler DM, Harris L, Rowland E. Calcium channel blockers and beta blockers: advantages and disadvantages of combination therapy in chronic stable angina pectoris. *Am Heart J* 1982;104:702–708.
3. Leon MB, Rosing D, Bonow MD, Lipson LC and Epstein SE. Clinical efficacy of verapamil alone and in combination with propranolol in treating patients with chronic stable angina pectoris. *Am J Cardiol* 1981;48:131–139.
4. Subramanian B, Boules MJ, Davies AD, Raftery EB. Combined therapy with verapamil and propranolol in chronic stable angina. *Am J Cardiol* 1982;49:125–132.
5. Winniford MD, Huxley R, Hillis LD. Randomized double blind comparison of propranolol alone and a propranolol–verapamil combination in patients with severe angina of effort. *Am J Cardiol* 1983;1(2 Pt 1):492–498.
6. Harris WS, Schoenfield CD, Brooks RH, Weissler AM. Effect of beta adrenergic blockade on the hemodynamic responses to epinephrine in man. *Am J Cardiol* 1966;17:484–492.
7. Houben H, Thien Th, de Boo Th, et al. Influence of selective and nonselective beta-adrenoceptor blockade on the haemodynamic effect of adrenaline during antihypertensive drug therapy. *Clin Sci* 1979;57(Suppl):397s–399s.
8. Van Herwaarden CKA, Fennis JFM, Binkhorst RA and van't Laar A. Haemodynamic effects of adrenaline during treatment of hypertensive patients with propranolol and metoprolol. *Eur J Clin Pharmacol* 1977;12:397–402.
9. Struthers AD, Reid JL, Lawrie CB, Rodger JC. Beta-adrenoceptor-linked Na/K ATPase: the effect of cardioselective and nonselective beta-blockade. *Drugs* 1983;25:253p.
10. Grifting GT, Coakley CE, Lessell S, Melby JC. Atenolol and timolol. *N Engl J Med* 1982;307:1344–1345.
11. Cass E, Kadar D, Stein HA. Hazards of phenylephrine topical medication in persons taking propranolol. *Can Med Assoc J* 1979;120:1261–1262.
12. Durao V, Prata MM, Goncalves LMP. Modification of antihypertensive effects of beta-adrenoceptor-blocking agents by inhibition of endogenous prostaglandin synthesis. *Lancet* 1977;2: 1005–1007.
13. Lopez-Orejero JA, Weber MA, Drayer JIM, Sealey JE, Laragh JH. Effects of indomethacin alone and during diuretic or beta-adrenoceptor-blockade therapy on blood pressure and the renin system in essential hypertension. *Clin Sci Mol Med* 1978;55 (Suppl):203s–205s.
14. Watkins J, Abbott EC, Hensby CN, Webster J, Dollery CT. Attenuation of hypotensive effect of propranolol and thiazide diuretics by indomethacin. *Br Med J* 1980;281:702–705.
15. Salvetti A, Arzilli F, Pedrinelli R, Beggi P, Motolese M. Interaction between oxprenolol and indomethacin on blood pressure in essential hypertension patients. *Eur J Clin Pharmacol* 1982;22:197–201.
16. Puddey IB, Beilin LJ, Vandongen R, Banks R, Rouse I. Differential effects of sulindac and indomethacin on blood pressure in treated essential hypertension subjects. *Clin Sci* 1985;69:327–336.
17. Kirch W, Schafer-Korting M, Axthelm T, Kohler H, Mutschler E. Interaction of atenolol with furosemide and calcium salts. *Clin Pharmacol Ther* 1981;30:429–435.
18. Dobbs JH, Skoutakis VA, Acchardio SR, Dobbs BR. Effects of aluminium hydroxide on the absorption of propranolol. *Curr Ther Res* 1977;21:887.
19. Regardh CG, Lundborg P, Persson PA. The effects of antacid,

metoclopramide and propantheline on the bioavailability of metoprolol and atenolol. *Biopharm Drug Dispos* 1981;2:79–87.
20. Kendall MJ, Quarterman CP, Jack DB, Beeley L. Metoprolol pharmacokinetics and the oral contraceptive pill. *Br J Clin Pharmacol* 1982;14:120–122.
21. Feely J, Wilkinson GR, Wood AJJ. Reduction of liver blood flow and propranolol metabolism by cimetidine. *N Engl J Med* 1981;304:692–695.
22. Donovan MA, Heagerty AM, Patel L, Castleden CM, Pohl JF. Cimetidine and bioavailability of propranolol. *Lancet* 1981;1:164.
23. Heagerty AM, Donovan MA, Castleden CM, Pohl JF, Patel L, Hedges A. Influence of cimetidine on pharmacokinetics of propranolol. *Br Med J* 1981;282:1917–1919.
24. Kirch W, Hohler H, Spahn H, Mutschler E. Interaction of cimetidine with metoprolol, propranolol or atenolol. *Lancet* 1981;2:531–532.
25. Spahn H, Kirch W, Mutschler E. The interaction of cimetidine with metoprolol, atenolol, propranolol, pindolol and penbutolol. *Br J Clin Pharmacol* 1983;15:500–501.
26. Heagerty AM, Castleden CM, Patel L. Failure of ranitidine to interact with propranolol. *Br Med J* 1982;284:1304.
27. Reimann IW, Klotz U, Frolich JC. Effects of cimetidine and ranitidine on steady-state propranolol kinetics and dynamics. *Clin Pharmacol Ther* 1982;32:749–757.
28. Patel L, Weerasuriya K. Effect of cimetidine and ranitidine on propranolol clearance. *Br J Clin Pharmacol* 1983;15:152p.
29. Bennett PN, John VA, Whitmarsh VB. Effect of rifampicin on metoprolol and antipyrine kinetics. *Br J Clin Pharmacol* 1982;13:387–391.
30. Herman RJ, Nakamura K, Wilkinson GR, Wood AJJ. Induction of propranolol metabolism in man by rifampicin. *Br J Clin Pharmacol* 1983;16:565–569.
31. Conway J, Lauwers P. Hemodynamic and hypotensive effects of long-term therapy with chlorothiazide. *Circulation* 1960;21:21–27.
32. Carney S, Gillies AI, Morgan T. Optimal dose of a thiazide diuretic. *Med J Aust* 1976;2:692–693.
33. Tobian L. Why do thiazide diuretics lower blood pressure in essential hypertension? *Annu Rev Pharmacol* 1967;7:399–408.
34. Pettinger WA. Minoxidil and the treatment of severe hypertension. *N Engl J Med* 1980;303:922–926.
35. Cleland JGF, Dargie HJ, McAlpine H, et al. Severe hypotension after first dose of enalapril in heart failure. *Br Med J* 1985;291:1309–1312.
36. Williams RL, Davies RO, Berman RS, Holmes GI, Huber P, Gee WL, Lin ET, Benet LZ. Hydrochlorothiazide pharmacokinetics and pharmacologic effect: the influence of indomethacin. *J Clin Pharmacol* 1982;22:32–41.
37. Kramer HJ, Dusing R, Stinnesback B, et al. Interaction of conventional and antikaliuretic diuretics with the renal prostaglandin system. *Clin Sci* 1980;59:67–70.
38. Davis JW, Davis RF. Lack of effect of indomethacin on diuretic effects and plasma levels of hydrochlorothiazide. *Clin Pharmacol Ther* 1979;25:220.
39. Steiness E, Waldorff S. Different interactions of indomethacin and sulindac with thiazides in hypertension. *Br Med J* 1982;285:1702–1703.
40. Favre L, Glasson P, Vallotton MD. Reversible acute renal failure from combined triamterene and indomethacin. *Ann Intern Med* 1982;96:317–319.
41. Favre L, Glasson PH, Riondel A, Vallotten MB. Interaction of diuretics and non-steroidal anti-inflammatory drugs in man. *Clin Sci* 1983;64:407–415.
42. Kauffman R, Azarnoff DL. Effect of colestipol on gastrointestinal absorption of chlorothiazide in man. *Clin Pharmacol Ther* 1973;14:886–890.
43. Brater DC. Increase in diuretic effect of chlorothiazide by probenecid. *Clin Pharmacol Ther* 1978;23:259–265.
44. Steele TH, Oppenheimer S. Factors affecting urate excretion following diuretic administration in man. *Am J Med* 1969;47:564–574.
45. Wilson TW, Rajput AH. Amantadine–dyazide interaction. *Can Med Assoc J* 1983;129:974–975.
46. Vlasses PH, Rotmensch HH, Swanson BN, Irvin JD, Lee RB, Koplin JR, Ferguson RK. Comparative antihypertensive effects of enalapril maleate and hydrochlorothiazide, alone and in combination. *J Clin Pharmacol* 1983;23:227–233.
47. Atkinson AB, Brown JJ, Lever AF, McAreavey D, Robertson JIS. Combined treatment of severe intractable hypertension with captopril and diuretic. *Lancet* 1980;2:105–107.
48. Case DB, Atlas SA, Laragh JH, et al. Clinical experience with blockade of the renin–angiotensin–aldosterone system by an oral converting enzyme inhibitor (SQ 14,225, captopril) in hypertensive patients. *Prog Cardiovasc Dis* 1978;21:195–206.
49. Lo TCN, Cryer RJ. Complete heart block induced by hyperkalaemia associated with treatment with a combination of captopril and spironolactone. *Br Med J* 1986;292:1672.
50. Lees KR, Reid JL. Lisinopril and nifedipine: no acute interaction in normotensives. *Br J Clin Pharmacol* 1988;25:307–313.
51. Donnelly R, Elliott HL, Meredith PA, Reid JL. An evaluation of the pharmacodynamics and pharmacokinetics of nicardipine combined with enalapril in essential hypertension. *J Cardiovasc Pharmacol* 1988;10:723–727.
52. White WB, Viadero JJ, Lane TJ, Podesta S. Effects of combination therapy with captopril and nifedipine in severe or resistant hypertension. *Clin Pharmacol Ther* 1986;39:43–48.
53. Mimran A, Ribstein J. Effect of chronic nifedipine in patients inadequately controlled by a converting enzyme inhibitor and a diuretic. *J Cardiovasc Pharmacol* 1985;7(Suppl 1):S92–S95.
54. Brouwer RM, Bolli P, Erne P, Conen D, Wolfgang IC, Buhler F. Antihypertensive treatment using calcium antagonists in combination with captopril rather than diuretics. *J Cardiovasc Pharmacol* 1985;7(Suppl 1):S88–S91.
55. Swartz SK, Williams GH. Angiotensin-converting enzyme inhibition and prostaglandins. *Am J Cardiol* 1982;49:1405–1409.
56. Ajayi AA, Campbell BC, Rubin PC, Reid JL. Effect of naloxone on the actions of captopril. *Clin Pharmacol Ther* 1985;38:560–565.
57. Ajayi AA, Rubin PC, Reid JL. Captopril and opiate antagonism in essential hypertension. *Br J Clin Pharmacol* 1986;21:543–545.
58. Mantyla T, Mannisto PT, Vuorela A, Sundberg S, Ottoila P. Impairment of captopril bioavailability by concomitant food and antacid intake. *Int J Clin Pharmacol Ther Toxicol* 1984;22:626–629.
59. Sluiter HE, Huysmans FThM, Thien ThA, Koene RAP. The influence of alpha$_1$-adrenergic blockade on the acute antihypertensive effect of nifedipine. *Eur J Clin Pharmacol* 1985;29:263–267.
60. Pasanisi F, Elliott HL, Meredith PA, McSharry DR, Reid JL. Combined alpha adrenoceptor antagonism and calcium channel blockade in normal subjects. *Clin Pharmacol Ther* 1984;36:716–723.
61. Meredith PA, Elliott HL, Pasanisi F, Kelman AW, Sumner DJ, Reid JL. Verapamil pharmacokinetics and apparent hepatic and renal blood flow. *Br J Clin Pharmacol* 1985;20:101–106.
62. Buhler FR, Hulthen UL, Kiowski W, Bolli, P. Greater antihypertensive efficacy of the calcium channel inhibitor verapamil in older and low renin patients. *Clin Sci* 1982;63:439s–442s.
63. Ohman KP, Weiner L, von Schenck H, Karlberg BE. Antihypertensive and metabolic effects of nifedipine and labetalol alone and in combination in primary hypertension. *Eur J Clin Pharmacol* 1985;29:149–154.
64. Kendall MJ, Jack DB, Laugher SJ, Lobo J, Rolf Smith S. *Br J Clin Pharmacol* 1984;18:331–335.
65. Keech AC, Harper RW, Harrison PM, Pitt A, McLean AJ. Pharmacokinetic interaction between oral metoprolol and verapamil for angina pectoris. *Am J Cardiol* 1986;58:551–552.
66. Pieper JA. Serum protein binding interactions between propranolol and calcium channel blockers. *Drug Intell Clin Pharmac* 1984;18:492.
67. Bloedow DC, Piepho RW, Nies AS, Gal J. Serum binding of diltiazem in humans. *J Clin Pharmacol* 1982;22:201–205.
68. Kleinbloesem CH, van Brummelen P, Hillers J, Moolenaar AJ, Breimer DD. Interaction between digoxin and nifedipine at steady state in patients with atrial fibrillation. *Ther Drug Monit* 1985;7:372–376.
69. Kirch W, Hutt HJ, Dylewicz P, Graf KJ, Ohnhaus EE. Dose-de-

pendence of the nifedipine–digoxin interaction? *Clin Pharmacol Ther* 1986;39:35–39.
70. Oyama Y, Fujii S, Kanda K, et al. Digoxin–diltiazem interaction. *Am J Cardiol* 1984;53:1480–1481.
71. Thiercelin JF, Hermann Ph, Warrington S, Thenot JP, Morselli PL. Interaction study between digoxin and calcium antagonists: verapamil and diltiazem. In: Lemberger I, Reidenberg M, eds. *Proceedings of the II World Conference on Clinical Pharmacology and Therapeutics,* Washington, DC, July 31–August 5. Bethesda, Maryland: American Society for Pharmacology and Therapeutics, 1984;47.
72. Klein HO, Lang R, Weiss E. The influence of verapamil on serum digoxin concentration. *Circulation* 1982;65:998–1003.
73. Pedersen KE, Dorph-Pederson A, Hvidt S, Klitgaard NA, Nielsen-Kudsk F. Digoxin–verapamil on interaction. *Clin Pharmacol Ther* 1981;30:311–316.
74. Klein HO, Kaplinsky E. Verapamil and digoxin: their respective effects on atrial fibrillation and their interaction. *Am J Cardiol* 1982;50:894–902.
75. Kirch W, Ramsch K, Janisch HD, et al. The influence of two histamine H_2-antagonists, cimetidine and ranitidine, on plasma levels and clinical effect of nifedipine and metoprolol. *Arch Toxicol* 1984;7(Suppl):256–257.
76. Kendall MJ, Laugher SJ, Wilkins MR. Ranitidine, cimetidine and nifedipine—a pharmacokinetic interaction study. *Gastroenterology* 1986;90:1490.
77. Smith MS, Benyunes MC, Bjornsson TD, Shand DG, Pritchett EKC. Influence of cimetidine on verapamil kinetics and dynamics. *J Clin Pharmacol Ther* 1984;36:551–555.
78. Back D, Blevins R, Kerner N, Rubenfire M, Edwardes DJ. The effect of verapamil on antipyrine pharmacokinetics and metabolism in man. *Br J Clin Pharmacol* 1986;21:655–659.
79. Bauer LA, Stenwall M, Horn JR, Davis R, Opheim K, Greene L. Changes in antipyrine and indocyanine green kinetics during nifedipine, verapamil and diltiazem therapy. *Clin Pharmacol Ther* 1986;40:239–242.
80. MacPhee GJA, McInnes GT, Thompson GG, Brodie MJ. Verapamil potentiates carbamazepine neurotoxicity: a clinically important inhibitory interaction. *Lancet* 1986;1:700–703.
81. Etoh A, Kohno K, Shimizu T. Studies on the drug interaction of diltiazem II. Effect of co-administered diltiazem on the bioavailability of propranolol. *J Pharm Soc Jpn* 1983;103:434–441.
82. Pochet JM, Pirson Y. Cyclosporin–diltiazem interaction. *Lancet* 1986;1:979.
83. Grino JM, Sabate I, Castelao AM, Alsina J. Influence of diltiazem on cyclosporin clearance. *Lancet* 1986;1:1387.
84. Simpson WG, Tseng MT, Anderson KC, Harty JI. Verapamil enhancement of chemotherapeutic efficacy in human bladder cancer cells. *J Urol* 1984;132:574–576.
85. Rogan AM, Hamilton TC, Young RC, Klecker RWJ, Ozols RF. Reversal of adriamycin resistance by verapamil in human ovarian cancer. *Science* 1984;224:994–996.
86. Trohman RG, Esks DM, Castellanos A, Palomo AR, Jyerburg RJ, Kessler KM. *Am J Cardiol* 1986;57:706–707.
87. Epstein SE, Rosing DR. Verapamil: its potential for causing serious complications in patients with hypertrophic cardiomyopathy. *Circulation* 1981;64:437–441.
88. Farringer JA, Green JA, O'Rourke RA, Linn WA, Clementi WA. Nifedipine-induced alterations in serum quinidine concentrations. *Am Heart J* 1985;108:1570–1572.
89. Lee TH, Friedman PL, Goldman L, Stone PH, Antman EM. Sinus arrest and hypotension with combined amiodarone–diltiazem therapy. *Am Heart J* 1985;109:163–164.
90. Valdiserri EV. A possible interaction between lithium and diltiazem: case report. *J Clin Psychiatry* 1985;46:540–541.
91. Price WA, Giannini AJ. Neurotoxicity caused by lithium–verapamil synergism. *J Clin Pharmacol* 1986;26:717–719.
92. Fries ED. Hydralazine in hypertension. *Am Heart J* 1964;67:133–134.
93. Pettinger WA. Minoxidil and the treatment of severe hypertension. *N Engl J Med* 1980;303:922–926.
94. Elliott HL, McLean K, Sumner DJ, Meredith PA, Reid JL. Immediate cardiovascular responses to oral prazosin—effects of concurrent beta-blockers. *Clin Pharmacol Ther* 1981;29:303–309.
95. Graham RM, Thornell IR, Gain JM, Bagnoli C, Oates HF, Stokes GS. Prazosin: the first-dose phenomenon. *Br Med J* 1976;2:1293–1294.
96. Seideman P, Grahnen A, Haglund K, Lindstrom B, von Bahr C. Prazosin first dose phenomenon during combined treatment with a beta-adrenoceptor blocker in hypertensive patients. *Br J Clin Pharmacol* 1982;13:865–870.
97. McLean AJ, Skews H, Bobik A, Dudley FJ. Interaction between oral propranolol and hydralazine. *Clin Pharmacol Ther* 1980;27:726–732.
98. Jack DB, Kendall MJ, Dean I, Laugher SJ, Zaman R, Tenneson ME. The effect of hydralazine on the pharmacokinetics of three different beta adrenoceptor antagonists: metoprolol, nadolol and acebutolol. *Biopharm Drug Dispos* 1982;3:47–54.
99. Rubin P, Jackson G, Blaschke T. Studies on the clinical pharmacology of prazosin. II. The influence of indomethacin and of propranolol on the action and disposition of prazosin. *Br J Clin Pharmacol* 1980;10:33–39.
100. Veterans Administration Cooperative Study Group on Antihypertensive Agents. Effects of treatment on morbidity in hypertension. *JAMA* 1967;202:1028–1034.
101. Henning M, Rubenson A. Evidence that the hypotensive action of methyldopa is mediated by central actions of methylnoradrenaline. *J Pharm Pharmacol* 1971;23:407–411.
102. Sannerstedt R, Varnauskas E, Werko L. Hemodynamic effects of methyldopa (Aldomet) at rest and during exercise in patients with arterial hypertension. *Acta Med Scand* 1962;171:75–82.
103. Houston MC. Clonidine hydrochloride. *South Med J* 1982;75:713–719.
104. Vernon C, Sakula A. Fatal rebound hypertension after abrupt withdrawal of clonidine and propranolol. *Br J Clin Pract* 1979;33:112,121.
105. Bruce DL, Droley TF, LEE JS. Pre-operative clonidine withdrawal syndrome. *Anesthesiology* 1979;51:90–92.
106. Bailey RR, Neale TJ. Rapid clonidine withdrawal with blood pressure overshoot exaggerated by beta blockade. *Br Med J* 1976;1:942–943.
107. Rosenthal T, Rabinowitz B, Biochis H, Elazar E, Brauner A, Neufeld HN. Use of labetalol in hypertensive patients during discontinuation of clonidine therapy. *Eur J Clin Pharmacol* 1981;20:237–240.
108. Nies AS, Shand DG. Hypertensive response to propranolol in a patient treated with methyldopa—a proposed mechanism. *Clin Pharmacol Ther* 1973;14:823–826.
109. White AG. Methyldopa and amitriptyline. *Lancet* 1965;2:441.
110. Reid JL, Porsius AJ, Zamboulis C, Polak G, Hamilton CA, Dean CR. The effect of desmethylimipramine on the pharmacological actions of alpha methyldopa in man. *Eur J Clin Pharmacol* 1979;16:75–80.
111. van Zwieten PA. Interaction between centrally acting hypotensive drugs and tricyclic antidepressants. *Arch Int Pharmacodyn Ther* 1975;214:12–30.
112. Clark WG, Pogrund RS. Inhibition of dopa decarboxylase *in vitro* and *in vivo. Circ Res* 1961;9:721–733.
113. Smith SE. The pharmacological actions of 3,4-dihydroxyphenyl-alpha-methylalanine (alpha-methyldopa), an inhibitor of 5-hydroxytryptophan decarboxylase. *Br J Pharmacol* 1960;15:319–327.
114. Peaston MJT. Parkinsonism associated with alpha-methyldopa therapy. *Br Med J* 1964;2:168.
115. Vaidya RA, Vaidya AB, Van Woert MH. Galactorrhea and Parkinson-like syndrome: an adverse effect of alpha-methyldopa. *Metabolism* 1970;19:1068–1070.
116. Gibberd FB, Small E. Interaction between levodopa and methyldopa. *Br Med J* 1973;2:90–91.
117. Thornton WE. Dementia induced by methyldopa with haloperidol. *N Engl J Med* 1976;294:1222.
118. Nadel I, Wallach M. Drug interaction between haloperidol and methyldopa. *Br J Psychiatry* 1979;135:484.
119. Chouinard G, Pinard G, Serrano M, Tetreault L. Potentiation of haloperidol by alpha-methyldopa in treatment of schizophrenic patients. *Curr Ther Res* 1973;15:473.
120. Dollery CT, Harington M, Hodge JV. Haemodynamic studies with methyldopa: effect on cardiac output and response to pressor amines. *Br Heart J* 1963;25:670–676.

Hypertension: Pathophysiology, Diagnosis, and Management, edited by J. H. Laragh and B. M. Brenner. Raven Press, Ltd., New York © 1990.

CHAPTER 146

Withdrawal of Drug Therapy

A Component of the Proper Management of the Hypertensive Patient

Michael H. Alderman and Bernard Lamport

Studies of Drug Withdrawal, 2302
Degree of Successful Withdrawal of Drug Treatment, 2303
Factors Influencing the Success of Withdrawal, 2303
Demographic Factors, 2303
Clinical Characteristics, 2303
Postwithdrawal Actions That May Extend Normotension, 2304
What Is the Mechanism of Postwithdrawal Normotension?, 2305
Resetting the Baroreceptor, 2305
Structural Regression, 2305
The Natural History of Blood Pressure Hypothesis, 2305
Potential and Real Hazards of Drug Withdrawal, 2305
Loss to Follow-Up, 2305
Withdrawal Syndrome, 2306
Unanticipated Loss of Cardioprotective Effect, 2306
Advantages of Drug Withdrawal, 2306
Medical, 2306
Economic, 2306
Conclusion, 2306
References, 2307

Soon after orally effective antihypertensive therapy became available, the question of whether successful treatment could be followed by sustained blood pressure control was raised. In 1962, Page and Dustan (1) reported that 9 of 27 (33%) controlled hypertensive patients remained normotensive for more than 1 year following drug withdrawal. They (1,2), as well as other early observers (3), chose to focus primarily upon the recidivism that characterized the course of most patients whose pharmacological intervention had been interrupted. But it was also clear that the return of high blood pressure was gradual in virtually all patients, and, for a minority of subjects, normotension was maintained for periods in excess of a year.

The stimulus to withdraw drugs relates to several aspects of antihypertensive treatment and to the admonition *primum non nocere.* Virtually all medication carries the potential of adverse (and sometimes unanticipated) consequences. Some unwanted effects of aspirin, for example, were first noted only decades after this seemingly innocuous drug was introduced. For patients with high blood pressure, the prospect of lifelong commitment to recently discovered and rather nonspecific therapy is particularly awesome. A second reason for physicians to resist unnecessary therapy derives from the realization that available drugs are not aimed at the "cause" of stroke or heart attack but are, instead, designed to modify a predisposing "risk" factor. Not all hypertensives are candidates for stroke or heart attack. In fact, most hypertensive persons would live a long and happy life even in the absence of therapeutic intervention. Since the benefit of drugs is realized by only a small minority of hypertensive persons, avoidance of unnecessary drug therapy certainly makes sense. To these considerations can be added a desire to avoid the "medicalization" of so large a segment of the population and thereby further escalate health care costs. Quite appropriately, therefore, the 1988 Joint National Committee Report on the "Detection, Evaluation, and Treatment of High Blood Pressure" (4) has recommended that all successfully treated hypertensives be exposed to the opportunity for drug withdrawal.

The goal of this chapter is to review the available data regarding the consequences of drug withdrawal in successfully treated patients and to suggest guidelines for application in clinical practice. Systematic study of drug withdrawal from hypertensive patients is relatively new, and, not surprisingly, there is insufficient information at present to make precise recommendations suitable for each clinical situation. General principles do, however, appear to be supportable on the basis of available evidence.

STUDIES OF DRUG WITHDRAWAL

Since the first report of Page and Dustan (1), there have been 18 studies of drug withdrawal as part of the course of hypertensive treatment (1–3,5–19). Four of these (5,11,16,17) will not be further considered because of small numbers of participants or short periods of observation. One study (9) is not included because it involved only subjects on a low-salt (i.e., <100 mEq/day) diet. The remaining 13 studies included 1647 patients (Table 1). Most had essential hypertension, although 25 patients with malignant hypertension, renal arterial stenosis, and/or renal parenchymal disease were included in several of the studies (1,2). The average age of patients was 54 years, and 60% were men. In most studies, the majority of participants were white. The "known" duration of hypertension varied from 0.5 to 22 years, and the time of drug treatment before withdrawal varied from 0.5 to 10 years, with a mean of 3.8 years. All classes of antihypertensive drugs in a variety of combinations were used. Levels of blood pressure (BP) control believed sufficient for a trial of withdrawal varied from 160/100 to 140/80 mmHg. In the Medical Research Council (MRC) study (18), withdrawal was arbitrarily undertaken after a specific period of treatment, regardless of BP level. The time of controlled BP on drugs before withdrawal varied from 0.5 to 5 years. Six studies were controlled (2,6,8,10,13,18); in five of them, the withdrawn drugs were replaced by placebo. The longest observed duration of normotension following withdrawal was 10 years (2). In two studies (13,14), drug withdrawal was accompanied by nutritional intervention (weight reduction and/or sodium restriction), and some studies were extensions of large-scale intervention trials (6,18).

After completion of the Veterans Administration study (6), in which the pretreatment average BP was 171/112 mmHg, 86 patients whose treated DBP had been ≤95 mmHg for 2 years or longer were entered into a study to determine the effect of drug withdrawal. These 86 patients were assigned by stratified randomization: 60 received placebo in a double-blind manner and 26 were continued on active medication. During the 72 weeks of follow-up, 51 of the 60 placebo-treated patients had to terminate the trial. Of this number, 42 experienced return of increased arterial pressure, six had major cardiovascular complications, and three were removed for unrelated reasons with regard to their BP. Among the 26 who were actively treated, there were no morbid events and only one patient had a gradually rising diastolic blood pressure (DBP). Nevertheless, at the end of the 18-month period, 15% of 60 patients whose pretreatment BP averaged 171/109 mmHg were still normotensive without active drug therapy.

A similar study followed completion of the MRC trial (18). Of 4286 early entrants who had completed $5\frac{1}{2}$ years of follow-up (active and placebo groups) before the end of the study, 2765 agreed to participate in a study of drug withdrawal. Patients who had been receiving bendrofluazide, propranolol, or a placebo were randomly assigned to continue their regimens or be withdrawn. The report described 2332 patients who completed 3 months of follow-up, 1422 who had completed 12 months, and 650 who had completed 2 years.

TABLE 1. *Drug withdrawal after treatment of hypertension*[a]

Study	Reference	Number of patients	BP at withdrawal ≥ 1 year	Percent of normotensive patients
1	1	27	<95	33
2	2	34	<95	6
		9[b]	<95	0
3	3	69	<90	23
4	6	60[b]	<95	15
5	7	20	<100	5
6	8	24[b]	<90	5
7	10	31[b]	<90	74
8	12	59	<85	64
9A	13	70	<180/95	45
B		89[c]	<180/95	35
10	14	44[d]	<90	50
11	15	66	<140/85[e] <150/90[f]	44
12	18	NA[b]	<90	52
13	19	95	<140/90	28
		Total: 1647		32

[a] NA, not available; BP, blood pressure.
[b] Placebo controlled.
[c] Patients were ≥120% above ideal weight.
[d] Alcohol intake <26 g/day.
[e] For patients <65 years of age.
[f] For patients ≥65 years of age.

The results are presented in Table 2. It can be seen that controlled pressure (DBP < 90 mmHg) was as likely to be maintained in patients withdrawn from active drugs as in those withdrawn from placebo. Thus, among these mildly hypertensive patients, withdrawal of active treatment for 9–12 months produced the same result in terms of blood pressure control as was reached among those withdrawn from placebo (Table 2). The authors reasonably concluded that long-term active drug use conferred no particular benefit. But, from the perspective of those interested in the consequences of drug withdrawal, it is important that 45–56% of those withdrawn from drugs were still normotensive 12 months later, as was realized also by those withdrawn from placebo (Table 2). This suggests that the explanation for prolonged drug-free normotension may have little to do with any effect produced by the active drug.

The effect of repeated withdrawal of antihypertensive drugs has not been studied. In patients who have had more than one period without drug treatment, the course of arterial pressure was reported to be similar each time (2). If this is confirmed, then the process of drug withdrawal can, and must be repeated. The overall potential of drug withdrawal will then be substantially increased.

DEGREE OF SUCCESSFUL WITHDRAWAL OF DRUG TREATMENT

In the reported studies (Table 1), the percentage of successful withdrawal of drug treatment (maintenance of normal blood pressure for more than 1 year) varied from 0% to 74%, with an average of 32%. Since all but one of these studies included selected patients and were not denominator based, they should not be used to estimate the percentage of all persons receiving BP medications who could manage without drugs.

One study (15) was, however, denominator based (Fig. 1). All 196 patients in a worksite-based hypertension control program were studied. To be eligible for the study, participants had to (a) be taking BP medication at the time of initial screening or (b) have an average of BP readings, on at least two separate pretreatment occasions, of ≥160/95 mmHg or higher; they were also required to have (c) a 6-month period of medication use and (d) no contraindication to drug withdrawal, such as angina or peripheral edema. The population investigated was predominantly female and white, with a mean age of 55.7 years. The BP criteria for drug withdrawal were at least two readings, during a 6-month period, of ≤140/85 mmHg for those younger than 65 years old and of ≤150/90 mmHg for those 65 and older. Of the 157 patients who met entry criteria, 88 (56.1%) met BP control criteria for withdrawal. It must be noted that if the criterion for BP control had been relaxed to ≤160/90 mmHg, then 98.6% of the entire group of patients would have been eligible for withdrawal. Sixty-six of these 88 patients actually had drugs withdrawn. Of these, 44 (67%) remained drug free for more than 1 year; and at the end of the second year, 18 of the available 35 patients (51.4%) were still controlled. In sum, more than 25% of all patients in this general hypertensive population remained normotensive without drugs for at least 1 year.

TABLE 2. *MRC study: patients withdrawn from therapy, with diastolic pressure < 90 mmHg 1 year later (%)*

Treatment	Status	Men	Women
Bendrofluazide	Continued	73	83
	Withdrawn	57	56
Propranolol	Continued	79	77
	Withdrawn	48	45
Placebos	Continued	53	52
	Withdrawn	52	53

FACTORS INFLUENCING THE SUCCESS OF WITHDRAWAL

No studies have been specifically designed to determine whether there are demographic, constitutional, or clinical features of hypertensive patients, or aspects of process of treatment, or characteristics of the process of drug withdrawal that determine the success or failure of drug withdrawal. However, assessment of the available data suggests that some general rules may apply.

Demographic Factors

Age

In the Veterans Administration (VA) study, the 25 patients under 50 years of age experienced a rise in BP sooner after drug withdrawal than did 35 patients above 50 (6). Several other observers also found that younger patients were less able to sustain post-treatment normotension than were older subjects (16,17). In one study, however, just the reverse occurred (8). Thus, on the basis of the data, it is not possible to determine what (if any) impact age has on the likelihood of successful withdrawal. What is clear, however, is that even older subjects, whose vascular systems might be expected to condone less variability and whose hypertension is more established, are able to interrupt medication and maintain normotension.

Race

In the VA study (6), after drug withdrawal the BP rose more quickly in 30 black patients than in 30 white patients. The authors suggest that this probably related to the level of pretreatment BP, which was higher in black patients than in white patients (DBP 112 and 106 mmHg, respectively).

Clinical Characteristics

Pretreatment BP Level

Not surprisingly, the likelihood of successful drug withdrawal, as well as the mean duration of sustained normotension, is strongly related to pretreatment levels. In vir-

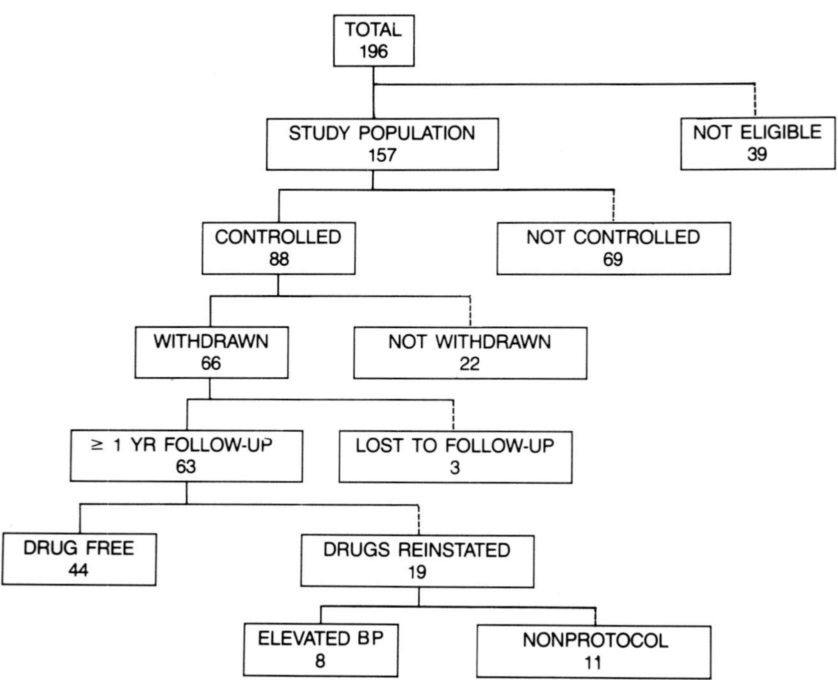

FIG. 1. Follow-up of withdrawal study population. (From ref. 15.)

tually all studies, those with milder levels maintained normotension longer than did those with higher levels. For example, in the VA study (6), pretreatment BP in successfully withdrawn patients was 153/102 mmHg, whereas those who relapsed had pre-study levels of 174/110 mmHg.

This observation is clearly consistent with the view that blood pressure varies widely and that, therefore, those closest to normal may have the best chance of achieving normality—at least on some occasions. In other words, regression toward the mean may account for some of the success observed after drugs are interrupted.

The Duration of Antihypertensive Therapy

This is of considerable importance, since it would be of considerable value to know how soon an attempt to discontinue drugs could be made. Page and Dustan (1) found that in eight hypertensive patients treated for less than 2 years, two (25%) remained controlled for 1 year after drug withdrawal, whereas in 10 patients treated for 2–6 years, eight (80%) remained normotensive, and in 12 patients treated for 5–9 years, nine (75%) remained normotensive. It has more recently been suggested that withdrawal of drugs in hypertension could be attempted after 6 months of control (20). Others have suggested that the period of treatment should be longer than 6 months but less than 5 years (21). In the absence of more precise data, there appears to be no contraindication with regard to attempting to remove drugs at any time. Moreover, despite the variety of their modes of action, there is no evidence that any particular drug treatment produces an important difference in post-treatment effect.

POSTWITHDRAWAL ACTIONS THAT MAY EXTEND NORMOTENSION (TABLE 3)

Nutritional interventions have been tested as means to extend the normotensive period after drugs. Since both sodium restriction and weight loss have been touted as effective means to reduce blood pressure, it is natural that

TABLE 3. *Influence of nutritional intervention on blood pressure after drug withdrawal: percent normotensive[a] at 1 year*

			Experimental		Control		
Reference	Weight status[b]	Intervention	Percent	Number of patients	Percent	Number of patients	Significance
13	Normal	Na[c] <40 mEq/day	53	68	45	70	NS[e]
	20% overweight	Na[c] <40 mEq/day	45	101	35	89	NS[e]
	20% overweight	4.5 kg weight loss[d]	59	87	35	89	<0.05
14	10–49% overweight	Na[c] <78 mEq/day + 1.8 kg weight loss[d]	69	97	50	44	<0.03 $\chi^2 = 4.73$

[a] <180/95 mmHg in ref. 13; <90 mmHg in ref. 14.
[b] By 1959 Metropolitan Life Insurance Tables for Desirable Body Weights.
[c] In addition, alcohol was restricted to <26 g/day.
[d] Group mean.
[e] NS, not significant.

they have also been recommended as adjuvants in the postwithdrawal phase.

In one uncontrolled study, it was suggested that sodium restriction was useful (9), since 75% of patients with salt restriction (i.e., <100 mEq/day) remained normotensive for 1 year after drug withdrawal, which appears to be higher than in studies not accompanied by salt restriction (see Table 1). In two controlled studies, the issue of nonpharmacological augmentation of drug withdrawal has been assessed (13,14). In one of these studies (14), 141 drug-withdrawn subjects were allocated to either alcohol restriction alone or in association with weight reduction *and* sodium restriction. It was found that the more comprehensively advised group did better (69% versus 50%, $p < 0.03$) than the alcohol-alone-restricted group at 1 year (Table 3).

A more discrete model was assessed among graduates of the Hypertension Detection and Follow-Up Program (HDFP) study (13) (Table 3). Participants were stratified into overweight and normal-weight categories. Normal-weight subjects were randomized to sodium-restricted or control groups after drug withdrawal. Of note is the fact that, overall, persons of normal weight had greater success than those who were obese. The overweight subjects were further randomized to either sodium-restricted, weight-loss, or control groups. Sodium restriction conferred no important advantage, but weight loss substantially increased the likelihood of success at 1 year.

The potential contribution to blood pressure containment that calcium, potassium, and/or fat intake might make has not been specifically evaluated. The value of physical exercise has not been assessed either.

WHAT IS THE MECHANISM OF POSTWITHDRAWAL NORMOTENSION?

Resetting the Baroreceptor

The notion that a change in carotid sinus baroreceptor setting could be responsible for postwithdrawal normotension was first suggested by Page and Dustan in 1962 (1). It had been previously shown that the carotid sinus of a Goldblatt dog lost the capacity to react by electric discharge to a further elevation of BP (22). Page and Dustan suggested that prolonged artificial normotension restored the ability of carotid baroreceptor to react to increased BP by lowering it. While attractive, this hypothesis lacks experimental validation.

Structural Regression

Vascular wall thickening (23) and left ventricular hypertrophy (LVH) (24) have long been recognized as consequences of sustained high blood pressure, although these morphological findings may sometimes precede the discovery of hypertension. Both these structural changes are also believed to play a role in sustaining hypertension. Following discovery of effective antihypertensive therapy, it was demonstrated that prolonged artificial reduction of blood pressure could reverse these structural changes (25–27). It was then noted, first in rats (28) and then in humans (11,29), that the maintenance of normotension after drug therapy withdrawal was related to the regression of the heart and blood vessel enlargement. There was, however, a study involving 24 patients in which it was found that left ventricular mass did not differ between patients whose pressure remained normal and those whose rose after drug withdrawal (8).

On balance, the weight of evidence supports the logical notion that some hypertrophy of vessels and heart play a role in the maintenance of blood pressure elevation. When corrected by therapy, this might contribute to sustained normotension. The "structural-regression" hypothesis suggests a potentially predictive sign of what might happen after drug withdrawal. Patients with pronounced regression, or absence of LVH and/or elevated total peripheral resistance index, would be promising candidates for successful withdrawal of drug treatment.

The Natural History of Blood Pressure Hypothesis

Blood pressure varies over each day and over time in all persons, both hypertensive and normotensive. Moreover, long-term studies of representative populations demonstrate that not all persons experience a rise in pressure over time. In fact, pressure often actually falls (30,31) (Table 4). Of 865 control subjects with initial DBP >160/95 mmHg, 40% had, after 5 years, BP <160/95 mmHg despite no treatment (31). In the Australian National Trial of Antihypertensive therapy (30), 48% of mild hypertensives who had been randomized to the control placebo group experienced a fall in pressure that persisted up to 3 years (30).

POTENTIAL AND REAL HAZARDS OF DRUG WITHDRAWAL

No studies of drug withdrawal in hypertension have reported any substantial adverse consequences. However, there are three possible areas of reasonable concern: loss to follow-up; withdrawal syndrome; and increased risk of cardiovascular disease (CVD) after withdrawal of drugs, even in normotensive subjects.

Loss to Follow-Up

Loss of follow-up has plagued hypertension control efforts since the dawn of the modern treatment era. Attrition is high even in regular drug treatment programs, and its

TABLE 4. *Spontaneous remission among persons with initial blood pressure >160/95 mmHg*

Reference	Number of patients	Follow-up (years)	Percentage of patients with blood pressure <160/95 mmHg
30	1963	3	48
31	865	5	40

increase after drug withdrawal seem a reasonable project (32). But, to our knowledge, no study has shown that dropouts increase after drugs are withdrawn. In fact, among patients withdrawn from drugs in one study (15), it was specifically noted that there was no increase in patient loss. Nevertheless, it is reasonable to be concerned that in this asymptomatic condition, some patients, lacking the need to refill a prescription, would permit their adherence to lapse. We believe, however, that patient adherence is central to all antihypertensive treatment and must be vigorously addressed in drug-treated patients as well as in withdrawn patients.

Withdrawal Syndrome

Three kinds of withdrawal syndrome have been noted to follow cessation of antihypertensive therapy (33): (i) BP remains relatively controlled or rises comparatively slowly, but the patient experiences signs and symptoms of sympathetic overactivity or experiences the occurrence of some morbid CVD event in predisposed patients, such as unstable angina, arrhythmias, acute myocardial infarction, or sudden death. (ii) There is sometimes a rapid return of BP to pretreatment levels, with symptoms and signs of sympathetic overactivity and sometimes encephalopathy, cerebrovascular and/or cardiovascular accidents. (iii) Sometimes observed is an "overshoot" of hypertension—a rapid rise of BP above pretreatment levels associated with subjective symptoms and signs of sympathetic overactivity and/or morbid cardiovascular events. These forms of withdrawal syndrome presumably may develop after cessation of treatment with all classes of antihypertensive drugs but have actually been seen to develop in only a few situations (i.e., after withdrawal of the central alpha-adrenoceptors clonidine and methyldopa) (34). Happily, in studies designed specifically to assess the impact of drug withdrawal, there has been no notice of any form of withdrawal syndrome. However, it certainly might occur and is a strong argument for continuing surveillance. Sufficient experience now exists, however, to make it exceedingly unlikely that an immediate catastrophic clinical event will immediately follow drug withdrawal. If reasonable precautions of gradual withdrawal are followed, risks should be minimal, particularly in mild or moderate hypertension.

Unanticipated Loss of Cardioprotective Effect

Some antihypertensive agents (i.e., beta-blockers) have cardioprotective effects beyond their hypotensive capacity (35). Perhaps their withdrawal could increase the risk of myocardial infarction. In view of the fact that in clinical trials of therapy for mild hypertension there was no cardioprotective effect of treatment, this seems more a theoretical than a practical concern.

By contrast, in the withdrawal study following the VA trial (6), which involved patients with average entry BP of 171/112 mmHg, the following was observed: Of 60 patients withdrawn from drug treatment, six developed severe cardiovascular complications (fatal myocardial infarction, nonfatal congestive heart failure, atrial fibrillation, and right bundle branch block), whereas none of 26 patients continuing drug treatment had such serious CVD complications. This difference did not attain significance; however, in view of the small sample size, its importance remains. It should be noted that these patients were severely hypertensive before treatment and, after withdrawal, were permitted to have pressures well above normal. Clearly, the conditions of drug reintroduction that characterized current practice were not applied in that study.

ADVANTAGES OF DRUG WITHDRAWAL

Medical

Antihypertensive drugs can adversely effect electrolyte, carbohydrate, and lipid metabolism (36–38). Withdrawal of drugs have been shown to normalize these metabolic shifts. Patients treated with diuretics have been shown to experience hyperuricemia, hyperglycemia, hyperlipidemia, and hypokalemia (36). It is hard to imagine that these metabolic rearrangements offer any particular medical benefit, although the actual extent of their adverse consequences is unknown. In a variety of studies (6,12,36), it has been shown that most metabolic alterations disappear or, at the very least, tend to regress toward pretreatment levels after drugs are withdrawn. Other adverse reactions to bendrofluazide and/or propranolol, such as impotence, dizziness, Raynaud's phenomenon, dyspnea, rash, lethargy, nausea, and headaches, also were rapidly reversible after withdrawal of these drugs (36). Moreover, drug discontinuation has a substantial psychological effect by providing patients with objective evidence of improvement (39).

Economic

About 33% of 60 million hypertensive patients in the United States, or about 20 million patients, are taking antihypertensive medication (40). Extrapolation from the small-denominator-based experience available (15) suggests that it may be possible to interrupt, for periods as long as 1 year, the drugs of 25% of these patients. This would translate into 5 million persons free of drugs and still normotensive.

The annual cost of drug treatment is about $200 ($140 for drugs and $60 for laboratory tests to detect drug complications) per patient (41). Elimination of this cost for 5 million patients would mean an annual savings of $1 billion.

CONCLUSION

What, then, are the reasonable recommendations for clinical practice that can be supported from the accumulated experience reviewed here? We believe that the data sustain several important conclusions. First, that discontinuation of antihypertensive drugs in successfully treated hypertensive patients is safe. In fact, there is little credible evidence that, even in patients whose pretreatment blood pressure levels were very high, there was any risk of dramatic sudden reversal of pressure or other adverse effects. Second, although blood pressure tends to rise in most patients after drug withdrawal so that by the end of a year, the majority again require pharmacological intervention, that rise is gradual, and a substantial minority remain normotensive for at least a year. Third, only the pretreatment level of pressure has been shown to predict the likelihood of successful withdrawal, and, not surprisingly, milder patients tend to do better than more severe hypertensives. Nevertheless, even patients with higher pressures do have the capacity to sometimes maintain normotension for prolonged periods of time. They also, therefore, deserve an attempt at withdrawal. The promising observation that regression of heart and blood vessel hypertrophy may predict successful withdrawal requires further assessment. Fourth, nonpharmacological measures may, in some patients, improve the chances for extending the period of normotension. This appears more likely when weight loss, rather than sodium restriction, is prescribed. Fifth, treatment-associated metabolic arrangements disappear in most patients following drug withdrawal. Finally, and disappointingly, it is not possible to explain why normotension persists in some patients whose drugs are removed, or why it fails in others. This should hardly be surprising, since neither the explanation for blood pressure elevation nor the determinants of its natural history are known.

In sum, the withdrawal of antihypertensive drug therapy deserves to become a standard dimension of the care of patients with high blood pressure. The notion that all hypertensive patients must remain on drugs for the rest of their lives is no longer consistent with available medical knowledge. Indeed, the regular attempt to reduce and, when possible, discontinue all medication should become a routine component of good medical practice for each and every patient. The goal of care is blood pressure control purchased with the least possible therapeutic intrusion. While the exact duration of successful control that should precede an attempt to discontinue drugs is unknown, it is generally felt that perhaps 6 months, or certainly a year, is a sufficient period to precede a trial of withdrawal of drug therapy with safety and with some chance of success. It should be done gradually and in combination with regular patient follow-up to ensure timely reintroduction of drug therapy.

If interrupted treatment becomes standard therapy, perhaps 25% of all treated hypertensives may be successfully managed without drugs for periods in excess of 1 year. Society will surely benefit through reduced drug costs. But more importantly, the real gainers will be large numbers of individual patients who, without sacrificing the benefits of normal blood pressure, will be freed of the discomfort, potential hazards, and expense of permanent drug dependence.

REFERENCES

1. Page IH, Dustan HP. Persistence of normal blood pressure after discontinuing treatment in hypertensive patients [Editorial]. *Circulation* 1962;25:433–436.
2. Dustan HP, Page IH, Tarazi RC, Frolich ED. Arterial pressure responses to discontinuing antihypertensive drugs. *Circulation* 1968;37:370–379.
3. Thurm RH, Smith WM. On resetting of "barostats" in hypertensive patients. *JAMA* 1967;201:85–88.
4. 1988 Joint National Committee. The 1988 Report of the Joint National Committee on detection, evaluation, and treatment of high blood pressure. *Arch Intern Med* 1988;148:1023–1038.
5. Perry HM, Schroeder HA, Catanzaro FJ, Moore-Jones D, Camel GH. Studies on the control of hypertension. VIII. Mortality, morbidity, and remissions during twelve years of intensive therapy. *Circulation* 1966;33:958–972.
6. Veteran Administration Cooperative Study Group on Antihypertensive Agents. Return of elevated blood pressure after withdrawal of antihypertensive drugs. *Circulation* 1975;51:1107–1113.
7. Boyle RM, Price ML, Hamilton M. Thiazide withdrawal in hypertension. *J R Coll Physicians Lond* 1979;13:172–173.
8. Levinson PD, Khatri IM, Freis ED. Persistence of normal BP after withdrawal of drug treatment in mild hypertension. *Arch Intern Med* 1982;142:2265–2268.
9. Fernandez PG, Galway AB, Kim BK, Granter S. Prolonged normotension following cessation of therapy in uncomplicated essential hypertension. *Clin Invest Med* 1982;5:31–37.
10. Maland LJ, Lutz LJ, Castle H. Effect of withdrawing diuretic therapy on blood pressure in mild hypertension. *Hypertension* 1983;5:539–544.
11. Jennings G, Korner P, Esler M, Restall R. Redevelopment of essential hypertension after cessation of long term therapy; preliminary findings. *Clin Exp Hypertens [A]* 1984;A6(1&2):493–505.
12. Finnerty FA. Step-down treatment of mild systemic hypertension. *Am J Cardiol* 1984;53:1304–1307.
13. Langford HG, Blaufox D, Oberman A, et al. Dietary therapy slows the return of hypertension after stopping prolonged medication. *JAMA* 1985;253:657–664.
14. Stamler R, Stamler J, Grimm R, et al. Nutritional therapy for high blood pressure. Final report of a four-year randomized controlled trial—the hypertension control program. *JAMA* 1987;257:1184–1191.
15. Alderman MH, David TK, Gerber LM, Robb M. Antihypertensive drug therapy withdrawal in a general population. *Arch Intern Med* 1986;148:1309–1311.
16. Smith SA, Mace JE, Litter WA. Felodipine, blood pressure, and cardiovascular reflexes in hypertensive humans. *Hypertension* 1986;8:1172–1178.
17. Ruoff G. Effect of withdrawal of terazosin therapy in patients with hypertension. *Am J Med* 1986;80(Suppl 5B):35–41.
18. Medical Research Council Working Party on Mild Hypertension. Course of blood pressure in mild hypertensives after withdrawal of long term antihypertensive treatment. *Br Med J* 1986;293:988–992.
19. Dannenberg AL, Kannel WB. Remission of hypertension. The 'natural' history of blood pressure treatment in the Framingham study. *JAMA* 1987;257:1177–1183.
20. Finnerty FA. Slowing the return of hypertension after stopping medication [Letter]. *JAMA* 1985;254:503.
21. Langford HG, Blaufox MD, Oberman A, Hawkins CM. In reply to FA Finnerty [Letter]. *JAMA* 1985;254:503.
22. McCubbin JW, Green JH, Page IH. Baroreceptor function in chronic renal hypertension. *Circ Res* 1956;4:205–210.
23. Berry C. Mechanical vascular changes and hypertension: pathological consequences. *Pathol Res Pract* 1985;180:336–337.
24. Frolich ED. The heart in hypertension: unresolved conceptual challenges. *Hypertension* 1988;11(Suppl 1):I-19–I-24.
25. Jennings GL, Esler MD, Korner PH. Effect of prolonged treatment on haemodynamics of essential hypertension before and after autonomic block. *Lancet* 1980;11:166–169.
26. Folkow B. The structural factor in primary hypertension: its relevance for future principles of treatment. *J Hypertens* 1987;5(Suppl 5):5611–5613.
27. Hartford M, Wendelhag I, Berglund G, et al. Cardiovascular and renal effects of long-term antihypertensive treatment. *JAMA* 1988;259:2553–2557.
28. Cadilhac M, Giudicelli JF. Myocardial and vascular effects of perindopril, a new converting enzyme inhibitor, during hypertension development in spontaneously hypertensive rats. *Arch Int Pharmacodyn* 1986;284:114–126.

29. Korner PI, Jennings GL, Esler MD, Broughton A. A new approach to the identification of pathogenetic factors and to therapy in human primary hypertension. *J Clin Hypertens* 1987;3:187–196.
30. A Report by the Management Committee of the Australian Therapeutic Trial in Mild Hypertension. Untreated mild hypertension. *Lancet* 1982;II:185–191.
31. Liu L, Ling Y, Jao S. A five year follow-up study of hypertension in 10,450 steel workers. *Chin Med J* 1979;92:719–722.
32. Smith WM. Resetting of barostat revised. *Arch Intern Med* 1982;142:2263–2264.
33. Houston MC. Abrupt cessation of treatment in hypertension: considerations of clinical features, mechanisms, prevention and management of the discontinuation syndrome. *Am Heart J* 1981;102:415–430.
34. Reid JL. Alpha-adrenergic receptors and blood pressure control. *Am J Cardiol* 1986;57:6E–12E.
35. Cohn JN. Role of drugs for systemic hypertension and their effect on the heart. *Am J Cardiol* 1987;60:72G–74G.
36. Report of Medical Research Council Working Party on Mild to Moderate Hypertension. Adverse reactions to bendrofluazide and propranolol for the treatment of mild hypertension. *Lancet* 1982;II:539–542.
37. Flamenbaum W. Metabolic consequences of antihypertensive therapy. *Arch Intern Med* 1983;98(part 2):875–880.
38. Stark RM. The atherogenic risk of antihypertensive therapy. *Am J Med* 1988;84(Suppl 1B):86–88.
39. Finnerty FA. Step-down therapy in hypertension. Importance in long-term management. *JAMA* 1981;246:2593–2596.
40. Hypertension prevalence and the status of awareness, treatment, and control in the United States. Final Report of the Subcommittee on definition and prevalence of the 1984 Joint National Committee. *Hypertension* 1985;7:457–468.
41. Stason WB. Opportunities for improving the cost-effectiveness of antihypertensive treatment. *Am J Med* 1986;81(Suppl 6C):45–49.

Hypertension: Pathophysiology, Diagnosis, and Management, edited by J. H. Laragh and B. M. Brenner. Raven Press, Ltd., New York © 1990.

CHAPTER 147

Medication-Taking in Hypertension

Peter Rudd and Gary Marshall

The Clinical Experiment, 2309
Chapter Overview, 2309
Definitions of Compliance, 2310
Alternative Terms, 2310
Assumptions, 2310
Forms of Improper Medication-Taking, 2310
Average Rates May Be Potentially Misleading, 2310
Regimen Components, 2310
Medication-Taking as a Continuous Variable, 2312
Medication-Taking Distributions, 2312
Summary, 2313
The Importance of Suboptimal Compliance, 2313
Extremes of Suboptimal Medication-Taking, 2313
The Dilemma of the Clinical Experiment, 2313
Consequences of Misclassifying Outcomes, 2313
Clinical Practice Settings, 2314
Clinical Trial Settings, 2314
Compliance Bias, 2314
Measures for Diagnosing Noncompliance, 2315
Measurement as Key, 2315
Direct, Biologic Measures, 2315
Indirect, Nonbiologic Measures, 2315
Comparative Performance Among Measures, 2317
Emergence of Medication Monitors, 2319
New Applications for the Medication Monitor, 2320
Recent Monitor Implementations in Clinical Trials, 2320
The Epidemiology of Compliance, 2320
Incidence and Prevalence, 2320
Natural History of Medication-Taking, 2321
Determinants/Predictors of Suboptimal Medication-Taking, 2321
Interventions to Enhance Medication-Taking, 2322
Guidelines for Clinicians and Investigators, 2323
Guidelines for Clinicians, 2323
Guidelines for Investigators, 2324
References, 2324

In light of what will be discussed in this chapter, we would like to quote the famous Greek physician Hippocrates, who, in his famous work *Aphorisms,* stated:

> Life is short, and the Art long; the occasion fleeting; experience fallacious; and judgment difficult. The physician must not only be prepared to do what is right for himself, but also to make the patient, the attendants, and externals cooperate.

THE CLINICAL EXPERIMENT

When treating hypertension with medication, the clinician performs a series of linked therapeutic experiments. He/she prescribes treatment, reviews the degree of achieving goal blood pressure, assesses other possible consequences of the treatment, and decides about optimal follow-up. This deceptively simple sequence contains hidden complexities, especially in interpreting the experiment's results. At each return visit, the clinician must decide whether the current treatment is appropriate, adequate, and advantageous, as compared to alternatives. We believe that the heart of the complexity centers on properly assessing compliance with the regimen.

CHAPTER OVERVIEW

This chapter summarizes much of what is known about medication compliance in hypertension. Often, the perspective of medication-taking behavior will be more useful than that of traditional "compliance." We shall address seven aspects relevant to both clinicians and investigators: (a) definitions of compliance; (b) the importance of suboptimal compliance; (c) measures for detecting and diagnosing noncompliance; (d) the epidemiology of compliance; (e) determinants and predictors of suboptimal compliance; (f) interventions for enhancing compliance; and (g) guidelines for clinicians and investigators. Since some of the biggest hurdles and most exciting developments are occurring in the area of measuring medication-taking, we shall place special emphasis there.

Our search will concentrate on aspects related to hypertension management whenever the reports support the distinction between hypertension and other medical conditions. We shall provide a critical and selective overview of the literature rather than trying to be comprehensive. For the interested reader, a number of relatively recent, balanced reviews with extensive bibliographies are available (1–8). When appropriate, we shall supplement the discussion with some of our unpublished data from a prospective comparison of multiple compliance measurements in an antihypertensive drug trial. Finally, we shall highlight unresolved areas, especially those in need of thoughtful future inquiry.

DEFINITIONS OF COMPLIANCE

Alternative Terms

The literature utilizes several terms for referring to *compliance,* most commonly defined as the extent to which a person's behavior (in terms of taking medications, following diets, or making other lifestyle changes) coincides with medical advice (9). An alternative term for the failure to comply is *defaulting.* Still other expressions for the concept have included *adherence* and *therapeutic alliance,* words which perhaps connote a more cooperative or interactive relationship between the clinician and the patient. The concept itself is nonjudgmental and assigns no specific blame for failure to any individual. The multiplicity of terms underscores the multifaceted nature of medication-taking.

Assumptions

This broad definition implicitly assumes a number of conditions (10,11). First, it assumes that the medical condition under consideration has been properly diagnosed. Second, the definition presupposes that effective treatment exists in a form shown to produce more good than harm. Third, it assumes that the clinician provides the recommendations in an understandable and achievable form. For example, suboptimal compliance might result if the prescription were offered in ambiguous language or at a cost prohibitive for a particular patient.

These assumptions are not trivial. They underscore the fact that compliance for medication-taking is situation-specific and subject to multiple influences. There is little sense to measure or to try improving adherence when the diagnosis is incorrect, since the treatment will prove to be generally harmful. For the specific case of hypertension, compliance represents the essential link between early detection/evaluation and subsequent long-term benefit (12).

Forms of Improper Medication-Taking

The forms of improper medication-taking may provide important management clues. Using verbal self-report from 357 outpatients, Hulka et al. (13,14) identified three predominant types of medication errors: inadvertent errors of commission, inadvertent errors of omission, and scheduling misconception. Much less commonly, they found deliberate scheduling noncompliance. The distinctions have implications for management. For example, there is a difference between (a) forgetting to take a pill despite knowing the proper regimen and (b) believing incorrectly that only two, rather than three, pills are needed daily. The causes and reinforcers of these four different forms are dissimilar. Whenever possible, therefore, the form(s) of medication-taking error should be specified in the definition of suboptimal compliance.

Average Rates May Be Potentially Misleading

Simple or composite averages for medication-taking may be misleading. Figure 1 summarizes some of our own data on mean intervisit compliance by pill count for the first 15 visits among 121 ambulatory hypertensives followed prospectively for up to 12 months (15). The sample size varies markedly by visit because many subjects could progress rapidly through dosage titration to maintenance level treatment. The group's mean rate of medication-taking varies little, although small sample sizes at any one visit tend to exaggerate the standard deviation. In contrast, Fig. 2 illustrates weekly pill count data from three of the subjects, each of whose average overall compliance rate closely approximated 100%. Nevertheless, their weekly rates varied wildly and without discernible pattern. Of special interest, after 14 weeks of weekly pill counts, the medication-taking rate was assessed only monthly. When the measurement interval lengthened, the apparent variability diminished, since under- and overcompliance phases compensated for each other. Thus, the time frame for assessing each regimen component should be specified.

Regimen Components

Meaningful definitions of compliance for medication-taking should separately assess each of the regimen's components. The behavioral demands of beginning a weight-loss exercise program are both qualitatively and quantitatively unlike those of starting antihypertensive medications. Initiating both components at once may inhibit adherence to both. Not surprisingly, the degree of compliance for one component may not correlate with that for another (16,17). The more numerous the prescribed new behaviors, the less likely that any one component will be followed (18). A patient may adhere rigidly to one ingredient and poorly to another, only to alter both patterns unexpectedly. Sometimes these changes may be linked to disruptive life events or to other alterations in routine.

Figure 3 demonstrates the poor correspondence among different drugs in the same regimen. Using pill-count compliance rates, we have graphed the medication-taking among 60 of the subjects for the interval between visits 14 and 15. The subjects received a primary study drug (hydralazine or pinacidil) alone or in combination with propranolol and/or hydrochlorothiazide. By pill count, the medica-

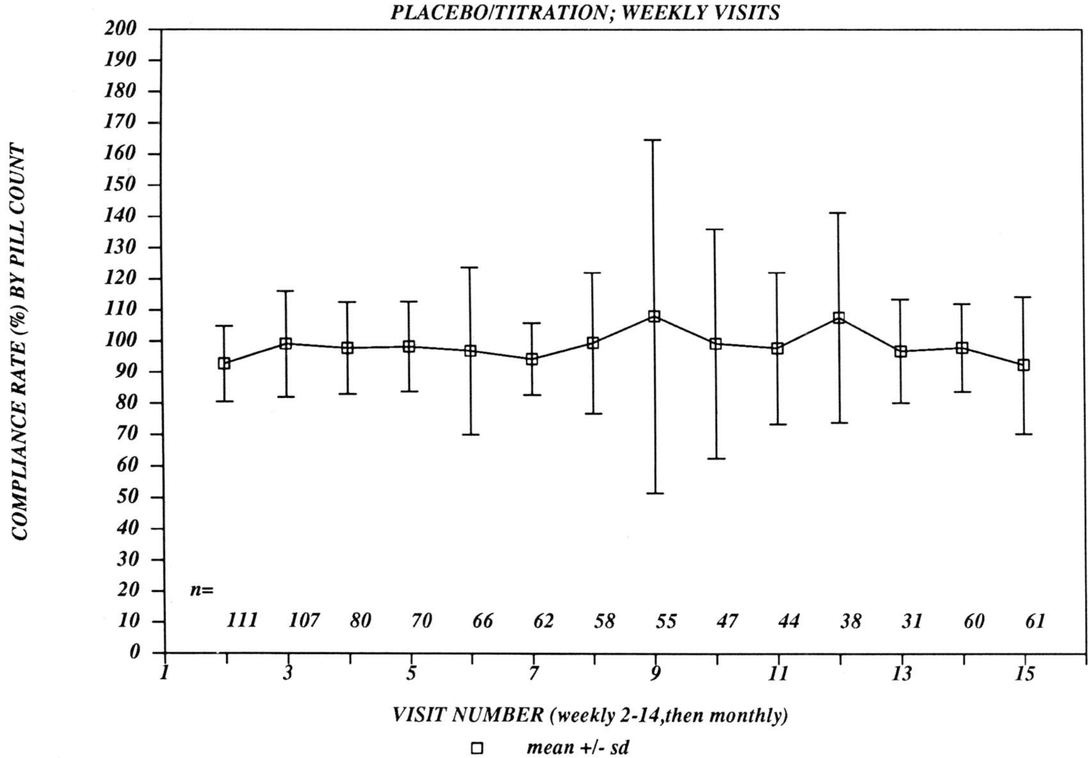

FIG. 1. Pill-count compliance in an ambulatory hypertensive drug trial. Initial cohort size = 121; there is a variable sample size at different visits because of rapid progression through titration for some subjects.

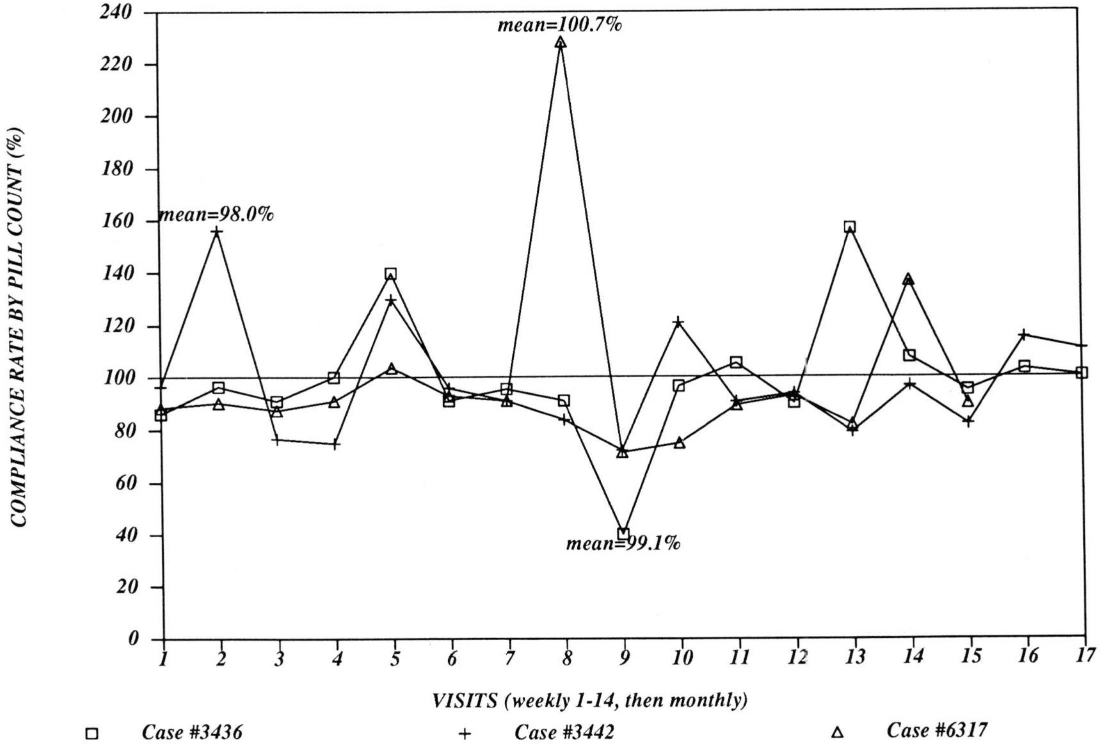

FIG. 2. Week-to-week variability in pill-count compliance. Compliance rate is calculated as the percentage of prescribed pills missing on return pill count of those which should have been taken.

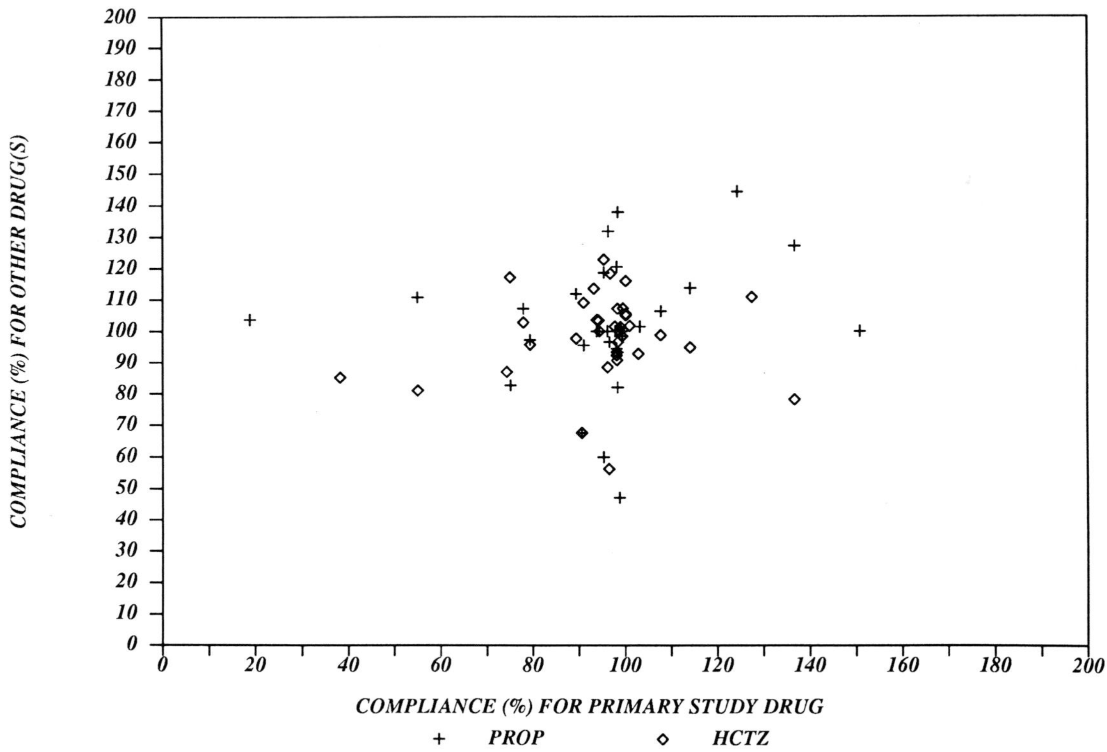

FIG. 3. Nonconcordance among pill counts according to regimen component. Each point represents the intersection of compliance rates by pill count for the primary study drug (pinacidil or hydralazine) and one of the secondary drugs (hydrochlorothiazide or propranolol).

tion-taking rates for the primary drug vary from 20% to 150%, with comparable spread for the other drugs. The scatter confirms that medication-taking behavior for one drug offers limited predictive value for any other drug in the regimen.

In addition, both simple and complex interactions may occur among regimen components. This includes both antihypertensive medications, medications for other conditions, and non-drug components. For example, complying with smoking cessation may prompt increased eating and weight gain, adversely affecting blood pressure control (19). Alternatively, careful adherence to a new prescription for a nonsteroidal anti-inflammatory agent may lead to fluid retention and blunting of antihypertensive drugs' efficacy (20). Behaviorally, a complying patient may then lose the reinforcing benefit of feedback that his/her blood pressure is well controlled. To be comprehensive, definitions must acknowledge the possibility of dynamic and dramatic shifts among compliance levels by component.

Medication-Taking as a Continuous Variable

The dynamic nature of medication-taking behavior favors description as a continuous (e.g., 75% versus 103%), rather than as a dichotomous (e.g., compliance versus noncompliance), variable. Once the clinical prescription is defined and the time frame is specified, we may quantify adherence to it using scales of proportion or percentage. Such metrics permit useful comparisons for the same patient over time or among different patients. Few clinical situations correspond to simplistic models of patients exhibiting either "good" or "bad" compliance (21). Such categories cover wide ranges of medication-taking behavior. Too many uncertainties prevail for dichotomous variables to suffice: (a) How much compliance is enough? (b) What is the relation between delivered dosage and therapeutic effect? (c) Is there a graded relationship or a discrete threshold for efficacy? Only continuous distributions allow searches and answers to such questions. Finally, simplistic categorizations obscure covariation between medication-taking behavior and the many factors that may influence it.

Medication-Taking Distributions

Populations of patients demonstrate a range of compliance rates, even for standardized, simple regimens. The observed distributions are rarely "normal" or bell-shaped. They therefore may be inadequately summarized by measures of central tendency (such as mean compliance rates) or by measures of variance (such as their standard deviation). Evaluating the full compliance distribution carries the additional benefit of identifying instances of overcompliance as well as of undercompliance (22).

Some instances of apparent overconsumption of medication may be an artifact of improper pill counts, whether by patient misrepresentation (e.g., pill-dumping prior to scheduled visits) or staff error. But others (23,24) have reported patient subgroups who systematically or periodically take more than they should, a practice with great potential dangers. The problem may be particularly ominous for the elderly, among whom impaired drug metabolism may combine with overcompliance to produce morbid consequences (25). Possible causes for such overcompliance may include forgetting that a dose was already taken and overcompensating for prior missed doses.

Summary

Simple definitions of compliance carry several critical assumptions. Most importantly, they assume the propriety of the clinical prescription and then seek the degree of concordance between prescription and patient behavior. The behavior itself is complex: multifaceted, capable of subtle or dramatic interaction among regimen components, and dynamic from interval to interval for most individuals and within groups of patients. Perhaps the most accurate definition incorporates the complexity: *Compliance* is the dynamic degree of correspondence between the clinical prescription for any regimen component and the patient's measured behavior in response to the prescription.

THE IMPORTANCE OF SUBOPTIMAL COMPLIANCE

Extremes of Suboptimal Medication-Taking

When we apply this definition to antihypertensive management, the importance of suboptimal compliance emerges. The vast majority of hypertensives, estimated at 98%, have primary hypertension or secondary hypertension of an incurable type (26). For them, long-term compliance with treatment is the essential method for controlling the disease. Most primary prevention trials confirm that consistent reduction in blood pressure is associated with parallel reductions in cardiovascular morbidity and mortality (27).

At the most simplistic level, low levels of medication-taking are likely to produce little blood pressure reduction and therefore less-than-maximal decreases in hypertensive and atherosclerotic complications. Economic analysis indicates that further expenditures for widespread screening and treatment programs are unjustified without substantial progress in reducing the high rates of dropping out of treatment and/or consuming suboptimal levels of medication (28). One telling case report noted that a wife brought in her dead husband's unused medications after his 3-year illness. Less than 100 capsules of the 3100 pills dispensed (3%) were missing from the medication vials (29). At the other extreme, taking more medication than prescribed may bring about drug-related toxicities and impair quality-of-life (30). Both extremes appear patently undesirable.

The Dilemma of the Clinical Experiment

Keeping these extreme possibilities in mind, we return to the dilemma of how best to interpret the clinical experiment, as posed in the first section of this chapter. For the particular case of hypertension management, the clinician seeks to help the patient achieve and maintain goal blood pressure. The clinician's interpretative problem, summarized by Taylor et al. (31) and Rudd and Marshall (32), centers on needing to assign the clinical response to one of four categories: (a) *high/good* (high compliance, with achieved good blood pressure control), corresponding to the ideal situation of correct diagnosis, full patient cooperation, and complete pharmacological response; (b) *high/poor* (high compliance, with non-achieved blood pressure control), suggesting an insufficiently vigorous regimen or perhaps pharmacologic resistance; (c) *low/good* (low compliance, with achieved blood pressure control), most consistent with either an incorrect diagnosis for a patient not needing antihypertensive treatment in the first place or perhaps overzealous prescription for mild disease; or (d) *low/poor* (low compliance, with non-achieved blood pressure control), corresponding to the classical noncomplier. The latter presumably does not need a more vigorous regimen, only the will and consistency to adhere to the existing prescription.

The interventions appropriate to each of the four categories are dissimilar. Unfortunately, the clinician is frequently unable to classify the clinical response with certainty. Sometimes, he/she will fail to consider the possibility that suboptimal medication-taking may account for the inability to achieve goal blood pressure. Fearing the risks of uncontrolled hypertension, the clinician may escalate the antihypertensive regimen to larger doses or more potent medications. The patient then undergoes the alternative risks of treatment-related toxicities.

Only limited data are available to suggest the relative frequency of misclassification. Taylor et al. (31) reported the outcomes among 134 hypertensive male steelworkers, providing pill counts (compliance measure) and casual blood pressures during a home visit 6 and 12 months after starting antihypertensive treatment. The investigators selected 80% compliance as the threshold for optimal medication-taking as a result of regression analysis, indicating that 80% was the minimal level of medication-taking associated with consistent reduction of blood pressure to the preselected goal level (11). They observed that only 23% had achieved goal blood pressure (defined as <90 mmHg) with high compliance (defined as ≥80% of the prescribed medication). In contrast, 12% of the subjects achieved goal blood pressure despite suboptimal medication-taking, whereas 34% showed uncontrolled blood pressure despite high compliance. The remaining 31% exhibited both uncontrolled blood pressure and low compliance. Thus, only 35% of the subjects achieved the goal blood pressure, and only 66% of these did so with near-optimal medication-taking.

Consequences of Misclassifying Outcomes

If we accept and generalize from these findings, several worrisome possibilities appear. We must cautiously conclude that up to two-thirds of patients might have their regimens adjusted incorrectly: Some incorrect adjustments might be due to clinicians failing to consider the possibility of suboptimal medication-taking as the cause of failure to achieve goal blood pressure, whereas some might be due to clinicians who ascribe all treatment failure to inadequate medication-taking. In such cases, they might reinforce the existing but inadequate regimen, offering the patient incomplete protection despite full cooperation. Very similar findings and distributions of patients were found in other ambulatory treatment settings (33). Inui et al. (34) observed that 40% of their well-controlled hypertensives were "noncompliant" by pill count, suggesting overmedication or misdiagnosis. We therefore believe the potential for misclassification to be a real issue and one of considerable magnitude. Improving assessment of patients' medication-taking behavior remains pivotal.

Clinical Practice Settings

In clinical practice, the dilemma becomes more complex, since a subgroup of individuals may spontaneously regress to normotensive levels. The clinician may then incorrectly conclude that the treatment is both successful and necessary. Among the Australian National High Blood Pressure Trial participants (27), fully 25% on inactive placebo treatment achieved goal blood pressure (<90 mmHg) and avoided cardiovascular complications over the 5-year study. The more worrisome error, of course, would be to aggressively augment the regimen for an individual who intermittently complies. Such a person would get less-than-optimal protection from cardiovascular morbidity and mortality, more-than-necessary exposure to drug effects, and major swings in blood pressure level.

One intriguing approach to quantify the potential for such distortion would be to define a "usefulness product" (UP) for each drug application. The UP represents the mathematical product of mean effectiveness for a given therapeutic goal (the average proportion of patients who respond pharmacologically to the drug for lowering blood pressure) and mean compliance for the particular medication (35). Such a composite score would allow setting preferences among alternative antihypertensive medications, taking into account both (a) the optimal effectiveness of each drug when taken as prescribed and (b) the likely clinical impact in real-world clinical settings in which medication-taking behavior is often suboptimal.

Clinical Trial Settings

In clinical drug trials, several other interpretative dilemmas occur. Many trials select relatively stable, uncomplicated hypertensive patients willing and able to comply with (a) the demanding constraints of multiple return visits, (b) frequent clinical and laboratory monitoring, and (c) the uncertainties of receiving investigational agents. Until recently, few studies even bothered to assess medication compliance. Soutter and Kennedy (36) reported that only 19% of 768 trials reported in the *British Medical Journal* or *Lancet* in 1969–1972 included any measure of adherence. Failure to do so runs the risks of erroneously concluding (a) that true differences do not exist, when inadequate medication-taking among those on the more effective treatment might account for no apparent difference, or (b) that similar drugs have differing efficacy, when the differences really reflect only the medication-taking rates.

High versus low compliers will differ quantitatively in the extent to which they exhibit a treatment response. Haynes and Dantes (37) reviewed several studies which indicate that the noncomplier (even to placebo treatment) may have other important differences, such as dying at nearly twice the rate as those who complied with placebo treatment in a coronary disease primary prevention trial ($p < 0.0001$). These observations underline the importance of including intensive follow-up and careful reporting of both noncompliers and compliers in any trial's analysis.

At the simplest level, noncompliance may increase within-group variance and diminish observed treatment effects enough to make acquisition of an adequate sample size an impractical matter. The minimal sample size required in order to achieve predetermined levels of statistical significance is directly proportional to the square of the standard deviation, itself an indication of the scatter around the mean. As mean compliance rates fall from 100% to 50%, the required sample size for each arm of a study may increase three- to fourfold (22).

Compliance Bias

Another issue involves distortion of the clinical trial's validity. As discussed by Feinstein (10,38) and Goldsmith (22) with hypothetical examples, *compliance bias* may result from different ways of handling suboptimal compliance in the design and analysis of trials. Often, the suboptimal compliance remains undetected or masked. The bias refers to several kinds of incorrect conclusions related to how subjects are selected, monitored, and/or analyzed. A *compliance sample* may arise when patients' willingness to cooperate is one entry criterion for participation. The resultant risk is that study subjects may be nonrepresentative of the patient population at large, thereby impairing generalizability to other groups.

A second type of bias is the result of association between medication-taking and other factors directly linked to one of the outcome variables. When present, this condition produces different outcome rates among those subjects who complied with the regimen than among those who did not, independent of the medication's effect itself. An ineffective regimen may then appear beneficial or deleterious to those who adhere to it, when compared to those who did not comply. Alternatively, an effective regimen may seem useless if the compliance rate is sufficiently low. Simple calculations confirm how compliance bias may lead to erroneous results (38), although some mathematical compensation is possible (39). Joyce (40) has provided one of the earliest demonstrations of how factoring in compliance levels minimizes misinterpretation of empiric trial results. Perhaps most usefully, analysis by compliance subgroup permits definition of a therapeutic gradient in which more adherence to a specified regimen may yield a proportional increase in benefit. The Lipid Research Clinics Coronary Primary Prevention trial provided one such demonstration (41).

MEASURES FOR DIAGNOSING NONCOMPLIANCE

Measurement as Key

The prior statements about consequences of suboptimal compliance were all predicted on knowing whether individuals were or were not consuming their medication. For compliance, as with many other aspects of science, measurement is the key. Measurement helps define the process, allows assessment of incidence and prevalence, permits a search for predictors, and enables evaluation of interventions. Without proper measurement, none of these things is possible. Both the pattern and rate of adherence are important. The specific measures we select, and the pattern with which we apply them, create a sampling of medication-taking behavior (42). We must still interpret the results of the sampling with circumspection.

Several excellent reviews have discussed the array of traditional measures of compliance as well as their relative advantages and disadvantages (32,43–46) (Table 1). The existing measures may be classified as either direct or indirect, biologic or nonbiologic.

Direct, Biologic Measures

The *direct measures,* like biologic assays of active drug or metabolite, confirm actual drug ingestion. If the details of dosing, possible interfering substances, pharmacokinetics, and pharmacodynamics are all known, one may make educated guesses about when drug ingestion last occurred (47). More realistically, clinicians and investigators rarely know all of these details. Many of the analytical techniques are complex, expensive, and, as yet, impractical for most ambulatory settings (48,49). A few successful applications are reported for a circumscribed number of antihypertensive drugs (50). The complexities of individual patients' metabolism further confound the effort. Even more importantly, biologic assays give little information about the consistency of medication-taking, especially back further than five half-lives for the index drug, the interval generally required for equilibrium to be achieved. To interpret individual drug concentrations, one may need to establish threshold criteria corresponding to optimal medication-taking. The criteria, in turn, will reflect arbitrary levels with trade-offs of sensitivity versus specificity. In sum, biologic measures often raise as many questions as they solve.

Markers have become a tempting but frustrating alternative to direct biologic assays (51). Most commonly, they consist of one of several biologically inert substances whose ingestion may be coupled, in some predictable way, with that of the active medication (52). Upon consumption, the marker may be monitored by semiquantitative urine assays or other direct assessment, free of the complexities surrounding the body's handling of the active drug. Several major problems remain. Existing regulatory agencies (e.g., Food and Drug Administration, Department of Agriculture) have not settled the question of how markers such as riboflavin should be considered. If the marker is a "drug," it must meet all FDA regulations for safety and efficacy, a laborious and expensive process. If it is a "food" or vitamin, still other guidelines would apply.

Most available data relate to riboflavin (53). Unfortunately, marked patient-to-patient variability in excretion patterns, interobserver variability in measuring urinary fluorescence, and interference from other riboflavin sources such as food supplements remain as unresolved issues (51,54). Other approaches include radioactive labeled markers (such as chromium-51) and stable isotopes (such as deuterium, oxygen-18, carbon-13, and nitrogen-15). Regardless of the specific marker, its data on adherence provide little assistance in reaching a behavioral diagnosis to explain suboptimal compliance or in reaching a basis for initiating and modifying interventions (55).

Indirect, Nonbiologic Measures

In contrast, *indirect measures* assess medication-taking without confirming that drug ingestion actually occurred. Such measures include the following: patient self-report (both prospective and recall); self-monitoring with a diary or log; pill count; monitoring prescription refills; clinician's opinion; therapeutic effect; and, most recently, a growing array of medication monitors. As a group, with the exception of the medication monitor and self-monitoring diaries, these measures assess compliance in a process distant in time and place from the actual medication-taking event. As a consequence, a variety of distortions may occur.

Self-report, in all its permutations, tends to exaggerate the adequacy of compliance (56,57). More rarely, close

TABLE 1. *Comparison of compliance measures*

Measure of medication-taking	Documentation of:							
	Intake	Dose	Frequency	Consistency	Duration	Objectivity	Practicality	Cost
1. Patient self-report	No	No	No	No	No	No	High	Low
2. Patient self-monitoring	No	±	±	±	±	No	High	Low
3. Pill count	No	±	±	±	±	Yes	±	Moderate
4. Biologic assay	Yes	±	±	±	±	Yes	±	High
5. Clinician opinion	No	No	No	No	No	No	High	Low
6. Therapeutic outcome	No	No	No	No	No	Yes	High	Low
7. Direct observation	Yes	Yes	Yes	Yes	Yes	Yes	Unacceptable	High
8. Medication monitor	No	±	Yes	Yes	Yes	Yes	High	Moderate to high

correlation between self-report and more objective measures such as medication count has been described (58). Patients may report the specifics of interdose intervals more accurately than the issue of whether or not they omitted particular doses (59). The longer the period of requested recall, the more likely the subject is to minimize deviation from the prescription. Scant published data are available to define the limit for accurate recall; it is probably less than 2 weeks (60). Beyond that interval, the inquiry will likely yield a simple estimate of average compliance, with little chance of an accurate, reproducible summary of specific doses taken versus doses missed. Much like difficulty in remembering what one has eaten or worn longer ago than 2 days previously, most patients can give valid recall of medication-taking events up to a period of 48 hr. Self-report may have further advantages in identifying individuals more likely to enhance their compliance when corrective interventions are applied (11). A compound decision rule combining blood pressure data and verbal inquiry yielded higher sensitivity (83%) than did self-report alone (55%) for detecting suboptimal compliance in an ambulatory, hypertensive population (34).

Pill counts are used extensively to estimate medication-taking in ambulatory drug trials, both for screening prior to study entry during placebo washout phases and for chronic monitoring of long-term medication-taking. As part of a drug trial, participating subjects quickly become accustomed to returning the pill supply at each visit, allowing surreptitious pill counts. Anecdotally, some subjects appear to cooperate by returning near-perfect pill counts or empty vials, while leaving many intact pills in clinic parking lots or waste containers. Pill counts can give only a putative average compliance rate for a particular interval. The longer the interval becomes (e.g., weeks instead of days), the more likely that important deviation will be obscured by the average compliance rate, as illustrated in Figs. 1 and 2.

Many investigators encounter logistical obstacles for pill counts, including subjects' forgetting to return pill vials, losing containers, sharing medication with other individuals, and storing medication in more than one place. In their usual application, pill counts require that patients/subjects remember to bring their medication container back at each visit. The very request to have them do this may prompt patients to conclude that medication-taking is under surveillance. Although simple reminders that compliance is important should be beneficial, any patient's concern about being judged may also induce duplicitous behavior, such as discarding some pills to simulate full adherence. These obstacles, in addition to the costs of the labor-intensive technique and the high probability of sensitizing patients to their medication-taking being monitored, make pill counts impractical for most nonresearch clinical settings (16).

Our own data on the 121 subjects in an antihypertensive drug trial illustrate several interesting features about pill counts (15). To continue in the study, the population had to meet entry criteria for both blood pressure and medication compliance and had to be willing to return at frequent intervals for monitoring of blood pressure and side effects. We observed that the compliance distribution for this highly selected population of chronic hypertensives was bell-shaped but skewed, centered close to 100%, as portrayed in Fig. 4.

Compliance rates by pill count frequently exceeded 100%. One possible explanation was patient dumping of medication, since patients generally received at least 50% more medication than would normally be required for the prescribed interval until the next scheduled visit. Thirty-three of the 1052 intervisit pill counts (3%) exceeded three standard deviations above the group mean (i.e., >135%), representing one to three visits with extremely high compliance rates among 24 subjects. Such improbably high rates likely represent a combination of (a) partial dumping of unused or lost pill supplies (increasing the compliance rate numerator) and (b) shorter-than-expected visit intervals (decreasing the denominator). Further indirect evidence for such pill dumping comes from our finding that 42 of 121 subjects (35%) showed >110% compliance by pill count on at least one visit (range: one to four visits).

Prescription refills may serve as a less sensitizing alternative to the pill count but may incorporate other shortcomings. The method is based on monitoring the prescribed dosing frequency and the interval between prescription renewals (61). In practical terms, patients may confound the technique by electing to obtain refills at more than one pharmacy. Some settings, such as prepaid health plans and military/institutional programs, may still use the approach because of centralized functions. Inui et al. (17) used prescription refill rates to track hypertensive outpatients in a Veterans Administration setting. They observed a U-shaped, rather than a bell-shaped, frequency distribution for patients' pattern of refills. The former presumably corresponds to most subjects faithfully filling nearly all, or nearly none, of their prescriptions. Possible confounding factors in "free care" settings may involve economic incentives for patients to share free or reduced-cost drugs with other individuals or may involve an absence of financial incentives so that patients will purchase only those medications which they will actually consume.

Clinicians' opinions sometimes appear in the literature as a measure of medication-taking. When carefully evaluated, they prove to be a disappointing measure of compliance (56,62). Early, seminal studies by Roth et al. (63,64) indicated that (a) more objective measures were essential and (b) most physicians performed little better than chance in predicting the degree to which suboptimal medication-taking occurred. As a rule, clinician opinion is highly specific (i.e., individuals whom they identified as likely to be noncompliant were usually not taking most of their prescribed medication) but relatively insensitive (56). Many patients they believed to be compliant were, in reality, suboptimal compliers. In these studies, more experienced clinicians did little better than did more junior trainees. Brody (65) has suggested that physicians may (a) be unaware of the importance of the relevant behavioral, psychological, and social aspects of care, (b) have insufficient time and/or skills to identify them, or (c) lack the skills or motivation to manage these problems.

Therapeutic impact is the measure perhaps most distal to the medication-taking event. For the particular case of hypertension, many confounding factors such as intercurrent

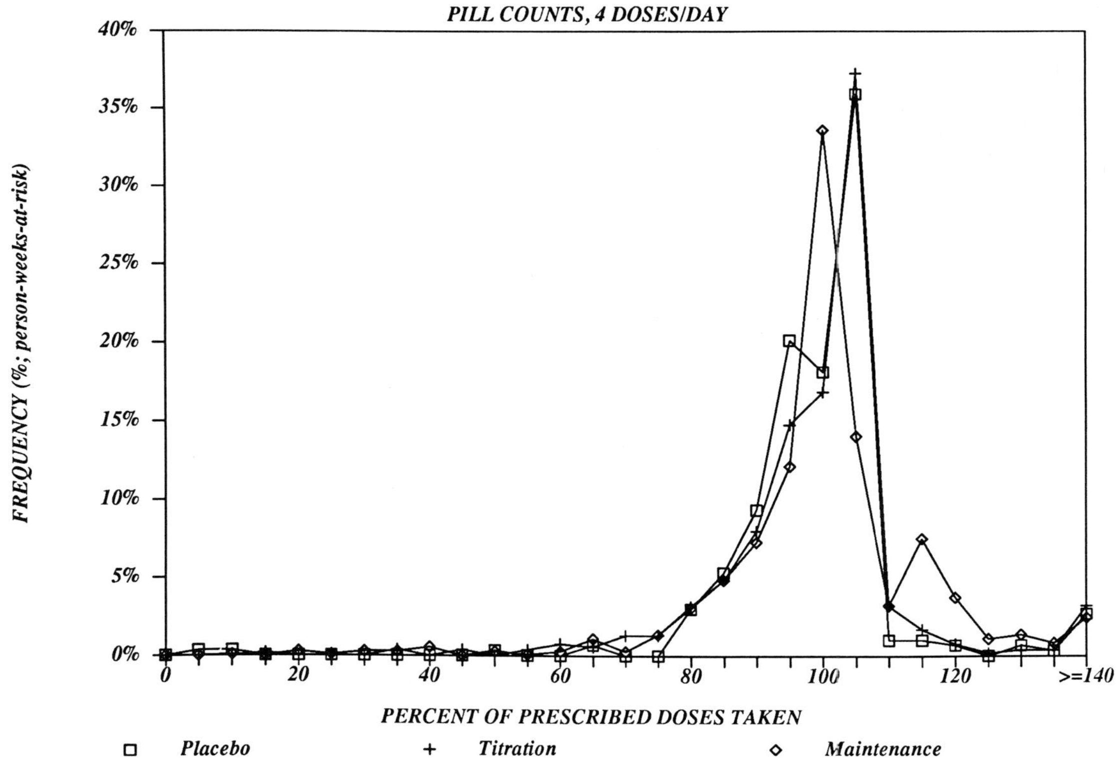

FIG. 4. Frequency distribution of doses taken according to pill count. Data for the primary study drug (pinacidil or hydralazine) administered four times daily among a survivor cohort of ambulatory hypertensive patients.

stresses, fluid status, or concomitant medications may interfere with consistent blood pressure control. A patient may faithfully take all prescribed medications and still fail to achieve or maintain blood pressure control. Nevertheless, higher levels of compliance by objective measures of adherence may correlate with achieved blood pressure level. Figure 5, taken from our drug trial (15), contrasts the mean blood pressures for subjects with near-optimal medication-taking (compliance rates: 80–119% by pill count) with those from subjects with more suboptimal rates (<80% or ≥120%). After the first three weekly visits on placebo, the near-optimal compliers exhibited significantly lower mean blood pressures ($p < 0.05$). Unfortunately, there was no significant correlation between an individual patient's change in blood pressure and his/her compliance rate by pill count. It was also impossible to predict compliance rate from blood pressure response.

Comparative Performance Among Measures

Few studies have compared simultaneous compliance measures for systematic distortion or concordance. Wandless et al. (24) assessed 81 elderly outpatients receiving a mean of 2.5 medications daily (range: 1–6), with a mean of 2.5 doses daily (range: 1–4). The investigators noted a correlation coefficient (r) of 0.47 ($p < 0.001$) between self-report and prescription refill rates; this accounts for less than 25% of the variance. Only 58% of those reporting near-perfect compliance (90–110%) by self-report exhibited equally desirable adherence rates on pill-count measures. When patient self-report and prescription refill rate agreed, the investigators found confirmatory, near-optimal pill counts in 69% of patients. When self-report and prescription refill both indicated suboptimal compliance (>10% deviation from prescription), pill count was confirmatory in 86% of cases. These data suggest that other objective measures, such as prescription refill rates, may be integrated with patient self-report to enhance its predictive value but that it is likely that no single, indirect measure of medication-taking is sufficient.

Fletcher et al. (16) compared patient interview (self-report), pill count, and serum drug concentration (biologic assay) among 173 outpatients prescribed digoxin. They noted that complete pill counts were possible for only 39% of subjects and that assay results were never available quickly enough to allow feedback during regular patient visits to clinic. While 83% of 138 subjects claimed perfect (100%) compliance, only one of 49 pill counts (2%) confirmed the perfect pill-taking. By criteria of cost, convenience, and remedial utility, the investigators concluded that patient interview was the best method.

Haynes et al. (66) evaluated 134 steelworkers during the first 6 months of their antihypertensive treatment. Patients' self-reports showed high correlation ($r = 0.74$; $p < 0.0001$) with compliance rates by pill count, but subjects overestimated their own compliance by an average of 17%. In contrast, 90% of those reporting suboptimal levels of medication-taking had pill counts consistent with the report. Interviews proved to be preferable in convenience and to be

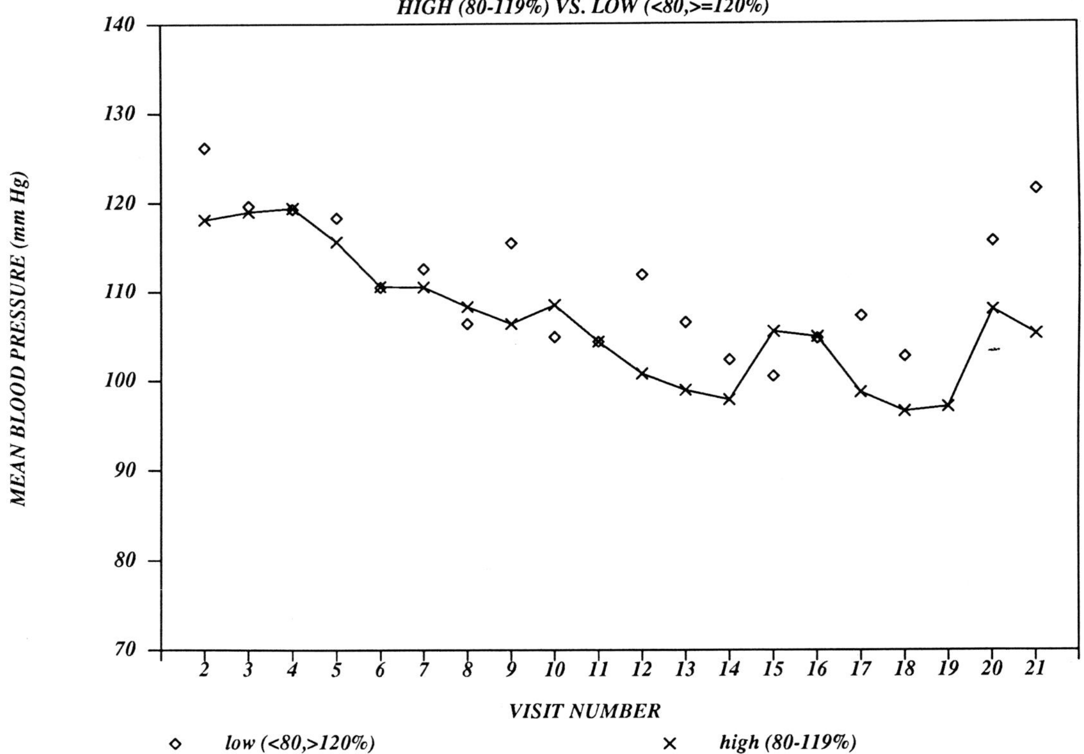

FIG. 5. Mean blood pressure according to compliance category. Mean blood pressure is calculated as the diastolic blood pressure plus (systolic − diastolic)/3. Compliance rate from pill counts, defining "high" compliance as rates 80–119% of the prescribed regimen and defining "low" compliance as all other rates. (From ref. 15.)

superior in correlation to pill counts, as compared to qualitative urinary drug assays, drug-induced metabolic changes, or blood pressure as alternative measures. Various combinations and permutations of alternative measures did not significantly improve the accuracy of interpreting patients' self-reports, using pill counts as a proxy gold standard.

Black et al. (67) applied self-report, pill count, and urinary chlorthalidone assay as procedures to 551 elderly hypertensives participating in the Systolic Hypertension in the Elderly Program. Overall compliance rates were high by all measures. Among 387 subjects claiming perfect compliance, pill-count data confirmed 100% adherence in 90% of patients. Urinary assay was similarly corroborating in 93% of 289 participants who provided adequate urine samples.

We examined various measures of medication-taking among a stable, "survivor cohort" of 121 chronic, ambulatory hypertensive patients (15). To proceed beyond randomization to two alternative antihypertensive medications, subjects had to have sustained hypertension and pill-count compliance rates of 75–125% over the 3-week placebo washout period. We collected six types of compliance measurement data: (a) *patient global self-report,* asking subjects what proportion of their usual medications do they take (on average) as prescribed: none (0%); few (1–24%); some (25–49%); many (50–74%); most (75–94%); all or almost all (95–100%); (b) *patient self-report by 48-hr recall,* specifying the precise number of prescribed doses taken in the preceding 48 hr; (c) *pill counts* of all study-related drugs, the ratio of missing and presumptively consumed pills to those prescribed for the interval; (d) *biologic assay* of plasma drug concentrations for patients prescribed pinacidil, using the values obtained after controlled dosing as the standard for comparison; (e) *clinicians' opinions* of average medication-taking rate over the course of the study; and (f) *therapeutic response* in terms of absolute and relative change in blood pressure (both systolic and diastolic) from baseline.

We observed limited correlation and concordance among the measures. Our task was hampered by the absence of a gold standard against which to compare any of the measures and thereby any one measure against another (32,60). The low level of correlation may, in part, have been artifact due to the limited variability from preselecting individuals with relatively high compliance rates. A more diverse population with a broad range of medication-taking patterns would increase the likelihood of detecting correlations, if they do exist.

Among the individual measures, several interesting patterns emerged. Although pill counts frequently exceeded 100%, the response categories of neither the patients' self-report nor the clinicians' estimates even mentioned compliance levels greater than 100%. This further weakened the correlative search. Patients' global self-report at baseline indicated near-perfect compliance, but requestioning a subsample of subjects 3 months later yielded a somewhat more modest estimate. The 48-hr recall provided the highest correlation with pill count among the self-report measures.

Biologic assay presented a number of other problems. Nearly 20% of the eligible subjects did not provide adequate blood specimens to establish an expected range of drug blood concentrations, projected from levels achieved by observed drug administration. Crude qualitative assessment confirmed that 29 of 30 eligible subjects consumed some of the study medication in the preceding several days. In addition, the consistency of bioassay class was poor: Only 41% of 17 subjects with "adequate" levels as defined above gave the same result 1 month later under identical conditions; 35% had lower values. Among the seven subjects with initially "low" levels, 57% had satisfactory values on repeat testing.

The data emphasize the high variability, both within and among subjects. This was particularly impressive for pill counts for which the largest data set was available. Figure 6 illustrates the distribution of variabilities, plotting mean compliance rates by pill count against the coefficient of variation (ratio of standard deviation to the mean value). Although the data plots are clustered near a mean value of 100% compliance, there is considerable scatter.

Since most measures occurred far in time and space from any specific medication-taking event, the poor correlation and concordance may be disappointing but is hardly surprising. All traditional measures of compliance proved imperfect. The advantages of cost, convenience, and acceptability must generally serve as counterweights to accuracy, nonreactivity, and comprehensiveness. No single measure offers all virtues; trade-offs are inevitable.

Emergence of Medication Monitors

Recent technological advances have generated several promising alternative measures of medication-taking. The alternatives focus on measuring the dispensing event with great accuracy. More specifically, the alternatives are medication-taking monitors, devices which record the precise time at which the medication vial is opened or at which the medication is actually dispensed (32,68,69).

Such medication monitors provide a time tracing, which then becomes the matrix on which the investigator places other observations, measurements, and potential predictors in search of associations. The monitors assess the medication-taking events on a dynamic, hour-to-hour basis. One limitation of the measure is that a patient might systematically open and close the medication monitor and not actually take the medication. Such an investment by a patient for deliberate deception seems unlikely. By providing detailed temporal data on medication-taking, one may use this type of measure to probe for factors which facilitate, cue, or inhibit specific occasions of dispensing (and presumably consuming) the medication. Medication monitors may also prove to be useful to validate alternative measures such as self-report, pill count, or biologic assay. Medication

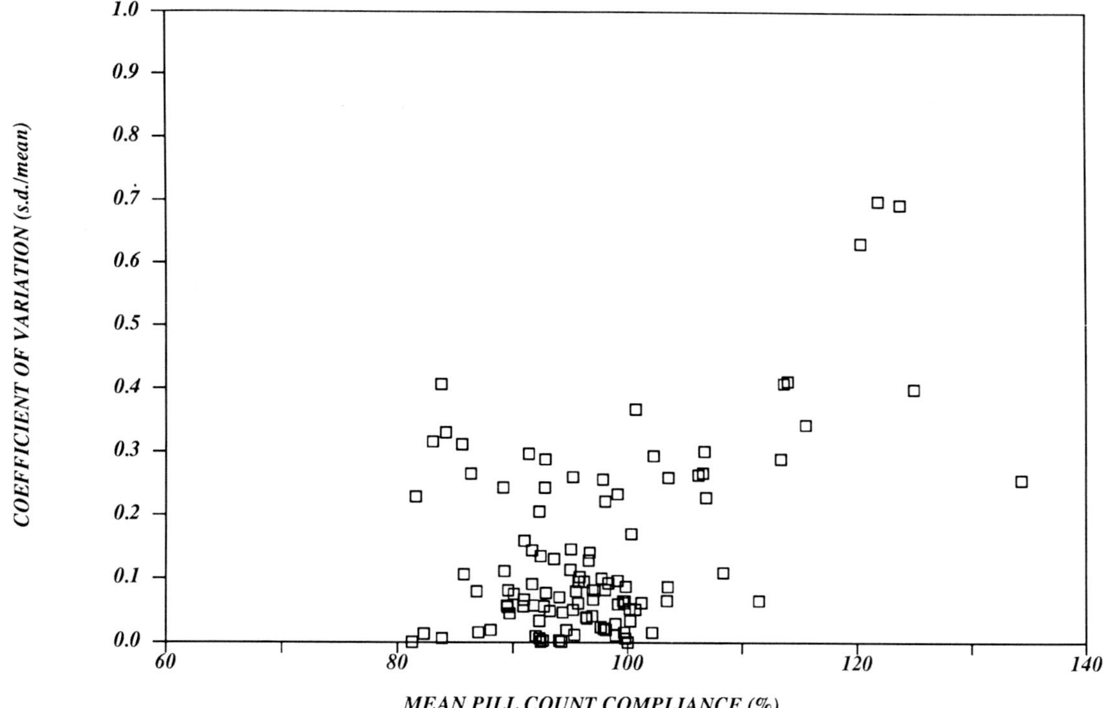

FIG. 6. Variability in compliance versus pill count among ambulatory hypertensives. Compliance rate is calculated as the percentage of prescribed pills missing on return pill count of those which should have been taken. Coefficient of variation (COV) is calculated as the ratio of (a) each individual's standard deviation of week-to-week compliance rate versus pill count to (b) his/her mean compliance rate. The higher the COV, the more variable was the compliance rate versus pill count.

monitors may permit less ambiguous interpretation of the clinical experiment. When a patient returns with uncontrolled blood pressure, the monitor allows better distinction between recent and chronic hypertension and between optimal and suboptimal compliance, thereby helping to distinguish among disease resistance, pharmacologic resistance, and adherence resistance.

New Applications for the Medication Monitor

With medication monitors in place, two new opportunities emerge (J. Urquhart, *personal communication,* December 14, 1987). First, the required sample size, and hence the cost of the trials, may decline. Subjects found by the monitor to be wildly deviant in their medication-taking can be readily excluded from analysis or analyzed separately, leaving the subpopulation of subjects with roughly comparable compliance rates. With similar medication inputs, the variability in therapeutic response should become more narrow. As the variability falls, the required sample size to achieve statistical significance also falls. The cost of the monitors and their analysis may then be balanced against the costs of the larger trial without monitors.

Second, the astute investigator may analyze the outcomes by subgroups, each with similar compliance patterns and rates. As reported by the Lipid Research Clinic trial (41), such analysis may reveal a gradient of therapeutic response rather than an all-or-none effect. On the one hand, we may then determine how high in dosage we should go with a patient to achieve a desired therapeutic response. On the other hand, we may get important, premarketing clues that "standard" doses may be excessive, if we observe that subjects taking only a fraction of the prescribed dose achieved full therapeutic response, often at lower levels of toxicity. The early decision to market some drugs at high dosage may be challenged earlier if better data on compliance becomes available. Examples of mistaken marketing probably include chlorthalidone and captopril, both initially released only in the 100- and 25-mg dose form, respectively. Soon it became clear that these doses were excessive for most patients. Better information at an earlier time might have spared many patients the dose-related toxicities. In sum, then, the medication monitor allows the investigator to "use" all participating subjects in a more precise way than do traditional compliance measures such as pill count or biologic assay, which leave much ambiguity.

Recent Monitor Implementations in Clinical Trials

After more than a decade of experimentation with alternative formats, several groups have implemented electronic devices possessing great accuracy. Some of the most imaginative work has occurred for monitoring antiglaucomatous eyedrop administration (45,56). Kass et al. (23) demonstrated great variability for interdose intervals. Many subjects compressed the timing of their four daily dosings; 30% of the patients allowed intervals averaging more than 12 hr between dosings. With 720 hours-at-risk during a month, 33% of the subjects had at least 23% of the hours "uncovered," given the known pharmacology of the medication. These data underscore the potential importance of ensuring pharmacological "coverage" and not merely dispensing the correct number of pills.

The monitors permit a degree of precision and details not available from traditional, indirect measures of medication-taking. Kass (M. A. Kass, *personal communication,* 1987) described the most common dosing patterns in decreasing order of frequency among 91 of his patients, allowing any individual to exhibit more than one pattern: (a) *near-optimal pill-taking* (49% of patients), producing an average compliance rate of 90–110% of prescribed doses; (b) *consistent underdosing* (40% of subjects), omitting 11–70% of the prescribed doses; (c) *drug holidays* (19% of subjects), consisting of ≥3 consecutive days without any dosing; (d) *abrupt jumps* (17%), involving major increases in dosing frequency from one day to the next; (e) *abrupt drops* (12%), involving major decreases in dosing frequency from one day to the next; and (f) *consistent overdosing* (10%), exhibiting 111–147% of the prescribed dose. Only one patient in 91 displayed the desirable dosing pattern of "perfect" compliance. The monitor's precision in tracking medication-taking over time represents its most impressive promise.

Data are also emerging from applying monitors in hypertension. Eisen et al. (70) reported medication-taking patterns among 24 outpatients receiving once-daily diuretic therapy, assessed with an electronic monitor. They observed that 84% of the doses were removed within ±12 hr of the prescribed time; the average deviation from consistent pill-taking was 4.1 hr. The proportion of prescribed doses that the patient removed in the month prior to blood pressure determination provided the best predictor of diastolic blood pressure ($r = -0.49$; $p = 0.0001$). Regression analysis for medication-taking over the entire month similarly and significantly predicted diastolic blood pressure at the end of the month ($p = 0.0002$). The individual with the worst compliance rate (60%) would have reduced diastolic blood pressure by an additional 16 mmHg, if he had taken all medications as prescribed when projected from the regression equation.

THE EPIDEMIOLOGY OF COMPLIANCE

The primitive measures of medication-taking available in the past have limited our knowledge of the epidemiology of compliance in general and medication-taking in particular. As a consequence, we must be cautious in interpreting published reports about incidence, prevalence, predictors, natural history, and interventional results.

Incidence and Prevalence

A large number of studies have addressed the frequency of suboptimal medication-taking. As a group, they have tended to distinguish acute from chronic conditions, symptomatic from asymptomatic diseases, and preventive from curative treatments (71). The trends of medication-taking for a variety of chronic conditions converge to approximately 50% of the prescribed regimen, with moderate variation. For the specific area of hypertension, Sackett (72) summarized the frequency of suboptimal compliance with several studies of ambulatory hypertensives using pill-count measures of medication-taking: (a) Only 53% of 240 steelworkers were taking ≥80% of their prescribed doses after 6 months of treatment; (b) only 20% of 49 outpatients consumed ≥90% of their prescribed regimen; and (c) only 47% of 100 hypertensive outpatients at a university hypertension clinic were taking ≥95% of their prescribed regimen. By all measures, the incidence and prevalence of suboptimal compliance for antihypertensive medication are high.

Several important epidemiologic qualifications are relevant. The behavior of *inception cohorts,* those patients who are newly diagnosed and starting therapy for the first time, may differ strikingly from that of *survivor cohorts,* those patients who stay under care and receive treatment for a prolonged time. By self-selection, the survivor cohort is more likely to have accepted the potential value of therapy and, hence, to adhere to the prescription. Kass et al. (23) used medication monitors to document that the mean compliance among an "inception" cohort of 184 ambulatory glaucoma patients was significantly lower (65% versus 76%) than among the "survivor" cohort ($p = 0.04$). Most studies of ambulatory hypertensive management indicate a high dropout rate in the first year after diagnosis, whether or not treatment begins (73). Those remaining comprise a survivor cohort, a population which provides the volunteers for most antihypertensive drug trials. One should be guarded in extrapolating to all hypertensives from the behavior of such survivors, even though the majority of American hypertensives have been previously diagnosed and treated (74).

Natural History of Medication-Taking

Few studies of the natural history of medication-taking have appeared. Sackett and co-workers (11,31) compared the medication-taking distributions of 134 ambulatory hypertensive steelworkers based on pill counts at 6 and 12 months after starting antihypertensive medications. The overall distribution of compliance rates changed little over the second 6-month follow-up. They observed a J-shaped distribution, with 15–30% taking none of the prescribed medications, 35–50% taking ≥80% of their doses, and the remainder falling in the mid-zone. The investigators, however, supplied no data on the mean net change in compliance rate over time by individual nor any comment on medication-taking rates surpassing 100%. Perhaps the out-of-pocket cost of medications among their patients served as a disincentive for medication-dumping.

Our own data from the previously cited comparison of compliance measures in a drug trial indicate marked inter- and intrasubject variability in medication-taking over time, using pill count as the most common measure (15). Starting with 121 individuals selected for high levels of compliance, we observed a skewed unimodal distribution at all phases of the trial (see Figs. 1, 3, and 5) rather than the J-shaped pattern reported by Sackett (11). Our selection criteria for study entry would have served to truncate the lower part of the distribution. The vast majority of our subjects represented a survivor cohort, who acknowledged an average of nearly 12 years of known hypertension prior to study entry.

DETERMINANTS/PREDICTORS OF SUBOPTIMAL MEDICATION-TAKING

Despite limited confidence in measures of compliance, many investigators have focused on variables definable at treatment's onset, in search of determinants and predictors of suboptimal medication-taking. The driving force behind the search consists of the desire to understand the phenomenon and to identify subgroups at high versus low risk for suboptimal compliance. Identifying a low-risk subpopulation at baseline would then allow clinicians' attention and effort to shift preferentially to the high-risk group and, hence, maximize their impact. There has been a reluctance to accept as inevitable and irreducible Charney's "rough-and-ready natural law . . . [that] the physician will be expected to prescribe with only approximate accuracy, and the patient will be expected to comply with only modest fidelity" (75).

Most of the early studies approached the problem with univariate searches, assessing the differential impact of single factors or gradations of single factors on outcome measures of medication-taking. Few investigators sought to quantify the relative contributions of multiple factors simultaneously or evaluated interactions among factors, which might augment or diminish their individual effects. Not surprisingly, a huge number of determinants were identified, each based on significant associations within particular populations. Haynes (76) performed a major service to the field by systematically assessing the existing studies, critiquing their methodologies, and extracting balanced conclusions from the most rigorous investigations.

Unfortunately, few determinants pass muster as important predictors of subsequent medication-taking levels (6). Among *sociodemographic features,* only extremes of age and abject poverty consistently point to suboptimal adherence. These features may be particularly powerful predictors of poor medication-taking in alternative treatment settings such as emergency rooms (77), or elsewhere when the cost of medications may be prohibitive (78). In contrast, providing "free" medical care enhances the consumption of antihypertensive medication and adherence to diet and smoking recommendations (79). Improved blood pressure control is another positive consequence. Other characteristics, such as gender, educational level, occupational status, marital status, income, ethnic background, and race offer little predictive value.

Somewhat more disappointing is the failure of *clinical features,* especially symptom level and objective signs of disease severity, to forecast the level of adherence. In particular, there is no study indicating that compliance improves as severity of symptoms increases. Greater levels of disability, however, are associated with higher adherence rates. Although no individual disease is immune from suboptimal compliance, patients with frank psychiatric disease most consistently demonstrated poor adherence. Other multivariate studies have shown that patients' self-perception as socially isolated and developing side effects from medications are associated with poor medication-taking, as indicated by self-report (80).

The *regimen's specifics* clearly affect compliance, particularly the dosing frequency and total number of regimen components (81). While the number of different medications prescribed is inversely proportional to the compliance rate, the number of daily dosings has a less clear effect (13). Patients unequivocally prefer once-daily dosing for asymptomatic conditions (82). However, direct comparisons between once-daily, twice-daily, and four-times-daily dosings show only marginally superior results for once-daily administration among outpatients (83). These results may be adversely affected by many patients' apparent misinterpretation of prescription instructions (84). Adherence rates fall as the prescribed duration of treatment increases (85). As a drug class, antihypertensive agents appear to induce intermediate medication-taking rates, as compared to other drug classes: higher than antacids, tranquilizers, and analgesics but lower than antidiabetic or cardiac medications (86). The use of child-resistant containers, especially among the elderly, may dramatically reduce medication-taking rates (87).

Patients' understanding of the regimen is obviously essential, but not sufficient, to ensure optimal medication-taking behavior (88,89). Their knowledge of the regimen is inversely proportional to the number of different medications prescribed (90). The level of understanding, in turn, may be linked, in a complex manner, with cognitive factors (such as memory) and psychosocial factors (such as satisfaction with the medical care provided) (91–93). Many patients may be particularly misinformed about the best action if a dose of medication is missed (94).

Medications' *side effects* may clearly affect compliance, yet they are cited as important obstacles to medication-taking by less than 10% of respondents in most surveys of patients' perceptions (76). Nevertheless, up to 15% of participants receiving active antihypertensive medications in the British Medical Research Council study (95) withdrew from the 5-year study because of intolerable side effects. Further indirect confirmation of the importance of side effects comes from Morisky et al.'s (96) finding of side effects as a predictor of blood pressure control over a 3-year follow-up. Several other studies have focused on antihypertensive medications' adverse effects on quality of life, thereby predisposing to suboptimal adherence (97).

Other *patient perceptions* may be critical in affecting medication-taking behavior. One of the most inclusive frameworks (and one of the most pervasive in the literature) is the "health belief model," which postulates that an individual's chances of following a recommended health action are dependent on four perceptions: (a) level of personal susceptibility to the particular condition, (b) degree of severity of the condition's consequences, (c) type of benefits from adhering to the health action, and (d) barriers to complying with the health action (98). When applied to hypertension, however, its predictive value for subsequent compliant behavior was not significant prior to treatment. After treatment was underway at least 6 months, the model provided limited ($r = 0.39$; $R^2 = 0.15$) prediction of medication-taking behavior by pill count (98). The patient's self-reported medication-taking further correlated with his/her perceived level of assistance at home to complete all prescribed regimen components with the health locus of control (99).

INTERVENTIONS TO ENHANCE MEDICATION-TAKING

The arena of interventions to enhance medication-taking remains an important barometer of assumptions and prejudices about compliance itself. Interventions remained modest in scope as long as suboptimal adherence was viewed as the unique responsibility of the patient. Compliance traditionally held little interest for the clinician, who gave priority to proper diagnosis and prescription. Failure to adhere to treatment—and, hence, failure to respond to it—lay as a clear consequence of patients' deliberate choices. Slowly and perhaps reluctantly, the field has come to acknowledge the finite contributions that clinicians and investigators can make to inhibit or impair medication-taking behavior. With the acknowledgment has come a growing sophistication about both determinants of compliance and the focuses for selective interventions (100). In contrast to short-term therapy for symptomatic disease, antihypertensive drug treatment requires intensive, sustained, and often clumsy reinforcement as long as medication-taking behavior is to be optimized (101).

In broad categories, the interventions readily fall into three groups: educational, behavioral, and system-based subtypes. The *educational interventions* start with the assumption that inadequate information lies at the heart of observed suboptimal compliance. If individuals better understood the potential seriousness of the condition, their personal susceptibility to be affected without proper treatment, the effectiveness of the therapy, its relative safety and convenience, and the particulars of the regimen, then all would be well.

The investigational data for educational interventions only partially support this perspective. Knowledge of medical diagnosis and drug purpose does not correlate with self-reported medication-taking behavior (102). As a group, most hypertensives seem well aware of the dangers of uncontrolled elevations of blood pressure and their individual risk status. In fact, exaggeration (or even reinforcement) of such fear messages in isolation appear to prompt patients' frank denial or simple evasion (103). Similarly, emphasis on the effectiveness of the treatment seems necessary, but not sufficient, as an enabling factor. Despite multifactorial designs, many studies demonstrated only modest changes in medication-taking behavior (104,105), although combinations of interventions were generally superior to single interventions (106). Others have found that combining written and oral instructions may create "information overload," especially among the elderly, whose complex regimens are easily confusing (107). Meta-analysis of 70 published evaluations of educational programs indicated that the largest impact occurred from one-to-one counseling, group education, or both in combination with audiovisual materials (108). Triaging among possible interventions may maximize impact and minimize cost or use of limited resources (109).

The *behavioral interventions* begin from a different perspective. It is acknowledged that many patients may not fully understand their medical condition but that compliant behavior may be induced and maintained by reinforcing behaviors (110). These have included the successful use of home blood pressure measurements, both to desensitize subjects to the blood pressure determination itself and to provide feedback about the consequences of taking, as opposed to not taking, their antihypertensive medications (111,112). One report confirmed that self-measurement of blood pressure was particularly effective (rise in compliance from 0% to 70%) among those initially showing "poor" compliance (113). Other efforts attempted contractual incentives by which the patient and clinician negotiate and sign contracts that specify the patient's compliant behavior in exchange for the clinician's consistent availability, punctuality, and thoughtful supervision of treatment (114).

Other forms of social support were similarly effective in enhancing medication-taking behavior and blood pressure control, including group therapy (115), patient-operated hypertension groups selecting their own medications under supervision (116), telephone counseling (117), and special worksite occupational nurses (118). Early efforts to employ special medication packaging yielded disappointing results (119,120), despite the ingenuity of some of the devices. Other efforts, especially when based on the concept of a drug calendar to remind patients to take the medications as prescribed, produced significant improvements in medication-taking behavior (121), including blister packaging rather than standard vials (122). As with the educational interventions, the behavioral maneuvers appeared most effective when applied serially and in combination rather than as single, poorly defined steps (123,124).

Some of the most successful interventions have employed this very strategy, combining *system-based* maneuvers. These efforts assume that no single interventive component will succeed with all subjects, given the complex determinants of compliant behavior. By providing a battery of components that range from educational or behavioral through logistical and philosophical, these studies seek less to prove the unique value of any component than to effect change by a variety of simultaneous mechanisms. One of the early feasibility studies confirmed that a dedicated clinic pharmacist could produce dramatic improvement in medication-taking and blood pressure control by soliciting drug-related side effects, adjusting the regimen in conjunction with prescribing physicians, and providing background information about hypertension (125). Mean compliance rates by pill count rose from 25% to 79% in the intervention group during the 5-month maneuver but returned promptly to baseline when the intervention was withheld. The study results underscored (a) the suboptimal communication that had previously existed between clinicians and patients and (b) the need for sustained reinforcement for improved medication-taking to continue. Similar, pharmacist-based interventions have significantly improved blood pressure control among ambulatory-"resistant" hypertensives (126).

A variety of other applications have employed less trained research assistants and aides to supplement the efforts of clinicians providing antihypertensive management. Perhaps the most famous of these endeavors, the series of linked studies by Sackett and coworkers (66,111,127), addressed hypertensive steelworkers at the Dofasco Foundry. They combined home self-monitoring of blood pressure and pill consumption, tailoring of medication-taking to reinforce daily events, and positive reinforcements, including money, to produce a 21% improvement in average compliance among the intervention group as compared to a 1% decline among controls. Similar programs have been successfully applied on a more modest scale in private practice settings (128).

GUIDELINES FOR CLINICIANS AND INVESTIGATORS

The interventions illustrate the kinds of initiatives clinicians and investigators can take to enhance medication-taking behavior. The full implications for clinicians and investigators may be somewhat different. We shall address each group separately.

Guidelines for Clinicians

Since Sackett's compliance practicum for the busy practitioner first appeared (129), a number of distinguished investigators and clinicians have proposed guiding principles (130–135). The majority are based on the limited available data and reflect a careful balance between the desirable and the possible. In simple terms, the behaviors may be subdivided into those for patients and those for clinicians. *Patients' behaviors* include (a) making the decision to control blood pressure, (b) following the therapeutic regimen as prescribed, (c) monitoring progress toward goal blood pressure, and (d) resolving problems that block blood pressure control. *Clinicians' behaviors* include (a) supporting the patient in his/her behaviors, (b) promoting adherence to the regimen, (c) monitoring progress to goal blood pressure, (d) problem-solving with the patient for all perceived obstacles, and (e) working collaboratively with other health care providers (131). Component actions may involve explaining events, reducing uncertainty, providing a basis for action, and strengthening the clinician–patient relationship (136). Somewhat more specifically, the guidelines for clinicians may include the following:

1. Monitor all hypertensive patients for clinic attendance and for blood pressure control, using specific follow-up appointment dates and an explicit goal blood pressure.
2. Follow up aggressively all those individuals who drop out of care or who fail to achieve goal blood pressure in a reasonable interval (e.g., 4–6 visits or 3–6 months), when given an appropriate antihypertensive regimen.
3. Inquire about compliance as a routine part of every visit; in a nonjudgmental way, ask about perceived obsta-

cles to optimal compliance and negotiate practical, evaluable solutions; address directly all perceived obstacles, including subtle symptoms attributed to the medications; and specify the actions the patient should take for missed doses.

4. Provide lavish praise and simple rewards for success; offer reassurance and constructive suggestions for failures in achieving blood pressure control.

5. Pay special attention to high-risk subgroups: the very old, the confused, those on complex or changing regimens, and those failing to achieve goal blood pressure.

6. Simplify antihypertensive regimens whenever possible, trying to avoid midday dosings.

7. Avoid introducing many changes in regimen all at once.

8. Ensure comprehension of the treatment plan, and provide verbal and written reinforcements as needed.

9. Consider suboptimal compliance as a plausible explanation for failure to achieve goal blood pressure before escalating the therapeutic regimen.

10. Adjust treatment-setting policies to minimize waiting times, facilitate patients' access for questions and concerns, enhance provider continuity, and encourage patients' participation in their own care.

11. Augment suboptimal compliance by increasing attention and supervision: more frequent outpatient visits and/or assistance by patients' significant others or health professionals (pharmacist or nurse).

12. Link medication-taking behavior to specific daily cues in patients' usual routines.

13. Progress to more complex and expensive behavioral interventions if simple efforts prove to be insufficient: e.g., patient–provider contracts, special cueing pill dispensers.

14. Offer verbal and written reinforcement for the specific regimen, seeking and correcting misinterpretations of dosing; specify the timing of each dose as precisely as possible; ensure legible, unambiguous instructions on the prescription label.

15. Establish and nurture a strong clinician–patient relationship.

Guidelines for Investigators

While most of the same principles are relevant to investigators designing and implementing specific regimens, a few additional guidelines are important:

1. Predetermine the most important aspects of compliance for the particular trial.
2. Design, implement, pilot-test, and modify more than one compliance measure, selecting ones suitable for (a) the study population, (b) the research question, and (c) the logistic constraints.
3. Analyze outcomes using compliance as both a continuous and dichotomous covariable.

The data in support of clinicians and investigators embracing such guidelines and applying them for their patients are disappointing. Much like patients, who may find the list of new behaviors somewhat daunting, clinicians and investigators may drift along old patterns. The knowledge base for hypertension management, including issues of medication-taking, appears to decline as the number of years since medical school graduation increases; reassuringly, focused educational interventions significantly increase the knowledge (137). More ambitious trials to enhance physicians' behaviors for improved medication-taking by patient have yielded inconsistent results (138,139).

The role of compliance in the management of hypertension has always been essential. Recent developments offer exciting promise of how to incorporate new perspectives and more specific data for (a) improving blood pressure control for individual patients and (b) enhancing the value and specificity of clinical trials.

REFERENCES

1. Blackwell B. Treatment adherence. *Br J Psychiatry* 1976;129:513–531.
2. Eraker SA, Kirscht JP, Becker MH. Understanding and improving patient compliance. *Ann Intern Med* 1984;100:258–268.
3. Evans L, Spelman M. The problem of non-compliance with drug therapy. *Drugs* 1983;25:63–76.
4. Glanz K, Scholl TO. Intervention strategies to improve adherence among hypertensives: review and recommendations. *Patient Counc Health Ed* 1982;4:14–28.
5. Haynes RB, Mattson ME, Chobanian AV, Dunbar JM, Engebretson TO, Garrity TF, Leventhal H, Levine RJ, Levy RL. Management of patient compliance in the treatment of hypertension; report of the NHLBI Working Group. *Hypertension* 1982;4:415–423.
6. Haynes RB, Taylor DW, Sackett DL, ed. *Compliance in health care.* Baltimore: Johns Hopkins University Press, 516 pp.
7. Luscher TF, Vetter H, Siegenthaler W, Vetter W. Compliance in hypertension: facts and concepts. *J Hypertens* 1985;3(Suppl 1):3–9.
8. Sackett DL, Haynes RB, Taylor DW. The problem of compliance with antihypertensive regimens. *Drugs* 1983;25(Suppl 2):12–18.
9. Haynes RB. Introduction. In: Haynes RB, Taylor DW, Sackett DL, eds. *Compliance in health care.* Baltimore: Johns Hopkins University Press, 1979;1–7.
10. Feinstein AR. Biostatistical problems in "compliance bias." *Clin Pharmacol Ther* 1975;16:846–857.
11. Sackett DL. Hypertension in the real world: public reaction, physician response, and patient compliance. In: Genest J, Koiw E, Kuchel O, eds. *Hypertension: physiopathology and treatment.* Baltimore: Johns Hopkins University Press, 1142–1149.
12. Sackett DL, Haynes RB, Gibson ES, Taylor DW, Roberts RS, Johnson AL. Hypertension control, compliance and science. *Am Heart J* 1977;94:666–667.
13. Hulka BS. Patient-clinician interactions and compliance. In: Haynes RB, Taylor DW, Sackett DL, eds. *Compliance in health care.* Baltimore: Johns Hopkins University Press, 1979;63–77.
14. Hulka BS, Cassel JC, Kupper LL, Burdette JA. Communication, compliance, and concordance between physicians and patients with prescribed medications. *Am J Public Health* 1976;66:847–853.
15. Rudd P, Byyny RL, Zachary V, LoVerde M, Titus C. Compliance variability with antihypertensive regimens. *Clin Res* 1986;34:835A.
16. Fletcher SW, Pappius EM, Harper SJ. Measurement of medication compliance in a clinical setting: comparison of three methods in patients prescribed digoxin. *Arch Intern Med* 1979;139:635–638.
17. Inui TS, Carter WB, Pecoraro RE, Pearlman RA, Dohan JJ. Variations in patient compliance with common long-term drugs. *Med Care* 1980;18:986–993.

18. Greenberg RN. Overview of patient compliance with medication dosing: a literature review. *Clin Ther* 1984;6:592–599.
19. Vandenbroucke JP, Mauritz BJ, De Bruin A, Verheesen JH, Heide-Wessel CV, Heide RM. Weight, smoking, and mortality. *JAMA* 252:2859–2860.
20. Clive DM, Stoff JS. Renal syndromes associated with nonsteroidal antiinflammatory drugs. *N Engl J Med* 1984;310:563–572.
21. Dirks JF, Kinsman RA. Nondichotomous patterns of medication usage: the yes–no fallacy. *Clin Pharm Ther* 1982;31:413–417.
22. Goldsmith CH. The effect of compliance distributions on therapeutic trials. In: Haynes RB, Taylor DW, Sackett DL, eds. *Compliance in health care.* Baltimore: Johns Hopkins University Press, 1979;297–308.
23. Kass MA, Meltzer DW, Gordon M, Cooper D, Goldberg J. Compliance with topical pilocarpine treatment. *Am J Ophthalmol* 1986;101:515–523.
24. Wandless I, Mucklow JC, Smith A, Prudham D. Compliance with prescribed medicines: a study of elderly patients in the community. *J R Coll Gen Pract* 1979;29:391–396.
25. Holmberg L, Bottiger LE. The drug-consuming patient and his drugs. II. The drugs. *Acta Med Scand* 1983;213:211–216.
26. Rudd P, Marton KI. Nontraditional problems of antihypertensive management. *West J Med* 1979;131:179–192.
27. Management Committee. The Australian Therapeutic Trial in mild hypertension. *Lancet* 1980;1:1261–1267.
28. Stason WB, Weinstein MC. Allocation of resources to manage hypertension. *N Engl J Med* 1977;296:732–739.
29. Goldberg LA. A hoard of capsules illustrating patient non-compliance. *Lancet* 1977;1:601.
30. Otten H, Schmieder R, Ruddel H. Disparate effects of initial antihypertensive therapy on well-being. *J Hypertens* 1987;5 (Suppl 1):S37–S40.
31. Taylor DW, Sackett DL, Haynes RB, Johnson AL, Gibson ES, Roberts RS. Compliance with antihypertensive drug therapy. *Ann NY Acad Sci* 1978;304:390–403.
32. Rudd P, Marshall G. Resolving problems of measuring compliance with medication monitors. *J Compliance Health Care* 1987;2:23–35.
33. Logan AG, Milne BJ, Flanagan PT, Haynes RB. Clinical effectiveness and cost-effectiveness of monitoring blood pressure of hypertensive employees at work. *Hypertension* 1983;5:828–836.
34. Inui TS, Carter WB, Pecoraro RE. Screening for noncompliance among patients with hypertension: Is self-report the best available measure? *Med Care* 1981;19:1061–1064.
35. Worthen DM. Patient compliance and the "usefulness product" of timolol. *Surv Ophthalmol* 1979;23:403–406.
36. Soutter BR, Kennedy MC. Patient compliance assessment in drug trials: usage and methods. *Aust NZ J Med* 1974;4:360–364.
37. Haynes RB, Dantes R. Patient compliance and the conduct and interpretation of therapeutic trials. *Contrib Clin Trials* 1987;8:12–19.
38. Feinstein AR. "Compliance bias" and the interpretation of therapeutic trials. In: Haynes RB, Taylor DW, Sackett DL, eds. *Compliance in health care.* Baltimore: Johns Hopkins University Press, 1979;309–322.
39. Halta M, McHugh R. Planning the size of a cohort study in the presence of both losses to follow-up and non-compliance. *J Chronic Dis* 1980;33:501–512.
40. Joyce CRB. Patient co-operation and the sensitivity of clinical trials. *J Chronic Dis* 1962;15:1025–1036.
41. Lipid Research Clinics Program. The Lipid Research Clinics Coronary Primary Prevention Trial results: I. Reduction in incidence of coronary heart disease. II. Relationship of reduction in incidence of coronary heart disease to cholesterol lowering. *JAMA* 1984;251:351–374.
42. Cordis L. General concepts for use of markers in clinical trials. *Contrib Clin Trials* 1984;5:481–487.
43. Caron HS. Compliance: the case for objective measurement. *J Hypertens* 1985;3(Suppl 1):11–17.
44. Dunbar J. Adherence measures and their utility. *Contrib Clin Trials* 1984;5:515–521.
45. Norell SE. Methods in assessing drug compliance. *Acta Med Scand (Suppl)* 1983;683:35–40.
46. Roth HP. Historical review: comparison with other methods. *Contrib Clin Trials* 1984;5:476–480.
47. Mollica JA. Monitoring compliance through analysis of drug and metabolite levels. *Contrib Clin Trials* 1984;5:505–514.
48. Nierenberg DW. Measuring drug levels in the office: rationale, possible advantages, and potential problems. *Med Clin North Am* 1987;71:653–664.
49. Prinoth M, Spahn H, Mutschler E. The development of reliable compliance tests for antihypertensive drugs. *Eur J Clin Pharmacol* 1986;29:535–539.
50. Jack DB, Dean S, Kendall MJ. Evaluation of a simple method to check compliance with antihypertensive drug therapy. *Br J Clin Pharmacol* 1980;10:183–184.
51. Insull W. Workshop summary. *Contrib Clin Trials* 1985;5:451–458.
52. Tempero KF. The potential use of markers for drug development. *Contrib Clin Trials* 1984;5:535–539.
53. Young LM, Haakenson CM, Lee KK, Van Eeckhout JP. Riboflavin use as a drug marker in Veterans Administration Cooperative Studies. *Contrib Clin Trials* 1984;5:497–504.
54. Dubbert PM, King A, Rapp SR, Brief E, Martin JE, Lake M. Riboflavin as a tracer of medication compliance. *J Behav Med* 1985;8:287–299.
55. Russell ML. Behavioral aspects of the use of medical markers in clinical trials. *Contrib Clin Trials* 1984;5:526–534.
56. Norell SE. Accuracy of patient interviews and estimates by clinical staff in determining medication compliance. *Soc Sci Med* 1981;15E:57–61.
57. Spector SL, Kinsman R, Mawhinney H, Siegel SC, Rachelsfsky GS, Katz RM, Rohr AS. Compliance of patients with asthma with an experimental aerosolized medication: implications for controlled clinical trials. *J Allergy Clin Immunol* 1986;77:65–70.
58. Smith NA, Seale JP, Shaw J. Medication compliance in children with asthma. *Aust Paediatr J* 1984;20:47–51.
59. Alfredsson LS, Norell SE. Spacing between doses on a thrice-daily regimen. *Br Med J* 1981;282:1036.
60. Rudd P. In search of the gold standard for compliance measurement. *Arch Intern Med* 1979;139:627–628.
61. Enlund H, Tuomilehto J, Turakka H. Patient report validated against prescription records for measuring use of and compliance with antihypertensive drugs. *Acta Med Scand* 1981;209:271–275.
62. Kass MA, Gordon M, Meltzer DW. Can ophthalmologists correctly identify patients defaulting from pilocarpine therapy? *Am J Ophthalmol* 1986;101:524–530.
63. Roth HP, Caron HS, Hsi BP. Measuring intake of a prescribed medication; a bottle cournt and a tracer technique compared. *Clin Pharmacol Ther* 1970;11:228–237.
64. Roth HP, Caron HS, Hsi BP. Estimating a patient's cooperation with his regimen. *Am J Med Sci* 1971;262:269–273.
65. Brody DS. Physician recognition of behavioral, psychological, and social aspects of medical care. *Arch Intern Med* 1980;140:1286–1289.
66. Haynes RB, Taylor DW, Sackett DL, Gibson ES, Bernholz CD, Mukherjee J. Can simple clinical measurements detect patient noncompliance? *Hypertension* 1980;2:757–764.
67. Black DM, Brand RJ, Greenlick M, Hughes G, Smith J. Compliance to treatment for hypertension in elderly patients: the SHEP pilot study. *J Gerontol* 1987;42:552–557.
68. Moulding TS. The unrealized potential of the medication monitor. *Clin Pharmacol Ther* 1979;25:131–136.
69. Rudd P. Medication packaging: simple solutions to nonadherence problems? *Clin Pharmacol Ther* 1979;25:257–265.
70. Eisen SA, Woodward RS, Miller G, Spitznagel E, Windham CA. The effect of medication compliance on the control of hypertension. *J Gen Intern Med* 1987;2:298–305.
71. Sackett DL, Snow JC. The magnitude of compliance and noncompliance. In: Haynes RB, Taylor DW, Sackett DL, eds. *Compliance in health care.* Baltimore: Johns Hopkins University Press, 1979;11–22.
72. Sackett DL. The hypertensive patient. 5. Compliance with therapy. *Can Med Assoc J* 1979;121:259–261.
73. Rudd P, Tul V, Brown K, Bostwick GH, Davidson SM. Hypertension continuation adherence: natural history and role as indicator. *Arch Intern Med* 1979;139:545–549.

74. Rowland M, Roberts J. Blood pressure levels and hypertension in persons aged 6–74 years: United States, 1976–80. *Advanced Data from vital and health statistics,* No. 84. DHHS Publication No. (PHS) 82-1250, 12 pp.
75. Charney E. Compliance and prescribance. *Am J Dis Child* 1975;129:1009–1010.
76. Haynes RB. Determinants of compliance: the disease and the mechanics of treatment. In: Haynes RB, Taylor DW, Sackett DL, eds. *Compliance in health care.* Baltimore: Johns Hopkins University Press, 1979;49–62.
77. Saunders CE. Patient compliance in filling prescriptions after discharge from the emergency department. *Am J Emerg Med* 1987;5:283–286.
78. Brand FN, Smith RT, Brand PA. Effect of economic barriers to medical care on patients' noncompliance. *Public Health Rep* 1977;92:72–78.
79. Keeler EB, Brook RH, Goldberg GA, Kamberg CJ, Newhouse JP. How free care reduced hypertension in the Health Insurance experiment. *JAMA* 1985;254:1926–1931.
80. Nelson EC, Stason WB, Neutra RR, Solomon HS. Identification of the noncompliant hypertensive patient. *Prev Med* 1980;9:504–517.
81. Haynes RB, Sackett DL, Taylor DW, Roberts RS, Johnson AL. Manipulation of the therapeutic regimen to improve compliance: conceptions and misconceptions. *Clin Pharmacol Ther* 1977;22:125–130.
82. Kubacka RT, Juhl RP. Attitudes of patients with hypertension or arthritis toward the frequency of medication administration. *Am J Hosp Pharm* 1985;42:2499–2501.
83. Taggart AJ, Johnston GD, McDevitt DG. Does the frequency of daily dosage influence compliance with digoxin therapy? *Br J Clin Pharmacol* 1981;1:31–34.
84. Mazzullo JM, Lasagna L, Griner PF. Variations in interpretation of prescription instructions; the need for improved prescribing habits. *JAMA* 227:929–931.
85. Hershey JC, Morton BG, Davis JB, Reichgott MJ. Patient compliance with antihypertensive medication. *Am J Public Health* 1980;70:1081–1089.
86. Closson R, Kikugawa C. Noncompliance varies by drug class. *J Am Hosp Assoc* 1975;49:89–93.
87. Sherman FT, Warach JD, Libow LS. Child-resistant containers for the elderly? *JAMA* 1979;241:1001–1002.
88. Greene JY, Weinberger M, Jerin MJ, Mamlin JJ. Compliance with medication regimens among chronically ill, inner city patients. *J Community Health* 1982;7:183–193.
89. Wartman SA, Morlock LL, Malitz FE, Palm EA. Patient understanding and satisfaction as predictors of compliance. *Med Care* 1983;21:886–891.
90. Brody DS. An analysis of patient recall of their therapeutic regimens. *J Chronic Dis* 1980;33:57–63.
91. Barsky AK. Nonpharmacologic aspects of medication. *Arch Intern Med* 1983;143:1544–1548.
92. Ley P. Doctor–patient communication: some quantitative estimates of the role of cognitive factors in non-compliance. *J Hypertens* 1985;3(Suppl 1):51–55.
93. Nagy VT, Wolfe GR. Cognitive predictors of compliance in chronic disease patients. *Med Care* 1984;22:912–921.
94. Ascione FJ, Kirscht JP, Shimp LA. An assessment of different components of patient medication knowledge. *Med Care* 1986;24:1018–1028.
95. Medical Research Council Working Party. MRC trial of treatment of mild hypertension; principal results. *Br Med J* 1985;291:97–104.
96. Morisky DE, Green LW, Levine DM. Concurrent and predictive validity of a self-reported measure of medication adherence. *Med Care* 1986;24:67–74.
97. Williams GH. Utility of behavioral science techniques in assessing adverse effects of antihypertensive agents. *Am J Kidney Dis* 1987;10(Suppl 1):61–65.
98. Becker MH, Maiman LA, Kirscht JP, Haefner DP, Drachman RH, Taylor DW. Patient perceptions and compliance: recent studies of the health belief model. In: Haynes RB, Taylor DW, Sackett DL, eds. *Compliance in health care.* Baltimore: Johns Hopkins University Press, 1979;78–109.
99. Lewis FM, Morisky DE, Flynn BS. A test of the construct validity of health locus of control: effects on self-reported compliance for hypertensive patients. *Health Ed Monogr* 1978;6:138–148.
100. Haynes RB. Strategies to improve compliance with referrals, appointments, and prescribed medical regimens. In: Haynes RB, Taylor DW, Sackett DL, eds. *Compliance in health care.* Baltimore: Johns Hopkins University Press, 1979;121–143.
101. Bond CA, Monson R. Sustained improvement in drug documentation, compliance, and disease control; a four-year analysis of an ambulatory care model. *Arch Intern Med* 1984;144:1159–1162.
102. Klein LE, German PS, McPhee SJ, Smith CS, Levine DM. Aging and its relationship to health knowledge and medication compliance. *Gerontology* 1982;22:384–387.
103. Leventhal H. Fear appeals and persuasion: the differentiation of a motivational construct. *Am J Public Health* 1971;61:1208–1224.
104. Glanz K, Kirscht JP, Rosenstock IM. Linking research and practice in patient education for hypertension; patient responses to four educational interventions. *Med Care* 1981;19:141–152.
105. Morisky DE, Levine DM, Green LW, Russell RP, Smith C, Benson P, Finlay J. The relative impact of health education for low- and high-risk patients with hypertension. *Prev Med* 1980;9:550–558.
106. Levine DM, Green LW, Deeds SG, Chwalow J, Russell RP, Finlay J. Health education for hypertensive patients. *JAMA* 1979;241:1700–1703.
107. Ascione FJ, Shimp LA. The effectiveness of four education strategies in the elderly. *Drug Intell Clin Pharm* 1984;18:926–931.
108. Mullen PD, Green LW, Persinger GS. Clinical trials of patient education for chronic conditions: a comparative meta-analysis of intervention types. *Prev Med* 1985;14:753–781.
109. Hatcher ME, Green LW, Levine DM, Flagle CE. Validation of a decision model for triaging hypertensive patients to alternate health education interventions. *Soc Sci Med* 1986;22:813–819.
110. Zifferblatt SM. Increasing patient compliance through the applied analysis of behavior. *Prev Med* 1975;4:173–182.
111. Haynes RB, Sackett EL, Gibson ES, Taylor DW, Hackett BC, Roberts RS, Johnson AL. Improvement of medication compliance in uncontrolled hypertension. *Lancet* 1976;1:1265–1268.
112. Johnson AL, Taylor DW, Sackett DL, Dunnett CW, Shimizu AG. Self-recording of blood pressure in the management of hypertension. *Can Med Assoc J* 1978;119:1034–1039.
113. Edmonds D, Foerster E, Groth H, Greminger P, Siegenthaler W, Vetter W. Does self-measurement of blood pressure improve patient compliance in hypertension? *J Hypertens* 1985;3(Suppl 1):31–34.
114. Steckel SB, Swain MA. Contracting with patients to improve compliance. *J Am Hosp Assoc* 1977;51:81–84.
115. Haehn KD. Psychological approaches to improve patient compliance. *J Hypertens* 1985;3(Suppl 1):61–64.
116. Nessman DG, Carnahan JE, Nugent CA. Increasing compliance; patient-operated hypertension groups. *Arch Intern Med* 1980;140:1427–1430.
117. Bertera EM, Bertera RL. The cost-effectiveness of telephone vs clinic counseling for hypertensive patients: a pilot study. *Am J Public Health* 1981;71:626–629.
118. Logan AG. Role of paraprofessionals in improving compliance with antihypertensive treatment. *J Hypertens* 1985;3(Suppl 1):65–68.
119. Crome P, Akehurst M, Keet J. Drug compliance in elderly hospital in-patients; trial of the Dosett box. *Practitioner* 1980;224: 782–785.
120. Eshelman FN, Fitzloff J. Effect of packaging on patient compliance with an antihypertensive medication. *Curr Ther Res* 1976;20:215–219.
121. Gabriel M, Gagnon JP, Bryan CK. Improved patient compliance through use of a daily drug reminder chart. *Am J Public Health* 1977;67:968–969.
122. Wong BSM, Norman DC. Evaluation of a novel medication aid, the calendar blister-pak, and its effect on drug compliance in a geriatric outpatient clinic. *J Am Geriatr Soc* 1987;35:21–26.
123. Levy RL. Social support and compliance: update. *J Hypertens* 1985;3(Suppl 1):45–49.
124. Spector R, McGrath P, Uretsky N, Newman R, Cohen P. Does

intervention by a nurse improve medication compliance? *Arch Intern Med* 1978;138:36–40.
125. McKenney JM, Slining JD, Henderson HR, Devins D, Barr M. The effect of clinical pharmacy services on patients with essential hypertension. *Circulation* 1973;48:1104–1111.
126. Morse GD, Douglas JB, Upton JH, Rodgers S, Gal P. Effect of pharmacist intervention on control of resistant hypertension. *Am J Hosp Pharm* 1986;43:905–909.
127. Sackett DL, Haynes RB, Gibson ES, Hackett BC, Taylor DW, Roberts RS, Johnson AL. Randomized clinical trial of strategies for improving medication compliance in primary hypertension. *Lancet* 1975;1:1205–1207.
128. Eismer DK, Gillum RF, Johnson CA, Becerra J, Johnson TH. Improving hypertension control in a private medical practice. *Arch Intern Med* 1982;142:297–299.
129. Sackett DL. A compliance practicum for the busy practitioner. In: Haynes RB, Taylor DW, Sackett DL, eds. *Compliance in health care.* Baltimore: Johns Hopkins University Press, 1979;286–294.
130. Becker MH, Maiman LA. Strategies for enhancing patient compliance. *J Community Health* 1980;6:113–135.
131. Coordinating Committee of the National High Blood Pressure Education Program. Collaboration in high blood pressure control: among professionals and with the patient. *Ann Intern Med* 1984;101:393–395.
132. Peck CL, King NJ. Increasing patient compliance with prescriptions. *JAMA* 1982;248:2874–2877.
133. RCP Working Party. Medication for the elderly. *Lancet* 1984;1:271–272.
134. Sbarbaro JA. Strategies to improve compliance with therapy. *Am J Med* 1985;79(Suppl 6A):34–38.
135. Working Group to Define Critical Patient Behaviors in High Blood Pressure Control. Patient behavior for blood pressure control; guidelines for professionals. *JAMA* 1979;241:2534–2537.
136. Coleman VR. Physician behavior and compliance. *J Hypertens* 1985;3(Suppl 1):69–71.
137. Evans CE, Haynes RB, Gilbert JR, Taylor EW, Sackett DL, Johnston M. Educational package on hypertension for primary care physicians. *Can Med Assoc J* 1984;130:719–722.
138. Cohen D, Berner U, Duback UC. Physician compliance in the management of hypertensive patients. *J Hypertens* 1985;3(Suppl 1):73–76.
139. Inui TS, Yourtee EL, Williamson JW. Improved outcomes in hypertension after physician tutorials; a controlled trial. *Ann Intern Med* 1976;84:646–651.

PART C

Future Horizons in Therapy

Hypertension: Pathophysiology, Diagnosis, and Management, edited by J. H. Laragh and B. M. Brenner. Raven Press, Ltd., New York © 1990.

CHAPTER 148

Clinical Development of Antihypertensive Drugs

Can We Perform Better?

Joël Ménard, Marc Bellet, and Hans R. Brunner

The Difficulties of Development of Antihypertensive Drugs, 2331
The Use of Normotensive Volunteers to Investigate Antihypertensive Drugs, 2332
Dose-Finding of Antihypertensive Drugs, 2335
The Definition of the Blood Pressure Baseline Value, 2335
The Definition of the Control Group, 2335
Constant Doses or Ascending Doses, 2335
The Cross-Over Designs, 2336
The Dose–Response Curve in Responders, 2338
The Methods for Measuring Blood Pressure, 2338
Conclusion, 2338
The Goals of a Phase III Program, 2338
Conclusion, 2339
Summary, 2340
References, 2340

Beginning with the early years when the first antihypertensive drugs (hexamethonium, hydralazine, reserpine, chlorothiazide) became available to physicians, before 1960 (1), and leading up to the present state of the art in antihypertensive therapy, a massive proliferation of drugs has occurred. Not only has the number of classes increased, but within some classes, more than 10 drugs have been made available for prescription. Since it has been necessary to register these drugs worldwide and to obtain their approval from the most stringent health regulatory authorities, one may imagine that the development of a new antihypertensive drug is nowadays a well-codified task, well known and well performed all over the world. This is certainly not the case, as shown by two examples.

THE DIFFICULTIES OF DEVELOPMENT OF ANTIHYPERTENSIVE DRUGS

Before 1960, the major error made during the development of antihypertensive drugs was the choice of an excessive daily dose. The use of too-high doses of hydralazine was well explained in 1951 by the severity of the disease in the patients treated at that time, as well as by the lack of knowledge as to how to conduct clinical trials according to rules which could only be established after learning more about hypertension treatment. The clinical development of hydralazine shows that the dose–response curve for severe adverse effects (lupus syndromes) is certainly as important as the dose–response curve for efficacy (2,3). Thiazide diuretics (4) have reinforced this need for a simultaneous evaluation of both the fall in blood pressure and the side effects (minor clinical side effects, biochemical changes, severe adverse effects). This evaluation was performed more than 15 years after the discovery of their efficacy in the treatment of hypertension (5) and is not yet completely integrated in the assessment of antihypertensive treatment (6). This has led to the unfortunate use of too-high doses in practice and in the large trials aimed at evaluation of the benefits of antihypertensive treatment (7). From the use of diuretics, we should have learned that a major part of the maximum effect of an antihypertensive drug is obtained at a relatively low dose, and that increasing the dose might provide a few millimeters less in blood pressure, but at the price of constant undesirable adverse effects (hypokalemia, hyperglycemia, hyperlipidemia, hyperuricemia, hypovolemia, hyperreninemia) or of frequent side effects (tiredness, muscular cramps, orthostatic hypotension). The lesson has never been learned: Alpha-methyldopa, propranolol, and clonidine were tested and initially used at a too-high dosage, and the major error which finally occurred during the clinical development of antihypertensive drugs concerns captopril. Severe dose-related (450–1200 mg/daily) side effects almost killed this major advance in drug treatment of hypertension (8). At that time, however, the early clinical pharmacology of this first ACE inhibitor had suggested, through the neutralization of the angiotensin I pressor effects, that 20 mg captopril was effective for more than 4 hr (9).

The second example of the lack of quality encountered in the development of new antihypertensive drugs will be built by the reader himself, and we hope that it will be an easy and profitable exercise. The major journals have recently published a series of papers which describe the main errors encountered during clinical trials. These errors either are described for all kinds of drugs (10–13), or are addressed specifically for antihypertensive drugs (14,15). After reviewing these extremely well written and useful papers, the reader should take the time to look at some of the numerous supplementary issues of various highly recognized journals which have recently been published (16–18). He or she will certainly have a chance to observe that all errors mentioned in refs. 10–15 are being permanently repeated and published.

Careful reading of six papers (10–15), as well as a review of the available guidelines for the development of antihypertensive drugs (19,20), could, in the future, improve the quality of the development of new antihypertensive compounds by leading to the following: (a) definition of the minimum effective dose at the time of peak effect and at the longest interval between doses, (b) dose proportionality of the side effects, (c) definition of the special subgroups either more likely to benefit from the new drug or at increased risk of severe adverse effects.

It will also make it possible to avoid the following errors:

1. describing patients included in a trial without mentioning (a) the percentage of previously treated patients, (b) the time they spent without active treatment before the initial placebo treatment period, (c) the dates of inclusion in the trial, and (d) the total population of hypertensives screened to find eligible patients;
2. providing blood pressure values without mentioning the exact time interval between the last dose intake and the blood pressure measurement;
3. forgetting a placebo-treated control group after an initial single-blind placebo administration to all included patients;
4. using a step-by-step increase of the drugs, which will bias the results in favor of the last and highest dose;
5. concluding that there is an absence of difference between two groups or two ages, with a statistical power inferior to 80%;
6. proposing as an original finding a correlation between the magnitude of the fall in blood pressure and baseline blood pressure.

In this context, we would now like to discuss, in more detail, some aspects of the process of clinical development of antihypertensive drugs which deserve more attention.

The Use of Normotensive Volunteers to Investigate Antihypertensive Drugs

As with all drugs, a new antihypertensive compound needs to go through Phase I studies to investigate its clinical and biological tolerability at doses which are initially selected according to the results of pharmacological studies and toxicological studies usually performed for 3 months, in two different species, after a pharmacokinetic investigation in these species. With the nontoxic dose in animals being known, the administration of single ascending doses to normotensive volunteers, followed by repeated administration of well-tolerated doses for several days, will allow (a) verification of the safety of the drug and (b) the initiation of pharmacokinetic studies.

A most challenging question is indeed whether the single objective of an antihypertensive drug—namely, to decrease blood pressure in hypertensive patients—can be predicted or detected in normotensive volunteers. The debate is created by the existence of two different views on hypertension and by the influence of the basal levels of blood pressure on the magnitude of a fall in blood pressure. If hypertension is a qualitative disorder, hypertensive patients will be basically different from normotensive subjects. They could have an abnormality in one or several of the multiple biological functions which control blood pressure levels. Therefore, they are extremely different from normotensive individuals and most probably comprise several subgroups which differ in their primary abnormality (21). If hypertension is a quantitative disorder, the difference between normotension and hypertension is only defined by norms, but there is no basic difference in the control of blood pressure in the so-called normotensives and hypertensives (22). Therefore, normotensive volunteers would be suitable if one is looking for a hypotensive effect, but the difficulty arises from the small magnitude of the decrease in blood pressure which can be detected when initial blood pressure values are low (23,24). Since a placebo effect exists in normotensives as well as in hypertensives, all studies in normal volunteers must be placebo-controlled and double-blind and are made difficult by the lack of sensitivity of the noninvasive blood pressure measurements to detect a fall of 5 mmHg, which can be biologically significant but clinically difficult to detect. For instance, a fall in blood pressure was not always detected in normotensive volunteers, in the recumbent position, on a normal-sodium diet, after the oral administration of converting-enzyme inhibitors (25–27). A pharmacodynamic effect of an orally active vasodilator, such as a calcium blocker or a hydralazine-related compound, may be more easily detected by the counterregulation induced by the peripheral dilatation on pulse rate or plasma renin than by the fall in blood pressure itself (28,29) (Fig. 1).

Although administration to normal volunteers will not lead to the introduction of delays in the availability of the drug to hypertensive patients, an innovative clinical investigation performed in normal volunteers at an early stage of the development, and then in parallel with the development in patients, is worthwhile for the clinical development of antihypertensive drugs. Let us take examples from the literature on converting-enzyme inhibitors and sympatholytics.

Investigation of Angiotensin-Converting-Enzyme (ACE) Inhibitors in Normal Volunteers

Fifteen years after the discovery of captopril, there are still uncertainties concerning the exact mechanism of the

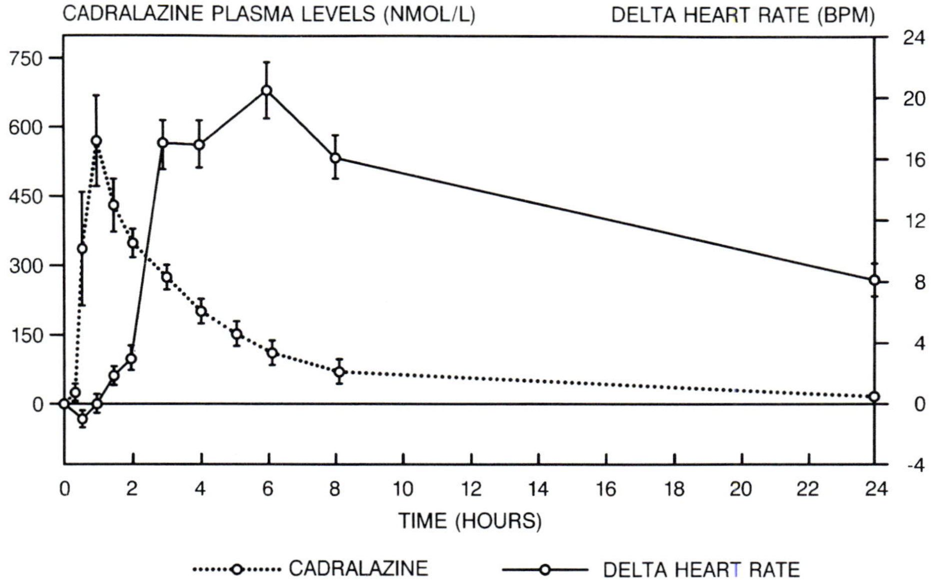

FIG. 1. This study was performed in 12 normal volunteers and showed the reactive increase in heart rate after a single dose of cadralazine (10 mg), a long-acting arteriolar vasodilator, despite the absence of a detectable fall in blood pressure. As predicted from these data, the fall in blood pressure in hypertensive patients treated with cadralazine was found to be maximal 4–6 hr after drug intake and was also found to persist for 24 hr. The pharmacokinetics of the drug in plasma did not correlate with its pharmacodynamic effects (29).

fall in blood pressure. Even if the hypotensive role of bradykinin is less frequently discussed now than in the past (30), the debate now concerns the sites where converting-enzyme inhibition is effective: The plasma and endothelial cells are the most likely (8), but the tissue renin–angiotensin system is also under investigation (31,32). Protocols performed on normal volunteers are helpful in addressing this question. In some studies, administration of ACE inhibitors to normal volunteers has led to a fall in blood pressure (25,33). This hypotensive effect was detected more easily than were the changes in blood pressure after diuretics and beta-blockers, whose antihypertensive properties cannot be predicted in normal volunteers. For these two classes of drugs, trials in normal volunteers have made it possible to provide dose–response curves for the diuretic properties and the beta-blocking effects (34,35), which are necessary to produce a fall in blood pressure in hypertensives; however, these data do not help in the quantification of the hypotensive effect. With ACE inhibitors, a fall in blood pressure was not always observed (27), and the magnitude of the fall was certainly less than that measured after administration of drugs which interfere with the sympathetic nervous system (36). Moreover, the state of salt balance and renin secretion influenced the blood pressure response. No precise dose–response curve could be drawn, but, as already mentioned, independently of the basal blood pressure levels, the intra-arterial measurement of angiotensin I pressor effects in normotensives following ingestion of captopril provided more relevant information on the captopril dose than did the clinical trials performed later. A scientific demonstration of the maximally effective antihypertensive dose of captopril, by a dose–response curve, was provided in 1984 (37). Initially, determinations of plasma ACE inhibition following captopril administration were not reproducible after storage of the plasma samples, and no method of measurement was available. These measurements were available at an early stage for enalapril and the other ACE inhibitors which were developed later, and they certainly made easier the choice of the dose for the initial studies in hypertensive patients. Using Ryan's method (38), a relationship was described between plasma ACE activity and the systolic blood pressure response to exogenous angiotensin I before and after the administration of these converting-enzyme inhibitors to normal volunteers (27). Plasma ACE activity must be reduced to less than 10% of its initial value to consistently abolish the pressor response to exogenous angiotensin I. Therefore, the minimum inhibiting dose should induce a more than 90% inhibition of converting-enzyme activity, measured by Ryan's method; moreover, a close correlation between plasma ACE inhibition and plasma enalaprilate levels has been demonstrated (39). Thus, in normal volunteers, it is possible to establish the minimum plasma concentration of inhibitor that is necessary to inhibit angiotensin I conversion adequately. The same doses are adequate to induce significant reductions in plasma angiotensin II and aldosterone (40), which reflect the inhibition of the renin–angiotensin system.

More impressive is the observation that some data published on the biochemical effects of ACE inhibitors (25) were able to explain why a major increase in the dose of an ACE inhibitor is unlikely to increase the fall in blood pressure, even if these data were not interpreted for that purpose. Manhem et al. (25) have shown that, 24 hr after dose intake, immunoreactive plasma angiotensin II and plasma aldosterone were not decreased, despite a permanent inhibition of plasma ACE, a constant finding with all ACE inhibitors (40). These authors gave doses of 5, 20, and 50 mg ramipril to their normal volunteers. This 10-fold increase in the dose was not more effective in decreasing the active product of the renin–angiotensin system, angiotensin II, 24 hr after dose intake. The modest reinforcement of plasma ACE inhibition (and probably also of endothelial ACE inhibition) induced a massive rise in plasma renin which led to an increase in angiotensin I, the substrate of ACE, to such an extent that the final product of the enzymatic reaction, angiotensin II, returned toward its initial levels (Fig. 2). More recently, Nussberger et al. (41) have demonstrated why it is so important to differentiate converting-enzyme inhibition from renin–angiotensin system inhibition. If this demonstration of the self-limitation of the renin–angiotensin system blockade after ACE inhibition had been realized earlier, finding of the optimum dose for many ACE inhibitors would have been different.

Investigation of Sympatholytics in Normal Volunteers

Another class of drugs that have been more carefully investigated through the use of normal volunteers are the *sympatholytics.* The effects of single and repeated oral doses of selective postsynaptic α_1-adrenoceptor antagonists (42–44) to normal volunteers of various ages (45) made it possible to predict (a) the hypotensive effects and risks of these drugs and (b) their consequences on the counterregulation systems, the sympathetic nervous system, and the renin–angiotensin system. Similarly, dose–response curves of the hypotensive, sedative, and salivary-flow effects have been drawn with clonidine and related compounds, allowing comparison between the magnitude of the hypotensive effect and the intensity of the side effects (36,46). Needless to say, hypotension in normal volunteers is not synonymous with an antihypertensive effect in patients; furthermore, at a very early stage of the clinical development of a potential antihypertensive drug, these carefully monitored investigations should also be performed in a small number of stable, hospitalized hypertensive patients before deciding the doses which will be used in placebo-controlled, double-blind studies. We should also bear in mind that (a) the single administration of a drug is not sufficient, (b) repeated administration is necessary, and (c) hospitalized patients

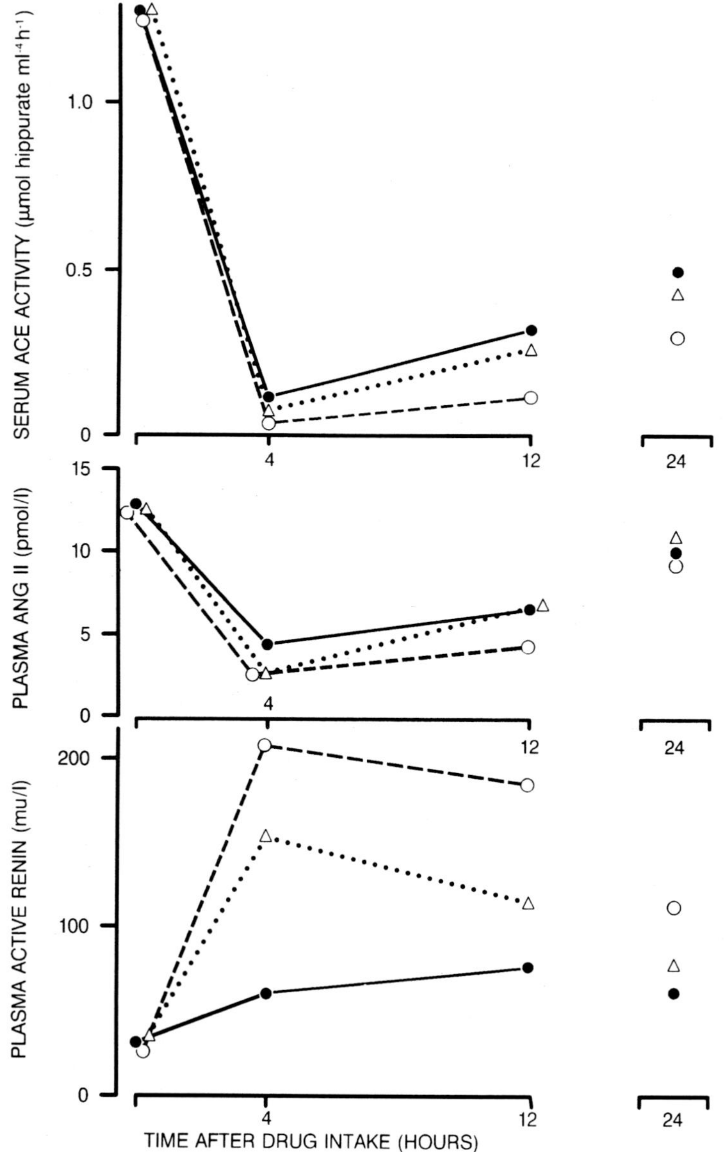

FIG. 2. A 10-fold increase in the dose of ramipril, administered to normal volunteers, moderately reinforces plasma ACE inhibition (**upper panel**), does not suppress angiotensin II 24 hr after drug intake (**middle panel**) but massively increases angiotensin I (**lower panel**), the substrate of ACE, in a first-order enzymatic reaction (25). (●) 5 mg; (△) 20 mg; (○) 50 mg.

exposed to the early administration of a new drug frequently have much more severe hypertension than do the mild to moderate hypertensive patients, who will be exposed to the drug as outpatients.

DOSE-FINDING OF ANTIHYPERTENSIVE DRUGS

There are many important issues in the dose-finding of an antihypertensive drug, which is the most essential, but also the most difficult, part of an antihypertensive drug development program.

The Definition of the Blood Pressure Baseline Value

A constant difficulty is the progressive decrease in blood pressure which occurs at successive visits to the physician's office, as shown, for instance, in the MRC trial and in the Australian trial (7,47). This fall in blood pressure is not due to the prescription of a placebo but, instead, to a decrease in the patient's reactivity to the medical environment. This adaption to the environment is included in the so-called "placebo" effect and seems to be diminished when ambulatory monitoring is performed (48). In an opposite direction, another difficulty encountered in obtaining a stable baseline blood pressure arises from the fact that in many trials the patients had been previously treated. They are offered a wash-out period, usually of 2–4 weeks, and then a placebo single-blind treatment period, also of 2–4 weeks. There is still a risk of a progressive rise in blood pressure resulting from the discontinuation of a previously effective treatment, which can minimize the effect of the investigational drug.

Still more inappropriate is the inclusion in trials of patients refractory to previous treatments. It might give the patient a chance to respond to a new therapy, but it certainly also exposes the new drug to (a) patients refractory to all treatments or (b) to noncompliant patients.

The Definition of the Control Group

After a single-blind placebo period (ideally 4 weeks), when it is demonstrated that diastolic and systolic blood pressures are permanently above certain values and fluctuate by less than 10 mmHg at two consecutive visits, the introduction of the active treatment still needs a placebo-treated control group. The repetition of the visits, even at this later stage of the trial, can still influence blood pressure and decrease it (47), which would overestimate the hypotensive effect of the new drug. Unfortunately, the placebo group is all too frequently omitted in many dose-finding studies, probably because of the risk that a cardiovascular complication of hypertension may occur in a patient maintained on placebo for a period whose length could be challenged from the ethical point of view. On the basis of the results of the large-scale trials of hypertension treatment (7,47,49–51), the risk of a major cardiovascular accident occurring during a 1-month placebo treatment has been calculated in Table 1. Moreover, a placebo treatment for a short period of time spares some patients an unnecessary active treatment if their blood pressure becomes normal within a few weeks.

TABLE 1. *Risk of cardiovascular event during a 1-month placebo treatment, according to blood pressure levels and age*

Diastolic blood pressure (mmHg) at inclusion	Circumstances of blood pressure measurement	Monthly risk (%)
115–129	In hospital (VA)	21
105–115	In hospital (VA)	4.9
99–119	Out patients, >60 (EWPHE)	1.1
95–109	Out patients, >60 (ANBPS)	0.4
90–109	Out patients, <60 (MRC)	0.1

Constant Doses or Ascending Doses

At the present time, no treatment is equally effective in all hypertensives (21). There are always fractions of a hypertensive group who are not sensitive to a given drug, either because of peculiarities in the pathophysiology of the disease or because of differences in the pharmacokinetics of the drug. The day-to-day practice of medicine is based on a stepwise increase in the dose of the marketed drugs in order to avoid a too rapid fall of blood pressure in sensitive subjects (especially in the elderly) and also to minimize side effects, by giving time to the patient to become familiar with the drug and its effects on the whole body, as well as with its hypotensive action. If the protocol of a placebo-controlled dose-finding trial allows for a titration consisting of two to four successive steps (Fig. 3), all patients resistant to this drug will receive the maximum dose. Therefore the conclusion of the trial will overestimate the effective dose, since it will take into account patients who should not have been treated with this drug and who, for this reason, received the maximum dose allowed by the protocol. Moreover, the influence of time on blood pressure always acts in favor of the last dose prescribed, which is the highest.

On the other hand, when the design consists of parallel groups, with no titration, the randomization process in each group, if they are sufficiently large, includes a similar number of sensitive and refractory patients (the drug-induced fall in blood pressure has a generally gaussian distribution). The average fall in blood pressure in each group will allow a true dose–response curve to be drawn and will possibly allow us to find the maximum effective dose. This implies that the groups are of sufficient size, that the range of the tested doses is wide, and that at least four groups are available, ideally more. We have found one dose–response curve published in the literature which almost fulfils these criteria (52), except for the absence of a placebo group, and this was justified by previous demonstration of the efficacy of the drug (lisinopril) versus a placebo (53). The tested doses ranged from 2.5 to 80 mg daily, which was only made possible because side effects of this compound were not dose-dependent within this range. Such a protocol would have been more difficult with antihypertensive drugs whose clinical side effects are strictly dose-related (calcium

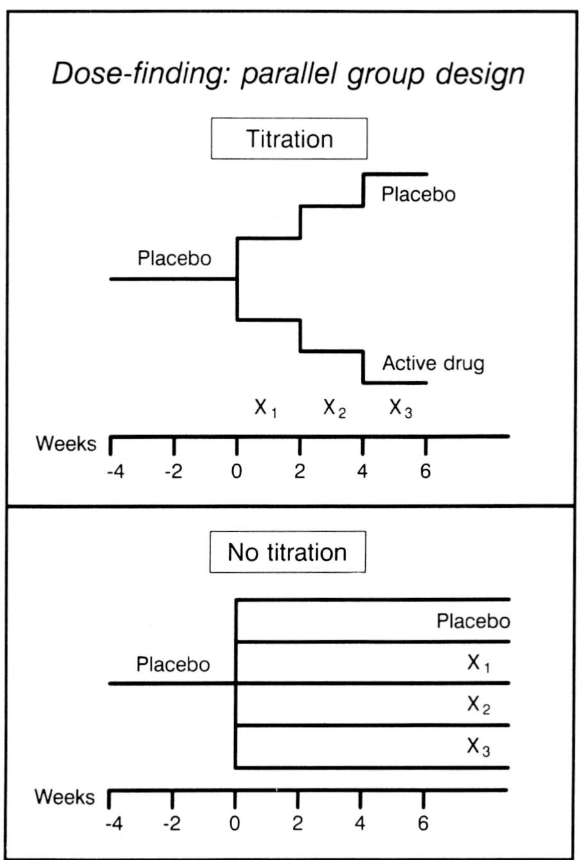

FIG. 3. Parallel group design, with and without titration.

blockers, for instance), and even in this case, it was indeed performed at a rather late stage of the development. The results of the study were analyzed at peak effect and at the time of least effect, 24 hr after dosing. It is possible to plot the results in a manner that is different from that of these authors, by assuming that the maximum fall in blood pressure is defined by the results obtained with the highest prescribed dose of 80 mg once a day (100%) (Fig. 4). This shows that (a) the increase in the dose from 2.5 to 10 mg once a day prolongs the duration of action as shown by the differences in the fall in blood pressure at peak effect and at 24 hr after dosing, (b) 10 mg and 20 mg once daily are not really different at peak effect, and (c) a major increase in the dose (80 mg) brings only a minor increase in the fall in blood pressure already obtained 24 hr after dosing with 20 mg once daily.

It is obvious that before deciding on such a difficult exercise, exploratory studies can be performed faster and easier, especially if a pharmacodynamic or biochemical basis has been provided from Phase I, in normotensive volunteers, to rationally select a potentially effective dose. With a power of 0.9 and an acceptable significance level of 0.05, 20 patients are sufficient in order to detect a fall in blood pressure of 21/10 mmHg in comparison to a placebo, if the standard deviations of the differences are around 14 mmHg for the systolic blood pressure and between 6 and 10 mmHg for the diastolic blood pressure (14).

In Table 2 are summarized the placebo effect on blood pressure observed during four different double-blind, placebo-controlled trials and its standard deviations (54–56). It shows that the standard deviation varies between 8 and 15 mmHg at the outpatient clinic, between 5 and 13 mmHg at the outpatient clinic with a 30-min recording of blood pressure by an automatic device (Sentron), and between 5 and 11 mmHg at home (self-blood pressure measurement and Remler). A reasonable planning of a trial can be based on the demonstration of a fall in diastolic blood pressure of 5 mmHg, either 12 or 24 hr after dosing, with a 10 mmHg standard deviation of the difference. The α-risk is usually established at 5%, and the β-risk is usually established at 20%. It is therefore difficult to find the most appropriate dose of an antihypertensive drug without two pivotal studies including 150–200 patients to test three or four doses versus a placebo and covering an eight-fold dose range. This is extremely difficult to perform, and the inclusion of several centers to recruit the appropriate number of patients may increase the standard deviation of the differences.

The Cross-Over Designs

In contrast to the parallel group design, a cross-over design exposes the same patient successively to various treat-

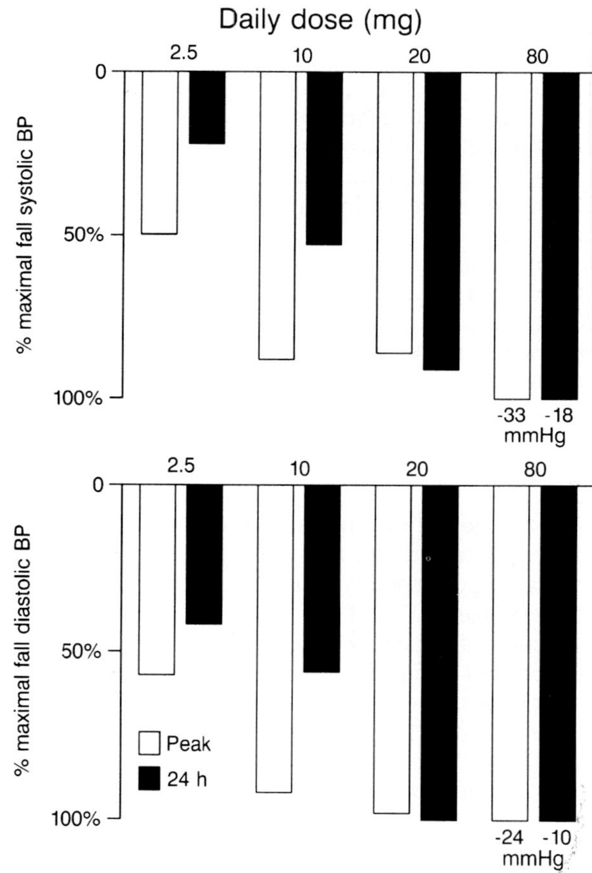

FIG. 4. The fall in systolic and diastolic blood pressure is expressed in terms of the percent of the antihypertensive effect of 80 mg lisinopril once a day. At peak effect, the gain is minimal between 10 and 20 mg, and 24 hr after dose intake, the gain is minimal between 20 and 80 mg (52).

TABLE 2. *Standard error of the difference in blood pressure during placebo treatment by using three different methods of blood pressure measurement*[a]

	Mercury manometer at the outpatient clinic		Automatic device (30 min, six measurements) at the outpatient clinic in the absence of physician		Self-blood pressure measurements at home	
	SBP	DBP	SBP	DBP	SBP	DBP
Permanent hypertension						
n = 100; 14 days (54)	−0.5 ± 8	−3 ± 8	−3 ± 12	−3 ± 13		
n = 20; 21 days (56)	−2 ± 11	0 ± 8	−1 ± 5	0 ± 5	−4 ± 9[b]	−3 ± 5[b]
Young hypertensives						
n = 17; 28 days (55)	−10 ± 11	−4 ± 9	−5 ± 7	−3 ± 6	−2 ± 6	−2 ± 7
Elderly hypertensives						
n = 18; 28 days (55)	−3 ± 15	−1 ± 10	+1.5 ± 13	+2 ± 9	−3 ± 11	−2 ± 5

[a] SBP, systolic blood pressure; DBP, diastolic blood pressure.
[b] Ambulatory blood pressure monitoring/Remler.

ments or various doses of the same treatment. The main limitations of this approach have been analyzed by Hills and Armitage for the two-period, two-treatment designs (57). A cross-over design can only be used (a) for a disease which is stable during the period of the trial, (b) with drugs which are immediately effective and whose effects disappear within a very short time, and (c) in the absence of an effect of the previous treatment period on the results obtained during a given period. For blood pressure trials, this "carry-over effect" might be due to the persistence of the biological effects of a drug. For instance, one does not know precisely how long it takes to normalize the sodium balance after discontinuation of a diuretic. This will be dependent on the dose of the diuretic, the sodium intake, and the delay in resetting the renin–angiotensin system. Furthermore, one does not know the time required for the blood pressure to return to its initial levels after normalization of the sodium balance, with this delay probably being very dependent on the duration of the diuretic therapy: The shorter it was, the shorter the time for the readjustment. A review of the data collected during the last 15 years by Chalmers' group (58) suggests that treatment periods (active or placebo) of 15 days might be sufficient to draw appropriate conclusions with diuretics, beta-blockers, ACE inhibitors, and calcium blockers. The absence of detectable carry-over effects is also supported by other studies (59). The estimation of the residual effects of treatment is a matter of debate, especially concerning (a) the power of the tests which are used (60) and (b) the most appropriate tests (61,62).

A cross-over design, when carefully performed in a single center by a single physician or nurse in order to standardize the conditions of blood pressure measurements, with patients actively participating in the trial, is certainly able to provide useful information (Fig. 5). At the end of the international development of benazepril, a converting-enzyme inhibitor, there was still doubt as to the efficacy of the once-daily dose of 10 mg, 20–24 hr after drug intake. A multiple-period (five) cross-over design was performed in 25 hypertensive patients to compare, 24 hr after dose intake, the blood pressure effects of 10 mg or 20 mg benazepril once a day with the effects of a placebo and with the effects of 10 mg and 20 mg of benazepril twice a day, 12 hr

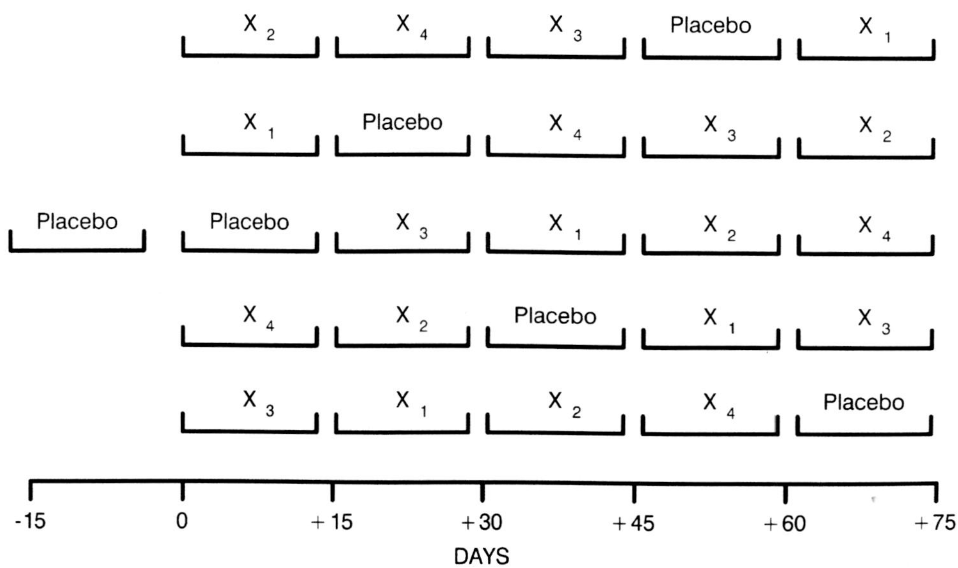

FIG. 5. Multiple-period cross-over design.

after dosing. A placebo period was included at random among the five 14-day treatment periods, as shown in Fig. 5. The efficacy of 10 mg once a day, 24 hr after drug intake, was easily demonstrated (Fig. 6). Blood pressure during the placebo period did not differ from baseline, which confirms that 2 weeks after discontinuation of the ACE inhibitor, blood pressure and active and total plasma renins were readjusted to their initial levels (63).

The Dose–Response Curve in Responders

At present, in any study designed to establish the dose of a new antihypertensive drug, complete nonresponders are pooled with the optimal responders for analysis. This corresponds to what will happen in practice, but it obviously reduces the average antihypertensive effect and thereby markedly decreases the resolution power of the analysis of the dose–response curve. It is a different issue to assess the overall efficacy of an antihypertensive drug, for which all nonresponders should be analyzed together with the responders (results are expressed in percentage of patients achieving the goal of blood pressure control), and to determine an "optimal therapeutic dose range." As in other fields of medicine, such as the use of β_2-agonists in the treatment of asthma, the dose range and the duration of action should be established in responders, since nonresponders should not be treated with the investigational drug, even if a major increase in the dose finally induces a small fall in blood pressure. The price for such a hypotensive effect is a high incidence of side effects and, later on, a rare, but severe, adverse reaction. Moreover, this procedure exposes such responders to treatment with an excessive dose of the drug. A precise definition of the optimal therapeutic dose range in responders would certainly decrease the average recommended dose of many currently available antihypertensive agents, which would have a beneficial influence on the incidence and severity of their clinical and biological side effects.

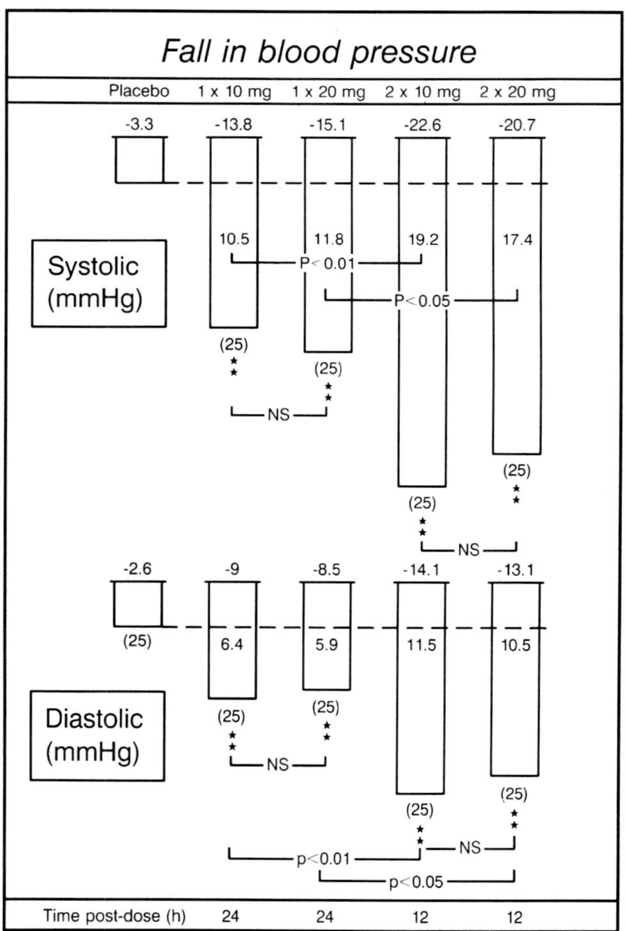

FIG. 6. In this multiple-period cross-over design, blood pressure on placebo is not statistically different from baseline blood pressure. Benazepril (10 mg), once daily, is effective 24 hr after drug intake; 10 mg benazepril and 20 mg benazepril, once a day, are equally effective 24 hr after drug intake during the once-daily treatment period and 12 hr after drug intake, during the b.i.d. treatment period.

The Methods for Measuring Blood Pressure

An increasing attention is rightly paid to the methods of blood pressure measurement (48,64–67), and some elementary recommendations should not be forgotten:

1. Whatever the method is, it should be well performed and well standardized.
2. The choice of the method depends on the goal which is set.
3. The statistical method for the evaluation of the results should be carefully defined before the trial (68).
4. The greater the number of measurements (such as in ambulatory blood pressure monitoring) (66,67), the better the accuracy, and the smaller the standard deviation, the lower the number of subjects needed to demonstrate a clinically relevant fall in blood pressure (59,66).

Conclusion

The dose-finding of an antihypertensive drug is so crucial that data should be obtained at peak effect and at the end of the dosing period by using several kinds of design (parallel groups, cross-over) and different methods of blood pressure measurement.

THE GOALS OF A PHASE III PROGRAM

When Phase II is concluded, the daily dose range of prescription of the new drug should be known, and the conventional objective of the next phase, the Phase III program, is the evaluation of the new drug in comparison with already existing antihypertensive drugs. This implies today a comparison with a diuretic, a beta-blocker, a calcium blocker, and a converting-enzyme inhibitor. In order to profile the new compound against competitors, these studies are frequently performed by means of comparison with two or three leading drugs of each of the prescribed classes. As already discussed, each treatment group should include around 50–75 patients so that it can have a 90% chance of picking up a difference of 5 mmHg for the fall in diastolic blood pressure. This is almost never achieved, and the conclusion reached is that no difference is found. Not only is such a conclusion exposed to a Type II error, but it is extremely dependent on the choice of the doses of the comparative drugs. Medicine is designed for individuals and not for groups. These kinds of results will not help the physician in his choice, except by providing him or her with a statistical guideline. Some patients might still be better treated by a drug which, in a large population, is generally less effective than other drugs with which it was compared (69).

As to side effects, in these comparative trials a large number of different complaints are reported which are difficult to interpret when they have no pharmacological explanation or a high incidence in the general population (tiredness and digestive disorders, for instance). Even with an appropriate number of patients, these trials will not detect a rare, but severe, side effect. If their conclusion is that in one treated group, treatment was stopped in 10% of the patients because of flush, tachycardia, pedal edema, or headache and in 3% of the patients because of cough or upper respiratory symptoms, what does this mean? Ninety percent of the patients in one group and 97% of the patients in the other group have no major side effects. The information tells the physician that with one of the two drugs he or she has a 10% risk of side effects as compared with a 3% risk with the other. On a probability basis, he or she might prefer to start the treatment with the second drug, but this does not solve any problem for the individual patient. A patient might prefer to take the risk of a harmless side effect in order to obtain the benefit of a drug, if this drug is more effective and better tolerated for him/her than are the others. From another viewpoint, if a serious side effect occurs in 0.1% of the patients, it might be better to prescribe the drug which produces benign side effects in 10% than the drug which gives a severe or more unpredictable troublesome side effect in 0.1% of the patients.

The registration dossiers, as well as the journals, are full of data collected from groups, but we strongly believe that these dossiers do not contain any useful information for the individual patient (21,69). The individualization of therapy is still a trial-and-error process and is an "N of 1" trial (70). Therefore, the goals of Phase III should be established in a different way. The primary goal of Phase III is to verify, in a large number of patients, the efficacy and tolerability of the new drug over a long period of time, not to systematically compare it with other drugs. However, in fact, all scientific evaluations have been based on comparisons. For this reason, all Phase II studies are performed versus a placebo, which is ethically possible because these studies are of short duration and are performed in mild to moderate hypertension. In Phase III, 3–12 months are necessary in order to prove that a long-term exposure to the drug does not make it ineffective (tolerance) or, on the contrary, excessively effective. Meanwhile, the clinical and biochemical adverse effects are monitored and analyzed. A comparative group is necessary, but because of the ethical impossibility of exposing to placebo for 1 year, hypertensive patients whose blood pressure is above 100 mmHg (or 95 or 105 mmHg, depending on the country), the comparative group is composed of patients actively treated with other drugs. The comparative group should only be considered as a standard reference for the purpose of ensuring that the efficacy and safety profile of the new drug is compatible with what is already available for the treatment of hypertension.

These trials are frequently expected to demonstrate that the new drug will be either more effective or better tolerated than the previous ones. This exercise has been repeated for 20 years with 10 diuretics, beta-blockers, alpha-blockers, calcium blockers, converting-enzyme inhibitors, and so on, and still there is a total lack of consensus among experts as to which drug is the best choice, with safety always being the most indisputable argument in favor of the older drug (71).

We therefore believe that one or two well-performed large-scale studies versus an accepted established treatment schedule in hypertension would be more convincing. This study should be 1 year in duration, with ascending doses of the investigational drugs (as in practice) and with the successive addition of a second and a third drug, when necessary, during the second and third month of the treatment. The comparative treatment could be diuretics + beta-blockers + vasodilators, beta-blockers + diuretics + ACE inhibitors, ACE inhibitors + diuretics + calcium blockers, calcium blockers + ACE inhibitors + diuretics, or ACE inhibitors + calcium blockers + diuretics. A similar 1-year study should be performed in patients over 65 years of age.

In the meantime, special studies could carefully analyze the additive, synergistic, or negative effect on blood pressure and tolerability of the new drug with other classes of antihypertensives, especially diuretics, as shown by the recent unexpected discovery of the cardiac risk induced by concomitant prescription of diuretics and ketanserin (72). The use of a factorial analysis of cross-over studies has been shown to be extremely useful and cost-effective in looking for partial or complete addition or synergism of the blood pressure effects of two drugs on a small number of patients (58).

Other separately designed trials to answer particular questions are obviously necessary in patients with renal insufficiency, coronary heart disease, vascular diseases, and metabolic disorders; pharmacokinetics and pharmacodynamics interaction studies with various drugs are also necessary.

CONCLUSION

Drug development should not be a business whereby quantity will try to make up for the lack of quality. Carefully collected data, based on innovative methods and rigorous protocols, performed in an adequate number of subjects, smaller than thought necessary in the past, provide more information than do studies performed by a multitude of poorly motivated trialists desperately trying to follow poorly designed protocols. The main steps of the clinical development of an antihypertensive drug are summarized in Table 3 and include, if feasible, the recent approach developed by Elliott and Meredith on drug concentration–effect relationship (73).

TABLE 3. *Recommended allocation of resources and efforts during the development of a new antihypertensive drug*

Phase I:	Precise and early biochemical, pharmacodynamic, and pharmacokinetic studies in normotensives
Phase II (the key phase):	More precise biochemical and pharmacodynamic studies in selected hypertensives
	Drug concentration–effect relationships in selected hypertensives
	More precise dose-finding (peak/duration) with cross-over and parallel-group designs
Phase III:	Minimum number of comparative trials with sufficient power
	Special studies in groups at risk (elderly patients; patients with renal insufficiency, diabetes, or complicated hypertension)
	Studies of combination therapy
Phase IV:	Careful drug monitoring in general populations

A crucial step is not reviewed in this chapter: the adequate monitoring of the drug when it is introduced on the market. One must remember that to be 95% confident of observing one unpredictable severe adverse reaction to a drug, investigators need to follow three times the reciprocal of the true adverse reaction rate (74). They should follow 3000 treated patients in order to be 95% confident of finding at least one such reaction, if its incidence is 1/1000 patients/year, which is roughly the rate at which patients on practolol developed eye damage and is equal to the beneficial effect of drug treatment of mild uncomplicated hypertension (7). For long-term treatments, safety remains the major objective; this makes so difficult the therapeutic research for lifelong diseases such as hypertension or hyperlipidemia, for which some of the available treatments have already been tested for more than 30 years.

SUMMARY

Even though the clinical trials performed during the international development of a new antihypertensive drug may include several thousands of patients, they do not always provide reliable data concerning the appropriate dose and dose interval which should be selected in practice. Drug safety always needs to be confirmed by means of careful large-scale careful drug monitoring studies in representative populations.

Errors in the study design easily explain the reasons why excessive doses of antihypertensive drugs were frequently prescribed in the past. The first major error was to use a titration procedure in parallel-group designs, where the highest dose was considered the most effective one because according to the protocol it was the last to be prescribed. As it was not fully understood to what an extent hypertension was heterogenous, another error was the inclusion of nonresponders in titration studies. These patients were exposed to the highest dose to obtain a minimal fall in blood pressure. Therefore, the prescription was oriented towards excessive doses for responders, the only ones who should have been treated with this drug and included in the trials.

Properly performed cross-over trials should be free from significant carry-over effects and allow for the comparative evaluation of a new drug in individuals. In addition to the usual statistical group analysis, a cross-over study offers the possibility to make an individual choice of the best drug for each patient. Cross-over designs can be used if the patients are in a steady state, if the drug has a rapid onset of action, and if there is no remanent effect on blood pressure, when the drug is stopped.

In the future, the whole antihypertensive drug development program should be organized with early scientifically-oriented studies to provide a more precise definition of the magnitude and the duration of the fall in blood pressure, an analysis of the mechanism of action of the drug and the counter-regulation triggered by its administration. More attention should be paid to the profile of those hypertensives who will most benefit from the new treatment and of those for whom the treatment will have risks. This strategy requires more Phase I and Phase II studies and fewer conventional Phase III multicenter comparative trials, and later on, will be completed, at a later stage, by a careful drug monitoring.

ACKNOWLEDGMENTS

The assistance of Dr. P. Levin in editing the manuscript and of Miss P. Herzog in typing it is greatly appreciated.

We thank Dr. John Laragh for his friendly contribution in the discussion of the issues described in the chapter.

REFERENCES

1. Page IH. Antihypertensive drugs: our debt to industrial chemists. *N Engl J Med* 1981;304:615–618.
2. Perry HM Jr, Schroeder HA, Catanzaro FJ, Moore-Jones D, Camel GH. Studies on the control of hypertension. 8. Mortality, morbidity, and remissions during twelve years of intensive therapy. *Circulation* 1966;33:958–972.
3. Cameron HA, Ramsay LE. The lupus syndrome induced by hydralazine: a common complication with low dose treatment. *Br Med J* 1984;289:410–412.
4. Freis ED, Wanko A, Wilson IM, Parrish AE. Chlorothiazide in hypertensive and normotensive patients. *Ann NY Acad Sci* 1958;71:450–455.
5. Bengtsson C, Johnsson G, Sannerstedt R, Werko L. Effect of different doses of chlorthalidone on blood pressure, serum potassium, and serum urate. *Br Med J* 1975;1:197–199.
6. Freis ED, Reda DJ, Materson BJ. Volume (weight) loss and blood pressure response following thiazide diuretics. *Hypertension* 1988;12:244–250.
7. Medical Research Council Working Party. MRC trial of treatment of mild hypertension: principal results. *Br Med J* 1985;291:97–104.
8. Brunner HR, Nussberger J, Waeber B. Effects of angiotensin converting enzyme inhibition: a clinical point of view. *J Cardiovasc Pharmacol* 1985;7:S73–S81.
9. Ferguson RK, Turini GA, Brunner HR, Gavras H, McKinstry DN. A specific orally active inhibitor of angiotensin-converting enzyme in man. *Lancet* 1977;1:775–778.
10. Charlson ME, Horwitz RI. Applying results of randomized trials to clinical practice: impact of losses before randomization. *Br Med J* 1984;289:1281–1284.

11. Pocock SJ, Hughes MD, Lee RJ. Statistical problems in the reporting of clinical trials. A survey of three medical journals. *N Engl J Med* 1987;317:426–432.
12. Freiman JA, Chalmers TC, Smith H Jr, Kuebler RR. The importance of beta, the type II error and sample size in the design and interpretation of the randomized control trial. Survey of 71 "negative" trials. *N Engl J Med* 1978;299:690–694.
13. Louis TA, Lavori PW, Bailar JC, Polansky M. Cross-over and self-controlled designs in clinical research. *N Engl J Med* 1984;310:24–31.
14. Freestone S, Silas JH, Ramsay LE. Sample size for short-term trials of antihypertensive drugs. *Br J Clin Pharmacol* 1982; 14:265–268.
15. Maxwell C. Clinical trials in hypertension: some general thoughts and some particular controversies. *Nephron* 1987;47:1–4.
16. Calcium antagonists in cardiovascular disease: rationale for 24 hours action. Proceedings of an official satellite symposium and papers on amlodipine presented at the 25th Anniversary International Symposium on Calcium Antagonists in Hypertension. Basel, Switzerland, February 11–12, 1988. *J Cardiovasc Pharmacol* 1988;12(Suppl 7).
17. Doxazosin: a distinctive approach to risk reduction of coronary heart disease in hypertensive patients. Proceedings of a symposium. Hamburg, West Germany, January 30, 1988. *Am Heart J* 1988;116:1707–1840.
18. A symposium: ramipril—a new angiotensin converting enzyme inhibitor. *Am J Cardiol* 1987;59:1D–176D.
19. Offerhaus L. Guidelines for evaluation of antihypertensive drugs in man. Report of a World Health Organization, Regional Office for Europe Scientific Working Group on the Harmonization of Guidelines for Clinical Trials and Drugs—Antihypertensive Drugs, Uppsala, April 24–25, 1978. *Eur J Clin Pharmacol* 1979;16:428–30.
20. FDC Reports. FDA's proposed guidelines for the clinical evaluation of antihypertensive drugs. June 6, 1988;9–10.
21. Laragh JH, Lamport B, Sealey J, Alderman MH. Diagnosis *ex juvantibus*. Individual response patterns to drugs reveal hypertension mechanisms and simplify treatment. *Hypertension* 1988; 12:223–226.
22. Pickering G. Hypertension. Definitions, natural histories and consequences. *Am J Med* 1972;52:570–583.
23. MacGregor GA, Rotellar C, Markandu ND, Smith SJ, Sagnella GA. Contrasting effects of nifedipine, captopril, and propranolol in normotensive and hypertensive subjects. *J Cardiovasc Pharmacol* 1982;4:S358–S362.
24. Sumner DJ, Meredith PA, Howie CA, Elliott HL. Initial blood pressure as a predictor of the response to antihypertensive therapy. *Br J Clin Pharmacol* 1988;26:715–720.
25. Manhem PJ, Ball SG, Morton JJ, Murray GD, Leckie BJ, Fraser R, Robertson JI. A dose–response study of HOE 498, a new nonsulphydryl converting enzyme inhibitor, on blood pressure, pulse rate and the renin–angiotensin–aldosterone system in normal man. *Br J Clin Pharmacol* 1985;20:27–35.
26. Hodsman GP, Zabludowski JR, Zoccali C, Fraser R, Morton JJ, Murray GD, Robertson JI. Enalapril (MK421) and its lysine analogue (MK521): a comparison of acute and chronic effects on blood pressure, renin–angiotensin system and sodium excretion in normal man. *Br J Clin Pharmacol* 1984;17:233–241.
27. Biollaz J, Burnier M, Turini GA, Brunner DB, Porchet M, Gomez HJ, Jones KH, Ferber F, Abrams WB, Gavras H, Brunner HR. Three new long-acting converting-enzyme inhibitors: relationship between plasma converting-enzyme activity and response to angiotensin I. *Clin Pharmacol Ther* 1981;29:665–670.
28. Lederballe-Pedersen O, Christensen NJ, Ramsch KD. Comparison of acute effects of nifedipine in normotensive and hypertensive man. *J Cardiovasc Pharmacol* 1980;2:357–366.
29. Brunel P, Lecaillon JB, Guyene TT, Imhof P, Menard J. Influence of the acetylator status on hemodynamics and pharmacokinetics in healthy volunteers after cadralazine. Manuscript in preparation.
30. Textor SC, Brunner HR, Gavras H. Converting enzyme inhibition during chronic angiotensin infusion in rats. Evidence against a nonangiotensin mechanism. *Hypertension* 1981;3:269–276.
31. Dzau VJ. Significance of the vascular renin–angiotensin pathway. *Hypertension* 1986;8:553–559.
32. Unger T, Ganten D, Lang RE, Scholkens BA. Is tissue converting enzyme inhibition a determinant of the antihypertensive efficacy of converting enzyme inhibitors? Studies with the two different compounds, Hoe498 and MK421, in spontaneously hypertensive rats. *J Cardiovasc Pharmacol* 1984;6:872–880.
33. MacGregor GA, Markandu ND, Roulston JE. Does the renin–angiotensin system maintain blood pressure in both hypertensive and normotensive subjects? A comparison of propranolol, saralasin and captopril. *Clin Sci* 1979;57:s145–s148.
34. Morgan T. The use of diuretic drugs and aldosterone antagonists in hypertension. In: Doyle AE, ed. *Handbook of hypertension, vol 5: pharmacology of antihypertension drugs.* Amsterdam: Elsevier, 1984;67–91.
35. Prichard BNC, Owens CWI. Beta-adrenoceptor blocking drugs. In: Doyle AE, ed. *Handbook of hypertension, vol 5: pharmacology of antihypertensive drugs.* Amsterdam: Elsevier, 1984;1947–1953.
36. Dollery CT, Reid JL. Double-blind comparison of the hypotensive, sedative and salivary flow effects of lofexidine and clonidine in normal subjects. *Arzneimittelforschung* 1982;32:984–987.
37. Low-dose captopril for the treatment of mild to moderate hypertension. I. Results of a 14-week trial. Veterans Administration Cooperative Study Group on Antihypertensive Agents. *Arch Intern Med* 1984;144:1947–1953.
38. Ryan JW, Chung A, Ammons C, Carlton ML. A simple radioassay for angiotensin-converting enzyme. *J Biochem* 1977;167:501–504.
39. Biollaz J, Schelling JL, Jacot-Des-Combes B, Brunner DB, Desponds G, Brunner HR, Ulm EH, Hichens M, Gomez HJ. Enalapril maleate and a lysine analogue (MK-521) in normal volunteers; relationship between plasma drug levels and the renin angiotensin system. *Br J Clin Pharmacol* 1982;14:363–368.
40. Nussberger J, Brunner DB, Waeber B, Brunner HR. True versus immunoreactive angiotensin II in human plasma. *Hypertension* 1985;7:1–7.
41. Nussberger J, Juillerat L, Perret F, Waeber B, Bellet M, Brunner HR, Menard J. Need for plasma angiotensin measurements to investigate converting enzyme inhibition in humans. *Am Heart J* 1989;117:717–721.
42. Nicholls DP, McNeill J, O'Connor PC, Harron DW, Leahey WJ, Shanks RG. Effect of indoramin, labetalol and alinidine on sympathetic function in normal man. *Br J Clin Pharmacol* 1984;18:215–221.
43. Wood AJ, Bolli P, Simpson FO. Prazosin in normal subjects: plasma levels, blood pressure and heart rate [Letter]. *Br J Clin Pharmacol* 1976;3:199–201.
44. Nicholls DP, Harron DWG, Shanks RG. Acute and chronic cardiovascular effects of indoramin and prazosin in normal man. *Br J Clin Pharmacol* 1981;12:s61–s66.
45. Elliott HL, Sumner DJ, McLean K, Reid JL. Effect of age on the responsiveness of vascular alpha-adrenoceptors in man. *Clin Sci* 1982;63:s305–s308.
46. Davies DS, Wing LMH, Reid JL, Neill E, Tippett P, Dollery CT. Pharmacokinetics and concentration–effect relationships of intravenous and oral clonidine. *Clin Pharmacol Ther* 1977;21:593–601.
47. A report by the Management Committee of the Australian Therapeutic Trial in Mild Hypertension. Untreated mild hypertension. *Lancet* 1982;1:185–191.
48. Gould BA, Mann S, Davies AB, Altman DG, Raftery EB. Does placebo lower blood-pressure? *Lancet* 1981;2:1377–1381.
49. Amery A, Birkenhager W, Brixko P, Bulpitt C, Clement D, Deruyttere M, De-Schaepdryver A, Dollery C, Fagard R, Forette F, et al. Mortality and morbidity results from the European Working Party on High Blood Pressure in the Elderly Trial. *Lancet* 1985;1:1349–1354.
50. Effects of treatment on morbidity in hypertension. Results in patients with diastolic blood pressures averaging 115 through 129 mm Hg. Veterans Administration Cooperative Study Group on Antihypertensive Agents. *JAMA* 1967;202:1028–1034.
51. Effects of treatment on morbidity in hypertension. II. Results in patients with diastolic blood pressure averaging 90 through 114 mmHg. Veterans Administration Cooperative Study Group on Antihypertensive Agents. *JAMA* 1970;213:1143–1152.
52. Cirillo VJ, Gomez HJ, Salonen J, Salonen R, Rissanen V, Bolo-

gnese JA, Nyberg R, Kristianson K. Lisinopril: dose–peak effect relationship in essential hypertension. *Br J Clin Pharmacol* 1988;25:533–538.

53. Gomez HJ, Cirillo VJ, Moncloa F. The clinical pharmacology of lisinopril. *J Cardiovasc Pharmacol* 1987;9:S27–S34.
54. Sassano P, Chatellier G, Billaud E, Alhenc-Gelas F, Corvol P, Menard J. Treatment of mild to moderate hypertension with or without the converting enzyme inhibitor enalapril. Results of a six-month double-blind trial. *Am J Med* 1987;83:227–235.
55. Jeunemaitre X, Ged E, Ducrocq MB, Alhenc-Gelas F, Corvol P, Menard J. Effects of transdermal clonidine in young and elderly patients with mild hypertension: evaluation by three noninvasive methods of blood pressure measurement. *J Cardiovasc Pharmacol* 1987;10:162–167.
56. Bellet M, Pagny JY, Chatellier G, Corvol P, Menard J. Evaluation of slow release nicardipine in essential hypertension by casual and ambulatory blood pressure measurements. Effects of acute versus chronic administration. *J Hypertens* 1987;5:599–604.
57. Hills M, Armitage P. The two-period cross-over clinical trial. *Br J Clin Pharmacol* 1979;8:7–20.
58. Wing LM, Chalmers JP, West MJ. Cross-over factorial studies with antihypertensive drugs. *Nephron* 1987;47:94–98.
59. Menard J, Serrurier D, Bautier P, Plouin PF, Corvol P. Cross-over design to test antihypertensive drugs with self-recorded blood pressure. *Hypertension* 1988;11:153–159.
60. Willan AR, Pater JL. Carry-over and the two-period cross-over clinical trial. *Biometrics* 1986;42:593–599.
61. Willan AR. Using the maximum test statistic in the two-period cross-over clinical trial. *Biometrics* 1988;44:211–218.
62. Abeyaskera S, Curnon RW. The desirability of adjusting for residual effects in a cross-over design. *Biometrics* 1984;40:1071–1078.
63. Guyene TT, Bellet M, Sassano P, Serrurier D, Corvol P, Menard J. Cross-over design for the dose-finding of a converting-enzyme inhibitor in hypertension. Manuscript in preparation.
64. Gould BA, Hornung RS, Kieso H, Cashman PM, Raftery EB. An evaluation of self-recorded blood pressure during drug trials. *Hypertension* 1986;8:267–271.
65. Mancia G, Bertinieri G, Grassi G, Parati G, Pomidossi G, Ferrari A, Gregorini L, Zanchetti A. Effects of blood-pressure measurement by the doctor on patient's blood pressure and heart rate. *Lancet* 1983;2:695–698.
66. Conway J, Johnston J, Coats A, Somers V, Sleight P. The use of ambulatory blood pressure monitoring to improve the accuracy and reduce the numbers of subjects in clinical trials of antihypertensive agents. *J Hypertens* 1988;6:111–116.
67. Waeber G, Beck G, Waeber B, Bidiville J, Nussberger J, Brunner HR. Comparison of betaxolol with verapamil in hypertensive patients: discrepancy between office and ambulatory blood pressures. *J Hypertens* 1988;6:239–245.
68. Marler MR, Jacob RG, Leholzky JP, Shapiro AP. The statistical analysis of treatment effects in 24-hour ambulatory blood pressure recordings. *Stat Med* 1988;7:697–716.
69. Menard J, Brunner HR, Waeber B, Plouin PF, Burnier M. Individualization of antihypertensive therapy [Letter]. *Hypertension* 1988;12:526–528.
70. Guyatt G, Sackett D, Taylor DW, Chong J, Roberts R, Pugsley S. Determining optimal therapy-randomized trials in individual patients. *N Engl J Med* 1986;314:889–892.
71. The 1988 report of the Joint National Committee on Detection, Evaluation, and Treatment of High Blood Pressure. *Arch Intern Med* 1988;148:1023–1038.
72. Prevention of atherosclerotic complications with ketanserin trial group. Prevention of atherosclerotic complications: controlled trial of ketanserin. *Br Med J* 1989;298:424–429.
73. Elliott HL, Meredith PA. Drug concentration–effect relationship in man. In: Turner P, VoPans JN, eds. *Recent advances in clinical pharmacology and toxicology*. Churchill Livingstone Lawson, 1989;4:19–37.
74. Sackett DL, Haynes RB, Tugwell P. *Clinical epidemiology. A basic science for clinical medicine.* Boston: Little, Brown and Company, 1985;226.

Hypertension: Pathophysiology, Diagnosis, and Management, edited by J. H. Laragh and B. M. Brenner. Raven Press, Ltd., New York © 1990.

CHAPTER 149

Specific Renin Inhibitors

The Concept and the Prospects

Edgar Haber and Kwan Y. Hui

Early Renin Inhibitors, 2344
Renin Inhibitors Based on the Substitution of Statine (or Its Variants) at the Scissile Bond, 2344
Other Substitutions at the Scissile Bond, 2345
Other Modifications, 2345
Prorenin Peptides, 2346
Species Specificity, 2346
Oral Activity, 2347
Principles of Renin Inhibition, 2347
Do Renin Inhibitors Have a Future as Clinically Effective Antihypertensive Agents?, 2347
References, 2348

Our image of the renin–angiotensin system has been transformed from being one of an academically interesting, but rather obscure, regulatory mechanism that may have contributed to an uncommon form of hypertension to being one of a potent regulator of cardiovascular homeostasis, the manipulation of which is now used to control the most prevalent types of hypertension and congestive heart failure. The clinical story of the manipulation of the renin–angiotensin system began in 1971 with saralasin, a competitive inhibitor of the angiotensin II receptor (1). Because this compound can be administered only by intravenous injection and has a very short half-life, however, its sole application is in the recognition of "angiotensinogenic" hypertension (2). Blockade of the renin–angiotensin system by direct inhibition of renin with renin-specific antibodies (3) and by inhibition of the angiotensin-converting enzyme with teprotide (a snake-venom peptide) (4) could be effected in experimental models of hypertension and in short-term clinical studies (5,6), but, as with saralasin, evaluations of long-term therapy could not be carried out because of the agents' limited half-lives and the need to administer them parenterally. In 1978, Gavras et al. (7) reported the first clinical trial of an orally administered converting-enzyme inhibitor, captopril. Soon thereafter, it became apparent that inhibition of the renin–angiotensin system was an effective treatment for essential hypertension, regardless of the patient's plasma renin concentration (8), and a means of ameliorating heart failure by reducing afterload (9).

The converting-enzyme inhibitors presently available for clinical use, captopril, enalapril, and lisinopril, are very effective and have low side-effect profiles. A question that an investigator or a clinician may ask is why any effort should be expended in seeking an alternative to converting-enzyme-inhibitor therapy. The purpose of this chapter is to address this question.

It appears that the major reason for looking beyond converting enzyme is its lack of specificity. In addition to its role as catalyst in the conversion of angiotensin I to II, the very same enzyme plays a role in the inactivation of bradykinin and, probably, in the inactivation of enkephalins as well as other biologically active peptides. As the degradation of bradykinin is inhibited, its plasma or tissue concentration may rise, resulting both in direct effects, such as vasodilatation, and in the stimulation of the production of eicosanoids. Some of the adverse effects of converting-enzyme inhibitors, such as the development of flushing or rash, have been attributed to the elaboration of bradykinin or prostaglandins (10). Other, more serious questions about the nonspecific action of converting-enzyme inhibitors surround their intrarenal effects: Is afferent renal arteriolar dilatation, with its significant effect on renal function, a consequence of the reduction of intrarenal angiotensin II concentration or of the production of bradykinin or prostaglandins within the kidney? Converting-enzyme inhibitors also cause renal failure in bilateral renal artery stenosis and appear to have beneficial effects in diabetic nephropathy. Will inhibition of the renin–angiotensin system in a more

TABLE 1. *Potential sites for inhibition of the renin–angiotensin system*

Step in the pathway	Agent
Renin biosynthesis	Transactivating factors (undiscovered)
Renin secretion	Beta-adrenergic blockers (nonspecific)
Renin activity	Antibodies
	Peptide inhibitors of renin
Converting enzyme	Captopril, enalapril, lisinopril
Angiotensin II receptor	Saralasin and similar peptides

selective manner avoid this both adverse and beneficial result?

The potential advantages of inhibitors whose effects are more specific may derive from the possibility of inhibiting tissue renin or of inhibiting renin within the central nervous system. There is now abundant evidence that renin is synthesized in tissues other than the kidney. In these tissues it may act locally, exerting a paracrine, rather than an endocrine, function. It is also not at all certain whether, in these tissues, converting enzyme is a necessary participant in angiotensin II formation. Thus the inhibition of renin rather than converting enzyme may be a better means of blocking angiotensin II formation in tissues.

Table 1 lists the potential targets for inhibition of the renin–angiotensin system. Among the presently accessible sites, the angiotensin II receptor and the enzyme renin itself provide opportunities for the most selective intervention. Angiotensin II receptor inhibitors are short-lived peptides that must be administered parenterally. Thus, as noted earlier, they have diagnostic, but not therapeutic, applications. There has been little advance in the development of long-lasting and specific blockers of the angiotensin II receptor. On the other hand, progress in the design of renin inhibitors has been considerable, and at present there is substantial research activity in the pharmaceutical industry as well as in academic laboratories.

EARLY RENIN INHIBITORS

Monoclonal antibodies are excellent experimental tools (11,12), but the necessity of parenteral administration and potential immunogenicity prevent their use in clinical trials: A small organic compound that was a specific renin inhibitor had to be found. The first low-molecular-weight inhibitor to block renin's action effectively *in vivo* was reported in 1980 (13). It was an analogue of an octapeptide that Skeggs et al. (14) had shown many years before to be the minimal substrate for renin. This substrate analogue was not very potent [inhibitory constants between 1.0 and 2.3 μM were reported (15,16)], and, although it was an effective hypotensive agent in the primate, at higher doses the analogue exhibited some lack of specificity (16,17).

RENIN INHIBITORS BASED ON THE SUBSTITUTION OF STATINE (OR ITS VARIANTS) AT THE SCISSILE BOND

More potent substrate analogue inhibitors have since been constructed by substituting various nonhydrolyzable residues for the scissile bond (the peptide bond renin cleaves in angiotensinogen). It had been noted that pepstatin, a potent inhibitor of pepsin, became a modestly potent, though nonselective, inhibitor of renin (pepsin and renin are both acid proteases) when pepstatin was modified to increase its solubility (18–20). Investigators then learned that the selectivity of renin substrate analogues could be increased by substituting the unusual amino acid statine (found in pepstatin and thought by some to be an analogue of the transition state of the peptide bond as it undergoes enzymatic hydrolysis) for the two amino acids on either side of the scissile bond region of the angiotensinogen sequence (21). Several variants of statine have been reported (Table 2). These include (3*S*,4*S*)-4-amino-3-hydroxy-5-phenylpentanoic acid (24) (AHPPA), (3*S*,4*S*)-4-amino-3-hydroxy-5-cyclohexylpentanoic acid (24) (ACHPA), di-

TABLE 2. *Scissile bond modifications with statine and its variants*

Statine variant	Example of renin inhibitor[a]	IC_{50} (nM)[b]	
Statine (21–23)	Iva—His—Pro—Phe—His—A—Ile—Phe—NH_2	1.9	(21)
	Boc—Phe—His—A—Ile—AMP	1.7	(22)
AHPPA (23,24)	Iva—His—Pro—Phe—His—B—Leu—Phe—NH_2	2.2	(24)
ACHPA (24–26)	Iva—His—Pro—Phe—His—C—Leu—Phe—NH_2	0.17	(24)
Difluorostatine	Boc—Phe—His—D—Ile—AMP	12	(22)
Difluorostatone (22,27)	Boc—Phe—His—E—Ile—AMP	0.52	(22)
2-Substituted statine	iBu—His—Pro—Phe—Phe—F—Leu—Phe—NH_2	1.7[c]	(28)
3-Amino-deoxystatine	Boc—His—Pro—Phe—His—G—Ile—His—NH_2	28	(29)
Difluoro-amino-deoxystatine	Boc—Phe—His—H—Ile—AMP	340	(30)

[a] A represents statine, or (3*S*,4*S*)-4-amino-3-hydroxy-6-methylheptanoic acid; B represents AHPPA, or (3*S*,4*S*)-4-amino-3-hydroxy-5-phenylpentanoic acid; C represents ACHPA, or (3*S*,4*S*)-4-amino-3-hydroxy-5-cyclohexylpentanoic acid; D represents difluorostatine, or (3*R*,4*S*)-4-amino-2,2-difluoro-3-hydroxy-6-methylheptanoic acid; E represents difluorostatone, or 4*S*-amino-2,2-difluoro-6-methyl-3-oxoheptanoic acid; F represents (2*R*,3*S*,4*S*)-4-amino-3-hydroxy-2-isobutyl-6-methylheptanoic acid; G represents 3-amino-deoxystatine, or (3*R*, 4*S*)-3, 4-diamino-6-methylheptanoic acid; H represents difluoro-amino-deoxystatine, or (3*R*,4*S*)-3,4-diamino-2,2-difluoro-6-methylheptanoic acid; Iva, isovaleryl; Boc, *tert*-butyloxycarbonyl; iBu, isobutyl; AMP, amino-methylpyridine.

[b] IC_{50} values are against human plasma renin.

[c] K_i value.

fluorostatine (22), difluorostatone (22), 2-substituted statine (28), and 3-amino-deoxystatine (29) and its difluoro analogue (30). This class of substrate analogues has proved to be very potent, with inhibitory constants in the nanomolar range (with the exception of the difluoro-amino-deoxystatine-containing inhibitors). Among these changes, the inclusion of a cyclohexylmethyl group as the statine side-chain is generally very effective in boosting potency.

OTHER SUBSTITUTIONS AT THE SCISSILE BOND

A number of modifications can be made to the scissile bond in order to prevent its hydrolysis by renin (Table 3). Substitutions include hydroxyethylene (also a transition-state analogue) (35, 36), a reduced peptide bond (secondary amine) (34), an olefine bond (43), an amino–alcohol bond (44), an ether linkage (40) [including thioether and its oxidized derivatives (41)], a retro–inverso amide formed by diamino-hydroxyalkanes (45, 46), and amino-hydroxyalkanoyl residues such as (2*R*,3*S*)-3-amino-2-hydroxy-5-methylhexanoic acid (31) [also called norstatine (33)]. In general, potency in this group of analogues relates directly to the number of amino acid residues on either side of the substituted scissile bond. However, a remarkable degree of activity has been reported for a dipeptide derivative (KRI-1230) that contains a scissile-bond substitution in conjunction with modifications at both termini (33).

OTHER MODIFICATIONS

Alterations to both the carboxyl and amino termini of the substrate analogue structure appear to be especially valuable for increasing the inhibitory potency of small peptides and peptide-like molecules. Table 4 summarizes the strategies reported. Some of these alterations include substituting an aldehyde (50, 52), an alcohol (51, 55), and polar or nonpolar amides (26, 53–57) for the carboxyl-terminal carboxylate, as well as substituting phenylalanine aminoadamantane for the entire carboxyl-terminal amino acid (56). Among the carboxyl-terminal modifications reported, the incorporation of an amino-methylpyridine seems to produce the most active analogue (53). Another approach is to substitute a statine-like carboxyl-terminal compound in place of the scissile-bond dipeptide (57–62). This shortens the length of the substrate analogue inhibitor and retains potency.

The amino termini of renin inhibitors are frequently protected by acetyl, isovaleryl, *tert*-butyloxycarbonyl, and benzyloxycarbonyl groups. To reduce the number of amino acid residues needed at the amino-terminal segment and to retain potency, bis[(1-naphthyl)methyl]acetyl (51) and 2-(1-naphthylmethyl)-3-(morpholinocarbonyl)propyl (33), which contain highly hydrophobic ring structures, have been used as the amino-terminal-protecting group.

Unusual amino acids substituted in conjunction with modifications at the scissile bond also appear to increase the analogue's inhibitory constant, as well as to impart other desirable properties such as a prolonged *in vivo* half-life. Examples include substitution of N^{α}-methylhistidine at the P2 position, N^{α}- or C^{α}-methylphenylalanine at the P2 or P3 position (47), and alpha-methylproline at the P4 position (48).

One of the favorable approaches in the design of enzyme inhibitors has been to construct conformationally restricted polypeptides. Several conformationally restricted renin inhibitory substrate analogues have been reported (63–67),

TABLE 3. *Scissile bond modifications with nonhydrolyzable pseudopeptides*

Pseudopeptide	Example of renin inhibitor[a]	IC_{50} (nM)[b]	
Secondary amine	Pro—His—Pro—Phe—His—Leu $\overset{R}{\text{——}}$ Val—Ile—His—Lys	10	(34)
Hydroxy isostere (35–39)	Boc—His—Pro—Phe—His—Leu $\overset{OH}{\text{——}}$ Val—Ile—His	6.9	(36)
Ether, thioether isosteres (40,41)	Pro—His—Pro—Phe—His—Leu $\overset{O}{\text{——}}$ Val—Ile—His—D—Lys	1700	(40)
Amino-hydroxyalkanoic acid (31–33,42)	NMP—His—Norstatine—$OCH(CH_3)_2$ (KRI-1230)	7.8	(33)
Olefinic amino acid	Leu[CH=CH]Gly—Val—Phe—OCH_3	400,000[c]	(43)
Amino alcohol	His—Pro—Phe—His—Leu(AA)Val—Ile—Phe—OCH_3	61[d]	(44)
Retro–inverso amide (45,46)	Boc—Phe—His—NH–[cyclohexylmethyl-substituted hydroxyalkyl chain, OH]–NH—$CO(CH_2)_2CH(CH_3)_2$	15[d]	(45)

[a] $\overset{R}{\text{——}}$, reduced peptide bond —CH_2—NH—; $\overset{OH}{\text{——}}$, hydroxyethylene —CH(OH)—CH_2—; $\overset{O}{\text{——}}$, ether linkage —CH_2—O—; Norstatine, (2*R*,3*S*)-3-amino-2-hydroxy-5-methylhexanoic acid (31–33); [CH=CH], trans carbon–carbon double bond; (AA), amino alcohol —CH(OH)—CH_2—NH—; Boc, *tert*-butyloxycarbonyl; NMP, 2-(1-naphthylmethyl)-3-(morpholinocarbonyl)propyl.

[b] IC_{50} values are against human plasma renin.

[c] K_i value against human amniotic renin.

[d] IC_{50} value against purified human kidney renin.

TABLE 4. *Other modifications to inhibitor structure*

Modification	Example of renin inhibitor[a]	IC_{50} (nM)[b]
Internal residue substitution		
N^{α}-Methyl and C^{α}-methyl amino acids (47,48)	Boc—Phe—MeHis—Statine—Ile—AMP	120 (47)
Hydrophobic residues (49–51)	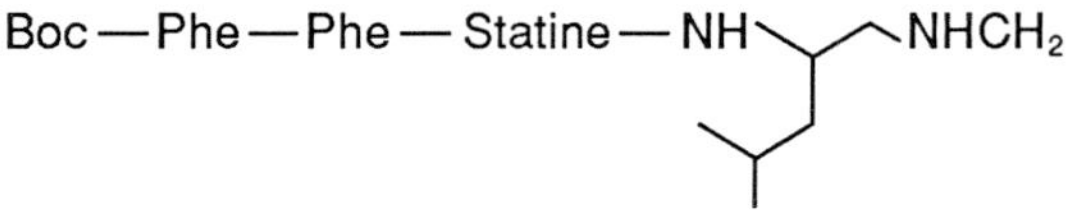 Boc—Phe—Phe—Statine—NH—(isobutyl-substituted)—NHCH$_2$	~1000 (49) 0.026[c] (49)
Carboxyl-terminal modification		
Peptide aldehyde and alcohol (50–52)	Z—[3-(1-naphthyl)Ala]—His—Leucinal	80[d] (50)
Polar and nonpolar amides (26,53–57)	Boc—Phe—His—ACHPA—Leu—AMP	0.047 (53)
Pseudostatine compounds (57–62)	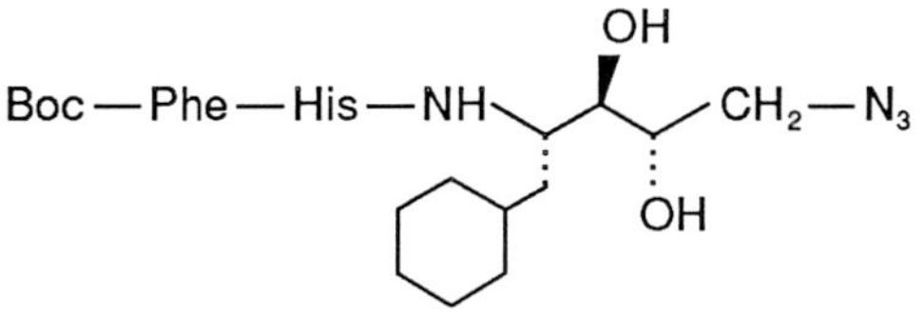 Boc—Phe—His—NH—(cyclohexylmethyl)—CH(OH)—CH(OH)—CH$_2$—N$_3$	0.4[e] (61)
Amino-terminal modification		
Hydrophobic ring structures (26,33,51)	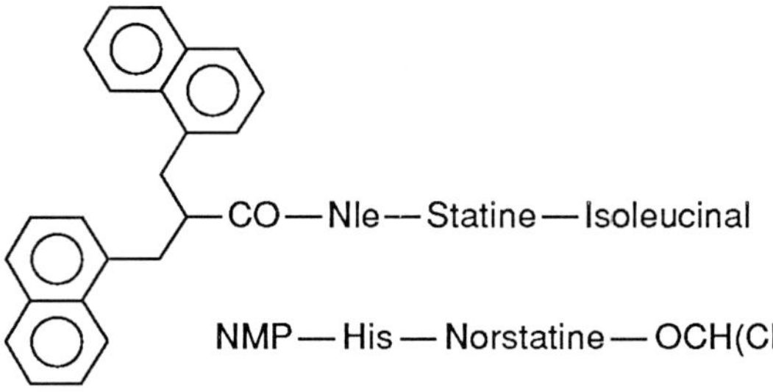 bis(1-naphthylmethyl)acetyl—CO—Nle—Statine—Isoleucinal	3 (51)
	NMP—His—Norstatine—OCH(CH$_3$)$_2$	7.8 (33)
Conformationally restricted analogues (63–67)	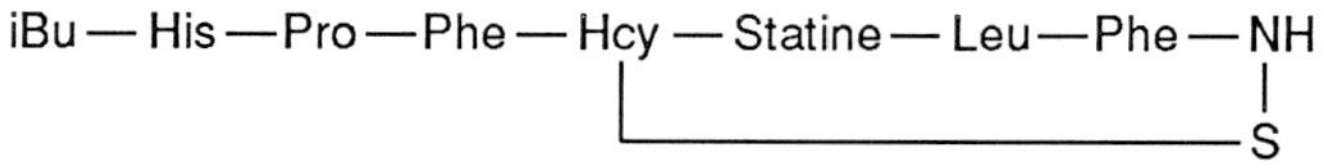 iBu—His—Pro—Phe—Hcy—Statine—Leu—Phe—NH (Hcy S–S linked to NH)	200[e] (63)

[a] Boc, *tert*-butyloxycarbonyl; Z, benzyloxycarbonyl; Statine, (3*S*,4*S*)-4-amino-3-hydroxy-6-methylheptanoic acid; ACHPA, (3*S*,4*S*)-4-amino-3-hydroxy-5-cyclohexylpentanoic acid; AMP, amino-methylpyridine; Hcy, homocysteine; iBu, isobutyl; Norstatine, (2*R*,3*S*)-3-amino-2-hydroxy-5-methylhexanoic acid (31–33).
[b] IC_{50} values are against human plasma renin.
[c] K_i value against purified human kidney renin using synthetic tetradecapeptide as the substrate.
[d] IC_{50} value against purified human kidney renin using sheep angiotensinogen as the substrate.
[e] IC_{50} value against purified human kidney renin.

although none has a potency in the nanomolar range. The creation of an irreversible renin inhibitor is an attractive concept. With this in mind, investigators have incorporated into substrate-like peptides epoxy groups that can react covalently with renin. One example is

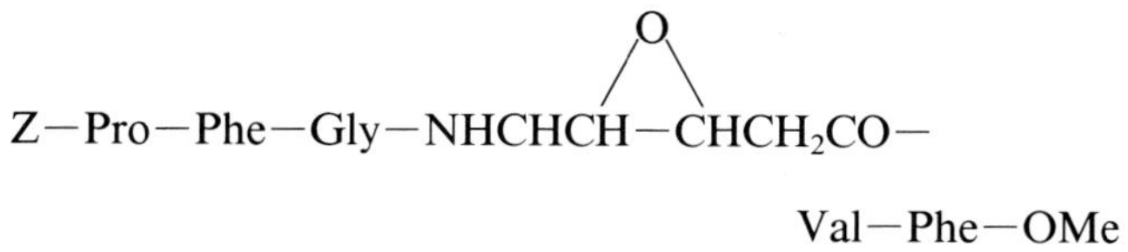

Z—Pro—Phe—Gly—NHCHCH—CHCH$_2$CO—Val—Phe—OMe (with an epoxide O bridging CH—CH)

which has an IC_{50} value of 7×10^{-5} M against human amniotic renin (68). Unfortunately, the inhibitory potency of this compound is too low for it to be of interest. This line of inquiry could, however, yield more interesting inhibitors.

PRORENIN PEPTIDES

Another approach to the development of renin inhibitors would be to modify the structure of prorenin, an inactive zymogen that becomes the active enzyme after cleavage of a peptide bond and subsequent loss of an amino-terminal peptide. Reasoning that the association of this peptide with renin would render the molecule inactive, investigators have thought that analogues of the prorenin peptide could act as inhibitors (69–71). However, these analogues have very low affinities for renin. Although the prorenin peptide analogue approach is highly innovative, it does not, for the present, appear to be a promising area for development.

SPECIES SPECIFICITY

Renin inhibitors vary greatly in potency—often by over several orders of magnitude—with respect to the species of renin against which they are tested. For obvious reasons, most work has focused on the development of inhibitors selective for human renin. Yet because of the rat's utility as an experimental animal (the availability of genetically determined models of hypertension make it particularly useful), efforts have been made to develop inhibitors selective for the renin of this species. (Renin inhibitors that are effective in humans or the primate are generally quite ineffective in the rat.) Several selective rat renin inhibitors have recently been reported (25, 72).

ORAL ACTIVITY

All the renin inhibitors discussed so far, although promising with respect to specificity and potency, are poorly absorbed by the gastrointestinal tract. Thus they would be of no use in investigations of the chronic illness for which they were designed—essential hypertension. As yet there is no general method for converting a pharmacologically active peptide into an equivalent compound that can be administered orally. However, several compounds have now been reported that are potent but have limited absorption (26, 33, 73, 74). Because absorption is still less than 20% of the administered dose, the likelihood of their being the subjects of clinical study is small. The main interest of these compounds lies in the hope they give to the search for an orally active renin inhibitor.

PRINCIPLES OF RENIN INHIBITION

As yet, our understanding of renin inhibitors has not reached a point equivalent to that of the masterful insight of Ondetti et al. (75), which generalized the principles of converting-enzyme inhibition and led to the commonly used antihypertensive drugs captopril, enalapril, and lisinopril. A detailed study of renin's catalytic site, either by the building of models based on the structure of related molecules (23, 76–79) or by the direct determination of human renin's three-dimensional structure by x-ray crystallography, may be required before the general principles of renin inhibition can emerge. Now that the human renin gene has been cloned (80) and expressed (81), a report of the crystallographic structure of the enzyme should follow shortly.

DO RENIN INHIBITORS HAVE A FUTURE AS CLINICALLY EFFECTIVE ANTIHYPERTENSIVE AGENTS?

Even though effective oral renin inhibitors may offer a more selective means of blocking the renin–angiotensin system, it is not certain whether they will offer significant clinical advantages over converting-enzyme inhibitors. One potential advantage of any new class of drugs is that it may eliminate adverse reactions associated with agents in current use. It remains to be determined, however, whether the adverse reactions common to captopril, enalapril, and lisinopril are the result of blockade of the target enzyme (angiotensin-converting enzyme and kininase II are the same) or whether they are the consequence of a general inhibition of the renin–angiotensin system that would be a feature of any class of drugs used to block it (10). Nonspecific effects of converting-enzyme inhibitors that could be independent of a reduction in angiotensin II concentration include increased bradykinin or prostaglandin concentrations, blunting of sympathetic activity, increased parasympathetic activity, effects on the central nervous system, and redistribution of blood flow. A potential advantage of renin inhibitors may derive from enhanced cellular penetration, so that tissue renins as well as extracellular renins could be blocked.

Renin-specific antibodies have proved to be excellent models for renin inhibitors, particularly with respect to the highly selective inhibition of the enzyme in extracellular fluid. Because of their molecular size, however, antibodies are unlikely to penetrate the cell membrane and thus cannot be used to address questions about potential intracellular effects. When a monospecific antibody for renin and teprotide, a converting-enzyme inhibitor, were compared in the sodium-depleted dog, their hemodynamic effects were identical (82). These results were confirmed later in the marmoset, in comparisons between monoclonal antibodies and enalaprilat (83, 84).

As soon as peptide inhibitors that were effective *in vivo* became available, they were compared with converting-enzyme inhibitors under a variety of circumstances. In normotensive dogs, as well as in hypertensive dogs subjected to renal artery constriction, Smith et al. (85) showed that a converting-enzyme inhibitor (enalaprilat) and a renin inhibitor (an ACHPA-containing peptide) were equipotent in lowering blood pressure (Fig. 1) and that the effects of both agents on glomerular filtration rate were identical. In the sodium-depleted primate, these two classes of compounds also lowered blood pressure to an equivalent degree (13, 36, 73, 86). Miyazaki et al. (87) reported similar results with another peptide renin inhibitor. And in mildly volume-depleted marmosets, Neisius et al. (88) showed that both

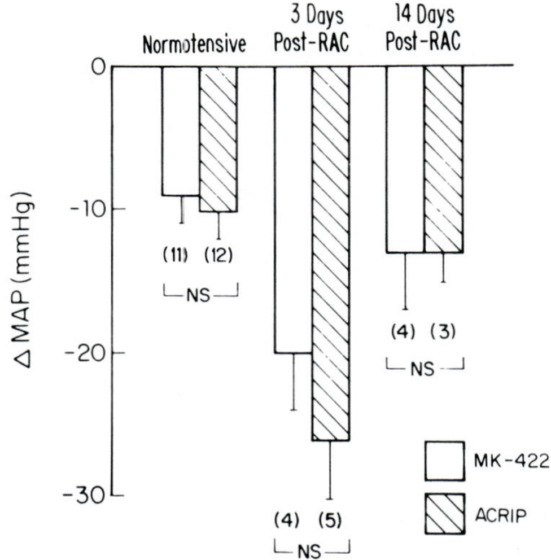

FIG. 1. An example of a comparison between a converting-enzyme inhibitor and a renin inhibitor in experimental hypertension. Shown are the maximal observed changes in mean arterial pressure (MAP) in dogs treated with either ACHPA-containing renin-inhibitory peptide (ACRIP) or enalaprilat (MK-422) at various stages in the development of one-kidney, one-clip hypertension. The values represent the mean ± SEM of the maximal changes at the indicated stage of renovascular hypertension. The number of animals per group is indicated in parentheses. NS, not statistically significant (at $p < 0.05$); RAC, renal artery constriction. (From ref. 85.)

renin and converting-enzyme inhibitors increase renal blood flow in an equivalent manner.

In a very interesting model of hypertension associated with normal renin levels in the marmoset, created by ligating a branch of one renal artery, Neisius and Wood (89) showed that a renin inhibitor and a converting-enzyme inhibitor lowered blood pressure equally. These reports are representative of many others that fail to demonstrate a convincing difference between renin and converting-enzyme inhibitors in acute systemic or renal hemodynamic studies. Other examples include those discussed in refs. 90–92.

Thus the notion that clear differences in effect exist between renin inhibitors and converting-enzyme inhibitors cannot be supported at present. Both systemic and local hemodynamic effects cannot be differentiated, making it difficult to define a role for kinin inhibition or eicosanoid release in the regulation of resistance vessels. Differences in tissue penetration have also not been demonstrated. It must, however, be emphasized that there are few truly chronic animal studies reported and that the effect of peptide renin inhibitors on human hypertension is as yet unknown. Before it can be concluded that there is no real difference between inhibiting renin and inhibiting converting enzyme, a great deal of additional work will be required.

REFERENCES

1. Pals DT, Masucci FD, Sipos F, Denning GS Jr. A specific competitive antagonist of the vascular action of angiotensin II. *Circ Res* 1971;29:664–672.
2. Streeten DHP, Anderson GH, Freiberg JM, Dalakos TG. Use of an angiotensin II antagonist (saralasin) in the recognition of "angiotensinogenic" hypertension. *N Engl J Med* 1975;292:657–662.
3. Dzau VJ, Kopelman RI, Barger AC, Haber E. Renin-specific antibody for study of cardiovascular homeostasis. *Science* 1980; 207:1091–1093.
4. Miller ED Jr, Samuels AI, Haber E, Barger AC. Inhibition of angiotensin conversion in experimental renovascular hypertension. *Science* 1972;177:1108–1109.
5. Sancho J, Re R, Burton J, Barger AC, Haber E. The role of the renin–angiotensin–aldosterone system in cardiovascular homeostasis in normal human subjects. *Circulation* 1976;53:400–405.
6. Gavras H, Brunner HR, Laragh JH, Sealey JE, Gavras I, Vukovich RA. An angiotensin converting-enzyme inhibitor to identify and treat vasoconstrictor and volume factors in hypertensive patients. *N Engl J Med* 1974;291:817–821.
7. Gavras H, Brunner HR, Turini GA, et al. Antihypertensive effect of the oral angiotensin converting-enzyme inhibitor SQ 14225 in man. *N Engl J Med* 1978;298:991–995.
8. Edwards CRW, Padfield PL. Angiotensin-converting enzyme inhibitors: past, present, and bright future. *Lancet* 1985;1:30–34.
9. Sutton FJ. Vasodilator therapy. *Am J Med* 1986;80(Suppl 2B): 54–58.
10. Brunner HR, Waeber B, Nussberger J. Pharmacology of converting enzyme inhibitors. *Clin Exp Theory Pract* 1987;A9:275–288.
11. Galen FX, Devaux C, Atlas S, et al. New monoclonal antibodies directed against human renin: powerful tools for the investigation of the renin system. *J Clin Invest* 1984;74:723–735.
12. Dzau VJ, Mudgett-Hunter M, Haber E. Monoclonal antibodies as molecular probes to study structural heterogeneity between human and animal renins and other aspartyl proteinases. *J Clin Endocrinol Metab* 1986;62:424–428.
13. Burton J, Cody RJ Jr, Herd JA, Haber E. Specific inhibition of renin by an angiotensinogen analog: studies in sodium depletion and renin-dependent hypertension. *Proc Natl Acad Sci USA* 1980;77:5476–5479.
14. Skeggs LT, Lentz KE, Kahn JR, Hochstrasser H. Kinetics of the reaction of renin with nine synthetic peptide substrates. *J Exp Med* 1968;128:13–34.
15. Cody RJ, Burton J, Evin G, Poulsen K, Herd JA, Haber E. A substrate analog inhibitor of renin that is effective *in vivo*. *Biochem Biophys Res Commun* 1980;97:230–235.
16. Pals DT, DeGraaf GL, Kati WM, Lawson JA, Smith CW, Skala GF. Cardiovascular effects of a renin inhibitor in relation to posture in nonhuman primates. *Clin Exp Theor Pract* 1985;A7:105–121.
17. Zusman RM, Burton J, Christensen D, Nussberger J, Dodds A, Haber E. Hemodynamic effects of a competitive renin inhibitory peptide in humans: evidence for multiple mechanisms of action. *Trans Assoc Am Phys* 1983;96:365–374.
18. Evin G, Castro B, Gardes J, Kreft C, Menard J, Corvol P. Soluble derivatives of pepstatin: new, potent, *in vivo* inhibitors of renin. In: Gross E, Meienhofer J, eds. *Peptides: structure and biological function. Proceedings of the Sixth American Peptide Symposium.* Rockford, IL: Pierce Chemical, 1979;165–168.
19. Eid M, Evin G, Castro B, Menard J, Corvol P. New renin inhibitors homologous with pepstatin. *Biochem J* 1981;197:465–471.
20. Guégan R, Diaz J, Cazaubon C, et al. Pepstatin analogues as novel renin inhibitors. *J Med Chem* 1986;29:1152–1159.
21. Boger J, Lohr NS, Ulm EH, et al. Novel renin inhibitors containing the amino acid statine. *Nature* 1983;303:81–84.
22. Thaisrivongs S, Pals DT, Kati WM, Turner SR, Thomasco LM, Watt W. Design and syntheses of potent and specific renin inhibitors containing difluorostatine, difluorostatone, and related analogues. *J Med Chem* 1986;29:2080–2087.
23. Hui KY, Carlson WD, Bernatowicz MS, Haber E. Analysis of structure–activity relationships in renin substrate analogue inhibitory peptides. *J Med Chem* 1987;30:1287–1295.
24. Boger J, Payne LS, Perlow DS, et al. Renin inhibitors. Syntheses of subnanomolar, competitive, transition-state analogue inhibitors containing a novel analogue of statine. *J Med Chem* 1985;28: 1779–1790.
25. Hui KY, Holtzman EJ, Quinones MA, Hollenberg NK, Haber E. Design of rat renin inhibitory peptides. *J Med Chem* 1988;31:1679–1686.
26. Nisato D, Lacour C, Roccon A, et al. Discovery and pharmacological characterization of highly potent, picomolar-range, renin inhibitors. *J Hypertens* 1987;5(Suppl 5):S23–S25.
27. Fearon K, Spaltenstein A, Hopkins PB, Gelb MH. Fluoro ketone containing peptides as inhibitors of human renin. *J Med Chem* 1987;30:1617–1622.
28. Veber DF, Bock MG, Brady SF, et al. Renin inhibitors containing 2-substituted statine. *Biochem Soc Trans* 1984;12:956–959.
29. Jones M, Sueiras-Diaz J, Szelke M, Leckie B, Beattie S. Renin inhibitors containing the novel amino-acid 3-amino-deoxystatine. In: Deber CM, Hruby VJ, Kopple KD, eds. *Peptides: structure and function. Proceedings of the Ninth American Peptide Symposium.* Rockford, IL: Pierce Chemical, 1985;759–762.
30. Thaisrivongs S, Schostarez HJ, Pals DT, Turner SR. α,α-Difluoro-β-aminodeoxystatine-containing renin inhibitory peptides. *J Med Chem* 1987;30:1837–1842.
31. Johnson RL. Renin inhibitors. Substitution of the leucyl residues of Leu-Leu-Val-Phe-OCH_3 with 3-amino-2-hydroxy-5-methylhexanoic acid. *J Med Chem* 1982;25:605–610.
32. Toda N, Miyazaki M, Etoh Y, Kubota T, Iizuka K. Human renin inhibiting dipeptide. *Eur J Pharmacol* 1986;129:393–396.
33. Iizuka K, Kamijo T, Kubota T, Akahane K, Umeyama H, Kiso Y. New human renin inhibitors containing an unnatural amino acid, norstatine. *J Med Chem* 1988;31:701–704.
34. Szelke M, Leckie B, Hallett A, et al. Potent new inhibitors of human renin. *Nature* 1982;299:555–557.
35. Szelke M, Jones DM, Atrash B, Hallett A, Leckie BJ. Novel transition-state analogue inhibitors of renin. In: Hruby VJ, Rich DH, eds. *Peptides: structure and function. Proceedings of the Eighth American Peptide Symposium.* Rockford, IL: Pierce Chemical, 1983;579–582.
36. Szelke M, Tree M, Leckie BJ, et al. A transition-state analogue inhibitor of human renin (H.261): test *in vitro* and a comparison

with captopril in the anaesthetized baboon. *J Hypertens* 1985;3: 13–18.

37. Kempf DJ, de Lara E, Stein HH, Cohen J, Plattner JJ. Renin inhibitors based on novel dipeptide analogues. Incorporation of the dehydrohydroxyethylene isostere at the scissile bond. *J Med Chem* 1987;30:1978–1983.
38. Thaisrivongs S, Pals DT, Kroll LT, Turner SR, Han FS. Renin inhibitors. Design of angiotensinogen transition-state analogues containing novel (2*R*,3*R*,4*R*,5*S*)-5-amino-3,4-dihydroxy-2-isopropyl-7-methyloctanoic acid. *J Med Chem* 1987;30:976–982.
39. Evans BE, Rittle KE, Ulm UH, Veber DF. A sterocontrolled synthesis of hydroxyethylene dipeptide isosteres using novel, chiral aminoalkyl epoxides: new renin inhibitor analogs. In: Deber CM, Hruby VJ, Kopple KD, eds. *Peptides: structure and function. Proceedings of the Ninth American Peptide Symposium.* Rockford, IL: Pierce Chemical, 1985;743–746.
40. TenBrink RE, Pals DT, Harris DW, Johnson GA. Renin inhibitors containing $\psi[CH_2O]$ pseudopeptide inserts. *J Med Chem* 1988;31:671–677.
41. Smith CW, Saneii HH, Sawyer TK, et al. Synthesis and renin inhibitory activity of angiotensinogen analogues having dehydrostatine, Leu$\psi[CH_2S]$Val, or Leu$\psi[CH_2SO]$Val at the P_1–P_1' cleavage site. *J Med Chem* 1988;31:1377–1382.
42. Johnson RL, Verschoor K. Inhibition of renin by angiotensinogen peptide fragments containing the hydroxy amino acid residue 5-amino-3-hydroxy-7-methyloctanoic acid. *J Med Chem* 1983;26: 1457–1462.
43. Johnson RL. Inhibition of renin by substrate analogue inhibitors containing the olefinic amino acid 5(*S*)-amino-7-methyl-3(*E*)-octenoic acid. *J Med Chem* 1984;27:1351–1354.
44. Dann JG, Stammers DK, Harris CJ, et al. Human renin: a new class of inhibitors. *Biochem Biophys Res Commun* 1986;134:71–77.
45. Rosenberg SH, Plattner JJ, Woods KW, et al. Novel renin inhibitors containing analogues of statine retro-inverted at the C-termini: specificity at the P_2 histidine site. *J Med Chem* 1987;30: 1224–1228.
46. Luly JR, Plattner JJ, Stein H, et al. Modified peptides which display potent and specific inhibition of human renin. *Biochem Biophys Res Commun* 1987;143:44–51.
47. Thaisrivongs S, Pals DT, Harris DW, Kati WM, Turner SR. Design and synthesis of a potent and specific renin inhibitor with a prolonged duration of action *in vivo*. *J Med Chem* 1986;29: 2088–2093.
48. Thaisrivongs S, Pals DT, Lawson JA, Turner SR, Harris DW. α-Methylproline-containing renin inhibitory peptides: *in vivo* evaluation in an anesthetized, ganglion-blocked, hog renin infused rat model. *J Med Chem* 1987;30:536–541.
49. Evans BE, Rittle KE, Bock MG, et al. A uniquely potent renin inhibitor and its unanticipated plasma binding component. *J Med Chem* 1985;28:1755–1756.
50. Kokubu T, Hiwada K, Murakami E, et al. Highly potent and specific inhibitors of human renin. *Hypertension* 1985;7(Suppl I):I-8–I-11.
51. Kokubu T, Hiwada K, Nagae A, et al. Statine-containing dipeptide and tripeptide inhibitors of human renin. *Hypertension* 1986;8(Suppl II):II-1–II-5.
52. Fehrentz JA, Heitz A, Castro B, Cazaubon C, Nisato D. Aldehydic peptides inhibiting renin. *FEBS Lett* 1984;167:273–276.
53. Bock MG, DiPardo RM, Evans BE, et al. Renin inhibitors. Synthesis and biological activity of statine- and ACHPA-containing peptides having polar end groups. In: Deber CM, Hruby VJ, Kopple KD, eds. *Peptides: structure and function. Proceedings of the Ninth American Peptide Symposium.* Rockford, IL: Pierce Chemical, 1985;751–754.
54. Bock MG, DiPardo RM, Evans BE, et al. Renin inhibitors. Statine-containing tetrapeptides with varied hydrophobic carboxy termini. *J Med Chem* 1987;30:1853–1857.
55. Hanson GJ, Baran JS, Lindberg T, et al. Dipeptide glycols: a new class of renin inhibitors. *Biochem Biophys Res Commun* 1985; 132:155–161.
56. Papaioannou S, Hansen D Jr, Babler M, et al. New class of inhibitors specific for human renin. *Clin Exp Theory Pract* 1985;A7: 1243–1257.
57. Natarajan S, Free CA, Sabo EF, et al. Tripeptide aminoalcohols: a new class of human renin inhibitors. In: Marshall GR, ed. *Peptides: chemistry and biology. Proceedings of the Tenth American Peptide Symposium.* Leiden: ESCOM, 1988;131–133.
58. Luly JR, Yi N, Soderquist J, et al. New inhibitors of human renin that contain novel Leu-Val replacements. *J Med Chem* 1987;30: 1609–1616.
59. Bolis G, Fung AKL, Greer J, et al. Renin inhibitors. Dipeptide analogues of angiotensinogen incorporating transition-state, nonpeptidic replacements at the scissile bond. *J Med Chem* 1987;30: 1729–1737.
60. Luly JR, Bolis G, BaMaung N, et al. New inhibitors of human renin that contain novel Leu-Val replacements. Examination of the P_1 site. *J Med Chem* 1988;31:532–539.
61. Rosenberg SH, Woods KW, Plattner JJ, Stein HH, Kleinert HD, Cohen J. Novel, subnanomolar renin inhibitors containing a postscissile site azide residue. In: Marshall GR, ed. *Peptides: chemistry and biology. Proceedings of the Tenth American Peptide Symposium.* Leiden: ESCOM, 1988;500–502.
62. Luly JR, Fung AKL, Plattner JJ, et al. Transition-state analog inhibitors of human renin. In: Marshall GR, ed. *Peptides: chemistry and biology. Proceedings of the Tenth American Peptide Symposium.* Leiden: ESCOM, 1988;487–489.
63. Boger J. Renin inhibitors. Design of angiotensinogen transition-state analogs containing statine. In: Hruby VJ, Rich DH, eds. *Peptides: structure and function. Proceedings of the Eighth American Peptide Symposium.* Rockford, IL: Pierce Chemical, 1983; 569–578.
64. Sham HL, Bolis G, Stein HH, et al. Renin inhibitors. Design and synthesis of a new class of conformationally restricted analogues of angiotensinogen. *J Med Chem* 1988;31:284–295.
65. Nakaie CR, Pesquero JL, Oliveira MCF, Juliano L, Pavia ACM. Renin inhibition by linear and conformationally restricted analogs of renin substrate. In: Deber CM, Hruby VJ, Kopple KD, eds. *Peptides: structure and function. Proceedings of the Ninth American Peptide Symposium.* Rockford, IL: Pierce Chemical, 1985; 755–758.
66. Thaisrivongs S, Pals DT, Turner SR, Kroll LT. Conformationally constrained renin inhibitory peptides: γ-lactam-bridged dipeptide isostere as conformational restriction. *J Med Chem* 1988;31: 1369–1376.
67. Sawyer TK, Pals DT, Smith CW, et al. "Transition state" substituted renin inhibitory peptides: structure–conformation–activity studies on N^{in}-formyl-trp and trp modified congeners. In: Deber CM, Hruby VJ, Kopple KD, eds. *Peptides: structure and function. Proceedings of the Ninth American Peptide Symposium.* Rockford, IL: Pierce Chemical, 1985;729–738.
68. Johnson RL. Synthesis of epoxypolypeptides as inhibitors of renin. In: Hruby VJ, Rich DH, eds. *Peptides: structure and function. Proceedings of the Eighth American Peptide Symposium.* Rockford, IL: Pierce Chemical, 1983;587–590.
69. Evin G, Devin J, Ménard J, Corvol P, Castro B. Synthesis of peptides related to the prosegment of renin precursor: a new way in the search for renin inhibitors. In: Hruby VJ, Rich DH, eds. *Peptides: structure and function. Proceedings of the Eighth American Peptide Symposium.* Rockford, IL: Pierce Chemical, 1983; 591–594.
70. Evin G, Devin J, Castro B, Menard J, Corvol P. Synthesis of peptides related to the prosegment of mouse submaxillary gland renin precursor: an approach to renin inhibitors. *Proc Natl Acad Sci USA* 1984;81:48–52.
71. Cumin F, Evin G, Fehrentz JA, et al. Inhibition of human renin by synthetic peptides derived from its prosegment. *J Biol Chem* 1985;260:9154–9157.
72. Sueiras-Diaz J, Jones DM, Evans DM, et al. Potent *in vivo* inhibitors of rat renin. In: Marshall GR, ed. *Peptides: chemistry and biology. Proceedings of the Tenth American Peptide Symposium.* Leiden: ESCOM, 1988;510–511.
73. Wood JM, Gulati N, Forgiarini P, Fuhrer W, Hofbauer KG. Effects of a specific and long-acting renin inhibitor in the marmoset. *Hypertension* 1985;7:797–803.
74. Pals DT, Thaisrivongs S, Lawson JA, et al. An orally active inhibitor of renin. *Hypertension* 1986;8:1105–1112.
75. Ondetti MA, Rubin B, Cushman DW. Design of specific inhibi-

tors of angiotensin-converting enzyme: new class of orally active antihypertensive agents. *Science* 1977;196:441–444.

76. Carlson W, Karplus M, Haber E. Construction of a model for the three-dimensional structure of human renal renin. *Hypertension* 1985;7:13–26.
77. Hemmings AM, Foundling SI, Sibanda BL, Wood SP, Pearl LH, Blundell T. Energy calculations on aspartic proteinases: human renin, endothiapepsin and its complex with an angiotensinogen fragment analogue, H-142. *Biochem Soc Trans* 1985;13:1036–1041.
78. Blundell TL, Cooper J, Foundling SI, Jones DM, Atrash B, Szelke M. On the rational design of renin inhibitors: X-ray studies of aspartic proteinases complexed with transition-state analogues. *Biochemistry* 1987;26:5585–5590.
79. Haber E, Hui KY, Carlson WD, Bernatowicz MS. Renin inhibitors: a search for principles of design. *J Cardiovasc Pharmacol* 1987;10(Suppl 7):S54–S58.
80. Hardman JA, Hort YJ, Catanzaro DF, et al. Primary structure of the human renin gene. *DNA* 1984;3:457–468.
81. Fritz LC, Arfsten AE, Dzau VJ, et al. Characterization of human prorenin expressed in mammalian cells from cloned cDNA. *Proc Natl Acad Sci USA* 1986;83:4114–4118.
82. Dzau VJ, Devine D, Mudgett-Hunter M, Kopelman RI, Barger AC, Haber E. Antibodies as specific renin inhibitors: studies with polyclonal and monoclonal antibodies and Fab fragments. *Clin Exp Hypertens* 1983;A5(7&8):1207–1220.
83. Michel J-B, Wood J, Hofbauer K, Corvol P, Menard J. Blood pressure effects of renin inhibition by human renin antiserum in normotensive marmosets. *Am J Physiol* 1984;246:F309–F316.
84. Wood JM, Heusser C, Gulati N, Forgiarini P, Hofbauer KG. Monoclonal antibodies against human renin. Blood pressure effects in the marmoset. *Hypertension* 1986;8:600–605.
85. Smith SG III, Seymour AA, Mazack EK, Boger J, Blaine EH. Comparison of a new renin inhibitor and enalaprilat in renal hypertensive dogs. *Hypertension* 1987;9:150–156.
86. Hui KY, Bernatowicz MS, Zusman RM, Carlson W, Haber E, Hartley LH. Statine-containing renin inhibitory peptides: hemodynamic effects in the primate. In: Deber CM, Hruby VJ, Kopple KD, eds. *Peptides: structure and function. Proceedings of the Ninth American Peptide Symposium.* Rockford, IL: Pierce Chemical, 1985;771–774.
87. Miyazaki M, Etoh Y, Toda N, Kubota T, Iizuka K. Hypotension caused by inhibitors of renin and converting-enzyme in monkeys [Abstract]. *Jpn J Pharmacol* 1987;43(Suppl):146P.
88. Neisius D, Wood JM, Hofbauer KG. Renal vasodilatation after inhibition of renin or converting enzyme in marmoset. *Am J Physiol* 1986;251:H897–H902.
89. Neisius D, Wood JM. Antihypertensive effect of a renin inhibitor in marmosets with a segmental renal infarction. *J Hypertens* 1987;5:721–725.
90. Hofbauer KG, Menard J, Michel JB, Wood JM. Inhibition of renin in the primate *Callithrix jacchus* (common marmoset). *Clin Exp Theory Pract* 1983;A5(7&8):1237–1247.
91. Takaori K, Hartley LH, Burton J. Hypotensive effects of the renin inhibitor (RI-78) and the converting enzyme inhibitor (teprotide) in conscious monkeys. *Clin Exper Theory Pract* 1987;A9(2&3):387–390.
92. Wood JM, Jobber RA, Baum H-P, Hofbauer KG. Comparison of chronic inhibition of renin and converting enzyme in the marmoset. *Clin Exp Theory Pract* 1987;A9(2&3):337–343.

Hypertension: Pathophysiology, Diagnosis, and Management, edited by J. H. Laragh and B. M. Brenner. Raven Press, Ltd., New York © 1990.

CHAPTER 150

The Discovery and Physiological Effects of a New Class of Highly Specific Angiotensin II-Receptor Antagonists

Pieter B. M. W. M. Timmermans, David J. Carini, Andrew T. Chiu, John V. Duncia, William A. Price, Jr., Gregory J. Wells, Pancras C. Wong, Ruth R. Wexler, and Alexander L. Johnson

Early Lead Compounds: S-8307 and S-8308, 2352
Newer Lead Compounds: EXP6155 and EXP6803, 2354
EXP7711: A Nonpeptide AII-Receptor Antagonist with Oral Activity, 2357
Concluding Remarks, 2359
References, 2360

The renin–angiotensin system (RAS) plays a pivotal role in the control of normal blood pressure regulation (1). The components and sources of this biochemical cascade include the following: (a) renin, from the kidney; (b) the renin substrate angiotensinogen, from the liver; and (c) angiotensin-converting enzyme (ACE), derived mainly from the capillary endothelium of the lung. Angiotensinogen is converted to the decapeptide, angiotensin I (AI), which is further cleaved by ACE to form the octapeptide, angiotensin II (AII). AII is the biologically active component of the RAS responsible for most, if not all, the peripheral effects of this system (2). The actions of AII are thought to be mediated by specific surface receptors on various target organs such as the adrenal cortex, blood vessels, kidney, noradrenergic nerve endings, and possibly others eliciting events such as aldosterone formation, vasoconstriction, renal sodium reabsorption, and norepinephrine release (3).

The RAS is a closed-loop, negative-feedback system reacting to a reduction in renal perfusion or excessive loss of sodium. Through the actions described above, the effector molecule of the system, AII, counteracts the initial stimulus that caused the release of renin. By restoration of arterial pressure and renal blood flow, the initial stimulus for renin secretion is turned off and the system is then returned to the original status.

Although there is still an incomplete understanding of the causal role of the RAS in the mosaic of essential hypertension, the RAS seems to be critically involved in the development and maintenance of hypertension as well as in congestive heart failure, where inappropriate control of this system is manifest. Ever since the 1950s, investigators have been exploring ways of blocking the RAS both as a means of further defining its role in hypertension and as a possible therapeutic mode in the treatment of this disorder. Evidence has been accumulated from the study of ACE inhibitors such as captopril (4) and enalapril (5) in experimental and human hypertension. These agents were initially introduced for treating severe and renal hypertension (i.e., those cases in which the RAS was commonly supposed to play a role). The success that they are now having in managing milder forms of essential hypertension as well as in managing heart failure suggests that the RAS plays a very relevant role in the pathophysiology of these disease states (6,7).

Acceptance of the notion that physiologically specific interruption of the RAS is therapeutically beneficial in certain circumstances has generated considerable interest in the development of novel pharmacological inhibitors of the RAS. Another potential approach to inhibition of the RAS is by blocking the action of renin on its substrate, angiotensinogen. Unlike ACE, which is a relatively nonspecific peptidyl-dipeptide hydrolase, renin may be a uniquely specific enzyme, with only one known natural substrate (8). Inhibition of the RAS by blockade at the renin reaction could be an extraordinarily specific pharmacological intervention (9). However, renin's substrate specificity has been questioned (10), and its rather widespread intracellular distribution is being increasingly appreciated (11). Nevertheless, the design and development of (orally active) renin inhibitors is vigorously pursued at present, and significant progress has been made (12–14).

Since AII is the effector molecule of the RAS, a more direct approach to blocking this system would be at the AII-receptor level to inhibit the hormone from binding. AII-receptor antagonists would represent an ideal species, because no matter how and where AII is produced, the system could be specifically turned off. However, AII-receptor antagonists have so far been limited to angiotensin-like peptides, and their usefulness as therapeutic agents and pharmacological tools has been hampered by their lack of oral bioavailability, short duration of action, and partial agonistic activity (15). Recently, some heterocyclic chemical structures have been disclosed which show promise as early leads in the design of therapeutically useful nonpeptide AII-receptor antagonists. In this chapter we wish to report on the advances which have been made toward the above objective, with emphasis on our work carried out at E. I. du Pont de Nemours & Company.

TABLE 1. *AII-antagonistic properties of some imidazole derivatives*[a]

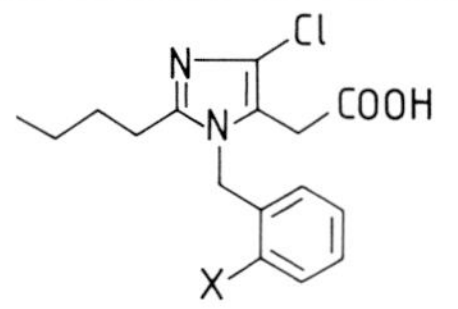

X	Concentration (μM)	Inhibition (%)
H	1	22[b], 55[c]
Cl	0.1	75[c]
NO_2	0.01	30[c]

[a] Antagonism is expressed as percentage inhibition of the contractile response of the isolated rabbit aorta to AII (4×10^{-9} M).
[b] Data from ref. 16.
[c] Data from ref. 17.

EARLY LEAD COMPOUNDS: S-8307 AND S-8308

The earliest reports documenting relatively small-sized chemical structures possessing AII-antagonistic properties are two patents granted to Furukawa et al. (16,17) of Takeda Chemical Industries, Ltd. (Osaka, Japan). Novel imidazole derivatives of the formula are given in Fig. 1, where: R_1 is lower alkyl or phenyl-$C_{1\text{-}2}$ alkyl which may be substituted with halogen or nitro; R_2 is lower alkyl, cycloalkyl, or phenyl; one of R_3 and R_4 is of the formula $-(CH_2)_n-COR_5$ (R_5 is amino, lower alkoxyl, or hydroxyl, n is an integer of 0, 1, or 2) and the other is hydrogen or halogen, provided that (a) R_1 is lower alkyl or phenethyl when R_3 is halogen, (b) n is 1, and (c) R_5 is lower alkoxyl or hydroxyl. The compounds were claimed to have AII-antagonistic activity as assessed *in vitro* against AII (4×10^{-9} M)-induced contractions of the isolated rabbit aorta. Table 1 lists the results obtained by Furukawa et al. (16,17) for some of these structures and indicates a remarkably high potential for antagonizing AII-induced vasoconstriction *in vitro.* Some of these imidazoles were also claimed to be active *in vivo.* Intravenous administration to anesthetized rats in which the blood pressure was elevated by approximately 45 mmHg by a continuous infusion of AII (20 ng/kg/min) was shown to attenuate this rise in blood pressure. As summarized in Table 2, the compounds were reported to be very effective and had a considerable duration of action. Subsequently, the compound with $R_2 = C_6H_5$ and $X = 3-CH_3,4-OCH_3$ was specifically reported by Takeda Research Laboratories (18) to exert hypotensive and diuretic effects in rats and dogs, but further details on the mechanism of action were not reported. To our knowledge, no further reports have been published by Takeda Research Laboratories on these structures.

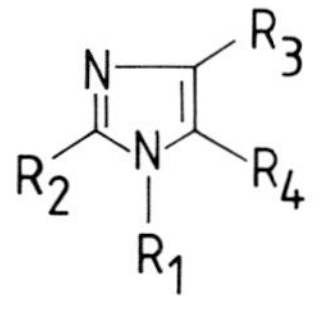

FIG. 1. General formula of imidazole derivatives reported to possess AII-antagonistic properties (see refs. 16 and 17).

We were intrigued by the claim in these patents that simple imidazole-5-acetic acid derivatives were antagonistic toward AII-induced vasoconstriction as well as by the reported degree of potency. However, it was unclear whether these agents were specific or nonspecific antagonists, since no mention of the specificity was made. We therefore examined two of these structures [i.e., S-8307 and S-8308 (Fig. 2)] in more detail (19,20).

In repeating the experiments reported by Furukawa et al. (16,17), mean arterial pressure of anesthetized normotensive rats was elevated by a constant infusion of AII. After blood pressure had stabilized, S-8307 or S-8308 was administered intravenously and their effect on mean arterial pressure and heart rate measured. Under these conditions, S-8307 and S-8308 at 100 mg/kg (intravenously) decreased mean arterial pressure by 53 and 45 mmHg, respectively, without influencing heart rate. At 10 mg/kg, both agents were without effect.

In the isolated rabbit aortic strips, S-8307 (3×10^{-6} to 3×10^{-4} M) and S-8308 (3×10^{-6} to 3×10^{-4} M) caused rightward parallel shifts of the AII-induced concentration–contractile-response curve without significantly affecting the maximum response to AII (Fig. 3). The slope of the Schild plots was not significantly different from unity, and pA_2 values of 5.49 and 5.74 were calculated for S-8307 and S-8308, respectively. The peptide AII-receptor antagonist, saralasin, displayed a noncompetitive type of inhibition in this preparation (20; also see ref. 21), with an apparent pA_2 of 9.47. At 10^{-4} M, S-8307 and S-8308 did not significantly reduce the aortic contraction to norepinephrine (10^{-7} M) and KCl (55 mM).

In the pithed rat preparation, S-8307 (30 and 100 mg/kg, intravenously) given 15 min prior to AII shifted the log-dose–vasopressor-response curve to this pressor agent par-

TABLE 2. *Antagonism of AII (20 ng/kg/min)-induced blood pressure increase in anesthetized rats by some imidazole derivatives following intravenous administration*[a]

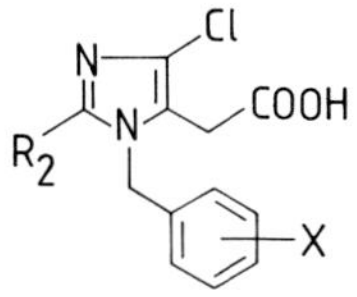

R_2	X	Dose (mg/kg, intravenously)	*n*	Inhibition (%) 10 min	30 min	90 min
n-C_4H_9	H	0.1	3	19.6 ± 1.5	64.3 ± 15.3	60.0 ± 21.5
		0.3	1	25	94	94
n-C_4H_9	2-Cl	0.1	1	38	100	86
C_6H_5	3-CH_3,4-OCH_3	0.5	4	33 ± 15	60 ± 18	62 ± 7

[a] Data taken from ref. 17.

allel to the right in a dose-dependent manner without depressing the maximum (19). S-8307 and S-8308, each administered at a dose of 100 mg/kg (intravenously), greatly inhibited the pressor response to AII (0.3 μg/kg) and slightly reduced the increase in diastolic pressure to sympathetic nerve stimulation at 3 Hz but had no significant effect on the responses to norepinephrine (1 μg/kg) and isoproterenol (0.1 μg/kg) (Fig. 4). This pattern of inhibition was mimicked by the peptide antagonist [Sar[1],Ile[8]]AII (Fig. 4). S-8307 and S-8308 also inhibited the heart rate responses to intravenous AII in pithed rats but did not change the responses to the other challenges (19).

In anesthetized normotensive rats, S-8307 did not influence the vasodepressor effects (−38 ± 5 mmHg) of bradykinin (1 μg/kg, intravenously) at the lower doses (12.5–50 mg/kg, intravenously) and slightly reduced it at 100 mg/kg (intravenously) (−26 ± 8 mmHg). Captopril (0.1 mg/kg, intravenously) potentiated the bradykinin vasodepressor response (−50 mmHg) (19).

Although our findings outlined above could not confirm the reported (16,17) potential of these two imidazole derivatives to act as antagonists of AII, the data clearly show that S-8307 and S-8308 are selective. Under *in vivo* and *in vitro* conditions, both derivatives markedly inhibited the responses to AII but did not change (or only slightly affected) the responses to various other challenges, thereby excluding numerous other properties, including inhibition of ACE. It is also noteworthy that S-8307 and S-8308 exhibited competitive antagonism in contrast to the noncompetitive behavior of saralasin.

Having established that S-8307 and S-8308 are weak (but specific) competitive AII-receptor antagonists, we then evaluated their antihypertensive potential in renal-artery-ligated rats. These animals were prepared by complete ligation of the left renal artery (22). Six days after ligation, hypertension is fully developed and is accompanied by a marked rise in plasma renin activity (23). The elevated blood pressure of these animals is primarily, if not exclusively, due to activation of the RAS, since captopril (5 mg/kg, intravenously) or saralasin (5 mg/kg, subcutaneously) restore the blood pressure to normotensive values (20,23). S-8307 and S-8308, each at 3 mg/kg (intravenously), did not alter mean arterial pressure in the renal-artery-ligated rats. At 10 mg/kg, both compounds lowered mean arterial pressure transiently by about 20 mmHg. Mean arterial pressure was rapidly reduced (by 35 mmHg) to normotensive values (99 ± 6 mmHg) by 30 mg/kg of S-8307 and was lowered (by 20 mmHg) by S-8308 (Fig. 5). The duration of the hypotensive effects was approximately 30 min. When S-8307 and S-8308 (Fig. 5) were given orally at 100 mg/kg, slight hypotensive effects were noted within 5 min, which reached their maximal effects (about −20 mmHg) 10 min after administration and lasted approximately 30 min (19,20). None of the treatments affected heart rate.

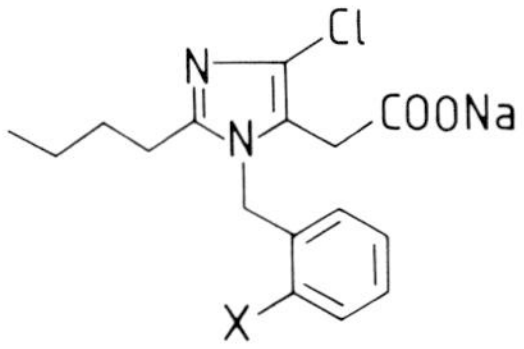

FIG. 2. Chemical structure of S-8307 (X = Cl) and S-8308 (X = NO_2).

The hypotensive effect of S-8307 was further characterized in furosemide-treated anesthetized rats in which S-8307 caused a dose-dependent decrease in mean arterial pressure (Fig. 6A). Furosemide pretreatment (20 mg/kg, intramuscularly) 30 min before anesthesia significantly increased plasma renin activity from 9.7 ± 3.3 to 30.1 ± 6.9 ng AI/ml/hr (n = 6) and enhanced the hypotensive response (Fig. 6A). Saralasin (10 μg/kg/min), captopril (5 mg/kg, intravenously), and bilateral nephrectomy (−18 to −24 hr) significantly reduced the hypotensive effect of S-8307 (Fig. 6B). On the other hand, a reduced mean arterial pressure, as produced by hydralazine (0.5 mg/kg, intravenously), did not influence the hypotension caused by S-8307 nor did pretreatment with indomethacin (5 mg/kg, intravenously) (19).

Taken together, we could show that these nonpeptide AII-receptor antagonists were hypotensive following intravenous administration. However, the duration of action is relatively short. Furthermore, only at a high oral dose did these compounds exhibit a (transient) hypotensive effect. Nevertheless, the decrease in mean arterial pressure pro-

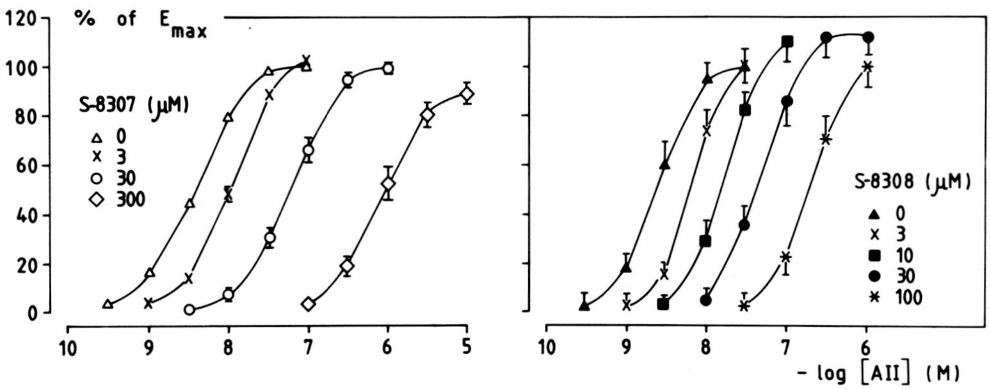

FIG. 3. Effect of S-8307 and S-8308 on the concentration–contractile-response curve for AII in isolated rabbit aortic strips. Values represent the mean ± S.E.M. (n = 3–6). (Modified after refs. 19 and 20.)

duced by these agents is partly due to interference with the RAS. This conclusion is based upon the observation that elimination of this system by three different approaches (i.e. saralasin, captopril, and nephrectomy) significantly reduced the magnitude of the hypotensive effect. Since these measures did not nullify the hypotensive action, it is likely that additional mechanisms contribute at these high doses. Since indomethacin was without effect, one of these possible mechanisms which is based on prostaglandins can be excluded.

In conclusion, the detailed pharmacological characterization of S-8307 and S-8308 described above identified this class of imidazole derivatives as *weak,* but *selective,* AII-receptor antagonists with a *competitive* mode of action. The modest potency (about 10,000-fold less than saralasin) did not discourage us, although it was obvious that appreciable improvements had to be made before these lead compounds could be considered useful probes, let alone therapeutic agents.

NEWER LEAD COMPOUNDS: EXP6155 AND EXP6803

Encouraged by the quality of the lead compounds S-8307 and S-8308, we embarked upon a synthetic program aimed at designing more potent antagonists while preserving their selective affinity for the AII receptor. To assist in the analysis, we used a radioligand binding assay (modified after refs. 24 and 25) in which the ability of the compounds to displace ^{3}H-AII from its specific binding affinity sites in rat isolated adrenocortical microsomes was determined. In this membrane preparation, a single population of high-affinity binding sites (B_{max} = 2.6 pmol/mg protein) was found for ^{3}H-AII, with an apparent dissociation constant (K_d) of 1.2 nM (26).

Using S-8307 and S-8308 as templates, structural modifications revealed some important features of the structure–affinity relationship (27). The chemical structures of the compounds of interest are depicted in Fig. 7.

Displacement curves of some analogues with respect to inhibition of the specific binding of ^{3}H-AII to rat adrenocortical microsomes are shown in Fig. 8. Table 3 lists the affinity, expressed as IC_{50}, of the various derivatives, including those of saralasin and S-8308 for comparison. Analogues lacking a free carboxyl functionality at the 5-position of the imidazole ring generally had lower affinities (i.e., higher IC_{50} values), especially when no other acidic group was present. This is illustrated by EXP6026, which had a threefold lower affinity than S-8308. Substitution at the para position of the benzyl group resulted in marked changes in affinity. When compared to S-8308, a nitro

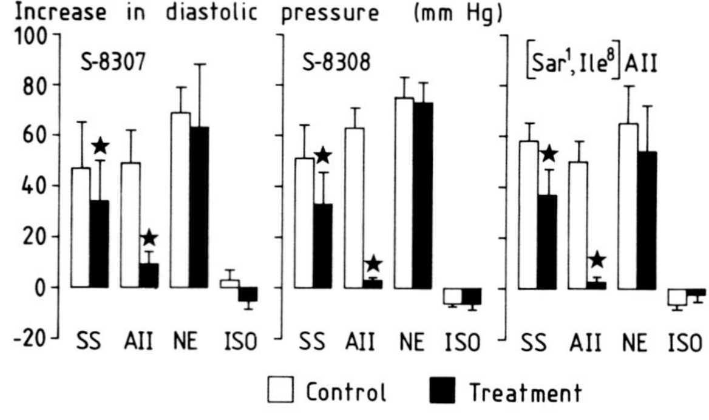

FIG. 4. Effect of S-8307, S-8308 (each at 100 mg/kg, intravenously), and [Sar[1], Ile[8]]AII (10 μg/kg/min, intravenously) on diastolic blood pressure of pithed rats in response to sympathetic nerve stimulation (SS, 3 Hz), AII (0.3 μg/kg), norepinephrine (NE, 1 μg/kg), and isoproterenol (0.1 μg/kg), all given intravenously. Values represent means ± S.E.M. (n = 4). Star denotes $p < 0.05$ (Student's paired t-test). (Modified after ref. 19.)

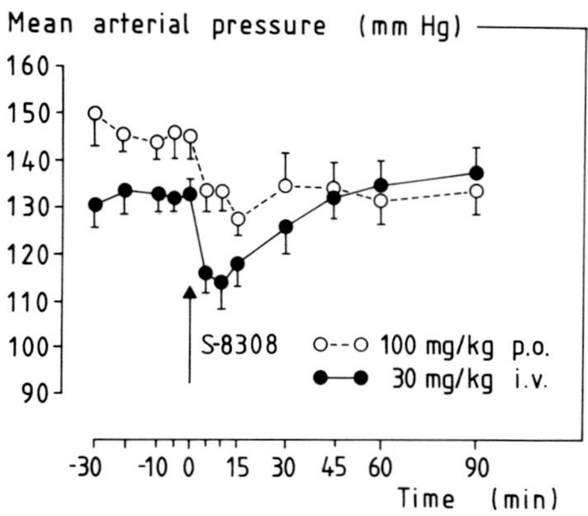

FIG. 5. Effects of S-8308 at 30 mg/kg (intravenously) and 100 mg/kg (orally) on mean arterial pressure of conscious renal-artery-ligated rats. Values represent means ± S.E.M. (n = 6). (From ref. 20.)

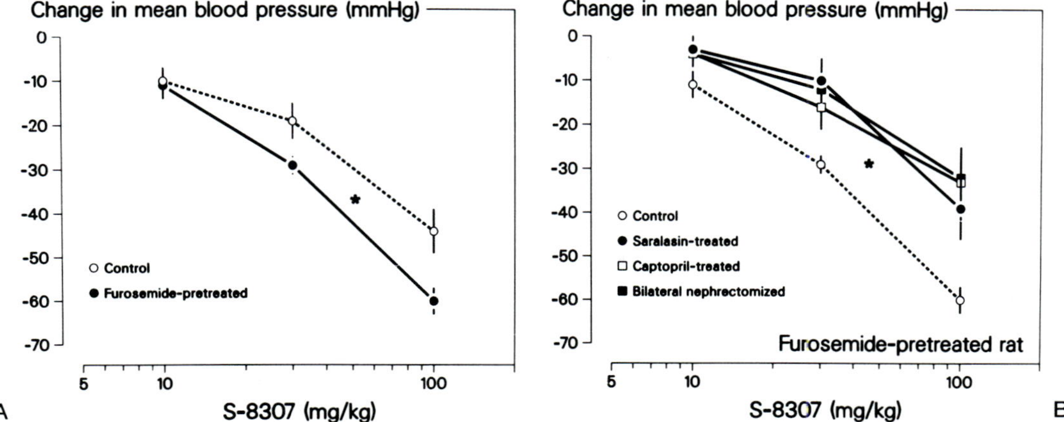

FIG. 6. A: Effect of furosemide (20 mg/kg, intramuscularly) on the hypotensive responses of intravenous S-8307 in anesthetized normotensive rats. Means ± S.E.M. (n = 6). **B:** Effects of saralasin (10 μg/kg/min), captopril (5 mg/kg, intravenously), and bilateral nephrectomy on the hypotensive responses to intravenous S-8307 in anesthetized normotensive rats. Means ± S.E.M. (n = 5–14). Star denotes $p <$ 0.05 with respect to control. (Modified after ref. 19.)

substituent at this position (EXP9993) caused a threefold loss in affinity, and the introduction of an amino group (EXP6151) reduced affinity even more. In contrast, a carboxylic acid functionality at this position (EXP6155) increased affinity ninefold over that of S-8308, and the 2-carboxybenzamido group (EXP6159) enhanced affinity 35-fold. Finally, modification at both positions led to EXP6803, which showed a 107-fold higher affinity than S-8308 for the AII-receptor binding sites in rat adrenocortical microsomes (26).

The radioligand-receptor binding studies discussed above showed that these nonpeptide AII-receptor antagonists exhibit appreciable affinity for AII-receptor binding sites in rat adrenal cortex and on rat smooth muscle cells. To evaluate whether these agents were indeed functional antagonists, their inhibitory effects on AII-induced $^{45}Ca^{2+}$ influx, an event subsequent to AII-receptor stimulation, were determined in rat aortic rings. AII, at a submaximal concentration of 3×10^{-8} M, promoted an influx of extracellular Ca^{2+} of 35.5 ± 3.2 μmol/kg tissue (n = 6) over the basal unstimulated control (26). This $^{45}Ca^{2+}$ influx produced by AII was effectively eliminated by saralasin as well as by the nonpeptide AII blockers in a concentration-dependent manner (Fig. 9).

The IC_{50} values are tabulated in Table 3. As can be seen, the order of inhibitory potency of the compounds, including saralasin, corresponds well with the order of affinity established in the two binding assays.

All compounds tested against AII-induced constriction of the isolated rabbit aorta *in vitro* behaved as true competitive antagonists. As illustrated by EXP6803 in Fig. 10, the log-concentration–contractile-response curve for AII was shifted progressively to the right in a parallel manner, whereas the maximum response was unaltered (26,28). The pA_2 values are reported in Table 3. The slope of the Schild plot for each compound was not significantly different from unity, except for saralasin (see above). EXP6803 was found to be the most potent, possessing a pA_2 value of 7.20,

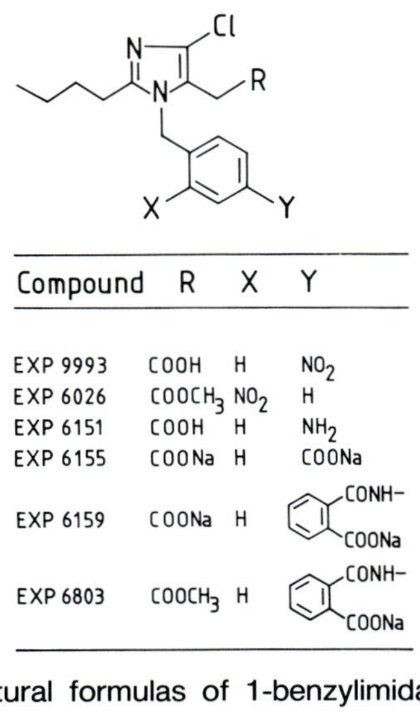

Compound	R	X	Y
EXP 9993	COOH	H	NO_2
EXP 6026	$COOCH_3$	NO_2	H
EXP 6151	COOH	H	NH_2
EXP 6155	COONa	H	COONa
EXP 6159	COONa	H	2-(CONH–)C$_6$H$_4$COONa
EXP 6803	$COOCH_3$	H	2-(CONH–)C$_6$H$_4$COONa

FIG. 7. Structural formulas of 1-benzylimidazole-5-acetate derivates defining some of the critical substituents (Y) on the phenyl ring.

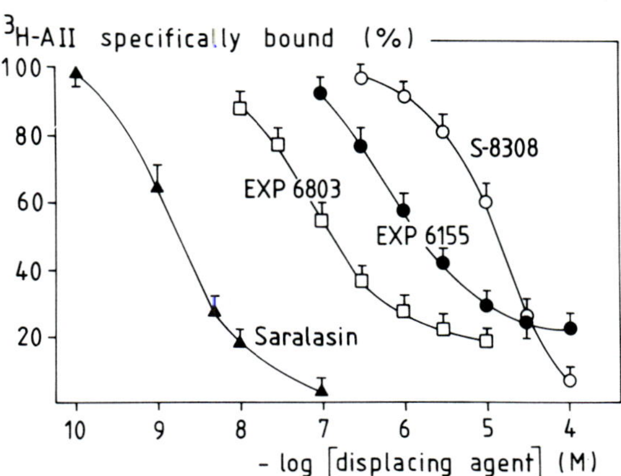

FIG. 8. Inhibition of the specific binding of ^{3}H-AII (2 nM) to rat adrenal cortical microsomes by saralasin and some nonpeptide AII-receptor antagonists. Symbols represent the mean ± S.E.M. of four to six separate determinations. (From ref. 26.)

TABLE 3. *Binding affinities to AII receptors and inhibitory potencies of AII-induced responses for some 1-benzylimidazole-5-acetate derivatives*

	IC_{50} (μM)			
Compound	Adrenocortical microsomes[a]	Smooth muscle cells[b]	pA_2[c]	IC_{50} (μM)[d]
S-8308	15	4.2	5.74	7.00
EXP9993	46	>10	ND	ND
EXP6026	42	>10	ND	ND
EXP6151	100	≫10	ND	ND
EXP6155	1.6	0.45	6.54	1.80
EXP6159	0.43	0.20	6.90	0.34
EXP6803	0.14	0.06	7.20	0.4
Saralasin	0.0018	0.0048	9.47	0.004

[a] Inhibition of specific binding of ^{3}H-AII (2 nM).
[b] Inhibition of specific binding of ^{125}I-AII (0.5 nM).
[c] Antagonism of AII-induced constriction of rabbit aorta.
[d] Inhibition of AII (3×10^{-8} M)-induced $^{45}Ca^{2+}$ influx in rat aorta.
[e] ND: not determined.

which is still two orders of magnitude less than the apparent pA_2 value of saralasin.

The specificity of this series of molecules was carefully analyzed. At concentrations of up to 10^{-4} M the compounds showed no affinity for sites other than AII receptors, such as alpha-1 adrenoceptors and calcium channels. They did not significantly alter the $^{45}Ca^{2+}$ influx elicited by KCl and norepinephrine nor did they affect the corresponding contractile responses, including those elicited by vasopressin *in vitro* as well as *in vivo.* At concentrations of up to 10^{-5} M, the compounds failed to alter (a) the kinetics of ^{14}C-hippurylhistidyl-leucine hydrolysis by rabbit lung converting enzyme and (b) the rate of AI generation by rat (plasma) renin (26). In addition, in the guinea-pig ileum, the derivatives did not change the contractile response to bradykinin, indicating the absence of ACE-inhibitory activity (28).

Since EXP6155 and EXP6803 represented truly novel leads with significant improvements over S-8307 and S-8308, the antihypertensive potential of both compounds was evaluated in more detail (26,28). Following intravenous bolus injections to conscious renal-artery-ligated hypertensive rats, EXP6803 produced a dose-dependent reduction in mean arterial pressure (Fig. 11) (26,28). The hypotensive effect was relatively short-lived at the lower doses, but it lasted for more than 2 hr for the 30-mg/kg dose. Heart rate was not significantly altered during the entire period of observation. EXP6155 was slightly less potent than EXP6803 in lowering mean arterial pressure following single intravenous bolus injections, and the duration of its hypotensive effect was shorter than that of EXP6803. It is important to note that neither EXP6803 nor EXP6155 caused an increase in mean arterial pressure following intravenous administration. This observation was verified in the conscious normotensive rat, in which these compounds lack a hypotensive response. As shown in Fig. 12, cumulative intravenous injections of EXP6155 at 3–100 mg/kg did not significantly affect mean arterial pressure (28). The absence of any pressor effect was also noticed for EXP6803 (3–100 mg/kg, cumulative intrave-

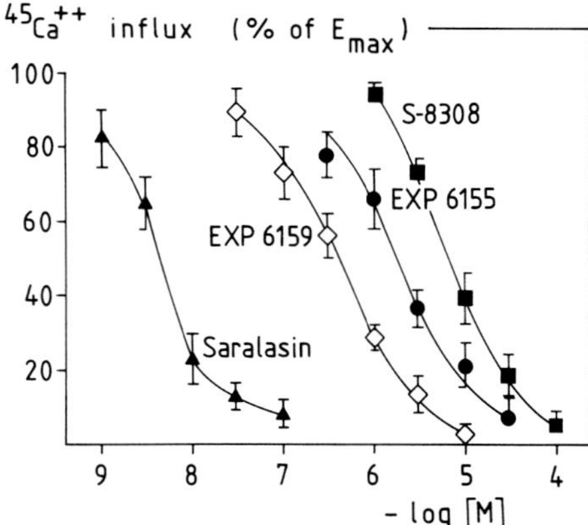

FIG. 9. Concentration-dependent inhibition of AII (3×10^{-8} M)-induced $^{45}Ca^{2+}$ influx by saralasin, EXP6159, EXP6155, and S-8308 in rat aortic smooth muscle rings. Values represent means ± S.E.M. (n = 6).

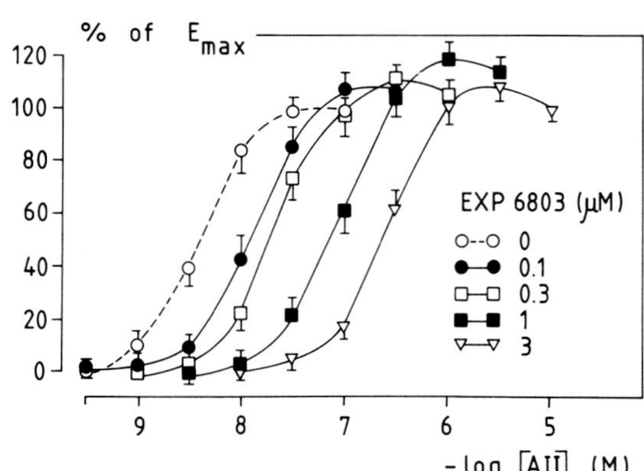

FIG. 10. Effect of EXP6803 (0.1–3 μM) on the log-concentration–contractile-response curve for AII in isolated helical strips of the rabbit aorta. Values represent the mean ± S.E.M. (n = 6). (From ref. 26.)

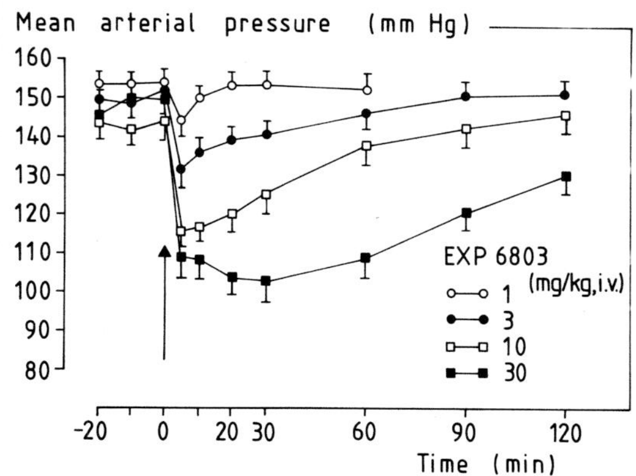

FIG. 11. Effect of intravenous bolus injections of EXP6803 (1–30 mg/kg) on mean arterial pressure of conscious renal-artery-ligated rats. Values represent the mean ± S.E.M. (n = 6). (From ref. 26.)

nously). This is in sharp contrast to saralasin, which produced an obvious increase in mean arterial pressure in normotensive (Fig. 12), as well as in renal hypertensive, rats (28).

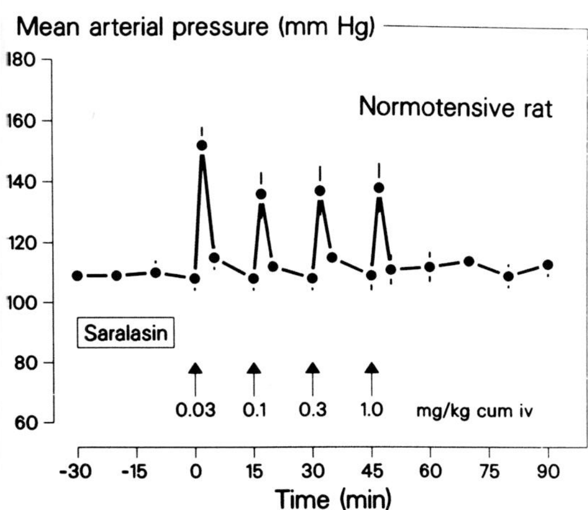

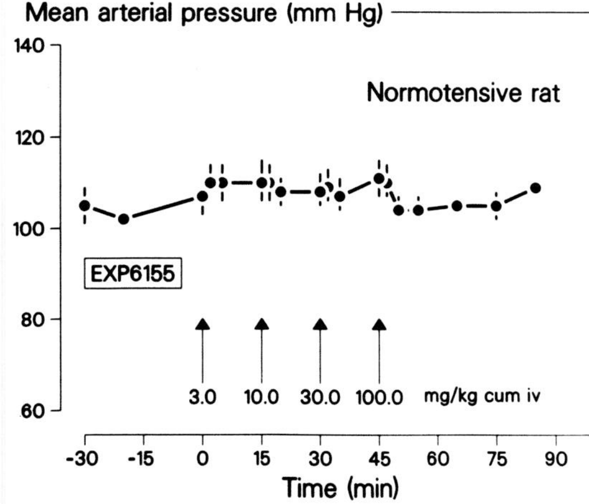

FIG. 12. Effect of saralasin (n = 6) and EXP6155 (n = 5) on mean arterial pressure of conscious normotensive rats following cumulative intravenous injection. Values represent the mean ± S.E.M. (From ref. 28.)

Despite the reasonable potency of EXP6155 and especially of EXP6803 in antagonizing AII-induced responses, as well as their attractive *in vivo* effects on cardiovascular parameters, both agents given orally in doses of up to 100 mg/kg to renal-artery-ligated rats were ineffective in lowering mean arterial pressure.

In conclusion, the findings described herein demonstrate that it is feasible to develop nonpeptide AII-receptor antagonists with reasonable affinity and a competitive mode of action without sacrificing specificity. It should also be obvious that partial agonism is not an intrinsic property of all AII-receptor antagonists, as is traditionally believed in the peptide arena. Although the most promising compound so far identified is still about 100-fold less potent in various test systems than the peptide blocker, saralasin, it may still be the preferred tool for studying the physiological role(s) of AII. Despite the lack of oral activity of EXP6803, it served as a challenge for further chemical refinement.

EXP7711: A NONPEPTIDE AII-RECEPTOR ANTAGONIST WITH ORAL ACTIVITY

As a result of investigations aimed at improving the oral bioavailability and duration of action of EXP6803, we found that after intravenous administration, this derivative is rapidly metabolized and secreted by the bile (29). However, the oral inactivity is the result of poor absorption rather than the result of first-pass metabolism. A series of compounds structurally related to EXP6803 was subsequently synthesized in which the amide (NHCO) linkage was replaced by a variety of groups of zero to three atoms in length. As the data listed in Table 4 show, a consistently high level of affinity was maintained in this series. Among the compounds in which X is a two-atom linkage, EXP6803 is more potent than the isosteric olefin (X = CH=CH) or ether (X = OCH_2). The compounds in which

TABLE 4. *Affinities of some nonpeptide AII-receptor antagonists structurally related to EXP6803 in which the amide linkage has been replaced by a series of linking groups of zero to three atoms in length*

X	IC_{50} (μM)[a]
CO	0.16
Single bond	0.28 (EXP7711)
O	0.40
S	0.40
OCH_2	0.92
NHCONH	2.4
CH=CH (trans)	5.4

[a] Inhibition of specific binding of ^{3}H-AII (2 nM) to rat isolated adrenocortical microsomes.

X is a zero-atom or one-atom linkage possess affinities comparable to that of EXP6803. Taken together, the data indicate that this class of nonpeptide AII-receptor antagonists is relatively flexible in the nature of the X-linker (30).

Further studies with this series of molecules identified EXP7711 as a particularly interesting AII-receptor blocker, since it showed a hypotensive action following oral administration (see below). EXP7711, which showed slightly less potency than EXP6803 in displacing ^{3}H-AII (2 nM) from its specific binding sites in rat isolated adrenocortical microsomes (Table 4), behaved as a competitive antagonist against AII-induced constriction of the rabbit isolated aorta. The pA_2 value was calculated to be 6.90; moreover, the slope of the Schild plot amounted to 0.96, which was not significantly different from unity. In concentrations of up to 10^{-5} M, EXP7711 did not alter the vascular effects of norepinephrine, KCl, vasopressin, and bradykinin, indicating its specificity and lack of ACE inhibition. Following intravenous administration to pithed normotensive rats, EXP7711 shifted the log-dose–vasopressor-effect curve for AII to the right in a parallel fashion without affecting the maximum. Three- and 10-fold rightward shifts were obtained following intravenous administration of 10 and 30 mg/kg (intravenously), respectively. In anesthetized normotensive rats, EXP7711 dose-dependently reduced the increase in mean arterial pressure to an intravenous bolus injection of 0.1 μg/kg of AII. The dose required to inhibit this response (46 ± 3 mmHg, $n = 6$) by 50% amounted to 4.4 mg/kg. Cumulative intravenous injection of EXP7711 (0.3–10 mg/kg) lowered mean arterial pressure in the awake renal-artery-ligated hypertensive rat in a dose-dependent manner without significantly affecting heart rate. The amount needed to decrease mean arterial pressure by 30 mmHg in this animal model was 3.7 mg/kg. It should be noted again that no indication of agonistic properties was observed in any of the test systems described above.

Upon oral administration of EXP7711 to conscious renal hypertensive rats, a dose-related drop in mean arterial pressure was observed. Figure 13 shows the results of these experiments. At an oral dose of 10 mg/kg, EXP7711 significantly reduced mean arterial pressure, whereas at 100 mg/kg the blood pressure of the animals was diminished close to normotensive values. None of these doses significantly influenced heart rate (Fig. 13). The hypotensive effect of EXP7711 lasted for over 3 hr. An oral dose of 100 mg/kg was without effect on blood pressure and heart rate in awake normotensive rats.

In the awake sodium-depleted (furosemide, 20 mg/kg, intramuscularly, −18 and −2 hr) dog, an intravenous injection of 10 mg/kg of EXP7711 produced a hypotensive response which lasted for approximately 90 min (Fig. 14). EXP7711 exhibited a slight, but longer-lasting, hypotensive effect following an oral dose of 30 mg/kg. The ACE inhibitor captopril, administered at an oral dose of 10 mg/kg, was

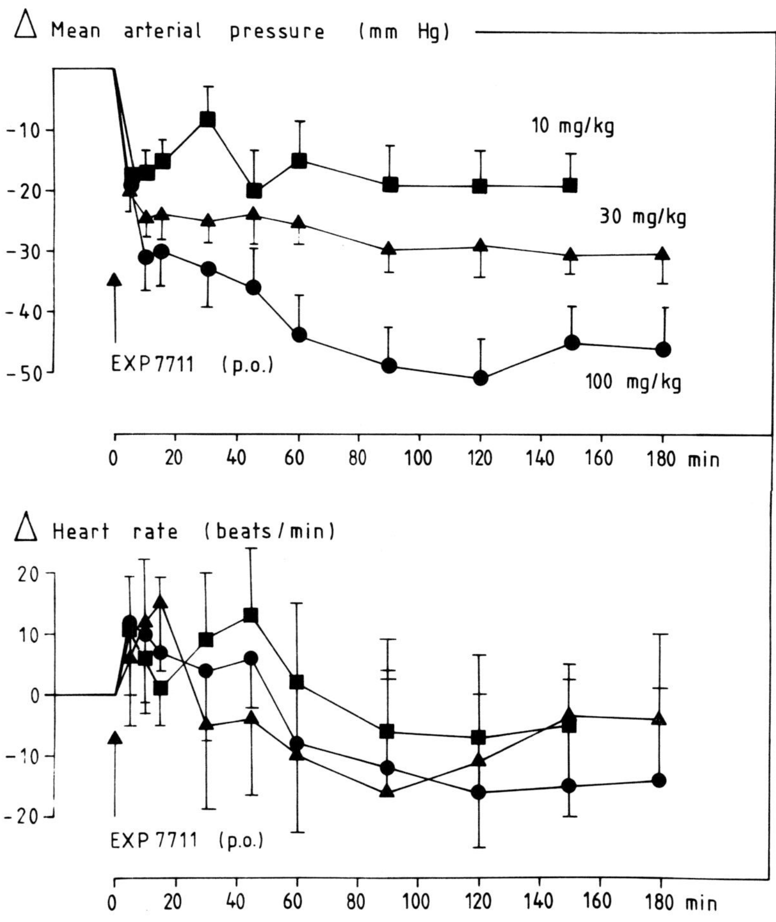

FIG. 13. Effect of EXP7711 on mean arterial pressure and heart rate following oral administration to conscious renal-artery-ligated hypertensive rats. Symbols represent mean values ± S.E.M. ($n = 6$).

mode of action, 2295
in normal volunteers, 2332–2334
parasympathetic nervous system, 2215
peripheral vascular disease, 2220
pheochromocytoma, 2218
plasma renin activity, 2173–2174
pregnancy, 1820–1821
prostglandin, 2212–2213
quality of life, 2222
renal circulation, 2216
renal disorder, 2219
renin-producing tumor, 2218
renin secretion, 2216
renomedullary interstitial cell, 843–844, 845, 846
renovascular hypertension, 2217–2218
respiratory disease, 2220
scintigraphy, 1524–1525
side effects, 2222–2223
angiotensin-converting enzyme activity per se, 2223
compound related, 2223
renin-angiotensin system, 2222–2223
sympathetic nervous system, 2214–2215
vasopressin, 2212
Angiotensin I, 1296, 1319–1321, 1325, 2210
angiotensin-converting enzyme, 1221
renin, hog vs. human, 1183
Angiotensin I-converting enzyme inhibitor, 1682
Angiotensin II, 583, 794, 1319–1322, 1324–1325, 1580, 1594, 1763, 1764, 1790, 1795, 1797, 2210
adenosine, 1111
adrenal gland, 1255–1260
adrenal function effects, 1255–1256
angiotensin II receptors, 1256
calcium homeostasis modulation, 1258–1259
G-protein, 1256–1257
guanine nucleotide regulatory protein, 1256–1257
phosphoinositide turnover, 1257–1258
signal transduction, 1256–1257
adrenal glomerulosa cell
A23187, 1258
arachidonic acid, 1259
atrial natriuretic peptide, 1259–1260
Ca^{2+} messenger system, 1259
cAMP messenger system, 1259
membrane potential, 1259
phospholipase A_2, 1259
aldosterone, 1300–1301, 1366
aldosterone biosynthesis, 1298
angiotensin-converting enzyme inhibitor, 2211
angiotensinogen, 1209–1210
arterial pressure, 1263
long-term control, 1121–1125
renal-body-fluid feedback, 1121–1123
arteriolar vasoconstriction, generalized, 1296–1297
atrial natriuretic factor, 867
antagonism, 867
blood pressure
potassium, 998–999
sensitivity to increase, 1124–1125
calcium homeostasis, 1250–1252
cathepsin G, 1200
cellular mechanisms of action, 1299
circumflex artery, 1014, 1015
converting-enzyme inhibitor, 1111
renal vascular response, 1359
coronary artery, 1014, 1015
diacylglycerol, 587, 588
acidification, 592
low temperature, 591
endothelium-derived relaxation factor, 1255
essential hypertension
altered responsiveness, 1356–1358
nonmodulation, 1356–1358
glomerular filtration rate, 1108–1110
autoregulatory mechanisms, 1109–1110
guanine nucleotide, 584, 585
hydrolysis products, 602
indomethacin, 1255
endothelium, 1255
inositol phosphate, 590
inositol trisphosphate, 586
calcium mobilization, 586
80-kDa protein phosphorylation of, 588
kidney, 1260–1265
blood pressure, 1260
extracellular fluid volume, 1260
glomerular mesangial cells, 1261–1262
intrarenal angiotensin II formation, 1261
renal hemodynamics, 1260–1261
renal sodium handling, 1262
tubule transport mechanism, 1264–1265
mesenteric artery, 584
metabolism, 1299
mitogenic effect, 544
myosin, 1253
peptide transmitter, 691–692
peritubular capillary dynamics, 1115–1116
phosphoinositide lipid, 604
physiologic effects, 1296–1299
postsynaptic effects, 2214–2215
potassium, 224
pregnancy, 1768
pressure natriuresis
long-term, 1123
renal escape, 1123–1124
presynaptic effects, 2214–2215
proximal convoluted tubule volume, 1264
receptor types, 583–584
renal hemodynamics, 1106–1112
angiotensin II blockade, 1107–1108
chronic renal failure, 1108
circulating angiotensin II, 1108–1110
glomerular filtration rate regulation, 1106
intrarenally formed angiotensin II, 1108–1110
preglomerular vessel constriction, 1110–1112
renal vascular resistance primary site, 1106
renovascular hypertension, 1108
tubuloglomerular feedback, 1106
renal tubular sodium reabsorption, 1298
renal vascular effects, 1297–1298
renin, 1295
renin-angiotensin-aldosterone system, 1443
salt balance in pregnancy, 1771
salt-loading renal function curve, 1035–1036
smooth muscle cell, 590
sodium, 1263
adrenal response, 1353
pressor response, 1353
renal response, 1353
sodium excretion, 1112–1121
aldosterone, 1113–1115
circulating angiotensin II mediation, 1119–1120
distal tubular effects, 1118–1119
internally formed angiotensin II mediation, 1119–1120
intrarenal actions, 1115
medullary hemodynamics, 1116–1117
natriuresis, 1120–1121
peritubular capillary dynamics, 1115–1116
proximal tubular effects, 1117–1118
sympathetic nervous system, 1112–1113
tubular reabsorption direct effects, 1117
SQ-14225, 1111
systemic vascular resistance, 998–999
testosterone biosynthesis, 1298–1299
thirst stimulation, 1298
urinary sodium excretion, 1263
vagal tone, 1298
vascular smooth muscle, 1247–1255
calcium homeostasis, 1250–1252
contractile proteins, 1253–1254
endothelium, 1254–1255
hydrogen ion metabolism, 1252
latch-bridge hypothesis, 1253
phosphoinositide metabolism, 1249–1250
prostaglandin, 1254–1255
receptor binding, 1249
receptors, 1248–1249
signaling pathways, 1252–1253
sodium ion metabolism, 1252
tone control, 1247–1248

Angiotensin II (*contd.*)
vascular smooth muscle receptor
G-protein, 1249
phospholipase C, 1249
vasoconstriction, 1296–1298
vasopressin, 1298
verapamil, vasodilator response, 2171
water drinking, 1298
Angiotensin II blockade
chronic renal failure, 1108
renovascular hypertension, 1108
Angiotensin II effector, G-protein, 1248
Angiotensin II receptor
cation, 584–585
G-protein, 1248
guanine nucleotide, 584–585
Angiotensin II-receptor antagonist, 2351–2360
lead compounds, 2352
Angiotensinogen, 1197–1212, 1295–1296
adrenal gland, 1207–1208
alpha-antitrypsin, 1204
amino-terminal amino acid sequence, 1203
angiotensin II, 1209–1210
antithrombin III, 1204
biosynthesis, 1204–1208
brain, 1206–1207
dog, 1198
erythropoietin, 1211–1212
estrogen, 1208–1209, 1295
glucocorticoid, 1209, 1295
heart, 1207
heterogeneity, 1200
high molecular weight. *See* High-molecular-weight angiotensinogen
hog, 1197–1198
vs. human, 1183
human, 1199–1203
purification, 1199
human amniotic fluid, 1201
inflammation, 1210–1211
intestine, 1208
kidney, 1207
larger molecular weights, 1200
liver, 1205–1206
synthesis, 1205
low molecular weight. *See* Low-molecular-weight angiotensinogen
lung, 1208
mesentery, 1208
nephrectomy, 1210
ovalbumin, 1204
ovary, 1208
ovine, 1198
pregnancy, 1200, 1201, 1766–1767
primary structure, 1203–1204
classic studies, 1203
recombinant cDNA studies, 1203–1204
processing, 1204–1208
production, 1666
prorenin, 1192
purification, 1198–1199
rabbit, 1198
rat, 1198–1199
regulation, 1208–1211
renin, 1295–1296
serpins, 1204
spleen, 1208
testes, 1208
thyroid hormone, 1210
thyroxine, 1210
tissue-specific differential regulation, 1211
triiodothyronine, 1210
vascular tissue, 1208
Angiotensinogen-converting enzyme, chloride, 1296
Animal pathophysiology, renovascular hypertension, 1539–1542
Anipamil, 492
Anterior pituitary hormone, atrial natriuretic factor, 869
Anteroventral third ventricle, sympathoadrenomedullary system, 717–718
Anthropometric measures, 1742
Anti-inflammatory drug, antihypertensive drug, 1905–1909
Antibiotic, calcium antagonist, 1014–1015, 1017
Antidiabetic agent, beta-blocker, 2202
Antidiuretic hormone, 798–799
hydrolysis products, 602
phosphoinositide lipid, 604
renal kallikrein-kinin system, 809
Antieclamptic therapy, 1819
magnesium sulfate, 1819
Antihypertensive drug, 113, 1402–1403, 1543, 1730, 1732–1733. *See also* Specific type
acute hypertension in pregnancy, 1816–1818
additive effects, 2291
age, 2173–2174
anti-inflammatory drug, 1905–1909
arterial compliance, 1413
beta blocker, 1644
cardiac output, 2128
cardiocerebrovascular complication, 2131–2132
cardiovascular hemodynamics, 2117–2119
changes in established hypertension, 2117
pressure-flow-resistance diagram, 2117
cerebrovascular pharmacology, 407–408
chronic hypertension in pregnancy, 1820–1821
compliance, 2132–2133, 2309–2313
development, 2098–2102, 2331–2340
ascending dose, 2335–2336
blood pressure baseline value definition, 2335
blood pressure measurement, 2338
constant dose, 2335–2336
control group definition, 2335
cross-over designs, 2336–2337
normotensive volunteers, 2332–2335
phase III program goals, 2338–2339
problems, 2331–2335
responder dose-response curve, 2338
dose-finding, 2335–2338
drug interaction, 2291–2298
efficacy testing, 2101–2102
excessive pressure reduction, 2138–2139
exercise, 1993–1994
hemodynamic profiles, 2127–2128
historical aspects, 2096–2099
interactions, 2063
J-shaped curve, 2138–2139
labile hypertension, 1424–1425
malignant hypertension
controlled trials, 2133, 2139
mortality, 2133
suboptimal effects, 2137–2138
metabolic side effects, 2132
mild hypertension
controlled trial, 2137
coronary disease, 2135–2137
diastolic pressure changes, 2135
five-year survival, 2135
major endpoint analysis, 2134–2137
mortality, 2135, 2136
prognosis improvement, 2134
stroke, 2135
suboptimal effects, 2137–2138
moderate hypertension
controlled trial, 2137
coronary disease, 2135–2137
diastolic pressure changes, 2135
five-year survival, 2135
major endpoint analysis, 2134–2137
mortality, 2135, 2136
prognosis improvement, 2134
stroke, 2135
suboptimal effects, 2137–2138
morbidity, 2131–2132
mortality, 2131–2132
nonsteroidal anti-inflammatory drug, 1905, 1906
nursing management, 2063–2064
pregnancy, 1815, 1816–1818, 1820–1821
angiotensin-converting enzyme inhibitors, 1820–1821
beta-adrenergic inhibitors, 1820–1821
clonidine, 1820
diazoxide, 1816–1818
hydralazine, 1816–1817, 1820
labetalol, 1816, 1818, 1820–1821
methyldopa, 1819–1820
nifedipine, 1816–1817, 1820
nitroprusside, 1816, 1818
prazosin, 1820–1821
thiazide diuretics, 1820–1822
quality of life, 2132–2133
race, 2173–2174

  renal hypertension, 2174–2175
  renal parenchymal disease, 1589–1590
  structural regression, 2305
  studies, 2303
  success of withdrawal, 2303
Antihypertensive neutral renomedullary lipid, 848
Antihypertensive polar renomedullary lipid
  acetyl glyceryl ether phosphorylcholine, 849
  platelet-activating factor, 849
Antiepileptic, calcium antagonist, 1014–1015, 1017
Antithrombin III, angiotensinogen, 1204
Anxiety
  borderline hypertension, 2086
  pheochromocytoma, 1643
Aorta, 1566–1567
  medial defect, 7
  potassium, 56
  pressure change, 577
  rat, 1799
  renin, 2173–2174
  renin inhibitor, 2347–2349
  risk, 1385
  selection, 2110–2114
    combining first-line drugs, 2113
    drug response, 2110
    high-renin patients, 2110–2111
    low-renin patients, 2111
    medium-renin patients, 2111–2113
    monotherapy, 2111–2113
    renin system patterns, 2110
  severe hypertension, 2174–2175
  side effects, 2063
  smoking, 1923–1924
  step down, 113–114
  structural cardiovascular change, 2132
  structural modulation, 577
  synergism, 2291
  total peripheral resistance, 2128
  toxicity, magnesium, 1010–1013
  vasodilator rule, 2128–2129
  withdrawal, 2301–2307
    acute use, 1865
    baroreceptor resetting, 2305
    chronic use, 1865
    cuff artifact, 1413
    development, 2107–2109
    dietary sodium restriction, 2016–2017
    historical background, 2107–2109
    natural history of blood pressure hypothesis, 2305
Aortic diastolic pressure, coronary vascular resistance, 576
Aortic dissection, hypertension, 381
  frequency, 380, 381
Aortic plaque, 1553
Aortic regurgitation, hypertension, 380
  frequency, 380, 381
Aortic valve, calcific deposits, 383
Aortic valve cusp, calcific deposits, 383
Aortogram, 1552, 1566
Aortorenal bypass, 1566
  children, 1570
Apical membrane, DOCA, 1281
Apolipoprotein-B, 132
Apoplexy, 7
Appedrine, 1913
Apresoline, adverse effects, 1898
Aprotinin, 808, 810–811
Apudoma, pheochromocytoma, 1646–1647
Aqueduct block, 59
Arachidonic acid
  endothelium-derived relaxation factor, 1255
  inositol phospholipid, 605
  linoleic acid, 257, 259
  metabolic pathways, 829–831
Arcuate wreath, 1780
Area postrema, 682
Arginine vasopressin, 798–799. *See also* Vasopressin
A.R.M. Allergy Relief, 1913
Arrhythmia, propranolol, 2197
Arterial baroreceptor resetting, beta-blocker, 2186–2187
Arterial baroreflex, 1462–1465
  blood pressure, 1463–1464
  cardiac output, 1464
  cardiopulmonary/baroreflex interaction, 1464
  heart rate, 1462–1463
    calculation, 1463
    variables, 1463
  humoral substance modulation, 1464–1465
  vascular resistance, 1463–1464
Arterial blood supply, placental bed, 1780
Arterial calcium accumulation, risk factors, 476–477
Arterial compliance, antihypertensive drugs, 1413
Arterial disease, 7–11
Arterial endothelial permeability, atherosclerosis, 512
Arterial hypertension
  intracranial pressure, 704–705
    acute elevation, 704–705
  renin-secretory response, 1098–1099
Arterial hypertrophy, potassium, 55
Arterial lesion, 34–35
  aminophylline, 40
  pathogenesis, 35
Arterial narrowing, hypertensive retinopathy, 447–450
Arterial necrosis, 35
Arterial occlusive disease, diabetes mellitus, 1709
Arterial pressure
  5-min intervals, 4, 5
  age, 13–14
  aldosterone, 1049
  anesthesia, 1681
  angiotensin II, 1263
    long-term control, 1121–1125
    renal-body-fluid feedback, 1121–1123
  antihypertensive treatment, 1724, 1732
  automatic recording, 4–5
  calcium, 234
  captopril, 1264
  cardiac output, 305
  cardiovascular-renal disease, 11
  central, 35
  cerebral hemorrhage, 10
  cerebral infarction, 10
  cyclo-oxygenase inhibitor, 1906–1907
  defense reflex, 6–7
  diabetes mellitus, 1695
  diurnal variations, 4
  doctor-caused rise, 6
  environmental factors, 3
  extracellular fluid volume, 1141
    angiotensin II, 1141
  filtration surface area, 1151–1152, 1157
  fluid volume, increased, 1037–1045
  genetics, 14
  glomerular filtration coefficient, 1046
  heart disease, 7
  hemodynamic events, 1588
  hypertension, pathogenesis, 1037–1045
  indomethacin, 1907
  intrarenal, 1544
  kidney, long-term regulation, 1029–1051
  lability, 1415–1425
  Leriche syndrome, 8
  life expectancy, 11
  lower-body negative pressure, 350
  major factors, 1004
  malignant hypertension, 10
  mean. *See* Mean arterial pressure
  as measured in clinic, 5–7
    conditions, 6
    replication, 6
  as measured in office, 18
  mortality, 3, 11
  natural history, 13–14
  nephron number, 1152–1153
  passive leg raising, 350
  polyenic inheritance, 14
  potassium, 1142–1146
  pressure control, renal-fluid volume mechanism, 1048–1050
  prostacyclin, 1905, 1906
  prostaglandin E_2, 1905, 1906
  regulation, 1585
  renal-body-fluid feedback, 1121–1123
  resistance, 573
  sleep, 3, 4–5
  stroke, 8
  total peripheral resistance, 1046
    afferent renal arteriolar resistances, 1047
  tubuloglomerular feedback
    acute change effect, 1081–1082
    autoregulation, 1081
    quantitation, 1081–1082
  variability, 3–5, 6

Arterial pressure (*contd.*)
  vascular bed, 573
  volume-loading hypertension, 1040
  water hardness, 1009–1010
Arterial pressure control
  aldosterone, 1032–1033
    feedback gain, 1032
  baroreceptor, 1032–1033
    feedback gain, 1032
  capillary fluid shift, 1032–1033
    feedback gain, 1032
  chemoreceptor, 1032–1033
    feedback gain, 1032
  conspicuous nondeterminants, 1033
  determinants, 1033
  net intake level, 1033
  renal function curve shift, 1033
  renin-angiotensin vasoconstriction, 1032–1033
    feedback gain, 1032
  stress relaxation, 1032–1033
    feedback gain, 1032
Arterial pulse, pounding, 383
Arterial sclerosis
  hypertensive retinopathy, 450, 452
  Wagener-Clay-Gibner classification, 440, 442
Arterial senescence
  calcium/magnesium ratio, 479
  calcium overload, 474–477
Arterial smooth muscle cell
  atherogenesis, 512
  hypertension, 512
  phenotypes, 512
  proliferation, 512
  replication, 512
Arterial sound, Korotkoff's categorization, 84
Arterial stiffness, cuff artifact, 1409–1411, 1413
Arterial tortuosity, hypertensive retinopathy, 450–451, 453
Arterial wall
  calcium, 471
  calcium-overload-induced sclerotic destruction, 493–507
  cholesterol, 471
  layers, 522
  lipid, 471
Arterial wall tension, blood pressure
  albumin, 120
  lipid, 120
Arteriography, 1551
  renal, 1569, 1575, 1576
Arteriolar hyalinosis, microalbuminuria, 1721
Arteriolar lesion, 27–29
Arteriolar lumen size, magnesium, 1016
Arteriolar nephrosclerosis, 1588
Arteriolar resistance, post-arteriolar constriction, 2098
Arteriolar spasm
  calcium antagonist, 490–493, 494
  ocular fundus, 490–493, 494
Arteriolar vasoconstriction, angiotensin II, 1296–1297
  generalized, 1296–1297
Arteriolar wall, blood pressure, 51–52
Arteriole
  diazoxide, circulatory effects, 2266
  efferent, 1555
  fibrinoid necrosis, 10, 393–394
  glomerulus, 1056
  hyaline arteriolosclerosis, 390–391
  hypertensive choroidopathy, 446
  myointimal hyperplasia, 392–393
  necrotizing arteriolitis, 393–394
Arteriosclerosis, 7, 10–11
  calcium, 471–508
  captopril, 504–507
  Dahl S rat
    calcium antagonists, 493–497
    mesenteric artery branches, 502
  Okamoto rat, calcium antagonists, 493–497
  spontaneously hypertensive rat, 498
    mesenteric artery, 499
Arteriosclerotic aneurysm, 7
Arteriovenous nicking, hypertensive retinopathy, 450, 451
Artery
  aging
    calcium affinity, 474–475
    cholesterol accumulation, 474–475
    elastic structure demolition, 475–476
  generalized narrowing, Wagener-Clay-Gibner classification, 440, 442
  pressure change, 577
  serotonin, 763
  structural modulation, 577
Artery branching angle, hypertensive retinopathy, 451–453
Aspartic acid, preprorenin, 1290
Aspartyl proteinase, 1179
Aspirin, 1907
  preeclampsia, 1800–1802, 1814
  spironolactone, 2063
Asthma
  angiotensin-converting enzyme inhibitor, 2220
  beta-blocker, 2189, 2199–2200
Atenolol
  alpha-blocking properties, 2119
  beta-1-adrenoceptor selectivity, 2119, 2183
  beta-blocking metabolites, 2183
  beta-blocking plasma concentration, 2183
  bioavailability, 2183
  blood pressure, 530
  cardiac output, 2121–2123
  cardiovascular hypertrophy, 530
  dosage, 2184
  dosage frequency, 2184
  equipotent single dose, 2184
  exercise, 1994
  heart rate, 2121–2123
  hemodynamics, 2186
  intrinsic sympathomimetic activity, 2119, 2183
  lipophilicity, 2183
  mean arterial pressure, 2121–2123
  membrane-stabilizing effect, 2183
  migraine, 2197
  mortality, 1975
  plasma half-life, 2184
  protein binding, 2183
  side effects, 201
  stroke volume, 2121–2123
  structure, 2182
  systolic pressure, 1975
  total peripheral resistance, 2121–2123
  vascular resistance, 2121
Atherogenesis
  activated T-cells, 527
  arterial smooth muscle cell, 512
  calcium, 471
  calcium channel antagonist, 511–517
  carotid artery, 514
    calcium channel antagonists, 514
  cholesterol, 527
  diet, 109
  growth-promoting factor, 527
  hypercholesterolemia, 512
  hyperlipemia, 527
  intimal cell mass, 526
  mechanisms, 526–527
  monoclonal hypothesis, 526
  neoplasm hypothesis, 526
  smooth muscle cell, 526
Atheroma, 7–8, 1545, 1546, 1553, 1554, 1555
  hypertension, 18
Atheroma elastosis, 11
Atheromatous renal artery stenosis, 1553
Atherosclerosis, 7, 1564
  arterial endothelial permeability, 512
  calcium antagonist, 512–513
    animal models, 512–513
  cholesterol, 512
  cholesterol-fed rabbit model, 513
  chondroitin sulfate, 513
  colcemid, 513
  collagen, 512
  diphosphonic acid derivative, 513
  early lesions, 512
  EDTA, 513
  elastin, 512
  guanethidine, 513
  heparin, 513
  hyperlipidemia, 512
    rabbit, 295
  hypertension, 422–423, 511–512, 521–533
    common elements, 511–512
    relationships, 119
  lanthanum, 513
  propranolol, 513
  proteoglycan, 512
  renal artery disease, 396, 1561–1563, 1565
  reserpine, 513
  smooth muscle cell, 512, 522
  vascular occlusion, 521

Atherosclerotic blood vessel, endothelium-dependent response, 642
Atherosclerotic cardiovascular disease, hypothyroidism, 1671–1672
Atherosclerotic lesion
  fatty infiltration, 525
  foam cell, 525
  initial lesion, 525
  intimal cell mass, 525
  macrophage, 525
  smooth muscle cell, 525
  smooth muscle replication, 525–526
Atherosclerotic renal artery disease, 1564–1565, 1568
Atherosclerotic vascular disease, 1668
Atherosis, acute, 1784
Atherothrombotic brain infarction
  cholesterol, 109
  hypertension, 102, 417–418
  systolic pressure, 417–418
Athlete, hypertension, 1995
Atrial natriuretic factor, 794–795, 861–877, 1631
  ACTH, 869
  aldosterone, 866–867
  amino acid sequences, 862, 863
  angiotensin-converting enzyme inhibitor, 2212
  angiotensin II, 867
    antagonism, 867
  anterior pituitary hormone, 869
  binding sites, 864
  biological actions, 865–869
  biosynthesis, 861–863
  blood pressure, 869
  cellular actions, 864–865
  central nervous system, 869
  cGMP, 625
  cirrhosis, 871
  congestive heart failure, 870–871
  cortisol, 868
  cytosolic free calcium, 864–865
  diabetes mellitus, 872
  diabetic hypertension, 1704
  effects, 861
  fluid compartmentalization, 868
  gene, 862
  glomerular efferent arteriole, 868
  glucocorticoid, 868
  gonadal steroid, 868
  guanylate cyclase, 868
  hematocrit, 868
  hemodynamics, 868
  human chorionic gonadotropin, 868
  hypertension, 629, 873–876
    hemodynamic responses, 875–876
    plasma levels, 873
    renal responsiveness, 875
    secretion alterations, 873–875
  infusion, 1541
  130-kDa glycoprotein, 625
  130-kDa molecular weight, 625
  luteinizing hormone, 868
  messenger RNA, 861–862
  nephrotic syndrome, 871
  nonedematous disorder, 872–873
  pathophysiological implications, 871–872
  peptide transmitter, 692–693
  physiological role, 869–870
  plasma volume, 868
  progesterone, 868
  receptor, 864–865
  receptor subtypes, 864
  renal failure, 872
  renal function, 865–866
  renin-angiotensin-aldosterone system, 866–867
  renin secretion, 866
  secretion regulation, 864
  sodium, 869
  steroid hormone, 867–868
  structure, 861–863
  supraventricular tachyarrhythmia, 872–873
  syndrome of inappropriate antidiuretic hormone secretion, 872
  thirst, 869
  thyroid hormone, 1667
  vascular smooth muscle, 868
  vasopressin, 869
  wall tension, 864
Atrial stretch, atrial natriuretic factor, 864
Atriopeptin, 794–795
Atrioventricular conduction defect, beta-blocker, 2189
Auscultation, anesthesia, 1894
Australian National Blood Pressure Study, 1945
  treatment effectiveness, 153
Australian Therapeutic Trial in Mild Hypertension, 18, 1878
  age, 198
  chlorothiazide, 197
  ischemic heart disease, 198
  methyldopa, 197
  mild, symptomless hypertension, 197
  pindolol, 197
  propranolol, 197
Automatic home blood pressure monitor, 1434–1435. *See also* Ambulatory recording
Autonomic dysfunction, sympathoadrenal system, 1422
Autonomic function, 711
  principles, 711
Autonomic nervous system
  borderline hypertension, 2084–2085
  cardiac index, stepwise blockade, 2084–2085
  hypertension, 2083–2089
  laboratory evaluation, 1461–1475
  prostaglandin, 832–833
Autonomic nervous system test
  carotid sinus hypersensitivity, 1470–1471
  clinical practice, 1469–1475
    patient selection, 1469
  hyperadrenergic dysautonomia, 1471–1475
  protocol, 1469–1470
Autonomic neuropathy, 1691
Autoregulation, 1040–1042
  cardiac output, 1040–1042
  cerebral circulation
    hypertensive adaptation, 403–405
    long-term antihypertensive treatment, 404–405, 406
  coarctation of the aorta, 1042
  hypertension, 1048
  long-term, 1042–1043
  non-tubuloglomerular feedback, 1081
  short-term, 1042–1043
  total peripheral resistance, 1040–1042
  tubuloglomerular feedback, 1081
  volume-loading hypertension, peripheral, 1048
Autotransplantation, 1570
Azathioprine, 1829
  cardiac transplant, 1830
Azepexole, characterization, 2236
Azotemia, 1556

B

B-HT 920, characterization, 2236
B-HT 933, characterization, 2236
Baroreceptor, arterial pressure control system, 1032–1033
  feedback gain, 1032
Baroreceptor control disturbance, hypertension, 707
Baroreceptor deafferentation, neurogenic hypertension, 734–735
Baroreceptor mechanism, reflex activity, 2238
Baroreceptor reflex, eicosanoid, 833
Baroreceptor signal, renin-secretory response, 1098–1099
Baroreflex, 1462–1465. *See also* Arterial baroreflex; Cardiopulmonary baroreflex
  age, 2172
  arterial function table, 1462
  arterial sensitivity, 1462–1465
  cardiopulmonary, 1465
  cardiopulmonary function table, 1465
  cardiovascular response, 1462–1465
  nifedipine, 2172
Bartter's syndrome, 1634, 1636, 1637
Basal body sodium, 211
  hypertension, 211–212
  primary aldosteronism, 211
  sodium homeostasis, setpoint, 1360–1361
Basal oxygen consumption, hypothyroidism, 1670
Basement membrane
  normal tubular, 1056
  proximal, 1056
Basolateral membrane
  aldosterone, 1282
  sodium-potassium ATPase, 1133
Bayliss reflex, 42
Behavioral factors, hypertension, 2083–2089
Bendrofluazide
  coronary event, 1947
  side effects, 201
  stroke, 1946, 1947, 1974

Bendroflumethiazide
  dosage, 2144
  dosage interval, 2144
  duration of action, 2144
  hypomagnesemia, 1009
  magnesium, 1009
Benign hypertension, smooth muscle proliferation, 528
  mass vs. number, 528–529
  therapy mass effects, 529
  therapy number effects, 529
1-Benzylimidazole-5-acetate derivative
  binding affinities, 2355–2356
  structural formula, 2354, 2355
Bergen Long-Term Study on Central Hemodynamics, 313–318
  ten-year follow-up, 313–314
    exercise, 314–315
    rest, 314–315
  twenty-year follow-up, 315–317
    hemodynamics, 316–317
    treated group, 317
    young vs. old hemodynamic pattern, 317–318
Beri-beri heart disease, 289
Beta-1 adrenoceptor, renin secretion, 1379–1380
Beta-2 adrenoceptor, renin secretion, 1379–1380
Beta-1-receptor blocker, renin, 1295
Beta-adrenergic blocker, 1656, 1668
  adverse effects, 1898
  arterial compliance, 1413
  development, 2100
  pregnancy, 1820–1821
Beta-adrenergic receptor, 1663
Beta-adrenergic stimulation, 1666
  renin secretion, 621
Beta blocker, 1549, 1564, 1656, 1727, 1728, 2121, 2181–2203, 2188. *See also* Specific type
  abrupt withdrawal, 2201–2203
  age, 2173–2174, 2193–2195
  alpha-1-blocker, 2246
    plus diuretic, 2246
  aluminum hydroxide gel, 2202
  aminophylline, 2202
  anesthesia, 2197
  angina, 2189
  angiotensin-converting enzyme inhibitor, 2221
  antidiabetic agent, 2202
  antihypertensive agent, 1644
  antihypertensive mode of action, 2185–2188
  arterial baroreceptor resetting, 2186–2187
  asthma, 2189, 2199–2200
  atrioventricular conduction defect, 2189
  beta-adrenoceptor blockade, 2188
  blood pressure, 530
  bradycardia, 2189
  bronchitis, 2189
  bronchospasm, 2189
  calcium-channel inhibitor, 2202
  cardiac output, 2186
  cardioselective, 1732, 1735
  cardioselective vs. nonselective, 2189–2190
  cardiovascular hemodynamics, 2119–2123
    acute hemodynamic effects, 2119–2120
    long-term hemodynamic effects, 2120–2121
  cardiovascular hypertrophy, 530
  central nervous system, 2187–2188
    side effects, 2201
  cimetidine, 2202
  clinical features, 2292
  clinical pharmacology, 2184–2185
  clonidine, 2189, 2192, 2202
  combination therapy, 2191–2193
  congestive heart failure, 2189
  contraindicated, 2199–2201
  coronary disease, 2109
  depression, 2189
  diabetes, 2189
    insulin-dependent, 2201
  dietary sodium restriction, 2017
  digitalis glycoside, 2202
  diltiazem, 2202
  diuretic, 2191, 2192
  drug interactions, 2201, 2202
  elderly, 2195
  epinephrine, 2202
  ergot alkaloid, 2202
  exercise, 1994, 2128
  eye, 2201
  gastrointestinal side effects, 2201
  glucagon, 2202
  guanethidine, 2192
  halofenate, 2202
  heart failure, 2199–2200
  hemodynamics, 323, 2186
  hyperlipidemia, 2189
  hypertension treatment, 1732
    cardiac arrhythmia, 2196
    complicated, 2195–2197
    diabetes, 2196
    ischemic heart disease, 2195–2196
    lipid disorder, 2196
    postmyocardial infarction, 2195–2196
    renal impairment, 2196
  hypertensive urgency, 2282–2283
  impotence, 2200–2201
  indomethacin, 2202
  insulin, 2189
  interactions, 2292–2293
    antihypertensive drugs, 2292–2293
  intermittent claudication, 2189
  intrinsic sympathomimetic, 2183, 2184
  intrinsic sympathomimetic activity, clinical relevance, 2190–2191
  isoproterenol, 2202
  levodopa, 2202
  lidocaine, 2202
  membrane-stabilizing effect, 2183, 2184
  metabolic side effect, 2132
  methyldopa, 2192, 2202
  migraine, 2189, 2197
  mode of action, 2292
  monoamine oxidase inhibitor, 2202
  mucous membrane, 2201
  muscle cramp, 2201
  myocardial infarction, 2109, 2197–2199
  nifedipine, 2192
  oculomucocutaneous syndrome, 2189
  overdose treatment, 2203
  peripheral vascular disease, 2201
  pharmacology, 2182–2183
  phenothiazine, 2202
  phenylpropranolamine, 2202
  phenytoin, 2202
  pheochromocytoma, 1657, 2189, 2195
    malignant, 1657
  plasma renin activity, 2173–2174
  plasma volume, 2188
  prazosin, 2192
  pregnancy, 2197
  pressure regulation, 1555
  prostaglandin, 2188
  quinidine, 2202
  Raynaud's phenomenon, 2189, 2200
  renal failure, 2189
  renin, 2193–2195
  renin release, 2186
  renovascular hypertension, 2195
  reserpine, 2192, 2202
  selection, 2110–2114
    clinical factors, 2189
  side effects, 2199–2201
  skin, 2201
  stroke volume, 2125
  structure, 2182
  sudden death, 2197
  sulfonylurea, 2189
  sympatholytic drug, 2192
  thyrotoxicosis, 2189
  tolerability, 2199–2201
  total peripheral resistance, 2125
  tricyclic antidepressant, 2202
  tubocurarine, 2202
  vasodilation, 2191
  vasodilator, 2191–2192
  verapamil, 2202
Beta-endorphin, 796
Beta-microglobulin, proximal tubular function, 1502
Beta-microglobulinuria, 1503
Beta-phenylethylamine, 1911
Beta thromboglobulin, 133
Betaxolol
  alpha-blocking properties, 2119
  beta-1-adrenoceptor selectivity, 2119
  intrinsic sympathomimetic activity, 2119
Bevantolol
  alpha-blocking properties, 2119
  beta-1-adrenoceptor selectivity, 2119, 2183
  beta-blocking metabolites, 2183
  beta-blocking plasma concentration, 2183

bioavailability, 2183
dosage, 2184
dosage frequency, 2184
equipotent single dose, 2184
intrinsic sympathomimetic activity, 2119, 2183
lipophilicity, 2183
membrane-stabilizing effect, 2183
plasma half-life, 2184
protein binding, 2183
Bezold-Jarisch-like reflex, serotonin, 763
Bilateral renal artery stenosis, 1550, 1551, 1555
Bilateral renal parenchymal disease, 1585–1591
neurogenic factors, 1586
Bilateral stenosis, renovascular hypertension, 1543–1545
Bilateral ureteral obstruction, 1603–1606
hypertension, 1605–1606
Binding protein, serotonin, 763
Binephrectomy, hypertension control, 1586
Binswanger's disease, 425–426
clinical correlates, 426
white-matter lesions, 426
Biochemical signaling pathway, 596
Biofeedback
hypertension treatment, 2088–2089
nursing management, 2067–2068
Biopsy
nonplacental bed, 1785
renal, 1719
uteroplacental bed, 1782, 1783
Biosynthesis, juxtaglomerular cell tumor, 1579–1580
Biotransformation
doxazosin, 2242
phenoxybenzamine, 2241
phentolamine, 2241
prazosin, 2241–2242
terazosin, 2242
trimazosin, 2242
urapidil, 2242
Bisoprolol
alpha-blocking properties, 2119
beta-1-adrenoceptor selectivity, 2119, 2183
beta-blocking metabolites, 2183
beta-blocking plasma concentration, 2183
bioavailability, 2183
dosage, 2184
dosage frequency, 2184
equipotent single dose, 2184
intrinsic sympathomimetic activity, 2119, 2183
lipophilicity, 2183
membrane-stabilizing effect, 2183
plasma half-life, 2184
protein binding, 2183
Black patient, 1154–1155. *See also* Race
alcohol, 280
calcium, 230, 234
sodium, 234
calcium antagonist, 2173–2174, 2175
child's blood pressure, 1858
defined, 1837
diltiazem, 2173–2174, 2175
hypertension, 159–173, 222, 1743, 1837–1848
cerebrovascular damage, 1841
clinical epidemiology, 167–170
education, 162
epidemiology, 1837–1838
genetics, 161–162
heart disease, 1838–1840
homogeneity, 161
inequality, 161
prevalence, 166–167
reasons for racial differences, 1841–1845
renal damage, 1840–1841
skin color, 161–162
socioeconomic status, 161
target organ damage, 1838–1841
vascular disease, 1838–1841
vs. African, 161, 1838
West Indian, 1838
Western Hemisphere vs. Africa, 1845
hypertension treatment
angiotensin-converting enzyme inhibitor, 1848
beta-blockers, 1847–1848
calcium-channel blockers, 1847
clonidine, 1848
combined alpha-beta blockers, 1847
cost, 1846
diuretics, 1846–1847
guanabenz, 1848
hydralazine, 1848
hydrochlorothiazide, 1846
methyldopa, 1848
nonpharmacologic therapy, 1846
pharmacologic therapy, 1846
prazosin, 1848
reserpine, 1848
side effects, 1846
left ventricular hypertrophy
education, 168–169
five-year mortality, 170
incidence, 169
mortality, 169
regression, 169
socioeconomic status, 169, 170
stepped-care program, 169–170
mortality, 1944
nicardipine, 2173–2174, 2175
nifedipine, 2173–2174, 2175
nitrendipine, 2173–2174, 2175
potassium, 49, 50, 217, 222
vs. white
environmental factors, 1842
genetic hypothesis, 1842–1845
pathogenetic hypotheses, 1842
reasons for racial differences, 1841–1845
Blood cell
human, 662–663
divalent ion concentrations, 663
hypertension, 662–663
Blood cell regulation
K^+
family history, 929
normotensives, 929
skin fibroblasts, 929
Na^+
family history, 929
normotensives, 929
skin fibroblasts, 929
Blood flow, skeletal muscle, 320
cardiac output, 320
early mild hypertension, 320
Blood lipid, coronary disease, 107–109
Blood pressure
acculturation adaptation, 139–140
varieties, 140
angiotensin-converting enzyme inhibitor, 530
adaptation, 138, 140
adoption study, 93–94
diastolic, 94
environment, 94
systolic, 94
alcohol, 277–291
hospitalized problem drinkers, 283–284
prospective studies, 283
alpha blocker, 530
angiotensin, 1354–1355
angiotensin II
potassium, 998–999
sensitivity to increase, 1124–1125
arterial baroreflex, 1463–1464
arterial wall tension
albumin, 120
lipid, 120
arteriolar wall, 51–52
atenolol, 530
atrial natriuretic factor, 869
beta blocker, 530
blood rheology, 334–335
experimental manipulations, 334–335
blood viscosity, 329–330
body weight, 1743
body weight change, 1744
calcium, 229–230, 249
28-day diet history, 232
24-hr recall, 230
animal studies, 234
calcium-regulating hormones, 235
calcium supplementation, 233–235
cellular effects, 235–236
dairy products, 230
dietary intake, 230–232
geographic patterns, 229–230
Guatemala, 234
hypertensive, 230, 234
Italy, 231–232
Japanese-American, 230
mechanisms, 235–236
Netherlands, 230–231
NHANES-I, 232

Blood pressure, calcium (*contd.*)
NHANES-II, 232
normotensive, 230, 234
population surveys, 230, 231
Puerto Rico, 232
renin-angiotensin, 235
rural Iowa, 231
salmon calcitonin, 233
South African black, 231
stanozolol, 233
upper-middle-class, 230
Western Electric Study, 232
calcium antagonist, 485–507
hypertensive animals, 485–490
calcium entry blocker, 530
calcium overload
normal, 474–485
pathogenic role, 474–485
captopril, 530, 1352–1353
cardiopulmonary receptor, 349–350
cardiovascular disease, 1942
casein, 251
changes without treatment, 18
characteristic distribution by sex, 87
children
black, 1858
body size, 1858–1859
measurement, 1853–1854
natural history, 1854–1859
normal, 1854–1856
race, 1858
sex, 1859
tracking, 1856–1858
white, 1858
clonidine, 530
comprehensive population-based studies, 86
continuous, 87
continuous frequency curves, 87
coronary atheroma, 120–121
counterregulation model, 1418
cross-cultural studies, 139–140
differential mortality, 140
overgeneralization, 140
cultural factors, 92–93
blacks, 92–93
Brazilian, 92–93
child, 92–93
Japanese-American, 92–93
Tecumseh, 92–93
Tokelau, 92–93
whites, 92–93
diabetes, 1724
experimental, 1018
diet, 248–250
dietary fiber, 249–250, 251
dietary Na/K molar ratio, 991
dietary potassium, 991, 1146–1147
dietary protein, 250–252
dietary sodium
black loading, 2003
clinical studies, 1999–2007
epidemiological studies, 2000
human loading, 2003, 2005
restriction in normal human, 2014
white loading, 2003
distribution, 87
diuretics, 530
ecological aspects, 137–143
endurance training, 1988–1993
blood pressure at rest, 1988–1991
blood pressure change mechanisms, 1992–1993
blood pressure during 24-hr period, 1992
blood pressure during exercise, 1991–1992
hemodynamic data, 1992
humoral data, 1992–1993
essential hypertension, 1352–1353, 1750
animal models, 334
evolutionary aspects, 137–143
assumptions, 137–138
definitions, 137–138
excessive reduction, 1949–1950, 1962, 2138
J-shaped relationship, 1962
myocardial infarction, 1962
exercise, 1985–1988
age, 1987
exercise-related sudden death, 1988
eye-fundus grade, 1987
maximal capacity, 1986–1987
prognostic significance, 1987
serum creatinine, 1987
Sokolow index, 1987
experimental situation, 306, 334–335
extracellular fluid volume, 58
familial aggregation
adults, 88–89
children, 89–90
extent, 88–90
first-degree relative, 86
historical aspects, 84
infants, 90
maternal-offspring, 89–90
newborn, 90
over time, 89
sibling, 88, 89–90
spouse pairs, 89
fat, 249, 257–273
felodipine, 530
fiber, 249–250, 251
furosemide, 530
genetic epidemiology, 81–98, 92–93
blacks, 92–93
Brazilian, 92–93
changes over time, 96
child, 92–93
developmentally regulated gene, 96–97
genetic mechanism, 95–96
genetic risk, 97–98
intermediate phenotypes, 96, 97
Japanese-American, 92–93
Mendelian locus, 97
Na-Li countertransport, 97
physiological processes, 96
Platt-Pickering controversy, 95–96
realistic genetic models, 95–97
sodium, 96
Tecumseh, 92–93
Tokelau, 92–93
whites, 92–93
genetics, 138, 902
Dahl rat gene structure, 959–961
F2 hybrids, 902–903
genomic DNA, 960, 961
molecular, 959–963
R renin gene restriction map, 960
renin allele co-segregation analysis, 961–963
restriction fragment-length polymorphism, 959
restriction fragment-length polymorphism generation mechanism, 959
S renin gene restriction map, 960
height, 45
hemodynamic methods, 306
hydralazine, 530
hydrochlorothiazide, 530
6-hydroxydopamine, 530
infant, 1854–1856, 1857
birth weight, 1856, 1857
insulin, 1749
intra-arterial method, 306
kidney, 1089
lability, 1408–1409
lead, 236–238
epidemiologic observations, 237
intracellular metabolic processes, 238
mechanisms, 237–238
NHANES II, 237
renin-angiotensin system, 238
level redefinition, 176–177
life expectancy, 189–190
magnesium, 229–230, 236, 249
geographic patterns, 229–230
low blood pressure, 236
magnesium deficiencies, 236
Newfoundland, 236
other nutrients, 236
magnesium metabolism, 2053–2054
measurement. *See* Blood pressure measurement
meat protein, 251
metallic ion intake, 229
methyldopa, 530
mortality, 180, 181
nature vs. nurture, 81–98
African, 83
black, 83–84
between population contrast, 83–84
Caribbean, 84
environmental components, 83
exercise, 83
family set method, 91
historical aspects, 81
lifestyle factors, 83
path analysis, 90–93
personality profile, 83
Polynesian, 83
smoking, 83
sodium, 83
stress, 83
Westernized lifestyle, 84
white, 83
neuropeptide, 791–800
in abnormalities, 799–800
angiotensin II, 791

blood vessels, 792–794
blood vessel walls, 792–793
bradykinin, 791
cardiac activity, 793, 794
cardiac function, 792–794
cardiac localization, 793, 794
central site, 792
heart, 792–794
insulin, 792
mechanism of action, 792–794
other neurotransmitter interactions, 793–794
other vasoactive hormone interactions, 793–794
parathyroid hormone, 791
peripheral site, 792
prolactin, 791
sauvagine, 792
vascular smooth muscle, 792–794
nifedipine, 530
non-Newtonian behavior, 330
non-Western population studies
measurement error, 138–139
research design, 138
sampling bias, 138
nonsteroidal anti-inflammatory drug, 833
norepinephrine, potassium, 998–999
obesity, 82–83
nature vs. nurture within-population contrast, 82–83
omega 3 fatty acid, 263–264
omega 6 fatty acid, 258–263
community-based studies, 268–270
dietary intervention studies, 264–271
epidemiologic studies, 270–271
free-living studies, 264–268
humans, 264–271
prostaglandin studies, 271–272
vegetarian diet, 270
phentolamine, 530
physical training, 1988–1993
plasma vasopressin, 780–781
baroreflexes, 780
concentrations, 780
constrictor effect, 780
direct pressor action, 780
sympathetic nervous system, 780–781
vasoactive hormone interaction, 780
polyunsaturated fat, 257
population biology, 140–142
cold stress, 141–142
heat stress, 141
high-altitude hypoxia, 140–141
potassium, 217–225
24-hr dietary recall, 217–218
24-hr urinary excretion, 218
angiotensin, 224
between-individual comparisons, 217
between-population comparisons, 217
blacks, 50, 217
cross-cultural comparisons, 217
effects, 219–223
eicosanoid metabolism, 224
England, 50
epidemiologic surveys, 217
hypertensives, 218
INTERSALT study, 218–219
intervention studies, 217
Japan, 50, 217
kallikrein-kinin system, 224
mechanisms of action, 223–224
migration studies, 217
natriuresis, 223
NHANES-I, 218
norepinephrine, 224
in normal human, 218, 220
northern Iran, 50
Norway, 50
primitive peoples, 50
protective effects, 220
renin-angiotensin system, 223
renin release, 223
sympathetic nervous system, 224
systolic pressure, 218
United States, 217
vasodilatation, 223
within-population surveys, 217
prazosin, 530
predictive value, 154
pregnancy, 1770
prevalence measurements, 175
propranolol, 530
prostaglandin, 258–263, 263–264
protein, 250–252
renal failure, 1709
renal involvement, 1719
renin-angiotensin-aldosterone system, 1288, 1443
sodium volume, 1303–1306
renin genotype, 962
renohepatic axis, 856–858
BW755C, 857
cytochrome-P450-dependent enzyme system, 857
isolated liver perfusion, 856–857
renoportal venous shunt, 856, 857
systemic circulation liver removal, 856, 857
reserpine, 530
rise with age, 87
Riva Rocci method, 306
saturated fat, 257
single-gene etiology, 86
smoking, 1918–1919
sodium, 205–212
epidemiological data, 205–208
physiological rationale, 2004–2005
sodium sensitivity, 2006–2007
genetic susceptibility, 2001
soya protein, 251
statistical characteristics, 87
strength training, 1993
stroke, 19
high, 412
treatment problems, 412
systolic pressure, tracking, 1857
thyroid hormone, 1661, 1665–1667
treatment decision. *See* Treatment decision
treatment continuance, 1972–1976
controlled trials, 1972–1973
J-shaped curve, 1973–1976
twin study, 93, 94–95
dizygotic, 95
monozygotic, 95
unimodal, 87
variability, 18
vasodilator, 530
vegetarian diet, 244–248
mechanisms of action, 252
Blood pressure measurement, 1976–1977
ambulatory, blood pressure measurement pressor effect, 1977–1978
blood variability, 1977
casual blood pressure, 1976–1977
clinic measurement accuracy, 1407–1413, 1429
cuff artifact, 1408–1411
iatrophobia, 1408
pseudonormotension, 1411–1413
white-coat syndrome, 1408
drawbacks, 1979–1980
exercise, 1976–1977
historical aspects, 2095
importance, 18
invasive techniques, 1977
mild hypertension, 18
noninvasive monitor, 1433–1439
noninvasive techniques, 1436–1438, 1977
nursing management, 2064–2065
clinic measurement, 2064–2065
home readings, 2065
office blood pressure, 1976–1977
physical examination, 1389
posture, 1976
repeated, 18
rest, 1976–1977
risk prediction, 1978–1979
therapy efficacy, 1978
Blood Pressure Study 180, 1979
Blood pressure variation, 1397–1403, 1408–1409, 1415–1425
antihypertensive treatment, 1402–1403
cardiac denervation, 1401
cigarette smoking, 1420
circadian rhythm, 1398–1399
dehydration/volume depletion, 1420
diurnal variation, 1397–1403, 1420
exercise, 1399, 1419
hypoglycemia, 1420
idiopathic orthostatic hypotension, 1401
menstrual cycle, 1420
mental activity, 1400
other sources, 1399–1403
pain, 1419
pathophysiology, 1416–1418
physical activity, 1399–1400
ingestion, 1400
physical factors, 1416
physiologic regulation, 1402
time course, 1402
postprandial alterations, 1419–1420
posture, 1419

Blood pressure variation (*contd.*)
psychological stress responses, 1420–1421
respiration, 1418–1419
seasonal variation, 1401, 1420
sexual intercourse, 1399
sleep, 1397–1398, 1400–1401, 1403
stages, 1397–1398
sleep apnea syndrome, 1401
sleep/arousal, 1418
temperature change, 1420
vascular compliance, 1416
wakefulness, 1397–1398
white-coat hypertension, 1419
Blood-retinal barrier, pathologic alterations, 435–436
Blood rheology, 330–331, 332
Blood sugar, hypertension, 103
Blood urea nitrogen, glomerular filtration rate, 1495
Blood vessel, serotonin, 763–765
Blood viscosity
blood pressure, 329–330
factors determining, 330–331
hematocrit, 330
hypertension
alpha-blocker, 335
alpha-methyldopa, 335
alprenolol, 335
atenolol, 335
beta-blocker, 335
calcium antagonist, 335
diuretics, 335
hematocrit variation, 332–333
ketanserin, 335
medication effects, 335
nicardipine, 335
oxprenolol, 335
plasma composition variation, 331–333
prazosin, 335
RBC aggregation variation, 333
RBC deformability variation, 333
timolol, 335
viscosity variation, 331–333
left ventricular hypertrophy, 334
plasma renin, 333
red blood cell, 330–331
shear rate, 330, 331
vascular response, 333
Blood volume
body weight, 341–342
cardiac output, 1745
central. *See* Central blood volume
clinical considerations, 340–341
diastolic pressure, 345
essential hypertension, 346
height, 341–344, 345
hypertension, 344–346
aldosterone profiling, 344
conflicting results, 345–346
renin profiling, 344
measurement, 340–341
BVA-100, 344
indicator dye dilution technique, 341
mean body hematocrit, 341
normal, 341–344
radioactive isotope, 341
measurements, 339–346
in normal human, 342
technical considerations, 340–341
Body fat distribution, 1744, 1746–1749
hyperinsulinemia, 1747–1748
Body mass index, 1741
Body-size correction, hemodynamic methods, 306
Body sodium, 210–211
components, 211
Body weight. *See also* Obesity
blood pressure, 1743
blood volume, 341–342
change, blood pressure effects, 1744
renin genotype, 962
Bombesin, 795
Bone, calcium, 983–984
Bopindolol
beta-1-selectivity, 2183
beta-blocking metabolites, 2183
beta-blocking plasma concentration, 2183
bioavailability, 2183
cardiac output, 2121–2123
dosage, 2184
dosage frequency, 2184
equipotent single dose, 2184
heart rate, 2121–2123
intrinsic sympathomimetic activity, 2183
lipophilicity, 2183
mean arterial pressure, 2121–2123
membrane-stabilizing effect, 2183
plasma half-life, 2184
protein binding, 2183
stroke volume, 2121–2123
total peripheral resistance, 2121–2123
Borderline hypertension, 1736
age, 175, 176
anxiety, 2086
autonomic nervous system, 2084–2085
cardiac output, 2086
cardiopulmonary reflex, 351–353
mortality, underweight, 183, 186
nervousness, 2086
office evaluation, 1388
peripheral circulation, 320
potassium, 220
prevalence, 175, 176
insured lives, 180
race, 175, 176
renal circulation, 320
sex, 175, 176
splanchnic circulation, 320
Bowman's capsule, kallikrein, 1063
Bradbury-Eggleston syndrome
HLA A:w32, 757
norepinephrine, 757
prognosis, 757
Bradycardia, beta-blocker, 2189
Bradykinin, 795, 805, 808, 819
analogues, 812
angiotensin-converting enzyme, 1221
endothelium-derived relaxing factor, 831, 1255
kinin antagonist, 811–812
kininase II, 1296
nitric oxide, 638
structure, 812
Bradykinin-containing peptide, 805
Brain
angiotensinogen, 1206–1207
hypertension, structural vascular changes, 403
renin, 1321
serotonin
ascending serotonin pathways, 767, 768
descending serotonin pathways, 768–769
level alteration, 767
serotonin-containing neuron
morphology, 766
projections, 766–767
third ventricle, 58–59
Brain stem
distortion in hypertension, 707
sympathoadrenomedullary system, 712–716
Branch retinal vein occlusion, 457
Breathing exercise, nursing management, 2067–2068
Bretylium, 2096
Bright's disease
classification, 38
vascular lesion, 38
Britain, systolic pressure, 147–148
BRL 34915, 2271
Bronchitis, beta-blocker, 2189
Bronchospasm, beta-blocker, 2189
Bruit, 1390–1391
Bucindolol, vasodilation, 2191
Buffer barrier, calcium, 553–555
Bumetanide
chemical structure, 2144
dosage, 2144
dosage interval, 2144
duration of action, 2144
BW755C, 857
Byrom, Frank, 33–47

C

Ca^{2+}, 471
Ca^{2+}-ATPase, 929
cell membrane transport pathway, 923–924
increased, cellular Na^{+} homeostasis, 930–931
Na^{+}-Ca^{2+}, 929
platelet, circulating factors, 929
regulation abnormalities, 929
Na^{+} abnormality, 930–932
Ca^{2+} antagonist, Mg^{2+}, 1019
Ca^{2+}-ATPase
Ca^{2+}, 929
essential hypertension
basal, 929
calmodulin, 929

Degradation, cAMP, synthesis, 619–620
Dehydration/volume depletion, blood pressure variation, 1420
Dehydrogenase
calcium, 970
mitochondria, 970
Dental abnormality, hyperkalemia, 1630
11-Deoxycorticosterone. *See* DOC
11-Deoxycorticosterone acetate. *See* DOCA
Depression
beta-blocker, 2189
centrally-acting antihypertensive agents, 2253
elderly, 201
Depressor compound, 1586
Des-arg-9-bradykinin, 819
Dexatrim, 1913
Diabetes, 12. *See also* Experimental diabetes
angiotensin-converting enzyme inhibitor, 2220
antihypertensive treatment
diabetic diets, 1728, 1730, 1732
pharmacological treatment, 1730–1733
arterial occlusive disease, 1709
arterial pressure, 1695
atrial natriuretic factor, 872
autonomic neuropathy, 758
beta-blocker, 2189
insulin-dependent, 2201
blood pressure elevation, 1724
calcium, 476–477
carotid artery occlusive disease, 1709
congestive heart failure, 1709
coronary disease, 1708–1709
health education, 1736
hypertension, 109, 1689, 1703
diagnosis and treatment, 1728–1735
epidemiology, 1705–1707
management, 1717–1718
pathogenesis, 1724, 1727
treatment, 1734
weight reduction, 1734
hypervolemia, 1689–1691
hypomagnesemia, 1011
experimental diabetes serum magnesium, 1012
insulin-dependent, 1011
red blood cell magnesium level, 1012
skeletal muscle magnesium level, 1012
urine magnesium level, 1012
insulin-dependent, 130, 1718
hypertension, 1696, 1697
mortality, 1733, 1735
juvenile-onset, 130
magnesium, 1010–1013
malignant hypertension, 1707
maturity-onset, 130–131
microangiopathy, 1683–1684
mortality, 183
myocardial infarction, 1709
nephropathy, 1718–1721
noninsulin-dependent, 130–131, 1718
elderly, 1737
essential hypertension, 1697
hypertension, 1696, 1697
obesity, 1690, 1692, 1693
proteinuria, 1706, 1707, 1708, 1710
renal hypertrophy, 1707
renal sodium handling, 1749
renin-angiotensin system, 1689, 1690, 1691–1692
renovascular hypertension, 1707
secondary hypertension, 1706–1707
sodium homeostasis, 1690
sodium hypertension, 1706–1707
sudden death, 112
systemic hypertension, 1677, 1680
type I, coronary atherosclerosis, 130
type II, 130–131
Diabetic nephropathy, 1710
Diabetic glomerulopathy, 1678
antihypertensive therapy, 1682–1683
filtration surface area, 1158
hypertension, 1680–1682
nephron number, 1157–1158
sodium, 1158
systemic hypertension, 1681
Diabetic glomerulosclerosis, 1710
Diabetic hyperfiltration, potential mediators, 1679
Diabetic hypertension
hemodynamic factors, 1695–1696
insulin, 1691–1694
metabolic control, 1694
nephropathy, 1696–1697
renin-angiotensin system, 1691–1692
sodium, 1689–1691
vascular reactivity, 1694–1695
Diabetic nephropathy, 1588, 1728
angiotensin-converting enzyme, 1730
antihypertensive treatment, 1732–1733
blood pressure changes, 1722
essential hypertension, 1724
microalbuminuria, 1719–1721
natural history, 1729
prevention, 1736–1737
proteinuria, 1737
renal function, 1733
sodium retention, 1722
Diabetic nephropathy stage, hypertension, 1705–1708
Diabetic renal disease
progression, 1680
type I diabetes, 130
Diabetic retinopathy, 1680
Diacylglycerol
angiotensin II
acidification, 592
low temperature, 591
antiogensin II, 587, 588
protein kinase C, 587–588
1,2-Diacylglycerol, 603
functions, 604–605
production, 603–604
Diagnosis, 14, 1963–1964. *See also* Treatment decision
differential diagnosis, 1385–1395
elderly, 1964
false negative consequences, 1407–1408
flow diagram, 1393
labeling, 1950, 2069
middle-aged patient, 1964
multiple visits, 1386
temporary hypertension drug therapy cessation, 1386
younger patient, 1964
Diagnosis *ex juvantibus*, 2110
Dialysis, 1586
extracellular fluid volume, 58
Diastolic filling
cardiac ventricle, 567
malignant hypertension, 312
Diastolic hypertension, pheochromocytoma, 1641
Diastolic pressure, 1796
age, 102, 104
blood volume, 345
calcium, 234
cardiac event, 1974
children, 1854
coronary disease, 1971
diagnosing hypertension, 1964
1,25-dihydroxyvitamin D, 2045
distribution, 1968
elderly, 191, 1870, 1871
insulin-dependent diabetes, 1723
magnesium, 2055
mortality, 183, 184, 1975–1976
English, 184
European, 184
myocardial infarction, 1975–1976
perinatal mortality, 1810
plasma renin activity, 2186, 2187
plasma volume, 345
propranolol, 2186, 2187
serum ionized calcium, 2045
sitting rest, 1985–1986
sodium, 2045
stroke, 1974
subscapular skinfold thickness, 105
supine rest, 1985–1986
taurine/creatinine, 300
treatment initiation, 1967–1969
type I diabetes, 130
urinary albumin excretion, diabetic nephropathy, 1726
waist/hip ratio, 132
worksite measurement, 1977
Diazoxide
arteriole, circulatory effects, 2266
cerebral circulation, 408
circulatory effects, 2270–2274
clinical features, 2297
emergency blood pressure lowering, 410
hypertensive emergency, 2279–2281
hypertensive emergency in child, 1865
interactions, 2297
antihypertensive drugs, 2297
metabolism, 2271
mode of action, 2270–2274, 2297
mode of use, 2271
pharmacokinetics, 2271
predominant hemodynamic effect, 2125

Diazoxide (*contd.*)
 pregnancy, 1816–1818
 side effects, 2271
 tolerance, 2271
 toxicity, 2271
Diet, 49–51, 241–253. *See also* Specific type
 atherogenesis, 109
 blood pressure, lowering dietary constituents, 248–250
 cerebral lesion, 296–297
  animal models, 296–297
 cholesterol, 245
 complex, 242–244
 coronary disease, 245
 cross-sectional observation studies, 243
 dietary change, 243–244
 dietary intervention trial, 242
 heart disease, 7
 high-potassium, 49–56
 high-protein, tubuloglomerular feedback, 1079
 high-salt
  converting-enzyme inhibition, 1359
  renal blood flow, 1359
 hypertension, 109, 245
 low-protein, urinary protein excretion, 1166
 low-sodium, 1446, 1447
  development, 2095
 methodological issues, 241–242
 migration study, 243
 Mormon, 246
 NIHONSAN study, 243
 population study, 242
 rural vs. urban areas, 243
 Samoan study, 142
 subcultures, 243
 types of data, 242
 unacculturated populations, 243
Dietac, 1913
Dietary calcium
 calcitonin-gene-related peptide, 2049
 central nervous system, 2049
 1,25-dihydroxyvitamin D, 2049–2051
 hypertension treatment, 2052–2056
  1,25-dihydroxyvitamin D, 2049–2051
  mechanism of action, 2049
  oral supplementation, 2046–2049
  parathyroid hormone, 2049–2051
  plasma renin activity, 2046, 2047
  rationale, 2039–2040
  salt-insensitive essential hypertensive subjects, 2046, 2048
  salt-sensitive essential hypertensive subjects, 2046, 2048
  serum ionized calcium, 2046, 2047
Dietary chloride
 Dahl S rat, 2021–2022
 DOCA hypertension, 2021
 essential hypertension, 2022
 salt-sensitive hypertension, 2021–2023
Dietary cholesterol, genetic differences, 295
Dietary fat, 1753
Dietary fiber
 blood pressure, 249–250, 251
 hypotensive response, 1753–1754
Dietary intake, sympathetic activity, 1751
Dietary intervention study, 114
 diet, 242
 nutrition, 242
Dietary Intervention Study in Hypertension, 2030
Dietary lipid, genetic differences, 295
Dietary magnesium
 cardiovascular-hypertensive disease, 1010
 hypertension, 2055–2056
  therapy rationale, 2052
 hypertension treatment, 2052–2056
Dietary magnesium deficiency
 hypertension, 1017
  arteriolar tone, 1017
  venular tone, 1017
 stress-induced hypertension, 1017
  arteriolar tone, 1017
  venular tone, 1017
Dietary sodium/potassium molar ratio, blood pressure, 991
Dietary potassium, 49–56
 adrenal regeneration hypertension, 991
 blood pressure, 991, 1146–1147
 DOCA salt hypertension, 991
 hypertension, kallikrein, 826
 kallikrein, 824–826
 renal kallikrein, 819–827
 renovascular hypertension, 991, 992
Dietary protein
 blood pressure, 250–252
 cardiovascular disease
  amino acids, 297
  lysine, 298
  mechanisms, 297–299
  methionine, 298
  sodium excretion, 298–299
  sympathetic nerve activity, 298
  taurine, 298
  urea, 298
  vascular hypertrophy, 297
 glomerular hemodynamics, 1164
 hypertension, 295–300
  epidemiologic studies, 299–300
  human, 299–300
  Japanese origin living in Hawaii, 299
  sodium/creatinine ratio, 299
  sulfate/creatinine ratio, 299
  urea/creatinine ratio, 299
  WHO-CARDIAC program, 299–300
 restriction, 1678, 1679
Dietary recall, 217–218
 problems, 217–218
Dietary sodium
 blood pressure
  black loading, 2003
  clinical studies, 1999–2007
  epidemiological studies, 2000
  human loading, 2003, 2005
  white loading, 2003
 extremely low intake, 2003–2004
 Framingham study, 2001
 high intake studies, 2000–2002
 industrialized cultures, 2000–2001
 infant, 2000
 Japan, 2000–2001
  programs to change, 2001
 methods of estimating, 1999–2000
 restriction, 1589, 2003–2004, 2005–2006
  hyperkalemia, 1636–1637
 urinary measurement, 1999
  urinary creatinine excretion, 1999
Dietary sodium restriction, 2011–2018
 adverse effects, 2017–2018
 angiotensin-converting-enzyme inhibitor, 2017
 antihypertensive drug treatment, 2016–2017
 beta-blocker, 2017
 blood pressure, in normal human, 2014
 calcium-channel blocker, 2017
 controlled trial, 2012–2013
  initial blood pressure differences, 2013
  statistical power, 2013
  study design, 2012–2013
 converting-enzyme inhibitor, 2017
 diuretics, 2016
 essential hypertension, 2011
 hypertension treatment, 2016–2017
 metoprolol, 2017
 nifedipine, 2017
 nitrendipine, 2017
 restriction level, 2018
 secondary hypertension, 2011
 verapamil, 2017
 weight loss, 2028–2033
  compliance, 2033
  floor effect, 2030
  vs. metoprolol, 2030
Digestive system disease, mortality, 183
Digital intravenous angiogram, 2062–2063
 arterial puncture, 2062
 indications, 2062
 nursing care after, 2062
Digital subtraction angiography, 1567
 renal artery stenosis, 1522, 1523
 renovascular hypertension, 1550
Digitalis glycoside
 beta-blocker, 2202
 digitalis-like factor, 941–942
 hemodynamics, 941–942
Digitalis-like factor, 940–945
 biochemical characterization, 940–941
 digitalis glycoside, 941–942
 endogenous, 942
 free fatty acid, 940
 hemodynamics, 941–942
 hypertension
  central nervous system studies, 945
  combined defect model, 943–944
  human blood cells, 944

    increased sodium permeability models, 942–943
    membrane transport studies, 942–945
    peripheral nervous system studies, 945
    pump inhibition model, 942–943
    steroid antagonists, 944–945
    vascular growth, 945
  lipid, 940
  natriuresis, 941
  plasma factor, 940
  plasmalogen, 940
  steroid, 940–941
  tissue distribution, 941
  unknown structural class, 941
  volume regulation, 941
Dihydralazine
  cerebral circulation, 408
  emergency blood pressure lowering, 410
Dihydropyridine, 966
  age, 2173–2174
  cardiovascular hemodynamics, 2127
  plasma renin activity, 2173–2174
1,4-Dihydropyridine, calcium antagonist, 1014–1015, 1017
Dihydrotachysterol
  calcium overload, 477–478
  magnesium, 478–480
Dihydroxyphenylserine, dopamine-beta-hydroxylase deficiency, 755–756
  biochemical effects, 755–756
  cardiovascular effects, 755–756
1,25-Dihydroxyvitamin D
  aldosteronism, 2043
  calcium homeostasis, 2039–2042
  diastolic pressure, 2045
  dietary calcium, 2049–2051
  essential hypertension, 2039–2042
  secondary hyperparathyroidism, 2043
  sodium, 2045
Dilantin, calcium antagonist, 1014–1015, 1017
Diltiazem
  age, 2173–2174, 2175
  beta-blocker, 2202
  black, 2173–2174, 2175
  calcium release, 556–557
  cardiovascular hemodynamics, 2126, 2127
  chemical structure, 472
  coronary artery, 480
  exercise, 1994
  nicotine, 483, 484
  norepinephrine, 556–557
  predominant hemodynamic effect, 2125
  race, 2173–2174, 2175
  renin, 2173–2174, 2175
  specificity, 472
  very-low-density lipoprotein, 514–515
  vitamin D_3, 479, 484
Diltiazem hydrochloride, side effects, 2065
Dipeptidyl carboxypeptidase, 1217
Diphenylmethylalkylamine, calcium antagonist, 1014–1015, 1017
Diphosphonic acid derivative, atherosclerosis, 513
Dipyramidole, coronary circulation, 320
Direct education, 156
Direct nerve recording, 725
Discrete stenosis, aorta, 1546
Displacement experiment, 584
Dissecting aneurysm, 7
Dissecting aortic aneurysm, 2285
  drugs of choice, 2283
Distal convoluted tubule
  diuretic, 2147
  nomenclature, 1274
  transport, 2146
Distal delivery, potassium, 1633
Distal nephron
  juxtaglomerular apparatus, 821, 1063
  post-macula densa, 822
Distal nephron flow rate
  glomerular filtration rate, 1140
    arterial pressure, 1140
    plasma potassium, 1140
  sodium excretion, 1141
Distal nephron lumen
  kallikrein, 810
  kinin, 810
Distal tubular function, renal concentrating capacity, 1502
Distal tubule
  angiotensin II, 1118–1119
  chloride, 1072
  chloride shunt, 1633–1634
  nomenclature, 1274
  sodium reabsorption, 1633
Diuretic, 1734. *See also* Specific type
  absorption, 2150
  acid-base homeostasis, 2149
  administration, 1589
  alpha 1-blocker, 2245–2246
    plus beta-blocker, 2246
  angiotensin-converting enzyme inhibitor, 2221
  antihypertensive action mechanism, 2150–2152
  antihypertensive efficacy, 2154
  beta-blocker, 2191, 2192
  blood pressure, 530
  calcium, 2154
  cardiovascular disease, 2154–2155
  cardiovascular hemodynamics, 2118–2119
  cardiovascular hypertrophy, 530
  cholesterol, 2157
  chronic therapy, 2148–2150
  clinical efficacy, 2154–2155
  clinical features, 2293
  connecting tubule, 2147–2148
  cortical collecting duct, 2147–2148
  dietary sodium restriction, 2016
  direct vasodilator effects, 2151–2152
  distal convoluted tubule, 2147
  divalent cation homeostasis, 2150
  dosage, 2158–2159
  drug interactions, 2157–2158
  exercise, 1993, 2128
  glucose intolerance, 2157
  half-life, 2150
  hemodynamics, 2151
  hypercalcemia, 2157
  hyperkalemia, 1636, 2156–2157
  hyperuricemia, 2149–2150, 2157
  hypokalemia, 1637
    management, 2159
  hypomagnesemia, 1009
  hyponatremia, 2149, 2155
  impotence, 2158
  interactions, 2293–2294
    antihypertensive drugs, 2293–2294
  kinin, 2154
  long-term treatment, 2143–2160
  magnesium, 1009
  magnesium wasting, 2157
  mechanism of renal actions, 2144–2148
  metabolic alkalosis, 2149
  metabolic side effects, 2132, 2155–2157
  metoprolol, 2191, 2192
  mode of action, 2150, 2293
  mortality, 1961
  nonsteroidal anti-inflammatory agent, 2158
  peripheral resistance, 2154
  pharmacology, 2150
  potassium homeostasis, 2149
  potassium wasting, 2155–2156
  preeclampsia, 1813
  pregnancy, 1820–1822
  propranolol, 2191, 2192
  prostacyclin, 2154
  proximal tubule, 2145
  renal-metabolic effects, 2148–2150
  renin, 1294
  renin-angiotensin-aldosterone system, 2152–2153
  response heterogeneity, 2152–2154
  salt depletion, 2150–2151, 2152
  selection, 2110–2114, 2158–2159
  side effects, 201, 1898
  sodium-volume homeostasis, 2148–2149
  spironolactone, 2158
  sudden death, 113
  sympathetic nervous system, 2153
  thick ascending limb of Henle's loop, 2145–2146
  toxicity, 2157–2158
  ventricular arrhythmia, 113
  volume depletion, 2155
    nonresponders, 2152
    responders, 2152
Diuril, adverse effects, 1898
Diurnal blood pressure rhythm, 1397–1403, 1420. *See also* Circadian blood pressure rhythm
  altering conditions table, 1401
  effects quantified, 1400
  normal and hypertensive subjects compared, 1400–1401
Divalent cation
  calcium antagonist, 1014–1015, 1017
  homeostasis, diuretic, 2150
Dizziness, 2244
  side effects, 201

DNA synthesis
  endothelin, 654
  vascular smooth muscle, 529
Dns-Ca-Gly-Phe, chloride, 1224
DOC
  adrenal hyperplasia, 73
  adrenal-regeneration hypertension, 69–71
    DOC oversecretion, 70
    exchangeable sodium, 70–71
    Long-Evans rat, 70
    peripheral plasma, 70
  Cushing's syndrome, 73
  essential hypertension, 73
  excess, 1620–1621
  structure, 64
  vascular lesion, 44
DOC-induced hypertension
  Long-Evans rat, 65
  pathogenesis, 64–66
  renin-angiotensin system, 64–65
  sex, 65
  sodium, 64
  sodium escape, 64
  Sprague-Dawley rat, 65
  strain, 65
  vasopressin, 65
  Wistar-Furth rat, 65
  Wistar rat, 65
DOCA
  Addison's disease, 63
  apical membrane, 1281
  cortical collecting tubule, 1276
  potassium, 1276, 1281
  sodium, 1281
  structure, 64
DOCA/salt hypertension, 45
  CNS role, 687–688
  dietary chloride, 2021
  dietary potassium, 991
  discovery, 63–64
  historical aspects, 63–64
  secondary hypertension, 736
Docosahexaenoic acid, 257
Dog, angiotensinogen, 1198
Dopamine, 726–727
  dopamine-beta-hydroxylase deficiency, 752–753
  monoaminergic mechanism, 688–690
Dopamine beta-hydroxylase, guanabenz, 2254
Dopamine-beta-hydroxylase deficiency, 749–758
  autonomic maneuver cardiovascular changes, 753
  biochemical measurements, 753
  clinical characteristics, 752
  diagnosis, 752–754
  dihydroxyphenylserine, 755–756
    biochemical effects, 755–756
    cardiovascular effects, 755–756
  dopamine, 752–753
  fludrocortisone, 754
  genes, 749
  metyrosine, 754–755
  neurotransmitter synthesis, 757
  norepinephrine, 756
  pathophysiology, 749–751
  pharmacologic intervention cardiovascular changes, 753
  phenylpropanolamine, 754
  plasma norepinephrine, 752–753
  presentation, 751–752
  prevalence, 756
  therapy, 754–756
Dopaminergic receptor, 1640
Doppler echocardiography
  left ventricle
    diastolic performance, 1488
    pump function, 1488
  renal artery stenosis, 1489
Dorsal motor nucleus, 680
Doxazosin
  biotransformation, 2242
  characterization, 2236
  chemical structures, 2234
  dosage, 2243–2244
  efficacy, 2243
  elderly, 2247
  hemodynamics, 323
  mode of action, 2239
  pharmacokinetics, 2242
  postural hypotension, 2244
Dristan, 1913
Drowsiness
  centrally-acting antihypertensive agents, 2253
  elderly, 201
Dry mouth, centrally-acting antihypertensive agents, 2253
Dry weight reduction, blood pressure control, 1590–1591
Dye-induced nephrotoxicity, 1550
Dysautonomia, 749. *See also* Hypoadrenergic dysautonomia
  acute, 758
  familial, 757–758
Dyslipidemia, 132–133, 134–135

E

Early hypertension, coronary circulation, 320
EC 3.4.15.1, 1217
Echocardiography, 1479–1490, 1543
  cost-effectiveness, 1489–1490
  examination, 1480–1482
  left ventricle, 1482–1488
    abnormal, 1485
    diastolic performance, 1488
    guidelines, 1483
    load, 1484–1485, 1486–1487
    pump function, 1488
    structure, 1482–1484, 1485
  principles, 1479–1482
Eclampsia, 1811, 1815–1816
  general approach, 1815–1816
  pituitary antidiuretic hormone, 33
Eclamptic uremia, 407
Ectopic tumor, aldosterone-producing, 1617
EDTA, atherosclerosis, 513
Education
  hypertension, prevalence, 166–167
  left ventricular hypertrophy, 168–169
  mortality, geographic distributions, 170–173
Effectiveness
  screening, 154–155
  vasodilator, 2266
Efferent arteriole, 1555
Eicosanoid, 1792
  baroreceptor reflex, 833
  chemoreceptor reflex, 833
  hypertension, 829–837
  preeclampsia, 1795–1803
  pregnancy, 1794–1795
  products, 1789–1794
  sodium, 832
  toxemia of pregnancy, 834
  water, 832
Eicosanoid metabolism, preeclampsia, 1813
Eicosapentaenoic acid, 257, 829
Eicosatetraynoic acid, endothelium-derived relaxing factor, 836
Ejection fraction, malignant hypertension, 312
Elastin, atherosclerosis, 512
Elderly patient
  alpha-blocker, 2246–2247
  beta-blocker, 2195
  blood pressure measurement, 1438–1439
  cardiovascular disease, 111
    systolic hypertension, 111
  cardiovascular mortality, 192, 193–194
  centrally-acting sympathetic inhibitor, 2258
  cerebral circulation therapy effects, 411
  clonidine, 2258
  demographics, 191
  depression, 201
  diastolic pressure, 191, 1870, 1871
  doxazosin, 2247
  drowsiness, 201
  Framingham Heart Disease Study, 191
  glucose tolerance, 200
  gout, 200
  guanabenz, 2258
  hypertension, 111, 1869–1884
    baroreceptor sensitivity, 1875
    cardiovascular disease risk, 1871–1872
    cardiovascular mortality, 192
    cellular sodium transport, 1876
    clinical assessment, 1877
    definitions, 1869–1870
    diagnosis, 1877
    diagnosis errors, 1877
    epidemiology, 191–202, 1870
    etiology, 1874–1877
    glomerular filtration rate, 1876
    hormonal changes, 1875
    hypertension risk, 1871–1872
    kidney, 1876

laboratory evaluation, 1877
left ventricular hypertrophy, 1878
measurement, 1877
mortality, 192
obesity, 1874
pathophysiology, 1872–1874
physical inactivity, 1876–1877
prevalence, 1870–1871
renin-angiotensin-aldosterone, 1875
secondary causes, 1877–1878
sex, 111
sleep apnea, 1877
sleep disorders, 1877
sympathetic nervous system, 1875–1876
target organ involvement, 111, 112
vascular changes, 1874–1875
Hypertension treatment, 1878–1883
adverse drug reactions, 1883
algorithm, 1883
alpha-1-adrenoreceptor blocker, 1881–1882
alpha-2-adrenoreceptor blocker, 1881
angiotensin-converting-enzyme inhibitor, 1882
Australian Therapeutic Trial in Mild Hypertension, 1878
calcium-channel blocker, 1882
clinical trials, 1878–1880
combination alpha-1- and beta-adrenoreceptor blocker, 1882
compliance, 1883
direct vasodilator, 1882
diuretic therapy, 1880–1881
drug treatment, 1880–1883
European Working Party on Hypertension in the Elderly, 1879–1880
guanadrel, 1882–1883
guanethidine, 1882–1883
Hypertension Detection and Follow-up Program, 1878
medication reduction, 1883
non-pharmacologic therapy, 1880
nondiuretic therapy, 1881–1883
reserpine, 1882
Veterans Administration Cooperative Study on Antihypertensive Agents, 1878
Hypertension treatment adherence, 200
Australian Therapeutic Trial in Mild Hypertension, 197–198
cardiovascular morbidity, 194
cardiovascular mortality, 194
congestive heart failure, 194
effect, 194–200
European Working Party on Hypertension in the Elderly, 198–199
Hypertension Detection and Follow-up Program, 197
hypertension-stroke cooperative study, 196–197
mild to moderate hypertension, 195–196
moderately severe hypertension, 195
observational studies, 195
randomized clinical trials, 195–200
Randomized Trial of Elderly Patients in Primary Care, 199
side effects, 200–201
stroke, 194
Systolic Hypertension in the Elderly Program, 199
Veteran's Administration Cooperative Study, 195–196
isolated systolic hypertension
cardiovascular mortality, 193–194
mortality, 193–194
lethargy, 201
methyldopa, 2258
mortality, 188, 189, 192, 193–194
all causes, 199, 200
cardiovascular mortality, 199, 200
stroke, 199, 200
nasal stuffiness, 200
NHANES II, 191
orthostatic hypotension, 201, 2246
peptic ulcer, 200
prazosin, 2246
pseudohypertension, 1438–1439
cuff artifact, 1409–1410
seizure, 200
side effects, 200
sleepiness, 200
stroke, 194
systolic hypertension, 1883–1884
systolic pressure, 191
terazosin, 2247
Electrical potential, cortical collecting tubule, 1280
Electrocardiography
abnormality in sudden death, 113
anesthesia, 1895
changes in pheochromocytoma, 1649
instrumental evaluation, 1392
laboratory evaluation, 1392
left ventricular hypertrophy
hypertension, 110–111
stroke, 112
myocardial infarction, 110–111
Electrolyte, aldosterone, 72
Electrolyte balance, 1762
Electron microscopy, renin juxtaglomerular cell tumor, 1577
Electroshock therapy, pheochromocytoma, 1646
Elschnig spot, 443, 445
healed stage, 446
Embolism, renal artery, 1563
Embryo transfer, 1763
Enalapril, 2210
cardiovascular hemodynamics, 2126
clinical features, 2295
cyclic nucleotide, 627
interactions, 2295
antihypertensive drugs, 2295
mode of action, 2295
nursing management, 2065
predominant hemodynamic effect, 2125
pregnancy, 2219
side effects, 2065
Enalaprilat, 2210
hypertensive urgency, 2282
Encephalitis subcorticalis chronica progressiva, 426
Endocrine adaptation, pregnancy, 1765
Endocrine gland, angiotensin-converting enzyme, 1226
Endocrine system, 805
Endogenous growth factor, vessel wall cell, 524
Endoplasmic reticulum, 1577
Ca-pumping ATPase, 971–972
calciosome, 971
calcium transport, 970–974
functional characteristics, 970–974
molecular characteristics, 970–974
calsequestrin, 971
hydrolysis products, 602
T system, 971
transverse tubular system, 971
Endoproteinase Lys-C, prorenin, 1192
Endothelial cell, potassium, 55–56
Endothelial-dependent remodeling factor, 531
Endothelial-derived relaxing factor, phosphoinositide lipid, 604
Endothelial injury, 18
Endothelin, 649–657, 795
amino acid sequence, 649, 650
biosynthetic pathway, 651
biphasic pressure response, 654
calcium flux, 653
cardiac effects, 654–655
cellular actions, 651–654
DNA synthesis, 654
epithelial effect, 654
gene expression, 649–651
glomerular microcirculation, 655
phospholipase C, 652–653
renal actions, 655
signal transduction pathway, 652–653
structural characteristics, 649–651
systemic hypertension, 656
transmembrane calcium flux, 653
vasoconstrictor response, 654
systemic, 654
vasodilatory response, 654
systemic, 654
in vivo actions, 654–655
volume homeostasis, 656
whole-kidney response, 655
Endothelin receptor, 653–654
Endothelium
angiotensin-converting enzyme, 1225
functional roles, 637
$5HT_1$-like receptor, 765
neuropeptide, vascular response, 799
nitric oxide, 638
prostacyclin, 638
Endothelium-dependent contraction, hypertension, 643–644
Endothelium-dependent relaxation, hypertension, 642–643

Endothelium-dependent response
  atherosclerotic blood vessel, 642
  hypertension, 642–645
    impaired response mechanism, 644–645
Endothelium-derived constricting factor, 639
Endothelium-derived relaxing factor, 55–56, 637–639, 836–837
  acetylcholine, 1255
  alpha-adrenergic receptor agonist, 1255
  angiotensin II, 1255
  arachidonic acid, 1255
  bradykinin, 1255
  cytochrome-P450 mono-oxygenase, 837
  eicosatetraynoic acid, 836
  histamine, 1255
  hypertension, 629
  metyrapone, 837
  nordihydroguariaretic acid, 836
  platelet function, 638–639
  serotonin, 1255
  SKF525A, 837
  superoxide dismutase, 837
  thrombin, 1255
  vasopressin, 1255
Endothelium-derived vasoactive substance, 637–647
Endothelium-derived vasoconstrictor peptide, 640
Endralazine, predominant hemodynamic effect, 2125
Endurance training, blood pressure, 1988–1993
  blood pressure at rest, 1988–1991
  blood pressure change mechanisms, 1992–1993
  blood pressure during a 24-hr period, 1992
  blood pressure during exercise, 1991–1992
  hemodynamic data, 1992
  humoral data, 1992–1993
Enterochromaffin cell, 772
Environment, office evaluation, 1389
Enzymatic deficiency, 1621
Epidemiologic study, 159–173
Epidermal growth factor
  phosphoinositide signaling system, 606
  thick ascending limb of Henle's loop, 1057
  vascular wall injury, 523
Epididymis, angiotensin-converting enzyme, 1225–1226
Epinephrine, 583
  adrenomedullary activity, 726
  beta-blocker, 2202
  essential hypertension, 731
  hyperadrenergic dysautonomia, 1471–1474
  monoaminergic mechanism, 684–688
    Dahl salt-sensitive rat, 689
    Goldblatt rat, 689
    Okamoto strain, 684–687
    renovascular hypertensive rat, 689
    spontaneously hypertensive rat, 684–687
  pathways, 684–688
  receptor subtypes, 583
  vascular lesion, 44
Epithelioid sarcoma, 1580
Epithelium, angiotensin-converting enzyme, 1225
Equipment evaluation
  ambulatory blood pressure monitoring, 1435–1438
  blood pressure measurement, 1429–1439
Ergot alkaloid, beta-blocker, 2202
Ergotamine, vascular lesion, 44
Erythrocyte
  Na^+-K^+ cotransport, 927
  Na^+-K^+ countertransport, Li^+ fractional renal clearance, 928
  Na^+-Li^+ countertransport, 927–928
  Na^+ pump, 925–926
Erythropoietin, angiotensinogen, 1211–1212
Essential fatty acid, conversion, 260
Essential hypertension, 13, 1616, 1670, 1697
  age, 2194
  aldosterone, diuretic-induced volume deficit, 1357
  angiotensin, 31
  angiotensin-converting enzyme inhibitor, 2217
  angiotensin II
    altered responsiveness, 1356–1358
    nonmodulation, 1356–1358
  benign phase, 5
    sleep, 5
  blood pressure, 1352–1353
  blood pressure regulation, 1750
  blood rheology, animal models, 334
  blood volume, 346
  Ca^{2+}-ATPase
    basal, 929
    calmodulin, 929
    erythrocytes, 929–930
    platelets, 929–930
  calcitonin, 2039–2042
  calcium-channel blockade, 2044
  cardiopulmonary reflex, 353, 354
    uncomplicated, 353, 354
  cardiovascular adaptation, 2169–2171
  catecholamine
    age, 731
    autonomic contribution, 730–731
    baroreflex, 733–734
    cardiovascular hypertrophy, 734
    cardiovascular stiffness, 734
    cerebrospinal fluid norepinephrine, 732
    epinephrine hypothesis, 731
    human, 730–734
    norepinephrine kinetics, 732
    plasma norepinephrine distribution, 730
    pressor responsiveness, 733–734
    salt sensitivity, 731–732
    stress responses, 732–733
  cell membrane alteration, 903–906
    human, 903–904, 906
    rat, 904–906
  cellular K^+, 928–929
  cellular Na^+, 928–929
  coronary circulation, 320
  coronary disease, treatment decision, 134
  diabetes, 1689, 1697
  diabetic nephropathy, 1724
  diagnosis, 11
  dietary chloride, 2022
  dietary sodium restriction, 2011
  1,25-dihydroxyvitamin D, 2039–2042
  DOC, 73
  downward structural resetting, 578
  environmental factors, 565
  epidemiology, 1692
  etiology, 558
  family history, 1546–1547
  filtration surface area, 1158
  genetics, 902–903
    rat, 902–903
  heart, 913–914
  hemodynamics
    blood volume, 321–322
    capacitance vessels, 321–322
    disturbance causes, 321–322
    left ventricle structural changes, 322
    sympathetic nervous system, 321
    therapeutic considerations, 322–323
  heterogeneity, 2109
  hormone, 906–908
    human, 906, 908
    rat, 906–908
  humoral factor, 906–908
  iatrogenic disease, 14
  intervention studies, 2011–2014
  ion transport, 923–932
  kidney function, 1503–1505
  kidney study methods, 1371–1372
    renal blood flow, 1371–1372
    transrenal humoral change, 1371–1372
  lipid disorder, familial, 132
  low potassium etiology, 222
  magnesium, 1007, 1008
  magnesium therapy, 2055
  malignant, 4–5, 34
  molecular mechanism, 903–906
    human, 903–904, 906
    rat, 904–906
  Na^+, 924–926
  Na^+-K^+ cotransport, 927
  Na^+-Li^+ countertransport, 927–928
  natriuresis, 1362
  natural history, 13–14
  nephron heterogeneity, 1089–1096
    abnormal renin responsiveness, 1094–1096
    abnormal renin-volume interactions, 1341
    dietary sodium changes, 1092–1094

zona fasciculata, 1618–1621
zona glomerulosa, 1613–1618
zona reticularis, 1621
Hypertension Detection and Follow-up Program, 18, 162, 1878, 1944–1945
age, 197
mortality, 197
prevalence estimates, 162–165
referred care, 197
stepped care, 197
treatment effectiveness, 153
Hypertension-Stroke Cooperative Study, 196–197
age, 196–197
mild to moderate hypertension, 196
stroke recurrence, 196
Hypertension treatment, 115–116, 153, 1590–1591, 1707, 1710–1712, 1735. *See also* Antihypertensive drug
age, 1951, 2173–2174
ancient beginnings, 2093–2094
anesthesia, 1898
arterial pressure, 1724, 1732
behavioral, 2088–2089
long-term results, 2089
beta-blocker, 2196
cardiac arrhythmia, 2196
complicated, 2195–2197
diabetes, 2196
ischemic heart disease, 2195–2196
lipid disorder, 2196
postmyocardial infarction, 2195–2196
renal impairment, 2196
biofeedback, 2088–2089
black patient
angiotensin-converting enzyme inhibitor, 1848
beta-blockers, 1847–1848
calcium-channel blockers, 1847
clonidine, 1848
combined alpha-beta blockers, 1847
cost, 1846
diuretics, 1846–1847
guanabenz, 1848
hydralazine, 1848
hydrochlorothiazide, 1846
methyldopa, 1848
nonpharmacologic therapy, 1846
pharmacologic therapy, 1846
prazosin, 1848
reserpine, 1848
side effects, 1848
calcium antagonist, 1711–1712
cardiocerebrovascular complication, 2131–2132
cardiovascular mortality, 115
child, 1864–1865
clinical trials, 1727–1728
compliance, 2132–2133, 2309–2313
coronary disease, 1948
cyclosporine-induced hypertension, 1833
calcium-channel blocker, 1833
converting-enzyme inhibitors, 1833
nifedipine, 1833
triple-drug immunosuppression, 1833
development, 2093–2103
diabetic glomerulopathy, 1682–1683
diabetic nephropathy, 1732–1733
dietary calcium, 893–894, 2052–2056
1,25-dihydroxyvitamin D, 2049–2051
mechanism of action, 2049
oral supplementation, 2046–2049
parathyroid hormone, 2049–2051
plasma renin activity, 2046, 2047
rationale, 2039–2040
salt-insensitive essential hypertensive subjects, 2046, 2048
salt-sensitive essential hypertensive subjects, 2046, 2048
serum ionized calcium, 2046, 2047
dietary magnesium, 2052–2056
dietary sodium restriction, 2016–2017
diuretic administration, 1591
drug therapy withdrawal, 2301–2307
baroreceptor resetting, 2305
natural history of blood pressure hypothesis, 2305
structural regression, 2305
studies, 2303
success of withdrawal, 2303
elderly patient, 1878–1883
adherence, 200
adverse drug reactions, 1883
algorithm, 1883
alpha-1-adrenoreceptor-enzyme inhibitor, 1882
alpha-2-adrenoreceptor-enzyme inhibitor, 1882
Australian Therapeutic Trial in Mild Hypertension, 197–198, 1878
calcium-channel blocker, 1882
cardiovascular morbidity, 194
cardiovascular mortality, 194
clinical trials, 1878–1880
combination alpha-1- and beta-adrenoreceptor blocker, 1882
compliance, 1883
congestive heart failure, 194
direct vasodilator, 1882
diuretic therapy, 1880–1881
drug treatment, 1880–1883
effect, 194–200
European Working Party on Hypertension in the Elderly, 198–199, 1879–1880
guanadrel, 1882–1883
guanethidine, 1882–1883
Hypertension Detection and Follow-up Program, 197, 1878
hypertension-stroke cooperative study, 196–197
medication reduction, 1883
mild to moderate hypertension, 195–196
moderately severe hypertension, 195
non-pharmacologic therapy, 1880
nondiuretic therapy, 1881–1883
observational studies, 195
randomized clinical trials, 195–200
Randomized Trial of Elderly Patients in Primary Care, 199
reserpine, 1882
side effects, 200–201
stroke, 194
Systolic Hypertension in the Elderly Program, 199
Veterans Administration Cooperative Study on Antihypertensive Agents, 195–196, 1878
excessive pressure, reduction, 2138–2139
experimental diabetes, 1681
follow-up, 1964
historical background, 2107–2109
hypertensive retinopathy, 453–456
hypertensive urgency, 2278
individualization, 1950–1951
initiation, 1967–1972
diastolic pressure, 1969–1972
J-shaped curve, 1973–1976
systolic pressure, 1969–1972
magnesium, 1018–1019
malignant hypertension
controlled trials, 2133, 2139
suboptimal effects, 2137–2138
mild hypertension
controlled trial, 2137
diastolic pressure changes, 2135
five-year survival, 2135
major endpoint analysis, 2134–2137
mortality, 2135, 2136
prognosis improvement, 2134
moderate hypertension
controlled trial, 2137
diastolic pressure changes, 2135
five-year survival, 2135
major endpoint analysis, 2134–2137
mortality, 2135, 2136
prognosis improvement, 2134
morbidity, 2131–2132
mortality, 2131–2132
mortality change, 1735
multiple risk factors, 1951
myocardial infarction, 412–413
nephropathy, 1727, 1728
nineteenth century, 2094
noncompliance, 2073, 2075–2076
non-pharmacological measures, 1964
optimal blood pressure, 1733
physician-patient interaction
clinical model, 2077–2080
clinical studies, 2075–2080
traditional role, 2075
traditional role and compliance, 2075–2076
potassium, 1146–1147
potential benefit, 1942–1943
potential harm, 1948–1950
preexisting end-organ damage, 1951
pregnancy, 1576

Hypertension treatment (*contd.*)
progressive muscular relaxation, 2088–2089
quality of life, 2132–2133
race, 1950–1951, 2173–2174
randomized controlled trials, 115
renin, 2173–2174
renin inhibitor, 2347–2349
salt sensitivity, 2015–2016
sex, 1950–1951
side effects, 1949
chemical changes, 1949
symptoms, 1949
stroke, 115, 412–413, 426–428
acute stroke hypertension management, 426–427
cerebral infarction, 426–427
intracerebral hemorrhage, 427
primary prevention, 426
subarachnoid hemorrhage, 427
structural cardiovascular change, 2132
therapeutic decision, 1950–1951
transcendental meditation, 2088–2089
treatment decision. *See* Treatment decision
vasodilator rule, 2128–2129
Hypertensive attack, pheochromocytoma, 1643
Hypertensive choroidopathy, 442, 446
arteriole, 446
choriocapillaris, 446
choroidal arteriole, 447
choroidal artery, 446
pathophysiologic mechanism, 443–444
Hypertensive crisis
acute, 2277–2278
angiotensin-converting enzyme inhibitor, 2221
surgical, 1654
Hypertensive emergency, 2275–2286
age, 2278
blood pressure elevation, 2275
defined, 2275
diazoxide, 2279–2281
drug treatment, 2279–2281
hypertension duration, 2278–2279
nitroprusside, 2279
oral vs. parenteral agents, 2279
sodium nitroprusside, 2279
trimethaphan camsylate, 2281
underlying medical conditions, 2279
volume status, 2278
vs. medical urgencies, 2275
Hypertensive encephalopathy, 34, 35, 2276, 2283, 2284
acute organic lesions, 40
breakthrough hypothesis, 44
capillary permeability, 40
cerebral blood flow
angiotensin, 44
autoregulation, 43–44
vasospasm, 44
cerebral blood flow change, 43
clip removal, 40
drugs of choice, 2283
focal cerebral edema, 43
focal spasm, 40, 41
headache, 407
mechanism, 40–42
overconstriction, 43–44
pathogenesis, 39–44, 407
forced vasodilation hypothesis, 407
vasospasm hypothesis, 407
regional blood flow, 44
Hypertensive gravida. *See* Pregnancy
Hypertensive lesion, 527
Hypertensive nephropathy, 394
Hypertensive ocular disease, pathophysiologic approach, 442–463
Hypertensive optic neuropathy, 460
lamina retinalis
acute phase, 461
resolution phase, 462
myelinated optic nerve, 461
acute, 461
resolution phase, 462
pathophysiologic mechanisms, 460–463
Hypertensive remodeling, mechanisms, 531–533
Hypertensive renal disease, dietary therapy, 1169–1170
Hypertensive retinopathy, 444–460
antihypertensive therapy, 453–456
arterial narrowing, 447–450
arterial sclerosis, 450, 452
arterial tortuosity, 450–451, 453
arteriovenous nicking, 450, 451
artery branching angle, 451–453
exudative phase, 434, 451–452
hyaline degeneration, 459
Keith-Wagener-Barker classification, 440, 442
Leishman classification, 443
modified Scheie classification, 443
pathophysiologic mechanisms, 455–459
plasmatic vasculosis, 457, 458
post-therapy, 453–455
previous classifications, 440–442
remodeling, 456
retinal exudative changes, 455
retinal vascular changes, 453–454
retinal vascular reactivity, 454–455
sclerotic phase, 446–451
tunica media, 459
vascular occlusion, 456
vasoconstrictive phase, 445
Hypertensive urgency, 2275, 2276
age, 2278
angiotensin-converting enzyme inhibitor, 2281–2282
beta-blocker, 2282–2283
calcium-channel blocker, 2282
captopril, 2281–2282
clonidine, 2283
drug treatment, 2280, 2281–2283
enalaprilat, 2282
hydralazine, 2282
hypertension duration, 2278–2279
hypertension treatment, 2278
labetolol, 2282–2283
methyldopa, 2283
minoxidil, 2282
nifedipine, 2282
oral vs. parenteral agents, 2279
reserpine, 2283
sympatholytic agent, 2282–2283
underlying medical conditions, 2279
vasodilator, 2282
verapamil, 2282
volume status, 2278
Hyperthyroidism
blood volume increase, 1664
cardiac contractility, 1664–1665
cardiac hypertrophy, 1665
cardiomyopathy, 1668
catecholamine excess, 1663
catecholamine secretion, 1666
incidence, 1667
nuclear medicine, 1529–1530
prevalence, 1667–1668
serum catecholamine, 1663
therapy, 1668–1669
Hypertonie essential, 2094
Hyperuricemia, diuretic, 2149–2150, 2157
Hypervolemia
diabetes, 1691
diabetes mellitus, 1689–1691
Hypoadrenergic dysautonomia, treatment recommendations, 1475
Hypoadrenergic orthostatic hypotension, 749
Hypoglycemia
blood pressure variation, 1420
pheochromocytoma, 1656
Hypokalemia, 993
diuretic, 1637
management, 2159
hypertension, pregnancy, 1774, 1775
pheochromocytoma, 1643
Hypokalemic alkalosis, 1613
Hypomagnesemia
bendroflumethiazide, 1009
chlorothalidone, 1009
chlorothiazide, 1009
congestive heart failure, 1013
diabetes, 1011
experimental diabetes serum magnesium, 1012
insulin-dependent, 1011
red blood cell magnesium level, 1012
skeletal muscle magnesium level, 1012
urine magnesium level, 1012
diuretics, 1009
experimental hypertension, 1007–1008
furosemide, 1009
hydrochlorothiazide, 1009
hypertension, 1006–1007
preeclampsia, 1013
stroke, 1013
thiazide, 1009
Hyponatremia, 1574
diuretic, 2149, 2155

Hypophyseal growth hormone, cardiovascular structural adaptation, 577–578
Hypophysectomy, adrenal-regeneration hypertension, 68
Hypoprostaglandism, 1634
Hypotension, 2244
  neuropeptide, 799–800
  opioid peptide, 799–800
  orthostatic. *See* Orthostatic hypotension
Hypotensive anesthesia, 412
Hypotensive effect, caloric restriction, 1752
Hypotensive medullary lipid, reduction, 38
Hypothalamic Na^+-K^+-ATPase inhibitor/Na^+-Ca^{2+} exchange hypothesis, 930–932
Hypothalamus, 682
  anterior, 683–684
  paraventricular nucleus, 682–683
  pressor regions, 682
  sympathoadrenomedullary system, 716–717
Hypothyroidism, 1663
  atherosclerotic cardiovascular disease, 1671–1672
  basal oxygen consumption, 1670
  cardiovascular manifestations, 1670
  hypertension, 1669–1670
  myxedema coma, 1671
  plasma renin, 1666
  prevalence, 1669–1670
  therapeutic response, 1670–1671
  vasopressin activity, 1667
Hypoxia, magnesium, 1005

I

Iatrophobia, 1408
Ibuprofen, 1907
ICS205-930, serotonin, 763
Idazoxan, characterization, 2236
Idiopathic hyperaldosteronism, 1614–1616
Idiopathic hypertension, sympathoadrenal system, 1423
Iliorenal bypass, 1567
Imaging, Cushing's syndrome, 1619
Imidazole derivative, angiotensin II antagonistic properties, 2352
  formula, 2352
Immunoreactive insulin, 1711
Immunoreactive renin, abnormal juxtaglomerular cell, 1772
Immunosuppressive treatment, renal transplantation, 1592, 1593
Impotence
  beta-blocker, 2200–2201
  diuretic, 2158
In vitro fertilization, 1763
Inbred strain, 955
Inbreeding, 955
Incipient diabetic nephropathy. *See* Diabetic nephropathy
Incretory function, 841
Indapamide
  dosage, 2144
  dosage interval, 2144
  duration of action, 2144
  salt depletion, 2150–2151, 2152
Inderal, adverse effects, 1898
Indicator dye dilution technique, 341
Indomethacin
  angiotensin II, 1255
    endothelium, 1255
  arterial pressure, 1907
  beta-blocker, 2202
  converting-enzyme inhibitor, 1907
  nonsteroidal anti-inflammatory agent, 2158
  phenylpropanolamine, 1914
  renin, 1908
Infant
  birth weight, 1856, 1857
  blood pressure, 1854–1856, 1857
  blood pressure measurement, 1438
  dietary sodium, 2000
  hypertension, 1860–1861
    causes, 1860–1861
    signs, 1860
Inflammation, angiotensinogen, 1210–1211
Inflow pressure, Dahl S rat, sodium excretion, 57
Informed consent, 2074
Ingestion, 1400
  blood pressure variability, 1400
Initial collecting tubule, aldosterone, basolateral membrane, 1282
Inositol, 585, 586
Inositol lipid, location, 601
Inositol phosphate
  angiotensin II, 590
  degradation, 1257
  hydrolysis products, 602
  lithium, 609
  smooth muscle cell, 590
  synthesis, 1257
Inositol phospholipid
  arachidonic acid, 605
  smooth muscle contraction, 605
Inositol triphosphate
  calcium release, 550–551
  sarcoplasmic reticulum, 973
Inositol trisphosphate
  angiotensin II, 586
  calcium mobilization, 586–587
Instrumental evaluation, 1391–1392
  catecholamine, 1392
  chest x-rays, 1392
  echocardiography, 1392
  electrocardiogram, 1392
  plasma renin, 1391
  renin-sodium profile, 1391, 1392
  serum potassium level, 1391
  urinary albumin, 1391
  urinary potassium, 1391
Insulin, 796
  beta-blocker, 2189
  blood pressure, 1749
  diabetic hypertension, 1691–1694
  glucose intolerance, 131
  hypertension, 130–131, 1749
  lipid abnormality, 131
  mitogenic effect, 544
  natriuretic capacity, 1750
  obesity, 131
  sympathetic nervous system, 1693, 1749–1750
  systolic pressure, 131
  thermogenesis, 1751
Insulin-like growth factor I, mitogenic effect, 544
Insulin pump treatment, 1726, 1727, 1729
Insulin resistance, 133, 1692, 1697, 1705, 1751
  abdominal obesity, 1748
  hyperinsulinemia, obesity, 1750–1751
Insulinopenia, 1679
Intermediate filament
  contraction, 594–595
  protein kinase C, 594–595
  second messenger, 595
Intermittent claudication
  beta-blocker, 2189
  ketanserin, 773
International Prospective Primary Prevention Study in Hypertension, 1947
Interstitial fibrosis, mild hypertension, 394–395
Interstitial nephritis, 12
  chronic, 34, 35
  nuclear medicine, 1530
  sulfonamide diuretic, 2158
Interview, anesthesia, 1890
Intestine
  angiotensin-converting enzyme, 1225
  angiotensinogen, 1208
Intima, vessel wall, 526
Intimal cell mass
  atherogenesis, 526
  atherosclerotic lesion, 525
Intimal fibroplasia, renal artery, 396–397
Intimal hyperplasia, 1545
Intimal injury, potassium, 55
Intra-arterial pressure measurement, 1429–1430
Intra-arterial tension, 41
Intracellular calcium, phosphoinositide lipid, 607
Intracellular ion defect, 923–932
Intracellular regulation, calcium, membrane carrier, 965–974
Intracerebral hemorrhage, 427
  hypertension, 423–425
    frequency, 380, 382
    primary, 382
Intracranial aneurysm, 7
Intracranial hemorrhage, 2284
  drugs of choice, 2283
Intracranial pressure
  arterial hypertension, 704–705
    acute elevation, 704–705
  chronic elevation, arterial pressure changes, 705

Intracranial pressure (*contd.*)
  hypertension, 703–705
    acute rises, 703
    Cushing response mechanism, 703–704
    experimental studies, 703
    raised pressure, 703–705
  prevention, 705
  vasopressor response, 703–704
Intracranial tumor, hypertension, 705–707
  antihypertensive drugs, 706
  clinical features, 706
  diagnosis, 706–707
  location, 706
  nature of lesion, 706
  radiotherapy, 706
  surgical removal, 706
  untreatable, 706
Intraerythrocytic sodium, 134
Intraglomerular pressure, 1163–1172
Intralobular artery
  myointimal hyperplasia, 392–393
  onion-skinning, 392–393
Intraocular pressure, choroidal circulation, 439–440
Intrarenal blood flow, 1374–1375
  age, renal fraction, 1374
  cortex, 1375
  renal vascular change, 1374–1375
Intrarenal blood flow measurement, inert-gas washout technique, 1372
Intravascular pressure, necrotizing arteritis, 39–40
Intravenous pyelogram, laboratory and instrumental evaluation, 1392
Invasive ambulatory recorder, 1435–1436
Iodine-123, doses, 1511
Iodine-131, doses, 1511
Ion channel, vascular muscle, 662
Ion specificity, 1072–1073
Ion transport, essential hypertension, 923–932
Ischemia, 2285
Ischemic heart disease, 120
  Australian Therapeutic Trial in Mild Hypertension, 198
  hypertension, treated, 122
  type-A behavior, 1013
  vegetarian diet, 245
Ischemic kidney
  renovascular hypertension, 1541–1542
  revascularization, 1554
  unclipping, 1541–1542
Ischemic vascular disease, 1672
Isogravimetric technique, 570
Isolated systolic hypertension, 103, 1706, 1971–1972
  elderly
    cardiovascular mortality, 193–194
    mortality, 193–194
  treatment initiation, 1971–1972
Isoprenaline, structure, 2182
Isoproterenol
  beta-blocker, 2202
  cyclic nucleotide, 626–627
  hyperadrenergic dysautonomia, 1471–1474
  structure, 2182
Isosorbide dinitrate
  metabolism, 2267
  pharmacokinetics, 2267
Isosorbide nitrate
  metabolism, 2267
  pharmacokinetics, 2267
Isotope renogram, 1550–1551
Isradipine, 472–473, 514
  high-density lipoprotein, 515
  low-density lipoprotein, 515
  predominant hemodynamic effect, 2125

J

J-shaped curve, 19, 1973–1976, 2138–2139
Japan
  cerebral hemorrhage, 10
  dietary sodium, 2000–2001
    programs to change, 2001
  systolic pressure, 147–148
Japanese-American, path analysis, 92–93
Joint National Committee on Detection, Evaluation and Treatment of High Blood Pressure, 177
  classifications, 177
Juxtaglomerular apparatus, 1053–1063
  distal nephron, 821, 1063
  innervation, 1061–1062
  kallikrein, 1063
  kinin, 1063
  monoaminergic nerve, 1061–1062
  mouse, 1054
  rat, 1054
  renin, 1063
  tubular component, 1053–1058, 1291
  tubulovascular relationships, 1062–1063
  vascular component, 1058–1061, 1291
Juxtaglomerular cell, 1053, 1058–1060, 1761
  renin, 1324
  sodium, 58
Juxtaglomerular cell tumor, 1574, 1583. *See also* Renin juxtaglomerular cell tumor
  angiotensin-converting enzyme inhibitor, 2218
  biosynthesis, 1579–1580
  diagnosis, 1575–1576
  unilateral renal parenchymal disease, 1583–1584
Juxtaglomerular granular cell
  afferent arteriole, 1060
  hypertension, 1059
  renovascular hypertension, 1059
Juxtamedullary nephron, feedback, 1070–1071

K

K^+
  blood cell regulation
    family history, 929
    normotensives, 929
    skin fibroblasts, 929
  cell membrane transport pathway, 923–924
  furosemide-sensitive cotransport, 926
  genetics, 928–929
  Na^+-K^+-ATPase, 924–926
  regulation abnormalities, 924–929
Kaiser Permanente study, alcohol, 278–279, 280–282
Kallidin, 224
Kallikrein
  afferent arteriole, 821
  anatomical distribution, 807
  Bowman's capsule, 1063
  connecting tubule, 820
    morphology, 823
  dietary potassium, 824–826
  distal nephron lumen, 810
  dominantly high urinary, 133–134
  glomerular basement membrane, 823
  Golgi apparatus, 822
  intracellular processing, 822–824
  juxtaglomerular apparatus, 1063
  kidney cortex, 824
  mineralocorticoid, 808–809
  nephron, 809
  plasma membrane, 822
  rough endoplasmic reticulum, 822
  secretion, 823
  sodium, 808–809
  spironolactone, 808–809
  substrate, 805
  ultrastructural features, 822
  vesicle, 822
Kallikrein-kinin
  activity evaluation, 806–807
  kininase II, 808
  other hormonal systems interrelationship, 807–809
Kallikrein-kinin system
  angiotensin-converting enzyme inhibitor, 2213–2214
  components, 2214
  pharmacological probes, 810, 811
  potassium, 224
  prostaglandin, 831–832
  renin-angiotensin-aldosterone system, 809
Kallikrein-like enzyme, anatomical distribution, 807
Kaposi's sarcoma, 522
Keith-Wagener-Barker classification system, 1389–1390
Kempner diet, 241, 244, 2003
  development, 2095
Kenya, systolic pressure, 147–148
Ketanserin
  chemical structure, 2234
  exercise, 1994
  hypertension, 773–775
    adverse effects, 773
    dosage, 773

elderly patients, 773
electrophysiologic effects, 774
mechanism of action, 774–775
intermittent claudication, 773
pharmacological properties, 2239
ritanserin, 775
serotonin, 763–764
serotonin antagonist, 770–771
ventricular tachycardia, 774
Ketoacidosis, 1736
Kidney
accessory circulation, 29
aldosterone, 1273–1283
action localization, 1273–1275
biochemical studies, 1274
mineralocorticoid action sites, 1274
morphological studies, 1274–1275
physiological actions, 1273–1283
receptor binding studies, 1273–1274
angiotensin-converting enzyme, 1225
angiotensin II, 1260–1265
blood pressure, 1260
extracellular fluid volume, 1260
glomerular mesangial cells, 1261–1262
intrarenal angiotensin II formation, 1261
renal hemodynamics, 1260–1261
renal sodium handling, 1262
tubule transport mechanism, 1264–1265
angiotensinogen, 1207
antihypertensive function, 844, 846
arterial pressure, long-term regulation, 1029–1051
arteriolar lesions, 51–52
blood pressure, 1089
chronic rejection, 1593
clamped, 35
excision effect, 37
glomerulus, 37
histology, 35
function
essential hypertension, 1503–1505
evaluation, 1493–1505
hypertension
arterioles, 390
historical aspects, 389
microvascular disease, 390
structure, 389–397
low sodium intake, 1309
nonclamped, 35, 36
afferent arterioles, 35
glomeruli, 35
lumen, 35
tubules, 35
nuclear medicine, 1511–1519
individual renal function, 1515–1516
orthoiodohippurate, 1513–1516
orthoiodohippurate clearance, 1515
orthoiodohippurate scintigraphy, 1514
orthoiodohippurate scintirenography, 1514
renogram, 1514
sodium Tc-99m pertechnetate, 1516
Tc-99m-labeled agents, 1516–1519
Tc-99m-dimercaptosuccinic acid, 1518–1519
Tc-99m-DTPA, 1516–1518
Tc-99m-glucoheptonate, 1518–1519
transit time, 1516
pathological changes, 34–38
plasma renin, 1089
preprorenin, 1322–1324
primary hypertension, 575
renin gene expression, 1322
separate function, 1500–1502
renography, 1501–1502
separate clearance, 1500–1501
sodium, excretion rate, 57
thyroid hormone, 1662
Kidney cortex, kallikrein, 824
Kidney mass
sodium, 1037, 1038
unequal size, 1544
Kidney renin system. *See* Renin-angiotensin system
Kidney transplant, cyclosporine, 1829
Kinin
converting-enzyme inhibitor, pharmacological effects, 812–813
distal nephron lumen, 810
diuretic, 2154
generating system, 805–806
juxtaglomerular apparatus, 1063
kininase II inhibitor, pharmacological effects, 812–813
prostaglandin, 832
structure, 806
Kinin antagonist, 811–812
bradykinin, 811–812
Kinin-destroying enzyme, 805
Kinin metabolism, 1679
Kinin-releasing enzyme, 805
Kininase I, kinin cleavage, 808
Kininase II, 1217
bradykinin, 1296
kallikrein-kinin, 808
kinin cleavage, 808
renin-angiotensin system, 808
Kininase II inhibitor, kinin, pharmacological effects, 812–813
Kininase inhibitor, 810
Kininogen, 805
Kininogenase inhibition, 810–811
Kininogenases, 805
Korotkoff Phase IV (6–8), pregnancy, 1809
Korotkoff signal, 1433
Korotkoff sound, 1430–1432
cuff size, 1430–1431
cuff vibrations, 1431
diastolic pressure, 1430
fourth, 1780
inaccuracies, 1430–1431
systolic pressure, 1430
technical error, 1431–1432

L

Labetalol
alpha-blocking properties, 2119
beta-1-adrenoceptor selectivity, 2119
chemical structures, 2234
emergency blood pressure lowering, 410
exercise, 1994, 2128
hypertensive emergency in child, 1865
hypertensive urgency, 2282–2283
intrinsic sympathomimetic activity, 2119
pharmacological properties, 2239
pregnancy, 1816, 1818
vasodilation, 2191
Labile hypertension, 102
office evaluation, 1388
Laboratory evaluation, 1391–1392
catecholamine, 1392
chest x-rays, 1392
echocardiography, 1392
electrocardiogram, 1392
plasma renin, 1391
renin-sodium profile, 1391, 1392
serum potassium level, 1391
urinary albumin, 1391
urinary potassium, 1391
Lacis, 1053, 1060–1061
Lacto-ovo-vegetarian, 244
Lacunar infarct, hypertension, 423–425
Lacunar softening, hypertension, 382
frequency, 380, 382
Lacune, 423
Lamina retinalis, hypertensive optic neuropathy
acute phase, 461
resolution phase, 462
Laminar flow, velocity profile, 330
Lanthanum
atherosclerosis, 513
calcium channel, 549
Laplace formula, 566–567
Laragh classification, 1670
Laryngeal stridor, Shy-Drager syndrome, 757
Lasix, adverse effects, 1898
Latch-bridge hypothesis, 594
Lead, blood pressure, 236–238
epidemiologic observations, 237
intracellular metabolic processes, 238
mechanisms, 237–238
NHANES II, 237
renin-angiotensin system, 238
Leak pathway, calcium, 548
Left ventricle
Doppler echocardiography
diastolic performance, 1488
pump function, 1488
echocardiographic dimension indexation, 360
echocardiography, 1482–1488

Left ventricle (*contd.*)
  hypertrophy. *See* Left ventricular hypertrophy
    abnormal, 1485
    diastolic performance, 1488
    guidelines, 1483
    load, 1484–1485, 1486–1487
    pump function, 1488
    structure, 1482–1484, 1485
  M-mode echocardiography, 1482–1485
    abnormal, 1485
    load, 1484–1485
    performance, 1484–1485
    structure, 1482–1484
  mass index, 360
  normal, 360
  two-dimensional echocardiography, 1485–1488
    load, 1486–1487
    performance, 1486–1487
    structure, 1486–1487
Left ventricular failure, 7, 2285
  drugs of choice, 2283
Left ventricular hypertrophy, 1407
  blacks
    education, 168–169
    five-year mortality, 170
    incidence, 169
    mortality, 169
    regression, 169
    socioeconomic status, 169, 170
    stepped-care program, 169–170
  blood viscosity, 334
  cardiac failure, obesity, 1745
  centrally acting sympathetic inhibitor, 2258–2259
  clonidine, 2259
  coronary atheroma, 124
  education, 168–169
  guanabenz, 2259
  hypertension, 359
    human prevalence, 360–361
  methyldopa, 2259
  prevalence, 168–169
  propranolol, 2259
  race
    education, 168–169
    five-year mortality, 170
    incidence, 169
    mortality, 169
    regression, 169
    socioeconomic status, 169, 170
Left ventricular mass
  afterload, animal models, 913
  normal limits, 360
  ventricular hypertrophy, 355
    hypertensive, 355
    normotensive, 355
Left ventricular mass index, systolic pressure, 1977
Left ventricular thickening. *See* Left ventricular hypertrophy
Leg
  nodular arteriosclerosis, 7
  passive raising. *See* Passive leg raising
Leriche syndrome
  arterial pressure, 8
  cholesterol, 8
  nodular arteriosclerosis, 7
Lethargy, elderly, 201
Leu⁵-enkephalin, angiotensin-converting enzyme, 1221
Leukotriene, 830
Levodopa, beta-blocker, 2202
Liddle's syndrome, 1636
Lidocaine, beta-blocker, 2202
Life expectancy
  arterial pressure, 11
  blood pressure, 189–190
  Dahl S rat, antihypertensive drugs, 497–504
  hypertension, 189–190
  spontaneously hypertensive rat, 497–504
    antihypertensive drugs, 497–504
    calcium antagonist, 497–504
Life expectancy table, 11, 12
Lifestyle factors, 83
  office evaluation, 1389
Light-microscopic study, 1577
Limbic cortex, 684
Limbic system, sympathoadrenomedullary system, 717
Linoleic acid, 257
  arachidonic acid, 257, 259
Lipid
  arterial wall, 471
  digitalis-like factor, 940
  mitogenic effect, 544
  vegetarian diet, 245
Lipid abnormality
  insulin, 131
  systolic pressure, 131
Lipid disorder, 2196
  essential hypertension, familial, 132
  inherited, genetics, 131–133
Lipid Research Clinics Prevalence Study, alcohol, 279–280
Lipoprotein, 18. *See also* Specific type
  calcium channel antagonist, 514
  mitogenic effect, 544
Lipoprotein metabolic pathway, calcium channel antagonist, 515–516
Lipoxygenase, 829–831
Lisinopril
  cardiovascular hemodynamics, 2126
  nursing management, 2065
  predominant hemodynamic effect, 2125
  side effects, 2065
Lithium, inositol phosphate, 609
Lithium clearance, proximal tubular function, 1502
Liver
  angiotensinogen, 1205–1206
    synthesis, 1205
  plasma angiotensinogen, 1295
  serotonin, 762–763
  thyroid hormone, 1662
Local load, 567
Local renin system. *See* Tissue renin system
Logistic equation, 1070
Long-Evans rat
  DOC-induced hypertension, 65
  potassium, 993
Loop diuretic
  cardiovascular hemodynamics, 2119
  chemical structure, 2144
  clinical features, 2293
  dosage, 2144
  dosage interval, 2144
  duration of action, 2144
  interactions, 2293–2294
    antihypertensive drugs, 2293–2294
  mode of action, 2293
Loop of Henle, 1634
  chloride, perfusion rate, 1072
  glomerular filtration rate, 1068–1071
    distal tubule, 1069, 1071
    feedback relationship, 1068–1069
    flow rate, 1068–1071
    juxtamedullary nephron feedback, 1070–1071
    loop of Henle microperfusion, 1068–1071
    loop of Henle perfusion techniques, 1068, 1069
    microinjection studies, 1068
    non-rat feedback, 1069–1070
    proximal tubule, 1069, 1071
    single-nephron glomerular filtration rate, 1068–1071
  thick ascending limb. *See* Thick ascending limb of Henle's loop
Low-density lipoprotein
  coronary disease, 107–109
  gene, 129
  isradipine, 515
  nifedipine, 515
Low-density lipoprotein receptor, hyperlipidemic rabbit, 295
Low-molecular-weight angiotensinogen, 1201–1203
  HepG2 cell, 1201
  pregnancy, 1201, 1202
Low-protein state, high-volume state, 1043–1044
Low-renin hypertension, 963
  cellular hypothesis, 2042–2044
  natriuretic hormone hypothesis, 947–949
  sodium, 212
  volume-regulation hypothesis, 947–949
Lower-body negative pressure
  arterial pressure, 350
  central venous pressure, 350
  heart rate, 350
  plasma renin activity, 350
LPC
  hemodynamics, 947
  hypertension, 947
  natriuresis, 947
  volume regulation, 947

Luminal signal, tubuloglomerular feedback
  distal sodium chloride concentration loop flow, 1071–1072
  ion specificity, 1072–1073
  sodium chloride concentration, 1072
  sodium chloride transport, 1073–1074
Lung
  angiotensinogen, 1208
  serotonin, 762–763
Lupus erythematosus, 1671
Lupus nephritis, 1679
Luteinizing hormone, 1762
  atrial natriuretic factor, 868
  prorenin, 1323
  renin, 1323
Lymphocytic thyroiditis, 1671
Lyon hypertensive rat, 977–978
Lyon hypertensive rat
  cell membrane alteration, 905
  hormone, 907
  humoral factor, 907
  molecular mechanism, 905
  neural mechanism, 912
Lys-bradykinin, 808
Lysil-bradykinin, 819
Lysine, 298
Lysophospholipid, 946–947
  hemodynamics, 947
  hypertension, 947
  natriuresis, 947
  volume regulation, 947

M

M-mode echocardiography, left ventricle, 1482–1485
  abnormal, 1485
  load, 1484–1485
  performance, 1484–1485
  structure, 1482–1484
Macrobiotic vegan, 244
Macrophage, atherosclerotic lesion, 525
Macula densa, 1053–1058, 1544
  basement membrane, glomerulus, 1056
  extraglomerular mesangium, 1055
  region, 1761, 1762
  renin, 1292
  renin secretion
    detector-effector mechanism, 1096
    sodium chloride, 1097
Magnesium, 1003–1020
  alcoholism, 1010–1013
  aldosterone, 1279–1280
  arteriolar lumen size, 1016
  bendroflumethiazide, 1009
  blood pressure, 229–230, 236, 249
    geographic patterns, 229–230
    low blood pressure, 236
    magnesium deficiencies, 236
    Newfoundland, 236
    other nutrients, 236
  cardioplegia, 1005
  chlorothalidone, 1009
  chlorothiazide, 1009
  cisplatin, 1011–1013
  cremaster muscle, 1016
  cyclosporine, 1011–1013
  daily requirement, 1010
  diabetes, 1010–1013
  diastolic pressure, 2055
  dietary. *See* Dietary magnesium
  dihydrotachysterol, 478–480
  diuretics, 1009
  drug toxicity, 1010–1013
  excitation-contraction coupling, 1005
  food supply, 1010
  furosemide, 1009
  hydrochlorothiazide, 1009
  hypertension, 103, 236, 1006–1009
    calcium, 236
    diuretics, 1009
  hypertension treatment, 1018–1019
  hypoxia, 1005
  mesentery, 1016
  spontaneously hypertensive rat, red blood cell level, 1007, 1008
  thiazide, 1009
  thick ascending limb of Henle's loop, 2146
  vascular tone
    Ca^{2+} cellular translocation, 1014–1015
    hormone and drug-receptor interactions, 1014
    humoral substance noninvolvement, 1015–1017
    membrane Ca^{2+}-ATPase alterations, 1017
    membrane Na^{+},K^{+}-ATPase alterations, 1017
    membrane permeability modulation, 1014–1015
    neurotransmitter noninvolvement, 1015–1017
  vegetarian diet, 1010
  verapamil, 481
  vessel reactivity
    Ca^{2+} cellular translocation, 1014–1015
    cyclic AMP, 1017
    hormone and drug-receptor interactions, 1014
    humoral substance noninvolvement, 1015–1017
    membrane Ca^{2+}-ATPase alterations, 1017
    membrane Na^{+},K^{+}-ATPase alterations, 1017
    membrane permeability modulation, 1014–1015
    neurotransmitter noninvolvement, 1015–1017
  vitamin D_3, 478–480
Magnesium deficiency
  cardiac bioenergetics, 1006
  type-A behavior, 1013
  vasospasm, 1013
Magnesium metabolism
  blood pressure, 2053–2054
  cellular effects, 2052–2053
  hypertension, 2052
Magnesium sulfate, antieclamptic therapy, 1819
Magnesium wasting, diuretic, 2157
Magnetic resonance imaging, 1489
Male pattern adiposity, 133
Malignant hypertension, 2276–2277, 2283–2284. *See also* Hypertension, malignant phase
  angiotensin-converting enzyme inhibitor, 2221
  antihypertensive drug
    controlled trials, 2133, 2139
    mortality, 2133
    suboptimal effects, 2137–2138
  arterial pressure, 10
  cerebrospinal fluid pressure, 407
  characterized, 10
  chronic interstitial nephritis, 34
  diabetes mellitus, 1707
  diastolic filling rate, 312
  drugs of choice, 2283
  ejection fraction, 312
  etiology, 2276
  extrarenal factor, 38
  five-year survival, 2134
  focal arterial necrosis, 40
  headache, 407
  hypertension treatment
    controlled trials, 2133, 2139
    suboptimal effects, 2137–2138
  left ventricular wall thickness, 312
  lesion pathogenesis, 27–29
  office evaluation, 1388
  pathogenesis, 10
  pathophysiology, 2276–2277
  pheochromocytoma, 1654
  pituitary basophilism, 38
  renal failure, 2277
  renal origin, 38
  renin, 31
  reversal, 10
  smoking, 1920
  smooth muscle proliferation, 527–528
    mass vs. number, 528–529
    onion skinning, 527
    therapy mass effects, 529
    therapy number effects, 529
  symptoms, 14
  two forms of vasoconstriction, 1336
  vascular lesion, 38
Malignant nephrosclerosis, pathogenesis, 35
Malignant sclerosis, 34
Malondialdehyde, 830
Marek's disease virus, 526
MDL72222, serotonin, 763
Mead's acid, 1796
Mean arterial pressure
  acebutolol, 2121–2123
  atenolol, 2121–2123
  bopindolol, 2121–2123
  pindolol, 2121–2123
  propranolol, 2121–2123
  renal plasma flow, 1372–1374

Mean arterial pressure (*contd.*)
  target organ damage, 1980
  ventricular hypertrophy, 355
    hypertensive, 355
    normotensive, 355
Meat protein, blood pressure, 251
Mecamylamine, smoking, 1928
Media education, 156
Medial dissection, renal artery, 396–397
Medial fibroplasia, 1562
  renal artery, 396–397
Medial hyperplasia, 1545
  renal artery, 396–397
Medial necrosis
  cerebral blood flow, 296
  vascular tissue, 296
Medical Impairment Study 1983, 183
Medical Research Council, 18
Medical Research Council Treatment Trial for Mild Hypertension, 1946
Medication, adverse effects, 1407
Medication monitor, compliance, 2319–2320
  clinical trials, 2320
Meditation, nursing management, 2067–2068
Medroxalol, vasodilation, 2191
Medulla, 680–682, 2085
Medullary hemodynamics, angiotensin II, 1116–1117
Medullary thyroid carcinoma, 1645
  pheochromocytoma, 1647, 1653
Medullipin, 841–858
  Goldblatt hypertensive animal, 852–856
    endocrine concept, 852–854
    Folkow's group, 852–854
    Masugi's group, 854
    Muirhead's group, 854
    renal venous effluent antihypertensive lipid, 854, 856
    Swales' group, 854
    unclipping, 852–854
    Vandongen's group, 854
Medullipin I
  biologic activity, 848, 851, 856
  glyceryl compound, 849–852
  hepatic effect, 848, 851
  vasodepressor effect, 848, 852
Melanocyte-stimulating hormone, 796
Melatonin, 762
Membrane-associated regulatory protein, 1248
Membrane mechanism, spontaneously hypertensive rat, 904–905
Membrane phosphoinositide metabolism, 541–543
Membrane potential
  calcium, 1144
  carotid artery, 1144
  potassium, 1144
  vascular muscle, 661–662
Membrane transport defect, 923–932
Mendelian inheritance, 956–957
Menstrual cycle
  blood pressure variation, 1420
  Rhesus monkey, 1781
Mental activity, 1400
  blood pressure variability, 1400
Mesenchymal cell, 1545
Mesenteric artery
  angiotensin, 43
  angiotensin II, 584
  calcium overload, 474
  overdistension, 42–43
  vascular reactions, 43
Mesentery
  angiotensinogen, 1208
  magnesium, 1016
Met^5-enkephalin
  angiotensin-converting enzyme, 1221
  substance P, 1221
Metabolic alkalosis, diuretic, 2149
Metabolic control, diabetic hypertension, 1694
Metabolism, 1792
Metabolite measurement
  DHPG, 725
  norepinephrine, 725
Metallic ion intake, blood pressure, 229
Methoxamine, characterization, 2236
Methoxyverapamil, renin, 1238
Methylclothiazide
  dosage, 2144
  dosage interval, 2144
  duration of action, 2144
Methyldopa, 2255–2256
  adverse effects, 1898, 2255
  beta-blocker, 2192, 2202
  blood pressure, 530
  cardiovascular hypertrophy, 530
  central nervous system, 2255
  clinical features, 2297
  dosage, 2255, 2256
  efficacy, 2255
  elderly, 2258
  hemodynamics, 2253
  hypertensive urgency, 2283
  interactions, 2297–2298
    antihypertensive drugs, 2297–2298
  left ventricular hypertrophy, 2259
  mode of action, 2297
  norepinephrine biosynthesis, 2255
  peripheral action, 2255
  pregnancy, 2197
  side effects, 2253
Metolazone
  chemical structure, 2144
  dosage, 2144
  dosage interval, 2144
Metoprolol
  alpha-blocking properties, 2119
  beta-1-adrenoceptor selectivity, 2119, 2183
  beta-blocking metabolites, 2183
  beta-blocking plasma concentration, 2183
  bioavailability, 2183
  cardiac output, 2121
  cholesterol-fed rabbit model, 514
  coronary event, 2109
  dietary sodium restriction, 2017
  diuretic, 2191, 2192
  dosage, 2184
  dosage frequency, 2184
  equipotent single dose, 2184
  exercise, 1994
  hemodynamics, 2186
  intrinsic sympathomimetic activity, 2119, 2183
  lipophilicity, 2183
  membrane-stabilizing effect, 2183
  migraine, 2197
  mortality, 1961
  plasma half-life, 2184
  protein binding, 2183
  thiazide, 1947–1948
  vascular resistance, 2121
Metoprolol Atherosclerosis Prevention in Hypertensives Study, 1947–1948
Metyrapone, endothelium-derived relaxing factor, 837
Metyrosine, dopamine-beta-hydroxylase deficiency, 754–755
Mg^{2+}. *See also* Magnesium
  Ca^{2+} antagonist, 1019
  circumflex artery, 1014
  coronary artery, 1014
  electrophysiologic actions, 1004–1005
  extracellular, 1005
    vascular tone, 1013–1014
    vessel reactivity, 1013–1014
  hemodynamics, 1005–1006
    intact, open-chest dog, 1005–1006
  intracellular, 1005
    vascular tone, 1013–1014
    vessel reactivity, 1013–1014
  myocardial effects, 1004–1005
  physiological roles, 1004
  umbilical artery, 1015
  umbilical vein, 1015
Mg^{2+} deficiency, vascular muscle membrane
  Ca^{2+} movement, 1019
  membrane leakiness, 1019
  permeability, 1019
Microalbuminuria, 1708
  arteriolar hyalinosis, 1721
  diabetic nephropathy, 1719–1721
  glycemic control, 1736–1737
  vascular disease, 1721–1722
Microalbuminuric diabetes, 1711
Microaneurysm, 9–10
Microangiopathy, 1691
Microvascular reconstruction, 1570
Midbrain, 682
Middle aortic syndrome, 1563
Migraine
  atenolol, 2197
  beta-blocker, 2189, 2197
  calcium antagonist, 2197
  metoprolol, 2197
  propranolol, 2197
Milan rat, 978
  cell membrane alteration, 905

normal, 1809–1810
eicosanoid formation, 1794–1795
pheochromocytoma, 1648
physiologic changes, 1781–1784
platelet activation, 1795
preeclampsia, 1810–1816
preeclampsia/eclampsia, 1811
pressure alterations, 1810
renin-angiotensin system, 1764–1775
renovascular hypertension, 1774
transient hypertension, 1812
Pregnancy-induced hypertension, 1576, 1796, 1797, 1798
Prehypertension, pathophysiology, 948–949
Prekallikrein, 805–806
Preload
afterload, 2098
cardiac design change, 575
Prenylamine
chemical structure, 472
specificity, 472
Preproendothelin cDNA, 649
amino acid sequence, 649, 650
nucleotide sequence, 649, 650
Preprorenin, 1193
amino acid sequence, 1180, 1290
aspartic acid, 1290
extrarenal renin-expressing tissues, 1322–1324
kidney, 1322–1324
post-translational processing, 1322–1323
Pressor, 1771
Pressor agent, 583–584
Pressor agent receptor, 583–584
Pressor compound, 1586–1587
Pressor hypersensitivity, 1634
Pressor response, 1797
Pressor substance, 31–32
labile hypertension, 1425
Pressure change
aorta, 577
artery, 577
vein, 577
Pressure control
renal-fluid volume mechanism, 1030–1037
arterial pressure, 1048–1050
body salt balance, 1031–1032
fluid intake output equilibration, 1031–1032
pressure diuresis, 1030
pressure natriuresis, 1030
renal function curve, 1031
volume mechanism
comparative pressure-controlling characteristics, 1032–1033
infinite gain characteristic, 1032–1033
Pressure diuresis mechanism, renal-body-fluid feedback, 1122
Pressure natriuresis, angiotensin II
long-term, 1123
renal escape, 1123–1124
Pressure natriuresis mechanism, renal-body-fluid feedback, 1122
Prevalence
blood pressure, measurements, 175
borderline hypertension, insured lives, 180
hypertension
insured lives, 180
trends, 179–180
left ventricular hypertrophy, 168–169
NHANES II, 175
Prevention
coronary disease, 1957–1961
beta-blocker, 1957–1961
myocardial infarction, beta-blocker, 2197–2199
sudden death, beta-blocker, 2197–2199
Primary adrenal hyperplasia, primary aldosteronism, 1616
Primary aldosterone deficiency, 1627. *See also* Aldosterone
Primary aldosteronism, 1616, 1774–1775
basal body sodium, 211
curable, 1392–1393
primary adrenal hyperplasia, 1616
saline infusion, 1615
subsets, 1614–1618
Primary amenorrhea, 1621
Primary arterial disease
stress, 46–47
vessel wall, 46–47
Primary hyperdeoxycorticosteronism, adrenal tumor, 1620–1621
Primary hypertension, 1706
anesthesia, 1899
catecholamine, 727–734
age, 727
cardiovascular hypertrophy prevention, 730
hypertension development prevention, 729
hypertensive rat baroreflex, 728
multiple loci of abnormalities, 728–729
spontaneously hypertensive rat, 727–730
stress, 727–728
kidney, 575
Primary intimal fibroplasia, 1562
Primary nephritis, chronic, 34
Primary reninism
biological study, 1579–1580
extrarenal renin-secreting tumor, 1578–1579
histology, 1576–1578
juxtaglomerular cell tumor, 1573
parameters, 1573–1574
medical treatment, 1574–1575
nephroblastoma, 1578
one-kidney one-clip model, 1574
parameters, 1573–1574
Prizidilol, vasodilation, 2191
Pro-atrial natriuretic factor, 861–862
Probe renography, 1501–1502
Procaine, calcium antagonist, 1014–1015, 1017
Progesterone, 1324, 1765, 1784
atrial natriuretic factor, 868
prorenin, 1323
renin, 1323
Progressive muscular relaxation, hypertension treatment, 2088–2089
Progressive systemic sclerosis, 1671
Prokallikrein, 819
Prolactin, 797
Prolamine, 1913
Pro-opiomelanocortin, 945
Propranolol
adverse effects, 1898
alpha-blocking properties, 2119
anesthesia, 2197
arrhythmia, 2197
atherosclerosis, 513
beta-1-adrenoceptor selectivity, 2119
beta-1-selectivity, 2183
beta-blocking metabolites, 2183
beta-blocking plasma concentration, 2183
bioavailability, 2183
blood pressure, 530
cardiac hypertrophy, 730
cardiac output, 2121
cardiovascular hypertrophy, 530
coronary event, 1947
cyclic nucleotide, 627
diastolic pressure, 2186, 2187
diuretic, 2191, 2192
dosage, 2184
dosage frequency, 2184
equipotent single dose, 2184
exercise, 1994, 2190
heart rate, 2190
hemodynamics, 2186
intrinsic sympathomimetic activity, 2119, 2183
left ventricular hypertrophy, 2259
lipophilicity, 2183
mean arterial pressure, 2121–2123
membrane-stabilizing effect, 2183
migraine, 2197
plasma half-life, 2184
plasma renin activity, 2186, 2187
protein binding, 2183
stroke, 1946, 1947, 1974
structure, 2182
systolic pressure, 2190
total peripheral resistance, 2121–2123
vascular resistance, 2121
Prorenin, 1188–1193
acid activation, 1190
angiotensinogen, 1192
chymotrypsin, 1192
closed form, 1325
endoproteinase Lys-C, 1192
estradiol, 1323
expression, 1190
factors affecting secretion, 1323–1324
extrarenal organs, 1324
kidney, 1324
function, 1762–1763
gonadotropin, 1324
inactive, 32

Prorenin (*contd.*)
  luteinizing hormone, 1323
  maturation mechanism, 621–622
  nephrectomy, 1322
  in normal subjects, 1454
  open form, 1325
  physiological role, 1194
  placenta, 1321–1322
  plasmin, 1192
  pregnancy, 1765–1766
  progesterone, 1323
  prosegment regions, 1193
  purification, 1190–1193, 1579
  renin, 1184–1185
  renin-angiotensin cascade, 1189
  reproductive organs, 1321–1322
    adrenal, 1321, 1325
    ovary, 1321, 1325
    testis, 1321, 1325
  reversible enzymatic activity, 1324–1325
  schematic representation, 1191
  tissue renin system, 1322–1324
    extrarenal organs, 1324
    kidney, 1324
    prorenin secretion, 1323–1324
  truncated derivatives, 1191
  trypsin, 1191–1192
  in vivo secretion, 1321, 1323
  zymogen, 1192
Prorenin-angiotensin system, 1325, 1764
Prorenin peptide, 2346
Prorenin secretion, 1580
Prostacyclin, 637–638, 1801
  acetylcholine, 638
  arterial pressure, 1905, 1906
  calcium ionophore A23187, 638
  diuretic, 2154
  endothelium, 638
  histamine, 638
  renin, 1905, 1906
  thrombin, 638
Prostaglandin, 257–258, 583, 1799, 1800
  angiotensin-converting enzyme inhibitor, 2212–2213
  autonomic nervous system, 832–833
  beta-blocker, 2188
  biology, 1789–1794
  biosynthesis pathways, 1905, 1906
  blood pressure, 258–264
  formation, 259
  hypertension, 834–835
    experimental, 834–835
    human, 834–835
  kallikrein-kinin system, 831–832
  kinin, 832
  as modulators, 831–833
  nonsteroidal anti-inflammatory drug, 1905, 1906
  omega 3 fatty acid, 263–264
  omega 6 fatty acid, 257–263, 264–272
    community-based studies, 268–270
    dietary intervention studies, 264–271
    epidemiologic studies, 270–271
    free-living studies, 264–268
    humans, 264–272
    prostaglandin studies, 271–272
    vegetarian diet, 270
  preeclampsia, 1795–1797
  renin
    first messenger, 1243
    second messenger, 1243
Prostaglandin E_2, 832–833, 834–835
  arterial pressure, 1905, 1906
  renin, 1905, 1906
Prostaglandin formation, 1790–1791, 1795–1797
  pregnancy, 1791–1794
    preeclampsia, 1795–1797
Prostaglandin I_2, 832–833, 834–835
Prostaglandin production, 1680
Prostaglandin synthesis, 2212
Prostaglandin system, renin-angiotensin-aldosterone system, 809
Prostanoid-like endothelium-derived constricting factor, 639–640
Prostate, angiotensin-converting enzyme, 1225–1226
Protein, 106
  blood pressure, 250–252
Protein kinase
  calcium release, 551
  cAMP, 619–620
  cGMP, 623
  hypertension, 628
Protein kinase C
  calcium, 605
  diacylglycerol, 587–588
  intermediate filament, 594–595
  phosphatidylserine, 605
  phosphoinositide lipid, 605
  phospholipase C, regulation, 590
Protein synthesis, 1763
Proteinuria, 1502–1503, 1711, 1712
  diabetes mellitus, 1706, 1707, 1708, 1710
  diabetic nephropathy, 1737
  hypertension, 1719
  preeclampsia diagnosis, 1811
  renin, 1298
  renovascular hypertension, 1547
  transient hypertension, 1812
  type I diabetes, 130
Proteoglycan, atherosclerosis, 512
Proximal tubule
  angiotensin II, 1117–1118
  diuretic, 2145
  function, 1632
    beta-microglobulin, 1502
    lithium clearance, 1502
    para-aminohippurate, 1502
Pseudohermaphroditism, 1621
Pseudohypertension, 1407–1413
  case presentations, 1410–1411
  clinical presentation, 1410–1411
  elderly, 1409
Pseudohypoparathyroidism
  adenylate cyclase, 619
  cAMP, 619
Pseudonormotension
  ambulatory pressure, 1411–1413
  case presentations, 1411–1413
  clinic pressure, 1411–1413
Pseudouremia, 40, 407
Psychological stress response, blood pressure variation, 1420–1421
Psychosocial stress, Samoan study, 142
Pulmonary artery pressure, anesthesia, 1895–1896
Pulmonary circulation
  mild hypertension, 320–321
  severe hypertension, 320–321
Pulmonary edema
  drugs of choice, 2283
  renovascular hypertension, 1547
Pulmonary hypertension, sympathoadrenal system, 1423
Pulse transit-time measurement technique, 1432
Pyelography, 1627
  hyperkalemia, 1628
  intravenous, 1548, 1550
Pyelonephritis, 12
  hypertension, 30
  nuclear medicine, 1530–1531
Pyrroxate, 1913

Q

Quality of life
  antihypertensive drug, 2132–2133
  assessment, 2076
  hypertension treatment, 2132–2133
Quanethidine, 2096
Quetelet's index, 1741
Quinidine, beta-blocker, 2202

R

Race. *See also* Specific type
  antihypertensive drug, 2173–2174
  antihypertensive drug withdrawal, 2303
  borderline hypertension, 175, 176
  calcium antagonist, 2173–2174, 2175
  defined, 1837
  diltiazem, 2173–2174, 2175
  hypertension, 159–173
    clinical epidemiology, 167–170
    controlled, 175, 176
    medicated, 175, 176
    prevalence, 166–167, 175, 176, 1838
    treatment, 178–179
  hypertension treatment, 1950–1951
  left ventricular hypertrophy
    education, 168–169
    five-year mortality, 170
    incidence, 169
    mortality, 169
    regression, 169
    socioeconomic status, 169, 170
  mortality, 1944
  nicardipine, 2173–2174, 2175
  nifedipine, 2173–2174, 2175
  plasma renin activity, 1445
  systolic hypertension, 176
  verapamil, 2173–2174, 2175

Radiation injury, renal arterial disease, 396
Radical, cellular defenses, 670
Radioactive isotope, 341
Radiography, preoperative localization, 1652
Radioisotope renography, 1501–1502
Ramipril, predominant hemodynamic effect, 2125
Random-zero sphygmomanometer, 1432
Randomized Trial of Elderly Patients in Primary Care, 199
Rash, side effects, 201
Rat. *See also* Specific type
  angiotensinogen, 1198–1199
  juxtaglomerular apparatus, 1054
Rauwolscine, characterization, 2236
Raynaud's phenomenon
  beta-blocker, 2189, 2200
  pheochromocytoma, 1644
Receptor-hormone complex, 1611
Receptor processing, phospholipase C, regulation, 590–591
Recombinant prorenin, 1179–1195
Recombinant renin, 1179–1195
Red blood cell, blood viscosity, 330–331
Referral, hypertension, 153
Reflex activity
  baroreceptor mechanism, 2238
  sympathetic nervous system, 2238
  vasodilator drug, 2238
Reflex tachycardia, 2244
  phenoxybenzamine, 2242
  phentolamine, 2242
Regional circulation, 318–319
  hypertensive encephalopathy, 44
  ultrasound, 1489
Regitine, characterization, 2236
Regulation abnormalities
  Ca^{2+} abnormalities, 930–932
  Na^{2+} abnormalities, 930–932
Rejection, 1593
  kidney
    acute, 1591–1592
    chronic, 1593
Relative weight, 1741, 1744
Relaxation therapy, nursing management, 2067–2068
Remnant kidney, post-transplant hypertension, 1591–1592
Renal ablation, glomerular hemodynamics, 1164
Renal adrenoceptor, renin secretion, 1378–1379
Renal afferent arteriolar resistance, peripheral resistance, 1045
Renal afferent arteriolar vasoconstriction, essential hypertension, 1089
Renal allotransplantation, 1568
Renal angioplasty, 1544
Renal antihypertensive endocrine function, 844
Renal arterial disease
  atherosclerosis, 396
  congenital anomaly, 396
  radiation injury, 396
  Takayasu's aortitis, 396
Renal arterial resistance, peripheral resistance, 1045
Renal arteriography, 1575, 1576
Renal arteriole, in local thickening variation, 1090–1091
Renal arteriovenous fistula, 1563
Renal artery
  anatomy, 1545–1546
  aortic ligation, 38
  clamp removal, 37
  clamped, untouched opposite kidney removal, 37–38
  diltiazem, 480
  dysplastic lesions, 396–397
  embolism, 1563
  extrinsic obstruction, 1563
  intimal fibroplasia, 396–397
  medial dissection, 396–397
  medial fibroplasia, 396–397
  medial hyperplasia, 396–397
  nodular arteriosclerosis, 7
  pathology, 1545–1546
  periarterial fibroplasia, 396–397
  perimedial fibroplasia, 396–397
  unclamped kidney excision, 37
Renal artery aneurysm, 1562–1563, 1564
Renal artery disease, 1565
  atherosclerosis, 1561–1563, 1565
  classification, 1561–1563
Renal artery embolism, nuclear medicine, 1530
Renal artery obstruction, 1569
Renal artery stenosis, 1549
  bilateral, 1543–1545
  digital subtraction angiogram, 1522, 1523
  Doppler echocardiography, 1489
  transplant, 1592–1593, 1594, 1595
  unilateral, 1543–1545, 1678
Renal artery thrombosis, 1563
Renal atrophy, 1602
Renal baroreceptor, renin, 1292
Renal baroreceptor mechanism, 1096–1097
Renal biopsy, 1719
Renal blood supply, angiotensin, 1352–1353
Renal-body-fluid feedback
  arterial pressure, 1121–1123
  infinite gain control system, 1122
  pressure diuresis mechanism, 1122
  pressure natriuresis mechanism, 1122
  sodium excretion, 1122
  water excretion, 1122
Renal bypass surgery, 1552
Renal cell carcinoma, 1578
Renal change, pregnancy, 1764–1765
Renal circulation, 1372–1374
  age, 1372–1374, 2170
    tubular extraction efficiency, 1373–1374
    xenon-washout technique, 1373–1374
  anesthesia, 1897
  angiotensin-converting enzyme inhibitor, 2216
  borderline hypertension, 320
  captopril, 1352–1353
  essential hypertension, 319, 1352–1353
  filtration fraction, 1499–1500
    normal values, 1500
  glomerular filtration rate, renal perfusion pressure, 1145
  high-salt diet, converting-enzyme inhibition, 1359
  inverse blood pressure height relationship, 1372–1374
  offspring from hypertensive parents, 320
  para-aminohippurate, 1498–1499
  renal blood flow, 1499
    normal values, 1500
  renal plasma flow, 1498
    normal values, 1500
  renal vascular resistance, 1499
  sodium, 1365
Renal concentrating capacity, distal tubular function, 1502
Renal disease
  angiotensin-converting enzyme inhibitor, 2219
  childhood hypertension, 1861
  end-stage, 1585, 1590–1591
  hypertension, progression, 1171
  lateralization, 1549
  progressive
    anemia, 1170
    antihypertensive therapy, 1167
    castration, 1170
    experimental models, 1165–1166
    hypophysectomy, 1170
    therapy, 1170–1171
    thyroidectomy, 1170
    triple therapy, 1167
  progressive nature, 1163–1164
  systemic hypertension, progression, 1165
  unilateral, 38
Renal electrolyte transport, aldosterone, 1275–1280
Renal failure
  angioplasty, 1553–1554
  atrial natriuretic factor, 872
  beta-blocker, 2189
  blood pressure control, 1709
  chronic, reversible, 1539
  filtration surface area, 1158
  hypertension, frequency, 380, 382–383
  malignant hypertension, 2277
  sodium, 1158
Renal-fluid volume mechanism, 1048–1050
  pressure control, 1030–1037
    body salt balance, 1031–1032
    fluid intake output equilibration, 1031–1032
    pressure diuresis, 1030
    pressure natriuresis, 1030
    renal function curve, 1031

Renal function
  atrial natriuretic factor, 865–866
  cardiopulmonary receptor, 350
  Dahl S rat, 910
  diabetic nephropathy, 1733
  essential hypertension, 908–911
    human, 909, 911
    rat, 909–911
  glomerular filtration rate, 1632
  hyperkalemia, 1632
  Milan rat, 910–911
  preeclampsia, 1813
  spontaneously hypertensive rat, 909
Renal function curve
  isolated kidney, 1034
    renin-angiotensin-aldosterone system, 1035
  net fluid intake level, 1031
  salt-loading
    predicting long-term arterial pressures, 1036–1037
    renin-angiotensin-aldosterone system, 1035
    renin-angiotensin system, 1033–1035
Renal hemodynamics
  angiotensin II, 1106–1112
    angiotensin II blockade, 1107–1108
    chronic renal failure, 1108
    circulating angiotensin II, 1108–1110
    glomerular filtration rate regulation, 1106
    intrarenally formed angiotensin II, 1108–1110
    preglomerular vessel constriction, 1110–1112
    renal vascular resistance primary site, 1106
    renovascular hypertension, 1108
    tubuloglomerular feedback, 1106
  filtration surface area, 1157
  sodium, 1156
Renal hilar fibrosis, 1566
Renal history, office evaluation, 1388
Renal hypertension. *See also* Renovascular hypertension
  adrenal cortex, 26
  adrenalectomy, 26
  antihypertensive drug, 2174–2175
  pathogenesis, vicious circle concept, 34–47
  renal vein, 26
  renin, 31–32
Renal hypertrophy, diabetes mellitus, 1707
Renal incretory function, 844
Renal injury
  functional adaptations, 1164–1165
  hydronephrosis, 1601
Renal insufficiency, renal parenchymal disease, 1589–1590
Renal ischemia, 30, 1539, 1555
Renal kallikrein, 819–824
  cellular localization
    human nephron, 820–822
    rat nephron, 819–820
  dietary potassium, 819–827
Renal kallikrein-kinin system, 809–810
  antidiuretic hormone, 809
Renal kallikrein system, 819
  functions, 819
Renal lesion
  potassium, 51–52
    arteriolar dimensions, 51–52
    Dahl S rats, 51
    dilation scores, 51
    glomerular lesion scores, 51
  severity, 36
Renal mass, reduced, salt-loading renal function curve, 1036
Renal medullary lesion, salt-loading renal function curve, 1036
Renal morphologic change, rat, 1678
Renal papilla
  crude extracts, 845–848, 850
  refined renomedullary extracts, 848
  renomedullary interstitial cell, 842–843
    cultured extracts, 848
Renal parenchymal disease, 1583–1591
  antihypertensive agent, 1589–1590
  bilateral, 1583–1584
  salt metabolism, 1589–1590
  unilateral, 1583–1584
Renal parenchymal hypertension, salt balance, 1585–1586
Renal perfusion pressure, natriuresis, 38
Renal plasma flow, 1371–1375
  constant-infusion technique, 1372
  creatinine clearance, 1375
  mean arterial pressure, 1372–1374
  renal circulation, 1498
    normal values, 1500
Renal renin release, normal mechanisms, 1096
Renal revascularization, 1565–1568
  autotransplantation, 1567–1568
Renal scan, 1550–1551
Renal secretion, glomerular filtration coefficient, 1046
Renal segmental infarction, renovascular hypertension, 1547
Renal sodium excretion
  Dahl S rat, 948
  hypertension, first-degree relatives, 948
  hypertension pathogenesis, 947
  potassium, 1142
Renal sodium reabsorption, 1749
Renal transplantation. *See also* Transplantation
  immunosuppressive treatment, 1592, 1593
  pathophysiology, 1591–1593
Renal tubular acidosis, 1627
Renal tubular disorder, 1636
Renal tubular physiology, 1637
Renal tubular sodium reabsorption, angiotensin II, 1298
Renal vascular pathology
  adrenergic system, 1377
  cardiac output, 1376
    vasoconstriction, 1376
    vasodilation, 1376
  functional mechanisms, 1376
  historical aspects, 22
  renin-angiotensin system, 1376
  sympathetic nervous system, 1377
  vascular lesion, 1376
  vasoconstriction, 1377
Renal vascular resistance, 1374
  renal circulation, 1499
Renal vein, renal hypertension, 26
Renal-vein renin angiogram, 2062–2063
  arterial puncture, 2062
  indications, 2062
  nursing care after, 2062
Renal-vein renin measurement, 1575
  renovascular hypertension, 1447–1450, 1549–1550
Renal vessel, structural autoregulation, 574
Renin, 1181–1188. *See also* Plasma renin activity
  adrenal gland, 1320–1321
  aldosterone, 1092–1094
  alpha-methyldopa, 1295
  amiloride, 1294
  amino acids, 1179
  amniotic fluid, 1321–1322
  angiotensin I, hog vs. human, 1183
  angiotensin II, 1295
  angiotensinogen, 1295–1296
  antihypertensive drug, 2173–2174
  assay, 1183–1185
  beta-1-receptor blocker, 1295
  beta-blocker, 2193–2195
  biosynthesis, 1289
  brain, 1321
  brain and pituitary, 1321
  calcium antagonist, 2173–2174, 2175
  cDNA, 1320
  characterization, 1185–1188
  charge isomers, 1187
  Chinese hamster ovary, 1184–1185
  chorionic tissue, 1324
  clonidine, 1295
  converting-enzyme inhibitor, 1294
  cyclic GMP, second messenger, 1243
  diltiazem, 2173–2174, 2175
  diuretics, 1294
  double-domain enzymes, 1179
  enhancer and regulatory elements, 1319–1326
  enzymology, 1194
  essential hypertension, 31–32
  estradiol, 1323
  ethacrynic acid, 1294
  expression, 1184–1185
  extrarenal tissue, 1320–1322
  function, 32
  furosemide, 1294
  H-142, 1188, 1189
  heart, 1320
  hypertension treatment, 2173–2174
  indomethacin, 1908

juxtaglomerular apparatus, 1063
juxtaglomerular cells, 1324
kidney, gene expression, 1322
luteinizing hormone, 1323
macula densa, 1292
macula densa baroreceptor interaction, 1292
malignant hypertension, 31
metabolism, 1289
methoxyverapamil, 1238
molecular biology, 1319–1320
  human gene, 1319–1320
  mouse gene, 1319
mRNA, 1320–1323, 1325
nephrectomy, 1322
nephron, 809
nicardipine, 2173–2174, 2175
nifedipine, 2173–2174, 2175
nitrendipine, 2173–2174, 2175
noncirculating, 32
normal role, 1351–1352
in normal subjects, 1454
ovary, 1321–1322
pepsinogen, 1319
peptide substrate, 1183
pharmacologic factors, 1293, 1294–1295
phorbol ester, 1324
physiologic factors, 1293–1294
physiological role, 1194
pituitary, 1321
placenta, 1321–1322
progesterone, 1323
properties, 1185–1188
prorenin, 1184–1185
prostacyclin, 1905, 1906
prostaglandin
  first messenger, 1243
  second messenger, 1243
prostaglandin E_2, 1905, 1906
proteinuria, 1298
purification, 1185, 1579
release mechanisms, 1289–1292
renal baroreceptor, 1292
renal hypertension, 31–32
reproductive organs, 1321–1322
  adrenal, 1321–1322
  ovary, 1321–1322
  testis, 1321–1322
second messenger
  calcium efflux, 1236
  calcium influx, 1237–1241
  calcium mobilization, 1237–1241
  calcium sequestration, 1236
  cyclic AMP, 1242–1243
  cyclic AMP-calcium interactions, 1243
  intracellular calcium receptors, 1241–1242
  intracellular calcium sequestration, 1237
  potential-operated calcium channels, 1237–1239
  primary active calcium transport, 1236
  receptor-operated ion channel, 1239–1241
  Sutherland's criteria, 1242–1243
spironolactone, 72
synthesis and release, 1666
testis, 1321–1322
tissue renin system, 1320–1322
uterus, 1321–1322
vasculature, 1320
vasoconstriction, 32
verapamil, 1238
Renin-aldosterone system, calcium, 2040–2042
Renin/angiotensin, direct vascular injury, 45
Renin-angiotensin-aldosterone system, 1351–1358, 1443, 1444, 1586
  aldosterone, 1443
  angiotensin
    adrenal, 1355–1356
    aldosterone secretion, 1352
    blood pressure, 1354–1355
    renal blood supply, 1352–1353
    vascular smooth muscle, 1355–1356
  angiotensin II, 1443
  atrial natriuretic factor, 866–867
  blood pressure, 1288, 1443
    sodium volume, 1303–1306
  clonidine, 2252
  components, 1443
  diuretic, 2152–2153
  historical background, 1287–1288
  kallikrein-kinin system, 809
  normal physiology, 1287–1311
  normal role of renin, 1351–1352
  potassium and sodium co-regulation, 1306–1310
  potassium homeostasis, 1443
  prostaglandin system, 809
  renin release, 1356
  salt-loading renal function curve, 1035–1036
  sodium, 1288, 1304–1306
  sodium homeostasis, 1443
  sodium-volume homeostasis, 1303–1304
  systemic vascular resistance, 997–998
  weight loss, 2031
Renin-angiotensin cascade, 1181
  prorenin, 1189
  zymogen, 1189
Renin-angiotensin system, 1319, 1377–1379, 1539, 1540, 1542, 1574–1575, 1577, 1697
  autonomic control, 1377–1379
  cerebral circulation, 401, 402–403
  components, 2210
  diabetes mellitus, 1689, 1690
  diabetic hypertension, 1691–1692
  DOC-induced hypertension, 64–65
  hypertension, 1584
    high-renin, 339–340
    low-renin, 339–340
    subdivision, 339–340
  kininase II, 808
  normal physiology, 1761–1764
  potassium, 223, 1142–1143
  potential inhibition sites, 2344
  pregnancy, 1764–1772
    hypertension, 1772–1775
  remnant kidney, 1591–1592
  renal vascular pathology, 1376
  renovascular hypertension, 1542, 1555
  tubuloglomerular feedback, 1074–1076
  zonation, 1609
Renin-angiotensin vasoconstriction, arterial pressure control system, 1032–1033
  feedback gain, 1032
Renin assay
  description, 1455
  selection, 1455–1456
Renin biosynthesis, 1579
Renin cDNA, 1184
Renin-expression organ, 1325–1326
Renin gene, 955–964
  genetics
    Dahl rat gene structure, 959–961
    genomic DNA, 960, 961
    low renin hypertension, 963
    molecular, 959–963
    R renin gene restriction map, 960
    renin allele co-segregation analysis, 961–963
    restriction fragment-length polymorphism, 959
    restriction fragment-length polymorphism generation mechanism, 959
    S renin gene restriction map, 960
Renin gene derepression, 1578
Renin gene expression, kidney, 1322
Renin genotype
  blood pressure, 962
  body weight, 962
  heart weight, 962
Renin inhibitor, 2343–2348
  antihypertensive drug, 2347–2349
  chemical structure, 1182
  early, 2344
  hypertension treatment, 2347–2349
  modifications, 2345–2346
  oral activity, 2347
  principles, 2347
  species specificity, 2346–2347
  statine, scissile bond modifications, 2344–2345
  in vitro activity, 1182
Renin-inhibitor complex, 1186, 1187
Renin juxtaglomerular cell tumor
  computerized tomography, 1576
  electron microscopy, 1577
  natural history, 1576
Renin modulator, normal, 212
Renin-producing tumor, angiotensin-converting enzyme inhibitor, 2218

Renin profiling, 339
  vs. blood volume measurement, 344–345
Renin release, 1356
  beta-blocker, 2186
  major mechanisms, 1096
Renin-responsive adenoma, aldosterone-producing, 1616
Renin-secreting tumor, 1580–1581, 1583–1584
  cell culture, 1580
Renin secretion
  abnormal renal, 1448
  activation, 1603
  adrenergic activity, 1378–1379
  alpha-adrenoceptor, 1379–1380
  alpha-1 adrenoceptor, 1379–1380
  alpha-2 adrenoceptor, 1379–1380
    isometric exercise, 1379–1380
  angiotensin-converting enzyme inhibitor, 2216
  atrial natriuretic factor, 866
  baroreceptor mechanisms, 1243–1244
  beta-adrenergic stimulation, 621
  beta-1 adrenoceptors, 1379–1380
  beta-2 adrenoceptors, 1379–1380
  calcium, second messenger, 1233–1243
  cAMP, 621
  catecholamine, 1378–1379
  essential hypertension, abnormal patterns, 1091–1092
  extrarenal mechanisms, 1244
  first messenger, 1233–1245
  intrarenal mechanisms, 1243–1244
  macula densa
    detector-effector mechanism, 1096
    mechanism, 1244
    sodium chloride, 1097
  nephron
    baroreceptor detectors, 1089
    determinants, 1089
    individual, 1097–1098
    macula densa, 1089
  neural control, 1378–1379
  physiological regulation, 1243–1244
  renal adrenoceptor, 1378–1379
  second messenger, 1233–1245
  serum renin, 1090
  sleep, 1378
Renin-secretory response
  arterial hypertension, 1098–1099
  baroreceptor signal, 1098–1099
Renin-sodium profile test, 1391, 1392, 2061
Renin-specific peptide, 1183
Renin substrate, 1453–1454
  factors affecting levels, 1453
  level interpretation, 1454
  in normal subjects, 1454
Renin system
  blockade, 1294–1295
  methodology, 1455–1459
  overview, 1288–1289
  Type I diabetes, 1704–1705
  Type II diabetes, 1704–1705
Renin test, role, 1446–1450
Reninism. *See* Primary reninism
Renocellular system, 841–844
Renography, 1501–1502, 1514
  captopril, 1551
  exercise, 1551
  renovascular hypertension, renal artery stenosis, 1521–1522
Renohepatic axis, blood pressure, 856–858
  BW755C, 857
  cytochrome-P450-dependent enzyme system, 857
  isolated liver perfusion, 856–857
  renoportal venous shunt, 856, 857
  systemic circulation liver removal, 856, 857
Renomedullary interstitial cell, 842
  antihypertensive actions, 843
  captopril, 846
  Dahl R rat, 847
  ladder-like arrangement, 842
  monolayer cell cultures, 842
  renal papilla, 842–843
    cultured extracts, 848
Renomedullary vasodepressor lipid, 841–858
Renoportal venous shunt, 856, 857
Renoprival hypertension, 45
Renorenal reflex, 1462
Renovascular hypertension, 21, 30. *See also* Goldblatt hypertension; Renal hypertension
  anesthesia, 1900
  angioplasty, 1552–1554
  angiotensin-converting enzyme inhibitor, 2217–2218
  angiotensin II blockade, 1108
  animal models, 1540–1542
    acute and chronic phases, 1540, 1541
  animal pathophysiology, 1539–1542
  beta-blocker, 2195
  bilateral stenosis, 1543–1545
  captopril test, 1548–1549
  children, 1547, 1568–1570
  clinical screening, 1563–1564
  clinical signs and symptoms, 1546–1547
  diabetes mellitus, 1707
  diagnosis, 1447–1450, 1548–1552
  dietary potassium, 991, 992
  digital subtraction angiography, 1550
  fibromuscular dysplasia, 1545–1546
  hormonal factors, 1545
  human pathophysiology, 1542–1545
  hydronephrosis, 1604–1605
  intrarenal hemodynamics, 1555
  juxtaglomerular granular cell, 1059
  nephroptosis, 1542–1543
  non-surgical treatment, 1552–1556
  nuclear medicine, 1511–1519
    differential diagnosis, 1521–1525
  one-kidney one-clip model, 1540–1541, 1543
  plasma renin activity, 1548
  potassium, 993
  pregnancy, 1774
  prevalence, 1546
  proteinuria, 1547
  pulmonary edema, 1547
  renal segmental infarction, 1547
  renal-vein renin determination, 1549–1550
  renal-vein renin measurement, 1447–1450
  renin-angiotensin system, 1542, 1555
  renin-value prediction, 1605
  renography, renal artery stenosis, 1521–1522
  retinopathy, 1547
  scintirenography, 1522
    false positive rate, 1522–1524
  secondary hypertension, 736
  smoking, 1546, 1547, 1920
  surgical treatment, 1561
    indications, 1564–1565
    methods, 1564–1568
    results, 1568
  two forms of vasoconstriction, 1336
  two-kidney one-clip model, 1540, 1541, 1542, 1543
  unilateral renal artery stenosis, 1549–1550
  unilateral stenosis, 1543–1545
Reproducibility, screening, 152
Reproductive organs
  prorenin, 1321–1322
    adrenal, 1321, 1325
    ovary, 1321, 1325
    testis, 1321, 1325
  renin, 1321–1322
    adrenal, 1321–1322
    ovary, 1321–1322
    testis, 1321–1322
Reserpine, 2256
  adverse effects, 1898
  atherosclerosis, 513
  beta-blocker, 2192, 2202
  blood pressure, 530
  cardiovascular hypertrophy, 530
  clinical features, 2297
  development, 2099
  dosage, 2256
  glomerular injury, 1167
  hemodynamics, 2253
  hypertensive urgency, 2283
  interactions, 2297–2298
    antihypertensive drugs, 2297–2298
  mode of action, 2297
  side effects, 2253
Resistance
  arterial pressure, 573
  vascular bed, 573
Resistance curve, 569
  vascular bed, 572
Resistance vessel, 567–568
  hemodynamics, 567, 571
  precapillary, 572
  variables, 571
  vascular smooth muscle, 568

Respiration, blood pressure variation, 1418–1419
Respiratory disease, angiotensin-converting enzyme inhibitor, 2220
Rest. *See also* Specific type
  blood pressure measurement, 1976–1977
Retina
  blood supply, 434
  retinal vascular changes, 453–454
  retinal vascular reactivity, 454–455
Retinal arterial macroaneurysm, 457
Retinal arteriole, 436
Retinal arteriosclerosis, complications, 452–453, 456, 457
Retinal artery, 34, 435
  anesthesia, 42
  focal arterial narrowing, 42
  hypertension, 42–43
  overdistension, 42–43
  systolic pressure, 42
  vascular spasm, 42–43
  vasoconstriction, labile, 42–43
Retinal basement-membrane thickening, 1683
Retinal capillary, 458
  pericyte, 435
Retinal circulation, 435
Retinal hyperperfusion, 1683
Retinal pigment epithelium, 443
Retinal vasculature
  angioarchitecture, 435–437
  intraocular pressure, 436–437
  metabolic mechanism, 436–437
  pacemaker cells, 436–437
  physiologic regulation, 435–437
  reactivity, 437
  sclerotic changes, defined, 446–451
  transmural pressure, 436–437
Retinopathy, 10, 1680, 1683, 1684
  diabetic, 1695
  nephropathy, 1721
  renovascular hypertension, 1547
  reversal, 10
Retrofacial nucleus, 681
Rheology, 330, 332
Rhesus monkey, menstrual cycle, 1781
Rheumatic valve disease
  coronary disease, 120
  syphilitic aortitis, 120
Riboflavin, vegetarian diet, 245
Rice diet, 2003
Rice-fruit diet, 241, 244
  development, 2095
Riley-Day syndrome, 757–758
Riodipine, 472–473
Risk differentiation, hypertension, 1386–1395
Ritanserin, ketanserin, 775
Rough endoplasmic reticulum, kallikrein, 822
Ryosidine, 472–473

S

S-8307, 2352–2354
  captopril, 2353, 2355
  chemical structure, 2352, 2353
  furosemide, 2353, 2355
  nephrectomy, 2353, 2355
  saralasin, 2353, 2355
S-8308, 2352–2354
  chemical structure, 2352, 2353
Sabra rat, 923
Saccular aneurysm of descending thoracic aorta
  hypertension, 381
  frequency, 380, 381
Saline infusion, primary aldosteronism, 1615
Saline injection experiment, 39–40
Samoan study
  diet, 142
  obesity, 142
  psychosocial stress, 142
  traditional population, 142
  Western lifestyle, 142
Saphenous vein graft, 1567
Sarafotoxin S6, amino acid sequence, 649, 650
Saralasin, 1575
  S-8307, 2353, 2355
Sarcoplasmic reticulum
  calciosome, 971
  calcium-ATPase, 553
  calcium-pumping ATPase, 971–972
  calcium release, mechanisms mediating, 550, 551
  calcium-release channel, 973–974
  calcium transport, 970–974
    functional characteristics, 970–974
    molecular characteristics, 970–974
  calsequestrin, 971
  inositol triphosphate, 973
  T system, 971
  transverse tubular system, 971
Saturated fat, blood pressure, 257
Sauvagine, 797
Scintigram, 1654
Scintigraphic localization, 1614
Scintirenography, renovascular hypertension, 1522
  false positive rate, 1522–1524
Scleroderma, 1671
Sclerosis, arterial, Wagener-Clay-Gibner classification, 440, 442
Screening, 151–155
  defined, 151
  effectiveness, 154–155
  efficiency, 154–155
  hypertension, 153
    disease natural history, 152
  predictive value, 153
  prerequisites, 151–153
  prevalence, 152
  renovascular hypertension, 1563–1564
  reproducibility, 152
  sensitivity, 152
  severity, 152
  specificity, 152
  test suitability, 152
  validity, 152
Second messenger
  actin, 595
  actin-binding protein, 595
  calcium
    calcium efflux, 1236
    calcium influx, 1237–1241
    calcium mobilization, 1237–1241
    calcium sequestration, 1236
    cyclic AMP, 1242–1243
    cyclic AMP-calcium interactions, 1243
    extracellular calcium, 1233–1236
    intracellular calcium, 1233–1236
    intracellular calcium receptors, 1241–1242
    intracellular calcium sequestration, 1237
    potential-operated calcium channels, 1237–1239
    primary active calcium transport, 1236
    receptor-operated ion channel, 1239–1241
    Sutherland's criteria, 1242–1243
  generation, 585–589
  intermediate filament, 595
  renin
    calcium efflux, 1236
    calcium influx, 1237–1241
    calcium mobilization, 1237–1241
    calcium sequestration, 1236
    cyclic AMP, 1242–1243
    cyclic AMP-calcium interactions, 1243
    intracellular calcium receptors, 1241–1242
    intracellular calcium sequestration, 1237
    potential-operated calcium channels, 1237–1239
    primary active calcium transport, 1236
    receptor-operated ion channel, 1239–1241
    Sutherland's criteria, 1242–1243
Secondary hyperparathyroidism
  aldosteronism, 2043
  1,25-dihydroxyvitamin D, 2043
Secondary hypertension, 1734
  causes, 1510
  diabetes mellitus, 1706–1707
  dietary sodium restriction, 2011
  DOCA/salt-induced hypertension, 736
  estrogen use, 1388
  intervention studies, 2011
  nuclear medicine, 1509–1510
  office evaluation, 1388
  pheochromocytoma, 735–736, 1388
  renal parenchymal disease, 1583, 1585
  renovascular hypertension, 736, 1388
Secretion, kallikrein, 823
Segregating population, 956–957

Seizure
  elderly, 200
  oxygen radical, 673
Selective breeding, 955–956
Selective mortality, population blood pressure, 150
Self-care, physician-patient interaction, 2077
Self-report, 2315–2316
Senile plethora, 2094
Sensitivity, screening, 152
Septal nucleus, 684
Septal wall thickness, ventricular hypertrophy, 355
  hypertensive, 355
  normotensive, 355
Serial renal angiography, 1561
Serosal membrane, 1611
Serotonin
  artery, 763
  Bezold-Jarisch-like reflex, 763
  binding protein, 763
  biosynthesis, 762
  blood vessel, 763–765
  brain
    ascending serotonin pathways, 767, 768
    descending serotonin pathways, 768–769
  cardiovascular effects, 763
  central nervous system, 766–769, 771
    ascending serotonergic neuron, 767
    blood pressure regulation, 767–769
    descending serotonergic neuron, 767
    ketanserin, 771
    morphology, 766
    prazosin, 771
  cocaine, 763
  coronary artery, 1014, 1015
  endothelium-derived relaxing factor, 1255
  experimental hypertension, 769–770
    baroreceptor reflexes, 769
    Bezold-Jarisch-like reflex, 769
    vascular constrictor and dilator effects, 769
  hypertension
    carcinoid syndrome, 772–773
    human, 772–775
    human blood concentration, 772
  ICS205-930, 763
  ketanserin, 763–764
  liver, 762–763
  lung, 762–763
  MDL72222, 763
  metabolic pathways, 762
  metabolism, 762
  monoaminergic mechanism, 690–691
  noradrenaline, 765–766
    sympathetic nerve terminal release inhibition, 763
  platelet, 763
  platelet-derived product, 641
  removal, 762–763
  source, 761
  vasoconstriction, 765–766
  vein, 763
Serotonin antagonist
  experimental hypertension, 770–771
  hypertension, 773
  ketanserin, 770–771
  prazosin, 770–771
Serotonin neuron
  ascending, 767
  blood pressure regulation, 767
  brain
    morphology, 766
    projections, 766–767
  descending, 767
  projections, 766–767
Serotonin receptor
  classification, 763
  location, 764
Serpasil, adverse effects, 1898
Serpins, angiotensinogen, 1204
Serum angiotensin-converting enzyme, 1226
Serum calcium, experimental genetic hypertension, 981
Serum creatinine, 1544
  glomerular filtration rate, 1493–1494
  normal values, 1494
Serum ionized calcium
  diastolic pressure, 2045
  sodium, 2045
Serum lipid, smoking, 1919
Serum magnesium
  essential hypertension, 1007
    intracellular red blood cell level, 1007, 1008
    red blood cell level, 1007, 1008
  spontaneously hypertensive rat, 1007, 1008
Serum potassium
  anesthesia, 1892
Serum renin, renin secretion, 1090
Seventh-Day Adventist, vegetarian diet, 245–247
Severe hypertension
  antihypertensive drug, 2174–2175
  hemodynamics, 311
  initial treatment, 411
  intensified treatment, 411
  pulmonary circulation, 320–321
  randomized treatment trials, 420–421
Sex
  borderline hypertension, 175, 176
  cardiovascular disease, 106–107, 108
  DOC-induced hypertension, 65
  heart disease, 7
  hypertension, 159–173
    awareness, 178–179
    controlled, 175, 176
    medicated, 175, 176
    prevalence, 175, 176, 1838
    treatment, 178–179
  hypertension treatment, 1950–1951
  mortality, 1944
  plasma renin activity, 1445
  systolic hypertension, 176
Sex hormone, fat distribution, 1748–1749
Sexual dysfunction, centrally acting antihypertensive agents, 2253
Sexual infantilism, 1621
Sexual intercourse, blood pressure variability, 1399
Shear rate, blood viscosity, 330, 331
Shock
  neuropeptide, 799–800
  opioid peptide, 799–800
Short stature, hyperkalemia, 1628–1629
Shy-Drager syndrome, 757
  Cheyne-Stokes respiration, 757
  laryngeal stridor, 757
  norepinephrine, 757
Side effects, 19
  atenolol, 201
  bendroflurazide, 201
  diuretics, 201
  dizziness, 201
  elderly patient, 200
  glucose tolerance, 201
  gout, 201
  hydralazine, 201
  hydrochlorothiazide, 201
  hyperglycemia, 201
  rash, 201
  syncope, 201
  thiazide, 201
  triamterene, 201
Signal amplification, cAMP, second messenger system, 620
Signal transduction pathway, endothelin, 652–653
Silent ischemia, sympathoadrenal system, 1422–1423
Singlet oxygen, 669–670
  sources, 669–670
Sitting at rest
  diastolic pressure, 1985–1986
  systemic vascular resistance, 1985–1986
  systolic pressure, 1985–1986
Skeletal muscle
  blood flow, 320
    cardiac output, 320
    early mild hypertension, 320
  potassium, 56
  thyroid hormone, 1662
SK&F 86466, characterization, 2236
SKF525A, endothelium-derived relaxing factor, 837
Skin, beta-blocker, 2201
Skin color, 1837
Sleep, renin secretion, 1378
Sleep apnea, 1407, 1877
  sympathoadrenal system, 1421
Sleep/arousal, blood pressure variation, 1418
Sleepiness, elderly, 200
Smoking, 83, 106. *See also* Nicotine
  anesthesia, 1891
  aorta, 1923–1924
  arterial lesion, 1923–1924

blood pressure, 1918–1919
  variation, 1420
calcium, 476–477
cardiovascular consequences, 1922–1924
cardiovascular disease, 1917–1929
  historical perspective, 1917–1918
cardiovascular risk factor, 1918
  atheromata, 1918
  atherosclerosis, 1918
  interrelationship with other risk factors, 1918–1920
cerebrovascular disease, 1923
cessation effects, 1926–1927
cessation techniques, 1927–1929
clonidine, 1928
coronary artery, 1922–1923
coronary event, 1947
cultural transmission, 129
family environment, 129
heart, 1922–1923
heart disease, 7
hematorrheology, 1919
high-density lipoprotein, 109
hypertension
  alcohol, 1922
  estrogen, 1922
  fibrinogen, 1921
  hematologic parameters, 1921–1922
  hematorrheology, 1921
  hormonal changes, 1922
  leucocyte counts, 1921
  multivariate logistic regression coefficients, 110
  obesity, 1921
  oral contraceptives, 1922
  platelet function, 1921
  prognosis, 1919–1920
  serum lipids, 1920
  therapy choice, 1920
malignant hypertension, 1920
mecamylamine, 1928
mortality, 184, 186
nursing management, 2066–2067
obesity, 1919
oral contraceptive, 1919
peripheral vascular disease, 1923–1924
renovascular hypertension, 1546, 1547, 1920
serum lipid, 1919
stroke, 1946
Smooth muscle, tunica media, 522
Smooth muscle cell, 521
  angiotensin II, 590
  atherogenesis, 526
  atherosclerosis, 512, 522
  atherosclerotic lesion, 525
  calcium leak, 550
  cAMP, 621–622
  differentiation signal, 522
  inositol phosphate, 590
  phospholipase C, 543
  plaque, 525
Smooth muscle cell proliferation
  flunarizine, 514
  nimodipine, 514
  verapamil, 514
Smooth muscle contraction
  calcium, 889–892
    agonist-induced increases, 889
    altered transport in hypertension, 890–892
    filamin-actin-desmin, 889
    phosphatidylinositol, 889
    transport mechanisms, 890
  inositol phospholipid, 605
Smooth muscle proliferation, 18
  benign hypertension, 528
    mass vs. number, 528–529
    therapy mass effects, 529
    therapy number effects, 529
  cell death, 524
  control, 522–525
  heparan sulfate, 523
  inhibitors, 523
  malignant hypertension, 527–528
    mass vs. number, 528–529
    onion-skinning, 527
    therapy mass effects, 529
    therapy number effects, 529
Smooth muscle relaxation, phosphoinositide system inhibition, 606
Smooth muscle replication, atherosclerotic lesion, 525–526
Socioeconomic change, obesity, 143
Socioeconomic status, hypertension, 159–173
  clinical epidemiology, 167–170
Sodium. *See also* Na^+
  aldosterone, 1049
  angiotensin II, 1263
    adrenal response, 1353
    pressor response, 1353
    renal response, 1353
  atrial natriuretic factor, 869
  blood pressure, 205–212
    epidemiological data, 205–208
    physiological rationale, 2004–2005
  calcium, 2002–2003
  connecting tubule, 2147
  converting-enzyme inhibitor, 1363
  cortical collecting duct, 2147
  cortical collecting tubule, 1276
  cultural transmission, 129
  Dahl S rat, 57
    glomerular filtration rate, 57–58
    mechanisms favoring retention, 57
  diabetic glomerulopathy, 1158
  diabetic hypertension, 1689–1691
  diastolic pressure, 2045
  1,25-dihydroxyvitamin D, 2045
  DOC-induced hypertension, 64
  DOCA, 1281
  eicosanoid, 832
  essential hypertension, 1158, 1361
    aldosterone, 210
    patterns, 210
    plasma renin activity, 210
    sensitivity frequency, 1351
  family environment, 129
  filtration surface area, 1157
  hypertension, 205–212, 1154–1156, 1350–1351
    aldosterone, 209
    angiotensin II, 209
    body sodium, 210–211
    calcium excreted, 209
    cardiac output, 209
    dopamine, 209
    epidemiological data, 205–208
    epinephrine, 209
    established, 208
    excretion, 210
    extracellular fluid volume, 209
    glomerular filtration rate, 209
    nonpeptide natriuretic hormone, 209
    norepinephrine, 209
    physiological adaptations, 209–210
    prostacyclin, 209
    renal hemodynamics, 1156
    restriction, 208
    sodium intake, 210–211
    sodium sensitivity, 208–209, 2006–2007
    sodium sensitivity frequency, 1351
    sodium sensitivity mechanism, 1351
    Strauss concept, 210–211
  intraerythrocytic, 134
  juxtaglomerular cell, 58
  kallikrein, 808–809
  kidney, excretion rate, 57
  kidney mass, 1037, 1038
  low-renin hypertension, 212
  molecular basis, 295
  natriuresis, 1363
  nonmodulation, 1362–1363
  plasma aldosterone, 1367
  plasma renin activity, 1367
  potassium, 1142–1146, 2002–2003
  potassium excretion, 1140, 1141
  pregnancy, 1770–1771
  renal blood flow, 1365
  renal failure, 1158
  renal hemodynamics, 1156
  renal parenchymal hypertension, 1585–1586
  renin, 1092–1094
  renin-angiotensin-aldosterone system, 1288, 1304–1306
  sensitivity
    blood pressure, 2006–2007
    hypertension, 2014–2015
    hypertension treatment, 2015–2016
    in normal human, 2014–2015
  serum ionized calcium, 2045
  signal transmission, 58–60
    aqueduct block, 59
    third brain ventricle, 58–59
  sodium chloride, 2022
  sodium citrate, 2022
  thyroid hormone, 1670
  urinary sodium excretion, 1092–1094

Sodium (*contd.*)
  vegetarian diet, 245
  weight loss, 2031–2032
Sodium bromide, 2023
Sodium-calcium exchange, 552, 967
Sodium chloride
  Dahl S rat, 56
    potassium, 56
  hypertension, 56–60
    evidence of relationship, 56–57
  sodium, 2022
  sodium citrate, 2022
Sodium citrate
  sodium, 2022
  sodium chloride, 2022
Sodium depletion, 2150–2151, 2152
  aldosterone excretion, 1307
  potassium, 1307
Sodium escape, 1611
  DOC-induced hypertension, 64
Sodium excretion, 1360
  angiotensin II, 1112–1121
    aldosterone, 1113–1115
    circulating angiotensin II mediation, 1119–1120
    distal tubular effects, 1118–1119
    internally formed angiotensin II mediation, 1119–1120
    intrarenal actions, 1115
    medullary hemodynamics, 1116–1117
    natriuresis, 1120–1121
    peritubular capillary dynamics, 1115–1116
    proximal tubular effects, 1117–1118
    sympathetic nervous system, 1112–1113
    tubular reabsorption direct effects, 1117
  captopril, 1264
  distal nephron flow rate, 1141
  potassium excretion, 1133
  renal-body-fluid feedback, 1122
Sodium homeostasis, 1358–1363
  basal body sodium, setpoint, 1360–1361
  central nervous system, setpoint, 1361
  diabetes mellitus, 1690
  mechanisms, 1365–1367
  renin-angiotensin-aldosterone system, 1443
Sodium intake
  blood pressure, genetic susceptibility, 2001
  determinants, 1359–1360
Sodium-lithium countertransport, 134, 1690
Sodium metabolism
  calcium metabolism, interaction, 2044–2046
  renal parenchymal disease, 1589–1590
Sodium nitroprusside
  cerebral circulation, 408
  circulatory effects, 2266–2267
  hypertensive emergency, 2279
    in child, 1865
  metabolism, 2267
  mode of action, 2266–2267
  mode of use, 2267
  pharmacokinetics, 2267
  predominant hemodynamic effect, 2125
  side effects, 2267
  toxicity, 2267
Sodium restriction, 1592, 1753
  hyperkalemia, 1635
  pregnancy, 1822
Sodium salt
  anionic component, 2022
  non-chloride-containing, 2022
Sodium thiocyanate, 2096
Sodium transport, 1749
  aldosterone, 1275–1276
Sodium-volume homeostasis
  diuretic, 2148–2149
  renin-angiotensin-aldosterone system, 1303–1304
Solitary kidney, 1554, 1556, 1564
  hydronephrosis, 1605–1606
  post-transplant hypertension, 1594, 1595
Somatostatin, 797
  neuropeptide, 800
Sotalol
  alpha-blocking properties, 2119
  beta-1-adrenoceptor selectivity, 2119, 2183
  beta-blocking metabolites, 2183
  beta-blocking plasma concentration, 2183
  bioavailability, 2183
  dosage, 2184
  dosage frequency, 2184
  equipotent single dose, 2184
  intrinsic sympathomimetic activity, 2119, 2183
  lipophilicity, 2183
  membrane-stabilizing effect, 2183
  plasma half-life, 2184
  protein binding, 2183
  structure, 2182
Soya protein, blood pressure, 251
Specificity, screening, 152
Sphygmomanometer
  development, 22
  historical aspects, 84
Spinal artery, maternal, 1786
Spinal cord, 679–680
  sympathoadrenomedullary system, 712
Spiral artery, 1785
  acute atherosis, 1784
Spironolactone
  adverse effects, 1898
  aldosterone, 1615–1616
  aspirin, 2063
  chemical structure, 2144
  diuretic, 2158
  dosage, 2144
  dosage interval, 2144
  duration of action, 2144
  kallikrein, 808–809
  renin, 72
  side effects, 2157
Splanchnic circulation
  anesthesia, 1896–1897
  borderline hypertension, 320
  established hypertension, 320
Spleen, angiotensinogen, 1208
Splenorenal bypass, 1566, 1567
  children, 1570
Split renal function test, 1551
Spontaneously hypertensive rat, 977–978
  arteriosclerosis, 498
    mesenteric artery, 499
  calcium antagonist
    distal mesenteric artery branches, 486
    mesenteric artery proximal part, 486
  cell membrane alteration, 904–905
  cytochrome-P450, 836
  glomerulosclerosis, 501
  hormone, 906–907
  humoral factor, 906–907
  hypertension, 296–300
    stroke-prone, 296–300
  life expectancy, 497–504
    antihypertensive drugs, 497–504
    calcium antagonist, 497–504
  magnesium, red blood cell level, 1007, 1008
  membrane mechanism, 904–905
  nephrosclerosis, 500
  neural mechanism, 911–912
  nisoldipine, 500, 501
  phenotypic variation, 977
  potassium, 52–55, 220, 992
  renal function, 909
  salt-loading renal function curve, 1036
  serum magnesium, 1007, 1008
  tubuloglomerular feedback, 1082
Sprague-Dawley rat
  DOC-induced hypertension, 65
  potassium, 220
SQ-14225, angiotensin II, 1111
St. Mary's study, 85–86
Statine, renin inhibitor, scissile bond modifications, 2344–2345
Stepped-care regimen
  development, 2107
  Hypertension Detection and Follow-up Program, 197
Steroid, digitalis-like factor, 940–941
Steroid hormone
  atrial natriuretic factor, 867–868
  biosynthetic pathway, 1610
Steroid hypertension
  stress, 46
  vessel wall, 46
Steroidogenesis
  adrenal cortex, 1609–1610
  regulation, 1610

Stilbestrol, adrenal-regeneration hypertension, 68
Stillbirth, captopril, 1771
Stimulus-response coupling mechanism, tubuloglomerular feedback, 1074–1076
  adenosine, 1075
  calcium ion, 1075–1076
  cyclic AMP, 1076
  prostaglandin, 1074–1076
  renin activation, 1074
  renin-angiotensin system, 1074
  renin secretion, 1074
  sodium chloride concentration, 1076
  sodium chloride osmolarity, 1076
Strain, DOC-induced hypertension, 65
Strength training, blood pressure, 1993
Stress, 1400
  age, 46
  blood pressure variability, 1400
  catecholamine, 727
  cholesterol, 245
  coronary disease, 245
  hypertension, 245
  primary arterial disease, 46–47
  steroid hypertension, 46
  sympathetic innervation, 45–46
  uremia, 46
  vascular hypertrophy, 45
  vessel wall, 45–47
  x-irradiation, 46
Stress-induced hypertension, dietary magnesium deficiency, 1017
  arteriolar tone, 1017
  venular tone, 1017
Stress relaxation, arterial pressure control system, 1032–1033
  feedback gain, 1032
Stretch-activated channel, 547
Striate artery, aneurysm, 9
Stroke, 18, 405–406, 2135, 2284–2285
  alcohol, 289–290, 2066
  antihypertensive treatment, 115, 412–413, 426–428
    acute stroke hypertension management, 426–427
    cerebral infarction, 426–427
    intracerebral hemorrhage, 427
    primary prevention, 426
    subarachnoid hemorrhage, 427
  arterial pressure, 8
  atherothrombotic, 405–406
  bendrofluazide, 1974
  black diet, 49
  blood pressure, 19
    high, 412
    treatment problems, 412
  Chinese diet, 49–50
  cholesterol, 19
  diastolic pressure, 1974
  drugs of choice, 2283
  elderly, 194
  electrocardiogram, left ventricular hypertrophy, 112
  epidemiological studies, 405
  European Working Party on Hypertension in the Elderly, 198
  historical aspects, 49
  hypertension, 101–102, 417–428
    antihypertensive treatment trials, 420–421
    atherosclerosis, 422
    epidemiologic evidence of risk, 417–420
    Finland, 419
    Framingham Heart Disease Epidemiology Study, 417–419
    Japan, 419
    Japanese descent, 419
    large-vessel disease, 422–423
    Netherlands, 419
    pathogenesis, 421–426
    plaque, 422
    relative risk, 101
    Rochester, Minn., 419–420
    small-vessel disease, 423–425
    stroke risk factor, 417–421
    treated, 122
    untreated, 122
  hypomagnesemia, 1013
  incidence, 419
  intracerebral hemorrhage, 405–406
  Japanese diet, 49–50
  lacunar, 405–406
  mortality, 113, 194
    geographic variation, 171–173
  potassium, deaths, 50–51
  prehistoric vs. present levels, 49
  prevention, 19
  propranolol, 1974
  recurrence prevention, 427–428
  Scots diet, 49
  smoking, 1946
  stroke-prone rat, 296–297
    diet, 296–297
  systolic pressure, 1973, 1974
    bendrofluazide, 1972
    propranolol, 1972
    smoking, 1972
  Tibetan diet, 49
Stroke volume
  acebutolol, 2121–2123
  atenolol, 2121–2123
  beta-blocker, 2125
  bopindolol, 2121–2123
  cardiac ventricle capacity, 567
Structural autoregulation, 527, 573
Structural modulation
  aorta, 577
  artery, 577
  vein, 577
Subarachnoid hemorrhage, 7, 406–407, 427
Subcortical arteriosclerotic encephalopathy, 425–426
Submandibular gland, glandular kallikrein, 806, 807
Subscapular skinfold thickness, 103–104, 107
  diastolic pressure, 105
  systolic pressure, 105
Substance P, 796
  met^5-enkephalin, 1221
Sucrets, 1913
Sudden coronary death, hypertension, frequency, 379–380
Sudden death, 112–113
  antihypertensive treatment, 112
  beta-blocker, 2197
  diabetes, 112
  diuretic, 113
  electrocardiogram abnormality, 113
  exercise-related, 1988
  hypertension, pathogenesis, 119
  MRFIT study, 113
  prevention, beta-blocker, 2197–2199
Sulfonamide
  coronary event, 2109
  interstitial nephritis, 2158
Sulfonylurea, beta-blocker, 2189
Sulindac, 1907
Super Odrinex, 1913
Superoxide
  acute hypertension, generation, 672
  oxygen, 668–669
  sources, 668
Superoxide dismutase, endothelium-derived relaxing factor, 837
Supine rest
  diastolic pressure, 1985–1986
  systemic vascular resistance, 1985–1986
  systolic pressure, 1985–1986
Supraventricular tachyarrhythmia, atrial natriuretic factor, 872–873
Surgical treatment, renovascular hypertension, 1561
Sympathectomy
  development, 2096
  surgical, 2096
Sympathetic activity, 1697
  cardiopulmonary receptor, 349–350
  dietary intake, 1751
Sympathetic innervation
  stress, 45–46
  vessel wall, 45–46
Sympathetic nervous system
  activity, 1753
  angiotensin-converting enzyme inhibitor, 2214–2215
  angiotensin II, 1112–1113
  blood pressure regulation, 1585, 1586
  cardiac output, 321
  cerebral circulation, 401
  direct nerve recording, 725
  diuretic, 2153
  heart rate, 321
  hypertension, brain lesions, 707
  insulin, 1693, 1749–1750
  norepinephrine, 1467–1469
    cerebrospinal fluid, 1468
    plasma, 1467–1468

Sympathetic nervous system, norepinephrine (*contd.*)
turnover, 1468–1469
urinary, 1467
opioid peptide, 796
oxygen consumption, 321
reflex activity, 2238
renal vascular pathology, 1377
renin secretion, 1762
sodium excretion, 1112–1113
Type I diabetes, 1704–1705
Type II diabetes, 1704–1705
vasoconstriction, two forms, 1340–1341
weight control, 1752, 1753
weight loss, 2031
Sympathoadrenal discharge abnormality syndrome
alcoholism, 1421
autonomic dysfunction, 1422
neurologic abnormality, 1421
panic attack, 1421–1422
postanesthesia hypertension, 1421
postsurgical hypertension, 1421
sleep apnea, 1421
withdrawal syndromes, 1421
Sympathoadrenal system, 1416–1424
blood volume control, 1416–1417
cardiopulmonary baroreflex, 1417
carotid baroreflex, 1417
central blood volume, 1417
central-volume-sympathoadrenal dysregulation syndromes, 1422–1424
chronic stress, 1420–1421
cigarette smoking, 1420
diurnal variation, 1420
exercise, 1419
hypoglycemia, 1420
life crises, 1420–1421
menstrual cycle, 1420
pain, 1419
perspiration, 1418–1419
postprandial alterations, 1419–1420
posture, 1417, 1419
seasonal change, 1420
sleep/arousal, 1418
systemic hemodynamics control, 1416–1417
temperature change, 1420
volume depletion, 1420
white coat hypertension, 1419
withdrawal syndromes, 1420–1421
Sympathoadrenomedullary system
adrenoceptor, 719–720
anteroventral third ventricle, 717–718
blood pressure arterial baroreflex homeostatic regulation, 712–713
brain stem, 712–716
cardiovascular adrenoceptor, 719–720
catecholamine release, 718–719
catecholamine synthesis, 718
central neural adrenoceptor, 720
circumventricular organ, 717–718
functional anatomy, 712–720
generalized activation pattern, 721–722
hierarchical organization, 712
hypothalamus, 716–717
limbic system, 717
mechanoreceptor reflexes, 714–715
resetting, 715
neural pathways, 713
norepinephrine, 719
local modulation, 719
reflexive modulation, 719
parasympathetic nervous system, 720–721
paraventricular nucleus, 717
spinal cord, 712
sympathetic nerve, 712
sympathetic neuroeffector junction, 718–720
sympathetic vasomotor tone origin, 715–716
ventrolateral medulla, 715–716
Sympatholytic drug
beta-blocker, 2192
hypertensive urgency, 2282–2283
in normal volunteers, 2334–2335
Syncope, side effects, 201
Syndrome of inappropriate antidiuretic hormone secretion, atrial natriuretic factor, 872
Syphilitic aortitis, rheumatic valve disease, 120
Systemic arterial pressure, phenylpropanolamine, 1913–1914
Systemic circulation, calcium
contractile vascular tone, 485
flow resistance, 485
Systemic flow resistance, essential hypertension, 329
Systemic hemodynamics
obesity, 2026–2027
weight loss, 2030–2031
Systemic hypertension, 1588–1589
angiotensin II, 1262–1263
diabetes, 1677, 1680
diabetic glomerulopathy, 1681
dietary therapies, 1169–1170
endothelin, 656
experimental models, 1165
pharmacologic therapy, 1167–1169
renal disease, progression, 1165
urinary protein excretion, 1166
Systemic lupus erythematosus, 1671
Systemic mastocytosis, histamine, 1424
Systemic precapillary resistance vessel
functional autoregulation, 573
structural autoregulation, 573
Systemic resistance vessel
biophysical aspects, 566–569
hypertrophic adaptation, 565–579
methodological aspects, 569–570
hemodynamic approach, 569–570
morphometric techniques, 569–570
structural changes, 570–575
cerebral vessel autoregulation, 575
coronary vessel autoregulation, 574–575
location, 572–574
renal vessel autoregulation, 574
Systemic vascular resistance
adrenergic nervous system, 997
angiotensin II, 998–999
exercise, 1986
exogenous hormone pressor responses, 998
renin-angiotensin-aldosterone system, 997–998
sitting rest, 1985–1986
supine rest, 1985–1986
transmembrane potential, 996–997
vasopressin, 997
Systolic hypertension, 11, 1668
age, 176
cardiovascular sequelae, 102, 104
elderly, 1883–1884
Type II diabetic, 1706
isolated, 1733
race, 176
sex, 176
Systolic Hypertension in the Elderly Program, 199
Systolic pressure
age, 102, 104
atenolol, 1975
atherothrombotic brain infarction, 417–418
blood pressure tracking, 1857
Britain, 147–148
cardiac event, 1974
controlled clinical trials, 1970–1971
converting-enzyme inhibitor, 1167–1168
coronary disease, 120, 1971, 1973
autopsy studies, 120
definitions, 1870, 1871
diagnosing hypertension, 1964
elderly, 191, 1964
epidemiological considerations, 1970
exercise, 1985–1986
insulin, 131
insulin-dependent diabetes, 1723
isolated systolic hypertension. *See* Isolated systolic hypertension
Japan, 147–148
Kenya, 147–148
left ventricular mass index, 1977
lipid abnormality, 131
mortality, 183, 184, 1973, 1975
English, 184
European, 184
nicotine, 1891
pindolol, 2190
potassium, 218
propranolol, 2190
retinal artery, 42
sitting rest, 1985–1986
stroke, 1973, 1974
bendrofluazide, 1972
propranolol, 1972
smoking, 1972

subscapular skinfold thickness, 105
supine rest, 1985–1986
taurine/creatinine, 300
treatment initiation, 1969–1972
pathological considerations, 1970
triple therapy, 1167–1168
type I diabetes, 130
urinary albumin excretion, 1731
diabetic nephropathy, 1725
waist/hip ratio, 132
worksite measurement, 1977

T

T system
endoplasmic reticulum, 971
sarcoplasmic reticulum, 971
Tabes dorsalis, 758
Tachycardia, nicotine, 1891
Takayasu's aortitis, renal arterial disease, 396
Takayasu's arteritis, 1546
Target organ damage, mean arterial pressure, 1980
Taurine/creatinine
diastolic pressure, 300
systolic pressure, 300
Technetium-99m, doses, 1511
Telephone transmission, home blood pressure monitors, 1435
Temperature change, blood pressure variation, 1420
Tension, vascular muscle, 661–662
Teprotide, 2210
Terazosin
biotransformation, 2242
cardiovascular hemodynamics, 2125–2126
characterization, 2236
chemical structures, 2234
dosage, 2244
efficacy, 2244
elderly, 2247
mode of action, 2239
pharmacokinetics, 2242
postural hypotension, 2244
predominant hemodynamic effect, 2125
Terminal artery
caliber changes, 41
spasm, 41
Testis
angiotensin-converting enzyme, 1226
angiotensinogen, 1208
renin, 1321–1322
Testosterone biosynthesis, angiotensin II, 1298–1299
Tetraethylammonium, 2097
hemodynamics, 2097
Tetraethylammonium chloride, 2096
TGF-beta, vascular wall injury, 523
Therapeutic alliance, 2310
Therapeutic nihilism, 2096
Thermogenesis
insulin, 1751
obesity, 1751–1752
thyroid hormone, 1662–1663
Thiamine deficiency, 289
Thiazide
adverse effects, 1898
cardiovascular hemodynamics, 2118–2119
chemical structure, 2144
cholecystitis, 2158
clinical features, 2293
development, 2099–2100
dosage, 2144
dosage interval, 2144
duration of action, 2144
hemodynamics, 323
hypomagnesemia, 1009
interactions, 2293–2294
antihypertensive drugs, 2293–2294
magnesium, 1009
metoprolol, 1947–1948
mode of action, 2293
side effects, 201
Thick ascending limb of Henle's loop, 1053
calcium, 2146
diuretic, 2145–2146
epidermal growth factor, 1057
magnesium, 2146
transport, 2146
Thirst, atrial natriuretic factor, 869
Thirst stimulation, angiotensin II, 1298
Thrombin
coronary artery, 642
endothelium-derived relaxation factor, 1255
norepinephrine, 641
prostacyclin, 638
Thrombosis, 521
Thromboxane, 1786, 1792
formation, 259
hypertension, 834–835
experimental, 834–835
human, 834–835
Thromboxane A_2, 830–831
biosynthesis pathways, 1905, 1906
glomerular filtration rate, 835
nonsteroidal anti-inflammatory drug, 1905, 1906
preeclampsia, 1798–1800
Thromboxane A_3, 835, 836
Thromboxane B_2, 833, 834–836
Thromboxane biosynthesis, 1801
Thyroid carcinoma, 1647
pheochromocytoma, 1645
Thyroid disease, 1671–1672
cardiovascular manifestations, 1662
hypertension, 1661
Thyroid hormone
aldosterone, 1667
angiotensinogen, 1210
atrial natriuretic factor, 1667
blood pressure regulation, 1661, 1665–1667
cardiovascular manifestations, 1668
cardiovascular system, 1663–1665
catecholamine, 1666
intracellular effects, 1661–1662
replacement, 1666, 1672
thermogenesis, 1662–1663
vascular resistance, 1664
Thyroid status, drug metabolism, 1663
Thyroid storm, 1669
Thyrotoxicosis, 1666
beta-blocker, 2189
Thyrotropin-releasing hormone, 797
neuropeptide, 800
Thyroxin, cardiovascular structural adaptation, 577–578
Thyroxine, angiotensinogen, 1210
Timolol
alpha-blocking properties, 2119
beta-1-adrenoceptor selectivity, 2119, 2183
beta-blocking metabolites, 2183
beta-blocking plasma concentration, 2183
bioavailability, 2183
cardiac output, 2121
dosage, 2184
dosage frequency, 2184
equipotent single dose, 2184
hemodynamics, 2186
intrinsic sympathomimetic activity, 2119, 2183
lipophilicity, 2183
membrane-stabilizing effect, 2183
plasma half-life, 2184
protein binding, 2183
structure, 2182
vascular resistance, 2121
Tissue kallikrein, characteristics, 806
Tissue renin system
hypertension, 1319–1326
adrenal gland, 1325
heart, 1325
kidney, 1325–1326
reproductive system, 1325
vasculature, 1325
prorenin, 1322–1324
extrarenal organs, 1324
kidney, 1324
prorenin secretion, 1323–1324
Tolazoline
characterization, 2236
chemical structures, 2234
Total peripheral resistance. *See also* Peripheral resistance
acebutolol, 2121–2123
antihypertensive drug, 2128
arterial pressure, 1046
afferent renal arteriolar resistance, 1047
atenolol, 2121–2123
autoregulation, 1040–1042
beta-blocker, 2125
bopindolol, 2121–2123
cardiac output, 305, 1046
afferent renal arteriolar resistance, 1047
hypertension, increasing, 1047

Total peripheral resistance (*contd.*)
pindolol, 2121–2123
propranolol, 2121–2123
volume-loading hypertension, 1040
late stage changes, 1040
Toxemia of pregnancy, eicosanoid, 834
Toxic principle, Goldblatt experiment, 28
Tractus solitarius nucleus, opioid peptide, 796
Traditional population
cardiovascular adaptation
cold stress, 141–142
heat stress, 141
high-altitude hypoxia, 140–141
Samoan study, 142
Transcendental meditation, hypertension treatment, 2088–2089
Transducin, 618
Transient ischemic attack, hemodynamic origin, 411–412
Transient left ventricular dysfunction, sympathoadrenal system, 1422–1423
Transluminal balloon dilatation, 1552
Transmembrane calcium flux, endothelin, 653
Transmembrane potential
systemic vascular resistance, 996–997
vascular smooth muscle cell, components, 996
Transplantation
cyclosporine, 1829
normal renal function, 1593
renal artery stenosis, 1592–1593
Transverse tubular system
endoplasmic reticulum, 971
sarcoplasmic reticulum, 971
Trasylol, 810–811
Treatment decision, 1967–1972
95 mmHg, 17
100 mmHg, 17
clinical trial evidence, 1956–1957
U.S. Joint National Committee report, 17
WHO recommendations, 17
Triaminic, 1913
Triaminic 12, 1913
Triaminicin, 1913
Triamterene
chemical structure, 2144
dosage, 2144
nonsteroidal anti-inflammatory agent, 2158
side effects, 201
Trichlormethazide
dosage, 2144
dosage interval, 2144
duration of action, 2144
Tricyclic antidepressant, beta-blocker, 2202
Tricyclic calcium antagonist, 1014–1015, 1017
Trifluoperazine, calcium antagonist, 1014–1015, 1017
Triglyceride, 106, 131–132
Triiodothyronine, angiotensinogen, 1210
Trimazosin
biotransformation, 2242
characterization, 2236
chemical structures, 2234
dosage, 2243
efficacy, 2243
mode of action, 2239
pharmacokinetics, 2242
Trimetaphan, cerebral circulation, 409
Trimethaphan camsylate
hypertensive emergency, 2281
nitroglycerin, 2281
phentolamine, 2281
Triple therapy
systolic pressure, 1167–1168
urinary protein excretion, 1167–1168
Trivalent cation, calcium antagonist, 1014–1015, 1017
Trophoblastic cell, 1785
Trophoblastic tissue, 1786
Trousseau's sign, 1613
Trypsin, prorenin, 1191–1192
Tryptophan, 762
chloride, 1224
Tubocurarine, beta-blocker, 2202
Tubular atrophy, mild hypertension, 394–395
Tubular component, juxtaglomerular apparatus, 1053–1058
Tubular electrolyte transport, aldosterone, mechanism of action, 1280–1282
Tubular function, 1502
Tubuloglomerular feedback, 1067–1087
arterial pressure
acute change effect, 1081–1082
autoregulation, 1081
quantitation, 1081–1082
carbonic anhydrase inhibitor, 1079
experimental hypertension, 1082–1083
external forcing, 1078, 1079
extracellular volume, 1079–1080
acute volume depletion, 1080
acute volume expansion, 1080
chronic extracellular volume increase, 1080
Goldblatt hypertension, 1082, 1083
high-protein diet, 1079
hypertension pathophysiology, 1082–1083
hypertonic sodium chloride, 1078–1079
integrated loop function, 1078–1083
luminal signal, 1071–1074
distal sodium chloride concentration loop flow, 1071–1072
ion specificity, 1072–1073
sodium chloride concentration, 1072
sodium chloride transport, 1073–1074
mechanism, 1071–1078
Milan rat, 1082
resetting, 1078, 1079, 1080–1081
interstitial pressure, 1080
luminal factors, 1081
plasma angiotensin, 1081
vascular resetting, 1080–1081
spontaneously hypertensive rat, 1082
stimulus-response coupling mechanism, 1074–1076
adenosine, 1075
calcium ion, 1075–1076
prostaglandin, 1074–1076
renin activation, 1074
renin-angiotensin system, 1074
renin secretion, 1074
sodium chloride concentration, 1076
sodium chloride osmolarity, 1076
transport alterations, 1078–1079
vascular effector mechanism, 1076–1078
flow resistance, 1078
glomerular plasma flow, 1077–1078
postglomerular resistance, 1078
preglomerular resistance, 1078
pressure gradients, 1076–1077
stop-flow pressure, 1076–1077
Tumor angiogenesis, 521–522
Tunica media
hypertensive retinopathy, 459
smooth muscle, 522
Tussagesic, 1913
Twin study, blood pressure, 93, 94–95
dizygotic, 95
monozygotic, 95
Two-detector renography, 1501–1502
Two-dimensional echocardiography, left ventricle, 1485–1488
load, 1486–1487
performance, 1486–1487
structure, 1486–1487
Two-kidney Goldblatt hypertension, 1681
Two-kidney one-clip model, renovascular hypertension, 1540, 1541, 1542, 1543
Type-A behavior
ischemic heart disease, 1013
magnesium deficiency, 1013
Type I diabetes, 1703
renin system, 1704–1705
sympathetic system, 1704–1705
Type II diabetes, 1703
hypertension, 1705, 1706
renin system, 1704–1705
sympathetic system, 1704–1705
Tyrosine hydroxylase, genes, 749
Tyrosine kinase system, phosphoinositide signaling system, 606

U

UK-14,304, characterization, 2236
Ultradian blood pressure rhythm, 1399
Ultrasound, 1551
lateral resolution, 1480
maximum frequency shift, 1480

  measurement techniques, 1432
  Nyquist limit, 1480
  physical principles, 1480
  regional circulation, 1489
  spatial resolution, 1480
Umbilical artery, Mg^{2+}, 1015
Umbilical vein, Mg^{2+}, 1015
Unilateral kidney disease, 38
Unilateral nephrectomy, 1583, 1584
Uninephrectomy, urinary protein excretion, 1166
Unsaturated fatty acid, hypertension, 835–836
Urapidil
  biotransformation, 2242
  cardiovascular hemodynamics, 2125–2126
  central hypotensive activity, 2240
  chemical structures, 2234
  dosage, 2244
  efficacy, 2244
  hemodynamics, 2240
  pharmacokinetics, 2242
  pharmacological properties, 2239
  predominant hemodynamic effect, 2125
  side effects, 2245
Urea, glomerular filtration rate, 1495
Uremia, 7
  arteriolar lesion, 27–29
  hypertension, untreated, 122
  stress, 46
  vascular lesion, 44
  vessel wall, 46
Ureteral obstruction
  bilateral, hemodynamic effects, 1603
  tubular effects, 1603
  unilateral
    hemodynamic effects, 1602–1603
    human observations, 1604–1605
    tubular effects, 1603
Ureterocaval anastomosis, 1541
Ureterovenous anastomosis, accelerated renoprival hypertension, 841
Urinary acidification, 1632
Urinary albumin, 1726, 1727
  diastolic blood pressure, diabetic nephropathy, 1726
  instrumental evaluation, 1391
  laboratory evaluation, 1391
  systolic blood pressure, 1731
    diabetic nephropathy, 1725
Urinary aldosterone, 1615
  assay description, 1457–1458
  blood collection, 1456–1457
  clinical laboratories, 1458
  commercial kits, 1458
  laboratory evaluation, 1392
  methods, 1456–1459
  plasma renin, 1091, 1092
  urinary sodium excretion, 1091, 1092, 1445
  urine collection, 1456–1457
Urinary catecholamine, pheochromocytoma, 1651
Urinary colic, 1602
Urinary creatinine
  normal values, 1494
  urinary sodium excretion, 1999
Urinary dopamine, 38, 726–727
Urinary excretion, 218
  measurement problems, 218
Urinary potassium, laboratory evaluation, 1391
Urinary protein excretion
  converting-enzyme inhibitor, 1167–1168
  low-protein diet, 1166
  systemic hypertension, 1166
  triple therapy, 1167–1168
  uninephrectomy, 1166
Urinary sodium
  aldosterone, 1049
  angiotensin II, 1263
  plasma renin, 1091, 1092
  plasma renin activity, 1445
  sodium, 1092–1094
  urinary aldosterone excretion, 1091, 1092, 1445
  urinary creatinine excretion, 1999
Urine, plasma aldosterone, 1450–1453
  factors, 1450–1451
  hypertension workup, 1451–1453
Urotensin I, 798
U.S. Public Health Service Hospital Study, 1943–1944
Uterine anatomy, 1780–1784
  pregnant uterus, 1781–1784
Uterine epithelium, 1782
Uterine nerve change, 1783–1784
Uteroplacental bed, 1786
  physiologic changes, 1787
Uteroplacental blood flow, 1771–1772
Uterus, renin, 1321–1322

V

Vagal tone, angiotensin II, 1298
Validity, screening, 152
Valsalva maneuver, hyperadrenergic dysautonomia, 1471–1474
Vascular bed, 567
  arterial pressure, 573
  norepinephrine, 571
  resistance, 573
  resistance curve, 572
Vascular disease
  calcium channel antagonist, 511–517
  hypertension, 30
  microalbuminuria, 1721–1722
Vascular effector mechanism, tubuloglomerular feedback, 1076–1078
  flow resistance, 1078
  glomerular plasma flow, 1077–1078
  postglomerular resistance, 1078
  preglomerular resistance, 1078
  pressure gradients, 1076–1077
  stop-flow pressure, 1076–1077
Vascular failure, high-volume state, 1044
Vascular hypertrophy
  essential hypertension, 914–915
  hypertension, non-kidney, 1047–1048
  stress, 45
  vessel wall, 45
Vascular injury, plasma renin, 1341–1344
  pressure hypothesis, 1343–1344
Vascular lesion, 38
  Bright's disease, 38
  deoxycorticosterone, 44
  epinephrine, 44
  ergotamine, 44
  malignant hypertension, 38
  pathogenesis, 39–44
  uremia, 44
  vasoactive agent, 44–45
  vasopressin, 44
Vascular muscle
  calcium influx, 662
  calcium release, 662
  electrophysiology, 661–664
  hypertension, 664
  ion channel, 662
  membrane potential, 661–662
  tension, 661–662
Vascular muscle membrane, Mg^{2+} deficiency
  Ca^{2+} movement, 1019
  membrane leakiness, 1019
  permeability, 1019
Vascular reactivity, 569
  diabetic hypertension, 1694–1695
Vascular remodeling
  biochemical mechanisms, 531
  hypertension, 521–533
  mechanisms, 529–531
Vascular resistance
  acebutolol, 2121
  alprenolol, 2121
  arterial baroreflex, 1463–1464
  atenolol, 2121
  cardiopulmonary receptor, 349–350
  metoprolol, 2121
  oxprenolol, 2121
  penbutolol, 2121
  pindolol, 2121
  practolol, 2121
  propranolol, 2121
  thyroid hormone, 1664
  timolol, 2121
Vascular response, pregnancy, 1770
Vascular smooth muscle
  angiotensin, 1355–1356
  angiotensin II, 1247–1255
    calcium homeostasis, 1250–1252
    contractile proteins, 1253–1254
    endothelium, 1254–1255
    hydrogen ion metabolism, 1252
    latch-bridge hypothesis, 1253
    phosphoinositide metabolism, 1249–1250
    prostaglandin, 1254–1255
    receptor binding, 1249
    receptors, 1248–1249
    signaling pathways, 1252–1253

Vascular smooth muscle, angiotensin II (*contd.*)
sodium ion metabolism, 1252
tone control, 1247–1248
atrial natriuretic factor, 868
Ca^{2+} metabolism
altered, 979–980
in hypertension, 979
intracellular, 978–979
whole-animal level, 978–979
calcium
entry pathways, 1019
response heterogeneity, 555–558
calcium metabolism, 978–979
intracellular, 978
whole-animal level, 978
calcium mobilization, 547–561
experimental hypertension, 558–561
hypertension etiology, 558–561
collagen, 574
collagen fibril, 574
DNA synthesis, 529
hyperplasia, 574
phasic contraction, 592–594
platelet, 929
potassium, 1143–1145
resistance vessel, 568
Vascular smooth muscle cell
cAMP, 621–622
connective tissue, 515
extracellular matrix, 515
transmembrane potential, components, 996
Vascular smooth muscle receptor
angiotensin II
G-protein, 1249
phospholipase C, 1249
calcium homeostasis, 1250–1252
Vascular tissue
angiotensinogen, 1208
medial necrosis, 296
Vascular tone
extrinsic, 1248
magnesium
Ca^{2+} cellular translocation, 1014–1015
hormone and drug-receptor interactions, 1014
humoral substance noninvolvement, 1015–1017
membrane Ca^{2+}-ATPase alterations, 1017
membrane Na^{+},K^{+}-ATPase alterations, 1017
membrane permeability modulation, 1014–1015
neurotransmitter noninvolvement, 1015–1017
Vascular wall histamine, 640
Vascular wall injury
epidermal growth factor, 523
platelet-derived growth factor, 523
TGF-beta, 523
Vasculature
primary genesis, 521–522
renin, 1320
Vasoactive agent, vascular lesion, 44–45
Vasoactive intestinal peptide, 798
neuropeptide, 800
Vasoconstriction
angiotensin II, 1296–1298
congestive heart failure, two forms, 1336–1337
cyclosporine, 1830
forms, 1331–1338
characteristics, 1333–1334
high-renin, cellular mechanisms, 1339–1340
low-renin, cellular mechanisms, 1339–1340
nephrotic syndrome, two forms, 1337–1338
renin, 32
renin-angiotensin-mediated form, 1331–1333
retinal artery, labile, 42–43
serotonin, 765–766
sodium-volume-mediated, 1334
sympathetic nervous system, two forms, 1340–1341
Vasoconstrictor, 1586
Vasoconstrictor hypertension, structural factor, 571
Vasoconstrictor response, endothelin, 654
systemic, 654
Vasoconstrictor tone, cardiopulmonary receptor, 349–350
Vasodilation
alpha-adrenoceptor-blocker, 2237–2239
beta-blocker, 2191
bucindolol, 2191
cAMP, 620
carvedilol, 2191
celiprolol, 2191
cold-induced, 142
diuretic, 2151–2152
labetalol, 2191
medroxalol, 2191
pindolol, 2191
potassium, 223
prizidilol, 2191
Vasodilator, 1693, 2263–2273. *See also* Specific type
beta-blocker, 2191–2192
blood pressure, 530
blood vessel type, 2265
cardiovascular hemodynamics, direct vasodilator, 2123–2125
classification, 2264–2265
clinical features, 2297
effectiveness, 2266
exercise, 1994
hemodynamics, 2265–2266
hypertensive urgency, 2282
interactions, 2297
antihypertensive drugs, 2297
mode of action, 2297
pregnancy, 1820
prostaglandin deficiency, 1634
reflex activity, 2238
vasodilation mechanisms, 2263–2264
Vasodilatory prostaglandin, 1602
Vasodilatory response, endothelin, 654
systemic, 654
Vasopressin, 583, 779–786, 798–799. *See also* Arginine vasopressin
angiotensin-converting enzyme inhibitor, 2212
angiotensin II, 1298
atrial natriuretic factor, 869
cardiopulmonary receptor, 350
circulatory homeostasis, 779
hydro-osmotic mechanism, 779
volumetric mechanism, 779
DOC-induced hypertension, 65
effects, 33
endothelium-derived relaxation factor, 1255
experimental hypertension
acute, 781–782
chronic, 782–784
hyperkalemia, 1636
treatment, 1636–1637
hypertension
human, 784–785
pathogenesis, 779–780
hypothyroidism, 1667
mitogenic effect, 544
neuropeptide, 800
peptide transmitter, 691
platelet-derived product, 641
receptor subtypes, 584
systemic vascular resistance, 997
vascular lesion, 44
vasospasm, 33
Vasopressinergic receptor
second messengers, 779
types, 779
Vasopressor response, intracranial pressure, 703–704
Vasospasm
cause, 33
lesions, 33
magnesium deficiency, 1013
vasopressin, 33
Vegetable, 49–50
Vegetable fiber, 245
Vegetarian diet
blood pressure, 244–248
mechanisms of action, 252
calcium, 245
historical aspects, 241
ischemic heart disease, 245
lipid, 245
magnesium, 1010
mild hypertension, 247–248
riboflavin, 245
Seventh-Day Adventist, 245–247
sodium, 245
vitamin B_{12}, 245
vitamin C, 245
Vein
nitroglycerin, circulatory effects, 2266
pressure change, 577

serotonin, 763
structural modulation, 577
Vena cava, 1653
Venous capacitance function, 567
Venous resistance, capacitance vessel, 568–569
Ventricular arrhythmia, diuretic, 113
Ventricular hypertrophy
central venous pressure, 355
hypertensive, 355
normotensive, 355
heart rate, 355
hypertensive, 355
normotensive, 355
left ventricular mass, 355
hypertensive, 355
normotensive, 355
mean arterial pressure, 355
hypertensive, 355
normotensive, 355
posterior wall thickness, 355
hypertensive, 355
normotensive, 355
septal wall thickness, 355
hypertensive, 355
normotensive, 355
Ventricular tachycardia, ketanserin, 774
Ventrolateral medulla, 680–681
afferent connections, 681
efferent connections, 681
sympathoadrenomedullary system, 715–716
Verapamil
age, 2173–2174
angiotensin II, vasodilator response, 2171
beta-blocker, 2202
calcium antagonist, 1014–1015, 1017
cardiovascular hemodynamics, 2126–2127
cardiovascular hypertrophy, 530
chemical structure, 472
cholesterol-fed rabbit model, 514
dietary sodium restriction, 2017
exercise, 1994
hypertensive urgency, 2282
magnesium, 481
plasma renin activity, 2173–2174
vasodilator response, 2171
predominant hemodynamic effect, 2125
race, 2173–2174, 2175
renin, 1238
side effects, 2065
smooth muscle cell proliferation, 514
specificity, 472
vitamin D_3, 481
Veratrum viride, 2098–2099
Very-low-density lipoprotein
coronary disease, 108
diltiazem, 514–515
Vesicle, kallikrein, 822
Vessel reactivity, magnesium
Ca^{2+} cellular translocation, 1014–1015
cyclic AMP, 1017
hormone and drug-receptor interactions, 1014
humoral substance noninvolvement, 1015–1017
membrane Ca^{2+}-ATPase alterations, 1017
membrane Na^+,K^+-ATPase alterations, 1017
membrane permeability modulation, 1014–1015
neurotransmitter noninvolvement, 1015–1017
Vessel wall
age, 46
intima, 526
platelet, 637–647
endothelium-derived vasoactive substance, 637–647
platelet-derived growth factor, 524
preexisting damage, 46–47
primary arterial disease, 46–47
steroid hypertension, 46
stress, 45–47
sympathetic innervation, 45–46
uremia, 46
vascular hypertrophy, 45
x-irradiation, 46
Vessel wall cell, endogenous growth factor, 524
Veterans Administration Cooperative Study Group, 1943, 2101–2102
treatment effectiveness, 153
Veterans Administration Cooperative Study on Antihypertensive Agents, 1878
Vision blurring, 460
Vitamin B_{12}, vegetarian diet, 245
Vitamin C, vegetarian diet, 245
Vitamin D, 982
calcium overload, 477–478
Vitamin D_3
diltiazem, 479, 484
femoral artery wall, 478
magnesium, 478–480
nicotine, 482, 483
Vitamin D metabolite
calcium, 892–893
parathyroid hormone, 892–893
Volume depletion, diuretic, 2155
responders, 2152
Volume-expanded hypertension, 781
Volume expansion therapy, pregnancy, 1818–1819
Volume homeostasis, endothelin, 656
Volume-loading essential hypertension, smooth muscle genetic theory, 1050–1051
Volume-loading hypertension, 1037–1038
arterial pressure, 1040
autoregulation, peripheral, 1048
cardiac output, 1039
circulatory filling pressure, 1039
circulatory hemodynamics, 1038–1039
early, 1043
fluid volume, 1038–1039
increases, 1043
late, 1043
total peripheral resistance, 1040
late stage changes, 1040
Volume regulation, pressure control
comparative pressure-controlling characteristics, 1032–1033
digitalis-like factor, 941
gamma-MSH, 946
infinite gain characteristics, 1032–1033
LPC, 947
lysophospholipid, 947
Volume status
hypertensive emergency, 2278
hypertensive urgency, 2278
von Hippel-Lindau's disease, 1646
von Recklinghausen's disease, 1646

W

Waist/hip ratio, 1746–1747
diastolic pressure, 132
systolic pressure, 132
Walking program, 2067, 2068
Wall shear stress, 18
Wall tension, atrial natriuretic factor, 864
Watanabe heritable hyperlipidemic rabbit, nifedipine, 513–514
Water
aldosterone, 1279–1280
eicosanoid, 832
Water drinking, angiotensin II, 1298
Water excretion, renal-body-fluid feedback, 1122
Water hardness, arterial blood pressure, 1009–1010
calcium concentration, 1009–1010
epidemiologic studies, 1010
magnesium concentration, 1009–1010
Water homeostasis, diuretic, 2149
Weight gain, centrally acting antihypertensive agents, 2253
Weight loss. *See also* Obesity
blood pressure, 1753
dietary sodium restriction, 2028–2033
compliance, 2033
floor effect, 2030
vs. metoprolol, 2030
endocrinic-adrenergic-metabolic changes, 2031–2032
fluid volume, 2030–2031
high-density lipoprotein, 109
insulin concentration levels, 2031
insulin resistance, 2031
Na^+-K^+-ATPase activity, 2031–2032
nursing management, 2066

Weight loss (*contd.*)
pheochromocytoma, 1643
renin-angiotensin-aldosterone system, 2031
sodium, 2031–2032
sympathetic nervous system, 2031
systemic hemodynamics, 2030–2031
Wernicke-Korsakoff syndrome, 758
Western diet, change, 243
Western lifestyle, Samoan study, 142
White-coat hypertension, 6, 18, 1408, 1416
blood pressure variation, 1419
suspected, 1408
White patient. *See also* Race
alcohol, 280
defined, 1837
hypertension, 159–173
Wilms' tumor, 1578, 1583. *See also* Nephroblastoma
Wistar-Furth rat, DOC-induced hypertension, 65
Wistar-Kyoto rat, phenotypic variation, 977
Wistar rat
DOC-induced hypertension, 65
potassium, 219
Withdrawal syndrome, 2306
sympathoadrenal system, 1421
Workup, 1386–1395
flow diagram, 1393
multiple visits, 1386
temporary hypertension drug therapy cessation, 1386
Worksite measurement
diastolic pressure, 1977
systolic pressure, 1977
Worksite screening program, 153–154

X
X-irradiation
stress, 46
vessel wall, 46

Y
Yohimbine
characterization, 2236
chemical structures, 2234

Z
Zimmerman pericyte, 1576
Zinc protease
angiotensin-converting enzyme, 1222, 1223
mechanistic comparisons, 1222, 1223
Zona fasciculata, 1610
17-deoxycorticosteroid pathway, 72
hypertension, 1618–1621
Zona glomerulosa, 1609, 1610
aldosterone, 1136
hypertension, 1613–1618
Zona reticularis, 1609, 1610
hypertension, 1621
Zonation, adrenal cortex, 1609–1610
Zymogen, 1179
prorenin, 1192
renin-angiotensin cascade, 1189

Author Index

A

Al-Bander, Hamoudi, 2021
Alderman, Michael H., 1941, 2301
Alexander, R. Wayne, 583
Altura, Bella T., 1003
Altura, Burton M., 1003
Amery, A., 1985
Anderson, Sharon, 1151, 1163, 1677
Angus, J.A., 761
Atlas, Steven A., 861, 2275
August, Phyllis, 1761
Aviv, Abraham, 923

B

Baker, Paul T., 137
Ballermann, Barbara J., 1247
Barajas, Luciano, 1053
Barber, Barry R., 901
Barron, William M., 1809
Beilin, Lawrence J., 241
Bell, Gordon M., 703, 1089
Bellet, Marc, 2331
Benjamin, N., 2263
Berglund, Göran, 1955
Biaggioni, Italo, 749
Bianchi, Giuseppe, 901
Bielen, E., 1985
Biglieri, Edward G., 1609
Birkenhäger, W.H., 1371
Black, Henry R., 1917
Blank, Seymour G., 1429
Blaufox, M. Donald, 1509
Blumenfeld, Jon D., 1089
Bolli, Peter, 2181
Bravo, Emmanuel L., 1911
Brenner, Barry M., 649, 1151, 1163, 1247, 1677
Briggs, Josephine P., 1067
Brooks, Bennie, 841
Brown, Peggy S., 841
Brownie, Alexander C., 63
Bruneval, P., 1573
Brunner, Hans R., 2209, 2331
Buckalew, Vardaman M., Jr., 939
Bühler, Fritz R., 637, 2169, 2181
Bukoski, Richard D., 977
Byers, Lawrence W., 841
Byyny, Richard L., 1869

C

Camilleri, J.P., 1573
Campbell, Gordon A., 1443
Carafoli, Ernesto, 965
Carini, David J., 2351
Carretero, Oscar A., 805
Chabanel, Anne, 329
Chalmers, J.P., 761
Chatellier, G., 1573
Chen, Yiu-Fai, 679
Cheung, Deanna G., 2251
Chien, Shu, 329
Chiesi, Michele, 965
Chiu, Andrew T., 2351
Churchill, Paul C., 1233
Coleman, Thomas G., 1029
Corvol, P., 1573
Curtis, John J., 1829

D

Dahlöf, Björn, 2131
de Leeuw, P.W., 1371
Devereux, Richard B., 359, 1479
Diederich, Dennis, 637
Dilley, Rodney J., 521
Dougherty, Rita M., 257
Doyle, Austin E., 119
Duncia, John V., 2351
Dunn, Michael J., 1583

E

Ehlers, Mario R.W., 1217
Erne, Paul, 661

F

Fagard, R., 1985
Feldschuh, Joseph, 339
Fernandez, Peter G., 2181
Ferrari, Alberto U., 349
Ferrari, Patrizia, 901
Field, Michael J., 1273
Fine, Eugene J., 1509
Fitzgerald, Desmond J., 1789
FitzGerald, Garret A., 1789
Fleckenstein, A., 471
Fleckenstein-Grün, G., 471
Folkow, Björn, 565
Freis, Edward D., 2093
Frey, M., 471

G

Galen, F.X., 1573
Garcia, Diego L., 1151
Gavras, Haralambos, 779
Gavras, Irene, 779
Gazzotti, Paolo, 965
Gelband, C.H., 547
Giebisch, Gerhard H., 1273
Gifford, Ray W., Jr., 1639
Goldblatt, Peter J., 21
Goldstein, David S., 711
Gordon, Richard D., 1625
Graettinger, William F., 2251
Granerus, Göran, 1493
Grassi, Guido, 349
Griendling, Kathy K., 583
Grim, Clarence E., 1837
Guo, Ji-Zhen, 1703
Gutzwiller, Felix, 147
Guyton, Arthur C., 1029, 1105

H

Haber, Edgar, 2343
Haddy, Francis J., 939
Hall, John E., 1029, 1105
Hamet, Pavel, 617
Hamlet, Stephen M., 1625
Hansson, Lennart, 2131
Harlan, Linda C., 229
Harlan, William R., 229
Hasslacher, Christoph, 1703
Hasstedt, Sandra J., 127
Heagerty, Anthony M., 601
Heinrikson, Robert L., 1179
Hermsmeyer, Kent, 661
Hespel, P., 1985
Hollenberg, Norman K., 1349
Hollister, Alan S., 749
Hopkins, Paul N., 127
Hui, Kwan Y., 2343
Hunt, Steven C., 127

I

Iacono, James M., 257
Irony, Ilan, 1609
Izzo, Joseph L., Jr., 1415

J

James, Gary D., 137
Jampol, Lee M., 433
Jennings, G.L., 761
Johnson, Alexander L., 2351
Julius, Stevo, 2083

K
Kannel, William B., 101
Kashgarian, Michael, 389
Kater, Claudio E., 1609
Keil, Ulrich, 147
Khalil, R.A., 547
King, Andrew J., 649
Klatsky, Arthur L., 277
Klein, Irwin, 1661
Klemm, Shelley A., 1625
Klotman, Paul E., 217
Kontos, Hermes A., 667
Kopin, Irwin J., 711
Krieger, Diane R., 1741
Kuida, Hiroshi, 127
Kumanyika, Shiriki K., 1837
Kurtz, Theodore, 2021

L
Lamport, Bernard, 2301
Landsberg, Lewis, 1741
Laragh, John H., 861, 1089, 1287, 1329, 1385, 2107
Lasker, Norman, 923
Ledingham, John M., 33
Lees, K.R., 2291
Lenz, Tomas, 1319
Lew, Edward A., 175
Lijnen, P., 1985
Linas, Stuart L., 989
Lindheimer, Marshall D., 1809
Ljungman, Susanne, 1493
Lodge, N.J., 547
Lovenberg, Walter, 295
Lund-Johansen, Per, 305
Lüscher, Thomas F., 637

M
Majesky, Mark W., 521
Man in't Veld, Arie J., 2117
Mancia, Giuseppe, 349
Manger, William M., 1639
Mann, Johannes, 1703
Mann, Samuel J., 2275
Manning, R. Davis, Jr., 1029
Marantz, Paul R., 1941
Marion, RoseMerie, 2061
Marsden, Philip A., 649, 1247
Marshall, Gary, 2309
McCarron, David A., 977
McGiff, J.C., 829
Meltzer, Jay I., 2073
Ménard, Jöel, 1573, 2331
Meyer, Philippe, 541
Minson, J.B., 761
Mitchell, Jerry R., 1461
Mogensen, C.E., 1717
Morris, R. Curtis, Jr., 2021
Muirhead, E. Eric, 841
Müller, Franco B., 1385, 2107
Murphy, Michael B., 1809

N
Novick, Andrew C., 1561
Nussberger, Jürg, 2209

O
Oates, John A., 1905
Ollerenshaw, J.D., 601
Omvik, Per, 305
Oparil, Suzanne, 679
Ostfeld, Adrian, 191

P
Pagny, J.Y., 1573
Paulson, Olaf B., 399
Pecker, Mark S., 1089, 2143
Petrin, Jurij, 2083
Phillips, Stephen J., 417
Pickering, Sir George, 3
Pickering, Thomas G., 17, 1397, 1429, 1539
Pinet, F., 1573
Pitcock, James A., 841
Plouin, P.F., 1573
Poorman, Roger A., 1179
Powers, Kenneth V., 1053
Preibisz, Jacek J., 1443
Price, William A., Jr., 2351

Q
Quilley, C.P., 829
Quilley, J., 829

R
Rapp, John P., 955
Reid, J.L., 2291
Reisin, Efrain, 2025
Resnick, Lawrence M., 2037
Riordan, James F., 1217
Ritz, Eberhard, 1703
Roberts, William C., 379
Robertson, David, 749
Robinson, Brian F., 2263
Rouse, Ian L., 241
Rudd, Peter, 2309
Ryan, Carolyn, 2061

S
Said, Sami I., 791
Saida, K., 547
Salido, Eduardo C., 1053
Savage, Daniel D., 1837
Schnermann, Jurgen, 1067
Schwartz, Stephen M., 521
Scicli, A. Guillermo, 805
Sealey, Jean E., 1089, 1287, 1319, 1329, 1443, 1761
Simpson, F. Olaf, 205
Sinaiko, Alan R., 1853
Smith, Michael C., 1583
Sommers, Sheldon C., 1089
Sosa, R. Ernest, 1601
Sowers, James R., 885
Spence, J. David, 1407
Staessen, J., 1985
Stern, Naftali, 1689
Strandgaard, Svend, 399
Stults, Barry M., 127
Svetkey, Laura P., 217
Swales, John D., 2011

T
Taylor, Addison A., 1461
Tewksbury, Duane A., 1197
Timmermans, Pieter B.M.W.M., 2351
Tobian, Louis, 49
Tremblay, Johanne, 617
Tso, Mark O.M., 433
Tuck, Michael L., 1689
Tunny, Terence J., 1625
Tuomilehto, Jaakko, 147
Tyroler, Herman A., 159

U
Ullian, Michael E., 989

V
van Breemen, Cornelis, 547
van den Meiracker, Anton H., 2117
Van Hoof, R., 1985
van Zwieten, Peter A., 2233
Vandam, Leroy D., 1889
Vanhees, L., 1985
Vanhoutte, Paul M., 637
Vaughan, E. Darracott, Jr., 1601
Vio, Carlos P., 819
Viscoli, C.M., 191

W
Waeber, Bernard, 2209
Wang, Sue-May, 955
Ward, Ryk, 81
Watkins, Laurence O., 1837
Weber, Michael A., 2251
Weinberger, Myron H., 1999
Weinstein, David B., 511
Wells, Gregory J., 2351
Wells, Thomas G., 1853
Wexler, Ruth R., 2351
Whisnant, Jack P., 417
Williams, Gordon H., 1349
Williams, Roger R., 127
Wong, Pancras C., 2351
Wu, Lily L., 127
Wyss, J. Michael, 679

Y
Yamori, Yukio, 295
Young, David B., 1131
Young, Eric W., 977

Z
Zanchetti, Alberto, 1967
Zemel, Michael B., 885
Zorn, J., 471
Zuspan, Frederick P., 1779